**LIPPINCOTT WILLIAMS & WILKINS'**

# Comprehensive Medical Assisting

EDITION

# LIPPINCOTT WILLIAMS & WILKINS'

# Comprehensive Medical Assisting

**Judy Kronenberger, PhD, RN, CMA(AAMA)**

Associate Professor and Program Director, Medical Assistant Program
University of Cincinnati Blue Ash
Blue Ash, Ohio

**Julie Ledbetter, CMA(AAMA), CMRS, CPC**

Adjunct Faculty, Medical Assistant Technology
Sinclair Community College
Dayton, Ohio

EDITION

5

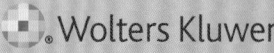 Wolters Kluwer

Philadelphia · Baltimore · New York · London
Buenos Aires · Hong Kong · Sydney · Tokyo

*Acquisitions Editor*: Jay Campbell
*Senior Product Development Editor*: Amy Millholen
*Production Product Manager*: David Saltzberg
*Editorial Assistant*: Tish Rogers
*Design Coordinator*: Joan Wendt
*Marketing Manager*: Shauna Kelley
*Compositor*: SPi Global

Fifth Edition

**Library of Congress Cataloging-in-Publication Data**
Lippincott Williams & Wilkins' comprehensive medical assisting / editors, Judy Kronenberger, Julie Ledbetter. — Fifth edition.
    p. ; cm.
    Comprehensive medical assisting
    Lippincott Williams and Wilkins' comprehensive medical assisting
    Preceded by: Lippincott Williams & Wilkins' comprehensive medical assisting. 4th ed. / Judy Kronenberger, Laura Southard Durham, Denise Woodson. c2013.
    Includes bibliographical references and index.
    ISBN 978-1-4963-0220-5
  I. Kronenberger, Judy, editor. II. Ledbetter, Julie, editor. III. Title: Comprehensive medical assisting. IV. Title: Lippincott Williams and Wilkins' comprehensive medical assisting.
    [DNLM: 1. Physician Assistants. 2. Clinical Medicine—methods. W 21.5]
    R697.P45
    610.73'72069—dc23
                                                                                            2015011509

**Disclaimer**
Care has been taken to confirm the accuracy of the information present and to describe generally accepted practices. However, the authors, editors, and publisher are not responsible for errors or omissions or for any consequences from application of the information in this book and make no warranty, expressed or implied, with respect to the currency, completeness, or accuracy of the contents of the publication. Application of this information in a particular situation remains the professional responsibility of the practitioner; the clinical treatments described and recommended may not be considered absolute and universal recommendations.

The authors, editors, and publisher have exerted every effort to ensure that drug selection and dosage set forth in this text are in accordance with the current recommendations and practice at the time of publication. However, in view of ongoing research, changes in government regulations, and the constant flow of information relating to drug therapy and drug reactions, the reader is urged to check the package insert for each drug for any change in indications and dosage and for added warnings and precautions. This is particularly important when the recommended agent is a new or infrequently employed drug.

Some drugs and medical devices presented in this publication have Food and Drug Administration (FDA) clearance for limited use in restricted research settings. It is the responsibility of the health care provider to ascertain the FDA status of each drug or device planned for use in their clinical practice.

The publishers have made every effort to trace the copyright holders for borrowed material. If they have inadvertently overlooked any, they will be pleased to make the necessary arrangements at the first opportunity.

To purchase additional copies of this book, call our customer service department at (800) 638-3030 or fax orders to (301) 223-2320. International customers should call (301) 223-2300.

Visit Lippincott Williams & Wilkins on the Internet: http://www.lww.com. Lippincott Williams & Wilkins customer service representatives are available from 8:30 am to 5:00 pm, EST.

This book is dedicated to all the people who have made an impact on my life including my husband Joe; my children Brian, Jennifer, Eric, and Brittany; and my grandchildren Arthur, Victor, Joseph, Hayden, Drew, and the newest granddaughter Eleanor, who is not here yet, but will no doubt fill my heart with even more love than it can hold! I would also like to acknowledge my mother-in-law, Alice Kronenberger, who unfortunately passed away during this revision. She will always be remembered for her kind words and encouragement of all my endeavors including this one! Special gratitude goes to Amy Millholen at Wolters Kluwer for her patience and encouragement during this edition—it was a pleasure to work with her!

JUDY KRONENBERGER

I wish to dedicate this edition to my husband, Larry, whose thoughtfulness and patience during this project were always appreciated and never unnoticed. Thank you for keeping up with family commitments in my absence and the many meals you provided just at the right time! My heartfelt thank you also goes to all the dedicated health care providers in my life, especially Dr. Janis Roberts. Your input was invaluable and your friendship priceless! I want to *especially* remember my dear friend, Pastor Rick Shoemaker, whose love of writing was an inspiration throughout this endeavor. I will always be grateful for the common bond of writing and friendship that we shared. Heaven gained a very talented author when you left us, but your wisdom and kind words will be forever engraved on my heart!

JULIE LEDBETTER

# About the Authors

### JUDY KRONENBERGER

Judy is currently an Associate Professor and Program Director in the Medical Assistant program at the University of Cincinnati, Blue Ash, Ohio. She is an active member of the American Association of Medical Assistants (AAMA) and enjoys serving this organization as an MAERB/CAAHEP site surveyor (since 2001) for medical assistant programs seeking accreditation or re-accreditation. Judy has served the Ohio State Society of Medical Assistants in various capacities, including State President (2011–2012). Her education includes an Associate Degree in Nursing (Sinclair Community College), a Bachelor of Arts degree in Human Development (McGregor School at Antioch University), a Master's of Science Degree in Education (University of Dayton), and a PhD in Higher Education (University of Dayton). Judy resides in Kettering, Ohio, with her husband of 35 years. She enjoys reading and spending time with her grandchildren and long-haired dachshund Schnitzel when she is not teaching.

### JULIE LEDBETTER

Julie is a Certified Medical Assistant and an active member in the Association of Medical Assistants (AAMA). She is also a Certified Professional Coder through the American Academy of Professional Coders, and a Certified Medical Reimbursement Specialist through the American Medical Billing Association. She has been a presenter at seminars for her local Montgomery County Chapter of Medical Assistants on administrative topics and is currently the chapter webmaster. Julie has several years' office management experience in medical specialty practices but has dedicated the last 12 years as an educator for medical assisting students as an adjunct instructor for the Medical Assistant Technology program at Sinclair Community College, Dayton, Ohio, where she earned the 2013–2014 Adjunct Excellence in Teaching Award for the Life and Health Sciences Division. She also teaches for the Health, Human, and Public Service Department at Clark State Community College, Springfield, Ohio. When not preparing for her classes, Julie enjoys reading, traveling, and spending time with her husband of 34 years, Larry, and her beautiful grandchildren.

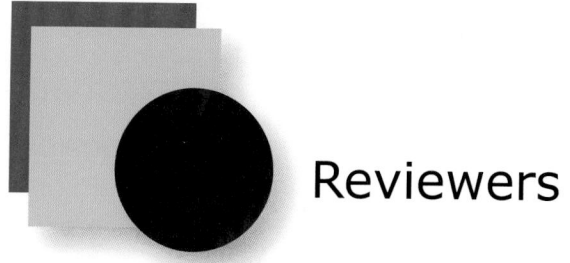

# Reviewers

**Michelle Adams**
MAA Instructor
Pima Medical Institute
Renton, Washington

**Ramona Atiles,** LPN
Clinical Coordinator
Allied Health
Career Institute of Health and Technology
Garden City, New York

**Linda J. Bird,** AS, RMA
Lead MA Instructor
Pima Medical Institute
Mesa, Arizona

**Suzanne Bitters-Woods,** RMA-NCPT/NCICS
Director of Education
Professional Medical Assisting
Harris School of Business
Upper Darby, Pennsylvania

**Cindi Brassington,** MS, CMA
Professor
Allied Health
Quinebaug Valley Community College
Danielson, Connecticut

**Alison L. Burchett,** MT(ASCP)
Curriculum Coordinator
Dayton Children's Hospital
Dayton, Ohio

**Desirae Carosi,** RMA, LMT
Medical Assistant Program Chair
Medical Assisting
Branford Hall Career Institute
Albany, New York

**Charles Chiaramonte,** CMA, CCMA
MAA Instructor
Pima Medical Institute
East Valley, Arizona

**Beth Collis,** CMA (AAMA), LXMO
Medical Assisting Program Coordinator
Academic Department
Rasmussen College
Bloomington, Minnesota

**Bobby Cox,** EMT/CMA
Instructor
Allied Health/Medical Assisting
Remington College—Memphis
Memphis, Tennessee

**Carlos Cuervo,** MD, USMLE
Teacher, Department Head
Allied Health
Florida National University
Miami, Florida

**Brenda Diaz,** MA
Allied Health Department Chair
Medical Assisting
Remington College
Nashville, Tennessee

**Trina Ellis,** ADN
Clinical Instructor
Health Sciences
Rasmussen College
Bloomington, Minnesota

**Pamela Fleming,** RN, BS, MPA
Professor
Medical Assisting
Quinsigamond Community College
Worcester, Massachusetts

**Todd Gervais,** AS
Curriculum Technician
Academic Affairs
San Joaquin Valley College
Visalia, California

Barbara Gibson, AAS–CRMA
Medical Assisting Coordinator
Medical Assisting
Southeastern College
Lakeland, Florida

Kathryn Goffard, BS, MS
Faculty
Allied Health
Waukesha County Technical College
Pewaukee, Wisconsin

Sally Haith-Glenn, RMA, AHI, MBA-HCM
Program Director
Medical Assistant and Medical Billing
Virginia College
Birmingham, Alabama

Jacquelyn Harris, MEd
Chair/Instructor
Allied Health
Wright Career Colleges
Wichita, Kansas

Joshua Henriot, AA
MA/MAA (Lead) Instructor
Pima Medical Institute
Business Office Supervisor
Swedish Medical Group
Seattle, Washington

Forrest Heredia, BSBA, CMAA, CPC-I
Lead MAA Instructor
Pima Medical Institute
Tucson, Arizona

Liz Hoffman, MA Ed, CMA (AAMA), CPT (ASPT)
Faculty
Medical Assistant
Henry Ford College
Dearborn, Michigan

Elizabeth Ingram, CCMA
MA/MAA Instructor
Pima Medical Institute
Albuquerque, New Mexico

Shirley Jelmo, BS, CMA (AAMA), RMA
Lead MA Instructor
Pima Medical Institute
Colorado Springs, Colorado

Beth Julsaint, BBA
Instructor
Medical Assistant
Concorde Career College
Grand Prairie, Texas

Donald J. Kennedy
MA Instructor
Pima Medical Institute
Mesa, Arizona

Sharyn Ketcham, MBA, MHSA
Medical Assisting Program Director
Health Professions
Phoenix College
Phoenix, Arizona

Jennifer Ketterling, PhD
Associate Dean
Medical Specialties Education
CollegeAmerica
Denver, Colorado

Judith Kline, CRMA
Instructor
Medical Assisting
Miami Lakes Educational Center
Miami Lakes, Florida

Juana LaBelle, MBA, BS
Adjunct Instructor
Medical Assistant Program
Brookline College
Phoenix, Arizona

Lora Lape, AS
Program Director
Medical Assisting
AmeriTech College
Provo, Utah

Linda Lee, RMA
Instructor/Program Director
Medical Assistant
Hamilton Technical College
Davenport, Iowa

Seantenia Lynch, BS
Program Chair/Lead Instructor
Allied Health
Lincoln College of Technology
Cleveland, Ohio

Sheniqua Maefau, DipBA, CMA
Instructor
Medical Assisting
Concorde Career College
North Hollywood, California

Christine Malone, MHA
Instructor
Health Sciences
Everett Community College
Everett, Washington

Benjamen McBride, AAS
Medical Assisting Program Director
Medical Assisting
AmeriTech College
Provo, Utah

Anthony McDonald, MA
Instructor
Medical Assisting
Concorde Career Institute
Miramar, Florida

Laura Melendez, BS, RMA, RT, BMO
Medical Assistant Instructor
Medical Assisting
Southeastern College
Lakeland, Florida

Helen Mills, RN, MSN, RMA, LXMO, AHI
Program Coordinator/Director of Student
    Services
Medical Assisting
Keiser University
Fort Lauderdale, Florida

Bonnie Nolen, AS/HCA, CCMA, CPT
Lead MA Instructor
Pima Medical Institute
Albuquerque, New Mexico

David Pintado, MD, MHA, CCMA
Faculty Externship Coordinator
Academics Affairs
Heald College—Concord
Concord, California

Carol Qare Carcar, DPM, CPT, RMA
Director of Healthcare
Medical Assisting, Office Administration, Billing
    and Coding, and Pharmacy Technology
Heald College
San Francisco, California

Patricia L. Rogers
Lead MAA Instructor
Pima Medical Institute
Denver, Colorado

Donna Rowan, MA, BA
Full Time Faculty
Health Para-Professionals
Community College of Baltimore County
Essex, Maryland

Karan Serowik, RMA-CCMA
Program Director Healthcare
Medical Assisting
Heald College
Portland, Oregon

Carrie Sharp, CMA, AAMA
Adjunct Instructor
Medical Assistant Program
Jackson Community College
Jackson County, Michigan

Prather Stinson, BSW, CMA (AAMA)
Lead MA Instructor
Pima Medical Institute
Renton, Washington

Margaret Swearingen
Lead MA Instructor
Pima Medical Institute
Denver, Colorado

Marybeth Wilson, BA
Instructor
Medical Specialties
CollegeAmerica
Denver, Colorado

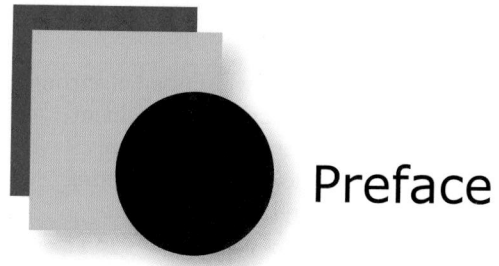

# Preface

Health care is changing; however, your role as the most versatile health care member is an important part of the successful physician practice and will continue to be integral as health care changes. Although the skills you perform may vary among medical offices, your education and training in the exciting field of medical assisting will prepare you for a variety of clinical and administrative skills, making you an essential part of the health care team.

*Lippincott Williams & Wilkins' Comprehensive Medical Assisting, Fifth Edition*, will provide you with the information and skills necessary to perform competently and with confidence. This edition has been updated to include the most current (2015) American Association of Medical Assistants (AAMA) curriculum standards for medical assistants in all three domains: cognitive, psychomotor, and affective. These standards are required for Commission on Accreditation of Allied Health Education Programs (CAAHEP)-accredited programs. This edition also includes the content and skills required by the American Medical Technologists (AMT) for Accrediting Bureau of Health Education Schools (ABHES)-accredited programs. These standards and competencies define your roles and responsibilities as a professional medical assistant, and this edition of the textbook and ancillary materials continue to support your education and training to fulfill these role responsibilities.

## Organization of the Text

As with previous editions, great care and concern were taken to organize this book in a logical and reader-friendly presentation. The fifth edition is divided into five sections:

- Part I, Introduction to Medical Assisting, consists of Unit One. Chapter 1 provides you with a brief history of the medical profession and the practice of medical assisting. Legal and ethical issues governing the medical community and your practice are discussed in Chapter 2. Chapter 3 helps you sharpen your communication skills, and Chapter 4 gives you the tools to deliver effective patient education.
- Part II, The Administrative Medical Assistant, consists of Unit Two (Chapters 5 through 10) and Unit Three (Chapters 11 through 15). Unit Two helps you master basic administrative skills and the basics of office management, whereas Unit Three explores financial management of the medical office.

- Part III, The Clinical Medical Assistant, consists of Units Four (Chapters 16 through 27) and Five (Chapters 28 through 39). Unit Four provides you with critical information regarding nutrition and wellness, aseptic techniques, infection control, patient assessment, vital signs, and assisting with the physical examination. You will also find an overview of pharmacology as well as information to help you properly prepare and administer medications. The final two chapters in this unit will give you the tools to recognize and respond to emergencies in the medical office and disaster preparedness. Unit Five focuses on specialty examinations, diagnostic tests, and therapeutic procedures for specific areas of medicine. Each chapter provides you with a brief overview of the system, typical therapeutic measures used to treat common disorders, and the role of the medical assistant in assisting the physician with diagnosis and treatment. The last two chapters in this unit focus on duties relating to special populations, including pediatrics and geriatrics.
- Part IV, The Clinical Laboratory, introduces you to the physician office laboratory. Chapters 40 through 45 will provide you with detailed information on maintaining a safe laboratory environment that operates in compliance with federal, state, and local regulations. Updated information includes information necessary to function in the physician office laboratory competently and with confidence. Skills included in this unit include competencies on collecting and processing specimens, handling the specimens in a manner that supports accurate testing, and following quality control protocols to monitor and evaluate testing procedures, supplies, and equipment.
- Part V, Career Strategies, includes Chapters 46 and 47. Chapter 46 gives information to help you make a smooth transition from the classroom environment to the workforce, and Chapter 47 is a comprehensive examination to assess your knowledge of the administrative and clinical information covered in this text.

## Features

Instructors should find the time invested to "link" the text and ancillary materials with the most current

CAAHEP and ABHES standards useful. Our goal is to make this textbook the most student-friendly resource available in the medical assisting field.

A variety of key chapter features are included to spark interest and promote comprehension, including:

- Chapter Outline
- Learning Outcomes specific to CAAHEP and ABHES standards
- Key Terms list
- Case Studies—NEW!
- Key points highlighted throughout the text
- Icons to indicate content that is part of the cognitive, psychomotor, and affective learning domains
- Checkpoint Questions
- Patient Education Boxes
- Ethical Tip Boxes
- Legal Tip Boxes
- What If? Boxes
- Triage Boxes
- Role Playing Activities—NEW!
- Video icons next to topics and procedures for which there is a skills video available in the online student resources
- Spanish Terms and Phrases
- Media Menu, containing information on videos, animations, and Internet resources
- Medication Boxes
- EMR Activities—NEW!
- Chapter Summaries
- Warm Ups for Critical Thinking
- Step-by-step procedure boxes

This textbook is fully supported with a robust teaching and learning package, each element of which is designed to help you and your instructor get the most out of the textbook. The resource package includes the following:

- Access to Harris CareTracker, a web-based electronic medical record (EMR) and practice management (PM) software. This fully integrated EMR and PM gives students the experience of documenting and tracking patient encounters from check in to check out for a real-world experience. Case Studies provided on thePoint walk students through the software helping them build proficiency and confidence in an EMR/PM environment and helping instructors meet the CAAHEP and ABHES EHR competency.
- A complete online instructor's resource kit includes a test generator, image bank, PowerPoint slides, lesson plans, answer keys for the text checkpoint questions and Study Guide, CAAHEP and ABHES competencies mapping spreadsheets linking the text and ancillary content to the competencies, and more.
- Online student resources, including certification exam preparation review questions, games and review activities, competency evaluation forms, work products, animations, videos, key terms audio glossary, and Spanish–English audio glossary.
- A separate student Study Guide is available for purchase to enhance learning and comprehension, with competency evaluation forms for each procedure in the textbook; critical thinking exercises; self-assessment exercises, such as matching and multiple choice; and study and work products.

Our hope is that this edition exceeds your expectations. May your career in medical assisting be challenging and fulfilling!

Judy Kronenberger, PhD, RN, CMA(AAMA)
Julie Ledbetter, CPC, CMRS, CMA(AAMA)

# User's Guide

This User's Guide shows you how to the put the features of *Lippincott Williams & Wilkins' Comprehensive Medical Assisting, Fifth Edition*, to work for you.

## Chapter Opening Elements

Each chapter begins with the following elements, which will help orient you to the material.

### Chapter Outline

This serves as your "roadmap" to the chapter content.

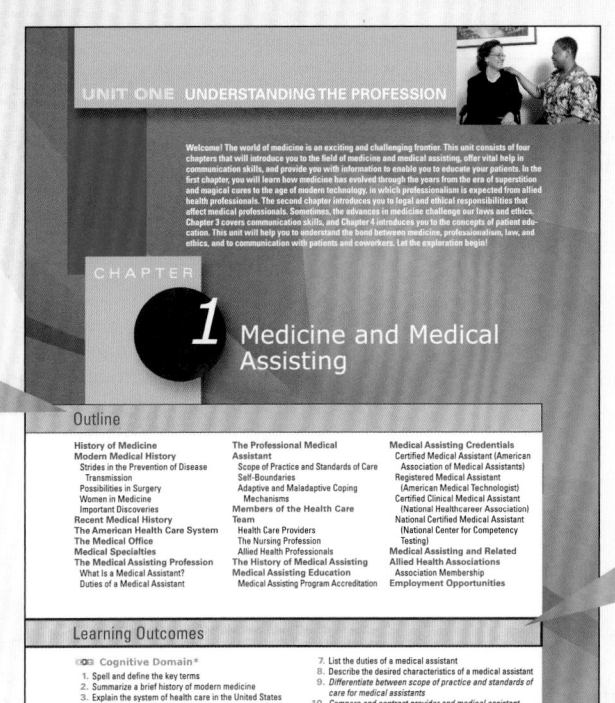

### Learning Outcomes

The Learning Outcomes list the skills learned, including the CAAHEP and ABHES Competencies specific to the chapter.

### Key Terms

The key terms that are defined in the chapter are listed for quick reference.

### Case Study

*R*ob Shelton, CMA, was recently hired as a clinical medical assistant at Great Falls Medical Center and has been told he will be responsible for giving all flu vaccines during his first week as ordered by the physicians. He will also be responsible for performing electrocardiograms for several patients scheduled for annual physical exams. Rob has also been told he will have to help with administrative duties when necessary. What are the clinical duties that Rob has been trained to do through his medical assisting education? What are the administrative responsibilities? Does giving injections fall within Rob's scope of practice? How is this determined? What does Rob have to do to maintain his CMA credential? Professional, credentialed medical assistants are invaluable to the physicians who employ them, and the job outlook continues to be excellent for individuals choosing this exciting career. In this chapter, you will learn what it takes to become a credentialed medical assistant and the skills necessary to earn a medical assisting credential. You will also learn about the benefits of joining a national organization as a professional medical assistant.

## Case Studies

New case studies challenge you to think through real-world situations and are tied to the EMR activities later in the chapter.

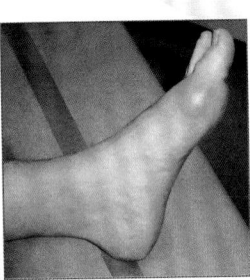
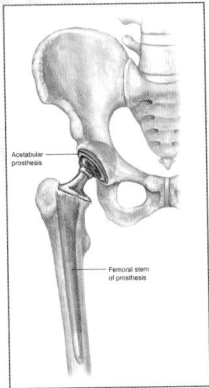

## Stunning Art Program

Full-color illustrations and photographs clarify clinical concepts and help you visually understand the topic.

 PROCEDURE 29-1

### Apply an Arm Sling

**PSY** Instruct and prepare a patient for a procedure or treatment; coach patients regarding disease prevention and treatment plans; coach patients appropriately considering cultural diversity, developmental life stage, and communication barriers; and document patient care accurately in the medical record.

**Purpose:** Correctly apply an arm sling

**Equipment:** A canvas arm sling with adjustable straps

| STEPS | PURPOSE |
|---|---|
| 1. Wash your hands. | Hand washing aids infection control. |
| 2. Assemble the equipment and supplies. | Be prepared before beginning any procedure. |
| 3. Greet and identify the patient and explain the procedure. Identify yourself including your credentials. | Identifying the patient prevents errors in the treatment. Explaining the procedure helps ease anxiety and ensure compliance. |
| 4. **AFF** Explain how to respond to a patient who does not speak English or speaks English as a second language (ESL). | Solicit assistance from anyone who may be with the patient or get another staff member who speaks his or her native language to interpret if available. If no interpreter is available, use hand gestures or pictures to explain the procedure to the patient. |
| 5. Position the affected limb with the hand at slightly less than a 90° angle so that the fingers are a bit higher than the elbow. | This position helps reduce swelling of the hand and fingers. |
| 6. Insert the arm into the pouch end of the sling with the elbow fitting into the pocket corner. | The elbow should fit snugly into the sling. |

## Procedure Boxes

Break procedures down into steps, showing you how to perform essential tasks properly. Needed equipment and supplies are listed. Reasons are given for the steps, so you understand not only how but also why each step is important.

 WHAT IF?

**A patient has been scheduled for a barium study at a local outpatient facility but calls your office to ask what to do if he ate breakfast this morning. What should you do?**

As a medical assistant, you must understand the reason for fasting before certain diagnostic procedures. In this situation, the patient should be instructed to call the diagnostic facility for further instructions, which will include rescheduling the procedure. Emphasize to the patient the importance of following all instructions carefully since not doing so will interfere with the procedure and/or the results. Not following instructions will result in further inconvenience of the patient and delay of a possible diagnose, further delaying treatment and outcomes for the patient.

## What If Boxes

Present a variety of real-life scenarios that you must be prepared to handle in the medical office. Each situation is clearly defined and explained.

 **PATIENT EDUCATION**

### Cast Care

Instruct patients with casts to do the following:

- Be aware of the initial warmth of the drying cast; this will diminish in 20 to 30 minutes.
- Keep a plaster cast dry.
- Avoid indentations by allowing the cast to dry completely before handling or propping it on a hard surface.
- Note that the fingers and toes are left uncovered to check for color, swelling, numbness, and temperature; report any impairment to the physician immediately.
- Report odors, staining, or undue warmth of the cast.
- Prevent swelling by elevating the limb for at least 24 hours after casting and as often as possible after that time.
- Never insert any object under the cast to scratch beneath it. Breaks in the skin may become infected and require that the cast be removed prematurely.

## Patient Education Boxes

Contain in-depth information on topics that you need to know in order to educate patients.

*español*

## Spanish Terminology

Help you communicate with Spanish-speaking patients.

### SPANISH TERMINOLOGY

**Voy a ponerle una tabilla en la pierna.**
I am going to put a splint on the leg.

**Voy a examinarle la pierna.**
I am going to examine your leg.

**Doble las rodillas, no la espalda.**
Bend your knees, not your back.

**¿Tiene dolor en sus articulaciones ó coyonturas?**
Do you feel pain in your joints?

**¿Tiene dolor en sus musculos?**
Do you feel pain in your muscles?

## Video Icons

Label topics for which there is a skills video available in the online student resources.

## Domain Icons

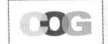  

Indicate content that is part of the cognitive (thinking), psychomotor (physical movement), and affective (emotional) learning domains.

 **CHECKPOINT QUESTION**

1. How does a luxation differ from a subluxation?

## Checkpoint Questions

Review questions appear throughout the chapter to ensure your understanding of the concepts from the section.

# Special Features (continued)

**ETHICAL TIP**

### Who Is Who?

It is important that medical assistants represent themselves honestly. Physicians often innocently refer to every employee as "the nurse." It is more accurate to say my assistant, my certified medical assistant, my registered medical assistant, or my clinical assistant. There are documented court cases involving misrepresentation of one's education and credentials. Protect yourself by referring to yourself appropriately to patients and coworkers. Do not identify yourself as "Dr. Smith's nurse." When patients refer to you as a nurse, you should correct them. The more your credentials are heard by patients and coworkers, the more understood and recognized they will be. You should be proud of your profession and your credentials. Let it be known.

## Ethical Tip Boxes

Offer guidelines to help you learn and abide by the ethical standards set forth by the AAMA (American Association of Medical Assistants).

## Media Menus

Located at the end of every chapter, the Media Menu contains information on video clips, animations, and Internet resources that are available to you.

**MEDIA MENU**

Student Resources on thePoint*
* **CMA/RMA Certification Exam Review**

Internet Resources
**Accrediting Bureau of Health Education Schools**
http://www.abhes.org
**American Board of Medical Specialties**
http://www.abms.org
**American Health Information Management Association**

## Legal Tip Boxes

Contain important legal information to help you understand the legal implications associated with your future profession.

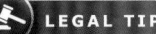

**LEGAL TIP**

### Assessing Circulation after a Cast Application

A cast that is applied improperly can lead to nerve and vascular damage, resulting in permanent loss of function to the extremity. In extreme situations, a surgical amputation may be required. To ensure proper care and to avoid lawsuits, it is essential that distal extremity circulation be assessed and documented before and after reductions and casting. Also, the patient should be taught to watch for and report signs of impaired circulation.

**ROLE-PLAYING ACTIVITY**

While waiting for the next patient to arrive, Rob Shelton, CMA, realizes that the receptionist is very busy and all of the phone lines are ringing at once. He immediately moves to a desk with another phone and begins assisting the receptionist by taking calls so she can give attention to the patients arriving to check in for their appointments. Later that day, another medical assistant approaches Rob and begins to complain about the practice being understaffed and comments that answering the phones is not specifically in his job description. She further complains about other staff members and even the office manager! How should

## Role-Playing Activities

New role-playing activities give you an opportunity to play the role of a medical assistant in responding to practice situations.

**AFF TRIAGE**

While working in the medical office, you begin the day by placing the following three patients into examination rooms:

A. Patient A, a new patient, arrives on time and was given the two-page medical history form to complete.
B. Patient B is an established patient who is scheduled to have his blood pressure checked today because he started a new antihypertensive medication last month.
C. Patient C is a 1-year-old baby who is scheduled to be seen today for a well-child checkup and immunizations.

**How would you sort these patients? Who should be seen first? Second? Third?**

Patient B should be called back first, since he will probably take the least amount of time. Unless this patient's blood pressure is not responding to the antihypertensive medication or he has unanticipated problems, this type of visit is typically conducted in a time-[...]
convenience to the pati[...]

## Triage Boxes

Triage boxes help you develop important skills for practice.

## EMR Activities

New hands-on EMR activities help you master content as you learn to use the software for patient scheduling, charting, coding, and billing.

**EMR Activity**

**HARRIS** CareTracker

Harris CareTracker is a web-based electronic medical record (EMR) application that you will use for the EMR activities included in this section at the end of each chapter. This application is actually used in physician offices, but is provided to you through the publisher, Wolters Kluwer Health, to give you hands-on practice working with EMRs. Your instructor will have more information about accessing your username, login, and Quickstart guide.

Prerequisite Activities in Harris CareTracker

* *The Getting Started and Quickstart documents and EMR Activities Step-by-Step Instructions are available at http://thePoint.lww.com/KronenbergerComp5e*

Activity Details

Using the "New ToDo" feature in the EMR, send yourself a message to research the local chapter of the American Association of Medical Assistants about the next scheduled meeting. This feature can be found on the *Home* module, *Messages* tab, and *Send Todo* button at the bottom of the screen. Choose the *Interoffice* category, *Practice Management* type, *Other* reason, *Medium* severity, and the *In Progress* status. Print your message to submit to your instructor.

## Chapter Summary

- The musculoskeletal system has many functions including the following:
  - Providing support and protection for vital organs
  - Allowing movement and mobility
  - Providing a frame (the skeleton) on which muscles are attached and the bones are held together at the joints
  - Providing stability and flexibility of the body
- Although the orthopedic physician specializes in the diagnosis and treatment of these conditions, you should expect to see patients with disorders of the musculoskeletal system in various medical offices, including pediatrics and family practice. In this chapter, you learned the following:
  - Common disorders of the musculoskeletal system including the upper and lower extremities
  - Diagnostic procedures including x-ray procedures that may be ordered by the physician to assist in diagnosing disorders of the musculoskeletal system

### Chapter Summary
Review key points from the chapter.

## Warm-Ups for Critical Thinking

1. Create a patient education brochure for the use of ambulatory aids. Be sure to include a brief description of the purpose of each aid along with the procedure steps.
2. The youth baseball league playoffs are coming to your town, and you are asked to staff the first aid station. What kinds of orthopedic injuries do you expect to see, and why? Develop a list of the first aid supplies that you want to have available and explain the reasons for your selections.
3. How would you respond to a patient with impaired circulation who tells you that he often uses a heating pad to relieve the pain in his legs although the physician has warned him not to do so?
4. Your patient with plantar fasciitis asks you why the pain is worse in the morning when first getting out of bed. Describe how you could explain this condition to a patient with limited understanding of human anatomy.
5. Using a drug reference book, look up several anti-inflammatory medications (naproxen sodium, ibuprofen). What gastrointestinal disorders may result from taking these medications, and how can these side effects be avoided?

### Warm Ups for Critical Thinking
Real-life scenarios that require you to develop, create, write, or search for more information.

# Additional Learning Resources

**This powerful learning tool also includes a companion Web site, which contains many helpful assets**

- Review activities and games
- Animations
- Videos
- Certification preparation question bank
- Competency evaluation forms

- An English-to-Spanish audio glossary and key terms glossary
- Student work products

The student companion site can be accessed at: http://thepoint.lww.com/kronenbergercomp5e

**Available for purchase separately:**

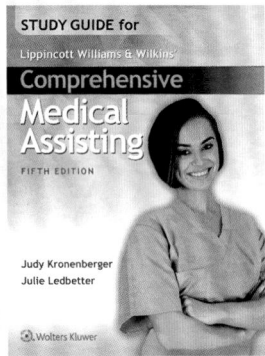

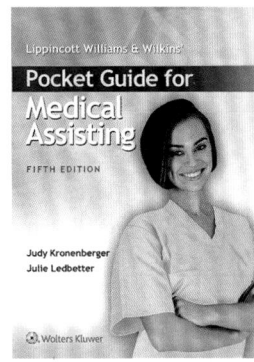

- *Study Guide for Lippincott Williams & Wilkins' Comprehensive Medical Assisting* comes with procedure skill sheets, case studies for critical thinking, and a variety of question types to meet the needs of different learning styles and to reinforce content and knowledge.

- *Lippincott Williams & Wilkins' Pocket Guide for Medical Assisting* gives step-by-step coverage of medical assisting procedures in both administrative and clinical settings. The small size makes it perfect for clinical and office use.

# Acknowledgments

This book would never have been successfully completed without the assistance, persistence, and hard work of many people. At the risk of leaving out others at Wolters Kluwer who made this book possible (we apologize in advance!), we would like to thank Amy Millholen, Senior Product Development Editor, and Jay Campbell, Acquisitions Editor, who were always there to offer support, insight, and guidance whenever needed. A special thank you should also go to Susan Caldwell (artist), Tish Rogers (Editorial Assistant), David Saltzberg (Production Product Manager), Beverly Ervin, PhD, and anyone else who may not be mentioned for making this book and ancillary materials a reality and supporting the education of medical assistants.

We would also like to thank Martha Armstrong-Benjamin, Ed Schultes, Freddie Patane, and Mark Lozier for their professionalism and expertise in making the photo and video shoots a success. A special thank you goes to the staff at CenterMed Family Practice and Wright State Physicians Health Center for providing the locations for the photo shoot and video shoot. Thanks also to Larry Ledbetter for helping out with additional photographs that added much clarity and value to this edition of the text! Of course, a huge thanks goes to all the family and friend "models" who agreed to participate in the photo and video shoot, especially medical assistant students from Sinclair Community College including Oakley Ooten, Angela Hanes, Mishalay Mabson, and Tonya Knoth.

# List of Procedures

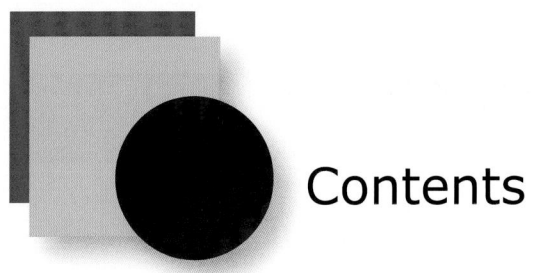

# Contents

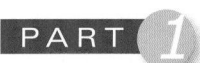
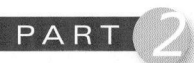

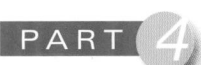

PART 4

# The Clinical Laboratory

## PART 5

# Career Strategies

# 1

# Introduction to Medical Assisting

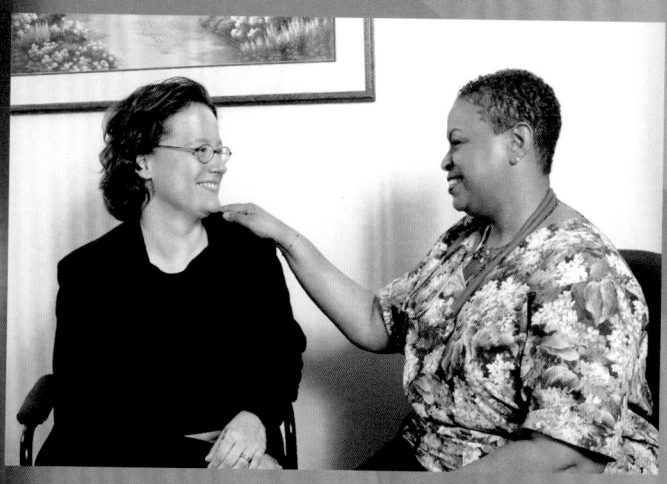

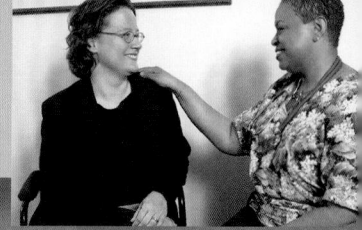

Welcome! The world of medicine is an exciting and challenging frontier. This unit consists of four chapters that will introduce you to the field of medicine and medical assisting, offer vital help in communication skills, and provide you with information to enable you to educate your patients. In the first chapter, you will learn how medicine has evolved through the years from the era of superstition and magical cures to the age of modern technology, in which professionalism is expected from allied health professionals. The second chapter introduces you to legal and ethical responsibilities that affect medical professionals. Sometimes, the advances in medicine challenge our laws and ethics. Chapter 3 covers communication skills, and Chapter 4 introduces you to the concepts of patient education. This unit will help you to understand the bond between medicine, professionalism, law, and ethics, and to communication with patients and coworkers. Let the exploration begin!

## CHAPTER

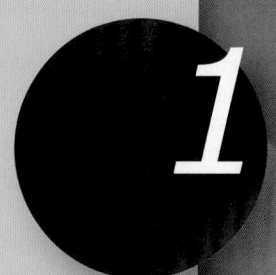

# 1 Medicine and Medical Assisting

## Outline

## Learning Outcomes

**COG Cognitive Domain***

1. Spell and define the key terms
2. Summarize a brief history of modern medicine
3. Explain the system of health care in the United States
4. Discuss the typical medical office
5. List medical specialties a medical assistant may encounter
6. List settings in which medical assistants may be employed

7. List the duties of a medical assistant
8. Describe the desired characteristics of a medical assistant
9. *Differentiate between scope of practice and standards of care for medical assistants*
10. *Compare and contrast provider and medical assistant roles in terms of standard of care*
11. Recognize the role of patient advocacy in the practice of medical assisting

*(continues on page 04)*

12. *Define a patient-centered medical home*
13. *Define the principles of self-boundaries*
14. *Differentiate between adaptive and nonadaptive coping mechanisms*
15. Identify members of the health care team
16. Explain the pathways of education for medical assistants
17. Discuss the importance of program accreditation
18. Name and describe the two nationally recognized accrediting agencies for medical assisting education programs
19. Explain the benefits and avenues of certification for the medical assistant
20. *Discuss licensure and certification as it applies to health care providers*
21. List the benefits of membership in a professional organization
22. *Identify the effect personal morals may have on professional performance*

### PSY Psychomotor Domain*

1. *Locate a state's legal scope of practice for medical assistants*
2. Perform within scope of practice
3. Practice within the standard of care for a medical assistant
4. *Develop a plan for separation of personal and professional ethics*
5. Respond to issues of confidentiality

### AFF Affective Domain*

1. Demonstrate awareness of the consequences of not working within the legal scope of practice
2. Apply ethical behaviors, including honesty and integrity, in the performance of medical assisting practice

3. *Recognize the impact personal ethics and morals have on the delivery of health care*
4. *Demonstrate the principles of self-boundaries*

***Note: AAMA/CAAHEP 2015 Standards are italicized.***

### ABHES Competencies

1. Comprehend the current employment outlook for the medical assistant
2. Compare and contrast the allied health professions and understand their relation to medical assisting
3. Understand medical assistant credentialing requirements and the process to obtain the credential. Comprehend the importance of credentialing
4. Have knowledge of the general responsibilities of the medical assistant
5. Define scope of practice for the medical assistant, and comprehend the conditions for practice within the state that the medical assistant is employed
6. Demonstrate professionalism by:
   a. Exhibiting dependability, punctuality, and a positive work ethic
   b. Exhibiting a positive attitude and a sense of responsibility
   c. Maintaining confidentiality at all times
   d. Being cognizant of ethical boundaries
   e. Exhibiting initiative
   f. Adapting to change
   g. Expressing a responsible attitude
   h. Being courteous and diplomatic
   i. Conducting work within scope of education, training, and ability
7. Comply with federal, state, and local health laws and regulations
8. Analyze the effect of hereditary, cultural, and environmental influences

## Key Terms

accreditation
administrative
certification
clinical
concierge
  medicine

continuing education
  units (CEUs)
inpatient
laboratory
medical assistant
multidisciplinary

multiskilled health
  professional
outpatient
Patient-Centered
  Medical Home (PCMH)
practicum

recertification
scope of practice
self-boundaries
specialty

## Case Study

$R$ob Shelton, CMA, was recently hired as a clinical medical assistant at Great Falls Medical Center and has been told he will be responsible for giving all flu vaccines during his first week as ordered by the physicians. He will also be responsible for performing electrocardiograms for several patients scheduled for annual physical exams. Rob has also been told he will have to help with administrative duties when necessary. What are the clinical duties that Rob has been trained to do through his medical assisting education? What are the administrative responsibilities? Does giving injections fall within Rob's scope of practice? How is this determined? What does Rob have to do to maintain his CMA credential? Professional, credentialed medical assistants are invaluable to the physicians who employ them, and the job outlook continues to be excellent for individuals choosing this exciting career. In this chapter, you will learn what it takes to become a credentialed medical assistant and the skills necessary to earn a medical assisting credential. You will also learn about the benefits of joining a national organization as a professional medical assistant.

Welcome to the field of medicine and to the medical assisting profession! You have selected a fascinating and challenging career, one of the fastest growing specialties in the medical field. The need for the **multiskilled health professional**—an individual with versatile training in the health care field—will continue to grow within the foreseeable future, and you are now a part of this exciting career direction.

To help you understand the significance of the medical knowledge and skills you will receive during your course of study, we begin by taking a chronological look at the history of medicine and then explore the profession of medical assisting.

## COG HISTORY OF MEDICINE

Tremendous achievements in the general health, comfort, and well-being of patients have been made just within the past 100 to 150 years, with the greatest advances occurring in the 20th century. The 21st century has brought continued advancement in cancer research, the human genome project, and the eradication of many diseases. Table 1-1 lists some of the important discoveries in the history of medicine. It is difficult to imagine health care without antibiotics, x-ray machines, or anesthesia, but these developments are fairly new to medicine. For example, penicillin was not produced in large quantities until World War II, and surgery was performed without anesthesia until the mid-1800s. The possibility of cures for some of the devastating diseases humans face gets closer with every research project, and there are many being conducted. Chances are good that the next great medical discovery will result from stem cell and cord blood research.

## COG MODERN MEDICAL HISTORY

The Renaissance was a period of enlightenment in all areas of art, science, and education, and it fostered great strides in medicine. The invention of the printing press and the establishment of great universities made the practice of medicine more accessible to larger numbers of practitioners. Great minds collaborated to advance medical and scientific theories and perform experiments that led to discoveries of enormous benefit in the fight against disease.

During this period, Andreas Vesalius (1514–1564) became known as the "Father of Modern Anatomy." He corrected many of Galen's errors and wrote the first relatively correct anatomy textbook. Soon afterward, William Harvey identified the pumping action of the heart. He described circulation as a continuous circuit pumped by the heart to carry blood through the body. Harvey studied the action of the heart using dogs, not humans.

The microscope was invented in the mid-1660s by a Dutch lens maker, Anton van Leeuwenhoek. He was the first person to observe bacteria under a lens, although he had no idea of the significance of the microorganisms to human health. His instrument also allowed him to accurately describe a red blood cell.

The stethoscope was invented by French physician Rene Laennec in 1816, which gave him insights into classifying respiratory conditions and lung diseases that are still being used today.

John Hunter (1728–1793) became known as the "Father of Scientific Surgery." He developed many surgical techniques that are still used today. Hunter also developed and inserted the first artificial feeding tube

## TABLE 1-1    Important Discoveries in Medicine

| Person(s) | Discovery |
| --- | --- |
| Andreas Vesalius (1514–1564) | Wrote the first relatively correct anatomy book. Known as the "Father of Modern Anatomy" |
| William Harvey (1578–1657) | Identified circulation as a continuous circuit pumped by the heart to carry blood through the body |
| Anton van Leeuwenhoek (1632–1723) | Invented the microscope |
| John Hunter (1728–1793) | Developed many surgical techniques still used today. Known as the "Father of Scientific Surgery" |
| Edward Jenner (1749–1823) | Developed the smallpox vaccine in 1796 |
| Benjamin Rush (1746–1813) | Known for efforts to improve the treatment of mentally ill patients. He wrote the first textbook on psychiatry in America. |
| Rene Laennec (1781–1826) | Invented the stethoscope |
| Ignaz Semmelweis (1818–1865) | Discovered hand washing to prevent childbed fever |
| Louis Pasteur (1822–1895) | Promoted using heat to sterilize surgical instruments. Also developed the rabies vaccine. Known as the "Father of Bacteriology" and the "Father of Preventative Medicine" |
| Florence Nightingale (1820–1910) | Founder of modern nursing |
| Elizabeth Blackwell (1821–1910) | First woman to complete medical school in the United States in 1849 |
| Clara Barton (1821–1912) | Founded the American Red Cross in 1881 |
| Joseph Lister (1827–1912) | Began applying antiseptics to wounds to prevent infections |
| Crawford Williamson Long (1815–1878) | Discovered modern anesthesia in 1842 |
| Marie Curie (1867–1934) | Together with her husband, Pierre Curie, discovered polonium and radium, which revolutionized the principles of energy and radioactivity |
| Wilhelm Konrad Roentgen (1845–1943) | Discovered x-rays in 1895 |
| Sir Alexander Fleming (1881–1955) | Discovered penicillin in 1928 |
| Jonas Edward Salk (1914–1995) | Discovered the polio vaccine in 1952 |
| Albert Sabin (1906–1993) | Discovered the oral polio vaccine in 1961 |
| John Gibbon (1903–1973) | Developed the first heart–lung machine in 1953 |
| C. Walton Lillehei (1918–1999) | Performed first successful open heart surgery in 1954. Known as the "Father of Open Heart Surgery" |

into a patient in 1778 and was the first to classify teeth in a scientific manner.

In 1796, Edward Jenner, a physician in England, overheard a young milkmaid explain that she could not catch smallpox because she had already had the very mild cowpox caught while milking her cows. Several weeks later, Jenner inoculated a small boy with smallpox crusts. The boy did not contract the disease, and the prevention for smallpox was discovered. Jenner's discovery of the smallpox vaccine led to more emphasis on prevention of disease rather than on cures.

Also during the early 1800s, the importance of the mind as a part of the health care process was becoming a recognized field of medicine. The first extensive work and writing on mental health was published in 1812 by Benjamin Rush, titled *Medical Inquiries and Observations upon Diseases of the Mind*. He advocated

humane treatment of the mentally ill at a time when most were imprisoned, chained, starved, exhibited like animals, or simply killed. Rush's influence began the separate field of study into the working of the mind that became modern psychiatry.

## Strides in the Prevention of Disease Transmission

The mid-1880s saw a surge in the study of disease transmission. Louis Pasteur (1822–1895) became famous for his work with bacteria. Pasteur discovered that wine turned sour because of the presence of bacteria. He found that, when the bacteria were eliminated, the wine lasted longer. Pasteur's discovery that bacteria in liquids could be eliminated by heat led to the process known as pasteurization. This finding led to using heat to sterilize surgical instruments. Pasteur has been called the "Father of Bacteriology" for this accomplishment. Pasteur also focused on preventing the transmission of anthrax and discovered the rabies vaccine and was honored with the title "Father of Preventive Medicine" for this work.

In the mid-1880s, Ignaz Semmelweis, a Hungarian physician, noticed that women whose babies were born at home with a midwife in attendance had childbed fever less often than those who delivered in well-respected hospitals with prestigious physicians at the bedside. He was ridiculed by the medical establishment and was fired from his position when he required medical personnel to wash their hands in a solution of chlorinated lime before performing obstetric examinations. He was right, of course, and hand washing is still the most important factor in the fight against disease transmission.

At about the same time, Joseph Lister began to apply antiseptics to wounds to prevent infection. The concept was not clearly understood, but before Lister's practices, as many patients died of infection as died of the primitive surgical techniques of the early part of the century.

In 1928, Sir Alexander Fleming, a bacteriologist, accidentally discovered penicillin when his assistant forgot to wash the Petri dishes Fleming had used for experiments. When he noticed the circles of nongrowth around areas of a certain mold, he was able to extract the prototype for one of our most potent weapons against disease. He won the Nobel Prize in 1945 for this accomplishment.

## Possibilities in Surgery

Modern anesthesia was discovered in 1842 by Crawford Williamson Long. The effects of nitrous oxide were known by the mid-1700s, but Long discovered its therapeutic use by accident when he observed a group of chemistry students inhaling it for amusement. Before this time, anesthesia consisted of large doses of alcohol or opium, leather straps for patient restraint, or the unconsciousness resulting from pain. Ether and chloroform came into use at about this time.

In 1952, the first successful open heart surgery was performed by C. Walton Lillehei, and the invention of the first heart–lung machine by John Gibbon paved the way for the first successful open heart surgery using the bypass machine in 1953.

## Women in Medicine

The 1800s brought the first notable records of the contributions of women to the medical field. Florence Nightingale (1820–1910) was the founder of modern nursing. She set standards and developed educational requirements for nurses.

Elizabeth Blackwell (1821–1910) became the first woman to complete medical school in the United States when she graduated from Geneva Medical College in New York. In 1869, Blackwell established her own medical school in Europe for women only, opening the door for a rapidly expanding role for women in the medical field.

Clara Barton (1821–1912) founded the American Red Cross in 1881 and was its first president. She identified the need for psychological as well as physical support for wounded soldiers in the Civil War.

Marie Curie (1867–1934), a brilliant science student, married Pierre Curie, and together, they discovered polonium and radium. Their discovery revolutionized the principles of energy and radioactivity. Marie and Pierre Curie shared the Nobel Prize for chemistry in 1903. Marie continued the research after Pierre's death and again won the Nobel Prize for physics in 1911.

## Important Discoveries

X-rays were discovered in 1895 by Wilhelm Konrad Roentgen when he observed that a previously unknown ray generated by a cathode tube could pass through soft tissue and outline underlying structures. Medical diagnosis was revolutionized, earning Roentgen a Nobel Prize in 1901 for his discovery. The therapeutic uses of x-rays were recognized much later.

Jonas Edward Salk and Albert Sabin discovered the vaccines for polio in the 1950s, which led to near eradication of one of the 20th century's greatest killers.

### CHECKPOINT QUESTION

1. How was penicillin discovered?

## RECENT MEDICAL HISTORY

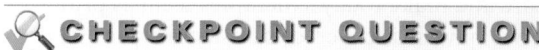

Throughout the next three decades, public health protection improved and advancements continued. Government legislation mandated clean water, and citizens reaped the benefits of preventive medicine and education about health issues.

In the 1980s, advancements in radiology gave doctors ways to see inside a patient with such accuracy that patients no longer had to have exploratory surgery. With computed tomography (CT) scans, radiologists can see tumors, cysts, inflammation, and so on, with cross-sectional slices of the patient's body. Magnetic resonance imaging (MRI) uses a strong magnetic field to realign ions to form an image on a screen. MRI is used to detect internal bleeding, tumors, cysts, and so on. Positron emission tomography (PET) has further revolutionized radiology. A "map" of the body shows the tissues in which the molecular probe has become concentrated and can be interpreted by nuclear medicine physicians or radiologists in the context of the patient's diagnosis and treatment plan. PET scans are increasingly read alongside CT scans or MRI scans, the combination giving both anatomic and metabolic information (what the structure is and what it is doing). PET is used in clinical oncology, showing tumors and determining areas where cancer has spread or metastasized. Researchers are using these scans in studying the human brain and the heart.

In July 1998, Ryuzo Yanagimachi of the University of Hawaii announced the cloning of mice when 7 of 22 mice were cloned from the cell of a single mouse. In December 1998, researchers from Kinki University in Nara, Japan, cloned 8 calves from a single cell.

In 2006, the final human genome papers were published. After years of work, a team of scientists from both the public and private sectors completed the identification and mapping of human genes. Mapping the sequence of the letters of the human genome that represent the handbook of a human being is a breakthrough that will revolutionize the practice of medicine by paving the way for new drugs and therapies. The achievement is one of the most significant scientific landmarks of all time. Many medicines that can be tailored to an individual's genetic makeup are on the market or in development. New discoveries will continue to expand the parameters of medicine as further research in recombinant DNA, transplantation, immunizations, diagnostic procedures, and so forth push back the boundaries of health care and make today's therapies seem as primitive as those we have just covered. You will be present during this fascinating evolution of health care.

Regenerative medicine is an area of research that has seen real progress in accelerating the healing process to fully restore the health of damaged tissues and organs. The goal of regenerative medicine is to one day be capable of maintaining the body in such a way that there will be no need to replace whole organs. These innovative medical therapies are showing great promise over traditional medical treatments. Stem cell procedures have restored sight to the blind, for example, in an Italian study published June 23, 2010, by the *New England Journal of Medicine* of three patients with alkali burns of the eyes. Figure 1-1 shows a printer used for printing skin cells.

Scientists at Wake Forest Institute for Regenerative Medicine in Winston-Salem, NC, were the first in the world to successfully implant a laboratory-grown organ into humans and, today, are working to grow more than 22 different organs and tissues in the laboratory. A series of child and teenage patients have received urinary bladders grown from their own cells. In addition, they are working to develop cell therapies that can help restore organ function. Figure 1-2 shows a bladder made in the laboratory from the patient's own cells.

Within the next decade, expect to see immunization against or cures for many of the illnesses that continue to plague us. And when we need a new kidney, we can make one in the laboratory!

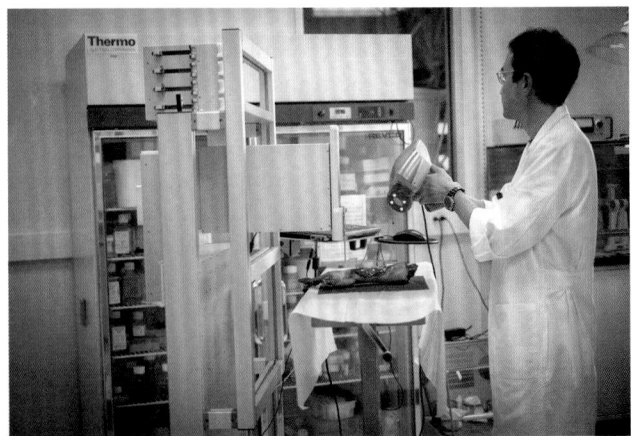

**Figure 1-1** • Scientists at Wake Forest Institute for Regenerative Medicine are using a specialized printer to print skin cells directly onto burns. Various types of skin cells are placed in vials, rather than in cartridges, and then "printed" directly on the wound. (Photo Courtesy of Wake Forest Institute for Regenerative Medicine.)

Your role as a **medical assistant**, the ultimate multiskilled health care professional, will expand as the need for highly trained, versatile medical personnel keeps pace with the ever-changing practice of medicine. Today, heart bypass surgeries and organ transplants are performed routinely. Researchers continue to search for the cures for cancer, acquired immunodeficiency syndrome,

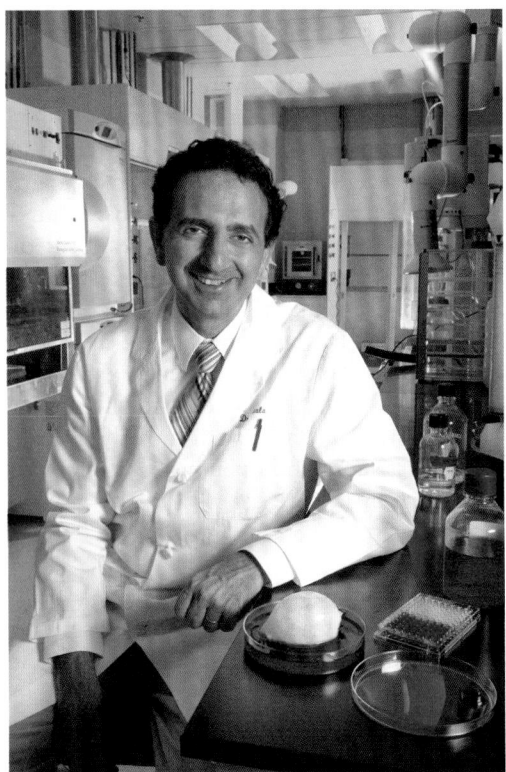

**Figure 1-2** • Dr. Anthony Atala of Wake Forest Institute for Regenerative Medicine and other scientists can now make a human bladder from the patient's own cells. (Photo courtesy of Wake Forest Institute for Regenerative Medicine.)

and many other ailments. Scientists are learning more about mutating organisms and ways to fight them. As a medical assistant, you will witness the progress made as you play a key role in caring for patients.

## ⚙️ THE AMERICAN HEALTH CARE SYSTEM

The American health care system is complex and has seen many changes in the past few decades. The enactment of the Patient Protection and Affordable Care Act (ACA) and the series of programs and regulations arising from the ACA will continue to be at the forefront of health care reform for many years. It is now even more important for the professional medical assistant to understand medical insurance as the ACA requires that all Americans, with few exceptions, have health insurance coverage in one form or another or pay a penalty (see Chapter 13). Understanding how health insurance may affect the health care of patients is necessary especially in terms of how managed care plans work. In today's world of managed care, which is discussed in the chapter on health insurance, many patients are a part of a group of covered members of a managed care plan called an HMO (health maintenance organization). In an HMO plan, patients must use the services of a primary physician who must get insurance authorization before referring patients to another physician (such as a specialist) or before providing many treatments in order for the insurance to cover the costs associated with those services. Although the doctor–patient relationship is one of trust and privacy, many people feel that in a managed care system, patients are treated as determined by the insurance companies. The purpose of care being directed by one physician and treatments to be approved by the insurance company is to control health care costs.

Health care costs are also monitored by the government for the Medicare and Medicaid systems through the Centers for Medicare and Medicaid Services (CMS). In the future, the percentage of office visits by patients 65 years of age and older will increase as baby boomers move into this age group. Many of those individuals will be covered under the Medicare system of insurance for the elderly.

As technology advanced the capabilities of medical facilities to operate electronically, the government responded with the Health Insurance Portability and Accountability Act of 1996 (HIPAA), which was passed to simplify the **administrative** process of transmitting insurance claims, receiving payments, and sharing private health information. HIPAA is discussed throughout the text and covered thoroughly in Chapter 8. The need to adhere to the rules and regulations of the government drives the management practices of the **outpatient**

medical facility. The allied health care arena has grown quickly. New professions have been added to the health care team, and each one is an important part of a patient's total care. As an allied health student, you have an exciting course of study ahead of you. Soon you will find yourself among a caring and conscientious group of health care professionals.

## ⚙️ THE MEDICAL OFFICE

Today's medical office is quite different from the office of the past, where patients were treated by their family physician, insurance was filed, and reimbursement was based on a percentage of the cost. Large corporations and hospitals now own many medical clinics, and physicians are their employees. Billing, collections, insurance processing, laboratory procedures, and other tasks performed in the medical office may be outsourced or handled in a central office for the corporation. Medical practices now have the capability to maintain a patient's record without a single piece of paper. Office employees need a general understanding of the many regulations of the government as well as insurance carriers. Every employee must be computer literate and should understand the legal aspects of the medical office. Although there are many medical specialties, the skills and basic functions of any medical office will be similar. With the new technology and the need for constant monitoring of regulations and changes, the medical office employee is now expected to acquire a formal education and certification.

The typical medical office employs one or more physicians. To assist with examining and treating patients, the physician may employ physician extenders such as physician assistants and/or nurse practitioners. All of these are the providers, and they need support staff. The goal of any medical practice is to provide quality care while maintaining sound financial practices within the laws and ethics of the medical profession. To achieve this goal, the physician needs a solid team. The administrative staff handles the financial aspects of the practice, and the clinical staff assists the providers with patient care. However, both aspects of the office must run smoothly as a team to reach the ultimate goal of the practice. The makeup of the team may differ among specialties. For example, an orthopedist may have an x-ray technologist on staff, or an obstetrician may have an on-site sonographer to perform ultrasounds on pregnant patients. Regardless of the mix of the team, the medical assistant is an integral part.

**Concierge medicine** is another type of health care delivery cropping up across the country. It involves a relationship between a patient and a primary care physician in which the patient pays an annual fee or retainer. This may or may not be in addition to other charges, and the patient's insurance may or may not cover some of the services provided in this type of arrangement. In exchange for the retainer, doctors provide enhanced care. Just as a concierge in a five-star hotel caters to the customer's needs, a physician practicing concierge medicine may see only seven to eight patients a day, attending to their particular health care needs.

The day-to-day operation of a medical office requires all the skills you learn in your curriculum. The patient's health care encounter can be pleasant or unpleasant, depending on the skills and the attitude of the team.

### CHECKPOINT QUESTION

2. What governmental agency monitors medical care finances?

## MEDICAL SPECIALTIES

After completion of medical school, physicians choose a **specialty**. Some prefer treating patients of all ages and will choose family medicine or internal medicine. Others choose surgery and further specialize in fields like cosmetic surgery or vascular surgery. Table 1-2 lists the most common surgical specialties. Table 1-3 lists specialists who may employ medical assistants.

### CHECKPOINT QUESTION

3. What is the specialty that treats newborn babies?

## THE MEDICAL ASSISTING PROFESSION

### What Is a Medical Assistant?

According to the Commission on Accreditation of Allied Health Education Programs (CAAHEP), medical assistants are multiskilled allied health professionals specifically educated to work in ambulatory settings performing administrative and clinical duties. The practice of medical assisting directly influences the public's health and well-being and requires mastery of a complex body of knowledge and specialized skills requiring both formal education and practical experience that serve as standards for entry into the profession.

**Administrative** tasks usually focus on office procedures. **Clinical** tasks generally involve direct patient care. Salaries depend on experience, size of practice or corporation, and geographic region. Hours and working conditions for medical assistants vary according to state laws regarding the medical assisting profession and the scope of the specialty of employer and job responsibilities. **Scope of practice** is defined as the procedures, actions, and processes that are permitted for a particular health care profession. State laws and regulations describe the particular requirements for education and training and define the scope of training for health care practitioners.

Because a medical assistant is not licensed, your scope of practice will depend on your physician–employer's delegation of duties according to state law regarding patient care (see Fig. 1-4). For signs that you are crossing the line, see Box 1-1.

### Duties of a Medical Assistant

The duties of a medical assistant are divided into three categories: general, administrative, and clinical, which includes **laboratory** duties. The ratio of administrative to clinical duties varies with your job description. For example, if you work in a family practice office, you may do mostly clinical work; a psychiatric practice will probably require primarily administrative duties.

### Administrative Duties

Performing administrative tasks correctly and in a timely manner will make the office more efficient and productive. Conversely, an office that is not managed correctly can result in loss of business, poor patient service, and

| TABLE 1-2   Common Surgical Specialties | |
|---|---|
| **Surgical Specialty** | **Description** |
| Cardiovascular | Repairs physical dysfunctions of the cardiovascular system |
| Cosmetic, reconstructive | Restores, repairs, or reconstructs body parts |
| General | Performs repairs on a variety of body parts |
| Maxillofacial | Repairs disorders of the face and mouth (a branch of dentistry) |
| Neurosurgery | Repairs disorders of the nervous system including brain and back surgery |
| Orthopedic | Corrects deformities and treats disorders of the musculoskeletal system |
| Thoracic | Repairs organs within the rib cage |
| Trauma | Limited to correcting traumatic wounds |
| Vascular | Repairs disorders of blood vessels, usually excluding the heart |

## TABLE 1-3  Specialists Who Employ Medical Assistants

| Specialty | Description |
| --- | --- |
| Allergist | Performs tests to determine the basis of allergic reactions to eliminate or counteract the offending allergen |
| Anesthesiologist | Determines the most appropriate anesthesia during surgery for the patient's situation |
| Cardiologist | Diagnoses and treats disorders of the cardiovascular system, including the heart, arteries, and veins |
| Chiropractor | Manipulates the musculoskeletal system and spine to relieve symptoms |
| Dermatologist | Diagnoses and treats skin disorders; may provide cosmetic treatments |
| Emergency physician | Usually works in emergency or trauma centers |
| Endocrinologist | Diagnoses and treats disorders of the endocrine system and its hormone-secreting glands, e.g., diabetes and dwarfism |
| Epidemiologist | Specializes in epidemics caused by infectious agents; studies toxic agents, air pollution, and other health-related phenomena; and works with sexually transmitted disease control |
| Family practitioner | Serves a variety of patient age levels, seeing patients for everything from ear infections to school physicals |
| Gastroenterologist | Diagnoses and treats disorders of the stomach and intestine |
| Gerontologist | Limits practice to disorders of the aging population and its unique challenges |
| Gynecologist | Diagnoses and treats disorders of the female reproductive system and may also be an obstetrician or limit the practice to gynecology, including surgery |
| Hematologist | Diagnoses and treats disorders of the blood and blood-forming organs |
| Immunologist | Concentrates on the body's immune system and disease incidence, transmission, and prevention |
| Internist | Limits practice to diagnosis and treatment of disorders of internal organs with medical (drug therapy and lifestyle changes) rather than surgical means |
| Neonatologist | Limits practice to the care and treatment of infants to about 6 weeks of age |
| Nephrologist | Diagnoses and treats disorders of the kidneys |
| Neurologist | Limits practice to the nonsurgical care and treatment of brain and spinal cord disorders |
| Obstetrician | Limits practice to care and treatment for pregnancy, the postpartum period, and fertility issues |
| Oncologist | Diagnoses and treats tumors, both benign (noncancerous) and malignant (cancerous) |
| Ophthalmologist | Diagnoses and treats disorders of the eyes, including surgery (an optometrist monitors and measures patients for corrective lenses, and an optician makes the lenses or dispenses contact lenses) |
| Orthopedist | Diagnoses and treats disorders of the musculoskeletal system, including surgery and care for fractures |
| Otorhinolaryngologist | Diagnoses and treats disorders of the ear, nose, and throat |
| Pain Management | Specializes in the treatment of patients with chronic pain |
| Pathologist | Analyzes tissue samples or specimens from surgery, diagnoses abnormalities, and performs autopsies |
| Pediatrician | Limits practice to childhood disorders or may be further specialized to early childhood or adolescent period |
| Podiatrist | Diagnoses and treats disorders of the feet and provides routine care for diabetic patients who may have poor circulation and require extra care |
| Proctologist | Limits practice to disorders of the colon, rectum, and anus |
| Psychiatrist | Diagnoses and treats mental disorders |
| Pulmonologist | Diagnoses and treats disorders of the respiratory system |
| Radiologist | Interprets x-rays and imaging studies and performs radiation therapy |
| Rheumatologist | Diagnoses and treats arthritis, gout, and other joint disorders |
| Surgeon | Performs surgical procedures (see Table 1-2, Common Surgical Specialties) |
| Urologist | Diagnoses and treats disorders of the urinary system, including the kidneys and bladder, and disorders of the male reproductive system |

**BOX 1-1** **Scope of Practice for a CMA (AAMA)**

It is important that you and your employers be familiar with the laws governing the practice of medicine in your state. Any limitations placed on allied health personnel would be found there. The American Association of Medical Assistants' (AAMA's) *Occupational Analysis of the CMA (AAMA)* outlines the knowledge and skills that define the profession of medical assisting. The scope of practice is addressed with a disclaimer that states, "this occupational analysis does not delineate delegable responsibilities" and directs specific questions regarding the legal scope of practice of the CMA (AAMA) to the Director and Legal Counsel of AAMA. Physicians who employ certified medical assistants do so with the understanding that the person holding those credentials has been through a formal training program that provides entry-level competence and has passed a comprehensive examination that evaluates the knowledge and critical thinking skills needed according to the standards of the profession.

loss of revenue. Following is a partial list of standard administrative duties:

- Managing and maintaining the waiting room, office, and examining rooms
- Handling telephone calls
- Using written and oral communication
- Preparing and maintaining medical records
- Bookkeeping
- Scheduling appointments
- Ensuring good public relations
- Maintaining office supplies
- Screening sales representatives
- Filing insurance forms
- Processing the payroll
- Arranging patient hospitalizations
- Sorting and filing mail
- Instructing new patients regarding office hours and procedures
- Applying computer concepts to office practices
- Implementing diagnostic and procedural coding for insurance claims
- Completing medical reports

## Clinical Duties

Clinical responsibilities vary among employers. As mentioned, state laws regarding the scope of practice for medical assistants also differ. In some states, medical assistants are not allowed to perform invasive procedures, such as injections or laboratory testing. Remember, states leave the responsibility for the medical assistant's actions with the physician–employer. Both the American Association of Medical Assistants (AAMA) and American Medical Technologists (AMT) have outlined the duties of a medical assistant. Following is a partial list of clinical duties:

- Preparing patients for examinations and treatments
- Assisting other health care providers with procedures
- Preparing and sterilizing instruments
- Completing electrocardiograms
- Applying Holter monitors
- Obtaining medical histories
- Administering medications and immunizations
- Obtaining vital signs (blood pressure, pulse, temperature, respirations)
- Obtaining height and weight measurements
- Documenting in the medical record
- Performing eye and ear irrigations
- Recognizing and treating medical emergencies
- Initiating and implementing patient education

## Laboratory Duties

A medical assistant may perform the following types of laboratory duties in the medical office:

- Low-complexity laboratory tests as determined by the Clinical Laboratory Improvement Amendments (CLIA) of 1988
- Collecting and processing laboratory specimens

## CHECKPOINT QUESTION

4. What are five administrative duties and five clinical or laboratory duties performed by a medical assistant?

 **PATIENT EDUCATION**

### The Health Care System

As a medical assistant, you play a key role in teaching patients not only about their health but also about the health care system. Some patients become confused and are overwhelmed by the number and variety of health care workers. You can help by providing the answers to these common questions:

- What is a multidisciplinary team?
- Who will conduct the examination (physician, physician's assistant, or nurse practitioner)?
- What is a medical assistant?
- What do medical assistants do?
- What kind of training is required for medical assistants?
- What does credentialing mean for a medical assistant?

When patients understand the health care field and know what to expect, they recover more quickly and are more comfortable asking questions about their health.

# AFF THE PROFESSIONAL MEDICAL ASSISTANT

Experts say that professionalism is the one quality all employers seek. An allied health care career holds excitement, variety, and prestige, but with that comes a responsibility to the patients being served. This requires professionalism and a strong work ethic. Work ethic refers to the commitment to your job and is a reflection that you place your job at high importance in your life. Table 1-4 focuses on the actions of an employee with a strong work ethic.

One sign of professionalism and seriousness of purpose is membership in a professional organization. The benefits of membership will be invaluable to you and your future. Participation in a professional organization keeps you abreast of changes and issues facing your profession. If you are a student member, continue as an active member. If not, consider joining. Many employers will pay dues and other expenses for professional activities. Information about joining these organizations can be found at their Web sites (see Media Menu).

Medical assistants play a key role in creating and maintaining a professional image for their employers. Medical assistants must always appear neat and well groomed. Clothing should be clean, pressed, and in good condition. Footwear should be neat, comfortable, and professional. If sneakers are approved by your supervisor, they should be all white. Only minimal makeup and jewelry should be worn. Tattoos and body piercings should not be visible. You should wear a watch with a second hand. Fingernails should be clean and, as per the CDCs guideline for and hygiene in health care settings, should be no longer than ¼ inch, and artificial nails should not be worn when there is direct patient contact. If polish is worn, it should be pale or clear (Fig. 1-3).

Medical assistants must be dependable and punctual (see Table 1-4). Tardiness and frequent absences are not acceptable. If you are not at work, someone must

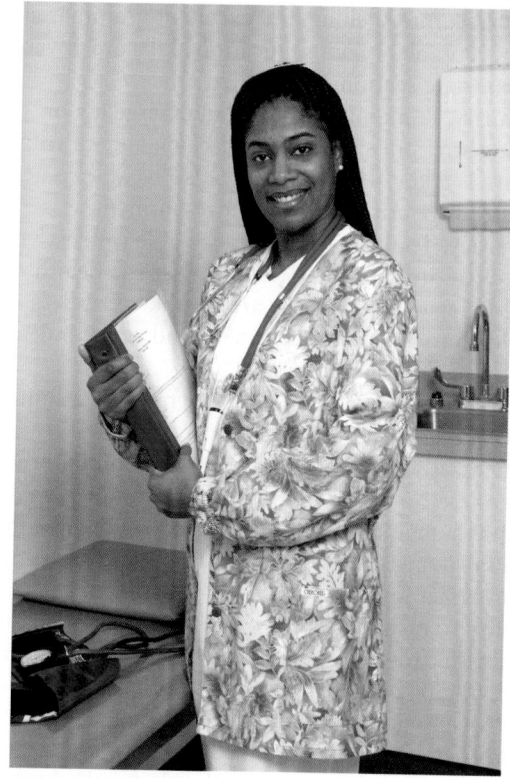

**Figure 1-3** • Medical assistants play a key role in creating and maintaining a professional image for their employers.

fill in for you causing an extra workload for the rest of the staff. Medical assistants must be flexible and adaptable to meet the constantly changing needs of the office. Weekend and holiday hours may be required in some specialties. You must be a team player and go the extra mile to make sure patients are receiving excellent care.

Additional characteristics vital to the profession include the following:

• Excellent written and oral communications skills. You will be required to interact with patients and other health care workers on a professional basis.

| TABLE 1-4 | Do You Have a Strong Work Ethic? |
|---|---|
| Always do the right thing | Your physician–employer has been in the papers lately for charges of tax evasion. Everywhere you go, people want to talk about it. You do *not* discuss it with anyone, saying, "Dr. Miller is my employer, and I am loyal to him." |
| Always try to exceed expectations | You are asked to head a committee to determine patient satisfaction. You complete the task with enthusiasm and see it as a chance to shine. |
| Be a team player | A coworker's mother is in the hospital, and your coworker needs to take a few days off. You were scheduled to be off, but you step in to cover for her knowing that patient care will be affected if both of you are out of the office. |
| Be self-motivated | The physician has seen his last patient. It's time to go home, but the autoclave needs to be emptied. You stay the few extra minutes it takes to put the sterilized items away. |
| Be committed to the organization | You overhear two patients complaining about their wait time. You offer your apologies and tell them you will pass on their concerns. You do just that and suggest that the problem of waiting times be discussed at the next staff meeting. Patient satisfaction is your goal because you are committed to the practice. |

Only accurate spelling and excellent grammar skills are acceptable. (Communication skills are covered in appropriate sections of this text.)

• Maturity. Remaining calm in an emergency or during stressful situations and being able to calm others is a key skill. You must also be able to accept constructive criticism without resentment.

• Accuracy. The physician must be able to trust you to pay close attention to detail because the health and well-being of the patients are at stake. Careless errors could cause harm to the patient and result in legal action against the physician.

• Honesty. If errors are made, they must be admitted, and corrective procedures must be initiated immediately. Covering up errors or blaming others is dishonest. So are using office property for personal business, making telephone calls during work time, and falsifying time records. Such practices can ruin your career and are to be strictly avoided.

• Ability to respect patient confidentiality. Few issues in health care can damage your career as profoundly as divulging confidential patient information, and the HIPAA privacy law mandates that patient privacy be protected at all costs.

• Empathy. The ability to care deeply for the health and welfare of your patients is the heart of medical assisting.

• Courtesy. Every patient who enters the office must be treated with respect and gracious manners.

• Good interpersonal skills. Tempers may flare in stressful situations; learn to keep yours in check and work well with all levels of interaction.

• Ability to project a positive self-image. If you are confident in your abilities as a professional, this attitude will reflect in all of your relationships.

• Ability to work as a team player. The patient's return to health is the most important objective of the office. Each staff member must work toward this goal.

• Initiative and responsibility. You must be able to move from one task to another quickly and without direct supervision. The entire team expects each of its members to perform assigned responsibilities.

• Tact and diplomacy. The right word at the right moment can calm and soothe anger, depression, and fear and relieve a potentially unsettling situation.

• High moral and ethical standards. Project for your profession the highest level of professionalism.

• Demonstration of adaptive coping mechanisms. The health care arena is constantly changing, and you must be able to see the positive in change.

## CHECKPOINT QUESTION

5. What are eight characteristics that a professional medical assistant should have?

## Scope of Practice and Standards of Care

Health professionals operate under a scope of practice— the specific activities allowed by state licensing boards and laws or by the practice itself. The term "scope of practice" refers to all medical professions, and staying within that scope is an important part of your work ethic. Figure 1-4 shows a decision-making tool for clinical professionals.

A handful of states specify scope of practice for medical assistants. However, in most of those states, medical assistants are barred from providing any type of direct patient care or procedure without the presence of a licensed medical professional on-site, which is typically a doctor, physician assistant, or nurse practitioner.

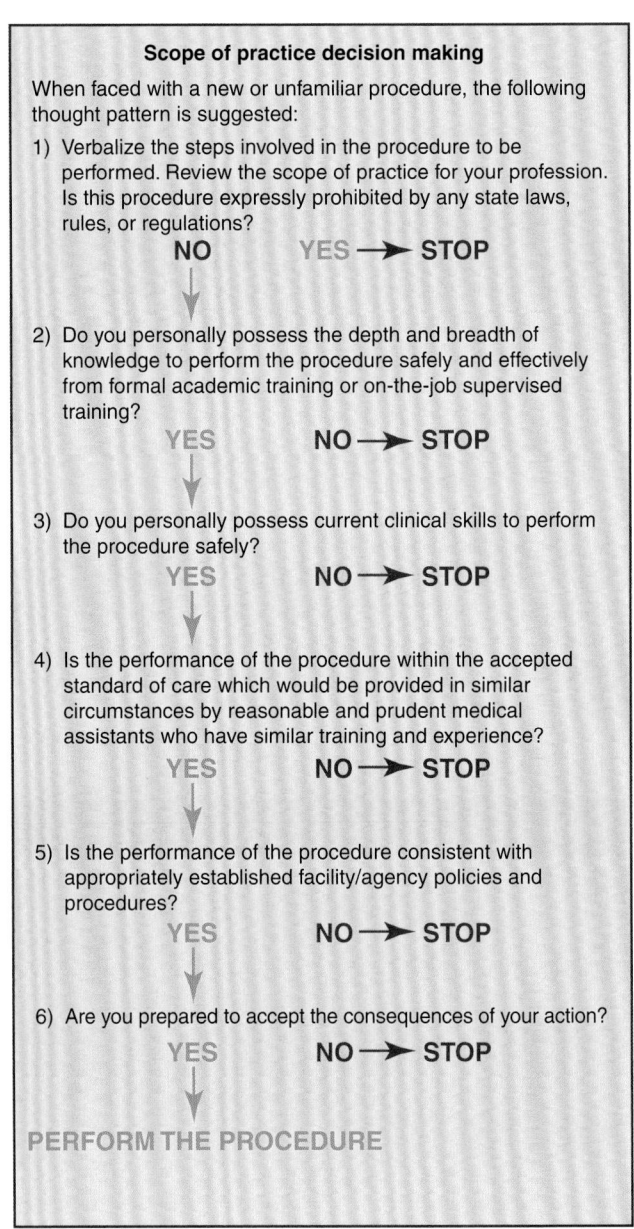

**Scope of practice decision making**

When faced with a new or unfamiliar procedure, the following thought pattern is suggested:

1) Verbalize the steps involved in the procedure to be performed. Review the scope of practice for your profession. Is this procedure expressly prohibited by any state laws, rules, or regulations?
   NO      YES ➤ STOP

2) Do you personally possess the depth and breadth of knowledge to perform the procedure safely and effectively from formal academic training or on-the-job supervised training?
   YES      NO ➤ STOP

3) Do you personally possess current clinical skills to perform the procedure safely?
   YES      NO ➤ STOP

4) Is the performance of the procedure within the accepted standard of care which would be provided in similar circumstances by reasonable and prudent medical assistants who have similar training and experience?
   YES      NO ➤ STOP

5) Is the performance of the procedure consistent with appropriately established facility/agency policies and procedures?
   YES      NO ➤ STOP

6) Are you prepared to accept the consequences of your action?
   YES      NO ➤ STOP

PERFORM THE PROCEDURE

**Figure 1-4** • Scope of Practice Decision-Making Tree. (Adapted from the Washington State Department of Health, Nursing Care Quality Assurance Commission, "Scope of Practice Decision Tree.")

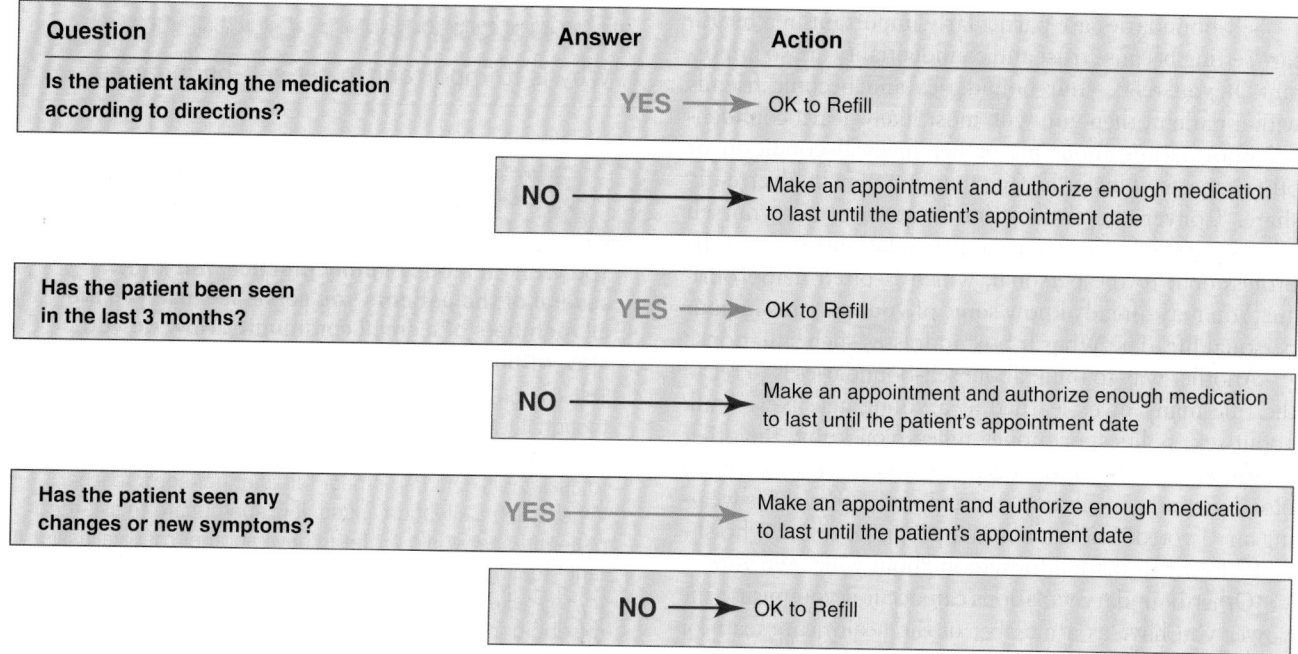

| Question | Answer | Action |
|---|---|---|
| Is the patient taking the medication according to directions? | YES ⟶ | OK to Refill |
| | NO ⟶ | Make an appointment and authorize enough medication to last until the patient's appointment date |
| Has the patient been seen in the last 3 months? | YES ⟶ | OK to Refill |
| | NO ⟶ | Make an appointment and authorize enough medication to last until the patient's appointment date |
| Has the patient seen any changes or new symptoms? | YES ⟶ | Make an appointment and authorize enough medication to last until the patient's appointment date |
| | NO ⟶ | OK to Refill |

**Figure 1-5 •** Sample flow sheet representing established protocol set by physician.

In states with no scope of practice, your duties as a medical assistant depend on those assigned by the physician, physician's assistant, or nurse practitioner who oversees you. A medical assistant's scope of practice is based on his or her education. The educational program that a medical assistant completes will determine what knowledge and skills the medical assistant possesses. Tasks that require medical judgment or interpretation are reserved for providers. In some cases, however, a provider will establish a specific protocol for certain patient encounters. For example, a patient's request for a refill on a narcotic medication may be handled by a medical assistant through the use of a flow chart. Figure 1-5 shows a typical tool used for such physician-delegated tasks. Protocols for decision guidelines are developed through experience working with your physician and are always approved by the physician before implementation.

Not only will you, the medical assistant, be held responsible for your actions, but the medical professional who oversees you will be held personally responsible for your actions as well. The provider can be sued for any actions you take that cross over into the practice of medicine or that may potentially harm a patient and can even result in losing his or her license. Even something as seemingly innocent as telling a patient over the phone not to worry about a symptom could be construed as "practicing medicine without a license."

In addition to practicing within the scope of your education, you must also be mindful of the standard of care you and your providers are giving. Standards of care refer to generally accepted guidelines and principles that health care practitioners follow in the practice of medicine. For instance, it is a standard of care that patients on blood thinners undergo blood coagulation labs at regular intervals. It is a standard of care that people with chronic obstructive pulmonary disease receive an annual flu vaccine and a pneumococcal vaccine as needed. Standards of care can involve tests used to diagnose or screen for diseases, such as mammograms for breast cancer, as well as treatment options. Legally, the standard of care is considered the manner in which other clinicians in the community typically practice.

Standards of care may come from evidence-based guidelines, decades of practice, community standards, and licensing and regulatory agencies, such as the Joint Commission and the Centers for Medicare and Medicaid Services. Hospitals and insurance organizations also set standards of care when they release practice guidelines, as do large medical organizations, such as the American Heart Association and the American Diabetes Association.

As a medical assistant, you must also adhere to accepted standards of care for any clinical services you provide. For instance, if you give an injection incorrectly, resulting in a problem for the patient, then the technique you used may be questioned as to whether it met the agreed-upon standard of care.

## PSY Self-Boundaries

What kind of person are you? Are you a friendly, outgoing person who immediately bonds with everyone you meet and has no problem sharing personal information? Or, are you more reserved, polite but private, maintaining strict boundaries between your personal and professional lives?

The answer is important because, when you work in the medical field, it is critical that you maintain what are called **self-boundaries**. This means setting limits on the relationships between yourself and your patients. Those limits, or boundaries, help delineate the personal from the professional and enable you to avoid inappropriate behavior with patients or even being perceived as displaying such inappropriate behavior.

Self-boundaries are particularly important in a health care setting because trust and confidentiality are so important. If you relax your boundaries and become friends with a patient, then you will, most likely, learn confidential information about his or her medical condition or other aspects of his or her life that you may inadvertently share. Conversely, sharing information about yourself with a patient begins to move that relationship from the professional to the personal, which is often inappropriate. You may already know some of your patients in your personal life. The What If box addresses such situations.

Another way to think about self-boundaries is to recall the rule many of us learned at a young age: Never talk about sex, politics, or money unless you know the other person *very* well. So, for instance, if you take a patient's blood pressure on election day and notice that she is wearing an "I voted" sticker, it is inappropriate to ask who she voted for or to share information about your own vote.

Other boundary violations can occur if you misuse the power you have as a member of the health care team or betray a patient's trust in any way. For instance, if you handle the billing for your office, and a patient calls to tell you that her husband just lost his job and she needs to delay payment, sharing that information with anyone other than your manager is a violation of the patient's trust.

Boundary violations also include not respecting the patient's religious, cultural, and social beliefs and values; neglecting the patient; and abusing the patient financially, verbally, emotionally, and physically. One of the worst boundary violations is crossing the sexual line. This could be as seemingly benign as remaining in the examining room as the patient undresses or as overt as inappropriately touching a patient or developing a sexual relationship with him or her. Box 1-2 outlines signs that you are crossing the self-boundary limits and offers suggestions for preventing boundary violations.

---

### BOX 1-2   Signs That You're Crossing Self-Boundary Limits

- Thinking about a patient when you're not at work
- Seeing the patient outside of work and/or sharing personal information
- Inappropriately touching the patient or the patient inappropriately touching you
- Keeping secrets with the patient
- Not sharing important aspects of the patient's behavior with the medical professionals in the office

**To prevent boundary violations:**

- Do not accept gifts from patients.
- Do not share personal information with patients.
- Do not develop personal relationships with patients.
- Do not accept invitations to personal parties or other social events from patients.

---

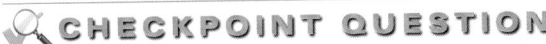

### CHECKPOINT QUESTION

6. Why is it important to set self-boundaries?

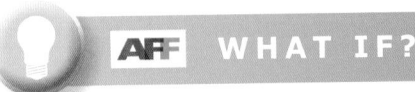   WHAT IF?

**You work in a busy family practice. You know several of the patients you serve because you are all members of a small community. How do you stay within your boundaries?**

This can be an uncomfortable and touchy situation. Even though it is understood that you will not share information acquired in the course of your duties, no one wants to assist with the Pap smear of his or her son's teacher. When such a situation arises, it is appropriate to ask the patient if she would prefer to have another medical assistant step in and assist the physician. If this is not possible, try to make the patient as comfortable as possible by making conversation to distract her. Remember, humor can be a valuable tool if used appropriately. Follow the lead of the patient. Many patients will understand that this is your job, and they will trust that you will be the professional you were trained to be. Maintaining a professional demeanor will help you stay within your boundaries.

## Adaptive and Maladaptive Coping Mechanisms

There is no doubt that the workplace—any workplace—is stressful. But a health care setting has stresses beyond the normal issues of workload, coworker interactions, and authoritarian supervisors. You're also dealing with sick, cranky patients and their commonly serious illnesses. How you cope with the stress and the situations that arise as a result will make a major difference in your professional success. For instance, suppose your office just installed a new electronic record management system. You not only have to learn the new system; you have to change nearly every aspect of how you work. Plus, you have to manually enter patient background information currently residing in paper files while continuing to function as medical office.

People with an adaptive coping mechanism would view the new system as an exciting learning opportunity, one that will add to their professional skills. They volunteer for extra training, view the need to enter the background information into the system as an opportunity to identify gaps in patient information, and restructure their workflow to reduce wasted time and identify opportunities for improvement.

Conversely, those with a maladaptive coping mechanism complain to their coworkers and patients about the extra work, convince themselves that the new system takes more time and effort, and do the bare minimum to maintain their jobs.

Now suppose that the transition to the new system is challenging, with the glitches and delays that are common with all new computer systems. At the end of one particularly difficult day, you feel drained. When you go home, do you go for a brisk walk to clear your head and stretch tight muscles? Or, do you get a spoon and devour a half gallon of butter pecan ice cream?

Obviously, the first choice is the more adaptive coping mechanism. Too often, people deal with stress by turning to food, alcohol, drugs, or other maladaptive behavior. Instead, consider

- Taking a candlelit bubble bath
- Meeting a friend for dinner
- Writing in a journal
- Going bowling
- Cleaning out a closet

Other aspects of adaptive coping behavior include the following:

- **Identifying ways to modify the stressor.** Maybe you cannot get rid of the new electronic records system, but you can ask for additional training.
- **Reframing the situation.** Instead of viewing the new system as cumbersome and time consuming, focus on how it will positively impact the office in a few months, when everyone is familiar with it, and patient medical information is just a few clicks away.
- **Creating boundaries.** Stay away from those in the office who are being negative about the new system; negativity is contagious.

When you develop tools to use when you must adapt in the workplace, you become a positive and valued member of the team.

## MEMBERS OF THE HEALTH CARE TEAM

As a medical assistant, you will work with a variety of health care workers. Today's health care team must be **multidisciplinary.** A multidisciplinary team is a group of specialized professionals who are brought together to meet the needs of the patient. Medical assistants are noted as being essential members of the **Patient-Centered Medical Home (PCMH) team** (see Chapter 13). This type of health care delivery model utilizes a team of providers to meet the needs of the patient including wellness, acute, and chronic care. Some patients will need the assistance of many individuals, whereas other patients may only need one or two members of the team; however, the professional medical assistant may be responsible for coordinating the care to make sure patients receive proper treatment in a manner that is timely, respectful, and with compassion.

### Health Care Providers

#### Physicians

Physicians generally are the team leaders. They are responsible for diagnosing and treating the patient. Minimum education for a physician consists of a 4-year undergraduate degree, often consisting of premedical studies, and 4 years of medical school, followed by a residency program usually concentrating on a certain specialty. The residency program can vary from 2 to 6 years based on the field of study. Physicians must pass a licensure examination for the state in which they wish to practice. A physician who chooses a specialty must pass an examination in that area of study and become board certified by the American Board of Medical Specialties (ABMS). The title "doctor" refers to a medical doctor (M.D.) or doctor of osteopathy (D.O.), but is also used to designate those who have received a doctoral degree in any discipline. For example, a podiatrist uses the title "Dr." He or she holds a doctorate degree in podiatric medicine or, a DPM. One who reaches the highest degree of education in his or her field receives a Ph.D. (Doctorate of Philosophy). Psychologists, educators, and others may hold doctoral degrees but are not medical doctors. In all instances, this title necessitates a degree of respect for the knowledge and hard work the recipient has shown.

### Physician Assistants

Physician assistants (PAs) are specially trained and usually licensed. They work closely with a physician and may perform many of the tasks traditionally done by physicians. What a physician assistant does varies with training, experience, and state law. Their scope of practice corresponds to the supervising physician's practice. In general, a physician assistant will see many of the same types of patients as the physician. The cases handled by physicians are generally the more complicated medical cases or those cases that require care that is not a routine part of the PA's scope of work. Close consultation between the patient, the PA, and the physician is done for unusual or hard to manage cases. Forty-nine states, the District of Columbia, and Guam have enacted laws that allow PAs to prescribe medications. Their educational levels vary from several months to 2 years, depending on the program and the individual's background in medicine. Most PA programs require a Bachelor's degree and 2 to 4 years of experience in the medical field.

National certification is available through the American Association of Physician Assistants. A physician assistant may also choose to become certified by the National Commission on Certification of PAs (NCCPA) and become a PA-C. This requires the PA to acquire 100 hours of continuing medical education every 2 years and take a **recertification** exam every 6 years.

### Nurse Practitioners

Nurse practitioners (NPs) are trained to diagnose patients and treat illnesses. In most states, NPs can write prescriptions, operate their own offices, and admit patients to hospitals. In other states, NPs work more closely with a physician. NPs are experienced RNs and, in most cases, have a master's degree in nursing with the addition of specialized training as an NP. In some states, NPs are regulated by the Board of Nursing. In five states, they are regulated by the Board of Nursing and the Board of Medicine. There has been a recent collaborative effort by the American Academy of Nurse Practitioners (AANP) to identify the Nurse Practitioners' Primary Care Competencies, which include adult, family, gerontology, pediatrics, and women's health.

## The Nursing Profession

Nurses are trained to work with physicians and implement various patient care needs in the **inpatient** or hospital setting. Their job descriptions vary according to their experiences, specialties, and certifications. There are several levels of education in nursing. A Bachelor of Science (BS) degree in nursing requires 4 years of college. A Licensed Practical Nurse (LPN) must complete a 1-year program. A nurse with an Associate in Applied Science (AAS) degree in nursing attends 2 years of college and becomes a Registered Nurse (RN). The nursing profession also monitors the education and provides the means for certification of the Certified Nursing Assistant (CNA I and CNA II). CNAs offer personal care and assist in nursing tasks. CNA programs usually last 4 to 6 weeks.

## Allied Health Professionals

Allied health care professionals make up a large section of the health care team. Box 1-3 lists and describes some

---

### BOX 1-3 Allied Health Care Professionals

Cardiovascular technologist—Assists in diagnostic process and treatment stage of all related heart and vascular problems

Dental assistant—Works under the supervision of dentists by doing a wide range of tasks in the dental office, ranging from patient care to administrative duties to laboratory functions

Dental hygienist—Trained and licensed to work with a dentist by providing preventive care

Electrocardiograph technician—Assists with the performance of diagnostic procedures for cardiac electrical activity

Electroencephalograph technician—Assists with the diagnostic procedures for brain wave activity

Electroneurodiagnostic technologist—Assists in the recording and study of the electrical activity of the brain and nervous system using a variety of techniques and instruments

Emergency medical technician—Trained in techniques of administering emergency care en route to trauma centers

Health information technologist—Trained in managing medical records, health care coding, and HIPAA regulations

Laboratory technician—Trained in performance of laboratory diagnostic procedures

Medical assistant—Trained in administrative, clinical, and laboratory skills for the medical facility

Medical coder—Assigns appropriate codes to report medical services to third-party payers for reimbursement

Medical office assistant—Trained in the administrative area of the outpatient medical facility

Medical transcriptionist—Trained in administrative skills; produces printed records of dictated medical information

Nuclear medical technician—Specializes in diagnostic procedures using radionuclides (electromagnetic radiation); works in a radiology department

Nutritionist—Addresses dietary needs associated with illness; assists and trains patients with special diets for weight control and supplementation needed for patients undergoing cancer treatment, etc.

Occupational therapist—Evaluates and plans programs to relieve physical and mental barriers that interfere with activities

Paramedic—Trained in advanced rescue and emergency procedures

Pharmacist—Prepares and dispenses medications by the physician's order

Phlebotomist—Collects blood specimens for laboratory procedures by performing venipuncture

Physical therapist—Plans and conducts rehabilitation to improve strength and mobility

Polysomnographer—Performs sleep diagnostics that are required for the diagnosis of sleep disorders

Psychologist—Trained in methods of psychological assessment and treatment

Radiographer—Works with a radiologist or physician to operate x-ray equipment for diagnosis and treatment. Radiography technologists may specialize in computed tomography/magnetic resonance imaging, nuclear medicine, mammography, etc.

Respiratory therapist—Trained to preserve or improve respiratory function

Risk manager—Identifies and corrects high-risk situations within the health care field

Sonographer—Uses high-frequency sound waves to image internal structures in the human body including abdominal organs, pelvic organs, small parts, and the vascular system

Speech therapist—Treats and prevents speech and language disorders

Surgical technician—Assists in the care of the surgical patient in the operating room and to function as a member of the surgical team

of these team members. The educational requirements and responsibilities vary greatly among these professionals. One thing they all have in common is the support of a professional organization. Medical assistants fall into this category.

## COG THE HISTORY OF MEDICAL ASSISTING

Medical assisting as a separate profession dates from the 1930s. In 1934, Dr. M. Mandl recognized the need for medical professionals who possessed the skills required in a medical office environment and opened the first school for medical assistants in New York City. Although medical assistants were employed before 1934, no formal schooling was available. Office assistants were trained on the job to perform clinical procedures, or nurses were trained to perform administrative procedures. The need for a highly trained professional with a background in administrative and clinical skills led to the formation of an alternative field of allied health care. In 1956, the AAMA, a professional organization for medical assistants, was founded during a meeting of medical assistants in Milwaukee, Wisconsin. The constitution and bylaws adopted by the group were commended by the American Medical Association (AMA), the professional association of licensed physicians. In 1959, Illinois recognized the AAMA as a not-for-profit educational organization. The national office was established in Chicago, with state and local chapters throughout the United States. In 1963, a certification examination for CMA was conducted that would set the standards required for medical assistant education. The first AAMA examinations were given in Kansas, California, and Florida. In the next two decades, the profession grew rapidly. The AMA collaborated in the development of the curriculum and **accreditation** of educational programs. In 1974, the U.S. Department of Health, Education, and Welfare recognized the AAMA Curriculum Review Board in conjunction with the American Medical Association's Council on Medical Education as an official accrediting agency for medical assisting programs in public and private schools.

In 1991, the Board of Trustees of the AAMA approved the current definition of medical assisting: Medical assisting is an allied health profession whose practitioners function as members of the health care delivery team and perform administrative and clinical procedures. Medical assistants continue to be vigilant for threats to their right to practice their profession. Each state mandates the actions of allied health professionals. It is the responsibility of medical assistants to be familiar with the laws of the state in

which they are working. Membership in the AAMA exceeds 20,000 medical assistants, with more than 300 local chapters in 43 states. A complete history of the AAMA is available at www.aama-ntl.org. Box 1-4 outlines important changes made by the House of Delegates of the AAMA.

---

### BOX 1-4 AAMA House of Delegate Changes

- In 1995, the American Association of Medical Assistants (AAMA) House of Delegates approved changing the eligibility pathway for candidates of the AAMA certification examination as follows: "Any candidate for the AAMA CMA Certification Exam must be a graduate of a CAAHEP-accredited medical assisting program." Before June 1998, medical assistants who had been employed by a physician for 1 year full-time or 2 years part-time were eligible to sit for the CMA Certification Examination.

- In 2001, AAMA made the decision to grant graduates of medical assisting programs accredited by the Accrediting Bureau of Health Education Schools immediate eligibility to sit for the certified medical assistant (CMA) examination beginning in January 2002.

- In January 2003, all CMAs employed or seeking employment were required to have current certification to use the CMA credentials in connection with employment.

- Effective January 2007, CMAs recertifying by continuing education method must attain 30 credits that are AAMA approved, with 10 recertification points in each content category: general, administrative, and clinical. Prior to 2007, 20 of the 60 continuing education units required had to be AAMA approved with 15 recertification points in each content category.

- In 2007, Certified Medical Assistant® became a trademark.

- In 2008, the CMA credentials changed to CMA (AAMA) in order to differentiate from other credentials being offered in the marketplace.

- In 2008, the Curriculum Review Board of the AAMA Endowment was officially changed to the Medical Assisting Education Review Board (MAERB).

---

### CHECKPOINT QUESTION

7. What prompted the establishment of a school for medical assistants?

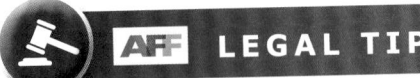

## LEGAL TIP

### Who's the Boss

Although a nurse's training involves inpatient or hospital care, some physicians choose to employ nurses in their offices. In some states, nurses working in physician offices are not allowed to supervise or delegate their authority to medical assistants. However, nurses and medical assistants work side by side in many instances because the medical assistant works under the supervision of the physician, not the nurse. For example, in the North Carolina law regarding this issue, the legislation refers to medical assistants as "unlicensed health care personnel." Medical assistants are certified, not licensed. There is a difference. **Certification**, by definition, indicates a higher level of competence. The legal issues involving licensure and certification are discussed in Chapter 2.

## MEDICAL ASSISTING EDUCATION

A medical assisting curriculum prepares individuals for entry into the medical assisting profession. Medical assisting programs are found in postsecondary schools, such as private business schools and technical colleges, 2-year colleges, and community colleges. Programs vary in length. Programs of 6 months to a year offer a certificate of graduation or a diploma, and 2-year programs award the graduate an associate degree. The 2-year curriculum usually includes general studies such as English, mathematics, and computer skills, in addition to the core courses, such as medical terminology and insurance coding. The curriculum in every accredited program must include the skills determined by the accrediting agency. Figure 1-6

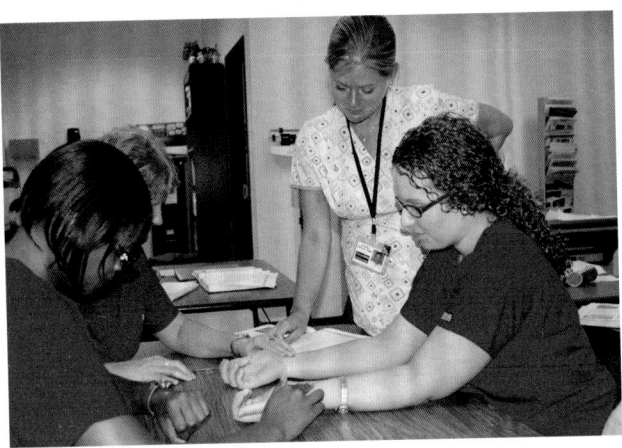

**Figure 1-6** • Students practice competencies taught in their medical assisting classes. Their scope of practice is determined by their training.

### BOX 1-5    AAMA Continuing Education

**Continuing education units (CEUs)** can be acquired by attending American Association of Medical Assistants (AAMA)-approved seminars, through articles in the organization's bimonthly publication, and by completing self-studies available through AAMA. Membership in AAMA is not required for maintaining the certified medical assistant credentials, but one of the member benefits is the maintenance of a CEU registry. Many state societies and local chapters offer AAMA-approved CEUs at their meetings.

shows students learning to take a patient's pulse rate. Box 1-5 specific requirements for an accredited program are discussed later.

Accredited programs must include a practicum. A **practicum** or externship is an educational course offered in the last module or semester during which the student works in the field gaining hands-on experience. It varies in length from 160 to 240 hours. Students are not paid but are awarded credit toward the degree (see the last chapter, *Making the Transition: Student to Employee*, for more detailed information). Some schools offer career placement services.

After you finish school, your education should not stop. You should continue to take courses on various related topics, and earning a medical assisting credential will require you to submit continuing education units (CEUs) to maintain your credential (see Box 1-4). These may include new computer programs, new clinical procedures, new laws and regulations, or pharmaceutical updates. Membership to professional organizations, such as the AAMA, gives opportunities to earn CEUs through seminars and conferences, and some employers pay for conferences (see additional information given in this chapter). In some situations, conference costs may be listed as a tax deduction when filing your income tax.

### Medical Assisting Program Accreditation

**Accreditation** is a nongovernmental professional peer review process that provides technical assistance and evaluates educational programs for quality based on pre-established academic and administrative standards. Medical assisting program accreditation is based on a school's adherence to the essentials of a sound education and services for students. The skills that medical assistants need to be successful in a job are taught and documented in a competency-based format. Entry-level competency is acquired and documented in a competency-based format that includes the specific skill to be mastered, the conditions under which you are to perform the skill (including equipment and supplies needed), and the standard of performance for the skill.

## The Commission on Accreditation of Allied Health Education Programs

The Commission on Accreditation of Allied Health Education Programs (CAAHEP), in collaboration with the Medical Assisting Education Review Board (MAERB), accredits medical assisting programs in both public and private postsecondary institutions throughout the United States. According to the CAAHEP Web site, CAAHEP is the largest programmatic accreditor in the health sciences field. In collaboration with its Committees on Accreditation, specifically the MAERB, CAAHEP reviews and accredits over 2,000 educational programs in 22 health science occupations. Its mission is to assure quality health profession education to serve the public interest. CAAHEP processes, actions, and strategies are guided by integrity, collaboration, accountability, and consensus.

## The Accrediting Bureau of Health Education Schools

The Accrediting Bureau of Health Education Schools (ABHES) accredits private postsecondary medical assisting programs. ABHES is nationally recognized by the U.S. Secretary of Education as a private, nonprofit, independent accrediting agency. ABHES enhances the quality of education and training and promotes institutional and programmatic accountability through systematic and consistent program evaluation. Its mission is to assure the quality of the programs it accredits and assist in the improvement of the programs. This quality determination is accomplished by rigorous and systematic evaluation based on valid standards.

The goals of ABHES focus on three key areas: recognition, resources, and service, all of which it believes to be essential and paramount to achieving its mission.

### CHECKPOINT QUESTION

8. What are the two accrediting agencies for medical assisting education programs?

 ## MEDICAL ASSISTING CREDENTIALS

Today, busy physician offices prefer to employ medical assistants who demonstrate competence through evidence of a credential such as certification. New laws and federal regulations such as the CMS ruling for the meaningful use payment incentive require physicians to hire only credentialed medical assistants for entering

orders into a computerized medical record. However, the types of medical assistant credentials available vary and not all credentials or their requirements for obtainment are alike. This section outlines the most common credentials, including recertification information if known.

## Certified Medical Assistant (American Association of Medical Assistants)

The CMA (AAMA) is the only credential sponsored by the American Association of Medical Assistants. Currently, only students who graduate from a CAAHEP (Commission on Accreditation of Allied Health Education Programs) or ABHES (Accrediting Bureau of Health Education Schools) accredited medical assistant program may sit for this certification examination. The exam was first offered in 1963 and has the distinction of having the National Board of Medical Examiners as test consultants. To maintain the credential, 60 continuing education units (CEUs) must be obtained every 5 years in three categories.

## Registered Medical Assistant (American Medical Technologist)

The RMA (AMT) credential is awarded by the American Medical Technologists, who also sponsors several allied health professions in addition to medical assistants. In addition to graduates from ABHES or CAAHEP accredited programs, others who may sit for the RMA exam include anyone who completes a medical assistant program in a postsecondary school or college that is regionally or nationally accredited and approved by the U.S. Department of Education, anyone who completes a formal training program that is part of the U.S. Armed Forces, anyone who has not received formal training but who has been employed in the profession of medical assisting for a minimum of 5 years, or anyone who has passed a medical assistant certification examination offered by another certification agency approved by the AMT Board of Directors.

To recertify, RMAs who received the credential prior to January 1, 2006, are encouraged to remain current; however, recertification is not required. Those who became certified after January 2006 are required to obtain 30 points every 3 years through a Certification Continuation Program (CCP).

## Certified Clinical Medical Assistant (National Healthcareer Association)

The CCMA exam was first offered in 1989. Like the AMT, the NHA certifies several allied health professions. To sit for this examination, the applicant must be at least 18 years of age, have a high school diploma (or equivalent), have successfully complete an allied health training program within the past year, *or* have 1 year of experience as a medical assistant. Ten continuing education hours is required from the NHA every 2 years to maintain this credential, and if certification expires, 10 CE credits, payment of the 2-year recertification fee, and a reinstatement fee are required.

## National Certified Medical Assistant (National Center for Competency Testing)

The NCMA credential is offered by the NCCT, which also offers exams for several allied health professions. Eligibility to sit for this examination includes a high school diploma or equivalent and either completion of an NCCT-approved medical assisting program within the last 10 years or 2 qualifying years (4,160 hours) of full-time employment (or equivalent part-time employment) within the last 10 years as a medical assistant.

 **CHECKPOINT QUESTION**

9. What is required to maintain current status as a certified medical assistant?

 **ETHICAL TIP**

### Who Is Who?

It is important that medical assistants represent themselves honestly. Physicians often innocently refer to every employee as "the nurse." It is more accurate to say my assistant, my certified medical assistant, my registered medical assistant, or my clinical assistant. There are documented court cases involving misrepresentation of one's education and credentials. Protect yourself by referring to yourself appropriately to patients and coworkers. Do not identify yourself as "Dr. Smith's nurse." When patients refer to you as a nurse, you should correct them. The more your credentials are heard by patients and coworkers, the more understood and recognized they will be. You should be proud of your profession and your credentials. Let it be known.

## MEDICAL ASSISTING AND RELATED ALLIED HEALTH ASSOCIATIONS

### Association Membership

You are not required to join a national organization to work as a medical assistant or to be eligible to take the certification examination. The associations have many

benefits, however, for members. These benefits include the following:

- Access to educational seminars
- Access to continuing education units
- Subscription to the professional journals that alert you to new procedures and trends in medicine
- Access to the annual conventions
- Group insurance plans
- Networking opportunities

For further information on these organizations, visit the Web sites listed at the end of the chapter. Contact your local chapter or speak with your instructor for the procedure for applying for membership. You can download applications and requirements from the AAMA Web site (http://www.aama-ntl.org/) and the AMT Web site (http://americanmedtech.org).

### American Association of Medical Assistants

The purpose of the AAMA is to promote the professional identity and stature of its members and the medical assisting profession through education and credentialing. *CMA Today*, which is published and distributed to members of the organization, includes articles of interest to the medical assistant to keep knowledge and skills current. Readers may take posttests at the end of articles and receive CEUs. Approved continuing education opportunities are available through the national organization, and free transcripts of acquired AAMA-approved CEUs are available online to members. Professional benefits, such as insurance, are also made available to AAMA members. Active members are CMAs, associate members are medical assistants who are not yet CMAs, and affiliate members are those interested in medical assisting. Students are encouraged to join and stay active in AAMA. Student members receive a reduced dues rate while in school and for 1 year following graduation. Figure 1-7 displays the logo for

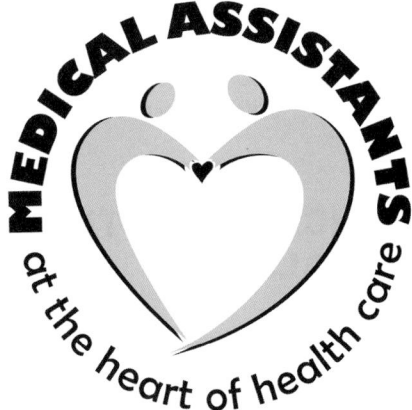

**Figure 1-7** • Logo for the American Association of Medical Assistants–sponsored Medical Assisting Recognition week. (Used with permission from AAMA.)

AAMA-sponsored Medical Assisting Recognition week, which falls on the third full week of October each year.

## American Medical Technologists

The AMT and its governing body are set up similarly to the AAMA, with local, state, and national affiliations, opportunities for continuing education, professional benefits, and a professional journal. Members include medical technologists, medical laboratory technicians, medical assistants, dental assistants, office laboratory technicians, phlebotomy technicians, laboratory consultants, and allied health instructors. To join AMT, you need to be certified or registered by meeting educational, professional experience, and examination requirements. Figure 1-8 displays the insignia of the AMT.

## Professional Coder Associations

The American Academy of Professional Coders (AAPC) was founded in 1988 to provide education and professional certification to physician-based medical coders and to elevate the standards of medical coding by providing student training, certification, ongoing education, and networking and job opportunities. Services to members include discounts on services and products and networking opportunities. AAPC certifications encompass the physician office (CPC®), the hospital outpatient facility (CPC-H®), payer perspective coding (CPC-P®), interventional radiology cardiovascular coding (CIRCC™), and medical coding auditor (CPMA™).

## American Health Information Management Association

The American Health Information Management Association (AHIMA) is a national professional organization dedicated to supporting the medical records or health information specialists. According to their Web site, health information management (HIM) is the body of knowledge and practice that ensures the availability of health information to facilitate real-time healthcare delivery and critical health-related decision making for multiple purposes across diverse organizations, settings, and disciplines. AHIMA administers the examination and awards the certified coding specialist (CCS) and certified coding specialists–physician based (CCS-P) through testing at a specified time and place.

---

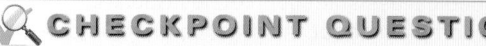 **CHECKPOINT QUESTION**

10. List six benefits of membership in a professional organization.

---

# EMPLOYMENT OPPORTUNITIES

The medical assisting profession has found its place in the allied health arena. Credentialed medical assistants are in great demand, salaries are going up, and employers appreciate the value of the skills trained medical assistants possess. Health care costs are a concern, and health care management consultants tout medical assistants as cost-effective employees in health care today. Because of the flexible, multiskilled nature of their education, medical assistants can work in a variety of health care settings. Medical assistants work under the direct supervision of a licensed health care provider. They perform many functions. Following are examples of the ambulatory settings where a medical assistant may work with a variety of responsibilities:

- Physicians' offices
- Chiropractors' offices
- Podiatrists' offices
- Physical therapy facilities
- Laboratories
- Imaging centers
- Research facilities
- Walk-in clinics
- Ambulatory surgical centers
- Insurance companies

---

**CHECKPOINT QUESTION**

11. Why is it important that medical assistants are multiskilled?

---

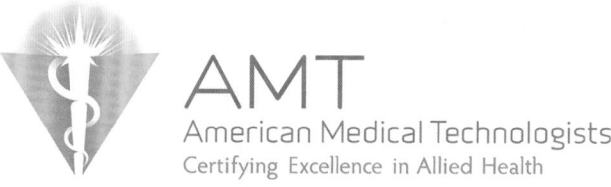

**Figure 1-8 •** Insignia of American Medical Technologists. (Used with permission from AMT.)

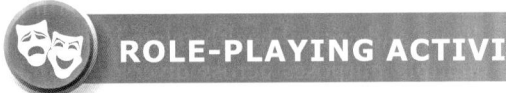

## ROLE-PLAYING ACTIVITY

While waiting for the next patient to arrive, Rob Shelton, CMA, realizes that the receptionist is very busy and all of the phone lines are ringing at once. He immediately moves to a desk with another phone and begins assisting the receptionist by taking calls so she can give attention to the patients arriving to check in for their appointments. Later that day, another medical assistant approaches Rob and begins to complain about the practice being understaffed and comments that answering the phones is not specifically in his job description. She further complains about other staff members and even the office manager! How should Rob handle this medical assistant's complaints? Is there anything Rob should say to the medical assistant to counteract her negativity? Role-play this scenario as the medical assistant, and think about how you would demonstrate professionalism and sensitivity to the complaining medical assistant. If you are the disgruntled medical assistant, think about why she might be having negative feelings. Is she tired or burned out? Your instructor will give you additional instructions for this activity.

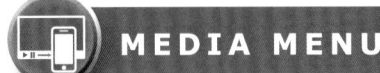

## MEDIA MENU

**Student Resources** on the Point°
- **CMA/RMA Certification Exam Review**

**Internet Resources**
**Accrediting Bureau of Health Education Schools**
http://www.abhes.org
**American Board of Medical Specialties**
http://www.abms.org
**American Health Information Management Association**
http://www.ahima.org
**American Medical Technologists**
http://americanmedtech.org
**Centers for Disease Control and Prevention**
www.cdc.gov
**Council on Accreditation of Allied Health Education Programs**
http://www.caahep.org
**American Association of Professional Coders**
http://www.aapc.com
**Regenerative Medicine Overview**
http://regenerativemedicine.net

## EMR Activity

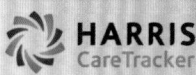

Harris CareTracker is a web-based electronic medical record (EMR) application that you will use for the EMR activities included in this section at the end of each chapter. This application is actually used in physician offices, but is provided to you through the publisher, Wolters Kluwer Health, to give you hands-on practice working with EMRs. Your instructor will have more information about accessing your username, login, and Quickstart guide.

Prerequisite Activities in Harris CareTracker

• *The Getting Started and Quickstart documents and EMR Activities Step-by-Step Instructions are available at* http://thePoint.lww.com/KronenbergerComp5e

Activity Details

Using the "New ToDo" feature in the EMR, send yourself a message to research the local chapter of the American Association of Medical Assistants about the next scheduled meeting. This feature can be found on the *Home* module, *Messages* tab, and *Send Todo* button at the bottom of the screen. Choose the *Interoffice* category, *Practice Management* type, *Other* reason, *Medium* severity, and the *In Progress* status. Print your message to submit to your instructor.

## Chapter Summary

- Medical history reveals 150 years of progress, with the most amazing strides made in the 20th century. New technologies continue to expand the possibilities of health care.
- Changes in the American health care system brought the necessity for highly trained professionals.
- The health care team works together to deliver quality patient care and remain financially sound.
- Professionalism is highly desired by employers. Medical assistants must understand their scope of practice.
- A graduate of an accredited medical assisting program can pursue certification or registration, which brings increasing marketability in the health care arena.
- By ensuring that educational levels are constantly enhanced and by continuing to grow professionally, the medical assistant graduate will prepare for the challenge of a lifelong career that is both fascinating and rewarding.

## Warm-Ups for Critical Thinking

1. Visit the Web site dedicated to regenerative medicine, http://regenerativemedicine.net, and determine the goals and accomplishments related to the field of regenerative medicine.
2. Review the list of characteristics for medical assistants. Which characteristics do you already have? How will you acquire the others? Are there additional characteristics that you have that will make you a good medical assistant?
3. Look at the list of physician specialties. Which type of physician would you want to work for and why? Which physician specialties would you least want to work with? Explain your response.
4. Visit www.aama-ntl.org and americanmedtech.org and determine which local chapter you would be a member of. How would membership benefit your career as a medical assistant?
5. How does certification or registration as a medical assistant impact scope of practice?
6. What is the importance of having adaptive coping mechanisms in place? Give an example of a situation in which such tools would be helpful.
7. How would you answer the question, "Legally, who is responsible for the actions of certified medical assistants or registered medical assistants as they perform their skills?"

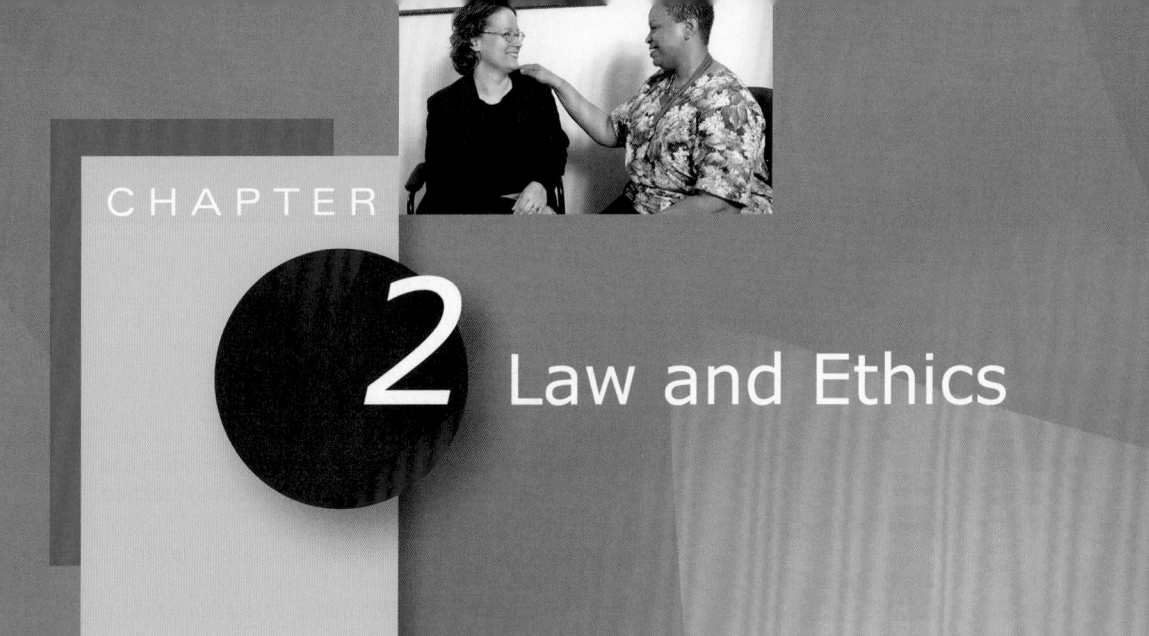

# CHAPTER

# 2 Law and Ethics

## Learning Outcomes

### COG Cognitive Domain*

1. Spell and define the key terms
2. Discuss all levels of governmental legislation and regulation as they apply to medical assisting practice, including FDA and DEA
3. *Compare criminal and civil law as it applies to the practicing medical assistant*
4. Provide an example of tort law as it would apply to a medical assistant
5. List the elements and types of contractual agreements and describe the difference in implied and express contracts
6. List four items that must be included in a contract termination or withdrawal letter
7. List six items that must be included in an informed consent form and explain who may sign consent forms

8. List five legally required disclosures that must be reported to specified authorities
9. Describe the four elements that must be proven in a medicolegal suit
10. Describe four possible defenses against litigation for the medical professional
11. Explain the theory of respondeat superior, or law of agency, and how it applies to the medical assistant
12. Outline the laws regarding employment and safety issues in the medical office
13. *Identify:*
    a. *Genetic Information Nondiscrimination Act of 2008 (GINA)*
    b. *Americans with Disabilities Act Amendments Act (ADAAA)*
14. Differentiate between legal, ethical, and moral issues affecting health care

*(continues on page 28)*

15. Define:
    a. Negligence
    b. Malpractice
    c. Statute of limitations
    d. Good Samaritan Act
    e. Uniform Anatomical Gift Act
    f. *Living will/advanced directives*
    g. *Medical durable power of attorney*
    h. *Patient Self-Determination Act (PSDA)*
16. List the seven American Medical Association principles of ethics
17. List the five ethical principles of ethical and moral conduct outlined by the American Association of Medical Assistants
18. *Define patient navigator*
19. *Describe the role of the medical assistant as the patient navigator*
20. Describe the purpose of the Self-Determination Act
21. Explore the issue of confidentiality as it applies to the medical assistant
22. *Describe components of the Health Insurance Portability and Accountability Act (HIPAA)*
23. Describe the implications of HIPAA for the medical assistant in various medical settings
24. *Summarize the Patients' Bill of Rights*
25. *Discuss licensure and certification as it applies to health care providers*
26. *Describe the following types of insurance:*
    a. *Liability*
    b. *Professional (malpractice)*
    c. *Personal injury*

### PSY  Psychomotor Domain*

1. Monitor federal and state health care legislation (Procedure 2-1)

2. *Apply HIPAA rules in regard to:*
   a. *Privacy (Procedure 2-5)*
   b. *Release of information (Procedure 2-5)*
3. *Apply the Patients' Bill of Rights as it relates to:*
   a. *Choice of treatment (Procedure 2-1)*
   b. *Consent for treatment (Procedure 2-1)*
   c. *Refusal of treatment (Procedure 2-1)*
4. Apply local, state, and federal health care legislation and regulations appropriate to the medical assisting practice setting (Procedure 2-3)
5. *Perform compliance reporting based on public health statutes (Procedure 2-2)*
6. *Report an illegal activity in the health care setting following proper protocol (Procedure 2-4)*

### AFF  Affective Domain*

1. *Demonstrate sensitivity to patient rights*
2. Recognize the importance of local, state, and federal legislation and regulations in the practice setting
3. Protect the integrity of the medical record

*Note: AAMA/CAAHEP 2015 Standards are italicized.*

### ABHES Competencies

1. Comply with federal, state, and local health laws and regulations
2. Institute federal and state guidelines when releasing medical records or information
3. Follow established policies when initiating or terminating medical treatment
4. Understand the importance of maintaining liability coverage once employed in the industry

## Key Terms

| | | | |
|---|---|---|---|
| abandonment | comparative negligence | fee splitting | negligence |
| advance directive | confidentiality | fraud | patient navigator |
| Americans with Disabilities Act Amendments Act (ADAAA) | consent | Genetic Information Nondiscrimination Act (GINA) | Patient Self-Determination Act (PSDA) |
| | contract | | plaintiff |
| | contributory negligence | implied consent | precedents |
| appeal | damages | implied contracts | protocol |
| assault | defamation of character | informed consent | registered |
| battery | defendant | intentional tort | res ipsa loquitur |
| bench trial | deposition | legally required disclosures | res judicata |
| bioethics | durable power of attorney | | respondeat superior |
| blood-borne pathogens | duress | libel | slander |
| breach | emancipated minor | licensure | stare decisis |
| certification | ethics | litigation | statute of limitations |
| civil law | expert witness | locum tenens | subpoena |
| common law | express consent | malpractice | tort |
| | express contracts | | |

## Case Study

As Derrick Moore, RMA, was gathering information for an established patient's visit at Great Falls Medical Center, he noted that the female patient had a large bruise on her cheek and appeared to be very anxious. Derrick also noted that there were several small cuts on the backs of her hands. The patient stated that her visit today was for birth control pills. When asked about the bruise on her face, she commented that she was "clumsy" and "fell into a wall yesterday." Later, she further confides in Derrick that she is having marital problems, but said she is working on them with her husband. Should Derrick note any of this information in the patient's medical record or just mention the reason for the patient's visit today? If information is documented about the noted injuries, what should be included? What is considered intimate partner abuse, and is anyone in the practice responsible for reporting suspected abuse? If so, when and who would be contacted and would you need signed authorization from the patient to release this information?

As health care workers, patients trust us to help them during their most vulnerable times and we must be their advocates in many situations. This chapter covers the medicolegal responsibilities of working in health care and the significance of laws and regulations in the health care environment.

During your career as a medical assistant, you will be involved in many medical situations with potential legal implications. You must uphold ethical standards to ensure the patient's well-being. Ethics deals with individual values and the concept of right and wrong. Laws are written to carry out these concepts. Physicians may be sued for a variety of reasons, including significant clinical errors (e.g., removing the wrong limb, ordering a toxic dose of medication), claims of improperly touching a patient without consent, or failure to properly diagnose or treat a disease. Medicare **fraud** (either knowingly or unknowingly concealing the truth) and falsifying medical records can also result in a lawsuit. Medical assistants and other health care workers are included in many of the suits brought to court. You may help to prevent many of these claims against your physician and protect yourself by complying with medical laws, keeping abreast of medical trends, and acting in an ethical manner by maintaining a high level of professionalism at all times.

## COG GOVERNMENTAL AND LEGISLATIVE REGULATION

There are many local, state, and federal laws that regulate health care in America, so it is essential to understand the components of our government. The US constitution provides for three branches of the federal government. The executive branch is headed by the President of the United States. The legislative branch comprises the Senate and the House of Representatives and is made up of representatives from each state who are elected by US citizens. This branch of government passes laws known as statutes through a series of steps beginning with an introduction of a bill in congress to its evolvement to an act. After an act is passed by congress, it becomes a statute when signed and approved by the President. The judicial branch is the court system, which includes the U.S. Supreme Court, Courts of Appeals, and District Courts. This branch of the government provides for laws known as case (or common) laws that are determined by the interpretation of judges on decisions made in previous cases (see "Sources of Law" below).

The federal government also establishes executive departments to regulate such areas as agriculture, commerce, defense, education, energy, transportation, homeland security, labor, etc. The executive department that regulates health care is the Department of Health and Human Services (DHHS). Within the DHHS is the Food and Drug Administration (FDA). The FDA regulates the manufacture and distribution of drugs, including drug quality and safety. The Drug Enforcement Agency (DEA) is a branch of the Department of Justice (DOJ) and regulates the sale and use of drugs. Providers who prescribe and/or dispense drugs are required to register with the DEA and are assigned a DEA number.

Of course, each state also has a government hierarchy that is similar to the federal government's legislative, judicial, and executive branches with the state governor as the head and state legislators that are elected by its citizens. Each state has laws and regulations that must be followed as well, so it is important to understand both the federal and state laws that govern your actions as a medical assistant. The various federal and state regulations associated with the practice of medical assisting are discussed throughout this textbook.

## ⊙ THE AMERICAN LEGAL SYSTEM

Our legal system is in place to ensure the rights of all citizens, and we depend on the legal system to protect us from the wrongdoings of others. Many potential medical suits prove to be unwarranted and never make it into the court system, but even in the best physician–patient relationships, **litigation** (lawsuits) between patients and physicians may occur. It is essential that you have a basic understanding of the American legal system to protect yourself, your patients, and your physician–employer by following the legal guidelines. You must know your legal duties and understand the legal nature of the physician–patient relationship and your role and responsibilities as the physician's agent.

### Sources of Law

Laws are rules of conduct that are enforced by appointed authorities. The foundation of our legal system is our rights outlined in the constitution and the laws established by our Founding Fathers. These traditional laws are known as **common law**.

Common law is based on the theory of **stare decisis**. This term means "the previous decision stands." Judges usually follow these **precedents** (previous court decisions) but sometimes overrule a previous decision, establishing new precedent.

Statutory laws are passed through legislation that are introduced as "bills" and go through a series of steps to become laws. Federal, state, or local legislators make laws or statutes, the police enforce them, and the court system interprets and administers justice. Administrative laws are created by executive departments, or governmental agencies, as authorized by legislature and called regulations. Regulations pertaining to Medicare, Medicaid, and the Food and Drug Administration are common examples of rules that must be followed in the medical profession.

### Branches of the Law

The two main branches that categorize laws are public laws and private or **civil laws**.

#### Public Law

Public law is the branch of law that focuses on issues between the government and its citizens. It can be divided into four subgroups:

1. **Criminal law** is concerned with issues of citizen welfare and safety. Examples include arson, burglary, murder, and rape. A medical assistant must stay within the boundaries of the profession. Treating patients without the physician's orders could result in a charge of practicing medicine without a license—an act covered under criminal law.
2. **Constitutional law** is commonly called the law of the land. The U.S. government has a constitution, and each state has a constitution with its own laws and regulations. State laws may be more restrictive than federal laws but may not be more lenient. Two examples of constitutional law are laws on abortion and civil rights.
3. **Administrative law** is the regulations set forth by governmental agencies. This category includes laws pertaining to, among others, the Food and Drug Administration, the Internal Revenue Service, and the Board of Medical Examiners.
4. **International law** pertains to treaties between countries. Related issues include trade agreements, extradition, boundaries, and international waters.

#### Private or Civil Law

Private or civil law is the branch of the law that focuses on issues between private citizens. The medical profession is primarily concerned with private law. The subcategories that pertain to the medical profession are contract, commercial, and tort law. Contract and commercial laws concern the rights and obligations of those who enter into contracts, as in a physician–patient relationship. Tort law governs the righting of wrongs or injuries suffered by someone because of another person's wrongdoing or misdeeds resulting from a **breach** of legal duty. Tort law is the basis of most lawsuits against physicians and health care workers and does not require that the action resulting in the lawsuit be intentional. Other civil law branches include property, inheritance, and corporation law.

### 🔍 CHECKPOINT QUESTION

1. Which branch of law covers a medical assistant charged with practicing medicine without a license?

## ⊙ THE RISE IN MEDICOLEGAL CASES

**Malpractice** refers to an action by a professional health care worker that harms a patient. A rise in the amounts of settlement awards has had a negative impact on the cost and coverage of malpractice insurance. With this rise, some physicians have actually changed the scope of their practice to reduce their costs. For example, an obstetrician may choose to limit practice to the care of nonpregnant women to avoid the high cost of malpractice insurance for physicians who deliver babies. In an attempt to protect professionals, legislation designed to limit the amount a jury can award has been introduced in congress. Legal issues involving the medical field are referred to as medicolegal, which combines the words medical and legal.

A government task force found four primary reasons for the rise in malpractice claims:

1. *Scientific advances.* As new and improved medical technology becomes available, the risks and potential for complications of these procedures escalate, making physicians more vulnerable to litigation.
2. *Unrealistic expectations.* Some patients expect miracle cures and file lawsuits because recovery was not as they hoped or expected, even if the physician is not at fault.
3. *Economic factors.* Some patients view lawsuits as a means to obtain quick cash. (In fact, the number of lawsuits filed has increased during economic recessions.)
4. *Poor communication.* Studies show that when patients do not feel a bond with their physician, they are more likely to sue. Attention to customer service helps develop a good rapport between patients, the provider, and the staff.

# PHYSICIAN–PATIENT RELATIONSHIP

## Rights and Responsibilities of the Physician

In any contractual relationship, both parties have certain rights and responsibilities. Physicians have the right to limit their practice to a certain specialty or a certain location. For example, patients may not expect a physician to treat them at home. Physicians also have the right to refuse service to new patients or existing patients with new problems unless they are on emergency room call, in which case they must continue to treat patients seen during this time. The subject of abandonment is discussed later. Doctors have the right to change their policies or availability as long as they give patients reasonable notice of the change. This can be done through a local newspaper advertisement and/or a letter to each patient. Box 2-1 lists the physician's responsibilities.

## Patients' Bill of Rights

In 1998, the U.S. Advisory Commission on Consumer Protection and Quality in the Health Care Industry adopted the Consumer Bill of Rights and Responsibilities,

---

**BOX 2-1   Responsibilities of the Patient and the Physician**

**Responsibilities of the Patient**

- Provide the physician with accurate data about the duration and nature of symptoms
- Provide a complete and accurate medical history to the physician
- Follow the physician's instructions for diet, exercise, medications, and appointments
- Compensate the physician for services rendered

**Responsibilities of the Physician**

- Respect the patient's confidential information
- Provide reasonable skill, experience, and knowledge in treating the patient
- Continue treating the patient until the contract has been withdrawn or as long as the condition requires treatment
- Inform patients of their condition, treatments, and prognosis
- Give complete and accurate information
- Provide competent coverage during time away from practice
- Obtain informed consent before performing procedures (informed consent is a statement of approval from the patient for the physician to perform a given procedure after the patient has been educated about the risks and benefits of the procedure)
- Caution against unneeded or undesirable treatment or surgery

---

also known as the Patients' Bill of Rights. Although the enactment of the Affordable Care Act (ACA) in 2010 created new patient rights, they primarily involve matters dealing with insurance companies. The original Patients' Bill of Rights still applies, however, and has three major goals:

1. To help patients feel more confident in the US health care system
2. To stress the importance of a strong relationship between patients and their health care providers
3. To stress the key role patients play in staying healthy by laying out rights and responsibilities for all patients and health care providers

The rights of the patient include the ability to choose a physician. This right may be limited to a list of participating providers under a patient's insurance plan. Patients have the right to determine whether to begin medical treatment and to set limits on that treatment. The patient also has the right to know in advance what the treatment will consist of, what affect it may have, and what dangers are to be expected. The concept of informed consent is discussed later in the chapter. Patients have the right to privacy. The Health Insurance Portability and Accountability Act of 1996 (HIPAA) outlines specific policies for protecting the privacy of electronic submissions of medical information. HIPAA is discussed at length in Chapter 8. Patients also have a right to emergency care. Box 2-2 outlines the Patients' Bill of Rights. It is important that you keep these rights in mind in all of your patient and physician encounters. Policies and procedures must incorporate these rights as well.

Some of the additional rights resulting from the ACA include requirements for insurance coverage for certain preventative screenings without charge to the patient, permitting young adults to stay on a parent's policy until 26 years of age if certain requirements are met, and banning lifetime limits on most new plan benefits (see Chapter 13).

## Contracts

A **contract** is an agreement between two or more parties with certain factors agreed on among all parties. The physician–patient relationship constitutes a contractual arrangement in which the patient seeks the expertise and care of a physician and the physician agrees to treat or determine the best course of action for the patient. All contractual agreements have three components:

1. Offer (contract initiation)
2. Acceptance (both parties agree to the terms)
3. Consideration (the exchange of fees for service)

A contract is not valid unless all three elements are present. A contract offer is made when a patient calls the office to request an appointment. The offer is accepted when you make an appointment for the patient. You have formed a contract that implies that for a fee, the physician will do all in his or her power to address the health concerns of the patient.

---

**BOX 2-2    Patients' Bill of Rights**

The bill covers eight key areas:

1. Information
   You have the right to accurate and easily understood information about your health plan, health care professionals, and health care facilities. If you speak another language, have a physical or mental disability, or just don't understand something, help should be given so you can make informed health care decisions.
2. Choice of Providers and Plans
   You have the right to choose health care providers who can give you high-quality health care when you need it.
3. Access to Emergency Services
   If you have severe pain, an injury, or sudden illness that makes you believe that your health is in danger, you have the right to be screened and stabilized using emergency services. You should be able to use these services whenever and wherever you need them, without needing to wait for authorization and without any financial penalty.
4. Taking Part in Treatment Decisions
   You have the right to know your treatment options and take part in decisions about your care. Parents, guardians, family members, or others that you choose can speak for you if you cannot make your own decisions.
5. Respect and Nondiscrimination
   You have a right to considerate, respectful care from your doctors, health plan representatives, and other health care providers that does not discriminate against you.

6. Confidentiality of Private Health Information
   You have the right to talk privately with health care providers and to have your health care information protected. You also have the right to read and copy your own medical record. You have the right to ask that your doctor change your record if it is not correct, relevant, or complete.
7. Complaints and Appeals
   In a health care system that protects consumer or patients' rights, patients should expect to take on some responsibilities to get well and/or stay well (for instance, exercising and not using tobacco). Patients are expected to do things like treat health care workers and other patients with respect, pay their medical bills, and follow the rules and benefits of their health plan coverage. You have the right to a fair, fast, and objective review of any complaint you have against your health plan, doctors, hospitals, or other health care personnel. This includes complaints about waiting times, operating hours, the actions of health care personnel, and the adequacy of health care facilities.
8. Consumer Responsibilities
   Having patients involved in their care increases the chance of the best possible outcomes and helps support a high-quality, cost-conscious health care system.

This Bill of Rights also applies to the insurance plans offered to federal employees. Many other health insurance plans and facilities have also adopted these values. Even Medicare and Medicaid stand by many of them.

Available at http://www.hcqualitycommission.gov/final

Certain individuals, such as children and those who are mentally incompetent or temporarily incapacitated, are not legally able to enter contracts. Patients in this category do not have the capacity to enter into a contract, and therefore, decisions about health care should be made by a competent party acting as a health care decision maker for the minor or incompetent person.

The two types of contracts between physicians and patients are implied and express.

## Implied Contracts

**Implied contracts**, the most common kind of contract between physicians and patients, are not written but are assumed by the actions of the parties. For example, a patient calls the office and requests to see Dr. Smith for an earache. The patient arrives for the appointment, is seen by the physician, and receives a prescription. It is *implied* that, because the patient came on his own and requested care, he wants this physician to care for him. The physician's action of accepting the patient for care *implies* that she acknowledges responsibility for her part of the contract. The patient *implies* by accepting the services that he will render payment even if the price was not discussed.

## Express Contracts

**Express contracts**, either written or oral, consist of specified details. A mutual sharing of responsibilities is always stated in an express contract. The agreement you have with your creditors is an express contract. These kinds of contracts are not used as often in the medical setting as implied contracts.

 **CHECKPOINT QUESTION**

2. What action should be taken when a physician makes a change in his services?

 **PATIENT EDUCATION**

### Legally Required Disclosures

Inform patients who have conditions that require legal disclosure about the applicable law. Assure them that you will protect their confidentiality. Educate them about why the disclosure is necessary, who receives the information, what particular forms will be completed, and any anticipated follow-up from the organization. For example, you are required to give the local health department the name, address, and condition of a patient with a sexually transmitted disease. The health department then contacts the patient to acquire the names of the patient's sexual contacts. These contacts are notified and counseled by the health department official. Patients who are educated about these legally required disclosures will better understand and accept the need to file official reports.

## Termination or Withdrawal of the Contract

A contract is ideally resolved when the patient is satisfactorily treated for the illness and the physician has been paid for the services. The patient may end the contract at any time, but the physician must follow legal **protocol** to dissolve the contract if the patient still seeks treatment, and the physician wishes to end the relationship.

### Patient-Initiated Termination

A patient who chooses to terminate the relationship should notify the physician and give the reasons. You must keep this letter in the medical record. After the receipt of this letter, the physician should then send a letter to the patient stating the following:

- The physician accepts the termination.
- Medical records are available on written request.
- Medical referrals are available if needed.

If the patient verbally asks to end this relationship, the physician should send a letter to the patient documenting the conversation and, again, offering referrals and access to the medical records. Clear documentation is essential.

### Physician-Initiated Termination

The physician may find it necessary to end the relationship. A physician may terminate the contract if the patient is noncompliant with treatment, does not keep appointments, has a delinquent account balance, or if the physician can no longer meet the needs or expectations of the patient. The physician must send a letter of withdrawal that includes the following:

- A statement of intent to terminate the relationship
- The reasons for this action
- The termination date at least 30 days from the date of receipt of the letter
- A statement that the medical records will be transferred to another physician at the patient's request
- A strong recommendation that the patient seek additional medical care as warranted

The letter must be sent by certified mail with a return receipt requested. A copy of the termination letter and the return receipt are placed in the patient's record. Figure 2-1 shows a sample letter of intent to terminate a physician–patient relationship.

## Abandonment

Once a patient has established a relationship with the physician, the physician is contractually obligated to care for the patient until treatment is no longer needed or the patient meets with one of the conditions necessary for termination of the relationship as mentioned above. If a contract is not properly terminated, the

Amy Fine, MD
Charlotte Family Practice
220 NW 3rd Avenue
Charlotte, NC 25673

October 11, 2012

Regina Dodson
Jones Hill Road
Charlotte, NC 25673

Dear Ms. Dodson,

Due to the fact that you have persistently failed to follow my medical advice and treatment of your diabetes, I will no longer be able to provide medical care to you. Since your condition requires ongoing medical care, you must find another physician within the next 30 days. I will be available to you until your appointment date with a new physician.

To ensure continuity of your care, I will make your records available to your new physician. As soon as you make an appointment with a new physician, please come by our office to sign an authorization form enabling us to send your records.

Sincerely,

Amy Fine, MD

Figure 2-1 • Letter of intent to terminate physician–patient relationship.

physician can be sued for **abandonment**. Abandonment may be charged if the physician withdraws from the contractual relationship without proper notification while the patient still needs treatment. Physicians must always arrange coverage when absent from the office for vacations, conferences, and so on. Patients may sue for abandonment in any instance that a suitable substitute is not available for care. Coverage may be provided by a **locum tenens**, a substitute physician.

Other examples of abandonment include the following:

- The physician abruptly and without reasonable notice stops treating a patient whose condition requires additional or continued care.
- The physician fails to see a patient as often as the condition requires or incorrectly advises the patient that further treatment is not needed.

## CHECKPOINT QUESTION

3. What five elements must be included in a physician's termination intent letter?

## Consent

The law requires that patients must **consent** or agree to being touched, examined, or treated by the physician or agents of the physician involved in the contractual agreement.

No treatment may be made without a consent given orally, nonverbally by behavior, or clearly in writing. Patients have the right to appoint a health care surrogate or health care power of attorney who may make health care decisions when the patient is unable to make them. A health care surrogate may be a spouse, a friend, a pastor, or an attorney. A **durable power of attorney** for health care gives the patient's representative the ability to make health care decisions as the health care surrogate. A patient's physician should be aware of the power of attorney agreement, and a copy of the legal documentation should be kept in the office medical record.

### Implied Consent

In the typical visit to the physician's office, the patient's actions represent an informal agreement for care to be given. A patient who raises a sleeve to receive an injection implies agreement to the treatment. **Implied consent** also occurs in an emergency. If a patient is in a life-threatening situation and is unable to give verbal permission for treatment, it is implied that the patient would consent to treatment if possible. As soon as possible, informed consent should be signed by either the patient or a family member in this type of situation. When there is no emergency, implied consent should be used only if the procedure poses no significant risk to the patient.

### Informed or Express Consent

The physician is responsible for obtaining the patient's **informed consent** whenever the treatment involves an invasive procedure such as surgery, use of experimental drugs, potentially dangerous procedures such as stress tests, or any treatment that poses a significant risk to the patient. A federal law discussed later requires that health care providers who administer certain vaccines give the patient a current vaccine information statement (VIS). A VIS provides a standardized way to give objective information about vaccine benefits and adverse events (side effects) to patients. The VIS is available online through the Centers for Disease Control and Prevention (CDC) in 26 languages. The Internet address can be found at the end of the chapter.

Informed consent is also referred to as **express consent**. Informed consent is based on the patient's right to know every possible benefit, risk, or alternative to the suggested treatment and the possible outcome if no treatment is initiated. The patient must voluntarily give permission and must understand the implications of consenting to the treatment. This requires that the physician and patient communicate in a manner understandable to the patient. Patients can be more active in personal health care decisions when they are educated about and understand their treatment and care.

A consent form must include the following information:

1. Name of the procedure to be performed
2. Name of the physician who will perform the procedure
3. Name of the person administering the anesthesia (if applicable)
4. Any potential risks from the procedure
5. Anticipated result or benefit from the procedure
6. Alternatives to the procedure and their risks
7. Probable effect on the patient's condition if the procedure is not performed
8. Any exclusions that the patient requests
9. Statement indicating that all of the patient's questions or concerns regarding the procedure have been answered
10. Patient's and witnesses' signatures and the date

As the medical assistant, you will frequently be required to witness consent signatures. A sample consent form is seen in Figure 2-2.

The informed consent form supplied for the patient's signature must be in the language that the patient speaks. Most physicians who treat multicultural patients have consent forms available in a variety of languages. Never ask a patient to sign a consent form if he or she:

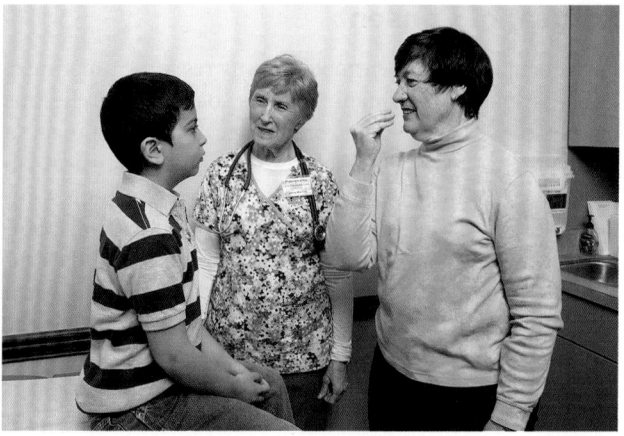

**Figure 2-3** • Using an interpreter, the CMA helps this patient understand the procedure.

- Does not understand the procedure
- Has unanswered questions regarding the procedure
- Is unable to read the consent form

Never coerce (force or compel against his or her wishes) a patient into signing a consent form. Figure 2-3 shows a certified medical assistant (CMA) obtaining consent from a hearing-impaired patient. The signing interpreter is assisting. Every patient has the right to be informed, and the medical assistant must be sure he or she understands.

### Who May Sign a Consent Form

An adult (usually someone over age 18) who is mentally competent and not under the influence of medication or other substances may sign a consent form. Depending on state law, a minor may sign a consent form if he or she is

- In the armed services
- Requesting treatment for communicable diseases (including sexually transmitted diseases)
- Pregnant
- Requesting information regarding birth control, abortion, or drug or alcohol abuse counseling
- Emancipated

An **emancipated minor** is under the age of majority but is either married or self-supporting and is responsible for his or her debts. The age of majority varies from state to state and ranges from 18 to 21 years. Minors may give consent if any one of the above-listed criteria is present.

Legal guardians may also sign consent forms. A legal guardian is appointed by a judge when the court has ruled an individual to be mentally incompetent. Health care surrogates may also sign consent forms. Health care surrogates are discussed later in the chapter.

---

I hereby authorize Dr. _____ , and such assistants as may be designated, to perform:

_____
(Name of treatment/procedure)

and any other related procedures or forms of treatment, including appropriate anesthesia, transfusions that they deem necessary for the welfare of:

_____
(Name of patient)

I consent to the administration of anesthesia and/or such drugs as may be necessary. I understand that all anesthetics involve risks of complications, serious injury, or rarely death from both known and unknown causes.

I consent to the examination and retention for educational, scientific and research purposes by the Medical Staff of

_____

of all body fluids, tissues and organs removed during the course of the above treatment/procedure with privilege of ultimate use and disposal resting with said medical staff.

The following has been explained to me and I understand:

A. The nature and character of the proposed treatment/procedure.
B. The anticipated results of the proposed treatment/procedure.
C. The recognized alternative forms of treatment/procedure.
D. The recognized serious possible risks and complications of the treatment/procedure and of the recognized alternative forms of treatment/procedure, including non-treatment.
E. The possible consequences of no treatment.
F. The anticipated date and time of the proposed treatment/procedure.

Additional M.D. comments: _____
_____
_____

My physician has offered to answer all inquiries concerning the proposed treatment/procedure. I understand that I am free to withhold or withdraw consent to the proposed treatment/procedure at any time.

| Witness | | | Signature of Person Giving Consent |
|---------|---|---|------------------------------------|
| Date Signed | Time | ☐ A.M. | Relationship to patient (if applicable) |
| | | ☐ P.M. | |

☐ Please check if this is a telephone monitored consent.
No treatment will be performed until this consent has been executed. This consent will be permanently filed in the patient's medical record.

| Pt. No. _____ | **Gastroenterology Associates** Anytown, PA |
|------------------|---------------------------------------------|
| Name _____ | |
| D.O.B. _____ | **Special Consent to Treatment** (Diagnostic & Surgical Procedures, Anesthesia, Medical Treatment & Other Procedures) |

**Figure 2-2** • Sample consent form.

---

### ✔ CHECKPOINT QUESTION

4. Under what circumstances should a patient never be asked to sign a consent form?

## Refusal of Consent

Patients may refuse treatment for any reason. Sometimes, patients make treatment choices based on religious or personal beliefs and preferences. For instance, a Jehovah's Witness may refuse a blood transfusion on religious grounds, or an elderly person may not want to undergo serious surgery because the potential complications may limit future lifestyle options. In this situation, the patient must sign a refusal of consent form indicating that the patient was instructed regarding the potential risks and benefits of the procedure as well as the risks if the procedure is not allowed. If the patient is a minor, the courts may become involved at the request of the physician or hospital and may award consent for the child. In this situation, the physician should follow legal counsel and document the incident carefully. In any instance that the patient refuses treatment, it should be documented in the patient's medical record to protect the physician. The physician has a legal right to refuse to perform elective surgery on a patient who refuses to receive blood if needed.

## Releasing Medical Information

The medical record is a legal document. Although the medical record itself belongs to the physician, the information belongs to the patient. Patients have the right to their medical information, and they have the right to deny the sharing of this information.

Requests for medical records are common. Other health care facilities, insurance companies, and patients themselves may need information from the medical chart. Staying within the law when releasing medical information is covered in Chapter 8.

## Legally Required Disclosures

Even though patients have the right to limit access to their medical records, health care facilities have a responsibility to report certain events to governmental agencies without the patient's consent, which are referred to as **legally required disclosures**. You and other health care providers must report to the department of public health the situations described in the following sections.

### Vital Statistics

All states maintain records of births, deaths, marriages, and divorces. These records include the following:

- Birth certificates.
- Stillbirth reports. Some states have separate stillbirth forms; other states use a regular death certificate.
- Death certificates. These must be signed by a physician. The cause and time of death must be included.

You may assist the physician in completing a death certificate and filing the finished report in the patient's chart.

### Medical Examiner's Reports

Each state has laws pertaining to which deaths must be reported to the medical examiner's office. Generally, these include the following:

- Death from an unknown cause
- Death from a suspected criminal or violent act
- Death of a person not attended by a physician at the time of death or for a reasonable period preceding the death
- Death within 24 hours of hospital admission

### Infectious or Communicable Diseases

These reports are made to the local health department. The information is used for statistical purposes and for preventing or tracking the spread of these diseases. Although state guidelines vary, there are usually three categories of reports:

- Telephone reports are required for diphtheria, cholera, meningococcal meningitis, and plague, usually within 24 hours of the diagnosis. Telephone reports must always be followed by written reports and forms are located on the health department's Web site for each state.
- Written reports are required for hepatitis, leprosy, malaria, rubeola, polio, rheumatic fever, tetanus, and tuberculosis. Sexually transmitted diseases must also be reported. Notification is usually required within 7 days of the date of discovery.
- Trend reports are made when your office notes an unusually high occurrence of influenza, streptococcal infections, or any other infectious diseases. Box 2-3 is a sample of reportable diseases and their time frames.

The CDC keeps a watchful eye on the public health. When necessary, the CDC establishes directives for the protection of the public. For example, when the public appeared to be at risk for contracting anthrax in 2001, the CDC mandated that documented anthrax cases be reported immediately. Fax machines and e-mail help facilitate such urgent public health communication.

### National Childhood Vaccine Injury Act of 1986

Health care providers who administer certain vaccines and toxoids must report to the U.S. Department of Health and Human Services (DHHS) the occurrence of any side effects listed in the manufacturer's package insert. In addition, health care providers must record in the patient's record the following information:

1. Date the vaccine was administered
2. Lot number and manufacturer of vaccine

---

### BOX 2-3 Reportable Conditions

Chapter 19—Health: Epidemiology
Subchapter 19a—Communicable Disease Control
Section .0100—Reporting of Communicable Diseases
.0101 Reportable Diseases and Conditions

(a) The following named diseases and conditions are declared to be dangerous to the public health and are hereby made reportable within the time period specified after the disease or condition is reasonably suspected to exist:

acquired immune deficiency syndrome (AIDS)—
    7 days
amebiasis—7 days
anthrax—24 hours
blastomycosis—7 days
botulism—24 hours
brucellosis—7 days
Campylobacter infection—24 hours
chancroid—24 hours
chlamydial infection (laboratory confirmed)—7 days
cholera—24 hours
dengue—7 days
diphtheria—24 hours
*Escherichia coli* infection—24 hours
encephalitis—7 days
food-borne disease, including but not limited to
    *Clostridium perfringens*, staphylococcal, and
    *Bacillus cereus*—24 hours
gonorrhea—24 hours
granuloma inguinale—24 hours
*Haemophilus influenzae*, invasive disease—24 hours
hepatitis A—24 hours
hepatitis B carriage—7 days
hepatitis non-A, non-B—7 days
HIV infection confirmed—7 days
legionellosis—7 days
leprosy—7 days
leptospirosis—7 days
Lyme disease—7 days

---

### BOX 2-4 Vaccinations Requiring Vaccine Information Statements

Anthrax
Chickenpox
Diphtheria, tetanus, and pertussis
*Haemophilus influenzae type b (Hib)*
Hepatitis A
Hepatitis B
Influenza
Lyme disease
Measles, mumps, and rubella
Meningococcal
Pneumococcal polysaccharide
Pneumococcal conjugate
Polio
Lymphogranuloma venereum—7 days
Malaria—7 days
Measles (rubeola)—24 hours
Meningitis, pneumococcal—7 days
Meningitis, viral (aseptic)—7 days
Meningococcal disease—24 hours
Mucocutaneous lymph node syndrome (Kawasaki
    syndrome)—7 days
Mumps—7 days

Excerpt from the North Carolina Administrative Code Regarding Reporting of Communicable Diseases.

---

3. Any adverse reactions to the vaccine
4. Name, title, and address of the person who administered the vaccine

Box 2-4 lists the vaccines and toxoids covered by the National Childhood Vaccine Injury Act.

## Abuse, Neglect, or Maltreatment

Abuse, neglect, or maltreatment of any person who is incapable of self-protection usually falls under this category and may include the elderly or the mentally incompetent. Each state has its own regulations regarding what must be reported. Patient confidentiality rights are waived when the law requires you to report certain conditions.

Abuse is thought to be the second most common cause of death in children under age 5. The Federal Child Abuse Prevention and Treatment Act mandates that threats to a child's physical and mental welfare be reported. Health care workers, teachers, and social workers who report suspected abuse are not identified to the parents and are protected against liability. State laws vary regarding the procedure for reporting abuse. Local regulations should be outlined in the policies and procedures manuals at any outpatient facility. If you suspect a child is being abused, relay your suspicions to the physician. The physician will make the formal report. When authorities receive a report from a health care provider, they follow up by investigating the situation. For assistance in reporting suspected child abuse, you may call the national 24-hour hotline at 800-4 A CHILD (800-422-4453).

Domestic violence is a significant problem in this country. Data from the CDC on "intimate partner violence" (IPV) show that the majority of victims are women, and often, many women and children are trapped in a cycle of abuse. Mothers who are financially dependent on their abusers may see no way out. You should record any information gathered in the patient interview or anything observed in the course of dealing with the patient that may indicate abuse. Report these observations to the physician. Most communities have anonymous safe places for victims of domestic abuse, and you should be familiar with these services. With proper referrals, you may be able to help break the cycle of domestic abuse.

This country is also undergoing a rise in elderly parents being cared for by their adult children who also have the responsibility of raising young children. This phenomenon can cause great stress among caregivers. Abuse of the elderly can be in the form of mistreatment (physical, emotional, or financial) or neglect (not providing appropriate care). You should pay attention to observations and information provided by your elderly patients. If mistreatment is suspected, alert the physician. Each state has Adult Protective Services laws to insure the well-being of the elderly population and local numbers to contact caseworkers when necessary. Support groups for those caring for the elderly are useful in dealing with the challenges of caring for others.

### Violent Injuries

Health care providers have the legal duty to report suspected criminal acts. Injuries resulting from weapons, assault, attempted suicide, and rape must be reported to local authorities.

### Other Reports

A diagnosis of cancer must be reported to assist in tracking malignancies and identifying environmental carcinogens. Just as the CDC keeps track of all communicable diseases reported, a database of treated tumors is kept in hospitals through a tumor registry. Some states also require that epilepsy (a seizure condition) be reported to local motor vehicle departments. The testing of newborns for phenylketonuria (PKU), which can cause mental retardation, is required in all states. Some states require positive PKU results to be reported to the health department so that close observation and follow-up care are ensured to prevent serious complications for the infant. Infantile hypothyroidism is also a reportable condition in some states.

### CHECKPOINT QUESTION

5. List six situations and conditions you are legally required to report.

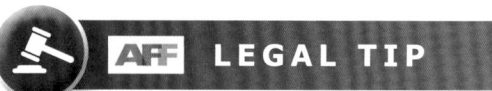

### LEGAL TIP

### Prescription Pad Safety Tips

- Keep only one prescription pad in a locked cabinet in the examining room. All other pads should be locked away elsewhere. Do not leave prescription pads unattended.
- Keep a limited supply of pads. It is better to reorder on a regular basis than to overstock.
- Keep track of the number of pads in the office. If a burglary occurs, you will be able to advise the police regarding the number of missing pads.
- Report any prescription pad theft to the police and alert local pharmacies of the theft. If the theft involves the loss of narcotic pads, the Drug Enforcement Agency must be notified.

## COG SPECIFIC LAWS AND STATUTES THAT APPLY TO HEALTH PROFESSIONALS

### Medical Practice Acts

Although each state has its own medical practice act, the following elements are usually included:

- Definition of the practice of medicine
- Requirements that the physician must have graduated from an accredited medical school and residency program and have passed the state medical examination
- Description of the procedure for **licensure**
- Description of the conditions for which a license can be suspended or revoked
- Description of the renewal process for licensure. Most states require the physician to have attended a certain number of continuing education hours.
- Personal requirements necessary to become a licensed physician. Generally, a licensed physician must be a state resident, of good moral character, a US citizen, and 21 years of age or older.

Medical practice acts are designed to protect the public by requiring licensure and standards of care for many health care professionals. A physician may have his or her license revoked or suspended by the Board of Medical Examiners in most states for a variety of reasons, including certain criminal offenses, unprofessional conduct, fraud, or professional or personal incompetence. Criminal offenses include but are not limited to murder, manslaughter, robbery, and rape. Examples of unprofessional conduct may include invasion of a patient's privacy, excessive use of alcohol or use of illegal drugs, and **fee splitting** (sharing fees for the referral of patients to certain colleagues). Fraud is a common reason for revoking a license. Fraud may include filing false Medicare or Medicaid claims, falsifying medical records, or professional misrepresentation. Examples of misrepresentation or fraud include advertising a medical cure that does not exist, guaranteeing 100% success of a treatment, or falsifying medical credentials. Incompetence is often a hard charge to prove. The three most common examples are insanity, senility, and other documented mental incompetence.

As a medical assistant, it is your responsibility to report illegal or unethical behavior or signs of incompetence in the medical office.

## Licensure, Certification, and Registration

As discussed in Chapter 1, medical professionals can be licensed, certified, or registered. Licensure is regulated by laws, such as medical practice acts and nursing practice acts. If a particular profession is a licensed one, it is mandatory that one maintain a license in each state where he or she works. Each state determines the qualifications and requirements for licensure of a particular profession. A state agency will be responsible for issuing and renewing licenses. Most professionals are licensed to practice their profession according to certain guidelines and are limited to specific duties. For example, nurses are licensed. As mentioned earlier, in North Carolina, the Nursing Practice Act specifically prohibits a nurse from delegating professional authority to unlicensed personnel.

The term registered indicates that a professional has met basic requirements, usually for education, has passed standard testing, and has been approved by a governing body to perform given tasks within a state. For example, x-ray technologists are registered as registered radiologic technologists. A national registry is available to verify a potential employee's status.

Certification is a voluntary process regulated through a professional organization. Standards for certification are set by the organization issuing the certificate. The certified medical assistant (CMA) and registered medical assistant (RMA) credentials are nationally recognized and do not require any action when moving from one state to another. Remember, you must adhere to the laws regarding the CMA or RMA in the state where you work.

As a medical assistant, you are working under the license of a physician who delegates certain duties to you to assist with taking care of his/her patients in the outpatient setting. The physician–employer has the sole responsibility of setting any limits on the duties of a medical assistant. Take a look back at Figure 1-4 in Chapter 1. A medical assistant's scope of practice is determined by his or her training and at the provider's discretion. Although most states do not require certification for employment, employers seek medical assistants with the CMA or RMA credential because certification indicates the achievement of certain standards of competence. Credentialed medical assistants are also very valuable to employers participating with Medicare and Medicaid's *Meaningful Use Incentive* because, as part of that payment incentive, only licensed health care providers (i.e., nurses) or credentialed medical assistants may enter computerized provider order entries (CPOE) into electronic health records (see Chapter 8). A few states require that you take a test or short course before performing certain clinical duties.

## Controlled Substances Act

The Controlled Substances Act of 1970 is a federal law enforced by the DEA. The act regulates the manufacture, distribution, and dispensing of narcotics and nonnarcotic drugs considered to have a high potential for abuse. This act categorizes drugs in five schedules (classifications) from those that are highly dangerous and addictive to drugs having a low potential for abuse. By placing drugs in one of the schedules, laws are created and enforced for each classification instead of having laws for specific drugs. These laws prohibit unauthorized possession and the illegal use of controlled substances to prevent substance abuse. The law also requires that any physician who dispenses, administers, or prescribes narcotics or other controlled substances be registered with the DEA.

Physicians who maintain a stock of controlled substances in the office for dispensing or administration must use a special triplicate order form available through the DEA. A record of each transaction must be kept and retained for 2 to 3 years and an inventory of drugs maintained must be available for inspection by the DEA at any time. The act requires that all controlled substances be kept in a locked cabinet out of the patients' view and that the keys be kept secure. Theft should be reported immediately to the local police and the nearest DEA office. Prescription pads used for prescribing controlled substances must remain in a safe place at all times. The Legal Tip box lists steps you can take to keep these prescription pads safe.

This act also requires a physician to return all registration certificates and any unused order forms to the DEA if the practice is closed or sold. Violation of this act is a criminal offense. Penalties range from fines to imprisonment.

## Good Samaritan Act

As the number of lawsuits against physicians began to rise, physicians feared that giving emergency care to strangers outside the office could lead to malpractice suits. To combat that fear, all states now have Good

Samaritan acts. Good Samaritan acts ensure that first responders in emergency situations are immune from liability suits as long as they give care in good faith and in a manner that a reasonable and prudent person would in a similar situation. Each state has specific guidelines. Some even set standards for various professional levels, such as one set of standards for a physician and another set of standards for emergency medical technicians. Your state's Good Samaritan Act will not protect you if you are grossly negligent or willfully perform negligent acts.

You are not covered by the Good Samaritan Act while you are working as a medical assistant, nor does it cover physicians in the performance of their duties. Liability and malpractice insurance policies are available to protect you in those situations. If you render emergency care and accept compensation for that care, the act does not apply.

The provisions only cover acts outside of the formal practice of the profession.

## BASIS OF MEDICAL LAW

### Tort Law

A tort is a wrongful act that results in harm for which monetary restitution is sought by the injured party. The two forms of torts are intentional and unintentional. An allegation of an unintentional tort means that the accuser (the **plaintiff**) believes a mistake has been made; however, the plaintiff believes the caregiver or accused party (the **defendant**) was operating in good faith and did not intend the mistake to occur. Consider the following scenario as an example of an unintentional tort: A medical assistant giving a patient a heat treatment for muscle aches inadvertently burns the arm of the patient because the equipment is faulty. This act was not intentional or malicious, but it caused damage to the patient. A large majority of suits against physicians fall into this category.

## Negligence and Malpractice (Unintentional Torts)

Most unintentional torts involve negligence. These are the most common forms of medical malpractice suits.

Negligence is performing an act that a reasonable health care worker or provider would not have done or the omission of an act that a reasonable professional or provider would have done. Failure to take reasonable precautions to prevent harm to a patient is termed **negligence**. If a physician is involved, the term usually used is malpractice. Malpractice is said to have occurred when the patient is harmed by the professional's actions. There are three types of malpractice:

- Malfeasance—incorrect treatment
- Misfeasance—treatment performed incorrectly
- Nonfeasance—treatment delayed or not attempted

In a legal situation, the standard of care determines what a reasonable professional would have done. Standards of care are written by various professional agencies to clarify what the reasonable and prudent physician or health care worker would do in a given situation. For example, a patient comes to an orthopedist's office after falling from a horse and complains of arm pain. The standard of care for orthopedists would require an x-ray of the injured extremity after trauma. Standards of care vary with the level of training and expertise of the professional. Every health care professional, including medical assistants, must practice within the scope of their training. The representing attorney may seek an **expert witness** to state under oath the standards of care for a specific situation. Expert witnesses may be used when parties involved in the court case, such as the court or jury, may not have knowledge about the subject matter. Expert witnesses may include physicians, nurses, physical therapists, or other specialized practitioners who have excellent reputations in their field.

Expert witnesses are always used in malpractice cases, except when the doctrine of **res ipsa loquitur** is tried. This doctrine means "the thing speaks for itself." In other words, it is obvious that the physician's actions or negligence caused the injury. A judge must preapprove the use of this theory in pretrial hearings. An example of a case tried under this doctrine might be a fracture that occurred when the patient fell from an examining table.

For negligence to be proved, the plaintiff's attorney must prove that the following four elements were present: duty, dereliction of duty, direct cause, and damage. The courts place the burden of proof on the plaintiff; the physician is assumed to have given proper care until proven otherwise.

### Duty

Duty is present when the patient and the physician have formed a contract. This is usually straightforward and the easiest of the elements to prove. If the patient presented to the physician's office and the physician sees the patient, there is duty.

### Dereliction of Duty

The patient must prove that the physician did not meet the standard of care guidelines, either by performing an act inappropriately or by omitting an act.

### Direct Cause

The plaintiff must prove that the derelict act directly caused the patient's injury. This can be difficult to prove if the patient has an extensive medical history that may have contributed to the injury.

## Damage

The plaintiff must prove that an injury or **damages** occurred. Documentation must be available to prove a diagnosis of an injury or illness.

## Jury Awards

There are three types of awards for damages:

1. *Nominal.* Minimal injuries or damages occurred, and compensation is small.
2. *Actual (compensatory).* Money is awarded for the injury, disability, mental suffering, loss of income, or the anticipated future earning loss. This payment is moderate to significant.
3. *Punitive.* Money is awarded to punish the practitioner for reckless or malicious wrongdoing. Punitive damages are the most costly. (Note: A physician may have committed a medical error, but if the patient suffered no injuries or damages, he or she cannot win the suit. Also, if the outcome was not as expected but the physician cannot be shown to be at fault, the patient will not be compensated.)

## CHECKPOINT QUESTION

6. What four elements must be proved in a negligence suit?

## Intentional Torts

An **intentional tort** is an act that takes place with malice and with the intent of causing harm. Intentional torts are the deliberate violation of another person's legal rights. Examples of intentional torts are assault and battery, use of duress, invasion of privacy, defamation of character, fraud, tort of outrage, and undue influence. These are described next.

## Assault and Battery

**Assault** is the unauthorized attempt or threat to touch another person without consent. **Battery** is the actual physical touching of a patient without consent; this includes beating and physical abuse. By law, a conscious adult has the right to refuse medical care. Care given without the patient's consent constitutes assault. An example of battery might be suturing a laceration against the patient's wishes.

## Duress

If a patient is coerced into an act, the patient can possibly sue for the tort of **duress**. Following is an example in which a patient may be able to sue successfully for assault, battery, and duress. A 22-year-old woman arrives at a pregnancy center. She is receiving public assistance and has five children. Her pregnancy test is positive. The staff persuades her to have an abortion. She signs the consent form, and the abortion is performed. Later, she sues, stating that she was verbally coerced into signing the consent form (duress) and that the abortion was performed against her wishes (assault and battery).

## Invasion of Privacy

Patients have the right to privacy. Remember, as part of the Privacy Rule, HIPAA regulates the sharing of information and requires that patients sign an acknowledgment of the Notice of Privacy Practices (NPP) on their first visit (this is further discussed in chapter 8). Patients are often asked to sign a release indicating how they may be contacted by the practice as well as authorization for others to receive their private health information (such as a spouse) if desired. It is the responsibility of the medical assistant to maintain patients' privacy at all times. This includes never leaving the medical record unattended where others may see the name of the patient or peruse the information in the chart. When using electronic health records, it is important to always lock the screen when finished making entries in a patient's record. Written permission must be obtained from the patient to:

- Release medical records or personal data
- Publish case histories in medical journals
- Make photographs of the patient (exception: suspected cases of abuse or maltreatment)
- Allow observers in examination rooms

For example, a 57-year-old woman is seen in your office for a skin biopsy. Her husband calls asking for information regarding the bill and asks for the biopsy report. You give the requested information and then find that the patient never signed a release form. She has a valid case for invasion of privacy.

## Defamation of Character

Making malicious or false statements about a person's character or reputation is **defamation of character. Libel** refers to written statements, and **slander** refers to oral statements. For example, a patient asks for a referral to another physician. She states that she has heard, "Dr. Rogers is a good surgeon." You have heard that he has a history of alcoholism. You tell the patient that he is probably not a good choice because of his drinking. That is defamation of his character, and you could be sued for saying it.

## Fraud

Fraud is any deceitful act with the intention to conceal the truth, such as:

- Intentionally raising false expectations regarding recovery
- Not properly instructing the patient regarding possible side effects of a procedure
- Filing false insurance claims

## Tort of Outrage

Tort of outrage is the intentional infliction of emotional distress. For this tort to be proved, the plaintiff's attorney must show that the physician:

- Intended to inflict emotional distress
- Acted in a manner that is not morally or ethically acceptable
- Caused severe emotional distress

## Undue Influence

Improperly persuading another to act in a way contrary to that person's free will is termed undue influence. For instance, preying on the elderly or the mentally incompetent is a common type of undue influence. Unethical practitioners who gain the trust of these persons and persuade them to submit to expensive and unnecessary medical procedures are practicing undue influence.

 CHECKPOINT QUESTION

7. What is the difference between assault and battery?

## The Litigation Process

The litigation process begins when a patient consults an attorney because he or she believes a health care provider has done wrong or becomes aware of a possible prior injury. The patient's attorney obtains the medical records, which are reviewed by medicolegal consultants. (Such consultants may be credentialed medical assistants, nurses, or physicians who are considered experts in their field.) Then, the plaintiff's attorney files a complaint, a written statement that lists the claim against the physician and the remedy desired, usually monetary compensation.

The defendant and his or her attorney answer the complaint. The discovery phase begins with interrogatories and depositions. During this phase, attorneys for both parties gather relevant information by formally documenting responses to questions from both parties involved (depositions) and through a subpoena (court order) for the patient's medical record.

Next, the trial phase begins. A jury is selected unless the parties agree to a bench trial. In a bench trial, the judge hears the case without a jury and renders a verdict (decision or judgment). Opening statements are given, first by the plaintiff's attorney and then by the defendant's attorney. The plaintiff's attorney presents the case. Expert witnesses are called, and the evidence is shown. Examination of the witnesses begins. Direct examination involves questioning by one's own attorney; cross-examination is questioning by the opposing attorney. When the plaintiff's attorney is finished, the defense presents the opposing arguments and evidence. The plaintiff's attorney may cross-examine the defendant's witnesses. Closing arguments are heard. Finally, a verdict is made.

If the defendant is found guilty, damages are awarded. If the defendant is found not guilty, the charges are dismissed. The decision may be appealed to a higher court. An appeal is a process by which the higher court reviews the decision of the lower court.

## Defenses to Professional Liability Suits

The objective of all court proceedings is to uncover the truth. Many defenses are available to a health care worker who is being sued. These include the medical record, statute of limitations, assumption of risk, res judicata, contributory negligence, and comparative negligence, discussed next.

### Medical Records

The best and most solid defense the caregiver has is the medical record. Every item in the record is considered to be a part of a legal document. Juries may believe a medical record regardless of testimony because they are tangible items from the actual time the injury occurred. There is a common saying in the medicolegal world: "If it's not in the chart, it did not happen." This means that even negative findings should be listed. For example, instead of saying that the patient's neurologic history is negative, the documentation might say the patient reports no headaches, seizures, one-sided weakness, and so on. Entries in the medical record refresh the memory of the defendant and provide documentation of care. As a medical assistant, you must make sure that all of your documentation is timely, accurate, and legible. (See Chapter 8 for specific information regarding charting practices.)

### Statute of Limitations

Each state has a statute that defines the length of time during which a patient may file a suit against a caregiver. When the statute of limitations expires, the patient loses the right to file a claim. Generally, the limits vary from 1 to 3 years following the alleged occurrence. Some states use a combination rule. Some states allow 1 to 3 years following the patient's discovery of the occurrence. States vary greatly when an alleged injury involves a minor. The statute may not take effect until the minor reaches the age of majority and then may extend 2 to 3 years past this time. Some states have longer claim periods in wrongful death suits.

## Assumption of Risk

In the assumption of risk defense, the physician will claim that the patient was aware of the risks involved before the procedure and fully accepted the potential for damages. For example, a patient is instructed regarding the adverse effects of chemotherapy. The patient fully understands these risks, receives the chemotherapy, and wants to sue for alopecia (hair loss). Alopecia is a given risk with certain forms of chemotherapy. A signed consent form indicating that the patient was informed of all of the risks of a procedure proves this point.

## Res Judicata

The doctrine of **res judicata** means "the thing has been decided." Once the suit has been brought against the physician or patient and a settlement has been reached, the losing party may not countersue. If, for instance, the physician sues a patient for not paying bills and the court orders the patient to pay, the patient cannot sue the physician for malpractice. The opposite may occur as well. If the physician is sued for malpractice and loses, he cannot countersue for defamation of character.

## Contributory Negligence

With the **contributory negligence** defense, the physician usually admits that negligence has occurred; he or she will claim, however, that the patient aggravated the injury or assisted in making the injury worse. For example, the patient's laceration is stitched with only three sutures when 10 were needed. The physician instructs the patient to limit movement of the arm. The patient plays baseball; the laceration reopens, causing infection; and subsequently, extensive scar tissue forms. Both the patient and the physician contributed to the postoperative damages. Most states do not grant damage awards for contributory negligence. If an award is granted, the courts assess **comparative negligence**.

## Comparative Negligence

In comparative negligence, the award of damages is based on a percentage of the contribution to the negligence. If the patient contributed 30% to the damage, the damage award is 30% less than what was granted. In the example in the previous paragraph, the courts may decide that the negligence is shared at 50%. Therefore, if the court assessed damages of $20,000, the physician would be responsible for $10,000.

In the past, contributory negligence, such as a patient not returning for appointments, was seen as absolute defense for the physician. This has changed over the years, however, and many defendants use the defense of comparative negligence, with the responsibility shared between the physician and the patient.

## COG DEFENSE FOR THE MEDICAL ASSISTANT

### Respondeat Superior or Law of Agency

The doctrine of **respondeat superior** literally means "let the master answer." This may also be called law of agency. This doctrine implies that physicians are liable for the actions of their employees, as discussed earlier. The physician is responsible for your actions as a medical assistant as long as your actions are within your scope of practice. If your actions exceed your abilities or training, the physician is not generally responsible for any error that you make. You must understand that you can be sued in this instance and that respondeat superior does not guarantee immunity for your actions.

For example, Mrs. Smith is a chronic complainer, calling your office frequently with minor concerns. Today, she calls complaining of tingling in her arms. The physician has left for the day, so you tell Mrs. Smith, "Don't worry about this; take your medication, and call us tomorrow." During the night, a blood vessel in Mrs. Smith's brain bursts. She has a cerebral hemorrhage (bleeding inside the brain) and dies. The family sues. The physician claims that you were instructed not to give advice over the telephone. You are not covered by respondeat superior because you acted outside of your scope of practice.

To protect yourself from situations such as this, have your job description in written form and always practice within its guidelines. Do not perform tasks that you have not been trained to do. Never hesitate to seek clarification from a physician. If you are not sure about something, such as a medication order, ask!

Malpractice insurance is available to allied health care professionals for further protection. Malpractice premiums are inexpensive and afford protection against losing any personal assets if sued. The insurance company would pay damages as assessed by a jury. Of course, as with any insurance policy, there will be conditions of coverage and maximum amounts the company will pay. The Legal Tip provides some additional advice for preventing lawsuits.

### CHECKPOINT QUESTION

8. What is the law of agency, and how does it apply to the medical assistant?

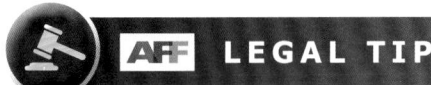

## LEGAL TIP

### You Can Avoid Litigation

- Keep medical records neat and organized. Always document and sign legibly.
- Stay abreast of new laws and medical technology.
- Become a certified or registered medical assistant (CMA or RMA, respectively).
- Keep both your cardiopulmonary resuscitation (CPR) and first aid certification current.
- Never give any information over the telephone unless you are sure of the caller's identity and you have patient consent.
- Keep the office neat and clean. Make sure that children's toys are clean and in good condition to avoid injuries. Perform safety checks frequently.
- Limit waiting time for patients. If an emergency arises, causing a long wait, explain the situation to waiting patients in a timely and professional manner.
- Practice good public relations. Always be polite, smile, and show genuine concern for your patients and their families.

## EMPLOYMENT AND SAFETY LAWS

### Civil Rights Act of 1964, Title VII

Title VII of the Civil Rights Act of 1964 protects employees from discrimination in the workplace. The Equal Employment Opportunity Commission (EEOC) enforces the provisions of the act and investigates any possible infractions. Employers may not refuse to hire, limit, segregate or classify, fire, compensate, or provide working conditions and privileges on the basis of race, color, sex, religion, or national origin. This act determines the questions that may be asked in a job interview. For example, a potential employee cannot be asked questions that would reveal age, marital status, religious affiliation, height, weight, or arrest record. It is acceptable, however, to ask if an applicant has ever been convicted of a crime. In the health care setting, employers can require a criminal records check and even drug screening to ensure the safety of the patients. The American Association of Medical Assistants (AAMA) has made recent changes to prohibit convicted felons from taking the CMA examination.

### Sexual Harassment

In recent years, Title VII has been expanded to include sexual harassment. Sexual harassment is defined by the EEOC as unwelcome sexual advances or requests for sexual favors in the workplace. The definition includes other verbal or physical conduct of a sexual nature when such conduct is made a condition of an individual's employment, is used as a basis for hiring or promotion, or has the purpose or effect of unreasonably interfering with an individual's work performance. If such behavior creates an intimidating, hostile, or offensive working environment, it is considered sexual harassment. In the past two decades, court decisions have confirmed that this form of harassment is a cause for both criminal prosecution and civil litigation.

In the medical office setting, the office manager must be alert for signs of harassment and should have in place a policy for handling complaints.

### Americans with Disabilities Act

Title VII also includes the Americans with Disabilities Act (ADA), passed in 1990, which prohibits discrimination against people with substantial disabilities in all employment practices, including job application procedures, hiring, firing, advancement, compensation, training, benefits, and all other privileges of employment. The ADA applies to all employers with 15 or more employees. The law covers those with impairments that limit their major life activities. The statute also protects those with AIDS or HIV-positive status and individuals with a history of mental illness or cancer. ADA also requires that employers provide basic accommodations for disabled employees. Those basic accommodations include extra-wide parking spaces close to the door, ramps or elevators, electric or easily opened doors, bathroom facilities designed for the disabled, an accessible break room, and a work area with counters low enough for a person in a wheelchair.

The ADA also takes safety into consideration. Employers are permitted to establish qualification standards that will exclude individuals who pose a direct threat to others if that risk cannot be lowered to an acceptable level by reasonable accommodations. In the medical field, technical standards are established that outline physical requirements of a certain job. For example, if a particular job requires adequate vision to see the dials on a piece of laboratory equipment, it is unreasonable to expect an employer to hire a person who is sight impaired. The law is designed to protect employees, not to require unreasonable accommodations.

The ADA also requires that all public buildings be accessible to physically challenged people. Following is a partial list of ways the medical office can comply with this act:

- Entrance ramps
- Widened restrooms to be wheelchair accessible
- Elevated toilet bowls for easier transferring from wheelchairs
- Easy-to-reach elevator buttons
- Braille signs
- Access to special telephone services to communicate with hearing-impaired patients

The definition of "disabled" was further defined in the ADA Amendments Act of 2008 to recognize and clarify impairments that may have been excluded under the ADA, such as individuals seeking employment who have recovered from a mental illness or cancer. The ADAAA further required the EEOC to amend its policies to reflect these changes.

## The Genetic Information Nondiscrimination Act

Some diseases have a genetic (hereditary) component, and genetic testing is available that may determine an individual's risk of contracting certain diseases. For example, there is genetic component to some cancers, such as breast and colon. The **Genetic Information Nondiscrimination Act (GINA)** is a federal law that was passed in 2008 to protect against employment discrimination based on a person's or their family's genetic information. It also prohibits health insurance plans from requiring genetic information in order to make decisions regarding health insurance coverage.

## Occupational Safety and Health Act

Employers must provide safe environments for their employees. In accordance with the Occupational Safety and Health Act of 1970, the Occupational Safety and Health Administration (OSHA) controls and monitors safety for workers. Specific OSHA rules and regulations are designed to protect the clinical worker from exposure to **blood-borne pathogens.** Blood-borne pathogens are microorganisms that can be spread through direct contact with blood or body fluids from an infected person. Universal or standard precautions are designed to protect health care workers from blood and body fluids contaminated with HIV, hepatitis, or any contagious "bugs" by requiring that those in direct contact with patients, use protective equipment (e.g., gloves, gowns, face mask). In the past, health care workers felt that they needed protection only from patients with known risk factors (sharing needles, having unprotected sexual intercourse). OSHA's regulations help to ensure protection from contracting a contagious disease from *any* body fluids handled.

Your medical assisting training will include an extensive study of safety issues and protection against accidental exposure to blood-borne pathogens. Box 2-5 outlines OSHA rules governing all free-standing health care providers. Box 2-6 outlines the laws governing employer and employee rights and responsibilities.

## Other Legal Considerations

The Clinical Laboratory Improvement Amendments (CLIA) of 1988 contain specific rules and regulations regarding laboratory safety. Laboratory procedures performed on patient specimens obtained in medical offices are typically waived CLIA tests because of their simplicity and low risk of error. A CLIA certificate of waiver, however, is required to be obtained by practices

---

**BOX 2-5   Occupational Safety and Health Act of 1970 Rules Governing Health Care Providers**

OSHA defines body fluids as semen, blood, amniotic fluids, vaginal secretions, synovial fluid (from joint spaces), pleural fluid (from the lungs), pericardial fluid (from the heart), cerebrospinal fluid (from the spinal cord), and saliva. OSHA employs inspectors who may conduct inspections and issue citations for violations and recommend penalties. Under specific rules, OSHA requires that health care facilities provide the following:

- A list of all employees who might be exposed to blood-borne diseases on either a regular or an occasional basis.
- A written exposure control plan that outlines steps to be taken in the event of an employee's accidental exposure to blood-borne pathogens.
- One employee who is responsible for OSHA compliance.
- Availability of protective clothing that fits properly.
- An employee training program in writing and records of sessions and participants.

- Warning labels and signs denoting biohazards (potentially dangerous materials).
- Written guidelines for identifying, containing, and disposing of medical waste, including housecleaning and laundry decontamination.
- Written guidelines and procedures to follow if any employee is exposed to blood or other potentially infectious materials as well as a policy for reporting incidents of exposure and maintaining records.
- Postexposure evaluation procedures, including follow-up testing of the exposed employee.
- Material safety data sheets (MSDS) listing each ingredient in a product used in the office. Manufacturers provide an MSDS for every product they sell. Information included in the sheets includes any hazards involved or necessary precautions that must be taken when handling materials.
- Hepatitis B vaccine free of charge to employees working with body fluids.

---

**BOX 2-6    Laws Governing Employer and Employment Rights and Responsibilities**

**Fair Labor Standards Act of 1939**

- Regulates wages and working conditions including:
- Federal minimum wage, overtime compensation, equal pay requirements, child labor, hours, and requirements for record keeping

**Civil Rights Act of 1964, Title VII**

- Applies to employers with 15 or more employees for at least 20 weeks of the year.
- Federal regulation forbids discrimination on the basis of race, color, sex, religion, or national origin. Some state laws also prohibit discrimination for sexual orientation, personal appearance, mental health, mental retardation, marital status, parenthood, and political affiliation.

**Americans with Disabilities Act of 1990**

- Applies to employers with 15 or more employees
- Prohibits discrimination against individuals with substantial impairments in all employment practices

**Age Discrimination in Employment Act of 1967**

- Applies to employers with 15 or more employees.
- Regulates discrimination against workers on the basis of age. Protects those who are 40 to 65 years of age

**Family and Medical Leave Act of 1993**

- Employees are covered after 1 year or 1,250 hours of employment over the past 12 months.
- Provides up to 12 weeks per year of unpaid, job-protected leave to eligible employees for certain family and medical reasons.

**Immigration Reform and Control Act of 1986**

- Applies to employers with four or more employees
- Prohibits employment of illegal aliens and protects legal aliens from discrimination based on national origin or citizenship

---

performing CLIA-waived tests through the Centers for Medicare and Medicaid Services (CMS).

Medical offices accredited by the Joint Commission (formerly known as the Joint Commission on Accreditation of Healthcare Organizations [JCAHO]) are a private organization that sets standards for health care settings (see Chapter 10). JCAHO accreditation is voluntary but requires standards to be maintained once accreditation is achieved. Each state also has specific laws regarding patient care, insurance billing, collections, and other such matters.

---

### CHECKPOINT QUESTION

9. What are blood-borne pathogens? Which government agency governs their control in the medical office?

---

## AFF MEDICAL ETHICS

Medical ethics are principles of ethical and moral conduct that govern the behavior and conduct of health professionals. These principles define proper medical etiquette, customs, and professional courtesy. Ethics are guidelines specifying right or wrong and are enforced by peer review and professional organizations. Laws are regulations and rules that are enforced by the government. Bioethics involves issues and dilemmas that result from emerging medical technology and advancements.

Many bioethical issues have arisen from the advances of modern medicine.

## American Medical Association Principles of Medical Ethics

A code of ethics is a "collective statement from a professional organization that depicts the behavioral expectations for its members. Additionally, a code of ethics allows the organization to set standards by which it may discipline its members." According to the AMA, "The Code of Medical Ethics is a living document, evolving as changes in medicine and the delivery of health care raise new questions about how the profession's core values apply in physicians' day-to-day practice. The Code links theory and practice." Box 2-7 outlines the AMA Principles of Medical Ethics.

Violations of these AMA principles may result in censure, suspension, or expulsion by the state medical board. Censure, the least punitive action, is a verbal or written reprimand from the association indicating negative findings regarding a specific incident. Suspension is the temporary removal of privileges and association with the organization. Expulsion is a formal discharge from the professional organization and is the maximum punishment. Many of these issues, however, deal with laws and the patient's rights as established by law. When violations of laws are involved, physicians may lose their license to practice, may be fined, or may be imprisoned. Serious consequences can arise from a breach of this code of ethics.

## BOX 2-7   AMA Principles of Medical Ethics

I. A physician shall be dedicated to providing competent medical care, with compassion and respect for human dignity and rights.

II. A physician shall uphold the standards of professionalism, be honest in all professional interactions, and strive to report physicians deficient in character or competence, or engaging in fraud or deception, to appropriate entities.

III. A physician shall respect the law and also recognize a responsibility to seek changes in those requirements that are contrary to the best interests of the patient.

IV. A physician shall respect the rights of patients, colleagues, and other health professionals and shall safeguard patient confidences and privacy within the constraints of the law.

V. A physician shall continue to study, apply, and advance scientific knowledge; maintain a commitment to medical education; make relevant information available to patients, colleagues, and the public; obtain consultation; and use the talents of other health professionals when indicated.

VI. A physician shall, in the provision of appropriate patient care, except in emergencies, be free to choose whom to serve, with whom to associate, and the environment in which to provide medical care.

VII. A physician shall recognize a responsibility to participate in activities contributing to the improvement of the community and the betterment of public health.

VIII. A physician shall, while caring for a patient, regard responsibility to the patient as paramount.

IX. A physician shall support access to medical care for all people.

## Medical Assistant's Role in Ethics

As an agent of the physician in the medical office, you are also governed by ethical standards and are responsible for:

• Protecting patient confidentiality
• Following all state and federal laws
• Being honest in all your actions

As a medical assistant, you must apply ethical standards as you perform your duties. You must realize that your personal feelings of right and wrong should be kept separate if they differ from the ethics of your profession. For example, a medical assistant who has a strong opinion against abortion would not be happy working in a medical facility that performs abortions. The care you give patients must be objective, and personal opinions about options must not be shared.

### Patient Advocacy

Your primary responsibility as a medical assistant is to be a patient advocate at all times. Advocacy requires that you consider the best interests of the patient above all other concerns. For example, medical assistants are often responsible for coordinating care for patients by scheduling appointments for ordered tests and referrals and seeking insurance authorization as necessary. Medical assistants must also be familiar with local social service agencies in order to provide contacts for patients needing assistance such as basic housing and food. As part of the Affordable Care Act, patient navigators are being used to help patients get the care they need (Box 2-8).

### Patient Confidentiality

**Confidentiality** of patient information is one of the most important ethical principles to be observed by the medical assistant. As discussed earlier, information obtained in the care of the patient may not be revealed without the

## BOX 2-8   Patient Navigators

The abundance of information that patients receive concerning their health care and health insurance may seem overwhelming to many people. **Patient navigators** are trained individuals who assist patients as they work through the health care system and receive the care they need. These patient advocates are in response to four provisions of the Affordable Care Act (ACA)

1. Prevention of disease: Navigators may help by encouraging patients to have routine screening tests by providing them available resources and education.

2. Health care access and coordination: To prevent delays in receiving health care services, navigators help patients with obtaining appointments and assist with transportation issues, if necessary. They may also be available to go to physician visits with them and provide patient education and cooperation for recommended therapies.

3. Health insurance coverage: The ACA's health insurance provision requires all Americans to have health insurance coverage. The role of patient navigators includes helping patients find affordable health insurance coverage and may involve helping with completion of paperwork so that coverage can begin. It is also important for navigators to help patients remain insured.

4. Diversity and cultural competency: Navigators may help with communication barriers between patients and their providers.

permission of the patient unless required by law. Whatever you say to, hear from, or do for a patient is confidential. Patients will reveal some of their innermost thoughts, feelings, and fears. This information is not for public knowledge. Family members, friends, pastors, or others may call the physician's office to inquire about a patient's condition. Many of these calls are made with good intentions; *no information*, however, should be released to anyone—friends, family, media, or insurance companies—without prior written approval from the patient (see Chapter 8).

## Honesty

One of the most important character traits for medical assistants is honesty. We all make mistakes at times; how we handle our mistakes is the indication of our ethical standards. If you make a mistake (e.g., giving the wrong medication), you must immediately report the error to your supervisor and the attending physician. The mark of a true professional is the ability to admit mistakes and take full responsibility for all actions. When speaking to patients concerning medical issues, be honest; give the facts in a straightforward manner. Never offer false expectations or hope. Never minimize or exaggerate the risks or benefits of a procedure. If you do not know the answer to a question, say, "I don't know, but I will find out for you," or refer the question to the physician. Treating the patient with dignity, respect, and honesty in all interactions will build trust in you and your professional abilities.

### CHECKPOINT QUESTION

10. What are the three ethical standards a CMA, as an agent of the physician, should follow?

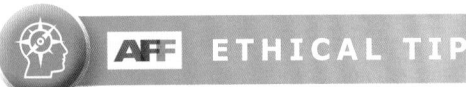

### AFF ETHICAL TIP

#### An Ethical Dilemma

How would you handle the following hypothetical ethical dilemma?

*You are the office manager for a well-respected family physician in a small town. He is 70 years old and is starting to show signs of senile dementia. He is forgetful and has even been disoriented and confused a few times. No one else seems to have noticed. Should you report your concerns? If so, to whom?*

The AMA Principles of Medical Ethics require that physicians, and medical assistants through the law of agency, report unethical behavior among colleagues. The medical profession is also governed by the patient's right to safety and quality care. It is your ethical responsibility to report the doctor's condition to the administration of the hospital where the physician has privileges or to the state board of medicine. The physician's family should be involved in the situation.

### BOX 2-9    Medical Assistants' Creed

The AAMA also has a written a creed for medical assistants. The creed of the AAMA is as follows:
I believe in the principles and purposes of the profession.
I endeavor to be more effective.
I aspire to render greater service.
I protect the confidence entrusted to me.
I am dedicated to the care and well-being of all patients.
I am loyal to my physician–employer.
I am true to the ethics of my profession.
I am strengthened by compassion, courage, and faith.

## American Association of Medical Assistants Code of Ethics

### Principles

The AAMA has published a set of five principles of ethical and moral conduct that all medical assistants must follow in the practice of the profession. They state that the medical assistant must always strive to:

1. Render services with respect for human dignity
2. Respect patient confidentiality, except when information is required by the law
3. Uphold the honor and high principles set forth by the AAMA
4. Continually improve knowledge and skills for the benefit of patients and the health care team
5. Participate in community services that promote good health and welfare to the general public

These principles are outlined in the AAMA creed seen in the Medical Assistants' Creed (Box 2-9).

According to the *AAMA's Disciplinary Standards and Procedures for CMAs*, CMAs who violate the disciplinary standards may face possible sanctions including denial of eligibility for the certification examination, probation, reprimand, temporary revocation of the CMA credentials, and permanent revocation of the CMA credential. For more information, see the AAMA Web site.

## COG BIOETHICS

Bioethics deals specifically with the moral issues and problems that affect human life. As a result of advances in medicine and research, many situations require moral decisions for which there are no clear answers. Abortion and genetic engineering are examples. The goal is to make the right decision in each specific instance as it applies to an individual's specific circumstances. What may be right for one patient may be wrong for another; that is the foundation of bioethics.

## American Medical Association Council on Ethical and Judicial Affairs

Because of the broad scope of medical ethics and bioethical issues, the AMA formed a subcommittee to review AMA principles and to interpret them as they apply to everyday clinical situations. This subcommittee is called the Council on Ethical and Judicial Affairs. The council has formulated a series of opinions on various medical and bioethical issues that are intended to provide the physician with guidelines for professional conduct and responsibilities. New ethical opinions are initiated through a series of discussion and research by the members of the council, and existing opinions are revised as needed for new technology and advances in medicine. These opinions are divided into four general categories:

- Social policy issues
- Relations with colleagues and hospitals
- Administrative office procedures
- Professional rights and responsibilities

The following discussion provides a summary of these opinions along with questions designed to promote your ability to use reasoning to examine difficult ethical issues. These issues are not within the scope of decisions for medical assistants, but you will be faced with their consequences at some time in your career.

## Social Policy Issues

The social policy section deals with various issues of societal importance and provides guidelines to aid the physician in making ethical choices. Five common societal topics and the opinion statements from the AMA Council on Ethical and Judicial Affairs follow.

### Allocation of Resources

The term *allocate* means to set aside or designate for a purpose. Allocation of resources in the medical profession may refer to many health needs:

- *Organs for transplantation.* Who gets the heart, the college professor or the young recovering addict whose heart was damaged by his lifestyle? Should lifestyle or perceived worth be considered in the decision?
- *Funds for research.* Which disease should receive more funding for research, cancer or AIDS?
- *Funds for health care.* For what should the money be spent, for keeping alive extremely premature infants or making preventive health care available for a greater number of poor children?

---

> **BOX 2-10   AMA Council on Ethical and Judicial Affairs Viewpoint**
>
> - When resources are limited, decisions for allocating health care materials should be based on fair and socially acceptable criteria. Economic or social position should not be a factor in the decision.
> - Priority care is given to the person or persons who are more likely to receive the greatest long-term benefit from the treatment. Patients with other disease processes or who are not good candidates for treatment for whatever reason will be less likely to receive treatment than otherwise healthy patients. For instance, a patient with cancer in other sites would not be considered for a liver transplant, whereas a patient whose liver was damaged by trauma but who has no other involvement would probably be a good candidate.
> - An individual's societal worth must not be a deciding factor during the decision process. A socially or politically prominent patient should not be considered a better recipient of treatment options than a young mother on welfare.
> - Age must not be considered in the decision process. If the age of the patient is not a contraindication for the treatment, all ages should be considered on an even basis for most medical resources.

---

- *Hospital beds and professional care.* With hospital care at a premium, who will pay for the indigent? How is it decided which patient is entitled to the last bed in the intensive care unit?

Box 2-10 outlines the judicial council's viewpoints on allocation of limited resources.

### Clinical Investigations and Research

Physicians are frequently involved in studying the effectiveness of new procedures and medications, often called clinical investigations or research. New drugs and treatments are tested on animals first and then considered safe for human testing. The council's viewpoint on research investigation of new drugs and procedures states:

- *A physician may participate in clinical research as long as the project is part of a systematic program with controls for patient evaluation during all phases of the research. At all stages of the testing and at the completion of the study, a protocol must be in place to evaluate the immediate and the long-term effects of the study.*
- *The goal of the research must be to obtain scientifically valid data. The objectives of the study must be available to the physician and the patient, results*

*must be provided to all participants on request, and the testing must serve a medically sound purpose to provide better patient care.*

- *Utmost care and respect must be given to patients involved in clinical research. They are entitled to be treated just as any other patient receiving health care.*
- *Physicians must obtain the patient's permission or consent before enrolling the patient in a research project.*
- *The patient's decision to participate in the program must be completely voluntary.*
- *The patient must be advised of any potential risks, side effects, and benefits of participating in the project.*
- *The patient must be advised that this procedure or drug is experimental. Patients must be made aware that research is not complete, that this is the purpose of the trials, and that the risks and benefits are not fully known at this time.*
- *The physician and the institution must have a check and balance system in place to ensure that quality care is always given and ethical standards are followed. Documentation of patient education and instruction for following testing guidelines and patient response to the treatment must be ongoing and thorough.*

## Obstetric Dilemmas

Advances in technology have created legal and ethical situations that have polarized opinions and are difficult to bring to consensus. Issues such as the beginning of life, genetic testing and engineering, sex determination, the rights of the fetus, ownership of the fertilized egg, and so forth will not be easily answered. The council formulated an opinion regarding obstetric issues as fairly as possible that states the following:

ABORTION. As the law now stands, a physician may perform an abortion as long as state and federal laws are followed regarding the trimester in which it is performed. A physician who does not want to perform abortions cannot be forced to perform the procedure; that physician, however, should refer the patient to other health care professionals who can assist the patient.

GENETIC TESTING. If amniocentesis is performed on a mother and a genetic defect is found, both parents must be told. The parents may request or refuse to have the pregnancy terminated. (Amniocentesis is a procedure in which a needle is inserted in a pregnant woman's abdomen to remove and test amniotic fluid. Many abnormalities and disorders can be diagnosed early in pregnancy by this procedure.)

ARTIFICIAL INSEMINATION. Artificial insemination involves the insertion of sperm into a woman's vagina for the purpose of conception. The donor may be the husband (artificial insemination by husband [AIH]) or an anonymous donor (artificial insemination by donor [AID]). The council states that both the husband and wife must consent to this procedure. If a donor is used, the sperm must be tested for infectious and genetic disorders. Complete confidentiality for the donor and recipient must be maintained.

 **CHECKPOINT QUESTION**

11. What is the opinion of the AMA's Council on Ethical and Judicial Affairs regarding abortion?

## Stem Cell Research

As we continue to find new technologies, ethical dilemmas continue to emerge. Stem cell research is an ethical issue resulting from our ability to program the immature and undifferentiated cells of a fetus to be muscle, liver, or cardiac cells. The implications of this ability have become a political issue in the last several years. Researchers have found that stem cells taken from the umbilical cord of a newborn are also useful. It is even possible for parents to have the umbilical cord of their infant frozen and stored for use in later years to cure any diseases encountered. Some people believe that the potential to cure such diseases as Parkinson disease and cystic fibrosis is worth using embryonic stem cells. Others believe that using fetal cells and tissue is immoral. The political debate about government funding of stem cell research continues. As discussed in Chapter 1, today's research has made it possible to use a patient's own stems cells to regenerate cells, tissue, and even organs. This makes the use of stem cells for treatment a less sensitive issue.

## Organ Transplantation

Organ transplantation became a medical option in the mid-1950s, although at that time, there were many problems with rejection of the organs by the recipient's immune system. When this postoperative complication was corrected by antirejection drugs, the practice became more common. Organs are viable (able to support life) for varying lengths of time, but most can be used successfully if transplanted within 24 to 48 hours. An organization in Richmond, Virginia, the United Network of Organ Sharing, coordinates local organ procurement teams that will fly to areas where organs are to be harvested to assist with the surgery if needed and to ensure the integrity of the organ. There are far fewer organs available than are needed, and every year, thousands of patients die who could have lived if an organ had been available.

The use of organs from a baby born without a brain (anencephaly) raises serious ethical issues. The council states that everything must be done for the infant until the determination of death can be made. For infant organs to be transplanted, both parents must consent.

The council's views on transplantation state:

- *The rights of the donor and organ recipient must be treated equally. The imminent death of the donor does not release the medical personnel from observing all rights that every patient is due.*
- *Organ donors must be given every medical opportunity for life. Life support is not removed until the patient is determined to have no brain activity and could not live without artificial support.*
- *Death of the donor must be determined by a physician who is not on the transplant team to avoid a charge of conflict of interest.*

- *Consent (permission) must be received from both the donor, if possible, and recipient before the transplant. Family members may give consent if the donor is unable to do so.*
- *Transplants can be performed only by surgeons who are qualified to perform this complex surgery and who are affiliated with institutions that have adequate facilities for the surgery and postoperative care.*

Box 2-11 highlights the Uniform Anatomical Gift Act.

## Withholding or Withdrawing Treatment

Physicians have a professional and ethical obligation to promote quality of life, which means sustaining life and relieving suffering. Sometimes, these obligations conflict with a patient's wishes. Patients have the right to refuse medical treatment and to request that life support or life-sustaining treatments be withheld or withdrawn. Withholding treatment means that certain medical treatments may not be initiated. Withdrawing treatment is terminating a treatment that has already begun. In 1991, congress passed the **Patient Self-Determination Act (PSDA)**, which gave all hospitalized patients or patients going into long-term care facilities the right to make health care decisions on admission. The PSDA requires all health care facilities to provide information to patients about their rights under their state laws in the event they become unable to make medical decisions for themselves. These decisions may be referred to as advance directives. An **advance directive** is a statement of a person's wishes for medical decisions prior to a critical event and includes living wills and health care powers of attorney. Living wills indicate the types of medical treatment desired, such as whether a ventilator can be used, whether CPR should be initiated, and whether a feeding tube should be inserted. The purpose of a health care power of attorney is to name someone to give him or her authorization to make health care decisions in the event the patient becomes unable to do so. Just completing an advance directive does not ensure that the patient's wishes will be carried out. It is important to make family members aware of these wishes. The patient's next of kin should keep a copy of the advance directive, and one should be placed in the medical office chart with special notation. Figure 2-4 is a sample of an advance directive.

---

### BOX 2-11 Uniform Anatomical Gift Act

Many organs can be transplanted, including the liver, kidney, cornea, heart, lung, and skin. To meet the growing need for organs and to allay the concern over donor standards, the National Conference of Commissioners for Uniform State Laws passed legislation known as the Uniform Anatomical Gift Act.

All acts include the following clauses:

- Any mentally competent person over age 18 may donate all or part of his or her body for transplantation or research.
- The donor's wishes supersede any other wishes except when state laws require an autopsy.
- Physicians accepting donor organs in good faith are immune from lawsuits against harvesting organs.
- Death of the donor must be determined by a physician not involved with the transplant team.
- Financial compensation may not be given to the donor or survivors.
- Persons wishing to donate organs can revoke permission or change their minds at any time.

In most states, the Department of Motor Vehicles asks applicants for a driver's license about organ donation and indicates their wishes on their license. In addition, an individual may declare the wish to donate all or parts of the body in a will or any legal document, including a Uniform Donor Card. Organ donors should make their families aware of their wishes to ensure they will be carried out.

---

## ✓ CHECKPOINT QUESTION

12. What is an advance directive? How can a patient be sure his or her wishes will be followed?

**ADVANCE DIRECTIVE**

UNIFORM ADVANCE DIRECTIVE OF [list name of declarant]

To my family, physician, attorney, and anyone else who may become responsible for my health, welfare, or affairs, I make this declaration while I am of sound mind.

If I should ever become in a terminal state and there is no reasonable expectation of my recovery, I direct that I be allowed to die a natural death and that my life not be prolonged by extraordinary measures. I do, however, ask that medication be mercifully administered to me to alleviate suffering, even though this may shorten my remaining life.

This statement is made after full reflection and is in accordance with my full desires. I want the above provisions carried out to the extent permitted by law. Insofar as they are not legally enforceable, I wish that those to whom this will is addressed will regard themselves as morally bound by this instrument.

If permissible in the jurisdiction in which I may be hospitalized I direct that in the event of a terminal diagnosis, the physicians supervising my care discontinue feeding should the continuation of feeding be judged to result in unduly prolonging a natural death.

If permissible in the jurisdiction in which I may be hospitalized I direct that in the event of a terminal diagnosis, the physicians supervising my care discontinue hydration (water) should the continuation of hydration be judged to result in unduly prolonging a natural death.

I herewith authorize my spouse, if any, or any relative who is related to me within the third degree to effectuate my transfer from any hospital or other health care facility in which I may be receiving care should that facility decline or refuse to effectuate the instructions given herein.

I herewith release any and all hospitals, physicians, and others for myself and for my estate from any liability for complying with this instrument.

Signed:

_____

[list name of declarant]

City of residence: _____

[city of residence]

County of residence: _____

[county of residence]

State of residence: _____

[state of residence]

Social Security Number: _____

[social security number]

Date: _____

_____

Witness

_____

Witness

STATE OF _____

COUNTY OF _____

This day personally appeared before me, the undersigned authority, a Notary Public in and for _____ County, _____ State,

_____    _____ (Witnesses)

who, being first duly sworn, say that they are the subscribing witnesses to the declaration of [list name of declarant], the declarant, signed, sealed, and published and declared the same as and for his declaration, in the presence of both these affiants; and that these affiants, at the request of said declarant, in the presence of each other, and in the presence of said declarant, all present at the same time, signed their names as attesting witnesses to said declaration.

Affiants further say that this affidavit is made at the request of [list name of declarant], declarant, and in his presence, and that [list name of declarant] at the time the declaration was executed, in the opinion of the affiants, of sound mind and memory, and over the age of eighteen years.

Taken, subscribed and sworn to before me by _____ (witness) and

_____ (witness) this _____ day of _____, 20_____.

My commission expires: _____

_____ Notary Public

**Figure 2-4** • Sample advance directive.

## WHAT IF?

**A well-meaning family member asks for information about her mother's condition. What should you say?**

Tell the family member that HIPAA's Privacy Rule does not allow you to discuss the patient without his or her permission. No information can be released to anyone—friends, family, media, or insurance companies—without prior written approval from the patient (see Chapter 8).

HIPAA also requires that each patient complete a form that establishes his or her wishes about giving information to family members and friends. If there is a particular family member who brings the patient to the office, the patient may sign a release form giving that person the right to receive information. Many physicians provide the patient with a short progress report including the patient's test results, diagnosis, treatment, and next appointment. A form could be designed for this purpose. This gives the patient the opportunity to share complete and accurate information if he or she chooses.

## AFF PROFESSIONAL AND ETHICAL CONDUCT AND BEHAVIOR

The council states that all health care professionals are responsible for reporting unethical practices to the appropriate agencies. No health care professional should engage in any act that he or she feels is ethically or morally wrong.

Additionally, the council states

- A physician must never assist or allow an unlicensed person to practice medicine.
- Hospitals and physicians must work together for the best care for patients. Hospitals should allow physicians staff privileges based on the ability of the physician, educational background, and the needs of the community. (Staff privileges allow physicians to admit their patients to a given hospital.) Issues of a personal nature must never be considered when accepting or declining a physician's application for privileges.
- It is unethical for physicians to admit patients to the hospital or to order excessive treatments for the sole purpose of financial rewards.

## CHECKPOINT QUESTION

13. What steps should be taken when a physician closes his or her practice?

## ROLE-PLAYING ACTIVITY

The EHR at Great Falls Medical Center has safeguards to ensure that only the minimum necessary information is available for the staff to perform their jobs effectively. For example, receptionists and schedulers do not have access to information in the clinical portion of patients' health records. Derrick Moore, RMA, assisted one of the physicians yesterday with a new patient and several tests were ordered including blood work and a cervical MRI. Today, Derrick was approached by the receptionist requesting information about the patient's visit because she said that patient was her sister. Is it appropriate to share this information with the patient's sister since the receptionist works at the practice? How should Derrick respond to the receptionist? Is this an ethical or a legal dilemma? Role-play this activity as the medical assistant responding to the receptionist in a professional manner. Consider factors that determine whether or not the patient's privacy would be violated. If you are playing the role of the receptionist, consider your emotions involved in wanting this information about your loved one. Your instructor will give you additional information about this activity!

## español SPANISH TERMINOLOGY

**¿Usted entiende la información que acaba de recibir?**
Do you understand the information I have given?

**¿Para estar seguro de que entendió la información que le acabo de dar, me podría repetir lo que le he dicho?**
To be sure that you understood the information given to you, can you repeat this to me?

**¿Nos autoriza usted a llevar a cabo este procedimiento médico?**
Do you give us permission to perform this procedure?

**¿Por favor, podría firmar aquí?**
Please, can you sign here?

**¿No sé exactamente cuáles son mis derechos como paciente, me podría imprimir un resumen?**
I don't know exactly what my rights are as a patient; can you please print out a summary for me?

**Necesitamos que firme este documento como testigo.**
We need you to sign this document as a witness.

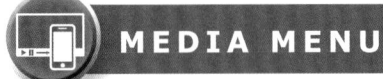

## MEDIA MENU

**Student Resources** on thePoint°

• **CMA/RMA Certification Exam Review**

**Internet Resources**
**Web sites to keep abreast of changes in the medical field:**
**Go to your state's home page and click on the link to the state legislature to view pending state legislation.**
**Go to the Library of Congress to view federal legislation to be considered in the coming week.**
http://Thomas.loc.gov

**Equal Employment Opportunity Commission**
http://www.eeoc.gov

**U.S. Department of Labor, Bureau of Labor Statistics**
http://stats.bls.gov

**To complete an advance directive**
http://www.legalzoom.com

**To download and print a Vaccination Information Statement**
http://www.cdc.gov/vaccines/pubs/vis/default.htm

**American Hospital Association**
http://www.aha.org

**AHA's Patient Care Partnership**
http://www.aha.org/aha/issues/Communicating-With-Patients/pt-care-partnership.html

**Reporting Child Abuse**
http://www.childwelfare.gov

**CLIA Web site to access certificate application**
http://www.cms.hhs.gov/cmsforms/downloads/cms116.pdf

**Controlled Substances**
http://www.deadiversion.usdoj.gov

**Intimate Partner Violence**
www.cdc.gov/violenceprevention

**Patients' Bill of Rights**
http://www.hcqualitycommission.gov/final

**National Center on Elder Abuse**
www.ncea.aoa.gov/Stop_Abuse

## EMR Activity

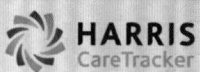

**HARRIS** CareTracker

Harris CareTracker is a web-based electronic medical record (EMR) application that you will use for the EMR activities included in this section at the end of each chapter. This application is actually used in physician offices but is provided to you through the publisher, Wolters Kluwer Health, to give you hands-on practice working with EMRs. Your instructor will have more information about accessing your username, login, and Quickstart guide.

Prerequisite Activities in Harris CareTracker

- *The Getting Started and Quickstart documents and EMR Activities Step-by-Step Instructions are available at* http://thePoint.lww.com/KronenbergerComp5e

Activity Details

The EMR can alert health care professionals to important patient information. Derrick Moore, RMA, just saw new patient Rachel Smith, who uses the help of a service animal due to a visual impairment. For this activity, first create a record for this new patient and then add a note regarding her service dog so that everyone in the practice will be alerted that this patient has a visual impairment.

## Chapter Summary

- The fields of medicine and law are linked in common concern for the patient's health and rights. Increasingly, health care professionals are the object of malpractice lawsuits.
- You can help prevent medical malpractice by acting professionally, maintaining clinical competency, and properly documenting in the medical record. Promoting good public relations between the patient and the health care team can avoid frivolous or unfounded suits and direct attention and energy toward optimum health care.
- Medical ethics and bioethics involve complex issues and controversial topics. There will be no easy or clear-cut answers to questions raised by these issues. As a medical assistant, your first priority must be to act as your patients' advocate, with their best interests and concerns foremost in your actions and interactions. You must always maintain ethical standards and report the unethical behaviors of others.
- Many acts and regulations affect health care organizations and their operations. A medical office must keep current on all legal updates.
- Most states publish a monthly bulletin that reports on new legislation. Every state has a Web site that will link you to legislative action. Read these on a regular basis.
- Each office should have legal counsel who can assist in interpreting legal issues.

## Warm-Ups for Critical Thinking

1. An acquaintance who knows you work in the medical field asks you to diagnose her rash. What do you say?
2. A patient owes a big bill at your office. She requests copies of her records. What do you do?
3. You suspect that a new employee in the office is misusing narcotics. What do you do?
4. Mrs. Rodriguez has bone cancer. Her doctor has estimated that she has 6 months to live. Mrs. Rodriguez wants the physician to withhold all medical treatments. She does not want chemotherapy or any life-sustaining measures. Her family disagrees. Should her family have any input into her health care decisions?
5. You are on your lunch hour from your job at a Planned Parenthood clinic. You run into the mother of a friend who happened to be seen earlier that day in your clinic. You say, "Hi, I just saw Heather this morning." Heather's mother says, "Oh, yes? And where did you see her?" What now? Discuss the need to think before you speak where confidentiality is concerned.

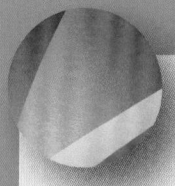

**PSY** PROCEDURE 2-1

## Obtaining an Informed Consent for Treatment

**PSY** Apply the Patient's Bill of Rights as it relates to:

a. Choice of treatment
b. Consent for treatment
c. Refusal of treatment

**Purpose:** To obtain written permission from a patient for a recommended treatment, including the risks and benefits, and giving an opportunity for questions to be answered and subsequent consent or refusal for the treatment

**Equipment:** Computer with word processing software, Internet connection, consent form, Vaccine Information Statement for Influenza from the CDC's Web site, 8-1/2 × 11 white paper

**Scenario:** Complete an informed consent for an adult patient receiving an inactivated (injectable) influenza vaccine

| STEPS | REASONS |
|---|---|
| 1. Upon receipt of the physician's order that a patient will receive an inactivated influenza vaccine, download and print the **most recent Vaccine Information Statement** from the CDC's Web site to give to the patient. | Information about the vaccine is necessary to make the patient aware of the risks and benefits of receiving the vaccine in order to make an informed decision. The most recent VIS form must be provided regardless of the age of the patient pursuant to the National Childhood Vaccine Injury Act. |
| 2. Complete an informed consent form for the inactivated influenza vaccine including the date of the VIS and the date it was given to the patient. | Providers are required by federal law to document VIS information about the vaccine being administered. |
| 3. Secure the patient's signature and date on the completed informed consent form. | The patient's signature is necessary to give the patient an opportunity to have any questions answered and for permission to receive or refuse the vaccine. |
| 4. File the informed consent in the patient's medical record. | Consents become part of the patient's medical record as evidence that the patient received information about the treatment, had an opportunity to ask questions, and gave permission for the vaccine to be administered. |
| 5. **AFF** Advise the patient on any follow-up procedures as instructed by the physician. | The patient must be made aware of potential reactions and follow-up if necessary. |

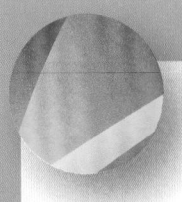

**PSY** PROCEDURE 2-2

# Reporting an Infectious Disease

**PSY** Perform compliance reporting based on public health statutes

**Purpose:** Recognize a reportable infectious disease and report it to the proper authority

**Scenario:** Search for your state's reporting requirements for a hepatitis B infection

**Equipment:** Computer with Internet connection, search engine, Web site list

| STEPS | REASONS |
|---|---|
| 1. Using a search engine, go to the Department of Health for your state. | State Departments of Health have information available to the public as well as physicians regarding health and safety matters. |
| 2. Access your state's list of reportable diseases. | It is the physician's responsibility to know and report infectious diseases. |
| 3. Search for your state's reporting requirements for hepatitis B. | Determine how, when, and to whom hepatitis B must be reported in your state. |
| 4. Interpret your state's requirement for reporting hepatitis B to the Centers for Disease Control. | Some infectious diseases must also be reported to the CDC. |
| 5. **AFF** How can you protect the patient's private health information in the medical record from being accessed by others? | The integrity of the medical record must be protected at all times. |

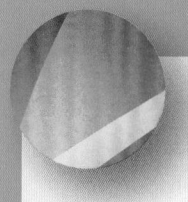

**PSY** PROCEDURE 2-3

## Monitoring Federal and State Regulations, Changes, and Updates

**PSY** Monitor federal and state health care legislation

**Purpose:** To ensure compliance with regulations by keeping abreast of changes and actions affecting medical assisting issues and health care legislation

**Equipment:** Computer, Internet connection, search engine, and Web site list

| STEPS | REASONS |
|---|---|
| 1. Using a search engine, input the keywords for your state legislature OR go to the home page for your state government. Example: http://www.nc.gov | The best source for legislative changes is a state's legislative Web site. |
| 2. Follow links to the legislative branch of your state. | The home page will give you the appropriate links. |
| 3. Search for such issues as health care finances, allied health professionals, outpatient medical care, Medicare, etc. | These general search words will lead you to information about current or pending legislation. |
| 4. Read and share information from the Centers for Disease Control and Prevention (CDC), Occupational Safety and Health Administration (OSHA), your state medical society, and the American Medical Association (AMA). | Information you receive from outside sources will keep you abreast of changes and trends. For example, OSHA informed providers about changes in the regulations for needle disposal. |
| 5. Create and enforce a policy for timely dissemination of information received by fax or e-mail from outside agencies. | OSHA and the CDC alert providers of vital information via fax or e-mail. |
| 6. Circulate information gathered to all appropriate employees with an avenue for sharing information. | Any information obtained should be shared. |
| 7. Post changes in a designated area of the office. | A break room or time clock area is a good place to display important information. |
| 8. **AFF** Explain what you would say to a fellow employee who responds to a change in a current law with: "I will just keep doing it the old way. Who is going to care?" | Health care professionals must stay current and abreast of any changes in the law. As the saying goes, "ignorance is no excuse" when it comes to changes in statutes and laws. You are legally obligated to obey the new law after the effective date. |

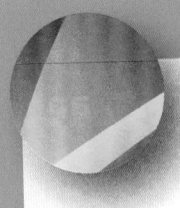

# Create an Office Policy to Report an Illegal Activity

**PSY** Report an illegal activity in the health care setting following proper protocol.

**Purpose:** To recognize an illegal activity and follow office policies to report to the proper authorities

**Scenario:** Create an office policy to report suspected case of child abuse according to local authorities when directed to do so by a physician

**Equipment:** Computer with word processing software, Internet connection, 8-1/2 × 11 white paper

| STEPS | REASONS |
|---|---|
| 1. Determine your state's statute that defines reportable child abuse. | All states have legal definitions and laws that require health care professionals to report suspected cases of child abuse and/or neglect. |
| 2. Identify the name and phone number of the Department of Health and Human Services to contact for cases of suspected child abuse and/or neglect. | State agencies have local child protective services available with direct numbers to contact child welfare or law enforcement personnel. |
| 3. Identify the employee who will be responsible for contacting the child welfare or law enforcement number when directed by a physician in cases of suspected child abuse and/or neglect. | Only one person, such as the office manager, is necessary to contact the agency and communicate instructions to the physician. |
| 4. List the steps for documenting the action taken and follow-up as directed by the child welfare agency. | Accurate documentation is necessary because it is necessary for future health care encounters and is a legal document. |
| 5. Indicate the title of the employee responsible for regularly updating and revising the policy as necessary. | Policy will be kept current. |
| 6. Provide the policy to every employee with signatures on an acknowledgment of receipt and of their understanding of the policy and/or revisions. | To make sure all employees are aware of the policy and/or revisions that have been approved by the physician(s) |

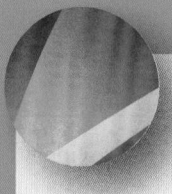

## **PSY** PROCEDURE 2-5

# Create an Office Policy to Protect Patient's Private Health Information

**PSY** Apply HIPAA Rules in regard to:

Privacy

Release of Information

**Purpose:** Recognize HIPAA requirements for protecting PHI

**Scenario:** Create an office policy to protect PHI and in compliance with HIPAA

**Equipment:** Computer with word processing software, Internet connection, 8-1/2 × 11 white paper

| STEPS | REASON |
|---|---|
| 1. Identify HIPAA's definition of *private health information (PHI)*. | Health Insurance Portability and Accountability Act (HIPAA) is a federal law that protects PHI. |
| 2. Research HIPAA privacy laws and patient rights regarding PHI in the medical record. | HIPAA laws require providers to have policies to protect patients' private health information. |
| 3. Identify the title of the employee who will be the HIPAA Privacy Officer. | HIPAA Privacy Rule requires medical offices to have at least one person to manage compliance and train staff in compliance. |
| 4. Address how the Notice of Privacy Practices will be distributed and how refusal of acknowledgments will be handled. | Providers are required to distribute NPPs to all patients at their first visit and obtain signature to acknowledge receipt of the practice's NPP. The NPP must contain the following elements:<br>**a.** How their PHI will be used and disclosed<br>**b.** The provider's responsibilities to protect the PHI<br>**c.** Patients' privacy rights including the right to file a complaint in the event they believe there has been a breach of privacy<br>**d.** How patients should contact the office to report and/or file a complaint for breach of privacy matters<br>Signatures should also be obtained as an acknowledgment of receipt. |
| 5. Determine how the paper medical record will be protected and the responsibilities of the employees. | Confidentiality and the integrity of the medical record must be maintained at all times. |
| 6. Determine how the electronic health record will be protected and the responsibilities of the employees. | Confidentiality and the integrity of the medical record must be maintained at all times. |
| 7. Identify (by titles) employees who will have access to the various portions of the medical record. | HIPAA requires providers to develop and implement "minimum necessary" standards based on employees' roles within the practice. |
| 8. List the requirements for releasing medical records upon a patient's request including fees (research your state's statutes for permissible charges for copies of medical records). | Release of medical records by patients for any reason should be in writing, with a second piece of identifying information noted and with specific documents requested to be released. State statutes may determine fees that may be charged for medical records. |

*(continues on page 62)*

## PROCEDURE 2-5 (continued)

| STEPS | REASON |
|---|---|
| 9. List the requirements for handling requests for medical records by individuals other than the patient. | Under the HIPAA Privacy Rule, health care providers may disclose PHI for a variety of reasons without written authorization from the patient. |
| 10. Indicate the title of the person responsible for updating and revising this policy as necessary. | Policy will be kept current. |
| 11. Provide the policy to all employees with an acknowledgment of receipt and their understanding of the policy and/or revisions. | To make sure all employees are aware of the policy and/or revisions that have been approved by the physician(s) |

# CHAPTER 3

# Communication Skills

## Outline

## Learning Outcomes

**COG Cognitive Domain\***

1. Spell and define the key terms
2. List two major forms of communication
3. *Identify styles and types of verbal communication*
4. *Identify types of nonverbal communication*
5. *Recognize barriers to communication*
6. *Identify techniques for overcoming communication barriers*
7. *Recognize the elements of oral communication using a sender–receiver process*
8. Identify resources and adaptations that are required based on individual needs, that is, culture and environment, developmental life stage, language, and physical threats to communication
9. Discuss examples of diversity:
   a. Cultural
   b. Social
   c. Ethnic

10. Discuss the role of cultural, social, and ethnic diversity in ethical performance of medical assisting practice
11. *Discuss the role of assertiveness in effective professional communication, and relate the following behaviors to professional communication:*
    a. *Assertive*
    b. *Aggressive*
    c. *Passive*
12. *Discuss the theories of:*
    a. *Erik Erikson*
    b. *Kübler-Ross*
13. Explain how various components of communication can affect the meaning of verbal messages
14. Define active listening
15. List and describe the six interviewing techniques
16. Give an example of how cultural differences may affect communication

*(continues on page 64)*

17. Discuss how to handle communication problems caused by language barriers
18. List two methods that you can use to promote communication among hearing-, sight-, and speech-impaired patients
19. Discuss how to handle an angry or distressed patient
20. List five actions that you can take to improve communication with a child
21. Discuss your role in communicating with a grieving patient or family member
22. Discuss the key elements of interdisciplinary communication
23. Explore issue of confidentiality as it applies to the medical assistant

### PSY Psychomotor Domain*

1. *Respond to nonverbal communication (Procedure 3-1)*
2. *Use feedback techniques to obtain patient information including the following:*
   a. *Reflection (Procedure 3-1)*
   b. *Restatement (Procedure 3-1)*
   c. *Clarification (Procedure 3-1)*
3. *Coach patients appropriately considering the following:*
   a. *Cultural diversity (Procedure 3-2)*
   b. *Developmental life stage (Procedure 3-2)*
   c. *Communication barriers (Procedure 3-2)*

### AFF Affective Domain*

1. *Demonstrate*
   a. *Empathy*
   b. *Active listening*
   c. *Nonverbal communication*
2. *Demonstrate respect for individual diversity including:*
   a. *Gender*
   b. *Race*
   c. *Religion*
   d. *Age*
   e. *Economic status*
   f. *Appearance*

3. Use appropriate body language and other nonverbal skills in communicating with patients, family, and staff
4. Demonstrate awareness of the territorial boundaries of the person with whom one is communicating
5. Demonstrate sensitivity appropriate to the message being delivered
6. Demonstrate awareness of how an individual's personal appearance affects anticipated responses
7. Demonstrate recognition of the patient's level of understanding in communications
8. Analyze communication in providing appropriate responses/feedback
9. *Demonstrate the principles of self-boundaries*
10. Respond to issues of confidentiality

*\*Note: AAMA/CAAHEP 2015 Standards are italicized.*

### ABHES Competencies

1. Identify and respond appropriately when working/caring for patients with special needs
2. Use empathy when treating terminally ill patients
3. Identify common stages that terminally ill patients go through and list organizations/support groups that can assist patients and family members of patients struggling with terminal illness
4. Advocate on behalf of family/patients, having ability to deal and communicate with family
5. Analyze the effect of hereditary, cultural, and environmental influences
6. Locate resources and information for patients and employers
7. Be attentive, listen, and learn
8. Be impartial and show empathy when dealing with patients
9. Communicate on the recipient's level of comprehension
10. Serve as liaison between the physician and others
11. Recognize and respond to verbal and nonverbal communication

## Key Terms

| | | | |
|---|---|---|---|
| anacusis | discrimination | messages | presbycusis |
| bias | dysphasia | mourning | reflecting |
| clarification | dysphonia | nonlanguage | stereotyping |
| cultures | feedback | paralanguage | summarizing |
| demeanor | grief | paraphrasing | therapeutic |

## Case Study

Natalie Garrett, CMA, is responsible for collecting information from new patients about their past medical history, family history, and social history at Great Falls Medical Center. The community is diverse, representing many cultures from around the world. There is also a large population of retired people. Natalie must be able to communicate effectively with everyone to gather information necessary to provide quality health care to patients. Today, Natalie must take a health history from a 65-year-old man who recently retired and is new to the area. What kinds of barriers might Natalie encounter when she interviews this patient and, specifically, what barriers to the communication process might the patient experience? What communication techniques might Natalie use to help her correctly understand the information this patient provides to her? In addition to language barriers, what other challenges might Natalie encounter as she works with new patients in the practice? What health problems associated with specific ethnic groups should she be aware of? Professional medical assistants must be aware of the cultural and development differences in patients. These questions and the importance of understanding professional communication are covered in this chapter.

Communication is sending and receiving **messages** (information), verbally or otherwise. Until the message is received accurately, communication has not taken place. The ability to communicate effectively is a crucial skill for medical assistants. In your role, you must accurately and appropriately share information with physicians, other professional staff members, and patients. When communicating with patients, you must be able to receive messages correctly, interpret them, and respond to the sender appropriately. Avoiding slang and using proper grammar are important! Although you may speak in an informal way with family and friends, you must speak in a professional manner while at work. The medical assistant is usually the first person the patient meets in the medical office. Thus, your positive attitude, pleasant presentation, and use of good communication skills will set the tone for future interactions.

### BASIC COMMUNICATION FLOW

Communication requires the following elements:

• A message to be sent
• A person to send the message
• A person to receive the message

During the act of communicating, two or more people will alternate roles as sender and receiver as they seek **feedback** (responses) and **clarification** (understanding) regarding the message. The process of message exchange is like a swing moving back and forth between two people. Figure 3-1 illustrates the flow of communication and its common components.

As a medical assistant, you will primarily be communicating in a therapeutic manner. This means that your communication will focus on conversations regarding pertinent topics relating to office procedures, policies, and patient care. Your other responsibilities for ensuring good communication include the following:

• Clarifying confusing messages
• Validating (confirming) the patient's perceptions

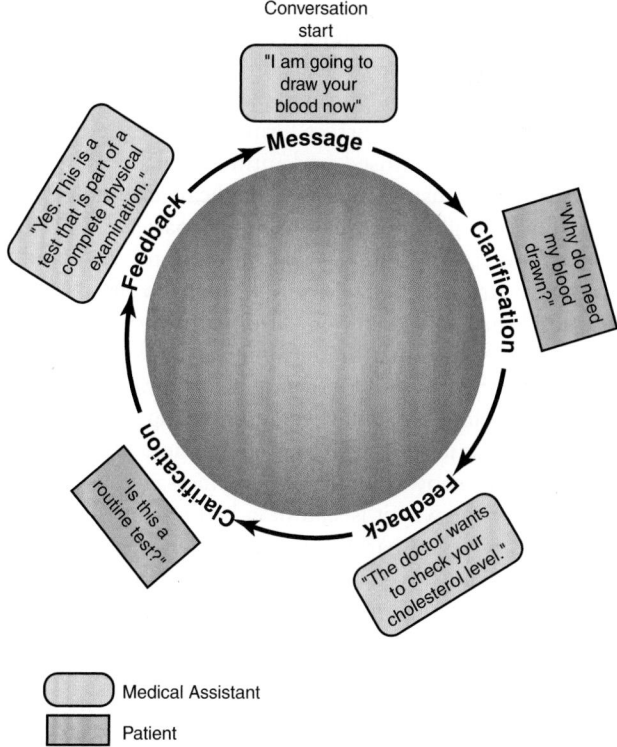

**Figure 3-1** • Flow of communication.

- Adapting messages to the patient's level of understanding
- Asking for feedback to ensure that the messages you sent were received by the patient or other persons as intended

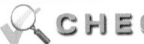 **CHECKPOINT QUESTION**

1. What three elements must be present for communication to occur?

## FORMS OF COMMUNICATION

### Verbal Communication

Verbal communication involves an exchange of messages using words or language; it is the most commonly used form and is usually the initial form of communication. You need good verbal communication skills when performing such tasks as making appointments, providing patient education, making referrals, and sharing information with the physician.

Oral communication is sending or receiving messages using spoken language. As a professional, you should use a pleasant and polite manner of speaking. Use proper English and grammar at all times; lapsing into slang and colloquialisms projects an unprofessional image.

You will have to adjust your conversation to accommodate the patient's developmental or educational level. Each stage of development has communication problems that must be addressed for accurate communication to occur (see below). An educated patient may resent your using other than the correct terms, yet a less educated patient may be confused and intimidated by the same phrases. Avoid using elaborate medical terminology if you think it might confuse or frighten a patient. Will this patient understand "myocardial infarction," or should you say heart attack? Do not talk down to the patient, but do phrase your communication appropriately.

Be aware, too, that the meaning of spoken messages may be affected by other components of oral communication, including paralanguage and nonlanguage sounds. The cliché that it's not what you say but how you say it is true. Research shows that the primary message is transmitted more by the way it is said than by the words that are used. This refers to paralanguage. **Paralanguage** includes voice tone, quality, volume, pitch, and range. **Nonlanguage** sounds include laughing, sobbing, sighing, grunting, and so on. Other nonlanguage clues to understanding can be found in a speaker's grammatical structure, pronunciation, and general articulation, which can indicate regional or cultural background and level of education. Knowing this information can help you adapt responses and explanations to the patient's level of understanding.

Main Street Pediatric Group
343 Main Street, Suite 609
King, NC 27021

**Instructions for Otitis Media**

Your child has an ear infection. It is easily treated with antibiotics. Get the prescription filled immediately. The first dose should be given as soon as you arrive home. Read the attached information on the antibiotic.

Here are some other important things to remember:

- Ear infections are not contagious.
- Symptoms usually resolve within 24 hours of beginning antibiotics. It is very important to make sure your child takes all of the prescription.
- If the pain persists for more than 48 hours, call the office.
- If you see any blood in the ear canal, call the office.

Make an appointment for a follow-up visit in 2 weeks.

_____          _____
Patient's signature                        Physician's signature

Written communication uses written language to exchange messages. The ability to write clearly, concisely, and accurately is important in the health care profession (see Chapter 7). Typically, patients receive oral instructions first, as you or the physician explain key points of concern. These verbal instructions are then reinforced with written instructions (Box 3-1).

If the instructions, oral or written, are not clear, the patient may misinterpret them. This misunderstanding can hinder treatment and recovery and possibly even require the patient to be admitted to the hospital. Here is an example of an unclear instruction: "Return to the office if you don't feel better." This provides the patient with no details. Clearer instructions would state, "If your fever and sore throat are not better in 24 hours, call the office to schedule a revisit." Even the most clearly outlined instructions can be misunderstood, particularly by those with deficient hearing or reading abilities. As a medical assistant, you are responsible for asking questions and receiving confirmatory feedback to verify that the patient has correctly understood the information. To verify that the patient understood these instructions, a good question to ask would be, "When should you call the office if you don't feel better?"

 **CHECKPOINT QUESTION**

2. List five examples of paralanguage.

## Nonverbal Communication

Nonverbal communication—exchanging messages without using words—is sometimes called body language. Body language includes several types of behaviors, such as kinesics, proxemics, and the use of touch. Kinesics refers to body movements, including facial expressions, gestures, and eye movements. A patient's face can sometimes reveal inner feelings, such as sadness, happiness, fear, or anger that may not be mentioned explicitly during a conversation. Gestures also carry various meanings. For instance, shrugging the shoulders can mean simple lack of interest or hopeless resignation. Eyes can often hint at what a person may be thinking or feeling. For example, a patient whose eyes wander away from you while you are talking may be impatient, lack interest, or not understand what you are saying.

Nonverbal communication may more accurately reflect a person's true feelings and attitude than verbal communication. In other words, people may say one thing but show a completely different response with their body language. For example, if the patient says, "The pain in my foot is not too bad," but the patient's face shows pain with each step, the nonverbal clues demonstrate an inconsistent message. Many patients mask their feelings, so you must learn to read their actions and nonverbal clues in addition to what they tell you. Be aware that patients are also acutely attuned to your facial and nonverbal reactions. Responding with an expression of disgust or shaking your head in a negative way can jeopardize communication and rapport between you and the patient.

How and where individuals physically place themselves in relation to others can affect communication as well. Proxemics refers to spatial relationships or physical proximity tolerated by humans. Generally, the area within a 3-foot radius around a person is considered personal space and is not to be invaded by strangers, although this area varies among individuals and people of various **cultures** (societies). To deliver care to a patient, physicians and medical assistants must enter a patient's personal space. After a patient task is completed, it is appropriate to take a few steps back and allow for more space between you and the patient. Because some individuals become uncomfortable when their space is invaded, it is essential to approach the patient in a professional manner and explain what you plan to do. Explanations help ease patient anxiety about what will happen.

Related to proxemics is the use of touch, which can be **therapeutic** (beneficial) for some patients. It can indicate emotional support and convey concern and feeling. For other patients, however, being touched by a stranger is an uncomfortable or even negative experience. Many patients perceive touch in a medical setting as a prelude to something unpleasant, such as an injection. To change this negative perception, try offering a comforting touch when nothing invasive or painful is imminent. Before

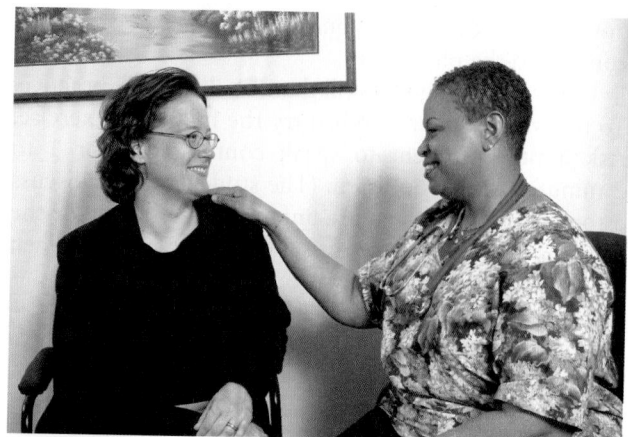

**Figure 3-2 •** Therapeutic touch conveys caring and concern.

comforting a patient by touching, assess the patient's **demeanor** (expressions and behavior) for clues indicating that touch would be acceptable. In Figure 3-2, the certified medical assistant's (CMA's) touch is comforting to the patient.

## Defense Mechanisms

The communication process can also be impeded by the use of defense mechanisms by patients and caregivers. *Merriam-Webster Collegiate Dictionary*, 11 ed., defines a defense mechanism as the process in the brain that makes you forget or ignore painful or disturbing thoughts, situations, etc. Patients and caregivers are often unaware that they are exhibiting these types of behaviors. For example, the defense mechanism of denial may be used when a patient refuses to accept an unfavorable diagnosis, such as cancer, or refusing to believe a diagnosis has been determined to be terminal. Table 4-2 in Chapter 4 describes common defense mechanisms. As patient advocates, medical assistants must be aware of various barriers to communication and respond appropriately.

## ACTIVE LISTENING

Active listening is important to ensure that messages are correctly received and interpreted. Failure to do so can result in poor patient care. To listen actively, you must give your full attention to the patient with whom you are speaking. Interruptions should be kept to a minimum. You need to focus not only on what is being said, but also on what is being conveyed through paralanguage, body language, and other aspects of communication. Occasionally, a patient's verbal messages may seem to conflict with the nonverbal messages. For example, a patient who is wringing his hands while telling you that everything is fine is sending conflicting signals that require further exploration. If a patient's verbal response does not correspond to your observations, convey your concern to the physician.

Active listening is a skill that develops with practice. To test your listening ability, try the following exercise. Ask another student to speak continuously for 1 to 2 minutes while you listen. (The student should discuss a topic with which you are unfamiliar.) When he or she finishes, wait silently for the same amount of time. Then try to repeat the message. If you have trouble doing this exercise, you need to practice listening.

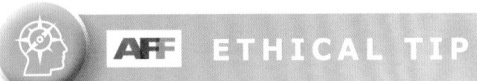

## Don't Let Your Mouth Get You in Trouble

All patient communication is confidential. Patient information is sometimes discussed unintentionally, however. To avoid breaching confidentiality, follow these guidelines:

- Do not discuss patients' problems in public places, such as elevators or parking lots. A patient's friends or family members might overhear your conversation and misinterpret what is said.
- Keep the glass window between the waiting room and the reception desk closed.
- Watch the volume of your voice.
- When calling coworkers over the office intercom, do not use a patient's name or reveal other information. Avoid saying something like, "Bob Smith is on the phone and wants to know if his strep throat culture came back." Instead, say "There's a patient on line 1."
- Before going home, destroy any slips of paper in your uniform pockets that contain patient information (e.g., reminder notes from verbal reports).

## INTERVIEW TECHNIQUES

As a medical assistant, you are typically responsible for gathering initial information and updating existing information about the patients. This task is accomplished by interviewing the patient. The interview will consist of you asking certain questions and then interpreting the patient's responses. The initial interview includes many areas. The key areas are the patient's medical and family history, a brief review of the body systems, and a social history. The main goal is to obtain accurate and pertinent information in each area for the physician. The interview for an established patient, however, is much different since the medical record already has the patient's past medical history and social history. You should review the established patient's chart to look at the patient's health problems, make a list of questions regarding the pertinent medical problems, and reconfirm medication usage and any specific treatments the patient is supposed to be

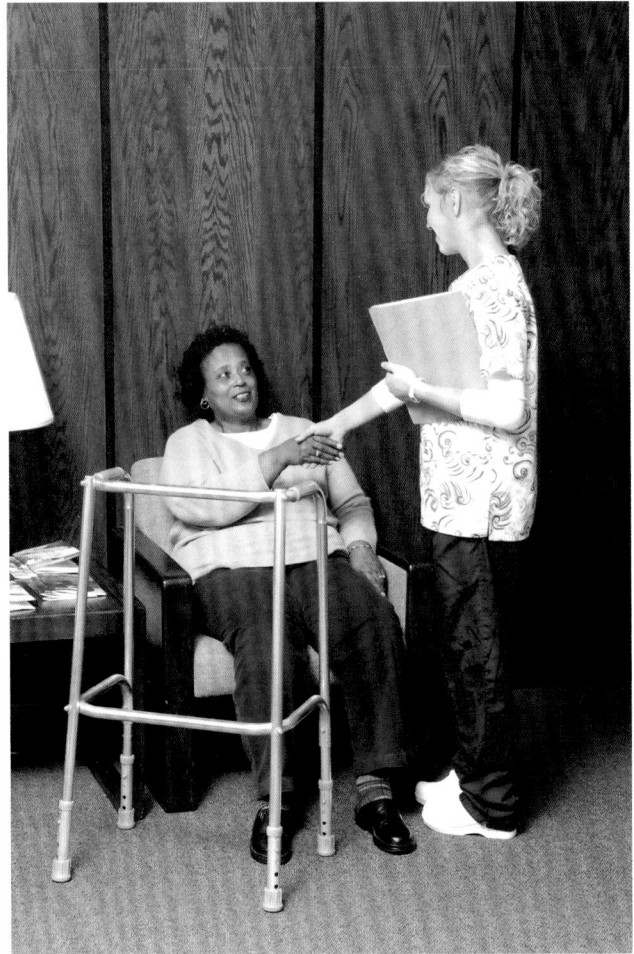

**Figure 3-3** • Begin the interview by introducing yourself.

doing. It is necessary to update every patient's medical record at every visit with known and any new allergies.

To conduct either type of interview, you must use effective techniques: listen actively, ask the appropriate questions, and record the answers. During the interview, you must demonstrate professionalism. Begin by introducing yourself (Fig. 3-3). Always conduct the interview in a private area and ask your patient to identify himself/herself. Know what questions you need to ask and in what order to ask them before you begin the interview. Be organized. It is also helpful to have an extra pen. And most important, do not answer phone calls or attend to other distractions until you have finished the interview. Last, when you leave the room, let patients know who will be in to see them and the approximate time, for example, "Dr. Sanchez will be in to see you in about 10 minutes."

The six interviewing techniques are reflecting, paraphrasing, clarification, asking open-ended questions, summarizing, and allowing silences.

### Reflecting

**Reflecting** is repeating what you have heard the patient say, using open-ended statements. With this technique, you do not complete a sentence but leave it up to the patient to do so. For example, you might say, "Mrs. Rivera, you were saying that when your back hurts you ...." Reflection encourages the patient to make further comments. It also can help bring the patient back to the subject if the conversation begins to drift. (Reflecting is a useful tool, but be careful not to overuse it, because some patients find it annoying to have their words constantly parroted back.)

## Paraphrasing or Restatement

**Paraphrasing** or restatement means repeating what you have heard, using your own words or phrases. Paraphrasing can help verify that you have accurately understood what was said. It also allows patients the opportunity to clarify their thoughts or statements. Typically, a paraphrased statement begins with "You are saying that ...," or "It sounds as if ...," followed by the rephrased content.

## Asking for Examples or Clarification

If you are confused about some of the information you have received, ask the patient to give an example of the situation being described. For instance, "Can you describe one of these dizzy spells?" The patient's example should help you better understand what the patient is saying. It also may give you an insight into how the patient perceives the situation.

## Asking Open-Ended Questions

The best way to obtain specific information is to ask open-ended questions that require the patient to formulate an answer and elaborate on the response. Open-ended questions usually begin with what, when, or how. For example, "What medications did you take this morning?" "When did you stop taking your medication?" "How did you get that large bruise on your arm?" Be careful about asking "why" questions, because they can often sound judgmental or accusing. For example, asking "Why did you do that?" or "Why didn't you follow the directions?" may imply to patients that you have already made a negative value judgment about their behavior, and they could become defensive and uncooperative. Instead, you might ask, "What part of the instructions did you not understand?" or "How can we help you follow these instructions?"

Avoid closed-ended questions that allow the patient to answer with one word, such as yes or no. For example, suppose you ask the patient, "Are you taking your medications?" The patient can easily say yes but may not be taking all of them. However, suppose you ask, "What medications do you take every day?" The patient's answer will give you a clearer understanding of whether the patient is taking the correct medications.

## Summarizing

Briefly reviewing the information you have obtained, or **summarizing**, gives the patient another chance to clarify statements or correct misinformation. This technique can also help you organize complex information or events in sequential order. For example, if the patient has been feeling dizzy and stumbling a lot, you might summarize by saying, "You told me that you have been feeling dizzy for the past 3 days and that you frequently stumble as you are walking."

## Allowing Silences

Periods of silence sometimes occur during the interview. These can be beneficial. Some people are uncomfortable with prolonged silences and feel a need to break the silence with words in an effort to jump-start a stalled conversation. Silences are natural parts of conversations and can give patients time to formulate their thoughts, reconstruct events, evaluate their feelings, or assess what has already been said. During moments of silence, gather your thoughts and formulate any additional questions that you may have.

## CHECKPOINT QUESTION

3. What are the six interviewing techniques?

## **COG** FACTORS AFFECTING COMMUNICATION

Sometimes, despite your best efforts, others may not receive your message accurately. A common occurrence that causes messages to be misinterpreted is the use of a cliché. For example, suppose you are teaching a patient to use crutches and she is having difficulty managing them. A cliché comment may be, "Don't worry. Rome wasn't built in a day. This takes time." The cliché is innocent and not meant to be demeaning, but the patient may misinterpret it to mean that she is slow, ancient. A more positive message would be, "I can see that you are making progress. Let's try walking down the hallway."

Here are some reasons for miscommunication:

1. The message may have been unclear or inappropriate to the situation. Keep in mind that most of your patients do not understand medical abbreviations and terms, so it is important to convey the message in terms that patients can understand. For example, "I have scheduled you for a PET scan in radiology tomorrow at 8 a.m." Positron emission tomography (PET) may be confused with computed tomography (CT). Also, where is radiology? A better message would be "The doctor wants you to have a test done tomorrow. It is called a PET scan; here is a brochure that explains it. Go to the second floor of the outpatient center on Main Street. Do you know how to get there?"

2. The person receiving the message may have been distracted, anxious, or confused. A common cause of distraction is pain. For example, teaching a patient how to use crutches cannot be done if the patient's ankle or knee still hurts. The concentration will be on the pain, not on what you are saying. Patients who have just received positive news can also be anxious to contact loved ones. This is commonly seen with patients who have just been told that they are pregnant. The patient's focus is on calling family members and not on your conversation.

3. Environmental elements, such as noise or interruptions, may also distort messages. Environmental noises from staff lounges or break rooms can easily be overheard. Keep the doors to these areas closed. Cleaning staff should not be vacuuming or emptying trash while patients are present.

In addition to these three items, other factors may affect communication. They are discussed next.

## Cultural Differences

The way a person perceives situations and other people is greatly influenced by cultural, social, and religious beliefs or firmly held convictions. Personal values (principles or ideals) are commonly developed from these same beliefs.

As a medical assistant, you will interact with people from varied ethnic backgrounds and cultural origins who bring with them beliefs and values that may differ from your own. Understanding those differences can aid communication and thereby improve patient care (Table 3-1). It is very important that you not form preconceived ideas about a given culture. Remember that each of your patients is unique and that their health care needs differ.

Some cultures may be offended by the types of intensely personal questions necessary for a medical history and may perceive them as an inexcusable invasion of privacy. If this occurs, your physician may be required to intervene to allay the patient's concerns.

Looking someone else directly in the eyes, or eye contact, is also perceived differently by people of various backgrounds. Eye contact occurs more often among friends and family members than among acquaintances or strangers. In the United States, someone who maintains good eye contact is usually perceived as being honest, believable, and concerned. In contrast, in some Asian and Mideastern cultures, direct eye contact is perceived as sexually suggestive or disrespectful. In other cultures, lack of eye contact or casting the eyes downward is a sign of respect.

In addition to cultural differences in values, many differences occur among individuals. Some people are just more reserved or shy than others and may feel less

| TABLE 3-1 | Cultural Factors That Affect Patient Care[a] | | |
|---|---|---|---|
| Cultural Group | Family | Folk and Traditional Healthcare | Common Health Problems |
| White | Nuclear family is highly valued<br>Elderly family members may live in a nursing home when they can no longer care for themselves | Self-diagnosis of illnesses<br>Use of over-the-counter drugs, especially vitamins and analgesics<br>Dieting, especially fad diets<br>Extensive use of exercise and exercise facilities | Cardiovascular disease<br>Gastrointestinal disease<br>Some forms of cancer<br>Motor vehicle accidents<br>Suicide<br>Mental illness<br>Substance abuse |
| African American | Close and supportive extended-family relationships<br>Strong kinship ties with nonblood relatives from church or organizational and social groups<br>Family unity, loyalty, and cooperation are important<br>Frequently matriarchal | Varies extensively and may include spiritualists, herb doctors, root doctors, conjurers, skilled elder family members, voodoo, faith healing | Hypertension<br>Sickle cell anemia<br>Skin disorders; inflammation of hair follicles, various types of dermatitis and excessive growth of scar tissue (keloids)<br>Lactose enzyme deficiency resulting in poor toleration of milk products<br>High rate of tuberculosis<br>Diabetes mellitus<br>Higher infant mortality rate than in the white population |

| Cultural Group | Family | Folk and Traditional Healthcare | Common Health Problems |
|---|---|---|---|
| Asian | Welfare of the family is valued above the individual person<br><br>Extended families are common<br><br>A person's lineage (ancestors) is respected.<br><br>Sharing among family members is expected. | Theoretical basis in Taoism, which seeks balance in all things<br><br>Good health is achieved through proper balance between yin (feminine, negative, dark, cold) and yang (masculine, positive, light, warm)<br><br>An imbalance in energy is caused by an improper diet or strong emotions<br><br>Diseases and food are classified as hot or cold, and a proper balance between them will promote wellness (e.g., treat a cold disease with hot foods)<br><br>Many Asian health care systems use herbs, diet, and application of hot or cold therapy<br><br>Many Asians believe some points on the body are on the meridians, or energy pathways; if the energy flow is out of balance, treatment of the pathways may be necessary to restore the energy equilibrium<br><br>*Acumassage:* Manipulation of points along the energy pathways<br><br>*Acupressure:* Technique for compressing the energy pathway points<br><br>*Acupuncture:* Insertion of fine needles into the body at energy pathway points | Tuberculosis<br><br>Communicable diseases<br><br>Malnutrition<br><br>Suicide<br><br>Various forms of mental illness<br><br>Lactose enzyme deficiency |
| Hispanic, Mexican American | Familial role is important<br><br>*Compadrazgo:* Special bond between a child's parents and grandparents<br><br>Family is the primary unit of society | *Curanderas(os):* Folk healers who base treatments on humoral pathology: basic functions of the body are controlled by four body fluids, or humors—blood, hot and wet; yellow bile, hot and dry; black bile, cold and dry; and phlegm, cold and wet<br><br>The secret of good health is to balance hot and cold within the body; therefore, most foods, beverages, herbs, and medications are classified as hot (caliente) or cold (fresco, frio); a cold disease will be cured with a hot treatment | Diabetes mellitus and its complications<br><br>Problems of poverty, such as poor nutrition, inadequate medical care, and poor prenatal care<br><br>Lactose enzyme deficiency |
| Hispanic, Puerto Rican | *Compadrazgo:* similar to Mexican American culture | Similar to that of other Spanish-speaking cultures | Parasitic diseases, such as dysentery, malaria, filariasis, hookworms<br><br>Lactose enzyme deficiency |
| Native American | Families large and extended<br><br>Grandparents are official and symbolic leaders and decision makers<br><br>A child's namesake may assume equal parenting author-ity with biological parent | Medicine men (shamans) are frequently consulted.<br><br>Heavy use of herbs and psychological treatments, ceremonies, fasting, meditation, heat, and massage | Alcoholism<br><br>Suicide<br><br>Tuberculosis<br><br>Malnutrition<br><br>Communicable diseases<br><br>Higher maternal and infant mortality rates than in most of the population<br><br>Diabetes mellitus<br><br>Hypertension<br><br>Gallbladder disease |

Reprinted from Taylor C, Lillis C, LeMone P. *Fundamentals of Nursing*, 2nd ed. Philadelphia, PA: Lippincott-Raven; 1996:122–125, with permission.

[a]The beliefs and practices vary within each group, and no assumptions should be based on a patient's cultural background alone. The factors in this table are merely a guide to some commonly observed and documented cultural factors.

comfortable in medical settings. To help avoid miscommunication and offending patients, you must be sensitive to these differences in all of your patient interactions.

## Stereotyping and Biased Opinions

Medical assisting deals with people of different ages, races, and sexual orientation. Sometimes, your values may be in stark contrast to those held by a patient, but you should not let your personal values or **biases** (opinions) affect your communication or treatment of a patient. All patients must be treated fairly, respectfully, and with dignity, regardless of their cultural, social, or personal values. To treat them in any other fashion is **discrimination**.

**Stereotyping** is holding an opinion of all members of a particular culture, race, religion, age group, or other group based on oversimplified or negative characterizations. It is a form of prejudice. Examples of negative stereotypes include "All old people are frail and senile" and "Those people are always dirty and never bathe." Stereotyping and prejudice are deterrents to establishing therapeutic relationships because they do not allow for patients' individuality and can prevent quality care from being given to everyone on an equal basis.

As a health care professional, you are expected to treat all patients impartially, to guard against discriminatory practices, remain nonjudgmental, avoid stereotypes, and have a professional demeanor. By doing so, you communicate to patients that you accept human differences and that quality health care will be provided to all those who seek it.

Let's suppose Ms. Henry arrives with her 3-year-old daughter for a checkup. The mother says, "I think she has gotten head lice from someone at the shelter." Which response would be most appropriate? "Don't worry about it. The shelter is full of people with lice. Do you know anyone with lice?" or "I will mention to the doctor that you are concerned that she may have lice. Is anyone else in your family being treated for lice?" The latter response demonstrates appropriate caring and concern. It also begins the dialogue for determining additional people who may need to be checked, which is key to preventing community outbreaks. The first response communicates stereotyping of a particular lifestyle and prevents collection of additional data.

## Language Barriers

Effective communication depends on the use of language, but some patients cannot speak or understand English well enough for good communication. Because it is crucial for you to give and receive accurate information, you will need to use an interpreter to help bridge any language barriers. A staff person might serve as the interpreter, or an English-speaking member of the patient's family may be able to help. In either case, be sure the interpreter fully understands what you are saying. In the absence of a reliable interpreter, a phrase book of common medical questions with lists of possible answers may be of help. If your area has a large population of non–English-speaking patients, your office should be equipped with an appropriate phrase book. (See Appendix B for a list of key health care phrases in English and Spanish.)

When choosing an interpreter, try to find someone of the same sex as the patient because certain cultures prohibit members of the opposite sex (even family members) from discussing personal issues about the body. Some cultures follow religious guidelines dictating how members of the opposite sex should interact with each other.

Use the following suggestions for communicating with non–English-speaking patients:

1. Do not shout. Raising your voice will not increase their understanding.
2. Demonstrate or pantomime as needed. Gestures are usually relatively universal.
3. If you are using an interpreter, speak directly to the patient, with the interpreter in your line of vision, so that the patient can read your facial expressions.
4. Speak slowly with simple sentences and phrases that require simple answers. The patient may comprehend some simple English.
5. Avoid slang; it may not translate well.
6. Avoid distractions and provide a relaxed, quiet interview space.
7. Learn some basic phrases of the most common language used in your area. Patients appreciate your effort.

## SPECIAL COMMUNICATION CHALLENGES

Many situations present special communication challenges. For instance, hearing- or sight-impaired patients, young children, patients with limited understanding, those who are too ill or sedated to comprehend, and those who are frightened or anxious require particular attention. In each instance, you will need to assess the situation and the patient's ability to comprehend. In some cases, a responsible family member or caregiver will be with the patient and can be included in the communication process. Never exclude the patient from the exchange, but do ensure that all needed information is communicated, whether you obtain the information through questions about the patient's condition or you give instructions for further care. Patients must feel that they are part of the process even if their condition requires involvement by family members or other caregivers.

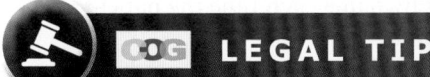

## LEGAL TIP

### Be Sure the Patient Understands

The patients' understanding of the risks and benefits of a proposed service or procedure is a basic right. It is the physician's legal responsibility to provide any accommodations necessary to be sure the patient understands his or her situation, options, descriptions of services and procedures, and benefits and risks regarding their care. Patients must be able to ask questions and get answers (see What If? box). Those who do not speak English, are hearing impaired, or have any other barrier to understanding may require special interpreters. If the patient cannot provide his or her own assistance, it is the legal responsibility of the physician and his agents to provide the means for effective communication. The American with Disabilities Act specifically requires auxiliary services, such as interpreters, be provided for qualified disabled individuals at no cost to the patient when necessary (see Chapter 2). In many cases, including language barriers, this person is a family member, friend, or church member.

## Hearing-Impaired Patients

There are many forms of hearing impairments. Impairments can vary from a partial loss to **anacusis**, complete hearing loss. The two types of impairments are conductive and sensorineural. Conductive hearing loss is caused by interference with sound in the external canal or the middle or inner ear. Sensorineural hearing loss is caused by lesions or problems with either nerves or the cochlea. The cochlea is a coiled tubular structure that turns vibrations into sounds. Most patients with anacusis are adept with communicating through sign language, interpreters, or other tools. However, patients with **presbycusis**, a common hearing impairment in older patients, often have a more difficult time communicating and tend to be in denial about their hearing abilities. Patients with presbycusis often benefit from hearing aids and other amplification devices.

To communicate with patients who have trouble hearing what you are saying, you need tact, diplomacy, and patience. These suggestions may help.

1. Touch the patient gently to gain his or her attention.
2. Talk directly face-to-face with the patient, not at an angle and certainly not with your back turned.
3. Turn to the most prominent light so that your face is illuminated.
4. Lower the pitch of your voice, since higher pitches are frequently lost with nerve impairment, but speak distinctly and with force. In most instances, shouting does not help and will only distort what might be heard.
5. Use note pads or demonstration as needed.
6. Pictograms are very helpful and should be readily available. A pictogram is a flash card that shows basic medical terms (Fig. 3-4).
7. Use short sentences with short words. Enunciate clearly, but do not exaggerate your facial movements.
8. Eliminate all distractions. Extraneous noises may confuse the patient.

If you need to call a hearing-impaired patient, keep in mind that patients can make and receive calls using a

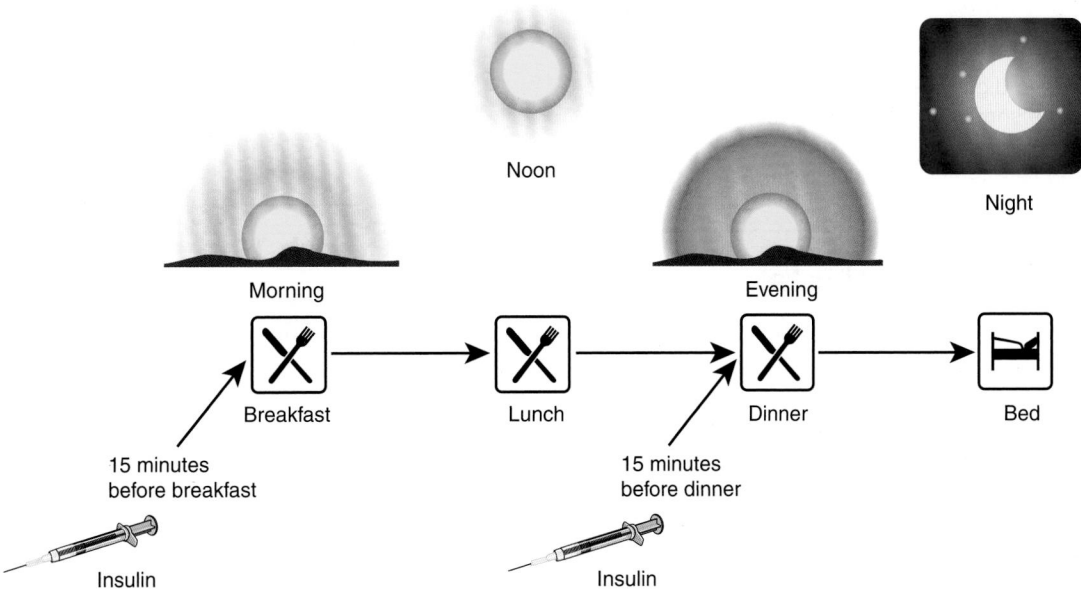

**Figure 3-4** • Pictogram for instructing a patient on medication routine.

special telephone with a service called converse communication center, which uses a system called telecommunication device for the deaf (TDD) or a text telephone (TTY). If your office has either of these types of phones, you call the patient and type in your message. The patient reads your message and types a response. If your office does not have one of these phones, your local telephone company can communicate with TDD/TTY users and nonusers. Check your telephone directory for more information. Most hospitals have TDD/TTY phones available.

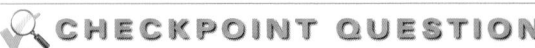

## CHECKPOINT QUESTION

4. How does the TDD system work?

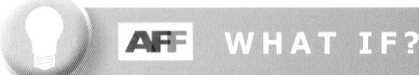

## WHAT IF?

**A patient is hearing impaired, and you cannot communicate with him to explain the procedure you are about to perform. What should you do?**

If the patient does not understand the procedure, he or she is not *informed*. Legally, you have not met your responsibilities to obtain informed consent if the patient does not understand the information you are trying to convey (see Legal Tip box; also see Chapter 2 for more information about informed consent).

Most community colleges offer courses in sign language. The Internet offers a site for the deaf community that will direct you to resources in your area. The American Sign Language alphabet chart is available online. It can be printed out for use with hearing-impaired patients. Handspeak is another Web site that provides a visual language dictionary. These Web sites are listed at the end of this chapter in the Media Menu. Medicine and technology promise to continue to improve communication for the deaf in the form of cochlear implants, computer software, and digital capabilities that we can only imagine. We should be doing everything we can to give the same experience to every patient. Prepare yourself to face the communication challenges you might encounter.

## Sight-Impaired Patients

Sight impairments range from complete blindness to blurred vision. The changes in vision tend to be slow and progressive. Some common medical conditions that can cause visual impairment include cataracts, glaucoma, macular degeneration, retinal detachment, hyperopia (farsightedness), myopia (nearsightedness), nyctalopia (night blindness), retinopathy, strabismus, and presbyopia. Patients who cannot see lose valuable information from nonverbal communication. To improve communication with a sight-impaired patient, try these suggestions.

1. Identify yourself by name each time the patient comes into the office.
2. Do not raise your voice; the patient is not hearing impaired.
3. Let the patient know exactly what you will be doing at all times, and alert him or her before touching.
4. Orient the patient spatially by having him or her touch the table, the chair, the counter, and so forth.
5. Assist the patient by offering your arm and escorting him or her to the interview room.
6. Tell the patient when you are leaving the room and knock before entering.
7. Explain the sounds of machines to be used in the examination (e.g., buzzing, whirring) and what each machine will do.

## Speech Impairments

Speech impairments can come from a variety of medical conditions. The medical term for difficulty with speech is **dysphasia**. Dysphasia is usually the result of a neurologic problem. A common neurologic condition that can result in dysphasia is a stroke. **Dysphonia** is a voice impairment that is caused by a physical condition, such as oral surgery, cancer of the tongue or voice box, or cleft palate. Stuttering is another medical condition that can impair the patient's ability to communicate.

Here are some suggestions to help you communicate with a patient who has a speech impediment:

- Allow such patients time to gather their thoughts.
- Allow plenty of time for them to communicate.
- Do not rush conversations.
- Offer a note pad to write questions.
- Discuss with the physician the potential benefits for getting a speech therapist referral for the patient.

## CHECKPOINT QUESTION

5. What is the difference between dysphasia and dysphonia?

## Mental Health Illnesses

Many mental illnesses and psychiatric disorders can impair a patient's ability to communicate. These illnesses produce a broad range of communication challenges. Some illnesses can cause the patient to have uncontrollable outbursts, whereas others can cause a mute condition in which the patient will not communicate at all. Some patients may hear voices that direct their communication to a given topic, whereas others may see objects that do not exist and will want confirmation from you that you see the objects. Communicating with patients with moderate to severe psychiatric disorders requires in-depth training. It is important to stress that not all patients with mental illnesses will be challenges. Most mental illnesses can be controlled and treated with medications and other therapies. Here are a few suggestions for communicating with patients who have mild mental illnesses:

- Tell the patient what to expect and when things will happen.
- Keep conversations focused and professional.
- Do not force or demand answers from patients who are withdrawn or mute.
- If you feel unsafe communicating with a given patient, speak to either your supervisor or the physician regarding your concerns.
- Do not confirm hearing voices or seeing nonexistent objects.
- Orient the patient to reality as appropriate.

Patients with a history of substance abuse, alcoholism, and other addictions can also present a communication challenge. Patients may have euphoria and communicate with a flight of ideas. Or they may demonstrate aggression and agitation while they are withdrawing from the addiction. Your responsibility in communicating with patients who have any of these conditions is to identify the reasons for today's visit and follow your regular assessment duties. It is not the role of the medical assistant to recommend treatments or counseling for these patients. Your communication should be professional, nonjudgmental, and encouraging when appropriate.

## Angry or Distressed Patients

Patients' emotions can run the spectrum from polite and cordial to angry and upset. There are numerous reasons for the latter. Prolonged waiting times, financial issues, and illness can spark untoward emotions. Do not take patients' anger or frustration personally. At some time in our lives, we all have had a cold, felt terrible, and snapped angrily at an innocent bystander. The key to communicating with upset patients is to prevent an escalation of the problem. Keep your patients informed about waiting times, billing and insurance changes, and other office policies that might trigger untoward emotions (Box 3-2).

It is understandable that patients will become upset on hearing sad or unfortunate news about their health.

---

**BOX 3-2** **AFF** **Case Scenario: Communicating with a Patient Who Is Upset**

Mr. Hunt, an elderly, long-time patient, calls the office and asks to speak to the doctor. When you inquire about the nature of his call, he begins to get louder and more upset.

*Note*: When patients ask to speak directly to the doctor, it is usually because they don't understand the workings of the office. Let the patient know that it is your job to screen the doctor's calls.

Mr. Hunt: "I just got this bill in the mail, and it says that I owe Dr. Smith $152.00. He is crazy if he thinks I'm paying this."

*Note*: Patients will say things they regret later. You may want to just let this one go.

Medical Assistant (MA): "I would be glad to help you with this, Mr. Hunt. Please hold while I look at your account."

*Note*: Putting the patient on hold may calm him down.

Mr. Hunt: "I'm not holding on very long."

*Note*: You can assure him that you will be right back.

MA: "I see that your balance is $152.00, Mr. Hunt, but you may make arrangements to pay this over several months."

*Note*: Giving the patient options may calm him down.

Mr. Hunt: "I'm not paying it at all because Dr. Smith didn't help me. I'm no better."

*Note*: A statement like this is upsetting, but you must remain professional.

MA: "I'm so sorry you are not feeling better, but Dr. Smith performed a service that you agreed to pay for. I will be happy to make you another appointment to come in and talk with him about a different course of treatment."

*Note*: Be firm but kind. Hopefully being firm will let the patient know who is in charge, but kindness will help defuse the anger.

Mr. Hunt: "I'll make an appointment, but I am not paying until I talk to the doctor."

*Note*: Again, you must not show your own feelings.

MA: "I will make a note of that on your account, and we can see you tomorrow at 9:30. Is that all right?"

*Note*: Documenting the patient's call will alert anyone working with the account. You would not want to add fuel to the flame by sending him another bill right away or making a collection call.

Mr. Hunt: "I'll be there, but you can tell that doctor that I'll have a thing or two to say to him."

*Note*: Document the conversation in the chart and be sure that the physician knows what to expect during the visit.

MA: "I hope we can resolve this, Mr. Hunt. We will see you tomorrow."

*Note*: You must remain calm and in control of the conversation.

## BOX 3-3   Stages of Human Development by Erik Erikson

| Age | Stage of Development | Considerations |
| --- | --- | --- |
| Infant 0–1 years | Trust versus mistrust | Provide a safe, amiable environment. |
| Toddler 2–3 years | Autonomy versus shame | Use simple words and give frequent praise. |
| Preschooler 3–6 years | Initiative versus guilt | Allow child to have some control and give frequent praise. |
| School age 6–11 years | Industry versus inferiority | Use child's vocabulary to teach about health care or treatment and give praise. |
| Adolescent 12–18 years | Identity versus role confusion | Use active listening to communicate effectively and assure confidentiality when appropriate. |
| Young adulthood 18–35 years | Intimacy versus isolation | Use active listening and be prepared to provide options for health or social services, as needed. |
| Middle adulthood 35–55 years | Generativity versus self-absorption | Use active listening. |
| Late adulthood 65 to death | Integrity versus despair | Use active listening and speak clearly. Be aware of a sense of sadness or fear. |

Most patients take sad news in a calm manner. It is important to offer assistance as needed. Provide written instructions and information for the patient to read later. This material should consist of information on the diagnosis, causes of the illness, treatment options, and phone numbers that the patient may call for additional information.

Here are some suggestions that will help you communicate with an angry or distressed patient.

- Take the patient to a private area and be supportive by using active listening skills.
- Stay calm and speak in a normal tone.
- Be open and honest in all communication.
- Do not provide false reassurances.
- Do not belittle the problem or concern.
- Ensure your own safety if the angry patient becomes aggressive or threatening.

## Developmental

It is essential that the professional medical assistant understand the stages of human development in order to communicate effectively with patients of all ages. Erik Erikson (1902–1994) was a developmental psychologist who developed the theory that there are eight stages of human development beginning with infants. As described in his book, *Childhood and Society,* as individuals age, they also develop psychosocially in stages throughout their lives. Each stage of life has its own communication problems that require certain accommodations to be made when interacting with patients. See Box 3-3 for a list of Erikson's eight stages of human development.

## Children

Levels of comprehension vary greatly during childhood, and therefore, communication needs must be tailored to the specific child's needs. The following suggestions will help facilitate communication:

1. Children are responsive to eye-level contact. Either raise them to your height or lower yourself to theirs (Fig. 3-5).
2. Keep your voice low pitched and gentle.
3. Make your movements slow and keep them visible. Tell children when you need to touch them.
4. Rephrase your questions until you are sure that the child understands.

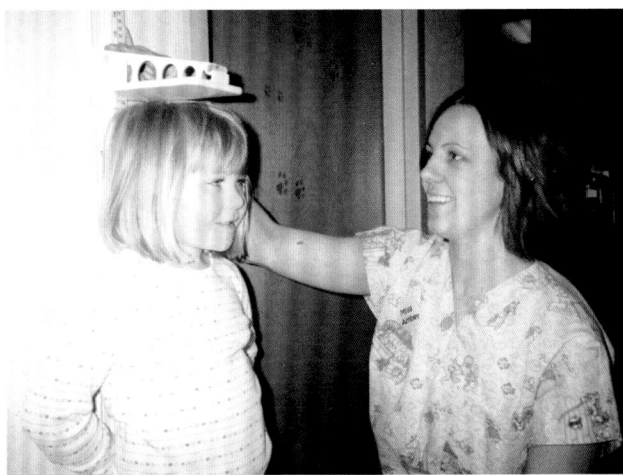

**Figure 3-5 •** The medical assistant communicates at the child's eye level.

5. Be prepared for the child to return to a lower developmental level for comfort during an illness. For example, a child may revert to thumb sucking during a stressful event.

6. Use play to phrase your questions and to gain the child's cooperation (e.g., if the child appears shy and does not want to talk, start by asking the child how a stuffed animal feels today:. "How does teddy feel today?" Follow up on the child's answer with "And how do you feel?" Offering to take the teddy's temperature first may lessen any fear of thermometers).

7. Allow the child to express fear, to cry, and so on.

8. As adolescents become independent, some teenagers may not want a parent in the room during the interview. Be aware of the possibility of confidential matters with adolescent patients, such as sexual activity, and assess the situation before including the parent.

9. Never show shock or judgment when dealing with adolescents; this will immediately close communication.

## 🔍 CHECKPOINT QUESTION

6. What is the stage of development in which trust versus mistrust is developed?

## 🔗 COMMUNICATING WITH A GRIEVING PATIENT OR FAMILY MEMBER

Occasionally, you will need to support patients who are in **grief** or great sadness caused by a loss. Grieving starts when a person experiences a significant loss, such as the loss of a loved one through death or the end of a relationship, a body part, or personal health. Grief includes such emotional responses as anger, sadness, and depression, and each emotion may trigger certain behaviors. For example, anger may result in outbursts, sadness may cause crying, and depression may lead to unusual quietness or isolation.

Dr. Elisabeth Kübler-Ross identified five distinct stages in the human grieving process. In her book *On Death and Dying*, she lists these stages that follow the realization that a person has a terminal illness: denial, anger, bargaining, depression, and acceptance. Dr. Kübler-Ross believed that these stages are also found in those experiencing change. Box 3-4 outlines these stages with examples. These stages may spread over months or years. It is possible to go through stages more than once. Sometimes, the collective signs of grief are referred to as **mourning**.

In medical settings, expect to see grief displayed in many ways. Know, too, that several factors can influence how a patient demonstrates grief and that different cultures and individuals demonstrate their grief in a variety of ways, ranging from stoic, impassive responses

| BOX 3-4 | The Five Stages of Grieving as Identified by Elisabeth Kübler-Ross |
|---|---|
| **Mechanism** | **Quote** |
| Denial | "The doctor must have read the test wrong." "I don't have cancer; I feel fine." |
| Anger | "I hate the doctor." "This is a terrible place." |
| Bargaining | "God, I will be the best person I can be if you take away this disease." |
| Depression | "I don't care if I live anymore." |
| Acceptance | "I understand that I have terminal disease and am going to die." |

to loud, prolonged wailing and fainting. Other responses may reflect religious beliefs about the meaning of death. Grieving is a unique and personal process. There is no set time period for grieving, and there is no "right" way to grieve. It is very important to remember that everyone grieves in their way at their own pace.

Grieving patients may want to talk about their feelings and review events. Terminally ill patients may want to discuss their fears of dying and concerns for surviving loved ones. Many times, it is too difficult to discuss dying with family members. Dying patients may want to spare their family's feelings. To support grieving patients, allow time for them to express themselves and actively listen to what they say. When appropriate, consider using touch to convey your understanding. If patients' concerns stem from a lack of understanding about their condition, provide pertinent education for them and for their caregivers (if appropriate). You should also become familiar with available community resources, such as grief or other counseling services and hospice care, so you can assist the patient and physician when these services are necessary.

It is normal for you to feel sad when a patient dies. It is important that your communication focuses on empathy, not sympathy. Many psychologists describe sympathy as feeling *for* someone and empathy as feeling *with* someone. In the health care setting, empathy means trying to understand what patients are feeling so you can help them. Empathy can help you recognize a patient's fear and discomfort so you can do everything possible to provide support and reassurance.

Sympathy, or pitying your patient, may compromise your professional distance and cause you to become personally involved. Box 3-5 offers suggestions for helping grieving patients.

BOX 3-5    Communicating with a Grieving Family Member or Patient

Patients and families faced with great loss can be helped through a variety of community resources. Hospice is a national program that offers support to patients and family members dealing with a terminal illness or loss. Hospice deals with all types of medical conditions and with people of all ages. The earlier the patient is introduced to a hospice program, the more beneficial. Hospice does have a palliative component. Hospice staff and volunteer grief counselors are trained to answer the questions, acknowledge the fears and anger, ease the transition, and offer respite for caregivers. A patient must never be forced to use hospice or other community resources. Grieving is an individual experience. Your local hospital may also have grief counselors or social workers who can help your patients. Other community resources may be available. The knowledgeable medical assistant will, with the physician's permission, direct the patient and the family to the proper organization.

## CHECKPOINT QUESTION

7. What are the five stages of grieving?

## 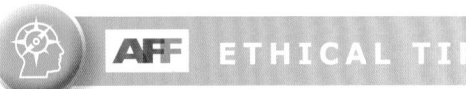 ESTABLISHING POSITIVE PATIENT RELATIONSHIPS

Your approach to patients conveys a message about who you are and how you feel about yourself and your profession. Medical assistants can be role models, earning the trust and admiration of patients. To establish and maintain positive relationships with patients, speak respectfully and exhibit an appropriate demeanor during all interactions. See Box 3-6 for guidance in communicating with patients on an individual basis.

### Proper Form of Address

The way you address patients provides clues about your attitude and how you will likely provide care. When greeting patients, use a proper form of address, for example, "Good morning, Mr. Jones!" or "How are you feeling, Mrs. Smith?" This type of address shows respect and sets a professional tone. In contrast, calling patients by pet names, such as sweetie, granny, gramps, or honey, can offend the person. These terms denigrate the individual's dignity and put the interaction on a personal, not professional, level. Always call patients by their last name unless and until they instruct you otherwise. Some people are bothered or offended by being addressed by

BOX 3-6        Check Your Behavior When Responding to Nonverbal Communications

Consider this scenario:

*You are interviewing a patient having a complete physical. You can sense that the 75-year-old man is nervous about his exam. He is obviously a shy man. He makes no eye contact. He keeps his arms folded on his chest. He asks that his 82-year-old wife remain with him. She provides the answers to your questions, and he seems to be more nervous as you progress through the patient history. His wife reports a previous head injury 5 years ago, and you realize that he is limited in his mental abilities.*

How will you communicate with this patient now that you know more about his individual situation?

1. Watch for nonverbal cues before touching him. He needs to be calmed, but his shyness may make the touch uncomfortable.
2. Because he depends on his wife for understanding, speak to both of them.
3. Speak slowly and calmly.
4. Use simple language.
5. Try to calm his nerves by explaining what he can expect.
6. Give written instructions and materials with contact information if they have questions later.

their first names; others prefer it. When patients indicate a preference or ask you specifically to use their first name, document this in the chart so others will know.

Other inappropriate forms of address include referring to the patient as a medical condition, such as "the gallbladder in room 2" or "the broken arm in the waiting room." Patients often come to the medical office feeling

## AFF    ETHICAL TIP

### "Come Along, Honey" Can Offend Some Patients

You must keep a professional distance in your patient encounters. Always treat each patient with respect. Patients of advanced age may be sensitive to the way they are spoken to. If you assume each older patient is feeble or hard of hearing, you tend to show it in your actions and tone. Speaking in a higher tone, using "baby talk" or calling a patient "sweetie" or "honey" can be seen as a sign of disrespect. Be friendly but respectful when speaking with each and every patient you encounter. Your encounters with your patients should be professional and pleasant for you *and* the patient.

anxious, so they may be particularly sensitive to everything they see and hear (or overhear). Referring to the patient as a medical condition sends the message that the staff values the patient as nothing more than an illness, which can lead to heightened anxiety.

## Professional Distance

As discussed in Chapter 1, you must stay within certain boundaries when dealing with patients. How people interact with each other is influenced by the level of emotional involvement between them. For instance, communication between a husband and wife is more intimate than the personal level of communication between friends or the social level of communication between acquaintances. In the health care setting, you must establish an appropriate level of communication to be effective. You should not become too personally involved with patients because doing so may jeopardize your ability to be objective. It is easy to become overly attached, especially to elderly patients who are lonely. For example, do not offer to drive patients to appointments, pick up prescriptions, or do their grocery shopping. Keeping a professional distance allows you to deal objectively with patients while creating a therapeutic environment. To keep this distance, avoid revealing intimate information about yourself (e.g., marital woes, financial troubles, family conflict) that might shift the dynamics of the relationship to a more personal level. Small talk may put a patient at ease, and you may need to distract a patient who is going through an unpleasant treatment or procedure, but be careful to choose general topics and keep the conversation light. Often, in an attempt to comfort a patient, we might say, "My grandmother was diagnosed with cancer too, but she is fine; it's not a big deal." Every situation is different. The patient may misinterpret this to mean that you don't think that his or her diagnosis of cancer is a big deal. But at that moment, it is a very big deal to the patient!

## Teaching Patients

One of the fundamental communication skills you will need is the ability to teach patients about their medical conditions (see Chapter 4). Teaching patients might involve something as relatively simple as explaining how often they should take a medication or instructing a newly diagnosed diabetic patient about self-injection. The guidelines listed below incorporate such key communication skills as interviewing and active listening. Follow these to provide effective patient education.

1. Be knowledgeable about current medical issues, discoveries, and trends.
2. Be aware of special services available in your area.
3. Have pertinent handouts or information sheets available.
4. Allow enough teaching time so that you are not interrupted or rushed.
5. Find a quiet room away from the main office flow if at all possible.
6. Give information in a clear, concise, sequential manner; provide written instructions as a follow-up.
7. Allow the patient time to process this new information.
8. Encourage the patient to ask questions.
9. Ask open-ended questions in a way that will allow you to know whether the patient understands the material.
10. Invite the patient to call the office with additional questions that may arise.

## COG PROFESSIONAL COMMUNICATION

### Assertiveness in Professional Communication

The line between being assertive and being aggressive is very thin. The key to effective communication in a professional setting is learning the difference between the two and ensuring that you never cross the line.

An assertive person:

- Sets clear boundaries for himself or herself and others
- Knows how to set limits
- Clearly and politely communicates his or her wants and needs
- Can say "no" without offending another person
- Understands the appropriate time for assertiveness versus passive compliance
- Refuses to be inappropriately dominated or "handled"
- Considers the feelings and roles of others
- Voices differences of opinion without being rude or overbearing
- Stands up for what he or she believes when appropriate
- Holds himself or herself with confidence and maintains eye contact
- Looks for compromise, not conflict
- Speaks firmly but pleasantly
- Respects others
- Understands when he or she is about to "step over a line" and pulls back
- Is honest and fair

An aggressive person, however, is hostile, threatening, demanding, loud, annoying, sarcastic, angry, and, often, mean. Aggressive employees want everything *their* way, and although they may listen to other people, they don't *hear* other people.

For instance, say your boss has asked you to work the last two weekends to process a backlog of claims and is now asking you to work next weekend as well. You do not want to work yet another weekend. A meek, unassertive person would swallow her anger and work the weekend, all the while building up resentment. An aggressive person would announce in front of his or her coworkers, "No, I'm not working one more weekend; it's not in my job description." An assertive person, however, would meet with his or her boss privately, explain his or her desire to return to normal business hours, and help find another solution to the claims backlog.

Which type of person are you?

## Communicating with Peers

Communication among your peers must remain professional and appropriate throughout the workday. Discussions of non–work-related topics should be kept to a minimum and occur only during designated break times. It is not appropriate to discuss last night's TV shows, family issues, shopping lists, and so on in front of patients. Excessive laughing, high-pitched voice tones, receiving calls or texting on your cell phone, and whispering can produce an unprofessional atmosphere.

During your career, you may come across a situation that requires communication with your supervisor about another peer's actions. Your communication must always be honest and accurate when reporting facts to a supervisor. Embellishing or hiding information can result in termination of your employment.

An excellent way to promote communication among your peers is to become active in your local professional organization. Your involvement at the local level can spread to national exposure. Involvement in local community organizations and support groups is also beneficial to promoting you and your profession.

## Communicating with Physicians

Physicians and other health care practitioners will rely on you to communicate pertinent information to patients in a timely manner to provide quality care. Your communication must always be professional. The physician should always be addressed as doctor unless he specifies otherwise. The use of inappropriate terms is never acceptable. When possible, the correct medical terminology should be used. If you are unsure of the correct medical term, however, explain the condition rather than use a term that you do not understand. For example, if a patient comes into the office with a chief complaint of difficulty urinating, simply say, "Mr. Bowen is complaining of trouble urinating." Never use a slang expression, such as "He is having trouble peeing."

Do not feel intimidated when speaking to a physician. Speak slowly and confidently and you will develop a professional rapport. Be honest. It is better to say, "I am not sure what to do with this specimen" than to assume and make a mistake.

Remember, there is a time and place for everything. The physician may be the biggest jokester or sports fan in the office, but it is not appropriate to draw on these topics in front of patients or family members.

## Communicating with Other Facilities

The medical administrative staff often makes referrals to other facilities or physicians. When contacting other facilities, follow these key points:

- Maintain patient confidentiality. Make sure you have appropriate patient consent.
- Observe all legal requirements for dispensing patient data.
- Use caution with fax machines, e-mail, and other electronic devices. Make sure the intended receiver is the one who gets the communication.
- Provide only the facts. Do not relay suspicions or assumptions.
- Always be nonjudgmental.
- Confirm that the message was received and that the referral will be handled.

 **ROLE-PLAYING ACTIVITY**

While taking a health history on a 32-year-old patient, Natalie Garrett, CMA, notices that the patient's eyes are red and she appears to be very sad. Natalie continues trying to gather important health information, and suddenly, the patient bursts into tears stating that her mother just passed away a month ago. She also shares that she doesn't think she is handling her mother's death very well because she is having trouble eating and sleeping. How should Natalie respond to this patient? Would it be appropriate to ask any questions about the death of the patient's mother? Should she touch her to comfort her? Role-play this activity as the medical assistant responding to this patient in a professional manner. What can Natalie say to calm this patient down and continue gathering information about her health history for the physician? Think about the significance of the family's health history as you continue to interview this patient. If you are playing the role of the patient, consider your emotions involved with this recent death of a loved one. Your instructor will give you additional information about this activity!

## *español* SPANISH TERMINOLOGY

**¿Podría hablar un poco más despacio por favor?**
Can you please speak slowly?

**Sí, hablo un poco de español.**
Yes, I speak a little bit of Spanish.

**No, no entiendo.**
No, I don't understand.

**¿Entiende?**
Do you understand?

**¿Cuándo?**
When?

**¿De qué tipo?**
What kind?

**¿Por Qué?**
Why?

**¿Cuántos?**
How many?

**¿Cuanto cuesta?**
How much?

**¿Qué?**
What?

**¿En qué puedo ayudarlo?**
Can I help you?

**¿Por favor me podría decir por qué esta aqui el dia de hoy?**
Can you please tell me, why are you here today?

**¿Cómo?**
How?

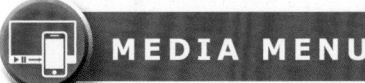

## MEDIA MENU

**Student Resources** on **thePoint**
• **CMA/RMA Certification Exam Review**

**Internet Resources**
**National Institute of Deafness and Other Communication Disorders**
http://www.nidcd.nih.gov

**National Association for the Deaf**
http://www.nad.org

**American Speech-Language-Hearing Association**
http://www.asha.org

**Hearing, Speech and Deafness Center**
http://www.hsdc.org

**National Hospice and Palliative Care Organization**
http://www.nhpco.org

**Handspeak: American Sign Language Online Dictionary**
http://www.handspeak.com

## EMR Activity

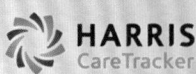
**HARRIS** CareTracker

Harris CareTracker is a web-based electronic medical record (EMR) application that you will use for the EMR activities included in this section at the end of each chapter. This application is actually used in physician offices but is provided to you through the publisher, Wolters Kluwer Health, to give you hands-on practice working with EMRs. Your instructor will have more information about accessing your username, login, and Quickstart guide.

Prerequisite Activities in Harris CareTracker

* *The Getting Started and Quickstart documents and EMR Activities Step-by-Step Instructions are available at* http://thePoint.lww.com/KronenbergerComp5e

Activity Details

Patients' past medical histories and immediate family health histories are entered into the EMR from a questionnaire completed by patients on paper or through an interview by the medical assistant. Natalie Garrett, CMA, must enter the health histories for new patient Marcus Stevens based on his answers on a paper questionnaire. Enter this new patient with a DOB of 09/27/1982 and note his health history of hay fever and depression in the appropriate area of the EMR. Also, accurately document in the family history portion of the EMR that he denies knowledge of any significant family history and that his mother and father are still alive and in good health.

# Chapter Summary

- Communication is a complex and dynamic process involving the sending and receiving of messages. It includes verbal and nonverbal forms of expression and is influenced by personal and societal values, individual beliefs, and cultural orientation.
- In the medical practice, important aspects of patient communication are interviewing and active listening.
- You will need to overcome many communication challenges to communicate with all patients. These challenges include patients with hearing, sight, and speech impairments.
- Children, angry or distressed patients, and patients with mental illnesses can also present a challenge to communication.
- To communicate effectively, you must understand the various factors that can affect the exchange of messages and use the communication techniques that are most appropriate for each individual situation.

# Warm-Ups for Critical Thinking

1. Dr. Hedrick has just told a patient that she has breast cancer. The words "breast cancer" can spark many emotions and fears. Write three sample questions that you could ask the patient to promote open communication about her feelings.
2. Dr. Yevin has just discharged a patient with specific instructions for crutch walking. How would you determine the patient's understanding of these instructions? Can nonverbal clues help you determine whether the patient is confused?
3. A mother brings in her 3-year-old child for a checkup. The child refuses to open her mouth so the doctor can examine her throat. How would you go about communicating the importance of this? What if the child was 6 years old?
4. A patient arrives in your office demanding to see the physician immediately. He is yelling and obviously very angry. The doctor is with another patient. Write three statements that you could say that might help the situation. Write three statements that would escalate the situation.
5. List five local resources that can assist a grieving patient or family member. Include the name of the agency, type of help that it offers, any special information, and its phone number.

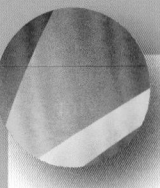

**PSY** PROCEDURE 3-1

## Recognizing Nonverbal Communication and Interview Techniques

**PSY** Respond to nonverbal communication. Use feedback techniques to obtain patient information including the following:

a. Reflection
b. Restatement
c. Clarification

**Purpose**: Use interviewing techniques to respond to nonverbal communication and a challenging communication situation.

**Scenario**: A patient arrives in the office without an appointment and waving a piece of paper that looks like an insurance document in the air demanding to see the physician immediately.

**Equipment**: None.

| STEPS | REASONS |
|---|---|
| 1. Observe the patient's behavior and tone of his voice to determine if there is an immediate problem. | Expressions of aggressive behaviors must be appropriately addressed to keep other patients and staff safe |
| 2. Take the patient to a private area. | To prevent an escalation of the problem and protect the disclosure of the patient's private health information |
| 3. Stay calm and maintain proper space between you and the patient. | To focus on what the patient wants to communicate without becoming defensive, but also keeping yourself safe |
| 4. Use active listening and ask open-ended questions to gather information about the patient's problem. | Gives the patient an opportunity to expand on details and avoid misunderstandings |
| 5. Use the *reflection* technique to gather additional information from the patient. | Encourages the patient to give additional information and keeps the conversation focused on the subject matter |
| 6. Use the *restatement* technique during the conversation with the patient. | Verifies that the information given by the patient has been correctly interpreted |
| 7. Ask a *clarification* question during the conversation with the patient. | To better understand something that the patient has communicated |
| 8. Allow *silence* during the conversation with the patient. | To give the patient an opportunity to think about and articulate the problem |
| 9. Observe the patient for signs of continued or increased agitation. | Seek assistance from others, such as the physician, if it becomes necessary |
| 10. **AFF** Demonstrate the principles of self-boundaries. | Avoid inappropriate or confrontational behavior |

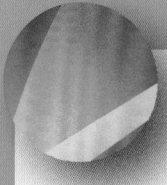

**PSY** PROCEDURE 3-2

## Understanding Barriers to Communication

**PSY** Coach patients appropriately considering:

a. Cultural diversity
b. Development life stage
c. Communication barriers

**Purpose**: Interview a patient with barriers to the communication process.

**Scenario**: Interview a new patient to obtain her health history. The patient is a 70-year-old female whose culture is different from your own and who speaks some English.

**Equipment**: Medical History Form.

| STEPS | REASONS |
|---|---|
| 1. Greet and identify the patient and explain what you need to ask. | Identifying the patient prevents errors; explaining what you need to ask promotes cooperation. |
| 2. Choose a private, quiet area, such as a treatment room, to begin the interview. | The patient may have hearing deficiencies due to her age; confidentiality must be maintained at all times. |
| 3. Sit facing the patient and maintain personal space. Observe nonverbal clues that indicate the patient is not comfortable with making eye contact. | To prevent inaccurate interpretations or misunderstandings by nonverbal communication. Be aware of cultural differences when making eye contact. |
| 4. Note on the Medical History Form the patient's affirmative response to any of the health history questions. | To gather accurate information about the patient's health history status. It may be necessary to use an interpreter, if available, or gestures to avoid misunderstandings. |
| 5. **AFF** Demonstrate respect for individual diversity including:<br>a. Gender<br>b. Race<br>c. Religion<br>d. Age<br>e. Economic status<br>d. Appearance | Patients have a right to considerate, respectful care from their health care providers. |

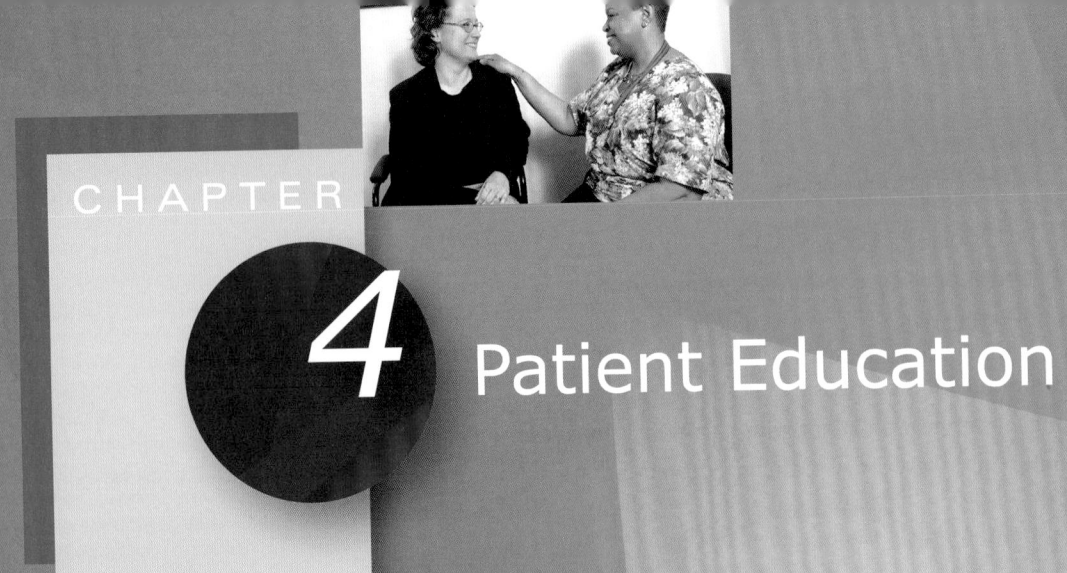

# CHAPTER 4

# Patient Education

## Learning Outcomes

### COG Cognitive Domain*

1. Spell and define the key terms
2. Explain the medical assistant's role in patient education
3. Define the five steps in the patient education process
4. Identify five conditions that are needed for patient education to occur
5. *Discuss the theories of:*
   a. *Maslow*
6. List five factors that may hinder patient education and at least two methods to compensate for each of these factors
7. Discuss five preventive medicine guidelines that you should teach your patients
8. Explain the kinds of information that should be included in patient teaching about medication therapy
9. Explain your role in teaching patients about alternative medicine therapies
10. List and explain relaxation techniques that you and patients can learn to help with stress management
11. Describe how to prepare a teaching plan
12. List potential sources of patient education materials
13. Locate community resources and list ways of organizing and disseminating information
14. *Recognize barriers to communication*
15. *Identify techniques for overcoming communication barriers*
16. *Define coaching a patient as it relates to:*
    a. *Health maintenance*
    b. *Disease prevention*
    c. *Compliance with a treatment plan*
    d. *Community resources*
    e. *Adaptations relevant to individual patient needs*
17. Identify resources and adaptations that are required based on individual needs, i.e., culture and environment, developmental life stage, language, and physical threats to communication

### PSY Psychomotor Domain*

1. Document patient education (Procedure 4-1)
2. *Develop and maintain a current list of community resources related to the patient's health care needs (Procedure 4-2)*

**3.** *Coach patients regarding:*
   **a.** *Health maintenance (Procedure 4-1)*
   **b.** *Disease prevention (Procedure 4-1)*
   **c.** *Treatment plan (Procedure 4-1)*
**4.** *Facilitate referrals to community resources in the role of a patient navigator (Procedure 4-2)*
**5.** *Report relevant information concisely and accurately (Procedure 4-1)*

### AFF Affective Domain*

**1.** *Use language/verbal skills that enable patients' understanding*
**2.** *Demonstrate respect for individual diversity including:*
   **a.** *Gender*
   **b.** *Race*
   **c.** *Religion*
   **d.** *Age*
   **e.** *Economic status*
   **f.** *Appearance*

**3.** *Demonstrate:*
   **a.** *Empathy*
   **b.** *Active listening*
   **c.** *Nonverbal communication*
**4.** *Explain to a patient the rationale for performance of a procedure.*
**5.** *Demonstrate sensitivity appropriate to the message being delivered*
**6.** *Demonstrate recognition of the patient's level of understanding in communications*
**7.** *Demonstrate sensitivity to patient rights*

*Note: AAMA/CAAHEP 2015 Standards are italicized.*

### ABHES Competencies

**1.** Identify and respond appropriately when working/caring for patients with special needs
**2.** Adapt to individualized needs
**3.** Communicate on the recipient's level of comprehension
**4.** Be impartial and show empathy when dealing with patients

## Key Terms

| | | | |
|---|---|---|---|
| alternative medicine | documentation | learning objectives | planning |
| assessment | evaluation | noncompliance | psychomotor |
| disseminates | implementation | placebo | stress |

## Case Study

*P*atient education is a primary responsibility for Dierdre Hall, RMA, at Great Falls Medical Center. The physicians rely on her to research and obtain information for patients on a variety of topics, such as women's health, preventative screenings, healthy lifestyle choices, and exercise for various chronic problems. Deirdre must also stay abreast of the community resources available so she can direct patients to information on accessing health care options or health care coverage as needed. Today, Dierdre has been asked by one of the physicians to apply a Holter monitor to a patient who has been experiencing an irregular heartbeat for the last couple of months. The patient has indicated that she is not sleeping well and is under a lot of stress at work. Where, in the office, should Dierdre instruct the patient on the use of the Holter monitor? What teaching aids can Dierdre use with the patient? What might hinder this patient's understanding of Dierdre's instructions? What community resources might be helpful to this patient? This chapter addresses how to give proper patient education, including choosing an environment that promotes patient learning.

In the current health care climate of short hospital stays, patients seen in the medical office typically have acute conditions requiring intensive and extensive education from their health care provider. Physicians rely extensively on medical assistants to help with patient education for a variety of topics in both the clinical and administrative areas. Medical assistants may be required to perform duties as a patient navigator to assist patients by providing guidance for insurance benefit questions or directing them to other available community health-related resources (see Chapter 2). This will be one of your most challenging and rewarding roles as a medical assistant. Of course, you will not be responsible for teaching patients everything they need to know about health care. Patient education is performed under the direction of the physician. The amount and types of education that you will be expected to do will vary greatly from office to office. This chapter will give you the foundation needed for providing patient education.

## THE PATIENT EDUCATION PROCESS

Patient education involves more than telling patients which medications they need to take or which lifestyle behaviors they need to change and expecting them to follow these instructions blindly. To educate patients effectively, you need to help them accept their illness, involve them in the process of gaining knowledge, and provide positive reinforcement. Ultimately, that knowledge should lead to a change in behavior or attitudes.

The process of patient education involves five major steps:

• Assessment
• Planning
• Implementation
• Evaluation
• Documentation

These five steps collectively produce the teaching plan. The plan may be formally written as the process is occurring or may be documented after the event. You must follow all these steps to achieve effective patient education.

### Assessment

Before you begin to teach, you must assess your feelings and attitudes about the patient and the topic to be taught. Sometimes in your career as a medical assistant, you may encounter situations or patients that make you feel uncomfortable. Your role as an educator, however, requires that you set aside your own personal feelings and life experiences to instruct the patient objectively and to the best of your ability. Always consider how your responses and actions will affect the patient, and be sure to treat each patient impartially.

Assessment requires gathering information about the patient's present health care needs and abilities.

In addition to knowing the present health care needs, you must also look at these other areas:

• Past medical and surgical conditions
• Current understanding and acceptance of health problems
• Needs for additional information
• Feelings about their health care status
• Factors that may hinder learning (covered in detail later in the chapter)

You may obtain this information from a number of sources. The most comprehensive source will be the medical record. The patient's medical record consists of all information regarding current diagnoses, treatments, medications, past medical history, and a variety of other documentation. The electronic health record allows you to run a report showing all of the patient's medical problems, and some paper medical records have a problem list on the inside cover. This will provide you with a snapshot of the patient and save you time from reading the entire document. Other sources of information will be the physician, family members, significant others, and other members of the health care team. When you have collected all of the assessment data, you are ready to start the next step of the education process: planning.

### CHECKPOINT QUESTION

1. What is the purpose of the assessment step during patient education?

### Planning

**Planning** involves using the information you have gathered during the assessment phase to determine how you will approach the patient's learning needs. If possible, involve the patient in this part of the process. Learning goals and objectives that are established with input from the patient are most meaningful. A patient's learning goal is what the patient and educator want to be the outcome of the program. The patient's **learning objectives** include procedures or tasks that will be discussed or performed at various points in the program to help achieve the goal. Make certain the objectives you establish are specific for each individual patient and are measurable in some manner. If the objectives are measurable, you will be able to evaluate when or whether the patient successfully completed them.

For example, consider a patient who needs to limit his fluid intake. Which of the following objectives is more specific and would allow you to evaluate the patient's progress? (1) The patient understands why he should limit his fluid intake, or (2) the patient is able to prepare a schedule for daily fluid intake and explain why it is important that he limit his fluids. The second objective is more specific and not only evaluates the patient's understanding but also requires the patient to demonstrate understanding. Having patients prepare their own schedule gets them involved in their health care. It allows them to customize the schedule to fit their lifestyle, which is likely to increase compliance.

## Implementation

After you establish the need for patient teaching and agree on the goals and objectives, you begin implementation. Implementation is the process used to perform the actual teaching. The teaching usually is carried out in several steps. Box 4-1 presents some commonly used teaching strategies. For example, you may start by telling the patient how to use crutches, followed by a demonstration, and finally, the patient may do a return demonstration. Patients also benefit from the use of teaching aids (drawings, charts, graphs, pamphlets) that they can take home and use as reference material. You can also use videos and CDs to supplement the implementation process.

Miscommunication or misinterpretation can lead to serious complications or injury. For example, assume you are teaching a patient to use crutches. It is very important that you stress to the patient that the crutch must not press directly into the axillary area. (There should be a two-finger distance between the crutch and the armpit.) If the patient does not comprehend the dangers of nerve damage to the axillary area from pressing the crutch into the armpit, a serious complication to the patient could occur. Miscommunication about medications can have fatal consequences. The implementation stage may occur once or over a longer period. The disease process and the patient's ability to comprehend information will dictate the length of teaching. For example, teaching a patient about diabetes takes place over multiple sessions. The first session may focus on what diabetes is, while subsequent teachings may include topics such as diet, foot care, glucose monitoring, and insulin injection.

After implementation of a given skill or knowledge, you must determine whether your teaching was effective. This step is called evaluation.

## Evaluation

Is the patient progressing? Did the teaching plan work? Does the plan need any changes? These are a few of the questions you may ask yourself when you begin to evaluate. Evaluation is the process that indicates how well patients are adapting or applying new information to their lives.

In the medical setting, where contact with patients is limited, part of the evaluation may have to be done by patients at home. For example, if office visits for direct observation are not scheduled, patients will be responsible for telephoning and reporting their status. In other words, can patients do the task they were taught, or are they having troubles? If they voice concern or appear unclear about their instructions, you should either redirect them on the phone or schedule them for an office appointment.

During the evaluation, you may discover **noncompliance**. Noncompliance is the patient's inability or refusal to follow a prescribed order. After determining that the given order is not being followed, your first step is to determine why the order is not being followed. It may be a misunderstanding. For example, a patient who is to take a certain medication twice a day may be taking it only twice a week because that is what he or she thought you said. If the noncompliance is because the patient refuses to follow these orders, however, you must notify the physician. Remember that the patient has the right to refuse medical treatment unless the patient is determined to be mentally incompetent. The physician will determine the next appropriate action in these cases. Evaluation is an ongoing process, so you should expect to update and modify your plan periodically.

---

### BOX 4-1  Implementation Strategies

Implementing the learning process should be individualized to the patient's best method of comprehension and retention. These may include the following:

1. *Lecture and demonstration.* This method presents the information in the most basic form but requires no patient participation for reinforcement and retention.
2. *Role playing and demonstration.* The patient watches you perform a medical procedure and then performs it to ensure understanding. Information is more likely to be recalled if the patient actively participates in the process.
3. *Discussion.* This two-way exchange of information and ideas works well for lifestyle changes (e.g., making dietary changes to lower cholesterol) rather than for medical procedures.
4. *Audiovisual material.* Audiocassettes or videos can often be taken home and reviewed by the patient and family members as needed. This allows for reinforcement of teachings and provides both visual and auditory stimulation.
5. *Printed material and programmed instructions.* All information should be discussed with the patient to clarify points and to elicit questions before assuming that the instructions are understood.

---

### CHECKPOINT QUESTION

2. What is the purpose of evaluation during patient education?

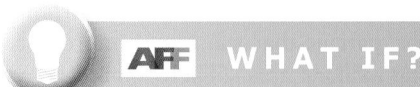

## WHAT IF?

**You are instructing a 60-year-old gentleman in the use of a Holter monitor (an ambulatory heart monitor) when he tells you that he has not been taking his heart medication because it makes him feel tired. You have heard Dr. Jones tell other patients that this particular medication can cause fatigue at first, but that the patient should keep taking it, and after several weeks, he will have more energy. Should you give the patient this information?**

As long as you are sure that your information is correct, you should share this with the patient. The patient then says that he still does not want to take the medication, but he asks that you not to tell the doctor because he may get angry. Since the patient needs this medication for a serious problem, the doctor must be notified. A physician cannot force a patient to take his medication, but he may be able to convince him to take the medication. Perhaps the patient could try another medication that may not have the same effect. Remember to document the details of the encounter in the patient's chart.

## Documentation

**Documentation** includes the recording of all teachings that have occurred. It should consist of the following information:

- Date and time of teaching.
- What information was taught, for example, "Diabetes foot care was discussed. It consisted of the proper method for toenail cutting and regular examination by a podiatrist."
- How the information was taught, for example, "ADA (American Diabetes Association) foot care video shown to the patient."
- Evaluation of teaching. For example, "Patient verbalized the need to make an appointment with a podiatrist."
- Any additional teaching planned, for example, "Patient will return on Monday to the office with his wife for glucose monitoring instructions."

Box 4-2 has a charting example for patient education. Your signature implies that you performed the teaching. If this is untrue or if another staff member assisted you in teaching, make sure that information is clearly noted. Also include the names of any interpreters who were used. You must also document all telephone conversations (e.g., "I spoke with this patient via the telephone today, and he said he is testing his blood sugar every morning without problems.").

Documentation is essential because, from a legal viewpoint, procedures are only considered to have been done if they are recorded. Documentation should become

---

### BOX 4-2   Charting Example

11/27/12
Patient arrived in the office for teaching on the glucose meter; brought meter from home. Following steps were demonstrated by me: calibration of meter strips, battery change, finger sticks, strip insertion into machine, and use of the patient logbook. Normal BGM ranges were reviewed along with the treatment of low blood sugar. Pt returned demonstration without problem. Reviewed glucose meter instructions manual with pt. Pt instructed to bring logbook to each MD appointment.
—Margaret Blackwell, CMA

---

second nature to you as you interact with patients each day. A complete and accurate medical record indicates good care and attention to detail.

## COG CONDITIONS NEEDED FOR PATIENT EDUCATION

Learning is the process of acquiring knowledge, wisdom, or skills through study or instruction. This process does not occur without certain conditions. Learning cannot occur without motivation or a perceived need to learn. For example, suppose you want to teach a patient about the need to adopt a low-sodium diet because of hypertension. Patients who feel that hypertension is not a problem, however, will not be motivated to learn the diet because they have not accepted the need for the teaching. For such patients to be taught, the following steps must occur:

1. The patient must accept that the hypertension has to be managed.
2. The patient must accept that there is a correlation between high sodium intake and hypertension.
3. The patient must accept and be willing to make this dietary change.

Only if these steps have occurred can teaching begin. In addition to patient motivation, basic human needs must be met first.

### Maslow Hierarchy of Needs

Abraham Maslow, an American psychiatrist, recognized that people are motivated by needs and that certain basic needs must be met before people can progress to higher needs, such as taking personal responsibility for their health (self-actualization). Maslow arranged human needs in the form of a pyramid, with basic needs

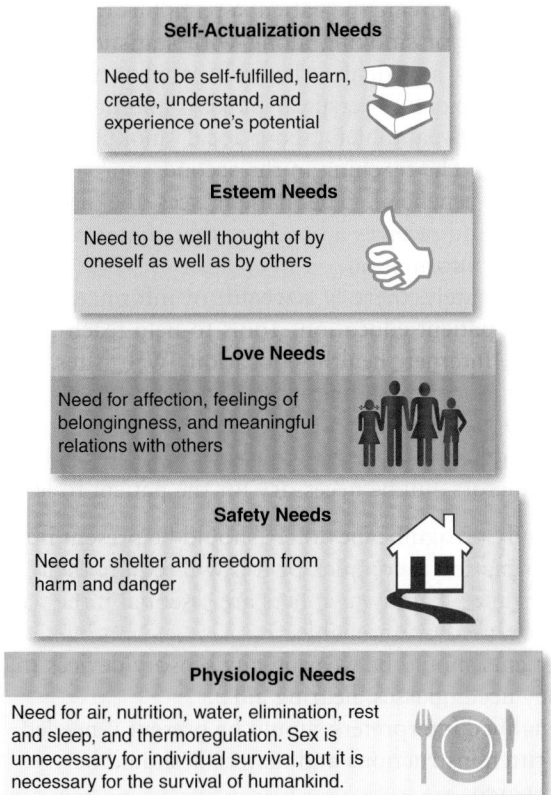

Figure 4-1 • Maslow hierarchy pyramid.

at the bottom and the higher needs at the top (Fig. 4-1). The patient progresses upward, fulfilling different levels of needs toward the highest level, which results in a state of health and well-being. In your responsibility as an educator, you need to be aware that patients must have the basic needs satisfied before they are willing or able to learn to take care of their own health. Not everyone will start at the bottom of the pyramid. Some patients will never reach the top, while others may be at the top and slide backward as a result of unfortunate circumstances.

*Physiologic needs* are air, water, food, rest, and comfort. If these basic needs are unmet, the patient cannot begin the process. Everyone has a different tolerance and expectation for these needs. For example, one person may expect that their food is served over three meals with full courses, while another person may accept that they will have one meal a day from a soup kitchen. If the patient perceives that these needs are met, we need to accept that and not judge the situation.

*Safety and security needs* include a safe environment and freedom from fear and anxiety. Patients are susceptible to fear and anxiety that accompany many medical conditions. For example, patients diagnosed with cancer may be so frightened that they are unable to think of anything but dying. Patients who have undergone some sort of trauma or disaster (hurricane, fire, motor vehicle accident) may place the need to feel safe above all other needs.

*Affection needs*, or the need for love and belonging, are essential for feeling connected and important to others. A sense of love or belonging can often be a powerful motivation for patients to try to regain good health.

*Esteem* needs involve our need to feel self-worth. Esteem can be self-generated, or it can come from those who admire us. If others value us or if we value ourselves, we are more likely to strive to maintain good health. Patients who lack self-esteem are less likely to want or accept education that targets improving their health. Thus, they will not see this as important information and will not be motivated to learn.

*Self-actualization* is the pinnacle of the pyramid, at which a person has satisfied all the other basic needs and feels personal responsibility and control over his or her own life. Self-actualized patients will strive to control their state of wellness by following all health directives and may even help others to achieve wellness. Not all patients will reach this level. Patients who have met this level will be ready to learn a multitude of health care skills and will strive to follow preventive health care maintenance guidelines.

After determining where on the pyramid the patient is, you can determine the appropriateness of education. For example, if the patient has not met the basic physiologic needs, you should help the patient meet these needs before beginning to teach. Patients who are in the middle levels may be able to focus and learn certain skills but may not be ready for complex teachings. If possible, you should involve family members or significant others in the teaching process.

## CHECKPOINT QUESTION

3. What are the basic physiologic needs outlined in Maslow's pyramid?

## Environment

The environment where you teach must be conducive to learning. The room should be quiet and well lit and have limited distractions. It is not appropriate to teach patients a skill in a hallway, waiting room, or other high-traffic area. These areas produce distractions and prohibit confidentiality.

For patients to acquire knowledge, they must feel relaxed and comfortable. For example, it would be inappropriate to attempt to teach a patient who is sitting on an examination table with the stirrups in place. She will not feel comfortable. Reset the stirrups and direct the patient to dress and have a seat in a chair. If the patient had a procedure done in the room and bloody dressings or suture equipment is still present, clean the area and then return for teaching.

## Equipment

A common type of education is teaching patients to perform a **psychomotor** skill. A psychomotor skill requires the participant to physically perform a task. Some examples include crutch walking, glucose monitoring, eye drop instillation, and dressing changes. The equipment for the skill must be present and functional. If possible, the equipment should be from the patient's home or be the exact replica of it.

The steps to teach a psychomotor skill are as follows:

1. Demonstrate the entire skill.
2. Demonstrate the skill step by step, explaining each step as you complete it.
3. Have the patient demonstrate the skill with your help.
4. Have the patient demonstrate the skill without your help.

Provide positive reinforcement throughout the steps. Always provide written step-by-step instructions. Always include instructions from the manufacturer for use and maintenance of any equipment.

## Knowledge

The person teaching the skill must have a solid knowledge of the material. Imagine how difficult it would be to learn to ski from an instructor who did not know how to put skis on. The same is true in medical assisting. If you are not comfortable or do not feel knowledgeable about the topic, ask for help before starting to teach a patient. Be reassured that you do not have to be an expert on the topic, but you do need to feel comfortable with the information. If you start teaching a given topic and the patient asks you a question that you are not able to answer, state that you are not sure about that specific piece but you will get the answer. Then, either research the answer or ask for help from another health care professional. Never guess or imply that you know something that you do not know.

## Resources

For patient education to be effective, it must consist of multiple techniques or approaches. The more techniques that are used, the more the patient will learn and retain. The three ways that we can learn are through auditory (hearing), visual (seeing), and kinesthetic (touch). Auditory learners prefer to listen to instructions; visual learners prefer demonstrations, written instructions, charts, etc.; and kinesthetic learners favor hands-on activities. If you can apply at least two of these senses in your teaching, your patient will be more stimulated to learn and will remember more information. For example, if you were teaching a patient about the dangers of smoking, which of the following would be more

effective: (1) Giving the patient a pamphlet that explains the dangers of smoking along with statistical data, or (2) Showing a patient a diagram of what a nonsmoker's lung looks like versus a smoker's and providing the patient with pamphlets about local smoking cessation programs? The teaching in the second approach would be more beneficial. The patient sees the dangers of smoking and receives a brochure that contains practical hands-on information.

Fortunately, there is a wealth of information available for patient education. Tools to help teach patients include Internet health education Web sites, video DVDs, food labels, manikins, models (heart, lungs), plastic food settings, pamphlets, and videos.

In addition to the five conditions already discussed, these factors will be necessary for the patient to learn:

- Family or significant others should be present if the information is complex or if it will require their assistance. Family members are essential if the patient is confused or unreliable.
- Patients should be wearing any sensory devices that they need (glasses, hearing aids).
- Qualified interpreters should be present if needed.
- Written instructions and materials should be prepared.

## COG FACTORS THAT CAN HINDER EDUCATION

Many factors or circumstances can hinder learning. It is important to recognize these factors and intervene as appropriate. In certain cases, teaching may have to be delayed, or your teaching plan may have to be revised.

### Existing Illnesses

The type of illness that patients have will play a large role in their ability and willingness to learn. Generally, patients with acute short-term illnesses will be motivated to learn a skill that will accelerate healing. Examples of short-term illnesses are orthopedic injuries (uncomplicated fractures, sprains), colds, and viruses.

These are six examples of illnesses or conditions that will affect learning:

- *Any illness in which the patient has moderate to severe pain.* Examples of these illnesses include neuropathies, bone cancer, kidney stones, and recent surgical procedures. The patient's pain level must reach a tolerable stage before teaching can start and the patient can concentrate on learning.
- *Any illness or condition with a poor prognosis or limited rehabilitation potential.* Examples include progressive neurologic disorders, certain cancers, and large traumatic events. It is important that you assess such patients' readiness to learn and their level of

acceptance of their illness before you proceed with your teaching.

- *Any illness or condition that results in weakness and general malaise as a primary symptom.* Examples include gastrointestinal disorders that cause vomiting and diarrhea, anemia, Lyme disease, and recent blood transfusion. For these patients, teaching should be limited to the essential information and expanded on as the patient regains strength.
- *Any illness or condition that impairs the patient's mental health or cognitive abilities.* Examples of these conditions include brain tumors, Alzheimer disease, substance abuse, and psychiatric disorders. In these patients, education should be provided to patients at their ability level. Family members or significant others should be brought in to complement the learning process.
- *Any patient who has more than one chronic illness.* For example, patients with diabetes often have cardiac, renal, and integumentary complications. In patients with multiple system failures, it is important to prioritize the learning needs. Focus your education on the main problem and work from there.
- *Any illness or condition that results in respiratory distress or difficult breathing.* Examples of these conditions include chronic obstructive pulmonary disease, pneumonias, lung cancer, and asthma. The priority goal is first to establish optimal oxygenation for the patient. Once this is met, you can begin teaching. These patients tend to become exhausted easily during acute exacerbations of their illnesses. Keep the teaching time short and to the point and expand teachings as their activity tolerance allows.

### 🔍 CHECKPOINT QUESTION

4. List six types of conditions or illnesses that may hinder your ability to educate patients effectively.

### ⚖️ AFF LEGAL TIP

#### Always Remember to Document Your Actions

There is a common saying in health care: "If it is not in the chart, it did not happen." In a court of law, the medical record is a health care professional's best defense. Always take special care to succinctly and accurately record every interaction with a patient and to give patients their instructions in writing. When patients receive a new diagnosis, provide educational materials about their disorder and direct them to appropriate Web sites. Document any instructions, information, or written materials given to the patient.

## Communication Barriers

Effective communication skills are essential for patient education. Any barriers to communication must be resolved before you can start teaching the patient. If an interpreter is needed for language translation or for hearing-impaired patients, schedule a time convenient to all parties (see Chapter 3).

## Age

The age of the patient plays a very important part in the amount and type of education that you can do. Small children need to be educated at an age-appropriate level (Fig. 4-2). For example, it would be inappropriate to teach a 2-year-old child how to assemble an asthma nebulizer. The parent or caregiver must be taught. It would be appropriate, however, to explain to the 2-year-old child that the nebulizer is not a toy and that it contains medication. Safety education is a prime teaching focus for small children and their parents. Box 4-3 presents some tips for communicating with and teaching children.

As children mature at different speeds, you should assess what information this child can handle and what information should not be shared with the child. Communication with the parents is essential. They know the child's developmental stage. For example, a 7-year-old child who has just been diagnosed with diabetes needs to know the signs and symptoms of low blood sugar and how to treat it. The child may not be ready, however, to learn about the long-term complications (e.g., blindness, renal failure). It is important to teach the child that the disease must be well controlled to prevent future problems, but not to the extent that the child develops fear.

The challenge in teaching adults is that they often have multiple responsibilities to their children, spouses, or aging parents. Obligations at work, school, church, and other activities may also limit their free time. These obligations and responsibilities

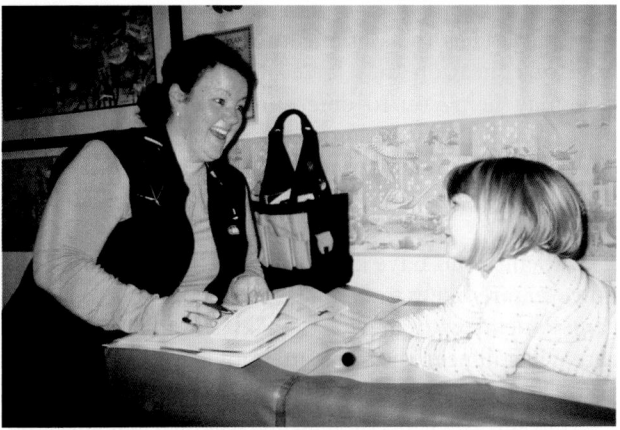

**Figure 4-2 •** Establishing rapport with the child.

---

**BOX 4-3    Tips for Teaching Children**

Children require special communication skills and different teaching strategies. Here are a few tips to help you:

- Encourage the child to be part of the teaching process.
- Speak directly to the child.
- Avoid confusing medical terms.
- Avoid using baby language.
- Teach only age-appropriate information.
- Discuss with the parents the child's knowledge base about the illness and any feelings the parent may have regarding what they want the child to know. (This should not be done in front of the child.)
- Demonstrate skills on stuffed animals or dolls.

---

can interfere with willingness to learn and attentiveness. Your teaching may have to occur in short sessions over long periods. This age group may benefit from electronic resources that they can access on their own time schedule.

Elderly patients can be a challenge to teach for a variety of reasons. These reasons include confusion, lack of interest, and overall poor health. Some older patients, however, can be the most attentive and curious learners. It is fairly common for this age group to address items that they have heard on the news. For example, a patient may hear an advertisement for a new medication for arthritis and request clarification from you regarding its effectiveness.

### CHECKPOINT QUESTION

5. What is the primary teaching focus for small children and their parents?

## Educational Background

Most initial health assessment forms ask patients what level of education they have obtained. This information may help you to determine the patient's ability to read. Caution is essential because graduation alone does not guarantee that the patient can read. You will need to use your tact and diplomacy to evaluate the situation.

Patients who have completed some college courses, however, are likely to be interested in preventive health care. Patients with an educational background in health care will still need the same attention and teaching from you. Do not assume that, since the patient is a nurse or a physician, you can skip teaching a skill. Their specialty may be in an unrelated area.

## Physical Impairments

Numerous physical impairments may hinder learning. For example, patients with severe arthritis in their hands may have difficulty performing certain psychomotor skills, like giving themselves insulin. An occupational therapist is the best resource to assist you. Speak to the physician to obtain the proper referrals.

## Other Factors

Other factors may hinder your ability to teach patients. The patient's culture may affect willingness to learn or the family's involvement in learning. Patients with financial troubles or confusion with health insurance benefits may not be ready to focus on learning new skills or knowledge. It is important that you assess the patient's readiness to learn and either try to remove or work around any obstacles that may be present.

## TEACHING SPECIFIC HEALTH CARE TOPICS

Your role in patient education will vary greatly. The topics that you will teach will depend on the patient, type of medical office, and physician's preferences. Staying well is a topic often discussed in the exam room. Medical assistants provide information and support about nutrition, exercise, and wellness. These topics are discussed in Chapter 16. Next are some other topics commonly taught by medical assistants.

## Preventive Medicine

Preventing health problems is the key to living a long, healthy life. But the advantages to good preventive medicine extend much further. There are huge economic benefits to preventing illnesses. Millions of people are hospitalized each year. Caring for sick and chronically ill patients costs approximately 75% of all U.S. health care expenses. These statistics affect everyone in higher taxes and increased health insurance premiums, so preventing illnesses and lowering health care costs are everyone's concern.

These are some commonly recommended preventive health care tips that you should teach all of your patients:

- Regular physical examinations for all age groups
- Annual flu and regular pneumonia vaccinations
- Adult immunizations for tetanus and hepatitis B
- Childhood immunizations
- Regular dental examinations
- Monthly breast self-examinations for women and regular physician examinations
- Cancer screening to include:

- Mammograms
- Colonoscopy
- Annual Pap tests
- Prostate-specific antigen blood tests for all men, along with need for regular digital rectal examinations

The frequency and age at which these procedures will be recommended to patients vary with the patient's medical history and genetics and the physician's preference. Patients with financial considerations should also be reminded that the Affordable Care Act addresses preventative care by mandating coverage of many preventative screenings. The law requires that all associated costs of certain preventative screenings be paid by insurance companies including Medicare. Many hospitals and clinics offer free preventive screenings to patients. Your office should have a list of which free screenings are available. Public health departments may also have this information available for your patients. Most providers and insurance coverage base the frequency and type of testing on the guidelines set forth by the American Cancer Society.

Your role as a medical assistant is to promote preventive screenings. The physician you work with will instruct you in his or her recommendations for these tests. If your practice is part of a patient-centered medical home model of care, you will be an important part of the medical team to address healthy lifestyle and wellness issues with patients (see Chapters 1 and 13).

Another large part of preventive medicine is teaching safety tips. Preventable injuries can arise from bicycle and car accidents, poisoning, fires, choking, falls, drownings, firearms, and lawn mowers. Toys can lead to injuries when they are broken or used by a child of an inappropriate age. The American Academy of Pediatrics (AAP) offers injury prevention tips for parents and health care providers. While working as a medical assistant, you will find valuable teaching tips to give to parents from their Web site. The AAP also provides numerous educational materials that can be mailed to physician offices and given to your patients.

According to the American Academy of Orthopaedic Surgeons (AAOS), falls cause 90% of the hip fractures that occur each year in the United States. By 2050, the AAOS estimates that the number of hip fractures per year will reach 650,000. Hip fractures require long hospitalizations and often rehabilitation in a nursing home. Most falls occur at home and are preventable. Fall prevention tips should be taught to all older patients or any patient who has a problem with maintaining balance or uses an ambulation device (cane, walker). Here are some tips that you can use to teach fall prevention:

- Encourage patients to remove all scatter rugs in their home. Remind patients to keep hallways clutter free.
- Instruct the patient to ensure adequate lighting in all rooms and hallways.

- Encourage the patient to avoid steps. Encourage one-floor living.
- Ensure that the patient has well-soled shoes or sneakers. Advise the patient to avoid wearing heels.
- Instruct the patient to place nonskid surfaces in bathtubs or purchase a shower chair.
- Instruct the patient to install handrails or grab bars in hallways and stairwells.
- Advise patients taking medications that lower their blood pressure to stand up slowly and get their balance, and then begin to walk.
- Advise patients to have regular eye examinations and have their glasses adjusted as needed.
- Encourage patients to have a plan for power outages and severe storms.

## Lifestyle Changes

In addition to instructing patients, in many cases, you will be asking them to make changes in their lifestyle. Change is difficult for anyone. It is easier to continue doing what you have always done. Some patients view illness as strong motivation to follow the physician's orders. Others are resistant to eating less and moving more to lose extra pounds or beginning a walking program to help their arthritis. You can help with the difficult process of change. Encouragement and close follow-up are effective ways to keep a patient on the right track. When a patient sees results from his changes, he is encouraged and wants to continue. Eventually, the changes become habits, and the patient has been successful in making a lifestyle change that will probably add years to his life. Giving up foods you love, pushing yourself to work hard, and resisting addictions are difficult and continuous battles. Patients should be reminded to strive for small successes at first, monitor their progress weekly, and take one day at a time.

## Healthy Community Program

To reduce and prevent chronic diseases such as heart disease, diabetes, obesity, etc., the Centers for Disease Control and Prevention (CDC) developed the Healthy Community Program to help communities address these growing problems. The CDC's Healthy Community Program (HCP) provides funding and technical assistance to communities desiring to implement strategies to promote a healthier population regardless of socioeconomic status. Health risk behaviors are identified that cause chronic diseases resulting in solutions at the local level. Extensive online public health resources are available free of charge through this program at the CDC's Web site.

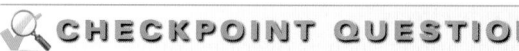

## CHECKPOINT QUESTION

6. To which patients should you teach fall prevention tips?

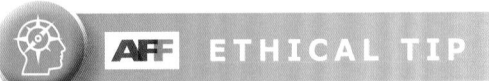

## ETHICAL TIP

### Be Supportive, Not Judgmental

Even with your best efforts, some patients do not follow the doctor's orders. It is hard to understand a lung cancer patient who is still smoking or a patient with high cholesterol levels who continues to eat fried food. As a health care professional, you should never judge a patient or offer your personal opinions. Avoid showing negative feelings or distaste for patients or their actions. Provide patients with as much information, support, and encouragement as possible. People respond to positive reinforcement, and your interest and concern may be just what they need to help them make difficult lifestyle changes.

## Medications

With the increasing number of medications available, the possibilities for teaching patients in this area are virtually endless. Pharmaceutical companies offer in-depth medication information for health care providers and patients concerning the chemical makeup of the drug, physiologic reactions in the body, prescribed dosage and route, and possible side effects. This information comes from the pharmaceutical companies either by mail or from the sales support team. In addition, some of this information will come in package inserts. If this information is not available, the patient may not understand the importance of the medication therapy, and this could lead to noncompliance, drug interactions, or other serious side effects. You may be responsible for gathering information about a patient's medication regimen, documenting all of the patient's medications including over-the-counter and vitamin supplements, and preparing teaching materials for your patients to help prevent such complications.

When preparing a medication therapy teaching tool, you must consider such factors as the patient's financial abilities, social or cultural demands, physical disabilities, and age. Be sure to include the following information in any teaching:

- Medication name (generic or brand)
- Dosage
- Route
- What the medication is for
- Why the medication must be taken as prescribed
- Possible changes in bodily functions (e.g., colored urine)
- Possible side effects
- Other medications, such as over-the-counter drugs, herbal supplements, and so on, that might interfere with the action of the medication
- Foods or liquids to be avoided or restricted

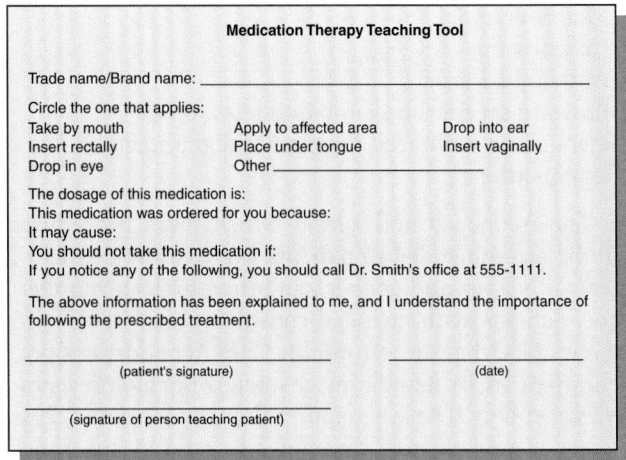

**Figure 4-3 •** Medication therapy teaching tool.

- Activities to be avoided
- Telephone number to call for any questions or concerns

Figure 4-3 shows a medication therapy teaching tool that incorporates all of these elements.

Medication teaching should also include any over-the-counter medications or herbal supplements the patient is taking. This information should consist of the same items listed above. Many patients have the misconception that over-the-counter medications (e.g., aspirin, ibuprofen, cough syrup) are 100% safe and no dangers are associated with them. Some of these medications may interact with their prescribed medications.

After assessing patients' understanding of all of their medications, you may find that scheduling is a prime concern. For example, the patient may be taking several types of medications at different times of the day or week. Before developing a medication schedule, evaluate the patient's daily routine to see how adhering to the schedule may affect the patient's lifestyle. For instance, you might ask the patient:

- How late do you sleep each morning?
- What time do you go to bed?
- When do you usually eat?

Once you have collected this information, you can create a scheduling tool to serve as a reminder to the patient about what medications to take when. Pillboxes can also help to remind patients to take their medication. Pillboxes are plastic containers prelabeled with the days of the week and times. You may instruct the patient in how to fill them. Pillboxes are sold in most pharmacies.

Another patient education area that falls under the category of medication therapy includes how to administer medications—orally, vaginally, rectally, and so on. This information will be taught in the clinical part of your curriculum. A patient's medication regimen should be reviewed at each visit to be sure the patient is taking the right medication in the right way. For more patient teaching information regarding safe and effective use of medications, you can contact the National Council on Patient Information and Education (NCPIE), a nonprofit organization, at 666 Eleventh Street, NW, Suite 810, Washington, DC 20001. NCPIE can provide you with literature and referrals to other sources.

## Alternative Medicine

Many ancient remedies that were once considered voodoo and dismissed by Western medicine have proven to be beneficial. Billions are spent yearly on **alternative medicine**, and surveys have shown that about 51% of all Americans have used some form of unconventional medicine. In 1998, a federal agency was created to evaluate and monitor alternative medicine therapies. That agency, the National Center for Complementary and Alternative Medicine (NCCAM), also conducts clinical trials and training programs for practitioners of alternative medicine.

There are numerous types of alternative medicine therapies. Following is a discussion of four of the most common therapies.

### Acupuncture

Acupuncture is one of the oldest forms of Chinese medicine. Acupuncture works on the principle that there are 2,000 acupuncture points in the human body. These 2,000 points are connected throughout the body by 12 pathways called *meridians*. The meridians conduct energy, or *qi*, in the body when they are triggered. The trigger comes in the form of a needle. When the meridian is stimulated, it prompts the brain to release certain chemicals and hormones.

Acupuncture is primarily used to treat addictions, fibromyalgia, osteoarthritis, asthma, and chronic back pain. It is sometimes used in treating children with attention-deficit/hyperactivity disorder.

In 1996, the Food and Drug Administration (FDA) required that all acupuncture needles be labeled for single use. Training and legal requirements vary among states.

### Acupressure

Acupressure is similar to acupuncture, except that it does not use needles. The practitioner applies pressure to the meridians through direct touch. This method has shown great success in treating nausea and vomiting associated with chemotherapy. Some hospitals and clinics offer acupressure on an outpatient basis to cancer patients. Studies have shown that acupressure may help alleviate chronic pains and may even boost the immune system. Requirements for licensure and training vary among states.

### Hypnosis

Hypnosis is portrayed on television as a magical method for reaching the inner workings of the brain. There is proof, however, that when conducted properly, it may provide some health care benefits. It is primarily used for weight reduction, for treatment of obsessive–compulsive disorders, and for smoking cessation. Hypnosis can be used for pain control and relaxation. Patients with anxiety disorders can be taught to do self-hypnosis. The training requirements vary greatly from state to state, and in most areas, licensure is not required.

### Yoga

Yoga has proved to be very beneficial for relieving stress and improving flexibility. Yoga consists of a comprehensive discipline of physical exercise, posture, breathing exercises, and meditation. There are a variety of types of yoga. Iyengar consists of motionless poses that emphasize posture and form. Once this method is learned, patients are able to practice this at home. This method may help patients who are recovering from injuries. Bikram consists of 26 poses that are conducted at 100°F. This method promotes muscle relaxation and stretching. Perspiration is thought to help cleanse the body of various toxins. Sivananda is a five-step system that focuses on breathing exercises, relaxation, diet, and meditation.

### Herbal Supplements

The use of herbal supplements is a multibillion-dollar business in the United States. The general public views herbal supplements as "natural," and hence safe. This is a misconception. Herbal supplements, vitamins, and similar substances are not regulated by the FDA. The patient or consumer must understand that, because there has been no formal government testing or approval of these substances, their dosages, side effects, interactions, and possible benefits are unclear. A classic example of an herbal supplement that has been shown to have dangerous side effects is ephedrine. This is the active ingredient in the herb ephedra and was once thought to be the weight-loss miracle. It can, however, cause heart attacks and strokes. The FDA issued many warnings about ephedrine's dangers and potential for abuse; in 2004, the FDA banned dietary supplements containing ephedra in the United States.

Other herbal supplements, such as Ginkgo, are taken to help with memory but also have anticoagulant properties. This is very dangerous for patients already taking an anticoagulant, such as Coumadin, as it increases the risk of bleeding.

Furthermore, since these products are not regulated, there is no guarantee that what the label claims is in the bottle is actually there. The quality and the purity of the herbal supplements have shown to vary greatly from manufacturer to manufacturer. Patients should be advised to purchase only supplements that are stamped with a U.S. Pharmacopeia bar code. This bar code means that the manufacture site has met certain standards for distribution but does not mean that the supplement has been tested for health care benefits. Box 4-4 provides some general teaching tips for any patient using an herbal supplement.

## BOX 4-4    General Teaching Tips for Herbal Supplements

Here are a few general teaching points on herbal supplements:

- Explain to patients the importance of always telling the physician or other health care provider about any herbal supplements that they are taking.
- Explain to patients that the fact that a product is "natural" does not mean it is safe. A good example is mushrooms. All mushrooms are natural, but some are very poisonous.
- Teach patients the importance of looking for the USP (United States Pharmacopeia) label. Teach patients to look for expiration dates on all supplements.
- Advise patients not to ask health store clerks for information on supplements but to speak to physicians or pharmacists.

- Advise patients to distrust advertisements that use words like magical or breakthrough or that claim to detoxify the whole body.
- Instruct patients to stop taking all herbal supplements at least 2 weeks prior to surgery and to tell their surgeon what supplements they have been using and how long. (Some supplements can increase bleeding time.)
- Warn diabetic patients that many supplements will interfere with blood sugar levels.
- Advise parents to avoid giving herbal supplements to their children unless approved by a physician.
- Advise pregnant or breast-feeding patients to consult with a pharmacist or physician before taking any supplements.

Some of these substances have evolved through folklore, various cultures, or clinical research. In some cases, there is an element of **placebo** action involved. Placebo is the power of believing that something will make you better when there is no chemical reaction that warrants such improvement. Other supplements actually have scientific studies to document their effects. Table 4-1 lists some commonly used herbal supplements and their reported benefits.

Your role as a medical assistant is to assess whether patients are using any alternative therapies. Your assessment should include the length of time they have used these treatments and any side effects or benefits that the patient has noted, and you should report such information to the physician. Patients should be advised to verify the training and credentials of the practitioner they are using and to ascertain that the practitioner is appropriately licensed. Patients should be encouraged to look at the National Center for Complementary and Alternative Medicine (NCCAM) Web site for safety updates and for more detailed information about alternative medicine. You should never recommend that a patient start taking herbal supplements or other alternative medicine therapies without a physician's approval.

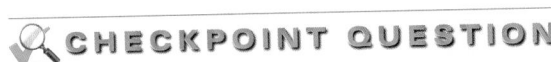 CHECKPOINT QUESTION

7. What is a placebo?

| TABLE 4-1    Herbal Supplements[a] | |
|---|---|
| **Supplement** | **Reported Benefits** |
| Alfalfa | Relief from arthritis pain; strength |
| Anise | Relief of dry cough; treatment of flatulence |
| Black cohosh root | Relief of premenstrual symptoms; rheumatoid arthritis |
| Chamomile | Treatment of migraines, gastric cramps |
| Cholestin | Lowers cholesterol and triglycerides |
| Echinacea | Treatment of colds; stimulates immune system; attacks viruses |
| Garlic | Treatment of colds; diuretic; prevention of cardiac diseases |
| Ginkgo | Increased blood flow to brain; treatment of Alzheimer disease |
| Ginseng | Mood elevator, antihypertensive |
| Glucosamine | Treats arthritis symptoms; improves joint mobility |
| Kava | Treatment of anxiety, restlessness; tranquilizer |
| Licorice | Soothes coughs, treats chronic fatigue syndrome |
| St. John's wort | Treats depression, premenstrual symptoms; antiviral |

[a]This box lists some commonly used herbal supplements and their reported benefits. Research is an ongoing process to document these findings. Some of these herbal supplements may have side effects or may interact with prescribed medications.

## ⚙ STRESS MANAGEMENT

Everyone is affected by an illness or injury at some time. Along with this often comes stress. **Stress** can come from forces such as fear, anger, anxiety, crisis, and joy. Stress may produce physiologic changes as well as psychological effects. When faced with illness or injury, a patient usually must confront

- Physical pain
- Inability to perform self-care
- Stress of treatments, procedures, and possible hospitalization
- Changes in role identity and self-image
- Loss of control and independence
- Changes in relationships with friends and family

Patients with chronic conditions may need more time to adjust than patients with acute illnesses. If patients are able to deal with stress factors, they are more likely to adapt and adjust to lifestyle changes.

Many other causes besides illness or injury can place patients under stress. The best way to cope with stress is by living a healthy lifestyle. When the body is healthy, it can handle stress more easily. Unfortunately, most of the reasons that hinder learning are the same factors that hinder patients' ability to comply with patient education. Patients who are not capable of coping with stress on their own or with the help of instruction provided by the medical office staff may need professional counseling.

### Positive and Negative Stress

Two types of stress affect all of us daily: positive stress and negative stress. Positive stress motivates individuals to work efficiently and perform to the best of their abilities. Examples of positive stress include working on a challenging new job or assignment, getting married, and giving a speech or performance. In fact, many people work best under positive stress. Under positive stress, the brain releases chemicals that increase the heart rate and breathing capacity. The body also releases stored glucose that gives an energy boost. Once the job (or wedding) is over, though, time must be taken to relax and prepare for the next project. If relaxation techniques are not incorporated into the daily routine, positive stress can become negative stress.

Negative stress is the inability to relax after a stressful encounter. Left unchecked, it can lead to such physiologic responses as:

- Headache
- Nausea, diarrhea
- Sweating palms
- Insomnia
- Malaise
- Rapid heart rate

Long-term physical effects of unrelieved stress include increases in blood pressure, glucose levels, metabolism, intraocular pressure, and finally exhaustion. There is also an increased risk of heart attack, stroke, diabetes, certain cancers, and immune system failure. If the stress is not relieved, patients will progress to higher anxiety levels and will require all of their energy and attention to focus solely on the problem at hand. Most mental and physical activity will be directed at relief of the stress to avoid the ultimate anxiety level known as panic—a sudden, overwhelming state of anxiety or terror.

It may be difficult to escape completely from stress-causing factors, but management of them is possible. For a patient suffering from the physiologic effects of negative stress, you can offer the following coping strategies:

- Encourage patients to attempt to reduce stressors but emphasize that it is not possible to remove all stressors. Warn them to avoid attempting to make everything perfect; perfectionism adds its own stress.
- Encourage patients to organize and limit activities as needed.
- Try to lessen patients' fear of failure so they just do the best they can.
- When patients are feeling anxious, encourage them to talk to someone about their problems and let off steam.

Any one of these tips may help patients to regain control over stressors. In addition, a number of relaxation techniques described in the following sections may help.

## Psychological Defense Mechanisms

Humans employ the use of defense mechanisms to cope with the painful and difficult problems life can bring. Freud's unconscious awareness theory says that we unconsciously avoid conflict and situations that cause us feelings of anxiety. Patients can use defense mechanisms to hide from or ignore their problems, especially those resulting from illness. We all use defense mechanisms from time to time, but psychologists say that the key to good mental health is to face our real conflicts and problems. You may encounter patients who are using such mechanisms to hide their true feelings. You must keep this possibility in mind as you attempt to understand and help patients. Table 4-2 outlines some common defense mechanisms.

## Relaxation Techniques

Patients can use any of several types of relaxation techniques. To determine what works best for them, they must first consider how much time they have and what type of relaxation they need. Next are three examples of relaxation techniques.

### Breathing Techniques

Breathing exercises can be done anywhere. Most people are shallow breathers and need to be instructed on deep-breathing techniques. To perform these breathing exercises, the patient should sit up straight with hands placed on the stomach and take a deep breath in through the nose, feeling the hands being pushed away by the

## TABLE 4-2 COMMON DEFENSE MECHANISMS

| Defense Mechanism | Explanation | Example |
|---|---|---|
| Denial | Refusing to acknowledge an unpleasant fact of life in order to delay facing it. Allowing yourself to believe that the problem does not exist. | A parent of a teen ignores or trivializes physical signs of drug abuse. |
| Displacement | Taking out your anger and frustration on someone other than the person responsible for the bad feelings. | A medical assistant is angry with her physician–employer. Later, she yells at her husband when he asks about dinner. |
| Intellectualization | Analyzing a difficult situation to try to make sense of it. | A daughter spends hours researching Alzheimer disease after her mother's diagnosis. |
| Projection | Blaming others for your unacceptable qualities. | A medical assisting graduate blames her teachers when she has trouble finding a job because of poor personal work history. |
| Rationalization | Using excuses for unacceptable behavior. | A patient says it is all right for him to smoke because he has a high-stress job. |
| Regression | Behaving in an immature way when faced with difficulty. | A patient pouts when she has to wait because the doctor has been called to the hospital. |
| Repression | Blocking out bad memories. | An abused wife remembers only "the good times" when she thinks about leaving her abuser. |
| Sublimation | Changing unwanted aggressive or sexual drives by finding an outlet through creative mental work. | A recovering abuser volunteers at a shelter and counsels abused spouses. |
| Withdrawal | Physically or emotionally pulling away from difficult situations. | A child sits alone on the playground because he is not as good at kickball as the others. |

stomach. (This may feel awkward because most people do just the opposite.) The patient holds the breath for a few seconds and then exhales through pursed lips as the hands are felt being pulled in. This exercise allows for good control of the rate of exhalation. Sometimes, getting the oxygen flowing through the body at a faster rate is all that is needed to relieve boredom, tension, and stress.

## Visualization

Visualization is a relaxation technique that involves allowing the mind to wander and the imagination to run free and focus on positive and relaxing situations. It is similar to daydreaming. It can "remove" the patient from a stressful situation and put him or her in a place where, if nothing else, the mind can relax. Instruct the patient to find a quiet place, close the eyes, and then visualize a soothing scene. Sometimes, background music helps. Remind the patient that it is important to choose appropriate times for this daydreaming technique. For example, it would be dangerous to use this technique when driving a car or operating heavy equipment.

## Physical Exercise

There is no better tranquilizer than physical exercise. Walking at least 30 minutes three times a week is a great stress reliever. Most people who exercise regularly say that it helps them reduce tension, relax, and rest better at night.

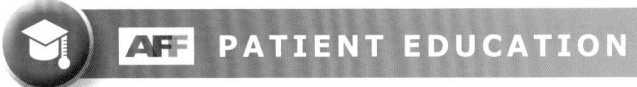 **AFF   PATIENT EDUCATION**

### Self-Relaxation Techniques

Here are two examples of self-relaxation techniques for you and your patients.

1. Sit with both feet on the floor, place your hands in your lap, and close your eyes. Visualize yourself standing at the top of a staircase with six steps. Now imagine that you are going down each step very slowly. With each step down, your body becomes more relaxed. When you feel completely relaxed for a minute or so, imagine going back up the steps. With each step up, you feel more alert and ready to take on the world. It takes practice, but after awhile, the process can be done in the time it takes to take a bathroom break. You will be refreshed and ready to sail through the rest of the day.

2. In a sitting position, concentrate on relaxing the muscles in your body. Beginning with the top of your head and moving down, concentrate on relaxing your shoulders, your arms, your hips, your legs, etc. Try this technique when you are having trouble getting to sleep or you're anxiously sitting in the dentist's chair.

## COG PATIENT TEACHING PLANS

### Developing a Plan

Because medical assistants are usually allotted only minimal time for patient teaching, you may often find yourself teaching without a written plan. To ensure that teaching is done logically, always use the education process to help you formulate a plan in your mind. Also remember to document in the patient's record whatever teaching you perform and the patient's response.

Many facilities use preprinted teaching plans for common problem areas, such as "Controlling Diabetes," "Living with Multiple Sclerosis," and "Coping with Hearing Loss." Although these save time, they are not individualized to the patient. If you use preprinted teaching plans, be sure to adapt them to your particular patient's learning needs and abilities.

If preprinted plans are not an option, consult teaching plan resource books, which contain the necessary information in outline form. You can take the plans from these sources and transfer them as needed to your facility-approved teaching plan format, adding your own comments to fit the patient's needs.

All teaching plans, no matter what the design, should contain the following elements:

- *Learning goal.* A description of what the patient should learn from implementation of the teaching plan.
- *Material to be covered.* All major topics to be discussed.
- *Learning objectives.* Steps or procedures the patient must understand or demonstrate to accomplish the learning goal.
- *Evaluation.* Appraisal of the patient's progress.
- *Comments.* Remarks concerning circumstances that may be preventing successful completion of the objectives.

Teaching plans must also include an area for documenting when the information was presented to the patient and when the patient successfully completed each objective. Figure 4-4 is an example of a teaching plan.

### Selecting and Adapting Teaching Material

An enormous amount of teaching material is available. Although the physician or institution may select much of the material you will use, you may be responsible for

**Teaching Plan:** 32-year-old female with Iron Deficiency Anemia
**Patient Learning Goal:** Increase patient's knowledge of Iron Deficiency Anemia, its complications and treatments
**Material to be Covered:** Description of disorder, complications, diet, medications, procedures

| Learning Objectives Comments | Teaching Methods/Tools | Procedure Explained/Demonstrated Date/Initial | PT Demonstrated/ Objectives Met Date/Initial |
|---|---|---|---|
| 1. Patient describes what happens when body's demand for oxygen is not met.<br>a. oxygen and hgb concentration decrease<br>b. signs/symptoms of anemia<br>c. anemia occurs only after body stores of iron are depleted | Instruction | | |
| 2. Patient describes complications caused by decrease of oxygen concentration<br>a. chronic fatigue<br>b. dyspnea<br>c. inability to concentrate, think<br>d. decrease in tissue repair<br>e. increase of infection<br>f. increase in heart rate | Instruction | | |
| 3. Patient discusses importance of diet in prevention of iron deficiency anemia<br>a. including iron-rich foods in diet (beef, poultry, green vegetables)<br>b. including foods that contain ascorbic acid to assist in absorbing iron in body (fruits)<br>c. importance of limiting large meals if fatigued; stress importance of several small meals | Instruction/Video: "Your Diet: Why It Is Important" | | |
| 4. Patient describes prescribed medication, its purpose, dosage, route, and side effects | Instruction/Pamphlet: *Taking Your Iron Supplements* | | |
| 5. Patient aware of importance of follow-up appointments for evaluation of prescribed plan of treatment | Instruction/Appointment slip with next scheduled appointment | | |

**Figure 4-4 •** Teaching plan.

selecting some teaching aids. Assess your patients' general level of understanding to choose materials appropriately. When using preprinted material, consider the format, headings, illustrations, vocabulary, and writing style for overall clarity and readability. Also, ensure that the information provided on commercial materials is truthful and in agreement with the policies and procedures of your facility. A good rule of thumb is to use commercial material only from nationally recognized organizations or government agencies.

Many patient education textbooks are available on the Internet or from your clinic library. There are many online sources that list addresses for other patient education materials available from companies or associations. The Centers for Disease Control and Prevention and state health departments are also good resources, and printed materials can often be ordered online at no charge on a variety of health-related topics. Use commercially prepared materials to start a patient teaching library in the physician's office so you will have information at your fingertips when needed.

## Developing Your Own Material

Sometimes, you may need to create your own teaching materials. Review available resources and teaching aids, and adapt the information to benefit your patients. When developing teaching material, remember to do the following:

- Indicate the objective of the information.
- Personalize the information so the patient wants to learn.
- Make sure information is clear and well organized.
- Use lists and outlines, which are easier to read and remember than paragraphs.
- Avoid medical jargon as much as possible.
- Focus on the key points.
- Select appropriate printing type.
- Use diagrams that are simple, clear, and well labeled.
- Include the names and telephone numbers of people or organizations that patients can call with further questions or concerns.

After patients have been using the material for a while, periodically evaluate its effectiveness and modify your teaching plan as needed.

Not all of the patient teaching materials you create will have to be in print form. Patients must be motivated to read, but many will be more receptive to audiovisual instruction. Take advantage of any opportunity to develop teaching materials in other media.

## CHECKPOINT QUESTION

8. List the elements of a written teaching plan.

## PSY Locating Community Resources and Disseminating Information

Patients have access to many services that sometimes they do not even realize are available. Many communities have a central agency that coordinates and **disseminates** or distributes information about many or all community resources. If this is not the case in your area, you will want to gather the information and create an information sheet for patients to take home. The patient and his family can then examine the resources, decide if they want to participate, and contact the appropriate community resource. Support groups not only provide assistance for patients and their families in coping with illness, but they also give the patient an opportunity to meet and exchange ideas with others who are experiencing the same issues such as Alzheimer disease, cancer, and diabetes.

Most local and online telephone directories include a section that outlines the agencies and resources available through the city and state. Information for patients who need financial assistance or assistance with transportation would be found in a telephone directory. The Internet is an excellent resource for local, state, and national agencies that provide information, support, and services to patients. Box 4-5 lists some of the agencies that might be available in your area. For information about local support, the Web sites of these agencies are listed as well.

### BOX 4-5   Community Resources

Council on Aging; http://www.ncoa.org
American Red Cross; http://www.redcross.org
Hospice; http://www.hospicefoundation.org
American Cancer Society; http://www.cancer.org
American Heart Association; http://www.heart.org
Civic organizations
Public health department
Social services
Home health agencies

Various support groups can be located in the telephone directory or local newspaper. Cancer centers would have information about the support they offer.

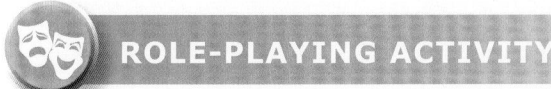

## ROLE-PLAYING ACTIVITY

A moderately obese patient was recently diagnosed by her physician at Great Falls Medical Center with type II diabetes mellitus. In addition to prescribing an oral medication, the physician asks Dierdre Hall, RMA, to educate the patient on the benefits of a healthy diet and exercise regimen to lose weight and, hopefully, lower her blood glucose level. The physician wants the patient to understand the benefits of eating a healthy diet and losing weight as well as the risks if her blood glucose levels are not managed. What resources can Deirdre use to obtain legitimate information on this topic? What factors should she consider before attempting to educate this patient, such as where and when? How should she approach the patient about this topic? If you are the patient, think about how you might feel if someone was giving you information about nutrition and exercise. Would you be encouraged or offended? How would you feel about your future health when given the information and risks of noncompliance? Your instructor will give you additional information about this activity.

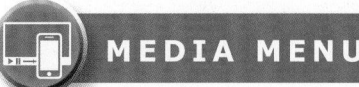

## MEDIA MENU

**Student Resources** on thePoint®
- **CMA/RMA Certification Exam Review**

**Internet Resources**
**American Academy of Pediatrics**
http://www.aap.org
**American Cancer Society**
http://www.cancer.org
**American Heart Association**
http://www.heart.org
**American Lung Association**
http://www.lungusa.org
**U.S. Food and Drug Administration**
http://www.fda.gov
**National Center for Complementary and Alternative Medicine**
http://www.nccam.nih.gov
**National Council on Patient Information and Education**
http://www.talkaboutrx.org
**Centers for Disease Control and Prevention**
http://www.cdc.gov/chronicdisease/resources/publications/
**The Community Guide**
www.thecommunityguide.org

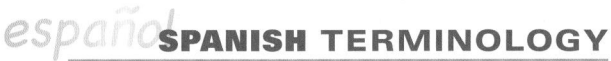

## *español* SPANISH TERMINOLOGY

**Tres veces al día**
Three times a day

**Cada ocho horas**
Every 8 hours

**Antes/después de las comidas**
Before/after meals

**Al acostarse**
At bedtime

**Tómela con los alimentos.**
Take this with food.

**Dele la medicina cada cuatro horas.**
Give him the medicine every 4 hours.

**Hola mi nombre es Maria, yo soy el asistente del Dr. Lewis.**
Hello, my name is Maria. I'm Dr. Lewis' Medical Assistant.

**Si no le entiende al doctor por favor digamelo para explicárselo de una manera más fácil para usted.**
If you do not understand the doctor, please let me know and I will explain in more detail.

**El doctor la (o) va a enviar con un especialista.**
The doctor will refer you to a specialist.

## EMR Activity

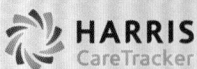
**HARRIS** CareTracker

Harris CareTracker is a web-based electronic medical record (EMR) application that you will use for the EMR activities included in this section at the end of each chapter. This application is actually used in physician offices but is provided to you through the publisher, Wolters Kluwer Health, to give you hands-on practice working with EMRs. Your instructor will have more information about accessing your username, login, and Quickstart guide.

Prerequisite Activities in Harris CareTracker

- *The Getting Started and Quickstart documents and EMR Activities Step-by-Step Instructions are available at* http://thePoint.lww.com/KronenbergerComp5e

Activity Details

Create and save a patient information brochure on a topic for a preventative screening using your computer word processing software. Upload it into the EMR for future reference using the *Patient Education Upload* feature in the *Clinical* tab of the *Administration* module.

## Chapter Summary

- Your role in teaching depends on the clinical setting in which you work. Never pass up an opportunity to teach.
- Encourage patients to ask questions.
- Periodically check to ensure that your teaching has been effective.
- Do not overstep your role as a medical assistant. The teaching you provide should clarify and complement information provided by the physician.
- A well-planned patient education program helps ensure that patients receive the high-quality health care they deserve.

## Warm-Ups for Critical Thinking

1. Look at the Maslow hierarchy pyramid. What level are you on? What steps can you take to reach the self-actualization level? If you are at that level, what steps can you take to ensure that you remain there?
2. Review the list of information that you should teach patients about their medications. Choose two medications, herbal supplements, or vitamins that you have taken. (The medication can be over the counter or prescribed.) Using all available resources, write the information for these two medications or supplements.
3. Review the material on fall prevention and preventing childhood injuries. Make a checklist of at least 10 safety tips for both groups. Take your list and visit an elderly family member, friend, or neighbor's home. Review these tips with the person. Inspect the home for safety. What improvements or recommendations were you able to provide?
4. Make a list of preprinted educational materials that every office should have. What professional organizations (e.g., American Heart Association, American Cancer Society) could help provide these materials?
5. From information found at the American Cancer Society's Web site, develop a patient education information sheet for the current guidelines for breast cancer screening.

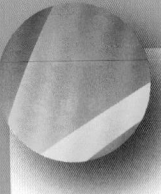

**PSY** PROCEDURE 4-1

## Document Patient Education

**PSY** Report relevant information concisely and accurately; and coach patients regarding:

a. health maintenance
b. disease prevention
c. treatment plan

**Purpose:** To record teaching that has occurred.

**Equipment:** Patient's chart, pen, student partner

| STEPS | REASONS |
|---|---|
| 1. Record the date and time of teaching. | To refresh the memory, make a legal and permanent note of your actions, and to facilitate the continuity of the patient's care. |
| 2. Record the information taught, for example, "Diabetes foot care was discussed. It consisted of the proper method for toenail cutting and regular examination by a podiatrist." | To refresh the memory, make a legal and permanent note of your actions, and to facilitate the continuity of the patient's care. |
| 3. Record the manner in which the information was taught, for example, "ADA (American Diabetes Association) foot care video shown to the patient." | To refresh the memory, make a legal and permanent note of your actions, and to facilitate the continuity of the patient's care. |
| 4. Record your evaluation of your teaching. For example, "Patient verbalized the need to make an appointment with a podiatrist." | To refresh the memory, make a legal and permanent note of your actions, and to facilitate the continuity of the patient's care. |
| 5. Record any additional teaching planned, for example, "Patient will return on Monday to the office with his wife for glucose monitoring instructions." | To refresh the memory, make a legal and permanent note of your actions, and to facilitate the continuity of the patient's care. |
| 6. Explain what you would do if you forgot to document an action you took during the patient education process. | Go back to the original entry and make the addition on a new line with today's date. For example: Current date. Addendum to 8/1/15 note: Also demonstrated back strengthening exercises. Patient voiced understanding and performed satisfactorily. Dierdre Hall, RMA
In an electronic record, you can edit the original entry with the above information. |

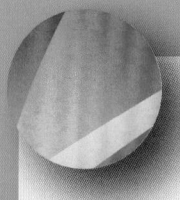

## PSY PROCEDURE 4-2

### Advocating on Behalf of Patients

**PSY** Develop and maintain a current list of community resources related to the patient's health care needs; and facilitate referrals to community resources in the role of a patient navigator

**Purpose:** To assist patients to identify and obtain assistance from available community resources

**Equipment:** Computer with Internet access

| STEPS | REASONS |
|---|---|
| 1. Assess the patient's needs. Does he or she need<br>  **a.** Education<br>  **b.** Health insurance coverage<br>  **c.** Financial information<br>  **d.** Support groups<br>  **e.** Home health needs | You must know what resources the patient needs. If there are several, organize the information to avoid confusion. |
| 2. Be prepared with materials already on hand. Create a resource for patients using Word or an Excel sheet, for example. | With each resource located, place the information in a manual so that you will have general information about the resources available to patients. |
| 3. Check the local telephone book or online directly for local and state resources. | Most telephone directories include a section for local, county, and state resources. Some patients do not have access to computers or the Internet. It is difficult for some patients to sort all of the information out. |
| 4. Check for Web sites for the city and/or county in which the patient lives. | Many patients do not have access to a computer, but phone numbers can be obtained from Web sites. |

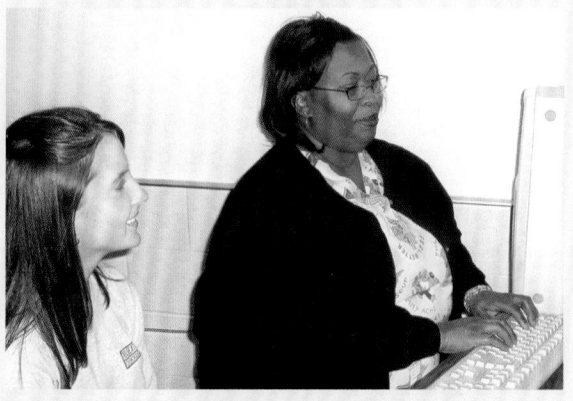

**Step 4:** Check Web sites for information.

| STEPS | REASONS |
|---|---|
| 5. Disseminate the information to patients at their level of understanding. | Remember that communication is not effective unless it is understood. |
| 6. Give the patient the contact information in writing. | Instructions for patients should be in writing to avoid any confusion or memory loss. |
| 7. Document your actions and the information you gave the patient. | If it's not in the chart, it did not happen. |
| 8. Instruct the patient to contact the office if there is any difficulty. | Always make sure the patient knows how to contact you. This is good customer service. |
| 9. Explain what suggestions or assistance you would offer to a patient who would benefit from online patient education resources but does not own a computer. | The patient can find insurance options at his or her state's Marketplace and could go to a public library, Internet cafe, or copy shop for public computer use. You could offer to print information for the patient if feasible. |

# 2

# The Administrative Medical Assistant

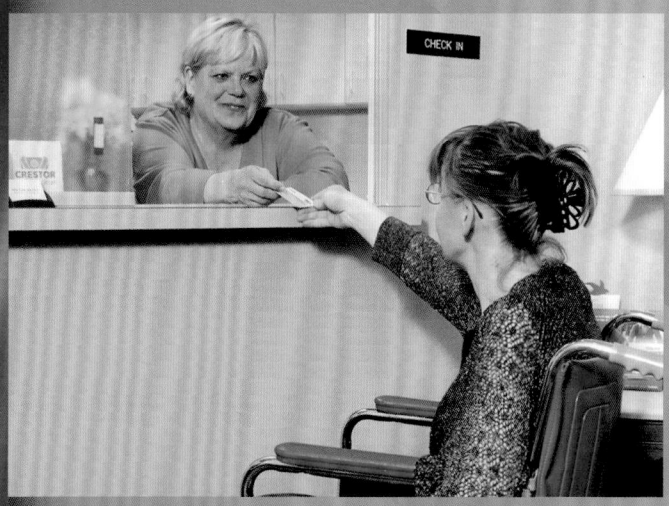

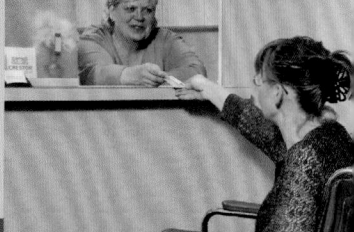

# UNIT TWO FUNDAMENTALS OF ADMINISTRATIVE MEDICAL ASSISTING

A well-run medical office requires that everyone works together as a team. Unit Two consists of six chapters that address administrative duties performed in the medical office. These duties include telephone and reception, appointment management, written communications, health information management, computer use, and medical office management. Some of these duties are shared with clinical personnel. This unit will help you to perform these duties whether you work in the front desk area or in the clinical area.

## CHAPTER

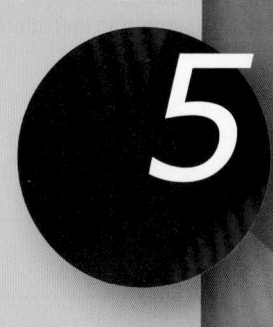

# 5

# The First Contact: Telephone and Reception

## Outline

**Professional Image**
Importance of a Good Attitude
The Medical Assistant as a Role Model
Courtesy and Diplomacy in the Medical Office
First Impressions
**Reception**
The Role of a Receptionist
Duties and Responsibilities of the Receptionist

Ergonomic Concerns for the Receptionist
The Waiting Room Environment
The End of the Patient Visit
**Telephone**
Importance of the Telephone in the Medical Office
Basic Guidelines for Telephone Use
Routine Incoming Calls
Challenging Incoming Calls

Triaging Incoming Calls
Taking Messages
Outgoing Calls
Services and Special Features
**Online Services**
Web Sites
Video Conferencing

## Learning Outcomes

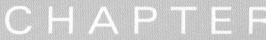 **Cognitive Domain\***

1. Spell and define the key terms
2. Explain the importance of displaying a professional image to all patients
3. List six duties of the medical office receptionist
4. List four sources from which messages can be retrieved
5. Discuss various steps that can be taken to promote good ergonomics
6. Describe the basic guidelines for waiting room environments
7. Describe the proper method for maintaining infection control standards in the waiting room
8. Discuss the five basic guidelines for telephone use
9. Describe the types of incoming telephone calls received by the medical office

10. Discuss how to identify and handle callers with medical emergencies
11. Describe how to triage incoming calls
12. List the information that should be given to an emergency medical service dispatcher
13. Describe the types of telephone services and special features
14. Discuss applications of electronic technology in effective communication

**PSY Psychomotor Domain\***

1. Demonstrate professional telephone techniques (Procedures 5-1 and 5-2)
2. Document telephone messages accurately (Procedures 5-1 and 5-2)

*(continues on page 112)*

3. Coach patients regarding (a) office policies (Procedure 5-3)
   - *Report relevant information concisely and accurately (Procedure 5-1)*

**AFF Affective Domain***

1. *Demonstrate empathy, active listening, and nonverbal communication*
2. Implement time management principles to maintain effective office function
3. *Show sensitivity when communicating with patients regarding third-party requirements*
4. Demonstrate awareness of the consequences of not working within the legal scope of practice
5. *Demonstrate sensitivity in communicating with both providers and patients*

6. *Demonstrate sensitivity to patient rights*
7. *Protect the integrity of the medical record*
8. *Recognize the physical and emotional effects on persons involved in an emergency situation*
9. *Demonstrate self-awareness in responding to an emergency situation*

*\*Note: AAMA/CAAHEP 2015 Standards are italicized.*

### ABHES Competencies

1. Use proper telephone technique
2. Receive, organize, prioritize, and transmit information expediently
3. Apply electronic technology

## Key Terms

| | | | |
|---|---|---|---|
| attitude | diplomacy | ergonomic | teletypewriter (TTY) |
| closed captioning | emergency medical service (EMS) | receptionist | triage |
| diction | | telemedicine | |

## Case Study

*A* deaf patient contacts Great Falls Medical Center using a telecommunications relay service (TRS) to schedule a new patient appointment. Landon Brown, CMA (AAMA), the new medical assistant working as the receptionist, takes the call. What is TRS, and how is it helpful for deaf patients using the phone? Can Landon receive the call if the office does not have a teletypewriter? Is this patient covered by the Americans with Disabilities Act? Are there any accommodations that must be made for this patient? The initial encounter between patients and receptionists often determines how patients will perceive their overall experience with the medical office. Providing good customer service to patients is a skill that requires a basic knowledge to handle all types of calls and good judgment that comes with experience. This chapter focuses on the tasks and responsibilities required of medical receptionists and how to perform these tasks efficiently.

As a medical assistant, you are the patient's primary contact with the physician. In certain situations, the patient may spend more time with you than with the physician. Your interaction with the patient sets the tone for the visit and directly influences the patient's perception of the office and the quality of care the patient will receive. Therefore, it is vital that you project a caring and competent professional image at all times. You will have responsibilities and duties that will vary among physician offices when working as a receptionist; however, proper telephone etiquette and use is an essential skill for *all* medical assistants. You must be able to handle incoming and outgoing calls correctly and efficiently.

The Health Insurance Portability and Accountability Act (HIPAA), which is discussed throughout this text, requires all health care settings to ensure privacy and security of patient information. HIPAA's Privacy Rule affects every area of the office. In waiting areas where conversations can be overheard or information can be seen by patients, you must take precautions to protect patient confidentiality.

## OG PROFESSIONAL IMAGE

### Importance of a Good Attitude

An **attitude** is a state of mind or feeling regarding some matter. It can be either positive or negative. Attitudes can be formed by past or present experiences; they can be transmitted from one person to another. How you feel influences how you act; thus, your attitude shapes your behavior. You transmit your attitude to others through your behavior, thereby influencing their attitudes and behaviors.

The medical assistant must be able to transmit a positive attitude to the patient. This requires acceptance of the patient as a unique individual who has the right to be treated with dignity and compassion in a nonjudgmental manner. Ask yourself how you would feel in a similar situation and how you would want to be treated. By demonstrating empathy, interest, and concern, you tell the patient that he or she is important to you and that you care. This exerts a positive influence on the patient's own attitude, behavior, and response.

For example, let's assume that you are working as a receptionist in a busy family practice office. It is the peak of the flu and cold season. Which of the following interactions between the medical assistant and the patient transmits a positive attitude to the patient?

- "I know you feel terrible, Mr. Smith, but so does everyone else in the waiting room. It's the flu season. Just have a seat, and the doctor will see you shortly."
- "I'm sorry you don't feel well. Do you feel well enough to sit in the waiting room for about 10 minutes? The doctor will be ready to see you then."

The second interaction shows the patient that you care about how he feels and reassures him that he will be seen by the physician shortly. In the first interaction, the attitude that was transmitted made Mr. Smith feel like just another sick patient. Your positive attitude will influence the patient's attitude, behavior, and response.

### The Medical Assistant as a Role Model

Another way in which you as a medical assistant influence the patient's perception of the medical office is your personal appearance. Good health and good grooming present a positive image to the patient. Taking care of yourself by eating well, exercising regularly, and getting enough rest is important not only for your appearance but also for your job performance. If you are tired or sluggish, you cannot give good patient care.

Pay particular attention to your personal hygiene to avoid offending your patients. A person who is ill is often acutely sensitive to odors, even those normally considered pleasant. A daily bath or shower is essential, followed by an unscented deodorant. Keep your hair clean and styled. Good oral hygiene is important, and during the day, you should avoid foods that may give an offensive odor. Keep your fingernails clean and trimmed, with clear or neutral polish. Long nails polished with vivid colors are not appropriate for the medical office, and natural nail tips must be less than a quarter inch long, according to the Centers for Disease Control and Prevention (CDC). Artificial nails may increase the potential for infection transmission to you and your patients. If you wear makeup, keep it natural, and apply it lightly. Do not wear perfume, cologne, scented lotion, hair spray, or anything with an odor that could be considered offensive to others as this could cause health problems such as a migraine headache in some patients and even an allergic reaction in others.

Most offices have a dress code that you will be required to follow, and whether you wear a uniform or street clothes, they should be clean, neat, and in good repair (Fig. 5-1). Wrinkles, missing buttons, split seams, torn hems, and stains project a negative image. Always wear clean, comfortable close-toed shoes. Stockings should be full length, of a neutral shade, and free from runs and holes. In addition to the dress code policy, most medical offices have a policy prohibiting visible tattoos and body piercings. These policies are designed to promote a professional image in the office and also are applicable for safety reasons. Jewelry such as dangling earrings, large rings, long chains, and ornate or multiple bracelets are not appropriate in the health care environment and could become hazardous when performing direct patient care.

### Courtesy and Diplomacy in the Medical Office

Being a medical assistant requires excellent human relations skills. In the course of a day, you will interact with a variety of personalities in a variety of situations, and you must be able to maintain a positive professional attitude regardless of how difficult the encounter may be.

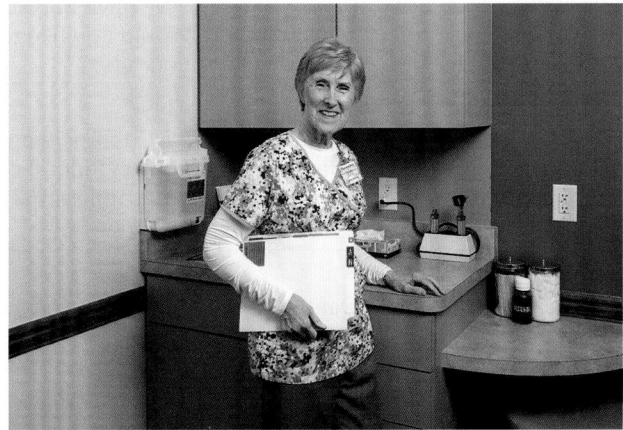

**Figure 5-1** • The properly dressed medical assistant presents a professional and positive image to patients.

For example, you may have to interact with a person who has recently been released from incarceration or is known to be abusive to others. It is important that you treat him or her with the same courtesy and respect that you offer all patients. Courtesy and diplomacy are fundamental to successful human relations.

Courtesy is based on sensitivity to the needs and feelings of others and demands that everyone be treated with respect and dignity. It is disrespectful to refer to physicians by first name or title only. Always use the title and last name. It is permissible to call a physician by his or her first name outside of clinical areas, but only if the physician so requests. Be courteous to your coworkers as well as your employer and your patients. Do not borrow supplies or use someone else's desk or computer without asking permission. Always knock before entering an office, even if the door is open.

**Diplomacy** is the art of handling people with tact and genuine concern. Use diplomacy in difficult situations. Patients may be curious about other patients; family members may want to know what the doctor said to the patient—such questions must be met with a polite refusal to disclose confidential information. Pain, worry, and waiting can make a patient unreasonable or irritable. You must exercise self-control and understanding and maintain your professional attitude. Never argue with a patient. Try to calm the patient by being attentive and listening to complaints in a nonjudgmental manner and communicate your desire to help. Table 5-1 lists three common problems with patients and the diplomatic way to control each situation.

## First Impressions

First impressions are lasting. Remember, you have only one chance to make a first impression on patients and other health care professionals. The patient's perception of the medical office is based in part on the impression you make. A negative perception can affect how patients perceive the entire health care encounter and may adversely affect their health. For example, a patient who has had a negative experience with the medical office may be reluctant to contact the office to seek medical attention if there is a health concern. A delay in treatment could potentially cause other health problems that could have been otherwise prevented. A positive perception contributes to a successful physician–patient relationship. Patients who feel positive about their relationship with health care providers are more likely to follow treatment regimens.

Patients want, expect, and deserve excellent customer service. Those who are not satisfied with their service may opt to leave, resulting in a loss of revenue for the practice. As a medical assistant, you play a key role in promoting a positive image for the physician's practice. It has been said that patients who have a negative experience will tell eight people. This can have a spiraling effect on your practice.

### CHECKPOINT QUESTION

1. What are four ways that you can demonstrate a professional image to patients?

## TABLE 5-1   PSY   Diplomatic Solutions to Common Challenges

| Common Problem | Example of What to Say | Example of What Not to Say |
|---|---|---|
| **Prolonged Waiting Time** | | |
| "My appointment was for 9:30, and it is now 10:00. When am I going to be seen?" | "The doctor will see you in about 30 minutes." <br> "We have had some emergencies. Would you like to wait or reschedule your visit?" | "It's flu season. Everyone is sick. Please sit down." <br> "We'll get to you when we get to you." |
| **Patient Confidentiality** | | |
| "I am worried about my neighbor. He was seen here yesterday and sent to the hospital by ambulance. What happened?" | "We appreciate your concern, but it is against federal privacy rules to give you confidential patient information." | "He was having some chest pain, but he is fine now." <br> "Yes, we sent him by ambulance because he was very sick." |
| **Patient Discomfort** | | |
| "I am in a lot of pain. I want to see the doctor now!" | "I can see that you are in pain. Please have a seat for 1 minute. I will find a room for you to lie down in." | "You are going to have to wait your turn. There are three patients ahead of you." |
| "I have been vomiting all day. I can't sit in the waiting room. I need to be seen now!" | "Please come with me. Here is a basin." | "I can see that you are sick. You'll still have to wait your turn. Here is a trash can." |

## 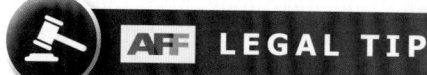 RECEPTION

### The Role of a Receptionist

The role of receptionist will vary greatly among offices. According to the 10th edition of *Merriam-Webster's Collegiate Dictionary*, a **receptionist** is a person employed to greet telephone callers, visitors, patients, or clients. In certain physician offices, the receptionist may be a nonmedically trained professional whose primary task is to greet patients and others coming into the office, alert staff members when patients are present, answer incoming calls, and possibly schedule appointments. If you are working in this type of setting, your role as a medical assistant will be to provide coverage while the receptionist is on break or at lunch.

In other office settings, however, you may work as the receptionist. These offices may also have multiple physicians but choose to have a medically trained person as the receptionist. No matter which type of office you work in, you will need to know and be able to assume the duties and responsibilities of a receptionist.

Some medical offices use self check-in at kiosks located in the reception area when patients and guests arrive. A receptionist or staff member may be available only to provide customer service support and assistance with kiosks as needed. Computers with touch-screen access allow patients to enter information about their arrival, which is then transmitted electronically to the correct person in the office. The computer will give instructions to visitors such as directing them to sit down until called back. Your role as the medical assistant in this office would be to greet patients when notified electronically of their arrival, check them in, and take them to exam rooms.

### Duties and Responsibilities of the Receptionist

The duties of the receptionist begin long before the first appointment of the day. Most offices have the receptionist arrive at least 30 minutes prior to the first appointment. Your first task will be to prepare the office for patient arrivals.

A waiting area and reception desk are places where confidentiality can be breached.

- Close the privacy window when you are not speaking with a patient.
- Never take patient information, demographic or clinical, at the front desk. Have the patient step to a more private area.
- Keep your voice down while discussing patients. Waiting patients may hear what you are saying.
- When making referral calls, use a telephone away from the reception area.

- Keep computer screens, printed appointment lists, appointment books, patient charts, etc., out of the view of patients at the window or around the reception area.
- Maintain the sign-in sheet in a manner that protects patients' privacy, such as obtaining signatures of patients upon arrival instead of leaving the sign-in sheet on the counter.
- Be mindful of patients' right to privacy as you go about your daily duties.

### Prepare the Office

As receptionist, you are responsible for preparing the office for patients and for other employee arrivals. These tasks should be done first:

- Unlock doors as appropriate.
- Disengage the alarm system.
- Turn on appropriate lights.
- Turn on computers, printers, copiers, and other electronic devices.
- If the office uses a drop box to leave specimens for evening pickups, check the box to ensure that the specimens were taken.
- Prepare a new patient sign-in sheet for the day.

After those tasks are done, do a systematic check of the office. The reception area should be clean and tidy. The reception desk should be free from clutter with confidential material safely out of sight. Restock your desk with necessary forms and office supplies before patients arrive. In smaller offices, you may be responsible for checking the examination rooms.

This process should not take long since the office should never be left messy or in disarray at the end of the day. Stocking of supplies and cleaning and disinfecting examination rooms should typically be done before the staff leaves at night. The office should be left in a professional manner.

## Retrieve Messages

Another responsibility you may have as a receptionist is to retrieve messages that were left while the office was closed. All physician offices have a method for communicating with patients after hours. Most offices leave a greeting message on their main incoming line that directs patients to call a given number (answering service) for acute medical problems or to go to the nearest hospital emergency room if the patient believes the illness or injury is life threatening. Usually, this message also instructs patients to leave nonemergency messages on the voice mail.

Messages may be obtained from four sources:

- Answering service
- Voice mail system
- Electronic mail
- Facsimile machine

No matter how a message has been sent, however, all information must be treated confidentially and handled according to HIPAA regulations. The Privacy Rule of HIPAA requires that you avoid inadvertently revealing electronically shared medical information. Box 5-1 provides suggestions to help you adhere to HIPAA's Privacy Rule.

Messages should be checked as soon as the office opens, at midday, after breaks, and periodically throughout the day. After retrieving the messages, forward them to the appropriate staff for resolution.

### Answering Service

Answering services receive calls from patients, hospital staff, and other physicians and communicate the emergency messages to the physician, generally by pager.

Other messages are left for the office staff to retrieve the following morning. Examples of messages that could be left are as follows:

- Patients calling the office for a sick appointment (not an emergency, such as an earache or flulike symptoms)
- Calls from hospitals or skilled nursing facilities about changes in patient status (new wounds or bed sores or patient falls without injury)

### Voice Mail Systems

A voice mailbox is a type of answering machine in which the caller can leave a detailed message on specific phone extensions. Most phone systems have voice mailbox capabilities with menu options for callers to choose the staff member to best handle their inquiry, such as the billing office. When retrieving messages for the receptionist, you will need to know the security code to access messages. After you obtain the messages, delete them from the recorder unless otherwise directed by office policy. Examples of messages that could be left here are as follows:

- Patients wishing to change or cancel their appointments
- Patients or pharmacies requesting prescription refills
- Family members or patients calling to ask for additional information or clarification about their medical care or test results

### Electronic Mail

The computer is a vital link for physicians to communicate with all health care professionals. E-mail messages are sent from other physicians, professional organizations, and hospital personnel. Some physician offices provide patients with their e-mail addresses, and other offices have patient portals via a personalized Internet Web site where patients can leave electronic messages as described below. Examples of messages left here are as follows:

- Memos from professional organizations
- Pharmaceutical representatives' updates or announcements
- Medical staff meeting minutes and announcements from hospital administration
- Upcoming continuing education courses for physicians
- Insurance representatives regarding billing issues
- Patient inquiries such as copies of medical records, tests results, prescription refills, etc.

### Facsimile Machines

All physician offices have a fax machine that is on a separate phone line apart from the main telephone numbers for the office. Because there is no guarantee that the information being faxed is going to be received by the correct recipient, anything faxed should have a fax

---

**BOX 5-1    Suggestions for Adhering to HIPAA's Privacy Rule**

1. Design office furniture to provide the most privacy around the front desk.
2. Keep monitors, fax machines, patient charts, etc., out of the sight of those at the front desk and in the waiting room.
3. Talk to patients about their private and protected health information in as private an area as possible.
4. Keep reception window closed when possible.
5. Be mindful that your conversations with coworkers can be heard by patients and others in the area.

cover sheet with a confidentiality statement at the bottom (see Chapter 7). The most common messages left here are as follows:

- Patient referrals
- Consultation reports
- Laboratory and radiology reports

## CHECKPOINT QUESTION

2. What four locations should you retrieve messages from?

## Prepare the Charts

Your next duty will be to gather charts. If using paper charts, gather them for the patients scheduled to be seen for the day and put them in chronological order by the scheduled appointment times. Review each chart to ensure that it is complete and up-to-date. Check that adequate clinical data sheets are available for the doctor to record any notes. Test results received since the patient's last appointment and any other new information are placed in the front of the chart for the doctor's review. If recent test results are missing, it is your responsibility to determine how to get those results before the patient's appointment. Make up a chart for each new patient and pull any referral information that may have been received. While many offices mail new patient registration paperwork well in advance of the scheduled appointments to be completed before the appointment, you must also have appropriate registration forms ready for patients to complete when they do not have the paperwork at the appointment (see *Register and Orient Patients* below). Once the charts are prepared, they are usually kept at the reception desk and given to the doctor or clinical medical assistant as each patient arrives, although some doctors prefer to have all charts on their desk at the start of the day (see Chapter 8).

## Welcome Patients and Visitors

Make every attempt to greet patients personally and by name, for example, "Good morning, Ms. Misko." A smile and cheerful greeting promote a positive image and make the patient feel welcome. Try to remember something personal about each patient, such as hobbies, pets, or special interests about which you can ask. Sometimes, you will not be at your desk when a patient arrives, so it is important to check the waiting room for new arrivals upon your return. Many offices install a bell or chime on the door and post a sign requesting patients to check in with the receptionist. Even if you cannot greet them immediately, acknowledge them with a smile and some sort of gesture, such as a nod, until you can help them. Acknowledging the presence of patients, even when you are busy, shows professionalism and courtesy that is a positive image for the entire practice. If it is your responsibility to greet patients, you should make this a top priority.

## Register and Orient Patients

Patients who are new to the office will have to complete registration paperwork that includes a demographics form, also called a patient information sheet. On this form, patients provide their name, address, telephone number, and possibly an e-mail address; the name, address, and telephone number of the insurance company or other party responsible for payment; employer names and addresses; marital status; spouse's name; social security number; and name of the person who referred the patient. Some information sheets include questions about medical history. Patient demographic forms must also be updated on a regular basis with established patients in order to have the most current information available. Current phone numbers are important if patients need to be contacted for scheduling conflicts, but collection efforts may become costly simply by not having current addresses to mail statements for outstanding account balances (see Chapter 15).

In accordance with HIPAA Privacy Laws, patients should also sign an Acknowledgment of Receipt of Privacy Practices for the office that should include how they would like to be contacted and where messages may be left such as e-mails, home phones, or cell phones. This notice should also explain how their private health information may be used as well as contact information for the person in the office handling matters involving potential violations of privacy. Most offices have patients fill in these forms themselves and ask for your help if questions arise. However, in some cases, it may be necessary to assist a patient with completion of the forms. Any assistance you may provide should always be done in a private area and away from others waiting in the reception area.

After registration, orient new patients to the office. Brochures that give the names of the doctor and staff, office hours, and contact information, such as telephone numbers and the practice e-mail, are helpful references for patients. (Keep in mind that they may also be given as a referral to your office to patients' friends and family!) Some offices also have a Web address with practice information and general patient education material that should also be noted in the office brochure. Explain any pertinent office policies or procedures, such as billing and financial policies, how to make or cancel appointments, and parking. Always give patients an opportunity to ask questions. Procedure 5-3 outlines the steps for explaining office policies to a new patient. There may be signs posted advising of the location of restrooms and water fountains, but you may have to direct patients when asked. However, it may be necessary for you to caution patients against using the restroom if there is a possibility that a urine specimen will be needed. Urine specimens are generally ordered for pregnant patients, patients with lower back or abdominal pain or back injuries, and patients being seen for drug or preemployment health examinations. At the appropriate time, you may be responsible for taking patients to the examination room unless another health care worker escorts the patients.

## Manage Waiting Time

Patients expect to be seen at the appointed time. Most patients are busy and have an allotted time in their schedule to see the doctor and do not want to be kept waiting. Unfortunately, one of the major complaints of patients is the length of time they must wait to see the physician. Advising patients if the doctor is behind schedule shows respect to patients and prevents unnecessary anxiety for lengthy wait times. If you expect the wait to be 30 minutes or more past the scheduled time, offer waiting patients some choices. Some choose to leave and come back later in the day, and some choose to reschedule the appointment for another day. Be honest with waiting patients. In some cases, it may be appropriate to tell patients why there is a delay. If the provider has been called away for an emergency, patients will respect the provider's dedication and appreciate the fact that if they need their doctor in an emergency, he or she will be there for them.

## Ergonomic Concerns for the Receptionist

For most of the day, you will be sitting at your desk performing these tasks. Occasional lifting of delivery boxes, paper supplies, and so on is required. The duties of the receptionist require you to twist from your primary desk to other areas to reach for files or to answer the telephone, which can lead to back injuries and other musculoskeletal disorders. Medical professionals are at high risk for such injuries. Having a good **ergonomic** workstation and good body mechanics, however, can prevent most injuries (see Chapter 10).

An ergonomic workstation is designed specifically to prevent injuries and often results in increased employee satisfaction and work efficiency. The Occupational Safety and Health Administration (OSHA) has many recommendations for preventing such injuries (Fig. 5-2). Here are some other suggestions to prevent injuries:

- Keep items that you must lift at waist level when possible. Keep the load close to the body. Bend at your hips.
- Instruct delivery people to place packages in locations that will not require movement.
- Carry only small loads of paper. Make additional trips as needed.
- Place items that you frequently use within easy reach. Moves from side to side are safer than twisting to a desk behind you. Avoid storing charts above chest level to limit reaching over your head. Use a step stool to reach high shelves instead of stretching.

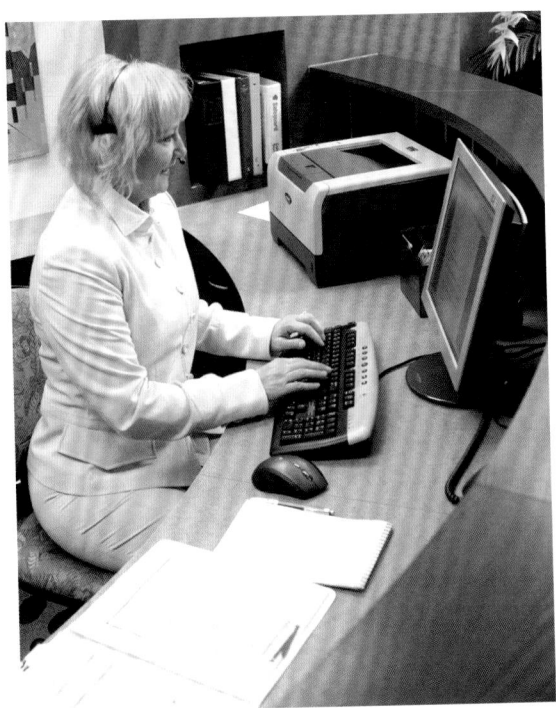

**Figure 5-2** • Use correct ergonomics when working on the computer to avoid injury.

- Telephones with headsets will keep your head upright and allow your shoulders to relax. If you use a stationary phone, a long handset cord can reduce muscle strain. Do not rest the telephone on your shoulder while talking, since this causes neck and back injuries.

## CHECKPOINT QUESTION

3. What is the purpose of having an ergonomic workstation?

## The Waiting Room Environment
### General Guidelines for Waiting Rooms

The reception area should be designed for the comfort, safety, and enjoyment of all patients. It should be kept clean and uncluttered, with the furniture arranged to allow ample room for walking. A coat rack and umbrella stand should be present. Restrooms and a water fountain should be easily accessible.

Furniture should be aesthetically pleasing, comfortable, and durable. Assessing the needs of the patients being served should be the primary consideration when choosing medical office furniture for the reception area. Chairs are preferable to sofas because they allow patients to maintain a degree of privacy and personal space. However, a specialty office, such as a gastroenterology practice that treats patients with gastric bypass surgery, may consider small sofas or oversized chairs for their patients. There should be a variety of soft chairs and firm chairs and chairs with and without arms. Some patients find it hard to stand up from a soft chair; others prefer the comfort. Some need chair arms to push themselves up, and others are more comfortable without chair arms. Pediatric furniture in the reception area may include a small table and chairs for the comfort of children.

A low-key color scheme is advisable. Muted pastels are preferable to bright primary colors, although the latter work well in pediatric offices (Fig. 5-3). Lighting should be bright but not harsh. The room should be well ventilated and kept at a comfortable temperature. Many offices provide soothing background music.

Landscapes, waterscapes, and floral and animal pictures make better wall décor than abstract art. Lamps and plants can add interest to corners. Keep plants in good condition, and remove any dead leaves, but keep in mind that some plants are toxic and should be kept away from small children. An office with dead or dying plants does not project a comforting image.

A good selection of reading material should be available. Have a variety of current magazines that are appropriate for your patients. The doctor's professional journals should not be included. The reception area is a good place to set out patient education materials.

Some offices provide television for patients who prefer not to read. Most patients find television relaxing and entertaining, but other patients find it annoying. Television can serve as an education tool. Here are a few tips that you should follow regarding television:

- The volume should be set to allow a group of people to hear the television but not at a distracting volume for the whole waiting room.
- A simple sign placed on the television, "Please do not touch the controls; see the receptionist for channel changes," will prevent patients from selecting inappropriate programs.
- Only family-oriented programs should be shown that is appropriate for the majority of patients being seen

in the office. It is acceptable to select a news channel. No shows with violence, strong language, or sexual content should be on. Soap operas are not suitable for medical office waiting rooms.

- Some offices leave the television off unless a patient asks to have it on.
- Patients with hearing impairments must be offered the option of **closed captioning** if they choose to watch television. (Closed captioning is the translation of the spoken word into a written format. Most televisions have this capability under their options menu.)

You should check the waiting room several times during the day to make sure it is clean and tidy. Also, check the entrance, hallways, and stairs for obstacles or hazards such as wet floors or light bulbs that are no longer working. Liability is a concern if patients slip or fall when coming into the office, and you should take care of hazardous conditions as soon as possible. If the problem is something you cannot take care of yourself, such as a burned out ceiling light fixture, it still remains your responsibility to contact someone responsible to resolve the problem immediately.

Regardless of how the furniture in the reception area is arranged, you must remain vigilant in keeping medical records, including computer screens, away from the view of patients. Remember, the privacy of all patients must be protected including the reception and waiting areas of the office (see Box 5-1).

 **PATIENT EDUCATION**

### Television as a Teaching Tool

A television in the reception area can entertain patients while they wait for an appointment, but it can also be a patient education tool. There are a variety of educational DVDs available. Here are some points to keep in mind:

- Be sure all material has been approved by the physician.
- Select DVDs and videos that are geared toward the specialty of the practice (e.g., a video about heart attacks is appropriate for a cardiologist's office but not for a dermatologist's office).
- Carefully assess the graphic nature of certain videos. (A film of the birth of a child may interest you, but it might be too much for some patients.)
- Keep in mind the age of the patients and family members who will be in the waiting room. Caution must be used if small children are often in the area. For example, a video about preventing sexually transmitted diseases may provide information appropriate for a family practice office, but it would not be appropriate to show the video in the reception area.

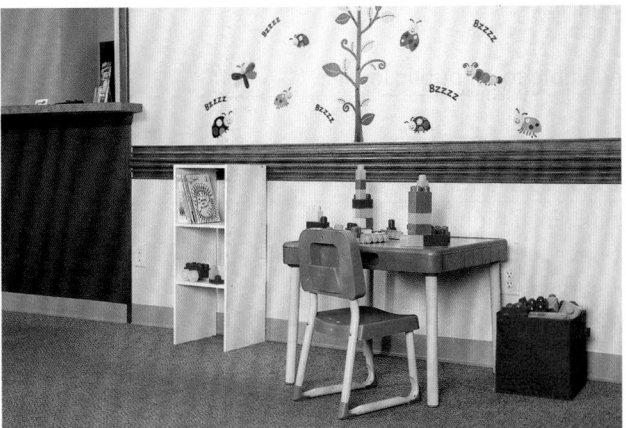

**Figure 5-3** • An example of an office waiting area that sees pediatric patients.

## CHECKPOINT QUESTION

4. What option should you offer hearing-impaired patients if they wish to watch television?

## Guidelines for Pediatric Waiting Rooms

Pediatric offices tend to be very busy practices with a multitude of reasons for patient visits. Generally, visits to the pediatrician can be divided into three types: well-child checks, sick-child visits, and follow-up visits. Although according to the American Academy of Pediatrics (AAP), no studies document the effectiveness of segregated waiting room areas, many pediatric waiting room areas are broken into two sections, one for well children and the other for sick children. Parents may have to be instructed by you as to which side of the waiting room they should sit in. The recommendation of the AAP is to move children with a communicable disease into an examination room as quickly as possible. Your employer will provide you with instructions and guidelines for dealing with sick children.

A children's play area must be closely watched and monitored. Toys should be kept away from the general seating area. Here are some guidelines for toys:

- Toys should be simple and easy to clean, without sharp edges.
- A policy must be in place for routine cleaning of these toys.
- Toys should be checked daily to ensure that they are not broken. Toys that are broken must be thrown away. Toys should never be glued or taped together.
- Battery-powered toys that make loud noises are not permissible.

- Toys can be a choking hazard. According to the American Heart Association, small children should never be given toys that can fit inside a standard toilet paper roll. Although older children would like to play with toys like Legos®, these toys should not be present. Older children should be expected to sit quietly while waiting for their appointment.

A good selection of books should be present for parents to read to their children. Books must be checked periodically to ensure that they are clean and no pages have been torn out. A small table and chairs will give children a place to read or color.

## Americans with Disabilities Act Requirements

The U.S. Department of Justice is responsible for ensuring that all people are treated without discrimination of any kind. The Americans with Disabilities Act (ADA) is a federal law that protects disabled individuals and prohibits discrimination on the basis of a person's disability. The ADA Title III Act requires that all public accommodations be accessible to everyone. This includes access into medical facilities. It is important that you be aware of the basic concept of the ADA rules. Table 5-2 lists some of the basic facility requirements. Additional information is available on the ADA Web site.

The existing structural dimensions are not something that you have control of, but you need to ensure that there is a clear path to the physician's office at all times. Here are some steps that you can take to ensure this:

- Check that deliveries are left in a safe place. They must not be left in the waiting area or block the door.

| TABLE 5-2    Summary of Americans with Disabilities Act Requirements for Public Buildings | |
|---|---|
| Area | Specifics |
| Access | Route must be stable, firm, and slip resistant. |
| | Route must be 36 inches wide. |
| Ramps | Ramps longer than 6 feet must have two railings. |
| | Railings must be 34–38 inches high. |
| | Ramp must be 36 inches wide. |
| | Ramps and elevators must be available to all public levels. |
| Entrance and door | Door must be 32 inches wide. |
| | Door handle must be no higher than 48 inches and must be operable with a closed fist. |
| | Interior doors must open without excessive force. |
| Miscellaneous | Carpeting must be no more than 0.5 inch high. |
| | Emergency egress system must have flashing lights and audible signals. |
| | Space for wheelchair seating must be available. |
| | Tables or counters must be 28–34 inches high. |
| Restrooms | Tactile signs must identify restrooms. |
| | Doorway must be at least 32 inches wide. |
| | All doors (including stall doors), soap dispensers, hand dryers, and faucets must be operable with a closed fist. |
| | Wheelchair stall is required and must be at least 5 feet by 5 feet. |

- Keep toys clear of entrance pathways.
- During the day, periodically check that chairs have not been moved in the reception area, thereby creating obstacles that might limit wheelchair accessibility.
- Ensure that doors are not blocked or propped opened with objects.
- Keep counters free of clutter and patient files (this may also violate HIPAA privacy laws!) that may limit all patients' access to you.
- Check the restroom regularly to make sure the entrance is open and not obstructed.

### CHECKPOINT QUESTION

5. What act prohibits discrimination of patients with disabilities?

## Infection Control Issues

To prevent the spread of disease, aseptic technique must be used in every aspect of work in the medical office. During the clinical portion of your training, you will learn detailed information about infection control. As a receptionist, however, you need to be aware of a few key points:

- Always follow standard precautions. This means that you must treat all body fluids with precautionary measures.
- Hand washing is the most important practice for preventing the transmission of diseases  You must wash your hands following all direct patient contact (touching the patient) (Fig. 5-4). Since it is not always possible to leave the desk to wash your hands, the CDC has approved the use of alcohol-based antiseptic hand washing solutions for health care providers.
- Patients are often told to bring specimens to the office. Never touch a specimen container without wearing proper gloves and personal protective equipment. Always wash your hands after removing gloves.
- Patients who arrive coughing and sneezing should be given tissues and instructed to cover their mouth and nose when coughing. Some offices may have disposable facemasks available for patients to prevent the spread of an infectious respiratory virus, such as the flu, to wear while waiting. Communicate with the clinical staff to have these patients taken directly into examination rooms. Patients who are vomiting, bleeding, or discharging other body fluids must not be left in the waiting room.

### Biohazard Waste

All body fluids must be considered infectious and be managed appropriately. All body fluid spills and blood-stained papers must be disposed of in accordance with federal, state, or local regulations. These spills must

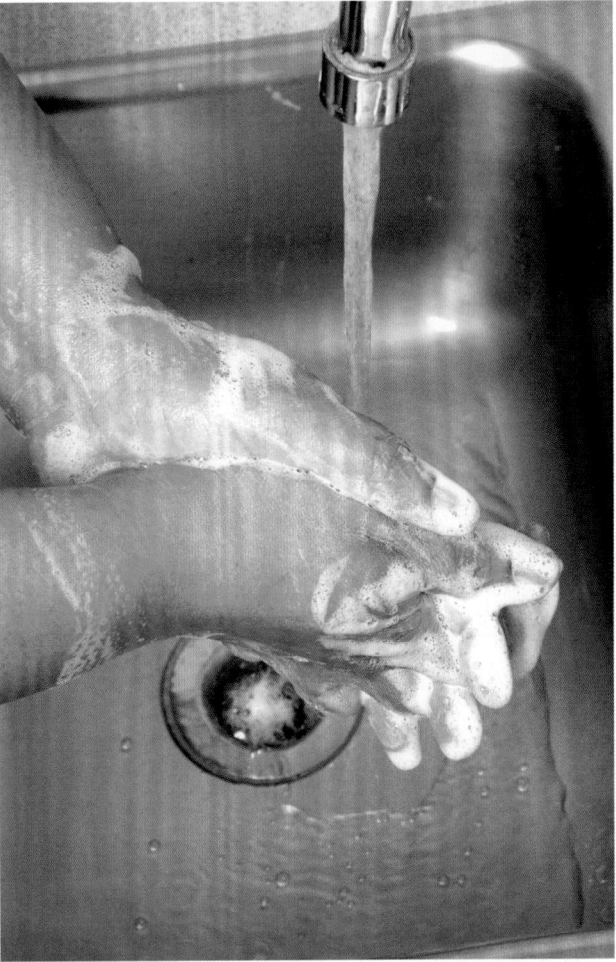

**Figure 5-4** • Good hand washing skills are essential to prevent disease transmission.

be cleaned with an approved germicidal solution. Although administrative medical assistants may have a minimal risk of exposure to biohazardous material, OSHA requires medical offices to provide Blood-Borne Pathogen Standard Training to new employees with training updated annually to all employees who may be exposed while on the job (see Chapter 17). If you have not been trained in handling such waste, do not touch it. Allow the clinical staff to handle the waste. If possible, contain the spill, such as placing an empty waste basket over it, and prevent other patients from touching the area. Here are some examples of biohazard waste that you may encounter:

- Dressing supplies with bloodstains from cuts or wounds
- Tissues from patients with acute nosebleeds
- Urine-saturated diapers left in the restroom
- Vomit
- Saturated tissues with sputum

### Communicable Diseases

Depending on the type of office you work in, the amount of exposure to communicable diseases will vary. Family

<table>
<tr><td>

**BOX 5-2**    **Patients Who Should Not be Left in the Waiting Room**

Patients with any of the following diseases or conditions should not be left in the waiting room. These patients should be taken to an examination room as soon as possible.

- Chickenpox
- Conjunctivitis
- Influenza
- Measles and rubella
- Meningitis (or suspected cases)
- Mumps
- Pertussis
- Pneumonia (if patient is coughing)
- Smallpox
- Tuberculosis
- Wounds (if open and draining)

</td></tr>
</table>

practice physicians and pediatricians, for example, treat acute communicable diseases regularly. If you work as a receptionist for a pediatrician, you will need to learn how to look at rashes and determine whether they are contagious. The physician will determine how to handle patients who may be contagious.

Good communication between you and the clinical staff is essential to manage patients with communicable diseases. The clinical staff is often aware of patients with such diseases and will communicate it to you. Most infectious diseases cannot be transmitted with routine physical contact (handshaking, talking, touching, sharing pencils, using the telephone). Examples of infectious diseases that cannot be transmitted by routine physical contact include HIV and hepatitis. Some diseases can be easily transmitted, however, and patients with these diseases should not be left in the waiting room. It is important to remember that frequent hand washing by everyone is the most important method to prevent the spread of infectious diseases. Box 5-2 lists patients who should not be left in the waiting room.

Patients who have an impaired immune system or are taking medications that hinder their immune system (chemotherapy agents) may require immediate placement in an examination room to prevent exposure to otherwise benign organisms. The clinical staff will alert you to these patients.

### CHECKPOINT QUESTION

6. What is the most antiseptic technique for preventing the transmission of diseases?

## The End of the Patient Visit

After physicians have completed the examination or other procedures, they generally direct patients to get dressed and wait for their discharge information. In some offices, physicians provide all discharge instructions, while in other office settings, medical assistants may be assigned to discharge patients and provide patient education as instructed by the physician. Chapter 4 discusses the information you need to teach your patients. After the medical portion is completed, patients are escorted to the front desk. It is generally at this time that any fees or copayments are collected by the receptionist. If the doctor has requested a follow-up visit, the appointment should be scheduled, and an appointment reminder card offered to the patient. You or other administrative personnel may do these tasks. You should bid the patient goodbye in a warm and friendly manner. As patients leave the office, they should feel they have been well cared for by a competent and courteous staff.

## COG TELEPHONE

### Importance of the Telephone in the Medical Office

The medical office is filled with expensive equipment used to assist in the diagnosis and treatment of disease, but one of the most important pieces of equipment is the telephone. It allows the patient rapid and easy access to medical care. A patient can schedule an appointment, seek medical advice, request prescription refills, obtain test results, question a bill, or report an emergency simply by picking up the telephone. The telephone also links the physician's office to the rest of the medical community, including hospitals, pharmacies, and other doctors.

You must be able to communicate a positive image of the physician and staff over the telephone without the aid of nonverbal cues such as appearance, facial expressions, body language, and gestures. You must be able to use the tone and quality of your voice and speech to project a competent and caring attitude over the telephone.

### Basic Guidelines for Telephone Use

Telephone communication is not effective if either party does not fully understand what is being said. Misunderstandings can be embarrassing, frustrating, or even life threatening. To have effective telephone communication, you must be able to overcome various obstacles, such as a noisy environment, a poor telephone connection, a patient's emotional distress, or a patient's hearing or speech impairments. Busy offices often provide cordless telephone headsets that allow mobility for receptionists as well prevent musculoskeletal problems from holding the phone while doing other tasks as already mentioned in this chapter.

## Diction

**Diction** refers to how words are spoken and enunciated. You should speak clearly and distinctly and use proper grammar. Talk clearly into the mouthpiece; do not prop the handset between your chin and shoulder. Never chew gum or eat while you speak on the telephone. Speak at a moderate pace to avoid slurring your words. Your grammar should be correct.

## Pronunciation

Make sure you pronounce words correctly to avoid misunderstandings. Avoid using unfamiliar words, slang, and idiomatic expressions. Most patients do not understand medical terminology, so it is best to use lay terms whenever possible. For example, do not ask the patient, "Are you dyspneic?" Instead ask, "Are you having trouble breathing?"

## Expression

Put a smile in your voice by sitting up straight and putting a smile on your lips. Speak with a modulated pitch and volume. Use proper inflection to avoid a droning, monotonous speaking style.

## Listening

Be an attentive listener. Focus on the conversation and ignore outside distractions. Guide the conversation to obtain the information you need from the caller, but do not interrupt the speaker. Some people tend to flood you with information, so in order to keep the call concise and to the point, you will need to direct the conversation without being rude. For example, Mrs. Jones calls for an appointment. When you ask her why she needs to see the doctor, she begins a detailed history of her headaches. You have what you need. You could say, "Mrs. Jones, let me interrupt you because I don't want you to have to repeat this to several people. The certified medical assistant will record all of this when you see the doctor." Although listening to the caller carefully is important, remember you are handling several telephone lines at the same time.

## Courtesy

Always speak politely and courteously. Address the caller by title and last name. Although many telephone calls interrupt your work, do not allow your voice to portray impatience or irritation. Using phrases such as "thank you" and "please" promotes a professional attitude (Fig. 5-5). Remember that you are there to help the patient.

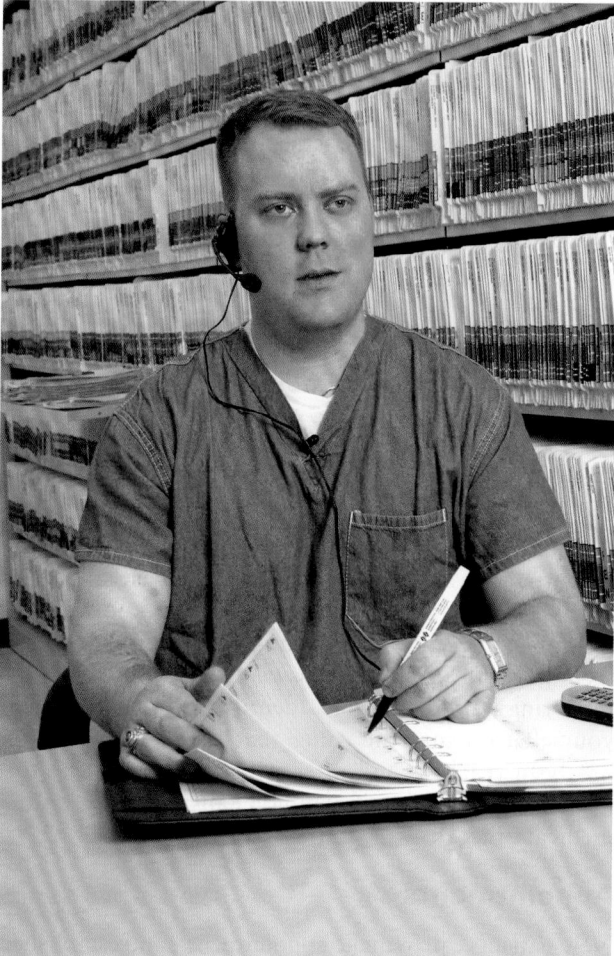

**Figure 5-5** • While speaking on the telephone, be courteous and professional.

Never answer the telephone and immediately put the caller on hold. If you need to answer another line or finish a task before you can engage in conversation, ask if the caller would mind holding. Courtesy demands that you wait for an answer before you place the call on hold. Also of great importance, you must determine whether the call is an emergency. If you are unable to take the call after 90 seconds, check back with the caller and ask whether he or she would like to continue holding. Again, wait for an answer before you place the call on hold. If the hold exceeds 3 minutes, you should apologize to the caller for the delay and offer to return the call as soon as you are available.

If you are already engaged in a telephone conversation and have to answer another line, ask the party with whom you are speaking if he or she would mind holding. Again, wait for a reply before answering the second call. Explain to the second caller that you are on the other line and need to complete that call. Do not handle the second call while the first party waits unless the second call is an emergency, a long distance call that cannot be referred to another worker, or a physician calling to speak with your physician.

Quite often, you will find that you are juggling the telephones and patients who are in the office. Exercise your best judgment in balancing the tasks. If the call is going to take a long time, ask the caller to wait a moment, address the needs of the patient in the office, and then return to the call. Remember, all information about and conversations with patients are confidential. Use caution when talking on the telephone in front of patients.

### CHECKPOINT QUESTION

7. What are the five basic guidelines for telephone use?

## Routine Incoming Calls

An incoming call should be given the same courtesy and attention as an arriving visitor. Just as you would not keep a patient waiting without acknowledging his or her presence, so too must you acknowledge an incoming call promptly. Answer the telephone by the third ring if at all possible. Identify both the office and yourself to assure the caller that the correct number has been reached, and offer your assistance. The following are examples of common calls that come into a medical office.

### Appointments

New patients call to make appointments, and established patients call to schedule return visits (see Chapter 6). It is important to always get current phone numbers from both new and established patients with every phone call received in the event that they will need to be contacted before their appointment.

### Billing Inquiries

In some offices, you may be responsible for handling routine inquiries concerning billing, fees, services, and insurance. You may be asked for specific information concerning the cost of services; do not quote exact prices, but tell the patient that costs depend on the type of examination and diagnostic tests performed. Sometimes, you may be requested to provide information to third-party payers for reimbursement purposes. This is permissible without the necessity of a signed release from the patient under the HIPAA provisions for release of information for treatment, payment, and operation purposes. However, only the specific information being requested should be released and only to the insurance company billed for that particular service (see Chapter 13).

### Diagnostic Test Results

Many laboratory and radiology reports are called in to the physician's office before the written copy is sent. Record the information and direct it to the certified

medical assistant or the physician as per office policy. If paper charts are being used, get the patient's chart and post the results on the front for the physician to review. If electronic medical records are used, a messaging system within the EMR may be used to notify the certified medical assistant or the physician of the test results. If the results are needed at once, bring the information to the physician's attention immediately upon receiving the report. Having at hand a blank laboratory slip or specially designed forms listing the most frequently ordered reports for your office will save time and make it easier to accurately record the results as they are relayed from the laboratory or radiology department. When diagnostic reports are received either in paper format or electronically, they must be signed by the physician indicating the results have been reviewed before being placed in the patient's medical record.

### Routine and Satisfactory Progress Reports

At the end of an office visit, a patient may be told to call in a progress report within a few days. If the patient says he or she is feeling better or getting stronger or the symptoms have resolved, take down the information, record it in the patient's chart, and place it on the physician's desk for review. You may also handle routine progress reports from hospitals, home health agencies, and other allied health professionals. For example, a home care nurse may call and report that a patient's blood pressure is now within normal limits, or a physical therapist may call the office and say that a patient's range of motion is improving. Again, record the information and place it on the physician's desk for review.

### Test Results

Patients often call for their test results, and many doctors allow the medical assistant to report favorable test results to patients. Your office will have a specific policy for handling these calls. It is illegal to give information to anyone other than the patient without the patient's specific consent. This consent should be in the form of written permission in the chart, in accordance with HIPAA regulations. Always document the call, as in Figure 5-6.

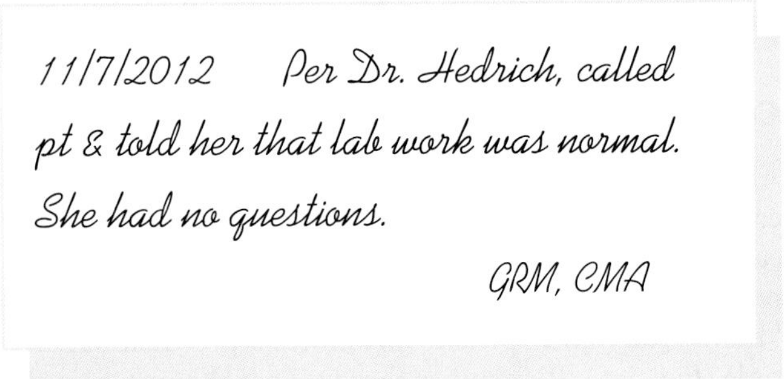

11/7/2012    Per Dr. Hedrich, called pt & told her that lab work was normal. She had no questions.

GRM, CMA

**Figure 5-6 •** Charting example.

## Unsatisfactory Progress Reports and Test Results

The doctor must speak with patients whose progress or test results are unsatisfactory. The urgency of the patient's condition determines whether the call requires the physician's immediate attention. The physician will discuss serious unsatisfactory test results with the patient. In less serious cases, the physician may ask you to speak with the patient. Never discuss unsatisfactory test results with a patient unless the doctor directs you to do so.

## Prescription Refills

As a medical assistant, you can handle requests for prescription refills if they are indicated on the chart. Most offices have an established protocol for refilling maintenance medications. If there is any doubt, tell the pharmacy or the patient that you will check with the doctor and call back.

## Other Calls

Other calls you ordinarily handle include requests for referrals to other physicians, clarifying instructions for patients, and calls concerning routine administrative matters.

Determining which calls the physician prefers to have transferred immediately and which calls can be returned later requires communication with the physician as well as experience in handling various types of incoming calls. Calls from other physicians should be directed to the physician immediately or according to office policy (Box 5-3). Physicians also receive personal calls and will usually tell you which calls should be put through immediately. Otherwise, take a message and tell the caller that the doctor will return the call.

# Challenging Incoming Calls
## Unidentified Callers

Sometimes, callers who ask to speak with the physician refuse to state their name or the nature of their business. In such instances, you should politely but firmly tell the caller that you cannot interrupt the physician and politely explain that you would be happy to take a message. If the caller persists, ask the caller to call back at a specific time when the physician will be available. Alert the physician that there will be a call for him or her at the specified time. Unidentified callers may be sales representatives.

## Irate Patients

When a caller is angry, you must be careful to keep your own temper in check. Try to calm the patient and offer assurance that you want to help. Listen carefully and take notes. If you cannot resolve the situation, let the patient know that you will take a message and see that it gets to someone who can help address the situation. Assure the patient that someone will call back and,

---

**BOX 5-3  AFF   Telephone Etiquette**

- When another physician calls, it is customary to give the call top priority. Many physicians instruct their receptionists to interrupt them. This shows the physician that you respect his time. Always ask the physician if you need to pull a patient chart before you get your doctor. If the call is about a patient, your doctor will need a chart. If it is a personal call or about something other than a patient, the calling doctor will say no. This way, you do not have to ask the nature of the call.
- Never put a patient on hold without first asking if they can hold and then waiting for a response.
- Include office extensions in the patient informational brochure so that patients do not have to listen to a long list of options. They can dial an extension to be put through immediately.
- Be respectful of the caller's time.
- Ensure that automated answering systems give the patient instructions to immediately bypass the recorded greetings in case of an emergency. For example, the first thing the caller should hear is "If this is an emergency, please dial '0' now."
- Make an effort to add the human touch to automated systems.

---

if possible, give a specific time frame such as this afternoon or within 24 hours. Depending on the staffing of the office, you may need to consult with the physician and offer to call back. Always tell the physician about complaints regarding medical treatment or care.

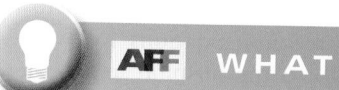

**AFF   WHAT IF**

**An upset patient calls with questions about her bill and demands to speak with the employee who handles accounts receivable, who is at lunch. What should you say?**

Patient: "Give me that woman who gets all of my money!"

Medical assistant (MA): "Mrs. Smith in the Accounts Receivable Department is out of the office for lunch. May I transfer you to her voice mailbox?"

Patient: "Absolutely not! Someone else there must know something about the billing."

MA: "I'll be glad to try and help you, Mrs. McGuire."

If you cannot answer Mrs. McGuire's questions, tell her exactly when she can expect a call from Mrs. Smith. Make sure that happens. By cross-training all employees to understand the billing process, you can give patients better service. Making notes in a memo area of your office computer's system will give every employee an opportunity to look at the patient's account and help patients when they call.

## Medical Emergencies

As a medical assistant, you must be able to differentiate between routine calls and emergencies. To do this, first try to calm the caller and ask specific questions concerning the patient's condition. Severe pain, profuse bleeding, respiratory distress, chest pain, loss of consciousness, burns, and a temperature above 102.0 °F are all emergencies. The professional medical assistant taking an emergency call will immediately gather appropriate information about the patient's condition in order to get the patient assistance as quickly as possible. Whenever possible, alert the physician of the emergency and, if the physician takes the call, get the patient's chart or pull it up on the EMR if you haven't already done so.

Determine the patient's name, location, and telephone number as quickly as possible in case you are disconnected or the patient is unable to continue the conversation. This will allow you to direct emergency personnel to the patient's aid. The office should have a policy for handling emergency calls when the doctor is not in the office. Most policies advise you to direct patients to go to the nearest emergency room or walk-in center.

Ask the physician to list instances that might constitute an emergency in his or her specialty and to describe how they should be handled. For example, if you work for a cardiologist, most of your emergency calls will be patients with chest pain and trouble breathing. The cardiologist may instruct you to ask the patient standard questions, have you instruct patients to take certain medications, and then instruct the patient to dial for an ambulance. If you are working for an obstetrician, your emergency calls will be related to patients who have labor concerns or sudden onset of bleeding. Most obstetricians have precise recommendations for when patients in labor should go to the hospital (e.g., contractions lasting more than 1 minute with a frequency of every 5 minutes). Once you have the list of the most common calls and what your response should be, put the list in a prominent place near the telephone.

## Triaging Incoming Calls

Usually, the office telephone has multiple lines, and frequently, several patients call at the same time. You must be able to **triage** (sort) them into a priority order. For example, any patient with a potentially life-threatening problem, such as chest pain, needs to be taken first. Follow your office policy for emergencies. Patients with serious but non–life-threatening problems should also be handled promptly according to office protocol. Callers who are upset or angry will become increasingly upset the longer they have to wait; handle these calls as quickly as possible. If you need to get back to the caller, do so in a timely manner. Do not leave messages unresolved.

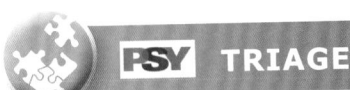
### TRIAGE

While answering the telephone, you must handle callers on four different lines:

**A.** Line 1 is a home care nurse calling the office with a patient status update.
**B.** Line 2 is a pharmacist questioning a prescription.
**C.** Line 3 is the mother of a 3-year-old child who has been vomiting for 24 hours.
**D.** Line 4 is a patient who is having trouble breathing.

#### How would prioritize these calls? Which one should be handled first? Last?

First, handle the patient on line 4. After gathering information about the patient's complaint and following office protocol, determine the best action. Instruct the patient to come in immediately or to report to the emergency department of a hospital. Next, handle Line 3 using office guidelines as mentioned earlier. Line 2 can be handled next. Even though the patient may be waiting at the pharmacy, the other two calls are more important since they involve the patients' conditions. Lastly, you may record the information on Line 1.

## Taking Messages

Taking messages for the physician or other health care professionals will be a large part of your daily responsibilities. Taking messages is easier using notepads designed for this task. Office supply companies have an assortment of pads, or your physician may choose to design his or her own. Carbonless copies give you a record of the messages taken during the day and the action taken.

The minimum information needed for a telephone message includes the name of the caller, date and time of the call, telephone number where the caller can be reached, a short description of the caller's concern, and the person to whom the message is routed.

Before you end the call, tell the patient when to expect a return call. Callback times vary from office to office. Some physicians return calls only at the end of the day, while others return calls randomly. Learn the policy of the office in which you are working.

The patient's chart must document all calls. If you return the call to the patient, document your conversation in the medical record. Some message pads are designed to be added to the progress note on the patient's chart when the call is complete. See Figure 5-5 for a charting example for documenting a call.

### CHECKPOINT QUESTION

8. What is the minimum information needed for taking messages?

# Outgoing Calls

## General Guidelines for Outgoing Calls

You will make outgoing calls as well as receive incoming calls. You should prepare for your calls carefully; have all information gathered and know what you want to say before you dial the number. If you are calling a patient to reschedule an appointment, be able to explain why the change is necessary and be prepared to offer a new appointment time.

At times, you may have to make long distance calls. You may be required to document calls for the office records. Keep in mind the difference in time zones; if you do not know the time zone of the city you are calling, check the front of the telephone directory. Long distance calls should be dialed directly, without operator assistance. If you dial a wrong number or become disconnected during the call, notify the long distance operator immediately to avoid charges. Never make a long distance call unless you are authorized to do so.

Your employer may ask you to place a conference call, which connects three or more people. Notify all parties of the date and time the call will be made to ensure that everyone will be available to participate. Participants should be given the access phone number and the access code in advance of the scheduled call.

## Calling Emergency Medical Services

Some patients will need immediate transport to a hospital. When emergencies occur in the physician's office, the clinical staff may be busy providing lifesaving procedures to the patient. As a receptionist, you will be directed to call the local **emergency medical services (EMS)** for transport. In most areas of the United States, the emergency number is 911; however, rural areas may have to dial the nearest emergency medical services. Prior to placing the call, obtain the following information:

- Patient's name, age, and sex (Age is important, especially if the patient is a newborn or child. This will allow the dispatcher to send the most appropriate responders.)
- Nature of the medical problem (chest pain, abdominal pain, bleeding)
- Type of service the physician is requesting. Generally, there are two levels of care: basic and advanced life support. Types of services will vary from community to community.
- Any specific instructions or requests the physician may have. Generally, patients are taken to the nearest hospital; the physician may have made arrangements for the patient to be admitted at a specific hospital, however, because of a condition or diagnosis. For example, a patient with a high-risk pregnancy may be sent to a hospital with an appropriate newborn nursery instead of the community hospital. It is important that this information be told to the dispatcher so the appropriate team can be sent.
- The location of the office and any specific instructions for access, for example, 92 Main Street, Medical Office Group, third floor, last door on the left. Keep in mind that hallways and doorways will need to be large enough to accommodate the stretcher, so another way to access the office other than the front entrance may need to be explained to the EMS.

After gathering the information, dial the emergency medical service number. Speak in a slow, calm voice to the dispatcher. Give the information. If the dispatcher has additional questions, answer them. Ask the dispatcher the approximate arrival time for the ambulance. Do not end the call until instructed to do so by the dispatcher (see Fig. 5-7).

After placing the call, alert the staff to the approximate arrival time and any other pertinent information. Ensure that the path for the ambulance personnel is unobstructed and accessible. Reassure other patients in the waiting room. If the patient has any family members present, offer them assistance and reassurance.

###  CHECKPOINT QUESTION

9. What patient information should you know before calling emergency medical services?

# Services and Special Features

The telephone system that is used for physician offices should be large enough to serve the needs of the office. For example, if you are working for a single dermatologist, two incoming phone lines may be enough. If you are a receptionist for a large family practice with multiple physicians and other practitioners, however, the number of incoming lines will be greater. Most offices also have unpublished incoming numbers or lines. Staff members, families, and other physicians primarily use these private lines. In addition, most offices have a direct line to the local hospital. A wide variety of communication equipment is available today, and communication consultants can help determine the appropriate services and equipment for your office. At minimum, the phone system should have recall, volume control, intercom, call forwarding, and caller identification.

An auto-attendant is the recorded message that answers your phones and instructs callers how to reach the person or department they are looking for. If an office has a high volume of calls, this may be important, or there may be value in having a real person

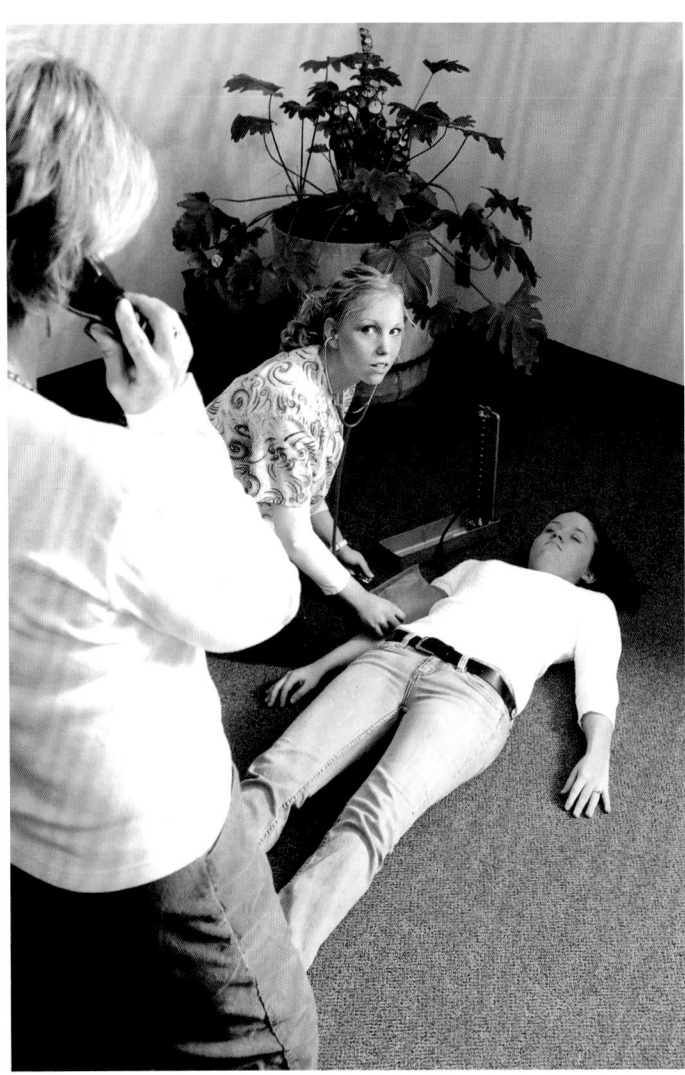

**Figure 5-7 •** No matter what role you play, an office emergency requires all employees to be prepared.

answer every call. You can help callers find the people they need with dial by name, dial by extension, or dial from directory services.

Phone sets themselves have more standard features, as well. Display phones have a small screen that shows information such as the name and extension of an internal caller, the duration of call, and in some cases, caller ID (identification). Speaker phones are familiar fixtures in many conference rooms but are also now standard on most new handsets. Speaker phones can be half duplex, which means that only one person on the call can be heard at a time, or full duplex, which lets both parties talk simultaneously, like a regular phone. Some phones also have a "listen-only" mode for speaker phone, which is useful for monitoring a conference call or while on hold. HIPAA guidelines for patient confidentiality must be considered when using speaker phone features. This should only be used in private areas of the office.

Most physicians have a cellular telephone with Internet access and text messaging available. This number should never be given to anyone, although it should be readily accessible for staff members. Physicians and other health care professionals also have pager systems. Most pager systems allow you to send typed messages to the recipient via the computer. These messages are displayed on the pager, for example, "Kate Larke's blood sugar was 420," or "Please call Dr. Harrison about Patrick Burke." Using technology to type messages directly to the physician is efficient and good time management. This feature is helpful when it is not necessary to speak with the person or a ringtone would be inappropriate.

## CHECKPOINT QUESTION

10. What is text messaging, and when might it be used?

## Telecommunication Relay Systems

Patients with hearing or speech impairments often have difficulty communicating with a standard telephone. The ADA requires that telephone companies have telecommunication relay systems (TRS) available 24 hours a day. A relay system allows the caller to type messages into a special telephone that transmits the message across the lines to the other party. The other party reads the message and types a response. The communication continues through written messages. A telephone with an attachment for typing messages is called a **teletypewriter (TTY)**. If the other party does not have the capabilities to read the message, an operator can be used to translate the message. Most physician offices have a TTY phone or access to one. The Federal Communications Commission has set minimum standards for TRS and TTY systems for public buildings. These standards can be found on its Web site.

- As the receptionist, you are the most visible and accessible representative of the medical practice. Duties and responsibilities of a receptionist vary among office settings.
- The key to being a good receptionist is to demonstrate tact and diplomacy in all interactions with patients. Providing a positive attitude will ease the patient's anxiety and ensure the best and most confident image of the practice is projected.
- Proper telephone etiquette and manners are essential for good patient care and to achieve effective communication among various health care providers. Triaging incoming calls is a skill that you must master if you are to be an effective receptionist.
- Excellent customer service is crucial to a successful medical practice.

## ONLINE SERVICES

### Web Sites

Some medical offices have a personalized Web site with information about the practice, such as contact information for various departments, practice policies, and patient education. Many offices use their Web sites to offer patients the convenience of online services including patient portals that so patients can ask general questions, request copies of medical records, etc., and receive a response within a short period of time from someone in the office. These patient portals offer the protection of privacy with a personal log-in and password. One of the duties of the medical assistant may be accessing, distributing, and responding to e-mails from patients'

or monitoring and responding to requests in the patient portals throughout the day (see Chapter 9).

## Video Conferencing

The use of technology in the medical office has made it very convenient for physicians to speak with other physicians and health care providers face-to-face via video conferencing. This type of technology may also be used to provide health care services remotely to some of their patients. Virtual office visits providing **telemedicine** services are becoming popular due to the flexibility and convenience they provide to physicians and patients alike. Although there are several services that offer telemedicine conferencing, they must be HIPAA compliant to maintain patients' privacy at all times. Working in a medical office utilizing telemedicine services may require you to log in to the service throughout the day and alert the physician to patients waiting to be seen online or to respond to patient e-mails through this service.

### CHECKPOINT QUESTION

11. What are some of the duties that may be required of the medical assistant working in a practice that utilizes telemedicine?

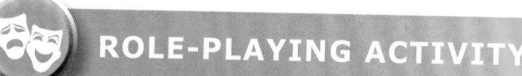

**ROLE-PLAYING ACTIVITY**

A patient arrives at Great Falls Medical Center for her appointment and has brought her three-year-old child who is unhappy about having to be at the doctor's office. Landon Brown, CMA(AAMA), is working at the reception desk and notices that the child has become very disruptive in the reception area by talking loudly and throwing magazines on the floor. While the mother is trying to keep the child quiet, she is not having much success, and the situation seems to be getting worse as several patients now seem annoyed. What should Landon say to the mother to calm the situation down in the reception area? What are some things he can do to distract the child? Role-play this scenario as the medical assistant, and think about how you would demonstrate professionalism and sensitivity in handling this child in way that will not offend the mother, but will give relief to the other patients waiting in the reception area. If you are the patient, think about how the mother might be feeling about her child's behavior. Embarrassment? Anger? Defensiveness? How do you think she might respond to Landon's intervention? Your instructor will give you additional information about this activity!

## *español* SPANISH TERMINOLOGY

**¡Hola!**
Hello!

**¿Cómo se llama usted?**
What is your name?

**¿En qué puedo servirle?**
May I help you?

**¿Por favor me podría dar su domicilio?**
Can you please tell me your address?

**¿Cuál es el código postal?**
What is the zip code?

**¿Cuál es su número de teléfono?**
What is your phone number?

**¿Fecha de nacimiento?**
What is your birth date?

**¿Cuántos años tiene?**
How old are you?

**¿Por favor podría tomar asiento en la sala de espera?**
Can you please have a seat in the waiting room?

**¿Podría hacerle unas preguntas?**
Can I ask you some questions?

**¿Por favor podría llenar estos documentos?**
Can you please fill out these documents?

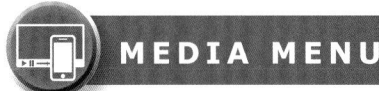

## MEDIA MENU

**Student Resources** on thePoint®
• **CMA/RMA Certification Exam Review**

**Internet Resources**
**American Academy of Pediatrics**
http://www.aap.org

**American Heart Association**
http://www.heart.org

**Centers for Disease Control and Prevention**
http://www.cdc.gov

**Federal Communications Commission**
http://www.fcc.gov/cib/dro

**Institute for Disabilities Research and Training**
http://www.idrt.com

**Online Yellow Pages**
http://www.yellowpages.com

**Occupational Safety and Health Administration**
http://www.osha.gov

**Telecommunications for the Deaf**
http://www.amrad.org/

**U.S. Department of Justice/Americans with Disabilities Act**
http://www.ada.gov

## EMR Activity

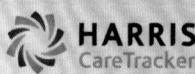

Harris CareTracker is a web-based electronic medical record (EMR) application that you will use for the EMR activities included in this section at the end of each chapter. This application is actually used in physician offices, but is provided to you through the publisher, Wolters Kluwer Health, to give you hands-on practice working with EMRs. Your instructor will have more information about accessing your username, login, and Quickstart guide.

Prerequisite Activities in Harris CareTracker

- *The Getting Started and Quickstart documents and EMR Activities Step-by-Step Instructions are available at* http://thePoint.lww.com/KronenbergerComp5e

Activity Details

Research a service in your area that provides sign language interpretation for hearing impaired patients. Using the *Mail* feature in Harris CareTracker EMR, send an email message with the details of your findings to your instructor. Include details available for the service, such as the cost.

## Chapter Summary

- As the receptionist, you are the most visible and accessible representative of the medical practice. Duties and responsibilities of a receptionist vary among office settings.
- The key to being a good receptionist is to demonstrate tact and diplomacy in all interactions with patients. Providing a positive attitude will ease the patient's anxiety and ensure that the best and most confident image of the practice is projected.
- Proper telephone etiquette and manners are essential for good patient care and to achieve effective communication among various health care providers. Triaging incoming calls is a skill that you must master if you are to be an effective receptionist.
- Excellent customer service is crucial to a successful medical practice.

## Warm-Ups for Critical Thinking

1. How would you calm an irate patient on the telephone? Identify some phrases that you might use to calm the caller. What phrases may make the situation worse?
2. Assume you are working in an obstetrician's office. What kinds of educational videos might be appropriate for the waiting room? What if you were working in an orthopedic office or for a surgeon?
3. Describe how you would handle a patient who is vomiting in the waiting room.
4. Assume you are working for a pediatrician. A mother arrives carrying an 18-month-old child with symptoms of a respiratory illness. As per office policy, you direct her to sit in the sick-child area. The mother refuses. What do you do?
5. A caller asks to speak to the office manager about a supply order on line 1, a patient is on line 2 complaining of chest pain, and line 3 is another patient needing a stronger pain medication. How would you handle these three callers?
6. A caller asks to speak to the physician directly. How would you respond?

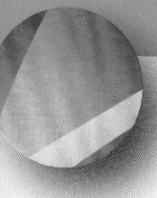

## PSY PROCEDURE 5-1

# Handling Incoming Calls

**PSY** Demonstrate professional telephone techniques; and report relevant information concisely and accurately.

**Purpose:** To receive calls into the practice and route them accordingly or take messages as appropriate

**Equipment:** Telephone, telephone message pad, writing utensil (pen or pencil), and headset (if applicable)

| STEPS | PURPOSE |
|---|---|
| 1. Gather the needed equipment. | Ensures that all materials are available and ready for use. |
| 2. Answer the phone within three rings. | Demonstrates professionalism and courtesy to the caller. |
| 3. Greet caller with proper identification (your name and the name of the office). | Demonstrates professionalism and courtesy to the caller. |
| 4. Identify the nature or reason for the call in a timely manner. | Allows the call to be appropriately managed. |
| 5. Triage the call appropriately. | Prompt identification of emergency calls is important for good patient care. |
| 6. Communicate in a professional manner and with unhurried speech. | Demonstrates compassion and caring for the patient. An unhurried speech pattern is reassuring to the patient. |
| 7. Clarify information as needed. | Prevents errors in communication. |
| 8. Record the message on a message pad. Include name of caller, date, time, telephone number where the caller can be reached, description of the caller's concerns, and person to whom the message is routed. | Promotes good communication between you and the recipient of the message. |

| FOR DOCTOR  Stephens | DATE  4/4/12 | URGENT  ☐ |
|---|---|---|
| PATIENT  Tommy Taylor | TIME  10 am | REFILL  ☐ |
| CALLER TEL.  312-462-5515 | AGE  42 | TEMP  N/A |
| MEDICATION  N/A | | WT.  N/A |
| MESSAGE  Per your instructions, pt. called to report improvement. He states he feels "a million times better." | | |
| PHARMACY / TELEPHONE  N/A | ALLERGIES  NKDA | RECEIVED BY  LF, CMA |

Step 8: Record the message.

*(continues on page 134)*

## PROCEDURE 5-1 (continued)

| STEPS | PURPOSE |
|---|---|
| 9. Give the caller an approximate time for a return call. | Provides reassurance to the patient that the call will be handled promptly and timely. |
| 10. Ask the caller whether he or she has any additional questions or needs any other help. | Confirms that the patient's needs have been met. |
| 11. Allow the caller to disconnect first. | Ensures that the caller has completed the communication. |
| 12. Put the message in an assigned place. | Having a certain place assigned ensures that the call will be handled correctly and the intended recipient gets the information. |
| 13. Complete the task within 10 minutes. | Ensures that the call is handled promptly and efficiently. |
| 14. **AFF** Explain how you would respond to a patient who is obviously angry. | You must remain calm yourself or you will make the patient more angry. Keep your voice calm and at a low volume. Have the patient go to an area away from waiting patients and listen carefully to their issue. Above all, remain calm. |

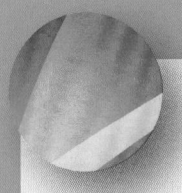

## **PSY** PROCEDURE 5-2

### Calling Emergency Medical Services

**PSY** Demonstrate professional telephone techniques

**Purpose:** To instruct a new patient about office policies based on their individual needs and level of comprehension

**Equipment:** Telephone, patient information, and writing utensil (pen, pencil)

| STEPS | REASONS |
|-------|---------|
| 1. Obtain the following information before dialing: patient's name, age, sex, nature of medical condition, type of service the physician is requesting, any special instructions or requests the physician may have, your location, and any special information for access. | Information is necessary for quick and correct dispatch of EMS personnel. Certain types of patients require special teams for transport. |
| 2. Dial 911 or other EMS number. | The call cannot be placed if the number is not dialed correctly. |
| 3. Calmly provide the dispatcher with the above information. | This allows information to be communicated quickly and professionally. |
| 4. Answer the dispatcher's questions calmly and professionally. | Allows dispatcher to obtain any additional information and verify the message |
| 5. Follow the dispatcher's instructions, if applicable. | Following instructions provides good patient care. |
| 6. End the call as per dispatcher instructions. | Ensures that all communication needs have been met |
| 7. Complete the task within 10 minutes. | Prompt access to EMS promotes good patient care and is essential for good outcomes. |
| 8. **AFF** Explain how you would respond to a family member who is getting in the way of performing this task. | If feasible, ask the family member to step outside the exam room. If not, explain to the family member and the patient that you need them to let you do your work so you can get the patient transported as quickly and safely as possible. |

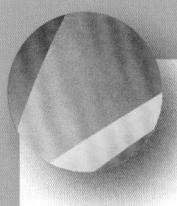

**PSY** PROCEDURE 5-3

## Explain General Office Policies

**PSY**  Coach patients regarding (a) office policies.

**Purpose:** To instruct a new patient about office policies based on the patient's individual needs and level of comprehension

**Equipment:** Patient's chart; office brochure

| STEPS | PURPOSE |
|---|---|
| 1. Assess the patient's level of understanding. | Patients may have hearing difficulties, mental deficiencies, inability to read, etc. |
| 2. Review important areas and highlight these in the office brochure. | Information about hours of operation, refill request procedures, etc., would be needed more than directions to the office, for example. |
| 3. Ask the patient if he or she understands or has any questions. | Ensures that the patient understood the information you provided and gives the patient an opportunity to clarify information or ask any additional questions |
| 4. Give the patient the brochure to take home. | Patients can read printed materials to refresh the memory. |
| 5. Put in place a procedure for updating information and letting patients know of changes. | A printed announcement of changes in hours, availability, services, etc., will keep patients informed. |
| 6. **AFF** Explain how you would instruct a hearing-impaired patient about office procedures. | Speak clearly in a normal volume. Face the patient when speaking to them. Do not exaggerate the movement of your mouth as you speak. Many hearing-impaired patients are lip readers. Be sure to give the patient complete information in writing as well. It is always helpful to have family members accompany the patient if possible. |

# 6 Managing Appointments

## Outline

## Learning Outcomes

**COG Cognitive Domain***

1. Spell and define the key terms
2. *Identify different types of appointment scheduling methods*
3. *Identify advantages and disadvantages of the following appointment systems:*
   a. *Manual*
   b. *Electronic*
4. Describe scheduling guidelines
5. Explain guidelines for scheduling appointments for new patients, return visits, inpatient admissions, and outpatient procedures
6. Recognize office policies and protocols for handling appointments
7. *Identify critical information required for scheduling patient procedures*
8. Discuss referral process for patients in a managed care program
9. List three ways to remind patients about appointments

10. Describe how to triage patient emergencies, acutely ill patients, and walk-in patients
11. Describe how to handle late patients
12. Explain what to do if the physician is delayed
13. Describe how to handle patients who miss their appointments
14. Describe how to handle appointment cancellations made by the office or by the patient

**PSY Psychomotor Domain***

1. *Manage appointment schedule, using established priorities (Procedure 6-1)*
   a. Schedule an appointment for a new patient (Procedure 6-1)
   b. Schedule an appointment for a return visit (Procedure 6-2)
2. *Schedule a patient procedure (Procedure 6-3)*
   a. Schedule an appointment for a referral to an outpatient facility (Procedure 6-3)
   b. Arrange for admission to an inpatient facility (Procedure 6-4)

*(continues on page 138)*

**3.** *Verify eligibility for services, including documentation (Procedure 6-3)*

**4.** *Obtain precertification, or preauthorization including documentation (Procedure 6-4)*

**5.** *Apply third-party managed care policies and procedures (Procedure 6-3 and Procedure 6-4)*

**6.** Use office hardware and software to maintain office systems (Procedure 6-2)

**7.** *Coach patients regarding:*
   **a.** *Office policies (Procedure 6-1)*

**AFF Affective Domain\***

**1.** Implement time management principles to maintain effective office functions

**2.** *Demonstrate:*
   **a.** *Empathy*
   **b.** *Active listening*
   **c.** *Nonverbal communication*

**3.** *Demonstrate respect for individual diversity including:*
   **a.** *Gender*
   **b.** *Race*
   **c.** *Religion*

**d.** *Age*
**e.** *Economic status*
**f.** *Appearance*

**4.** Communicate in language the patient can understand regarding managed care and insurance plans

**5.** Demonstrate recognition of the patient's level of understanding in communications

**6.** *Display sensitivity when managing appointments*

*\*Note: AAMA/CAAHEP 2015 Standards are italicized.*

**ABHES Competencies**

1. Schedule and manage appointments
2. Schedule inpatient and outpatient admissions
3. Be impartial and show empathy when dealing with patients
4. Apply third-party guidelines
5. Obtain managed care referrals and precertification
6. Apply computer application skills using a variety of different electronic programs including both practice management software and EMR software
7. Communicate on the recipient's level of comprehension
8. Serve as liaison between the physician and others

## Key Terms

| | | | |
|---|---|---|---|
| acute | constellation of symptoms | precertification | streaming |
| buffer | consultation | providers | wave scheduling system |
| chronic | double booking | referral | |
| clustering | matrix | STAT | |

## Case Study

*R*onnie Wilson, RMA, is handling the scheduling duties for the next week for all of the physicians at Great Falls Medical Center while the scheduler is on vacation. The practice currently uses the appointment scheduling feature in their electronic medical record. In addition to scheduling many appointments for patients with acute illnesses, Ronnie must also block off next Thursday afternoon and all day next Friday for personal leave time for one of the physicians, Dr. Kyle Dunn. The office manager has also asked him to matrix the appointment schedule for the upcoming American Medical Association (AMA) conference in 3 months, which all of the physicians have decided to attend. What is matrixing the appointment schedule? What does Ronnie need to know, and how will he accomplish this task? Does Ronnie need any scheduling guidelines? Are there different types of appointment scheduling options? How should he handle patients who cancel their appointments? An office that has an efficient scheduling system not only alleviates stress for everyone involved, including the physicians, but also promotes patient satisfaction. This chapter focuses on managing patient appointments to keep the schedule moving forward in an orderly manner.

Responsibility for scheduling and managing the flow of patient care in a medical office or clinic is one of the most important duties assigned to a medical assistant. As appointment manager, you make the first, last, and most durable impression on the patient and **providers**. Depending on your demeanor and actions, that impression can be favorable or unfavorable. A properly used appointment system helps maintain an efficient office. If improperly used, it can mean confusion and chaos; more important, it can waste precious time for the patient, the provider, and the staff.

To use the office facilities and the physician's availability most efficiently, determine which patients will be seen, when they will be seen, and how much time to allot to each of them, depending on their problems. Of course, every practice will have occasional delays and emergencies. Your responsibility is to manage all of this while maintaining a calm, efficient, and polite attitude.

# APPOINTMENT SCHEDULING SYSTEMS

There are two systems of appointment scheduling for outpatient medical facilities: the manual system, which uses an appointment book, and a computerized scheduling system. The choice of systems will depend on the size of the practice, how many providers' schedules must be managed, and the preferences of the staff responsible for the daily schedule. Whether a medical office uses a manual or computerized system, many of the guidelines for effectively scheduling the workday discussed in this chapter are the same.

## Manual Appointment Scheduling

Medical offices may choose to use a manual appointment scheduling system even if the other administrative functions in the office are computerized.

### The Appointment Book

If your medical office uses a manual system of scheduled appointments for patient office visits, you will need an appointment book. These are relatively inexpensive and may be purchased through an office supply store and available in a variety of formats. The typical appointment book provides space for noting appointments for an entire year. It may have a single sheet for each day and a separate page for each provider or show an entire week on two facing pages. Some offices prefer an appointment book with pages showing only one day at a time; others may want to see a whole week at a glance. A different color page for each day may also be desired.

The more information required for scheduling, the larger the pages should be. Make sure the book has enough space for all pertinent information (e.g., patient's name, telephone number, reason for visit), is divided into time units appropriate for your practice (e.g., 10- or 15-minute intervals), can open flat on the desk where it will be used, and fits easily into its storage place when not in use.

One of the limitations to using an appointment book is that it may only be accessed by one person at a time. When one person is scheduling, another person must wait until the book is available before scheduling another patient. Another limitation is searching for an appointment that has been scheduled in advance but has been misplaced by the patient. The medical assistant must look on several pages to locate where the appointment is scheduled.

Once you have acquired and prepared an appointment book (see *Establishing a Matrix* below), it is not enough to schedule a time and date for a patient visit and hope everything will run smoothly. Before actually making an appointment, you should review the schedule carefully, evaluating the needs of each patient and considering the physician's preferences and availability of the office facilities. At the beginning of each day, copies of the schedule should be distributed to all staff members. Along with the notations in a patient's chart, the pages of the appointment book provide documentation of a patient's visits and any changes, such as cancellations and rescheduled appointments. This provides further legal documentation to protect the physician and the patient in case of a dispute, as discussed in Chapter 2.

## Computerized Appointment Scheduling

Medical management software designed to assist with administrative functions includes systems for appointment scheduling. Although electronic health records are primarily for patient records, many also have scheduling capabilities. Computerized scheduling is more expensive than is using an appointment book; however, there are many advantages to using this technology. For example, information used to establish a matrix (e.g., hospital rounds 7:30 to 8:30, lunch 12:30 to 1:30) has to be entered only once. The schedule can also be accessed by more than one person at a time, allowing multiple people to assist patients with their appointments.

Any medical office software will have an appointment toolbar that requires one click to add a patient, add to the waiting list, see a calendar, or search for available times. Many software packages offer an advanced search that defines the resources required for a certain type of appointment.

This quick method allows you to search for available appointment times. Typically, you enter the desired date, and the computer displays the schedule for that day, showing any available time slots. Another feature allows you to search the appointment database for the next available time slot. For example, a patient is instructed to return in 3 months and has a preference for the time of day. You can search for the first available afternoon appointment with that particular provider.

Depending on the specific software, you can also print numerous documents, such as the daily or weekly appointment schedule, appointment reminders, or billing slips. Once the daily schedule is printed, this important document is referred to as the daily activity sheet or the day sheet and is the guide for everyone involved in the flow of patient care. Figure 6-1 shows a computer-generated daily activity sheet.

An important advantage to computerized appointment scheduling is the easy access to billing information. For example, a patient may call for an appointment, and the medical assistant can inform the patient that he needs to pay his balance due of $32 when he comes in to be seen. Credit and collections are discussed in Chapter 12.

### Establishing a Matrix

Before you begin using either scheduling system, you will have to set up a **matrix**. A matrix is established by crossing out times that providers are unavailable for patient visits (Fig. 6-2). For example, the physician may have a breakfast meeting and not be in the office until 10:00 AM on certain days of the week. This is indicated by crossing out the blocks from 8:00 to 10:00 AM with the first appointment that can be scheduled available at 10:00 AM Write in the reason for crossing off the space (e.g., vacation, meeting, hospital rounds). Some practices reserve specific times or even days for certain types of appointments, such as physical examinations and surgery. Also, some physicians may instruct you to block off 15 to 30 minutes each morning and afternoon to accommodate emergencies, late arrivals, and other delays. Some physicians want their professional or personal obligations noted on the appointment schedule so

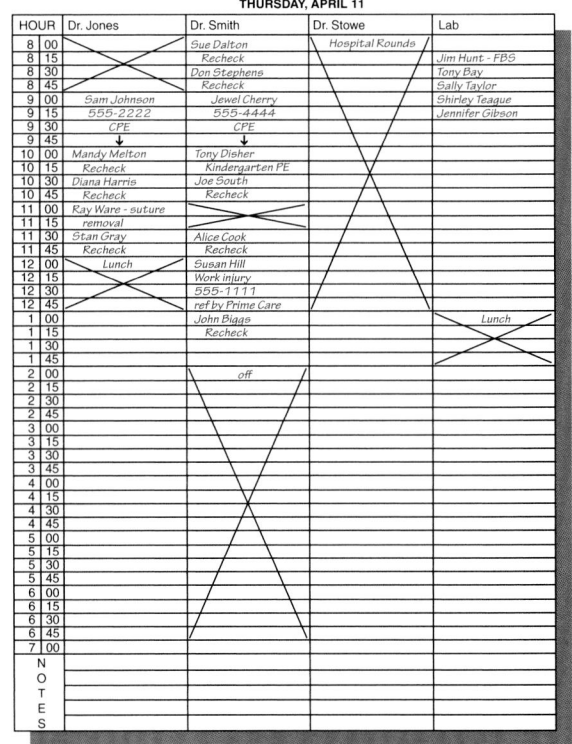

**Figure 6-2 •** Sample page from manual appointment book.

that patients are not booked immediately before these times. Always be sure to follow office policies to determine when to block the schedule.

### CHECKPOINT QUESTION

1. What is the purpose of a matrix?

## TYPES OF SCHEDULING

### Structured Appointments

Most medical offices use a system of structured or scheduled appointments for office visits. Each patient is assigned a time on the schedule and allotted a specific period of time for examination and treatment depending on the reason necessitating the visit. Box 6-1 shows examples of time allotment. The advantages of this system include good time management and optimum use of the office facility. Additionally, a daily schedule may be developed, and traditional charts may be prepared in advance of patient arrival. The medical assistant may also have time to be sure that results of tests or other information are available before the patient arrives for the appointment.

A disadvantage of this system is that a patient may need more of the physician's time than you have scheduled. Therefore, it is important that you ask the

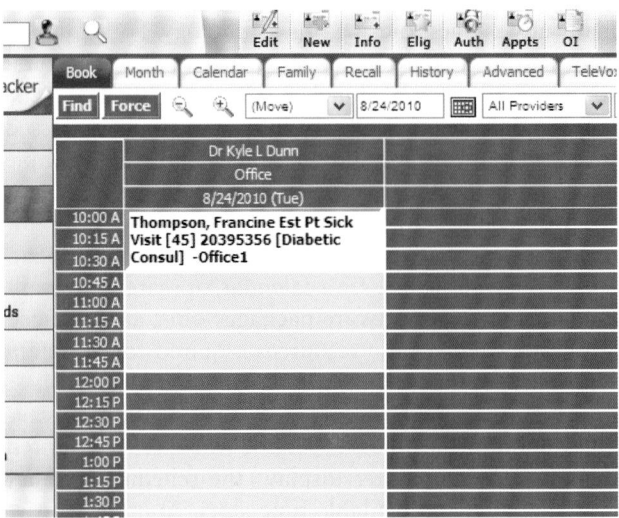

**Figure 6-1 •** A computer-generated appointment schedule. Courtesy of Ingenix® CareTracker.™

## BOX 6-1   How Much Time Do I Allot?

Every outpatient medical facility has variables that determine the time allotted for each service. Factors like the number of providers, the number of examination rooms, and the size of the office must be considered when establishing the appointment scheduling guidelines. This partial list of typical outpatient services shows an estimate of the time needed for each.

| | |
|---|---|
| Complete physical examination | 1 hour |
| School physical | 30 minutes |
| Recheck | 15 minutes |
| Dressing change | 10 minutes |
| Blood pressure check | 5 minutes |
| Patient teaching | 30 minutes–1 hour |

proper questions at the time the appointment is made to anticipate the time needed. Such questions might include "Why do you need to see the doctor?" The patient's reply will tell you how many issues will be addressed. "Do you have a form to be completed for your physical?" The answer to this question will tell you whether this is a school physical or a complete physical.

The practice of adding **buffer** time to the schedule gives extra time to accommodate emergencies, walk-ins, and other demands on the provider's daily time schedule that are not considered direct patient care. Such tasks include returning phone calls, reviewing records, and transcribing reports. For example, some office policies allow you to cross off 30 minutes at the beginning and end of the daily schedule to be used as a buffer.

Methods of scheduling patients include clustering, wave, modified wave, stream, and double booking.

### Clustering

**Clustering** is grouping patients with similar problems or needs. For example, an obstetrics and gynecology practice may see all pregnant patients in the morning and other patients in the afternoon. A pediatrician may schedule vaccinations on certain days of the week. Special tests like sigmoidoscopies may be scheduled one morning a week. Advantages to clustering include maximum use of special equipment, ease in maintaining control of the schedule, the ability to provide many patients with information about their particular situation at the same time, and efficient use of employees' time.

### Wave

Outpatient medical facilities may use the **wave scheduling system** or modify the wave system in ways that work for their particular specialty. With the wave system, several

patients are scheduled the first 30 minutes of each hour. They are seen in the order that they arrive at the office. The second half of each hour is left open. This technique works well in large facilities with several departments giving medical care. For example, several patients may arrive for a 9:00 appointment, be seen by the physician, be sent to the laboratory for blood work, and return to the physician 20 minutes later. The physician has the second part of the hour to see these patients after their testing. That second half of each hour is used as a buffer or extra time that can be used for emergencies, walk-ins, returning phone calls, and tasks other than direct patient care. Modifications to this system may include seeing new patients who will have complete physical examinations on the hour with three or four rechecks scheduled on the half hour. For example, a 75-year-old man being seen for a complete physical would be scheduled at 9:00 AM, with a 22-year-old being seen for a follow-up of strep throat and a 6-year-old being seen for recheck of an ear infection scheduled at 9:30 AM.

### Fixed Scheduling

Fixed scheduling is the most commonly used method. It divides each hour into increments of 15, 30, 45, or 60 minutes. The reason for each patient's visit will determine the length of time assigned. Patients who are late or do not report for their appointment can cause major problems in the flow of the day. It is helpful to schedule chronically late patients at the end of the day. Another tactic is to tell the patient to arrive 30 minutes prior to the time you schedule.

### Streaming

**Streaming** is a method that helps minimize gaps in time and backups. Appointments are given based on the needs of the individual patient. If a patient is being seen for a complete physical, 1 hour may be allotted. The next patient seen may need a blood pressure recheck, which would be allotted a 15-minute slot. Although this method ensures a smooth work flow, the medical assistant scheduling the appointment must understand the procedures and guidelines for deciding the time that should be allotted. Box 6-1 outlines examples of services and their probable time allotments.

### Double Booking

With **double booking**, two patients are scheduled for the same period with the same physician. This is considered poor practice and should be avoided if at all possible. The medical assistant must determine if there is a need for another appointment to be scheduled in an already full schedule and notify the physician of the situation. One solution would be to add the patient's name to a cancellation list to contact him/her if another appointment becomes available.

## Flexible Hours

Offices that operate with flexible hours are open at different times throughout the week. For example, Monday, Wednesday, and Friday office hours might be from 8:00 AM to 5:00 PM, and Tuesday and Thursday office hours might be from 8:00 AM to 8:00 PM. Some offices may also be open on Saturdays for all or part of the day. Patients still have scheduled appointments, but this greater range of available appointment times better accommodates work and family schedules. Your main challenge with flexible hours is to determine which patients really need to be scheduled for these special times. For example, Saturday appointments may be reserved only for patients whose work schedules do not permit weekday appointments. Flexible hours are most often used by clinics, group practices, and family physicians.

## Open Hours

A medical office that operates with open hours for patient visits is open for specified hours during the day or evening. Patients may arrive at any time during those hours to be seen by the physician in the order of their arrival; there are no scheduled appointments. This system is commonly seen in urgent care clinics and eliminates patient complaints such as "I had an appointment at 2:00 PM but had to wait until 3:00 PM to be seen." Open-hour scheduling, however, has some clear disadvantages:

- Effective time management is almost impossible.
- The facilities may be overloaded at some times and empty at other times.
- Charts must be pulled and prepared as each patient arrives.

So that patients are seen in the order in which they arrive, many offices use sign-in sheets. The Health Insurance Portability and Accountability Act of 1996 (HIPAA) provides for incidental disclosures of private information for the purposes of sign-in sheets in medical waiting rooms. However, no medical information about any patient should be noted on the sign-in sheet as this would be considered a breach of confidentiality.

### CHECKPOINT QUESTION

2. What are the three systems that can be used for scheduling patient office visits?

# FACTORS THAT AFFECT SCHEDULING

## Patients' Needs

People express their needs in varied ways. A patient might be feeling uncertainty, embarrassment, shyness, or fear. With a patient in an emotional state, even the slightest real or imagined miscommunication can lead to negative response from the patient. Be courteous and maintain your professionalism.

Before scheduling an appointment, you should determine the following:

- Why the patient wishes to see the physician
- How long the patient has had the symptoms
- Whether the problem is **acute** (abrupt onset) or **chronic** (long-standing)
- The most convenient time for the patient to come in (e.g., early morning or evenings)
- Any special transportation services the patient requires (community or hospital van services operate only during certain hours)
- Whether the patient needs to see other office staff
- Any third-party payers' constraints
- Receipt of necessary documentation for referrals when the patient is enrolled in a program that requires such documentation (third-party payers are discussed further in Chapter 14)

Control of the appointment schedule is your responsibility. Strive to accommodate a patient's requests whenever possible but not if it will overload the schedule. For example, if a patient requests a 2:00 PM appointment this Tuesday and you already have patients in that time slot, politely explain that you cannot schedule the appointment then unless you have a cancellation. You might offer a later time on Tuesday or on another day at 2:00 PM You can also ask if the patient wishes to be put on a cancellation list to be notified if an earlier appointment opens up. In other words, you control the schedule. Do not let it control you. The entire medical office team depends on a well-managed schedule.

## Providers' Preferences and Needs

The management of the practice depends on the desires and requirements of the providers working in it. Providers in a medical practice may include the physician, nurse practitioner, or physician's assistant. Some providers often run behind schedule; others are extremely punctual. Recognize your providers' habits, and communicate any problems to the physician or office manager. The physician may allow you to adjust the schedule to accommodate his or her habits. If you are employed to assist the physician with clinical duties (e.g., removing sutures, performing electrocardiograms, giving injections), the schedule can be adjusted to accommodate a larger number of patients while still allowing the provider enough time to give each patient personal attention.

As discussed earlier, the physician also needs time to receive and return telephone calls, review laboratory and pathology reports, dictate chart notes or correspondence, and so on. If your physician is on the staff of a teaching hospital, you may also have to block off time for clinic conferences and other teaching duties.

The physician will need time to meet with unscheduled office visitors other than patients. Such visitors might include other physicians and sales representatives from medical supply or pharmaceutical companies. You should determine in advance how the physician wants you to handle these visitors. For example, the physician may want to be notified immediately if another physician comes to the office. With salespersons or pharmaceutical representatives, however, the physician may have another staff member meet with them or may request that an appointment be scheduled for a more convenient time.

## Physical Facilities

The physical facilities available in the medical office will affect the management of the appointment schedule. Consider these points: How many providers use the facility? How many examination rooms are there? Is it necessary to sterilize instruments between procedures, or is more than one set of instruments available? You would not want to schedule two sigmoidoscopies at the same time, for example, if the office has only one appropriately equipped examination room. You must thoroughly understand the requirements for procedures to be performed in the office to schedule appointments accurately.

 **CHECKPOINT QUESTION**

3. What are three factors that can affect appointment scheduling?

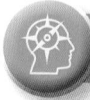 **ARF ETHICAL TIP**

### Think before You Speak

As discussed throughout the text, it is illegal and unethical to release patient information without the patient's consent. You may be breaching confidentiality without even realizing it. Consider this: You are a receptionist in a busy obstetrics/gynecology practice. A former classmate comes in for a pregnancy test. While you are making her return appointment, she tells you that the test was positive. Later, while having lunch at a nearby restaurant, you see her mother. You congratulate her on her new grandchild and quickly realize that she does not know about her daughter's pregnancy yet. You have just breached the patient's confidentiality.

What if the scenario had been like what follows? "Hi, Mrs. Roberts. What a coincidence; I just saw Susie this morning." Mrs. Roberts says, "Where did you see her?" You reply, "At work." You have just told Mrs. Roberts that her daughter was at an obstetrics/gynecology office. This innocent exchange is a serious violation of the Privacy Rule of HIPAA. Most employers consider this to be reason for immediate dismissal. Be careful.

# SCHEDULING GUIDELINES

Whether the patient is making an appointment by telephone or in person, be pleasant and maintain a helpful attitude. Always write the patient's telephone number on the schedule when making appointments. Emergencies and delays are unavoidable, and schedule corrections can be made quickly if the telephone number is handy. Invariably, problems will arise (e.g., late patients, emergencies) and disrupt the regular appointment schedule. If possible, leave some time slots open during each day to allow the schedule to catch up. Also, patients calling for appointments will not appreciate being told that no time is available for 2 or 3 weeks. Open slots can be used to schedule brief appointments as needed. Procedure 6-1 describes the steps for scheduling appointments for new patients.

## New Patients

Most appointments for new patients are made by telephone; however, some offices have online scheduling features in the patient portal in their practice Web site. The information you exchange at this encounter is crucial, and entering the patient's data accurately is imperative. The first encounter with a new patient is discussed in Procedure 6-1.

Practice Web sites conveniently offer many options for patients including practice information and new patient forms to complete online. They may also be downloaded, printed, and completed before the appointment. An office brochure can also be mailed to the patient in advance of the appointment. Some offices send new-patient forms to be filled out and brought in at the appointment. When scheduling an appointment for a new patient, follow these guidelines:

1. Allow an adequate amount of time for the appointment. To do so, obtain as much information as possible from the patient:
   - Full name and correct spelling
   - Mailing address
   - Day and evening telephone numbers
   - Reason for the visit
   - Name of the referring physician or individual
   - Responsible party and third-party payer (insurance plan)
2. Explain the office's financial policy. Most offices require full or partial payment at the time of an initial visit, and patients must understand this policy. Instruct patients to bring all pertinent insurance information.
3. Be sure patients know your office location; if needed, give them concise directions. You may also want to tell patients how long they can expect to be at the office.
4. Some patients are sensitive about messages left on an answering machine or given to a coworker. To avoid violating confidentiality, ask the patient if it is permissible to call at home or at work and include this information in the patient's chart.

5. Before ending the call, confirm the time and date of the appointment. You might say, "Thank you for calling Mr. Brown. We look forward to seeing you on Tuesday, December 10, at 2:00 PM"

6. Always check your appointment system or book to be sure that you have placed the appointment on the correct day in the right time slot.

7. If the patient was referred by another physician, you may need to call that physician's office in advance of the appointment for copies of laboratory work, radiology and pathology reports, and so on.

Remember, the patient does not need to give authorization to release medical documents for treatment and continuity of care (see Chapter 9). Give these reports to the physician prior to the patient's appointment.

## Established Patients

Established patients will be given return appointments when necessary. Most return appointments are made before the patient leaves the office. Procedure 6-2 describes the steps for scheduling a return appointment.

When making a return appointment, follow these guidelines:

1. Carefully check your appointment book or screen before offering an appointment time. If a specific examination, test, or x-ray is to be performed on the return visit, avoid scheduling two patients for the same examination at the same time.

2. Offer the patient a specific time and date. For example, you might say, "Mrs. Hernandez, I have next Tuesday, the 15th, available at 3:30 PM" (Avoid asking the patient when he or she would like to return, as this can elicit indecision.) If the offered appointment is not convenient, offer another specific time and date.

3. Write the patient's name and telephone number in the appointment book, or enter in the information on the appointment screen.

4. Transfer the pertinent information to an appointment card and give it to the patient. Computerized systems print an appointment card. Repeat aloud the appointment day, date, and time to the patient as you hand over the card (Fig. 6-3).

5. Double-check your book or screen to be sure you have not made an error.

6. End your conversation with a pleasant word and a smile.

## COG PREPARING A DAILY OR WEEKLY SCHEDULE

In most offices, as medical assistant, you are responsible for preparing a daily and possibly a weekly schedule of appointments. Make a copy for the providers and

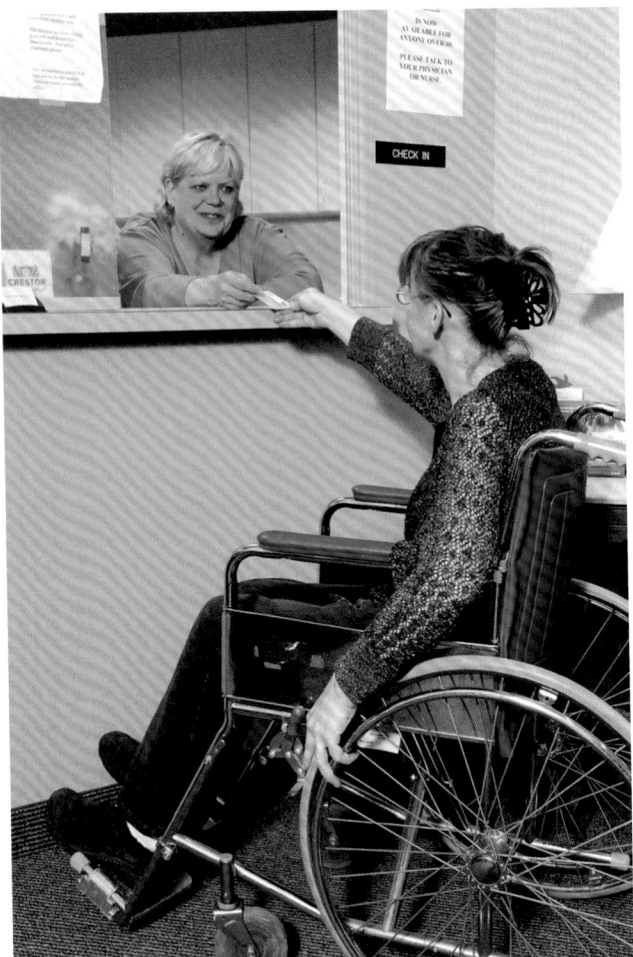

**Figure 6-3 •** An appointment card will help the patient remember his or her appointment and reduce no-shows.

other office staff members. When there are changes in the schedule, ensure that corrections are made on all copies. Place the next day's schedule on the physician's desk before he or she leaves for the day. Give the next week's schedule to the physician before he or she leaves on Friday. Schedules should include not only patients' appointments but also hospital rounds, surgeries, meetings, and any personal engagements on the schedule. Computer systems print a daily or weekly schedule, but you must remember to make changes manually as the day progresses.

## PATIENT REMINDERS

Offices use various kinds of reminders to tell a patient about an appointment that should be made or to remind them that an appointment has been made on a specific date and time. These reminders are the appointment card, the telephone call, and the mailed card.

## Appointment Cards

An appointment card is given to the patient when he or she leaves the office. It should have the following information:

- Patient's name
- Day, date, and time of the return visit
- Physician's name and telephone number

If the patient requires a series of appointments, try to make them on the same day of the week and at the same time of day. This will make it easier for the patient to remember the appointments. Unless your appointment card allows you to list the complete series of appointments, however, give the patient a card for the next appointment only and repeat this procedure after each subsequent visit. When the patient has to save several cards, they can easily be lost or cause confusion. If using a manual system, write on the card with ink so that it cannot be altered. Computer appointment scheduling software provides appointment cards that can be printed on special perforated paper.

## Telephone Reminders

All new patients and patients with appointments scheduled in advance should receive a telephone reminder the day before their appointment. Computer systems can place the call to the programmed number and remind the patient of the appointment with a prerecorded message. Remember, do not call a patient at work or leave a message unless you have been given permission to do so. Make the telephone reminder simple. Identify your office and yourself, and state the date and time of the appointment. For example, you might say, "This is Ms. Sprinkle from Dr. Yokley's office. I'm calling to confirm your appointment for tomorrow, Thursday, February 10, at 3:30 PM." Unless the patient has a question, then say, "Thank you and goodbye." This reminder helps jog the patient's memory, and if the patient must cancel or reschedule an appointment, you will have time to fill the slot. Keep a list with the names and phone numbers of patients who have asked to be called or who need to be seen sooner than their next appointment. This list may be called a cancellation list, a waiting list, or a move-up list. Make a notation on the appointment schedule, such as confirmed, left message, or no answer. Figure 6-4 shows a sample appointment card.

## Mailed Reminder Cards

Some offices send reminder cards instead of making phone calls. Reminder cards are also used to remind patients who could not be reached by phone that it is time to keep an upcoming scheduled appointment. These should be mailed at least a week before the date of the appointment. In addition, reminder cards are sent after

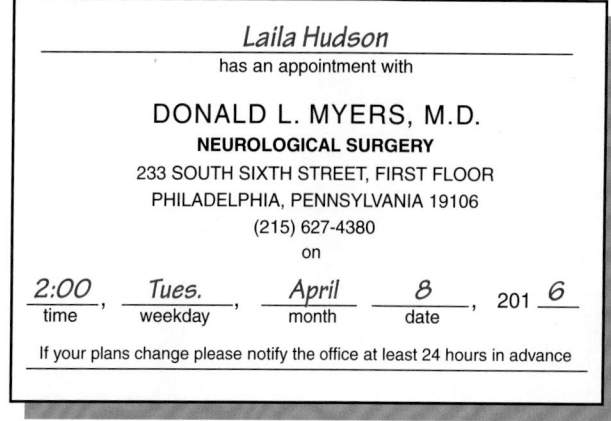

*Laila Hudson*
has an appointment with

**DONALD L. MYERS, M.D.**
**NEUROLOGICAL SURGERY**
233 SOUTH SIXTH STREET, FIRST FLOOR
PHILADELPHIA, PENNSYLVANIA 19106
(215) 627-4380
on

| 2:00 | Tues. | April | 8 | 201 6 |
|------|-------|-------|---|--------|
| time | weekday | month | date | |

If your plans change please notify the office at least 24 hours in advance

**Figure 6-4** • Sample reminder postcard.

a set period since a patient's last appointment. Reminder cards are often used to alert patients to the need for annual examinations (e.g., Pap smears, mammograms, prostate examinations).

To handle this kind of reminder, keep a supply of preprinted postcards in the office. The cards should have a simple one- or two-sentence message, such as, "According to our records, you are due for your annual physical. If you would kindly call the office, we will be glad to arrange an appointment for you." The physician's name, address, and telephone number should be printed on the card. Mail the card at the appropriate time. Most medical management software packages produce a list that can be used to alert you of the need for patient reminders.

## Electronic Reminders

Technology is an important part of many peoples' lives today and is invaluable in keeping track of busy schedules and appointments. Smart phones have Internet capabilities, and some patients may want to be contacted through an email or a text message of any appointment reminders or changes. These messages are professional communications and should never include slang or abbreviations (see Chapter 7) and should be concise and accurate. Always maintain patient confidentiality when sending any message, and verify that the phone number or email address is correct before sending your message.

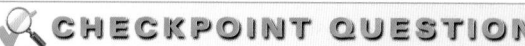

## CHECKPOINT QUESTION

4. What are the three types of patient reminders?

# ADAPTING THE SCHEDULE

## Emergencies

When a patient calls with an emergency (Fig. 6-5), your first responsibility is to determine whether the problem can be treated in the office. The office should have a

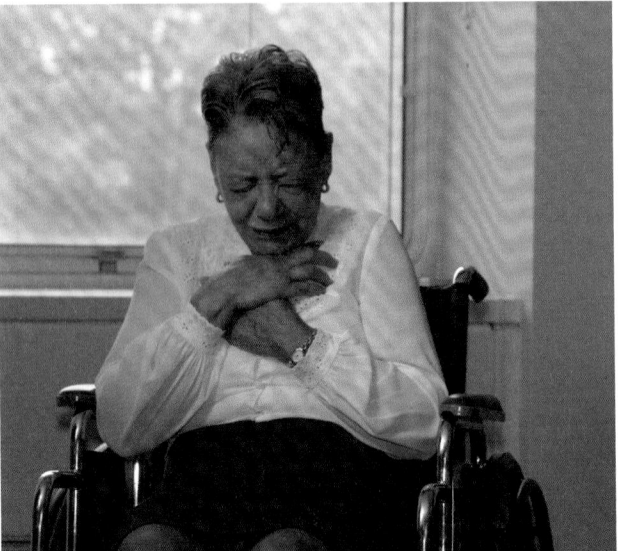

Figure 6-5 • When a patient calls with chest pain, you may need to call 911.

policy for evaluation of the situation. The word **STAT** is used in the medical field to indicate that something should be done immediately (Box 6-2). You also should have a list of appropriate questions to ask the patient, such as "Are you having chest pain? Are you having difficulty breathing? How long have you had the symptoms?" (Box 6-3). When several symptoms occur together, they may indicate a particular problem. This group of complaints is referred to as a **constellation of symptoms**. One group of symptoms found to indicate a certain disorder is severe right lower quadrant pain, nausea, and fever. A physician who sees this constellation of symptoms considers appendicitis. Medical

---

**BOX 6-2    When Does the Patient Need to Be Seen _Now?_**

When the patient calls with any of the following complaints:

- Shortness of breath
- Severe chest pain
- Uncontrollable bleeding
- Large open wounds
- Potential accidental poisoning
- Bleeding in a pregnant patient
- Injury to a pregnant patient
- Shock
- Serious burns
- Severe bleeding
- Any symptoms of internal bleeding (dark, tarry stools; discoloration of the skin)

Note: Remember to check with the physician for proper procedures concerning triage.

---

**BOX 6-3    When a Patient Could Be Having a Heart Attack**

When a patient calls complaining of the following constellation of symptoms, you should assume that this is a potential heart attack:

- Shortness of breath
- Chest pain
- Arm or neck pain
- Nausea and/or vomiting

Just one of these symptoms alone may not indicate a cardiac event, but when there is more than one, you should be alert to the fact that this may be a heart attack. Studies have shown that, in women, early symptoms of a heart attack are different from those in men. These symptoms include jaw, neck, and back pain and severe fatigue. Keep this in mind when questioning the patient. Call 911, and stay on the line with the patient. Do not advise the patient to drive to the hospital. Follow office policies for such an emergency.

---

assistants must work with their physicians to determine what constitutes an actual emergency situation.

## Patients Who Are Acutely Ill

Patients who are acutely ill often have serious, although not life-threatening, conditions. These patients need to be seen as soon as possible but not necessarily on that same day. Obtain as much information about the patient's medical problem as you can so your message to the physician will allow him or her to decide how soon the patient should be seen. Place the chart with a note in the location selected by the physician, and tell the patient you will call back as soon as the physician makes a decision.

## Walk-in Patients

Walk-in patients are those who arrive at the office without a scheduled appointment and expect to see the physician that day. Typically, the physician will have a set protocol, or prescribed list of steps, for handling such situations. In general, you must first determine the reason for the walk-in. Patients with medical emergencies need to be seen immediately. Other patients can be asked to have a seat in the waiting room while you inform the physician of the patient's presence. The physician can then make the decision to see the patient or not.

If the patient is to be seen, explain that you will work him or her into the schedule as soon as possible for a brief examination. When the patient leaves the office, you might apologize for the delay and then ask the patient to schedule an appointment for the next visit.

If the physician decides not to see a walk-in patient, you will have to ask the patient to schedule an appointment and to return later.

## Late Patients

Patients who are late cause problems in the schedule. You should gently but firmly apologize for any delay but tell the patient, "You were late, and Dr. Wooten is seeing another patient now. The doctor should be able to see you in about 15 minutes." Patients who are routinely late should be politely advised that "According to our office policy, patients who are more than 15 minutes late will have to be rescheduled." Some offices have found that scheduling the habitually late patient at the end of the day is helpful. In addition, ask patients to call the office if they know ahead of time that they are going to be late.

## Physician Delays

Of course, sometimes the physician calls in to say he or she has been delayed and will be in the office later. If office hours have not yet begun, call patients with appointments scheduled early, and give them the option of coming in later in the day or rescheduling the appointment for another day. If patients are waiting in the office, inform them immediately if the physician will be delayed. For example, you might say, "Dr. Franklin has been delayed and will probably be 20 to 30 minutes late. Would you like to wait, or would you prefer to reschedule for another time?" Always keep your patients informed; most people will understand if they know you have not ignored or forgotten them. Most patients appreciate the fact that the physician would also be available to them in an emergency. If you reschedule an appointment, note in the patient's chart the reason for the cancellation or rescheduling.

## Missed Appointments

A missed appointment, or no-show, occurs when a patient neglects to keep an appointment and does not notify the office. When this happens, call the patient to try to determine why the appointment was missed and to reschedule for another time. If you are unable to reach the patient by telephone, send a card asking the patient to call the office to reschedule. Note in the patient's chart the missed appointment and that you have either rescheduled the appointment or mailed a card to schedule another appointment. Even if the office does not routinely remind patients of appointments, be sure to call and remind habitually late patients the day before the appointment.

Continued failure to keep appointments should be brought to the attention of the physician, who may want to call the patient personally (particularly if the patient is seriously ill) or send a letter expressing concern for the patient's welfare. In extreme cases, the physician may

### BOX 6-4  Charting Example

05/12/16–1530
Mrs. Parrish was called regarding missing scheduled appointment for today at 9:30 AM. Patient said she forgot about the appointment. Appointment was rescheduled for 05/14/16 at 10:00 AM. Patient was advised of the need to have regular prenatal checkups. Patient verbalized understanding. Dr. Wong was notified that appointment was missed and rescheduled.
—Tamara Dorsett, RMA

choose to terminate the physician–patient relationship. See Chapter 2 for the proper procedure for this action. Notations of all actions and copies of any letters sent to the patient should become a permanent part of the individual's medical record. Box 6-4 is an example of a chart note.

## CANCELLATIONS

### Cancellations by the Office

You may have to cancel a patient's appointment if the physician is ill, has an emergency, or has personal time off. Patients who must be rescheduled need not be told the specific reason for the physician's absence. These cancellations should be noted in the patient's medical record.

When you have advance notice, write a letter to patients with appointments you must cancel, indicating

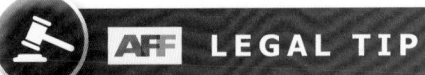

### LEGAL TIP

#### Document, Document, Document!

When a patient does not show up for his or her appointment, you must make an entry in the chart. Because your physician has a legal contract with the patient, he or she has an obligation to treat the patient as long and as often as necessary. If the patient does not report for scheduled appointments, the patient is breaking the contract. This would be an important factor in a court cases involving a physician being sued for abandonment. The chart is the physician's defense. Being diligent with documentation is not optional. Example:

10/07/16. Mr. Quinn did not report for his appointment at 10:00 AM today. I called him at 11:00 AM, and he stated that he did not want to reschedule. He says he is doing fine and will call next week to reschedule.
—Tracy Amaral, CMA

that the physician will be away from the office but will return by a certain date. Patients should be alerted to cancellations a week before their appointments. Ask the patient to call the office to reschedule. If you have to cancel on the day of the appointment, call the patient and explain. For example, you might say, "Dr. Flora has been called out of the office unexpectedly. Would it be convenient to reschedule your appointment for sometime next week?" If the patient arrives at the office before you can contact him or her, apologize and politely explain the situation. Most patients will be understanding. When a physician is unavailable for an extended period, another physician must cover the practice or be on call. Everyone in the office should have a list of names and addresses of on-call physicians, and you should give this information to your patients, according to your office policy. When a locum tenens, or substitute physician, is employed, the office appointments will not be interrupted (see Chapter 2).

## Cancellations by the Patient

When a patient cancels an appointment, ask the reason for the cancellation and mark it on your appointment schedule and in the patient's chart. Offer to reschedule at another time. If the patient is being seen for a continuing problem, be sure he or she understands the necessity for the follow-up visit. If the patient wants to call back for an appointment, make a note to yourself to check on the callback in a few days. If a patient cancels appointments frequently, bring this to the physician's attention.

If a patient cancels an appointment and you have a full schedule, no action is needed. If your schedule is light, however, refer to your cancellation list to try to fill the vacancy.

# MAKING APPOINTMENTS FOR PATIENTS IN OTHER FACILITIES

## Referrals and Consultations

When the provider requests assistance from another physician in **consultation**, makes a **referral** to another physician, or sends a patient to another facility for testing, make certain that the referral meets the requirements of any third-party payers. Managed care companies like health management organizations have strict requirements regarding **precertification** and documentation for referrals to specialists and other facilities. If the patient's third-party payer requires a referral form, you will need to complete it with the referral approval number that you must obtain from the insurance company. Figure 6-6 is a sample referral form (see Chapter 13). Be sure the physician you are calling is on

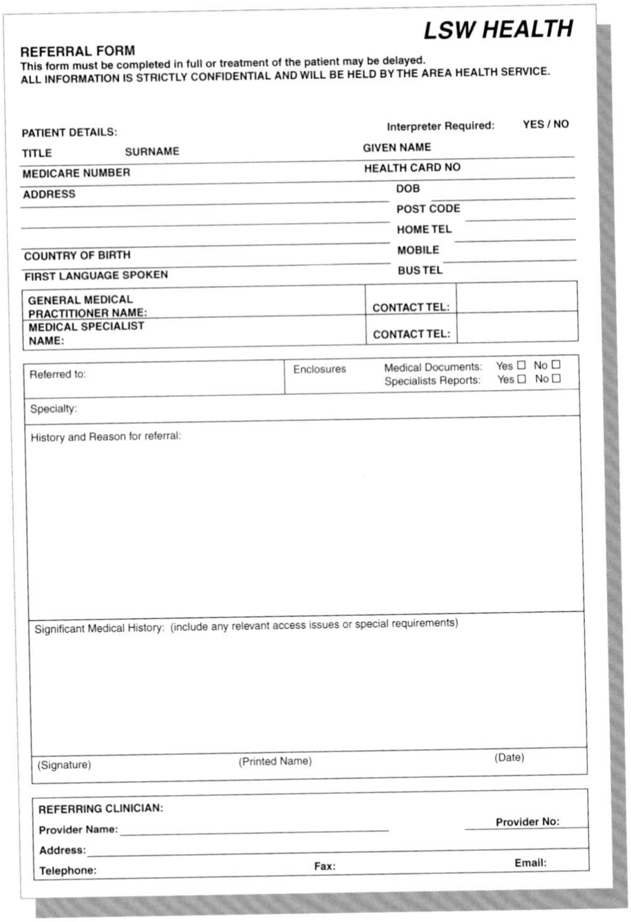
LSW HEALTH
REFERRAL FORM
This form must be completed in full or treatment of the patient may be delayed.
ALL INFORMATION IS STRICTLY CONFIDENTIAL AND WILL BE HELD BY THE AREA HEALTH SERVICE.

PATIENT DETAILS: Interpreter Required: YES / NO
TITLE SURNAME GIVEN NAME
MEDICARE NUMBER HEALTH CARD NO
ADDRESS DOB
POST CODE
HOME TEL
COUNTRY OF BIRTH MOBILE
FIRST LANGUAGE SPOKEN BUS TEL

| | |
|---|---|
| GENERAL MEDICAL PRACTITIONER NAME: | CONTACT TEL: |
| MEDICAL SPECIALIST NAME: | CONTACT TEL: |

Referred to: Enclosures Medical Documents: Yes ☐ No ☐ Specialists Reports: Yes ☐ No ☐
Specialty:
History and Reason for referral:
Significant Medical History: (include any relevant access issues or special requirements)
(Signature) (Printed Name) (Date)

REFERRING CLINICIAN:
Provider Name: Provider No:
Address:
Telephone: Fax: Email:

**Figure 6-6** • Sample referral form.

the preferred provider list for the patient's insurance company. Patients should be given a choice when being referred to a specialist.

When calling another physician's office for an appointment for your patient (Procedure 6-3), provide the following information:

- Physician's name and telephone number
- Patient's name, address, and telephone number
- Reason for the referral
- Degree of urgency
- Insurance information

Record in the patient's chart the time and date of the call and the person who received your call. Tell the person you are calling that you wish to be notified if your patient does not keep the appointment. If this occurs, be sure to tell the physician and enter this information in the patient's record.

Write the name, address, and telephone number of the referral doctor on your office stationery and include the date and time of the appointment. Give or mail this information to your patient. The patient may call the referring physician to make his or her own appointment. If this is the situation, ask the patient to call you with the appointment date and document it in the chart.

## Diagnostic Testing

Sometimes, patients are sent for diagnostic testing or treatment at another facility. Such testing includes laboratory tests, radiology, computed tomography, magnetic resonance imaging, and nuclear medicine studies. These appointments are usually made while the patient is still in the office. Before scheduling, determine the exact test or tests the physician requires and how soon the results are needed. (Be sure to indicate to the facility if the results are needed immediately, or STAT.) Also, check with the patient for any time restrictions he or she may have. Give the facility the patient's name, address, telephone number, the exact test or tests required, and any other special instructions from the physician. Give the patient a laboratory or x-ray referral slip with the time and date of the appointment and the name, address, and telephone number of the outside facility.

Some laboratory studies or x-ray tests require advance preparation by the patient. Give your patient a written and verbal explanation of the required preparation, and be sure he or she understands the importance of following the instructions. On the patient's chart, note the name of the outside facility and the date and time of the appointment. Also set a reminder on your appointment schedule to be sure the test results are received as requested (see Procedure 6-3).

## Surgery

You also assist with the scheduling of procedures in a hospital operating room or an outpatient surgical facility. Determine the patient's need for precertification with the insurance carrier. You may have to call the number on the back of the patient's insurance card for a precertification number. Call the participating facility chosen by the patient and specify the time and date the physician has requested. The operating facility will need to know the exact procedure, the amount of time needed, the type of anesthesia required, and any other special instructions your physician may have. The facility will also need the patient's name, age, address, telephone number, insurance information, and the precertification number if required.

If the hospital has supplied your office with preadmission forms, give a copy to the patient and make sure he or she understands the need to complete and return the form in a timely manner. Follow the policies of the surgical facility regarding preadmission testing, which may include laboratory studies, x-rays, or autologous blood donation (donation of a person's own blood in advance). Write down all appointment dates, times, and locations for the patient and be certain he or she understands where to go and when.

Finally, note in the patient's record the name of the operating facility and the date and time the surgery is scheduled. You may also need to arrange for hospital admission by providing the same information to the hospital admitting department (Procedure 6-4).

### CHECKPOINT QUESTION

5. What information should be readily available when calling to schedule a patient for surgery in another facility?

## COG  WHEN THE APPOINTMENT SCHEDULE DOES NOT WORK

No appointment schedule runs smoothly all the time, and an occasional glitch is to be expected. If, however, you find that your schedule is chaotic nearly every day, you should determine the cause. The medical assistant's responsibility is to help the physician manage the schedule, so it may be necessary to evaluate the schedule over period of time. For example, make a list of all patients seen, their arrival times, the amount of time they spent with the physician, the time they left, and the amount of time needed to perform each examination or treatment. Since the workflow of the office affects every staff member, involve all employees in your study.

Office meetings are an ideal way to identify scheduling problems. Your evaluation may reveal that many of your patients are arriving late or that you have not allotted enough time for certain procedures. Sometimes, a habitually delayed physician is the problem. You may find that too many staff people are making appointments. If this is the case, you can assign only one staff person to handle all scheduling. Some problems may never be completely solved. If they are identified, however, you can often make adjustments to avoid causing frustration for both patients and office personnel.

### ROLE-PLAYING ACTIVITY

The appointment schedule at Great Falls Medical Center has been very busy lately with patients needing appointments for acute illnesses. Lately, Dr. Kyle Dunn has been very behind requiring his medical assistant, Ronnie Wilson, RMA, to work an extra two hours every evening to help him see all of his patients. Although Ronnie does not mind the overtime, he has other obligations after work and is finding that this is becoming a problem for him. A time management analysis by Ronnie revealed that Dr. Dunn is beginning about an hour late every day and is taking a longer lunch break than the other physicians. Should Ronnie bring this problem to Dr. Dunn's attention? If so, how can he approach the physician with this dilemma and communicate what he believes to be the problem in a tactful manner? What solutions can Ronnie offer to Dr. Dunn to alleviate the scheduling problems to keep from getting behind every day? If you are playing the role of Dr. Dunn, think about how you might feel if an employee questioned your handling of patient appointments. Will he be angry, or will he appreciate Ronnie's help? Your instructor will give you additional information about this activity.

## *español* SPANISH TERMINOLOGY

**¿Me podría decir cuál es el motivo de su visita el dia de hoy?**
Can you tell me why you are here today?

**¿Por qué necesita ver al doctor?**
Why do you need to see the doctor?

**¿Desde cuándo se siente mal?**
How long has this been going on?

**¿Prefiere la cita en la mañana ó por la tarde?**
Would you prefer your appointment in the morning or in the afternoon?

**Le llamaremos para recordarle su cita con nosotros.**
I am calling to remind you of your appointment.

**Le voy a dar una cita para que vea al doctor nuevamente.**
I will give you another appointment to see the doctor for a follow-up.

**Para su próxima visita, por favor traiga su tarjeta del seguro médico y todas las medicinas que está tomando.**
Please bring your insurance card and medicine bottles with you for your next appointment.

| Dias de la semana | La una y media |
|---|---|
| Days of the week | 1:30 |
| **Domingo** | **Las dos en punto** |
| Sunday | 2:00 |
| **Lunes** | **Son las dos y media** |
| Monday | 2:30 |
| **Martes** | **Tres en punto** |
| Tuesday | 3:00 |
| **Miércoles** | **Son las tres y media** |
| Wednesday | 3:30 |
| **Jueves** | **Las siete en punto** |
| Thursday | 7:00 |
| **Viernes** | **Son las siete y media** |
| Friday | 7:30 |
| **Sábado** | **Ocho en punto** |
| Saturday | 8:00 |
| **Las horas del día** | **Son las ocho y media** |
| Times of the day | 8:30 |
| **Mañana** | **Nueve en punto** |
| Morning | 9:00 |
| **Tarde** | **Son las nueve y media** |
| Afternoon | 9:30 |
| **Mediodía** | **Son las diez y cuarto** |
| Noon | 10:15 |
| **Noche** | **Once y cuarenta y cinco** |
| Night | 11:45 |
| **La un** | |
| One o'clock | |

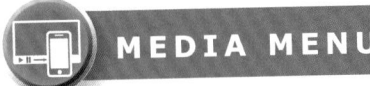

**MEDIA MENU**

**Student Resources** on thePoint®
- *Video:* Scheduling an Appointment for a New Patient (Procedure 6-1)
- *Video:* Scheduling an Appointment for a Return Patient (Procedure 6-2)
- *Video:* Making an Appointment for a Referral to an Outpatient Facility (Procedure 6-3)
- *Video:* Arranging for Admission to an Inpatient Facility (Procedure 6-4)
- **CMA/RMA Certification Exam Review**

## EMR Activity

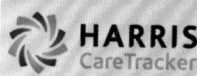

Harris CareTracker is a web-based electronic medical record (EMR) application that you will use for the EMR activities included in this section at the end of each chapter. This application is actually used in physician offices but is provided to you through the publisher, Wolters Kluwer Health, to give you hands-on practice working with EMRs. Your instructor will have more information about accessing your username, login, and Quickstart guide.

Prerequisite Activities in Harris CareTracker

• *The Getting Started and Quickstart documents and EMR Activities Step-by-Step Instructions are available at* http://thePoint.lww.com/KronenbergerComp5e

Activity Details

Dr. Dunn is planning a vacation during the first 2 full weeks next month, therefore, you must matrix the appointment schedule accordingly. To block off Dr. Dunn's vacation time in the schedule, you first must build the schedule for him following the instructions provided in the *EMR Activities Step-by-Step Instructions.*

## Chapter Summary

- The outpatient medical facility can be chaotic without an efficient appointment system. Moving patients through the facility while treating each person equally and thoroughly is one of the biggest challenges in the medical office.
- It is difficult for a busy practice to run smoothly all of the time. You need structure, but you must be flexible. Available times, equipment and room usage, and personnel coverage must be considered when finding just the right formula for a well-run and efficient office.
- The goals of the outpatient medical facility are to provide quality patient care and maintain financial stability. To reach those goals, an office must have a plan for the efficient scheduling and carrying out of the daily activities.
- Appointment scheduling systems include manual systems using appointment books and computerized systems that render helpful reports and daily activity sheets. The size of a practice, the number of physicians, the types of services, and so on are considered when establishing an appointment scheduling system.
- Sick patients calling to make appointments should be given priority, and there are established guidelines for determining the urgency of a patient's problem. Other functions, such as phone calls, reviewing records, and lunch breaks, are also scheduled into the daily activities of the office.
- An established protocol or list of steps should be in place to handle pharmaceutical representatives and other visitors to the office. As the medical assistant at the front desk, you will be one of the most important factors in the daily operation of the outpatient medical facility.
- As a medical assistant, you will make appointments, document encounters with patients that deal with appointments, and make referrals to other health care facilities. Learning the issues involved in successful appointment scheduling will help you make sure your facility runs smoothly.

## Warm-Ups for Critical Thinking

1. Assume that you are the office manager in a physician's office. Create a policy and procedure for scheduling patients.
2. Sign-in sheets can cause a breach in patient confidentiality. What other methods could you use that would limit the potential for invasion of patient privacy?
3. You notice that patients typically wait 30 to 45 minutes past their scheduled appointment times because of the physician. How would you approach a physician who chronically runs late?

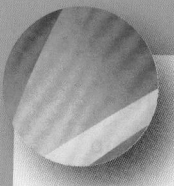

## PSY PROCEDURE 6-1

# Making an Appointment for a New Patient

**PSY** Manage appointment schedule using established priorities; and coach patients regarding: a) office policies.

**Purpose:** To secure an allotted time for a patient who is new to your facility to see the provider

**Equipment:** Patient's demographic information, patient's chief complaint, appointment book or computer with appointment software

| STEPS | REASONS |
|---|---|
| 1. Obtain as much information as possible from the patient, such as:<br><br>• Full name and correct spelling<br>• Mailing address (not all offices require this)<br>• Day and evening telephone numbers<br>• Reason for the visit<br>• Name of the referring person | To stay on schedule, you must allow enough time for the appointment. This information will help determine appointment needs and save time at the first visit. |
| 2. Determine the patient's chief complaint or the reason for seeing the physician. | The reason for the visit will determine the time allotment, use of special rooms or equipment, etc. |
| 3. Enter the appointment on a date and for the amount of time established by the office policies for a new patient. | The office policy may require clustering for scheduling new patients. |
| 4. Explain the cancellation and financial policies of the practice. Most offices require a minimum of 24 hours for a cancellation as well as payment at the time of an initial visit. | Patients must understand these policies if they are to follow them. Instruct patients to bring all pertinent insurance information. |
| 5. Be sure patients know your office location; give directions if needed. You may also want to give patients an idea of how long they can expect to be at the office. | Helps patients arrive on time and lets them concisely budget their time. |
| 6. To avoid violating confidentiality, ask the patient if it is permissible to call at home or at work. | HIPAA's Privacy Rule prohibits leaving messages on an answering machine or giving any information to another individual who has not been named by the patient. |
| 7. Before ending the call, confirm the time and date of the appointment. Say, "Thank you for calling, Mr. Brown. We look forward to seeing you on Tuesday, December 10, at 2:00 PM." | Repeating the appointment time will ensure that effective communication has taken place and increase the likelihood that the patient will be there on time. |
| 8. Always check your appointment schedule to be sure that you have placed the appointment on the correct day in the right time slot. | Failure to record every appointment in the proper location can cause overbooking, frustrated physicians and staff, and irate patients. |
| 9. If the patient was referred by another physician, you may need to call that physician's office before the appointment for copies of laboratory work, radiology, pathology reports, and so on. Give this information to the physician prior to the patient's appointment. | |
| 10. **AFF** Explain how you would respond in a situation in which a patient does NOT give permission to phone him or her at work. | Make sure that information is recorded prominently so all will know. Do not call the patient at work under any circumstances. Call only the number the patient gave you permission to call. |

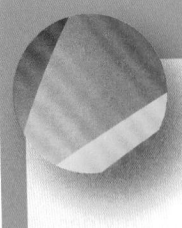

# PROCEDURE 6-2

## Making an Appointment for an Established Patient

**PSY**   Schedule an appointment for a return visit; and use office hardware and software to maintain office systems.

**Purpose:** To secure an allotted time for a patient who is returning to your office as an established patient

**Equipment:** Appointment book or computer with appointment software, appointment card

| STEPS | REASONS |
|---|---|
| 1. Determine what will be done at the return visit. Check your appointment book or computer system before offering an appointment. | If a specific examination, test, or scan is to be performed, you will want to avoid scheduling two patients for the same examination at the same time. |
| 2. Offer the patient a specific time and date. Avoid asking the patient when he or she would like to return, as this can cause indecision. | Give the patient a choice, and if neither time is convenient, offer another specific time and date. Giving a patient a choice is good practice. "Mrs. Chang, we can see you next Tuesday, the 15th, at 3:30 PM, or Wednesday, the 16th, at 9:00 AM." |
| 3. Write the patient's name and telephone number in the appointment book or enter it in the computer. | Writing the phone number in the appointment book or making a notation in the computer will give you a quick reference if you need to call the patient to change the appointment. |
| 4. Transfer the pertinent information to an appointment card and give it to the patient. Repeat aloud the appointment day, date, and time to the patient as you hand over the card (see Fig. 6-4). | Repeating the information reinforces the patient's memory and helps ensure that the appointment will be kept. |
| 5. Double-check your book or computer to be sure you have not made an error. | Errors in appointments waste the patient's, staff's, and physician's time. |
| 6. Whether in person or on the phone, end your conversation with a pleasant word and a smile. | A smile always feels good to a patient who may be apprehensive about needing to return to the doctor. |
| 7. **AFF** Explain how you would respond to a patient who insists on coming for a return appointment at a time when the doctor is in surgery. | Explain that the doctors have certain hours that they see patients, but he or she is welcome to see another provider in the practice. |

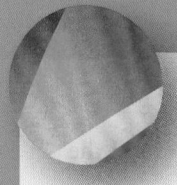

## PROCEDURE 6-3

# Making an Appointment for an Outpatient Facility

**PSY** Schedule a patient procedure; schedule an appointment for a referral to an outpatient facility; apply third-party managed care policies and procedures, and verify eligibility for services including documentation.

**Purpose:** To secure an allotted time for a patient who needs to have a screening colonoscopy

**Equipment:** Patient's chart with demographic information; physician's order for services needed by the patient and reason for the services; patient's insurance card with referral information, referral form, and directions to office

| STEPS | REASONS |
|---|---|
| 1. Make certain that the requirements of any third-party payers are met. | It is important to contact the patient's insurance company to determine if they are eligible to receive benefits for the services or referral being requested. Telephone numbers for insurance eligibility and preauthorization inquiries will be printed on the back of the insurance card. Some insurance plans require only the patient's primary care physician or gatekeeper make referrals. Notify the patient if he or she is ineligible for insurance benefits for the requested services, and document on the form approved by the office manager or physician for insurance authorizations. |
| 2. Refer to the patient's insurance company to determine if the outpatient facility and the physician performing the procedure participates (has a contract) with the patient's insurance company. | Managed care companies have strict requirements for patients not seeking services within the approved network of providers. The patient may be responsible for all charges if the provider and/or facility is not in his/her insurance network of approved providers (see Chapter 13). |
| 3. Have the following information available when you make the call to schedule the procedure:<br><br>• Physician's name and telephone number<br>• Patient's name, address, and telephone number<br>• Reason for the call<br>• Degree of urgency<br>• The patient's insurance information and precertification number. | The physician performing the procedure and the outpatient facility needs to know these things to serve the patient well. |
| 4. Advise the patient verbally and in writing of the following information as soon as possible:<br><br>• The date, time, and location of the procedure<br>• Any specific restrictions or requirements to prepare for the procedure<br>• Be sure the information is complete, accurate, and easy to read. | The patient must be instructed on any preparation involved prior to having the procedure as well as when it is scheduled. Both communication formats reinforce the patient's memory and prevent miscommunication that might occur and possibly delay the procedure. It is important that the patient keeps his or her appointment. |

*(continues on page 156)*

## PROCEDURE 6.3 (continued)

| STEPS | REASONS |
|-------|---------|
| 5. Record in the patient's chart the time and date of the call and the name of the person who received your call. | This is necessary for proper documentation of the patient's care. |
| 6. Tell the person you are calling that you wish to be notified if your patient does not keep the appointment. If this occurs, be sure to tell your physician and enter this information in the patient's record. | The physician is responsible for the patient's care and should know if the appointment is not kept. Anyone in the office who needs this information will have it. |
| 7. **AFF** Explain how you would handle the following situation: The patient is an elderly male who is severely hearing impaired. How can you make certain that he understands the information about the procedure accurately? | You could make sure you have his attention and speak slowly and in a louder tone than you would normally use for other patients. Patient confidentiality must be maintained, so this should be done in a private area. With his authorization, you may also give this information to someone else, such as a spouse or caregiver. |

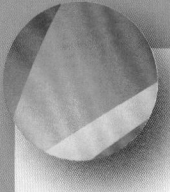

## PROCEDURE 6-4

# Arranging for Admission to an Inpatient Facility

**PSY** Arrange for admission to an inpatient facility; apply third-party managed care policies and procedures; and obtain precertification, including documentation

**Purpose:** To arrange admission to an inpatient facility providing all necessary information including insurance precertification, and to provide instructions to the patient

**Equipment:** Physician's order with diagnosis, patient's chart with demographic information, contact information for inpatient facility

| STEPS | REASONS |
|---|---|
| 1. Determine the place that the patient and/or physician wants the admission arranged. | Physicians may have privileges at one hospital or several hospitals. The patient's insurance carrier may have a preferred facility list as well. |
| 2. Gather information for the other facility, including demographic and insurance information. | Having the patient's demographic and insurance information handy avoids delays. |
| 3. Determine any precertification requirements. If needed, locate contact information on the back of the insurance card and call the insurance carrier to obtain a precertification number. | Most insurance carriers must be notified in advance of an admission to an inpatient facility. Telephone numbers for insurance eligibility and precertification inquiries will be printed on the back of the insurance card. You will be given a precertification number that must be given to the hospital admissions department. This number will follow the patient through the claims later filed for that admission. Document on the form approved by the office manager or physician for insurance authorizations or in the patient's medical record. |
| 4. Obtain from the physician the diagnosis and exact needs of the patient for an admission. | The hospital admissions department will need the patient's exact diagnosis. They will also need to know of any special requirements, such as a private room, isolation, etc. |
| 5. Call the admissions department of the inpatient facility and give information from Step 2. | The admissions department handles all preliminary information, insurance information, etc. before assigning the patient a room. |
| 6. Obtain instructions for the patient and call or give the patient instructions and information. | Patients should be given complete information in writing if possible. Patients may be afraid and emotional when they are being admitted to a hospital. Be sure they understand their instructions. |
| 7. Provide the patient with the physician's orders for his or her hospital stay, including diet, medications, bed rest, etc. | If the patient is not at your office, the physician must call in this information. Most hospitals prefer that patients bring this information. |
| 8. Document time, place, etc. in patient's chart, including any precertification requirements completed. | Any appointments made for the patient must be documented in the patient's chart. This provides the information to anyone in the office who needs it. |
| 9. **AFF** Explain how you would respond to a patient who is visibly shaken about finding that he or she is being admitted to the hospital. | Remain calm yourself. Be patient and do not rush the patient, if possible. Reassure the patient that he or she will receive excellent care. Be careful not to make promises of any outcomes. |

# CHAPTER 7 Written Communications

## Learning Outcomes

### COG Cognitive Domain*

1. Spell and define the key terms
2. *Recognize elements of fundamental writing skills*
3. Discuss the basic guidelines for grammar, punctuation, and spelling in medical writing
4. *Organize technical information and summaries*
5. Discuss the 11 key components of a business letter
6. Describe the process of writing a memorandum
7. List the items that must be included in an agenda
8. Identify the items that must be included when typing minutes
9. Cite the various services available for sending written information
10. Discuss the various mailing options
11. Identify the types of incoming written communication seen in a physician's office
12. Explain the guidelines for opening and sorting mail
13. *Discuss applications of electronic technology in professional communication*

### PSY Psychomotor Domain*

1. *Compose a professional correspondence utilizing electronic technology (Procedure 7-1)*
2. Open and sort mail (Procedure 7-2)
3. *Report relevant information concisely and accurately (Procedure 7-1)*

### AFF Affective Domain*

1. Use language/verbal skills that enable the patient's understanding
2. Demonstrate empathy in communicating with patients, family, and staff
3. Demonstrate sensitivity appropriate to the message being delivered
4. Demonstrate recognition of the patient's level of understanding in communications

*Note: AAMA/CAAHEP 2015 Standards are italicized.*

**ABHES Competencies**

1. Perform fundamental writing skills including correct grammar, spelling, and formatting techniques when writing prescriptions, documenting medical records, etc.
2. Apply electronic technology
3. Adapt communications to individual's ability to understand
4. Respond to and initiate written communications
5. Utilize electronic technology to receive, organize, prioritize, and transmit information
6. Use correct grammar, spelling, and formatting techniques in written word

## Key Terms

| | | | |
|---|---|---|---|
| agenda | enclosure | margin | semiblock |
| annotation | font | memorandum | template |
| BiCaps | full block | proofread | |
| block | intercaps | salutation | |

## Case Study

*S*ophie Taylor, CMA, has the responsibility of writing many of the physicians' letters concerning day-to-day operations at Great Falls Medical Center. The letters she writes include requests for release of medical records, patient collection letters, appeals to denials by insurance companies, and responses to patient e-mails on the patient portal in the electronic medical record. She also attends the quarterly board of directors meetings and takes the minutes. Is there a certain format that Sophie should use to compose business letters? What are the "minutes" and is there a format she should use for documenting them? What rules should she follow when writing professional correspondence? Is it appropriate to respond to patients' e-mails using text message language and abbreviations? This chapter addresses all of these questions and many others concerning written communications in the medical office.

Good written communication skills are important for success. In the medical office, written communication is generated in several forms, such as reports (Table 7-1) and letters. Medical assistants commonly compose collection letters, patient reminders, and notifications of test results. You may also have an opportunity to produce memoranda, agendas, and minutes for meetings. Another important form of written communication is the handwritten entry in a patient's medical record. No matter which form it takes, your written communication must be clear, concise, and correct. Poorly written documents reflect negatively on you, the practice, and the physician. Written communication may be sent or received through facsimile machines, electronic mail, delivery services, or United States postal service. As discussed throughout this text, the Health Insurance Portability and Accountability Act of 1996 (HIPAA) Privacy Rule protects the confidentiality of all medical communication. Sending and receiving written communication according to the rules of confidentiality are also discussed. This chapter discusses guidelines for composing letters, writing memoranda, and composing agendas and minutes with proper grammar, spelling, and punctuation.

| TABLE 7-1 Medical Reports | |
|---|---|
| **Medical Office Documents** | **Hospital Documents** |
| The most common documents generated in a medical office are | Documents generated in the hospital setting include |
| • History and physical examination (H&P) reports<br>• Consultation reports<br>• Progress reports<br>• Diagnostic test reports (if the practice offers diagnostic tests) | • H&Ps<br>• Consultation reports<br>• Radiology and pathology reports<br>• Transfer summaries<br>• Discharge and death summaries<br>• Autopsy reports |
| Other types of documents in outpatient facilities include | |
| • Reports of minor surgical procedures<br>• Legal abstracts<br>• General office correspondence | |

Hospital (inpatient) documents and medical office (outpatient) documents are different. You need to become familiar with the reports generated in a hospital because they become a part of the office chart and are needed for patient care, coding insurance claims, etc. Appendix F contains samples of typical reports generated in a hospital or inpatient setting.

## GUIDELINES FOR PRODUCING PROFESSIONAL AND MEDICAL DOCUMENTS

### Basic Grammar and Punctuation Guidelines

Professional writing requires that you follow the appropriate rules of grammar and punctuation. Box 7-1 provides a helpful list of key rules you will need to know.

### Basic Spelling Guidelines

Spelling, according to *Merriam-Webster Collegiate Dictionary,* 11th ed., is the act of forming words from letters. Good spelling skills take time to acquire, but learning to spell correctly is indispensable to the written communication process. Successful communication requires that the information received is understood by the recipient, and that process may be hindered or misunderstood if words are not used correctly or are misspelled (see Chapter 3). Box 7-2 lists basic tips for spelling. Many words sound exactly alike but are spelled differently and have different meanings. Be very careful with these words. Which of the following sentences has a spelling error?

• Wound cultures were taken from the left lower leg site.
• Wound cultures were taken from the left lower leg cite.

The first sentence is correct. Site and cite sound alike, and both are spelled correctly, but in the second sentence, the wrong word was used.

Spell check in word processing programs can be a great asset, but it has limitations. Medical terminology spell check software should be added to your computer

and be updated frequently. You can add medical terms into your computer's spell check dictionary, but make sure that any word you add is spelled correctly! Spell checks can never be 100% stocked with all the needed terms, especially in the medical profession, as new technologies, medications, and treatments arise daily.

Remember, spell check will not recognize words that are spelled correctly but misused. Even if you use spell check, you should proofread your document for other errors.

For example, the following sentence would pass spell check but is incorrect.

• The patient has inflammation of the prostrate.

Prostrate is an adjective that means face down. "The patient was in a prostrate position." The patient has inflammation of the *prostate*, the male sex gland.

• The physician received a plague.
• The physician received a plaque.

There is a big difference between plaque (commemorative item) and plague (bacterial disease)! These types of errors occur as a result of poor word usage and poor spelling. Box 7-3 lists some commonly used medical words that can easily be misspelled or misused.

### Accuracy

Many of the medical documents or letters that you will write contain information that requires precision, accuracy, and careful attention to details. Inaccurate information in some letters can lead to injury of a patient and lawsuits and can harm the physician's practice. Some of your letters will be placed in the patient's permanent medical record. Most letters will start with the physician

## BOX 7-1 Basic Grammar and Punctuation Tips

### Punctuation

- Period (.)—Used at end of sentences and following some abbreviations.
- Comma (,)—Used to separate words or phrases that are part of a series of three or more. The final comma before the "and" may be omitted. A comma can also be used after a long introductory clause or to separate independent clauses joined by "and," "but," "yet," "or," and "nor."
- Semicolon (;)—Used to separate a long list of items in a series and to separate independent clauses not joined by a conjunction (e.g., and, but, or).
- Colon (:)—Used to introduce a series of items, to follow formal salutations, and to separate the hours from minutes indicating time.
- Apostrophe (')—Used to denote omissions of letters and to denote the possessive case of nouns.
- Quotation marks (" ")—Used to set off spoken dialogue, some titles (e.g., journal articles, newspaper articles, television, and radio program episodes), and words used in a special way (Table 7-2).
- Parentheses [( )]—Used to indicate a part of a sentence that is not part of the main sentence but is essential for the meaning of the sentence. Also used

to enclose a number, for confirmation, that is spelled out in a sentence.
- Ellipsis (…)—Used in place of a period to indicate a prolonged continuation of a conversation or list. Also used to display individual items or to connect phrases that are loosely connected.
- Diagonal (/)—Used in abbreviations (c/o), in dates (2003/2004), in fractions (3/4), and to indicate two or more options (AM/FM).

### Sentence Structure

- Avoid long, run-on sentences.
- A verb must always agree with its subject in number and person.
- Ensure that the proper pronoun (he or she) is used.
- Adjectives should be used when they add an important message. Don't overuse adjectives or adverbs. Remember, double negatives used in one sentence make the sentence positive.

### Capitalization

- Capitalize the first word in a sentence, proper nouns, the pronoun "I," book titles, and known geographical names.
- Names of persons, holidays, and trademark items should be capitalized.

### TABLE 7-2 The Use of Other Punctuation with Quotation Marks

| Rule | Example |
| --- | --- |
| Place commas and periods inside quotation marks. | "Your bill," explained the patient, "has not come in the mail." |
| Place colons and semicolons outside quotation marks. | She said, "The doctor told me to come back on Friday"; however, he has no openings. |
| Place other punctuation inside quotation marks only if they belong in the quotation. | The student asked, "Is that going to be on the test?" |
| Place commas and periods outside quotation marks when used with single letters or single words. | Even though she earned an "A," she felt it was not her best work. |

asking you to draft a letter. The physician may or may not give you some notes to follow. He or she may dictate the letter. Either way, your responsibility in typing the letter is to be as accurate as possible and to question anything about which you are unsure. Here are some examples of inaccuracy:

- You wrote, "The patient was started on the MVP chemotherapy regimen." The physician, however, had written "MVPP." These are two completely different regimens. MVP is used for treating lung cancer, and MVPP is used for Hodgkin lymphoma.

- The nurse practitioner dictated, "Patient was told to take Dristan Cold tablets." You rearranged the sentence, however, and typed, "The patient had a cold and was told to take Dristan tablets." Dristan Cold contains an antihistamine medication that plain Dristan does not. Never edit a physician's sentence unless you are sure that it will not affect the meaning.
- The physician said, "There is no reason for him to start radiation therapy at this time." You wrote, "Per Dr. Smith, there is reason for him to start radiation therapy at this time." The simple elimination

## BOX 7-2   Basic Spelling Tips

When in doubt about the spelling of a word, always use a dictionary or a spell check. Keep in mind that a computer spell check will check for spelling but will not alert you to inappropriate word usage.

Remember this rhyme: I comes before e, except after c, or when sounded like a as in neighbor and weigh. Examples: achieve, receive. (The exceptions are either, neither, weird, leisure, and conscience.)

- Words ending in -ie drop the e and change the i to y before adding -ing. Examples: die, dying; lie, lying.
- Words ending in -o that are preceded by a vowel are made plural by adding s. Example: studio, studios; trio, trios. Words ending in o that are preceded by a consonant form the plural by adding es. Examples: potato, potatoes; hero, heroes.
- Words ending in -y preceded by a vowel form the plural by adding s. Examples: attorney, attorneys; day, days. For words ending in -y that are preceded by a consonant, change the y to i and add es. Examples: berry, berries; lady, ladies.
- The final consonant of a one-syllable word is doubled before adding a suffix beginning with a vowel. Examples: run, running; pin, pinning. If the final consonant is preceded by another consonant or by two vowels, do not double the consonant. Examples: look, looking; act, acting.
- Words ending in a silent -e generally drop the e before adding a suffix beginning with a vowel. Examples: ice, icing; judge, judging. The exceptions are dye, eye, shoe, and toe. The e is not dropped, however, in suffixes beginning with a consonant unless another vowel precedes the final e. Examples: pale, paleness; argue, argument.
- For all words ending in -c, insert a k before adding a suffix beginning with e, i, or y. Examples: picnic, picnicking; traffic, trafficker.

## BOX 7-3   Commonly Misused or Misspelled Medical Terms

- anoxia and anorexia
- aphagia and aphasia
- bowl and bowel
- emphysema and empyema
- fundus and fungus
- lactose and lactase
- metatarsals and metacarpals
- mucus and mucous
- parental and parenteral
- postnatal and postnasal
- pubic and pubis
- rubella and rubeola
- serum and sebum
- uvula and vulva

### CHECKPOINT QUESTION

1. What are three consequences that could arise from inaccurate information in a business letter?

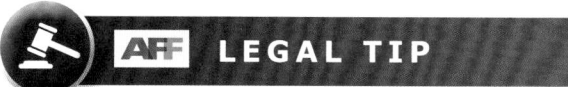

## LEGAL TIP

### Be Cautious When Using Abbreviations

Here are some abbreviations that could be misinterpreted:

- The physician wrote, "The patient had good BS." You assumed that BS meant bowel sounds, so you typed "The patient had good bowel sounds," but the physician meant the abbreviation BS to mean breath sounds.
- Do not change < or > signs to *less than* or *greater than* unless you are sure of what the statement is saying. For example, "The patient will not be admitted to the hospital until her hemoglobin is less than 13." If you made a mistake and typed "greater than 13," confusion and patient safety would occur.
- The symbols for male (♂) and female (♀) are commonly used in handwritten notes, but you should replace these symbols with words when writing a business or professional letter.

## Capitalization

It is important to know when to capitalize and when to use lowercase letters. Following standard guidelines for using capital letters applies to most correspondence, but there are some exceptions and additional rules when typing medical documents. Never change how a word is capitalized unless directed to do so. Ask for clarification and mark the proof letter with a question mark for the physician to assist.

of the word "no" completely changes the meaning of the sentence and can lead to errors in patient care.

- The physician's assistant dictated, "Hospitalization is needed because the patient continues to be violent." However, you typed, "Hospitalization is needed because the patient continues to be violet." The meaning of the sentence has been changed by the elimination of one "n" in violent.

Use capital letters:

1. For headings: CHIEF COMPLAINT or Chief Complaint.
2. For eponyms (terms formed using the name of a person, usually the name of the researcher or physician who identified a disorder or the inventor of equipment, instruments, supplies, and so on); the second word in the phrase is not capitalized. *Note:* Recent revisions in punctuation guidelines eliminate the possessive apostrophe.

   Down syndrome
   Foley catheter
   Healy clamp
3. For trade or brand names of drugs and products. Do not capitalize generic names of drugs and products.

   diazepam Valium
   tissue Kleenex
4. For the genus of an organism. An example of this classification system of living organisms is *Staphylococcus aureus*. *Staphylococcus* is the genus, and *aureus* is the species. A singular genus is capitalized and italicized. If the genus is plural or used as an adjective, it is lowercase and not italicized. Use lowercase letters and italics for the species.

   As noun: *Staphylococcus aureus*
   As adjective: staphylococcal infection
5. For a department name when the name is the proper title of a place, but not for department names within a facility.

   The patient was taken to the emergency room.
   The patient was taken to the Forsyth Medical Center Emergency Room.
6. For proper names of languages, races, and religions. Do not capitalize informal designations such as white or black.

   She is a 23-year-old Hispanic woman.
7. For acronyms (words formed from initials of words in a phrase).

   NKDA (no known drug allergies)
   CABG (coronary artery bypass graft)
8. To draw attention to vital information, such as allergies.

   ALLERGIES: The patient is allergic to PENICILLIN.
9. **Intercaps** or **BiCaps** are abbreviations, words, or phrases with unusual capitalization. Note that the accepted format should be used. For example, m-BACOD is a very different medication regimen from M-BACOD.

   pH, RhoGam, rPA, ReoPro, aVR

## Abbreviations and Symbols

Abbreviations and symbols can save time in long handwriting and with word processing documents. When you use abbreviations in medical documents, your reader must be able to recognize or translate the abbreviation; however, professional correspondence should avoid abbreviations and spell words in their entirety. The possibility of confusion is not worth the time saved by using an abbreviation. When in doubt, spell it out. Abbreviations are also discussed in Chapter 8.

Medical facilities and practices accredited by The Joint Commission are required to "standardize" the abbreviations, acronyms, and symbols used by their employees. Standardization includes having a process to identify accepted abbreviations and then making sure all employees are informed of and have access to a list of these approved abbreviations. The list should be updated regularly. In cases where there may be more than one definition of an established abbreviation, you must identify the definition to be accepted by the facility. The Joint Commission also requires facilities to make and communicate a "do not use" list, which should include abbreviations and symbols that could be ambiguous. (See Chapter 8 and Appendix D for more information.)

Some medical practices have abbreviations that are commonly used and specific to the practice. Like words in English, many abbreviations have two meanings. Some abbreviations have become accepted because they are used more than the long form. BP has come to be easily recognized as blood pressure when used in the vital sign section of the medical documentation.

Most doctors' offices use standard abbreviations when writing in patient charts, but when you are typing a formal report, it is risky to use abbreviations. If it is the policy of your practice to use abbreviations in letters and formal reports, spell out the words the first time the abbreviation is used, with the abbreviation following in parentheses. For example, "The patient had a coronary artery bypass graft (CABG) in 1987." Become familiar with the abbreviations and symbols that are used where you work. Appendix D lists the most common abbreviations.

## Plural and Possessive

Converting words to plural or possessive form can be tricky in English. Most medical terms have a Latin or Greek origin and have their own set of rules for pluralization. Box 7-4 shows the rules for pluralizing most medical terms. When writing in a medical chart, you should be accurate because mistakes can cause confusion. It is best to avoid contractions. For example, "The patient's coming in Monday to be taught to give herself allergy injections. This will require the patient's undivided attention." The contraction in the first sentence should be written out. The second sentence shows the proper usage of the apostrophe.

To show possession, use an apostrophe and add an S to the word: "The patient's appointment is tomorrow."

## BOX 7-4   Rules for Pluralizing Medical Terms

| | |
|---|---|
| A add an E | bulla becomes bullae |
| UM changes to A | ovum becomes ova |
| US changes to I | bronchus becomes bronchi |
| ON changes to A | phenomenon becomes phenomena |
| IS changes to ES or IDES | testis becomes testes, epididymis becomes epididymides |
| AX or IX: change the X to C and add ES | thorax becomes thoraces |
| EX changes to ICES | index becomes indices |
| EN: drop the EN and add INA | lumen becomes lumina |
| MA changes to MATA | carcinoma becomes carcinomata |
| NX or YNX change to NGES | phalanx becomes phalanges, larynx becomes larynges |

To show possession in a plural word, place the apostrophe after the S: "The medical assistants' credentials are verified before they are hired."

It is common in the medical environment to hear possessive units of time: "The patient will return in 2 weeks' time." or "Tuesday's patients will have to be rescheduled."

## Numbers

In general, numbers one to nine should be spelled out, except when used with units of measurement (e.g., 5 mg), and numbers 10 and over may be expressed as a numeral. When several numbers are used in a sentence, this rule is ignored in order to maintain consistency. All numbers in the sentence should be written in the same form. For example, "There are 21 students in the 2-year medical assisting program."

Here are some important tips you will need to remember about numbers:

- Numbers referring to an obstetrical patient's medical history are not written out: "The patient is a gravida 3, para 2." Do not convert these numbers.
- Watch decimal point placement. There is a huge difference in medication between 12.5 mg and 1.25 mg.
- Double-check that you have not transposed numbers. For example, you typed, "The patient's red blood cell count was 5.1," but it was actually 1.5. A red blood cell count of 1.5 is incompatible with life.

- Roman numerals should never be changed to words. For example, "lead II of the patient's electrocardiogram" should never be changed to "lead two of the patient's electrocardiogram."
- Many health care professionals use military time. Time that is written in military style does not have to be changed if the recipient of the letter is familiar with it (doctors, nurses). If the letter is going to a patient or other person who may not be able to interpret it, however, either convert the time or express the standard time in parenthesis; for example, "The patient's next appointment is at 1430 hours (2:30 PM)." No colons are used in military time.
- Temperatures must always have the correct symbol for Celsius or Fahrenheit included (98.6°F or 37°C).
- Telephone numbers should include the area code in parentheses or followed by a hyphen, then the number with a hyphen. Add extensions to the number by placing a comma after the last digit of the number, then type Ext. and the number: (800) 555-0000, Ext. 6480. Periods may replace hyphens and parentheses: 800.555.0000.

## CHECKPOINT QUESTION

2. Why should all numbers in a sentence be written in the same way regardless of the rule?

## PROFESSIONAL LETTER DEVELOPMENT

Professional writing is different from writing letters or sending e-mails or text messages to your friends or family members. The goal of professional writing is to get information communicated in a concise, accurate, and comprehensible manner. Slang or idiomatic terms that are commonly used in writing to friends are not appropriate for business letters. For example, "Drop by and say hi" is not suitable for a professional letter, even if you know the recipient personally.

Writing effective business letters is a skill that requires practice and careful attention to detail. To write a professional business letter, you must

- Understand the components of a letter
- Use the correct letter format
- Ensure that the message is clear, concise, and accurate

Word processing has replaced the typewriter for written correspondence and medical reports. Documents can be saved and retrieved, and editing applications make it easy to produce professional documents. Form letters can be used and correspondence merged with a mailing list to make communicating with patients easy

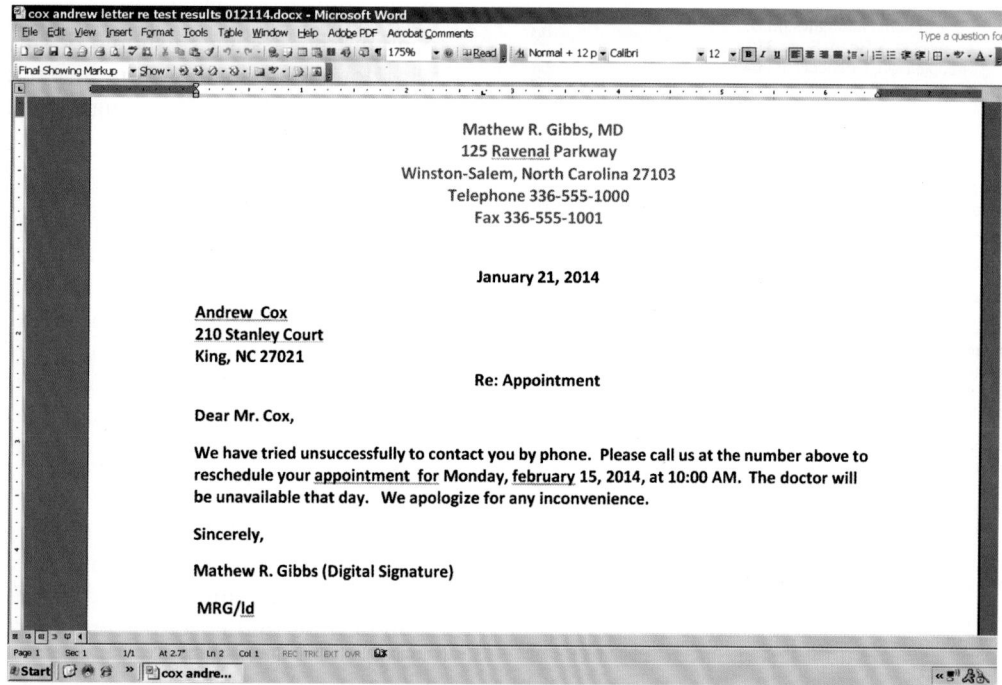

**Figure 7-1** • A document generated in Microsoft Word. Note the four errors marked by spell and grammar check. The letter uses a digital signature line supplied with the software license.

and efficient. Grammar and spell check applications mark errors by underlining the incorrect item in green or red. Figure 7-1 shows a letter generated in Microsoft Word.

These skills are described in the following sections.

## Components of a Letter

A typical business letter has 11 components. We will explore each one, beginning at the top of the page. For easy reference, Figure 7-2 displays a sample business letter with these components marked.

1. *Letterhead*. The letterhead consists of the name of the practice or physician, address, telephone number, fax number, and possibly an e-mail address and Web site for the practice. The letterhead may also have the company logo with everything embossed in color and centered on the top of the page. The letterhead may also be preset into a **template**. (Templates are discussed later in the chapter.)
2. *Date*. The date includes the month, day, and year. It should be positioned two to four spaces below the letterhead. The date must be typed on only one line, and abbreviations should not be used.
3. *Inside address*. The inside address refers to the name and address of the person to whom the letter is being sent. A nine-digit zip code should be used if available. The inside address is placed two

spaces down from the date unless the letter is being mailed with a window envelope, and it will not be aligned correctly. Never abbreviate city or town names. States can be abbreviated. (See Appendix C for a list of abbreviations approved by the postal service.) Never abbreviate business titles (e.g., President, Chief Executive Officer). Here are some other points to remember:

- If the letter is going to a business, type the name of the addressee, followed by his or her title, the name of the business on the next line, and then the address.
- If the letter is being addressed to two or more people at different addresses, type the individual address block one line space under the other or place the addresses side by side.
- If the letter is going to two people at the same address but with different last names, type them in alphabetical order by last names with each name listed below the other and then the address.

4. *Subject line*. The subject line, an optional component, is used to state the intent of a letter or to indicate what the letter is regarding. It is placed on the third line below the inside address and is written as Re: (an abbreviation for regarding) followed by the subject. For example, Re: Blood tests.
5. *Salutation*. The **salutation** is the greeting of the letter. It is placed two spaces down from the inside

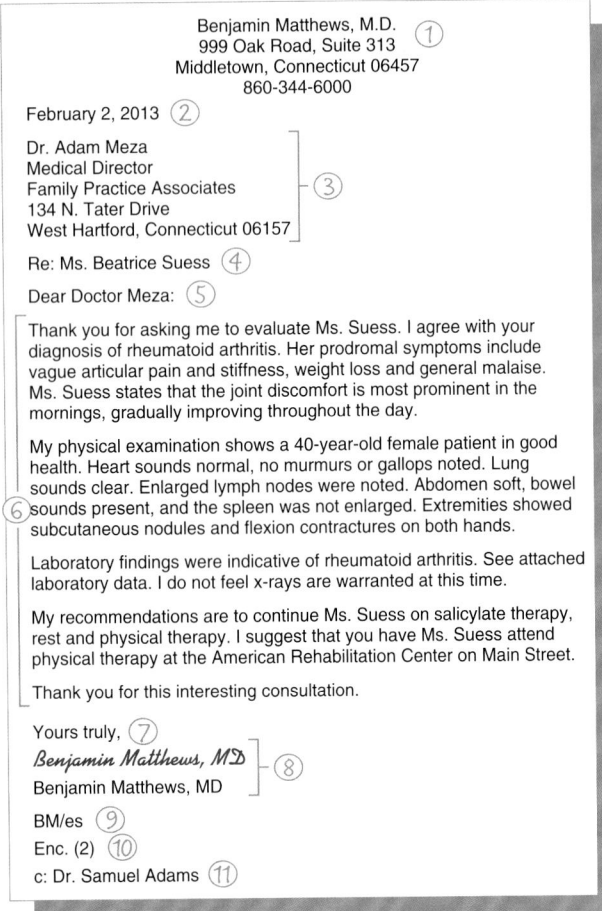

Benjamin Matthews, M.D. ①
999 Oak Road, Suite 313
Middletown, Connecticut 06457
860-344-6000

February 2, 2013 ②

Dr. Adam Meza
Medical Director
Family Practice Associates ③
134 N. Tater Drive
West Hartford, Connecticut 06157

Re: Ms. Beatrice Suess ④

Dear Doctor Meza: ⑤

Thank you for asking me to evaluate Ms. Suess. I agree with your diagnosis of rheumatoid arthritis. Her prodromal symptoms include vague articular pain and stiffness, weight loss and general malaise. Ms. Suess states that the joint discomfort is most prominent in the mornings, gradually improving throughout the day.

My physical examination shows a 40-year-old female patient in good health. Heart sounds normal, no murmurs or gallops noted. Lung sounds clear. Enlarged lymph nodes were noted. Abdomen soft, bowel ⑥ sounds present, and the spleen was not enlarged. Extremities showed subcutaneous nodules and flexion contractures on both hands.

Laboratory findings were indicative of rheumatoid arthritis. See attached laboratory data. I do not feel x-rays are warranted at this time.

My recommendations are to continue Ms. Suess on salicylate therapy, rest and physical therapy. I suggest that you have Ms. Suess attend physical therapy at the American Rehabilitation Center on Main Street.

Thank you for this interesting consultation.

Yours truly, ⑦
*Benjamin Matthews, MD* ⑧
Benjamin Matthews, MD

BM/es ⑨
Enc. (2) ⑩
c: Dr. Samuel Adams ⑪

**Figure 7-2** • Components of a business letter. This letter is done in full block format and contains the following elements: (1) letterhead, (2) date, (3) inside address, (4) subject line, (5) salutation, (6) body, (7) closing, (8) signature and typed name, (9) identification line, (10) enclosure, and (11) copy.

address or the subject line. Capitalize the first letter of each word in the phrase, and end the phrase with a colon. It is permissible to eliminate the salutation if the letter is informal or if a subject line has been used. Always use professional titles, if known, such as "Dr. Jones" in your salutations. Here are other recommendations when writing salutations:

- If the letter is going to one person and the gender is known, write "Dear Mr. Rogers."
- If the letter is going to one person and the gender is *not* known, write "Dear Pat Smith" (use the person's first name).
- If the letter is going to a woman and a man with different last names, always address the woman first: "Dear Ms. Ray and Mr. Oscar."
- If the letter is going to several people, place them in alphabetical order: "Dear Mr. Andersen, Mr. Cats, Ms. Dart, and Mr. Raymond."
- To Whom It May Concern, Dear Sir, or Dear Madam should not be used.

6. *Body of the letter*. The body of the letter contains the message. It should be single spaced with double spacing between the paragraphs. Here are some guidelines for writing the body of the letter:

- If the letter is more than one page long, try to avoid dividing a paragraph at the end of a page. If you must, leave at least two sentences at the bottom of the first page. Use the automatic page break feature in your word processor program to prevent single lines in a paragraph from appearing at the bottom of a page or the top of a page. This may be conveniently accomplished through the widow and orphan control feature in your word processing software.
- Tables and graphs should not be broken. They should appear on one page only.
- Web addresses and e-mail addresses should fit on one line and never be continued to another page.
- If the letter is more than one page long, page numbers should be used.
- Use a bulleted format to highlight key points for the reader. For example, "The possible side effects of this medication are:" (then list them vertically with a bullet symbol).
- The letterhead is used only on the first page of the letter. The second page should be a blank page, but the same quality paper as the letterhead. Start the second page with a continuation line (name of person the letter is going to and the date of the letter). Continue the letter two lines down from the continuation line. Your **margins** must be the same as those on page 1. Most templates type the continuation line for you.

7. *Closing*. The closing concludes the letter and comes just before the writer's signature. Some common closings are Sincerely, Yours truly, Regards, Respectfully, and Cordially yours. Only the first word is capitalized, and a comma follows the phrase. Closings are placed two spaces down from the end of the letter. Never put the closing alone on a page.

8. *Signature and typed name*. The name of the person sending the document is typed four spaces below the closing, with the person's title typed directly below. The physician will read and sign the letter above the typed name. If you are instructed to sign the letter, sign the physician's name followed by a slash mark and your name, e.g., Susan James, MD/Raymond Smith, RMA.

9. *Identification line*. The identification line, an optional component, indicates who dictated the letter and who wrote it. It consists of abbreviations

only. The initials of the person who dictated the letter are capitalized (generally the physician); the initials of the writer of the letter are in lowercase (generally these will be yours). The identification line can also be called the *reference line*. The dictator can sign off on the document electronically by using a digital signature provided in the word processing software. In the letter in Figure 7-1, a digital signature is used.

10. *Enclosure*. An **enclosure** is something that is included with a letter. It is abbreviated Enc. and is placed two spaces down from the identification line. The number of documents included is placed in parentheses; if only one document is included, just the abbreviation Enc. is used.

11. *Copy*. The abbreviation c is used to indicate that a duplicate letter has been sent. It is typed two spaces below the enclosure line. Usually, letters are copied to managers, supervisors, or to the physician who requested that the given information be dispersed.

## Letter Formats

There are three basic types of letter formats: **full block**, **semiblock**, and **block**. Office policy or the physician preferences will dictate which format you use. Full block is shown in Figure 7-2, which shows the components of a business letter. The elements of the block letter are seen in Figure 7-3, and the semiblock format

William Erikson, MD
Storrs Family Practice
22 Maple Avenue
Storrs, Connecticut 06268

August 15, 2012

Ms. Karen Roberts
Office Manager
ABC Copier
Fifth Avenue
Storrs, Connecticut 06268

Dear Ms. Roberts:

We are pleased to announce that we have selected your firm to meet our copying needs for 2013.

Please forward a contract to us, including the stipulations that were previously discussed. After reviewing the contract, I will contact you to arrange for a date and time for a staff orientation session on using the new copier.

I look forward to working with you and ABC Copier.

Sincerely,

Jenny Jacobs, RMA

WE/jj

c: William Erikson, M.D.

**Figure 7-3** • Sample block letter.

Elizabeth Jones, M.D.
750 East Street, Suite 205
Hialeah, Florida 33013
305-311-2666

June 12, 2013

Margaret Trent
18 Cambridge Street
Hialeah, Florida 33013

Dear Ms. Trent:

As per our phone conversation, your blood glucose level remains elevated. It is essential that we stabilize your blood sugar level.

In order to achieve normal blood sugar levels, you must follow the enclosed diet. A meeting with a Registered Dietitian can be arranged for you to discuss any dietary concerns you may have.

I am also enclosing patient education instructions for the use of a glucometer. You must test your blood sugar every morning and keep a diary of your results. Glucometers can be purchased from any pharmacy. If you need assistance in using the glucometer, please contact Raymond Smith, CMA, at 555-6423.

Presently, I do not wish to prescribe any medications. If we are unable to get your blood sugar under control, I will prescribe an oral diabetic medication.

Please call my office and schedule an appointment for the week of June 20 for a blood draw and a follow-up visit.

Sincerely,

Elizabeth Jones, M.D.

EJ/rs

enc. (2)

**Figure 7-4** • Sample semiblock letter.

is seen in Figure 7-4. Semiblock is also referred to as *modified block*.

## Composing a Business Letter

To create a professional business letter, follow these three steps: preparation, composition, and editing. Box 7-5 gives you some guidelines for starting to write a letter.

### CHECKPOINT QUESTION

3. Whose address is typed as the inside address? What is the purpose of the salutation? What is the purpose of the identification line?

### Composition

The goal of composition is to ensure that your message is transmitted clearly, concisely, and accurately to your reader. As you did during preparation, focus on the message, not on the mechanics.

A clear message ensures that your reader knows precisely what is expected; an unclear message is poor communication that leaves room for doubt, thereby causing confusion.

*Unclear*: Please contact me.
*Clear*: Please contact me by Thursday, October 1.

**BOX 7-5**  **PSY** **How to Start Writing a Letter**

By determining the answers to these four questions, you can better prepare the message of your letter.

1. Who is my reader?

   It is very important that you use proper gender identification. Be especially careful with names that can be used for males or females (e.g., Sam, Kelly, Ronnie, Alex, Tracy). Determine the reader's comprehension level. Letters to physicians will be more technical and will use medical terminology. Letters to patients will be less technical and use medical terminology sparingly.

2. What do I want my reader to do?

   This is your call to action; make it clear and specific. For example, you might write, "Please complete the enclosed insurance form (two pages). Be sure to include all necessary information and sign your name. Place the form in the enclosed envelope, and return it to our office by June 15, 2003." Avoid using "at your earliest convenience"; include a date for the required action. If possible, include a response mechanism, such as a self-addressed, stamped envelope.

3. What do I want to say?

   Briefly list the necessary information. To help you remember all of the necessary information, ask yourself who, what, where, when, why, and how.

4. How will I organize my message?

   Here are three basic ways that you can organize your message:

   • Chronological: Discuss items in a sequential manner, beginning with the earliest date and proceeding to the most recent date. For example, when discussing the physician's career, list his or her earlier experiences before the most recent career achievements.
   • Problem oriented: Let the reader know about a specific problem and provide instructions for correcting the problem. For example, if a patient's blood work came back with abnormal findings, a letter would be sent identifying the problem (e.g., low hematocrit) and advising the patient on the possible causes, treatments, and follow-up procedures.
   • Comparison: Evaluate the effectiveness of two or more items. For example, as an office manager, you may have to write to the physician comparing two service contracts or two sample computer software packages.

*Unclear:* You need to make an appointment for blood work.
*Clear:* Call Temple Hospital laboratories (555–4010) and make an appointment for a blood glucose test on March 13.

A concise message is short and to the point. Wordy phrases with many adjectives should not be used.

*Not concise:* Please enclose a check in an envelope for exactly $50.
*Concise:* Please enclose a $50 check.

An accurate message includes the correct date, time, figures, and information. Inaccurate messages cause delays and confusion and can lead to poor patient outcomes as well as public relation problems. Letter templates are good tools for messages that are often repeated, such as collection letters, but they may have to be modified to become suitable for a specific situation. Many electronic health records have templates available to create letters concerning patients that may include clinical information abstracted from their medical record.

## Editing

After you have composed the letter, edit it for both grammatical errors and factual information. Editing is a key step in making your letter a success. Editing entails two steps: proofreading and corrections.

### Proofreading

Whenever possible, have a colleague **proofread** (read text and check for accuracy) your letter and provide constructive criticism. Be sure to maintain confidentiality. Consider printing out a hard copy of your document for proofreading; some individuals find it difficult to proofread a document on the computer screen. It is also important to use an easy-to-read font for business letters. Check for the following items:

• Accuracy of all information
• Clarity and conciseness
• Grammar
• Spelling
• Punctuation
• Paragraphs appropriate in length and limited to one subject
• Capitalization
• Logical organization and flow

Use proofreader marks (Box 7-6) to speed up the editing process. These are standard marks used to indicate corrections. You should become familiar with the basic marks. Letters generated using the electronic health records must also be carefully proofread in order to prevent accidental disclosures of patients' private information.

## BOX 7-6 Standard Proofreader Marks

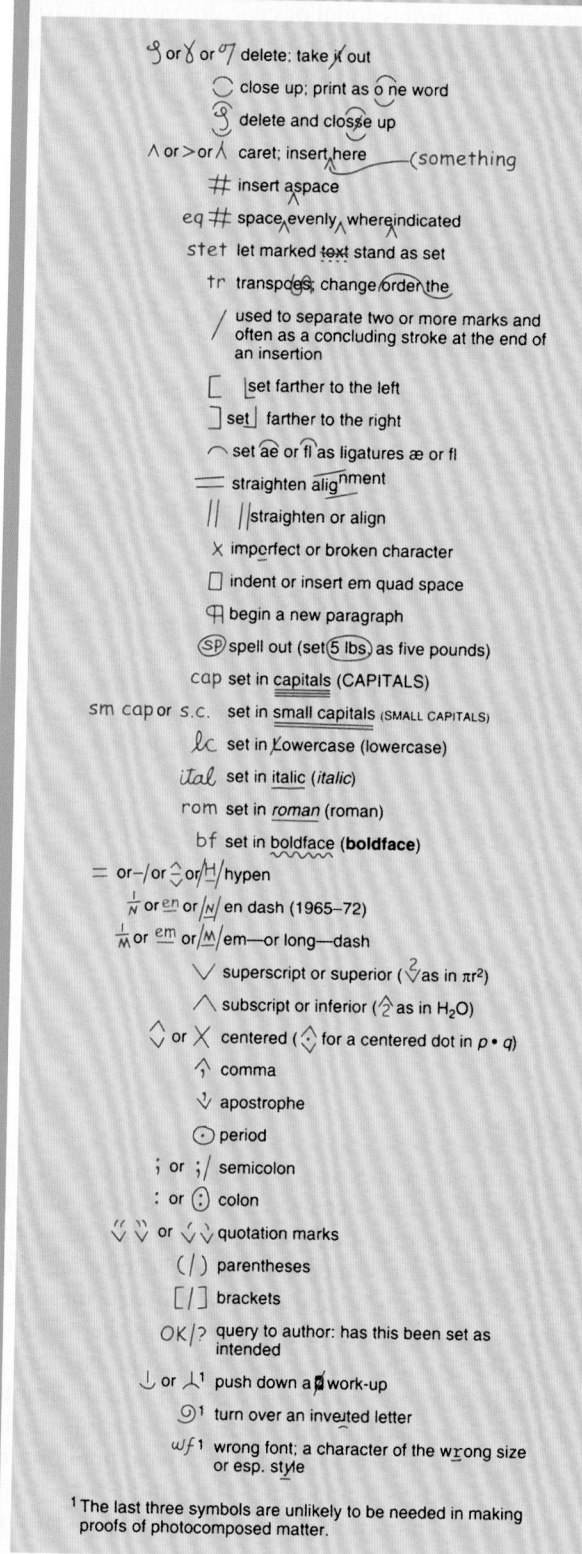

$^1$ The last three symbols are unlikely to be needed in making proofs of photocomposed matter.

4. What is the purpose of proofreading?

### Corrections

After making corrections, print a final copy of the letter. Remember, a computer spell check should be used with caution because it highlights misspelled words but not incorrectly used words.

## Types of Business Letters

You will be asked to create and type various letters. Letters that you write will be sent to patients, insurance companies, other health care providers, pharmaceutical companies, and various businesses. Here are some common types of letters that you may write:

- Letters welcoming new patients to the practice
- Letters to patients regarding their test results
- Consultation reports to other health care professionals
- Workers' compensation letters verifying the patient's injury or treatment
- Justification or explanation of treatments to insurance companies
- Cover letters for transferring patients' records to another practice
- Clarification or explanation to patients regarding fees or billing concerns
- Thank you letters to sales representatives
- Physician changes for on-call schedules (generally sent to the hospital and covering physicians)
- Announcements of new services, hours, or office location changes
- Discharge letters to patients

## COG MEMORANDUM DEVELOPMENT

A **memorandum** (often called a memo) is for communication within the office or with another department only; it is never sent to patients. It is less formal than a letter and is generally used for brief announcements such as changes in policies or an upcoming event.

## Components of a Memorandum

A memorandum contains the standard elements in the following list. Use these guidelines to complete each element. Figure 7-5 shows a sample memorandum.

1. *Heading.* The word "Memorandum" is typed across the top of the page.
2. *Date.* Use the same rules for letters when typing the date for memorandums.
3. *To.* List the names of all recipients in either alphabetic or hierarchic order. If the memorandum is going to a particular group (e.g., all department managers, all employees), it can be addressed to the group.

Franklin Dermatology Center
123 Main Street
Rockfall, Kansas
913-755-2600

**Memorandum**

**To:**    All Medical Assistants
**From:**  Patty Stricker, Office Manager
**Date:**  12/03/12
**Re:**    Holiday time

Please notify me by December 10 of any requests you have for taking time off during Christmas or New Year's. Remember that holiday requests will be based on seniority. The office will be closed at noon on December 24. The office will be closed on the 25th and reopen on the 26th. The office will also close on December 31st at noon. The office will be closed on January 1, reopening on the 2nd.

If you have any questions, please e-mail me.

**Figure 7-5 •** Sample memorandum.

4. *From.* List the name and title of the person sending the memorandum.
5. *Subject.* Insert a brief phrase describing the purpose of the memorandum.
6. *Body.* Write the message of the memorandum here.
7. *Copy (c).* Use the same rules as for letters when sending duplicate copies of memorandums.

Salutations and closings are not used in memorandums. All lines in a memorandum are justified left, and 1-inch margins are used. Writing a memorandum entails the same steps (preparation, composition, editing) as writing a business letter. The memorandum should be read and initialed by the physician before it is distributed. Your computer software will have a memorandum template.

 **CHECKPOINT QUESTION**

5. What are memorandums used for?

## COMPOSING AGENDAS AND MINUTES

Two other forms of written communication are agendas and minutes.

### Agendas

The purpose of an **agenda** is to outline briefly the topics to be discussed at a meeting. It allows the meeting participants to prepare any necessary reports before the meeting and to anticipate questions. Agendas usually begin with a call to order, followed by a review of previous meeting minutes, old business updates, and then new business. Adjournment is the last item on the agenda. The format and amount of detail included in an agenda is determined by the type of group that is meeting. Figure 7-6 shows an appropriate format for the meeting of a professional or civic organization. Your physician may take a leadership role in an organization, and you would be asked to prepare an agenda for the meetings.

 **ETHICAL TIP**

### Be Careful What You Record in the Minutes

Remember, you are recording the happenings of a meeting that will stay on record for years. The minutes of a meeting should not include personal opinions or any information that is not relevant to the *business* of the group. The purpose of minutes is to record the *actions* that took place at the meeting, not this:

*Tracy Amaral made a motion to have a bake sale for the scholarship fund. Anna Hylton seconded the motion. Discussion followed: Tracy told the group not to tell Rebecca about the bake sale. Judy reminded the group about Rebecca's ginger cookies that broke Shelby's tooth that time. Everybody got a good laugh. The motion passed.*

A more appropriate entry is as follows:
*A motion was made by Tracy Amaral to hold a bake sale on November 2nd at the community college from 7:00 AM until 3:00 PM with proceeds going to the scholarship fund. The motion was seconded by Anna Hylton. Discussion followed. The motion passed.*

### Minutes

The minutes of a meeting outline the actions of the group. Members may need to refer back to the minutes of a previous meeting. In organizations with officers, the secretary takes notes and/or records the meeting. For other meetings such as committee or board meetings, someone is assigned the task of preparing the minutes. You should type the minutes of a meeting as soon as possible. Record only motions, seconds, and the results of a vote. You may include a brief discussion of the motions but do not include unrelated items, opinions, or individual members' statements. The minutes of a meeting become an important document in the association's history. Include the following information:

• List of members present
• List of members absent
• Date and time the meeting was called to order
• Statement regarding the acceptance of the previous minutes

**Forsyth-Stokes-Davie Chapter of Medical Assistants**
**Winston-Salem NC**
**Meeting Agenda**
**September 13, 2013**

**Welcome**
*President*
**Introductions**
*Members*
**Introduction of Speaker**
*Program Committee Chair*
**Speaker**
*Roberta Williams, BSN, OSHA Update*
**Call to Order**
*President*
**Reading of the Minutes of October Mtg.**
*Secretary*
**Officers' Reports**
**Committee Reports**
**Membership Campaign**
**New Business**
**Announcements**
**Newsletter Deadline Dec. 1**
**Adjournment**

**Figure 7-6** • Sample meeting agenda.

- Motions made and the name of the person making the motion.
- Brief report of discussion
- Results of voting, whether the motion passed or not
- List of reports that were submitted
- Date and time of the next meeting
- Adjournment time
- Signature of the person who prepared the minutes and the chairperson's signature

## SENDING WRITTEN COMMUNICATION

After the document has been written, proofread, and signed, it is ready for you to send it to its receiver. Fold the letter in thirds, and place it in an envelope. Most professional letters are sent through the postal service. Other types of written communications are sent through facsimile machines or by electronic mail. Here are two key steps to remember when sending any type of written communication:

- All attempts must be made to ensure patient confidentiality. The outside of envelopes should be marked confidential when the correspondence contains information about a patient. Send letters only to known or confirmed addresses.
- Return addresses must be used so that mail can be returned if the recipient is no longer at the given address.

## Facsimile Machines

Facsimile, or fax, machines allow the medical office to send and receive printed material over a phone line. These machines offer a convenient and cost-effective way to transmit records, orders, prescriptions, test results, and other materials that require quick receipt. Always use a cover sheet (Fig. 7-7) when sending papers through a fax machine. At minimum, a cover sheet should have the following information:

- Name, address, telephone, and fax number of the physician's practice
- Name of the intended receiver of the fax
- Number of pages being sent, counting the cover sheet
- Telephone number of the fax machine of the intended recipient
- Date and time the fax was sent

Cardiology Associates
Maria Sefferin, MD
897 Bayou Drive
Philadelphia, PA
215-112-9999

**facsimile transmittal**

| To: | Fax: |
|---|---|
| From: | Date: |
| Re: | Pages: |
| CC: | |

☐ Urgent ☐ For Review ☐ Please Comment ☐ Please Reply ☐ Please Recycle

Comments:

**CONFIDENTIAL INFORMATION**
The information in the facsimile message and any accompanying documents is confidential. This information is intended only for use by the individual or entity name above. If you are not the intended recipient of this information you are hereby notified that any disclosure, copying or distribution of this information is strictly prohibited. Please notify the sender immediately by telephone.

**Figure 7-7** • Sample fax cover sheet.

• Confidentiality statement (e.g., "The information in the facsimile message and any accompanying documents is confidential. This information is intended only for use by the individual or entity name above. If you are not the intended recipient of this information, you are hereby notified that any disclosure, copying, or distribution of this information is strictly prohibited. Please notify the sender immediately by telephone.")

When you receive a fax, forward it to the appropriate person. The fax machine should be checked regularly throughout the day, and all items should be sorted quickly.

Sometimes when you fax a letter, the fax machine may be busy, or the number dialed may be busy. If the documents did not get faxed, it is not acceptable to leave them in the machine for redial unless you are sure that no one else will have access to that document. Never leave documents unattended.

## Electronic Mail

Electronic mail, or e-mail, allows computer-to-computer communication, whether within the same facility or anywhere throughout the world. The communication occurs through the Internet with computers linked to an online service provider. Chapter 9 discusses electronic mail in more detail. Here are a few things you should remember about sending letters via electronic mail:

• Confidentiality cannot be guaranteed.
• Follow the usual steps of preparation, composition, and editing. Never use abbreviated text message language, terms, or symbols in a professional e-mail.
• You can attach letters to an e-mail by clicking on the file attachment icon, locating the letter, and inserting it. It is always a good idea to open the attachment to make sure that you are attaching the correct letter or version.

## United States Postal Service

Written communication is commonly sent via the United States Postal Service (USPS). Envelopes must be correctly prepared so that the optical character readers (OCR) used by the USPS can sort the mail quickly and efficiently. The OCR reads the envelope, scanning for information. The OCR scans all envelopes using these margins: 1/2 inch on either side and 5/8 inch from the top or bottom of the envelope. Addresses or notations outside of these margins will not be read.

### Addressing Envelopes

The standard business envelope is no. 10. USPS regulations state that the minimal size of an envelope is 3 1/2 × 5 inches. It must be rectangular and no less than 0.007 inch thick. The standard no. 10 business envelope is 4 1/8 × 9 1/2 inches.

The requirements for addressing an envelope are necessary because the postal service uses OCRs, which quickly and efficiently sort the mail. As the mail travels through the scanning devices, it is sorted electronically.

The return address is placed in the upper left hand corner. It should not exceed five lines. The return address is typed with the same guidelines as for letters and is single spaced. Often, medical offices have the return address preprinted on the envelope.

The recipient's address is approximately 2 1/2 inches from the top of the envelope and about 4 inches from the left side of the envelope, which is almost centered on the face of a standard no. 10 envelope. All words of the address should be capitalized. Only postal abbreviations for states should be used, and no punctuation is used between the postal abbreviation and the zip code. All addresses must include the five-digit zip code; whenever possible, the four-digit expanded zip code should also be used. The expanded zip code allows the USPS to sort and route the mail faster and more accurately. Envelopes should not be handwritten, as this does not portray a professional image. The entire address should not exceed five lines. Your software may allow you to insert a USPS PostNet bar code. This is generally inserted two to three lines below the address. This bar code accelerates USPS sorting. Always check your software to make sure it is certified by the USPS.

Special notations such as "confidential" or "personal" are placed on the left-hand side of the envelope two lines below the return address. Notations for hand canceling and special delivery are made in the upper right-hand corner of the envelope below the postage. Nothing should be printed in the right lower corner of the envelope because the USPS uses that space for its bar codes. Figure 7-8 displays a properly addressed envelope.

Here are some additional things to remember regarding envelopes:

• Be sure that graphics or logos do not impede the OCR's ability to read the address.
• Do not use fancy **fonts** that may impede the OCR's ability to read the address.

PIEDMONT INTERNAL MEDICINE
1050 S MAIN STREET
ASHEBORO NC 26092-1050

SEAMSTER JANITORIAL SERVICE
P O BOX 5030
RALEIGH NC 25532-5030

**Figure 7-8** • Sample envelope.

- A minimum of eight-point type is recommended by the USPS.
- USE ALL CAPS.
- Do not use dark envelopes.
- White or tan envelope with black type is preferred.
- Do not use the # sign; if it cannot be avoided, leave one space between the # sign and the number (this is a USPS recommendation).
- If you are using an envelope with a window frame, there should be an 8-inch clearance around the address.

### CHECKPOINT QUESTION

6. What does an optical character reader do?

## Affixing Postage

Proper postage must be affixed to the envelope by a stamp, permit imprint, or a postage meter machine. Postage meter machines are in-house machines that are regulated by the USPS. They contain a prepaid amount of postage and can imprint the postage stamp either directly on the envelope or onto an adhesive tape that is applied to the envelope. Some machines weigh, stuff, and seal the envelopes. The date on the postage machine must be changed daily, and the ink roller must be kept full.

The physician may opt to use the USPS permit imprint program. In this case, you take the mail, sealed and ready to be sent, to the post office. The postal clerk passes your letters through the USPS machine, and a permit stamp is placed on the envelope. The postal clerk deducts the postage charges from your prepaid account. The advantages to this system are that it saves time and does not require the office to care for the postal meter machine.

## United States Postal Service Mailing Options

Mail can be sent in a variety of ways based on its urgency and value. The following is a brief description of the services offered by the USPS:

- Priority Mail Express, the fastest service, ensures delivery of your package by 1-day or 2-day expedited service 7 days a week. Express mail is automatically insured for $100. Additional insurance is available.
- Priority mail, the second fastest service, offers 2-day delivery to most destinations. The maximum weight is 70 pounds, and the rate is based on the distance of where the package is being sent and weight of the package. There is no cost for tracking your priority letter or package, and insurance may be purchased when sending valuable items.
- First-class mail is the service used for sending standard mail (letters and postcards) weighing up to 13 ounces. Mail weighing more than 13 ounces will be considered priority mail.

- Standard mail is used by companies for bulk mail service for sending newsletters and flyers. This service has a discounted rate but requires a minimum of 200 items or 50 pounds. A permit is also required by the post office.
- Postal rates, fees, and services are subject to change. You must stay abreast of the latest information. Use the USPS Web site for additional information and updates.

## United States Postal Service Special Services

A certificate of mailing is used to prove that a document was mailed. No record is kept at the post office. It does not provide proof that the letter was received by the addressee.

Certified mail provides a mailing receipt and a record of the mailing at the local post office (Fig. 7-9). This service is available only for first-class and priority mail. Return receipts can be purchased in conjunction with this. Return receipts are used to prove that the recipient received the document (Fig. 7-10).

Registered mail provides the most protection for valuables. It is available only for priority and first-class mail. The maximum insurance that can be obtained is $25,000. This service can be combined with return receipts. International rates are available from your local post office. Type the address as discussed earlier, and type the name of the country on the last line without abbreviations (Japan, Korea). All physician offices should have a supply of express and priority mail envelopes along with a current fee schedule.

## Other Delivery Options

Many other companies specialize in document and package delivery, particularly with next-day or second-day delivery services. Examples of these companies include Federal Express and United Parcel Service (UPS). Fees vary, so you may have to contact each company for

**Figure 7-9 •** Certified mail receipt.

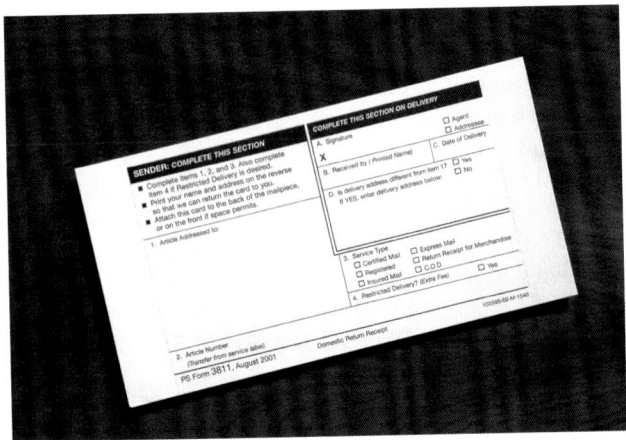

**Figure 7-10** • Return receipt.

prices and available services. These companies offer services such as tracking, pick-up services, money back guarantees, and proof of delivery. The tracking service can be done online through their Web sites.

## ⬚ RECEIVING AND HANDLING INCOMING MAIL

Part of the daily routine for a medical assistant is handling the incoming mail. Sort the mail quickly and promptly to ensure efficient functioning of the office.

### Types of Incoming Mail

Many types of mail are received daily in a physician's office:

- Advertisements
- Bills for office services
- Consultation letters
- Hospital communications and newsletters
- Laboratory and radiographic reports
- Office supply magazines
- Patient correspondence
- Payments from insurance companies and patients
- Professional journals
- Literature from professional organizations
- Samples (drugs, laboratory test kits)
- Waiting room magazines

### Opening and Sorting Mail

Each medical office will have an individual policy on which mail you should open and how you should process it. Any mail marked urgent should be handled first, followed by mail about patient-related issues. Promotional materials should be handled last. Some physicians will have you sort, file, and respond to mail without their review. In some practices, however, all mail is placed in

a special file folder and handled only by the physician or office manager. Procedure 7-2 outlines the steps for opening and sorting the mail. Most physicians will open and handle their own e-mail. If the physician is on vacation, he or she will apply an auto reply response to his or her e-mail address.

When the physician is away, personal mail is placed on his or her desk and left for the physician to handle. Mail that pertains to patient care issues should be opened and handled appropriately. If the mail requires an urgent response, the covering physician should be contacted unless otherwise directed. Mail should never be allowed to accumulate in outside mailboxes because patient information is confidential.

 **CHECKPOINT QUESTION**

7. What mail must be opened first?

### Annotation

Some physicians request that letters be annotated. **Annotation** involves reading a document and highlighting the key points. If the letter is very detailed, a summary of the key points should be written in the margins. The summary should be factual and not editorialized.

 **ROLE-PLAYING ACTIVITY**

A medical assistant at Great Falls Medical Center drafted a form letter welcoming all new patients to the practice and has asked Sophie Taylor, CMA, to proofread it for him. Unfortunately, the letter is not very professional and has several misspelled words, text message abbreviations, etc. It also does not include other pieces of important information that Sophie knows would be helpful to patients new to the practice, such as basic directions to the office, and the office financial policy. The medical assistant is known in the office for not handling criticism very well, but Sophie knows this letter cannot go to patients because of the reflection it will have on the entire practice. How can Sophie address these problems with him in a nonjudgmental way that will help him edit and correct the letter to be more professional? Are there other areas that could be considered not professional in written communications besides the ones that have been mentioned? What resources could Sophie suggest to the MA to help with his writing skills? If you are the medical assistant who wrote the letter, think about how you would feel if someone gave you constructive criticism of a letter you just wrote. Would you be grateful? Resentful or angry? Consider your emotions, if any, toward someone offering suggestions to improve your writing. Your instructor will give you additional information about this activity!

## *español* SPANISH TERMINOLOGY

**¿Me podría decir donde está la oficina de correos?**
Where is the post office?

**Necesito enviar esta carta por correo.**
I need to mail this letter.

**¿Cuanto cuestan las estampillas?**
How much does the postage cost?

**Necesitamos enviar esta información al paciente por correo certificado.**
We need to send this information to the patient by certified mail.

**El doctor va enviar su receta a la farmacia por medio de la computadora.**
The doctor will send your prescription to the pharmacy online.

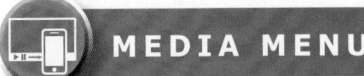

## MEDIA MENU

**Student Resources** on thePoint®
- **CMA/RMA Certification Exam Review**

**Internet Resources**
**Federal Express**
http://www.fedex.com/us
**Medical dictionary**
http://www.medical-dictionary.com
**Merriam-Webster's Dictionary**
http://www.merriam-webster.com
**United Parcel Service**
http://www.ups.com
**United States Postal Service**
http://www.usps.com

## EMR Activity

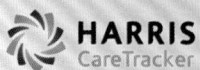

Harris CareTracker is a web-based electronic medical record (EMR) application that you will use for the EMR activities included in this section at the end of each chapter. This application is actually used in physician offices, but is provided to you through the publisher, Wolters Kluwer Health, to give you hands-on practice working with EMRs. Your instructor will have more information about accessing your username, login, and Quickstart guide.

Prerequisite Activities in Harris CareTracker

- *The Getting Started and Quickstart documents and EMR Activities Step-by-Step Instructions are available at* http://thePoint.lww.com/KronenbergerComp5e

Activity Details

Sophie Taylor, CMA, has been asked to generate a standard letter that welcomes new patients to Great Falls Medical. In addition to presenting the basic policies of the practice, this letter should also include the patient information sheet with instructions for patients to complete and bring with them to their appointment. Using the *Clinical Letter Editor* feature under the *Clinical* tab in the *Administration* module, generate this letter in the *Letter Template* builder that will be used to send all new patients in the future. In the letter, instruct patients to bring their insurance cards with them at their appointment and include any other pertinent information.

## Chapter Summary

- As a medical assistant, you need excellent written communication skills.
- Careful attention to detail is essential. Your documentation in a medical office could become part of a lawsuit!
- Medical information is crucial to patient care and must be prepared with proper grammar, punctuation, and spelling.
- You will write letters, memorandums, and other correspondence with patients, physicians, and businesses.
- After preparing your document, you must be able to select the appropriate service for mailing your letters.
- Medical information is confidential and must be handled according to HIPAA guidelines.
- Your primary goal with all written communication is to get your message across in a clear, concise, and accurate manner.

## Warm-Ups for Critical Thinking

1. Create a business letter. Include all the components and use the full block format. Print your unedited copy and, using proofreader marks, indicate your corrections. Make the corrections and reprint a final copy. Ask your instructor to review both copies.
2. Write 10 sentences using terms from Box 7-3. Use some terms correctly and others incorrectly. Exchange your sentences with another student. Correct your peer's sentences.
3. Collect five pieces of mail that you have received at home. What method of affixing postage did they use? Go to your local USPS office. Obtain either a priority mail or express mail envelope. Correctly address the envelope.
4. Suppose the physician told you to read his e-mails while he was on vacation. In doing so, you come across a personal piece of information that you know he would not want you to see. How would you handle it? Would you tell anyone that you saw it? Would you question the physician about it?

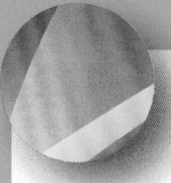

## PSY PROCEDURE 7-1

## Composing a Professional Business Letter

Compose a professional correspondence utilizing electronic technology; and report relevant information concisely and accurately

**Purpose:** To construct a clear and concise business letter using proper grammar and punctuation

**Equipment:** Computer with word processing software, 8 1/2 × 11 white paper, no. 10–sized envelope

**Scenario:** Type a letter from Dr. Tom Chandler (1200 West Main Street, Suite 103, Danberry, VA 24451) to patient James Heffernan (1010 Chestnut Street, Danberry, VA 24451). The letter is in reference to the denial of his insurance claim by Unique Comprehensive Medical Benefits. The denial letter, dated May 28th of the current year, states that the procedure planned by Dr. Chandler has been deemed as medically unnecessary. The letter should inform Mr. Heffernan of his insurance company's decision. Dr. Chandler instructs you to advise the patient that he has every intention of writing a letter to appeal this decision.

| STEPS | REASONS |
|---|---|
| 1. Move the cursor down two lines below the letterhead and enter today's date, flush right. | Use the date that the letter was dictated or constructed by the sender, not the date it was typed. |
| 2. Flush left, move the cursor down two lines, and enter the inside address using the name and address of the person to whom you are writing. | Check the incoming correspondence or directory for the exact spelling of the name of the recipient. |
| 3. Double space and enter a reference line. | At a glance, the reader will know what or who the letter is about. Those filing the letter have a quick reference as well. |
| 4. Double space and type the salutation followed by a colon. | Using a proper salutation and colon denotes professionalism. |
| 5. Double-space between paragraphs. | This is block letter style. |
| 6. Double-space and flush right, enter the complimentary close. | The close should be professional in a business letter. "Later" would not be an appropriate closing. |
| 7. Move cursor down four spaces and enter the sender's name. | This leaves space for the sender's signature. |
| 8. Double-space and enter initials of the sender in all caps. | Reference initials let the sender and recipient know who composed and dictated the letter. |
| 9. Enter a slash and your initials in lowercase letters. | Lowercase initials indicate the person who typed the letter. If necessary, that person can be identified in case of error, omission of enclosures, etc. |
| 10. Enter c: and the names of those who get copies of the letter. | In the days of carbon paper and typewriters, cc: meant carbon copy. Using a single c: is now acceptable to indicate that a copy of this letter was also sent to the person listed. |
| 11. Enter Enc: and the number and description of each enclosed sheet. | If there are enclosures, the reader can see what the sender intended to be included in the envelope with the letter. These enclosures may or may not be mentioned in the body of the letter. |

## PROCEDURE 7.1 (continued)

| STEPS | REASONS |
|---|---|
| **12.** Print on letterhead. | Letterhead gives the correspondence a professional look. If no letterhead is available, you may construct it using the name, address, and phone number of the sender. |
| **13.** Proofread the letter. | This is the most important step in this procedure. No matter how well written a letter is, errors indicate a lack of professionalism. |
| **14.** Attach the letter to the patient's chart. | When the sender of the letter receives the letter for signature, he or she may need to refer back to the information used to compose the letter. |
| **15.** Submit to the sender of the letter for review and signature. | The sender should review the letter carefully. It is the sender who is ultimately responsible for the content and condition of the correspondence. |
| **16.** Make a copy of the letter for the patient's chart. | Medical documentation guidelines require you to keep copies of every transaction and communication with or on behalf of a patient. |
| **17.** Address envelopes using all caps and no punctuation. | In order for the USPS OCR equipment to read an envelope, it should be typed in all capital letters or written in block with no punctuation. |
| **18.** **AFF** Explain how you would respond in this situation: your physician reviews the letter you prepared and asks you to insert a comma where you know a comma is not required. | Respectfully tell the physician that your resources do not suggest a comma in this instance. You may even show him or her the resource. |

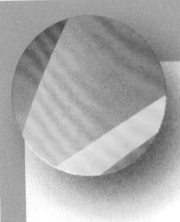

## PSY PROCEDURE 7-2

# Opening and Sorting Incoming Mail

**Purpose:** To efficiently and accurately open and sort mail to be distributed to the appropriate persons in the office

**Equipment:** Letter opener, paper clips, directional tabs, date stamp

| STEPS | REASONS |
|---|---|
| 1. Gather the necessary equipment. | An efficient medical assistant has his or her tools at his or her fingertips. |
| 2. Open all letters and check for enclosures. | If the letter states that enclosures were sent but they are not in the envelope, contact the sender and request them. Indicate on the letter that the enclosures were missing and the name of the person you contacted. |
| 3. Paper clip enclosures to the letter. | Paper clipping enclosures to a letter reduces the chance of misplacing. |
| 4. Date-stamp each item. | Stamping each piece of correspondence with the date it was opened gives more authenticity to a letter. It also lets the reader know when action should be taken. |
| 5. Sort the mail into categories and deal with it appropriately. Generally, you should handle the following types of mail as noted:<br><br>*Correspondence regarding a patient:*<br>a. Use a paper clip to attach letters, test results, etc. to the patient's chart.<br>b. Place the chart in a pile for the physician to review.<br>*Payments and other checks:*<br>a. Record promptly all insurance payments and checks and deposit them according to office policy.<br>b. Account for all drug samples and appropriately log them into the sample book. | Using these guidelines helps ensure the proper handling of all incoming mail. |
| 6. Dispose of miscellaneous advertisements unless otherwise directed. | Dispose of items only when instructed to do so by the recipient of the mail. Your idea of junk mail and the recipient's may be different. |
| 7. Distribute the mail to the appropriate staff members. For example, mail might be for the physician, office manager, office manager, billing clerk, or other personnel. | Take care that the appropriate person gets each piece of mail. Many times, a letter has the name of someone who is not really the person in the office who should get this type of information. Determine the right person to receive the correspondence. |
| 8. **PSY** Explain how you would handle a letter marked "Personal and confidential." | Do not open the letter. Place it on the top of the addressee's stack of mail. |

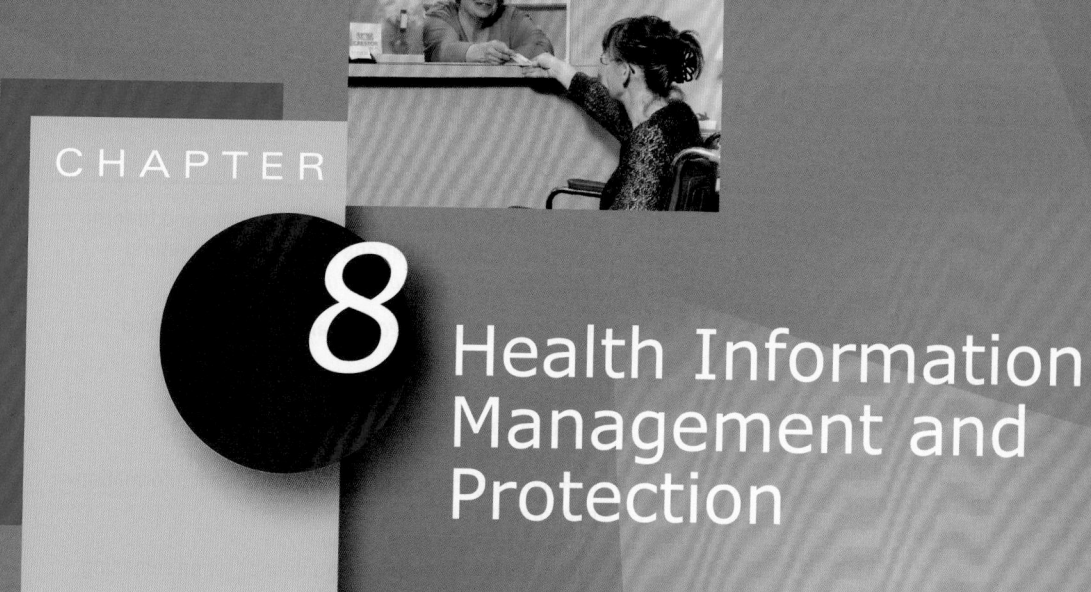

# CHAPTER

# 8 Health Information Management and Protection

## Learning Outcomes

**COG Cognitive Domain***

1. Spell and define the key terms
2. Explain the requirements of the Health Insurance Portability and Accountability Act relating to the sharing and saving of personal and protected health information
3. Identify types of records common to the health care setting
4. Describe standard and electronic health record systems
5. Explain the process for releasing medical records to third-party payers and individual patients
6. Discuss principles of using an electronic medical record
7. *Define types of information contained in the patient's medical record*
8. *Identify methods of organizing the patient's medical record based on:*
   a. Problem-oriented medical record (POMR)
   b. Source-oriented medical record (SOMR)

9. Explain how to make an entry in a patient's medical record, using abbreviations when appropriate
10. Explain how to make a correction in a standard and electronic health record
11. Discuss pros and cons of various filing methods
12. *Describe filing indexing rules*
13. Discuss filing procedures
14. *Identify equipment and supplies needed for medical records in order to:*
   a. Create
   b. Maintain
   c. Store
15. Explain the guidelines of sound policies for record retention
16. Describe the proper disposal of paper and electronic protected health information
17. Explore issue of confidentiality as it applies to the medical assistant

*(continues on page 182)*

18. Describe the implications of HIPAA for the medical assistant in various medical settings
19. *Explain the importance of data backup*
20. *Explain meaningful use as it applies to EMR.*

**PSY Psychomotor Domain***

1. *Create and organize a patient's medical record (Procedure 8-1)*
2. *File patient medical records (Procedure 8-2)*
3. Maintain organization by filing (Procedure 8-2)
4. Respond to issues of confidentiality (Procedure 8-3)
5. Apply HIPAA rules in regard to privacy/release of information (Procedure 8-3)

**AFF Affective Domain***

1. *Demonstrate sensitivity to patient rights*
2. Demonstrate awareness of the consequences of not working within the legal scope of practice

3. Recognize the importance of local, state, and federal legislation and regulations in the practice setting
4. *Protect the integrity of the medical record*

***Note: AAMA/CAAHEP 2015 Standards are italicized***

**ABHES Competencies**

1. Perform basic clerical functions
2. Prepare and maintain medical records
3. Receive, organize, prioritize, and transmit information expediently
4. Apply electronic technology
5. Institute federal and state guidelines when releasing medical records or information
6. Efficiently maintain and understand different types of medical correspondence and medical reports

# Key Terms

alphabetic filing
chief complaint
chronological order
clearinghouse
covered entity
cross-reference
demographic data

electronic health records
(EHRs)
flow sheet
Health Information Technology
for Economic and Clinical
Health (HITECH) Act
medical history forms

microfiche
microfilm
narrative
numeric filing
present illness
problem-oriented medical
record (POMR)

protected health
information (PHI)
reverse chronological
order
SOAP
subject filing
workers' compensation

# Case Study

Great Falls Medical Center is eligible to participate in the Centers for Medicare and Medicaid Services Meaningful Use incentive, which requires implementation of an electronic medical record (EMR) for their patients. The staff have been given adequate training on using the new EMR, and Kayla Murphy, RMA, has been chosen to troubleshoot problems as they are encountered throughout the day. She is also the Health Insurance Portability and Accountability Act (HIPAA) privacy officer and is responsible for releasing medical records, both paper and electronic, as they are requested. What is "meaningful use" and how does it affect implementing the EMR in the medical office? What changes, if any, need to be made by the practice in terms of transitioning from paper medical records to an EMR system? Does being a HIPAA privacy officer require Kayla to have special training or knowledge? This chapter answers these questions and provides information about documenting patient encounters and the release of that documentation in compliance with the law.

Medical records have a vital role in ensuring quality patient care. The medical record contains clinical information such as the health history, observations, and findings for patient encounters. It also contains personal information about patients necessary for billing purposes and communication and further provides for continuity of care between health care professionals. Whether information is maintained on paper or in electronic form, proper management of the medical record requires adherence to certain legal, moral, and ethical standards. If these standards are disregarded, a breach of contract between patient and physician may occur, exposing the patient to potential embarrassment or harm and making the physician vulnerable to fines and/or lawsuits (see Chapter 2).

A thorough and accurate medical record furnishes documented evidence of the patient's evaluation, treatment, change in condition, and communication with the physician and staff. Medical records have many other uses as well, including research, quality assurance, and patient education. Information gathered from medical records aids the government in planning for future health care needs and protecting the health of the public. Due to the personal and sensitive information contained in medical records, in 1996, the Health Insurance Portability and Accountability Act (HIPAA) was enacted to provide for privacy of patients' health information. It was also concerned with providing consumers with greater access to health care insurance and to promote more standardization and efficiency in the health care industry.

# THE HEALTH INSURANCE PORTABILITY AND ACCOUNTABILITY ACT OF 1996

Congress addressed the need for reform in the health care industry by passing HIPAA. The act includes five "titles." The titles of HIPAA and their subject matter are outlined in Table 8-1.

HIPAA's goals include the following:

- Simplifying the health insurance claims process and speeding up the process of reimbursement
- Providing greater access to health care insurance when individuals change employers
- Addressing issues dealing with funds set up by employers to pay for health care costs
- Requiring ease of electronic transmissions by establishing a Standard Unique Employer Identifier, which provides complete but coded information about the holder of the code.
- Protection of communication of health information between physicians and insurance companies

In addition to these issues addressed by HIPAA, the rapid advancement of technology in medical information maintenance caused the need for strict regulations to keep electronically transmitted and stored protected health information (PHI) safe from unauthorized releases. Confidentiality has always been required in the medical

| TABLE 8-1  Titles of HIPAA | |
|---|---|
| Title | Action |
| Title I, Health Insurance Access, Portability, and Renewal | Amended the Employee Retirement Income Security Act of 1974 (ERISA) and the Public Health Act. |
| | Changed the rules about preexisting condition exclusions by insurance companies. |
| | Prohibited discrimination based on health status by insurance companies. |
| Title II, Preventing Health Care Fraud and Abuse | Is concerned with how health care providers interact with the insurance network. Includes the Privacy Rule. |
| | Prevents fraud and abuse in the delivery of and payment for health care. |
| | Improves the Medicare program and others. |
| | Establishes standards and requirements for all electronic transmission of certain health information. |
| Title III, Tax-Related Provisions | Deals with MSAs (Medical Savings Accounts). |
| | Consumers deposit money into the account and withdraw it as needed for medical bills only. |
| | The money deposited is tax free. |
| | Concerned with how employers handle these funds. |
| Title IV, Group Health Plan Requirements | Amends earlier legislation regarding group insurance. |
| | Allows people to carry the same health insurance coverage to a new job. |
| | Avoids starting over again with waiting periods for preexisting conditions. |
| | Costs are high without employer's contribution. |
| Title V, Revenue Offsets | Changes to the Internal Revenue Code of 1986 to generate more revenue to offset the HIPAA-required costs. |

world, but each state had its own laws regarding the exchange of medical information. HIPAA also addresses important new issues that arose after medical facilities became computerized. The use of the Internet brought concerns about hackers obtaining personal health information.

Physician offices are required to take appropriate steps to ensure that any company they are associated with also follows HIPAA regulations. Physician offices often have a variety of business partnerships that help keep the office flowing professionally and effectively. Some examples of business partnerships are cleaning services, document-shredding companies, laboratory and specimen transport personnel, temporary staffing agencies, and educational facilities. Contracts among physicians and their business partners should reflect that the business adheres to HIPAA regulations. For example, computer technicians hired by the practice for the purpose of repairing or installing computers for the practice must sign a business associate agreement prior to being permitted to work on the computers in the practice. Students completing practicums are also required to sign confidentiality agreements.

## Covered Entities

HIPAA uses the language "**covered entity**" to describe those who must adhere to these regulations. A covered entity is defined as health insurance plans, health care **clearinghouses** (entities that receive, review, send, and manage insurance claims for physicians), and health care providers who use electronic billing, funds transfers, and **electronic health records** (EHRs). In some instances, HIPAA identifies covered entities as those meeting the criteria above with more than 25 employees. Civil and criminal penalties are set by the federal act, but each state has enacted regulations governing insurance companies. Covered entities are subject to individual state laws, but if state and federal laws are different, you must follow the strictest laws. In the medical office, you will be concerned with the administrative simplification and privacy rules.

## Administrative Simplification

There are four parts to HIPAA's Administrative Simplification section. They include electronic transactions, privacy requirements, security requirements, and national identifier requirements.

## The HIPAA Officer

Each health care provider must have certain policies in place to comply with the rulings. In most cases, as long as reasonable care is taken to comply with the intent of the ruling and that effort is documented, providers are considered compliant with HIPAA. HIPAA requires that at least one employee be designated as the HIPAA officer and one as a privacy officer. This requirement varies with the size of the practice or business. The HIPAA officer coordinates and oversees the various aspects of compliance. Covered

---

**BOX 8-1    Responsibilities of a HIPAA Officer**

1. Assess, establish, and review policies and procedures to ensure continuous HIPAA compliance.
2. Coordinate mandatory training of employees including specific rules and regulations, reporting any event that might compromise the protection of information, explanation of privacy issues, etc. For example, proper log-in and log-off procedures.
3. Monitor the access to health information by periodically checking for security threats or gaps when changes occur in equipment or software.
4. Ensure sound practices by the human resources department as employees leave the workforce or move from one department to another. Passwords and access to certain information should be adjusted as employees change responsibilities according to the minimum necessary information needed as stated in the privacy rule. For example, does the appointment secretary need access to the entire chart in order to schedule an appointment?
5. Maintain the integrity of the system by ensuring data and information have not been altered or destroyed in an unauthorized manner by designing and monitoring tracking reports.

---

entities are subject to inspections by representatives of the Centers for Medicaid and Medicare Services (CMS). Any audits would be coordinated through the HIPAA officer. The privacy officer keeps track of who has access to protected health information. The responsibilities of these employees are listed in Box 8-1. These duties should be listed on the job descriptions of these appointed employees.

## HIPAA's Forms

The Notice of Privacy Practices must be provided to patients at the first office visit (Fig. 8-1). HIPAA also requires you to obtain patients' written acknowledgment that notice has been received and file the acknowledgment in the patient record. A patient's refusal to sign the acknowledgment should be documented and filed in the patient record. A sample Notice of Privacy Practices can be downloaded and tailored to reflect your practice's policies and your state's privacy laws. State privacy laws should continue to be followed if they are more stringent than the HIPAA regulations.

The following information is required to be included in the Notice of Privacy Policies:

- How the covered entity may use and disclose protected health information about an individual
- The individual's rights with respect to the information and how he or she may exercise these rights, including how to make a complaint to the physician's office

**Southern Arundel OBGYN**
**3008 Pryson Avenue, Severn, Maryland 21140**
**Privacy Official: Jessica Pyrtle, CMA**
**Telephone: 410-966-2100**

## Authorization for Use or Disclosure of Health Information

Patient Name: _____

[print or type]

Patient's Date of Birth: _____ Patient's Identification/Chart No.: _____

I hereby authorize the use and disclosure of individually identifiable health information relating to me as described below:

**Specific Description of the Information to be Used or Disclosed Including (If Practicable) the Dates of Service(s) Related to Such Information:** _____

_____

The above information will be called "Authorized Information" throughout the rest of this form.

**Persons or Class of Persons Authorized to Make the Use or Disclosure of Authorized Information:**

_____

_____

**Persons or Class of Persons to Whom the Use or Disclosure of Authorized Information May be Made:**

_____

_____

**Authorized Information will be used and/or disclosed for the following purposes:**
[ ]  At the request of the individual (check box if applicable)
[ ]  Other *(Please list each purpose of the use(s) or disclosure(s) in the space provided.)*:

_____

- I understand that if the person or entity receiving Authorized Information is not a health plan or health care provider covered by federal privacy regulations, the authorized information may be re-disclosed by the recipient and may no longer be protected by federal or state law.

- I understand that I may revoke this authorization at any time by notifying _____ [NAME OF PRACTICE] in writing. However, if I choose to do so, I understand that my revocation will not affect any actions taken by

_____
[NAME OF PRACTICE] before receiving my revocation.

- I understand that I may refuse to sign this authorization and that my refusal to sign in no way affects my treatment, payment, enrollment in a health plan, or eligibility for benefits.

[ALTERNATIVE, IF APPLICABLE: I understand that _____ [NAME OF PRACTICE] may require me to sign an authorization prior to receiving research-related treatment or treatment solely for the purpose of creating health information for another party and that _____ [NAME OF PRACTICE] will not provide such research-related treatment unless I provide this authorization. **NOTE:** If this provision is applicable, the third party for whom the information is being created must be listed under "Persons or Class of Persons to Whom the Use or Disclosure of Authorized Information May be Made." Also, the purpose for which the information is to be created and disclosed must be listed under "Authorized Information will be Used or Disclosed for the Following Purposes."

- [FOR MARKETING AUTHORIZATIONS ONLY, IF APPLICABLE] I understand that the person or entity I am authorizing to use and/or disclose Authorized Information for marketing purposes may receive either direct or indirect compensation for doing so.

**This authorization expires at the earlier of** _____ **OR the date the following event occurs:** _____

_____
[describe event or write "not applicable"]

Signature of Patient or Patient's Personal Representative: _____ Date: _____

For Personal Representative of the Patient (if applicable): _____

Print Name of Personal Representative: _____

Describe Personal Representative Relationship/Authority to Act for the Individual (parent, guardian, etc.): _____

**Figure 8-1** • A sample Notice of Privacy Practices required by HIPAA.

- The physician's office's legal duties with respect to information, including a statement that the covered entity is required by law to maintain the privacy of protected health information
- Whom patients can contact for further information about the office's privacy policies

Although not specifically required by HIPAA, it is recommended that you use a Patient Authorization for Disclosure of PHI in your practice. This authorization form specifies methods by which a patient agrees to let your practice use his or her protected information for routine treatment, payment, or health care operations (TPO) purposes. It may also state how the patient may be contacted such as whether or not a message may be left on their answering machine. Should a patient complain that his or her privacy rights have been violated, a signed authorization form may afford you an extra measure of protection if your practice is investigated for HIPAA noncompliance.

HIPAA privacy regulations do not require you to obtain patients' consent to use their PHI for routine disclosures such as those related to TPO. However, the regulations do mandate that you obtain written patient consent before releasing their information for any reason other than TPO (e.g., disclosure of psychotherapy notes). To comply, you'll need to identify situations in your practice where special authorization is needed and develop an authorization form for patients to sign. HIPAA also mandates that practices provide patients with an accounting of the disclosures of their PHI upon request. A signed copy or documentation of the patient's refusal to sign any authorization for release of PHI should be retained in the patient record. Figures 8-1 through 8-3 show samples of the necessary forms.

## Releasing Medical Records

The protection of personal information is crucial to the privacy of patients. Although the physical medical record legally belongs to the physician, the information belongs to the patient. Any release of records must first be authorized by the patient or the patient's legal guardian. When releasing a medical record, provide a copy only. *Never* release the original medical record except in limited circumstances.

Insurance companies, lawyers, other health care practitioners, and patients themselves may request copies of medical records. All requests should be made in writing, stating the patient's name, address, and social security number, and must contain the patient's *original* signature authorizing the release of records. Never release information over the telephone. You will have no way of verifying that the person with whom you are speaking is actually the person who has authorization.

State laws allow physicians to charge a fee for providing copies of the medical record. The American Medical

I, _____, give my permission for _____ to release information generated in my medical record between the dates of _____ and _____ to _____.

Signature _____ Date _____
Witness _____ Date _____

Or

I, _____, give my permission for _____ to release information in my medical record regarding the care and treatment of _____ to _____.

Signature _____ Date _____
Witness _____ Date _____

**Figure 8-2 •** A proper authorization for release of information.

Association (AMA) has also published guidelines for physicians to ensure ethical business practices. They recommend a reasonable fee for reproduction of records. Charges for copies of medical records may also be

Mamie Parrish

| 10/17/14 | Pt. Called c/o fever, sore throat. Asked to speak to Dr. Johnson. Instructed patient to come in for exam; explained that Dr. Johnson cannot treat her over the phone. Given appt for tomorrow at 10:00 a.m. |
| 10/18/14 | Pt. called and stated that she felt "90% better". Appt. canceled. |
| | Jennifer Wise, CMA |

| 12/05/14 | Office Visit |
| SUBJECTIVE: | Pt presents c/o of bad pain in RLQ x 2 days. |
| OBJECTIVE: | Vital signs: T-101.3, P-94, R-16, BP-112/76. Urine pregnancy test was done, negative. Urine dip was negative for blood and WBC, pH 7.0, Urine was clear. Blood was sent to the laboratory for CBC with diff. |
| ASSESSMENT: | Pain in RLQ. Possible appendicitis vs. ovarian cyst. |
| PLAN: | Tylenol 650 mg suppository given now. Will await lab results and notify patient with further instructions at that time. |
| | James Owens, MD |

| 12/16/14 | Lab work normal. Called pt. Per Dr. Johnson and instructed to notify us if her fever is not gone tomorrow. Patient states, "I guess I feel some better." Pt. will call office p.r.n. |
| | Melissa Hurley, RMA |

**Figure 8-3 •** Sample page from patient's chart.

determined by state laws, and in addition to charges for the actual copies, administrative costs may also be added for record retrieval costs, postage, and other expenses.

## HIPAA's Privacy Rule

HIPAA provides protection of the sharing of what is referred to as PHI. PHI is any information that can be linked to a specific person. A diagnosis alone without a full name is not identifiable, but a first and last name associated with a diagnosis is identifiable; therefore, it is protected health information. For example, the Centers for Disease Control and Prevention (CDC) publishes information to cite statistics about communicable diseases. Since the names of the people who have been diagnosed with the diseases are not published, this information is not protected.

The privacy rule establishes safeguards to protect the confidentiality of medical information. Covered entities must

- Share health information for health purposes only
- Provide the minimum amount of information necessary
- Adopt written privacy procedures
- Designate a privacy officer
- Train employees

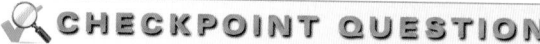

## CHECKPOINT QUESTION

1. What is the purpose of HIPAA?

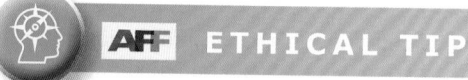

### HIPAA Says Patients Have Rights

Through HIPAA, the federal government recognizes that it is ethical to give patients certain rights. HIPAA protects the rights of patients by allowing them to

- Ask to see and get a copy of their health records
- Have corrections added to their health information
- Receive a notice that tells them how their health information may be used and shared
- Decide if they want to give permission before their health information can be used or shared for certain purposes such as for marketing
- Get a report on when and why their health information was shared for certain purposes
- File a complaint with the provider or health insurer if they believe their rights have been denied or their health information is not being protected
- File a complaint with the U.S. government

Patients can learn about their rights, including how to file a complaint, from the Web site at http://www.hhs.gov/ocr/privacy/hipaa/understanding/consumers/index.html or by calling 1-866-627-7748.

## COG RELEASING RECORDS TO PATIENTS

As discussed previously, releasing medical records is an important part of any medical facility. When patients request copies of their own records, the doctor makes the decision about what to copy. Except for emancipated minors, patients aged 17 years and under cannot get copies of their own medical records without a signed consent from a parent or legal guardian. However, they may obtain certain services independently (check your state's law regarding treatment of minors); in such cases, under the law, you are not permitted to contact the parent or guardian. Some states allow minors to seek treatment for sexually transmitted diseases and birth control without parental knowledge or consent. Sometimes, the parent or guardian may still be billed for these services without the bill being itemized. The billing statement should include only the treatment dates and amount due.

### Subpoena Duces Tecum

An original record may be released when it is subpoenaed by a court of law. In such situations, the physician may wish to have the judge sign a document stating that he or she will temporarily take charge of the medical record. This signed document should be filed in the medical office until the record is returned. To further ensure the record's safety, a staff member can transport the original record to court on the day it is requested and then return the record at the end of the court session that day. As soon as it is known that a record will be part of a court case, the record should be kept in a locked cabinet. When the court orders that a record be submitted to the court at a given date and time, the legal order is termed *subpoena duces tecum*.

### Abbreviations? When in Doubt, Spell It Out

The Joint Commission is charged with monitoring and accrediting inpatient and some outpatient medical facilities. Recent changes in standards regarding some ambiguous handwritten abbreviations reflect the growing feeling that many commonly used abbreviations are overused, used incorrectly, open to interpretation, or easily confused with another abbreviation. For instance, the abbreviation BS might stand for bowel sounds, breath sounds, or blood sugar. In addition to requiring facilities to keep a list of acceptable abbreviations used in the facility, The Joint Commission issues a "Do Not Use" list that can be found at http://www.jointcommission.org. Even though some abbreviations can be confusing and should not be used, many continue to be used. Appendix D has a general list of commonly used abbreviations. The Joint Commission is covered in more detail in Chapter 10.

## Proper Authorization

You must follow certain guidelines even with a signed release form (see Fig. 8-3). The authorization form must give the patient the opportunity to limit the information to be released. Patients may release only information relating to a specific disorder, or they may specify a time limit. They may not, however, ask that the physician leave out information pertinent to the situation.

References to mental health diagnoses or treatments, drug or alcohol abuse, HIV, AIDS, or any other sexually transmitted disease may not be released without specific mention on the signed authorization form. If such information is not specifically requested by the patient, place a piece of blank white paper over any such areas of information when you are copying the record. Never whiteout these areas on the original document or mention what these blank areas included.

Protected health information can be shared with proper authorization by the patient. By signing an appropriate authorization, the patient gives permission for the health care provider to share their personal health information with anyone they designate. The form must include the name of the person to receive the information, the name of the provider releasing the information, and the dates of service and/or certain conditions covered by the authorization. It is recommended that there also be a witness signature. Figure 8-3 is a sample of a proper authorization form.

### CHECKPOINT QUESTION

2. What is required for a legal disclosure of a patient's HIV status?

## Legally Required Disclosures

As previously discussed in Chapter 2, in certain situations, the law requires reporting information to particular authorities. Requirements for reporting vary among states.

As with most laws, there are exceptions to the privacy rule. Certain information is crucial to the patient, needed for the protection of the public, or involves criminal activity and is released without the patient's permission. Such disclosures include the following:

- Vital statistics
- Child and elder abuse or maltreatment
- Emergency circumstances
- Identification of body of deceased person
- Cause of death
- Public health needs, such as communicable diseases
- Research
- Judicial and administrative proceedings
- Law enforcement concerns such as violent criminal activities
- Activities related to national defense and security

### CHECKPOINT QUESTION

3. Why is some information released without a patient's permission?

## PATIENT EDUCATION

### Protect Your Patients by Teaching Them to Read What They Are Signing

Many patients feel inadequate when it comes to understanding the intricacies of the laws that are designed to protect them. Patients are often ready to sign a form handed to them without even reading it. Patients trust and depend on their health care provider to protect their rights to privacy. Whatever form, authorization, or consent the patient is handed should be accompanied by a verbal explanation of what they are signing.

For example, legal experts advise that some forms designed for patients to give their authorization to release their personal information are too general and are not even considered legally binding. Proper authorization should include the elements in Figure 8-2. Patients should understand that it would be improper to sign a form like this:

I, _____, give my permission for the release of my medical records.

Signature: _____.

This blanket permission opens patients up to the possibility of any and all of their information being shared with anyone at anytime. Each time patients need or want their information to be released, they must sign a new authorization outlining the specific information to be released by who and to whom. Help them understand the importance of knowing what they are signing, and tell them to ask questions if they need any clarification.

## STANDARD MEDICAL RECORDS

Even though our expanding technology gives today's medical office the ability to store health information in electronic form, some medical offices still use the paper medical record with or without the electronic health record. Outpatient medical offices that are not electronic accumulate mounds of paper every day. A medical facility has a variety of options for standard or manual record keeping. The best systems are those that have been tried, revised, and revised again. No matter how the records are stored, make sure that the information is

- Easily retrievable
- Kept in an orderly manner
- Complete

- Legible
- Accurate
- Brief

Whether a record is on paper or stored electronically, all medical records have the same contents.

## COG CONTENTS OF THE MEDICAL RECORD

A paper medical record in an outpatient facility, often called a chart or a file, contains confidential clinical information about the patient's health and treatment in addition to the billing and insurance information discussed in Chapter 15.

General information, such as name, address, telephone number, date of birth, social security number, credit history, and next of kin, is vital to a complete chart but should never be intermingled with the clinical information. Metal fasteners can be used to keep certain pages on one side of the chart.

The following information is typically found in the clinical section of the medical chart:

- *Chief complaint*—A description of the symptoms that led the patient to seek the physician's care. This information is supplied by the patient during the interview at the beginning of the visit. It is usually stated in the patient's own words in quotation marks. For example, the patient complains of "something stuck in my throat."
- *Present illness*—A more specific account of the chief complaint, including time frames and characteristics. For example: "The patient says it started 2 days ago. She describes the pain as severe and stabbing and reports taking Tylenol with no relief."
- *Family and personal history*—A review of any major illnesses of family members, including grandparents, parents, siblings, aunts, and uncles. Any previous major illnesses and surgeries of the patient are listed under personal history.
- *Review of systems*—A systematic review of the body's 10 systems to detect problems not yet identified. For example, problems with the integumentary system (skin) may be identified if the patient reports a rash, areas of discoloration, or change in a mole.
- *Progress notes*—Documentation of each patient encounter, including information obtained in phone calls and refills of prescriptions.
- *Radiographic reports*—Reports of any radiologic studies with the most recent filed on top is filed in this section of the medical record after the ordering physician has reviewed and initialed the report and released it for filing.
- *Laboratory results*—A copy of the results of any laboratory work done in the office or a report from an outside facility.

- *Consultation reports*—Any reports from other physicians regarding consultations with the patient.
- *Medication administration*—This information is included as part of the clinical documentation for the present illness; however, some facilities may also use a separate sheet to log medications given in the office. If an opioid is given, still another form is completed, as discussed in Chapter 2.
- *Diagnosis or medical impression*—The most recent entry on the progress note will contain the provider's opinion of the patient's problems.
- *Physician's and/or medical assistant's identification and signature*—Experts have suggested that you sign your entire name instead of initials, with your credentials written after the name, for example, Susan Jones, CMA. A signature log should be kept and maintained by the office manager listing the full names of everyone, including their credentials, who are permitted to make entries into the medical records. Signatures and initials would be made by everyone beside their printed name on the log; however, it is important that a new log be updated and signed as employees are added to the list of authorized signatures. This is very helpful during an audit situation to identify authorized personnel who have made entries into the medical records.
- *Documented advance directives, such as living will and power of attorney for medical care*—A copy of any instructions from the patient regarding end-of-life decisions or the appointment of another person who can give consent for treatment for the patient.
- *All correspondence pertaining to the patient*—Any letters or memos generated in the facility and sent out are copied and placed in the chart. Correspondence from other physicians is also included in the chart.

Appendix F contains samples of the reports common to the typical medical record.

### CHECKPOINT QUESTION

4. What is meant by the heading *chief complaint*?

## COG ELECTRONIC HEALTH RECORDS

Medical records that store information using computer software have many advantages over the paper medical record. Searching for a medical record that has been misplaced (or misfiled!) is not a problem when using electronic records, and more than one person may access the record at any given moment. By 2017, most physicians who see patients covered by Medicare or Medicaid programs must be using some type of electronic health record.

Although electronic medical record (EMR) and electronic health record (EHR) are often used interchangeably, there is a difference in how the information may be accessed and the ease of sharing clinical information. Health information stored in an EMR is restricted only for use in that office or practice, while the same information stored on an EHR is easily shared with other health providers such as the hospital, laboratories, and other physicians.

## The Health Information Technology for Economic and Clinical Health Act

As part of the push by the federal government for greater use of information technology (IT), the American Recovery and Reinvestment Act of 2009 included provisions outlined in The Health Information Technology for Economic and Clinical Health (HITECH) Act to provide support and financial incentives for providers to use electronic health records. HITECH also addressed privacy and security concerns associated with the electronic exchange of health information already in place through HIPAA laws by increasing the civil and criminal penalties for privacy and security violations.

## Meaningful Use

Under HITECH, eligible physicians, hospitals, and other providers may earn significant financial payments by meeting specific objectives using electronic health records as defined by the Centers for Medicaid and Medicare Services. These objectives require providers to demonstrate that they are using their EHR technology to its fullest potential to improve quality, accuracy, and efficiency in the delivery of health care and in patient safety. There are three stages for reporting and documenting meaningful use of EHRs to receive incentive payments to eligible physicians as they adopt, implement, upgrade, or demonstrate meaningful use of certified EHR technology. Physicians who prove meaningful use of EHRs will receive payments up to $44,000 in the three stages to help with associated expenses.

Another part of this move to EHRs is the Patient-Centered Medical Home (PCMH). Box 8-2 outlines the concepts of this approach to medical care using EHRs.

---

### BOX 8-2    Patient-Centered Medical Home

NCQA's Initial Physician Practice Connections®—Patient-Centered Medical Home™ (PPC-PCMH) program reflects the input of the American College of Physicians, American Academy of Family Physicians, American Academy of Pediatrics and American Osteopathic Association, and others in the revision of Physician Practice Connections® to assess whether physician practices are functioning as medical homes. Building on the joint principles developed by the primary care specialty societies, the PPC-PCMH standards emphasize the use of systematic, patient-centered, coordinated care management processes.

NCQA's PCMH 2011 is an innovative program for improving primary care. In a set of standards that describe clear and specific criteria, the program gives practices information about organizing care around patients, working in teams, and coordinating and tracking care over time. The NCQA PCMH standards strengthen and add to the issues addressed by NCQA's original program.

The PCMH is a health care setting that facilitates partnerships between individual patients, and their personal physicians, and when appropriate, the patient's family. Care is facilitated by registries, information technology, health information exchange, and other means to assure that patients get the indicated care when and where they need and want it in a culturally and linguistically appropriate manner.

There are six PCMH 2011 standards, including six must-pass elements, which can result in one of three levels of recognition. Practices seeking PCMH complete a Web-based data collection tool and provide documentation that validates responses.

The below resources provide detailed information on the PCMH from primary care specialty societies and the organizations dedicated to promoting the advancement of the medical home.

The new PCMH 2011 standards build on the success of earlier standards and make the program even more responsive to patients' needs. Although the standards have always pointed practices toward using systems—including electronic health records—to support tracking care, the new program aligns closely with many specific elements of the federal program that rewards clinicians for using health information technology to improve quality (CMS Meaningful Use [MU] Requirements).

The Patient-Centered Primary Care Collaborative (PCPCC) believes that, if implemented, the PCMH will improve the health of patients and the viability of the health care delivery system. One of the key elements of the PCMH is that IT is utilized appropriately and in a meaningful way to support optimal patient care, performance measurement, patient education, and enhanced communication. Health IT can play a significant role in providing a foundation for many key elements of the PCMH. Specifically, health IT can provide critical information about the patient to the entire care coordination team across all stages of care, support physician–patient communication, enable more timely and accurate performance measurement and improvement, and improve accessibility of the physician practice to the patient.

*Source*: http://www.pcpcc.net.

Learn more about this collaborative at http://aama-ntl.org/PCMH.aspx.

## Features and Capabilities of Electronic Health Records

The goal of EHRs is to improve patient care while boosting efficiency in the medical office. Some of the key features of electronic health records are discussed in the following list:

- *Point-of-care charting*—Touch screens make inputting easy, and drop-down menus takes less time than handwriting notes, improving quality and productivity in charting.
- *Improved documentation*—Problems with illegibility are eliminated, decreasing errors. Physicians can also include drawings to support documentation and use graphing features to transfer numeric data (height, weight, vital signs, etc.) into chart form.
- *Data collection from multiple sources*—Data from the hospital, pharmacy, laboratory, radiology, and other departments are stored in EHRs for quick retrieval.
- *Medication management*—Computerized prescription order entry helps prevent medication errors by providing warnings about patient allergies, contraindications, or possible interactions. It also avoids problems at the pharmacy due to poor handwriting by the prescriber.
- *Assistance with clinical decision making*—Alerts, reminders, and patient care recommendations give providers valuable information at their fingertips.
- *Improved communication*—Easy access to information enhances communication among medical office staff, as well as with patients and other health care entities.
- *Support for administrative, financial, and operational functions*—Electronic health records assist with storage of patient **demographic data**, appointment scheduling, insurance billing and coding (see next section), accounting procedures, and inventory and supply tracking, among other tasks. EHRs may even help increase revenue by (eventually) allowing the practice to eliminate the file room and turn the extra space into exam rooms or office space. EHRs also reduce medical transcription costs.

Electronic health records do have some disadvantages, however, including cost, potential software or hardware damage or failure, and the need for in-depth staff training. The task of inputting data from hundreds or thousands of charts into the computer is time consuming but must be done before the system is used. Sometimes, in the beginning stages, implementing EHR can actually reduce physician and staff productivity instead of increasing it. But over time, the benefits should outweigh the drawbacks.

## **COG** BILLING AND CODING USING ELECTRONIC HEALTH RECORDS

In later chapters, you will learn the world of coding. Selecting the various levels of patient visits to the office is based on many factors. Physicians must choose the level based on the amount of information gathered, the extent of the physical examination performed, and the level of decision making the patient's care required. Many EHR software companies include drop-down lists and preset menus to help providers select the appropriate code based on the information entered for that visit. This is an important feature because every office that accepts Medicare and/or Medicaid is subject to government audits. These audits are designed to verify that the level of office visit charged to the patient is consistent with the criteria outlined by the CMS. If discrepancies are found, the office may be fined. Software that assists with these coding issues can have many benefits, such as avoiding returned claims, preventing insurance fraud, decreasing staff data entry errors, reducing the possibility of an audit, and increasing revenue through streamlined and timely billing processes.

### The Medical Assistant's Role

As a medical assistant, you have the same roles and responsibilities related to EHRs as with paper records. The difference is that you will perform more of your regular tasks using the computer. Two of your main responsibilities are data collection and patient care. Electronic health records allow you to quickly and accurately record chart notes, look up test results, call in medication orders, and so on. With computers in exam rooms, no time is wasted looking for missing patient data; records are easily stored and retrieved. EHRs may also help you gather more complete patient information by prompting you to ask questions that might otherwise be missed before allowing you to move on to the next screen. Tools such as tickler messages can also remind you to provide patient teaching on topics such as vaccines, yearly checkups, blood pressure checks, mammograms, and so on. Medical practices participating in the CMS Meaningful Use incentives are also required to permit only licensed professionals and credentialed medical assistants to enter orders into the computer.

Medical assistants can also provide assurance to patients about the safety and security of their health information. In order to comply with HIPAA, electronic health record systems have built-in features to decrease the risk of stolen or misused data. These safeguards include password protections, electronic firewalls that block access by unauthorized users, audit trails that can track who accessed a record and when, data encryption, and more. By explaining the privacy safeguards integrated into EHRs, you promote patient confidence in the medical practice. (See Electronic Health Record Security section for more details about EHR security.)

**What if the EHR system goes down due to a power outage?**

If the lights go out, return to the old paper system, and then input the data when the electricity comes back on again. Use backup reports and schedules that were printed ahead of time. Backup tapes should be done at the end of every workday to save information in case a problem occurs. Always have contingency plans for data backup, disaster recovery, or other emergencies ready to be implemented if needed.

## Electronic Health Record Security

AMA and many risk management companies have published guidelines for the EHR. Following are suggestions and guidelines based on HIPAA's requirements for practices using computers to transfer or store patient information. Experts advise physicians and office managers considering software programs to look for the following capabilities:

- User-friendly commands that allow users to move easily within the system.
- Spell check and free text fields for inserting corrections and late entries. The electronic record is corrected by using the same rules as in the standard record. Entries are not deleted but corrected, with an explanation to avoid the appearance of hiding information.
- Security levels to limit entry to all functions. For example, a receptionist does not need access to patient diagnoses or the physician's personal taxes.
- A system, including encryption, to repel hackers. Evidence shows that persons with access to technology can invade patients' records stored on computer databases. This is a breach of confidentiality and is illegal.

To maintain security, facilities are urged to do the following:

- Keep all computer backup storage (tapes, disks, etc.) in a safe place away from the practice such as a bank safe-deposit box.
- Use passwords with characters other than letters and encrypt the passwords.
- Change log-in codes and passwords every 30 days.
- Prepare a backup plan for use when the computer system is down.
- Turn terminals away from areas where information may be seen by patients.
- Keep the fax machines and printers that receive personal medical information in a private place.

- Ensure that each user is restricted to the information needed to do his or her job.
- Train employees on confidentiality and each person's responsibility to adhere to HIPAA's Privacy Rule.
- Design a written confidentiality policy that employees sign.
- Conduct routine audits that produce a trail of each employee's movement through the EHR system.
- Include disciplinary measures for breaches of confidentiality including sharing passwords.

Providers may use a handheld personal data device (PDA), laptop, electronic notebook, or personal computer (PC) in central areas or examination rooms. The same security measures apply to these items. Patients should not have access to computer screens in the examination room. The physician should take care in keeping a personal data system, just as he or she protects the prescription pad. The PDAs and laptops may contain the entire *Physicians' Desk Reference*, giving the provider information needed for prescribing drugs at the fingertips. Other applications of such portable devices include downloading patient education materials and documenting and transferring information about patient encounters when the office is closed. In this era of paperless medical offices, care must be taken to protect the privacy of the patient as carefully as in the world of paper.

## MEDICAL RECORD ORGANIZATION

Information in the paper medical record is usually organized in a standard chart order and placed in a specially designed folder. The order in which documents are placed in the medical record depends on the physician's preference. As mentioned earlier, the demographic information is kept separate from the clinical information. The clinical portion of the medical record is organized in either a source-oriented or a problem-oriented format. In source-oriented medical records, all similar categories or sources of information are grouped together. The typical groupings are as follows:

- Billing and insurance information
- Physician orders
- Progress notes
- Laboratory results
- Radiographic results (magnetic resonance imaging, computed tomography, ultrasound)
- Patient education

All documentation in these categories is placed in **reverse chronological order**; that is, the most recent documents are placed on top of previous sheets.

# Provider Encounters

Whether the patient is new or established or seen by a physician assistant, nurse practitioner, or physician, the visit must be documented. It may be handwritten, typed, or entered into a computer, but in any event, it must be recorded. In the paperless office, you will complete the information gathered at the patient's visit by choosing items from a drop-down box that appears when you click on a particular field.

Some offices record new patients' encounters in the history and physical format. Visits of established patients returning for follow-up are documented in a different format. Although some offices use the same format for new and established patients, the most common formats used to document each established patient encounter are narrative, SOAP, and POMR.

## Narrative Format

Some providers document visits in the narrative form. **Narrative** is the oldest documentation form and the least structured. It is simply a paragraph indicating the contact with the patient, what was done for the patient, and the outcome of any action. In the sample page shown in Figure 8-3, the chart entries made are in narrative format.

## SOAP Format

The **SOAP** (subjective–objective–assessment–plan) format is one of the most common methods for documenting patient visits. The *subjective* component is a statement of what the patient says. Whenever possible, actual quotations by the patient should be used. The *objective* component is what is observed about the patient when the medical assistant begins the assessment and when the provider does the examination. The *assessment* portion is a phrase stating the impression of what is wrong or the patient's diagnosis. If a final diagnosis cannot be made yet, the provider lists possible disorders to be ruled out, called the differential diagnosis. The *plan* is a list of interventions that are to be carried out. In Box 8-3, the second note is written in the SOAP format.

## POMR Format

The **problem-oriented medical record (POMR)** lists each problem of the patient, usually at the beginning of the folder, and references each problem with a number throughout the folder. This method was developed by Dr. Lawrence Weed and is a common method of compiling information because of its logical flow and the ease with which information can be reviewed. In group practices where patients may be seen by more than one physician, the POMR format makes it easier to track the patient's treatment and progress. For instance,

---

**BOX 8-3  SOAP Method to Document Patient Information**

Jennifer Mosley states that her daughter, Marcia, has been vomiting all night. She also states that Marcia had diarrhea for 2 days before her appointment and has only eaten crackers and bananas since 6:00 PM last night. Dr. Gibson's notes indicate that Marcia has lost 3 pounds since her last visit and that she appears pale, weak, and slightly dehydrated. He suspects a viral infection.

Dr. Gibson ordered a stool culture along with a complete blood count (CBC) with differential. He prescribed the BRAT (bananas, rice, applesauce, and toast) diet and suggested that Mrs. Mosley give Marcia Imodium A-D for the next 48 hours. He also told Mrs. Mosley to call the office if Marcia's symptoms worsen and to bring her back for a recheck if the symptoms are not cleared up by the end of the week.

**S:** According to the patient's mother, the patient has been vomiting all night and has had diarrhea for the past 2 days. She has eaten only crackers and bananas since 6:00 PM the night before.

**O:** The patient appears pale, weak, and slightly dehydrated and has lost 3 pounds since her last visit.

**A:** Possible viral infection.

**P:** Stool culture, CBC with differential, BRAT diet, and Imodium for the next 48 hours. Call office if symptoms worsen; return to office if patient not well by the end of the week.

---

if Mr. Jones has hypertension and hyperglycemia, each diagnosis will be assigned a problem number as soon as the diagnosis is made:

2/4/9 #1. Hypertension
2/4/9 #2. Hyperglycemia

At each subsequent visit made by Mr. Jones, these problems will be referenced by these numbers. If a problem develops and is resolved, the problem number will be terminated by a single strikethrough with a date beside it or by adding an X to a heading that indicates resolution of problems. Chronic problems, such as hypertension and hyperglycemia, will be retained by number for as long as the patient remains with the practice. These may be divided by headings of acute and chronic or short-term and long-term for convenience.

POMR documents are divided into four components:

1. *Database.* This contains the following:
   - Chief complaint (Fig. 8-4 shows charting for a chief complaint and history of present illness)
   - Present illness
   - Patient profile

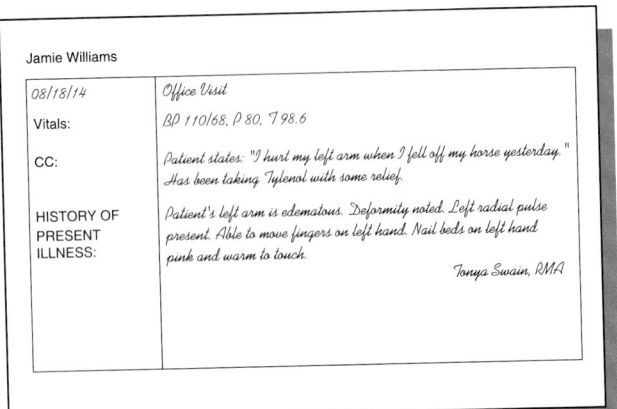

Jamie Williams

| 08/18/14 | Office Visit |
|---|---|
| Vitals: | BP 110/68, P 80, T 98.6 |
| CC: | Patient states: "I hurt my left arm when I fell off my horse yesterday." Has been taking Tylenol with some relief. |
| HISTORY OF PRESENT ILLNESS: | Patient's left arm is edematous. Deformity noted. Left radial pulse present. Able to move fingers on left hand. Nail beds on left hand pink and warm to touch. |
| | Tonya Swain, RMA |

**Figure 8-4** • Charting a chief complaint and history of present illness.

- Review of systems
- Physical examination
- Laboratory reports
2. *Problem list.* This includes every problem the patient has that requires evaluation, including social, demographic, medical, and surgical problems. (Demographic problems relate to statistical characteristics of certain populations.)
3. *Treatment plan.* This includes management, additional workups that may be necessary, and therapy.
4. *Progress notes.* These are structured notes corresponding to each problem.

## CHECKPOINT QUESTION

5. What are three common formats used to document patient–provider encounters?

## Documentation Forms

Using printed forms and flow sheets in the medical record saves space and time and allows for easy retrieval of information. They are usually customized to meet the needs of the individual practice. Some forms, like vaccination records, are required by federal law. In the paperless office, these forms are completed by the patient and transferred to the patient's electronic record by data entry, and then the completed form is shredded.

### Medical History Forms

**Medical history forms** are commonly used to gather information from the patient before the visit with the physician (see Chapter 18, Fig. 18-1). Some medical offices mail these forms to new patients and have them bring the completed form to their visit. This gives the patient the opportunity to concentrate on the questions, gather information about the family history, and give a more complete history. Whether the patient brings the completed form or fills out the history form in the office, you will review the information with the patient to clarify any questions and add additional information gathered in the interview. Specialty practices use forms designed to gather the type of information they will need to manage the patient's care. For example, an orthopedist's history form might include fields for prior orthopedic injuries, accident information, and physical therapy visits.

## Flow Sheets

The **flow sheet** is designed to limit the need for long, handwritten care notes by allowing information to be recorded in either graphic or table form. Generally, flow sheets are designed for a given task. Color-coded sheets for medication administration, vital signs, pediatric growth charts, and so on eliminate the need to read through the pages of a chart to retrieve information. For example, if the physician asks you what the baby weighed 3 months ago, you find the pink growth chart, which saves time and frustration. An advantage of using electronic health records is the capability of converting such information to charts, graphs, and flow sheets. In an electronic health record, clicking an icon for a growth chart takes you to a screen that allows you to enter the information. The software transfers the numbers to a graph. Figure 8-5 shows the growth chart that appears on the screen. When you refill a patient's daily blood pressure medication, you enter the information into the computer record, and it is transferred to the medication record. The record of all entries related to the patient's medications can then be easily retrieved by clicking on the medication icon. Figure 8-6 is an example of a medication flow sheet from a fictitious patient's electronic chart.

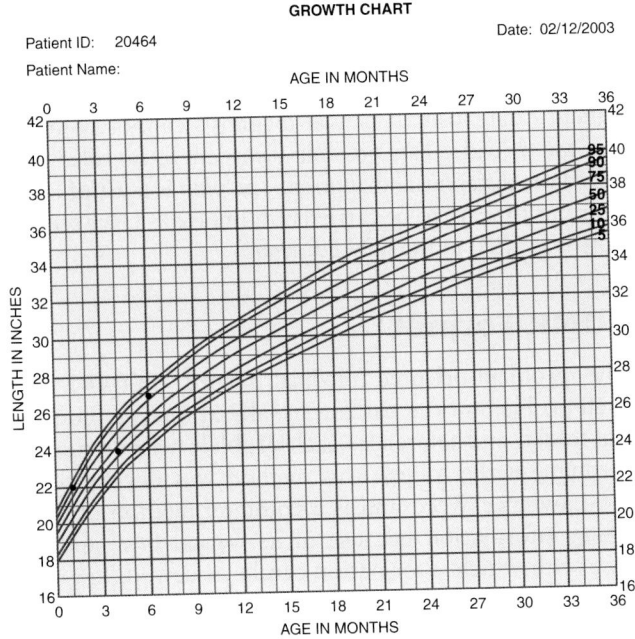

**Figure 8-5** • Growth chart from electronic health records.

**Ardmore Family Practice, P.A.**
2805 Lyndhurst Avenue
Winston-Salem, NC 27103
PHONE: 336-659-0076
FAX: 336-659-0272

**Patient:**  MICHAEL FIELDS                    **Date:**  02-12-2014 9:06 AM

## MEDICATIONS

| Date | Drug Name | Strength/Form | Dispense | Refill | Sig | Last Dose/ Disc Date | Status |
|------|-----------|---------------|----------|--------|-----|----------------------|--------|
| 1/28/14 | SINGULAIR | 10 MG TABS | 5 | 0 | 1 PO BID | | NEW |
| 1/28/14 | ZITHROMAX | 200 MG/5ML SUSR | 5 | 0 | 1 P.O Q DAY | | NEW |
| 1/22/14 | ACCUPRIL | 10 MG TABS | 34 | 4 | 1 PO QD | 1/28/14 | CONTINUE |
| 1/22/14 | ADVIL | 200 MG TABS | 1 | 1 | 1/2 Q A.M. | 1/25/14 | NEW |
| 1/22/14 | ALTACE | 5 MG CAPS | 60 | 5 | ONE TWICE DAILY | 1/28/14 | CONTINUE |
| 1/22/14 | MACROBID | 100 MG CAPS | 14 | 0 | 1 PO BID | 1/28/14 | CONTINUE |
| 8/26/13 | ALTACE | 5 MG CAPS | 60 | 5 | ONE TWICE DAILY | | CONTINUE |
| 8/7/13 | PRECOSE | 25 MG CAPS | 60 | 0 | 1/2 B.I.D. | 10/5/13 | NEW |
| 5/2/12 | ACCUPRIL | 10 MG TABS | 34 | 4 | 1 PO QD | | NEW |
| 5/2/12 | ACCUPRIL | 20 MG TABS | 30 | 0 | 1 PO QD | | NEW |
| 5/2/12 | ACCUPRIL | 40 MG TABS | 30 | 5 | 1 PO QD | | NEW |
| 4/25/12 | ACCUPRIL | 20 MG TABS | 30 | 0 | 1 PO QD | 4/25/12 | NEW |
| 4/25/12 | ACCUPRIL | 40 MG TABS | 30 | 5 | 1 PO QD | | NEW |
| 4/25/12 | MACROBID | 100 MG TABS | 14 | 0 | 1 PO BID | 5/1/12 | NEW |
| 3/2/12 | ACIPHEX 20 MG | TABS | 30 | 6 | 1 PO QD | | NEW |
| 3/2/12 | ACTOS 30 MG | TABS | 30 | 2 | 1 PO QD | | NEW |
| 1/23/12 | ENTEX PSE | 120-600 MG TB12 | 45 | 0 | 1 PO BID | | NEW |
| 1/23/12 | NASONEX | 50 MCG/ACT SUSP | 1 | 3 | 2 SPRAYS EACH NOSTRIL QD | | NEW |
| 8/24/10 | ADALAT CC | 60 MG TBCR | 34 | 5 | 1 PO QD | 8/24/10 | NEW |
| 7/8/10 | NITROGLYCERIN | 0.4 MG/DOSE AERS | 100 | 1 | 1 TAB SL Q 5 MIN X 3, IF CHEST PAIN PERS | 7/8/10 | NEW |
| 6/26/10 | CLARITIN | 10 MG TABS | 30 | 5 | ONE EVERY MORNING | | NEW |
| 6/23/10 | CELEBREX 100 MG | CAPS | 90 | 3 | 1 PO Q AM AND 2 PO Q PM | | NEW |
| 6/3/10 | GLUCOPHAGE | 850 MG TABS | 90 | 6 | ONE 3 TIMES DAILY | 6/3/10 | NEW |
| 6/3/10 | HYTRIN | 5 MG CAPS | 30 | 6 | ONE EVERY DAY | 6/3/10 | NEW |

**Figure 8-6** • Medication administration flow sheet.

## Progress Notes

Progress notes are statements that document the various aspects of patient encounters. The entries in Figure 8-4 are typical progress notes. Some facilities use a lined piece of paper with two columns. The left column is used to document the date and time, and the right column is used to write the note. Others use a plain or lined piece of paper without columns. The progress notes will reflect each encounter with the patient chronologically, whether by phone, by e-mail, or in person. In the electronic health record, you will record vital signs, information given by the patient, etc. The results of lab work done in one area of a practice can be entered into the computer. The computer screen in the examination room will then display the results. This immediate availability makes patient care more efficient and convenient for the physician and the patient. No matter what form is used for documenting, you must always include the date, time, your signature, and your credential. The electronic health record has a feature that allows you to assign your signature electronically. A typical user message might say "press enter to sign."

 **CHECKPOINT QUESTION**

6. List three advantages of using flow sheets in a medical chart.

## COG MEDICAL RECORD ENTRIES

Proper medical record entries are necessary for efficient communication and for legal considerations. The medical record allows health care practitioners to communicate among themselves and therefore provide the best care possible for the patient. Good communication fosters continuity of patient care.

The medical record is a legal document that can be subpoenaed in a malpractice suit. If the documentation is accurate, timely, and legible, it can help win a lawsuit or prevent one altogether. If the documentation is messy, inaccurate, or improperly done, however, it can raise questions that might cause the practice to lose a malpractice suit. Figure 8-7 is a charting example that shows the difference between a well-written chart note and one that leaves what really happened in question. It has been said that if it is not documented, it was not done. The reality is that it is very difficult to prove what was done if the patient information is incomplete. Therefore, all patient procedures, assessments, interventions, evaluations, teachings, and communications must be documented. Box 8-4 lists guidelines for documenting in patients' medical records.

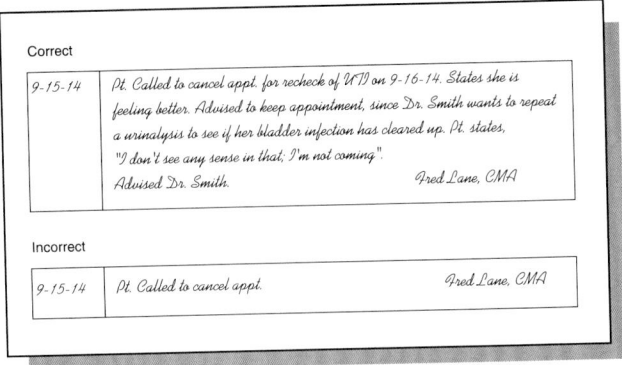

**Figure 8-7 •** Charting example showing correct and incorrect entries.

## Charting Communications with Patients

As discussed earlier, in addition to documenting patient visits to the facility, other encounters and communications may occur and should become a part of the permanent record. To ensure continuity of care and patient safety, charts should contain a progress sheet or some sort of tool to record each communication with a patient. Actions taken by the physician or employees as directed by the physician on behalf of the patient should be charted. For example, when a prescription is phoned to a pharmacy, the action is recorded. The physician may give instructions to be carried out regarding a patient, such as calling the patient with normal test results. This should be concisely explained in the chart. These entries should appear in **chronological order**. Dates that are out of order and gaps between entries may confuse the reader and give the appearance of poor service. For this reason, entries should be made immediately after communications with the patient.

Telephone or electronic communications with patients are typically recorded in a narrative manner. When a patient calls or e-mails the office, the conversation must be documented in the chart immediately. Phone calls should be documented with the time and date of the call, patient's problem or request, and actions taken by the person making the entry. If special telephone message pads are used, a copy should be placed in the patient's chart. E-mails from patients should be printed and kept in the chart. Replies to a patient's e-mail should be printed out and included with the progress sheet. Remember, care must be taken to adhere to HIPAA's Privacy Rules to ensure protection of the patient's privacy when using electronic means to communicate.

## Additions to Medical Records

Any additions to a medical record, such as laboratory results, that are smaller than the standard 8.5 × 11 inches should be transcribed onto a full sheet of paper or

## BOX 8-4   Documentation Guidelines

1. Make sure you know the office policy regarding charting. Find out who is allowed to write in the chart and the procedures for doing so.
2. Make sure you have the correct patient chart. If the patient's name is common, ask for a birth date or social security number as a double check.
3. Document in ink.
4. Sign your complete name and credential.
5. Always record the date of each entry. Some outpatient facilities record the time as well. Using military time will eliminate the need to use AM and PM (Fig. 8-8).
6. Write legibly. Printing is more legible than cursive writing.
7. Check spelling, especially medical terms, before entering them into the chart. Chapter 7 offers help with spelling.
8. Use only abbreviations that are accepted by your facility. Because abbreviations can cause confusion and errors in patient care, the use of certain handwritten abbreviations has been prohibited by The Joint Commission. (See Legal Tip: Abbreviations? When in Doubt, Spell It Out.)
9. When charting the patient's statements, use quotation marks to signify the patient's own words. For example, "My head is killing me."
10. Do not attempt to make a diagnosis. For example, if the patient says, "My throat is sore," do not write pharyngitis. It is not within the scope of your training to diagnose.
11. Document as soon as possible after completing a task to promote accuracy.
12. Document missed appointments in the patient's chart. Chart your attempts to reach the patient to remind him or her of the appointment.
13. Document any telephone conversations with the patient in the chart.
14. Be honest. If you have given a wrong medication or performed the wrong procedure, as soon as the appropriate supervisor is notified, document it, and then complete an incident report (see Chapter 11). State only the facts; do not draw any conclusions or place blame.
15. Never document for someone else, and never ask someone else to document for you.
16. Never document false information.
17. Never delete, erase, scribble over, or white-out information in the medical record because this can be construed as attempting to cover the truth and tampering with a legal document. If you do make an error, draw a single line through it, initial it, and date it. Then write the word "correction" and document the correct information (Fig. 8-9).

You can click on an icon to make a correction in the electronic chart, but the original information is not deleted. For example, if you discover that you have entered the wrong date of birth after the patient's information has been saved, you can correct it, but most systems allow only certain users to make changes in the saved database.

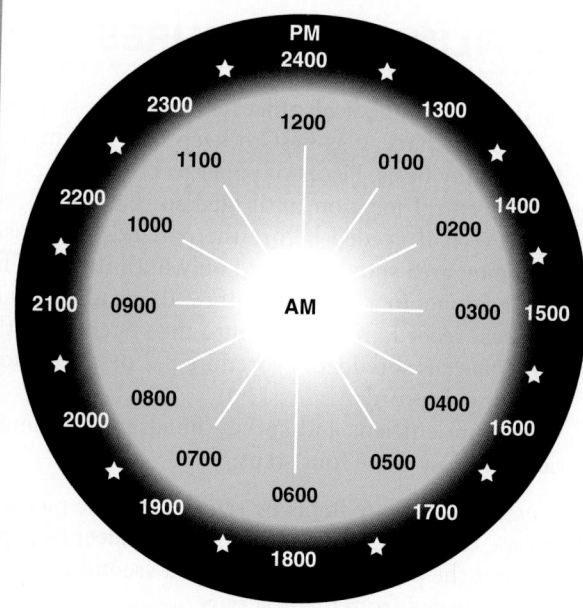

**Figure 8-8** • Military time.

When correcting a charting error, draw a single line through the error, initial it, date it, and document the correct information.

*left 05/15/14 TW*
*05/15/14  Patient presents today complaining of pain in ~~right~~ eye. Tracy Wiles, CMA*

**Figure 8-9** • Correcting an error in a medical record.

shingled and placed in the appropriate area of the chart. Shingling is taping the paper across the top to a regular-size sheet. Each sheet is then added under the current one with a piece of tape across the top. Each sheet can be lifted to view the entire document. Most laboratory reports are computer generated and will come ready to insert into the chart. Paper records that are received may be scanned and uploaded into the patient's electronic health record if necessary. All additions to the medical record (e.g., laboratory results, radiographic reports, consultation reports) should be read and initialed by the physician before you put them in the chart.

### CHECKPOINT QUESTION

7. What three qualities must a medical record have to be helpful in a lawsuit?

## WORKERS' COMPENSATION RECORDS

From time to time, a patient who is active in your practice may seek treatment for a **workers' compensation** case or an injury or illness related to employment. The government requires employers to provide insurance for care when an injury occurs at work. Workers' compensation is discussed in Chapter 13. When this occurs, do not simply add the information to the patient's medical record. Instead, start a new record. A workers' compensation medical record actually belongs to the employer, so the data in that record can be reviewed by the employer's insurance carrier. Information about the patient's previous health or family history that is not pertinent to the workplace incident should *not* be made available to the insurance carrier.

Depending on the diagnoses covered under workers' compensation claims, cases may be kept open for a minimum of 2 years after the last date of treatment for any follow-up care that may be required. After that time, care may not be covered under the same case. Even after the care is complete, the separate record is kept with the patient's other record, and information is incorporated into the original record as needed.

### CHECKPOINT QUESTION

8. Why is it necessary to make a new chart for an established patient who is being seen for an injury sustained at work?

## STORING MEDICAL RECORDS

Using electronic health records eliminates the need for filing, but manual records must be prepared and kept in a way that promotes easy retrieval. Since the medical record is the foundation for patient care, much care and attention is given to the process of storing and retrieving medical charts.

### Medical Record Preparation

To start filing, you need folders, labels, and any other appropriate supplies. Keep these supplies on hand and follow the same steps every time you put together and file a medical record. Procedure 8-1 outlines the steps for establishing and maintaining a medical record. Over the course of many years, you may have to replace worn-out folders or peeling labels and stickers. Do so before the folder tears or the labels fall off.

After preparing the folders, you may also want to prepare several out guides, that is, plastic sheets with a tab (projection) and a pocket for index cards. Type "Out guide" on the tabbed edge of the sheet. Then, when you remove a chart, write the date, name of the patient, your initials, and where the chart can be found on an index card. Place the card inside the out guide, and put the out guide in the spot in the file cabinet where the chart was. An out guide indicates that the chart has been removed and where it can be found. Hospitals and larger clinics often use bar codes to keep track of charts and radiographs. When a chart arrives in a certain location, a wand is passed over a bar code. When the patient's number is entered into the computer, the screen shows the location of the patient's chart at the moment. If it is in the file cabinet, that is also indicated.

### CHECKPOINT QUESTION

9. What is the purpose of an out guide?

## FILING PROCEDURES

Every day in the medical office, information is added to a patient's chart. It is best to keep this information filed on a daily basis. Pieces of paper to be added can be kept in a central location until filed so that employees can retrieve it if needed before the patient's next visit. This holding area should be used only until the daily filing can be done. In a paperless office, these additions to the medical record are scanned into the system, and the original paper is shredded. Procedure 8-2 describes how to file manual records.

To ensure efficient and speedy filing and document retrieval, follow these four steps:

1. *Condition.* Prepare items by removing loose pieces of tape or paper clips. Make sure each sheet of paper includes the patient's name in case a second page gets separated from the first page.
2. *Index.* Separate business records from patient records.
3. *Sort.* Put each group of records in proper order to be filed on shelves, either alphabetic or numeric. This makes actual filing go much faster because you are not moving up and down and back and forth to find the proper letter area; you will just move down in order.
4. *Store.* Place each record in the proper storage area, as described next.

# FILING SYSTEMS

The two main filing systems are alphabetic and numeric. In some practices, you may use both systems, each for different types of files.

## Alphabetic Filing

As the name implies, **alphabetic filing** is a system using letters. Begin alphabetic filing by distinguishing the first, second, and third unit as described in Box 8-5. (A unit is each part of a name or title that is used in indexing.) Using the first letter of the first unit, place your records in small groups in order from A to Z. After that, take each small group and gradually work through the second and consecutive letters to put the small groups in order. Using this process allows you to work in a progressive order as you add records to existing files.

If the entire first unit is the same, move onto the second unit. If the second unit is still the same, move onto the third unit. Occasionally, you will have records whose units one, two, and three are identical. In such cases, it does not matter which one is filed first; use extreme caution, however, when retrieving records with identical units to prevent errors. Asking the patient to provide his or her birthday will ensure that you have the right patient and avoid confusion.

With alphabetic filing, color coding may also be used. Letters of the alphabet are color coded and affixed to each folder, or a color-coded bar is placed next to the label with the patient's name. For example, names beginning with A to F may be blue; G to L, green; M to T, yellow; and U to Z, purple. Using this system, Michele Beals would have a blue strip, Laurie Palmer would have a yellow strip, Lauren Kayser would have a green strip, and Dana Warbeck would have a purple strip. Finding misfiled charts is easier. With one glance at the cabinet, for example, you can spot one purple tab in the middle of the green ones.

## Numeric Filing

**Numeric filing** uses digits, usually six. The digits are typically run together but read as three groups of two digits. For example, the record filed as 324478 is read as 32, 44, 78. Commas are not placed or any separation used when applying the labels to the tabbed edge of the file folder. The records are placed in numeric order without concern for duplication, which may sometimes happen with the alphabetic system. If you use this technique, it is called straight digit filing because you are reading the number straight out from left to right.

Sometimes, the file label will look the same, 324478, but will be read in the reverse order: 78, 44, 32. This technique is called terminal digit filing; that is, the groups of numbers are read in pairs from right to left. Be careful not to mix the two filing systems. If using both techniques within your office, be sure to keep them separate by changing the folder color or some other means to prevent errors. The chart is filed by using the last pairs of digits.

Numeric filing plays an important role in the medical office. With HIPAA's Privacy Rule requirements, the use of numeric filing makes sense. When this technique is used, it is important to keep a **cross-reference** in a secure area, away from patient areas, listing the numeric code and the name of the patient. Such a reference is

---

> **BOX 8-5** **Indexing Rules for Alphabetic Filing**
>
> When filing records alphabetically, use these indexing rules to help you decide the placement of each record. Indexing rules apply whether you use the title of the record's contents or a person's name.
>
> File by name according to last name, first name, and middle initial, and treat each letter in the name as a separate unit. For example, Jamey L. Crowell should be filed as Crowell, Jamey L. and should come before Crowell, Jamie L.
>
> - Make sure professional initials are placed after a full name. John P. Bonnet, D.O., should be filed as Bonnet, John P., D.O.
> - Treat hyphenated names as one unit. Bernadette M. Ryan-Nardone should be filed as Ryan-Nardone, Bernadette M. not as Nardone, Bernadette M. Ryan.
> - File abbreviated names as if they were spelled out. Finnigan, Wm. should be filed as Finnigan, William, and St. James should be filed as Saint James.
> - File last names beginning with Mac and Mc in regular order or grouped together, depending on your preference, but be consistent with either approach.
> - File a married woman's record by using her own first name. Helen Johnston (Mrs. Kevin Johnston) should be filed as Johnston, Helen, not as Johnston, Kevin Mrs.
> - Jr. and Sr. should be used in indexing and labeling the record. Many times, a father and son are patients at the same facility.
> - When names are identical, use the next unit, such as birth dates or the mother's maiden name. Use Durham, Iran (2-4-94) and Durham, Iran (4-5-45).
> - Disregard apostrophes.
> - Disregard articles (a, the), conjunctions (and, or), and prepositions (in, of) in filing. File *The Cat in the Hat* under Cat in Hat.
> - Treat letters in a company name as separate units. For ASM, Inc., "A" is the first unit, "S" is the second unit, and "M" is the third unit.

called a master patient index. This way, a limited number of people know who the patient is, which maintains privacy. Boxes 8-6 and 8-7 describe how to file patient records alphabetically or numerically.

## Other Filing Systems

The medical office keeps files other than patient records. An office manager keeps files on employees, insurance policies, accounts payable, and so on. For this type of filing, systems include **subject filing**, in which documents are arranged alphabetically according to subject (e.g., insurance, medications, referrals); geographic filing, in which documents are grouped alphabetically according to locations, such as state, county, or city; and chronological filing, in which documents are grouped in the order of their date.

A well-kept, complete, and accurate medical record and the ability to quickly retrieve information are reflections of the quality and efficiency of the medical facility in which they are generated.

### CHECKPOINT QUESTION

10. What are the two main filing systems? Briefly describe each.

---

### BOX 8-6    Alphabetic Filing Examples

The following patient records are to be filed alphabetically:

Mary P. Martin
Floyd D. Huey, Sr.
Susan Bailey
Ellen P. Parrish
Karen Hart
Susan Roberts-Hill
Amy Dalton
Amy Roberson
Clayton A. Parker, MD
Mrs. John Moser (Donna)

The correct order is as follows:

Susan Bailey
Amy Dalton
Karen Hart
Floyd D. Huey, Sr.
Mary P. Martin
Donna Moser
Clayton A. Parker
Ellen P. Parrish
Amy Roberson
Susan Roberts-Hill

---

### BOX 8-7    Numeric Filing Examples

The following patient records are to be filed numerically:

| Ramsey, LeRoy | 213456 |
|---|---|
| Flora, Curtis | 334387 |
| King, Sharon | 979779 |
| Moore, Cathy | 321138 |

In straight digit filing, the proper order is as follows:

213456
321138
334387
979779

In terminal digit filing, the proper order is as follows:

321138
213456
979779
334387

With files in which one or two groups of numbers are the same numbers, you refer to the second or third groups of numbers. For example, in straight digit filing (reading from left to right), the number 003491 comes before 004592. The first group of numbers (00) is the same for both files, so you determine the order of filing by the second group of numbers; in this case, 34 comes before 45.

In terminal digit filing (reading from right to left), 456128 would come before 926128. The first two groups of numbers (28 and 61) are the same for both files, so you go to the third group of numbers; in this case, 45 comes before 92.

## COG STORING HEALTH INFORMATION

Whether a facility uses an electronic form, a manual system, or a combination of both, the records used in the delivery of health care must be stored safely and privately. A goal of a good system includes easy retrieval of the information. Logical organization and policies that ensure that information is safe, secure, and easily accessed make for an efficient medical office.

### Electronic Data Storage

The paperless medical office must consider storage of data other than using paper and folders. HIPAA's Administrative Simplification section addresses the issues involved in storing electronically generated transmissions and storage. Backup copies of computerized records must be made daily and stored in a safe, fireproof location. Security experts advise storing backup disks off-site. HIPAA mandates that offices establish a disaster plan that includes emergency storage of data and security and safety of that data. Any computer infrastructure should allow for chart availability in a disaster situation. A medical office may choose to outsource the off-site storage of their data. Health information stored off-site may be classified as "hot," which means the records are accessible and usable. A storage backup would need activation for use. The speed of computer technology and government involvement promises changes and new practices. In order to optimize efficiency, you must keep abreast of these new regulations and technologies.

## Storage of Standard Medical Records

Medical offices use a variety of storage methods for active files that are used on a daily basis. Shelf files are stationary shelves. Shelving units are stacked on each other or placed side by side. These shelves may also be custom-ordered to the width you need. Records are stored horizontally, and labels are read from the side. Figure 8-10 shows an example of shelving units.

Drawer files are a type of filing cabinet. The drawer pulls out for easy access and visibility of all records. This type of filing system allows you easier access to all sides of files, which can help in searches for missing files that may have been pushed to the back or behind other files. Drawer files also allow easier filing because you can read from above the files, rather than squatting to read the labels from the sides as you work your way down to the lower shelves. A disadvantage is that these files take up a great deal of space.

Rotary circular or lateral files allow records to be stored in units that either spin in a circle or stack one behind the other, enabling you to rotate different units to the front. This system allows for maximum use of office space and is suggested for a medical office with large quantities of records to be stored. With shelf or

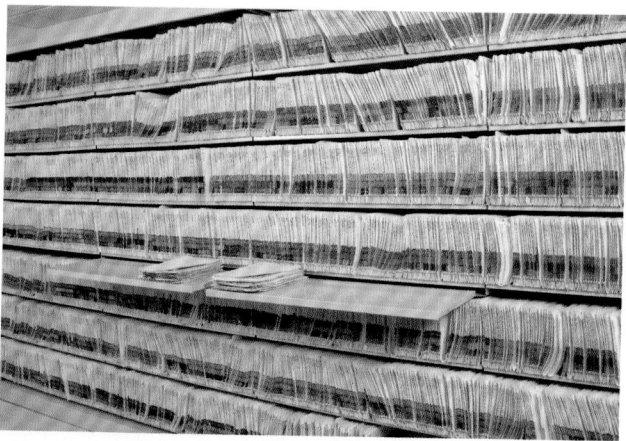

**Figure 8-10** • File cabinets.

drawer units, more wall space is needed to spread out each unit, but with rotary files, less wall space is needed.

## Classification of Medical Records

For the purpose of storing records, they may be classified in three categories: active, inactive, or closed. Active records are those of patients who have been seen within the past few years. The exact amount of time is designated within each practice; it usually ranges from 1 to 5 years. Keep these records in the most accessible storage spot available because you will be using them regularly.

Inactive records are those of patients who have not been treated in the office for a set time. Most offices consider files inactive after 2 to 3 years. You will still keep inactive records in the office, but they do not have to be as accessible as the active files. Usually, they are placed on bottom shelves to eliminate constant bending when reaching for active files, or they may be stored in another room within the office. They can be stored in the office in an out-of-the-way area, such as a basement or attic. They may even be kept in the physician's home. This practice is permitted because the records belong to the physician, but it is not recommended because, at any time, the office staff may need access to these records. "Inactive" patients have not formally terminated their contact with the physician, but they have either not needed the physician's services or have not informed the office regarding a move, change in physician, or death.

Closed records are those of patients who have terminated their relationship with the physician. Reasons for such termination might include the patient moving, termination of physician–patient relationship by letter, no further treatment necessary, or death of the patient.

Many practices use document imaging technology, such as scanning paper records into a computer database, **microfilm** or **microfiche**, to store closed records. Archiving medical records by scanning documents requires that the information be stored in some type of electronic media system or into a secure online database. Both ways provide for quick access and retrieval of patient information. Microfilm and microfiche are ways to photograph documents and store them in a reduced form. Microfilm, a popular method for storing large volumes of records, particularly in hospitals and clinics, uses a photographic process that develops medical records in miniature on film. Information is stored on cards holding single film frames or in reels or strips for projection on compact electric viewers

Microfiche is a miniature photographic system that stores rows of images in reduced size on cards with clear plastic sleeves rather than on film strips. Information can be handled manually, examined on a viewer that enlarges the record, or reproduced as hard copy on a high-speed photocopier. A standard microfiche card holds more than 60 pages of information. The microfiche process allows 3200 papers to be reduced to fit on a single 4- to 6-inch transparency.

# **∞** **MEDICAL RECORD RETENTION**

As discussed in Chapter 2, the statute of limitations is the legal time limit set for filing suit against an alleged wrongdoer. The time limit varies from state to state. You must observe the statute of limitations in your particular state to know how long medical and business records should be kept in storage.

It is recommended that medical records be stored permanently because, in some states, malpractice lawsuits can be filed within 2 years of the date of discovery of the alleged malpractice. The statute of limitations for minors is extended until the child reaches legal age in every state; the time given past the legal age varies, however. It is considered good practice to check with the physician's malpractice insurance company to determine how long to retain all medical records.

When a health care provider's practice ends, either from retirement or death, notice to all patients with records stored in the facility is required. This notice can be in the form of a letter to each patient and/or a newspaper notification advising patients of the closing of the practice and giving them a reasonable length of time in which to pick up their records. Since the facility no longer exists, you may release the original record to the patients. As discussed previously, the record itself belongs to the facility, but the information in the record belongs to the patient. Since the facility no longer exists, it is felt that the record now belongs to the patient. Retiring physicians or the families of deceased physicians may ask a colleague to maintain storage of any patient records that are not claimed. This location should be given to the patients in their written notification. Of course, the statute of limitations for legal action and the need for these records should be taken into consideration. Most risk management experts advise that the records should be kept in some form forever, but this is not always feasible. At the least, every reasonable attempt should be made to notify patients and disseminate the information maintained by the retiring or deceased physician.

---

## BOX 8-8 **North Carolina Medical Board's Position Statement**

The North Carolina Medical Board supports and adopts the following language of Section 7.05 of the American Medical Association's current Code of Medical Ethics regarding the retention of medical records by physicians.

### 7.05: Retention of Medical Records

Physicians have an obligation to retain patient records which may reasonably be of value to a patient. The following guidelines are offered to assist physicians in meeting their ethical and legal obligations:

1. Medical considerations are the primary basis for deciding how long to retain medical records. For example, operative notes and chemotherapy records should always be part of the patient's chart. In deciding whether to keep certain parts of the record, an appropriate criterion is whether a physician would want the information if he or she were seeing the patient for the first time.

2. If a particular record no longer needs to be kept for medical reasons, the physician should check state laws to see if there is a requirement that records be kept for a minimum length of time. Most states will not have such a provision. If they do, it will be part of the statutory code or state licensing board.

3. In all cases, medical records should be kept for at least as long as the length of time of the statute of limitations for medical malpractice claims. The statute of limitations may be 3 or more years, depending on the state law. State medical associations and insurance carriers are the best resources for this information.

4. Whatever the statute of limitations, a physician should measure time from the last professional contact with the patient.

5. If a patient is a minor, the statute of limitations for medical malpractice claims may not apply until the patient reaches the age of majority.

6. Immunization records always must be kept.

7. The records of any patient covered by Medicare or Medicaid must be kept at least 5 years.

8. In order to preserve confidentiality when discarding old records, all documents should be destroyed.

9. Before discarding old records, patients should be given an opportunity to claim the records or have them sent to another physician, if it is feasible to give them the opportunity.

Please Note:

a. North Carolina has no statute relating specifically to the retention of medical records.

b. Several North Carolina statutes relate to time limitations for the filing of malpractice actions. Legal advice should be sought regarding such limitations.

*(Adopted 5/98)*
Reprinted with permission from NC Medical Society.

##  DISPOSAL OF MEDICAL RECORDS

Before a paper medical record is destroyed, the owner of the information should be given the opportunity to pick up the record. If this is not possible, and/or the record will not be needed for continuity of care in the future, then the record can be destroyed. Paper medical records should *never* be placed in a regular trash can or a dumpster. There are cases of companies being fined for illegally discarding medical records in dumpsters. These records contained patient names, birth dates, social security numbers, and other protected health information.

Before protected medical records can be thrown out, they should be shredded or burned. Many medical facilities outsource this task to a record disposal company. Keep small trash cans labeled "TO BE SHREDDED" at each work station to encourage employees to comply.

Electronic PHI is less likely to require disposal. However, if your office uses any type of removable or portable electronic media such as floppy disks, CDs, or flash drives, be sure to erase, delete, or reformat any information that is no longer needed. Be sure to remove information from the hard drive of computers that are no longer in use or being sold in such a way that prevents the data from being recovered. Box 8-8 is the position statement of the North Carolina Medical Society. It is designed to assist physicians in adopting medical record retention and disposal practices.

### CHECKPOINT QUESTION

11. What is the primary basis for deciding how long a record should be kept?

### WHAT IF?

**You work in a family practice office where your physician treats many children. How long should you keep the children's records? The statute of limitations in your state is 3 years from the date of the last treatment.**

By law, when a physician treats an adult, the record should be kept until the statute of limitations expires. A minor has the right to bring suit against a health care provider when he becomes of legal age. Therefore, the minor's records should be kept at least 3 years past the 18th birthday.

###  ROLE-PLAYING ACTIVITY

Great Falls Medical Center has an extensive medical records department for active patients. There is an office policy requiring everyone to use out guides when taking medical records from the cabinet; however, several medical records are now missing with no out guides to indicate where they might be located. Kayla Murphy, RMA, is responsible for filing, maintaining, and releasing medical records and has determined which staff member she believes is responsible for not using out guides when taking medical records from the cabinet. What is the best approach that Kayla should use to discuss this problem with the employee? Can Kayla be sure that she has the correct person responsible for not following office protocol when taking medical records? If you are playing the role of the medical assistant, think about other options you might offer to the employee to assist with following this policy in the future. If you are playing the role as the staff member, think about how you might feel if confronted with this and accused of not following the office policy. Would you feel embarrassed? Angry? Defensive? Your instructor will give you additional information about this activity!

## *español* SPANISH TERMINOLOGY

**Vamos a necesitar copias de su historial médico de su médico anterior.**
We will need copies of your medical records from your previous doctor.

**Al firmar aquí, usted nos da permiso de compartir su información médica con su compañía de seguro.**
By signing here, you are giving us permission to share your medical information with your insurance company.

**Toda su información referente a su historial médico está protegida por la ley de HIPAA (Ley de Portabilidad y Contabilidad de Seguros de Salud de 1996).**
All your medical information is protected under a federal law known as HIPAA.

**Nosotros somos los dueños de su expediente médico pero usted es el dueño de la información en el. Usted puede solicitar una copia en cualquier momento.**
We own your medical record, but you own the information in it. You have the right to ask for a copy anytime.

**Por favor asegurese de que toda la información en su historia clínica sea verídica, esto es muy importante para que su médico pueda diagnosticarle correctamente.**
Please make sure that all the information posted in your medical history is accurate; this will help your doctor to diagnose correctly.

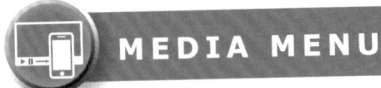

## MEDIA MENU

**Student Resources** on thePoint®

• **CMA/RMA Certification Exam Review**

**Internet Resources**

**U.S. Department of Health and Human Services, CMS, HIPAA—General Information**
http://www.cms.gov/HIPAAGenInfo

**U.S. Department of Health and Human Services, CMS, National Provider Identifier Standard**
http://www.cms.gov/NationalProvIdentStand

**Office of the National Coordinator for Health Information Technology**
http://www.healthit.gov

**American Health Information Management Association**
http://www.ahima.org

**Health Level Seven (HL7)**
http://www.hl7.org

**Certification Commission for Health Information Technology**
http://www.cchit.org

**Office of the National Coordinator for Health Information Technology**
http://www.hhs.gov/healthit/hithca.html

# EMR Activity

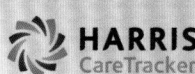

Harris CareTracker is a web-based electronic medical record (EMR) application that you will use for the EMR activities included in this section at the end of each chapter. This application is actually used in physician offices, but is provided to you through the publisher, Wolters Kluwer Health, to give you hands-on practice working with EMRs. Your instructor will have more information about accessing your username, log-in, and Quickstart guide.

Prerequisite Activities in Harris CareTracker
- *The Getting Started and Quickstart documents and EMR Activities Step-by-Step Instructions are available at* http://thePoint.lww.com/KronenbergerComp5e

Activity Details

It was an unusually busy day at Great Falls Medical Center yesterday, and several new patients were registered and entered into the electronic medical record. Although everyone signed the Notice of Privacy Practices, it was not noted in one of the patient's electronic medical record. Document in the EMR for new patient Joshua Thompson that he received the NPP at his visit in the *Demographics* tab of the EMR.

## Chapter Summary

- Medical records are not only a means of communication among health care providers but also legal documents depicting the quality of patient care.
- HIPAA ensures confidentiality of all medical information. The patient's privacy must be protected at all times.
- You must adhere to strict guidelines when sharing protected health information electronically and releasing any information in patients' medical records.
- You must use sound practices when entering information into a patient's medical record.
- To ensure efficient recording and retrieval, you must be familiar with the varied documentation forms as well as the different kinds of filing systems.
- The system of storage of medical information used by a provider must ensure the safety, security, and confidentiality of the patient's protected health information.
- You must follow applicable laws and sound guidelines regarding the retention and disposal of records in order to safeguard the patient's rights to their personal medical information.
- The quality, use, and care of the medical record are reflections of the quality of the medical facility itself.

## Warm-Ups for Critical Thinking

1. Interview a fellow student with a hypothetical illness. Document the visit with the chief complaint.
2. Compare and contrast alphabetic filing with numeric filling. Which system do you think works better? Explain your response.
3. Role play with a fellow student who is requesting his or her medical records for a new doctor. Construct a proper authorization for release of information form and have the "patient" complete it.
4. Write an office policy for maintaining confidentiality with electronic modalities, such as fax machines, printers, laptops, and computer screens.
5. You work for an orthopedist who is retiring in 3 months. He asks you to construct a letter to be sent to all of the patients informing them of his retirement and instructing them to come in and pick up their records. List the hours the office will be open and the deadline for picking up the records. Include in the letter the location of the records after that deadline.

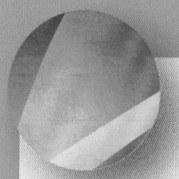

**PSY** PROCEDURE 8-1

# Establishing, Organizing, and Maintaining a Medical File

**PSY** Create and organize a patient's medical record

**Purpose:** To create a file that will organize and save a patient's medical information, including records of transactions and interactions with the office and its staff

**Equipment:** File folder, metal fasteners, hole punch, five divider sheets with tabs, title, year, and alphabetic or numeric labels

| STEPS | REASONS |
|---|---|
| 1. Decide the name of the file (a patient's name, company name, or name of the type of information to be stored). | Properly naming a file allows for easy retrieval. |
| 2. Type a label with the title *in unit order* (e.g., Lynn, Laila S., *not* Laila S. Lynn). | Typing the label in unit order helps avoid filing errors. |
| 3. Place the label along the tabbed edge of the folder so that the title extends out beyond the folder itself. (Tabs can be either the length of the folder or tabbed in various positions, such as left, center, and right.) | This ensures easy readability when the folder is in a storage cabinet. |

**Step 3:** Place label along tabbed edge of folder.

| | |
|---|---|
| 4. Place a year label along the top edge of the tab before the label with the title. This will be changed each year the patient has been seen. *Note:* Do not automatically replace these labels at the start of a new year; remove the old year and replace with a new one only when the patient comes in for the first visit of the new year. | Doing this makes removing inactive files more time efficient. At the beginning of each new year, you can easily spot the records that are years beyond your storage time limit in the active file area. Doing this also can help you locate inactive files if patients return years later. (By determining the last year the patient was seen, you can narrow your search to files with a matching year label.) |
| 5. Place the appropriate alphabetic or numeric labels below the title. | This aids in accurate filing and retrieval. |

*(continues on page 208)*

## PROCEDURE 8-1 (continued)

| STEPS | REASONS |
|---|---|
| **6.** Apply any additional labels that your office may decide to use. | Labels noting special information (e.g., insurance, drug allergies, advanced directives) act as quick and easy reminders. |

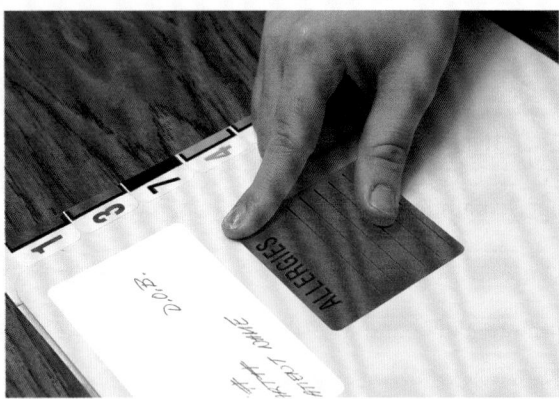

**Step 6:** Apply additional labels as needed.

**7.** Punch holes and insert demographic and financial information using top fasteners across the top.

General information should not be intermingled with clinical information.

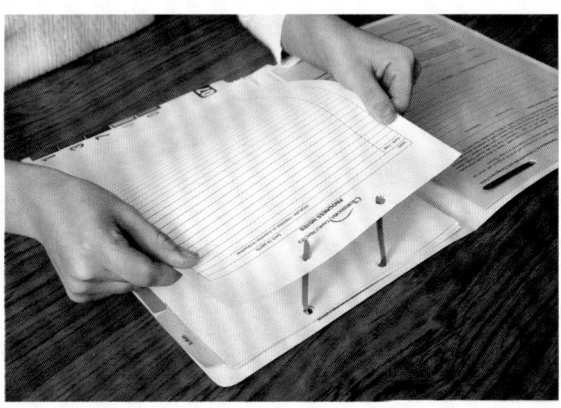

**Step 7:** Punch holes and insert pages in chart.

**8.** Make tabs for: Ex. H&P, Progress Notes, Medication Log, Correspondence, and Test Results.

This will allow quick and easy retrieval of specific information.

**9.** Place pages behind appropriate tabs.

Misplacing charts or sheets out of charts creates big problems for everyone.

**10.** **AFF** Explain what you would do when you receive a revised copy correcting an error on a document already in a patient's chart.

Attach the revised document to the old one. The new one should be marked "revised" and placed on top of the old one. In an electronic record, the new document should be scanned into the patient's record and the old document can be deleted. In other words, you are replacing the document altogether.

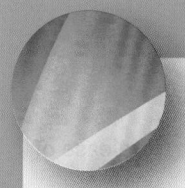

**PSY** PROCEDURE 8-2

# Filing Medical Records/Maintain Organization by Filing

**PSY** File patient medical records

**Purpose:** To place medical information in a designated location that will facilitate easy retrieval and the safety of the record

**Equipment:** Simulated patient file folder, several single sheets to be filed in the chart, file cabinet with other files

| STEPS | PURPOSE |
| --- | --- |
| 1. Double-check spelling of names on the chart and any single sheets to be placed in the folder. | To prevent an error that may cause a breach in a patient's private health information that is misfiled. |
| 2. Condition any single sheets, etc. | Removing staples, paper clips, and tape will keep paper from getting torn. |
| 3. Place sheets behind proper tab in the chart. | Organizing documents and placing tabs allows for easy retrieval of specific information. |
| 4. Remove out guide. | The out guide will serve as a double check for the proper placement of the chart. |
| 5. Place the folder between the two appropriate existing folders, taking care to place the folder between the two charts. | It is easy to accidentally place a folder within a folder. |
| 6. Scan color coding to ensure none of the charts in that section are out of order. | Color-coded tabs enable you to spot a misfiled chart easily. |
| 7. **AFF** Explain what you would do when you find a chart out of order. | If a chart is out of order, the efficiency of patient care is affected. At the least, it should be mentioned at the next office meeting. |

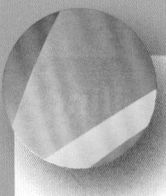

**PSY** PROCEDURE 8-3

## Releasing Medical Records

**PSY**  Respond to issues of confidentiality; and apply HIPAA rules in regard to privacy/release of information

**Purpose:** To correctly respond to a request for medical records.

**Scenario:** A patient's insurance company requests documentation for a specific date of service in order to process a medical claim

**Equipment:** Simulated patient medical record (paper or electronic)

| STEPS | REASONS |
|---|---|
| 1. Verify the patient's name and another piece of identifying information in order to pull the correct medical record | Confirming the patient's name and another identifying piece of information, such as the date of birth, prevents releasing PHI to unauthorized parties |
| 2. Determine if a release of medical records must be signed before the records can be released. | HIPAA does not require a signed release of information for treatment, payment, or operations. |
| 3. Choose the correct document(s) to be released and provide a *copy* of the documentation if it is not sent electronically. | Only release the documentation for the date of service being requested. Never release an original document from the patient's medical record. |
| 4. Determine whether or not a fee should be assessed for copies of the medical record. | There would be no charge assessed for sending medical records to the patient's insurance for TPO; however, state laws may determine the amounts that may be charged for records requested by other entities. |
| 5. **AFF** Explain how you would handle copying the requested medical documentation when using a copier located near the reception door. | Remove the documentation from the patient's medical record in a private area and away from patients and take it to the copier in an unmarked folder so that private health information is not disclosed. This is necessary to protect the integrity of the medical record. |

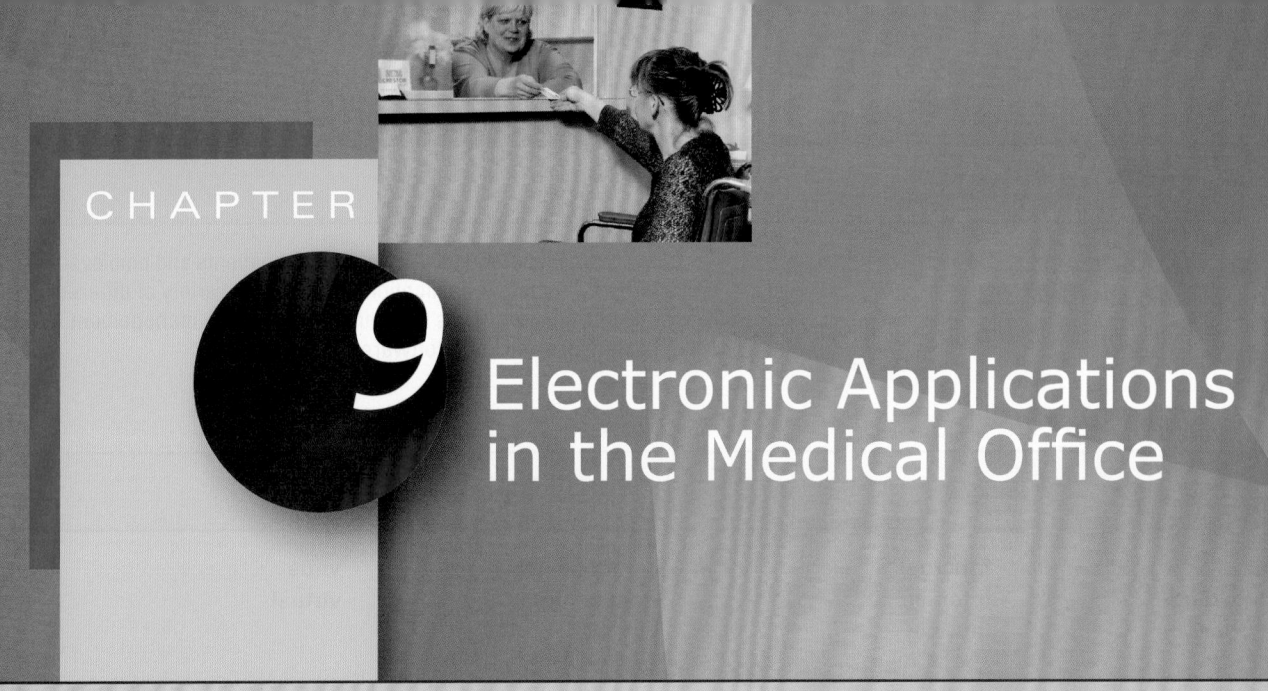

# CHAPTER 9

# Electronic Applications in the Medical Office

## Outline

**The Computer**
Hardware
Peripherals
Care and Maintenance of the System
and Equipment
**Internet Basics**
Getting Started and Connected
Security of Electronically Shared
Personal Health Information
Internet Security
Viruses
Downloading Information

Working Offline
**Electronic Mail**
Access
Attachments
Opening Electronic Mail
**Medical Applications of the Internet**
Search Engines
Professional Medical Sites
Patient Teaching Issues Regarding the
Internet
**Intranet**

**Medical Software Applications**
Clinical Applications
Administrative Applications
**Adopting Electronic Health Records Technology**
Making the Transition
**Purchasing a Computer**
**Training Options**
**Cell Phones and Texting**
**Computer Ethics**

## Learning Outcomes

### COG Cognitive Domain*

1. Spell and define the key words
2. Identify the basic computer components
3. *Explain the purpose of routine maintenance of administrative and clinical equipment*
4. Explain the basics of connecting to the Internet
5. Discuss the safety concerns for online searching
6. Describe how to use a search engine
7. List sites that can be used by professionals and sites geared for patients
8. Describe the benefits of an intranet and explain how it differs from the Internet
9. Describe the various types of clinical software that might be used in a physician's office
10. Describe the various types of administrative software that might be used in a physician's office
11. *Discuss applications of electronic technology in professional communication*
12. Describe the considerations for purchasing a computer
13. Describe various training options
14. Discuss the adoption of electronic health records

15. Describe the steps in making the transition from paper to electronic records
16. Discuss the ethics related to computer access
17. *Differentiate between electronic medical records (EMR) and a practice management system*

### AFF Affective Domain*

1. Apply ethical behaviors, including honesty and integrity, in the performance of medical assisting practice

### PSY Psychomotor Domain*

1. *Perform routine maintenance of administrative or clinical equipment* (Procedure 9-1)
2. Use the Internet to access information related to the medical office (Procedure 9-2)
3. *Input patient data utilizing a practice management system* (Procedure 9-3)

*Note: AAMA/CAAHEP 2015 Standards are italicized.*

*(continues on page 212)*

## ABHES Competencies

1. Apply electronic technology
2. Receive, organize, prioritize, and transmit information expediently
3. Locate information and resources for patients and employers
4. Apply computer application skills using a variety of different electronic programs including both practice management software and EMR software

## Key Terms

| | | | |
|---|---|---|---|
| cookies | Ethernet | literary search | virus |
| downloading | Internet | search engine | virtual |
| encryption | intranet | | |

## Case Study

Great Falls Medical Center uses a variety of electronic applications in the administrative and clinical areas of the practice. Colton Smith, CMA, troubleshoots technological problems in the office. He was involved in the selection of the computer hardware and peripherals when the practice purchased the electronic medical record system and is responsible for updating all software, including virus protection, and backing up the computers on the company's networked server. Once a month, he also backs up the entire computer network on a secure cloud storage. What is computer hardware, and how is it different from peripherals? What are computer viruses, and how are they transmitted? Is the practice information safely stored when it is on a cloud? These and other questions are covered in this chapter.

Computers play a major role in keeping the physician office running efficiently and serve many functions in both the clinical and administrative areas. Software applications that primarily run the business of the practice, such as scheduling and medical billing, are known as practice management applications. These applications are crucial for organizing and transmitting large amounts of data. Clinical software, on the other hand, records clinical information about patients' health care encounters and is known as the electronic medical or electronic health record (see Chapter 8). Computers are also used to search the Internet on a variety of health-related topics and connect health care workers to invaluable resources such as other health care facilities, educational materials, and government agencies involved in the delivery of health care. You will need excellent computer skills to work as a medical assistant. This chapter will help you to improve your existing skills. It provides a basic review of computer components. You will learn how the Internet is used in health

care settings and some precautions. Various medical software applications will also be discussed. You will learn about training options and governmental regulations associated with electronic health records.

## THE COMPUTER

A computer system is roughly divided into two areas, hardware and peripherals.

### Hardware

Computer hardware consists of several key elements (Fig. 9-1). Here is a review of their parts:

- *Central processing unit.* The central processing unit (CPU), or microprocessor, is the circuitry imprinted on a silicon chip that processes information. The CPU consists of a variety of

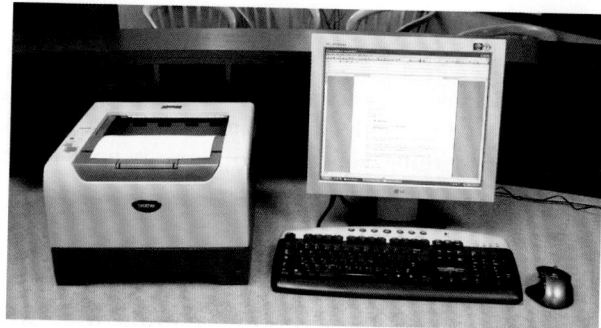

**Figure 9-1** • The computer consists of the CPU, keyboard, monitor, hard drive, printer, and secondary storage systems. Additional peripherals include the mouse, battery backup, and modems.

electronic and magnetic cells. These cells read, analyze, and process data and instruct the computer how to operate a given program. All CPUs function basically the same way, but chips differ dramatically in capabilities and speeds. Your CPU has many ports to connect the printer, mouse, and speakers. At minimum, it has multiple universal serial bus (USB) ports. USB ports allow you to connect to peripherals (see below).

- *Hard drive.* The hard drive provides storage for programs, data, and files. The capacity of a hard drive (i.e., the quantity of program and data it can hold) is measured in binary units and is commonly measured today in gigabytes or terabytes.
- *Secondary storage systems.* All computers have multiple methods for saving data including storage on the computer's hard drive as well as removal flash drives that are inserted in a USB port. When saving any type of data, remember that good organization skills are essential. Name your files appropriately and place files in properly identified folders. Most computers have preset timing systems that automatically save data. Check your default setting and readjust as needed.

## CHECKPOINT QUESTION

1. What do the CPU cells do?

## Peripherals

Computers can have many peripheral connections. Three key computer peripherals that you need to know are

- *Keyboard.* The keyboard is the primary means by which information is entered into the computer. Besides the typical letter and number keys, you will find special function keys that provide increased capabilities. Examples of special function keys are Alt, Ctrl, Insert, and Esc. Each of these keys has a

specific function that is determined by the software program. These functions may include searching for and replacing words, moving blocks of text, indenting or centering text, and spell checking.

- *Monitor.* The monitor, also called a visual display terminal, is often referred to as the computer screen. They come in various sizes and connect to the computer with a cable; however, they are part of the computer system in portable computers such as laptops and notebooks. Most monitors are LCD screens due to their smaller size, the quality of graphics, and their decreasing cost.
- *Mouse.* The mouse can be used to control the cursor on the display screen. Although you cannot type in characters using the mouse, you can move or delete individual characters, words, or entire blocks of text with it. The track ball is an alternative to a mouse. Your finger rotates the ball to move the pointer. It takes less space than does a mouse and is used based on personal preference.
- *Battery backup.* A battery backup allows the computer system to function in the event of a power failure. Batteries come in various sizes depending on the size of your computer and the amount of work to be done during a power failure.
- *Modem.* A modem is a communication device that connects your computer with other computers, including the Internet, online services, and electronic mail systems. Modems may be connected through cable systems or through the telephone. Digital subscriber line (DSL) is similar to a cable system and allows for fast transfer of data. It is the preferred method, but both the cable and DSL connection require your computer to have an **Ethernet** port or an Ethernet interface card before you can connect to an Internet service provider.
- *Printer.* The printer transfers information stored electronically to paper (hard copy). Printers use various technologies, operate at various speeds, and print in either black and white or color. The cost of printers varies depending on the needs of the practice, and printers range from the inexpensive inkjet printers to the more expensive laser printers. They also may be purchased as a combination with other office equipment such as a printer/scanner/fax machine/copier.
- *Scanner.* A scanner allows you to take a picture of a document and read it into the computer. In offices with no paper charts, it may be necessary to scan laboratory reports, radiology reports, discharge summaries, letters, and other paper documents into a patient's medical record. Patient education materials can also be scanned into the computer and then adjusted to meet the needs of your office. Keep in mind that you need to adhere to copyright laws.

- *External storage systems.* The HIPAA Security Rule specifically requires that any electronic protected health information (PHI) be accessible on demand. In this era of electronic health records, it is important to always back up data on a regular basis. External hard drives may be used and, for further safeguards, stored in a location away from the office. An online storage service is another option in which data are stored on a third party's database. This is also known as **cloud storage**.

## CHECKPOINT QUESTION

2. What is an Ethernet, and why should your computer have an Ethernet port or Ethernet interface card?

## Care and Maintenance of the System and Equipment

As with any piece of equipment in the medical office, it is necessary to maintain your computer on a regular basis. Some maintenance agreements require that a service representative clean and inspect the system on a regular basis. Each employee should take the responsibility of taking care of the equipment in an office. A computer and its accessories will last longer and perform better with care and maintenance. Most equipment in a medical office is very expensive. Its accuracy is crucial. Imagine the inefficiency that would be created if a physician's office could not make copies or receive faxes because of equipment failure. Just as the human body performs better with health maintenance, computer hardware and other equipment and machinery perform better when care and maintenance are carried out. A messy desk (Fig. 9-2) can be a disaster for the hardware components of a computer. Procedure 9-1 outlines the general care guidelines for a computer.

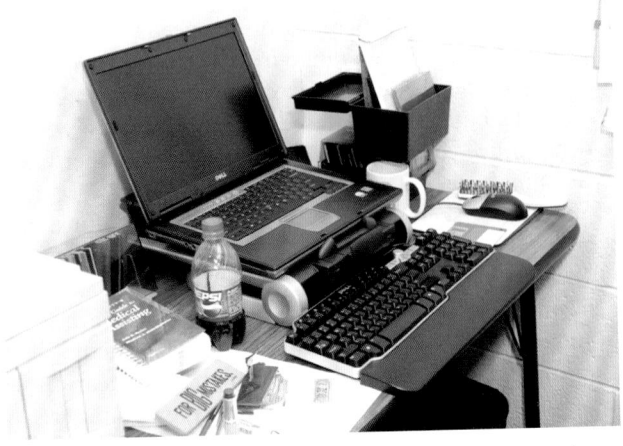

**Figure 9-2 •** A messy desk can be a disaster for the hardware components of a computer.

## INTERNET BASICS

Most physicians' offices can connect to the **Internet**. The Internet is used for both clinical and administrative reasons. The first thing you need to know is how to get your computer connected.

## Getting Started and Connected

The Internet is used for access to the World Wide Web (WWW) and for electronic mail (e-mail). To get connected, you will need an Internet connection company and appropriate Internet software.

There are three ways that your computer can connect to the Internet. One is an Internet service provider (ISP). The ISP is a company that connects your computer's modem to the Internet through the phone line. The slowest and cheapest method is known as a dial-up service. The second option is your cable television company. This system provides a faster connection. The third option is a DSL. This is the fastest connection but is not available in all areas. If you need to download large files through the Internet, you should use either a DSL or cable connection. A different connection or ISP may be needed if you experience problems accessing the Internet due to slow service or connection troubles. Wireless technology is imbedded in most newer computers that allow Internet access to users on a wireless network.

Second, your computer will need a Web browser. A Web browser is software that communicates with your computer and the Internet. There are several browsers available, but two common examples are Internet Explorer and Mozilla Firefox. Most computers are preloaded with a Web browser; however, they may also be downloaded into individual computers at no cost. It is important to always follow your office policies before downloading anything on company computers. Clicking on the Web browser icon makes the actual connection to the Internet. Depending on how your system is set up, you may have to use a password.

## CHECKPOINT QUESTION

3. Which two types of Internet connections are recommended for downloading large files?

## Security of Electronically Shared Personal Health Information

As previously discussed, the federal government regulates the sharing and storage of protected health information. The Health Insurance Portability and Accountability Act of 1996 (HIPAA) legislation mandates that, when a health care provider and health plan transmit and receive PHI ( protected health information) electronically, the transmission must comply with certain standards. There are code sets to identify the physician's specialty, training, and payment policies, the status of a claim, why claims have been denied or adjusted, types of health plans, benefits, patient eligibility, provider organization types, and disability types. This simplification of information exchange ultimately results in increased efficiency and available cash flow.

The HIPAA Security Rule requires covered entities to implement policies and procedures designed to prevent, detect, and contain any breaks in security. The HIPAA Officer in a physician's practice is required to monitor the security of their electronic information by conducting a risk analysis. This analysis includes following the path of each type of transmission or movement of data to look for problems. They also periodically check for security threats or gaps by reviewing audit logs and other security tracking measures.

## Internet Security

If you choose correct sites and follow some general safety tips, the Internet is a safe way to obtain and transfer patient information. Here are a few key points:

- Never send any patient information over the Internet to a site that does not have a secure sockets layer (SSL). This scrambles your information as it leaves your computer and unscrambles it when it arrives at its designated address.
- Look for a lock icon on the status bar.
- Set limits on your Web browser for **cookies**. A cookie is a tiny file from a Web site left on your computer's hard drive without your permission. By examining your cookies, a Web site can learn what sites you

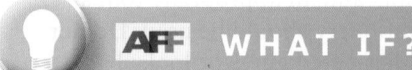 **WHAT IF?**

**Parents ask you how to keep their child safe on the internet. What should you say?**

First and foremost, explain to the parent that direct parental observation is the best method. Encourage parents to have an open and honest discussion with their child regarding the dangers on the Internet. Computers should be kept in living rooms or family rooms. Advise parents not to let children have a computer with Internet access in his or her bedroom. Parents can require a password to be entered for Internet access. This prevents access when the parent is not present. Most Web browser programs let the parent allow access only to "safe" sites. A few sites can add filters or safety nets to a child's computer. These sites are Net Nanny (http://www.netnanny.com), Internet Guard Dog (http://www.mcafee.com/us), and CyberPatrol (http://www.cyberpatrol.com).

have visited, products for which you have been searching, and files that you have downloaded. You may control your computer's cookies by setting limits on your Web browser software. Limit setters can generally be found on your toolbar under Internet options, then under either privacy or security.

## Viruses

**Virus** protection is an important security issue. A virus is a dangerous invader that enters your computer through some source and can destroy your files, software programs, and possibly even the hard drive. A worm is a specific type of virus that affects e-mail. Most computers come with virus protection software. This software will identify and stop harmful transmission. However, virus protection is not 100% guaranteed. Some ways that you can protect your computer are

- Do not open any attachments from unknown or suspicious sites.
- Update your virus protection software regularly. Most virus protection programs offer an updating service. Virus protection updates address new worms, as well.
- Remember, new viruses are detected daily.

## Downloading Information

The Internet is filled with great patient teaching resources and other information. You may decide to copy some of this material into your computer. This is **downloading**. Downloading transfers information from an outside location to your computer's hard drive. Download only files that pertain to work. Do not download screen savers, news releases, recipes, or other personal information. Do not assume that you can photocopy any material that you have downloaded and distribute it. Always ask for permission from the author. Some government and professional medical Web sites state that their material can be freely copied and used. A good example of this is the U.S. Department of Agriculture (USDA) Web site, which allows the food pyramids to be copied and used for teaching.

## Working Offline

It is possible to access Web pages without connecting your computer to the Internet. To do this, save your commonly accessed sites on your Web browser. (If you are unsure how to do this, search your help topics for working offline). Then, to view the pages offline, click on the connection icon, select work offline, and locate your file. Remember, Web pages are regularly updated, and a page that you have saved to view offline may not be the latest version. Periodically view the online site and resave the site.

## 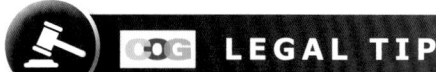 ELECTRONIC MAIL

Electronic mail provides many benefits to the health care system. E-mail promotes good patient care, enhances communication, promotes teamwork, eliminates phone tag, and provides written documentation of messages. Since e-mail messages cannot be guaranteed to provide confidentiality, you must use reasonable measures to ensure compliance with HIPAA's Privacy Rule when handling e-mails from patients. When an e-mail is received from a patient or another sender about a patient, the message should be recorded in the patient record and then deleted from the computer. If you are using a manual or paper chart system, print the e-mail and either enter the information in the record or place the correspondence in the chart. Once the information is recorded in the chart, any paper copies should be shredded. Be sure to document any action taken or reply sent. Issue passwords for those who need access to e-mails from patients.

Here are some general tips for using e-mail:

- Use the office e-mail address only to send work-related messages. Do not send personal messages.
- Do not participate in chain letters.
- Download your e-mail and read it offline unless you are using a DSL or cable connection.
- All e-mail messages should be professional.
- Read your e-mail's **encryption** feature and activate it. Encryption is a process of scrambling messages so that they cannot be read until they reach the recipient.
- Always leave a message on your e-mail system when you will be out of the office for a vacation or other reason. This message is automatically sent to the incoming e-mail senders. This alerts the sender that you will not be reading their message. Include the date when you will be returning to the office and instructions on who they should contact in case of emergencies. This feature is often called the "out-of-office assistant." Following is an example of a good message: "I will be out of the office from 1/20 through 1/28. If this e-mail requires immediate attention, please forward it to Barbara Smith. I will respond to your e-mail when I return."

### 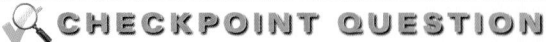 CHECKPOINT QUESTION

4. What does the encryption feature do?

## Access

Access to your e-mail account is through either the Internet or intranet. The intranet is discussed later in the chapter. To access your e-mail, locate the mail icon, double-click it, and then enter appropriate information. A password is generally required. See the Legal Tip for some guidelines for password use.

---

### LEGAL TIP

#### Password Guidelines to Ensure Security

- Establish written policies for the assignment and use of passwords to protect personal health information.
- Make unique passwords (combine letters and numbers).
- Do not use your initials, birth date, or phone number.
- System-wide passwords that allow access to the computer should be changed after an employee leaves the practice.
- Do not share your password with your colleagues.
- Do not tape your password on the computer monitor or leave it on your desk.
- Have additional password verifications for certain secure sites (laboratory reports).

### Composing Messages

When composing a message, follow the guidelines in Chapter 7 for writing business letters. Here are a few additional tips:

- Check your spelling, grammar, and punctuation before sending any messages.
- Keep messages short, concise, and to the point.
- Flag messages of high importance. This will alert the recipient that the message is important and should be read first. Do not overuse this feature. Flag only messages that warrant immediate response or attention. Never send an e-mail about a patient who is having an emergency. Always call or page the physician instead. The following is an example of an inappropriate e-mail: "Ms. Smith's water broke. Do you want her to go the hospital or come into the office?"
- Use appropriate fonts and an appropriate font size.
- Generic or plain stationery should be used. Do not use stationery that has cute figures or looks busy.
- Always complete the subject line. Keep the subject line short and use only a few key words, for example, *Staff meeting tomorrow*.
- It is a good idea to restrict e-mail messages to only one topic.
- Paragraphs are not indented on e-mail messages. Skip a line between paragraphs.
- You can add a permanent signature to all outgoing e-mails. Your signature should include your name, credentials, and phone number with extension.
- Never use text message abbreviations or symbols when sending an e-mail message.

### Address Books

Your e-mail software will allow you to create address books. An address book is a collection of e-mail addresses. Additional information, such as phone numbers, fax numbers, and street addresses, can be added. A few tips regarding address books are

- Keep your addresses up to date.
- Organize your addresses in folders or categories. For example, one folder may contain all the cardiologists in the area, and another may contain just insurance-related addresses.

## Attachments

An attachment is a file that is sent along with an e-mail. You attach a single file (letter) or several documents at one time. Remember these guidelines:

- When you receive an e-mail with an attachment, open the attached file or letter. File it in an appropriate place on your computer. If appropriate, print the attachment and distribute it as needed.
- If you are sending an e-mail and need to attach a file, compose your message first. Then, attach the file by going into the tool bar and locating the menu for file attachments. Click Browse to find the file on your computer, and then click to attach it. It is a good idea before sending the attachment to open it to be sure that you have selected the correct file or version of the document.

## Opening Electronic Mail

Some general guidelines regarding opening an e-mail message follow:

- Open only your own e-mail messages unless otherwise instructed.
- After reading the e-mail, either delete it or place it in a folder. Do not allow multiple e-mails to clog your inbox.
- Always open flagged messages first and respond to them immediately.
- If you receive a message that you cannot address or resolve, forward the message to your supervisor and alert the sender that the message has been forwarded.
- If you start receiving bulk mail, either block the sender or ask to be deleted from that mailing list. This can be accomplished by clicking on "unsubscribe," usually at the end of the message.

### CHECKPOINT QUESTION

5. List three steps to take to ensure the privacy of an e-mail from a patient.

##  MEDICAL APPLICATIONS OF THE INTERNET

Besides e-mail, the Internet offers the World Wide Web, which provides health care professionals with great resources and information. Navigating through the Web quickly and efficiently takes skill and practice. Unorganized surfing can be time consuming and unproductive.

Before surfing for information, you need to remember one important rule: Not all of the information on the Web is accurate or truthful. Anyone can post anything or make any claim. Since the information that you obtain from the Web will affect patient care, all steps must be taken to ensure that only accurate information is found and used. First, look for the logo of a verification program such as the HON (Health on the Net) seal. Verification does not guarantee that the information is correct or truthful but does certify it is a good starting point. Keep in mind that many good sites, for example, government sites, do not have this seal. The Patient Education Box provides some guidelines for selecting safe sites.

### PATIENT EDUCATION

#### Guidelines for Selecting Safe Web Sites

Remember these key points when recommending the Internet to a patient:

- Beware of phrases like breakthrough, medical miracle, and secret formula.
- Avoid sites that advertise that they have cured a disease.
- Use caution when you see the phrase "ancient remedy."
- Use caution when you find a site that will treat a whole list of diseases with the same treatment.
- Do not believe every testimonial that you read.
- If the site claims that the government is hiding information to cure a disease, use extreme caution.
- Use caution when the treatment can "only be bought here."
- If the site suggests that you not tell your doctor about it, stay away.
- See http://www.quackwatch.com.
- You can send complaints to the Federal Trade Commission at http://www.ftc.gov about sites that provide information that is misleading and wrong.
- Do not try to learn lifesaving skills, such as cardio-pulmonary resuscitation, on the Internet. No matter how good the information or site is, you need to take a professional class.

## Search Engines

A **search engine** allows you to find sites that have the information that you need. There are numerous search engines (Google, Yahoo, Lycos, Excite, Dogpile, Bing).

These sites are best used for searching out general information. Once you arrive at the search engine page, you must enter some key words. Your key words should be focused to limit the number of responses or "hits" that you will get. For example, if you type in the key word "heart," you will get thousands of sites that pertain to the heart. Some of these sites will be referring to the heart as an organ, and other sites will address how to mend a broken heart. If you had selected your key words to be "heart attack," however, you would narrow your search tremendously. To further narrow your search, use the advanced search feature. Click on advance search, and use the key words "heart and attack and prevention." By doing this, you will obtain the information you want faster and more efficiently. Unless you are using a medical search engine, avoid using medical terms. For example, use the word lung instead of pulmonary. When you need to find medical information, use a medical search or a megamedical site with links. Procedure 9-2 lists the steps necessary to search the Internet. See the listing of Web sites at the end of this chapter for some good places to start searching for medical information.

 **CHECKPOINT QUESTION**

6. What is a search engine?

## Professional Medical Sites

At the end of the chapters in this book, you see various Web addresses listed that provide you with more information on that chapter's content. These are good starting points for professional topics. But keep in mind that Web addresses change frequently. If you are unable to access a site, try eliminating the letters and symbols after a slash (/). Use the primary site address. For example, suppose you want to enter this site: http://www.fda.gov/cder/drug/consumer/buyonline/guide.htm. If you cannot access that site, try http://www.fda.gov and advance from there. Most sites will link you automatically to a new home page. Also, depending on your Web browser, you may not have to type in www. In this case, you would just type in fda.gov.

The Internet can help you communicate with patients who speak a foreign language. Some Web sites translate phrases and words. Box 9-1 lists sites that physicians are most likely to use. All medical specialties have their own special site. Hospitals have their own sites also. When you start working as a medical assistant, learn the Web addresses of the specialty of your physician. For example, if you work for a neurologist, you will frequently use http://www.aan.com (American Academy of Neurology).

These sites will help you translate between English and Spanish:

- AltaVista—http://www.altavista.com (click on translate)
- Free English to Spanish translations—http://www.freetranslation.com

### BOX 9-1    Sites Physicians Use

Physicians and other health care professionals are likely to use these sites:

**Journal of the American Medical Association**
http://jama.ama-assn.org
**New England Journal of Medicine**
http://www.nejm.org
**The Lancet**
http://www.thelancet.com
**Annals of Internal Medicine**
http://www.annals.org
**American Medical Association**
http://www.ama-assn.org
**The Joint Commission**
http://www.jointcommission.org
**Centers for Disease Control and Prevention**
http://www.cdc.gov
**Clinical trials**
http://www.clinicaltrials.gov

The Centers for Disease Control and Prevention site is also available in Spanish. You can give the following address to patients who want to view the site in Spanish: http://www.cdc.gov/spanish.

## Literary Searches

According to the American Medical Association, approximately 80% of practicing physicians regularly surf the Internet for medical research information. Most research information is found through a **literary search**. A literary search involves finding journal articles that present new facts or data about a given topic. Physicians who specialize in a given area and have conducted a controlled research study write these articles. Various databases can be used to do a literary search:

- OVID will search for articles as far back as 1966. It contains access to more than 4,000 professional journals. Its address is http://gateway.ovid.com.
- PubMed will search for journal articles back to 1966 from the National Library of Medicine.
- CINAHL contains journal articles published since 1982. It has primarily journals for nurses and other allied health care professionals.

Most literary search databases require an annual subscription fee. Once you arrive at the site, you can start to search for the information. First, enter your key words. To narrow the search, you can request journal articles from all countries or limit it to the United States. You can also limit the search by selecting a time line, such as the past 6 months. Once you have done your search, a list of articles will be displayed, and you can highlight the ones you wish to see. You will be asked whether you want to see the whole article or only the abstract. An abstract is a summary of the article. It is always a good idea to print only the abstracts and allow the physician to decide which full articles he or she will want to see. Fees for downloading the complete journal article vary. Abstracts can generally be downloaded free. Your local hospital librarian is often available to assist you with literary searches and may be able to get the article for free. Some libraries will do searches for physicians on staff at no charge. Use this service if it is available.

 **CHECKPOINT QUESTION**

7. How is a literary search different from a search on an Internet Web site?

## Health-Related Calculators

The Web has numerous calculators that can be used for various health care topics:

- Due date calculator—http://www.babycenter.com/pregnancy-due-date-calculator
- Ovulation calculator—http://www.babycenter.com/ovulation-calculator
- Target heart rate—http://www.webmd.com/hw-popup/target-heart-rate-20512
- Body mass index (or BMI)—http://www.cdc.gov/healthyweight/assessing/bmi/index.html

## Insurance-Related Sites

The insurance world can seem like an endless maze of papers and regulations. The Internet can help you sort through and clarify some information. Your first stop should be the patient's insurance company. Its Web address is usually listed on the back of the patient's insurance card. Bookmark these sites. Chapter 13 will get into more details on this issue. Following are a few sites that can also help you and your patients:

- For information on buying health insurance online at the Health Insurance Marketplace: https://www.healthcare.gov/quick-guide
- The Medicare site (http://www.medicare.gov) discusses the basics of Medicare programs, eligibility, enrollment, drug assistance programs, and many frequently asked questions. This site will link you to various other options. You will also find links to report Medicare fraud and abuse.
- Patients who express concern about their health records being red flagged because of an illness (HIV, cancer) can check a database that alerts insurance companies to "red-flagged" patients. This site is http://www.mib.com. There is a fee for using this site.

## Patient Teaching Issues Regarding the Internet

Some of your patients will be very skilled at using the Internet. As discussed in Chapter 4, they can find enormous amounts of information regarding their disease, treatment options, and medications. The guidelines discussed in the Patient Education Box pertain to patients who surf the Internet. You cannot stop or limit the information that patients will search and find. Keep in mind that patients often turn to the Internet when they feel confused or hopeless about their disease or anger about the medical profession. If a patient communicates any such feelings, alert the physician.

Teach patients to acquire reliable medical information and advise them of the dangers on the Web. Some physician offices print brochures with recommended Web addresses. This is a very good education tool for patients. Some areas you should be aware of are discussed in the following sections.

### Buying Medications Online

As the cost of prescription medications soars, patients look for options. It is possible to buy prescription medications over the Internet. A good Internet pharmacy will provide information on what the medication is used for, possible side effects, dosage recommendation, and safety concerns. If patients want to purchase prescriptions online, advise them to use only sites that are certified by the Verified Internet Pharmacy Practice Site (VIPPS). This certification comes from the National Association of Boards of Pharmacy and indicates that the site has been checked and is monitored for safety and quality care. Advise patients to purchase only medications that have been prescribed by the physician. For consumer safety tips, advise patients to use http://www.fda.gov/Drugs/default.htm.

 **CHECKPOINT QUESTION**

8. If you find misleading or erroneous information on a product Web site, who can you notify?

### Financial Assistance for Medications

In 2006, after many years of debate, the federal government provided drug coverage for Medicare beneficiaries. Part D Medicare provides seniors and people with disabilities with a comprehensive prescription drug benefit under the Medicare program. The Patient Protection and Affordable Care Act (ACA) in 2014 began requiring insurance plans available in states' Health Insurance Marketplaces to have essential benefits including prescription drug coverage. However, specific medications to be covered are still determined by individual states. If a patient's coverage does not include a certain prescribed medication, there are many resources available to discount the cost or to completely pay for the medication if necessary. First, you should advise patients to search the drug company's homepage, for example, http://www.pfizer.com/home, to determine if they qualify for the company's patient assistance program. A good source for all pharmaceutical patient assistance programs is located on the site http://www.needymeds.org, which helps patients research and download the correct forms. Another site for patient assistance programs is at http://www.rxhope.com/home.aspx, which is also useful for physicians to find local financial resources for patients. Patients on Medicare will find assistance on http://www.medicare.gov/prescription/home.asp.

### Medical Records

Patients may choose to create their own "medical records" and store personal health information on sites. Patients who travel frequently may opt for this. Microsoft and Google are two companies who offer such a service. Patients can store information about their medications, immunizations, laboratory tests, surgeries, and so on. Remind patients that this information is not secure and could be accessed by unauthorized people. A more secure way to keep this information is to download medical record forms, complete the printed copy, and store them safely.

### Medical Record Forms

The American Health Information and Management Association provides forms online for patients to record their health histories. These are available at http://www.ahima.org. The American College of Emergency Physicians has an emergency consent form (www.acep.org) that parents can sign giving permission for another person to consent to their child to be treated in case of an emergency. This is valuable for parents who travel on business and have their child stay with a relative or friend.

Advance directives and legal forms for medical power of attorney are also available online. Patients should be advised to seek legal counsel and speak to the physician before completing these forms. The federal government has cards available online for patients to complete and carry with them regarding their wishes to be an organ and tissue donor at this Web site: http://www.organdonor.gov.

### Injury Prevention

Injuries are a leading cause of death for children. The American Academy of Pediatrics (http://www.aap.org) has reference materials that can help parents with safety tips. The federal government sites (http://www.cdc.gov and http://www.nih.gov) also have good information that you can direct parents to search. The National Safe Kids Foundation is another excellent resource (http://www.safekids.org). Questions regarding product recalls can be found at http://www.cpsc.gov.

## INTRANET

An **intranet** is a private network of computers that share data. Intranets, sometimes called *internal Webs*, are used in large multiphysician practices. An intranet is more secure than the Internet. The only people with access to an intranet homepage are people with an affiliation to the practice. Access may be limited to those within the offices or may allow for access from home computer systems. The benefits of an intranet are enhanced communication, quick access to needed information, increased productivity, and enhanced security. Common examples of data found on an intranet are

- Policy and procedure manuals
- Marketing information
- Minutes from meetings and upcoming agendas
- Staff schedules
- Local hospital announcements or information
- Commonly used forms
- Internal newsletters
- Internal job postings
- Employee directory
- Videoconference support
- Links to specialty sites

### CHECKPOINT QUESTION
9. What are the benefits of an intranet?

## MEDICAL SOFTWARE APPLICATIONS

The types of medical software applications and their possibilities are endless. Every day, thousands of new software packages are released into the market. Upgrades and new versions of existing packages are also released daily. Each type of software program will have good benefits and will lack some features. The type of software that you will use will vary among different physician offices. The selection of software is based on the size of the practice, number of physicians, specialty, and the affiliated hospital's software. If the hospital software is compatible, interchanging information is relatively easy. Physician and office manager preferences play a role in the software selection. Other factors include how many users can use software at one time, can the software be used with multiple windows open, how often does the company plan to update it, and is the software HIPAA compliant with regard to security and code sets.

Never buy or install a new software program or update an existing version without permission from either the office manager or the physician.

Learning to use a particular software program and navigate quickly and efficiently through its features takes time. Most programs come with a tutorial program. On-site training is often included in the purchase price of major software applications. Training options will be discussed later in the chapter.

Medical software applications can be divided into two main groups: clinical and administrative. Clinical software packages help the physician or health care professional provide the best possible medical care to patients. Administrative software packages focus on tasks to keep the office flowing efficiently and financially strong. Many clinical software applications include practice management software, but if they are different, it may be necessary to purchase an interface to connect them so the two systems can communicate. The next sections introduce you to what types of software capabilities are available and most commonly used. Keep in mind that new technologies are emerging every day.

## Clinical Applications

As discussed in Chapter 8, clinical software is designed to help the physician, medical assistant, or other health care professional provide the most efficient, safest, and most reliable health care available. Here are some examples of the benefits that clinical software programs can bring into the physician's office:

1. Create an electronic medical record also known as a **virtual** patient chart. A virtual chart is a paperless chart in which all documentation is stored on the computer. Some offices create dual charts (virtual and paper), and other offices will keep one or the other.

   The advantages to a virtual charting system are that it saves filing space, increases access to patients' charts for all staff members, eliminates hunting for misplaced charts, and keeps the charts better organized and neater. Since the charting is done through keyboarding, the notes are always readable.

2. Clinical software can maintain an up-to-date list of clinical tasks organized by employee's name. For example, suppose you just discharged a patient and made a note on his chart that you need to check his laboratory tests tomorrow. The task manager would automatically assign this task to your list of duties for tomorrow. Or a physician may discharge a patient and want you to call that patient in the morning for a follow-up. The physician could assign this task to your list. This promotes organization and decreases the potential for tasks to get overlooked or forgotten.

3. The software available for prescription management and drug information is tremendous. The ability

of a prescriber to write and transmit prescriptions electronically is known as **e-prescribing**. This method allows prescriptions to be transmitted directly to a patient's pharmacy. At minimum, the software should enable the physician to find the patient's name in a database, virtually write the prescription, and download it immediately to the patient's pharmacy. Increased patient satisfaction results because this allows the pharmacist to fill the prescription before the patient arrives. Thus, the patient gets the medication much faster. More important, since most prescription filling errors are due to physicians' poor handwriting, this potentially lethal error is prevented. Most medication software packages red flag the physician if the prescription is contraindicated for the patient. Medications can be contraindicated because of a particular disease (e.g., asthma or diabetes), interaction with other medications the patient is taking, or an allergy. For example, assume the physician has written a prescription for Bactrim, which contains a sulfonamide. The software would find in the patient's medical record that the patient is allergic to sulfonamides. The computer would alert the physician, and the physician would select a different medication. Software also allows the physician to save the patient money. Each insurance company and hospital has a formulary of medications that it reimburses. If the physician orders a medication that is on the patient's insurance formulary, the patient saves money. If the physician selects a medication outside the formulary, the insurance company may refuse to pay some or all of the cost of the medication.

4. Computer programs can insert laboratory reports directly into the patient's records. This is more time efficient than faxing or manually recording the results. It also eliminates transcription errors. Most software will alert the physician when a new laboratory report has been received. Laboratory reports of serious or life-threatening findings will still be telephoned to the office.

5. Perhaps one of the greatest technologies is the importing of the actual imaging study into a patient's chart. Some software allows the physician to see the radiograph or computed tomograph from the office. Without this program, the physician gets a typed written report, such as "chest radiograph shows left lower lobe infiltrate." With this technology, the physician can see the radiograph itself and thus make better clinical decisions.

6. Plastic surgeons use a wide variety of image reconstruction programs in their office. This software allows the physician to insert a picture of the patient and contrast it with the expected outcomes of the surgery. This helps patients both to decide whether the surgery is warranted and to develop realistic expectations of the surgery.

7. Many physicians' offices have a special defibrillator called an automated external defibrillator (AED). Once the AED is used on a patient, the information from the machine must be downloaded to the patient's chart for legal documentation. After use, the AED is attached to a desktop computer, and the AED sends the report into the computer and then into the patient's record. If the patient's chart is not on the computer, the data can be printed on paper and placed in a conventional chart.

8. Some programs can help you with telephone triage. Triage is sorting patients according to their need for care. The software allows you to select a caller's topic and displays a list of relevant questions. The software also provides you some instructions for the patient. For example, assume you have a caller with abdominal pain. You type the key words "abdominal pain," and a list of questions appears. These programs log the calls with the date, time, and instructions, which provides legal protection for you.

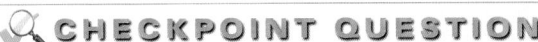

## CHECKPOINT QUESTION

10. What is a virtual chart?

## Administrative Applications

There are hundreds of administrative software packages available for physician offices. Most practice management systems have a combination of features. Some examples of benefits administrative software can bring to the physician's office follow:

1. Appointment making and tracking are more efficient with a computer program than with a book format. As discussed in Chapter 6, good appointment software will allow you to enter appointments quickly and make changes more easily. It should allow for an unlimited comment area near the patient's name. The comment area allows you to add special notes, such as "patient is requesting a pregnancy test." Appointment software can keep a waiting list of patients who are looking for appointments or wanting to move their appointment date and time to the first available time. Appointment software can also automatically print notices to remind patients of the need to make appointments. For example, the program can be set to alert patients who have an annual Pap smear to be sent a letter each year reminding them when it is time for the next one. Some appointment software applications can be integrated with other physicians' offices to allow you to have access to their appointment books. This allows you to see when the next available appointment is. For example, assume your physician makes a referral

for Mr. Kearns to see a dermatologist. You would be able to view the schedule of the dermatologist and see when he could get an appointment and then later see if he went for his appointment. Software programs allow clustering appointments to be made when necessary (see Chapter 6). For example, the patient needs a biopsy that is done with a particular laser machine. The machine is available only on Tuesdays, so the program would automatically set the appointment for the patient on a Tuesday.

2. Software can allow you or the office manager to track patient flows. This can be helpful to adjust staff scheduling needs, with more help at the busiest hours or days and less staff on slower days. It can alert managers to the productivity of staff members. For example, one physician may average 45 minutes per patient, while another may average 30 minutes. This allows you to schedule appointments at various intervals and thus promotes patient flow. It can track the time patients wait in the waiting room or examination room. Examining such information allows the staff to change the office flow to decrease waiting times or to indicate the need for additional staff. It can also highlight the days when patients are most likely to cancel their appointments. Patient demographics can be obtained, used for marketing, and allow the office to apply for special funding based on these demographics.

3. Software programs are needed to send insurance claims electronically. You will be able to send claims and track their progress. This allows for faster reimbursement to the practice and can identify problems of reimbursement earlier. The programs that you will use should have access to numerous plans and can be updated frequently and easily.

4. Software programs can allow integration with insurance companies and other businesses to allow for automatic quick payment and posting. This saves time and is less complicated to use than traditional accounting books.

5. Physicians' offices should have software that allows for credit card authorization. A variety of card types should be available (Visa, MasterCard, American Express).

6. Insurance software can allow you to check for patient eligibility. Most programs have enough room for the addresses and phone numbers of the primary, secondary, and tertiary providers. Case manager names should be added when available. Software can also allow for preadmission certifications to be completed and electronically submitted. Preadmission or preauthorization allows you and the patient to verify that the insurance company will cover the procedure or admission. Some software programs come with codes (ICD-9 and ICD-10, CPT, HCPCS) preinstalled.

7. Again, programs must aim to comply with HIPAA's Privacy Rule; these programs allow you to document your adherence to these rules and regulations.

8. Other programs alert you to send collection letters. These programs have a variety of template collection letters. Always double-check the information before sending a collection letter. More information on how to collect past due accounts is discussed in Chapter 13.

9. A variety of financial software programs track accounts receivable and accounts payable. You may need to adjust the billing cycles to meet the needs of the office in which you are working. Software programs can also automate the tickler system (see Chapter 10).

10. Automated payroll software can automatically calculate tax deductions and other deductions. You will be able to arrange for direct deposit of employee checks through these software programs.

11. You will find transcription systems in most physicians' offices. These programs help you transcribe various medical reports quickly and effectively.

12. A medical office cannot run effectively without a word processing system. These systems help you write letters and other types of documentation.

13. An important part of any administrative software is the section that handles the personnel records. Contracts, disciplinary reports, performance evaluations, and so on can all be stored in a virtual personnel record.

## CHECKPOINT QUESTION

11. What items may be included in a virtual personnel record?

## ADOPTING ELECTRONIC HEALTH RECORDS TECHNOLOGY

The *Meaningful Use* incentive by the Centers for Medicare and Medicaid Services (CMS) requires eligible providers and hospitals to use EHRr products that have been certified in order to receive funding under the American Recovery and Reinvestment Act (ARRA). One of the ARRA provisions is the HITECH Act that was established to encourage and reward eligible providers to use computers for collecting, maintaining, and storing patient data (see Chapter 8). Providers must use EHR software that meets the standards established by the Certification Commission for Health Information Technology (CCHIT). CCHIT is an independent, nonprofit organization that certifies ambulatory electronic health record

(EHR) products as well as other health care information technology products. In 2006, CCHIT was named a "Recognized Certification Body" by the U.S. Department of Health and Human Services. (For more information and a list of certified products, visit http://www.cchit.org.)

Issues concerning health care reform are discussed further in Chapter 10.

Changing from a paper-based office environment to one using advanced technology takes time, money, careful decision making, and staff education, among other factors. One of the first steps in the process involves choosing a vendor. Again, the Medicare and Medicaid Incentive programs require that vendors be certified, and their products must meet stringent criteria. Below are some examples of criteria to consider (in addition to CCHIT certification) when purchasing EHR products:

- The vendor's reputation and history (check references or speak with current customers)
- The vendor's understanding of how your medical office plans to use the EHR including the requirements for incentive payments under the *Meaningful Use* provisions of the HITECH Act (see Chapter 8)
- The product's use of customizable technology
- Easy access to product support
- Regular product maintenance and updates
- Ability to automate office workflow
- Ease of training and implementation
- Ability to send and receive electronic data to and from other health care entities, such as laboratories or hospitals
- Security of patient information

## Making the Transition

Besides computer workstations, printers, and Internet access, the amount and kind of equipment required for EHR depends on the medical office's needs and budget. Other commonly used devices may include laptops and tablet computers, which allow greater physician mobility and require less space in exam rooms than do desktop computers. Whatever equipment setup is ultimately chosen, it should not physically impede the physician–patient relationship. For example, avoid setups in which the physician must turn his or her back to patients when inputting information, which might make the physician appear detached or uninterested.

Changeover to EHR usually occurs in stages. To avoid problems, the medical office should not eliminate paper charts until the EHR system is consistently working as intended. Integration of paper charts and other records can be accomplished in various ways, depending on office goals and the amount of data to be input. Some facilities keep hybrid records; personnel scan and index medical records into the system and then store paper copies in the office for a few months before destroying them.

Other facilities transfer old paper records to microfiche or another permanent record storage system then destroy the paper sources. Off-site medical record storage facilities can house the records until time of disposal or indefinitely, whatever the physician wants. Keep in mind that implementing EHR will not eliminate the need to maintain paper documents right away. It can take months or years to fully complete the transition.

To work productively with EHR, medical assistants need training and practice. Graduating from an accredited medical assisting program, which includes training in coding, billing, and computer skills, ensures baseline preparation. Adequate education about the specific EHR system used by the medical office is also required. Medical assistants and other office staff usually undergo 1 to 2 days of initial training; after that, daily practice with EHR in the medical office allows users to get comfortable with the system. Workflow will be set by the facility according to their policies and procedures for EHR. One key point to remember is that when implementing new technology, everyone must be willing to change. Staff may need to adjust some processes so that EHR can work effectively for the office.

## PURCHASING A COMPUTER

Purchasing a new office computer system or updating an existing one is a very important business decision. All key members of the staff should be consulted prior to such a purchase and should be actively involved in selecting the hardware and software. Here are some general guidelines to follow when shopping for a computer and software:

- Determine your specific needs. For example, do you need both clinical and administrative applications? If you have separate practice management and electronic health record software, it may be necessary to purchase an interface.
- Visit physicians' offices and clinics to see what other medical office staff are using. Ask questions: How user-friendly are the programs? How long did it take to educate the staff? What does the staff like and dislike about the programs?
- Try out many software packages. Most have online demonstrations or disks that can be used to evaluate the system.
- Interview and compare different computer vendors.

  Find out:

  1. If the company and its products are certified by the federal government
  2. How long they have been in service
  3. How many service representatives they have and whether they are available 24 hours a day

4. Specifics of the system
5. Specifics of any service and warranty contracts they provide
6. What training they provide and at what additional cost
7. How to transfer data into the new system
8. How much the system costs
9. Whether the software can be customized and at what cost
10. What is their response time for service or technical support calls
11. Whether their programs are HIPAA compliant

Independent computer consultants can be hired to evaluate your particular office and make specific recommendations. This option is often more expensive initially but can save money in the long run.

## TRAINING OPTIONS

To achieve the optimal benefit from any computer or software package, you must be trained in its use. There are a number of ways that this can be accomplished:

- The company from which the computer was purchased may provide personnel to train you and other staff members.
- A user manual will come with your system. You can refer to it when you have problems.
- Help screens installed with every software package allow the user to self-teach. The disadvantage of this method is that it is often time consuming.
- Most software packages come with a tutorial. This is an on-screen short course on the use of the software. Many also offer online tutorials that can be viewed from any computer with Internet service.
- Most computer manufacturers and software programs will have a service called a help desk, which provides technical support. It is usually accessed by calling a toll-free number and is manned by computer professionals who can answer your questions concerning the system.

A combination of these methods is the best approach to learning about your computer and software.

## CELL PHONES AND TEXTING

In the past, medical office personnel depended on telephone answering services to communicate with physicians. The use of cellular telephones has made wireless communication an optimal way to contact providers. You can send a text message to providers right in the office or when they are out of the office. Again, you must always keep in mind that confidentiality is an issue. Consider the following guidelines when creating a text message:

1. Refrain from using identifying information such as patients' names or medical record numbers.
2. Keep communications businesslike. For example, avoid abbreviations such as "lol" (laugh out loud).
3. Keep communications brief and to the point. For example, "please call office ASAP" or "you are needed in ICU."

With the advances in technology and more federal regulations, possibilities for electronic communication are bound to emerge and change. A good rule of thumb is to keep all communications professional and always remember to protect your patient's privacy.

## AFF COG COMPUTER ETHICS

The computer is a must in all physicians' offices. Its capabilities are endless. It can, however, lead to invasion of patients' privacy and unethical behavior. Some key points to keep in mind are

- Never give out your login password. New employees must be issued their own passwords.
- Never leave a screen open with patient information and walk away from the computer. Lock or exit the file.
- Only key people need access to sensitive patient information. Some programs, such as those with laboratory results, should have individual passwords.
- Physicians can often access patient data (e.g., radiology and laboratory reports) from the hospital computers. The hospital gives the physician a special code. It is not appropriate for the physician to share this with staff members. Never use another person's password to get patient information unless instructed to do so by a supervisor. You should be given your own code by the administrator of the program.
- Do not use the office Internet access for anything other than work-related tasks. It is inappropriate to surf the Internet for personal reasons while at work.
- E-mails should be read only by the person to whom they were sent. To avoid conflicts, the physician should have his or her own e-mail account, and the practice should have a generic e-mail address. It is never appropriate for you to receive personal e-mail messages on the office's e-mail address. It is also inappropriate to access your personal e-mail while at work.

- Sensitive patient data should not be sent via e-mail from one office to the other unless it is clearly known that the recipient of the e-mail is the only one with access to it. It is a common practice to send patient information to the consulting physician. This information may include cancer diagnosis, HIV testing, and drug abuse reports. Extreme caution must be used.
- If you are allowed access to local laboratories to obtain laboratory results, it is to be used only on patients in your practice. It is unethical and illegal to obtain other people's reports. For example, if your son had a throat culture done at the pediatrician's office and sent to the laboratory you have access to, you should not look up his results.
- Do not take advantage of your position in the medical field. Remember, you have a legal and ethical responsibility to protect patient information.

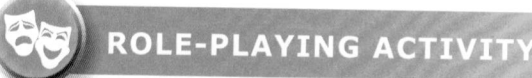

## CHECKPOINT QUESTION

12. What is a tutorial?

## ROLE-PLAYING ACTIVITY

Carla, a part-time staff member at Great Falls Medical Center, asked Colton Smith, CMA, to open the EHR so she could see a patient's private information. Carla is unable to access the practice management system and said she had noticed her neighbor waiting in the reception area earlier today. Carla also said that she had heard at the last neighborhood barbeque that the patient was having serious personal financial problems, had recently lost her job, and was separated from her husband. How should Colton respond? Based on what you know, is there any information that Colton can share with the staff member? What information should he use to support his decision? In this activity, role-play the MA who is being asked to share a patient's private information with a staff member. Consider the potential problems with releasing this information as you think about how to respond. If you are playing the role of the staff member, think about how you could persuade the MA to allow you to see the patient's private information. How would you justify your request? Your instructor will give you additional information about this activity!

## español SPANISH TERMINOLOGY

**Asegúrese de buscar los iconos en el sitio de web para asegurarse de su credibilidad.**
Be sure you look for the icons on a Web site to ensure its credibility.

**Tenga cautela al comprar medicamentos en el Internet.**
Be careful if you buy medications online.

**Nuestro sistema computarizado es seguro y privado.**
Our computer system is secure and private.

**Su medicina será enviada a la farmacia por el Sistema e-receta.**
Your medication will be sent to the pharmacy by e-prescription.

**La información médica que necesita está en un sitio de Internet seguro y profesional que se llama_____.**
The medical information that you need is in a safe and professional Web site named_____.

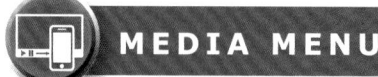

## MEDIA MENU

**Student Resources** on thePoint®

• **CMA/RMA Certification Exam Review**

**Internet Resources**
**Occupational Safety and Health Administration**
**Safety and Health Topics: Ergonomics**
http://www.osha.gov/SLTC/ergonomics/index.html

**Typing Injuries Frequently Asked Questions**
http://www.tifaq.com

**U.S. Department of Health and Human Services**
http://www.healthfinder.gov

**Medline Plus**
http://www.nlm.nih.gov/medlineplus

**HealthCentral**
http://www.healthcentral.com

**WebMD**
http://www.webmd.com

**Mayo Clinic**
http://www.mayoclinic.com

**FamilyDoctor**
http://familydoctor.org/online/famdocen/home.html

**Rare Disease Search Engine**
http://www.raredisease.org (this site has a database of over 1,000 rare diseases and over 900 drugs that can be used to treat rare diseases)

## EMR Activity

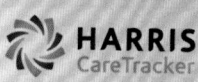

Harris CareTracker is a Web-based electronic medical record (EMR) application that you will use for the EMR activities included in this section at the end of each chapter. This application is actually used in physician offices, but is provided to you through the publisher, Wolters Kluwer Health, to give you hands-on practice working with EMRs. Your instructor will have more information about accessing your username, login, and Quickstart guide.

Prerequisite Activities in Harris CareTracker

• *The Getting Started and Quickstart documents and EMR Activities Step-by-Step Instructions are available at* http://thePoint.lww.com/KronenbergerComp5e

Activity Details

An information packet from a new patient, Connie Meyers, was received in the mail today at Great Falls Medical Center (GFMC) and Colton Smith, CMA, is responsible for entering it into the practice management system. GFMC uses an electronic medical record (EMR) that has a practice management application. Enter Ms. Meyers' demographics information given in the *EMR Activities Step-by-Step Instructions* into the EMR.

## Chapter Summary

- Computers are an essential piece of technology in the medical office.
- As a medical assistant, you will use the computer for both clinical and administrative tasks. Computers will help you perform your job more efficiently, timely, and professionally.
- You will take precautions to comply with HIPAA's Administrative Simplification, Security, and Privacy Rules.
- Computers promote good patient care.
- You will be able to communicate with various health care professionals by using electronic mail.
- The Internet plays a key role in medicine.
- Patients, physicians, and medical assistants use the Internet to find new medical cures and for seeking current information about various health topics.
- You will need to be able to navigate the Web quickly and safely.
- It is essential that you stay abreast of computer technology, as it changes and improves daily.

## Warm-Ups for Critical Thinking

1. Log on to the Internet and locate a search engine. Search for a medical topic. It can be administrative or clinical. What are your key words? How many sites are listed? Now, using the same key words, use the advanced search engine. How many sites are listed? What are the benefits of using the advanced search method?
2. Select any five Web addresses listed in this chapter, and view the homepage. What benefits do the sites offer? What information or topics were missing?
3. Review the Patient Education Box about selecting Web sites safely. Find three Web sites that use these types of phrases or words. Do you think these sites are misleading? Do you think they pose a danger to patients?
4. Your office manager asks you to serve on a committee to purchase an electronic medical record system. Formulate a list of questions that you can ask a vendor before buying a computer system.
5. List five Web addresses for a patient who has just been diagnosed with type 2 diabetes.

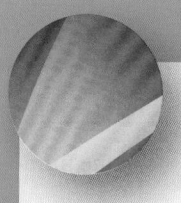

**PSY** PROCEDURE 9-1

## Caring for and Maintaining Computer Hardware

**PSY** Perform routine maintenance of administrative or clinical equipment

**Purpose:** To prolong the life of computer hardware by following certain guidelines and performing preventative maintenance

**Equipment:** Computer CPU, monitor, keyboard, mouse, printer, duster, simulated warranties

| STEPS | REASONS |
|-------|---------|
| 1. Place the monitor, keyboard, and printer in a cool, dry area out of direct sunlight. | Sunlight can damage casings, and heat and cold are also harmful to hardware. |
| 2. Place the computer desk on an antistatic floor mat or carpet. | Static electricity can cause memory loss, inaccurate data collection, and other adverse reactions. |
| 3. Clean the monitor screen with antistatic wipes. | Glass cleaner is not recommended. |
| 4. Use dust covers for the keyboard and the monitor when they are not in use. | Dust can accumulate and cause the keyboard and mouse to stick and malfunction. |
| 5. When moving the computer, lock the hard drive. | This will protect the CPU and disk drives. |
| 6. Keep keyboard and mouse free of debris and liquids. Dust and/or vacuum the keyboard periodically to eliminate dust particles under the key pads. | Dust and debris can be hazardous to the keyboard and cause the keys to stick, etc. Never eat or drink when using the computer. |

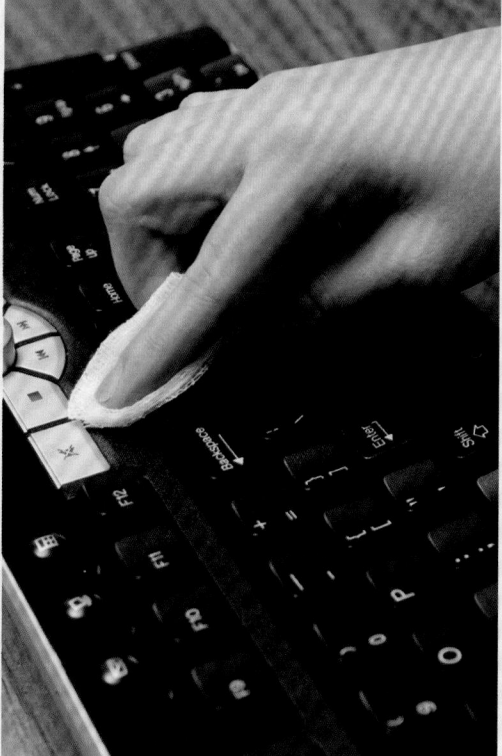

**Step 6:** Keep the keyboard free of dust and debris.

*(continues on page 230)*

## PROCEDURE 9-1 (continued)

| STEPS | REASONS |
|---|---|
| 7. Create a file for maintenance and warranty contracts for the computer system. | This will allow quick and easy retrieval of phone numbers, etc. if a representative is needed. |
| 8. Handle data storage disks and flash drives with special care. | Scratches, fingerprints, etc., can corrupt data. |
| 9. **AFF** If you were the office manager, explain how you would respond to an employee who continued to spill soft drinks on her keyboard. | Prohibit eating and drinking at employee work stations. A break room should be available for eating and drinking. |

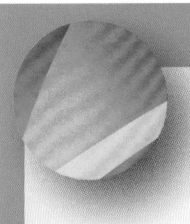

**PSY** PROCEDURE 9-2

## Searching on the Internet

**PSY** Use Internet to access information related to the medical office

**Purpose:** To quickly and effectively search the Internet, resulting in good time management

**Equipment:** Computer with Web browser software, modem, and active Internet connection account

| STEPS | PURPOSE |
|---|---|
| 1. Connect your computer to the Internet. | An Internet connection is necessary to search the Internet. |
| 2. Locate a search engine. | A search engine is necessary to find information on the Internet. |
| 3. Select two or three key words and type them at the appropriate place on the Web page. | Key words tell the search engine what to look for. |
| 4. View the number of search results. If no sites were found, check spelling and retype or choose new key words. | The search engine was unable to find sites that can provide the information you requested. |
| 5. If the search produced a long list, do an advanced search and refine your key words. | Reading through numerous sites is not time efficient. |
| 6. Select an appropriate site and open its home page. | This allows you to view the information on the Web site. |
| 7. If you are satisfied with the site's information, either download the material or bookmark the page. If you are unsatisfied with its information, either visit a site listed on the results page or return to the search engine. | Downloading or bookmarking the information gives you access to it in the future. |
| 8. **AFF** You sit down to use your office computer to search for information with a patient when a coworker's Facebook page pops up. You are embarrassed at the unprofessionalism this displays in front of the patient. Explain how you would respond in this situation. | Speak to the coworker in person about personal use of the office computers. Refer her to the computer use policy of the office. If this does not make an impact, you could tell the office manager. |

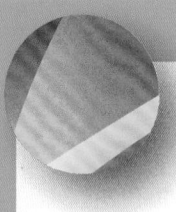

### **PSY** PROCEDURE 9-3

## Entering Patient Demographics into a Practice Management System

**PSY** Input data utilizing a practice management system

**Purpose:** To accurately transfer a new patient's demographic information into a practice management system

**Equipment:** Computer, a completed patient demographics form, and a practice management system such as Caretracker

| STEPS | PURPOSE |
|---|---|
| 1. Open the practice management application and verify that the patient is not already in the system. | Prevents duplication of patients. This could cause problems with reimbursement or patient care if more than one record is in the system for a patient. |
| 2. Open the "patient" module and enter all of the patient's personal information on the "demographics" tab including emergency contact information. | Accurately transfer the information on the patient demographics form to the electronic format. Note: Chart numbers are generated automatically by the software. |
| 3. Enter the insurance/subscriber information for the primary insurance. | Accurate information is necessary to bill the patient's insurance company for services rendered. |
| 4. Enter the patient's employer information, if available. | This may be left blank if unavailable. |
| 5. Click on "save." | Stores information on the patient database for future retrieval |
| 6. Verify if correct information has been entered from the patient information form. | Accuracy is ensured for future reference and for billing purposes. |
| 7. **AFF** While entering the patient's demographic information, you are interrupted by the physician and walk away from your computer. What choices could you have made to protect the patient's private information? | Always lock your computer any time you leave your desk to prevent unauthorized users from entering data. Leaving an unlocked computer is a security violation that puts the entire electronic health record in jeopardy of being compromised. Immediately reset your password. |

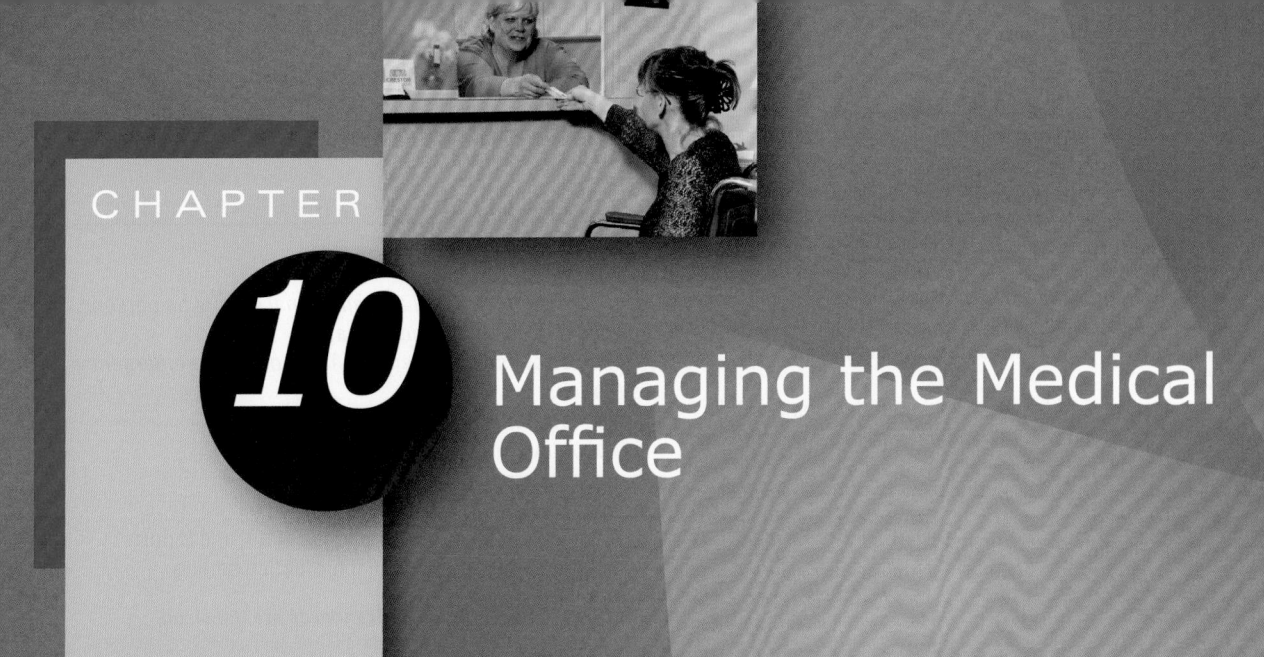

# CHAPTER 10

# Managing the Medical Office

## Outline

**Overview of Medical Office Management**
Organizational Structure
The Medical Office Manager
**Responsibilities of the Medical Office Manager**
Communication
Staffing Issues
Policy and Procedures Manuals
Developing Promotional Materials
Financial Concerns
Office Maintenance
Management of Inventory and Supplies
Education

**Risk Management**
Waste Management
Liability Insurance
Reporting Occupational Injuries and Illnesses
**Regulatory Agencies**
Centers for Medicare and Medicaid Services
Occupational Safety and Health Administration
The Joint Commission
The National Committee on Quality Assurance

**Developing a Quality Improvement Program**
Seven Steps for a Successful Program
**Safety in the Medical Office**
Body Mechanics
Ergonomics
Evaluating the Medical Office for Safety Issues
Fire Safety in the Medical Office
**Medical Office Emergencies**
Emergency Medical Kit
Evacuation Plan for the Physician Office

## Learning Outcomes

### COG Cognitive Domain*

1. Spell and define the key terms
2. Describe what is meant by organizational structure
3. List seven responsibilities of the medical office manager
4. Explain the five staffing issues that a medical office manager will be responsible for handling
5. List the types of policies and procedures that should be included in a medical office's policy and procedures manual
6. List five types of promotional materials that a medical office may distribute
7. Discuss financial concerns that the medical office manager must be capable of addressing
8. Describe the duties regarding office maintenance, inventory, and service contracts
9. Discuss the need for continuing education
10. Describe liability, professional, personal injury, and third-party insurance

11. List three services provided by most medical malpractice companies
12. List six guidelines for completing incident reports
13. List four regulatory agencies that require medical offices to have quality improvement programs
14. Describe the accreditation process of The Joint Commission
15. Describe the steps to developing a quality improvement program
16. Identify safety techniques that can be used to prevent accidents and maintain a safe work environment
17. *Describe the purpose of Safety Data Sheets (SDS) in a health care setting*
18. *Discuss fire safety issues in an ambulatory health care environment.*
19. Explain the evacuation plan for a physician's office
20. Discuss requirements for disposing of hazardous material
21. *Identify principles of:*
    a. *Body mechanics*
    b. *Ergonomics*

*(continues on page 234)*

22. List and discuss legal and illegal applicant interview questions
23. Discuss all levels of governmental legislation and regulation as they apply to medical assisting practice
24. Apply local, state, and federal health care legislation and regulation appropriate to the medical assisting practice setting
25. Describe the process in compliance reporting:
    a. Unsafe activities
    b. Errors in patient care
    c. Conflicts of interest
    d. Incident reports

### PSY Psychomotor Domain*

1. Create a policy and procedures manual (Procedure 10-1)
2. *Perform an inventory with documentation (Procedure 10-2)*
3. *Report relevant information concisely and accurately (Procedures 10-3 and 10-4)*
4. *Evaluate the work environment to identify unsafe working conditions (Procedure 10-3)*
5. *Complete an incident report related to an error in patient care (Procedure 10-4)*
6. Apply local, state, and federal health care legislation and regulation appropriate to the medical assisting practice setting (Procedure 10-3)

### AFF Affective Domain*

1. *Recognize the physical and emotional effects on persons involved in an emergency situation*
2. *Demonstrate self-awareness in responding to emergency situations*
3. *Demonstrate:*
    a. *Empathy*
    b. *Active listening*
    c. *Nonverbal communication*
4. Recognize the importance of local, state, and federal legislation and regulation in the practice setting

*Note: AAMA/CAAHEP 2015 Standards are italicized.*

### ABHES Competencies

1. Perform routine maintenance of administrative and clinical equipment
2. Maintain inventory, equipment, and supplies
3. Maintain medical facility
4. Serve as liaison between the physician and others
5. Interview effectively
6. Comprehend the current employment outlook for the medical assistant
7. Understand the importance of maintaining liability coverage once employed in the industry
8. Perform risk management procedures
9. Comply with federal, state, and local health laws and regulations

## Key Terms

| | | | |
|---|---|---|---|
| body mechanics | expected threshold | mission statement | procedure |
| budget | incident reports | organizational chart | quality improvement |
| compliance officer | job description | policy | task force |
| ergonomics | | | |

## Case Study

*B*en Larson, RMA, is the medical office manager for Great Falls Medical Practice and has much responsibility in this position. He is the primary contact for hiring clinical and administrative staff and is responsible for handling office emergencies. He is also responsible for inventory control and ordering all office and medical supplies. What questions may Ben ask when interviewing perspective applicants when hiring for the medical practice? What kinds of medical emergencies may be encountered in the medical office, and what form(s) will Ben need to have completed in the event of an accident in the office? What is inventory control, and how will Ben accomplish this task? This chapter covers some of the important duties involved with managing a medical office and the responsibilities associated with the office manager.

A successful and safe medical practice needs an effective medical office management process. This process must be a team effort among the physicians, medical assistants, and the office manager. A medical practice must manage risk and engage in ongoing quality improvement procedures. It is important that medical office personnel recognize unsafe conditions, understand fire safety issues, and guide patients and staff calmly in the event of an evacuation of the medical office. This chapter provides an overview of medical office management, a medical office manager's specific responsibilities, as well as a discussion of risk management and quality improvement.

## OVERVIEW OF MEDICAL OFFICE MANAGEMENT

Each medical office is organized in a slightly different manner, depending on the size and complexity of the setting. It has been said that change is the only constant in our lives, and the health care arena is no exception. Federal, state, and local laws must be followed, and ignorance of the law is not a defense when noncompliance results in a lawsuit. There are also governmental and private regulations for medical offices to follow. For example, in an attempt to reform the complexity of the US health care system, the provisions and programs arising from the Patient Protection and Affordable Care Act (ACA) must be explored and understood by medical office management in order to meet the needs of the patients served by the providers.

## Organizational Structure

The medical office's organizational structure, or chain of command, is depicted in an **organizational chart**, a flow sheet that allows the manager and employees to identify their team members and to see where they fit into the team. Figure 10-1 displays a sample organizational chart for a physician's office in which there is a partnership between two physicians. In this example, it is assumed that the physicians have an equal partnership in the practice.

### CHECKPOINT QUESTION

1. What is the purpose of an organizational chart?

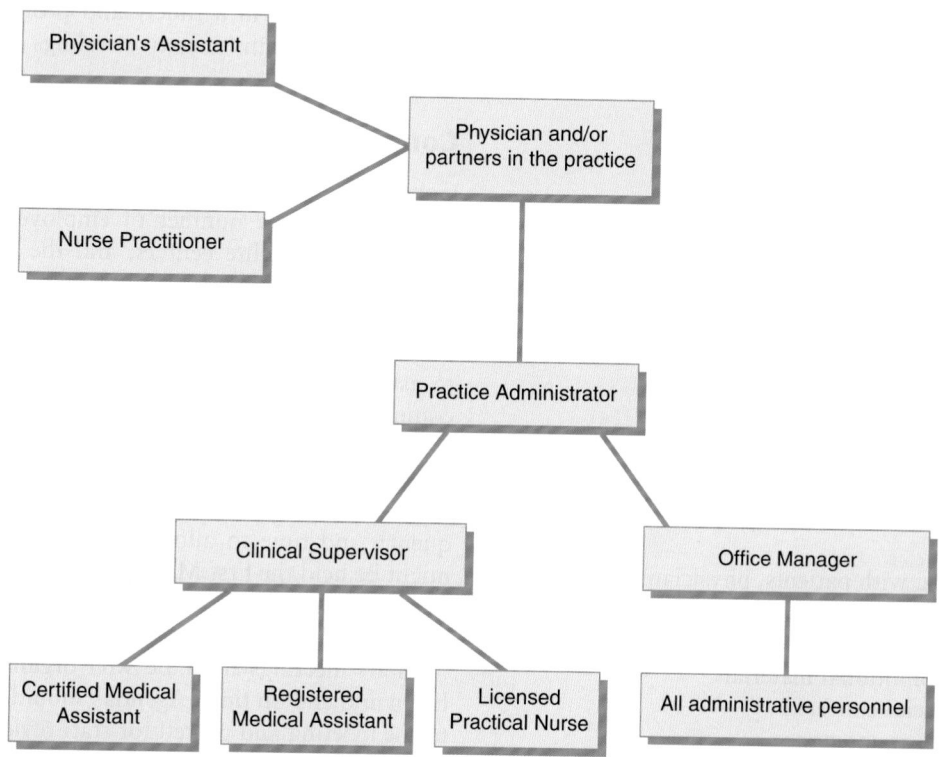

**Figure 10-1** • Sample organizational chart.

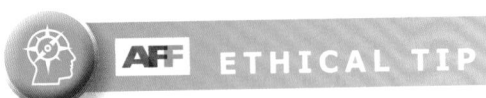

## Tough Spot

Consider this scenario: A coworker tells you that a newly hired employee says she is a certified medical assistant (CMA), but you have a mutual friend who says this person never passed the exam. Should you share this information with anyone? *Yes.* This would constitute fraud. Unfortunately, some people are dishonest and unethical. It would be unethical for you to ignore the information. Tell the office manager who can then verify the employee's stated credentials by calling the appropriate certification registry. You can check the validity of any license or certification by contacting the licensing agency or professional organization that awards the credential. A CMA's status can be obtained by calling 1-800-ACT-AAMA. Many state medical assisting societies also have certification registries. Try going to the particular profession's Web site.

## The Medical Office Manager

The medical office manager must be multiskilled, multitalented, and able to prioritize a variety of issues, juggle responsibilities, and communicate effectively with patients, staff, and physicians. In some settings, the medical office manager may be referred to as the business manager. Managers may be clinical or administrative support personnel. Although the qualifications and educational requirements for the position vary greatly among health care organizations, a successful medical office manager must be

- Flexible
- A positive role model for employees
- Honest and fair
- A good communicator
- A resource person for employees
- Supportive of all management decisions
- Well organized
- Able to focus on a given task
- Able to resolve conflicts
- Able to see the big picture
- A lifelong learner

A medical office manager's responsibilities include varied tasks:

- Communicating with patients, physicians, and staff
- Handling staffing issues
- Writing and revising policy and procedures manuals
- Developing promotional materials
- Handling financial concerns
- Handling office maintenance
- Managing supplies and inventory
- Ensuring that the staff receives appropriate education

- Maintaining budgets
- Enforcing HIPAA regulations and other accrediting agency regulations

A medical office manager also must keep abreast of important legal issues, such as medical practice acts, employment and safety laws, patient care laws, billing and insurance regulations, and more. See Chapter 2 for more details on these topics.

## RESPONSIBILITIES OF THE MEDICAL OFFICE MANAGER

### Communication

Perhaps one of the hardest and yet most important aspects of being an effective manager is being able to communicate with fellow employees, colleagues, physicians, and patients. (The techniques for effective communication are discussed in Chapter 3.) You must be a good listener, have good interpersonal skills, and be aware of your own nonverbal language.

### Communicating with Patients

Communication with patients on a management level can often be challenging. Patients come to you with a variety of complaints, such as incorrect billing, poor care, or long waits to see physicians. Of course, you must always be diplomatic. Your goal should be to correct the problem in a timely and professional manner and to alleviate any negative feelings the patient may have.

### Communicating with Staff

Communication with staff members can be difficult, depending on the number of employees, number and locations of satellite centers, and the variety of shifts that are in place. There are three ways to promote communication with staff members: staff meetings, bulletin boards, and communication notebooks. It is a good idea to ask your staff for input in deciding the best way to communicate with them.

#### Staff Meetings

Staff meetings should be scheduled at a predictable frequency and time to allow the staff to plan (e.g., they might be held the first Monday of every month at 8 AM). *Meetings should never be canceled except in a true emergency.*

Staff meetings must be well organized and should begin and end on time. Agendas should be created prior to the meeting and posted for staff review. (See Chapter 7 for information on agendas.) The agenda should be followed as closely as possible. Individual staff concerns or complaints should not be handled during a general

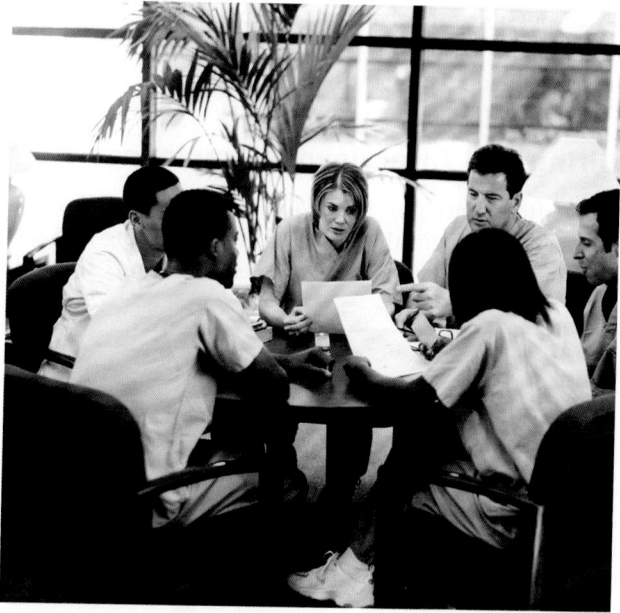

**Figure 10-2** • Staff meeting being conducted in a private area.

staff meeting; the meeting should remain focused and constructive and not turn into a battleground for staff disagreements. Minutes should be taken and distributed to staff or kept in a notebook for staff to review as needed. (See Chapter 7 for information on minutes.)

Staff meetings should be conducted in a private area out of patients' sight and hearing (Fig. 10-2). All interruptions, except for emergencies, should be avoided.

Have the telephone covered by an answering service or a prerecorded message informing callers of the time the staff will be unavailable. Lock the door, and place a sign with the time the office will reopen. Of course, you will give clear instructions to callers or visitors who have an emergency. The personnel manual should clearly state the attendance policy for staff meetings. In addition, some offices include attendance as a duty in each employee's **job description** (statement of work-related responsibilities). To improve attendance at staff meetings, consider serving food or including an educational presentation. Involve staff as much as possible when setting the meeting agenda.

## Bulletin Boards

Bulletin board postings allow employees to get a quick and easy look at new policies or procedures. To encourage staff members to read the postings, make sure the bulletin boards are attractive, well organized, and updated regularly. It is a good idea to have employees initial all messages on the bulletin board after reading them.

## Communication Notebooks

A simple notebook can serve as a two-way communication tool: You can write messages to employees, and they can write back to you. Such a notebook is usually

kept in the staff lounge. Again, staff members should initial any important messages after reading them. If the message is directed to you, be sure to respond as soon as possible. One medical office places a notebook with pertinent information for employees in staff restrooms and titles it "Potty Training."

### Communicating Electronically

E-mail has become popular and is an easy and time-saving way to communicate with staff. Messages can be printed and kept in a binder for easy reference. E-mail messages eliminate the need for memos that must be posted or circulated. Your e-mail system will provide you with an address book that can be customized to include groups such as all employees, all clinical employees, employees and physicians, and so on.

Sometimes, the stress of daily duties prevents managers from communicating with staff members on a personal level. To be an effective manager, you should communicate not only bad news but also positive messages to your employees. You can communicate positive messages through birthday and holiday cards and employee recognition awards. Send thank you notes to the staff to compliment them when they go above and beyond the call of duty. Genuine, positive communication is also effective in maintaining good morale among the staff that leads to less absenteeism and higher productivity.

 **CHECKPOINT QUESTION**

2. What are three ways to promote communication with staff members?

## Staffing Issues

Staffing issues will occupy most of your time as an office manager. These concerns include writing job descriptions, hiring new employees, evaluating present employees, taking disciplinary actions, handling terminations, and scheduling. Sometimes, an office manager also becomes a coach and a counselor.

## Writing Job Descriptions

Each job must have a description. The purpose of a job description is to inform the employee about the essential job duties and expectations for a given position. Job descriptions also help you in interviewing applicants and evaluating existing employees.

Each employee should receive a copy of his or her job description at the time of hiring and after any revisions to the description are made. Some medical offices have a policy requiring the employee to read and sign the job description at the time of hiring and for each annual evaluation. An accurate job description is also essential when questions or concerns arise regarding the scope of practice for employees. Medical assistants must never perform any task, clinical or administrative, that they do not feel comfortable or without proper training.

Formats for writing job descriptions vary among offices. In general, the following elements are included: job title, supervisor, position summary, hours, location, employment requirements, physical requirements, duties, and the evaluation process (Fig. 10-3). The description should also include the date it was written and date of any revisions.

If possible, involve staff members in writing and revising their job descriptions. Employee participation leads to greater cooperation.

## Hiring and Interviewing Employees

Only after creating or reviewing an existing job description can you begin the process of interviewing and hiring a new employee. You can seek applicants through

---

### Job Description

**Title:** Medical Assistant

**Supervisor(s):** Clinical Supervisor
Office Manager for Administrative Duties

**Position summary:** This is a 40-hour position that will require the employee to perform various duties including administrative, clinical, and laboratory procedures. Scheduling will be variable to meet the needs of the office.

**Hours:** Hours will vary to meet the needs of the office. Hours will rotate from 8:00 AM to 4:30 PM and 10:00 AM to 6:30 PM. You will be expected to work one Saturday per month.

**Location:** Our main office is located at 129 South Main Street. The satellite office is located at 56 West Road, Suite 102. This position will primarily require you to work at our main office. However, occasional days may be assigned at the satellite office.

**Employment Requirements:** The employee must have graduated from a Medical Assisting Program. CMA or RMA is preferred. The employee must have a current CPR and First Aid card. One year of experience or completion of an externship is preferred.

• *Language skills:* The employee must be able to read and interpret documents and respond appropriately (verbally and/or in writing). Must be able to document in a professional manner.

• *Mathematical skills:* The employee must be able to add, subtract, multiply, and divide whole numbers and fractions.

**Physical requirements:** The following are physical requirements for this job: Standing: 6–8 hours/day; Sitting: 6–8 hours/day; Lifting: 50 pounds; Twisting and rotating: 45 degrees; Squatting: As needed to assist patients or to perform office tasks.

**Duties:** You will be expected to perform the following duties after completing the orientation process. This is a partial list; and other duties can be added as necessary.

**Administrative:**
Scheduling appointments
Transcribing documents
Filing
Completing insurance forms

Processing mail
Operating the telephone
Providing patient education

**Clinical/Laboratory:**
Operating centrifuge
Performing phlebotomy
Performing HCT/HGB/CBC
Performing pregnancy and monospot tests
Obtaining visual acuities

Obtaining vital signs
Administering vaccines and other medications
  as ordered
Providing patient education
Assisting the physician as directed

**Evaluation process:** Three evaluations will be conducted in the first year. 30 days from start date, 90 days from start date, and then at the 1-year anniversary date. Following the first year of employment, annual evaluations will be done.

I have read my job description, and I understand what is expected of me. I am able to physically perform all the required duties.

Signature of Employee: _____    Date: _____

Signature of Supervisor: _____    Date: _____

Signature of Supervisor: _____    Date: _____

**Figure 10-3 •** Sample job description.

online employment Web sites, advertising in local newspaper classified sections, career placement personnel at local schools that offer medical assisting programs, networking, and local employment agencies.

All applicants should complete an application. State laws vary regarding the types of questions that can be asked on applications. In general, you must avoid any questions pertaining to an applicant's age, sex, race, national origin, religion, and physical or mental disabilities. If your medical facility requires a criminal background check and drug testing, the form should include this information with a place for the applicant to give necessary permission with a signature. Any employee application form should be reviewed by legal counsel prior to its use. It is always a good idea to request that the applicant bring a résumé to the interview.

Before interviewing an applicant, prepare a list of questions. Again, use caution; under law, you are not permitted to ask about some topics. Ask only questions that are job related. Ask questions like, "Tell me about a time when you disagreed with your supervisor. How did you handle it?" This type of "behavioral interviewing" will give the interviewer the most information about the candidate's job knowledge and behavior. During the interview, assess the applicant's ability to do the following:

• Perform technical skills
• Treat patients in a caring manner
• Fit into your organization
• Communicate in a professional yet friendly manner
• Remain flexible

Be consistent and fair when selecting the best candidate.

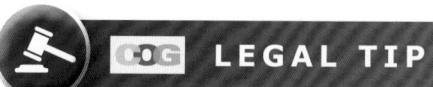

## LEGAL TIP

### Make Sure Your Interview Questions are Appropriate

Title VII of the Civil Rights Act prohibits discrimination in the workplace. To ensure that hiring practices are fair and nondiscriminatory, be careful and consistent in the types of questions asked in an interview. You may ask work-related questions like, "Are you proficient in typing?" Avoid questions that might give the appearance of discrimination. You may not ask applicants their age, race, religion, or marital status. You cannot ask about children, day care, or plans for future children.

## Evaluating Employees

All employees must be evaluated annually. The evaluation should be a positive experience for the employee. Employee evaluations must be fair, accurate, and objective.

Some type of written evaluation should be given to the employee to read, sign, and comment on. Most forms ask employees to list their objectives and goals for the coming year. Figure 10-4 displays a sample evaluation form. Some organizations call evaluations performance appraisals.

New employees should be evaluated 1 month after their start date, again in 90 days, and then at their 1-year anniversary date. This process helps new employees gain confidence and improve weaknesses. Coaching and counseling should occur throughout the year. The employee should know what will be said during the feedback because the manager has communicated with them throughout the year. An employee should never be surprised by the feedback.

## Taking Disciplinary Action

Most offices have policies regarding documentation of disciplinary action. Disciplinary actions can be verbal or written. Verbal warnings are generally done for a first-time minor occurrence (e.g., not showing up for work and not calling in). A note should go into the employee's file stating that a verbal warning was given, the date, any actions that were taken, and any comments that the employee made.

Written notices are used for more serious problems (e.g., breaching patient confidentiality, substance abuse) or recurrent minor ones. Employees should sign any written warning notices. These documents can be used as evidence in the event that the person is fired and brings a lawsuit for wrongful discharge. Figure 10-5 shows a sample written disciplinary action form. Determine whether the employee's credentialing agency should be notified of serious infractions.

## Terminating Employees

Having to terminate (fire) an employee is never an easy or pleasant task. It is essential that policies regarding termination be followed precisely. All disciplinary actions must be clearly and objectively stated and documented. Terminating employees for unlawful reasons or failing to follow the organization's termination policy can result in lawsuits against you and the office. When disciplining an employee, make sure to ask yourself if other employees have committed the same policy violations. Have they all been treated the same? Some reasons for termination include the following:

• Excessive tardiness or absenteeism
• Inappropriate dress or behavior
• Alcohol or drug use
• Endangering patients
• Lying or stealing
• Falsifying medical records or time sheets
• Breaching patient confidentiality

**Employee Evaluation Form**

Employee: _Jackie England_
Evaluation Date: _5/2/13_
Job Title: _CMA_
Ratings:

| Traits | Score |
|---|---|
| Appearance | 5 |
| Communication Skills | 3 |
| Attendance | 4 |
| Quality of work | 5 |
| Reliability | 4 |
| Initiative | 4 |
| Other: _Willingness to work as a team_ | 5 |
| Total Score: | 30 |

Rating scale:
5—Excellent
4—Above average
3—Meets job expectations
2—Below job expectations
1—Does not meet job expectations
Supervisor comments:
_Is an excellent CMA. She is shy with patients + co-workers, but improving._

Employee goals for the next year (to be completed by employee):
_I will continue to attain CEU's for recertification. I plan to take class on being assertive._

Employee Comments:
_I love working here and appreciate having good + fair bosses._

Supervisor Signature: _Diane Hall_          Date: _5/2/13_
Employee Signature: _Jackie England_        Date: _5/2/13_

**Figure 10-4** • Sample employee evaluation form.

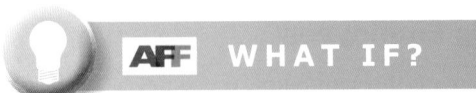 **WHAT IF?**

**You receive a call requesting a reference for an employee who was fired. What should you say?**

Be careful! This situation can turn into a legal and ethical nightmare if not handled appropriately. If you give a wonderful report to the potential employer and say, "She was great; we never had any problems," you and the office may be sued by the former employee for wrongful discharge. In court, you would be asked, "If she was so wonderful, why did you fire her?" On the other hand, if you say, "She was a terrible employee, and we fired her," you can be sued for defamation of character. Because of the legal concerns in providing employment references, most organizations have a policy stating that the only information to be released is verification of employment dates and job titles. When in doubt, give no information. Ask for the caller's name and phone number, discuss the issue with the physician in charge, and then return the phone call.

## Scheduling

The primary goal of scheduling is to meet the needs of the office. The secondary goal is to meet the requests of your employees. You must be fair in scheduling and always follow your organization's policies for weekend and holiday or personal day requests. If possible, employees should be given time off with pay when attending seminars and meetings of their professional organization. This practice will keep morale high and encourage employees to stay current with their skills. Depending on the number of employees that you have to schedule and the complexity of the hours or shifts, you can either schedule by hand or use a computer program. If your organization is small and cohesive, you may want to assign a senior staff member to do the scheduling, or you might allow the employees to self-schedule. No matter what scheduling format is used, you are ultimately responsible for ensuring that the appropriate number and type of employees needed are scheduled.

**Discipline Record**

Employee Name: _Brenda Elliott_      #: _26_      Date of Warning: _5/28/13_

**Warning**

Date of Violation: _5/28/13_      Time: _9:15 AM_  Place: _Exam Room 1_

Description of Violation:

_Brenda was assisting Dr. Baymor in surgery. She took no action when the sterile field was compromised. The possibly contaminated field was not reset. She told no one. It was questioned by the patient._

_____ Verbal Warning
_____ Written Warning
__✔___ Probation __30__ Days
_____ Suspension _____ Days
_____ Termination
_Dana Hudson, CMA_
Supervisor's Signature

Action To Be Taken:
_Brenda is placed on probation for 30 days. Another occurrence will mean possible dismissal._

Date

**Employee's Remarks**

Do you agree with the details above:      Yes: _✔_      No: _____

Comments: _I understand the seriousness of my error. It will never happen again._

Employee's Signature: _Brenda Elliott_           Date: _5/28/13_

**Figure 10-5 •** Sample disciplinary action form.

Requests for time off should be put in writing. Depending on the size of the organization, such requests may have to be received by a given date or time according to office policies. For example, the policy may read, "A request for a day off in May should be submitted by April 15. Any requests for time off filed after the cutoff date will be approved whenever possible." This eliminates repeated adjustment of the staffing schedule.

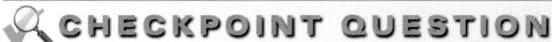

## CHECKPOINT QUESTION

3. What is the medical office manager's primary goal in scheduling?

## Policy and Procedures Manuals

Every business needs written rules and regulations to ensure that its practices are within legal and ethical boundaries. Employees need written procedures to ensure consistency in the practices of the business. In the outpatient medical facility, these written policies and procedures are *required* by regulatory and accrediting agencies.

It is the office manager's responsibility to coordinate the orientation and training of any new employee. A personnel manual that includes the organization's policies and outlines step-by-step procedures for each task performed in the facility becomes the new employee's information source. Even veteran employees may have to refer to the proper procedure for a task. As new procedures become available or existing procedures are changed, this is added to the procedures manual. Tips regarding policy and procedures manual are detailed in Box 10-1.

Most organizations create a policy and procedures manual that is written, maintained, and regarded as one document. A **policy** is a statement regarding the organization's rules on a given topic. A **procedure** is a series of steps required to perform a given task. Policies and procedures must be written in a clear, concise, and understandable format. Each policy or procedure is signed by the employees, indicating they have read, understand, and will adhere to the policy or procedure. Policies regarding medical office management are signed by the physician and supervisory staff.

### Types of Policies and Procedures

There are many types of policies and procedures. In general, the following areas are included in a policy and procedures manual:

1. Mission statement
2. Organizational structure

## BOX 10-1    Tips Regarding Personnel Manuals

- Form a personnel committee. If staff members help develop the policies and procedures, they are more likely to follow them.
- Determine the rules and regulations of the office with the physician and managers.
- Contact local organizations, medical offices, or ambulatory care centers and ask for copies of their personnel manuals including policies and procedures.
- Research state and federal laws that regulate the medical office.
- Ensure compliance by appointing a **compliance officer**.
- Keep personnel manuals in a central location so they are available to each employee for review.
- Review all policies and procedures annually to make sure they are up-to-date and accurate.

3. Human resources or personnel
4. Quality improvement and risk management
5. Clinical procedures
6. Administrative procedures
7. Infection control
8. Safety measures
9. Emergency preparedness

### Section 1: Mission Statement

A **mission statement** describes the goals of the practice and whom it serves. Often, a mission statement provides a philosophical look at an organization. It is generally one to two paragraphs long that is created and/or approved by the physician(s) or owner(s) of the practice (Fig. 10-6).

The mission statement should not only be included in the policy and procedures manual; it should also be available to patients. Often, it is framed and placed in the waiting room or printed in the practice brochure.

North Shore Family Practice is a group practice dedicated to providing quality care through compassion, innovation, performance, and education. It is our goal to provide medical care to the community of Rochester, New York. The physicians, nurse practitioners, and all staff members are committed to working together as a team to provide the patient with the best care possible.

**Figure 10-6** • Sample mission statement.

### Section 2: Organizational Structure

The organizational chart is included in this section along with policies regarding the following:

- Chain of command
- How and when to contact various members of the team
- Coverage for managers
- Physician on-call policies

### Section 3: Human Resources or Personnel

This section consists of policies relating to staff responsibilities, benefits, and rules and regulations for employees. Box 10-2 lists the kinds of policies found in this section of the manual. A sample human resources policy is displayed in Figure 10-7.

### Section 4: Quality Improvement and Risk Management

This section includes policies outlining who is in charge of **quality improvement**, the steps for developing a quality improvement plan, and explanations of incident reporting, discussed later.

## BOX 10-2    Types of Human Resource Policies

Absentee policies
Cafeteria plans
Confidentiality policy
Continuing education requirements
Disciplinary action procedures
Emergency procedures
Employee benefits (health and dental insurance)
Evaluation and performance appraisals
Grievance procedures
Grooming, uniforms, appearance
Holiday coverage and compensation for holidays
Jury duty
Office hours
Orientation
Overtime reports
Parking
Payroll
Personal phone calls
Resignations
Sexual harassment
Sick leave and family leave
Staff meetings
Tardiness
Termination process
Time recording
Vacation days

**Benjamin William, MD**
**2295 Matthews Drive**
**Boca Raton, Florida 33432**
**POLICY AND PROCEDURE MANUAL**

**Policy title:** Human Resources, Absences
**Purpose:** The purpose of this policy is to advise all employees of the policy for absences and to prewarn employees regarding the disciplinary steps that will be taken as a result of not complying with this policy.
**Equipment/Forms necessary:** No equipment or forms are required.
**Explanation:**

- If you are going to call in sick, you must call in two hours prior to your assigned time. Messages should be left with the answering service if the office is not open.
- If you have personal days accrued, you can use them for compensation.
- If you are going to be out sick for more than three consecutive working days, you will need to obtain a physician's note to document the illness.
- Employees are allowed six (6) absences per year without disciplinary action. Seven (7) absences will result in a verbal warning regarding attendance. Eight (8) absences will result in a written warning. Nine (9) absences will result in termination. Exceptions to disciplinary action will be reviewed on an individual basis and are at the joint discretion of the office manager and physician.

_____                          _____
Susan Rogers, RMA                                Benjamin William, MD
Office Manager

_Date: original policy - 06/96, revised 01/00, 02/03, 02/06, 02/10, 02/13_
_HR: 14_

**Figure 10-7 •** Sample human resources policy.

## Section 5: Clinical Procedures

Any task that requires intervention with a patient should be listed in this section. (Some offices separate laboratory procedures into a different section for convenience.) In addition, clinical procedures should include specific infection control guidelines for the particular procedure, patient education guidelines, and instructions for documentation. Sample documentation forms should be included in this section. It is a good idea to complete the sample form correctly so that it can serve as a model. In the medical office, these procedures may vary slightly to meet the needs of the office, physicians' requests, or manufacturers' guidelines.

## Section 6: Administrative Procedures

This section includes procedures on all tasks that the administrative office staff must perform. Sample forms should also be included and updated as necessary. Examples of administrative tasks are as follows:

- Accounting and bookkeeping
- Appointment scheduling
- Collections
- Computer care and operations
- Insurance filings
- Medical records management
- Mail and postal machine operations

## Section 7: Infection Control

Depending on the length of this section, some offices opt for a separate manual dedicated to infection control and prevention. Examples of these policies are as follows:

- Types of personal protection equipment available
- Biohazardous waste disposal
- Handling of various disease identities
- Handling of employee exposures and needlesticks
- Documentation required by the Occupational Safety and Health Administration (OSHA)
- Employee education for infection control

## Section 8: Emergency Preparedness

Most offices have a separate binder for handling emergencies and disasters. The information in this binder should be reviewed annually by all employees in order to prepare everyone with assisting patients, coworkers, and the community, if necessary, during a disaster (see Chapter 27 for specific instructions on emergency preparedness).

### CHECKPOINT QUESTION

4. Which seven elements must be included when writing a policy or procedure?

## Developing Promotional Materials

The medical office manager is often responsible for developing and distributing promotional literature for the practice. Depending on the budget, promotional materials can be created and produced at commercial printing shops or done in the office with desktop publishing programs. Examples of promotional materials follow:

• Education pamphlets and booklets for patients. Be sure to use educational information that has been accredited or approved by an appropriate authority (Fig. 10-8).
• Practice brochures (Box 10-3)
• Practice Web site
• Newsletters (printed and/or online)
• Holiday cards
• Birthday cards (usually used by pediatricians)
• Newspaper articles
• Yellow pages
• Direct mail
• Business cards

Follow these guidelines when creating promotional materials:

• Double-check all spelling and grammar.
• Ensure accuracy.
• Use clear and specific language.
• Avoid abbreviations and complex medical terms.
• Use brightly colored materials.
• If you are using a commercial printer, be sure to review the proofs carefully before the final printing.

---

### BOX 10-3    Information to be Included in an Office Brochure

A well-written, attractive informational brochure will help the office run efficiently and reduce patient questions and confusion. Having this important information in one handy place will not only help patients but also provide confidence that you are giving all patients complete and consistent information.

A patient information brochure should include the following information:

• Name and address of practice with directions.
• Office hours.
• Providers' names, credentials, and specialties.
• Physician's assistants, nurse practitioners, counselors, etc., and their credentials.
• Services provided.
• Payment policies, insurance claim filing information, and major third-party payers accepted.
• Phone numbers and extensions for all departments, including emergency numbers.
• Procedures for reaching providers after hours.
• A statement about how the office handles phone calls, medication refills, triage, etc.
• Be sure to update information as changes occur.
• If space allows, you may include all employee names and positions, short biographies of the physicians, etc.

---

## Financial Concerns

### Budgets

A **budget** is a financial planning tool that helps an organization estimate its anticipated expenditures and revenues. Budgeting has many purposes for an organization:

• Forcing the manager and physician to plan
• Causing managers and staff to become cost conscious
• Promoting communication among staff and managers
• Helping the organization achieve a financial goal

The medical office generally has both an operating and a capital budget. Operating budgets consist of all costs to run the office. These include but are not limited to payroll, office and medical supplies, education, promotional materials, electricity, telephone services, etc. Capital budgets consist of large outlays of money. These include large purchases (usually over $500), building maintenance, property management, and equipment.

Developing and writing a budget takes practice and instructions from the financial officer, accountant, or physician. In general, the previous year's expense report is reviewed, revenues are projected for the following year, and figures are assigned to ensure that income balances with the outgoing expenses.

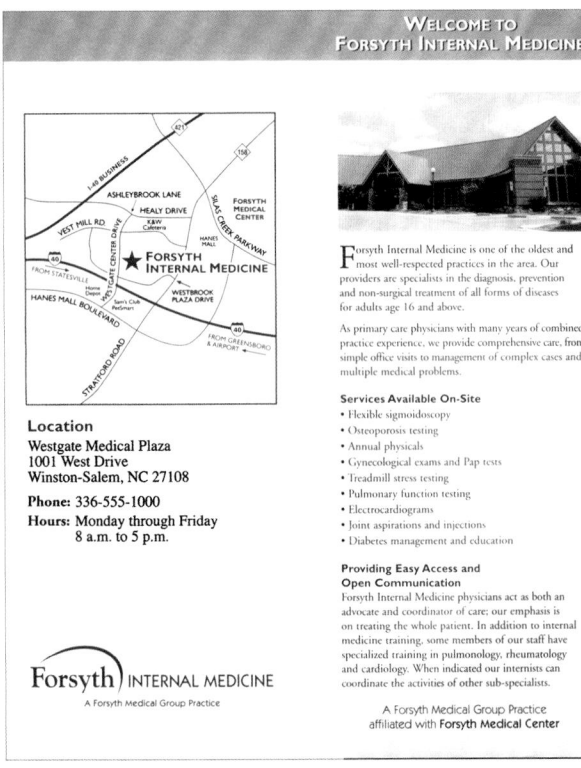

**Figure 10-8** • Sample patient brochure.

5. What is the definition of a budget?

## Payroll

Another financial concern for the manager is payroll. All employees expect to receive the correct amount of pay on time, and those expectations must be met. Payroll is a complex task that must satisfy state and federal laws regarding deductions for Social Security and other withholding taxes. Timely and accurate reporting and payment of taxes that have been withheld from employees' pay is necessary to prevent late fees and fines by federal, state, and local governments. Because of this and because payroll is so time consuming, some offices outsource this service.

## Office Maintenance

One of the medical office manager's key responsibilities is to keep the office neat, clean, safe, efficient, and well organized. Most offices have outside agencies to clean and maintain the lobby, examination rooms, and offices, to do laundry and landscaping, to manage heating and air conditioning, etc. OSHA requires that you use a licensed vender for biohazardous waste disposal. Office manager duties include managing and scheduling these service vendors. These services would be considered accounts payable, which is covered in Chapter 14.

A well-lit, attractive entrance and waiting area reflect quality throughout the facility. Staff should be encouraged to check the lobby periodically for neatness and to assist in routine cleaning and straightening. Remember, special attention to waiting room toys is necessary because they can pose a safety threat to children (see Chapter 5).

## Management of Inventory and Supplies

Extensive supplies, including clinical and office equipment, are necessary for running an efficient medical office that meets the needs of its patients. Ordering and receiving supplies is an important part of the office manager's job that may be delegated to another staff member; however, there should be a policy outlining who is responsible for ordering supplies and the procedure for ordering. There also must be some process to track orders and check that deliveries of supplies are complete and accurate. Most medical management software has a feature for keeping up with supplies, but when using a manual system, a tickler file can be used. A tickler file system has a file divider for every month as well as dividers for the days of the month (1 through 31) that are placed behind each monthly divider. As a medical office manager, you must develop a logical system to keep track of supplies. A manual reminder system can be used to organize vendor information, supply lists, reorder information, etc. Many computer systems have inventory control and accounts payable capabilities. A spreadsheet can easily be constructed to save information about vendors, dates supplies were ordered, etc. Ordering supplies and accounts payable are covered more thoroughly in Chapter 14.

Although it is best if the person who orders supplies also receives them, other office staff members who receive the supplies must check the packing slip against the actual contents to ensure that all supplies are in the shipment. The person should initial the packing slip, which shows that all goods were received. When it is time to issue checks for payables, the administrative medical assistant responsible for paying bills can then pay the invoice or bill with confidence that all of the items ordered were received. These receipts or packing slips should be placed in a bills pending file for payment.

## Service Contracts

The medical office manager is responsible for keeping track of all service contracts. A service contract is an agreement between the medical organization and a service company in which the company agrees to perform regular inspections of and care for a specific piece of equipment. Service contracts are usually obtained for copiers, computers, fax machines, and other large and expensive pieces of equipment.

## Education

### Staff Education

The medical office manager must keep the staff up-to-date on medical procedures, drugs and vaccines, insurance coding and billing regulations, and any other topics that promote good patient care. In addition to these topics, annual education is usually conducted on cardiopulmonary resuscitation (CPR), infection control, and fire and electrical safety. Most allied health professionals are required to accumulate continuing education units (CEUs). CMAs must receive 60 CEUs every 5 years to retain the CMA credential. The office manager may choose to keep a file for each employee with the necessary documentation. This will assist the staff in the recertification process.

As the medical office manager, you should select an educational topic for each month. In some offices, the educational topic is covered during the monthly staff meetings, whereas other offices have separate educational programs. After choosing the monthly topic, select an appropriate presenter. Suggestions for presenters include colleagues, physicians, sales representatives, local hospital staff development coordinators, and specialists. Presenters for CPR classes must be CPR instructors who are approved by a national organization.

To promote attendance, create informative flyers and distribute them to all staff members. Keep attendance records for all classes given.

In addition to formal educational programs, there are other ways to keep your staff up-to-date. For instance, educational videos and DVDs can be rented or purchased for staff viewing; consider developing a posttest to assess for comprehension. Also, many professional magazines have continuing education articles on various topics, usually accompanied by a posttest. Finally, staff members should be sent to one or two seminars a year. Outside seminars help increase employee productivity, self-esteem, and retention.

## PATIENT EDUCATION

All members of the health care team must constantly contribute to educating patients. As a manager, you may not provide patient education directly, but you are responsible for assisting the staff in performing this task. You can help the staff with patient education by creating booklets, developing posters, and teaching your staff how, when, and what to teach patients and families.

Patient education brochures should be colorful and easy to read. Close attention to spelling, grammar, punctuation, and accuracy is essential. All patient educational material should be reviewed by a physician. Depending on your office's clientele, the brochures should be printed in various languages. Refer to Chapter 4 for more details on creating patient education brochures.

### Manager Education

Managers should attend workshops and conferences and read appropriate printed materials to enhance their knowledge and skills in managing a medical office. All new managers can benefit from courses on time management, stress management, solving personnel conflicts, and budget preparation. Memberships in professional organizations can also assist the new office manager. Two such organizations are

Medical Office Management Association, 1355 South Colorado Boulevard, Suite 900, Denver, CO 80222-3331

Professional Association of Health Care Office Management, 2929 Langley Avenue, Suite 102, Pensacola, FL 32504-7355

## RISK MANAGEMENT

Risk management is an internal process geared to identifying potential problems before they cause injury to patients or employees. Potential problems are related to risk factors. A risk factor is any situation or condition that poses a safety or liability concern for a given practice. Examples of risk factors are poor lighting, clutter, unlocked medication cabinets, failure to dispose of needles properly, and faulty patient identification procedures. Such factors may lead to patient falls, medication errors, employee needlesticks, and mistakes in therapeutic intervention. Risk factors for a particular health care organization are identified through a study of patterns. As discussed later, by tracking information obtained in incident reports, risks can be identified and managed. For example, tracking of incident reports might identify particular days of the week when most negative events happen. If most events occur on Friday afternoons, perhaps staffing on Friday afternoons should be reevaluated.

## Waste Management

The medical office generates waste described as regular trash or biohazardous waste, and office managers are responsible for making sure that policies are in place for handling both types. Office managers will have to contract certain vendors for weekly trash removal service in addition to a company to regularly remove and dispose of biohazardous waste such as used needles in a sharps container. Compliance with OSHA regulations for proper handling and disposal of biohazardous waste is mandatory (see below), so office managers must understand existing requirements as well as new regulations as they develop. The removal and disposal of biohazardous waste is very expensive, so the staff should be advised and periodically reminded of what is acceptable as biohazard waste (see Chapter 5 for more information on biohazard waste).

## Liability Insurance

Doctors today face challenges that those of a generation ago never imagined. As discussed in Chapter 2, physicians are at risk for malpractice suits and must use sound practices to decrease this risk. New medical procedures, treatments, and drugs require regular review to ensure each practice meets high standards of safety and care. Physicians need malpractice insurance to protect them from financial loss in the event of a successful lawsuit or settlement. Clinical staff may also be covered under the physicians' malpractice insurance; however, many allied health professionals are now opting for their own coverage as well.

Many malpractice insurance companies offer services such as teaching employees to take preventative measures and to identify problems before they become threats. They also conduct risk inspections, supply self-auditing tools, and provide bulletins. Malpractice insurance Web sites have many helpful tools for office managers.

A medical office is not just subject to liability regarding patients; since it is a public place, any visitor to the office could slip and fall on a wet floor or be hurt by a picture falling from a wall. As office manager, you should periodically review the liability insurance policy and assess the coverage needs including the needs of the employees.

## CHECKPOINT QUESTION

6. Why do physicians need malpractice insurance?

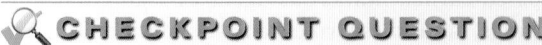

## LEGAL TIP

### Reporting Occupational Injuries and Illnesses

Medical and dental offices are currently exempt from maintaining an official log of reportable injuries and illnesses under the federal OSHA recordkeeping rule; however, some states may require such records. You should be familiar with the laws in the state where you work and comply with any laws as necessary. All employers, including medical and dental offices, must report any work-related fatality or the hospitalization of three or more employees in a single incident to the nearest OSHA office.

## Reporting Occupational Injuries and Illnesses

### Incident Reports

**Incident reports,** sometimes referred to as occurrence reports, are written accounts of negative patient, visitor, or staff events. Such events may be minor or life or limb threatening. The insurance company that provides the institution's liability insurance often requires incident reports.

An incident report is written or completed by the staff member involved in or at the scene of the incident on a preprinted form and is usually given to the office manager or the physician. They may also be sent to a central location in a larger medical practice. Depending on the type of event and organizational policy, a physician may or may not document the event on the incident report. If an unusual event happens to a patient, however, the physician should assess the patient and document the findings on the incident report. Figure 10-9 is a sample incident report.

### When to Complete an Incident Report

Even in the safest settings, undesirable things can happen to anyone. These events sometimes result from human error (e.g., giving the wrong medication), or they may be idiopathic. Idiopathic means that something occurred for unknown reasons and was unavoidable (e.g., an allergic reaction). Incident reports must be completed even if no injury resulted from an event. A few examples of situations requiring an incident report are

**Figure 10-9 •** Sample incident report.

- All medication errors
- All patient, visitor, and employee falls
- Drawing blood from a wrong patient
- Mislabeling of blood tubes or specimens
- Incorrect surgical instrument counts following surgery
- Employee needlesticks
- Workers' compensation injuries

The rule of thumb is when in doubt, always complete an incident report.

### Information Included in an Incident Report

Although every practice has its own form, the following data are always included in an incident report:

- Name, address, and phone number of the injured party
- Date of birth and sex of the injured party
- Date, time, and location of the incident
- Brief description of the incident and what was done to correct it
- Any diagnostic procedures or treatments that were needed
- Patient examination findings, if applicable

- Names and addresses of witnesses, if applicable
- Signature and title of person completing form
- Physician's and supervisor's signatures as per policy

### Guidelines for Completing an Incident Report

When completing an incident report, follow these guidelines:

1. State only the facts. Do not draw conclusions or summarize the event. For example, if you walk into the reception room and find a patient on the floor, do not write, "Patient tripped and fell in reception area," because that draws a conclusion. Instead, document the incident as follows: "Patient found on the floor in the reception area. Patient states that he fell."
2. Write legibly and sign your name legibly. Be sure to include your title.
3. Complete the form in a timely fashion. In general, incident reports should be completed within 24 hours of the event.
4. Do not leave any blank spaces on the form. If a particular section of the report does not apply, write n/a (not applicable).
5. Never photocopy an incident report for your own personal record.
6. Never place the incident report in the patient's chart. Never document in the patient's chart that an incident report was completed. Only document the event in the patient's chart. (By writing in the medical record that an incident report was completed, it opens the potential for lawyers to subpoena the incident report, should there be a lawsuit.)
7. After incident reports are completed, review and track to highlight specific patterns. The resulting statistical data can be used to identify problem areas, which can be corrected through quality improvement (QI) programs.

### WHAT IF?

**You give the wrong medication, and the patient has a bad reaction to it. Would you be better off not documenting the medication error?**

*No!* By not documenting the incident, you place yourself at risk. These risks can include allegations of falsifying medical records, tampering with medical records, and failing to follow reporting policies and procedures. On the incident report, do not say, "I gave the wrong medication"; just state the facts: "X medication was ordered. I gave Y medication." Then, document whom you told and when, what you were advised to do, and any other pertinent information. Your supervisor or the risk manager may call the medical office's insurance company to alert them to the incident. If the incident results in a malpractice lawsuit, an accurately completed incident report can prove helpful to your organization's attorney.

## REGULATORY AGENCIES

One of the most challenging problems for risk managers is to prevent noncompliance with regulatory agencies. As discussed earlier, numerous agencies regulate health care settings, and these rules and regulations change frequently. You can stay up-to-date with new changes by reading newsletters from these organizations, attending your state and local professional meetings, and frequently visiting various professional Web sites. Most states publish a monthly bulletin that reports new legislation. Every state has a Web site that will link you to legislative action. Read these regularly. Each office should have legal counsel who can assist in interpreting legal issues. It is important for a new manager to meet with the medical office's attorney to discuss legal concerns for the practice. These regulatory agencies monitor medical practices to ensure quality of care, protection of employees, and sound practices.

### Centers for Medicare and Medicaid Services

The Centers for Medicare and Medicaid Services (CMS), a division of the U.S. Department of Health and Human Services, regulates and runs various departments and programs, including Medicare and Medicaid. This federal agency is assigned to monitor and follow two key regulations that will affect your job as a medical assistant. These two laws are the Clinical Laboratory Improvement Amendments Act (CLIA) and the Health Insurance Portability and Accountability Act (HIPAA). See Chapter 8 for information on HIPAA.

### Occupational Safety and Health Administration

The Occupational Safety and Health Administration (OSHA) and the Occupational Safety and Health (OSH) Act of 1970 guarantee your right to a workplace that is free from serious hazards. The OSH Act also requires that your employer comply with occupational safety and health standards. Many states also have occupational and safety regulations that your office must follow. Unlike with those of The Joint Commission, compliance with OSHA regulations is not voluntary. Noncompliance with OSHA regulations can result in fines and closure of the health care organization. OSHA also requires that QI programs be in place to protect the health and welfare of patients and employees.

As it does with every profession, OSHA has identified safety hazards specific to medical offices. Examples are rules for blood-borne pathogen protection, use of personal protective equipment (PPE), tuberculosis prevention, management of biohazardous waste, ergonomics, and laser protection. Laser protection is needed if you are working with a physician who is operating a laser in the office. These rules and other guidelines can be found on the OSHA Web site. It also provides specific guidelines that offices must implement to ensure employee and patient safety.

The first step is to make sure that your office has an OSHA poster located in a place routinely accessed by employees, such as the break room or bathroom wall. This poster explains the rights of employees regarding a safe workplace and includes instructions on how to file a complaint if necessary. If you do not have this poster for your office, a free copy can be downloaded or ordered from OSHA's Web site at http://www.osha.gov. OSHA and its requirements are discussed throughout this chapter.

 **CHECKPOINT QUESTION**

7. What is the mission of OSHA?

## The Joint Commission

The Joint Commission is a private agency that sets health care standards and evaluates an organization's implementation of these standards for health care settings. Prior to the mid-1990s, the primary focus of The Joint Commission was on evaluating hospitals and inpatient care institutions such as nursing homes. In 1996, The Joint Commission expanded its jurisdiction to outpatient and ambulatory care settings. This change was, in part, due to the shift of patient care from inpatient to outpatient services such as ambulatory and office-based surgery centers. As mentioned in Chapter 8, The Joint Commission sets standards and evaluates the care in the various health care settings. Box 10-4 lists various types of freestanding facilities for which The Joint Commission sets standards and provides accreditation.

The Joint Commission surveys these centers and then assigns them an accreditation title. A survey is an on-site evaluation of the organization's facility and policies. Participation in The Joint Commission is voluntary for health care organizations; without accreditation, however, the health care organization may not be eligible to participate in particular federal- and state-funded programs, such as Medicare and Medicaid. In addition, accreditation indicates to the community that an organization has met basic practice standards, which is important for marketing its services.

## The National Committee on Quality Assurance

The National Committee on Quality Assurance (NCQA) surveys and accredits 60% of all managed care organizations, which cover 85% of all insured lives in this country. To fulfill its mission "to improve the quality of health care," NCQA works with federal and

---

**BOX 10-4   Types of Facilities**

The Joint Commission accredits a variety of health care settings. These are some types of centers that can be accredited:

- Ambulatory care centers
- Birthing centers
- Chiropractic clinics
- Community health organizations
- Corporate health services
- County jail infirmaries
- Dental clinics
- Dialysis centers
- Endoscopy centers
- Group practices
- Imaging centers
- Independent practitioner practices
- Lithotripsy centers
- Magnetic resonance imaging centers

Oncology centers
Ophthalmology surgery centers
Pain management centers
Podiatry centers
Physician offices
Rehabilitative centers
Research centers
Sleep centers
Student health centers
Women's health centers

---

state lawmakers and executive agency personnel. The NCQA Public Policy team provides information and comment letters for its government partners. NCQA also works in coalition with other involved organizations to advance policies that will improve the quality and efficiency of the health care system. At the federal level, NCQA accreditation and performance measures are valued components of health care policy. The new health care reform law has many provisions that connect to NCQA's mission and capabilities. The law builds on many of NCQA's successful activities over the past 20 years and challenges us to take more steps to work with federal and state policymakers to improve quality and value through measurement, accountability, and transparency. In 2008, NCQA established the PPC-PCMH (Physician Practice Connections) standards for offices to participate in and be recognized for by the government and insurance carriers as a PCMH (Patient-Centered Medical Home).

 **CHECKPOINT QUESTION**

8. What are the benefits of being accredited by The Joint Commission?

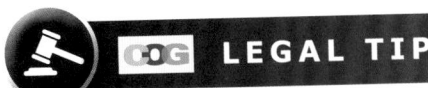

## LEGAL TIP

### The Impact of the Affordable Care Act on Future Office Management

Understanding the changes resulting from the provisions and regulations of the ACA is necessary for effective medical office management. Quality patient care is a major emphasis of the ACA, and one way patient care will be improved is through utilization of the electronic health record. Using the EHR in a meaningful way, such as electronic communication with patients, e-prescribing, etc., gives providers payment incentives through CMS. In addition, telemedicine capabilities (see Chapter 5) are now a reality giving patients an option for virtual office visits. Communication will be carried out through e-mail, and virtual office visits will be a possibility. "The Patient-Centered Medical Home" is a team-based model of care led by a personal physician who provides continuous and coordinated care throughout a patient's lifetime to maximize health outcomes. The PCMH is a health care model that facilitates partnerships between individual patients, patients and their personal physicians, and, when appropriate, the patient's family (Source: http://www.ncqa.com).

## DEVELOPING A QUALITY IMPROVEMENT PROGRAM

The size and complexity of an organization's QI program depends on the organization's particular needs. In large facilities, numerous committees may be assigned to monitor and implement QI plans. Examples of QI plans are fall prevention, needlestick surveillance, and laboratory contamination rates. The committees will consist of staff members, including physicians. Most facilities have a specific person assigned to oversee all of these committees.

In the medical office and ambulatory care settings, QI programs tend to be more informal. Usually, the office manager or senior physician is responsible for monitoring and implementing QI plans. As more outpatient centers become accredited by The Joint Commission, however, QI programs have become more structured. A few examples of quality issues that can be monitored in the physician offices are

- Patient waiting times
- Unplanned returned patient visits for the same ailment or illness
- Misdiagnosed illnesses that are detected by another partner in the practice
- Patient or family complaints
- Timely follow-up telephone calls to patients
- Patient falls in physician's office or office building
- Mislabeled specimens sent to the laboratory
- Blood specimens that are coagulated or contaminated

## Seven Steps for a Successful Program

The following seven steps are essential for creating an effective QI program:

1. *Identify the problem or potential problem.* All organizations can improve their delivery of patient care. Suggestions for improving care can come from many resources, including the following:
   - Office managers
   - Physicians (recommendations and complaints)
   - Other employees (e.g., medical assistants and administrative staff)
   - Patients (interviews or surveys)
   - Incident report trending (discussed earlier)

   The person responsible for QI in the medical office reviews all QI problems or potential problems and selects the one to be addressed first. Problems given top priority are those that are high risk (most likely to occur) and those that are most likely to cause injury to patients, family members, or employees.

2. *Form a task force.* A **task force** is a group of employees with different roles within the organization brought together to solve a given problem. In a medical office, the task force usually consists of a physician, medical assistant, and office manager.

3. *Assign an expected threshold.* The task force establishes an **expected threshold** (numerical goal) for a given problem. Thresholds must be realistic and achievable. For example, if the problem is needlestick injuries, the expected threshold is a realistic number of employee needlestick injuries that the task force considers acceptable in a given period. For instance, the threshold may be one employee stick per month. It is not realistic to set the goal at zero; this may be optimal but is not achievable.

4. *Explore the problem and propose solutions.* The task force investigates the problem thoroughly to determine all potential causes and possible solutions. After various solutions are discussed, the task force decides what solution or solutions are to be implemented.

5. *Implement the solution.* The key to successful implementation of the solution is staff education. All staff members must be taught about the problem and the plan to decrease the problem. The type of implementation will be based on the problem. For example, if the problem is patients falling at the entrance to the building, fixing the problem is likely to be complex and expensive. It may involve reengineering and construction of new walkways. If the problem is mislabeling or misspelling patients' names on laboratory specimens, the implementation will be simpler, possibly printing labels from the computer database.

6. *Establish a QI monitoring plan.* After implementation, the solution must be evaluated to determine whether it worked and, if so, how well. QI monitoring plans have three elements:
   - Source of monitoring, that is, where the numerical data will be obtained (e.g., medical record review, incident reports, laboratory reports, office logs)
   - Frequency of monitoring, that is, how often the data will be monitored and tallied (e.g., once a week, once a month)
   - Person responsible for monitoring, that is, who collects the data and presents the results in graphic form, allowing for easy comparison of data from before and after implementation of the solution

7. *Obtain feedback.* The members of the task force must review the graphs in relation to their expected threshold. Did they meet the threshold? If yes, the problem has been resolved. If the threshold was not met, the task force must determine whether the expected threshold was unrealistic or the solutions were inadequate. In either case, the problem has not been resolved; therefore, the task force must review each of the steps and make appropriate changes.

## CHECKPOINT QUESTION

9. What are the three elements of a QI monitoring plan?

# SAFETY IN THE MEDICAL OFFICE

As a medical assistant, you must be aware of safety issues and practice safety measures in the medical office environment. Patients, staff, and visitors will look to you for leadership and guidance during an emergency situation. It is important for you to recognize unsafe conditions, understand fire safety issues, and guide patients and staff calmly in the event of an evacuation of the medical office. Anticipating an emergency situation and having a written plan to deal with possible emergencies is one way to assure that everyone in the office knows what to do in the event of a local or community emergency. Whether performing a routine task or assisting during an emergency, you must also practice basic personal safety through the use of proper body mechanics to minimize or avoid injury to yourself during an emergency.

## Body Mechanics

Understanding and using principles of proper body mechanics and ergonomics can help you avoid both short- and long-term injury as you carry out your routine medical assisting duties. In the event of an emergency, practicing and using these principles will help prevent injury to you as you assist others who will be relying on you for guidance. Proper body mechanics—using the correct muscles and posture to complete a task safely and efficiently—involves following basic principles when standing, moving, lifting, or reaching. According to OSHA (http://www.osha.gov/SLTC/ergonomics/index.html), risk factors that may contribute to the injury of health care workers include the following:

- Force—the amount of physical effort required to perform a task (such as heavy lifting) or to maintain control of equipment or tools
- Repetition—performing the same motion or series of motions continually or frequently
- Awkward postures—assuming positions that place stress on the body, such as reaching above shoulder height, kneeling, squatting, leaning over a bed, or twisting the torso while lifting

Excessive exposure to these risk factors can result in a variety of musculoskeletal disorders in the medical assistant. Conditions that may result from poor body mechanics include low back pain, sciatica, rotator cuff injuries, epicondylitis, and carpal tunnel syndrome. Your genetic makeup, gender, age, and physical activity outside the workplace may also contribute to the development of musculoskeletal injuries. Although some injuries develop gradually over time, others may result from single events such as lifting something heavy. Following these basic principles when standing, moving, lifting, or reaching for objects may prevent injury:

1. Maintain correct body alignment.
2. Maintain a stable center of gravity.
3. Maintain the line of gravity.
4. Maintain a strong base of support.

In the clinical area, proper body mechanics is important when performing any patient care activities such as helping a patient on and off an examination table or into a chair or pushing a patient in a wheelchair. Proper body mechanics is also essential when performing administrative activities, such as lifting, carrying, or reaching for equipment and office supplies. To avoid physical strain that can lead to injury, use these proper mechanics:

- When standing: Make sure to wear comfortable shoes with good arch support to protect your feet, provide a firm foundation, and prevent slipping. When standing, keep your feet flat on the floor about 12 inches apart. Keep your back straight and stand with one foot slightly in front of the other.
- When walking: Keep your back straight as you walk. If helping another person walk, you may need to place one arm around the back of the person. Keep the other arm at your side, ready to help if necessary.

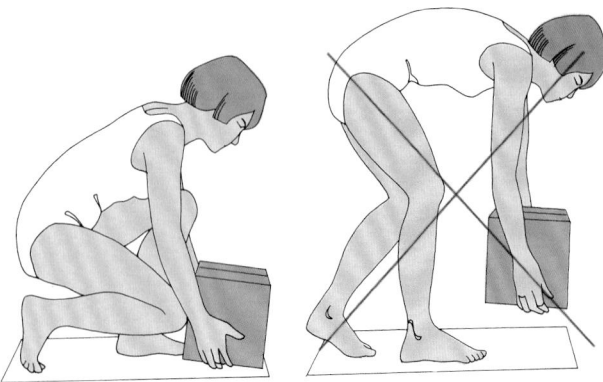

**Figure 10-10** • Proper and improper lifting techniques.

- When lifting an object: Maintain a wide base for maximum stability. In a standing position, keep feet shoulder-width apart. Lower you body and keep your back straight to get close to the object. Bend from your hips and knees (never the waist), grip the object by putting your hands around it, and keep it close to you (Fig. 10-10). Then, keeping your knees bent and your back straight, lift using arm and leg muscles—never your back muscles. Lift straight upward in one smooth motion. If the object is too heavy, get help.
- When pushing or pulling: If possible, push instead of pull, and use the weight of your body, especially your legs to push (or pull) an object. Your feet should be about 12 inches apart with your back straight. Lower your body to get close to the object. Bend from your hips and knees (never your waist). If the object or person is too heavy, get help.
- When reaching: If you are reaching for an object that is low, such as reaching into a bottom file drawer, squat and avoid twisting or bending. When reaching for an object that is high, reach only as high as is comfortable; otherwise, use a small step stool. Never use an office chair to stand and reach objects.

## Ergonomics

Workplace ergonomics is the study of the "fit" between workers and their work environment. Short-term health problems, such as fatigue and discomfort, and long-term health problems, such as carpal tunnel syndrome and tendonitis, can often be avoided by using proper ergonomics. Equipment manufacturers, architects, and workspace planners consider ergonomics when designing devices and workstations. Consider the following techniques to reduce strain and fatigue as you work:

1. Adjust your chair:
   - Adjust your chair height so your feet are flat on the floor. Use a footrest if necessary.
   - Sit upright in the chair with your lower back and your shoulders against the backrest.
   - If the chair has armrests, your elbows and lower arms should rest lightly to avoid circulatory or

nerve problems. Also, adjust armrests so that you can rest your arms at your side and relax your shoulders while working.
   - Adjust the backrest to support the natural inward curvature of your lower back. Use a rolled towel or lumbar pad for extra support.
2. Adjust your desktop:
   - Organize your desk to avoid excessive reaching.
   - If you are using a document holder, place it at the same height as the monitor and at the same distance from your eyes to reduce eye movement and strain.
3. Adjust your computer monitor:
   - Adjust the brightness and contrast to optimum comfort.
   - Position the monitor directly in front of you at arm's length.
   - Position the top of the screen at eye level.
   - Tilt the monitor back 10 to 20 degrees.
   - To reduce glare, angle the monitor away from windows and direct lighting, or use a filter.
   - Make sure the monitor screen is clean.
4. Adjust your keyboard and mouse:
   - Adjust the keyboard height so that your shoulders can relax and let your arms rest at your sides (a swiveling keyboard tray can be helpful).
   - Position the keyboard close enough to prevent excessive reaching and high enough for your forearms to be level.
   - Position the mouse beside and at the same height as the keyboard.
   - Avoid reaching for the keyboard mouse. Wrists should be in a neutral position (not excessively flexed or extended).
   - Rest your hands in your lap when not entering data, not on the mouse.
5. Adjust your lighting:
   - Close drapes or blinds and adjust lighting to reduce glare.
   - Angle the monitor away from windows.
   - Reduce overhead lighting.
   - Use indirect or shielded lighting where possible.

## CHECKPOINT QUESTION

10. What conditions can be prevented by using good body mechanics and principles of ergonomics?

## Evaluating the Medical Office for Safety Issues

Most of us don't think about our work environment being dangerous, but every year, nearly 8 out of 100 employees in hospitals, 9 out of every 100 employees in long-term care facilities, and 2 out of every 100 people who work in physician offices are injured on the job. Threats such as fires, floods, weather-related emergencies, violence, and crime are just as possible when you are at work as they are when you are at home. Other threats that can jeopardize your safety in a medical office include chemical spills, radiation leaks from x-ray machines, and needlesticks that could spread blood-borne pathogens. You could even trip over a stack of files and break your ankle! It is very important that you learn to evaluate your work environment regularly for safety issues that could affect you, other staff, visitors, and patients.

## Personal and Employee Safety Plans

A personal safety plan is designed to protect you and other employees as well as your patients. The steps that OSHA requires in a personal safety plan are listed below for each category. You can use this information to develop a safety plan for your office.

1. Blood-borne pathogens
   - Have a written exposure control plan that is updated annually and explains the rationale for the equipment chosen for your office.
   - Use universal precautions and consideration of safer, engineered needles and sharps.
   - Use engineering and work practice controls and appropriate PPE (gloves, face and eye protection, gowns).
   - Provide free hepatitis B vaccines to employees exposed to blood-borne pathogens.
   - Provide medical follow-up in the event of an exposure incident.
   - Use labels or color coding for items such as sharps disposal boxes and containers for regulated waste, contaminated laundry, and certain specimens.
   - Provide regular employee training on preventing pathogen exposure.
   - Properly contain and dispose all regulated waste.
2. Hazard communication

The hazard communication standard is sometimes called the "employee right-to-know" standard. It requires that employees have access to information about hazards in the workplace. The basic requirements of this standard include

- A written hazard communication plan
- A list of hazardous chemicals such as alcohol, disinfectants, anesthetic agents, sterilants, and mercury that may be stored in the office
- A copy of the Safety Data Sheets (SDS) for each chemical used or stored in the office (The SDS describes the appropriate manner in which these items should be handled, stored, and contained in the event of an emergency [Fig. 10-11A and B].) Safety Data Sheets are formerly known as Material Safety Data Sheets (MSDS), but updated in a standardized 16-section format in compliance with OSHA's updated Hazard Communication Standard.
- Employee training on office-based chemical hazards

3. Ionizing radiation

If your office has an x-ray machine or other radiation-emitting equipment, there should be a list of the type of radiation used in the office. In addition, areas of potential radiation exposure should be restricted to limit employee exposure. Rooms containing radioactive material should be labeled and equipped with caution signs as needed. Employees working in these restricted areas must wear personal radiation monitors such as film badges (refer to Chapter 25).

4. Exit routes

Your office must provide safe and accessible exits from the building in case of fire or other emergencies. Although you may want to consult with your local fire/police department and insurance company for additional information, the basic responsibilities required by OSHA include
   - Exit routes sufficient for the number of employees in any occupied space
   - A diagram of evacuation routes posted in a visible location

5. Electrical safety

The electrical safety standards are required to protect employees in the medical office and apply to electrical equipment and wiring in hazardous locations. If your office uses flammable gases, you may need special wiring and equipment installed. Again, you should check with your local fire department or insurance company for additional information specific to your office.

 **CHECKPOINT QUESTION**

11. Who is protected by a personal safety plan?

## Fire Safety in the Medical Office

A fire in a health care environment can be devastating. Fires not only spring up quickly but also move quickly, destroying everything in their path. Of course, health care facilities including medical offices also have vulnerable patients who may be disabled and incapable of moving quickly to escape life-threatening smoke and flames.

Numerous agencies mandate a variety of fire safety issues in health care facilities including local and state licensing agencies and OSHA. Although you may be aware of the fire safety issues in your home, it is also important that you be aware of fire safety issues in your work environment. These include the following:

- *Fire alarm and detection systems*: All health care facilities should have hardwired, battery backup smoke detectors in every room and hallway. These are designed to detect smoke and heat and may provide information back to a communication center regarding their location.

# MATERIAL SAFETY DATA SHEET

Revision #: 03

## Section 1 - Product Identification & Use

| | |
|---|---|
| Product Name: | **Advance-12A Chlorine Bleach** |
| Synonyms: | Liquid Swimming Pool, 12% Chlorine Bleach, Sodium Hypochlorite Solutions, Javel Water, Advance12-FP |
| Chemical Family: | Hypochlorite solutions |
| Chemical formula of Active: | NaOCl |
| Product Use: | Disinfectant, sanitizer, odour control, water purification, textile bleaching, commercial laundry applications. |
| WHMIS Classification: | Class C, Oxidizing Material<br>Class D, Div. 2, Toxic Liquid, Skin Sensitizer<br>Class E, Corrosive Liquid |
| TDG Classification: | Hypochlorite Solutions UN 1791, Class 8, packing group III |
| D.I.N. | 02229425 |
| REGISTRATION NO. | 24922  PEST CONTROL PRODUCTS ACT |
| Manufacturer: | Advance Chemicals Ltd.<br>2023 Kingsway Ave<br>Port Coquitlam, BC  V3C 1S9<br>Phone: (604)945-9666,<br>Fax: (604)945-9617 |
| Emergency phone: | CANUTEC 24 hrs: (613) 996-6666 |

## Section 2 - Hazardous Ingredients

| Hazardous Components | %(w/w) | C.A.S. No. | $LD_{50}$ & $LC_{50}$ |
|---|---|---|---|
| Sodium Hypochlorite | 10-12 | 7681-52-9 | (oral, mouse)5800 mg/kg<br>ACGIH TLV 2 mg/m$^3$ |

## Section 3 - Physical Data

| | |
|---|---|
| Physical state: liquid | Boiling point: decomposes at 40°C |
| Density: 1.160-1.170 g/mL | Freezing point: -6°C (5% aq. sol'n.) |
| pH: 12.5-13.5 @ 20°C | Vapour pressure:17.5mmHg @ 20°C |
| Solubility in water: 100% | Evaporation rate: no data |

**Odour & Appearance:**  The product is a clear, light green to golden yellow liquid. There is a chlorine like odour above the open liquid. The odour is due to the normal, slow but gradual decomposition process**.** See storage and handling conditions.

## Section 4 - Fire or Explosion Hazard

**Flammability:**  The product is not considered to be flammable.

**Extinguishing media:** Use an extinguishing media for surrounding the fire,  or all purpose foam by manufacturer's recommended techniques for large fires. Use water to cool fire exposed containers to prevent vapour build-up and rupture. Water may also be used to flush spills away from dangerous exposures.

**Hazardous Combustion Products:**  This product decomposes thermally above 40°C. Hazardous and toxic decomposition products may include chlorine gas, oxygen and sodium chlorate. Unvented containers will build-up internal pressure and may rupture causing a product leak.  When Advance-12 is heated or comes into contact with acids, chlorine gas may be released. Vigorous reaction with oxidizable and organic materials may result in fire.

## Section 5 - Reactivity Data

**Stability:**  Under normal conditions of storage and use, this product will slowly decompose over time. The long term decomposition products are not dangerous if the product is stored in a cool, dry, well ventilated area away from direct exposure to sunlight. See also section 7, Preventative Measures.

**Thermal Stability:**  This product will begin to decompose above 40°C. Container may rupture from excessive pressure build-up. Open cap slowly to release any pressure. Hazardous and toxic decomposition products may include chlorine gas, oxygen and sodium chlorate.

**Incompatible substances:**  All acids, ammonium salts and aqueous ammonium hydroxide solutions, metals, oxidizers, nitrogen compounds,  and methanol.

**Polymerization:** Will not occur.

**Conditions to Avoid:**  High temperatures, open flame, direct sunlight (UV radiation initiates decomposition). When Advance-12 is heated, contacted with acids, contacted with oxidizers, or contacted with organic materials, a vigorous reaction may release chlorine gas and heat, resulting in a fire hazard. Allow any paper towels or rags used to wipe up spills to dry or rinse with water before discarding in an approved manner.

## Section 6 - Toxicological Properties

**Acute Toxicity:**  No data found.

**Carcinogenicity:**  The ingredients in this product are; not classified as carcinogenic by the American Conference of Governmental Industrial Hygienists (ACGIH), or the International Agency for Research on Cancer (IARC); not regulated as carcinogens by the Occupational Health and Safety Administration (OSHA); and not listed as carcinogens by the National Toxicology Program (NTP).

**Respiratory & Skin Sensitization:**  May cause skin sensitization and other allergenic responses. Sensitization is the process whereby a biological change occurs in the individual because of previous exposure to a substance, and as a result, the individual reacts more strongly when subsequently exposed to the product. Once sensitized, an individual can react to extremely low airborne levels, even below the TLV, or to skin contact.

**Effects of Exposure:**

**Skin contact:**  Prolonged and repeated exposure often causes irritation, redness, pain, drying and cracking of the skin. Concentrated solutions may cause severe burns to the skin.

**Eye contact:**  This product will cause irritation, redness and pain. May cause corneal damage and conjunctivitis (inflammation of the mucous membrane between the eyeball and inner eyelid).

**Inhalation:**  This product is irritating to the nose, throat and respiratory tract.

**Ingestion:**  This product causes severe burning and pain in the mouth, throat and abdomen. Vomiting, diarrhea and perforation of the esophagus and stomach lining may occur.

## Section 7 - Preventative Measures

Recommendations listed in this section indicate the type of equipment which will provide protection against overexposure to this product. Conditions of use, adequacy of engineering or other control measures, and actual exposures will dictate the need for specific protective devices at your workplace.

**Skin protection:** Gloves and protective clothing made from natural rubber, neoprene or nitrile rubber should be impervious under normal conditions of use. Prior to use, user should confirm impermeability.

**Eye protection:**  Safety glasses with side shields are recommended. Use chemical safety goggles if there is a potential for eye contact.

**Other Personal Protective Equipment:**  Avoid contact with product by wearing chemical protective clothing and rubber boots if necessary. Eye wash fountains and safety shower facilities should be provided nearby for emergency use.

**Figure 10-11 • A.** An SDS for bleach—front page. (From OHSAH MSDS Database: http://msds.ohsah.bc.ca/Default.aspx)

# Advance-12 - MSDS Continued

**Respiratory protection:** No specific guidelines available. Use an NIOSH or MSHA approved air purifying respirator equipped with chlorine cartridges for concentrations up to about 8-10ppm. An air supplied or self contained breathing apparatus should be used if concentrations are exceptionally high or unknown.

**Ventilation Requirements:** This product should be used in a well ventilated area at all times. Local exhaust ventilation may be required and must be corrosion proof. Do not use this product in a poorly ventilated or confined area without approved respiratory protection.

**Storage Requirements:** Store Advance Bleach in a cool, well ventilated area. Keep away from heat, sparks and open flames. Store away from exposure to direct sunlight. Do not expose sealed containers to temperatures above 40°Celcius.

**Action to take for spills & leaks:** Wear chemical protective clothing, rubber gloves and suitable respiratory protection. SMALL SPILLS should be wiped up with absorbent material and disposed of in government approved waste containers. Paper towels may become extremely hot when saturated with this product and cause a secondary fire hazard. Rinse out absorbent materials used in small spill recovery with plenty of water, (see section 5, reactivity data).

LARGER SPILLS should be contained by diking with sand, soil or other absorbent, non-combustible material, then transferred into approved waste containers for proper disposal. Keep product out of sewers, storm drains, surface run-off water and soil. Harmful to aquatic life at low concentrations. Can be dangerous if allowed to enter potable water intakes. Wear appropriate respiratory protection and restrict access to non-protected personnel. Comply with all government regulations on spill reporting, and handling and disposal of waste.

**The contained bleach spill can be effectively neutralized as follows;**

1. Wear respiratory protection and protective clothing, gloves, glasses, etc.
2. Very slowly and cautiously, apply a dilute aqueous solution of Sodium Sulphite, or Sodium meta-Bisulphite to the spill. Mix well. This neutralizes the available chlorine content while reducing the pH to about pH 4. Check with a pH meter or test strip paper. Chlorine gas is a dangerous by-product of this reaction procedure.
3. Increase the pH of the contained spill to about pH 7 by slowly adding a dilute aqueous solution of Soda Ash or Sodium Bicarbonate. Check pH frequently.
4. The bleach spill should be neutral, with a pH of 7. Check with the appropriate local, provincial or federal agencies for proper and correct disposal methods for this product. If available, use a field test kit to check for levels of residual chlorine in the treated waste water.

**Disposal methods:** Dispose of contaminated product and materials used in cleaning up spills or leaks in a manner approved for this material. Consult appropriate federal, provincial and local regulatory agencies to ascertain proper disposal procedures.
**Note:** Empty containers can have residues, gases and mist s, and are subject to proper waste disposal as mentioned above.
**Repair and Maintenance Precautions:** Do not cut, grind, weld or drill in, on or near this container. Do not re-use the original container for any other product, substance, food or drink.

### Section 8 - First Aid Measures

**If inhaled:** Remove victim to fresh air. Give artificial respiration if not breathing. Get immediate emergency medical attention.

**In case of eye contact:** Immediately flush eyes with clean water for at least fifteen (15) minutes, lifting the upper and lower eye lids occasionally. If irritation persists, repeat flushing and GET IMMEDIATE EMERGENCY MEDICAL ATTENTION.

**In case of skin contact:** Immediately flush skin with plenty of clean running water for at least fifteen (15) minutes. Remove contaminated clothing and shoes. If irritation persists, flush skin again and seek medical attention. Wash and launder clothes before re-use. If irritation persists after washing, get immediate medical attention.

**In case of ingestion or swallowing:** If victim is conscious and not convulsing, rinse mouth out with water, and give a glass of water to dilute stomach contents. NEVER GIVE ANYTHING BY MOUTH TO AN UNCONSCIOUS VICTIM. Immediately contact local poison control centre. Vomiting should only be induced under the direction of a physician or poison control official. If spontaneous vomiting occurs, have patient lean forward with head down to avoid breathing in the vomitus. Rinse mouth out and administer more water. GET IMMEDIATE EMERGENCY MEDICAL ATTENTION.

**Emergency Medical Care:** Treat symptomatically

### Section 9 - Preparation Information

Advance Chemicals Limited expressly disclaims all expressed or implied warranties of merchantability and fitness for a particular purpose with respect to the product provided. The information contained herein is offered only as a guide to the handling of this specific product, and has been prepared in good faith by technically knowledgeable personnel. This M.S.D.S. is not intended to be all inclusive, and the manner and conditions of use may involve other and additional considerations.
Revised: 19 October 2006, 24 May 2007; 17 February 2010

**Figure 10-11 • B.** An SDS for bleach—back page. (From OHSAH SDS Database: http://msds.ohsah.bc.ca/Default.aspx)

- *Firefighting equipment*: A variety of fire extinguishers should be placed throughout the medical practice along with hose reels and fire blankets in larger facilities. In compliance with OSHA requirements, fire extinguishers must be visible and accessible and employees must be properly trained regarding the locations and types of extinguishers available. Annual inspections must be performed on all fire extinguishers to ensure they are in working order if needed. All medical offices should have automated sprinkler systems and emergency escape lighting.
- *Fire drills*: Medical offices should regularly hold fire drills according to state licensing requirements. At

the minimum, medical offices should hold one fire drill per year.
- *Training*: All staff should receive fire safety training including employee responsibilities, use of a fire extinguisher, types of fires, fire alarms, detecting and reporting a fire, and evacuating in the event of a fire. As in Figure 10-12, employees should be allowed to use an extinguisher *before* an emergency. Local fire departments offer training in the use of fire extinguishers.
- *Hazardous materials*: In addition to oxygen tanks, other materials in the medical office that may be hazardous include electrical equipment and medical waste.

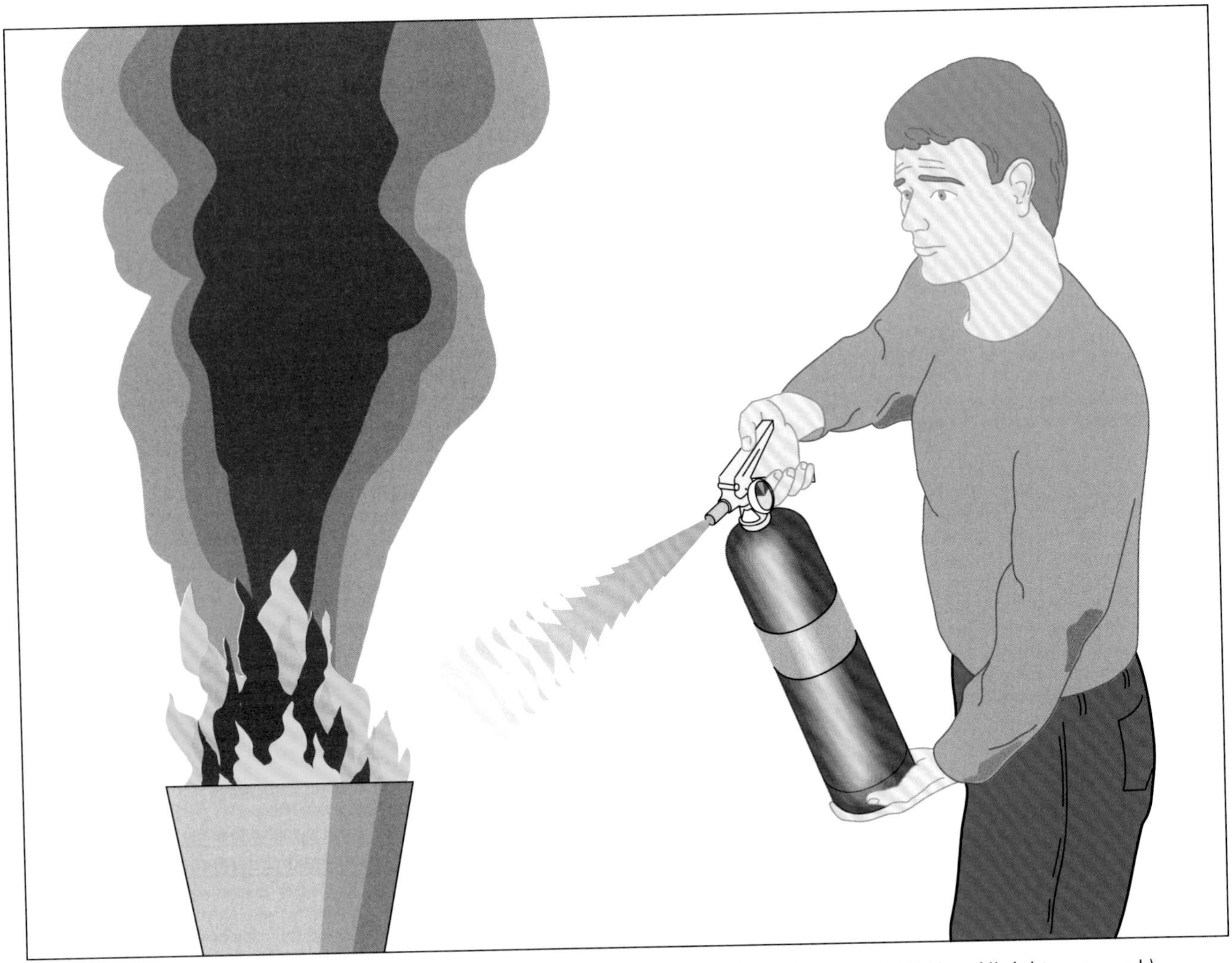

**Figure 10-12** • Fire extinguisher use. (LifeART image copyright © 2012 Lippincott Williams & Wilkins. All rights reserved.)

- *Safe exits*: All medical offices should have enough exits in enough locations to get everyone out of the building safely if necessary. Fire doors must be kept clear and unlocked, stairwells must be uncluttered and well lighted, and signs for alternative exits clearly posted in the event of a fire (Fig. 10-13). Exit signs should also be lighted in order to be seen through smoke.

   Knowing the basics of fire prevention is an important aspect of your role as a professional medical assistant. To prevent fire in a medical office:

- Keep items that could fuel a fire such as paper, linen, clothing, etc., away from heat-producing devices such as lamps.
- Dispose of construction or remodeling items (oily rags, flammable liquids, sawdust, wood shavings) and other fire hazards that tend to accumulate in maintenance and storage areas.

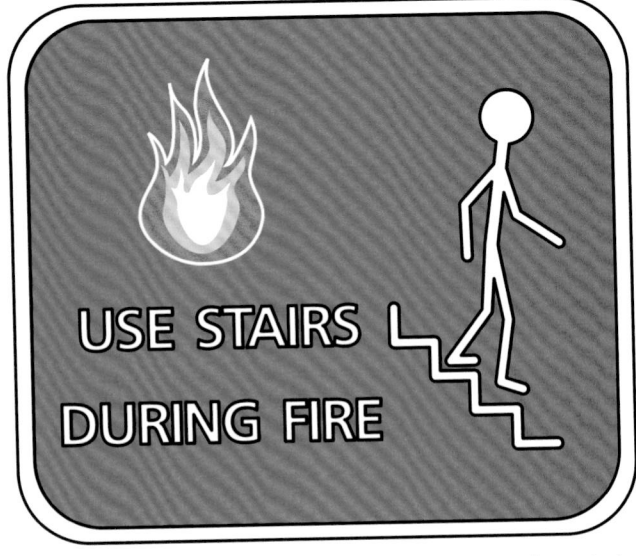

**Figure 10-13** • Fire safety signs should be properly posted in the medical office.

- Ban items that emit sparks from areas that contain supplemental oxygen.
- Store cylinders or tanks that contain flammable gases or liquids away from patients and keep them capped when not in use.
- Clear hallways and stairways of trash or other items that could ignite or impede escape.

## MEDICAL OFFICE EMERGENCIES

Situations in the medical office may develop into emergencies without warning and could occur during a typical workday in the medical office. During a crisis, you should be prepared to assist not only patients and coworkers but also the community at large.

Potential emergencies that could happen in the normal course of the day include medical emergencies such as breathing problems. In addition, natural disasters that are outside of human control can occur forcefully and abruptly. Some examples of natural disasters include

- Earthquake
- Epidemics
- Flood
- Hurricane
- Tornado
- Snowstorm
- Storms

Other emergencies may be caused by or controlled by humans. These include accidents involving multiple vehicles, plane crashes, or train derailments. (See Chapter 27 for more information on disaster preparedness.)

### Emergency Medical Kit

Proper equipment and supplies should be readily available in a medical emergency, and the office manager may be responsible for maintaining the contents of the emergency medical kit and replacing medical supplies that have been used or expired. Although the office's equipment and supplies vary with the medical specialty, emergency equipment and supplies are fairly standard. This equipment should be kept in a designated location that is accessible to all staff. Standard supplies for a medical emergency kit are listed in Box 10-5.

### Evacuation Plan for the Physician Office

Although it is not as involved as the scene in a hospital or nursing home, evacuating a physician office still requires planning and practice. It is important that you be familiar with the key elements of such an evacuation

---

**BOX 10-5  Emergency Medical Kit and Equipment**

The following are standard supplies that can be used to make up an emergency medical kit:

- Activated charcoal
- Adhesive strip bandages, assorted sizes
- Adhesive tape, 1- and 2-inch rolls
- Alcohol (70%)
- Alcohol wipes
- Antimicrobial skin ointment
- Chemical ice pack
- Cotton balls
- Cotton swabs
- Disposable gloves
- Elastic bandages, 2- and 3-inch widths
- Gauze pads, 2 × 2- and 4 × 4-inch widths
- Roller, self-adhesive gauze, 2- and 4-inch widths
- Safety pins, various sizes
- Scissors
- Syrup of ipecac
- Thermometer
- Triangular bandage
- Tweezers

In addition to these contents, the following equipment should be available:

- Blood pressure cuff (pediatric and adult)
- Stethoscope
- Bag valve mask device with assorted size masks
- Flashlight or penlight
- Portable oxygen tank with regulator
- Oxygen masks
- Suction unit and catheters

Additional equipment that may be available includes

- Various sizes of endotracheal tubes
- Laryngoscope handle and various sizes of blades
- Automatic external defibrillator
- Intravenous supplies (catheters, administration set tubing, assorted solutions)
- Emergency drugs including atropine, epinephrine, and sodium bicarbonate

---

plan because you will, by necessity, play an important role in any emergency evacuation.

The first step is to know what constitutes an emergency requiring evacuation. This could be a fire, a chemical spill, impending weather-related emergencies, a threat of violence, or even a highly infectious patient. You should discuss the specific situations that might trigger an evacuation order in your office with your physician, office manager, and other staff and develop a policy to guide the process.

In addition to the key elements given in Chapter 27, other items to be considered for a physician office include the following:

- Communicating the evacuation. This may be done verbally, through an e-mail or text message, or with an alarm. Include how patients will be notified of the evacuation before, during, and after the event.
- Determining who is responsible for giving the evacuation order. This will most likely be a physician or the office manager.
- Identifying specific staff responsibilities including who will be in charge of evacuating patients currently in the office, both those patients who are well bodied and those who are disabled.
- Determining how patient records will be protected and/or transported.
- Identifying available transportation for the evacuation.
- Determining a meeting place for all employees once the evacuation is complete.
- Identifying exit routes from your work area. There should be at least two.
- Identifying any employees with disabilities who may require special attention during an evacuation. It should be clarified how these individuals will be assisted.
- Determining how the office will be secured during and after the evacuation.
- Identifying what, if anything, should be taken from the office and who should be responsible for seeing that the item or items are removed and secure.
- Identifying who will communicate with emergency personnel.
- Determining if any personnel should remain behind after the primary evacuation.

- Identifying a way to account for employees during and after the evacuation.
- Identifying the person who will be responsible for notifying the public utilities (electricity, telephone, water, gas, etc.) that the building or office has been evacuated.
- Identifying and obtaining any special equipment that may be required for evacuation such as safety goggles, masks, gloves, etc.

 **ROLE-PLAYING ACTIVITY**

Ben Larson, RMA, is in the process of hiring a new receptionist at Great Falls Medical Center. This very busy practice requires someone with the ability to greet patients and visitors as well as handle a variety of incoming calls in a professional manner. The receptionist must also handle patient payments throughout the day and be flexible to make appointments when the scheduler is unavailable. The position also requires someone who is punctual and dependable. What kinds of questions may Ben ask during an interview with an applicant? What questions should he avoid asking in order to not violate any laws concerning the patients' privacy? In this activity, role-play as the MA interviewing the applicant and think about the questions that would be important to ask during an interview. If you are playing the part of the applicant, think about how you will respond to various types of questions, including those that may violate your right to privacy. Your instructor will give you additional information about this activity!

## *español* SPANISH TERMINOLOGY

**Ando buscando trabajo.**
I am looking for a job.

**¿Tiene usted algún empleo disponible?**
Do you have any jobs available?

**¿Dónde están las aplicaciones?**
Where are the applications?

**Yo soy el director.**
I am the manager.

**¿Vió usted lo que pasó?**
Did you see what happened?

**¿Se cayó?**
Did you fall?

**¿Está usted lastimado?**
Are you hurt?

**¿Quiere usted ver un doctor?**
Do you want to see a doctor?

**Usted necesita que le tomen una radiografía.**
You need an x-ray.

**¿Tiene dolor?**
Do you have pain?

**¿Tiene dificultad para respirar?**
Are you having any problem breathing?

**¿Cuando ocurrió el accidente?**
When did the accident happen?

**Cálmese, por favor. La ambulancia está en camino.**
Calm down, please. The ambulance is on the way.

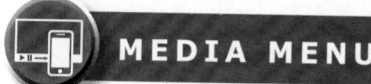

## MEDIA MENU

**Student Resources** on thePoint®
• **CMA/RMA Certification Exam Review**

**Internet Resources**
**Medical Group Management Association**
http://www.mgma.com

**Physicians Practice Group**
http://www.physicianspractice.com/home

**Family Leave Act/Department of Labor**
http://www.dol.gov

**Americans with Disabilities Act/U.S. Department of Justice**
http://www.justice.gov

**Centers for Medicare and Medicaid Services**
http://www.cms.gov

**Clinical Laboratory Improvement Amendments Act**
http://www.cms.hhs.gov/clia

**Health Care Report Cards**
http://www.healthgrades.com

**Health Insurance Portability and Accountability Act**
http://www.cms.gov/HIPAAGenInfo

**Occupational Safety and Health Administration**
http://www.osha.gov

**National Committee on Quality Assurance**
http://www.ncqa.org

**Medscape Today from Web MD**
http://www.medscape.com/medscapetoday

**American Heart Association**
http://www.heart.org

**American Red Cross**
http://www.redcross.org

**American Safety and Health Institute**
http://www.hsi.com/

**National Safety Council**
http://www.nsc.org/Pages/Home.aspx

## EMR Activity

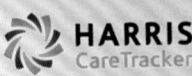

Harris CareTracker is a Web-based electronic medical record (EMR) application that you will use for the EMR activities included in this section at the end of each chapter. This application is actually used in physician offices, but is provided to you through the publisher, Wolters Kluwer Health, to give you hands-on practice working with EMRs. Your instructor will have more information about accessing your username, log-in, and Quickstart guide.

### Prerequisite Activities in Harris CareTracker

- *The Getting Started and Quickstart documents and EMR Activities Step-by-Step Instructions are available at* http://thePoint.lww.com/KronenbergerComp5e

### Activity Details

A large, unused storage room was recently remodeled at Great Falls Medical Center in order to create two new exam rooms. The office manager, Ben Larson, RMA, must add the two new rooms to the *Room Maintenance* application in the EMR. This feature allows the location of patients to be monitored in the EMR within the practice from the moment of their arrival until they are discharged after being seen by the provider. Add exam room 3 and exam room 4 in the *Room Maintenance* application found under the *Setup* tab of the *Administration* module of the EMR.

## Chapter Summary

- Effective management of the medical office is essential for a health care organization to succeed in the competitive marketplace.
- A good manager must be able to perform a variety of tasks in an organized and efficient manner.
- An office manager will be communicating simultaneously with patients and staff, handling staffing issues, developing policy and procedures manuals, creating promotional materials, preparing budgets, and overseeing educational programs.
- The medical office manager must keep current on legal requirements related to office operations.
- QI programs have many benefits to health care organizations. They can identify potential problems for patients and employees.
- After identifying the problem, a task force can create solutions to resolve them.
- QI programs are also required by various agencies. Four important agencies are The Joint Commission, OSHA, CMS, and your state health department. You must stay alert to new regulations from these agencies. Patients place trust in all health care workers and health care settings. We must all work hard to provide good quality care to all patients every time they are treated.
- Dealing with a medical emergency in the office or community will require you to
- Communicate clearly and calmly
- Recognize the need for immediate medical intervention
- Perform emergency procedures immediately and competently
- Provide first aid and life support measures that can mean the difference between life and death
- Reassure the patient and family members
- Work with the physician and other health care team members efficiently and with confidence

## Warm-Ups for Critical Thinking

1. Review the list of qualities that a manager should have. Which ones do you have? How would you acquire the others? Should any other qualities be listed?
2. Review the types of sections that are often included in policy and procedures manuals. Now, assume that you are to help a physician set up a practice. How would you organize your policy and procedures manual? Create one sample sheet for each section of your manual. Be sure to include all necessary elements when you write your policies and procedures.
3. Create a list of potential patient or employee problems that could be solved with a QI program. Be sure to include some administrative, clinical, and laboratory examples. Then, select three problems and develop a list of solutions for each problem.
4. Plan a mock fire drill for a medical office: assign employees to certain tasks, and design a form to document the drill.

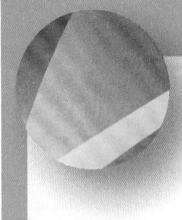

## PSY PROCEDURE 10-1

# Create a Procedures Manual

**PSY** Create a policy and procedures manual

**Purpose:** To communicate the proper policies and procedures to be used by all employees in a practice in order to ensure consistent, accurate, and efficient patient interaction and care

**Equipment:** Word processor, three-ring binder, paper; choose any procedure approved by your instructor

| STEPS | REASONS |
|---|---|
| 1. Check the latest information from key governmental agencies, local and state health departments, and health care organizations, such as OSHA and the CDC, to make sure that the policies and procedures being written comply with federal and state legislation and regulations. | Serious consequences can occur if you are not conscientious about keeping abreast of changes in the medical and legal worlds. This information can be found on the Internet and in published reports. |
| 2. Gather product information; consult government agencies, as needed. If the procedure is for new equipment, ask the sales representative for training pamphlets. | This ensures that you are using products and equipment according to the manufacturer's usage suggestions and that you are practicing within legal and ethical boundaries. |
| 3. Title the procedure, for example, Infection Control Procedure for Hand Washing. | A logical, easily identifiable format will allow easy retrieval. |
| 4. Number the procedure, for example, "HR 14" means human resource section, policy 14. | All policies and procedures should be numbered to allow for easy access and identification. |
| 5. Define the overall purpose of the procedure. This should be a sentence or two at most, explaining the intent of the procedure. | Provides the staff with a rationale for the procedure |
| 6. List any necessary equipment or forms. Include everything needed to complete the task. Also indicate if no special equipment or forms are necessary. | The employee will be prepared before beginning the procedure if he or she has everything needed at hand. |
| 7. List each step with its rationale. The steps must be complete and in order. Never assume the reader knows how or when to perform a given step such as hand washing. The employee will be able to follow specific steps, ensuring patient safety. | Listing the steps in order promotes compliance and accuracy for procedure completion. |
| 8. Provide spaces for signatures for the employee, office manager, and possibly the physician. | The employee's signature will verify that he or she has read and understands the procedure. |
| 9. Record the date the procedure was written. If changes are needed, the procedure is rewritten, signed, and dated again. The previous dates also are generally listed. | By recording the date, you ensure that you are reading the most current revision. It will also help you know when a new revision should be considered. |
| 10. **AFF** Describe how you would explain to employees why they were asked to work in a group to create a procedures manual. | It is important to work effectively with a group to accomplish the task of creating a procedures manual. Employees from different areas of the practice will bring different perspectives to the task. |

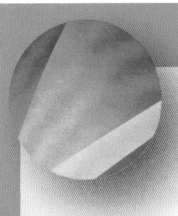

## PSY PROCEDURE 10-2

# Perform an Office Inventory

**PSY** Perform an inventory with documentation

**Purpose:** To maintain a sufficient amount of supplies needed to perform daily administrative, clinical, and laboratory duties involved in patient care

**Equipment:** Inventory Form, Reorder Form

| STEPS | REASONS |
|---|---|
| 1. Using forms supplied by your instructor, count and record the amounts of specified supplies. | Established forms will promote consistency. |
| 2. Record amount of each item. | As always, accuracy is important. |
| 3. Compare amount on hand with amount needed. | These amounts will be established based on usage. |
| 4. Complete reorder form based on these numbers. | You must also consider the time it will take for the ordered supplies to arrive to avoid running out. |
| 5. Submit reorder forms to office manager. | Although many individuals may count supplies, the duty of ordering should be placed on one or two employees, usually a supervisor. |
| 6. Document your actions per the ordering procedure. | Proper documentation prevents duplication in ordering. |
| 7. **AFF** Explain how you would respond to an employee who continually takes a vacation day when the office plans to take inventory. | Explain to the employee that this is an important part of having an efficient workplace. Everyone must do their part as a member of the team. Being a team player is essential. |

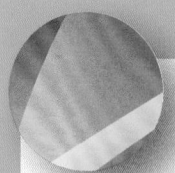

**PSY** PROCEDURE 10-3

## Medical Office Safety Checklist

**PSY** Evaluate the work environment to identify unsafe working conditions

**Purpose**: Identify hazards throughout the medical office and prioritize action to be taken according to the risks involved

**Scenario**: Determine hazards and safety concerns during a visual inspection of all areas of a medical office

**Equipment**: Office Safety Checklist, pen

| STEPS | REASONS |
|---|---|
| 1. Obtain a floor plan of the medical office before beginning the inspection. | To ensure a thorough inspection of the entire office |
| 2. Perform a general visual inspection of every room/area in the medical office for potential hazards. | Corrective action can be taken after potential safety hazards are identified. |
| 3. Inspect office equipment in the medical office for potential hazards. | Corrective action can be taken after potential safety hazards are identified. |

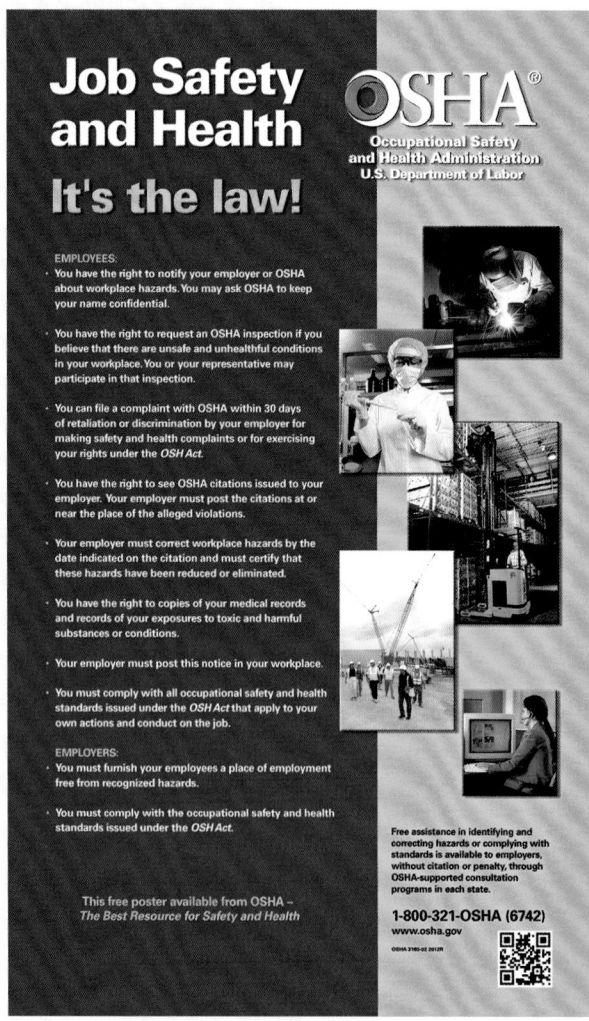

## PROCEDURE 10.3 (continued)

| STEPS | REASONS |
|---|---|
| 4. Examine all fire extinguishers and determine that they are in their appropriate places, fully charged and operating properly. | Fire extinguishers must be unobstructed and in working condition. |
| 5. Check for posted emergency evacuation routes in every room and lighted exit signs are working. | Required by OSHA in order to exit the building safely and orderly in the event of an emergency evacuation |
| 6. Is the OSHA poster (publication 3165) displayed in a prominent location? | Every workplace is required by OSHA to display this poster to explain workers rights to a safe workplace and how to file a complaint. |
| 7. Are the Safety Data Sheets accessible to all employees in a prominent location? | This is required as part of OSHA's *Hazard Communication Standard*. |
| 8. **AFF** Advise the physician of any hazardous situations that you may find that need corrective action. | The physician is responsible for a safe work environment for all employees. |

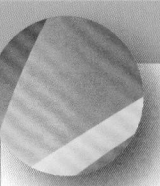

**PSY** PROCEDURE 10-4

# Complete an Incident Report

**PSY** Perform an incident report related to an error in patient care

**Purpose**: Recognize that error was made when private health information was recorded in another patient's medical record, and complete the documentation required as a result of this error

**Scenario**: After documenting a patient's chief complaint and vital signs, you realize that you did not properly identify the patient and erroneously recorded the information in the wrong patient's medical record.

**Equipment**: An incident form.

| STEPS | REASONS |
|---|---|
| 1. Recognize the error in patient care (i.e., recording of PHI in the wrong medical record) because you did not get another piece of identifiable information from the patient being seen. | Ethically, you must acknowledge the error and take the steps necessary to correct both patients' medical records. |
| 2. After correcting the error appropriately in the wrong patient's medical record, complete an incident report. | Follow office policies and procedures for making corrections in the medical record and documenting the error. |
| 3. Sign and date the incident report form and file with the office or practice manager. | The incident report should not be placed into the patient's medical record. |
| 4. **AFF** What steps can be taken to ensure that the correct medical record is used in the future? | Always have at least two identifiable pieces of information for patients to ensure the correct medical record is available for the visit. |

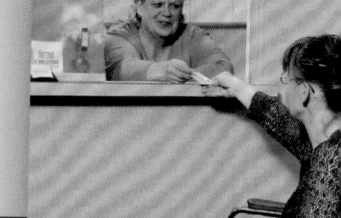

Good management of finances is essential for a medical practice to succeed. This unit introduces you to various aspects of medical office finances beginning with an introduction to diagnostic and procedural coding and health insurance reimbursement. Next, you will learn bookkeeping and banking skills as well as other accounting responsibilities and will complete the reimbursement process with a chapter dedicated to collecting medical fees. A financially strong practice is good for the patients, the community, and you.

CHAPTER

# 11

# Diagnostic Coding

## Outline

## Learning Outcomes

### COG Cognitive Domain*

1. Spell and define the key terms
2. Describe the relationship between coding and reimbursement
3. Name and describe the coding system used to describe diseases, injuries, and other reasons for encounters with a medical provider
4. Explain the format of the ICD-9-CM
5. Give four examples of ways E codes are used

6. *Describe how to use the most current diagnostic coding classification system*
7. Describe the ICD-10-CM/PCS version and its differences from ICD-9

### PSY Psychomotor Domain*

1. *Perform diagnostic coding (Procedure 11-1)*
2. *Utilize medical necessity guidelines (Procedure 11-1)*

*(continues on page 268)*

**AFF Affective Domain***

1. Work with the physician to achieve the maximum reimbursement
2. *Utilize tactful communication skills with medical providers to ensure accurate code selection*

*Note: AAMA/CAAHEP 2015 Standards are italicized.*

**ABHES Competencies**

1. Apply third-party guidelines
2. Perform diagnostic and procedural coding
3. Comply with federal, state, and local health laws and regulations

## Key Terms

advance beneficiary
notice (ABN)
audit
conventions
cross-reference
E codes

eponym
etiology
inpatient
International Classification
of Diseases, Ninth or
Tenth Revision, Clinical

Modification (ICD-9-CM
or ICD-10-CM)
late effects
main terms
medical necessity
outpatient

primary diagnosis
service
specificity
truncated
V codes

## Case Study

Working in the billing department at Great Falls Medical Center requires Tonya Little, CMA, to verify diagnosis codes as necessary when the billing software indicates that there is a problem with coding. She is also responsible for management of the denied claims, including investigating the reason for the denials and resubmitting the claims in a timely manner. Lately, Tonya has noticed that insurance companies have denied several claims due to "truncated coding" errors. What is diagnosis coding, and what books are used to find diagnosis codes? What does the term "truncated coding" mean? Does it matter which edition of the diagnosis coding book Tonya uses in her search for the correct code? Proper selection of a diagnosis code is important to accurately describe a patient's health status. Incorrect codes not only cause problems with reimbursement of health care encounters but also may affect the patient's medical outcome because they determine the medical necessity for requested services and procedures. This chapter covers the types of diagnostic coding and the procedures for accurately choosing a diagnosis code.

Proper selection of diagnoses codes is important in order to accurately describe a patient's health status. Incorrect codes not only cause problems with reimbursement for health care encounters but also may affect the patient's medical outcome since they determine the medical necessary for requested services and procedures. This chapter covers the types of diagnostic coding and the process for accurately choosing a diagnosis code.

Coding, at its simplest, is the assignment of a number to a verbal statement or description. **The International Classification of Diseases** is a system for transforming verbal descriptions of diseases, injuries, conditions, and inpatient procedures into numeric codes. In compliance with the Health Insurance Portability and Accountability Act of 1996 (HIPAA), the Centers for Medicare and Medicaid Services (CMS) mandated that all health care providers use the International Classification of Diseases, Ninth Revision, Clinical Modification (ICD-9-CM) code set to report inpatient and outpatient diseases, injuries, conditions, etc. The ICD-9-CM is updated and revised annually and is being replaced with the tenth revision (ICD-10-CM). Health care providers must begin using ICD-10-CM to code the reasons for patient encounters and ICD-10-PCS for coding hospital and inpatient procedures in the near future, and the current implementation date set by the CMS may be found on their Web site at www.cms.gov/ICD10. It is essential that the physician and medical assistant work together to achieve accurate documentation, code assignment, and reporting of diagnoses and procedures. Use of standardized codes makes it easier for third-party payers to understand the reason for the patient's encounter with the health care provider and increases the likelihood of timely processing of claims and prompt payment when appropriate.

Coding is a way to standardize medical information for purposes such as collecting health care statistics, performing a medical care review, and indexing medical records. It is also used for health insurance claims processing (see Chapter 13). Because coding is the basis for reimbursement, it is imperative that you code patient visits accurately and precisely. Incorrect, insufficient, or incomplete coding on claims forms can lead to nonpayment for the physician as well as incorrect information in the insurance companies' databases, which may affect the patients' insurability. For example, if a patient complaining of chest pain is coded as having "acute myocardial infarction" instead of "chest pain," that patient may be incorrectly labeled as having heart disease. The Current Procedural Terminology (CPT) codes, which are used to report services and procedures performed by health care providers, determine the amount paid (see Chapter 12), but the code assigned to the diagnosis or reason for the service or procedure provides the medical necessity for the services or procedures so that claims are paid. The third-party payer needs to know why the service was performed to assess **medical necessity**. Medical necessity means the procedure or service would have been performed by any reasonable physician under the same or similar circumstances. The ICD-9 and ICD-10 diagnosis codes convey this information. Is a chest radiograph medically necessary for a patient who has gout? No, but it may be necessary for a patient with acute bronchitis. The diagnosis justifies or supports the procedure.

Since Medicare considers certain procedures medically necessary only at certain intervals, having the patient sign an advance beneficiary notice (ABN) will ensure payment of treatments and procedures that will likely be denied by Medicare. An example is a Pap smear for a low-risk woman, which will be paid for once every 2 years. If the physician considers it not to be medically necessary, but the patient wants a Pap test, the patient will be responsible for payment and must sign an ABN.

## CHECKPOINT QUESTION

1. What is meant by medical necessity?

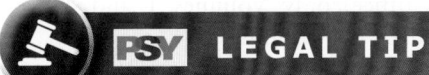

### LEGAL TIP

### Does Everyone Need to Know?

Remember that diagnosis codes placed on the CMS-1500 are confidential and should be protected as much as any other medical information. Forms left lying in common areas in the office may be seen by other patients. Keep printers and copies of these forms in a private place, and share the diagnosis codes only with those who need the information to carry out their duties. Patients have the right to keep their diagnoses private.

## DIAGNOSTIC CODING

The ICD-9-CM is a statistical classification system based on the ICD-9, developed by the World Health Organization (WHO). The CM, which stands for *clinical modification*, addresses the intent of these codes to describe the clinical picture of the patient. These codes are much more precise than those needed for statistical grouping and trend analysis found in the ICD-9 and used in hospital coding.

The new ICD-10 diagnosis codes classification system provides significant improvements over ICD-9-CM with more detailed and current information. The new system will provide for expansion and increased specificity to more accurately describe diseases, injuries, and conditions. These alphanumeric codes are three to seven digits long and always begin with a letter followed by a number. The remaining digits (three through seven) can be alpha or numeric. There are approximately 70,000 diagnosis codes and 72,000 procedure codes in the ICD-10-CM.

Until recently, the ICD-9-CM has been the most comprehensive statistical classification of its kind. These numeric codes have three to five digits and supplementary codes that begin with a letter followed by up to four digits. Containing more than 13,000 diagnoses codes and less than 4,000 procedure codes, it consists of three volumes:

- Volume 1: Tabular List of Diseases
- Volume 2: Alphabetic Index of Diseases
- Volume 3: Tabular List and Alphabetic Index of Procedures (Inpatient)

The ICD-9-CM and ICD-10-CM codebooks are available in different formats, such as manuals, computer software, or a Web-based format, and may be purchased from several publishers. Although the presentation of the material may be different, the content must be the same. Depending on the publisher, these three volumes may be included within one book.

In the physician's office, only Volumes 1 and 2 are used. Volume 3 is used by hospitals.

The diagnostic classification systems in Volumes 1 and 2 are maintained by a federal government agency, the National Center for Health Statistics (NCHS); the procedure classification (Volume 3) is maintained by the CMS, the federal agency that regulates health care financing. All three volumes are updated regularly, with codes being added, revised, and sometimes deleted. Changes in the ICD-9-CM are published by the NCHS and CMS with the approval of the WHO. Both the American Health Information Management Association (AHIMA) and the American Hospital Association (AHA) advise and assist in keeping the classification system current.

 **CHECKPOINT QUESTION**

2. What organization must approve any changes in the disease classification system?

## Inpatient versus Outpatient Coding

There is a big difference between coding medical claims in a hospital or other inpatient facility and coding for the physician in an outpatient medical practice. The systems and references used to assign codes to third-party claims are only one difference in the coding requirements and practices of the physician and the inpatient medical facility. Volumes 1 and 2 of the ICD-9-CM are used to report the diagnostic code that justifies physician services whether those services are provided in the office or in the hospital. Hospital coders use Volume 3 to report inpatient procedures, services, and supplies, as well as the reasons for the services.

The UB-04 (uniform bill) is used by institutions to report inpatient admissions and outpatient and emergency department services and procedures. These charges are for nursing services, building maintenance, and all costs associated with running the institution. These charges do not include physician services. The CMS-1500 (universal claim form) is used to report physician services, regardless of whether or not the physician sees the patient in the office, emergency department, hospital, or nursing home. The place where the physician provided service will be reported using a place of service code (see Chapter 13, Procedure 13-1).

The term **outpatient** is used to describe patients treated in the following places:

- Health care provider's office
- Hospital clinic
- Emergency department
- Hospital same-day surgery unit or ambulatory surgical center that releases the patient within 23 hours
- Observation status in a hospital (the patient is admitted for a short time for observation only, and the physician bills for his or her service during the stay)

The term **inpatient** refers to a patient who is admitted to the hospital for treatment with the expectation that the patient will remain in the hospital for 24 hours or more.

Hospital coders code only services provided by the hospital and hospital employees. Coders who are employed by the physician practice are concerned with the services provided by the physician no matter where the services are provided. For example, the hospital room, meals, and laboratory testing that a patient receives are billed and coded by the hospital billing department. The daily visits the physician makes to the patient are billed and coded by the physician's office.

Since the focus of this textbook is medical assisting, we concentrate on outpatient coding.

**CHECKPOINT QUESTION**

3. Name and give uses for the three volumes of the ICD-9-CM.

## **COG THE DIAGNOSIS CODEBOOK**

Coding books are available from several publishers, such as Ingenix and Medicode. The American Medical Association(AMA) Press also publishes coding books and training materials. The classification system is also available as part of a medical software package; one of these packages is CodeManager from the AMA. Although each publisher offers special features and helpful aids, the format remains the same. Some coders become comfortable with certain special features (i.e., AMA publications are spiral bound) and, since the content is the same, can choose among the various publications based on organization, illustrations, tabs, bullets, and color coding.

To become an expert medical coder, you need general knowledge of human anatomy and medical terminology. In addition to using a codebook, you will need reference materials such as a medical dictionary and/or medical dictionary software.

To ensure accurate coding, always use current ICD-CM (9th or 10th edition, whichever is mandated by the CMA) codebooks and software to begin implementation of the new or revised codes that are published in late summer and effective every October 1. It is also important to update your coding books and software as needed throughout the year. (Updates and addenda can be purchased from the publisher of your coding book.) You must update codes on superbills (preprinted bills listing a variety of procedures) or any other forms you use. Experts have estimated that millions of dollars in reimbursement have been lost because an incorrect code was taken from an encounter form that had not been updated.

4. How often is the ICD-CM updated? When is the use of the new codes required?

## Tabular List of Diseases

Both ICD-9-CM and ICD-10-CM have tabular lists that contain the classification of diseases (conditions) and injuries by code numbers. This is known as Volume 1 for ICD-9-CM. Both code sets have chapters that list codes in bold print in numeric or alphanumeric order and are indented. Figure 11-1 shows the chapters from the table of contents of both code sets. There are 17 chapters in ICD-9-CM and 21 chapters in ICD-10-CM

that cover groupings of diseases and injuries by **etiology** or cause (e.g., infectious diseases) and by anatomic system (e.g., digestive, respiratory). Figure 11-2 is a sample page from the ICD-9-CM tabular list showing each level of classification. Note that each chapter has a heading or title [e.g., 16, Symptoms, Signs, and Ill-Defined Conditions (780 to 799)]. Following the title in parentheses is the range of three-digit categories included in that chapter. In each chapter, you will find subtitles in large type followed by a range of three-digit categories in parentheses [e.g., 16, Symptoms (780 to 789)]. These sections describe general disease. Three-digit codes followed by a title, the category codes, describe specific diseases (e.g., 780, general symptoms). The fourth digit further breaks down the category (e.g., 780.0, alteration

| ICD-9-CM | | |
|---|---|---|
| Chapter | Title | Category Range |
| 1 | Infectious and Parasitic Diseases | 001–039 |
| 2 | Neoplasms | 140–239 |
| 3 | Endocrine, Nutritional, and Metabolic Diseases and Immunity Disorders | 240–279 |
| 4 | Diseases of the Blood and Blood-forming Organs | 280–289 |
| 5 | Mental Disorders | 290–319 |
| 6 | Diseases of the Nervous System and Sense Organs | 320–389 |
| 7 | Diseases of the Circulatory System | 390–459 |
| 8 | Diseases of the Respiratory System | 460–519 |
| 9 | Diseases of the Digestive System | 520–579 |
| 10 | Disease of the Genitourinary System | 580–629 |
| 11 | Complications of Pregnancy, Childbirth, and the Puerperium | 630–679 |
| 12 | Diseases of the Skin and Subcutaneous Tissue | 680–709 |
| 13 | Diseases of Musculoskeletal System and Connective Tissue | 710–739 |
| 14 | Congenital Anomalies | 740–759 |
| 15 | Certain Conditions Originating in the Perinatal Period | 760–779 |
| 16 | Symptoms, Signs, and Ill-Defined Conditions | 780–799 |
| 17 | Injury and Poisoning | 800–999 |
| Supplemental Classification: V Codes | | |
| Supplemental Classification: E Codes | | |

| ICD-10-CM | | |
|---|---|---|
| Chapter | Title | Category Range |
| 1 | Certain Infectious and Parasitic Diseases | A00–B99 |
| 2 | Neoplasms | C00–D49 |
| 3 | Disease of the Blood, Blood-forming organs and Certain Immune Disorders | D50–D89 |
| 4 | Endocrine, Nutritional, and Metabolic Diseases | E00–E89 |
| 5 | Mental and Behavioral Disorders | F01–F99 |
| 6 | Diseases of the Nervous System | G00–G99 |
| 7 | Diseases of the Eye and Adnexa | H00–H59 |
| 8 | Disease of the Ear and Mastoid Process | H60–H95 |
| 9 | Diseases of the Circulatory System | I00–I99 |
| 10 | Diseases of the Respiratory System | J00–J99 |
| 11 | Diseases of the Digestive System | K00–K94 |
| 12 | Diseases of the Skin and Subcutaneous | L00–L99 |
| 13 | Diseases of the Musculoskeletal & Connective Tissue | M00–M99 |
| 14 | Diseases of the Genitourinary System | N00–N99 |
| 15 | Pregnancy, Child-birth, and the Puerperium | O00–O9A |
| 16 | Certain Conditions Originating in the Perinatal Period | P00–P96 |
| 17 | Congenital Malformations, Deformations, and Chromosomal Abnormalities | Q00–Q99 |
| 18 | Symptoms, Signs, and Abnormal Clinical & Laboratory Findings NEC | R00–R99 |
| 19 | Injury, Poisoning, and Certain Other Consequences of External Causes | S00–T88 |
| 20 | External Causes of Morbidity | V01–Y99 |
| 21 | Factors Influencing Health Status and Contact with Health Services | Z00–Z99 |

**Figure 11-1** • Table of contents from ICD-9-CM, Volume 1, and ICD-10-CM.

✓5ᵗʰ 780.5    **Sleep disturbances**
      **EXCLUDES**    *that of nonorganic origin (307.40-307.49)*

    780.50    **Sleep disturbance, unspecified**

    780.51    **Insomnia with sleep apnea**
        DEF: Transient cessation of breathing disturbing sleep.

    780.52    **Other insomnia**
        Insomnia NOS
        DEF: Inability to maintain adequate sleep cycle.

    780.53    **Hypersomnia with sleep apnea**
        DEF: Autonomic response inhibited during sleep; causes insufficient oxygen intake, acidosis and pulmonary hypertension.

    780.54    **Other hypersomnia**
        Hypersomnia NOS
        DEF: Prolonged sleep cycle.

    780.55    **Disruptions of 24-hour sleep-wake cycle**
        Inversion of sleep rhythm
        Irregular sleep-wake rhythm NOS
        Non-24-hour sleep-wake rhythm

    780.56    **Dysfunctions associated with sleep stages or arousal from sleep**

    780.57    **Other and unspecified sleep apnea**

    780.59    **Other**

✓4ᵗʰ 780    **General symptoms**

✓5ᵗʰ 780.0    **Alteration of consciousness**
      **EXCLUDES**    *coma:*
            *diabetic (250.2-250.3)*
            *hepatic (572.2)*
            *originating in the perinatal period (779.2)*

    780.01    **Coma**
        DEF: State of unconsciousness from which the patient cannot be awakened.

    780.02    **Transient alteration of awareness**
        DEF: Temporary, recurring spells of reduced consciousness.

    780.03    **Persistent vegetative state**
        DEF: Persistent wakefulness without consciousness due to nonfunctioning cerebral cortex.

    780.09    **Other**
        Drowsiness     Stupor
        Semicoma     Unconsciousness
        Somnolence

    780.1    **Hallucinations**
        Hallucinations:     Hallucinations:
          NOS          olfactory
          auditory      tactile
          gustatory
        **EXCLUDES**    *those associated with mental disorders, as functional*
            *psychoses (295.0-298.9)*
          *organic brain syndromes (290.0-294.9, 310.0-310.9)*
          *visual hallucinations (368.16)*

        DEF: Perception of external stimulus in absence of stimulus; inability to distinguish between real and imagined.

✓5ᵗʰ 779.8    **Other specified conditions originating in the perinatal period**

    779.81    **Neonatal bradycardia**
        **EXCLUDES**    *abnormality in fetal heart rate or rhythm*
              *complicating labor and delivery*
              *(763.81-763.83)*
           *bradycardia due to birth asphyxia (768.5-768.9)*

    779.82    **Neonatal tachycardia**
        **EXCLUDES**    *abnormality in fetal heart rate or rhythm*
              *complicating labor and delivery*
              *(763.81-763.83)*

    779.89    **Other specified conditions originating in the perinatal period**

**Figure 11-2** • Sample page from ICD-9-CM, Volume 1, showing categories, subheadings, and so on.

| TABLE 11-1   ICD-9-CM Appendices | |
| --- | --- |
| *The following five appendices are found in Volume 1.* | |
| **Title** | **Description** |
| Appendix A: Morphology of Neoplasms | This appendix is used in conjunction with Chapter 2 in ICD-9-CM when coding neoplasms. It lists the five-digit alphanumeric codes used to identify the morphology of a neoplasm. For example, in the morphology code M8070/3, the 8070 indicates that the morphology is squamous cell carcinoma. The "/3" indicates that it is the primary site. |
| Appendix B: Glossary of Mental Disorders | Alphabetic list of mental disorders, including detailed descriptions of each disease. |
| Appendix C: Classification of Drugs by American Hospital Formulary Service (AHFS) List Number and the ICD-9-CM Equivalents | This appendix lists the AHFS list number (e.g., 24:04 for cardiac drugs) and the ICD-9-CM code number for each one (e.g., 24.04 cardiac drugs would be equivalent to category 972.9, the ICD-9-CM category of "other and unspecified agents primarily affecting the cardiovascular system"). |
| Appendix D: Classification of Industrial Accidents by Agency | This includes codes that can be used as a supplement to describe types of equipment or materials that may be responsible for an industrial accident or illness. |
| Appendix E: List of Three-Digit Categories | This is a list of all three-digit categories in ICD-9-CM. |

*Note*: Appendices A through D are not recognized by most government programs, such as Medicare and Medicaid. As previously mentioned, ICD-9-CM has other uses, however, and you may find that you need the appendices to track such things as disorders treated.

of consciousness), and the fifth digit is the highest level of definition (e.g., 780.01, coma). Volume 1 also includes five appendices, which are outlined in Table 11-1.

In both ICD-9-CM and ICD-10-CM, you must always code a diagnosis to its highest level of specificity. Using a diagnosis code when another, more accurate, code is available is considered **truncated coding** resulting in claim denials and lost revenue for the practice.

## Supplementary Classifications

Supplementary classifications in ICD-9-CM Volume 1 include V and E codes. These supplementary classifications have been replaced in ICD-10-CM with Chapter 20, *External Causes of Morbidity*, and Chapter 21, *Factors Influencing Health Status and Contact with Health Services.*

### Factors Influencing Health Status

**V codes,** which range from V01 to V82 in ICD-9-CM and Z00 to Z99 in Chapter 21 in ICD-10-CM, provide a means of indexing the reason for medical services for other than current or genuine illness, such as a personal or family history of illness and immunizations. An example of using a code from this supplementary code section would be for a person with a personal history of a malignant neoplasm of the stomach. Because of this history, it would be important for this patient to have regular checkups. You would not want to code the visit neoplasm of the stomach, because that would imply the

patient has the malignant neoplasm at this visit. These supplementary codes may be used alone if no disease diagnosis is appropriate or as the second or third code to help better explain the reason for the visit. Chapter 21 in ICD-10-CM gives many additional codes to use along with other diagnoses codes to further explain the reason for medical encounters including codes for lifestyle problems such as tobacco use (Z72.0) or lack of physical exercise (Z72.3).

### External Causes of Injury

**E codes,** which range from E800 to E999 in ICD-9-CM and Chapter 20 in ICD-10-CM, are used to classify external causes of injuries and poisoning. These codes are used in conjunction with other diagnosis codes to help to provide information of interest to industrial medicine, insurance underwriters, national safety programs, public health agencies, and others concerned with causes of injuries (e.g., auto accidents, accidents caused by heavy industrial machinery). These codes do not affect reimbursement.

ICD-9-CM, Volume 2, Section 3, has a separate index to access E codes, the Alphabetic Index to External Causes of Injury and Poisoning.

## CHECKPOINT QUESTION

5. List four reasons for using supplemental codes.

## Alphabetic Index to Diseases

ICD-9-CM and ICD-10-CM have an Alphabetic Index to Diseases and Injuries. Both code sets list main terms in bold and in alphabetical order with subterms listed alphabetically and indented underneath the main terms. Always check all indentations in the index under the condition to ensure that you have the one most appropriate to the diagnosis you intend to code.

The alphabetic index is organized into two sections for both ICD-9-CM and ICD-10-CM; however, ICD-9-CM also has a third section for *External Causes* that has been replaced by Chapter 20 in ICD-10-CM:

- Section 1, Alphabetic Index to Diseases and Injuries, is organized by main terms printed in boldface type. Section 1 is used for reporting the reason for patient encounters for most insurance claims. Following the main term is a code number, which refers you to the tabular listing. You must not accept this number as the correct code without a cross-reference or check of the tabular list. Never code directly from the alphabetic index. This could result in an incomplete or incorrect coding assignment. For example, if you have a patient with fluid overload and you look under fluid, it may seem logical to code the first code under fluid, which is abdomen, but your patient is generally retaining fluid. If you use the alphabetic index only, you do not know that the correct ICD-9-CM code is actually 276.6, fluid overload, which excludes ascites, 789.5, and localized edema, 782.3. Box 11-1 outlines several exceptions to the main term rule.
- Section 2, Table of Drugs and Chemicals, includes an extensive listing of drugs, chemical substances, and toxic agents. It also shows E codes and American Hospital Formulary Service (AHFS) list numbers, which are in the table under the main term *Drug*.
- Section 3 in ICD-9-CM is an Alphabetic Index to External Cases of Injuries and Poisonings that leads you to codes that describe circumstances of injuries, accidents, and violence. These codes are not used for medical diagnoses. Main entries in this section usually are a type of accident or violence (e.g., assault, fall, collision). These codes can supplement the diagnostic code, but they should never be used alone or as principal diagnosis codes. E codes are frequently used with these codes. For example, a person who fractured a tibia in a fall off a sidewalk curb would be given a code from Chapter 17, Volume 1, in the ICD-9-CM for the injury (e.g., fracture of the tibia, closed, is 823.80), and an additional code, E880.0, indicates that the accident was a fall off a sidewalk curb. Again, this section has been replaced with Chapter 20 in ICD-10-CM.

### CHECKPOINT QUESTION

6. What are Supplementary codes to classify Factors Influencing Health Status used for?

---

**BOX 11-1    Tips Regarding Personnel Manuals**

Sometimes, you have to think outside the box. Most of the time, locating the condition instead of the location works well, but sometimes a diagnosis will stump you:

1. Obstetric conditions may be found under the main terms *Delivery*, *Pregnancy*, and *Puerperal*.
2. Complications of medical or surgical procedures or primary diagnoses can be found under complications. For example, complications of pneumonia would be found under *Complications*—not *Pneumonia*.
3. Conditions arising from an earlier problem or procedure are called "late effects" and can be found under the words *Late effects*, *Due to ...*, *As a result of ...*, *Residual*, etc.
4. Lacerations can be found under *Wounds*.
5. V codes are codes used for patients who are not sick. They may be found by looking for terms such as *Admission, Examination, History of ..., Observation, Problem with ..., Status, Vaccination, Encounter for ..., Follow-up*, etc.

## Inpatient Coding

ICD-9-CM, Volume 3, the Tabular List and Alphabetic Index of Procedures, is used in inpatient facilities and is based on anatomy, not surgical specialty. There are no alphabetic characters in these procedure codes. The codes are two-digit categories with a maximum of two decimal digits where necessary. Most refer to surgical procedures, and the rest cover miscellaneous diagnostic and therapeutic procedures. An example of a procedure code is 31.61, larynx laceration suture. Volume 3 is used for inpatient coding only. As previously mentioned, this volume has been replaced by ICD-10-PCS.

## COG LOCATING THE APPROPRIATE CODE

Box 11-2 outlines CMS guidelines for diagnostic coding. These are explained next.

### Using the Diagnosis Coding Conventions

Figure 11-3 lists the conventions used in the ICD-9-CM indexes. **Conventions** are rules that apply to the assignment of codes, and many of the conventions remain

## BOX 11-2 CMS Diagnostic Coding Guidelines

CMS defines specific guidelines that provide the basic knowledge necessary to apply the correct diagnosis codes. Although these guidelines were developed for use in submitting government claims, most insurance companies have also adopted them. Many variations exist among the private insurance companies; therefore, care must be taken in recognizing the different requirements for each third-party payer. Most coders operate on the assumption that the government regulations are the strictest, and following those guidelines will satisfy most third-party payers.

1. Identify each service and procedure, or supply with a diagnosis code to describe the diagnosis, symptom, complaint, condition, or problem.
2. Identify services or visits for circumstances other than disease or injury, such as follow-up care after chemotherapy, with supplementary codes provided for this purpose.
3. Code the reason for the visit first and code any coexisting conditions that affect the treatment of the patient for that visit or procedure as supplementary information. Do not code a diagnosis that is no longer applicable.
4. Code to the highest degree of specificity. Carry the numeric code to the highest number of digits possible for the specific diagnosis.
5. Code a chronic diagnosis as often as it is applicable to the patient's treatment.
6. When only ancillary services are provided, list the appropriate supplementary code for the reason for the visit (V code from ICD-9 or Chapter 21 from ICD-10) first and the problem second.
7. For ambulatory or outpatient surgical procedures, code the diagnosis applicable to the procedure. If the postoperative diagnosis is different from the preoperative diagnosis, use the postoperative diagnosis.

## WHAT IF?

**You need to code a condition described as acute, chronic, or both. What code should you use?**

When a particular condition is described as both acute and chronic, code it according to the subentries in the alphabetic index for the condition. If there are separate entries listed for *acute*, *subacute*, and *chronic*, use both codes. The first code listed should be for the acute condition, the reason the patient came to the office today. Respiratory and orthopedic conditions tend to be acute and chronic. That is, a patient with emphysema will always have underlying symptoms of progressive disease, but during the spring, pollen may aggravate the condition and cause acute breathing problems.

## Main Term

When trying to locate a diagnosis with more than one word, look first under the main term or condition. Often, a diagnosis may be an **eponym** (e.g., Ménière disease or syndrome). These terms can be found under the main term *Disease* or *Syndrome*. In the diagnosis of breast cyst, the main term is *Cyst*. Find the condition, not the location. Imagine how large any diagnosis codebook would have to be to list every condition possible for the leg, the arm, or any other location. Instead, the condition is listed, and the arm or leg would be found under that term. For example, the diagnosis code for fracture of the left tibia would be found by looking up the main term fracture, not tibia.

## Additional Digits

In many instances, additional digits have been added to a category to provide more detail or **specificity**. These are subcategory codes. In ICD-9-CM, some codes have a fourth or fifth digit because of the need to code to a higher specificity, and in ICD-10-CM, there can be four to seven additional digits. Only digits that are not further subdivided are considered actual codes in ICD-10-CM. Figure 11-4 shows samples of fifth-digit classifications from the ICD-9-CM, Volumes 1 and 2. The code 807.1 tells the third-party payer that the patient was seen for an open fracture of a rib. The fifth digit is added to describe how many ribs. A patient who fractured two ribs would be assigned the code 807.12. This gives a more thorough picture of the patient's problem and enables the payer to determine whether the treatment is medically necessary. Figure 11-5 is an example of the seven-digit classifications from the ICD-10-CM for an initial encounter for an open fracture of a rib. When coding from this section, note that a letter must be added as the seventh character to identify the encounter and the type of fracture.

the same for ICD-10-CM. They are found throughout both the Index to Diseases and the Tabular List and include general notes using specific terms, cross-references, abbreviations, punctuation marks, symbols, typeface, and format. They direct and guide the coder to the appropriate code and should be strictly adhered to. Each publisher uses these same conventions, and many add more to assist coders in providing the most complete and accurate reason for the encounter. For example, when you locate the word *Itch*, you will find "See pruritus," the medical term for severe itching. This is a helpful tool for coders who are unfamiliar with medical terminology.

## Conventions

**Brackets [ ]**   Brackets enclose synonyms, alternate wording, or explanatory phrases.

**Colon :**   A colon is used after an incomplete term that needs one or more of the modifiers that follow to make it assignable to a given category.

**Parentheses ( )**   Parentheses enclose supplementary words that may be present or absent in the statement of a disease or procedure, without affecting the code number to which it is assigned.

**NEC (not elsewhere classifiable)**   Alerts the coder that the specified form of the condition is classified differently.  Codes following NEC should be used only when the coder lacks the information necessary to code the term in a more specific category.

**NOS (not otherwise specified)**   The coder should continue to look for a more specific code.

**"Includes"**   Indicates separate terms as adjectives that further modify sites and conditions or to further define or give examples of the content of a certain category.

**"Excludes"**   A box with "excludes" in italics draws the reader's attention to instructions that direct the coder to the proper code.  This convention is found in the Tabular List.

**"See," "See Also," and "See Category"**   Direct the coder to other terms or sections that should be considered.  ALWAYS follow these instructions.

**"Use additional code"**   This directs the coder to add another code to further explain and give the third-party payer a better understanding of a diagnosis.

**"Code First Underlying Disease"**   This direction is used in the tabular list when a reason for an encounter results from another disorder.  The coder is instructed to indicate the underlying disease that caused the current problem or symptom that brought the patient to the office.

## Index to Disease Example

478.1    Other diseases of nasal cavity and sinuses

Abscess  
Necrosis  } Of nose (septum)  
Ulcer

422.92   Septic myocarditis  
Myocarditis, acute or subacute:  
    Pneumococcal  
    Staphylococcal  
Use additional code to identify infectious organism [e.g., Staphylococcus 041.1]

See above example 478.1 (septum) may or may not be present in the diagnosis given.

Infection  
    Streptococcal NEC 041.00  
        Group  
            A 041.01  
            B 041.002

As soon as the bacterium is identified, code for specific infection.

At the time of the service, it has not been established whether a neoplasm is benign or secondary, for example  Remember, you are coding for a date of service with the information documented for that date of service.

INCLUDES   Allergic rhinitis (nonseasonal)  
477 Allergic rhinitis (seasonal)  
Hay fever

EXCLUDES   Allergic rhinitis with asthma (bronchial) (493.0)

Itch (see also Pruritus) 698.9

See 422.92 examples above.

362.72   Retinal dystrophy in other systemic disorders and syndromes  
        Code first underlying disease, as:  
            Bassen-Kornzweig syndrome (272.5)  
            Refsum's disease (356.3)

**Figure 11-3 •** Conventions used in diagnostic coding.

## Primary Codes

In outpatient coding, the **primary diagnosis** is simply the patient's chief complaint or the reason the patient sought medical attention today. It may be a routine follow-up visit, or there may be a new problem. The primary code is listed first on the CMS-1500.

## When More Than One Code Is Used

The revised CMS-1500 version 02-12 form allows the reporting of twelve different diagnosis codes (see Chapter 13). In many cases, more than one code is used for a single patient visit. When patients have more than one diagnosis, it is necessary to convey an accurate picture of the patient's total condition. For example, an elderly patient may have

the following diagnoses listed each time she visits the doctor: degenerative arthritis, type 2 diabetes mellitus, macular degeneration, hypertension, and pernicious anemia. If any of these conditions is related to or affects her treatment, they should be listed as supplementary information. If she visits the doctor because she has influenza and her other diagnoses are not addressed at the visit, it is not necessary to list all the diagnoses given. The primary diagnosis is her reason for coming to the office (symptoms of influenza). But the fact that she is diabetic will affect her treatment and makes her visit medically necessary. Multiple codes should be sequenced with the proper service or procedure code on the proper line of the CMS-1500. Figure 11-6 shows the proper sequencing for another patient's CMS-1500. On Line 1 of Section 24 on the CMS-1500, you place the code and charge for the visit. In Block 24E, the diagnosis

✓4ᵗʰ **807 Fracture of rib(s), sternum, larynx, and trachea**

The following fifth-digit subclassification is for use with codes 807.0-807.1:

0   **rib(s), unspecified**
1   **one rib**
2   **two ribs**
3   **three ribs**
4   **four ribs**
5   **five ribs**
6   **six ribs**
7   **seven ribs**
8   **eight or more ribs**
9   **multiple ribs, unspecified**

✓5ᵗʰ 807.0   **Rib(s), closed**                                    `MSP`
✓5ᵗʰ 807.1   **Rib(s), open**                                      `MSP`
807.2   **Sternum, closed**                                        `MSP`
DEF: Break in flat bone (breast bone) in anterior thorax.

807.3   **Sternum, open**                                          `MSP`
DEF: Break, with open wound, in flat bone in mid anterior thorax.

807.4   **Flail chest**                                            `MSP`
807.5   **Larynx and trachea, closed**                             `MSP`
Hyoid bone                   Trachea
Thyroid cartilage

807.6   **Larynx and trachea, open**                               `MSP`

**A**

**Fracture** — *continued*
multiple — *continued*
skull, specified or unspecified bones, or
face bone(s) with any other bone(s) —
*continued*

Note — *Use the following fifth-digit
subclassification with categories 800, 801,
803, and 804:*

0   *unspecified state of consciousness*
1   *with no loss of consciousness*
2   *with brief [less than one hour] loss
of consciousness*
3   *with moderate [1-24 hours] loss of
consciousness*
4   *with prolonged [more than 24 hours]
loss of consciousness and return to
pre-existing conscious level*
5   *with prolonged [more than 24 hours]
loss of consciousness, without
return to pre-existing conscious level*

Use fifth-digit 5 to designate when a
patient is unconscious and dies
before regaining consciousness,
regardless of the duration of the
loss of consciousness

6   *with loss of consciousness of
unspecified duration*
9   *with concussion, unspecified*

with
contusion, cerebral 804.1
epidural hemorrhage 804.2
extradural hemorrhage 804.2
hemorrhage (intracranial) NEC
804.8
intracranial injury NEC 804.4
laceration, cerebral 804.1
subarachnoid hemorrhage 804.2
subdural hemorrhage 804.2

**B**

**Figure 11-4** • Samples of fifth-digit classifications from ICD-9-CM.**(A)**
Volume 1. **(B)** Volume 2.

code for the ankle injury appears first as referenced on Line 21, Item A, because that is what brought the patient to the office today. On Line 2 of 24A, the laboratory work is listed but is also referenced to the diagnosis on Line 21, Item B, which is the proper code for the patient's diabetes; this is also referenced on the second line of Block 24E. If the patient did not have diabetes, the laboratory work would not be considered reasonable for a patient with an ankle injury. If this procedure were not followed, the laboratory work would be seen as medically unnecessary, and the physician would not be reimbursed.

## Late Effects

**Late effects** are symptoms or conditions arising from an acute illness. The effects are present after treatment for the acute illness or injury has ended. Proper coding sequence requires that you list the code number

| | | | |
|---|---|---|---|
| **S22** | **Fracture of rib(s), sternum and thoracic spine** | | |
| | The appropriate 7<sup>th</sup> character is to be added to each code from category S22 | | |

**S22**   **Fracture of rib(s), sternum and thoracic spine**
The appropriate 7$^{th}$ character is to be added to each code from category S22
A fracture not identified as open or closed should be coded to closed

| | | |
|---|---|---|
| A | initial encounter for closed fracture |
| B | initial encounter for open fracture |
| D | subsequent encounter for fracture with routine healing |
| G | subsequent encounter for fracture with delayed healing |
| K | subsequent encounter for fracture with nonunion |
| S | sequela |

**S22.0**       **Fracture of thoracic vertebra**

**S22.000  Wedge compression fracture of unspecified thoracic vertebra**

**S22.001  Stable burst fracture of unspecified thoracic vertebra**

**S22.002  Unstable burst fracture of unspecified thoracic vertebra**

**S22.008  Other fracture of unspecified thoracic vertebra**

**S22.009  Unspecified fracture of unspecified thoracic vertebra**

**Figure 11-5** • Samples of seventh-digit classification from ICD-10.

identifying the residual or current condition first, with the code number identifying the cause or original illness or injury listed second. Keywords used in the patient's medical records defining late effects include "late," "due to an old injury," "due to a previous illness/injury," "due to an illness or injury occurring a year or more ago," "sequela of ...," "as a result of ...," "resulting from ...," and so on. Patients who are status postcerebrovascular accident (CVA) may have residual effects from their original stroke, for example, and may have a diagnosis of left hemiparesis as a result of CVA 3 years ago. Figure 11-7 is a sample listing of a late effect from the ICD-9-CM.

## Coding Suspected Conditions

In the inpatient setting, coders list conditions after the patient's testing is complete. In other words, they are coding with complete information. In outpatient settings, however, the coder reports the reason for the patient visit as it occurs. When filing claims, the coder is limited by the information and documentation on hand at the time of the patient visit. If at the end of the visit the diagnosis is not confirmed, the physician may indicate "rule out," "suspected," or "probable." For example, a patient who comes in complaining of headache may be sent for magnetic resonance imaging (MRI) of the head because the physician suspects a serious disorder. On the patient's encounter form, the physician may list the diagnosis as "rule out brain tumor." It is not accurate to code the visit as brain tumor before it is confirmed by MRI. On this first visit to the physician's office, the reason for being seen is headache. The patient's symptom (headache) is the only confirmed reason for the encounter at this point. On the second visit to the doctor, the MRI has confirmed a glioma in the frontal lobe. For the second and all subsequent visits, glioma is coded as the reason for the encounter.

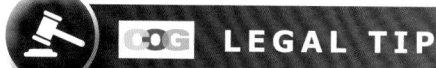

## CHECKPOINT QUESTION

7. When coding a visit on a date before a definitive diagnosis is made, what is coded?

**LEGAL TIP**

### Don't Give Patients a Disease They Don't Have!

It is important that you use the code that explains the patient's situation accurately. Coding AIDS before that diagnosis is made could be construed as defamation of character and even libel. Some patients just want to be tested for HIV, but there are no signs or symptoms.

The ICD-9-CM and ICD-10-CM code sets offer a variety of supplementary codes for HIV testing. For a patient who has the test simply because he or she wants to know, you will use ICD-9 supplementary code V72.6, which is simply "laboratory examination." The code used for a patient who has known exposure is V01.79, which is "contact with or exposure to communicable diseases and/or other viral diseases." For patients who want to be tested because they are worried about exposure, V69.2 is used. This code is "high-risk sexual behavior." In this case, two codes would be used: V69.2 and V01.79. This approach will ensure that a patient is not assigned a diagnosis code for a problem he or she does not have.

## Documentation Requirements

As discussed throughout this chapter, you should choose the code assigned to any given claim for a service or

# HEALTH INSURANCE CLAIM FORM

APPROVED BY NATIONAL UNIFORM CLAIM COMMITTEE (NUCC) 02/12

[ ][ ] PICA

| | | | | | | | | |
|---|---|---|---|---|---|---|---|---|

1. MEDICARE [X] (Medicare#)   MEDICAID [ ] (Medicaid#)   TRICARE [ ] (ID#/DoD#)   CHAMPVA [ ] (Member ID#)   GROUP HEALTH PLAN [ ] (ID#)   FECA BLK LUNG [ ] (ID#)   OTHER [ ] (ID#)

1a. INSURED'S I.D. NUMBER   (For Program in Item 1)
**001000101A**

2. PATIENT'S NAME (Last Name, First Name, Middle Initial)
**DISHMAN NAOMI A**

3. PATIENT'S BIRTH DATE   MM 04 DD 14 YY 24   SEX M [ ] F [X]

4. INSURED'S NAME (Last Name, First Name, Middle Initial)
**SAME**

5. PATIENT'S ADDRESS (No., Street)
**405 CAROLINA AVE**

6. PATIENT RELATIONSHIP TO INSURED
Self [X]  Spouse [ ]  Child [ ]  Other [ ]

7. INSURED'S ADDRESS (No., Street)

CITY  **DANVILLE**   STATE **VA**

8. RESERVED FOR NUCC USE

CITY   STATE

ZIP CODE  **24540**   TELEPHONE (Include Area Code) **( 434 ) 555-5555**

ZIP CODE   TELEPHONE (Include Area Code) ( )

9. OTHER INSURED'S NAME (Last Name, First Name, Middle Initial)

10. IS PATIENT'S CONDITION RELATED TO:

11. INSURED'S POLICY GROUP OR FECA NUMBER
**NONE**

a. OTHER INSURED'S POLICY OR GROUP NUMBER

a. EMPLOYMENT? (Current or Previous)
[ ] YES   [X] NO

a. INSURED'S DATE OF BIRTH   MM DD YY   SEX M [ ] F [ ]

b. RESERVED FOR NUCC USE

b. AUTO ACCIDENT?   PLACE (State)
[ ] YES   [X] NO

b. OTHER CLAIM ID (Designated by NUCC)

c. RESERVED FOR NUCC USE

c. OTHER ACCIDENT?
[ ] YES   [X] NO

c. INSURANCE PLAN NAME OR PROGRAM NAME

d. INSURANCE PLAN NAME OR PROGRAM NAME

10d. CLAIM CODES (Designated by NUCC)

d. IS THERE ANOTHER HEALTH BENEFIT PLAN?
[ ] YES   [X] NO   If yes, complete items 9, 9a, and 9d.

**READ BACK OF FORM BEFORE COMPLETING & SIGNING THIS FORM.**
12. PATIENT'S OR AUTHORIZED PERSON'S SIGNATURE I authorize the release of any medical or other information necessary to process this claim. I also request payment of government benefits either to myself or to the party who accepts assignment below.

SIGNED **SOF**   DATE **06/01/2015**

13. INSURED'S OR AUTHORIZED PERSON'S SIGNATURE I authorize payment of medical benefits to the undersigned physician or supplier for services described below.

SIGNED **SOF**

14. DATE OF CURRENT ILLNESS, INJURY, or PREGNANCY (LMP)   MM DD YY   QUAL.

15. OTHER DATE   QUAL.   MM DD YY

16. DATES PATIENT UNABLE TO WORK IN CURRENT OCCUPATION
FROM MM DD YY   TO MM DD YY

17. NAME OF REFERRING PROVIDER OR OTHER SOURCE
**DK   JOSEPH G NORTH MD**

17a.
17b. NPI  **9876512344**

18. HOSPITALIZATION DATES RELATED TO CURRENT SERVICES
FROM MM DD YY   TO MM DD YY

19. ADDITIONAL CLAIM INFORMATION (Designated by NUCC)

20. OUTSIDE LAB?   $ CHARGES
[ ] YES   [ ] NO

21. DIAGNOSIS OR NATURE OF ILLNESS OR INJURY  Relate A-L to service line below (24E)   ICD Ind. [ ]
A. **S93.402A**   B. **W10.9**   C. **E11.9**   D.
E.   F.   G.   H.
I.   J.   K.   L.

22. RESUBMISSION CODE   ORIGINAL REF. NO.

23. PRIOR AUTHORIZATION NUMBER

| 24. A. DATE(S) OF SERVICE From MM DD YY | To MM DD YY | B. PLACE OF SERVICE | C. EMG | D. PROCEDURES, SERVICES, OR SUPPLIES (Explain Unusual Circumstances) CPT/HCPCS | MODIFIER | E. DIAGNOSIS POINTER | F. $ CHARGES | G. DAYS OR UNITS | H. EPSDT Family Plan | I. ID. QUAL | J. RENDERING PROVIDER ID. # |
|---|---|---|---|---|---|---|---|---|---|---|---|
| 1  05 28 15 | 05 28 15 | 11 | | 99213 | | A | 100 00 | 1 | | NPI | 9876512344 |
| 2  05 28 15 | 05 28 15 | 11 | | 82947 | | C | 25 00 | 1 | | NPI | 9876512344 |
| 3 | | | | | | | | | | NPI | |
| 4 | | | | | | | | | | NPI | |
| 5 | | | | | | | | | | NPI | |
| 6 | | | | | | | | | | NPI | |

25. FEDERAL TAX I.D. NUMBER   SSN EIN
**54-0111111**   [ ] [X]

26. PATIENT'S ACCOUNT NO.

27. ACCEPT ASSIGNMENT? (For govt. claims, see back)
[X] YES   [ ] NO

28. TOTAL CHARGE
$ **125** 00

29. AMOUNT PAID
$

30. Rsvd for NUCC Use

31. SIGNATURE OF PHYSICIAN OR SUPPLIER INCLUDING DEGREES OR CREDENTIALS (I certify that the statements on the reverse apply to this bill and are made a part thereof.)
SIGNED **SOF**   DATE **6/1/2015**

32. SERVICE FACILITY LOCATION INFORMATION
1111 GRAYSON STREET
DANVILLE VA  24540

a. NPI   b.

33. BILLING PROVIDER INFO & PH # ( 434 ) 255-0422
JOSEPH G. NORTH MD
1111 GRAYSON STREET
DANVILLE, VA  24540

a. NPI   b.

NUCC Instruction Manual available at: www.nucc.org   PLEASE PRINT OR TYPE   APPROVED OMB-0938-1197 FORM 1500 (02-12)

**Figure 11-6** • Sample CMS-1500 claim form indicating proper sequencing.

**LATE EFFECTS OF INJURIES, POISONINGS, TOXIC EFFECTS, AND OTHER EXTERNAL CAUSES (905-909)**

Note: These categories are to be used to indicate conditions classifiable to 800-999 as the cause of late effects, which are themselves classified elsewhere. The "late effects" include those specified as such, or as sequelae, which may occur at any time after the acute injury.

**✓4ᵗʰ 905 Late effects of musculoskeletal and connective tissue injuries**

905.0 **Late effect of fracture of skull and face bones**
Late effect of injury classifiable to 800-804

905.1 **Late effect of fracture of spine and trunk without mention of spinal cord lesion**
Late effect of injury classifiable to 805, 807-809

905.2 **Late effect of fracture of upper extremities**
Late effect of injury classifiable to 810-819

905.3 **Late effect of fracture of neck of femur**
Late effect of injury classifiable to 820

905.4 **Late effect of fracture of lower extremities**
Late effect of injury classifiable to 821-827

905.5 **Late effect of fracture of multiple and unspecified bones**
Late effect of injury classifiable to 828-829

905.6 **Late effect of dislocation**
Late effect of injury classifiable to 830-839

905.7 **Late effect of sprain and strain without mention of tendon injury**
Late effect of injury classifiable to 840-848, except tendon injury

905.8 **Late effect of tendon injury**
Late effect of tendon injury due to:
open wound [injury classifiable to 880-884 with .2, 890-894 with .2]
sprain and strain [injury classifiable to 840-848]

905.9 **Late effect of traumatic amputation**
Late effect of injury classifiable to 885-887, 895-897
**EXCLUDES** *late amputation stump complication (997.60-997.69)*

**A**

**Late**

**Late** — *continued*
effect(s) (of) — continued
tuberculosis — *continued*
genitourinary (conditions classifiable to 016) 137.2
pulmonary (conditions classifiable to 010-012) 137.0
specified organs NEC (conditions classifiable to 014, 017-018) 137.4
viral encephalitis (conditions classifiable to 049.8, 049.9, 062-064) 139.0
wound, open
extremity (injury classifiable to 880-884 and 890-894, except .2) 906.1
tendon (injury classifiable to 880-884 with .2 and 890-894 with.2) 905.8
head, neck, and trunk (injury classifiable to 870-879) 906.0

**B**

**Figure 11-7 •** Sample section of late effects in ICD-9-CM. **(A)** Volume 1. **(B)** Volume 2.

procedure based on the documentation available in the patient's record at the time of the service. An audit may be conducted by the government, a managed care company, or a health care organization to determine compliance and to detect fraud. Audits may also be initiated by the practice as part of an ongoing compliance plan to verify and make necessary corrections in the billing process (not the medical documentation!) to maintain accurate billing and coding. Remember, if it's not in the chart, it did not happen. Auditors verify the codes used based on information recorded in the chart on the date of service.

## COG THE FUTURE OF DIAGNOSTIC CODING: INTERNATIONAL CLASSIFICATION OF DISEASES, CLINICAL MODIFICATION, TENTH REVISION

With the impending implementation of the International Classification of Diseases, Tenth Revision (ICD-10), investing time now to learn this important code set is vital to the financial health of the practice. Although both ICD-9-CM and ICD-10-CM have similarities in their structure, the vast amount of codes added by ICD-10-CM and increased detail of codes will require the professional medical assistant to review anatomy and human diseases to better understand code selections. The new codes will enable providers and payers to track and analyze information about patient encounters such as the health status of a certain population. A basic knowledge of ICD-9-CM, however, still remains valuable and necessary for claim submission and follow-up for dates of service prior to the implementation of ICD-10-CM codes.

## Conventions

Many of the same conventions will be used. One major difference deals with the use of "Excludes" notes. With ICD-10-CM, there will be two types of excludes notes: *Excludes1* and *Excludes2*. "Excludes1" means not coded here and does not allow for exceptions. It means that the two codes in question cannot be used together. "Excludes2" indicates that if medical documentation supports both conditions, both may be coded. For example:

Excludes1: Intestinal malabsorption (K90) sequelae of protein–calorie malnutrition (E64.0)
Excludes2: Nutritional anemias (D50 to D53) starvation (T73.0)

In the above example, you are told that for the malnutrition codes in the range of E40 to E46, you *cannot* use codes in the K90 category or in the E64.0 category. However, for the malnutrition codes in the range of E40 to E46, you *can* include nutritional anemias in the range of D50 to D53 and starvation, T73.0, provided that both conditions exist and are well documented by the physician in the medical record.

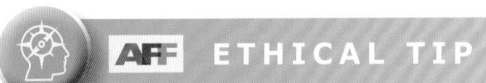

### ETHICAL TIP

### Don't Break the Rules

Imagine an unethical patient asking a physician to break the rules. Unfortunately, it happens. Some insurance companies still offer limited coverage when the patient is not sick. Routine exams and tests may be covered at a reduced rate or not at all. For this reason, some patients may think that if the doctor codes the claim with a diagnosis, then that makes the service medically necessary, and their insurance will pay. Coding based on anything other than what the documentation proves is wrong. It is not only unethical, it is illegal. If a patient asks you to be dishonest, explain that this would be unethical. Tell the patient that random audits are often carried out by the CMS to ensure that the medical chart indicates that the services and procedures on claims were actually performed and the reasons were legitimate.

## Placeholder "X"

In ICD-9-CM, coders are instructed to use a fifth digit when applicable. With the addition of more characters, some disorders will require a seventh character in ICD-10-CM. In some cases, there will be no fifth or sixth digit used, but a seventh digit is required. Coding for this type of diagnosis necessitates the use of a placeholder "X" to fill in the missing digits up to the seventh digit that is required by the specific code. For example:

032.1: Maternal care for breech presentation

The seventh character is either 1 for a single gestation or 1 to 9 for multiple gestations. Each fetus must be identified in the record so that consistent designation can be made to the correct fetus:

0: Not applicable or unspecified
1: Fetus 1
2: Fetus 2
3: Fetus 3
4: Fetus 4
5: Fetus 5
9: Other fetus

Therefore, if the maternal care is for a single gestation, the correct code is 032.1XX0. If the "X" placeholder is not there and 032.10 is assigned, the code is incorrect.

## Special Codes

As mentioned above, E codes and V codes are no longer located in a supplemental listing. In ICD-10-CM, these types of codes have been placed into their own chapters. Category Y93 includes activity codes, which are used with other diagnoses codes to indicate that the reason for the encounter was a result of some sort of activity, such as an injury that occurred while riding a roller coaster. These new codes are used together with an external cause code and place of occurrence code. Seventh characters specify if the activity was work related, non–work related, student activity, or military activity.

In ICD-10-CM, the codes for diabetes mellitus will change considerably. They provide more detail than does the current 250 category in ICD-9-CM. Box 11-3 outlines the new, more specific diabetes codes.

Medical coders must learn to use the new ICD-10-CM codebooks and will find training opportunities through the various coding professional organizations and the CMS. It will be a challenge to learn, but the new system promises to enhance efficiency and accuracy and will ultimately improve the important process of coding claims.

### CHECKPOINT QUESTION

8. How will the implementation of ICD-10-CM improve the coding of reasons for services?

## BOX 11-3    Diabetes Mellitus Codes in ICD-10-CM

Categories E08 to E13 are as follows:

E08:    Diabetes mellitus due to underlying conditions

E09:    Drug- or chemical-induced diabetes mellitus

E10:    Type 1 diabetes mellitus

E11:    Type 2 diabetes mellitus

E13:    Other specified diabetes mellitus

As you can see, these three-character codes do not provide full information. To provide further detail, a fourth digit describes underlying conditions, and the fifth and sixth digits provide even more specificity. Just as in ICD-9-CM, you must take the code to the last character provided within the category.

For example, for a diagnosis of diabetes mellitus type 2 with moderate nonproliferative retinopathy without macular edema, the code will be chosen from the following:

E11.3:    Type 2 diabetes mellitus with ophthalmic complications

E11.33:    Type 2 diabetes mellitus with moderate non-proliferative diabetic retinopathy

E11.331:    Type 2 diabetes mellitus with moderate non-proliferative diabetic retinopathy with macular edema

E11.339:    Type 2 diabetes mellitus with moderate nonproliferative diabetic retinopathy without macular edema

*Source*: Excerpted from Falen TJ. *Learning to code with ICD-9-CM 2011*. Baltimore, MD: Lippincott Williams & Wilkins; 2010.

 ## ROLE-PLAYING ACTIVITY

While reviewing denied claims, Tonya Little, CMA, noted that most of the diagnosis coding problems were coded by only one of the three billers in the office. This biller consistently had truncated coding errors, and Tonya must address them with her to correct the problem and prevent future denials of claims. How can Tonya handle this in a professional manner? What attitude should Tonya have when she approaches the biller? Are there any reference materials she should have available when they meet? If you are playing the part of the biller, how would you feel if someone brought a problem to your attention indicating you were causing claim denials and reimbursement problems? How would you respond to Tonya? Your instructor will give you additional information about this activity!

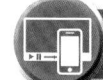 ## MEDIA MENU

**Student Resources** on thePoint®

• **CMA/RMA Certification Exam Review**

**Internet Resources**
**World Health Organization**
http://www.who.int/en

**U.S. Department of Health and Human Services**
http://www.hhs.gov

**Centers for Medicare and Medicaid Services**
http://www.cms.gov

**American Health Information Management Association**
http://www.ahima.org

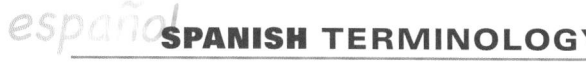 ## SPANISH TERMINOLOGY

**¿Que significan estas cantidades? ¿Es esta la factura?**
What are all these numbers? Is that my bill?

**No, estos números son códigos que su compañia de seguros necesita para procesar su reclamo.**
No, these numbers are codes required and used by your insurance company to be able to process the claim.

**Se les llaman números de codificación.**
These are called coding numbers.

**¿Por favor podría verificar que la información en la factura es correcta?**
Can you please verify that the information in the bill is accurate?

## EMR Activity

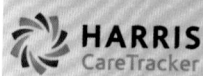

Harris CareTracker is a Web-based electronic medical record (EMR) application that you will use for the EMR activities included in this section at the end of each chapter. This application is actually used in physician offices but is provided to you through the publisher, Wolters Kluwer Health, to give you hands-on practice working with EMRs. Your instructor will have more information about accessing your username, log-in, and Quickstart guide.

### Prerequisite Activities in Harris CareTracker

• *The Getting Started and Quickstart documents and EMR Activities Step-by-Step Instructions are available at* http://thePoint.lww.com/KronenbergerComp5e

### Activity Details

Tonya Little, CMA, needs to review the Great Falls Medical Center encounter form to update current diagnostic codes. Locate the *GFMC encounter* form located in Harris CareTracker, and using the most current edition of the ICD-CM (ICD-9 or ICD-10), review the diagnosis codes to determine which codes need to be updated or replaced.

## Chapter Summary

- Medical outpatient diagnostic coding involves the use of numbers to describe diseases, injuries, and other reasons for seeking medical care. ICD-9-CM and ICD-10-CM provide an index to report and track diseases. Diagnostic coding is linked to reimbursement because it assures that the physician's service or procedure was medically necessary.
- As a medical assistant, you must understand the format and guidelines for assigning a code or reason for each encounter, treatment, and/or service.
- ICD-10-CM will replace the current version with different code formatting. The implementation date may be found on the CMS Web site at www.cms.gov.

## Warm-Ups for Critical Thinking

1. Tom Barksdale has been seen by the physician for controlled non–insulin-dependent type 2 diabetes mellitus for about 10 years. While being seen for a routine check of his blood sugar, he complains of numbness and tingling in his left lower leg and foot. An x-ray of both legs is performed because poor circulation in the extremities can be a complication of diabetes. The x-ray confirms the diagnosis of peripheral neuropathy. Which ICD-9-CM code should be listed with the office visit? Which ICD-10-CM code should be listed with the office visit? Which code indicates the reason for the x-ray? Which code should be placed on the CMA-1500 first as the primary diagnosis or reason for the visit?

2. Determine the main term for the following multiple word diagnoses: gestational diabetes; amyotrophic lateral sclerosis; benign, localized hyperplasia of prostate; and nursemaid's elbow.

3. A patient calls complaining of pain and swelling in the right hand since awakening this morning. The patient comes in, sees the doctor, and returns to the front desk with an encounter form that states that his diagnosis is "gout." In order to make this diagnosis, the physician would need to know the patient's uric acid level. You know that the patient just had blood drawn for the test. It is a test that must be sent to an outside lab. Do you still code today's visit as "gout?" What would you do?

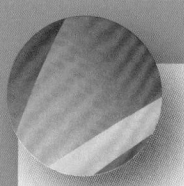

**PSY** PROCEDURE 11-1

## Locating a Diagnostic Code

**PSY**   Perform diagnostic coding; utilize tactful communication skills with medical providers to ensure accurate code selection

**Purpose:** To quickly and accurately locate a code based on reasonableness for the medical service or procedure performed

**Equipment:** Diagnosis, ICD-9-CM Volumes I and II or ICD-10-CM Codebook, medical dictionary

| STEPS | PURPOSE |
|---|---|
| 1. Using the diagnosis "chronic rheumatoid arthritis," choose the main term within the diagnostic statement. If necessary, look up the word(s) in your dictionary (main term is *Arthritis*). | In a diagnosis that has more than one word, choosing the condition, not the location, helps find the code quickly. If you don't know what the word(s) means, you cannot make the most accurate choice. |
| 2. Locate the main term in Volume 2. | The alphabetic list is in Volume 2 of ICD-9-CM and in the alphabetic index in ICD-10-CM. This generally identifies the condition or disease with the corresponding diagnosis code. |
| 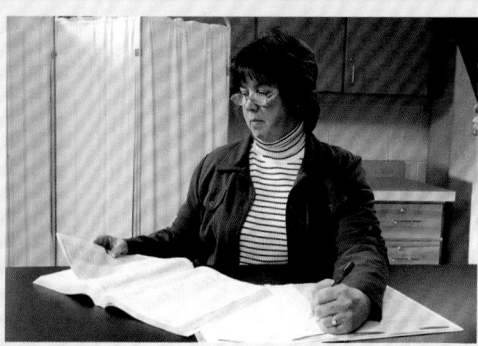 **Step 2.** Locate the main term. | |
| 3. Refer to all notes and conventions under the main term. | These notes and conventions are there for a reason. In order to find the correct code, you should pay close attention to them. |
| 4. Find the appropriate indented subordinate term (appropriate indented subordinate term is *rheumatoid*). | The indented terms go with the terms above them. |
| 5. Follow any relevant instructions, such as "See also." | If the book wants you to see another code, you should go there to determine if the code you have chosen is the correct code. |
| 6. Confirm the selected code by cross-referencing to the Tabular List (Volume 1 in ICD-9-CM). Make sure you have added any necessary additional digits. | The tabular list indicates if additional digits are needed to further specify a diagnosis. Remember, if there are additional digits, they must be used. |
| 7. Assign the code. | Without an appropriate code to explain the medical necessity of a service, insurance will not pay! |
| 8. **AFF** Your physician instructs you to assign a diagnosis code to a claim for a patient that is not documented in the medical record. What would you do? | |

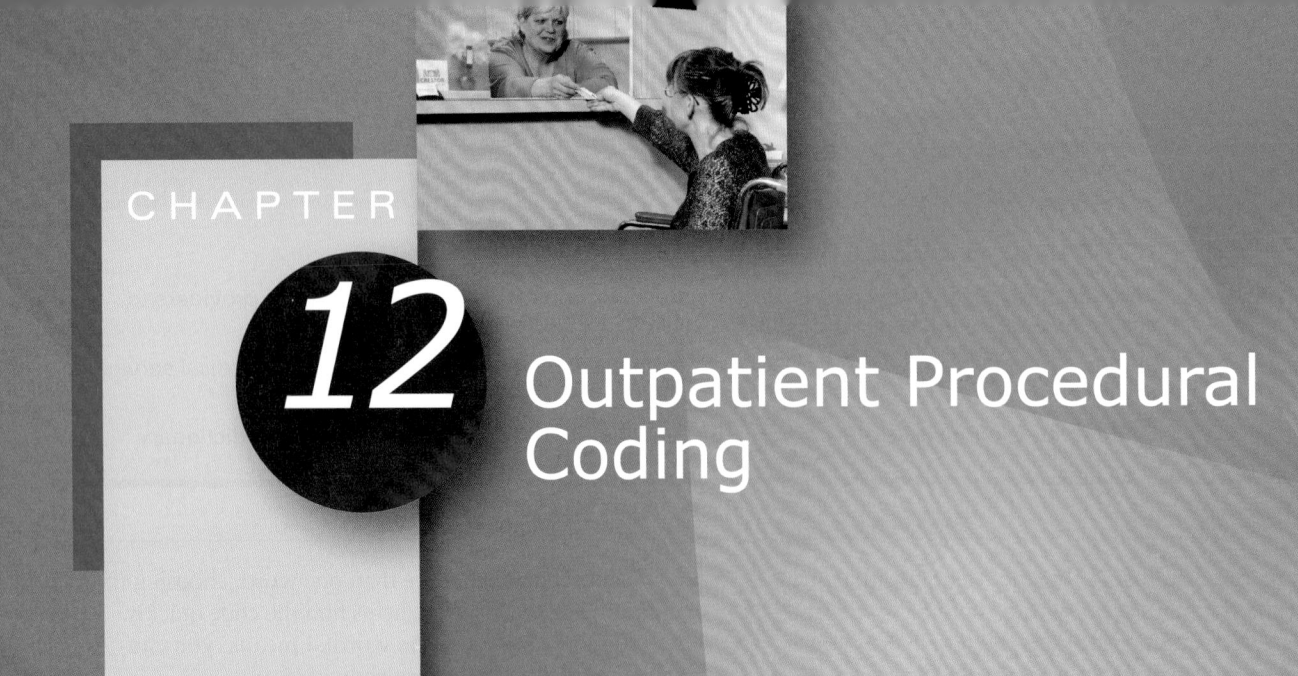

# 12 Outpatient Procedural Coding

## Outline

## Learning Outcomes

### COG Cognitive Domain*

1. Spell and define the key terms
2. Explain the Healthcare Common Procedure Coding System (HCPCS), levels I and II
3. Explain the format of level I, Current Procedural Terminology (CPT-4) and its use
4. Describe the relationship between coding and reimbursement
5. *Describe how to use the most current procedure coding system*
6. Discuss the effects of the following:
   a. Upcoding
   b. Downcoding
7. *Describe how to use the most current HCPCS coding*
8. Describe the concept of RBRVS
9. Define both medical terms and abbreviations related to all body systems
10. *Define medical necessity as it applies to procedural coding*

### PSY Psychomotor Domain*

1. *Perform procedural coding (Procedure 15-1)*

### AFF Affective Domain*

1. Work with physician to achieve the maximum reimbursement
2. *Interact professionally with third-party representatives*
3. *Display tactful behavior when communicating with medical providers regarding third-party requirements*
4. *Utilize tactful communication skills with medical providers to ensure accurate code selection*
5. Apply ethical behaviors, including honesty/integrity in performance of medical assisting practice

***Note: AAMA/CAAHEP 2015 Standards are italicized.***

### ABHES Competencies

1. Apply third-party guidelines
2. Perform diagnostic and procedural coding
3. Comply with federal, state, and local health laws and regulations

## Key Terms

## Case Study

*T*he office manager at Great Falls Medical Center has asked Janae Baker, RMA, to verify procedure codes for patients seen in the office yesterday. In addition to some who had routine office visits, one patient had a preoperative visit for an outpatient surgery scheduled tomorrow morning. Several patients received injections for influenza immunizations, and others were given antibiotics injections. Tests waived by the Clinical Laboratory Improvement Amendments (CLIA) were also performed in the office for six patients, and one patient had a 12-lead electrocardiogram done. Where will Janae find the codes necessary to bill these procedures? Are medications and vaccines found in the same coding manual? Can tests be billed for specimens collected and tested in the office? Are all of these services billable? Should modifiers be used on any of the codes when billing? This chapter discusses billing for procedures and services in the outpatient setting and provides guidance for answering these important questions.

As discussed in Chapter 11, coding is a way to standardize medical information for purposes such as collecting health care statistics, performing a medical care review, and indexing medical records. It is also used for health insurance claims processing (see Chapter 13 for more information). Because coding is linked to reimbursement, you must code accurately and precisely. Incorrect, insufficient, or incomplete coding on claims forms can lead to improper reimbursement for the physician as well as recording and possibly passing along inaccurate patient information. Because learning to code is an ongoing process, continuing education is vital. This can be accomplished by attending workshops in your geographic area or by joining a local association of coders, which may also sponsor coding clinics. Two professional coding organizations are the American Academy of Professional Coders (AAPC) and the American Health Information Management Association (AHIMA). Other sources are local medical societies and your school.

### HEALTHCARE COMMON PROCEDURE CODING SYSTEM

The **Healthcare Common Procedure Coding System** (HCPCS) is divided into two principal subsystems, referred to as level I and level II. Level I of the HCPCS comprises Current Procedural Terminology, Fourth Edition (CPT-4), a

five-digit numeric coding system maintained by the American Medical Association (AMA). Level II of the HCPCS is a standardized coding system developed primarily for Medicare but used by other carriers to identify products, supplies, and certain services not included in the CPT-4 codes. These codes include items such as ambulance services, durable medical equipment, prosthetics, orthotics, and supplies when used outside a physician's office. Box 12-1 describes level II codes. Level III codes, also referred to as local codes, were established when an insurer preferred that suppliers use a local code to identify a service, for which there was no level I or level II code. In the interest of standardizing code sets, The Health Insurance Portability and Accountability Act of 1996 (HIPAA) required the elimination of level III local codes, which took effect on December 31, 2003.

### CHECKPOINT QUESTION

1. What are level II codes? List their sections.

### PHYSICIAN'S CURRENT PROCEDURAL TERMINOLOGY

HCPCS level I codes, or the Physician's **Current Procedural Terminology** (CPT), is a comprehensive listing of medical terms and codes for the uniform coding

## BOX 12-1    HCPCS Level II Codes

Because Medicare and other insurers cover a variety of services, supplies, and equipment that are not identified by CPT codes, the level II HCPCS codes were established for submitting claims for these items. The development and use of level II of the HCPCS began in the 1980s. Level II codes are also referred to as alphanumeric codes because they consist of a single alphabetical letter followed by four numeric digits, whereas CPT codes are identified using five numeric digits. The HCPCS level II code listing comes out once a year in the National Coding Manual, which can be ordered from the American Hospital Association, American Medical Association, or other publishers of the CPT coding book. It includes the following sections:

• Chemotherapeutic drugs
• Dental services
• Durable medical equipment
• Medications for injections
• Ophthalmology services
• Orthotics
• Some pathology and laboratory and rehabilitation supplies
• Vision care

of procedures and services provided by physicians. The fourth edition, CPT-4, contains more than 7,000 new codes and is updated annually with new editions available in the fall before implementation of deleted, revised, or new codes are required on January 1. It is important that providers purchase the newest edition of the CPT-4 manual every year to prevent denials of medical claims because of inaccurate coding. The AMA is also responsible for revising and updating vaccine product codes listed in the *Medicines/Vaccines and Toxoids* section, and those codes are released semiannually and become effective 6 months later. CPT books are available in both the traditional book format and the electronic format using computer software. The CPT-4 allows insurance companies to

• Communicate easily with one another
• Compare reimbursable amounts for procedures
• Speed claims processing

## PERFORMING PROCEDURAL CODING

Every code means something unique and is used only to describe a specific **procedure**, service, or medical supply provided by physicians to their patients. Codes

and descriptions are updated, revised, or changed annually, so if your physician's office uses an encounter form or preprinted routing slip that lists the procedures performed, you must update this form yearly and work with your software vendor to update your computer software. The CPT-4 code selected will be placed on the CMS-1500 universal claim form in Section 24, Box D, along with any modifiers used. Procedure 12-1 outlines the steps in performing procedural coding. The National Uniform Claim Committee (NUCC) is responsible for maintaining the CMS-1500 claim form, and the most recent version (02–12) began implementation in April 2014 (see Chapter 13). Figure 12-1 is a sample universal claim form showing the proper placement of codes for consultation and chest radiography. The general layout and features of the CPT-4 book published by the American Medical Association are user friendly. There are definitions, diagrams, simple explanations, examples, and instructions.

## The Layout of CPT-4

CPT-4 is divided into six major sections: Evaluation and Management, Anesthesia, Surgery, Radiology, Pathology and Laboratory, and Medicine. These are the largest collection of procedural codes and are sequenced numerically with guidelines for usage at the beginning of every section. There are also unlisted procedure codes listed at the beginning of every section in the event a service or procedure is not covered (see *Unlisted Procedures and Special Reports* below).

Category I codes are followed by explanations and listings of the Category II and Category III codes. Descriptions of all three CPT-4 categories are explained in Box 12-2.

Next are the appendices. The appendices most widely used in the outpatient arena are Appendices A through C. Appendix A is a listing of the modifiers available to help further explain a code. Appendix B is a summary of the additions, deletions, and revisions made since the last edition of the CPT-4. Appendix C includes clinical examples designed to assist providers in the selection of Evaluation and Management levels.

## The Alphabetic Index

The CPT alphabetic index is located in the back of the book and is organized by main terms like the ICD-9-CM book (Fig. 12-2). Unlike the ICD-9 index, you can locate codes by finding the procedure, the location, or the condition. For example, the code for removal of a colon polyp could be found under *Removal*, *Colon*, or *Polyp*. When you find the service or procedure, you will see either one code or a range of codes. Cross-reference by finding this section in the tabular section to be sure you have the correct code.

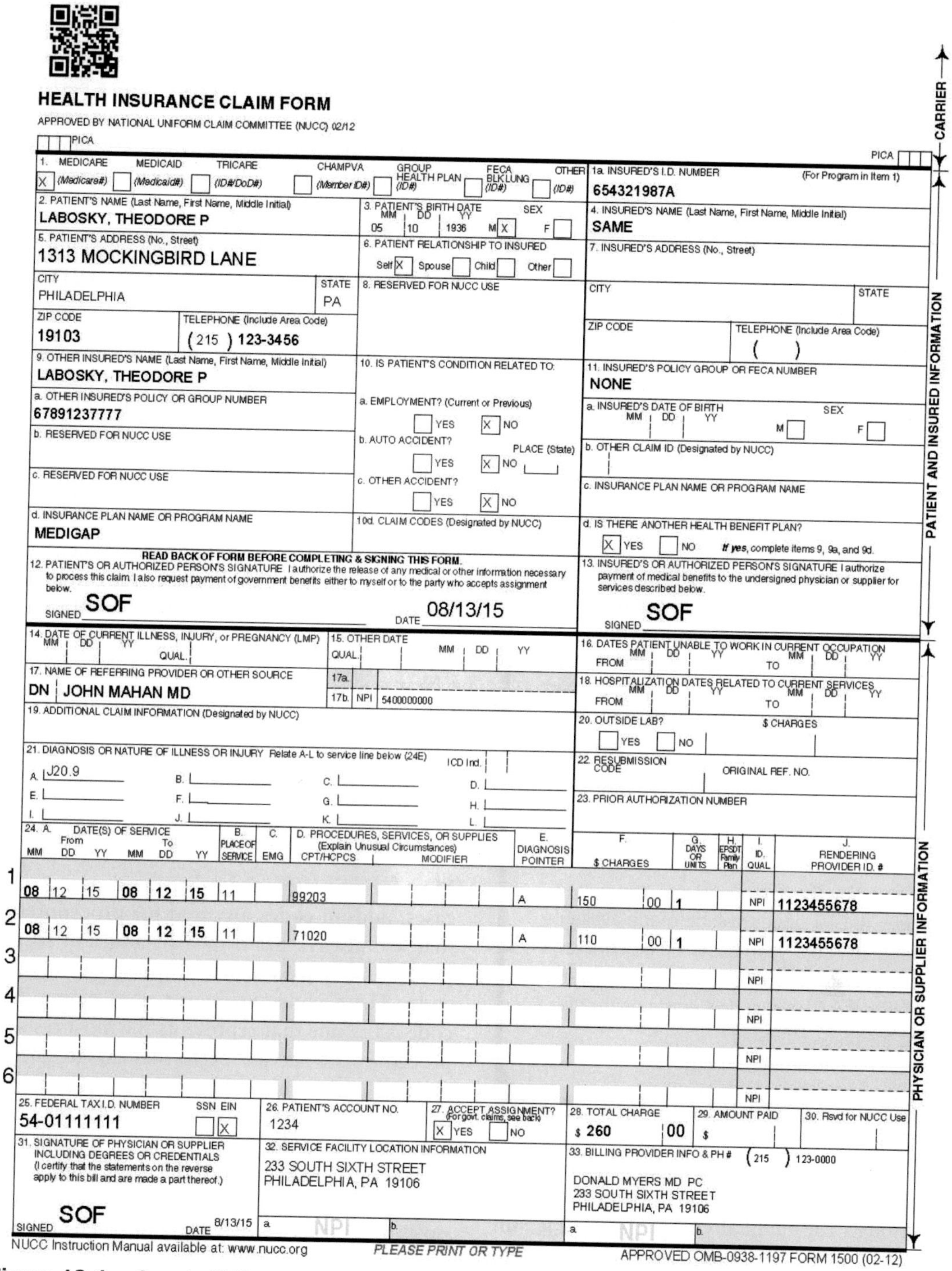

**Figure 12-1** • Sample CMS claim form for consultation and chest radiography.

## Reading Descriptors

When reading a code's **descriptor**, or description, you will read up to the semicolon and then look down for any indentations using the same words before the semicolon. Figure 12-2 is a sample page from a CPT-4 book. Refer to Figure 12-2, and locate the code for incision and drainage of an infected bursa. The proper code is 27604. It is indented under the code 27603. Read up to the semicolon in the code above. The descriptor for 27603 reads, "Incision and drainage, leg or ankle; deep abscess or hematoma." If the incision and drainage was done in an infected bursa of the leg or ankle, then the code is 27604. This descriptor is "Incision and drainage, leg or ankle; infected bursa." You would use 27603 for an incision and drainage of a leg or ankle for a deep abscess or a hematoma. Use of the indentation and

## BOX 12-2    CPT-4 Categories

CPT-4 includes three categories of codes. Category I codes include all current U.S. Food and Drug Administration–approved physicians' procedures and services. The AMA developed it in collaboration with various other health organizations.

Category I CPT codes describe a procedure or service identified with a five-digit CPT code and descriptor nomenclature. The inclusion of a descriptor and its associated specific five-digit identifying code number in this category of CPT codes is generally based upon the procedure being consistent with contemporary medical practice and being performed by many physicians in clinical practice in multiple locations.

Category II CPT codes are intended to facilitate data collection by coding certain services and/or test results that are agreed upon as contributing to positive health outcomes and quality patient care. This category of CPT codes is a set of optional tracking codes for performance measurement. These codes may be services that are typically included in an E/M service or other component part of a service and are not appropriate for Category I CPT codes. The use of tracking codes for performance measures will decrease the need for record abstraction and chart review, thus minimizing administrative burdens on physicians and survey costs for health plans.

Once approved by the Editorial Panel, the newly added Category III CPT codes will be made available on a semiannual (twice a year) basis via electronic distribution on the AMA/CPT Web site. The full set of Category III codes will be included in the next published edition for that CPT cycle.

*Source*: http://www.ama-assn.org

the semicolon organizes the codes in a way that also saves space and keeps the CPT books from becoming too large. Although the manual coding process is still widely used, CPT software is available and is growing in popularity.

 **CHECKPOINT QUESTION**

2. What is the significance of the semicolon in a CPT descriptor?

## Place of Service

The CPT-4 book begins with "Place of Service Codes for Professional Claims." Most payers require that place of service codes be placed on each line of Section 24,

Column B of the CMS-1500 claim form. Because the CMS maintains place of service codes, you should make sure that a certain payer recognizes the codes listed in CPT-4. For example, if a procedure is performed in the physician's office, the place of service code recognized by most payers including Medicare and Medicaid is 11. The most commonly used place of service codes are found in Table 12-1.

## Section Guidelines and Symbols

Each section begins with its own specific guidelines and a listing of specific procedures and services applicable in that field. The guidelines contain definitions, explanatory notes, a listing of the previously unlisted procedures found in that particular section, directions on how to file a special report, modifiers for use in that particular section, and definitions to assist the coder.

Symbols are used throughout CPT-4 to help provide additional information about codes. When a code has one of these symbols beside it, the coder can look at the bottom of the page to see what the symbol means. Some of the most common symbols found in CPT are as follows:

- New code
- Revised code
- New or revised text
- Add-on code

## Primary and Add-On Codes

Most of the CPT codes are used alone; but in some cases, **add-on codes** are used for procedures or services that are always performed in addition to the primary procedure. A plus sign (+) appears next to an add-on code. These codes are never used alone. The **primary code** is the one that represents the most resource-intense procedure or service performed at an encounter. The primary code is listed first on the CMS-1500 form. The add-on code is listed on the line under the primary code. For example, a dermatology coder uses the code 11100 for a biopsy on a lesion. If the doctor biopsies more than one lesion, 11100 is listed on the first line, and the add-on code +11101 is used to report each additional lesion.

## Unlisted Procedures and Special Reports

CPT provides unlisted codes at the beginning of each section for use when an unusual, variable, or new procedure is done. Before using an unlisted CPT code, the medical assistant must first look in the Category III section for temporary codes and use a code from that section, if available. When an unlisted code is used, however, you must submit a copy of the procedure report with the claim. Each section's guidelines list the

## Leg (Tibia) and Fibula) and Ankle Joint

### Incision

27600    Decompression fasciotomy, leg; anterior and/or lateral compartments only

27601      posterior compartment(s) only

27602      anterior and/or lateral, and posterior compartment(s)

     (For incision and drainage procedures, superficial, see 10040-10160)

     (For decompression fasciotomy with debridement, see 27892-27894)

27603    Incision and drainage, leg or ankle; deep abscess or hematoma

27604      infected bursa

27605    Tenotomy, percutaneous, Achilles tendon (separate procedure); local anesthesia

27606      general anesthesia

27607    Incision (eg, osteomyelitis or bone abscess), leg or ankle

27610    Arthrotomy, ankle, including exploration, drainage, or removal of foreign body
       *CPT Assistant* Nov 98:9

27612    Arthrotomy, posterior capsular release, ankle, with or without Achilles tendon lengthening
       *CPT Assistant* Nov 98:8

     (See also 27685)

### Excision

27613    Biopsy, soft tissue of leg or ankle area; superficial

27614      deep (subfascial or intramuscular)
       *CPT Assistant* Nov 98:8

     (For needle biopsy of soft tissue, use 20206)

27615    Radical resection of tumor (eg, malignant neoplasm), soft tissue of leg or ankle area

27618    Excision, tumor, leg or ankle area; subcutaneous tissue

27619      deep (subfascial or intramuscular)

27620    Arthrotomy, ankle, with joint exploration, with or without biopsy, with or without removal of loose or foreign body

27625    Arthrotomy, with synovectomy, ankle;
       *CPT Assistant* Nov 98:8

27626      including tenosynovectomy

27630    Excision of lesion of tendon sheath or capsule (eg, cyst or ganglion), leg and/or ankle

27635    Excision or curettage of bone cyst or benign tumor; tibia or fibula;

27637      with autograft (includes obtaining graft)

27638      with allograft

27640    Partial excision (craterization, saucerization, or diaphysectomy) bone (eg, osteomyelitis or exostosis); tibia

27641      fibula

27645    Radical resection of tumor, bone; tibia

27646      fibula

27647      talus or calcaneus

### Introduction or Removal

27648    Injection procedure for ankle arthrography

     (For radiological supervision and interpretation, use 73615. Do not report 76003 in addition to 73615)

     (For ankle arthroscopy, see 29894-29898)

### Repair, Revision, and/or Reconstruction

27650    Repair, primary, open or percutaneous, ruptured Achilles tendon;

27652      with graft (includes obtaining graft)

27654    Repair, secondary, Achilles tendon, with or without graft

27656    Repair, fascial defect of leg

27658    Repair, flexor tendon, leg; primary, without graft, each tendon
       *CPT Assistant* Nov 98:8

27659      secondary, with or without graft, each tendon

27664    Repair, extensor tendon, leg; primary, without graft, each tendon
       *CPT Assistant* Nov 98:8

27665      secondary, with or without graft, each tendon
       *CPT Assistant* Nov 98:8

27675    Repair, dislocating peroneal tendons; without fibular osteotomy

27676      with fibular osteotomy

27680    Tenolysis, flexor or extensor tendon, leg and/or ankle; single, each tendon
       *CPT Assistant* Nov 98:8

27681      multiple tendons (through separate incision(s))
       *CPT Assistant* Nov 98:8

27685    Lengthening or shortening of tendon, leg or ankle; single tendon (separate procedure)
       *CPT Assistant* Nov 98:8

27686      multiple tendons (through same incision), each
       *CPT Assistant* Nov 98:8

= Revised code      = New code      = Contains new or revised text      = References: see p xv for details

**Figure 12-2** • Sample page of 2014 CPT book.

information to be included in a special report. This information includes the following:

1. Definition or description of the nature, extent, and need for the procedure

2. Time, effort, and equipment necessary to provide the service

3. Complexity of symptoms

4. Final diagnosis

5. Pertinent physical findings

6. Diagnostic and therapeutic procedures

7. Concurrent problems

8. Follow-up care

| TABLE 12-1 | Place of Service Codes Used in Physician Coding | |
| --- | --- |
| **Place of Service** | **Code** |
| Physician's office | 11 |
| Patient's home | 12 |
| Assisted living facility | 13 |
| Urgent care facility | 20 |
| Inpatient hospital | 21 |
| Outpatient hospital | 22 |
| Emergency room–hospital | 23 |
| Ambulatory surgical center | 24 |
| Skilled nursing facility | 31 |
| Hospice | 34 |

These two-digit codes are placed on each line of Section 24, Column B.

*Source*: Current Procedural Terminology, CPT 2014 Professional Edition; American Medical Association.

## ⊙OG EVALUATION AND MANAGEMENT CODES

Evaluation and Management (E/M) codes are five-digit numbers that begin with the number 9. These are the most frequently used codes in the medical office. E/M codes describe various patient histories, examinations, and decisions physicians must make in evaluating and treating patients in various settings (e.g., office, outpatient, hospital). In essence, the E/M codes address what the physician does when interacting with the patient. For this reason, the physician's documentation must meet standards so the physician and coder (medical assistant) can decide which level or type of code to use for a specific patient–physician encounter.

### Key Components

To code the services described in the E/M section, you must be sure that the patient's medical record indicates that certain **key components** are present. Two of three key components are required for established patients, and three of three are required for new patients. New patients are those who have not received services from the provider or anyone of the same speciality in the practice within the last 3 years. These components are the elements that make up the visit. All E/M codes contain the following components:

- History
- Physical examination
- Medical decision making
- Counseling

- Coordination of care
- Nature of presenting problem
- Time

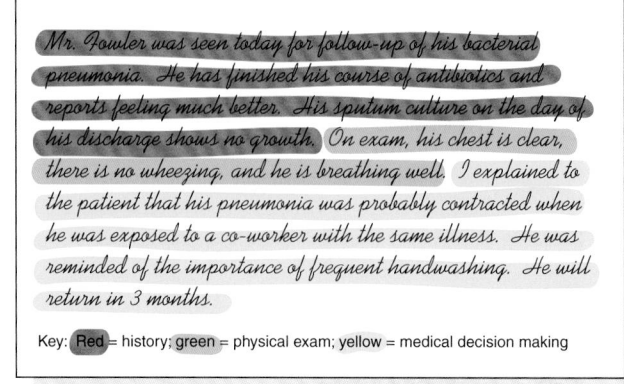

Mr. Fowler was seen today for follow-up of his bacterial pneumonia. He has finished his course of antibiotics and reports feeling much better. His sputum culture on the day of his discharge shows no growth. On exam, his chest is clear, there is no wheezing, and he is breathing well. I explained to the patient that his pneumonia was probably contracted when he was exposed to a co-worker with the same illness. He was reminded of the importance of frequent handwashing. He will return in 3 months.

Key: Red = history; green = physical exam; yellow = medical decision making

History, physical examination, and medical decision making are three key components for a visit.

### History

The amount of history documented in a patient's record determines which of the four classifications or levels is assigned. The classifications of the type of history taken from the patient are as follows:

- Problem focused
- Expanded problem focused
- Detailed
- Comprehensive

Table 12-2 lists the classifications and gives a general description and examples of each. The provider must select one of these based on the documentation in the patient's record. Note that the times listed in the table are not regulated; they are used only for describing a typical level.

### Examination

The examination levels are the same as for the history taken. A review of systems is a systematic way to obtain additional information by questioning the patient to before or during a physical exam. The level of an examination depends on how many body systems were examined. CPT recognizes the following body systems: eyes; ears, nose, mouth, and throat; cardiovascular; respiratory; gastrointestinal; genitourinary; musculoskeletal; skin; neurologic; psychiatric; and hematologic/immunologic (laboratory tests). Analyze the following chart note to assign the proper level of exam.

At this visit, the patient had an expanded problem-focused examination. The doctor examined her eyes, nose, and throat (her problem area) and also did a urinalysis to confirm that an earlier treatment took care of her previous urinary tract infection. Note that even

**TABLE 12-2  History and Physical Examinations**

The physician or provider must select which history and physical examination code to use. You, however, should have a basic understanding of each category. It is important to note that there are separate codes for each category and separate codes for both new and established patients.

| Type of History and Physical Examination | Patient Problems and Physician Time Required | Examples |
|---|---|---|
| Problem focused | Patient problems are self-limited and minor. Physician time: usually 10 minutes | A 9-month-old patient with diaper rash<br>A 40-year-old patient with sunburn<br>An 18-year-old patient with poison ivy<br>A 60-year-old patient with a routine blood pressure check |
| Expanded problem focused | Patient problems are mild to moderate. Physician time: 15–20 minutes | A 55-year-old patient with recurrent urinary tract infection<br>A 16-year-old patient with chronic asthma presenting with a cold<br>A 76-year-old patient with osteoarthritis<br>A 56-year-old patient with a stomach ulcer |
| Detailed | Patient problems are moderate to severe. Physician time: usually 30 minutes | An 18-year-old patient with first Pap smear and contraceptive education<br>A 67-year-old patient with the new onset of dysuria<br>An 18-month-old patient with delayed motor skill development<br>A 34-year-old patient with diabetes requiring insulin dose changes |
| Comprehensive | Patient problems are moderate to severe. Physician time: usually 45 minutes | A 36-year-old patient with infertility<br>An 8-year-old patient with new onset of diabetes<br>A 65-year-old patient with history of left-sided weakness and confusion |

if the doctor examined the patient's skin, arm strength, etc., if it is not in the chart note, it cannot be considered in the selection of the level of her examination.

> *Patient presents with complaints of runny nose and sore throat x 3 days. Patient states the urinary tract infection we treated two weeks ago is better. On examination her eyes are red, nose is boggy, throat is red and swollen. Patient reports no more urinary problems since finishing the Bactrim DS. Urinalysis is clear.*

## Medical Decision Making

The third key component, medical decision making, is defined in CPT-4 as follows:

- Straightforward
- Low complexity
- Moderate complexity or
- High complexity

Medical decision making refers to the kinds of things the physician must do to establish a diagnosis for the patient. A provider must consider and determine the number of diagnoses and/or management options

available, the amount and complexity of any data to be reviewed, and the risk of complications or other problems the patient has. To use a particular decision-making level, the physician must document the information to justify his level selection. For example, a doctor may write a chart note like this:

> *Mr. Jones presents today for follow-up of his severe back pain. He is no better. I offered him several options, including physical therapy, anti-inflammatories, and surgery. I reviewed 35 pages of records from his surgery in Baltimore, MD, five years ago. He has cardiac problems that may make another surgery too risky.*

This visit would qualify for a level of moderate complexity. The documentation states the number of management options and the amount of data reviewed and lists the patient's other problems.

## Time

Time is not considered a key component unless more than half of the visit is spent counseling the patient. Time spent with a patient (e.g., counseling or coordinating care) is sometimes the key component in determining E/M codes. When time spent with the patient is more than 50% of the typical time for the visit, time becomes the deciding factor in choosing an E/M code. For example, if a physician spends an additional 15 minutes' counseling a patient in what would normally be only a 10-minute expanded problem-focused history and physical examination, the counseling was more than 50% of the typical 25-minute face-to-face time. The appropriate E/M code is one with a 25-minute time frame (10 minutes and an extra 15 minutes for counseling).

### 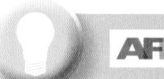 CHECKPOINT QUESTION

3. List three things a physician must consider when assigning a level of medical decision making.

 **WHAT IF?**

**What if a patient's visit turns out to be mostly counseling?**

A 42-year-old established patient with a family history of alcoholism sees her family doctor for an annual exam. She tells the doctor that she is doing fine, but her exam reveals some tenderness over her liver, and there is a faint odor of vodka on her breath. After a few minutes, the patient admits to the doctor that she is having marital problems and has been drinking excessively lately. The rest of the visit is spent explaining the dangers of drinking and the effects of alcohol on the liver. The doctor spends time giving her information about Alcoholics Anonymous and other resources. The chart notation reads: "Visit began at 9:15 AM. Patient states she is doing well. On palpation of the liver, there is guarding and tenderness. There is a faint odor of ETOH. I spent 30 minutes of a 45-minute appointment counseling the patient and arranging a referral to Southside Drug and Alcohol Rehabilitation Center. Her husband was given several brochures, information about Al-Anon (an arm of Alcoholics Anonymous for family members of alcoholics), and hints about finding online resources. She left in the care of her husband who was instructed to take the patient to the rehab center now. Time 10:00 AM."

Time is the only factor when selecting the level for this office visit. Remember, the documentation must clearly state that more than half of the visit was spent counseling a patient face to face. According to CPT, the time counted can be with the patient and/or family members or caretaker. Using the times listed in the descriptors in CPT, locate the proper category (office visit for established patient), and find the level that describes the amount of time the physician spent with the patient. The chart states the entire visit was 45 minutes; therefore, the correct code would be 99215.

## OTHER CATEGORIES OF EVALUATION AND MANAGEMENT CODES

As a medical assistant, you will be responsible for ensuring accurate billing for your provider–employer. Although many of these services are performed in the medical office, physicians also visit and care for patients in other places. You will assist the physician in assigning codes for these visits and procedures. Other categories in the E/M section include observation codes and hospital inpatient services including initial care and subsequent care. There is a section for consultations ordered by other physicians.

Emergency department service codes are used only when the service is rendered in a 24-hour hospital-based facility that specializes in providing treatment of unscheduled events. Nursing homes, rest homes, and home visits are listed. Critical care, preventive medicine, and newborn care are other sections used by physicians for their direct care of patients. For a complete list of the subsections and categories, refer to the CPT codebook.

### CHECKPOINT QUESTION

4. To code for a service in the E/M section, what three key elements are considered?

### Anesthesia Section

Anesthesia codes are five-digit codes that begin with 0. Anesthesia codes are divided by anatomic site and by specific type of procedure. For example, head, neck, and thorax are anatomic sites, and the codes in each section represent the specific procedure, such as plastic repair of cleft lip. Medical assistants in an anesthesiology practice code anesthesia procedures provided in the hospital setting, even though the office is an outpatient facility.

Two types of **modifiers** (letters or numbers added to a code to add detail to the code) are used in the anesthesia section. One type is the standard modifier that is found in all sections of CPT. The other type is the physical status modifier, a two-digit code beginning with the letter P and ending in a number from 1 to 6. These physical status modifiers indicate the patient's condition at the time of anesthesia and the corresponding complexity of services (e.g., P1 indicates a normal, healthy patient, and P5 indicates a patient who is not expected to survive without the procedure).

### Surgery Section

The surgery section is organized by body systems. Surgery codes begin with numbers 1 through 6. Many of the CPT-4 codes in this section include surgery packages. This means that when there is a decision for surgery, the CPT-4 code surgery code includes a preoperative evaluation and management visit, the surgical procedure; normal, uncomplicated follow-up care; and local infiltration, metacarpal, metatarsal, or digital block or topical anesthesia. General anesthesia must be given by an anesthesiologist. The fee for the surgery includes everything in the "package" under normal conditions and without unforeseen complications.

Insurance company benefits determine what surgical packages include, but most major procedures cannot have the preoperative and postoperative visits billed separately unless you use a modifier to explain the circumstances. For example, a patient has a cholecystectomy (gallbladder removal). Under the patient's insurance plan benefits, the CPT code billed for the surgery covers three postoperative office visits after the surgery. Between the first and the second visit, the patient develops symptoms associated with appendicitis. The doctor can charge for this office visit because it is not related to the cholecystectomy. The surgery package does not apply.

The Centers for Medicare and Medicaid Services (CMS) has defined the surgical package for Medicare recipients somewhat differently. According to CPT-4, no complications or problems related to the surgery are included in the surgical package. If additional procedures are performed to correct or alleviate these problems, they should be coded separately. According to CMS, however, complications that do not require a revisit to the operating room are included in the price of surgery.

Third-party payers have different rules about what constitutes a surgery package, so the coder must check with the relevant third-party payers. Some insurance carriers have a set number of follow-up days that is consistent for all surgical services. Check with the carrier to learn what these are so you can bill for the additional office, outpatient, or hospital visits. The fees for fracture care and deliveries also include the care given before and after the service.

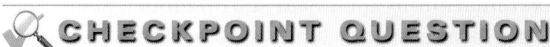

### CHECKPOINT QUESTION

5. What items are included in a surgical package?

## Content of the Surgery Section

The subheadings in the surgery section are as follows: integumentary system, musculoskeletal system, respiratory system, cardiovascular system, hemic and lymphatic system, urinary system, digestive system, male genital system, intersex surgery, female genital system, maternity care and delivery, endocrine system, nervous system, eye and ocular adnexa, and auditory system. Each subheading contains subsections that organize the procedures by location and type. For example, in the musculoskeletal system section, the subcategories begin with the head and move down the body. The first heading is "Head." Under

| TABLE 12-3 | Medical Terminology Refresher | |
|---|---|---|
| Words that end in the following suffixes are related to surgical procedures. | | |
| CPT Subcategory | Suffix | Meaning |
| Incision | -tomy | Incision into |
| Excision | -ectomy | Surgical removal |
| Repair, revision, or reconstruction | -pexy | Surgical fixation |
| | -plasty | Surgical repair |
| | -rrhaphy | Suture |

this heading are the following procedures that are done to the head: incision; excision; introduction or removal; repair, revision, and/or reconstruction; skull, facial, and nasal fractures and/or dislocations, etc. The next heading is "Neck (Soft Tissues) and Thorax," which begins with incision, excision, and so on.

It is helpful to be familiar with the suffixes and definitions related to surgical procedures. Table 12-3 provides a refresher on these words and word parts.

## Radiology Section

The radiology section of CPT-4 is divided into the following seven subsections:

- Diagnostic radiology/diagnostic imaging
- Diagnostic ultrasound
- Radiologic guidance
- Breast, mammography
- Bone/joint studies
- Radiation oncology
- Nuclear medicine

All radiology codes are five-digit numbers that begin with 7. They are generally arranged by anatomic site, from the top of the body to the bottom and can be found by searching the alphabetic index for the type of service, such as x-ray, then the numerical index. Many radiology codes indicate the number of views for a particular study. Obviously, the facility must be reimbursed for film, developer, and the radiology technologist's time and service.

Some radiologic tests require the administration of a contrast medium that enhances the image. The descriptors for such tests specify "with contrast" or "without contrast." "With contrast" refers to contrast medium that is given in a vein, in an artery, or in the subarachnoid space of the spinal cord. If the contrast medium is given orally or rectally, you use the code "without contrast."

Coding guidelines are provided with specific radiology codes to advise when other CPT codes should and should *not* be used. For example, if a physician performs a procedure and supervises and interprets an imaging procedure (e.g., injects contrast medium and then supervises and interprets), two codes may be required, and a written report in the patient's medical record is necessary for billing these codes. The code for the procedure can be found in the surgery, medicine, or radiology section, and the code for supervision and interpretation is found in the radiology section. If two physicians are participating (e.g., a surgeon and radiologist), the radiology portion is billed by the radiologist.

## Pathology and Laboratory Section

All codes in pathology and laboratory work are five-digit numbers that begin with 8. These codes are divided into sections for panels of tests, drug testing, consultations with pathologists, urinalysis, chemistry testing, hematology and coagulation, antibody testing, cytopathology, and so on. The last part of the pathology and laboratory section includes services and procedures provided by a pathologist, including gross (can be seen by the naked eye) and microscopic examination of tissue removed in surgery. Each tissue specimen is submitted under a different identifying code for diagnosis by the pathologist. The codes represent the level of the physician's work. Postmortem examination or autopsy is performed by a pathologist, and CPT-4 provides codes to report such examinations.

Medical assistants are typically responsible for obtaining specimens from patients in the office. For the routine collection of blood, bill the venipuncture CPT code 36415; however, note that codes 36400-36410 may be used as indicated based on the age of the patient. If the specimen is going to an outside lab, the venipuncture code should be appended with the modifier-90 (*Reference, [outside ] laboratory*).

Certain tests may be performed on specimens collected in the physician office laboratory (POL) pursuant to the Clinical Laboratory Improvement Amendments Act of 1988 (CLIA). Tests that have been determined to be simple and involve few steps are considered *CLIA waived* and may be performed with a Certificate of Waiver (see Chapter 2). When billing for these tests for Medicare patients, you must append the CPT code with the HCPCS level II modifier *QW* indicating it is a CLIA-waived test.

Physicians often order a series of tests to be performed on a specimen in order to help correctly diagnose or treat a patient appropriately. The section for *Organ or Disease-Oriented Panels* has a CPT code for a collection of tests listed under the code, and each test has its own separate CPT code. These collections of tests are commonly performed together and are considered *bundled* under the main CPT code for that panel and may not be reported separately when all tests are performed for a specific panel.

Also of note are the terms *qualitative* and *quantitative* used in the drug screening section. Patients who are on certain medications, such as digoxin for the heart or Dilantin for seizures, have regular drug levels tested to be sure the amount of drug in the blood is at the proper therapeutic level. These tests are quantitative because the doctor is looking for the amount of drug in the blood. When testing for illegal drugs, however, the amount does not matter. The mere presence of the drug makes the test positive and provides the information wanted. This is qualitative information.

## Medicine Section

Like the E/M codes, medicine codes are five-digit numbers that begin with 9. Like the other five sections of the CPT-4, this section includes guidelines for appropriate coding.

One of the first subsections in the medicine section is for immunization injections. Typically, immunization injections are given when the patient comes to the physician's office either for a routine physical examination or for a minor problem, such as a sore throat. When the injection is given at the time of such a visit, use two codes—one for the service (usually an E/M code) and one for the immunization injection. For example, an established patient may come into the physician's office for a brief examination for a minor problem (e.g., controlled hypertension blood pressure check). The patient's blood pressure may be taken by the medical assistant and, while the physician is in the office, may also be given an immunization for poliomyelitis as ordered by the physician. The codes for this are as follows:

1. 99211, office and other outpatient visit for the evaluation and management of an established patient, which may not require the presence of a physician. Usually, the presenting problems are minimal. Typically, 5 minutes are spent performing or supervising services. (This code is generally used for examination by a clinical staff member, such as the medical assistant while a physician is in the office but not performing the examination.)
2. 90471, immunization administration.
3. 90713, poliomyelitis vaccine.

Therapeutic or diagnostic subcutaneous or intramuscular injections are also listed in this section of CPT. In order to be reimbursed for the medication itself, an additional, more specific code is necessary. Other than vaccines and toxoid injection codes that are listed in this section of CPT-4, other medications to be injected begin with a J and can be found in the HCPCS level II codes. This section of CPT-4 also includes infusions and chemotherapy (see Box 12-1). Using the most specific codes for injectable substances and supplies while keeping invoices to document actual cost helps verify charges submitted for these services.

The medicine section also includes codes used by psychiatrists and codes for biofeedback; dialysis; esophageal procedures; eye surgery and other ophthalmologic services; speech and hearing services including cochlear implants; cardiac diagnostic testing, such as electrocardiography and echocardiography; CPR; vascular studies like cardiac catheterization; allergy testing; electroencephalography; sleep studies; and other miscellaneous services and procedures.

 **CHECKPOINT QUESTION**

6. Why is it necessary to use two codes for an injection?

 **AFF** ETHICAL TIP

### Be Diligent About Accuracy

Even if you pay attention to detail and strive for accuracy, there are still times when you will make mistakes. Insurance companies are valuable resources for coding questions and information on how to submit accurate claims that will be processed and reimbursed in a timely manner. Although coding mistakes occasionally happen, it is important, not to make the same error twice. Carefully examine every remittance advice or explanation of benefits for problems, and develop a system to remember and track rejected claims. Do what it takes to correct any coding problems as quickly as possible in order to get reimbursement. When a claim is pending, patients usually receive a letter from their insurance company telling them that they have asked for additional information from their doctor. Often, patients receive this letter before you receive the request for information. Be as prompt as possible in answering these requests. Patients will depend on you to assist them with their claims. It is your ethical responsibility to take care in getting the proper reimbursement.

## HCPCS LEVEL II CODES

The HCPCS level II coding system was developed to process Medicare claims and is maintained by the Center for Medicare and Medicaid Services (CMS). It is used to report certain services, medical supplies, medications, durable medical equipment, and other procedures not listed in CPT-4. They are alphanumeric codes that begin with a letter followed by four digits. Many carriers use sections of the HCPCS level II codes including the "*J*" codes for reporting medications that are injected, such as antibiotics, on the CMS-1500 claim form.

The medical assistant performing coding in the office must remember that there may be a CPT code *and* a HCPCS level II code for certain procedures. Many of these services are for screenings, and when billing for a Medicare (or Medicaid) patient, you must always use the HCPCS level II code even when there is a code for that service. For example, billing for a Medicare patent's sigmoidoscopy for colorectal cancer screening would be done by reporting the HCPCS code G0104 instead of the CPT 45330.

## COG **MODIFIERS**

There are two types of modifiers—one for level I HCPCS (CPT-4) and one for level II HCPCS. Both levels have two-digit modifiers to give additional information about a procedure, and a hyphen is generally placed between the procedure code and the modifier to separate them.

There are two ways to report modifiers on the CMS-1500 claim form. You can write the five-digit code followed by the two-digit modifier in the first Modifier field. Hyphens are never used on the CMS-1500 claim form. If multiple modifiers are necessary, write the five-digit code with the modifier 99 in the first modifier field and list all of the modifiers in block 19 on the CMS-1500 claim form. It is also best to check with payers to determine the order of multiple modifiers as some directly influence reimbursement. Of course, the modifier can never appear on the claim form by itself because it refers to the procedure being billed.

Box 12-3 provides a few examples of modifiers. The modifiers used for certain sections are listed in the section guidelines. A separate listing of available modifiers can be found in both Appendices A of CPT-4 and HCPCS level II codes. Check Appendix A first; then go to the guidelines of the appropriate section to verify that the modifier may be used with the specific code. Failure to use an appropriate modifier causes database and reimbursement errors.

---

**BOX 12-3   Examples of CPT-4 Modifiers**

Here are just a few examples of CPT-4 modifiers. A complete list can be found in Appendix A of CPT-4.

- *23 unusual anesthesia*: This modifier signifies that anesthesia was used in a procedure that normally would not require it.
- *26 professional component*: This modifier signifies that there are two components to the procedure, a professional one and a technical one; for example, a physician who does not perform a particular test, but interprets the test and dictates a report.
- *51 multiple procedures*: This modifier signifies that more than one procedure, other than an evaluation and management, has been performed at the same visit.

**CHECKPOINT QUESTION**

7. What are modifiers?

## FRAUD AND CODING

Billing for services not performed, using another patient's coverage to receive reimbursement, and falsifying records are examples of blatant fraud. Millions of dollars have been budgeted to investigate fraud and abuse. The attorney general of the United States has jurisdiction over such cases, and in most states, the Office of the Inspector General investigates reports of possible fraud. In cases of suspected fraud, peer review organizations have been authorized by CMS to obtain medical records of Medicare beneficiaries for review.

Less severe and nondeliberate fraudulent practices also cause misuse of health care dollars, and CMS remains vigilant by conducting audits. Medicare Administrative Contractors (organizations under contract with the US government to handle Medicare claims) randomly review and compare the documentation in the record with the information and codes received and report their findings on the particular providers.

Even though the physician may already have been paid for a claim, the medical office may still be audited and everyone in the billing process, including the physician, held accountable for fraudulent billing practices. As a federal program, Medicare has the same authority as the Internal Revenue Service to audit claims and may do so retroactively. This means that an audit can occur even a couple of years after payment has been received for claims. If the medical practice is found to be in error, the physician may be required to repay an amount owed plus interest. Even worse, such errors can jeopardize the physician's ability to participate in Medicare-funded programs.

When submitting Medicare or other insurance claims, do not bill for services the physician has not performed, and do not bill more than the proper fee for a service (**upcoding**). Investigations involving upcoding claims to receive a higher reimbursement is a serious offense and have resulted in prosecution of both the physician and the members of the billing staff. Just as problematic, **downcoding** is done by providers who are fearful of submitting claims at the more accurate higher level reimbursement code because of the possibility of payer investigations or audits. Routinely downcoding claims results, of course, in decreased revenue to the practice and does not accurately reflect the level of care being given. Billing for services using codes based on the documentation is the solution to prevent upcoding and downcoding problems.

Another area of concern by payers is the determination as to whether or not medical care being given meets

**BOX 12-4   False Claims Act**

Under the Civil Monetary Penalties Law, sanctions can be against any person *who engages in a practice or pattern of presenting or causing to be presented a claim:*

- *For an item or service that was not provided as claimed and is based on a code for a service that the person knows **or should know** will result in greater payment*
- *For a medical or other item or service and the person knows **or should know** the claim is false or fraudulent*
- *Is for a pattern of medical or other item or service and the person knows **or should know** are not medically necessary*

a generally accepted medical standard. Care that does not meet that standard does not meet the medical necessity requirements. Meeting these requirements means that the medical services are determined by the payer to be reasonable and necessary based on the patient's diagnoses and other medical conditions and based on the care of other providers of the same specialty (see Chapter 11). Payers have coverage guidelines for procedures and services available online that should be regularly accessed and reviewed for compliance. It is up to the medical assistant to assist the physician to submit accurate claims and be vigilant with laws and regulations surrounding medical coding and reimbursement. Although the physician is ultimately responsible for coding and billing for his/her services, Box 12-4 addresses those who may also be held responsible under the false claims act.

 **LEGAL TIP**

### Be Careful

To avoid costly errors, be certain that you can justify your coding:

- Keep adequate, accurate, and complete documentation in medical and billing records.
- Use the proper tools to code. Codebooks are updated yearly. Always use the most recent book.
- Follow the coding rules.
- Stay abreast of new rules, and keep up to date on any changes to existing ones. Medicare has regional updates, usually at no charge, and provides one of the best sources of information.
- Work closely with the provider, and never code anything about which you are not sure.

 # INPATIENT PROCEDURAL CODING

The ICD-10-PCS Procedure Classification System developed by the CMS and the National Center for Health Statistics is a replacement for Volume 3 of the ICD-9 and is used in the United States exclusively for inpatient hospital settings. The new procedure coding system uses seven alpha or numeric characters, whereas the ICD-9-CM coding system uses only three to five numeric digits. The use of this new system will roll out in conjunction with implementation of the ICD-10-CM requirements (see Chapter 11).

## ROLE-PLAYING ACTIVITY

Janae Baker, RMA, works in the billing department at Great Falls Medical Center and just reviewed benefits for a patient who has an order to receive another steroid injection into her right knee. Unfortunately, Janae found out that the patient's insurance has determined that only one injection every 6 months is medically necessary for her diagnosis of osteoarthritis and her last injection was 3 months ago. The patient is scheduled to come in today to meet with Janae to discuss her insurance benefits and to schedule this procedure. How can Janae communicate the lack of benefits for this procedure to the patient? What other options does Janae have in order to attempt to get approval for this to be covered by the insurance company. What options, if any, can Janae offer the patient in order to get this procedure scheduled? If you are playing the role as the patient, think about how you would feel if you were in pain and needing to have a procedure that your insurance would not cover. Your instructor will give you additional information about this activity!

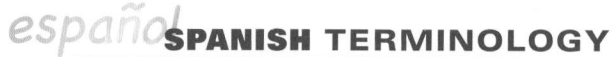 ## español SPANISH TERMINOLOGY

**Usted necesita contactar la oficina de Medicare para actualizar la lista de sus beneficiaries.**
You need to contact Medicare to update your beneficiaries.

**El doctor tiene unos precios muy altos para nuestras necesidades.**
The doctor has a fee for service list that is too expensive for our needs.

**Medicare no le cubre este procedimiento diagnóstico.**
Medicare does not cover your diagnostic procedure.

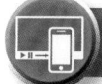 ## MEDIA MENU

**Student Resources** on thePoint®
• **CMA/RMA Certification Exam Review**

**Internet Resources**
**Medical Billing Association**
http://www.e-medbill.com

**American Health Information Management Association**
http://www.ahima.org

**American Medical Association**
http://www.ama-assn.org

## EMR Activity

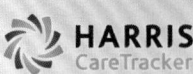

Harris CareTracker is a Web-based electronic medical record (EMR) application that you will use for the EMR activities included in this section at the end of each chapter. This application is actually used in physician offices but is provided to you through the publisher, Wolters Kluwer Health, to give you hands-on practice working with EMRs. Your instructor will have more information about accessing your username, log-in, and Quickstart guide.

Prerequisite Activities in Harris CareTracker

• *The Getting Started and Quickstart documents and EMR Activities Step-by-Step Instructions are available at* http://thePoint.lww.com/KronenbergerComp5e.

Activity Details

Janae Baker, RMA, is responsible for updating charges for services to be sure they exceed the highest payer's reimbursement fee schedule. In the *Administration* module, *Setup* tab, search for the procedure code for a new patient office visit (procedure code 99203) in the *GFMC Fees* Schedule, and update the fee to $200.00. Also search for the chest x-ray (2 views) (procedure code 71020) and update the fee to $30.00.

## Chapter Summary

- Medical coding involves the use of numbers to describe diseases, injuries, and procedures.
- The purposes of coding include indexing medical records, performing medical care reviews, deriving health statistics, and reimbursing physicians and hospitals for services.
- As a medical assistant, you are responsible for knowing the format and usage of CPT-4 and HCPCS level II codes, the system used to report services and procedures by the physician.
- Accurate and thorough coding is essential to ensure appropriate reimbursement.
- You must assist the physician in making sure the proper documentation is available to substantiate the codes used on a claim.
- As in all other aspects of patient contact and care, coding of patients' records is covered by the Health Insurance Portability and Accountability Act of 1996 (HIPAA). Only those with a need to know should have access to patient records.

## Warm-Ups for Critical Thinking

1. How would you handle a physician who you think overbills for procedures? To whom would you report this? How might you collect documentation of fraud?
2. Using a CPT-4 codebook, find as many different main terms as you can for "Removal of earwax" (69210). Remember, the medical term for earwax is *cerumen*. Hint: When thinking of the ear, think, "auditory canal."
3. By attempting to locate the code for the procedure in the scenario that follows, make a list of any further information needed to select the correct code. A 12-year-old girl presents for headaches. She reports that when she has a headache, she cannot see well. The physician orders an electroencephalogram.

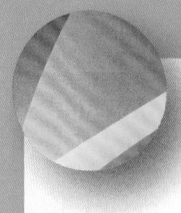

**PSY** PROCEDURE 12-1

## Locating a CPT Code

**PSY** Perform procedural coding; utilize medical necessity guidelines

**Purpose:** To assign the most accurate code for services and procedures rendered by a physician or other provider in order to communicate with a third-party payer

**Equipment:** CPT-4 codebook and patient chart

| STEPS | PURPOSE |
|---|---|
| 1. Identify the exact procedure performed (*right hip joint injection*). | This will ensure accuracy. |
| 2. Obtain the documentation of the procedure in the patient's chart. | The documentation must match the code assigned. |
| 3. Choose the proper codebook. | CPT level I and II codes are listed separately. |
| 4. Using the alphabetic index, locate the procedure. | The alphabetic index is a quick reference. |
| 5. Locate the code or range of codes given in the tabular section. | The index lists ranges of codes in many cases. You must select the correct code by cross-referencing to the codes themselves. |
| 6. Read the descriptors to find the one that most closely describes the procedure. | Reading the descriptors carefully ensures accuracy. |
| 7. Check the section guidelines for any special circumstances. | These guidelines are helpful in staying within the coding rules for each section. |
| 8. Review the documentation to be sure it justifies the code. | |
| 9. Verify the diagnosis for the procedure and determine if it meets medical necessity standards for the procedure.<br><br>The diagnosis must justify the reason for performing the procedure or service. | In the event of a chart audit, the documentation must match the code. |
| 10. Determine if any modifiers are needed. | If there are any unusual circumstances, modifiers will explain. |
| 11. Select the code and place it in the appropriate field of the CMS-1500 form (accurate code is 20610). | Accurate completion of the CMS-1500 form produces clean claims. |
| 12. **AFF**  Your physician is helping you find a code in the CPT-4 codebook. He chooses a code based on what the surgery entailed, but the operative report does not support what he says he did. How would you advise the physician to correct the problem and proceed? | |

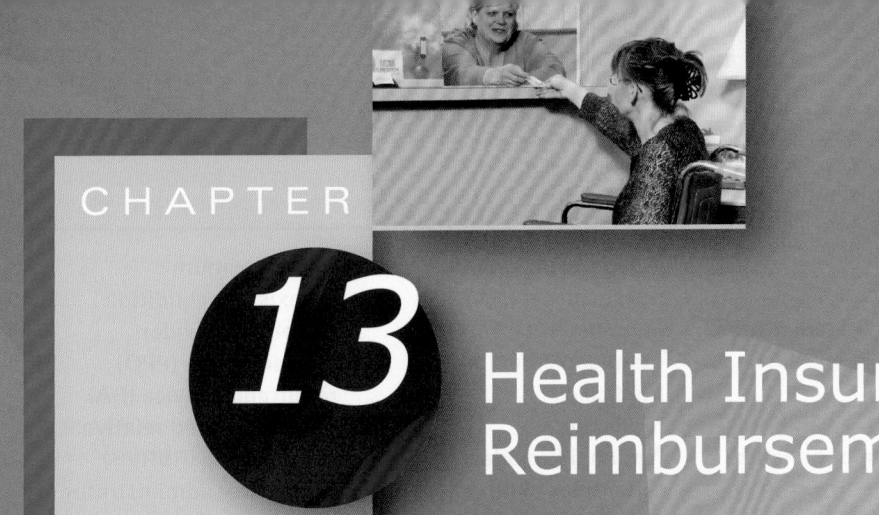

# 13

# Health Insurance and Reimbursement

## Outline

## Learning Outcomes

**COG Cognitive Domain***

1. Spell and define the key terms
2. *Identify*
   a. *Types of third-party plans*
   b. *Information required to file a third-party claim*
   c. *The steps for filing a third-party claim*
3. Discuss workers' compensation as it applies to patients
4. Describe procedures for implementing both managed care and insurance plans
5. Discuss utilization review principles
6. *Outline managed care requirements for patient referral*
7. Compare processes for filing insurance claims both manually and electron*ically*
8. Describe guidelines for third-party claims
9. Discuss types of physician fee schedules
10. Describe the concept of RBRVS
11. Define diagnosis-related groups (DRGs)
12. Name two legal issues affecting claims submissions
13. *Describe processes for:*
    a. *Verification of eligibility for services*
    b. *Precertification*
    c. *Preauthorization*
14. *Define a Patient-Centered Medical Homes (PCMH)*
15. *Differentiate between fraud and abuse*

**PSY Psychomotor Domain***

1. Complete an insurance claim form (Procedure 13-1)

2. Apply both managed care policies and procedures (Procedure 13-1)
3. Apply third-party guidelines (Procedure 13-1)
4. *Interpret information on an insurance card (Procedure 13-2)*
5. *Obtain precertification or preauthorization including documentation (Procedure 13-2)*
6. *Verify eligibility for services including documentation (Procedure 13-2)*
7. *Utilize medical necessity guidelines (Procedure 13-2)*

**AFF Affective Domain***

1. *Interact professionally with third-party representatives*
2. *Display tactful behavior when communicating with medical providers regarding third-party requirements*
3. Communicate in language the patient can understand regarding managed care and insurance plans
4. *Show sensitivity when communicating with patients regarding third-party requirements*
5. Apply ethical behaviors, including honesty/integrity, in the performance of medical assisting practi*ce*

***Note: AAMA/CAAHEP 2015 Standards are italicized.***

**ABHES Competencies**

1. Prepare and submit insurance claims
2. Serve as liaison between physician and others
3. Comply with federal, state, and local health laws and regulations

# Key Terms

accountable care
  organizations
Affordable Care Act (ACA)
assignment of benefits
balance billing
birthday rule
capitation
carrier
claims
claims administrator
coinsurance
coordination of benefits
copayments
crossover claim

deductible
dependent
diagnosis-related groups
  (DRGs)
eligibility
employee
explanation of benefits
  (EOB)
fee-for-service
fee schedule
group member
health care savings
  account (HSA)
health insurance

independent practice
  association (IPA)
insured
managed care
Medicaid
Medicare
National Provider
  Identifier (NPI)
out-of-pocket
Patient-Centered Medical
  Homes (PCMH)
peer review organization
physician hospital
  organization (PHO)

plan maximum
preexisting condition
preferred provider
  organization (PPO)
remittance advice (RA)
resource-based relative
  value scale (RBRVS)
third-party administrator
  (TPA)
usual, customary, and
  reasonable (UCR)
utilization review (UR)

# Case Study

*T*he medical billing department at Great Falls Medical Center is short of staff due to a change in the billing system, and Alex Zeller, CMA (AAMA), has agreed to help with claims preparation today. As he reviews the encounter sheet for the first patient's claim, he notices that there are two insurance companies listed, with both insurance cards scanned into the emergency medical record (EMR). The patient has group insurance through his employer, with a $1,000 annual deductible that has not been met, and a group insurance plan through his wife's employer. What is a deductible and which insurance company will he bill first? What is the correct form he must use to complete a paper claim? What other pieces of information will he need to complete an accurate claim form, and how should the form be completed? This chapter addresses various types of insurance coverage and the language used by payers in the medical reimbursement process.

In the United States, **health insurance** is funded by a combination of employer and employee contributions and tax-funded coverage. In addition to the numerous Blue Cross and Blue Shield plans, health benefits also are provided by other insurance companies, self-funded group plans, and government plans such as Medicare and Medicaid. The benefits vary with each plan and from state to state. According to the 2010 Federal Census Bureau, approximately 80% of Americans are enrolled in health benefit plans of one sort or another. Consequently, most of the patients you will encounter in the physician's office have some type of health insurance. With so many different companies and plans, it would be impossible for you to know each patient's insurance plan requirements, but as a medical assistant, you will need to know where and how to obtain such information so that you can complete and file claim forms appropriately. You must keep abreast of changes as you are notified. You will also need to learn the special terminology associated with health insurance claims. In addition, you may need to instruct patients about insurance matters.

# ☁ HEALTH BENEFIT PLANS

## The Affordable Care Act

The Patient Protection and Affordable Care Act (ACA) was signed into law in March 2010 in order to provide uninsured Americans with affordable health coverage. This law also gave new rights, benefits, and protections regarding health insurance to all Americans. Some of the important features of the law include coverage for required preventative and wellness services. The ACA requires all individuals to have some sort of health coverage effective May 1, 2014, or pay a tax penalty. Online Health Insurance Marketplaces were created to enable individuals to compare and enroll in health insurance plans and to allow for premiums for health insurance purchased through the Marketplace to be subsidized for qualified individuals (Box 13-1). However, using the Marketplace is optional and individuals may still purchase their own individual health plans through other methods. Although there are some benefits that are required for health insurance plans to be ACA compliant, coverage of other benefits varies, so it is very important for the medical assistant to understand what types of insurance patients have as well as coverage and benefits provided in their plans.

## Group Health Benefits

Group health benefits are sponsored by an organization, such as an employer, a union, or an association. A person covered by group health benefits is either an employee or a **group member** who, by virtue of employment or membership in an organization, may participate in and receive benefits from a health plan. Coverage in health plans differs greatly, so you need to know the **eligibility** of the patient for services being provided by your office. Although the ACA requires insurance policies to have basic coverage including preventative care for men, women, and children, employers may offer several different plans from which employees may choose with a variety of services that are covered under each plan.

Employer health benefits may be either **insured** or self-funded. Commonly, health benefits are referred to as insurance. It is, however, important to distinguish between the actual benefits and the vehicle used to fund and provide them.

With insured benefits, the employer, employee, or both pay a monthly premium to an insurance company. The insurance company, in turn, is obligated to pay for any eligible health benefits. Self-funded benefits on the surface appear the same as insured benefits. They are paid for in the same manner as group health benefits, but instead of the employer paying the insurance company to invest the money to cover payments, they invest it themselves. They pay an insurance company or other agency to process **claims** and make payments on their behalf. Any payment for medical services that are not paid by the patient or physician is said to be paid by a *third-party payer*. In this case, the payer is an agent for the self-funded plan and is, therefore, known as a **third-party administrator (TPA)**. The Department of Insurance for each state determines and regulates how employers may choose to self-fund their group benefit plans rather than insure them through an insurance company.

For a group benefit plan to cover (pay for) eligible expenses, the patient must meet several criteria, called eligibility requirements. These are defined in the policy or plan document and may include a minimum number of hours worked per week and a waiting period from the date of employment before benefits become effective.

The eligibility of a **dependent** (spouse, children) is based on the employee's eligibility. Certain eligibility limitations apply to dependent children. Eligibility usually requires that children be the unmarried natural or adopted children of the employee, unmarried stepchildren, or children for whom the employee has legal guardianship and eligibility may be extended if the child is disabled.

To confirm a patient's eligibility, check the back of the patient's identification (ID) card (Fig. 13-1) for a Web address or phone number to contact the **claims administrator** for the health benefit plan.

Group and individual health benefits describe contractual agreements and how the policies are paid. Both groups and individuals can choose from many different types

---

### BOX 13-1   The Affordable Care Act

On March 23, 2010, the ACA was signed into law by President Obama for comprehensive health insurance reforms and to require everyone to get health insurance as of January 1, 2014. The state or federal government's Health Exchange (Health Insurance Marketplace) allows patients to compare coverage for qualified health insurance plans. Some individuals may also qualify for subsidized or reduced health insurance premiums, but only if insurance is purchased through the Marketplace.

Patients may check for eligibility to purchase health insurance through the Marketplace and to determine if they qualify for subsidized or reduced health insurance premiums during open enrollment, which is from November 15 through February 15 of the following year. Under certain circumstances, patients may qualify to obtain coverage during a *special enrollment period* as determined by the Marketplace.

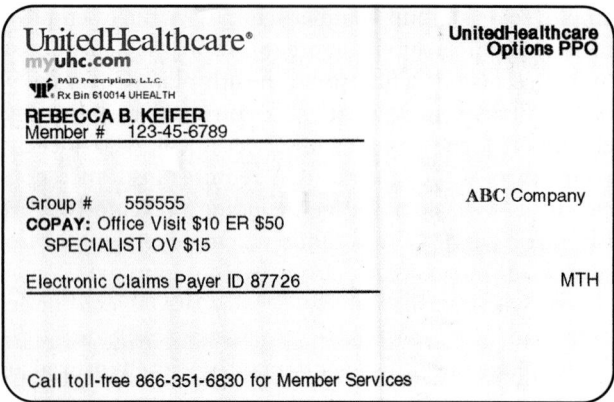

**Figure 13-1** • Patient identification card.

of plans, such as traditional, HMO (health maintenance organization), and PPO (preferred provider organization). These types are further discussed later in this chapter.

## Health Care Savings Accounts

**Health care savings accounts (HSAs)** are often offered as an employee benefit. Employees save money through payroll deduction to accounts that can only be used for medical care. Money is put into a health savings account before it is taxed and can be withdrawn instantly for qualified medical expenses as needed; any dollars remaining can be carried over to be spent in future years or invested to accumulate savings for health needs after retirement. HSAs are not designed to replace a regular health insurance policy but work in conjunction with a high-health insurance policy, usually a PPO, which costs less. In effect, an employee would pay for medical care, using his or her tax-free HSA dollars, until he or she spends up to the deductible. A **deductible** is the predetermined amount the policyholder must incur before the insurance begins paying. Once the deductible is met, the health insurance pays for most or all of the employee's medical expenses for the rest of the year.

 **CHECKPOINT QUESTION**

1. Under what circumstances is a dependent eligible for coverage by a parent's insurance policy?

## Individual Health Benefits

Individual health benefits policies are purchased by an individual from an insurance company. The individual pays premiums directly to the insurance company, and the insurance company pays either the doctor or the hospital directly if they are a participating provider or reimburses the individual for eligible medical expenses.

For patients with individual health benefits, the criteria for completing and filing claims are the same as for patients with group health benefits. Individual health policies commonly have less generous coverage, however, than group health plans have. An individual policy may also have a rider that limits or eliminates benefits for certain illnesses or injuries based on the determination of the underwriter at the time the policy was issued. The Health Insurance Portability and Accountability Act of 1996 (HIPAA) includes a provision to protect employees changing jobs from being denied benefits for preexisting conditions (see Appendix A). Although a provision of the ACA prohibits insurance companies from denying coverage to individuals who have a preexisting condition, there are still plans that are exempt from this mandate. (See section on filing claims for more information.) Therefore, it may also be necessary for the medical assistant to determine if a patient has a plan that does not cover certain conditions.

With the cost of health care skyrocketing and more insurance companies limiting what they will cover, many people have more than one health care insurance policy. It is extremely important that you know which insurance you bill first (primary) and which to bill the remainder of the charges (secondary). This is called **coordination of benefits**, and it is the responsibility of patients with more than one insurance to indicate which insurance is primary, secondary, tertiary, etc. (See section of filing claims for more information.)

## Government-Sponsored (Public) Health Benefits

Government-sponsored benefit programs are funded and regulated by the federal government or individual states. Government programs have been developed over the years to assist persons who do not otherwise have health benefits, such as the elderly, the indigent, and others unable to obtain benefits. Government programs include Medicare, Medicaid, TRICARE/CHAMPVA, and workers' compensation.

## Medicare

In 1965, the Social Security Act established **Medicare** to provide health insurance for the elderly. Elderly persons were defined as Social Security recipients age 65 or older. In 1972, amendments to the Social Security Act expanded Medicare coverage to two additional high-risk groups: disabled persons who have been receiving Social Security benefits for 24 months and persons suffering from end-stage renal disease.

Medicare Part A covers hospital expenses and is provided at no additional charge to persons eligible for Social Security benefits. Medicare Part B pays for physician fees, both inpatient and outpatient, diagnostic testing, certain immunizations (influenza and pneumonia), and specific screening tests (PSA, mammograms, Pap smears, bone density testing, colorectal screening). Part B Medicare is optional, and the participant is charged a premium for Part B coverage. The premium is usually deducted from the monthly Social Security benefits.

Persons signing up for or receiving Social Security benefits are automatically enrolled in both Part A and Part B Medicare when they reach age 65 years. If they do not wish to participate in Part B, they must decline it. Both Part A and Part B of Medicare have deductibles and copayments, and as with most health insurance policies, these generally increase yearly.

Patients with Medicare coverage who are actively employed and covered by their employer's plan may have secondary Medicare benefits. A retired person age 65 or older who has health insurance in addition to Medicare may have primary or secondary Medicare benefits as outlined in the Medicare Secondary Payer (MSP) rules.

After the deductible has been met, Medicare Part B has an 80/20 coinsurance, which means that Medicare reimburses the physician 80% of the Medicare-approved charges. The patient is responsible for the remaining 20% of the Medicare-approved fee. Under certain circumstances, if paying the 20% causes undue financial hardship, the physician may not charge the remaining 20%, but there must be signed documentation from the patient stating the necessity for the inability to pay the remaining amount that is the patient's financial responsibility. The Centers for Medicare and Medicaid Services (CMS) can provide forms with the requirements, and the forms should always be used.

In addition to Medicare, the Social Security Act of 1965 established Medicaid, a program of health care coverage for the poor. If patients are financially unable to pay the 20%, they may be eligible for Medicaid. This is referred to as a **Medi–Medi claim** because the patient is eligible under both Medicare and Medicaid. After Medicare pays on a Medi–Medi claim, it is forwarded to Medicaid to processing without the necessity of completing another claim form. This is known as a **crossover claim**. Physicians participating in Medicare are required to submit claims on behalf of Medicare patients, and these claims must be filed within one year of the time the service is incurred. (See section on filing claims for more information.) Most providers must file Medicare claims electronically; however, Medicare will accept original paper claims on the CMS-1500 version 02/12 from providers who are exempt from the electronic filing requirement under certain limited conditions.

The Centers for Medicare and Medicaid Services (CMS), which was known as the *Health Care Financing Administration (HCFA)* prior to July 1, 2001, is a government agency that oversees the financial aspects of health care in the United States (Box 13-2). The CMS contracts with Medicare Administrative Contractors (**MAC**s) to process Part A and Part B claims in various regions of the United States. In addition to processing claims, MACs also serve to educate providers in matters related to medical billing for Medicare and Medicaid services. CMS requires that all claims be submitted to MACs with certain code sets, such as the Current Procedural Terminology (CPT) coding system (see Chapter 12), but the CMS has also established another code set for Part B services that may be used for claims known as the Healthcare Common Procedure Coding System (HCPCS) codes (see Chapter 12). For proper reimbursement, it is important for the medical assistant performing billing duties to understand when to use the HCPCS codes when billing for Medicare services.

It is important to ask the patient about supplemental or secondary coverage provided as a benefit for retirement or purchased individually. These policies

---

**BOX 13-2   What is the CMS?**

The CMS is the federal agency that administers Medicare, Medicaid, and the State Children's Health Insurance Program (SCHIP). The CMS also performs quality-focused activities, including regulation of laboratory testing, development of coverage policies, and quality-of-care improvement. The CMS maintains oversight of the survey and certification of nursing homes and continuing care providers, including home health agencies and intermediate care facilities for the mentally retarded. It makes available to beneficiaries, providers, researchers, and state surveyors information about these activities and nursing home quality.

To ensure public and expert involvement in running their programs, the CMS maintains a number of chartered advisory committees. These committees, whose meetings are open to the public, provide advice or make recommendations on a variety of issues relating to CMS's responsibilities and activities.

usually cover the deductible and charges not covered by Medicare. In this case, it is often necessary to file a second claim to that insurance attaching Medicare's **remittance advice** (formerly the explanation of benefits) that shows reimbursement details from the payer. (See section on explanation of benefits for more information.)

 **CHECKPOINT QUESTION**

2. What is the difference between parts A and B of Medicare coverage?

## Medicaid

**Medicaid** provides health benefits to low-income or indigent persons of all ages. Often, eligibility for Medicaid is based on a patient's eligibility for other state programs, such as welfare assistance. Medicaid is governed by both federal and state statutes and rules and then implemented on a state and local level. Although the federal government stipulates the minimum health care coverage, states can provide coverage beyond the minimum. The ACA also provides a method for states to increase eligibility requirements for Medicaid coverage in order to receive funding from the federal government to cover the cost of expanding coverage, for example, increasing coverage to include eligible adults without children who fall within the Federal Poverty Level. Not all states participate in this Medicaid expansion; therefore, Medicaid eligibility and benefits vary from state to state. At a minimum, Medicaid provides 100% coverage for the following:

- Inpatient hospital care
- Outpatient treatment and services
- Diagnostic services
- Family planning
- Skilled nursing facilities
- Diagnostic screenings for children

Many states use a managed care type of Medicaid coverage in which recipients make a copayment based on their income and are assigned a primary care physician as a "gatekeeper." This is a cost-effective method that prevents misuse or overuse of health care services.

Since circumstances that make recipients eligible for coverage change from month to month (i.e., employment), standard Medicaid patients receive a new ID card each month. Make a photocopy of the card for the patient's file on the first visit of each month. However, Medicaid managed care plans may issue one card that is very similar to a private insurance card, so it is very important for the medical assistant to always verify eligibility at every visit. Most states have online eligibility and authorization verification capabilities. Because reimbursement is considerably less than other insurances, not all physicians accept Medicaid patients, nor are they required to do so. If Medicaid patients are accepted, you need to be familiar with Medicaid as administered in your state.

 **CHECKPOINT QUESTION**

3. List six types of medical expenses that are covered at 100% by Medicaid.

 **AFF   WHAT IF?**

**What if a patient comes in to see the physician but does not have her Medicaid card?**

Most states offer Medicaid providers the ability to verify eligibility on any given date of service online. By searching for the Department of Human Services on the Web in almost any city, you can be directed to this feature. This is especially helpful since Medicaid eligibility is managed on a monthly basis, and sometimes, patients will not receive their cards before the first day of a new month. Before this capability existed, many times, patients were sent away if they did not have their cards with them. As long as you have an ID number or Social Security number, you can verify eligibility instantly.

## TRICARE/CHAMPVA

TRICARE is administered by the U.S. Department of Defense and provides medical coverage for dependents of active service personnel, dependents of service personnel who died during active duty, and retired service personnel. When Congress realized that CHAMPUS costs could be controlled with managed care, they mandated that HMOs and PPOs (discussed later in this chapter) be added to the coverage. This three-part system is now called TRICARE. This system requires that participants be assigned a primary care manager (PCM). The PCM is named on the beneficiary's card.

If a patient lives within 40 miles of a uniformed services hospital and that facility is unable to handle the needs of patients covered by TRICARE, a statement of unavailability is required for treatment by a physician's office or civilian hospital. Patients who live more than 40 miles from a uniformed services hospital do not need this statement to be treated in a physician's office or civilian hospital and for the physician or hospital to be reimbursed.

The Civilian Health and Medical Program of the Veterans Administration (CHAMPVA) covers dependents of veterans who have total and permanent service-connected disabilities. CHAMPVA is administered by the area Veterans Administration hospital. Once admitted to the CHAMPVA program, patients select their own physician; this allows them the same benefits as private insurance.

## ☰ MANAGED CARE

Health care costs in the United States have grown at about twice the general rate of inflation. As a result, the United States now spends more for health care services than any other industrialized nation, both as a percentage of gross national product and per person. In the United States, most people obtain health coverage through their employer. The exceptions are Medicare for the elderly, TRICARE for retired military personnel and their dependents, Medicaid for low-income Americans, and those who buy their own health insurance.

The rapid rate of healthcare inflation encouraged employers to begin offering **managed care** programs, which are typically less costly than traditional insurance coverage systems. Managed care programs vary greatly, but all involve a different relationship between the insurer, health care provider, and covered individual from that of traditional insurance programs. To understand this difference, we first discuss the traditional insurance system.

In traditional insurance systems, the covered patient may seek care from any provider. Normally, the patient and physician decide what care is needed. Then, services are rendered, and the insurer pays a portion of the provider's bills (after deductibles and coinsurance). The insurer has no relationship with the provider.

In managed care systems, however, the insurer has a contractual relationship with the provider. The contract usually establishes what prices will be charged for each service and the conditions under which a service would be covered. Most managed care programs contain the following elements:

- *Precertification of hospital admissions* (often also called *utilization management [UM]* or **utilization review [UR]**). A patient can be admitted to a hospital for certain conditions only if that admission has been certified (approved) by the insurer. The goal of this requirement is to ensure that a patient's care is provided in the most cost-effective setting. For example, many surgical procedures that used to require an inpatient hospital stay can now be performed in an outpatient setting if proper education and support are available to the patient. Conflict between a UR guideline and the physician's requirements for the patient can be appealed to an impartial **peer review organization** composed of physicians and specialists who will review the case and make the final recommendation.
- *Approved referrals*. As discussed in Chapter 6, in many managed care plans, a specialty physician can provide services to a managed care patient only on referral from the patient's primary care physician. The purpose is to ensure that the services provided by the specialist are medically necessary and, again, provided in the most cost-effective setting. Payment of a claim depends on the completion of the appropriate form.

- *Network*. A network consists of providers (physicians, hospitals, pharmacies, and other providers and suppliers) who have signed contracts with the insurer or **health maintenance organization (HMO)** to provide services to covered persons in individual, group, or public health plans. A patient is normally required to use network providers to receive full coverage. The financial penalties (lost coverage) are often very high if a patient does not use these providers.
- *Assignment of benefits*. By contract, the network provider cannot bill the patient for any amounts not paid by the insurer (no **balance billing**) except for copayments, coinsurance, and deductibles. If payment for a service provided by a network physician or hospital is denied by the insurer because it was not properly authorized, the provider cannot bill the patient for these services unless the contract does not contain a hold-harmless clause for the patient. This puts teeth in the control features of the managed care program.

Most physicians have contracts with more than one managed care program, and each of these programs has its own requirements and reimbursement schedules. So that the physician can provide the patient with needed health care services, while ensuring that the physician is paid for his or her services, it is necessary to consider the requirements of each patient's program. UM or precertification requirements are extremely important. Check the patient's ID card for details (see Fig. 13-1). UM requirements may apply to inpatient services or to a variety of outpatient and doctor office services.

Until you are very familiar with the requirements of each of your patient's managed care programs, you should call the number on the ID card before a patient is admitted to a hospital (on a nonemergency basis), referred to another physician, or scheduled for specific laboratory, radiologic, or other tests or evaluations. For inpatient admissions, the UM firm may ask for the diagnosis, the procedure or procedures to be performed, and other related information before approving the admission. Once the procedure is approved, the UM firm may only approve a specified length of stay in the hospital. Failure to comply with the precertification requirements results in a financial penalty for the patient and possibly also for the physician and the hospital.

It is important to be familiar with physicians within the network. The physician, hospital, laboratory, or other provider you normally refer a patient to may not be in the patient's managed care network. By calling the UM number to check, you can avoid penalties and improve the satisfaction of the patient with your services by advising them of any **out-of-pocket** expenses they may have to incur due to out-of-network referrals. Many times, these requirements can be met electronically as companies improve their technology.

4. What are the four key elements of a managed care program?

## Health Maintenance Organizations

It is easiest to understand how an HMO functions if we contrast it with a traditional health insurance program. In the traditional insurance system, the relationship between the covered individual and the insurer or self-insurer is purely financial. In return for receiving a paid monthly premium, the insurer promises to reimburse (indemnify) the individual if he or she incurs certain types of covered medical expense. There are often limits to coverage (exclusions and limitations), and normally, the coverage has a deductible (amount below which services are not reimbursable) and coinsurance (the patient pays a percentage of the medical expense after the deductible is satisfied). For example, the patient pays the first $200 (deductible) in physician charges each year starting January 1; then, insurance pays 80% of covered charges, and the patient must pay the other 20%.

The covered individual seeks medical services and thereby incurs an expense. The individual, not the insurer, must pay for this expense. If the medical treatment is covered as defined in the insurance policy, the insurer will reimburse the patient a portion of the amount incurred after deductibles and coinsurance.

In contrast to traditional insurance companies, an HMO promises to provide covered services rather than pay for them. In this respect, the HMO acts as both an insurer and a provider of service. HMO policies are written differently from insurance policies. The HMO policy lists the medical services that the member is entitled to receive and the physicians and hospitals that will provide these services. The HMO has a contract with both the patient and provider. It must provide covered services to the member either directly from its own physician staff and hospitals or indirectly from physicians and hospitals contracted to provide the services promised to the member. The HMO, rather than the patient, is responsible for the costs of medical services as long as patients' care remains with the providers in the HMO network.

This is one reason HMOs do not normally use deductibles and coinsurance, which are standard features of health insurance programs. A patient does not receive a provider's bill, so deductibles and coinsurance cannot apply. Instead, HMOs use predetermined copayments (e.g., $10 per physician office visit) to reduce premium prices.

HMOs come in many forms. An HMO contracts with employers to cover their employees. The medical group and hospitals contract with the health plan to provide the services required in the health plan's contract with employers. Rather than paying for these services on a fee-for-service basis, a company pays the physicians per employee. Consistent with its history, the health plan does not pay the medical group a fee for each service provided. Instead, it pays each party based on the number of members enrolled in the health plan. This is often called capitation because there is one payment per member. Capitation payments are also used by other types of HMOs.

As group model HMOs developed (they were called prepaid group practices until 1973 federal legislation changed their names), nongroup physicians are organized into an entity called an independent practice association (IPA). The early IPA HMOs were often sponsored by a local medical society and were developed to allow independent physicians to compete with prepaid group practices.

IPA HMOs contract with employers in the same manner as group model HMOs, and their members receive covered services from IPA physicians. The HMO's contracts with physicians are different, however, because these physicians are not organized into a single multispecialty group practice. IPA physicians are paid in a number of ways. Some are paid on a capitation basis, and some may be paid on a fee-for-service basis using a fee schedule established by the HMO. Often, a portion of any reimbursement is withheld by the HMO and paid only if the HMO's total medical expense is within budget; this encourages the physician to be cost conscious in caring for patients.

In some of these HMOs, the IPA is a separate corporation, often owned by physicians. With this structure (still called an IPA HMO), the IPA contracts with physicians, and the HMO contracts with the IPA instead of directly with each physician.

Over the years, HMOs have continued to evolve, and many are now a mixture of these discussed models. As a medical assistant, you must know what type of relationship the practice has with an HMO before you can determine how the practice is reimbursed. Most HMOs require claims to be submitted even if payment is capitation rather than fee-for-service.

Although requirements vary, a gatekeeper provision is common with HMOs. A gatekeeper is a primary care physician who participates within the HMO network of providers. Participants are required to see a primary care physician (PCP) for all nonemergency services, and the PCP will either treat the patient or refer the patient to a specialist within the HMO network. Before the patient may be seen, however, the PCP must seek preauthorization from the HMO for the referral (see Box 13-3). Preauthorizations for services are typically for *outpatient* diagnostic and surgical services and are essentially advising the HMO of the medical necessity for the treatment and

## BOX 13-3  Referrals Are More Than Just Phone Calls

As discussed in Chapter 6, when a patient has third-party coverage that requires preauthorization for a referral to a specialist, you must follow the steps and complete the proper forms in order for the patient to be covered for the specialist's services. You will know the patient's requirements by looking at the card or going to a Web site listed on the card. For example, your physician employer is Mr. Smith's primary care physician (PCP) or gatekeeper. Mr. Smith's policy requires preauthorization for referrals. Mr. Smith is complaining of frequent and severe headaches. Your doctor wants him to see a neurologist to rule out migraine headaches. Before calling to make an appointment with the neurologist, you must contact the third-party payer for approval. They will want to know the patient's situation, the physician's plans for him, the rationale for the referral, etc. If the referral is approved, they will give you a referral approval number that must be provided to the neurologist in order to be reimbursed for the referral services.

## PATIENT EDUCATION

### Help Patients Understand Their Obligation

As discussed in Chapter 2, the contract between a physician and his patient implies that the *patient* will pay the physician for his services, not the patient's insurance company. When a physician participates with an insurance company, he may be required to file a patient's claims, but this is not the case with all third-party payers. Although patients have the ultimate responsibility of paying the physician, they tend to think that a physician should wait for their insurance to pay. A physician who does not choose to participate with a particular third-party payer is not obligated to extend credit to a patient. Of course, most practices choose to offer filing the patient's claim as a courtesy. Because of the nature of a physician's work, most physicians are willing to make reasonable credit arrangements, but patients should understand that their physician may not be legally obligated to file their claims or extend credit.

Understanding their insurance benefits will give patients the opportunity to take a more active role in their physician's reimbursement. Direct patients to their insurance company's Web site, keep abreast of changes, and be willing to discuss these matters openly. Help patients understand their obligations to the physician and their insurance company's obligations to them. This approach will not only benefit the patients but will also improve your collection ratio.

confirming it is a covered benefit with the patient's insurance plan.

Some services may need **precertification**, which is similar to preauthorization in that it also confirms medical necessity and covered benefits, but it also hospital inpatient services (such as the number of days the patient may need to be hospitalized). Some outpatient surgical services are required to be precertified as well, so it is important to always check with the insurance company when in doubt. Both preauthorizations and precertifications are often handled online on the HMOs Web site, but some companies may have a specific form to be completed and faxed or emailed.

The gatekeeper provision seeks to reduce the plan cost of specialists. For example, without such a provision, a patient might see a specialist first at a more costly fee, even though the condition may have been adequately treated by a less costly primary care physician. The gatekeeper approach also encourages patients to establish a relationship with a primary care physician, who is then in a position to manage the patient's care.

## CHECKPOINT QUESTION

5. How does an HMO differ from a traditional health insurance program?

## Preferred Provider Organizations

Whereas HMOs promise to provide services and have a financial risk in their relationships with subscribers, a **preferred provider organization (PPO)** is a type of health benefit program whose purpose is simply to contract with providers and then lease this network of contracted providers to health care plans. The PPO network is not risk bearing; it does not have any financial involvement in the health plan. PPOs are typically developed by hospitals and physicians as a vehicle to attract patients, although some are developed and managed by insurance **carriers**.

PPOs contract with participating providers, including hospitals and physicians. These contracts allow the PPO to contract with insurers and other purchasers of health care services on behalf of the participating providers, who typically accept less than their normal charges and agree to follow the UM and other administrative protocols as specified by the PPO.

Typically, a health plan with a PPO offers benefits at two levels, commonly referred to as in network and out of network. Unlike in an HMO, patients may visit any provider they wish for services. If the provider is in network (a participating provider), the levels of benefit

Example of a Health Plan with a PPO

| Benefit | In-network | Out-of-network |
|---|---|---|
| Deductible | $100 | $300 |
| Coinsurance | 90% | 70% |
| Routine care | $200 per calendar year | -0- |
| Mental health | 80% | 50% |
| Office visit | $10 co-pay; no deductible | 70% |

**Figure 13-2 •** A health plan with a PPO.

for the patient are greater than if the patient receives services from an out-of-network (nonparticipating) provider.

A typical health plan with a PPO may look like the breakdown shown in Figure 13-2.

As you can see from the example, each time the patient sees an in-network provider, he or she receives significantly better benefits. A primary difference between an HMO and PPO, therefore, is that with PPO plans, patients can see any physician of their choice and receive benefits; they simply have an incentive in the form of higher benefits when they see an in-network provider. HMO plans, on the other hand, are more restrictive and do not pay benefits unless patients seek care from in-network providers.

As part of your responsibilities, you should identify the PPOs with which the physician has contracted and determine the administrative requirements set forth by each PPO in the contract. To understand the necessary administrative procedures agreed to by the physician, review all managed care contracts carefully. Also, be aware that most PPOs have a provider relations representative who works with the contracted providers (physicians) to answer questions and clarify procedures. The PPO is typically operated by a group of hospitals or physicians or by an insurance company or independent organization. Physicians agree to participate in PPOs to serve their existing patients who now have PPO plans and sometimes to gain additional patients who seek the services of a PPO physician.

Participating physicians have agreed to perform certain administrative services for PPO patients. Commonly, the physician's office must accept assignment of benefits and provide claims filing services for the patient. The physician agrees to accept the reimbursement by the claims administrator as payment in full and agrees not to bill the patient for any difference between the physician's usual charge and the PPO-negotiated charge for the service. The participating physician is responsible for collecting any copay amount at the time of service. The physician also agrees to comply with any precertification requirements stipulated by the plan.

**CHECKPOINT QUESTION**

6. What is the primary difference between an HMO and a PPO?

## Physician Hospital Organizations

Physicians and hospitals have become more active in developing managed care alternatives. A **physician hospital organization (PHO)** is a coalition of physicians and a hospital contracting with large employers, insurance carriers, and other benefit groups to provide discounted health services. There are numerous variations of PHOs. A PHO may look much like a PPO with no risk-bearing elements, in which case the network of providers constituting the PHO are under no financial obligation to subscribers. Alternatively, a PHO may be more like an HMO, wherein the participating providers in the PHO do have a risk-bearing contract and assume responsibility for the overall medical budget of subscribing units. Physician organizations (POs) are such groups consisting of physicians only. As with any managed care program, it is important to know and understand the particulars of each managed care contract and the requirements of the provider and obligations to patients and the managed care entity.

## Accountable Care Organizations

Although HMOs, PPOs, and increasingly PHOs are the most common managed care programs, many others cover patients today, and still more are being developed. **Accountable Care Organizations (ACOs)** are groups of providers, including primary care physicians, specialists, and hospitals, who have joined together to provide coordinated care to patients. The goal of an ACO is to reduce unnecessary health care costs by helping patients get health care services when needed and avoiding duplication of services when multiple providers are involved. Payment incentives are given to providers participating in an ACO, including Medicare's ACOs Shared Savings Program, as health care savings are achieved while maintaining the quality of patient care that is rendered. ACOs do not require gatekeepers; however, primary physicians in an ACO may also participate in Patient-Centered Medical Homes (PCMH) described below.

## Patient-Centered Medical Homes

**Patient-Centered Medical Homes (PCMH)** is a concept similar to a gatekeeper in which the primary physician assumes responsibility for a patient's overall health care and coordination of health services. The primary feature for a PCMH is a relationship between the patient and the primary physician who will direct the patient's care as necessary to improve patient outcomes. Depending on the individual needs of patients, the primary physician uses a variety of health care professionals in a team approach. As patient advocates, medical assistants are being given the responsibility to communicate and handle the coordination of care for patients in practices participating in a PCMH (see Chapter 8).

## ⊕◯Ⓖ WORKERS' COMPENSATION

Workers' compensation benefits were developed to cover the expenses resulting from a work-related illness or injury. In the event of a work-related illness or injury, claims submitted to the group or individual health benefit plan will be returned with instructions to file with the workers' compensation administrator, who determines the validity of the claim and reimburses accordingly. Because your practice will likely be taking care of the patient for both routine medical care and work-related illness or injury, it is important to determine at the time services are rendered whether the illness or injury is work related and, if so, to account and file for those services separately.

You are responsible for knowing your state's workers' compensation regulations and procedures. Consult your state's office for workers' compensation or your state's designated claims administrator of the workers' compensation program for specific information.

## ⊕◯Ⓖ FILING CLAIMS

Completion of accurate claim forms is crucial to the financial health of the practice. In addition to patient encounter forms (see Chapter 14), patient demographics and copies of insurance card(s) must be updated at each visit (see Chapter 5) to make sure claims are completed as accurately as possible. In addition, as part of the HIPAA Simplification Standard, all providers must have their own 10-digit **National Provider Identifier (NPI)** number to submit on claim forms. This number identifies each provider, and a database is kept by CMS for all NPI numbers known as the National Plan and Provider Enumerator System (NPPES).

If the provider requires patients to make full payment at the time of the visit, the physician may still submit a claim on the patient's behalf; however, the patient may need to submit claims to the claims administrator for reimbursement. Most providers accept assignment of benefits as a requirement for most insurance participation contracts, however. To do this, the patient must give written authorization for the claims administrator to reimburse the physician for billed charges. As a medical assistant, you may be responsible for obtaining all necessary claims information from the provider and the patient and then submitting a claim for payment to the claims administrator.

As discussed in Chapter 5, the patient's ID card is a source of information necessary for complete and accurate claims submission. Keep a copy of this card in the patient's file and be sure to update it at least yearly and preferably at each visit, since the patient's employment and eligibility may change.

In addition, a patient may be covered by more than one group plan. For example, a patient may be covered both on an employer's group plan and as a dependent on his or her spouse's group plan. The primary plan—the one that pays first—is the plan provided by the patient's employer. Any unpaid amount is then considered for payment by the spouse's group plan, which is considered secondary. This is called **coordination of benefits**.

Dependent children may be covered under one or two parents' plans. Unless the plans state otherwise, the plan of the parent whose birthday occurs first each calendar year (not necessarily the oldest parent) is the primary plan. This is known as the **birthday rule**. This rule is commonly used by benefit plans and claims administrators to coordinate the benefits of dependent children covered by two plans. If the parents are legally separated or divorced, however, the primary plan is the plan of the parent who has custody or, in some instances, is subject to a court order or divorce decree.

After establishing the primary plan and the claims submission destination, you prepare the claim for filing. The CMS-1500 was developed by the National Uniform Claim Committee (NUCC) consisting of members from the American Medical Association and CMS in order to standardize an acceptable paper claim form for different plans and different claims administrators (Fig 13-3). Most payers have electronic claim filing capabilities; however, there are exceptions, and some providers may continue to bill for services using the most recent version of CMS-1500 claim form. This claim form is accepted by most claims administrators, including Blue Cross and Blue Shield, Medicare, Medicaid, and TRICARE/CHAMPVA. Procedure 13-1 explains how to complete a CMS-1500 claim form.

Some insurance plans include a clause that excludes coverage for a stated period (usually 12 months) for a condition that existed before the plan's effective date; this is known as a **preexisting condition**. For example, a patient with a diagnosis of depression before the effective date of his or her plan would be covered for all other conditions from the effective date forward but would not be covered for services related to the diagnosis or treatment of depression for the preexisting exclusion period (in this example, 12 months). Although the ACA has a preexisting coverage mandate that prevents insurance companies from denying coverage or increasing the cost of coverage to patients with a preexisting condition, some insurance plans that were in place before March 23, 2010, are exempt from this mandate. Patients with a preexisting condition that is not covered under the ACA mandate will be responsible for charges incurred to treat that condition.

Many pieces of information are needed for timely and efficient claims processing. The insurance company or managed care plan cannot process claims with incomplete or inaccurate information and will return them to the provider for completion, correction, and resubmission. This lengthens the time the provider must wait for reimbursement, making accurate claims submission

## HEALTH INSURANCE CLAIM FORM

APPROVED BY NATIONAL UNIFORM CLAIM COMMITTEE (NUCC) 02/12

PICA | PICA

CARRIER

1. MEDICARE (Medicare#) | MEDICAID (Medicaid#) | TRICARE (ID#/DoD#) | CHAMPVA (Member ID#) | GROUP HEALTH PLAN (ID#) | FECA BLK LUNG (ID#) | OTHER (ID#)

1a. INSURED'S I.D. NUMBER (For Program in Item 1)

2. PATIENT'S NAME (Last Name, First Name, Middle Initial)

3. PATIENT'S BIRTH DATE MM DD YY — SEX M F

4. INSURED'S NAME (Last Name, First Name, Middle Initial)

5. PATIENT'S ADDRESS (No., Street)

6. PATIENT RELATIONSHIP TO INSURED — Self Spouse Child Other

7. INSURED'S ADDRESS (No., Street)

CITY | STATE

8. RESERVED FOR NUCC USE

CITY | STATE

ZIP CODE | TELEPHONE (Include Area Code) ( )

ZIP CODE | TELEPHONE (Include Area Code) ( )

9. OTHER INSURED'S NAME (Last Name, First Name, Middle Initial)

10. IS PATIENT'S CONDITION RELATED TO:

11. INSURED'S POLICY GROUP OR FECA NUMBER

a. OTHER INSURED'S POLICY OR GROUP NUMBER

a. EMPLOYMENT? (Current or Previous) YES NO

a. INSURED'S DATE OF BIRTH MM DD YY — SEX M F

b. RESERVED FOR NUCC USE

b. AUTO ACCIDENT? YES NO PLACE (State)

b. OTHER CLAIM ID (Designated by NUCC)

c. RESERVED FOR NUCC USE

c. OTHER ACCIDENT? YES NO

c. INSURANCE PLAN NAME OR PROGRAM NAME

d. INSURANCE PLAN NAME OR PROGRAM NAME

10d. CLAIM CODES (Designated by NUCC)

d. IS THERE ANOTHER HEALTH BENEFIT PLAN? YES NO *If yes*, complete items 9, 9a, and 9d.

**READ BACK OF FORM BEFORE COMPLETING & SIGNING THIS FORM.**

12. PATIENT'S OR AUTHORIZED PERSON'S SIGNATURE I authorize the release of any medical or other information necessary to process this claim. I also request payment of government benefits either to myself or to the party who accepts assignment below.

SIGNED ____ DATE ____

13. INSURED'S OR AUTHORIZED PERSON'S SIGNATURE I authorize payment of medical benefits to the undersigned physician or supplier for services described below.

SIGNED ____

PATIENT AND INSURED INFORMATION

14. DATE OF CURRENT ILLNESS, INJURY, or PREGNANCY (LMP) MM DD YY QUAL.

15. OTHER DATE QUAL. MM DD YY

16. DATES PATIENT UNABLE TO WORK IN CURRENT OCCUPATION FROM MM DD YY TO MM DD YY

17. NAME OF REFERRING PROVIDER OR OTHER SOURCE | 17a. | 17b. NPI

18. HOSPITALIZATION DATES RELATED TO CURRENT SERVICES FROM MM DD YY TO MM DD YY

19. ADDITIONAL CLAIM INFORMATION (Designated by NUCC)

20. OUTSIDE LAB? YES NO $ CHARGES

21. DIAGNOSIS OR NATURE OF ILLNESS OR INJURY Relate A-L to service line below (24E) ICD Ind.

A. B. C. D.
E. F. G. H.
I. J. K. L.

22. RESUBMISSION CODE ORIGINAL REF. NO.

23. PRIOR AUTHORIZATION NUMBER

| 24. A. DATE(S) OF SERVICE From MM DD YY | To MM DD YY | B. PLACE OF SERVICE | C. EMG | D. PROCEDURES, SERVICES, OR SUPPLIES (Explain Unusual Circumstances) CPT/HCPCS | MODIFIER | E. DIAGNOSIS POINTER | F. $ CHARGES | G. DAYS OR UNITS | H. EPSDT Family Plan | I. ID. QUAL. | J. RENDERING PROVIDER ID. # |
|---|---|---|---|---|---|---|---|---|---|---|---|
| 1 | | | | | | | | | | NPI | |
| 2 | | | | | | | | | | NPI | |
| 3 | | | | | | | | | | NPI | |
| 4 | | | | | | | | | | NPI | |
| 5 | | | | | | | | | | NPI | |
| 6 | | | | | | | | | | NPI | |

25. FEDERAL TAX I.D. NUMBER SSN EIN

26. PATIENT'S ACCOUNT NO.

27. ACCEPT ASSIGNMENT? (For govt. claims, see back) YES NO

28. TOTAL CHARGE $

29. AMOUNT PAID $

30. Rsvd for NUCC Use

31. SIGNATURE OF PHYSICIAN OR SUPPLIER INCLUDING DEGREES OR CREDENTIALS (I certify that the statements on the reverse apply to this bill and are made a part thereof.)

SIGNED DATE

32. SERVICE FACILITY LOCATION INFORMATION

a. b.

33. BILLING PROVIDER INFO & PH # ( )

a. b.

PHYSICIAN OR SUPPLIER INFORMATION

NUCC Instruction Manual available at: www.nucc.org **_PLEASE PRINT OR TYPE_** APPROVED OMB-0938-1197 FORM 1500 (02-12)

**Figure 13-3** • CMS-1500 version 02-12 claim form. This is known as the *universal claim form*.

| TABLE 13-1 Frequent Causes for Claim Denial and Corrective Actions | |
| --- | --- |
| Causes for Claim Denial | Corrective Actions |
| The patient cannot be identified as a covered person. | Confirm that coverage information on file is current, including insurance company and group number, and that the Social Security number is accurate. |
| Coding is deemed inappropriately necessary. | Review provided services and recode as for services provided. |
| The patient is no longer covered by the plan. | Bill the patient for the charges. The patient may provide confirmation of new coverage. |
| The data are incomplete. | Complete the required data and resubmit the claim. Flag it as a resubmission. |
| Services are not covered by the plan. | Bill the patient for the charges unless there is a basis for an appeal. |

a critical aspect of your responsibilities. Table 13-1 describes the most frequent causes for denial of a claim and the corrective actions that you can take.

## Electronic Claims Submission

Although some practices continue to submit claims on paper through the mail and most claims administrators continue to accept this practice, most practices submit at least their Medicare and Medicaid claims electronically using the electronic HIPAA 837P claim. Remember, HIPAA requires covered entities to submit electronic information safely and confidentially. The physician's medical billing software includes the CMS-1500 format for convenient and automated claims filing. With a computer and Internet capabilities (or a modem), electronic health claims can be filed immediately, reducing the time for the reimbursement cycle. You will need to work closely with your practice's software vendor to ensure compatibility with the insurance companies' computer systems if the practice is not using the services of a clearinghouse.

Several regional and national clearinghouses receive health benefits claims and electronically direct them to the appropriate claims administrators. This system allows you to file all electronic claims through one clearinghouse rather than filing separately with each claims administrator. Not only do clearinghouses process and transmit electronic claims in a timely, HIPAA-compliant manner; they are also a cost-effective method to determine whether or not claims have been submitted properly from the provider (i.e., verify each patient's eligibility status, incorrect insurance ID numbers, etc.) before submitting to the payer electronically.

The clearinghouse system requires that all fields on the electronic claim form be completed and in the required format. If the claim is incomplete or inaccurate, the system will not transmit the claim and a report with unprocessable claims will be generated by the clearinghouse and sent electronically to the

provider before the claim is sent to the payer. You can complete or correct the form online, allowing the form to be transmitted. Claims submitted electronically that do not meet the plan's criteria will be rejected by the clearinghouse and must be submitted by mail. In addition, claims that are particularly complicated or cumbersome, have attachments, or are otherwise unsuitable for electronic submission should be filed on paper with the claims administrator. Figure 13-4 is a screenshot of an electronic insurance information "form."

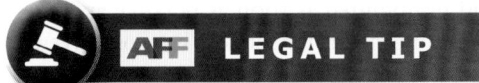

### LEGAL TIP

### Signature on File

Keeping patient information confidential is a primary concern in all medical practices. Releasing private health information (PHI) with a patient or guardian's written consent is a breach of confidentiality and a HIPAA violation. To adhere to HIPAA's regulations, you should not release any information about the patient to any party. Although HIPAA allows the release of PHI for treatment, payment, and operations (TPO), it is a good idea to always obtain a written authorization to release information to the patient's insurance company from each patient on his or her first visit to the practice. This insurance authorization should also include language that allows the physician to file claims on behalf of the patient without necessitating signatures on every claim form by allowing the physician's office to place the words "signature on file" on claim forms. Keep this signature in the patient's file, and update the signature every year by having patients sign a new authorization at the patient's first visit of the year. This written authorization for the release of information only pertains to the insurance company specified. Only such information as is pertinent to the claim and necessary for the processing of that claim should be released.

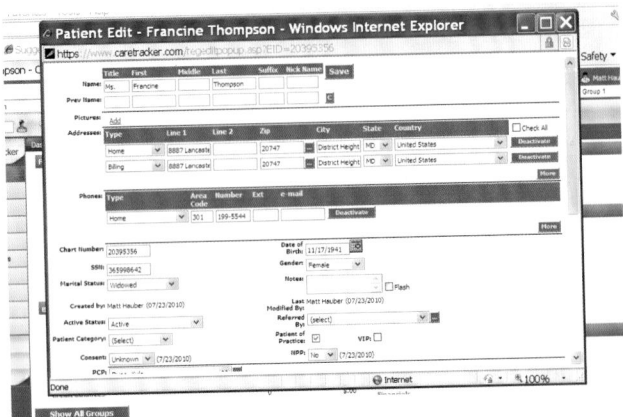

**Figure 13-4** • Screenshot of insurance information "form" in an electronic version. (Courtesy of Ingenix®CareTracker™.)

## Explanation of Benefits

When the claims administrator settles a claim, that is, makes or denies a payment, an **explanation of benefits (EOB)** is issued to both the provider and the patient (Fig. 13-5). The EOB tells how the payment was made, including deductible and coinsurance information, and includes reasons for denials, if necessary. Some EOBs include information for several claims on several patients that may have been processed during a particular period. You must check the EOB to be sure that all payments made to the physician are for the appropriate procedures and in the correct amounts. Claims that are denied should be corrected and resubmitted as soon as possible as there are time limits on filing claims for services by most payers.

## REIMBURSEMENT

### Diagnosis-Related Groups

In Chapter 11, you will learn to assign diagnosis codes. The diagnosis code is provided to a third-party payer to tell them why a service or procedure was provided. **Diagnosis-related groups (DRGs)** categorize inpatients according to the similarity of their diagnoses, treatments, and length of hospital stays. Initially, these categories were developed by researchers at Yale University in the mid-1970s to aid the process of UR. Some 13,000 codes were run through a computer and grouped according to their clinical similarities (including similarities in resources used). Today, DRGs are used to determine reimbursement for Medicare patients' inpatient services. The fee attached to each DRG is based on the national average of all Medicare charges and is adjusted for regional differences in hospital wages and updates. Hospitals are paid a set amount for each DRG regardless of actual costs for treating the patient. For example, if a hospital uses fewer resources to care for a patient and discharges that patient in less time, it may keep the difference between its actual cost and the DRG payment. Conversely, if the

patient stays longer than usual and requires more services, the hospital absorbs the loss. A patient who has an unusually long stay or a complicated case is considered an *outlier*, and the hospital may be paid more than the standard DRG rate if the added expenses can be justified. The hospital coder uses ICD-10-CM codes to pick the appropriate DRG. The more information the hospital has prior to admission, the more accurate the coding; for example, for a patient admitted with chest pain, the hospital coder needs to know that the patient also has hypertension and diabetes.

You may be asked to schedule a patient for admission to the hospital. Assigning the correct diagnostic code from the outpatient practice will influence the DRG to which the patient will be assigned. The hospital coder selects the proper DRG based on these factors:

- Principal diagnosis
- Surgeries
- Complications and comorbid conditions

Physicians can help with coding in the following ways:

- Record the appropriate documentation to identify each patient's problems, complaints, or other reasons for the encounter or visit.
- Work with the medical records or the office coding and billing staffs to determine the proper diagnosis to code, using terminology that includes specific diagnoses, symptoms, problems, or reasons for the encounter (ICD-10-CM codes describe all of these).

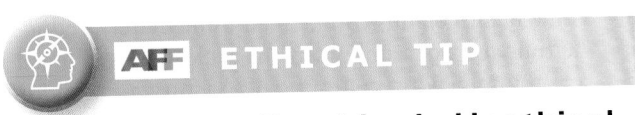

## When a Provider Is Unethical

The following scenario may occur in a medical office:

*While you are filing an insurance claim, the physician tells you to "adjust" the laceration length from 4 to 9 cm. (The physician can bill more for a 9-cm laceration.) When you question him about this, he says, "Don't worry. The patient isn't paying the difference, the insurance company is, and they have plenty of money."*

How should you handle this situation?

Ethically and legally, you cannot change the length of a laceration on the medical record or the bill. This is fraud. You must explain to the physician that you are uncomfortable with this request and that you are ethically and legally bound to truthful billing. Any requests to alter or misrepresent the medical records or claims of a patient must be firmly denied.

A physician who operates in an unethical manner should be reported. If he or she is a partner in a practice, alert the other physicians about the suspect actions. You can also contact your state medical association, the American Medical Association, or the institutional review board at the hospital where your physician is affiliated.

## Explanation of Benefits

Employee Name:   Joe Doe

SSN: 555-55-5555   (1)

Group No. 55555

Patient Name: Joe Doe

Date of Service: 6-15-2013

Provider: Dr. Jones

Provider TIN: 35-5555555

| Date of Service (2) | Comment Code (3) | Amount of Charge (4) | Amount Allowed (5) | At (6) | Amount Paid (7) |
|---|---|---|---|---|---|
| 6-15-2009 | 57 | 87.00 | 82.00 | 80% | 65.60 |
| | | | | | |

| | | |
|---|---|---|
| Total (8) | | 65.60 |
| Less Deductible (9) | | 25.00 |
| Amount Paid (10) | | 40.60 |

Payable to:   Dr. Jones
              Address

Comment Code:

57 - The amount charged exceeds Usual and Customary

### Reading the EOB (Explanation of Benefits)

After the claim has been processed, an EOB will be issued. Although each payer has his or her own EOB format, this sample EOB illustrates the key points included in an EOB. The terms used may differ, and the formats differ widely.

(1) The top section typically includes the name of the employee and the Social Security number (SSN) or other identifying number, as well as the name of the patient, the group number, the date of service and provider name, and employer identification number (EIN) (Federal identification number assigned to the physician).

(2) The date of service is included and is shown as the date the service is actually rendered, not the date that was posted or billed.

(3) The Comment Code is a tool used on many EOBs to indicate a coded comment that is on the bottom as exceeding "Usual and Customary." In this situation, the claim will be processed on the Usual and Customary amount. The difference between the amount charged ($87.00) and the amount allowed ($82.00) is $5.00. Unless the physician is contractually bound by an agreement with a managed care plan that forbids the practice of balance billing, that difference of $5.00 may be billed to the patient.

(4) Amount of Charge shows the amount that the physician's office billed for the service.

(5) Amount Allowed shows the amount of charge upon which the claim processing will be based (in this example, it is the amount of Usual and Customary).

(6) This indicates the percentage of co-insurance payable by the plan.

(7) Amount Paid shows the amount payable by the plan after co-insurance has been applied, but is not necessarily the amount that is actually paid (see #10).

(8) The Total shows the total submitted and payable after the claim has been processed.

(9) After all processing on the claim has been completed, any deductible is applied. In this example, Joe still had $25.00 to be applied to his annual deductible. Therefore, $25.00 is deducted from the amount paid and the actual reimbursement to the physician is $40.60. The amount applied to the deductible should be billed to the patient.

(10) The amount actually reimbursed.

**Figure 13-5** • Explanation of benefits.

## Resource-Based Relative Value Scale

As part of the 1989 Omnibus Budget Reconciliation Act (OBRA), the U.S. Congress stipulated that reimbursement to physicians for Medicare services is based on a fee schedule. This fee schedule sets a maximal fee for each service with the **resource-based relative value scale (RBRVS)**. The goal of RBRVS is to reduce Medicare Part B costs and to establish national standards for payment based on CPT-4 codes. (Remember, Part B of Medicare covers physicians' services; Part A covers hospital expenses.)

Fee calculations are based on the following factors:

- Intensity of the service
- Time required
- Skills needed
- Overhead expenses
- Malpractice premiums

The particular fee is adjusted by a geographical practice cost index (GPCI), which reflects the difference in health care costs in different parts of the country. This determines the relative value unit (RVU). Finally, a national conversion factor is assigned annually. The formula looks like this: CPT code 99205 has an RVU of 4.58, and the national conversion factor is 36.7856. The Medicare allowed charge would be $168.48. RVU × national conversion factor = Medicare allowed amount.

 **CHECKPOINT QUESTION**

7. Why are DRGs used?

## POLICIES IN THE PRACTICE

Managed care contracts and negotiated services affect many practice policies. You must be knowledgeable and precise in administering practice policies, especially with regard to assignment of benefits and balance billing.

Assignment of benefits is a service the practice may provide. If assignment of benefits is accepted, the patient's signature must be on file, authorizing the claims administrator to reimburse the physician. Managed care plans require physicians to accept assignment, although many physicians do not accept assignment for insurance plans in which they do not participate. If assignment is not accepted, the patient is responsible for paying all charges and filing a claim with the claims administrator for reimbursement directly to the patient.

Participating providers in a health insurance company requires physicians to be responsible for collecting balances that are the patient's responsibility as determined by insurance benefits. However, physicians cannot charge the patient the difference between the physician's usual charge and the allowable charge specified by the contract. For insurance plans in which the provider does not participate, however, balance billing is not restricted, and the practice may bill the patient for any difference between the physician's charged fee and the amount allowable by the plan according to **usual, customary, and reasonable (UCR)** tables.

A few national firms provide UCR data to claims administrators who use that information to determine the maximum amount payable for any given service (the **plan maximum**). UCR data are calculated from surveys of the amount physicians charge for each service or procedure. That amount is calculated on a geographic basis to reflect regional variations in health care costs. Non–managed care plan physician reimbursements are based on a maximum allowable charge as specified in the UCR data. The physician may choose to bill the patient for the difference between the amount charged and the UCR amount.

 **ROLE-PLAYING ACTIVITY**

After submitting a batch of electronic claims to the clearinghouse, Alex Zeller, CMA (AAMA), received a report that there is a problem with an established patient's primary insurance. The report states that the patient's coverage was terminated two weeks ago. What should Alex do to get this matter straightened out? What are some of the reasons that the coverage may have been terminated? Role-play this scenario as the medical assistant, and consider how this should be handled to demonstrate professionalism and tactfulness. If you are the patient, think about how you might feel if you received a call that your insurance coverage was no longer in effect. Would you be embarrassed? Angry? How would you respond to someone who displays these emotions? Your instructor will give you additional information about this activity.

## *español* SPANISH TERMINOLOGY

**¿Tiene usted seguro médico?**
Do you have medical insurance?

**¿Cuál es el nombre del seguro?**
What is the name of the insurance?

**¿Cuál es el número de su póliza?**
What is the number of your policy?

**¿Cubre el hospital?**
Will it pay for the hospital?

**¿Tiene Medicare?**
Do you have Medicare?

**¿Tiene su tarjeta de Medicare?**
Do you have your Medicare card?

**Su visita de hoy requiere de un co-pago.**
Your visit today requires a copayment.

**Su enfermedad es una condición preexistente.**
Your illness is a pre-existing condition.

**Su cheque de reembolso será enviado por correo.**
Your reimbursement check will be send to you by mail.

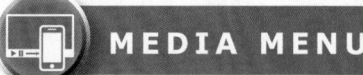

## MEDIA MENU

**Student Resources on thePoint®**

• **CMA/RMA Certification Exam Review**

**Internet Resources**
**Centers for Medicare and Medicaid Services**
http://www.cms.gov
**Medicare for Recipients**
**HIPAA Administrative Simplification, Transactions and Code Sets**
http://www.Medicare.gov
**BlueCross BlueShield Association**
http://www.bluecares.com
**Local Medical Review Policies**
http://www.lmrpdata.com
**American Medical Association**
http://www.ama-assn.org
**All Government Agencies, Federal, and State**
http://www.usa.gov
**U.S. Census Bureau**
http://www.census.gov
**Health Insurance Marketplace**
http://www.healthcare.gov
**National Plan and Provider Enumerator System**
http://nppes.cms.hhs.gov

## EMR Activity

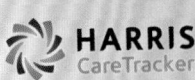

Harris CareTracker is a Web-based electronic medical record (EMR) application that you will use for the EMR activities included in this section at the end of each chapter. This application is actually used in physician offices, but is provided to you through the publisher, Wolters Kluwer Health, to give you hands-on practice working with EMRs. Your instructor will have more information about accessing your username, login, and Quickstart guide.

### Prerequisite Activities in Harris CareTracker

- *The Getting Started and Quickstart documents and EMR Activities Step-by-Step Instructions are available at* http://thePoint.lww.com/KronenbergerComp5e

### Activity Details

When registering all new and established patients for appointments, it is essential that financial obligations are also verified and updated at every visit. Alex Zeller, CMA, checked in established patient Connie Meyers today, and she informed him that her insurance had changed from Blue Cross Blue Shield to Aetna U.S. Healthcare and presented a new card. After scanning the card into the EMR, her new insurance information in the Demographics application must also be updated with the new ID #6098YY23, effective on the first day of the current month.

## Chapter Summary

- Most patients in the physician's office have some type of health care plan.
- Types of plans include group, individual, and government-sponsored health benefits, such as Medicare or Medicaid.
- Many physicians have contracts with managed care plans, such as HMOs and PPOs.
- Each type of plan has certain requirements regarding eligibility and claims submission, and you must be knowledgeable about those requirements.
- In particular, one of your primary duties is to file claims in a timely and accurate manner to ensure appropriate reimbursement for the physician.
- When filing claims, you must be careful to maintain patient confidentiality and to avoid fraud.

## Warm-Ups for Critical Thinking

1. Jane and Joe are married, and both are employed and cover themselves and their two children on their health plans. Jane's birthday is July 23, and Joe's birthday is August 9. Joe is 2 years older than Jane. When claims are submitted for their two children, which spouse's plan is primary? Show which plan is primary and secondary for each family member.
2. The requirements for Medicaid vary from state to state. How do you determine the Medicaid requirements for your particular state? Locate the name, address, and telephone number of your state's resource.
3. As discussed in Chapter 8, HIPAA requires certain procedures and practices when transmitting insurance claims electronically. Search the HIPAA law for these guidelines and create a procedure for ensuring compliance regarding electronic claims filing. You can find this information by going to the U.S. Department of Health and Human Services Web site and review the Transactions and Code Sets in the HIPAA's Administrative Simplification section.

|         | Primary | Secondary |
|---------|---------|-----------|
| Jane    |         |           |
| Joe     |         |           |
| Child 1 |         |           |
| Child 2 |         |           |

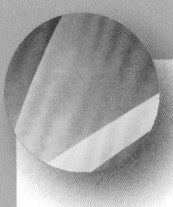

**PSY** P R O C E D U R E  1 3 - 1

# Completing a CMS-1500 Claim Form

**Purpose:** To ensure competency in completing a CMS-1500 claim form accurately and completely using managed care policies and procedures and third-party guidelines

**Equipment:** Case scenario, completed encounter form, blank CMS-1500 claim form, pen

**Scenario:** Naomi A. Dishman is an established diabetic patient who was seen in your office on June 20, 2016, 30 minutes after falling down the steps of her home. She is complaining of pain and swelling in her right ankle. Her charges and codes for the visit are Established Patient Office Visit Level III (99213) and x-ray, right ankle, two views (73600). Her diagnosis is listed as left ankle sprain.

| STEPS | PURPOSE |
|---|---|
| 1. Using the information provided in Figure 13-5, complete the demographic information in lines 1 through 11d. | This section includes vital information to identify the policyholder and start the process of paying the claim. |
| 2. Insert "SOF" (signature on file) on lines 12 and 13. Check to be sure there is a current signature on file in the chart and that it is specifically for the third-party payer being filed. | It is fraudulent to say there is a signature on file if there is not one in the chart. Patients should sign a separate authorization for each recipient of their information. If there is no SOF, you must call the patient to come in and sign one or mail them a form to be signed and sent back. |
| 3. If the services being filed are for a hospital stay, insert information in lines 16 and 18. | These fields are used for hospital services only. |
| 4. If the services are related to an injury, insert the date of the accident in line 14. | If the date of accident field is not completed and an ICD-10 code for an injury is used, the payer's computer system will reject the claim. |
| 5. Enter the name of the referring provider and his/her NPI with the appropriate qualifier in lines 17 and 17b. If unknown, enter the name of the ordering provider rendering the care. | Enter the qualifier to the left of the dotted vertical line in block 17 to indicate the role of the physician: DN for referring provider, DK for ordering provider, and DQ for supervising provider. |
| 6. Insert dates of service. Each line may be a different date of service. | You must be accurate with the dates of service. |
| 7. Using the encounter form, place the CPT code listed for each service and procedure checked off in column D of lines 21–24 on the form. | The codes on the encounter form are current and accurate because the form has been reviewed before using any revised or new codes every January. |
| 8. List the reason(s) for the encounter on line 21A-L and any other diagnoses listed on the encounter form that relate to or affect the services or procedures. | All diagnoses or concurrent conditions that will affect the current treatment should be communicated to the third-party payer. For example, diabetes should be listed for a podiatric service. |
| 9. Reference the code where the service was rendered on all lines listing a CPT code in block 24, column B (i.e., place of service code number "11" is for the office). | The place of service (POS) code tells the payer where the services were rendered such as medical office, ambulatory surgical center, urgent care, walk-in retail clinic, etc. (see Chapter 12). |
| 10. Reference the codes placed in lines 21 (A-L) to each line listing a different CPT code by placing the corresponding letter in line 24, column E. | Each line that lists a CPT code must also list a reason for that particular service or procedure. This reason will justify the medical necessity of the service or procedure. |

## PROCEDURE 13-1 (continued)

| STEPS | PURPOSE |
|---|---|
| 11. Enter the number of units on all lines listing a CPT code in line 24, column G. | The unit price charge for each CPT code being billed will be multiplied by the number of units in line 24 column G to reflect the total for that service on line 24, column F. |
| 12. Reference the NPI number for the provider rendering the service on each line that is billed in the lower unshaded portion of 24J. | The NPI accurately identifies the provider who rendered the service(s) being billed. |
| 13. Enter the federal tax ID number (EIN) for the practice on line 25 if incorporated. If not, use the provider's Social Security Number, and check the appropriate box. | Reimbursement of claims submitted without this information may be denied. |
| 14. Check the "Accept Assignment" box on line 27. | Reimbursement will be sent to the provider and not to the patient or guarantor. |
| 15. Enter the total charges on line 28. | Add all of the charges in column 24F |
| 16. Enter SOF on line 31 | The physician should sign the insurance authorization after the patient's signature (see above step 2) to allow all claims to be filed without necessitating the physician's signature on every claim. |
| 17. Enter the address of the location where the service was provided for the dates of service being billed. | This must be done for all Medicare claims even if it is the same address given on line 33. |
| 18. Enter the name of the rendering provider, address, and phone number where payments are to be sent. | The rendering provider's name must match the NPI number given in blocks 24J. |
| 19. **AFF** You notice that Ms. Dishman has no signature on file, but the box on line 12 of her claim form says she does. Explain how you would respond. | Correct the error immediately. Do not file the claim until the signed form is in her record. Mail the patient an authorization with a self-addressed, stamped envelope and a letter explaining that you need this for her record. You could also flag her account with a note to obtain a signed authorization at her next visit. |

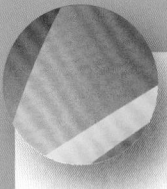

## PROCEDURE 13-2

### Obtain Preauthorization for Services

**PSY**  Interpret information on an insurance card, verify eligibility for services including documentation, utilize medical necessity guidelines, and obtain precertification or preauthorization for services

**Purpose:** To ensure competency in completing the preauthorization process for medical services

**Equipment:** Case scenario with patient's demographic information including insurance card information, a physician's order for treatment, preauthorization form, and pen

**Scenario:** Dr. Kyle Dunn requested authorization for his patient, Gerald Tackett, to undergo a polysomnography testing that is in a facility with a technician present to confirm a diagnosis of obstructive sleep apnea. The patient has a comorbid condition of moderate congestive heart failure and has a complaint of severe insomnia for the last 7 months. The CPT code for the polysomnography is 95807.

| STEPS | REASONS |
| --- | --- |
| 1. Verify the physician's order for the polysomnography and the patient's demographics with a copy of the front and back of the patient's insurance card. | Identifying the order with the correct patient prevents errors. |
| 2. Complete the preauthorization form (preauth form) as provided by the insurance company or the practice's form with details involving the requested services including the date the preauthorization is being requested. | Accurate information provides the medical necessity for the services ordered by the physician. This form can be online or a hard copy to be faxed as required by the insurance company, or it can be a generic form for use by the office. |
| 3. Contact the insurance company's preauthorization department by calling the number listed on the back of the patient's insurance card to verify the patient's eligibility for the services and document on the preauth form. | Determining whether or not the patient is eligible for services is the first step before seeking authorization. Documentation of eligibility for services may prevent confusion in the event there is a future reimbursement question or problem. |
| 4. Determine whether or not the patient's insurance benefits require preauthorization or precertification from the insurance company for the requested service. | Insurance benefits determine what services must be preauthorized and are specific to each patient's plan. |
| 5. Note the name or identification of the insurance preauthorization representative on the preauth form. | Documentation with accurate details including specific details may prevent confusion in the event there is a question or problem in the future. |
| 6. Provide details noted on the completed preauthorization form for the requested services and/or treatment to the insurance preauthorization representative. | Medical documentation provides medical necessity for the services being preauthorized. Having all of the information available prevents a delay in authorization and ordered services and/or treatment. |
| 7. Accurately document the preauthorization number given for the service or treatment on the preauth form. This information must be given to the provider performing the authorized services. | The claim form submitted to the insurance company for the authorized services must have the preauthorization number in order to be reimbursed. |

## PROCEDURE 13-2 (continued)

| STEPS | REASONS |
|---|---|
| 8. Sign the preauthorization form as the person who got the authorization, and file it in the patient's medical record. | The person who got the services or treatment authorized may need to be contacted if there is a question or problem in the future with reimbursement. The completed preauth form is a record of how the preauthorization was obtained. |
| 9. **AFF** Describe how you would handle advising a patient that his/her insurance benefits did not cover the ordered service or treatment. | Before contacting the patient, advise the physician about the insurance denial to see if there is another recommended course of action that may be recommended to the patient. Also, find out how much the denied coverage for services will cost the patient and if there are payment options. Contact the patient and speak with him/her in a private area either by telephone or in the office and explain that the services are non-covered as per benefits in his/her plan. Offer solutions to help the patient get the services necessary (such as a payment plan), or depending on the situation, you may offer to help with an appeal process at the insurance company. Above all, be professional in all matters in dealing with patients and insurance companies regardless of how you feel about the denial of coverage. |

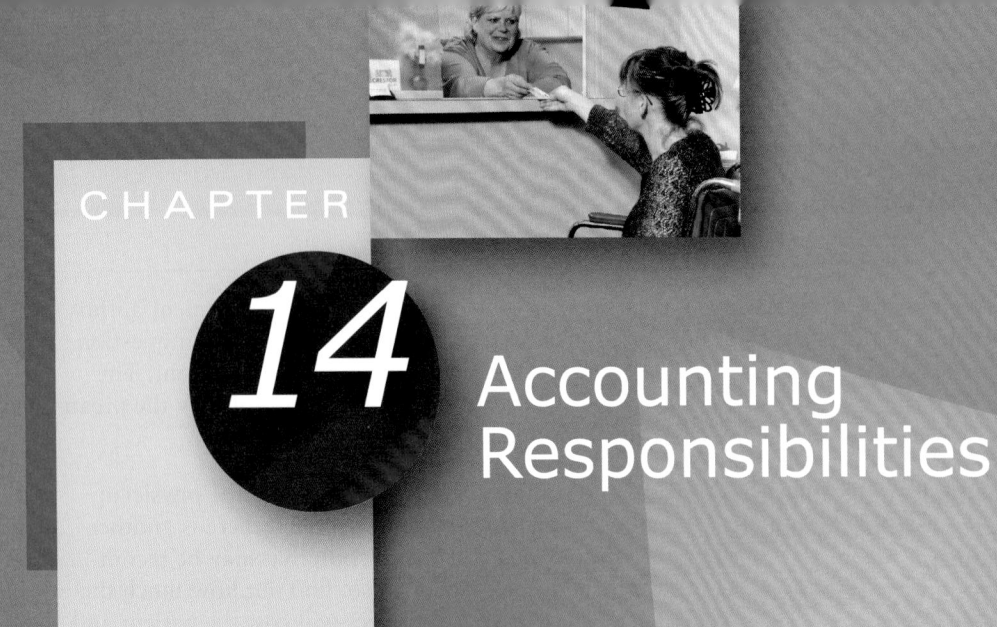

# CHAPTER 14

# Accounting Responsibilities

## Learning Outcomes

**COG Cognitive Domain\***

1. Spell and define the key terms
2. *Define the following bookkeeping terms:*
   a. *Charges*
   b. *Payments*
   c. *Accounts receivable*
   d. *Accounts payable*
   e. *Adjustments*
3. Explain the concept of the pegboard bookkeeping system
4. Describe the components of the pegboard system
5. Identify and discuss the special features of the pegboard daysheet
6. Describe the functions of a computer accounting system
7. List the uses and components of computer accounting reports
8. Explain banking services, including types of accounts and fees
9. Describe the accounting cycle
10. Describe the components of a record-keeping system

11. Explain the process of ordering supplies and paying invoices
12. *Explain basic booking computations*
13. *Differentiate between bookkeeping and accounting*
14. *Describe banking procedures as related to the ambulatory care setting*
15. *Identify precautions for accepting the following types of payments:*
    a. Cash
    b. Check
    c. Credit card
    d. Debit card
16. Compare types of endorsements
17. Differentiate between accounts payable and accounts receivable
18. Compare manual and computerized bookkeeping systems used in ambulatory health care
19. Describe common periodic financial reports
20. *Explain patient financial obligations for services rendered*

21. Identify types of information contained in the patient's billing record
22. Describe types of adjustments made to patient accounts including:
    a. Nonsufficient funds (NSF) check
    b. Collection agency transaction
    c. Credit balance
    d. Third party

### PSY Psychomotor Domain*

1. Prepare a bank deposit (Procedure 14-9)
2. Perform accounts receivable procedures to patient accounts including:
    a. Posting charges(Procedure 14-1)
    b. Posting payments (Procedure 14-2)
    c. Posting adjustments (Procedures 14-4 to 14-6)
    d. Processing a credit balance (Procedure 14-3)
    e. Processing refunds (Procedure 14-4)
    f. Posting nonsufficient fund (NSF) checks (Procedure 14-7)
    g. Posting collection agency payments (Procedure 14-6)
3. Balance a daysheet (Procedure 14-8)
4. Reconcile a bank statement (Procedure 14-10)
5. Maintain a petty cash account (Procedure 14-11)
6. Order supplies (Procedure 14-12)
7. Write a check (Procedure 14-13)

### AFF Affective Domain*

1. Apply ethical behaviors, including honesty and integrity in performance of medical assisting practice
2. Apply local, state, and federal health care legislation and regulation appropriate to the medical assisting practice setting
3. Display sensitivity when requesting payment for services rendered
4. Demonstrate professionalism when discussing patient's billing record

*Note: AAMA/CAAHEP 2015 Standards are italicized.

### ABHES Competencies

1. Prepare and reconcile a bank statement and deposit record
2. Post entries on a daysheet
3. Perform billing and collection procedures
4. Perform accounts receivable procedures
5. Use physician fee schedule
6. Establish and maintain a petty cash fund
7. Post adjustments
8. Process credit balance
9. Process refunds
10. Post nonsufficient funds (NSF)
11. Post collection agency payments
12. Use manual or computerized bookkeeping systems

# Key Terms

| | | | |
|---|---|---|---|
| accounting | charge slip | Internal Revenue Service (IRS) | posting |
| accounting cycle | check register | invoice | profit-and-loss statement |
| accounts payable | check stub | ledger card | purchase order |
| accounts receivable | credit | liabilities | returned check fee |
| adjustment | daysheet | packing slip | service charge |
| audit | debit | payroll | summation report |
| balance | encounter form | | take-back |
| bookkeeping | | | |

# Case Study

Great Falls Medical Center uses a computerized bookkeeping system, and Toby Dickerson, RMA, is responsible for accurately documenting the financial transactions for the practice. Unfortunately, the computer system is down this afternoon, but daily transactions must still be entered. In addition to payments from insurance companies, Toby has checks and cash payments from patients to be applied to their account balances. What forms does he need to post charges to patients' accounts? What forms are required to post patient payments? In this chapter, you will learn the importance of keeping accurate financial records and correctly posting accounts receivable as well as accounts payable.

Bookkeeping and banking are important facets of medical office management. In most medical practices, bookkeeping and banking involve maintaining both patient and office account records, including petty cash, **accounts receivable** (money owed to the practice), and **accounts payable** (money owed by the practice). Most medical practices use computer bookkeeping systems, although some smaller practices and satellite offices still use manual systems. When a computerized system is down, the pegboard serves as a backup. Although daily bookkeeping practices are handled in the office, an accountant receives the reports of the daily financial functions in order to summarize and analyze the results to determine the practice's overall financial health. It is important that accurate financial records are maintained to ensure there is sufficient money to meet the obligations necessary to continue to provide health care services to the patients and community served by the practice.

## ACCOUNTING AND DAILY BOOKKEEPING

**Accounting**, as defined by the 11th edition of *Merriam-Webster's Collegiate Dictionary*, is a method of tracking, recording, analyzing, and reporting the results of financial transactions during a specific period in time. Financial reports that summarize the results of financial transactions are created by an accountant who specializes in analyzing and advising the owners of the practice regarding financial matters.

The foundation of accounting is this equation:

$$\text{Assets} = \text{liabilities} + \text{equity}$$

Assets are all things of value owned by or relating to the practice. Liabilities are monies owed. Equity refers to the amount of capital the physician has invested in the practice. Because the two sides of the accounting equation must always **balance** (be equal), each transaction requires a **debit** (charge) on one side of the equation and a **credit** (payment) on the other side of the equation; the amount of the debit and credit must be equal. Double-entry systems are usually used by accounting firms and corporations.

Most medical facilities use the *cash basis* type of accounting, which means that income is considered as income only when money is collected and that payables (money owed) are considered expenses only when money is paid. The process of bookkeeping is the recording of financial transactions throughout the day and is part of the accounting process. **Bookkeeping** is defined as an organized and accurate record-keeping system of financial transactions for a business. The daily financial transactions of a medical office include patient payments that arrive through the mail, patient payments from patients seen in the office, and patient charges that are added

to the accounts receivable. Most medical practices use the single-entry bookkeeping system. The most popular formats for daily bookkeeping are the manual pegboard system and computer systems.

## MANUAL ACCOUNTING

### Pegboard Bookkeeping System

Medical assisting educators across the country continue to debate the merits of teaching the seemingly old-fashioned ways of a manual bookkeeping system. It is important, however, for you to understand the bookkeeping process of entering charges and payments in a manual way so you will understand the workings of a computerized system. The pegboard, or write-it-once, bookkeeping system uses a board with pegs running down the left side. The pegs hold a **daysheet**, or daily journal, in place on the board. All transactions for the day are recorded on this daysheet. Each patient has a **ledger card** (record of the patient's financial activities). When a patient transaction occurs, the bookkeeper places the ledger card over the daysheet and the **charge slip** (also called an encounter sheet) over the ledger card on the next available entry line and makes the appropriate entry on the ledger card. Figure 14-1 is a sample daysheet.

Daysheets come with a sheet of carbon paper or some other specialized paper that duplicates entries as they are entered. This system permits entries for daily transactions to be entered once, but recorded on multiple financial documents as necessary. For example, when a charge is entered for services rendered to patient, the entry is recorded on the charge slip, the patient's account ledger card, and on the daysheet at the same time by posting the transaction only one time. As the day progresses, each patient's ledger card is placed on the next available line on the daysheet, so that the day's entries appear consecutively. At the end of the day, all of the transactions are totaled to verify the remaining accounts receivable balance.

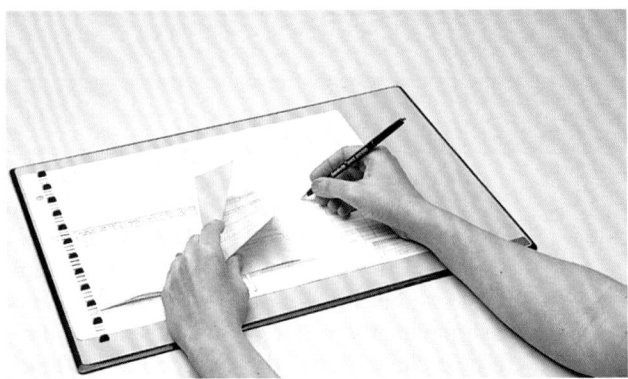

**Figure 14-1 •** Sample daysheet with ledger card and charge slip (to fill in before sending). (Courtesy of Control-o-fax, Waterloo, IA.)

The various components used in a pegboard system and the specific steps for recording patient transactions are discussed in greater detail next.

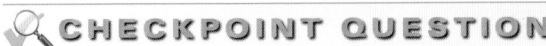

## CHECKPOINT QUESTION

1. What is an asset?

## Daysheet

The daysheet keeps track of daily patient transactions, such as charges for services to patients, payments received from patients and insurance carriers, and adjustments to patient accounts. A daysheet should be kept for each day that the physician sees patients; on busy days or for practices with more than one physician, more than one daysheet may be required.

The daysheet has several sections: a deposit slip, distribution columns, a section for payments, a section for adjustments, and a section for **posting** proofs (a method of checking for errors so that corrections can be made immediately).

The deposit slip is a detachable portion of the daysheet. All payments received are noted on the deposit slip, and at the end of the day, it is separated from the daysheet and deposited with that day's payments.

The distribution columns are used to assign charges for various services. How these columns are used depends on the needs of the individual practice. In a group practice, each practitioner has his or her own column. Some practices may assign columns to the various insurance plans they accept. Finally, these columns can be used to provide information on quality improvement issues. The distribution columns, regardless of how they are assigned, provide the physician with important information about how the practice earns its income.

An **adjustment** is an entry to change an account balance. The adjustments section allows for reductions in office fees, as with professional courtesy discounts and insurance disallowances. The adjustments section also allows for crediting an account for uncollectible monies without using the payment column. It can also be used to return charges to an account if the patient's payment has been returned by the bank for insufficient funds.

The posting proofs section is where the day's totals are entered and the daysheet is balanced, much as one would balance a checkbook. Once the daysheet is complete, each column or section is totaled individually. It is best to total each column twice to make sure that no errors have been made. After all the columns have been totaled, the posting proofs section is filled out.

If the posting proofs do not balance, an error has been made on the daysheet. To locate the error, go over each transaction one by one. Add the previous balance to the fee or subtract the payment from the previous balance to check whether the new balance listed is correct. If the posted charges are correct, total each column

again. Do not erase or white-out errors; draw a line through the erroneous entry and enter the transaction on a new line. When you reenter a transaction on the daysheet, use the ledger card again.

The daysheet is important because it keeps track of accounts receivable. The accounts receivable total changes every time a charge, payment, or adjustment is made to an account. You should perform a trial balance at the end of each month. Add the totals of each ledger card with an outstanding balance. The total should match the running total kept on the daysheet. This practice ensures the accuracy of your financial records.

Completed daysheets are filed chronologically in a ledger (a book of accounts) with the most recent daysheet on top. Completed daysheets are important legal documents and must be kept for at least 7 years for tax purposes. They should be stored in a safe, dark area to avoid loss or fading.

## CHECKPOINT QUESTION

2. What are five sections of a pegboard daysheet?

## Ledger Cards

The ledger card is a financial record for each patient. Most ledger cards include areas for the responsible person's name, address, telephone number, and insurance information. Figure 14-2 is a sample ledger card. Patient information appears on the top of the ledger card; the bottom portion is used to record the patient's financial activities.

| DATE | DESCRIPTION | CHARGES | CREDITS PYMNTS. | ADJ. | BALANCE | |
|---|---|---|---|---|---|---|
| | | BALANCE FORWARD ➔ | | | 20 | 00 |
| 5/2/13 | OV | 50 00 | | | 70 | 00 |
| 2/10/13 | BC/BS ck (5/2) | | 60 00 | 10 00 | -0- | |
| 5/25/13 | OV, Lab | 120 00 | | | 120 | 00 |

FORM MR 10        PLEASE PAY LAST AMOUNT IN BALANCE COLUMN ➔

**Figure 14-2 •** Sample ledger card.

A photocopy of an individual's ledger card is often sent as a bill when a remaining account balance becomes the patient's responsibility. If you use a copy of the ledger card for billing, make sure that no information other than the billing name and address is visible through the window of the envelope. Allowing other information to be visible is a breach of privacy.

The ledger card is a legal document and should be kept for the same length of time as the patient's medical record. Ledger cards are filed alphabetically in a ledger tray. A medical practice may require more than one ledger tray. Ledger cards with outstanding balances are kept separate from paid ledger cards; this makes it easier to photocopy the monthly bills or find a ledger card when a patient calls about an outstanding bill. If the office uses only one ledger tray, the ledger cards with outstanding balances are filed alphabetically in the front of the ledger tray, with the paid ledger cards filed alphabetically in the back.

### Encounter Forms and Charge Slips

The **encounter form** and the charge slip are preprinted patient statements that list codes for basic office charges and have sections for the patient's current balance and next appointment. Most encounter forms and charge slips have three-part copies:

1. The first copy is kept by the facility for auditing purposes (all are numbered).
2. The second copy is given to the patient for insurance filing (if the patient files the insurance claims).
3. The third copy, which has a carbon line at the top to match your ledgers and daysheets, is given to the patient as a receipt of services.

Charge slips are smaller versions of an encounter form and are designed to be used in conjunction with ledger cards. They often have different-colored no-carbon-required (NCR) copies. Figure 14-3 shows a computer-generated encounter form and a charge slip used in a manual system. You can see the same information found in a computerized system in the screen shot in Figure 14-4.

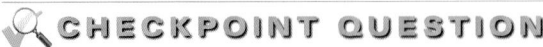
### CHECKPOINT QUESTION

3. What is an encounter form?

## Posting a Charge

The charge column of the daysheet is for original charges incurred for services received by the patient from the physician or staff on a specific date. Examples include office visits, electrocardiograms, blood work, hospital visits, consultations, and fees for returned checks. As discussed previously, charges in a medical office are based on a fee schedule or list of charges determined by the usual, customary, and reasonable charges of similar providers in similar localities who practice under similar circumstances. Procedure 14-1 outlines the steps for posting a charge.

## Posting a Payment

Payments received by the practice may include insurance checks received in the mail, money orders, credit card payments, or cash received from patients. Procedure 14-2 outlines the steps for posting payments and adjustments.

## Processing a Credit Balance

Sometimes, an account is overpaid, either by the patient or the insurance company. Such an overpayment is termed a credit (money owed to the patient or insurance carrier). This will show on the patient's ledger card as the last balance, with brackets (e.g., [25]) indicating a credit (Procedure 14-3). Brackets indicate the opposite of the column's usual meaning. For example, the balance column normally shows patients' debits, or amounts patients owe to the doctor. Brackets around an amount indicate the opposite, namely, that the doctor owes the patient or the patient's insurance company money.

## Processing Refunds

Credits are handled in one of two ways: (1) the credit stays on the account and is subtracted from the charges on the patient's next visit or (2) the patient is mailed a refund for the amount of the overpayment. How an overpayment is handled depends on office policy and the amount of the overpayment. Generally, overpayments under $5 are left on account as a credit, whereas overpayments over $5 are refunded. Procedure 14-4 indicates how to process refunds.

## Posting a Credit Adjustment

The adjustments section is used to indicate nonstandard office fees and to credit an account for uncollectible monies. Below are three specific situations that require a credit adjustment.

*Example 1.* The physician wishes to give a registered nurse a 25% professional discount on charges incurred for an office visit. You enter the fee from the fee schedule in the charge column, show in the description column an office visit with a professional discount of 25%, and put the 25% in the adjustment column. Assume an office visit is $40. You put $40 in the charge column and $10 (25% of $40) in the adjustment column. The patient owes your facility $30 for this visit.

*Example 2.* Most medical offices participate with certain insurance groups, which means the physician has signed an agreement with the insurance carrier to

Patient Name: _____

Patient ID #: _____ DOB: _____ Sex: _____

PCP: _____

SSN: _____ Financial Class: _____

Phone: _____ (home) _____ (work)

Medical Record #: _____ Date of Service: _____

Benefit Pkg: _____ Copay $ _____

Encounter #: _____

Service Provider: _____

Appt. Status: ☐ Scheduled  ☐ Same Day  ☐ Walk-in

Check-in Time: _____ Check-out Time: _____
Escorted to Exam Room: _____ Time Patient Seen: _____
Appointment Time: _____

Is Patient Being Seen in Relation to:
☐ Motor Vehicle Accident  ☐ Workman's Compensation

Appointment Failure Reason:
☐ Patient Cancel  ☐ No Show  ☐ Walk Out  ☐ PHA Cancel

## TYPE OF VISIT

| ✓ | CODE | DESCRIPTION | FEE | ✓ | CODE | DESCRIPTION | FEE | ✓ | CODE | DESCRIPTION | FEE | ✓ | CODE | DESCRIPTION | FEE |
|---|------|-------------|-----|---|------|-------------|-----|---|------|-------------|-----|---|------|-------------|-----|
| | | **OFFICE VISITS-EST.** | | | | **OFFICE VISITS-NEW CONT.** | | | | **PREVENTATIVE, NEW** | | | | **COUNSELING** | |
| | 99211 | Minimal | | | 99204 | Compreh. | | | 99385 | E&M 18-39 | | | 99401 | 15 Min. | |
| | 99212 | Focused | | | 99205 | Comp. & Complex | | | 99386 | E&M 40-64 | | | 99402 | 30 Min. | |
| | 99213 | Expanded | | | | **NURSE VISIT** | | | 99387 | E&M 65 & over | | | 99403 | 45 Min. | |
| | 99214 | Detailed | | | 99211 | Minimal | | | | **CONSULTATION** | | | 99404 | 60 Min. | |
| | 99215 | Compreh. | | | | **PREVENTATIVE, EST.** | | | 99241 | Focused | | | | | |
| | | **OFFICE VISITS-NEW** | | | 99395 | E&M 18-39 | | | 99242 | Pre-Op Consult | | | | | |
| | 99201 | Focused | | | 99396 | E&M 40-64 | | | 99244 | 2nd Opinion | | | | | |
| | 99202 | Expanded | | | 99397 | E&M 65 & over | | | | | | | | | |
| | 99203 | Detailed | | | | | | | | | | | | | |

## PROCEDURES

| ✓ | CODE | DESCRIPTION | FEE | ✓ | CODE | DESCRIPTION | FEE | ✓ | CODE | DESCRIPTION | FEE | ✓ | CODE | DESCRIPTION | FEE |
|---|------|-------------|-----|---|------|-------------|-----|---|------|-------------|-----|---|------|-------------|-----|
| | 88170 | Aspiration - Cyst | | | 11200 | Skin Tag Removal | | | | **IMMUNIZATIONS/INJECTIONS** | | | | **IMMUNIZATIONS/INJECTIONS CONT.** | |
| | 20600 | Aspiration - Joint (Small) | | | 20550 | Trigger point/Tendon Inj. | | | G0009 | Administration Fee - Pneumovax | | | J2203 | Triamcinolone Inj. | |
| | 20605 | Aspiration - Joint (Interm.) | | | | | | | G0010 | Administration Fee - Hepatitis B | | | J3420 | Vitamin B₁₂ | |
| | 20610 | Aspiration - Joint (Large) | | | | **SPECIALTY SERVICES** | | | 95115 | Allergy Injection Single | | | | **IN-HOUSE LABORATORY** | |
| | 16020 | Burn Dressing | | | 99070 | Ace Bandage | | | 95117 | Allergy Injection Multiple | | | 89050 | Cell Count, except blood | |
| | 69210 | Ear Irrigation | | | E0110 | Crutches | | | 90788 | Antibiotic IM | | | 89060 | Crystalanalysis | |
| | 10120 | Foreign Body Removal, Skin | | | 29130 | Finger Splint | | | J2910 | Aurothioglucose | | | 82948 | Glucose | |
| | 10060 | I&D Abscess, simple | | | 29125 | Wrist Splint | | | G0008 | Flu Vaccine | | | 85013 | HCT | |
| | 90780 | IV Infusion Therapy | | | 99080 | Form Completion | | | J1600 | Gold Injection | | | 85018 | Hemoglobin Screen | |
| | 12001 | Laceration Repair, Simple | | | | **TESTING/SCREENING** | | | 90731 | Hepatitis B | | | 81025 | Pregnancy | |
| | 13160 | Laceration Repair, Extens. | | | 95004 | Allergy - Skin Test | | | 90741 | Immune Globulin | | | 81002 | Urinalysis, Dipstick | |
| | 64450 | Medial Nerve Infiltration | | | 92557 | Audiometry | | | 90724 | Influenza | | | 81000 | Urinalysis, Full | |
| | 17110 | Molluscum/Wart Rmvl | | | 93000 | EKG | | | J9217 | Lupron 3.75 mg | | | G0001 | Venipuncture | |
| | 94640 | Nebulizer | | | 92506 | Hearing Screen | | | J9217 | Lupron 7.5 mg | | | | **OTHER PROCEDURES** | |
| | 82270 | Stool for Blood (Hemocult) | | | 86580 | PPD | | | J9250 | Methotrexate 2-5 mg | | | | | |
| | 12001 | Suturing, Superficial | | | 94010 | Pulmonary Function | | | 90732 | Pneumovax | | | | | |
| | 13100 | Suturing, Complex | | | 94760 | Pulse Oximetry, Single | | | 90718 | Td | | | | | |
| | 11050 | Skin Les./Wart Cautery | | | 45330 | Sigmoidoscopy, Flexible | | | 90782 | Therapeutic SQ or IM | | | | | |

P = PRIMARY   S = SECONDARY   S1-S9 = NUMBERED SECONDARY

## DIAGNOSIS

| ✓ | CODE | DESCRIPTION | ✓ | CODE | DESCRIPTION | ✓ | CODE | DESCRIPTION |
|---|------|-------------|---|------|-------------|---|------|-------------|
| | 789.0 | Abdominal Pain | | 780.6 | Fever | | 462 | Pharyngitis (sore throat) |
| | 879.8 | Abrasion/Laceration | | 704.8 | Folliculitis | | 486 | Pneumonia |
| | 995.3 | Allergic Reaction | | 535.5 | Gastritis | | V70.3 | Pre-Marital Testing |
| | 477.9 | Allergic Rhinitis | | 558.9 | Gastroenteritis | | V72.81 | Pre-op Cardiac Exam |
| | 285.9 | Anemia | | 274.9 | Gout | | V72.83 | Pre-op Exam, Other |
| | 413.9 | Angina | | V72.3 | Gyn Exam | | 601.0 | Prostatits |
| | 300.00 | Anxiety | | 784.0 | Headache | | 600 | Prostatism |
| | 716.90 | Arthritis | | 389.9 | Hearing Loss | | 782.1 | Rash |
| | 427.9 | Arrhythmia | | 536.8 | Heartburn/Indigestion | | 569.3 | Rectal Bleeding |
| | 493.90 | Asthma | | 573.3 | Hepatitis | | 530.81 | Reflux |
| | 611.72 | Breast Lump | | 455.6 | Hemorrhoids | | V81.2 | Screening for Cardiac Condition |
| | 490 | Bronchitis | | 553.9 | Hernia | | 780.3 | Seizure Disorder |
| | 727.3 | Bursitis | | 401.9 | Hypertension (NOS) | | 473.9 | Sinusitis |
| | 354.0 | Carpal Tunnel Syndrome | | 272.4 | Hyperlipidemia | | 848.9 | Strain/Sprain |
| | 682.9 | Cellulitis | | 242.00 | Hyperthyroidism | | 438 | Stroke |
| | 786.50 | Chest Pain | | 251.2 | Hypoglycemia | | 305.90 | Substance Abuse |
| | 575.1 | Cholecystitis | | 380.4 | Impacted Cerumen | | 099.9 | STD |
| | 372.3 | Conjunctivitis | | 780.52 | Insomnia | | 727.00 | Tenosynovitis, Tendonitis |
| | 496 | COPD | | 564.1 | Irritable Bowel Syndrome | | 451.9 | Thrombophlebitis |
| | 414.9 | Coronary Artery Disease | | 719.40 | Joint Pain | | 246.9 | Thyroid Disease |
| | 290.9 | Dementia | | 592.0 | Kidney Stones | | 435.9 | TIA |
| | 311 | Depression | | 464.0 | Laryngitis | | 463 | Tonsillitis |
| | 692.9 | Dermatitis | | 724.2 | Low Back Pain | | 011.90 | Tuberculosis |
| | 250.01 | Diabetes, IDDM | | 710.0 | Lupus | | 465.9 | Upper Respiratory Infection |
| | 250.00 | Diabetes, NIDDM | | V70.0 | Medical Exam/Physical | | 599.0 | Urinary Tract Infection |
| | 558.9 | Diarrhea | | 346.9 | Migraine | | V04.8 | Vaccination, Flu |
| | 562.10 | Diverticular Disease | | 278.0 | Obesity | | V03.9 | Vaccination, Pneumovax |
| | 780.4 | Dizziness | | 382.9 | Otitis Media | | 616.10 | Vaginitis |
| | 995.2 | Drug Reaction | | 614.9 | Pelvic Inflammatory Disease | | 424.9 | Valvular Heart Disease |
| | 782.3 | Edema | | 533.9 | Peptic Ulcer Disease | | 079.9 | Viral Syndrome |
| | 780.7 | Fatigue/Tiredness/Malaise | | 443.9 | Perpheral Vascular Disease | | | |

*Comments:*

| PREVIOUS BALANCE | $ |
|---|---|
| TODAY'S CHARGES | $ |
| PAYMENT | $ |
| **BALANCE** | $ |

RETURN APPOINTMENT:
_____ Days  _____ Weeks  _____ Months
APPT. LENGTH: _____  PROVIDER: _____

APPT. REASON:

PROVIDER SIGNATURE:

**Adult**

Philadelphia
Health Associates
Tax ID #23-2350500
PHA Group # PH75923

☐ 3550 Market Street
Philadelphia, PA 19104
(215) 823-8660

☐ The Bourse Building
111 S. Independence Mall
East • 7th Floor
Philadelphia, PA 19106
(215) 625-9100

## OTHER DIAGNOSIS

| ✓ | CODE | DESCRIPTION | ✓ | CODE | DESCRIPTION |
|---|------|-------------|---|------|-------------|
| | | | | | |
| | | | | | |

PHA-019 (6/95)

**Figure 14-3** • Sample encounter form and charge slip.

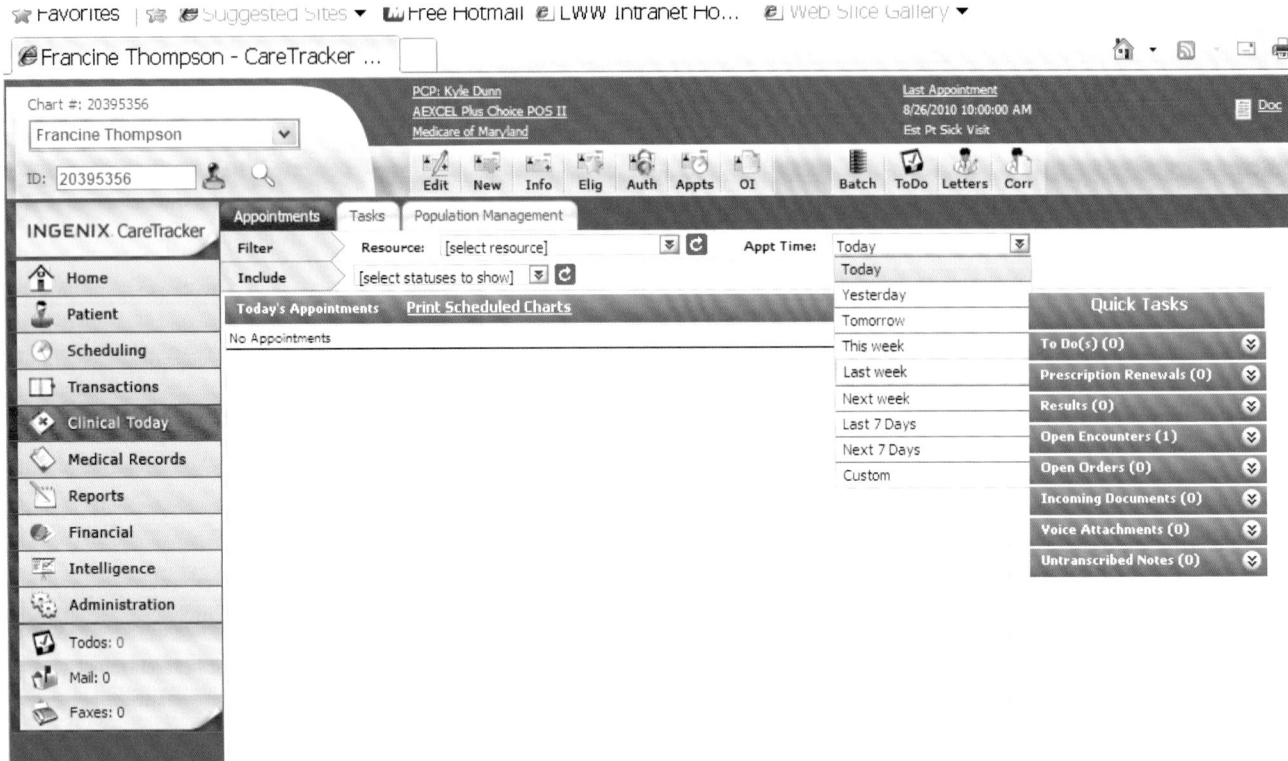

**Figure 14-4** • Computerized patient encounter screen. (Courtesy of Ingenix® CareTracker™.)

accept the fee for services set by that carrier instead of the physician's normal fee. Again, you must charge the same fee for the procedure. When payment is received, however, the explanation of benefits from that carrier will show the agreed-on amount, also called the allowed amount, for that procedure. You will post the payment in the normal way, but you must write off the difference between the physician's standard fee for this procedure and the allowed amount. Assume the doctor charged $40 for an office visit and the insurance carrier's agreed-on amount was $35. You would post $40 in the payment column and $5 in the adjustment column to arrive at the agreed-on amount.

*Example 3.* Most facilities require that you write off the balance of an account when you turn it over to a collection agency to keep better control of the accounts receivable. Therefore, if the patient's balance is $1,200, you would show "collection agency" in the description column of the ledger and put the $1,200 in the adjustment column, which would bring the balance to 0. Procedures 14-5 and 14-6 list the steps for posting an adjustment and collection agency payment.

## Posting a Debit Adjustment

Generally, a credit adjustment reduces the patient's account balance, whereas a debit adjustment adds to the patient's account balance. Below are three specific situations that require a debit adjustment.

*Example 1.* You receive a nonsufficient funds (NSF) check from the bank today. The check was given to you by a payment made earlier in the month and posted as such to his account (see What If? box). The previous payment is no longer valid. Therefore, you must eliminate that payment because the patient now owes it again. Because this is not an original charge, you may not use the charge column for this entry. To post this debit adjustment to the patient's account, you will show NSF in the description column and the amount of the NSF check in the payment column with brackets. Procedure 14-7 describes the steps for processing NSF checks.

*Example 2.* Assume that you have turned over an account to a collection agency and the patient comes in later to pay the amount owed. You must first put the money back on the account, or you will create a credit balance. Place the ledger card on the daysheet, and in the description column, write "reverse collection." Again, this is not an original or new charge, so you do not use the charge column. Show the amount in the adjustment column in brackets because you are adding the amount to the patient's balance. You may now show the payment in the payment column.

*Example 3.* Your office requires that you refund all money over $5 to the patient or insurance carrier. You must also post this to eliminate the credit balance on the account. Place the ledger card on the daysheet, and in the description column, write "refund to patient" (or insurance carrier). To eliminate a credit balance, you must debit the account. You put the amount of the refund in the adjustment column in brackets, indicating that it is a debit, not a credit adjustment. Procedure 14-4 describes the steps in processing refunds.

## CHECKPOINT QUESTION

4. How does a credit adjustment differ from a debit adjustment?

## PATIENT EDUCATION

### Physician Charges: What Happens to the Difference?

The concept of writing off the difference in the amount the physician charges and the amount a third-party payer pays is often misunderstood by patients. Many patients think that this means the physician has overcharged them. You can help clear up confusion by saying something like this: "The doctor charges $50.00 for a level 1 exam. When we file a claim with your insurance company, they only 'allow' $40.00 for that particular exam. The doctor has made an agreement with your insurance company to accept less in exchange for being your choice of physician."

Let's say a patient's coverage requires her to pay 20% of the bill. Insurance will pay their portion of what they allowed, which would be 80% of $40.00 or $32.00. The patient pays $8.00. This would leave a balance of $10.00, which is the difference in what was charged and what was allowed. This $10.00 is adjusted off of the account. This amount is written off only when the doctor is a participating provider with the insurance company. If you break it down, most patients will understand and appreciate the lesson.

## Posting to Cash-Paid-Out Section of Daysheet

Some insurance carriers adjust for money overpaid to your facility by holding that amount out of money they are paying your facility for other patients. This is known as a **take-back** and, although you are posting the correct amounts in the payment column for each patient, the check amount from the insurance carrier is short the refund or kept-out money. You write this in the cash-paid-out section of the daysheet, explaining, "insurance refund on account of [patient's name]." It is also a good idea to make a copy of the explanation of benefits and staple it to the back of your daysheet for future reference. Procedure 14-8 describes how to balance a daysheet.

# COMPUTERIZED ACCOUNTING

Most medical office accounting software available today is easy to use and requires a minimum of computer skills. Computer programs fulfill many of the same functions as a pegboard system but do so much faster. Instead of recording entries on a daysheet, you key entries into a computer. You can print out invoices and receipts for patients and insurance companies. Since most practices have computer stations in several locations, the patient's account can be quickly and easily retrieved in all areas of the office, enabling everyone involved in the patient's care to access information about third-party coverage, co-payments required, and so on.

Computer bookkeeping programs have a variety of advantages over pegboard bookkeeping. Computer programs work as expanded calculators and perform the arithmetic functions, such as balancing individual accounts and the day's totals. Many bookkeeping programs also can write checks, and many programs manage electronic banking between the office and bank. The office may have computerized many functions, including bookkeeping, medical billing, and medical management; therefore, it is essential that data stored on the computer be backed up in a reliable way in case the computer crashes. Figure 14-5 shows a screenshot of the equivalent of the patient's ledger card.

## Posting to Computer Accounts

If you understand the fundamentals of accounting and how to post entries manually, you will be able to use a computer system with ease. When you post charges into the computer database, in most systems, you use a local or access code to indicate a certain procedure or service. For example, you may enter 211 to post a level 2 office visit for a new patient. When the information prints on the claim form, the CPT (Current Procedural Terminology) code 99212 will appear (see Chapter 12). Figure 14-6 is a screenshot showing a charge posted to a patient's computerized account.

To post payments, first retrieve the patient's account. The software will take you through the process. You enter the source and amount of the payment, the allowed amount for the service, and any necessary adjustments. As in a manual system, this information is provided on the insurance carrier's explanation of benefits (EOB). Calculations are automatic and error free. Figure 14-7 shows a screenshot for posting an insurance payment in a computerized system.

## Computer Accounting Reports

Depending on the software package, you can easily generate daily, monthly, and yearly reports on transactions of an individual physician in a group practice. Daily and weekly reports provide the same information found on

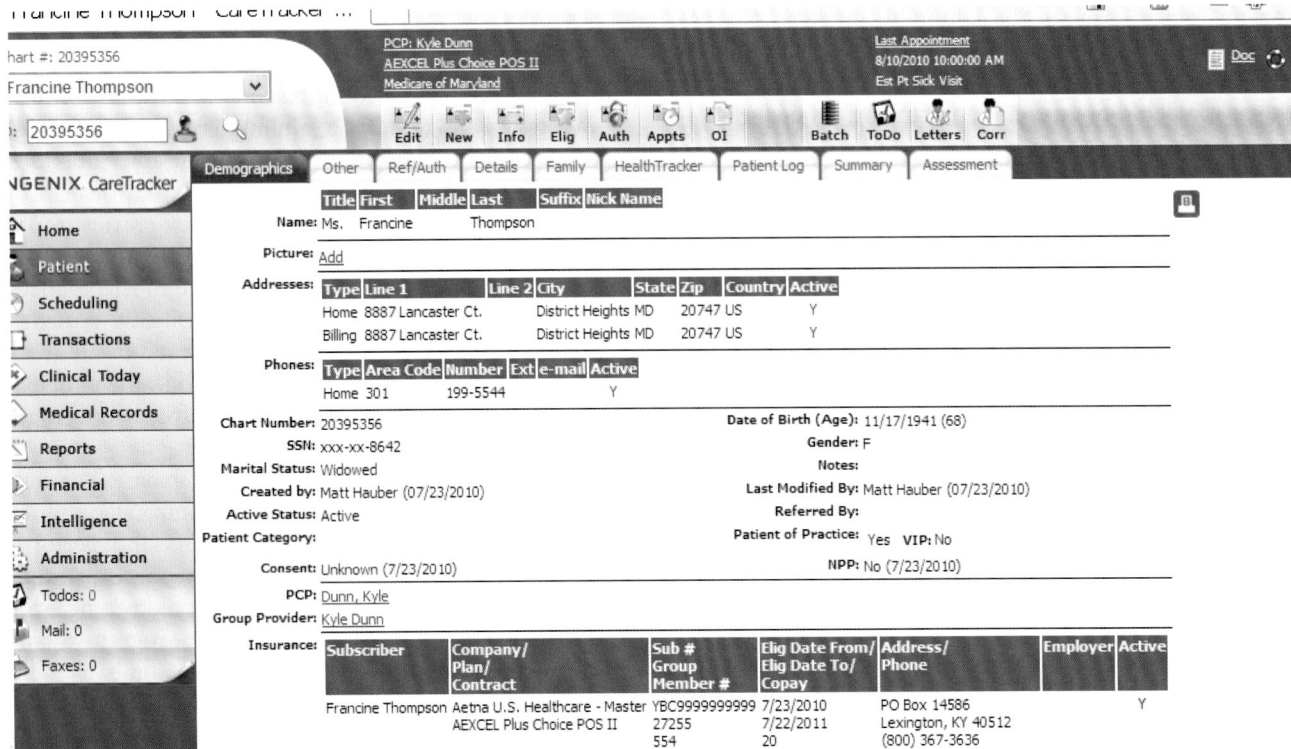

Figure 14-5 • Patient account screenshot. (Courtesy of Ingenix® CareTracker™.)

the bottom of a daysheet in a manual accounting system. At any given time, you can request a report that displays the practice's period-to-date and year-to-date financial status.

Computer systems record the daily activities described earlier for the manual system, and bookkeeping software enables you to create a closing report that prints a list of the day's financial activities. You may run a trial daily report or a final daily report. In a trial report, the information keyed in that day is printed for review. You correct any errors before running a final report. As on the daysheet, you categorize receipts as cash, check, and so on. A check register report can print the amount of the daily deposit and a list of checks for the day.

## CHECKPOINT QUESTION

5. What is a local or access code?

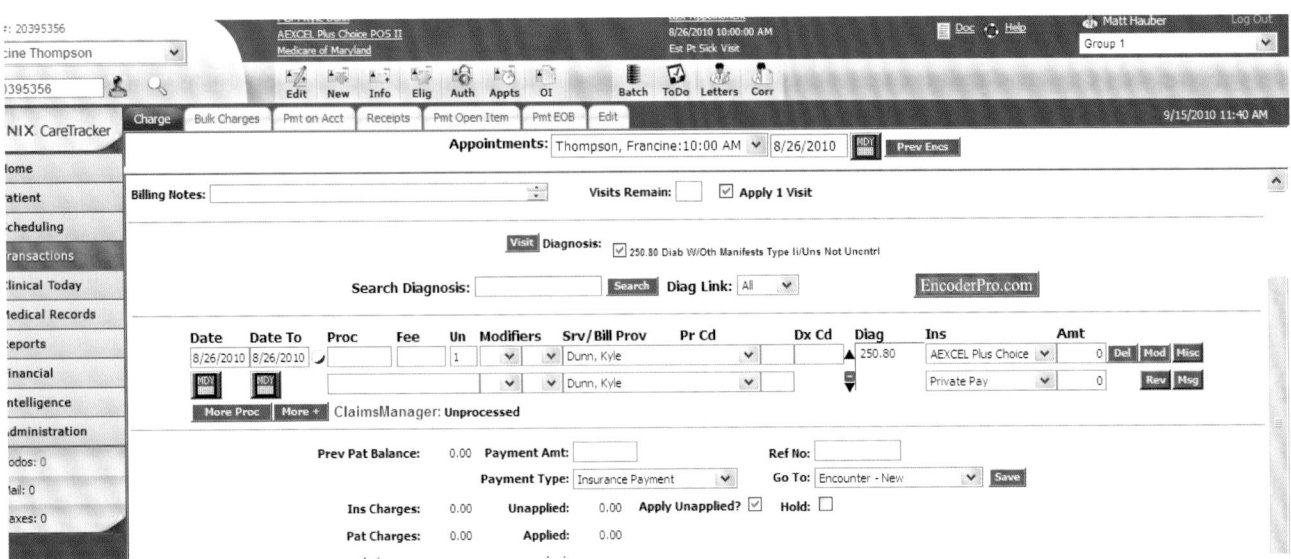

Figure 14-6 • Charge posting screenshot. (Courtesy of Ingenix® CareTracker™.)

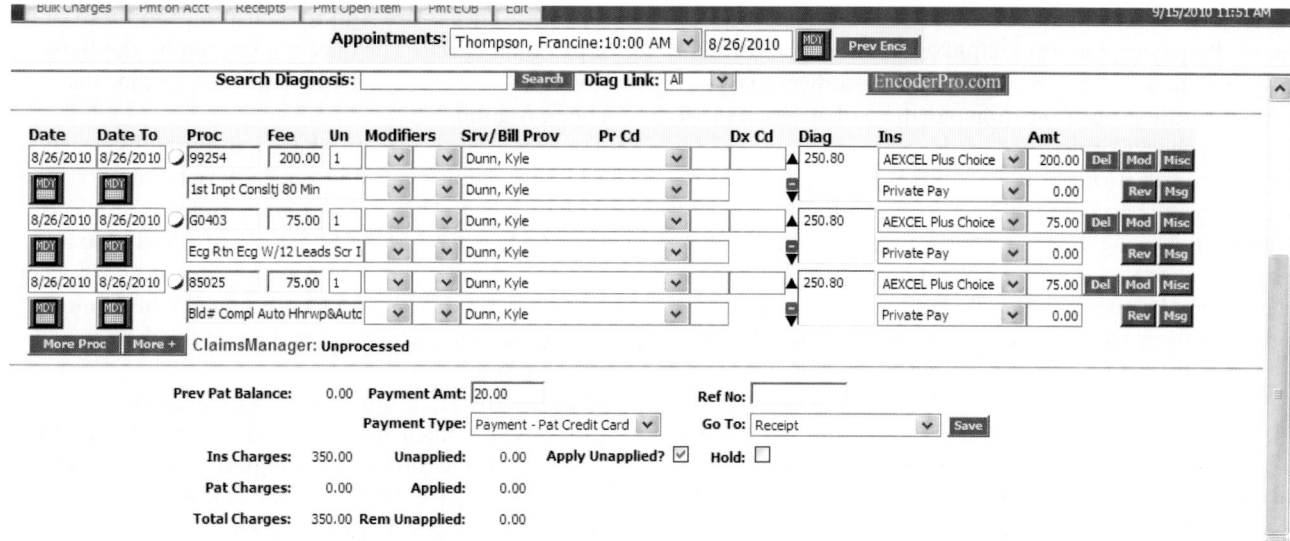

**Figure 14-7** • Insurance payment posting screenshot. (Courtesy of Ingenix® CareTracker™.)

# ⛓ BANKS AND THEIR SERVICES

## Types of Accounts

Besides physical location, several factors are important when choosing a bank for the office business account. These factors include the monthly service fees, overdraft protection programs (protection against bouncing checks), interest-bearing accounts, and returned check fees.

## Checking Accounts

A checking account allows you to write checks for funds that are deposited in the account. Each day, you will deposit to a checking account the money collected in the office. At the time a new checking account is opened, checks are ordered with a check order form. The administrative medical assistant must maintain the checkbook and ensure that checks are reordered as needed.

Banks offer a variety of options for checking accounts. Variables include monthly service charges, maximum amounts of checks written, minimum balance requirements, and so on. Interest-bearing checking accounts pay interest if the balance is kept above a certain amount. Most banks set the minimum checking account balance at $500 to $2,500. The bank pays this interest in exchange for the use of your money for loans and other transactions. If you drop below the minimum balance, however, you will not earn interest. Most banks also charge a monthly service fee and a fee for each check written for the period the balance was below the limit. Some banks waive the monthly service fee if the office agrees to maintain a minimum balance in another account, such as a savings account.

## Savings Accounts

The medical practice may use a savings account for money that is put aside for long-term plans or money that is not needed for writing checks. A savings account pays interest at a higher percentage rate than a checking account, allowing the money to grow. Funds can be transferred to the checking account as needed.

## Money Market Accounts

Money market accounts are a combination of a savings account and an interest-bearing checking account. The minimum balance is usually much higher than that of a checking account (as much as $2,500), but the interest rate also is much higher. These accounts offer limited check-writing privileges, including an initial deposit of $2,000 and minimum balance of $500 per check.

## Bank Fees

Banks charge fees for services. In an effort to get new business, banks offer special services and plans for small business, including the medical office.

### Monthly Service Fees

Bank policies concerning monthly fees or service charges vary widely. A **service charge** is a fee charged monthly for using an account. The charge can be a fixed amount or may be an individual charge for each check written on the account. As discussed, some banks do not levy a service charge if a specific minimum balance is maintained for the account.

### Overdraft Fees and Protection

According to NYtimes.com, in 2010, banks generated $20 billion in overdraft fees. As of July 1, 2010, the Federal Reserve requires that banks obtain a customer's consent before they can charge overdraft fees for automatic teller machine transactions and debit purchases instead of automatically paying the transaction and charging customers overdraft fees. Banks now encourage customers to opt in for overdraft protection to avoid the embarrassment of returned checks or declined cards.

Overdraft protection guarantees that checks written against the account will be paid even when there is not enough money in the account at the time. Usually, the bank pays the checks and retrieves the money owed to it when the account balance is restored. Many banks offer overdraft protection as a "loan," and the customer is charged a fee.

### Returned Check Fee

Some banks charge a **returned check fee,** which is a fee charged for any check that is deposited into the checking account but that is later returned to the bank because the account it was issued from had insufficient funds with which to pay the check. Such a check is often referred to as a bounced check. Since checks to be deposited are endorsed (as described below), the practice assumes responsibility if the bank account upon which the check is drawn is insufficient. If the check bounces, therefore, the bank charges a fee to the practice and most facilities charge this amount to the patient. Because this is an original charge, the bad check fee is listed in the charge column of the patient ledger and daysheet, with the amount of the check being recorded as a debit adjustment.

## WHAT IF

**What if a patient's check is returned for nonsufficient funds?**

As a courtesy, you may call the patient and explain that the check has been returned for nonsufficient funds. Many times, the patient will instruct you to send the check back through the bank. You will need to make a separate deposit slip from the daily deposit of money taken in that day.

If this is not an option, then the patient should come into the office and pay the amount of the check plus any fees your office charges for a returned check. The returned check would then be given back to the patient since he or she has now paid cash for the amount. It is a good practice to flag the patient's account and even to demand cash only for future payments. Some businesses use a check service that electronically approves a check. There is a fee for this service.

## Types of Checks

Most medical offices use the standard business check, but when certain circumstances require, there are other types available:

- Certified checks are stamped and signed by the bank to verify that the amount of the check is being held in the account for payment. The check is written from the customer's account.

- Cashier's checks are sold to a customer for cash or a personal check. The check is written by the bank, giving the recipient the added guarantee that the check is good.
- Traveler's checks are purchased and used like cash when traveling but, unlike cash, may be replaced if stolen or lost. They are available in denominations of $10, $20, and $50 and are used for individuals who do not want to use an ATM or credit card when traveling. Traveler's checks are signed when bought and are countersigned (signed again) in the presence of the payee.
- Money orders, although not checks, can be purchased with cash from a bank or the U.S. Postal Service. Money orders, which guarantee payment to the recipient, are often used for mailing payments because it is not safe to mail cash.

Box 14-1 highlights other terms used in the language of banking.

---

**BOX 14-1   Common Banking Language**

**ABA number:** A number originated by the American Bankers Association to identify the bank on which the check is written. It is written in the form of a fraction and is usually found above or below the check number. The top number of the fraction indicates the geographic location, and the bottom number identifies the bank.

**ATM:** Automated teller machines (ATM) have made 24-hour banking possible. With the use of a card you insert into a slot and a personal identification number (PIN), you can make deposits, withdrawals, and transfers at an ATM. If your bank owns the ATM, this convenience is usually free. If you use any other ATM, a service fee of up to $3.50 is charged. The ATM screen gives you the opportunity to cancel the transaction if you are not willing to pay the service fee.

**Debit card:** A card with a magnetic strip that is presented for payment directly from your checking account. When a transaction occurs, you record it in your check registry.

**Online banking:** Electronic or online banking gives you the opportunity to view your account at any time. Withdrawals and deposits are listed and can be printed, and transfers can be made.

**Stale check:** A check that has not been cashed within a certain time, usually 6 months. Some checks must be cashed within a shorter time, but that requirement must be printed on the check.

## ⊙⊙ BANKING RESPONSIBILITIES

### Writing Checks for Accounts Payable

Another financial responsibility of the medical assistant may be to handle accounts payable or pay the bills. The accounts payable in a medical office usually include rent, utilities, taxes, salaries, vendors of supplies and services, patient refunds, and petty cash reimbursement. The accounts are usually paid by check. Banks require signature cards for each person authorized to sign checks. In some cases, this is limited to the physician or physicians. Some medical offices require two signatures, especially if the check is over a certain amount. Bookkeeping computer systems allow you to enter information in the proper field and print checks while keeping track of every transaction using a check. When using a manual system, type or write legibly in black ink. Use the current date and write the amount of the payment in both figures and words and the name of the payee. Complete the memo line for reference. Record the date, check number, amount of the check, and payee on the check registry. Post this transaction to the appropriate account in the general ledger or apply it to the proper category in a computer system by entering the type of payment on the proper screen. Recording transactions in the proper account or category is important when preparing the office taxes. Subtract each amount from the check register balance.

### Receiving Checks and Making Deposits

When checks are received in the office, they are first endorsed. To endorse a check requires writing (or rubber stamping) on the back of the check the name and number of the account into which it will be deposited (Fig. 14-8). This way, if the payments are lost or stolen, no one else can cash them. It also ensures that the bank deposits the payments to the correct account and makes the practice responsible for the amount of the check in the event there is insufficient funds in the payer's bank account. An endorsement stamp can be purchased from your bank or an office supply store.

Checks may also be submitted directly into the practice bank account electronically. Insurance companies offer incentives to providers to bill for services and receive payments electronically such as faster claims processing and faster reimbursement. Deposits made electronically must be posted on the daysheet, but will not, of course, be taken to the bank with a deposit slip (see Chapter 13).

After all payments are posted, total all of the checks and all cash received that day. This total should match

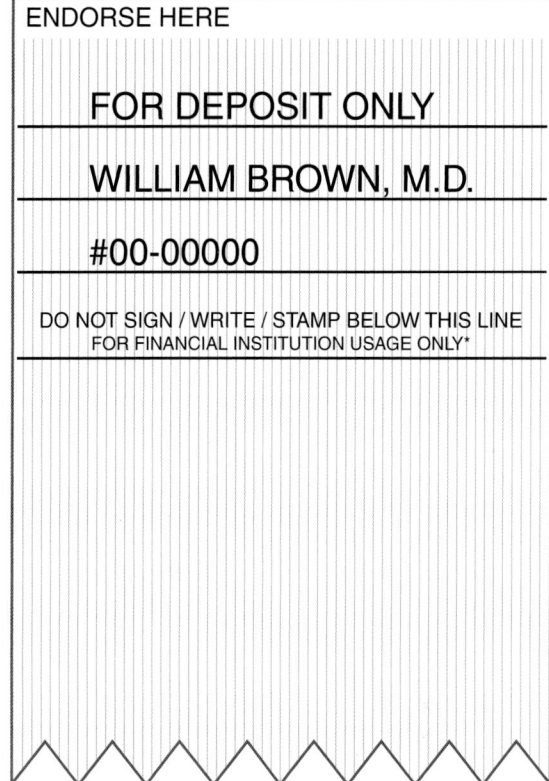

ENDORSE HERE

**FOR DEPOSIT ONLY**

**WILLIAM BROWN, M.D.**

**#00-00000**

DO NOT SIGN / WRITE / STAMP BELOW THIS LINE
FOR FINANCIAL INSTITUTION USAGE ONLY*

**Figure 14-8 •** An endorsed check.

the totals of the payments column on your daysheet. Detach the deposit sheet from the daysheet and stamp the back with the endorsement check stamp. If a computer program is used, print out a deposit slip. Wrap the deposit slip around the checks and complete a bank deposit slip for the account to which the deposit is made. The deposit can be hand delivered or mailed to the bank.

A hand-delivered deposit may be taken to a teller, who will issue a deposit receipt, or dropped in a depository. If the deposit is mailed, make sure sufficient postage has been affixed to the envelope. Never include cash payments in a deposit that is mailed or placed in a depository. Cash deposits should always be hand delivered, and a teller's receipt should always be obtained. Procedure 14-9 describes how to make a bank deposit.

### Reconciling Bank Statements

All banks mail monthly statements to account holders on which are listed all transactions since the last closing date. This bank statement must be reconciled, or compared for accuracy, with your records each month.

The statement consists of a list of all checks written and their amounts, all deposits made and their amounts, any electronic transactions, and any service charges. Verify that all checks and deposits are listed correctly. Make a check mark on the checkbook stub of each check that has been paid by the bank. On the

1.  Subtract any fees or charges that appear on this statement from your checkbook balance.
2.  Add any interest paid on your checking account to your checkbook balance.
3.  List the checks you have written that have not been paid (these checks did not yet appear on your bank statement). You can also include in this list any withdrawals you have made since the ending date of the banking statement that do not appear on the statement.

| Check Number | Amount |
| --- | --- |
| 6217 | 32.94 |
| 6218 | 50.00 |
| 6219 | 119.24 |
| Total | 202.18 |

4.  If you have entered deposits or other additions to your checkbook that do not appear on the statement, list them here:

| Date | Amount |
| --- | --- |
| 12-8-13 | 592.00 |
| Total | 592.00 |

5.  Enter the ending balance from your statement here:  9542.91
    Add the total deposits from Step 4:                + 592.00
    Subtract the total from Step 3:                    − 202.18
    Total (this should equal your checkbook balance):    9932.73

If these balances do not equal your checkbook balance:
*   Check the addition and subtraction in your checkbook
*   Check the amount of each transaction in your checkbook with the amount shown on your statement
*   Check to see that all transactions from your previous statement have been accounted for
*   Call your bank manager for assistance

**Figure 14-9** • Completed reconciling worksheet.

back of the statement is a worksheet that explains how to balance the account (Fig. 14-9). Following the steps listed on the worksheet makes balancing the account fairly easy. The steps for reconciling a bank statement are listed in Procedure 14-10.

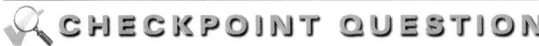

### CHECKPOINT QUESTION

6. What information is found on a bank statement?

## COG PETTY CASH

A petty cash account is a cash fund kept in the office specifically for small purchases, such as buying postage stamps or office supplies. The value of the petty cash account should always remain the same. A petty cash fund is always a designated sum of money. When money is taken from the fund, a voucher (Fig. 14-10)

or receipt is placed in the fund to verify the purchase. The remaining cash and the sum of the vouchers should always equal the designated sum; for example, a petty cash fund of $40 with $13 in actual cash should have receipts that amount to $27.

Petty cash funds should be kept separate from patient cash payments. All cash should be kept in a securely locked area, and one person should be designated to maintain the petty cash fund and issue vouchers. A voucher with an attached receipt should always be placed in the petty cash box, both to provide proof of the purchase and to keep the account balanced. The petty cash fund normally is replenished when the cash is low, which is usually once a month. To replenish the fund, cash a check in the amount of the total of the vouchers. The money is placed in the fund, and the vouchers are removed and filed (Procedure 14-11).

Some offices keep a petty cash expense record. This record is similar to a checkbook that keeps track of the account balance as checks are written, such as personal checkbook. This expense record also categorizes

```
              PETTY CASH RECEIPT

                        12/1    20 13
  _____
  Supplies:
                        14.  32
  _____
  Postage:
                         1.  17
  _____
  Travel Expenses:
                          ⌀
  _____
  Other:
    fish food
                         4.  00
  _____
  Approved    12/1/13
                      TOTAL   19.49
    L. Davis, CMA

              Received Above Amount
                  19.49              HP, CMA
```

**Figure 14-10** • Completed petty cash receipt.

purchases so that they can be included with the monthly office expenses. Purchases such as stamps and office and medical supplies can be deducted as office expenses and added to the accounts payable expense record.

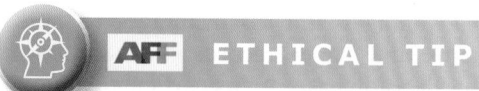

### CHECKPOINT QUESTION

7. List six guidelines for managing petty cash.

### ETHICAL TIP

#### Honesty Is the Best Policy

Physician-employers put their trust in their employees every day. In the clinical area, they trust that their assistants will be conscientious and careful. In the administrative area, they trust that employees will be completely honest and trustworthy. Borrowing $5.00 out of petty cash for lunch is not acceptable. When handling money for the facility, follow established procedures to the letter. "Cross every 't' " and "dot every 'i' " so there will be no reason to doubt you. Fortunately, most physicians and their medical assistants enjoy a mutual respect and loyalty. By following the rules, you will prove to your employer that you are worthy of his or her trust.

## OVERVIEW OF ACCOUNTING

Accounting is the compilation of a business's financial records. It is necessary for assessment of the practice's financial history and current financial stakes, which serves as the basis for sound financial management. The medical office, like other businesses, requires strict adherence to sound record-keeping practices. Records must be maintained in an orderly fashion so you can retrieve financial information at any time and to present an organized picture of the business's finances. A system of checks and balances is an integral part of record management. Generally, the check-and-balance status of accounts is examined monthly by comparing the total of all accounts with outstanding balances against the running total taken from the daily logs of all financial transactions. The practice's accountant will also closely scrutinize these records at scheduled intervals for tax-reporting purposes.

Although manual accounting systems are still used, computer accounting is available as part of most medical software packages, and the many advantages include efficient tracking and analysis of critical information, improved productivity, and smarter business decisions. General ledger, payables, receivables, inventory, purchasing, cash flow, bank reconciliation, collections, fixed assets, and many other applications integrate with each other so you can manage the office's core processes efficiently and effectively.

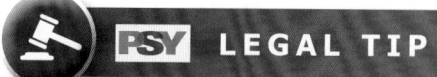

### LEGAL TIP

#### Correct It Correctly

It is illegal to falsify any financial documents. Accurate record keeping is essential. The Internal Revenue Service will examine the practice's financial records. You may be held liable for errors or omissions to these documents. White-out is a great product but should not be used in a medical office. There are documented cases of suspected fraud when financial records were corrected with white-out. Corrections to ledger cards, daysheets, petty cash records, etc., are made just as they are in the medical record. Draw a single line through the wrong number, and place the correct one above or below. You should be able to see the item being corrected. If the space is too small for this, cross out the entire transaction and start a new one. Initial the correction.

## Accounting Cycle

The finances of medical practices operate in one of two 12-month intervals or durations. The office **accounting cycle** follows either a fiscal year (a consecutive 12-month period starting with a specified date) or a calendar year (January through December). The yearly interval used depends on the way the practice's accountant has structured the business. For example, the medical practice can exist as a sole proprietorship, which typically uses the calendar year, or as a professional corporation with a fiscal year that begins at any time for a 12-month period. Once a tax return is filed for the business, however, the practice must get permission from the federal **Internal Revenue Service (IRS)** to change a tax year.

The **IRS** examines a business's income statements for the amount of profit and owed tax four times a year by quarterly estimated tax returns. The practice's annual tax return is a summary of the quarterly returns and reports the final year-end profit or loss (income minus expenses equals profit or loss) for the fiscal or calendar reporting period. If financial records are scrupulously maintained all year, preparation of the annual income tax return should merely be a summation of existing accounting facts. Well-maintained office records not only facilitate IRS returns but also provide data that define the practice's business picture.

There are many reasons for a physician along with an accountant to review financial data on a regular basis. Financial records reflect growing expenditures and growth in the business. Conclusions drawn from financial data can affect future financial decisions. For example, analysis of the practice's accounts receivable can predict the amount of salary increases. Tax records must be available in case of an IRS inquiry or **audit** (review of accounts). Records such as receipts should be retained for 7 years, but records such as bank statements, canceled checks, and IRS tax returns should be kept for the duration of the business.

## RECORD-KEEPING COMPONENTS

The practice's financial records should include a running record of income, accounts receivable, and total expenditures, including **payroll** (employee salaries), cash on hand, and **liabilities** (amounts the practice owes). Expenditures can be broken down into categories (Box 14-2). This is important because it enables the record keeper to track the practice's expenses and provide the physician and accountant with a cohesive picture of the practice's expenses at tax time.

Categories can be accommodated by several types of bookkeeping systems; a simple business checkbook does not allow this. Pegboard systems allow the bookkeeper to write the check once over the **check register** (a place to record checks) or the ledger sheet and then have multiple pages with columns to distribute an expense into categories, including a back sheet for payroll. These columns are totaled and balanced at the completion of

---

**BOX 14-2   Categories of Expenditures**

- Office supplies: items used by the facility's employees, such as paper, pencils, daysheets, and ledger cards
- Medical supplies: items used for patients, such as examination gowns, electrocardiograph paper, syringes, and tongue depressors
- Drugs: drug purchases, such as injectables; some facilities keep a separate column for these purchases, and others put this amount in the medical supplies category
- Payroll: gross amount paid to employees
- Taxes: taxes paid, such as the Federal Insurance Contributions Act tax, Medicare, federal withholding, state withholding (listed separately)
- Rent: amount paid to rent the facility
- Utilities: gas, electric, telephone
- Maintenance: routine care of the facility, such as cleaning personnel
- Travel: physician's car lease payment, gas mileage if paid to employees, and so on
- Personal: any money used personally by the physician

---

each check register sheet and can be subtotaled monthly, quarterly, and annually (discussed later in the chapter). Keeping a monthly accounts payable disbursement sheet lets the administrative medical assistant easily compare past years' expenses for the same part of the year.

Software packages offer the most sophisticated way to maintain financial records, not just for the categorization of expenses but also for the rapid formation of financial reports. Automating accounts payable does, however, require a personal computer (PC), software, and the training to use it.

There are advantages and disadvantages to both computer systems and paper records. Each practice should make this decision based on its particular volume and needs. Either system (pegboard or computer) can provide the practice and its accountant with the ability to pay and track expenses and to furnish the financial data necessary to create reports.

Multiple **summation reports**, such as the payroll report, itemized category report, account balances, and the **profit-and-loss statement**, must be prepared for the practice's accountant. If financial data are entered diligently into the bookkeeping system, preparing monthly, quarterly, or yearly reports should not be a daunting task. Income tax accounting cycles are divided into quarters: January through March, April through June, July through September, and October through December. Payroll reports show the amount of taxes being withheld and made monthly, quarterly, or annually. Normally, the practice's accountant will send you necessary reports and have you mail the checks.

## 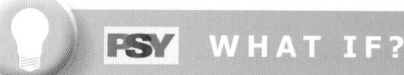 ACCOUNTS PAYABLE

### Ordering Goods and Services

There are many economical ways to purchase office supplies or equipment. For instance, purchasing cooperatives (co-ops) offer bulk rate discounts by allowing physicians to order in a pool with other purchasers. Vendors may offer discounts for buying in volume or for paying promptly. Large warehouse-type merchandisers and companies with discount catalogs also offer competitive prices. Researching and cost-comparing office products and medical supplies can be time consuming, but it is worth the effort, especially for items used frequently. Compare past invoices with prices in new catalogs.

Besides cost, other considerations come to bear when purchasing office supplies. For example, office supply companies often provide free delivery, but office warehouse chains may charge a fee or require a minimum order for free delivery. Quality also plays a role. Supplies should be of standard quality as well as economical. It is common to use several office supply vendors according to quality or pricing of specific goods. Also, it is important when buying in bulk that considerations be made for the storage of supplies when received.

Office supplies or equipment can be ordered in a number of ways. Once an account is set up, offices can place orders by telephone, fax, mail, or e-mail. These orders can be paid monthly by check or by credit card. It is preferable to pay for supplies by check or credit card rather than by cash, but when cash purchases are necessary, retain a detailed receipt for tax purposes. Credit card purchases can be made online, over the telephone, or by mail, but for security reasons, credit card account numbers should not be faxed.

When placing orders for supplies, give the office's account number to the vendor or write it on the order form. It is a good idea to use a **purchase order** that lists the supplies ordered and their order numbers, so that order numbers for frequently ordered items can be pulled from the previous purchase order; this saves time with subsequent orders. Be sure to record the charges for your order and verify them against the bill later. It is also handy to keep a list of all vendors, telephone numbers, and account numbers. Procedure 14-12 lists the steps for ordering supplies.

### CHECKPOINT QUESTION

8. When purchasing office supplies, what factors besides price should you consider?

### Receiving Supplies

When goods are delivered to the office, a receipt or **packing slip** listing the enclosed items should always accompany the order. The office staff member who receives the supplies must check the packing slip against the actual contents to ensure that all supplies are in the shipment.

The person should initial the packing slip, which shows that all goods were received. When it is time to issue checks for payables, the assistant can then pay the **invoice** or bill with confidence that all items purchased have been received. These receipts or packing slips should be placed in a bills pending file, so that they may be compared to the bill when it arrives. If the bill has already been paid by check or credit card, the invoice should be placed in the appropriate account's paid file; there should be such a file for each fiscal or calendar year.

### PSY   WHAT IF?

**What if all of the supplies ordered from a particular vendor are not in the shipment?**

Check the packing slip to see that the item was actually sent (Fig. 14-11). The form should indicate whether the item or items are being shipped separately, out of stock, or discontinued. If the item is listed on the form as having been shipped, you will need to call the supplier. The supplier will need an order number from the packing slip. The missing item may have just been left out. Be sure to document the date, findings of the call, and name of the person you spoke with. Place a reminder on your calendar to follow up if the item is not there when promised. Do not pay for something you do not get.

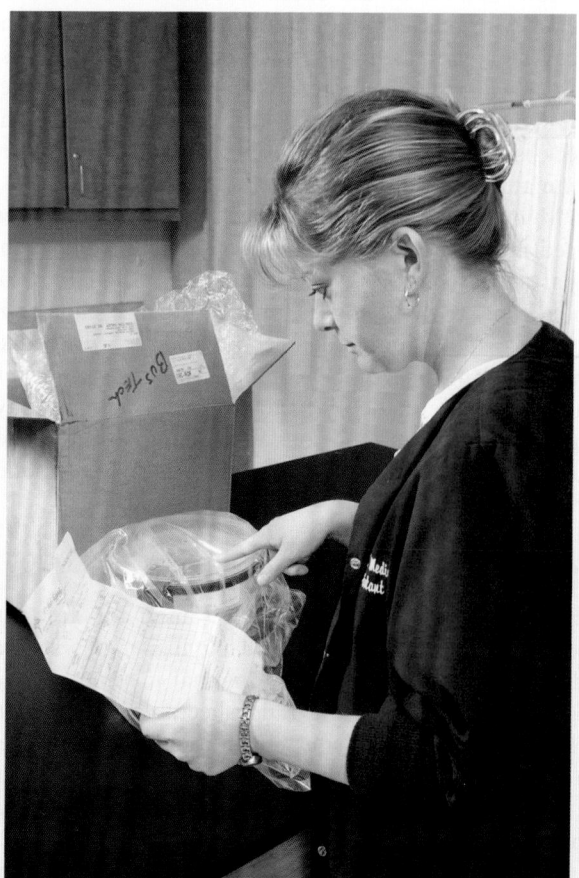

**Figure 14-11 •** The medical assistant should be sure supplies are received and checked carefully.

## Paying Invoices

Invoices for supplies and other types of bills payable by the practice should be kept together in a bills pending file to avoid loss or misplacement of a bill. Bills can be paid daily, weekly, biweekly, or monthly.

### Manual Payment

Manual payment of bills requires a checkbook and checks (Procedure 14-13). The practice's accountant may recommend use of a log or record book into which is entered information about each check, such as payroll taxes or the breakdown of expenses for a monthly credit card bill. The large checks and checkbooks available from banks and business printers offer more space for writing memos or itemizing a check. Each check, once written, is detached from a **check stub**, which remains in the checkbook. If you make a mistake while writing a check, void the check and stub and staple the voided check to the stub. Never make corrections on the facility's checks. Check stubs should be filed with other fiscal or calendar year records and kept for the life of the practice.

The information recorded on the check stub includes the check number, the date the check was issued, the payee (the party to whom the check was written), and the full amount of the check. Notes should be written on both the memo section of the check and on the check stub. For example, when entering the purchase of a new pager, the note might read, "payee: Office Communications" or "new pager for Dr. Smith." The check is then attached to the bill or invoice and signed by an authorized individual.

Memos or notations on check stubs can be referenced later if a question arises concerning payment by a particular check. A log or record book enables the bookkeeper to make entries for each expense, categorize expenses, and maintain detailed payroll records. Unlike one-write (pegboard) or computer systems, multiple entries must be made by hand to track office bill paying. This can seem laborious when compared to other bookkeeping systems, but it may be ideal for smaller practices.

### Pegboard Payment

The same pegboard system that is used for accounts receivable may be used for bill paying; it has several advantages over the ordinary manual method of paying bills. Instead of using a daysheet, a **check register** (also referred to as a disbursement journal) page is used to record the checks that have been written. The check is then aligned on the pegboard over the register page and is filled out as with any other check (Fig. 14-12). Pegboard checks have a carbon or transfer strip, and on this strip is written the date, the payee, the check number, and the amount. The information written on

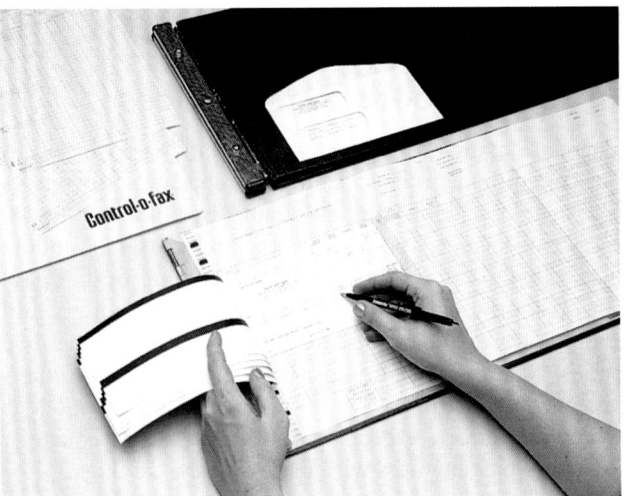

**Figure 14-12 •** Sample pegboard check and check register. (Courtesy of Control-o-fax, Waterloo, IA.)

the strip is recorded automatically on the check register. These check-writing systems are referred to as one-write systems for this reason. The check can be addressed directly beneath the payee line and mailed in a window envelope, which saves the time it would take to address an envelope.

The pegboard check register has approximately 20 columns that can be used to categorize expenses, such as rent, insurance, office supplies, utilities, service contracts, postage, and any other applicable categories. All entries on the check register are totaled when the register is completed; these totals are carried forward to the new register page. Each fiscal or calendar year begins with a new first page (page 1), and the last check register page will have totals for the entire year. The check register provides a system of checks and balances even before the bank statement arrives because the check register must be balanced, as with a bank statement.

The check register also allows entries for bank deposits, and the back page of the register is used for payroll record keeping. As with pegboard accounts receivable, completed pegboard check registers are filed in a separate binder in chronological order, with the most recent register on top.

### Computer Payment

A computer accounts payable system has all the advantages that a pegboard system offers: access at a glance to check registers, itemized categories and their totals, payroll records, and entries for bank deposits. To use such a system, you must have a PC, accounts payable program software, printer, and bank checks that are compatible with the software and printer. The initial expense with a computer system is much higher than that of manual or pegboard systems. Office personnel will need computer training to use the program. Also, since it runs on electricity, a computer may not work during power failures. A good computer accounting program will, however, provide functions for both accounts receivable and accounts payable. Financial data should be recorded in three forms: on the computer's hard drive, on a magnetic tape or CD, and in printout form (hard copy).

Although entering data in the computer may be time consuming at first, this becomes less of a concern with practice. Furthermore, financial reports can be compiled and printed in a fraction of the time required with manual or pegboard systems. The computer program can also perform the record-keeping arithmetic; as a result, mathematical errors are practically nonexistent.

Paying bills by computer requires using the software to open the check-writing file. Checks are presented on the computer screen in the same way that a paper check would normally appear, and the information that is required to appear on the check is entered on the computer keyboard. The information is stored, and the check is printed out; the computer program automatically subtracts the amount of the check from the account's balance. The bookkeeper can print one check at a time or a batch of checks together.

The computer can "memorize" checks so that the information on them can be recalled and reprinted without reentering it; this is especially helpful with payroll checks. A good accounting program also allows for bill and backup reminders. Of course, it is essential to back up financial data in case of computer problems.

### 🔍 CHECKPOINT QUESTION

9. Whether using a manual, pegboard, or computer accounts payable system, two steps must always occur when ordering and receiving supplies. What are they?

## 🆔 PREPARATION OF REPORTS

The bookkeeper must also prepare reports for the practice's accountant or the IRS based on financial data stored in the office's bookkeeping system. For this reason, care should always be taken when recording financial data.

The manual system, when assisted by the use of a log or record book, should be able to provide monthly, quarterly, and annual summaries for income, expenditures, and payroll. It is advisable to have subtotals and totals for these periods for tax payment purposes.

The pegboard system is also practical for providing summaries of income, expenses, and payroll and can be

totaled monthly, quarterly, and yearly. Each daysheet, check register, and payroll journal is individually totaled, with all balances forwarded to the next page. These records are stored in binders and kept for future reference.

A computer system of accounting offers all of the previously mentioned reports along with other more complicated reports that generally require more advanced accounting skills. The great advantage with a report generated by a computer is that the computer will perform all of the mathematical calculations for the time frame requested.

## 🆔 ASSISTING WITH AUDITS

An audit may be informal (in-house) and used to assist the practice's accountant with tax preparation, or it may be a formal audit by the IRS. If meticulous attention to record keeping has been paid throughout the year, the preparation time needed for such an audit should be minimal. It is important to save all bank statements, copies of annual and quarterly tax returns, and receipts for expenditures. Canceled checks and payroll records should be readily available.

Manual and pegboard systems can provide spending category and payroll summaries in addition to examination of the actual entries for the period being audited. A computer accounting system can provide all of this plus reports such as profit-and-loss statements, which normally would be compiled by an accountant.

 **ROLE-PLAYING ACTIVITY**

A new patient with Great Falls Medical Center recently wrote a check for services rendered that was subsequently returned by the bank as NSF. Toby Dickerson, RMA, is the medical assistant responsible for handling the financial matters of practice and must contact the patient to advise that the check has bounced and, as per office policies, payment must be replaced immediately with cash. In addition, the patient is now responsible for the $50 NSF bank fee. What should Toby say to the patient to get the NSF check replaced plus the NSF fee paid? Role-play this scenario as the medical assistant responsible for handling this matter and another student as the patient. If you are the medical assistant, think about how you would demonstrate professionalism and sensitivity when discussing the financial situation with the patient. If you are the patient, think about the emotions a "real" patient might display when confronted about his/her financial situation. Embarrassment? Anger? Defensiveness? What would be behaviors associated with these emotions? How would you respond to someone who displays these emotions? Your instructor will give you additional information about this activity!

## *español* SPANISH TERMINOLOGY

**Tenemos que deducir sus impuestos de su salario bruto.**
Taxes must be taken out of your paycheck.

**Usted necesita llenar estas formas.**
You need to complete these forms.

**Gracias por su pago.**
Thank you for your payment.

**Gracias por su cheque.**
Thank you for your check.

**Este es su recibo.**
This is your receipt.

**Esta cantidad es lo que usted todavía debe.**
This is your balance.

**Este es su crédito.**
This is your credit.

**No pague esta factura.**
Do not pay this bill.

**Su cheque ha sido devuelto por fondos insuficientes.**
Your check was returned for insufficient funds.

**Su cuenta ha sido enviada a una agencia de colección.**
Your account has been sent to a collection agency.

**En caso de que su cheque no tengas fondos, el banco y nosotros le cobraremos una cantidad extra.**
In case that your check has no funds, the bank will charge you a fee and we will also.

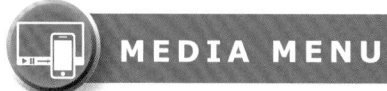

## MEDIA MENU

**Student Resources** on thePoint®

• **CMA/RMA Certification Exam Review**

**Internet Resources**
**Superbill Forms and Creations**
http://www.physicianshelp.com

**Comptroller of Currency Administrator of National Banks**
http://www.occ.treas.gov

**The Accounting Library**
http://www.accountinglibrary.com

**QuickBooks Online**
http://payroll.intuit.com/index.jsp;
http://www.quickbooks.intuit.com

**Microsoft Business Solutions**
http://www.microsoft.com/en-us/dynamics/default.aspx

**Internal Revenue Service**
http://www.irs.gov

## EMR Activity

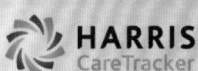

Harris CareTracker is a Web-based electronic medical record (EMR) application that you will use for the EMR activities included in this section at the end of each chapter. This application is actually used in physician offices but is provided to you through the publisher, Wolters Kluwer Health, to give you hands-on practice working with EMRs. Your instructor will have more information about accessing your username, log-in, and Quickstart guide.

Prerequisite Activities in Harris CareTracker

• *The Getting Started and Quickstart documents and EMR Activities Step-by-Step Instructions are available at* http://thePoint.lww.com/KronenbergerComp5e.

Activity Details

The accountant for Great Falls Medical Center has advised that fiscal period for last month may now be closed. In the *Administration* module, *Practice* tab, of Harris CareTracker, change the *Open* status for last month's fiscal period to *Closed*.

# Chapter Summary

- Accounting is a complex process involving many legal issues. As a medical assistant, you must keep neat and well-organized accounting records.
- Whether a medical practice uses a manual bookkeeping system, such as the pegboard system, or a computer system, you may be responsible for keeping records of accounts payable, accounts receivable, and petty cash.
- You may also be responsible for banking functions, such as receiving checks, making deposits, and reconciling monthly bank statements. To carry out these responsibilities effectively, you must record all transactions accurately and promptly.
- Computers have made the daily bookkeeping practices much easier, but you must understand the principles of accounting applied in the manual system if you are to use the computer system.
- Using the appropriate banking services will allow the day-to-day financial operations to be efficient, accurate, and secure.
- Managing the supplies and equipment in a practice, ordering goods and services efficiently and economically, and paying invoices are important duties of a medical assistant.
- With the computer being used for many administrative medical office functions, it is imperative that you keep abreast of changes and new opportunities to make this process more efficient and up-to-date.

# Warm-Ups for Critical Thinking

1. Your daysheet deposit slip and your posting proofs do not agree. How do you find the error?
2. Your office is considering going from a pegboard system to a computer bookkeeping system. What features should you look for in the software?
3. Explain the advantages of using computerized accounting systems.
4. When might a manual bookkeeping system using a pegboard be used?
5. A vendor continually mixes up your orders, and the physician asks you to look for a new vendor. How do you decide which one to recommend? What factors influence your choice of one office supply vendor over another?
6. The physician asks you, the office manager, how much money is owed to him. How do you gather the information needed to answer his question?

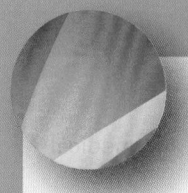

**PSY** PROCEDURE 14-1

## Post Charges on a Daysheet

**Purpose:** To keep a daily and running account of all charges to patients in the medical practice

**Equipment:** Pen, pegboard, calculator, daysheet, encounter forms, ledger cards, previous day's balance, list of patients and charges, fee schedule

**Computer and medical office software:** Follow the software requirements for posting credits to patient accounts

| STEPS | PURPOSE |
|---|---|
| 1. Place a new daysheet on the pegboard and record the totals from the previous daysheet. | A new sheet should be used each day. Transferring the totals from the day before enables you to keep a running total. |
| 2. Align the patient's ledger card with the first available line on the daysheet. | Each line should be used. It is easy to accidentally overlap entries. |
| 3. Place receipt to align with the appropriate line on the ledger card. | Proper alignment makes neat and legible entries. |
| 4. Record the number of the receipt in the appropriate column. | This enables you to cross-reference and provides two forms of tracking. |
| 5. Write the patient's name on the receipt. | This is the section that will appear in the name section. |
| 6. Record any existing balance the patient owes in the previous balance column of the daysheet. | This total must be added to any charges because this amount is already owed. |
| 7. Record a brief description of the charge in the description line. | This will tell you and the patient what the charges were for. |

| Statement | | | | | |
|---|---|---|---|---|---|
| DATE | DESCRIPTION | CHARGES | CREDITS PYMNTS. | ADJ. | BALANCE |
| | BALANCE FORWARD → | | | | |
| | OV, Lab | | | | |
| | | | | | |
| | | | | | |
| | | | | | |

**Step 7.** Write a description in the proper line of the daysheet.

| STEPS | PURPOSE |
|---|---|
| 8. Record the total charges in the charge column. Press hard so that marks go through to the ledger card and the daysheet. | Totaling the charges for a visit saves room on the ledger cards and the daysheets. |
| 9. Add the total charges to the previous balance and record this number in the current balance column. | The current balance is what is already owed plus the new charges. |
| 10. Return the ledger card to appropriate storage. | Cards should be returned promptly for quick and easy retrieval. |

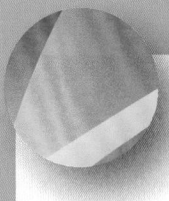

**PSY** PROCEDURE 14-2

# Post Payments on a Daysheet

**Purpose:** To keep a daily and running account of all payments made to accounts in the medical practice

**Equipment:** Pen, pegboard, calculator, daysheet, encounter forms, ledger cards, previous day's balance, list of patients and charges, fee schedule

**Computer and medical office software:** Follow the software requirements for posting credits to patient accounts

| STEPS | PURPOSE |
|---|---|
| 1. Place a new daysheet on the pegboard and record the totals from the previous daysheet. | A new sheet should be used each day. Transferring the totals from the day before enables you to keep a running total. |
| 2. Align the patient's ledger card with the first available line on the daysheet. | Proper alignment makes neat and legible entries. |
| 3. Place receipt to align with the appropriate line on the ledger card. | Each line should be used. It is easy to accidentally overlap entries. |
| 4. Record the number of the receipt in the appropriate column. | This enables you to cross-reference and provides two forms of tracking. |
| 5. Write the patient's name on the receipt. | This is the section that will appear in the name section. |
| 6. Record any existing balance the patient owes in the previous balance column of the daysheet. | This total must be added to any charges because this amount is already owed. |
| 7. Record the date of service being paid for, source, and type of the payment in the description line. | Such information makes tracking the payment easier and gives vital information that can be easily retrieved. |
| 8. Record appropriate adjustments in adjustment column. | In many cases, it is illegal not to write off certain adjustments. |
| 9. Record the total payment in the payment column. Press hard so that marks go through to the ledger card and the daysheet. | Because you are using a write-it-once system, your marks must go through three thicknesses. |
| 10. Subtract the payment and adjustments from outstanding/previous balance, and record the current balance. | Subtracting these amounts will give you the current amount owed. |
| 11. Return the ledger card to appropriate storage. | Cards should be returned promptly for quick and easy retrieval. |

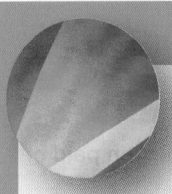 **PSY** PROCEDURE 14-3

## Process a Credit Balance

**Purpose:** To determine and record monies that have been paid on an account beyond what is owed

**Equipment:** Pen, pegboard, calculator, daysheet, ledger card

**Computer and medical office software:** Follow the software requirements for processing a credit balance in patient accounts

| STEPS | PURPOSE |
|---|---|
| 1. Determine the reason for the credit balance and be sure it is recorded in the explanation column of the ledger card. | An explanation will help you discuss the account with the patient. |
| 2. Place brackets around the balance indicating that it is a negative number. | Brackets indicate the opposite of the usual action of a certain column. For example, when totaling the daysheet, a number in brackets would be subtracted instead of added. |

| Statement | | | | | |
|---|---|---|---|---|---|
| DATE | DESCRIPTION | CHARGES | CREDITS PYMNTS. | ADJ. | BALANCE |
| | BALANCE FORWARD ——→ | | | | |
| | | | <47 00> | | |
| | | | | | |
| | | | | | |
| | | | | | |

**Step 2.** Place brackets around number.

3. Write a refund check by following the steps in Procedure 14-4.

A credit indicates that a patient's account has been overpaid.

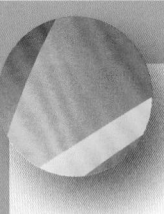

## PSY  PROCEDURE 14-4

### Process Refunds

**Purpose:** To return money to the proper person or company when more money has been paid on an account than is owed

**Equipment:** Pen, pegboard, calculator, daysheet, ledger card, checkbook, check register, word processor letterhead, envelope, postage, copy machine, patient's chart, refund file

| STEPS | REASONS |
|---|---|
| 1. Determine who gets the refund—the patient or the insurance company. | The explanation of benefits will list the patient's responsibility. |
| 2. Pull patient's ledger card and place on current daysheet aligned with the first available line. | Proper alignment makes neat and legible entries. |
| 3. Post the amount of the refund in the adjustment column in brackets, indicating it is a debit, not a credit, adjustment. | The brackets will instruct you to perform the opposite action of the column. |
| 4. Write "Refund to Patient" or "Refund to _____" (name of insurance company) in the description column. | This information will be needed to discuss the account with the patient. |
| 5. Write a check for the credit amount made out to the appropriate party (see Procedure 14-13). | Refunds should be made in a timely fashion. It is unethical to keep money that does not belong to the practice. |
| 6. Record the amount and name of payee in the check register. | This follows proper procedure for writing a check. |
| 7. Mail check with letter of explanation to patient or insurance company. | Place any identifying numbers in the letter to help match the refund to the proper person. Again, this should be done as soon as possible after writing the check. |
| 8. Place copy of check and copy of letter in the patient's record or in refund file. | You must keep complete and accurate records of all transactions. |
| 9. Return the patient's ledger card to its storage area. | Cards should be returned promptly for quick and easy retrieval. |

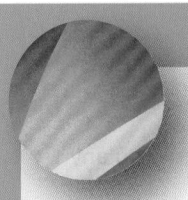

## PSY PROCEDURE 14-5

# Post Adjustments to a Daysheet

**Purpose:** To keep a daily and running account of all adjustments made to patients' accounts in the medical practice

**Equipment:** Pen, pegboard, calculator, daysheet, encounter forms, ledger cards, previous day's balance, list of patients and charges, fee schedule

**Computer and medical office software:** Follow the software requirements for posting credits to patient accounts

| STEPS | REASONS |
|---|---|
| 1. Pull the patient's ledger card and place on current daysheet aligned with the first available line. | Proper alignment makes neat and legible entries. |
| 2. Post the amount to be written off in the adjustment column. Press hard so that marks go through to the ledger card and the daysheet. | Because you are using a write-it-once system, your marks must go through three thicknesses. |
| 3. Subtract the adjustment from the outstanding/previous balance, and record in the current balance column. | Subtracting these amounts will give you the current amount owed. |
| 4. Return the ledger card to appropriate storage. | Cards should be returned promptly for quick and easy retrieval. |

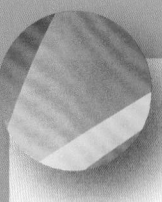

**PSY** PROCEDURE 14-6

## Post Collection Agency Payments

**Purpose:** To apply payments made to collection agencies to patients' accounts, adjusting any amount paid to the collection agency

**Equipment:** Pen, pegboard, calculator, daysheet, patient's ledger card

| STEPS | REASONS |
|-------|---------|
| 1. Review check stub or report from the collection agency explaining the amounts to be applied to the accounts. | There may be more than one patient's account paid in a single check. You must determine the amount for each individual account. |
| 2. Pull the patients' ledger cards. | Pulling all cards that are needed will minimize interruptions. |
| 3. Post the amount to be applied in the payment column for each patient. | This amount should be subtracted from the outstanding amount for a particular date of service. |
| 4. Write "payment from collection agency" in the explanation column. | This makes tracking the amount owed easier. |
| 5. Adjust off the amount representing the percentage of the payment charged by the collection agency. | Subtracting the amount paid to the collection agency clears out the outstanding balance. |

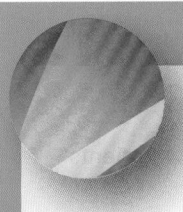

**PSY** PROCEDURE 14-7

## Process NSF Checks

**Purpose:** To document, record, notify patients, charge back amount "paid," assess fees, and retrieve funds when the medical practice has a check returned due to nonsufficient funds (NSF)

**Equipment:** Pen, pegboard, calculator, daysheet, patient's ledger card

| STEPS | PURPOSE |
|-------|---------|
| 1. Pull patient's ledger card and place on current aligned with the first available line. | Proper alignment makes neat and legible daysheet entries. |
| 2. Write the amount of the check in the payment column in brackets indicating it is a debit, not a credit, adjustment. | Brackets tell you to do the opposite action of that expected in a particular column. Normally, the payment column is subtracted from the outstanding balance. Brackets instruct you to add the amount instead. |
| 3. Write "Check Returned for Nonsufficient Funds" in the description column. | An explanation will make it easier to track transactions and determine specific reasons. |
| 4. Post a returned check charge with an appropriate explanation in the charge column. | If the office charges a returned check fee, it should be posted here. This amount is designed to discourage returned checks and to cover administrative costs. |
| 5. Write "Bank Fee for Returned Check" in the description column. | If the bank charges the practice with a fee, then you will pass this charge along to the patient. |
| 6. Call the patient to advise him or her of the returned check and the fee. | The patient should be notified immediately in order to rectify the situation. |
| 7. Construct a proper letter of explanation and a copy of the ledger card and mail to patient. | Even though the patient is notified by phone, details should also be recorded in writing. |
| 8. Place a copy of the letter and the check in the patient's file. | A copy of the letter placed in the patient's chart proves the communication with the patient actually happened. |
| 9. Make arrangements for the patient to pay cash to cover the check and fees. | Requiring cash will eliminate the possibility of another returned check. |
| 10. Flag the patient's account as a credit risk for future transactions. | It is helpful to know of possible future problems with payment of an account. |
| 11. Return the patient's ledger card to its storage area. | Cards should be returned promptly for quick and easy retrieval. |
| 12. **AFF** You see a patient whose check was returned for nonsufficient funds out at a soccer game. He whispers to you to keep quiet about the bad check. Explain how you would respond. | Assure him that you do not discuss patients outside of the office. |

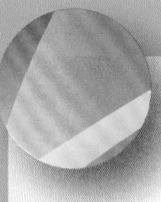

**PSY** PROCEDURE 14-8

## Balance a Daysheet

**Purpose:** To ensure an accurate daily total of charges, payments, and adjustments to patients' accounts in the medical practice

**Equipment:** Daysheet with totals brought forward, calculator, pen

| STEPS | PURPOSE |
|---|---|
| 1. Be sure the totals from the previous daysheet are recorded in the column for previous totals. | You must have these previous totals in order to keep a running balance of the accounts receivable. |
| 2. Total the charge column and place that number in the proper blank. | |
| 3. Total the payment column and place that number in the proper blank. | |
| 4. Total the adjustment column and place that number in the proper blank. | |
| 5. Total the current balance column and place that number in the proper blank. | |
| 6. Total the previous balance column and place that number in the proper blank. | |
| 7. Take the grand total of the previous balances, add the grand total of the charges, and subtract the grand totals of the payments and adjustments. This number must equal the grand total of the current balance. | This will prove that the daysheet is balanced and there are no errors. |
| 8. If the numbers do not match, calculate your totals again, and continue looking for errors until the numbers match. | The daysheet must be accurate before moving on to a new daysheet. |
| 9. Record the totals of the columns in the proper space on the next daysheet. | You will be prepared for balancing the new daysheet. |

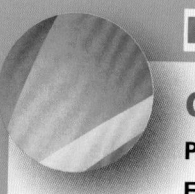

**PSY** PROCEDURE 14-9

## Complete a Bank Deposit Slip and Make a Deposit

**Purpose:** To place money collected in the medical practice into a safe and secure bank account

**Equipment:** Calculator with tape, currency, coins, checks for deposit, deposit slip, endorsement stamp, deposit envelope

| STEPS | PURPOSE |
|-------|---------|
| 1. Separate the cash from the checks. | These will be recorded separately on the deposit slip. |
| 2. Arrange bills face up and sorted with the largest denomination on top. | Most bill counters in banks are loaded in this manner. Sorting the bills is also a courtesy to the bank. |
| 3. Record the total in the cash block on the deposit slip. | |
| 4. Endorse the back of each check with "For Deposit Only." | This is one safety practice to reduce the possibility of fraud and/or forgery. |
| 5. Record the amount of each check beside an identifying number on the deposit slip. | This helps ensure the identity and accuracy of each check. |
| 6. Total and record the amounts of checks in the line on the deposit slip labeled "total of checks." | This amount will be added to the amount of cash. |
| 7. Subtotal and record the amount of cash and checks for the total deposit. | Add the amount of cash and the amount of checks. |
| 8. Record the total amount of the deposit in the office checkbook register. | This step will keep the checkbook balance accurate and current. |
| 9. Make a copy of both sides of the deposit slip or office records. | Keeping records helps you prove any errors for future discrepancies. |
| 10. Place the cash, checks, and completed deposit slip in an envelope or bank bag for transporting to the bank for deposit. | Deposits should be made as soon as possible to prevent loss or theft. If using a night deposit box, pay close attention to your surroundings and stay safe. |

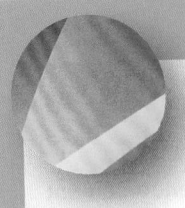

**PSY** PROCEDURE 14-10

# Reconcile a Bank Statement

**Purpose:** To ensure the accuracy and sound financial practices of the bank accounts of the medical practice

**Equipment:** Bank statement, reconciliation worksheet, calculator, pen

| STEPS | PURPOSE |
|---|---|
| 1. Compare the opening balance on the new statement with the closing balance on the previous statement. | You must know where your last bank statement ends and where the current one begins. |
| 2. List the bank balance in the appropriate space on the reconciliation worksheet. | Since there is no standard format for a reconciliation statement, be sure you are using the proper blank. |
| 3. Compare the check entries on the statement with the entries in the check register. Place a check mark beside each check listed as paid on the statement. | This will help you identify the outstanding checks. |

| Withdrawals / Debits | | | |
|---|---|---|---|
| DATE | AMOUNT | DESCRIPTION | REFERENCE # |
| 02-12 | 38.90 | Food Lion | ✓ 436674796 |
| 02-12 | 500.00 | Melton Custodial Servic | ✓ 426580282 |
| 02-13 | 1200.00 | Lewis Realty | ✓ 446480157 |
| 02-13 | 22.00 | John Little | ✓ 456974902 |
| 02-14 | 150.00 | HS Brown, Florist | ✓ 466748392 |

**Step 3.** Place check marks next to checks listed as paid.

| STEPS | PURPOSE |
|---|---|
| 4. List the amounts of the checks without checkmarks (outstanding checks). | These have not cleared the bank. |
| 5. Total outstanding checks. | |
| 6. Subtract from the checkbook balance items such as withdrawals, automatic payments, or service charges that appear on the statement but not in the checkbook. | These transactions are reflected in the bank statement but not in the checkbook. |
| 7. Add to the bank statement balance any deposits not shown on the bank statement. | This gives you the proper current balance in the account. |
| 8. Make sure that the balance in the checkbook and the bank statement agree. | This will ensure the accuracy of the current balance in the account. |

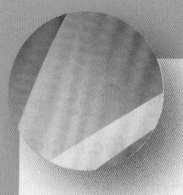

## PSY PROCEDURE 14-11

# Maintain a Petty Cash Account

**Purpose:** To keep a small amount of cash on hand to cover expenses such as postage due, reimbursement for emergency supplies, etc.

**Equipment:** Daysheet and an exercise from the workbook about establishing and maintaining a petty cash fund

| STEPS | REASONS |
|---|---|
| 1. Count the money remaining in the box. | This amount will remain in the box. |

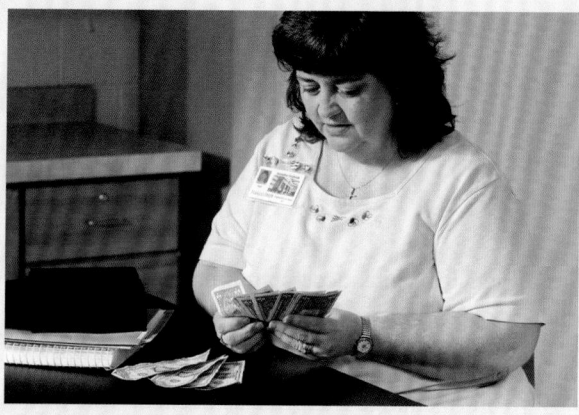

Step 1. Count the cash from the box.

| STEPS | REASONS |
|---|---|
| 2. Total the amounts of all vouchers in the petty cash box to determine the amount of expenditures. | This total will represent the amount of money used. |
| 3. Subtract the amount of receipts from the original amount in petty cash. | This should equal the amount of cash remaining in the box. |
| 4. When the cash has been balanced against the receipts, write a check only for the amount that was used. | You will keep the same amount of petty cash unless instructed otherwise. |
| 5. Record totals on the memo line of the check stub. | This is proper procedure for writing a check. |
| 6. Sort and record all vouchers to the appropriate practice accounts. | The next step in the accounting is to post the amounts to the individual accounts of the practice. |
| 7. File the list of vouchers and receipts attached. | Records of all business transactions must be kept. |
| 8. Place cash in petty cash fund. | Added to the amount already in the box, this will replenish the petty cash box. |
| 9. **AFF** A coworker asks to borrow money from petty cash for bus fare home. She promises to pay it back tomorrow. Explain how you would respond. | Absolutely refuse her request. Perhaps you could find another way to help her. |

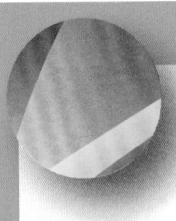

## PSY PROCEDURE 14-12

# Order Supplies

**Purpose:** To maintain the materials and supplies needed to operate a medical practice efficiently

**Equipment:** 5 × 7 index cards, file box with divider cards, computer with Internet (optional), medical supply catalogs

| STEPS | PURPOSE |
|---|---|
| 1. Create a list of supplies to be ordered. Knowing what supplies you are ordering will help you know what catalogs will be needed. Making a list of all the needed items will help you organize the ordering process. | Employees will report supply needs as they occur. |
| 2. Create an index card for each supply on the list by placing the name of the supply in the top left corner and including name and contact information of vendor(s) and product identification number. | This establishes a record of the supplies used in the facility. |
| 3. File the index cards in the file box with divider cards alphabetically or by product type. | This allows for quick access and makes reordering easier. |
| 4. Record the current price of the item and how the item is supplied. Make a note of any price breaks on larger quantities, etc. | The price should be written in pencil because this allows you to change the price as needed. You will save money by taking advantage of special discounts for larger quantities. |
| 5. Record the reorder point. This is the point where you reorder an item. | When supplies on hand reach half of the amount you need, you will know to reorder. |

## PSY PROCEDURE 14-13

## Write a Check

**Purpose:** To disperse money to individuals or companies from the medical practice by preparing checks from a checking account

**Equipment:** Simulated page of checks from checkbook, scenario giving amount of check, check register

| STEPS | PURPOSE |
|---|---|
| 1. Fill out the check register with the following information:<br>  a. Check number<br>  b. Date<br>  c. Payee information<br>  d. Amount<br>  e. Previous balance<br>  f. New balance | This is all crucial information and must be recorded accurately. |
| 2. Enter the date on the check. | Dates are also crucial to a bookkeeping system. |
| 3. Enter the payee on the check. | Without a payee, the check is nonnegotiable. |
| 4. Enter the amount of the check using numerals. | This is the amount paid by the bank. It will be compared to the written amount below, ensuring that the amount has not been tampered with. |
| 5. Write out the amount of the check beginning as far left as possible and making a straight line to fill in space between dollars and cents. | This practice creates a double check system that helps to verify the authenticity of the check. |
| 6. Record cents as a fraction with 100 as the denominator. | According to banking guidelines, this is the customary way to write a check. |
| 7. Obtain appropriate signature(s). | Many offices require more than one signature to help reduce the possibility of employee theft. |

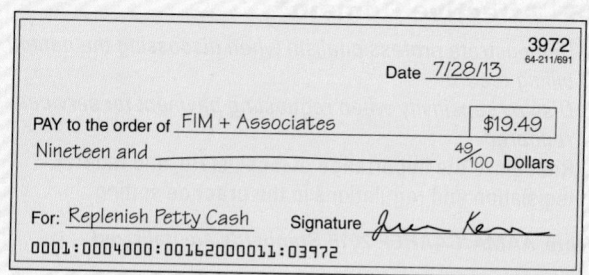

| | |
|---|---|
| 8. Proofread for accuracy. | **Step 7.** A properly completed check.<br><br>Accuracy is important in everything a medical assistant does. |

# CHAPTER 15 Credit and Collections

## Learning Outcomes

### COG Cognitive Domain*

1. Spell and define the key terms
2. Discuss physician's fee schedules
3. *Identify precautions for accepting the following types of payments: a, cash; b, check; c, credit card; d, debit card*
4. *Identify types of information contained in the patient's billing record*
5. Discuss the legal implications of credit collection
6. *Explain patient financial obligations for services rendered*
7. Discuss procedures for collecting outstanding accounts
8. Describe the impact of both the Fair Debt Collection Act and the Federal Truth in Lending Act of 1968 as they apply to collections
9. Describe the concept of RBRVS
10. Describe the implications of HIPAA for the medical assistant in various medical settings
11. Discuss all levels of government legislation and regulation as they apply to medical assisting practice, including FDA and DEA regulations

### PSY Psychomotor Domain*

1. Evaluate and manage a patient account (Procedure 15-1)
2. *Inform a patient of financial obligations for services rendered* (Procedure 15-1)
3. Write a collection letter (Procedure 15-2)

### AFF Affective Domain*

1. *Demonstrate professionalism when discussing the patient's billing record*
2. *Display sensitivity when requesting payment for services rendered*
3. Recognize the importance of local, state, and federal legislation and regulations in the practice setting

*Note: AAMA/CAAHEP 2015 Standards are italicized*

### ABHES Competencies

1. Perform billing and collection procedures
2. Use physician fee schedule

## Key Terms

| | | | |
|---|---|---|---|
| adjustment | credit | installment | patient co-payment |
| aging schedule | executor | limiting charge | professional courtesy |
| collections | hardship | participating providers | write-off |

## Case Study

Great Falls Medical Center, a busy family practice where Sally Thomas, CMA (AAMA), works, has recently determined that they have a 74% collection percentage rate. An analysis of payments made by patients at the time of service was done, and it was discovered that many patients had outstanding balances but were not being asked for payment when they were in the office even when accounts were more than 90 days delinquent. What is the collection percentage rate, and what would be a good rate? Why is it important to have financial policies in the medical office? What steps can be taken to improve the collection percentage rate? This chapter discusses the importance of understanding how fees are billed and reimbursed for medical services and the process for collection from patients when an account balance becomes their responsibility.

The medical practice must operate in a financially sound manner to continue to serve the patients and the community. The office depends on the fees generated by patient visits, laboratory work, and in-office procedures, and without these fees, the medical office would be unable to pay for staff, office space, and supplies. Therefore, collecting fees from insurance companies, patients, and guarantors as well as other sources is essential for the medical practice to succeed. Box 15-1 shows how to determine whether your office is collecting fees satisfactorily.

### BOX 15-1 Determining a Practice's Collection Percentage

Medical practices should evaluate their method of collections periodically to determine the effectiveness of their practices. A collection analysis lets you identify the strengths and weaknesses of the system.

To do a collection analysis, determine the monthly accounts receivable for charges billed from the first day of each month to the last day. This will be the total charges posted to all patients' accounts. Next, determine the revenues the practice received. Computer systems will automatically total payments received during a specified time. Divide revenue by production to determine the collection percentage. Analysis of the collection percentage should reveal the percentage of the collection of all outstanding debts to the practice.

Collection percentage = monthly revenue received monthly ÷ accounts receivable

Most medical practices average 8% to 20% loss yearly. Experts consider a collection percentage above 80% to be reasonable. Performing a 2-year collection percentage comparison analysis will help you evaluate past collection effectiveness.

## FEES

### Fee Schedules

Generally, the physician is responsible for setting charges for services and procedures such as office visits, laboratory work, and in-office procedures. Several factors are used to determine charges, such as the normal fees charged by other physicians for the same service and the amounts that insurance companies will reimburse for each service. Reimbursement from insurance companies, however, is determined by a couple of different methods. One method is the UCR concept: (1) U (usual) for fair value of the service, (2) C (customary) for competitive rates charged by other physicians of the same specialty in that geographical area, and (3) R (reasonable) for services that are more extensive or require more resources than does the typical procedure. The RVS (relative value scale) is another method in which similar services are assigned a value that is determined by the skill and training required to do the service, the expenses incurred by the practice for providing the service (such as rent, supplies, and payroll for employees), and the malpractice liability expenses. The reimbursement methodology used by Medicare is the resource-based relative value scale (RBRVS), by which fees are based on the relative value of a particular service and adjusted for geographical differences. (See Chapter 13 for more information about UCR fees and RBRVS.) A list of the services and procedures offered in an office along with descriptions, procedure codes, and prices must be available to patients. Federal regulations require that a sign to this effect be posted in the office.

The practice will have several reimbursement fee schedules for different insurance companies. **Participating providers** are doctors who agree to participate with managed care contracts and other third-party payers in exchange for building a solid patient base. Patients covered under participating plans will

| CPT CODE | PAR FEE | NON-PAR FEE | LIMITING CHARGE |
|---|---|---|---|
| 99211 | $19.08 | $18.13 | $20.85 |
| 99212 | $41.94 | $39.84 | $45.82 |
| 99213 | $70.61 | $67.09 | $77.15 |
| 99214 | $104.36 | $99.14 | $114.01 |
| 99215 | $139.97 | $132.97 | $152.92 |

**Figure 15-1 •** Sample Medicare fee schedule.

have a different fee schedule from patients who are self-pay (paying with no money from insurance). Each managed care plan, government payer, such as Medicare and Medicaid, and workers' compensation has a different fee schedule. (See Chapter 13 for further discussion of third-party payers.)

A participating fee is an amount agreed upon between an insurance company and the physician to be reimbursed for services and procedures. Physicians who do not sign an agreement with an insurance company are considered nonparticipating and, therefore, do not have a contracted reimbursement fee schedule from that company. Depending on the patient's out-of-network benefits, the physician may receive payment from the insurance company, but the patient is still responsible for the balance remaining after any insurance payment is applied. However, special rules apply when charging Medicare patients for services as a nonparticipating provider. A **limiting charge** is the amount a nonparticipating physician can charge a Medicare patient. (See Chapter 13 for more information on the Medicare limiting charge.) Figure 15-1 is a sample Medicare fee schedule.

 **CHECKPOINT QUESTION**

1. Great Falls Medical Center is a participating provider for Medicare. What is meant by "participating provider?"

## Discussing Fees in Advance

It is always a good policy to discuss fees with patients in advance. This ensures that patients are aware of the charges and may plan for any out-of-pocket expenses for which they are responsible. Patients will need to know in advance whether the medical office is a participating provider with their insurance carrier. Managed care companies usually require that the patient pay a certain share of the bill, known as the **patient co-payment**, or co-pay. A good and easy way to initiate a discussion of fees is by providing an office brochure that lists not only the office's address, telephone number, and hours but also the practice's financial policies such as when payments are due, third-party payments and how they are handled, when accounts are considered delinquent, and the collections process. The office policy regarding the discharge of patients with delinquent accounts should

also be noted. Patients should understand that co-pays are to be paid at the time of service. Many offices post a sign in the waiting area stating the office financial policies.

Ideally, you should collect the entire amount due from a new patient on the first visit. Obviously, the less credit you extend, the lower your accounts receivable and the better the cash flow. As discussed in Chapter 5, many problems associated with collection (acquiring funds that are due) come from patients who move and leave no forwarding address or those who go from one practice to another. Be sure you get complete information including the names, numbers, and relationships of contacts able to give you information about a patient's new location. You should also get a picture identification, such as a driver's license, on a patient's first visit. (See Chapter 5, The First Contact: Telephone and Reception.)

## Forms of Payment

Depending on the medical office's policies, patients can usually pay for services in several ways: cash, personal check, debit card, or credit card (e.g., Visa, MasterCard, Discover). If a new patient is paying by check, get two forms of identification.

By agreeing to accept a credit card payment, the medical office also agrees to pay the credit card company a fee for each transaction at rates that vary depending on each lender usually in the form of a percentage of the total charge. There may also be a monthly fee associated with the acceptance of debit or credit cards. Although this may seem costly, it is sometimes more cost-effective to receive payment by credit card than to receive it in installments—or not at all—from the patient.

 **CHECKPOINT QUESTION**

2. List four forms of payments accepted by most physician offices.

## Payment by Insurance Companies

By far, the largest proportions of fees are paid by insurance companies. Therefore, it is imperative that patients' insurance information be kept current. Most medical practices require that a patient submit a medical insurance card for each visit; this way, changes in insurance can quickly and easily be noted. Remember, always make a copy of both sides of the patient's insurance card and place it in the appropriate section of the chart for billing reference or scan it to place in the appropriate section of the electronic medical record. Most insurance companies offer online services such as checking coverage, eligibility for procedures, co-pays, etc.

## Adjusting Fees

Sometimes, **adjustments** (changes in a posted account) must be made to account balances, as when the medical office accepts a contractual insurance fee schedule for a service. You must charge the patient the regular fee for the service; when the insurance carrier sends payment, however, the explanation of benefits (EOB) will show how the reimbursement was made with details of the patient's insurance benefits. If the provider participates with the insurance company and has a contracted fee schedule, the difference between the physician's normal fee and the insurance carrier's allowed fee will be adjusted in the credit adjustment column on the patient's account. Nonparticipating providers are not obligated to make insurance adjustments because there is no contractual fee schedule.

Other fee adjustments include **professional courtesy** fees, in which other health care professionals are charged a reduced rate. The physician may choose not to charge a fee at all; this too is considered a professional courtesy and should not be confused with writing off a fee. (A **write-off** is cancellation of an unpaid debt; these generally can be claimed as deductions on the practice's federal taxes.) Again, you charge the regular fee and then adjust the designated amount in the adjustment column with "professional courtesy" in the description column. Some practices offer discounts for paying in full. You would handle this as earlier described for adjustments (charge the full amount and adjust off the discount).

### CHECKPOINT QUESTION

3. What is the difference between a fee adjustment and a write-off?

##  CREDIT

### Extending Credit

It is not always possible for patients to pay the entire bill when costs are incurred. Depending on the medical office's financial policy, **credit** may be extended to patients on an installment plan. Collection experts have estimated that billing one patient costs the practice about $8 per month. This total includes the resources necessary to collect the bill, such as the time it takes to

prepare the statements, the supplies needed, and so on. Extension of credit to a patient is a decision that is sometimes made solely by the physician and may be handled in house or with financing through a bank or other lending facility. If the credit is extended by the practice without the use of a third party, credit to a patient should be extended only after checking the patient's credit history (Box 15-2). Many offices outsource their credit and billing functions. There are medical billing companies that manage the practice's accounts receivable, prepare the insurance claims, offer training to the employees, and provide other related services.

## Legal Considerations

When a medical practice extends credit to a patient, it may charge interest on the patient's unpaid balance. If interest is going to be charged or if there are more than three loan payment installments, the medical office is legally required to disclose this information to the patient, along with any other fees or charges incurred by the patient's acceptance of credit. The patient must be given a completed settlement statement as required by the Truth in Lending Act. This legal document must be filed in the patient's medical chart (Fig. 15-2).

Different states have different laws concerning the extension of credit. Generally, credit cannot be denied based on age, gender, race, marital status, religion, national origin, or source of income (e.g., if a patient receives public assistance). If your facility has given credit to one patient, you typically may not refuse the same arrangement to another patient. Some states have laws limiting the amount of interest that can be charged. The practice's accountant should be able to provide the information required by the state and municipality.

### CHECKPOINT QUESTION

4. On what grounds would it be illegal to deny credit?

**Bruce C. Collin, M.D.**                                    305 Madison Avenue
                                                             Anderson, Indiana 46027

I agree to pay $_____ per week/month on my account balance of $_____.

Payments are due by the _____ of each _____ and will begin _____.
                                          (week/month)              (date)

Interest will/will not be charged on the outstanding balance (see Truth-in-Lending form below for rate of interest).

I agree that if payments are not made in the full amount stated above or if payments are not received on time, the entire account balance will be considered delinquent and will be due and payable immediately.

I agree to be responsible for any reasonable collection costs or attorney fees incurred in collecting a delinquent account.

_____          _____
Date                                    Signature

This disclosure is in compliance with the Truth-in-Lending Act.

_____          _____
Patient's Name                          Address

_____          _____
Responsible Party (if other than patient)    City, State, Zip Code

| | | |
|---|---|---|
| 1. | Cash Price (Medical and/or Surgical Fee) | $ |
| | Less Cash Down Payment (Advance) | $ |
| 2. | Unpaid Balance of Cash Price | $ |
| 3. | Amount Financed | $ |
| 4. | FINANCE CHARGE | $ |
| 5. | Total of Payments (3 + 4) | $ |
| 6. | Deferred Payment Price (1 + 4) | $ |
| 7. | ANNUAL PERCENTAGE RATE | % |

The "Total of Payments" shown above is payable to Bruce Collin, M.D. at the address shown above in _____ weekly/monthly installments of $_____, the first installment being payable on this date _____, and all subsequent installments are due on the same day of each consecutive week/month until paid in full.

_____          _____
Date                                    Signature

**Figure 15-2** • Truth-in-lending form.

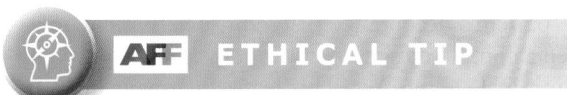

**AFF ETHICAL TIP**

### Paying the Doctor with Eggs?

There was a time when patients paid for their medical care with eggs from their farm. Those days are long gone. In today's complicated financial world, it is necessary for a physician practice to behave as any other business. Although it is legal to charge patients reasonable interest rates, finance charges, and late payment fees, risk managers suggest avoiding them. Even the American Medical Association, which advises physicians on matters such as ethical principles and finances, warns that patients may be put off by their doctor charging these fees. Doctors are in the business of taking care of people, but they must pay their bills. These charges may create bad will or be seen as a conflict from a caring and helpful physician. You must use empathy and treat patients with respect—even the ones who have trouble paying.

## COG COLLECTIONS

When a patient has an unpaid bill or has not paid an installment per a credit extension agreement, those funds must be collected. **Collection** is defined as the process of acquiring funds that are owed. Collecting an unpaid debt is costly to any business and can also be time consuming. Collection practices are regulated by a variety of consumer protection laws and many medical practices outsource their billing to companies specializing in billing and debt collection.

### Legal Considerations

The Fair Debt Collection Act of 1996 requires debt collectors and creditors to treat debtors fairly. It prohibits harassment, misrepresentation, threats, disseminating false information about the debtor, and engaging in unfair or illegal practices in attempting to collect a debt.

Certain procedures should be followed when attempting to collect a debt. A debt collector—in this case, the medical assistant or billing clerk—must exercise reasonable restraint when contacting a patient about a bill. Attempting to collect a debt from a patient's estate requires working with the executor of the estate and filing forms in the probate court in the patient's home jurisdiction. When a guarantor files bankruptcy, all collection activity including sending monthly statements must be ceased, and a form should be filed with the bankruptcy court as an unsecured creditor.

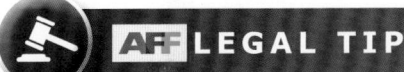

## Be Careful When Leaving Messages on Answering Machines

Patients are required to sign an authorization form for a general release of information at their first visit to a medical office. In order to comply with the Health Insurance Portability and Accountability Act of 1996 Privacy Rule, also referred to as HIPAA, this authorization form can be designed to give permission to leave a message on their answering machines or cell phones. Because many people may be unavailable to receive calls during the day, you may need to leave a message for the patient to call you back. This is fine if they have given you permission. Because you cannot be sure who will retrieve the message, you must protect patients' rights. HIPAA prohibits disclosing information that would link the patient to a particular physician or medical treatment. Your message must not include any such information. For example, it would be improper to leave a message asking for payment on a past due account. It would be within the law, however, to ask the person to call you back. You should only give your first name and telephone number. Do not state the nature of the call.

## Collecting a Debt

### Monthly Billings

The easiest way to collect a debt or an installment is by monthly billing. Once a month, the medical office sends bills to its patients who have unpaid balances. Larger offices set up a billing cycle and divide the alphabet, sending statements once a week to each selected group. For example, patients with names beginning with the letters A to G might be billed on the 1st of the month, H to N on the 8th, O to S on the 15th, and T to Z on the 22nd. If your facility changes a billing cycle, you are legally required to notify patients of the change three months before the change takes effect.

The uncomputerized office normally just copies the ledger cards of the patients who owe balances to send as patient statements. It is important to make each entry on the ledger card with consistency and provide a key for office codes or abbreviations. The patient should be able to understand each entry. When a practice is computerized, the staff can easily send statements using the medical billing software, which often gives the option of printing a separate message at the bottom of patient statements. For instance, you may add "Happy Holidays" to every patient's December statement or "Time for your flu shot" in the September statements.

If the account is on an **installment** plan, the patient's statement should always reflect the total account balance and any third-party payments or adjustments applied to the account for the date(s) of services being billed. If the patient is being charged interest on an account balance, the current monthly payment amount should be noted with the total account balance. This way, the patient has the option of paying more than is due for that particular month (and thereby reducing the amount of any interest charged) and is aware of the current balance.

### Aging Accounts

Unpaid accounts must be monitored to determine how far overdue they are. You will base your actions on the age of the account by determining the amount of time between the date of the first bill sent to the patient and the date of the last payment. Note that it is calculated from the first date of billing, not by the procedure or service date. For example, a patient has an office visit on April 5 and the first statement is sent on May 1. The account will be 30 days old on June 1.

In a computerized accounting system, an **aging schedule** lists the patient's name, balance, any payments, and comments, such as reminders or second notices sent. In a manual system, such a schedule can be kept on a large sheet of paper. Figure 15-3 is a sample of a manual report. Figure 15-4 shows a computerized billing screen.

Aging of accounts is a measure of the practice's ability to collect its fees. Nearly all fees (80%) should be collected within 30 days. If the aging shows a high percentage (50%) of fees being collected 30 days or more after billing, the practice's billing and collection procedures should be reviewed. Procedure 15-1 outlines the steps in aging accounts.

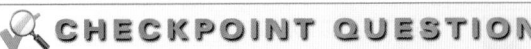

### CHECKPOINT QUESTION

5. What is meant by aging of accounts?

## Collecting Overdue Accounts

There are many reasons why patients allow unpaid account balances with physicians to become delinquent, and communication with the patient is vital to successful collection efforts. The three most common ways of collecting an overdue account are sending an overdue notice to the patient, telephoning the patient to let him or her know the

## Aging of Accounts Receivable Report: April 30, 2013

| Patient Name | Account Number | Due Date | Amount |
|---|---|---|---|
| **Accounts 30 Days Past Due:** | | | |
| Doe, John C. | 000-00-0000 | 3/6/13 | 625.00 |
| Graham, Paula R. | 000-00-0000 | 3/29/13 | 450.00 |
| O'Toole, William Q. | 000-00-0000 | 3/13/13 | 25.00 |
| Parker, Mary W. | 000-00-0000 | 3/25/13 | 299.00 |
| Reeves, Chris A. | 000-00-0000 | 3/11/13 | 58.00 |
| South, Cheryl C. | 000-00-0000 | 3/8/13 | 385.00 |
| Yarkony, Ralph M. | 000-00-0000 | 3/11/13 | 108.00 |
| **Accounts 60 Days Past Due:** | | | |
| Forest, Patricia L. | 000-00-0000 | 2/19/13 | 476.00 |
| Heany, Beverly O. | 000-00-0000 | 2/13/13 | 57.00 |
| Thomas, Walter T. | 000-00-0000 | 2/27/13 | 185.00 |
| **Accounts 90 Days Past Due:** | | | |
| Glick, Rhonda K | 000-00-0000 | 1/4/13 | 28.00 |
| Payne, Robert A. | 000-00-0000 | 1/25/13 | 456.00 |
| **Accounts 120 Days or More Past Due:** | | | |
| Baird, Jane C. | 000-00-0000 | 10/3/12 | 45.00 |
| Wallace, Michael S. | 000-00-0000 | 12/15/12 | 349.00 |
| **Total Overdue Accounts Receivable** | | | **$3,546.00** |

**Figure 15-3** • Manual aging schedule.

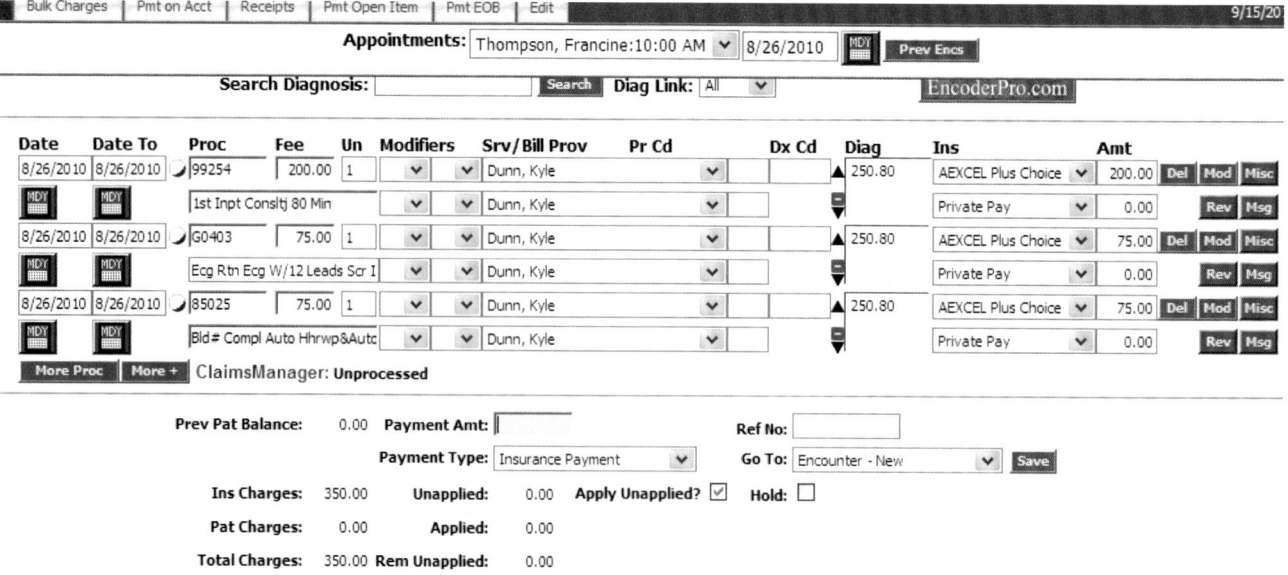

**Figure 15-4** • Computerized billing screen. (Courtesy of Ingenix® CareTracker™.)

account is overdue, and informing the patient at his or her next office visit. It is always important, however, to follow federal and state credit and collection laws when attempting to collect unpaid or delinquent account balances.

### Overdue Notices

With a manual system, overdue notices are fairly simple to prepare. Often, they consist of a copy of the patient's monthly billing with the words "overdue" or "second notice" stamped in red. Alternatively, a form letter with spaces for the patient's particulars may be sent. Figure 15-5 is a sample collection letter. If a computer billing program is used, the computer often can automatically generate overdue notices. Procedure 15-2 describes how to compose a collection letter.

### Telephoning the Patient

If written notices bring no response, you may have to telephone the patient to inquire about an overdue account. Be specific about the reason for the call when speaking with the patient or guarantor, and use active listening skills to determine if there is a **hardship** involved. There may be legitimate reasons preventing the patient from paying on an account balance such as the loss of employment or another unforeseen financial emergency. While you may be sympathetic to a patient's financial situation, you must also remember that the medical office is a business and must have a consistent cash flow to pay its own obligations. It is important to have payment options available to give the patient

an opportunity to work with you and get the account balance paid as quickly as possible. Always ask when payment may be forthcoming and document the reply on the patient's account. If payment is not received as promised, contact the patient again. (See Legal Tip.)

### In-Office Reminders

A patient can be reminded of an overdue balance when he or she comes to the office to see the physician. To handle this situation discreetly, simply give the patient a copy of the most recent overdue notice. Once again, ask when payment may be forthcoming and follow through. Computer systems may offer the option of a message on the computer screen when the patient's overdue account is retrieved. This alerts anyone working with the patient either to discuss payment or to refer the patient to someone in the office who will explain that payment is expected. The more contact you have with the patient, the more likely he or she will pay. If payment is not mentioned, the patient may believe that you are not worried about it. Some physicians prefer not to discuss fees and accounts with patients; others will want to know when a patient's account is past due and will feel comfortable mentioning it to the patient.

 **CHECKPOINT QUESTION**

6. What is the proper and legal way to leave a message on a patient's answering machine or voice mail?

---

 **LEGAL TIP**

### Stay Within the Law with Collection Attempts by Phone

When attempting to collect a debt by telephone, a debt collector should *never* do the following:

- Contact the patient before 8:00 a.m. or after 9:00 p.m.
- Contact the patient at his or her place of employment if the employer objects
- Contact the patient at all if the patient's account has been turned over to a collection agency or the patient has filed for bankruptcy
- Harass or intimidate the patient; that is, use abusive language, provide false or misleading information, or pose as someone other than a debt collector
- Make threats of actions on the account without taking the action (e.g., you tell the patient that you are going to turn the account over to a collection agency if payment is not received by a certain date; payment is not received, but you do not turn the account over)
- Tell anyone other than the patient or responsible party about a debt without court authorization

Remember that even though the patient owes you money, you must treat him or her with courtesy and respect.

---

Elkin Neurologic Center
1222 Brook Blvd
Edenton South Carolina 22617
331-561-8821

June 20, 2013

Christine Stultz
149 Fourth Street
Reedtown, SC 22617

Dear Mrs. Stultz,

This is to inform you that your account is more than 90 days past due. I know that you value your good credit rating, and I would like to speak with you as soon as possible about taking care of this obligation.

I will expect your payment of the balance of $250.00 by Friday, June 30, 2013.

I look forward to hearing from you.

Sincerely,

Tiffany Stone, CMA
Credit Manager

**Figure 15-5** • Sample collection letter.

## Collection Alternatives

Sometimes, it is more cost effective for collections to be handled outside the medical office. Three common options include collection agencies, small claims court, and credit bureaus.

### Collection Agencies

Collection agencies specialize in collecting debts. For either a fee or a percentage of the debt, the collection agency attempts to collect the monies due by the methods listed earlier. In addition, the collection agency can represent the medical practice in small claims court (in some courts) and can have the bad debt listed with credit-reporting agencies. Many practices choose to use the services of a collection agency because of staff limitations and cost-effectiveness.

### Small Claims Court

The medical practice can, of course, sue patients in small claims court and report patients with delinquent accounts to credit bureaus themselves. Filing small claims court proceedings are designed to be less expensive and less complicated than formal collection litigation; however, filing rules, such as minimum and maximum debt limits, vary from state to state and even within municipalities. Depending on the small claims court rules, some courts do not allow legal representation at hearings. Advance preparation and accurate documentation are necessary in order to successfully secure a judgment against the debtor.

## CLAIMS AGAINST ESTATES

In most cases, an outstanding account balance becomes the financial obligation of the estate upon the death of a patient. A formal estate proceeding is usually filed with the probate court in the county in which the patient resided at the time of death, and creditors are listed and subsequently notified by the court advising them of the name of the **executor**, the individual responsible for handling the patient's affairs after death. In order to be considered to receive any payment from the estate, it is necessary to file a claim with the probate court and attach an itemized statement of the account. This should be done as soon as possible in order to stay within the timely filing limits and statutes governing claims on estates.

## BANKRUPTCIES

Upon receipt of notification that a bankruptcy has been filed by a patient with an outstanding balance, all communication must cease in an attempt to collect said debt including telephone calls and sending monthly statements. If an account has been sent to a collection agency, the agency should be notified immediately of the bankruptcy proceeding. Claims must be filed with the bankruptcy court and itemized statements attached for payment consideration. Payments, if any, are made according to the type of bankruptcy filed and may include an extended and/or reduced payment plan.

---

**CHECKPOINT QUESTION**

7. What are three ways of collecting overdue accounts?

---

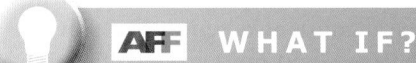

**WHAT IF?**

**What should you do if you need to collect a debt from a patient's estate?**

Collecting debts from an estate requires professionalism and tact. When a patient dies, give the family time to grieve. Never contact the family regarding a debt immediately after a patient's death. Most offices have a policy stating that family members of deceased patients will not be contacted until at least a week after the funeral. At the appropriate time, call the next of kin listed in the patient's chart. Offer your sympathy and ask for the name of the patient's executor. The executor may be an attorney, spouse, friend, or other relative. Call the executor, introduce yourself, and verify where a final statement may be sent for the patient's estate. It is important that all claims on a patient's estate be made promptly. If the estate does not have enough funds to meet all of its debts, the probate court will decide the priority list and percentages for debt collection. If your bill is not in the list of debts, it will not be paid.

 **ROLE-PLAYING SCENARIO**

Sally Thomas, CMA(AAMA), is working at the reception desk at Great Falls Medical Center, and today, a patient comes in for an appointment who has an account balance that is delinquent. What should Sally say to this patient to collect payment today? What are some of the payment options she could offer the patient to get the account to a zero balance as quickly as possible? Role-play this scenario as the medical assistant asking for payment and another student as the patient. If you are the medical assistant, think about how you would demonstrate professionalism and sensitivity when discussing the financial situation with the patient. If you are the patient, think about the emotions a "real" patient might display when confronted about his/her financial situation. Embarrassment? Anger? Defensiveness? What would be behaviors associated with these emotions? How would you respond to someone who displays these emotions? Your instructor will give you additional information about this activity!

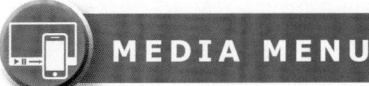 **MEDIA MENU**

**Student Resources** on thePoint®
- **CMA/RMA Certification Exam Review**

**Internet Resources**
**Collections & Credit Risk**
http://www.collectionscreditrisk.com
**Fair Debt Collection Practice/Federal Trade Commission Statutes**
http://www.ftc.gov
**National Credit Systems**
http://www.nationalcreditsystems.com
**Experian**
http://www.experian.com
**Transunion**
http://www.transunion.com
**Equifax**
http://www.equifax.com/home/en_us

## español SPANISH TERMINOLOGY

**Necesito cobrar el monto total de su deuda con nosotros.**
I need to collect the balance owed on your account.

**¿Podría usted hacer pagos parciales de su deuda?**
¿Can you pay some of your balance?

**Este es un requerimiento de cobro.**
This is a collection letter.

**Usted le debe dinero a esta oficina.**
You owe money to this office.

**Hay un costo for revisar su nivel de crédito.**
There is a charge for checking your credit score.

**Si usted no paga a tiempo, su crédito se puede ver afectado por años.**
If you do not pay on time, your credit can be affected for years.

## EMR Activity

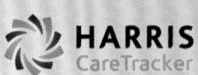

Harris CareTracker is a Web-based electronic medical record (EMR) application that you will use for the EMR activities included in this section at the end of each chapter. This application is actually used in physician offices but is provided to you through the publisher, Wolters Kluwer Health, to give you hands-on practice working with EMRs. Your instructor will have more information about accessing your username, log-in, and Quickstart guide.

Prerequisite Activities in Harris CareTracker

- *The Getting Started and Quickstart documents and EMR Activities Step-by-Step Instructions are available at* http://thePoint.lww.com/KronenbergerComp5e

### Activity Details

The billing manager at Great Falls Medical Center would like an aging schedule, or aged accounts receivable (A/R) report. Although your Harris CareTracker training account does not contain sufficient patient data to generate an aged A/R report, this activity will introduce you to the location of this report in Harris CareTracker and provide basic instructions on how to initiate a search of patient financial data to produce such a report.

## Chapter Summary

- The financial status of a medical office is based on the ability of the staff to collect the physician's fees.
- Fee collection must be done in a professional manner and in accordance with state and federal laws. Technology affords the medical office the ability to streamline procedures, and collection practices are more efficient with computer systems.
- Aging accounts and communicating with patients in a fair and professional manner ensures a constant cash flow and success in managing the finances of the outpatient medical practice.
- Keeping the delicate balance between taking care of people and running a business can be a challenge.

## Warm-Ups for Critical Thinking

1. Write a script for leaving a message on a patient's answering machine asking the patient to return your call.
2. A patient has an overdue account balance. She is coming in for a visit today. What would you say to her?
3. A patient tells you that he does not believe he owes the amount on his statement. He says his insurance will pay. You have received a statement from his insurance indicating that he owes the balance on the account. What do you say to him?
4. Create a collection letter that you would send to a patient's executor or patient's estate.
5. A patient promises to come by and bring you $100.00 on Friday. The payment is now 5 days late. What will you say when you call the patient?

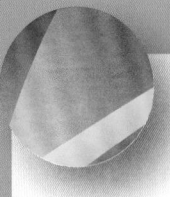

## PSY PROCEDURE 15-1

# Evaluate and Manage a Patient's Account

**PSY** Inform a patient of financial obligations for services rendered.

**Purpose:** To monitor the activity on a patient's credit account in order to keep the collection ratio at a maximum rate

**Equipment:** Simulation including scenario; sample patient ledger card with transactions; yellow, blue, and red stickers:

Yellow for accounts 30 days past due
Blue for accounts 60 days past due
Red for accounts 90 days past due

**Scenario:** Stephen Hill was seen first on March 3, 2008. His total bill that day was $250.00 for a level 2 consultation. He paid $50.00 as he was leaving. He returned to the office on April 9, 2013, for a revisit. His limited office visit was $50.00. He paid nothing that day. He has no insurance. It is now May 4, 2013. Post the charges and payment on a ledger card. Make a copy of the ledger card and place the appropriate sticker.

| STEPS | PURPOSE |
|---|---|
| 1. Review the patient's account history to determine the "age" of the account. If payment has not been made between 30 and 59 days from today's date, the account is 40 days past due, and so on. | Aging accounts lets you know what action to take. |
| 2. Flag the account for appropriate action. Place a yellow flag (sticker) on accounts that are 30 days old. Place a blue flag on accounts that are 60 days old. Place a red flag on accounts that are 90 days old. | Color coding the ledger cards lets everyone know the status of the account. In a computerized accounting system, the status of the account is determined automatically. |
| 3. Set aside accounts that have had no payment in 91 days or longer. | You will write collection letters to these patients (see Procedure 11-2). |
| 4. Make copies of the ledger cards. | These copies will serve as the patient's monthly statement. |
| 5. Sort the copies by category: 30, 60, or 90 days. | Keeping each type together will make the next step quicker and easier. |
| 6. Write or stamp the copies with the appropriate message, for example, "30 days past due" or, "Your account is 30 days past due, please remit." | The messages you placed on the accounts will hopefully generate payment. The messages will be designed to become stronger as the account ages. In these cases, the patient may need more than a gentle nudge. |
| 7. "Mail" the statements to the patients. | Patient is advised of balance owed. |
| 8. Follow through with the collection process by continually reviewing past due accounts. | Following up on collection attempts and promises is the most important part of the process. Patients need to know that there will be continuous and consistent attempts to receive payment. They will be more apt to pay. |
| 9. **AFF** When you call a patient with a seriously past due account, he informs you that he has not paid because his wife passed away and he can hardly get through the day. Explain how you would respond. | Express your sympathy and the sympathy of the entire office. Be calm and gentle in your speech. Explain to the patient that arrangements must be made to pay the account. Give him a specific date and amount to pay. Send him a self-addressed, stamped envelope. |

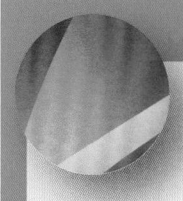

## PSY  PROCEDURE 15-2

## Composing a Collection Letter

**Purpose:** To obtain payment from a patient whose account is more than 90 days old

**Equipment:** Ledger cards generated in Procedure 15-1, word processor, stationery with letterhead

| STEPS | PURPOSE |
|---|---|
| 1. Review the patients' accounts and sort the accounts by age. | Sorting the accounts will make the task quicker and easier. |
| 2. Design a rough draft of a form letter that can be used for collections. | A rough draft gives you the opportunity to review and edit your letter. |
| 3. In the first paragraph, tell the patient why you are writing. | Let the patient know that you are attempting to collect a debt. |
| 4. Inform the patient of the action you expect. Example: "To avoid further action, please pay $50.00 on this account by Friday, May 1, 2013." | Being specific will let the patient know exactly what you expect and enable you to follow up more efficiently. |
| 5. Proofread the rough draft for errors, clarity, and accuracy, and then retype. | Errors in a letter may translate to the patient as inattention to detail and, therefore, to your collection follow-through. |
| 6. Take the collection letter to a supervisor or physician for approval. | Since you are serving as an agent of the facility, you should be sure the contents of the letter are appropriate. |
| 7. Fill in the appropriate amounts and dates on each letter. Ask for at least half of the account balance within a 2-week period. | Each letter will have a different amount based on the account activity. |
| 8. Print, sign, and mail the letter. | |
| 9. **AFF** You are helping a coworker get her collections letters in the mail. You notice several errors in the letters. Explain how you would respond. | Show her the errors and joke about your spelling capabilities. Offer to proofread for her in the future. |

# The Clinical Medical Assistant

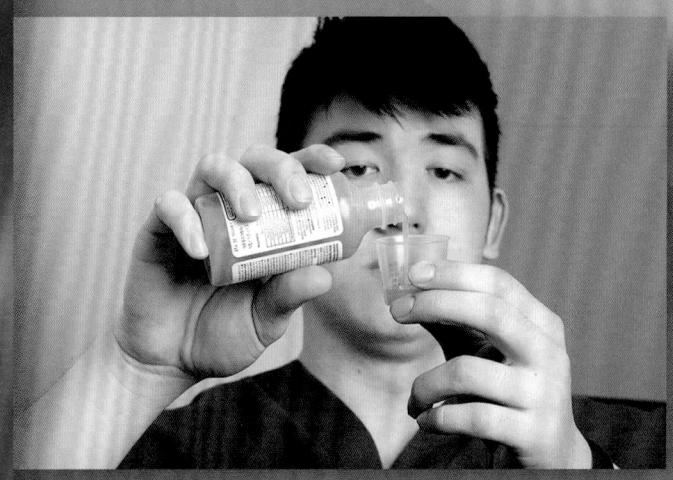

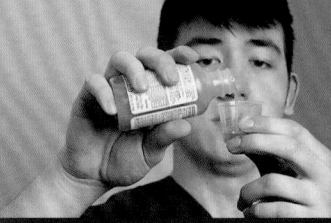

CHAPTER

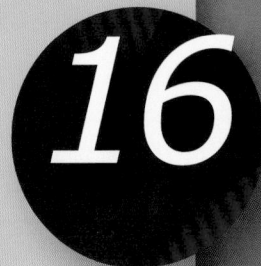

# 16 Nutrition and Wellness

## Outline

## Learning Outcomes

**COG Cognitive Domain***

1. Spell and define the key terms
2. *Identify body systems*
3. *List major organs in each body system*
4. *Identify the anatomical location of major organs in each body system*
5. *Describe the normal function of the digestive system*
6. *Analyze health care results as reported in graphs and/or tables (BMI)*
7. Describe dietary nutrients including carbohydrates, fats, proteins, minerals, electrolytes, vitamins, fiber, and water. Discuss the body's basal metabolic rate and its importance in weight management
8. Explain how to use the food pyramid and MyPlate guides to promote healthy food choices
9. Read and explain the information on food labels
10. Identify the special dietary needs for weight control, cardiovascular disease, and hypertension
11. Define the function of dietary supplements
12. List the components of physical fitness
13. Discuss suggestions for a healthy lifestyle
14. Explain the importance of disease prevention

15. List and describe the effects of the substances most commonly abused
16. Recognize the dangers of substance abuse

**PSY Psychomotor Domain***

1. Teach a patient how to read food labels (Procedure 16-1)
2. *Document patient care accurately in the medical record*
3. *Develop a meal plan utilizing the basic principles of nutrition (Procedure 16-2)*
4. *Instruct a patient according to the patient's special dietary needs (Procedure 16-2)*
5. *Coach patients appropriately considering a. cultural diversity, b. developmental life stage, and c. communication barriers*

**PSY Affective Domain***

1. *Incorporate critical thinking skills when performing patient assessment*
2. *Incorporate critical thinking skills when performing patient care*
3. *Show awareness of a patient's concerns regarding dietary changes*

*(continues on page 378)*

4. *Protect the integrity of the medical record*
5. *Demonstrate a. empathy, b. active listening, and c. nonverbal communication*
6. *Demonstrate the principles of self-boundaries*
7. *Demonstrate respect for individual diversity including a. gender, b. race, c. religion, d. age, e. economic status, and f. appearance*
8. *Explain to a patient the rationale for performance of a procedure*

*\*Note: AAMA/CAAHEP 2015 Standards are italicized.*

### ABHES Competencies

1. Comprehend and explain to the patient the importance of diet and nutrition
2. Effectively convey and educate patients regarding the proper diet and nutrition guidelines
3. Identify categories of patients who require special diets or diet modifications
4. Document accurately

## Key Terms

| | | | |
|---|---|---|---|
| anabolism | calories | essential amino acids | metabolism |
| basal metabolic rate (BMR) | catabolism | euphoria | minerals |
| body mass index (BMI) | dental cavities | guided imagery | predisposed |
| | endorphins | homeostasis | |

## Case Study

*J*ack Stone, CMA (AAMA), has been working at Great Falls Medical Center since graduating from a 1-year medical assisting program in his community 5 years ago. Recently, his office has seen several elementary school–aged children whose parents are concerned about reports from the school nurse regarding increased body mass index (BMI) in their children. The parents are questioning this assessment and its implications for the overall health of their children. What does the BMI measure? Are there current or future health risks that may be experienced by children with a high BMI? What does this assessment mean for adults? This chapter addresses issues related to weight, including nutrition and maintaining good health.

The human body requires certain things such as regular exercise and a balanced diet to maintain its efficiency. Together, diet and exercise offer important benefits for overall health maintenance and disease prevention for people of all ages. Psychological wellness is also crucial to a balanced, healthy life. Avoiding harmful substances and unhealthy practices is as important to overall health as diet and exercise. As a medical assistant, you should consider yourself a role model for your patients. Throughout your career, you will have many opportunities to teach patients the essentials of good health and disease prevention by knowing how behaviors affect short-term and long-term health.

## DIGESTION AND METABOLISM

Digestion consists of both the physical and chemical breakdown of complex food into simpler substances that the body can use for energy. When you swallow, food travels from the mouth, through the esophagus, into the stomach, and through the small and large intestines. The process of digestion begins in your mouth as the enzymes in your saliva start to break down the food as you chew. As the partly digested food passes through the remainder of the digestive tract, enzymes continue to break down food, and, in the small intestines, the process of absorption allows these nutrients to be absorbed into the bloodstream. Once in the bloodstream, the nutrients are taken to the liver to be further broken down and filtered before making their way to every cell in the body. Any nutrients not needed are eliminated from the body or stored as fat for future energy use. The process whereby food is broken down, absorbed, used by the cells, or stored by the body is known as **metabolism**.

There are two phases in the process of metabolism, **catabolism** and **anabolism**. Catabolism is the destructive phase of metabolism in which larger molecules are converted into smaller molecules. An example of catabolism includes the conversion of glycogen into pyruvic acid. This process releases energy, which is measured in **calories**. This energy is needed for cell growth and heat production. In some cases, nutrients are broken down and reassembled by the body to produce substances needed by the body. This process is known as anabolism, which is considered the constructive phase of metabolism as the smaller molecules are converted to larger molecules. An example of anabolism is the conversion of amino acids into specific proteins. The speed of these metabolic processes is particular to each individual, which explains why some people seem to be able to eat more and maintain a healthy weight, whereas others consume the same amount of food and gain weight.

## ESSENTIALS OF NUTRITION

Although many factors influence **homeostasis**, making healthy food choices gives you the best chance at maintaining a state of wellness including homeostasis. When the body is working efficiently and in balance, it is considered to be homeostatic. Eating a diet that includes all nutrients in adequate amounts increases your body's ability to maintain wellness.

### Nutrients

Nutrients include the elements found in the food we eat that are important for all aspects of health maintenance. Essential nutrients include vitamins, minerals, carbohydrates, proteins, fiber, and certain fats. Micronutrients are elements that are needed in trace amounts. The consumption of water is also important to metabolic processes and general good health.

### Carbohydrates

Carbohydrates are chemical substances that are broken down by the body into simple sugars (glucose), which provide energy to all cells of the body. Foods that contain carbohydrates include those made from grain products, fruits, vegetables, legumes, and sugars. Chemically, carbohydrates are made of carbon, hydrogen, and oxygen atoms, and, depending on the structure of these elements in the carbohydrate molecule and how easily digested by the body, they are considered complex or simple. Complex carbohydrates take longer to digest and therefore provide long-term energy to the body. Examples of these types of carbohydrates include starches that are found in grains, legumes, potatoes, and pasta. Simple carbohydrates are unrefined sugars found in fruits and plants, which are easily broken down and absorbed by the body. Refined sugars have a high caloric value but no nutritious value and should be kept to a minimum. Carbohydrates consumed but not used by the body for energy are converted to fat and stored in the adipose tissue of the body.

### Proteins

When broken down, proteins are made up of amino acids, which provide energy, build and repair tissue, and assist with antibody production in the body. There are approximately 80 amino acids found in nature, but the human body only needs 20 of them. The body produces 11 of these on its own; the other nine are known as **essential amino acids** and come from your diet. Some animal proteins provide all the necessary amino acids and are called *complete proteins*. Examples of foods that contain complete proteins include milk, cheese, eggs, fish, and meat from animals or poultry. Other proteins do not contain all of the nine essential amino acids and are considered *incomplete proteins*. Plants, such as beans, legumes, nuts, and seeds, are natural sources of incomplete proteins. A combination of both types of proteins, complete and incomplete, will ensure a proper amount of protein in the diet.

### Fats

Fats, also known as lipids, serve as a concentrated source of heat production and energy and provide essential fatty acids. Many tissues, including heart and skeletal muscle, derive energy from fatty acids. Chemically, fats are composed of carbon, hydrogen, and oxygen but in different proportions than those found in carbohydrates. Food must supply essential fatty acids that are necessary for nutritional well-being. If the body has inadequate supplies of glucose to break down for energy, it will catabolize, or break down, fats. Fats have important functions within the body including providing a cushion for internal organs, providing insulation to maintain normal body temperature, and assisting cells to function properly. Because the body can store fat reserves for future energy use in adipose tissue, an excess of fat in the diet will result in weight gain. Although food labels

## TABLE 16-1    The Good and Bad Fats

| Type of Fat | What Does It Do? | Where Is It Found? |
| --- | --- | --- |
| Monounsaturated (MUFA) fat | Does not raise "bad" cholesterol levels | Olive oil and canola oil |
| Omega-3 fatty acid | May protect against heart disease | Salmon, albacore tuna, mackerel, sardines, herring, and trout |
| Polyunsaturated (PUFA) fat | Contains some essential fatty acids; does not raise "bad" cholesterol levels | Natural oils found in certain fish and nuts; vegetable oils such as corn oil, soybean oil, and sunflower oil |
| Saturated fat | Raises "bad" cholesterol levels, increases risk of heart disease | Meat, poultry, dairy products, processed and fast foods |
| Trans fat or hydrogenated fat[a] | Raises "bad" cholesterol levels, increases risk of heart disease | Cookies, cakes, margarine, crackers, and some fried foods |
| Triglycerides | Excess amounts increase risk of heart disease when coupled with other risk factors | Main form of fat in foods, produced by the body and stored as fat from excess calories |

[a]Trans fats are created by adding hydrogen to vegetable oil. This process, called *hydrogenation*, increases the shelf life of certain products. Hydrogenation turns liquid vegetable oils into solid fats.

*Source*: http://www.fda.gov/AboutFDA/Transparency/Basics/ucm194310.htm

often list information about fats, these labels can be confusing. Table 16-1 lists the types, characteristics, and sources of fats.

## Vitamins

Vitamins are organic substances that enhance the breakdown of proteins, carbohydrates, and fats. Some vitamins are used in the formation of blood cells and hormones as well as in the production of neurochemical substances necessary for life. Eating a diet that contains all of the nutrients usually means that the vitamins necessary to maintain good health are consumed in adequate amounts. However, many people supplement their intake of food with a daily multivitamin to make sure they are getting a proper amount of each vitamin in the appropriate amounts.

Vitamins are categorized as either *fat soluble* or *water soluble*. Fat-soluble vitamins include vitamins A, D, E, and K. These vitamins are usually absorbed with foods that contain fat and are stored in the liver, kidneys, and body fat. Bile, which is formed in the liver, breaks down fat-soluble vitamins. The consumption of additional fat-soluble vitamins should be avoided because the body stores these vitamins, and an excess can result in serious illness.

Water-soluble vitamins include vitamin C and the B-complex vitamins such as thiamin (B1), riboflavin (B2), niacin (B3), and folic acid. The body does not store these vitamins, and they must be provided daily through the diet. Any excess water-soluble vitamins taken in will not be stored but excreted by the body.

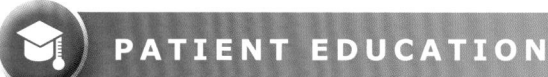

## PATIENT EDUCATION

### Women and Folic Acid

Folate, one of the B vitamins, has been found to reduce the risk of neural tube defects in developing fetuses. These types of defects, like spina bifida and anencephaly, affect the fetus's brain and spine during early pregnancy. Neural tube defects can cause paralysis and, in extreme cases, death. In 1998, the March of Dimes, in its dedication to wiping out birth defects, began a national campaign to get the word about folate out to women of childbearing age who may become pregnant. The March of Dimes joined forces with other agencies to provide education, training, and vitamin distribution to women across the nation. Since that time, women have become more aware of the importance of folic acid, and physicians provide more information and assistance to patients.

A daily intake of 400 mcg per day of synthetic folate or folic acid from fortified foods or supplements is recommended for women of childbearing age who may become pregnant. Women are encouraged to eat foods naturally rich in folate including liver, avocado, orange juice, boiled asparagus, spinach, and green, leafy vegetables. Vegetables should be eaten raw or lightly steamed as cooking may destroy the vitamins. Many breakfast cereals and breads are fortified with folic acid. Women of childbearing age are also encouraged to read labels to see if the amount of folic acid in products meets their daily requirement. The March of Dimes campaign has played a significant role in decreasing the occurrence of neural tube defects by 50% to 70%.

## CHECKPOINT QUESTION

1. Based on what Jack Stone, the medical assistant at Great Falls Medical Center, knows about vitamins, why is it important to follow the recommended dosage of a fat-soluble vitamin?

## Minerals

Minerals are inorganic substances used in the formation of hard and soft body tissue, muscle contraction, nerve conduction, and blood clotting. As with vitamins, you get minerals from the foods you eat. Examples of minerals necessary for good health include sodium, potassium, calcium, phosphorus, magnesium, iron, and iodine. Because the body uses minerals in differing amounts, those minerals that are only required in small amounts are known as *trace minerals*. Minerals that are only needed in trace amounts include fluorine, zinc, copper, cobalt, and chromium.

## Cholesterol

All animals produce a substance known as *cholesterol*, which is necessary for the body to function properly. Foods such as meat, poultry, seafood, eggs, and dairy products are considered animal products and therefore contain cholesterol. Egg yolks and organ meats, such as liver, are particularly high in cholesterol. Vegetables and vegetable products do not contain cholesterol; however, they may contain oils and fats.

The body requires cholesterol to maintain good health, and it is manufactured in sufficient amounts by the body. Unfortunately, the consumption of animal products also provides cholesterol and can result in an unhealthy amount of cholesterol in the bloodstream. Any excess cholesterol in the blood can result in plaque buildup inside the blood vessels, eventually causing occlusion or blockage of the blood vessel. According to the National Cholesterol Education Program (NCEP), it is recommended that adults consume fewer than 300 mg of dietary cholesterol each day to avoid this problem and less than 200 mg a day to lower known elevated cholesterol blood levels.

## Lipoproteins

Lipoproteins are substances composed of lipids (fats) and proteins that transport cholesterol between the liver and arterial walls. Food sources do not contain lipoproteins; they are found only in the body. The amounts and types of lipoproteins found in the blood are a good indicator of the risk of heart disease. There are two types of lipoproteins categorized as *low-density lipoproteins (LDLs)* and *high-density lipoproteins (HDLs)*.

LDLs transport cholesterol from the liver to the walls of large- and medium-sized arteries. Excess LDLs in the blood can cause plaques to form, which reduce the flow of blood within the affected artery. Circulation becomes impaired, and, as LDL levels rise above the normal range, the risk of heart disease increases. Due to these risks, LDL is occasionally labeled "bad" cholesterol. Factors that contribute to an unhealthy increase in LDL levels include excess body fat and a diet high in saturated fat and cholesterol. An LDL level above 160 mg/dL indicates an increased risk for heart disease. The optimal blood level of LDLs is less than 100 mg/dL.

HDLs are responsible for carrying cholesterol away from arterial walls back to the liver, which then removes cholesterol from the body. High levels of HDL have been linked to a reduction in the risk of heart disease. For this reason, HDL is sometimes called "good" or "healthy" cholesterol. Regular exercise helps increase HDL levels. An HDL level above 60 mg/dL indicates a lower risk for heart disease. HDL levels less than 40 mg/dL is a major heart disease risk factor according to the National Health Institute.

## CHECKPOINT QUESTION

2. A parent of one of the children seen at Great Falls Medical Center asks Jack Stone, CMA(AAMA), about complete proteins and where are they found. How should he answer this question?

## Fiber

Fiber is necessary in the diet to help the body with elimination of waste products in the digestive system. Foods that are high in fiber content include all vegetables, raw and cooked fruits, and whole-grain foods, such as breads, grains, and cereals. Patients with chronic colitis, ileitis, or diverticulitis may be instructed to follow a low-fiber diet, avoiding fresh fruits and vegetables and consuming only broiled, boiled, or baked meats, fish, and poultry; pastas; dairy products; well-cooked vegetables; fruit and vegetable juices; and canned fruit. A high-fiber diet may be recommended for patients with constipation or to regulate bowel movements. These patients would be told to avoid fatty foods and eat whole-grain cereals and breads. There are many brands of over-the-counter fiber supplements that can be added to a liquid for daily regularity. When discussing diet and nutrition topics with your patients, do not forget to discuss healthy food preparation and the importance of fiber in the diet (Box 16-1).

## Nutritional Guidelines

The U.S. Department of Health and Human Services (DHHS), the U.S. Department of Agriculture (USDA), the National Academy of Sciences, and the Food and

## BOX 16-1    Healthy Food Preparation Tips

Here are a few guidelines on how to prepare healthy foods that you can share with your patients:

- Broil, boil, bake, roast, or grill meat, poultry, and fish.
- Trim the fat from beef.
- Use a cooking rack so that fat drips away from the meat.
- Remove the skin from chicken. Use caution with raw chicken. Wash hands and cutting surfaces immediately.
- Cook homemade soups or gravies and then chill them. Skim the fat off and then reheat.
- Use unsaturated oils (canola, corn, safflower).Use nonstick spray when possible. Avoid saturated oils (e.g., butter, lard).

Nutrition Board are all involved in establishing the guidelines recommended for a healthy diet. All of these organizations have Web sites that can give you more information on nutrition and how to maintain a healthy diet.

## MyPyramid and MyPlate Guidelines

The USDA developed a food guidance system in 1992 called MyPyramid, to help people maintain healthy diets and sufficient exercise levels. In 2005, MyPyramid was updated to reflect the Dietary Guidelines for Americans (Fig. 16-1). The categories of food in this guidance system include oil and five main food groups:

1. Grains
2. Vegetables
3. Fruits
4. Milk
5. Meat and beans

Figure 16-2 is a sample food pyramid based on a 2,000 calorie diet. In 2010, the USDA updated the dietary guidelines for Americans and, in 2011, provided a new, simplified visual reference to communicate these guidelines to the public. This concept, known as MyPlate, is based on the same food groups and recommendations for healthy eating as MyPyramid (Fig. 16-3). Although MyPlate does not give specific information about serving sizes, it is a reminder to Americans to choose reduced portions at meals, include a plate

# Anatomy of MyPyramid

**One size doesn't fit all**
USDA's new MyPyramid symbolizes a personalized approach to healthy eating and physical activity. The symbol has been designed to be simple. It has been developed to remind consumers to make healthy food choices and to be active every day. The different parts of the symbol are described below.

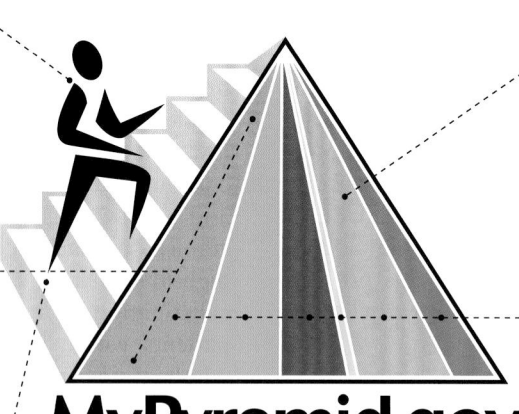

**Activity**
Activity is represented by the steps and the person climbing them, as a reminder of the importance of daily physical activity.

**Moderation**
Moderation is represented by the narrowing of each food group from bottom to top. The wider base stands for foods with little or no solid fats or added sugars. These should be selected more often. The narrower top area stands for foods containing more added sugars and solid fats. The more active you are, the more of these foods can fit into your diet.

**Personalization**
Personalization is shown by the person on the steps, the slogan, and the URL. Find the kinds and amounts of food to eat each day at MyPyramid.gov.

**Proportionality**
Proportionality is shown by the different widths of the food group bands. The widths suggest how much food a person should choose from each group. The widths are just a general guide, not exact proportions. Check the Web site for how much is right for you.

**Variety**
Variety is symbolized by the 6 color bands representing the 5 food groups of the Pyramid and oils. This illustrates that foods from all groups are needed each day for good health.

**Gradual Improvement**
Gradual improvement is encouraged by the slogan. It suggests that individuals can benefit from taking small steps to improve their diet and lifestyle each day.

## MyPyramid.gov
### STEPS TO A HEALTHIER YOU

USDA  U.S. Department of Agriculture Center for Nutrition Policy and Promotion April 2005 CNPP-16

GRAINS   VEGETABLES   FRUITS   MILK   MEAT & BEANS

USDA is an equal opportunity provider and employer.

**Figure 16-1 •** Anatomy of MyPyramid.

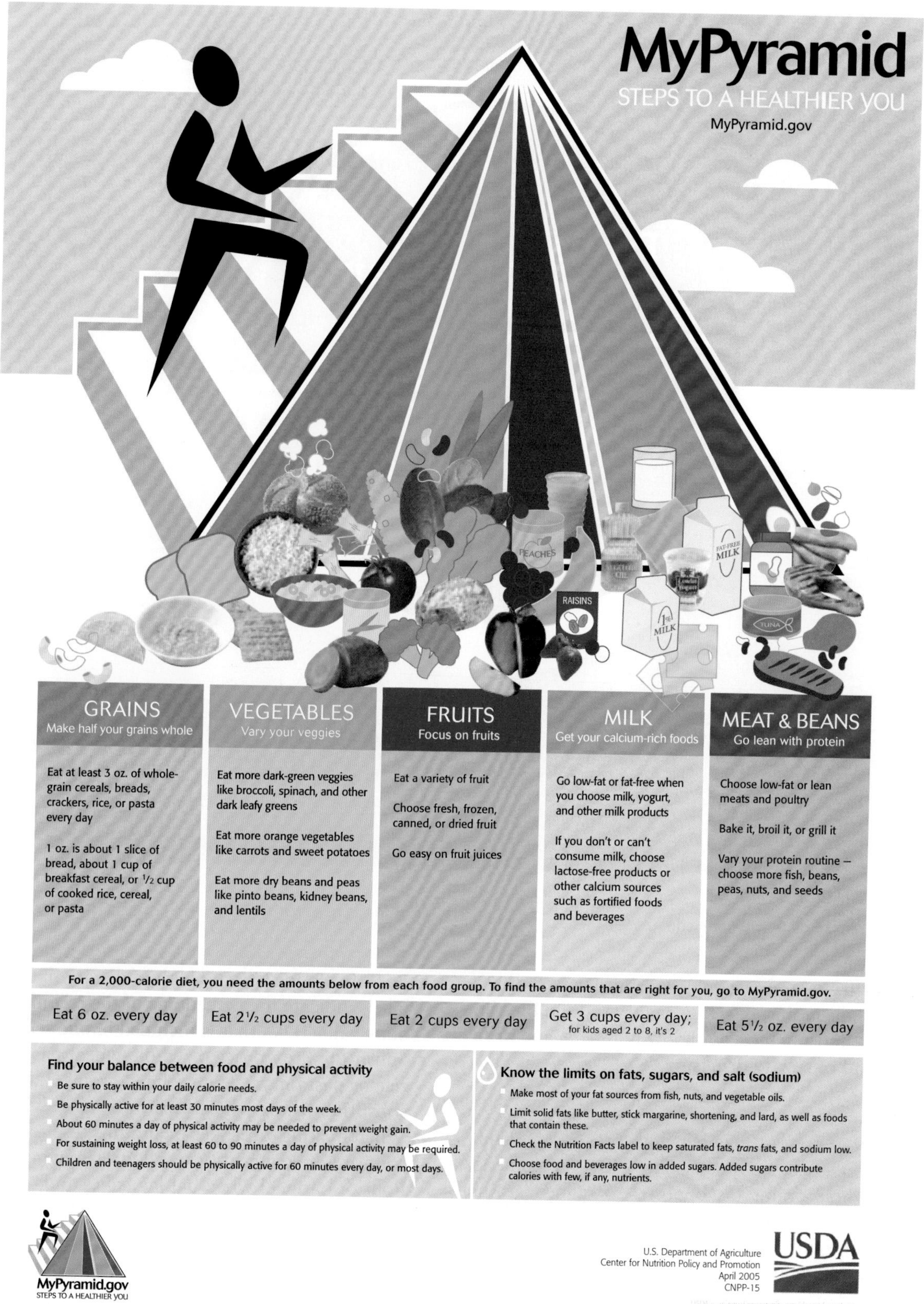

# MyPyramid
## STEPS TO A HEALTHIER YOU
### MyPyramid.gov

| GRAINS | VEGETABLES | FRUITS | MILK | MEAT & BEANS |
|---|---|---|---|---|
| Make half your grains whole | Vary your veggies | Focus on fruits | Get your calcium-rich foods | Go lean with protein |
| Eat at least 3 oz. of whole-grain cereals, breads, crackers, rice, or pasta every day<br><br>1 oz. is about 1 slice of bread, about 1 cup of breakfast cereal, or ½ cup of cooked rice, cereal, or pasta | Eat more dark-green veggies like broccoli, spinach, and other dark leafy greens<br><br>Eat more orange vegetables like carrots and sweet potatoes<br><br>Eat more dry beans and peas like pinto beans, kidney beans, and lentils | Eat a variety of fruit<br><br>Choose fresh, frozen, canned, or dried fruit<br><br>Go easy on fruit juices | Go low-fat or fat-free when you choose milk, yogurt, and other milk products<br><br>If you don't or can't consume milk, choose lactose-free products or other calcium sources such as fortified foods and beverages | Choose low-fat or lean meats and poultry<br><br>Bake it, broil it, or grill it<br><br>Vary your protein routine — choose more fish, beans, peas, nuts, and seeds |

For a 2,000-calorie diet, you need the amounts below from each food group. To find the amounts that are right for you, go to MyPyramid.gov.

| Eat 6 oz. every day | Eat 2½ cups every day | Eat 2 cups every day | Get 3 cups every day; for kids aged 2 to 8, it's 2 | Eat 5½ oz. every day |

**Find your balance between food and physical activity**
- Be sure to stay within your daily calorie needs.
- Be physically active for at least 30 minutes most days of the week.
- About 60 minutes a day of physical activity may be needed to prevent weight gain.
- For sustaining weight loss, at least 60 to 90 minutes a day of physical activity may be required.
- Children and teenagers should be physically active for 60 minutes every day, or most days.

**Know the limits on fats, sugars, and salt (sodium)**
- Make most of your fat sources from fish, nuts, and vegetable oils.
- Limit solid fats like butter, stick margarine, shortening, and lard, as well as foods that contain these.
- Check the Nutrition Facts label to keep saturated fats, *trans* fats, and sodium low.
- Choose food and beverages low in added sugars. Added sugars contribute calories with few, if any, nutrients.

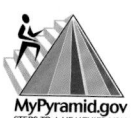

**MyPyramid.gov**
STEPS TO A HEALTHIER YOU

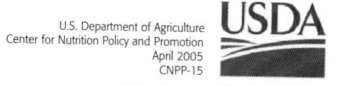

U.S. Department of Agriculture
Center for Nutrition Policy and Promotion
April 2005
CNPP-15

**USDA**

**Figure 16-2 •** MyPyramid guide based on a 2,000-calorie diet.

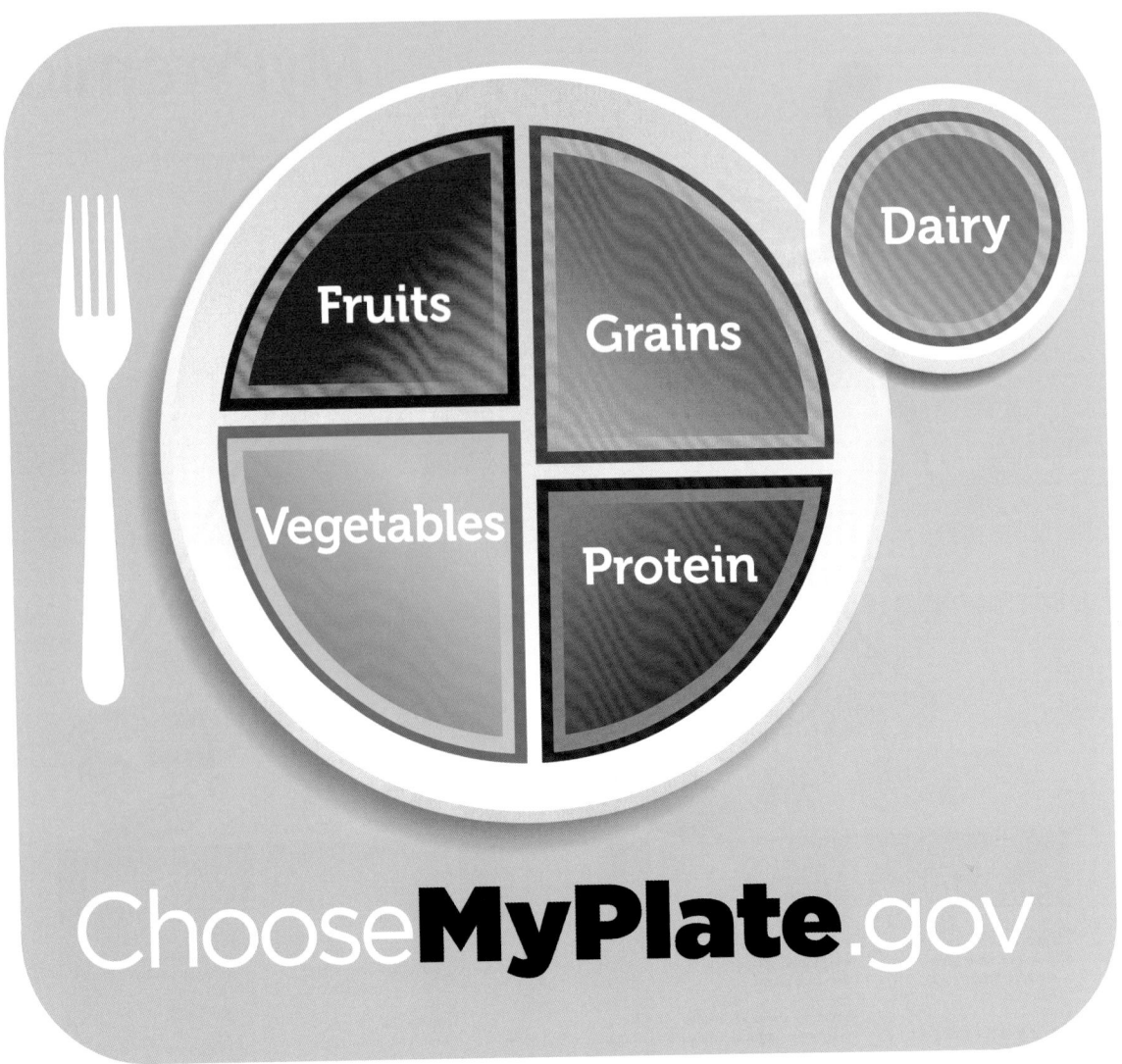

**Figure 16-3** • MyPlate icon.

of one-half fruits and vegetables, drink fat-free or 1% milk, eat whole grains, decrease dietary sodium by comparing and choosing those with low numbers, and drink water instead of sugary drinks.

### Grains

Foods in the grain food group include bread, cereal, oatmeal, crackers, rice, and pasta. The USDA recommends choosing whole grains (as opposed to refined grains) for at least half of your daily servings. Whole grains are made with the entire grain kernel and contain nutrients such as fiber, certain vitamins, carbohydrates, proteins, and antioxidants. Refined grains, on the other hand, only include part of the grain kernel. These types of grains lack fiber, iron, and some vitamins. Here are some tips to follow when selecting foods from this group:

- Look at the product's ingredient list. Foods with ingredients such as "whole wheat," "bulgur," "whole-grain corn," "oatmeal," "whole oats," or "wild rice" at the beginning of the list indicate whole grains.

- Look for foods that are high in dietary fiber. Nutrition labels indicate the percentage of the recommended daily value (DV) that is included in one serving.
- Substitute brown rice or whole-wheat pasta for white rice or pasta made from refined grains. Likewise, substitute whole-wheat bread for white bread.
- When making pancakes or muffins, use recipes that call for whole wheat or oat flour. Use whole-grain flour or oatmeal when baking cakes and cookies.
- Choose whole-grain snacks, such as baked tortilla chips or air-popped popcorn (without added salt or butter), instead of potato chips.
- Eat whole-grain cereals, such as muesli or toasted oat cereal.

### Vegetables

The vegetables group is subdivided into five categories: dark green vegetables, orange vegetables, dry beans and peas, starchy vegetables, and other vegetables. The key to choosing foods within this group is to select a variety of vegetables from different categories. Other tips include the following:

- Eat fresh seasonal vegetables. Fresh vegetables have more flavor and generally cost less than do processed vegetables (e.g., canned or frozen vegetables). Processed vegetables may also contain sauces or seasonings that add sodium and fat.
- When buying canned vegetables, look for foods without added salt. Choose vegetables labeled "no salt added," or check the sodium content on the nutrition label.
- Choose foods with high levels of potassium, such as sweet potatoes, tomato paste, beet greens, white potatoes, white beans, soybeans, lima beans, and spinach.
- Eat a green salad with lunch or dinner each day. Add only a small amount of salad dressing.
- Prepare vegetable main dish meals, such as soups, stews, and stir-fries. Include potatoes in soups and stews for added texture and nutrients.

### Fruits

The fruits food group includes 100% fruit juice as well as fresh, frozen, dried, and canned fruit. Here are some tips for selecting foods from this group:

- Get most of your daily servings from whole fruit instead of juice. Whole or cut-up fruit contains dietary fiber, while most juices do not. When buying packaged fruit, look for items that do not contain added sugar. For example, select canned fruit stored in 100% juice or water instead of syrup. Eat a wide variety of fruits to obtain the greatest nutritional benefit. Prune juice, bananas, and dried apricots supply potassium. Pears, raspberries, and blackberries provide dietary fiber. Guava, kiwi, and oranges are good sources of vitamin C. Add fresh berries, peaches, or bananas to your cereal at breakfast and drink a glass of 100% orange or grapefruit juice. Snack on cut-up or dried fruit. Cut-up fruit is often sold in convenient single-serving packages, and dried fruit can be stored in a bag or desk drawer. One-fourth cup of dried fruit is equal to one-half cup of other fruit. When baking cakes, substitute applesauce for some of the oil in the recipe.

### Milk

Also referred to as the "milk, yogurt, and cheese group," this food group includes all milk and milk products that retain their calcium content. Found in this food group are liquid milk (including lactose-free milk), milk-based desserts (such as pudding and ice cream), hard and soft cheeses, and yogurt. Not included in this group are milk products such as butter and cream cheese, which do not provide calcium. In choosing foods from this group, it's important to select low-fat or nonfat items. Other tips include the following:

- Drink a glass of low-fat or fat-free milk with meals. Have pudding made from low-fat or fat-free milk for dessert. When making hot cereals or oatmeal, use low-fat or fat-free milk instead of water. Also, substitute milk for water when preparing condensed cream soups. Snack on low-fat or fat-free yogurt topped with fresh fruit. Add low-fat cheese to soups, stews, and casseroles. Top vegetables with melted low-fat cheese, or add low-fat or fat-free yogurt to baked potatoes. For those who are lactose intolerant, choose lactose-free or lower lactose milk products. Although soy milk, orange juice, and other products may be calcium fortified, these foods do not provide all the essential nutrients supplied by foods within the milk group.

### Meat and Beans

The meat and beans group includes all foods made from meat, poultry, eggs, dry beans, peas, nuts, and seeds. The high fat and cholesterol content of some foods in this group (such as beef or egg yolks) makes varying your food choices important. It is also crucial to select a variety of foods to obtain the greatest nutritional benefit. For example, sunflower seeds and almonds are high in vitamin E; salmon and trout contain omega-3 fatty acids; clams and oysters provide iron; and beef, lamb, pork, poultry, fish, shellfish, and eggs are good sources of protein.

Here are some guidelines to use when choosing foods from the meat and beans group:

- For vegetarians, alternate protein sources include eggs, beans, nuts, peas, and foods made from soybeans, such as tofu. Select lean cuts of beef (round steaks, roasts, top loin, top sirloin) and pork (pork loin, tenderloin, ham). When buying ground beef, look for packages labeled "90% lean," "93% lean," or "95% lean." Choose boneless skinless chicken breasts and turkey cutlets, or remove the skin from poultry before cooking. Prepare meat, poultry, and fish without adding fat. First, trim off any visible fat and then broil, grill, roast, or boil foods, being careful to drain off excess fat during cooking. Add little or no breading, and avoid using gravies or sauces that are high in fat. Prepare meatless main dishes containing dry beans or peas. For example, use kidney or pinto beans to make chili, cook split pea soup or minestrone, add chickpeas or garbanzo beans to a salad, or prepare tofu or veggie burgers. Eat fish more often than you eat meat or poultry. Salmon, trout, and herring are excellent sources of omega-3 fatty acids. Substitute nuts in dishes containing meat or poultry. Add pine nuts instead of chicken to pesto sauce; substitute peanuts or cashews for meat in vegetable stir-fries; and add walnuts, almonds, or pecans to green salads instead of meat or chicken.

### Oils

One additional category is oils. Included in this category are fats that maintain a liquid form at room temperature including vegetable oils and oils that come from other natural plant and fish sources. Fats that are solid at room temperature, such as butter, shortening, and beef or chicken fat, are not considered oils. The recommended daily servings for this category are relatively small, usually several teaspoons, depending on a person's age, gender, and level of physical activity. Therefore, the most important guideline to use when choosing foods in this category is to avoid exceeding recommended amounts. Most people consume enough oils in the foods they eat (e.g., olives, avocados, nuts, fish, cooking oils, and salad dressing).

 **CHECKPOINT QUESTION**

3. Who publishes the MyPyramid and MyPlate food guidance systems and why?

 **LEGAL TIP**

### US Government Is Concerned about Americans' Eating Habits

The US government is dedicated to improving America's nutritional needs, and this is evident when you consider the many bills passed and programs provided by the agencies of the federal government. Based on data concerning dietary intake and evidence of public health problems, experts say that Americans have formed some poor eating habits. Studies have shown that Americans consume too many calories per day as well as unhealthy amounts of saturated and trans fat, cholesterol, added sugars, and sodium. In addition, most people do not meet the recommended daily intakes for a number of nutrients. The federal government says most manufacturers must list the nutrients and their amounts in food packaging. The U.S. Food and Drug Administration (FDA) mandates the information included on a food label. A recent mandate requires manufacturers to list the amount of trans fats in their products.

In the 1960s, the federal government instituted the Presidential Physical Fitness Award, which outlined specific physical programs for school physical fitness programs. The USDA regulates the public school lunch programs and requires lunches to satisfy the recommended daily dietary requirements. Head Start is a federal preschool program that has an excellent food program, ensuring that disadvantaged children get at least one nutritious meal a day. Their food programs, along with agricultural extensions across the nation, train parents in proper nutrition and food preparation through regular workshops and training.

### Understanding Food Labels

The Nutritional Labeling and Education Act was passed in 1990 to help consumers identify nutritional content in food products. Most food manufacturers (except meat and poultry) are required to list the nutritional information prominently on the package. The FDA regulates this information. Mandatory food labeling was designed to help consumers make informed food choices. Even fast-food restaurants are including labeling as consumers become more health conscious.

Currently, food labels must include measurements of calories, fat content, cholesterol, sodium, carbohydrates, dietary fiber, protein, vitamins, calcium, and any other nutrients contained in the product. Foods that only have a few of certain nutrients are not required to list them on the label. It is important to pay attention to the serving size noted on the label because the amount of a particular nutrient noted on the label is specific to that size. In addition to the amount of nutrients, the percentage of the total daily intake is listed on the right side of the label. This information on the food label helps you choose the daily allowances of the good nutrients like fiber, protein, vitamins, and minerals and a minimal amount of the things that are harmful like fats, cholesterol, sodium, and sugar. A DV of 0% is listed for those things that should be kept to a minimum. The calories listed on the label measure how much energy is received from one serving, including how many of those calories are from fat. Calories will be discussed in greater detail later.

To get the full benefit of food labels, patients must understand how to read them. You can help your patients understand how to use this information by becoming familiar with reading food labels and adapting the way you present this information based on the needs of the individual patient. Figure 16-4 is a sample food label with an explanation of each component. Procedure 16-1 outlines the steps in instructing a patient to read food labels.

 **CHECKPOINT QUESTION**

4. Jack Stone explains to a parent that food labels contain nutritional information about the food or product. What information is listed on the right side of a food label?

 **PATIENT EDUCATION**

### Vegetarian Diets

Patients may ask you about vegetarian diets including the types, benefits, and concerns about overall health for those following a vegetarian diet. There are three types of vegetarian diets, each varying in the types of animal products permitted. A *lacto-ovo-vegetarian* diet means that the diet of vegetables is supplemented with milk, eggs, and cheese. A *lacto-vegetarian* diet means the diet is supplemented only with milk and cheese. A *pure vegetarian* diet is only vegetables and fruits and excludes all foods of animal origin. It is possible to eat healthy and obtain necessary nutrients with all three vegetarian diets. The USDA provides guidelines educating vegetarians about appropriate foods that provide essential nutrients.

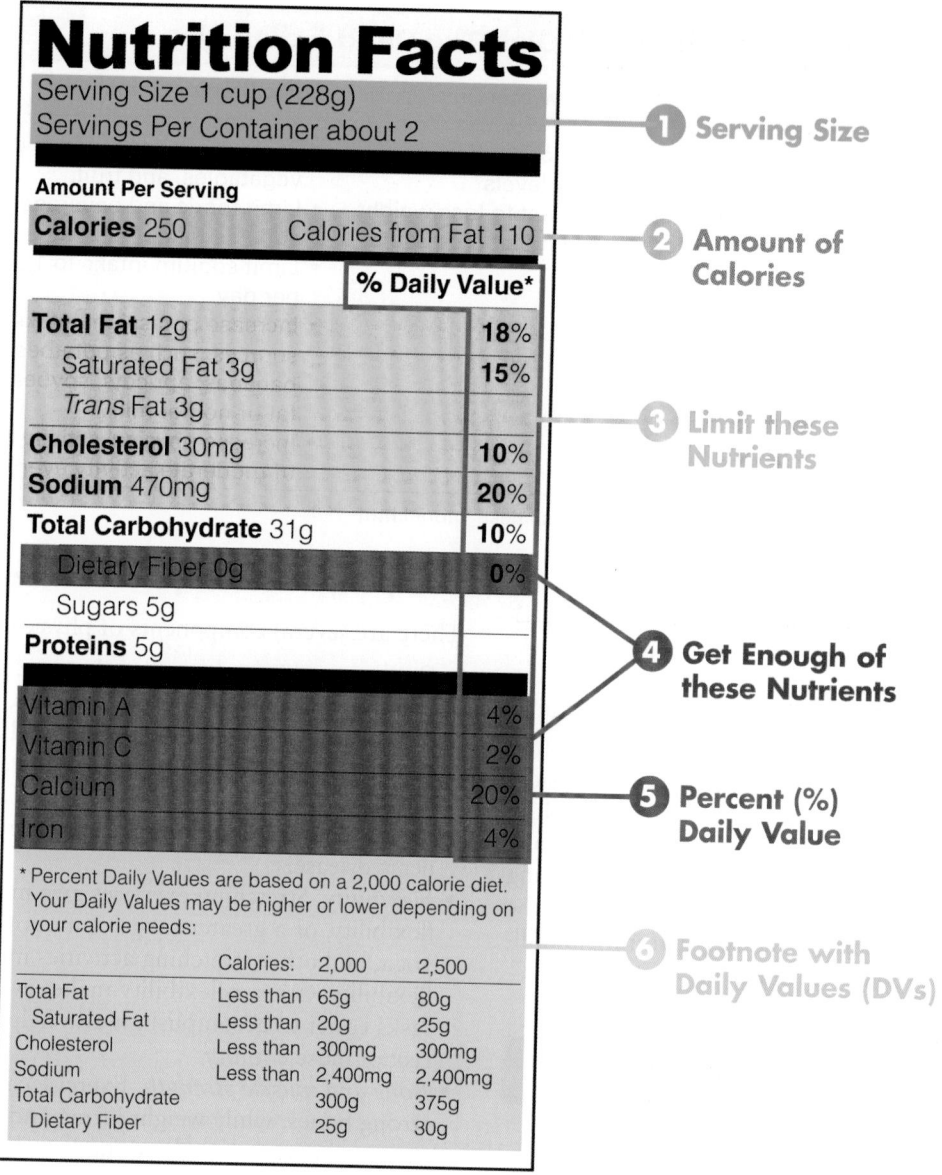

**Nutrition Facts**
Serving Size 1 cup (228g)
Servings Per Container about 2

**Amount Per Serving**

**Calories** 250          Calories from Fat 110

% Daily Value*

**Total Fat** 12g                                    18%
 Saturated Fat 3g                             15%
 *Trans* Fat 3g
**Cholesterol** 30mg                            10%
**Sodium** 470mg                                   20%
**Total Carbohydrate** 31g                  10%
 Dietary Fiber 0g                                 0%
 Sugars 5g
**Proteins** 5g

Vitamin A                                                 4%
Vitamin C                                                 2%
Calcium                                                  20%
Iron                                                          4%

\* Percent Daily Values are based on a 2,000 calorie diet.
 Your Daily Values may be higher or lower depending on
 your calorie needs:

|  | Calories: | 2,000 | 2,500 |
|---|---|---|---|
| Total Fat | Less than | 65g | 80g |
| Saturated Fat | Less than | 20g | 25g |
| Cholesterol | Less than | 300mg | 300mg |
| Sodium | Less than | 2,400mg | 2,400mg |
| Total Carbohydrate |  | 300g | 375g |
| Dietary Fiber |  | 25g | 30g |

**①** Serving Size
**②** Amount of Calories
**③** Limit these Nutrients
**④** Get Enough of these Nutrients
**⑤** Percent (%) Daily Value
**⑥** Footnote with Daily Values (DVs)

For educational purposes only. This label does not meet the labeling requirements described in 21 CFR 101.9.

**Figure 16-4** • Sample food label.

## Therapeutic Nutrition

Although each part of the lifespan brings different nutritional needs, sometimes, a patient's medical condition or situation will require diet restrictions and special foods. In these situations, the physician will order a therapeutic diet, and you may be responsible for teaching the patient how to follow the guidelines. Because therapeutic diets are used to treat specific conditions, you should never recommend a therapeutic diet or any dietary changes without instructions from the physician to do so. You must also avoid giving advice about taking dietary supplements without the physician's knowledge and approval as this may be viewed as practicing medicine and outside the scope of a medical assistant or licensed health care provided authorized by state law to diagnose and prescribe patient treatments.

Chronic conditions that require special diets include diabetes and heart disease. Patients such as those who are confined to bed or those recovering from surgical procedures may also be required to eat certain foods such as high protein or low carbohydrates. Regardless of the reason for the therapeutic diet, the purposes include facilitating the healing process, promoting healthy weight, assisting with chewing and swallowing, and/or influencing the components found in blood, such as cholesterol or blood glucose levels. Table 16-2 shows an example of a special diet that may be prescribed to treat or prevent high blood pressure. This special diet is referred to as the *Dietary Approaches to Stop Hypertension (DASH)* eating plan.

### CHECKPOINT QUESTION

5. List four possible reasons for a patient's need for a special therapeutic diet.

| TABLE 16-2   Example of a Therapeutic Diet: The DASH Eating Plan | | |
|---|---|---|
| **What Does This Diet Accomplish?** | **Who May Follow This Diet?** | **Basic Dietary Guidelines** |
| • Lowers blood pressure<br>• Reduces the risk of developing hypertension<br>• Lowers "bad" cholesterol (LDL's)<br>• Decrease body weight | • Adults with blood pressure above normal levels<br>• Adults who want to lose weight and avoid high blood pressure | • Consume more servings of grains, vegetables, and fruit.<br>• Limit foods and beverages containing added sugars.<br>• Limit sodium intake to 1,500–2,300 mg per day.<br>• Increase potassium intake from natural sources, such as potatoes, spinach, bananas, apricots, soybeans, and low-fat or nonfat milk.<br>• Increase physical activity to 30 minutes of moderate activity every day |

*Source*: http://www.nhlbi.nih.gov/health/public/heart/hbp/dash/dash_inbrief.htm

## ☺☰G  WELLNESS

### Physical Fitness

Physical fitness is characterized by endurance, flexibility, and strength. Along with a healthy and balanced diet, regular exercise is necessary for maintaining physical fitness. Physical movement helps maintain a healthy musculoskeletal system, a normal weight, and a positive mental attitude. Studies have shown that exercising regularly improves the immune system and causes the production of **endorphins**, the body's "natural painkillers" that tend to produce **euphoria**, or "good feelings."

## PATIENT EDUCATION

### Calculating Target Heart Rate

Patients who are starting an exercise program may need to learn how to calculate their target heart rate. Aerobic activities, such as running, bike riding, rowing, and swimming, are most effective when target heart rate is maintained. Target heart rate should be anywhere between 60% and 90% of a patient's maximum heart rate. To find a patient's target heart rate, follow these steps:

1. Subtract the patient's age (in years) from 220 (beats/minute) to calculate the maximum heart rate. For example, a 35-year-old patient would have a maximum heart rate of 185.

$$220 - 35 = 185$$

2. Multiply the maximum heart rate by the desired intensity level (60% to 90% of the maximum heart rate) to obtain the target heart rate. A patient with a maximum heart rate of 185 who would like to exercise at 70% intensity would need to maintain a target heart rate of 129.5.

$$185 \times 0.70 = 129.5$$

### Components of Physical Fitness

There are several components of physical fitness:

- *Cardiovascular health and endurance.* Regular exercise, particularly aerobic activities, can improve cardiovascular system functioning and endurance. Benefits of a healthy heart include lowered blood pressure, lower cholesterol levels, and a reduced risk for developing conditions such as type 2 diabetes or heart disease.
- *Flexibility.* Stretching exercises give muscles increased flexibility, or a greater range of motion. Calisthenics, yoga, and other stretching activities improve flexibility. Greater flexibility makes everyday physical tasks easier to accomplish; it also helps decrease the risk of muscle injury.
- *Bone and muscle strength.* Exercise can help build strong bones, while weight lifting and resistance training increase muscle strength and endurance.

### 🔍 CHECKPOINT QUESTION

6. What types of physical activities promote cardiovascular health and endurance?

### Weight Management

The rate of obesity in the United States has doubled in the past two decades. Nearly one-third of the adult population is obese, and an estimated 17% of children and young adults ages 2 to 19 years are overweight. Excess body fat can result in a higher risk of certain health conditions, such as hypertension, heart disease, type 2 diabetes, gallbladder disease, respiratory disorders, and certain kinds of cancers.

In the last 20 years, the obesity rate has doubled among children and tripled among adolescents. Because obesity in childhood often leads to obesity in adulthood, it is important to find ways to slow the unhealthy rate of weight gain while maintaining normal growth and development. Involving both parents and children in managing body weight is essential for compliance with any prescribe dietary plan. Simple methods for managing body weight include eating more nutritious, lower calorie foods and increasing physical activity. Even losing a small amount of weight is beneficial to overall health and preventing future weight gain.

## Physiologic Issues

Reducing and maintaining a healthy weight depends on a familiar formula—increased physical activity + taking in fewer calories = reduction in body weight. The energy that the body expends burns the calories you consume. Knowing how many calories your body requires based on age and gender is necessary for calculating the amount of calories required to lose or maintain weight. To do this, you must understand the three basic ways the body expends energy. These include

- **Basal metabolic rate (BMR)** (or how many calories the body uses to perform basic functions, such as respiration and heartbeat, while in a resting state)
- Energy expended during physical activity
- The thermic effect of food (or how much energy the body expends while processing different foods)

The body's daily caloric needs are most accurately determined by taking into account all three of these factors. Each of these is discussed in the following sections.

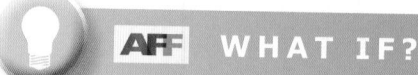

### WHAT IF?

**A patient who is a young mother of three says that she would like to stay fit, but she has no time for a fitness plan. What are some ways she can incorporate exercise into her busy schedule?**

Remind her that exercise does not have to consist of a 30-minute walk or an hour in the gym. Give her some suggestions for creative ways to be physically active every day. For example, take the stairs instead of the elevator. Take two steps at a time for leg and buttock strengthening. On weekends, take a long walk or run around with the children at the park. Doing yard work is another way to be physically active; mowing the lawn with a push mower and raking leaves are ways to stay active while accomplishing necessary chores. While watching television in the evening, jog in place or do jumping jacks. Do calf raises while waiting in line at the grocery store. While talking on the phone, walk up and down stairs or do leg lifts. A simple trip to the grocery store provides exercise by walking and lifting. While driving in the car, tense up various muscle groups for a few seconds and then release. Do leg lifts with your child sitting across your feet. Even a hearty laugh works the abdominal muscles.

The benefits of regular physical activity go beyond maintaining a healthy level of physical fitness. Being active also helps relieve stress. By taking small steps to be more active every day, you will eventually progress to a point where you will want to engage in more physical activity. Then, perhaps you can hire a babysitter and go take a kickboxing class. Meanwhile, just move more!

### Basal Metabolic Rate

As mentioned earlier, metabolism is the process of digesting and processing food consumed into energy to be used by the body or stored in adipose tissue as fat reserves. An individual's BMR refers to the amount of energy used in a unit of time to maintain vital functions by a fasting, resting subject. Approximately 60% to 70% of the body's energy is expended through BMR basic activities, such as respiration, heartbeat, and maintaining body temperature.

### Level of Physical Activity

The second way that your body expends energy is through physical activity, which makes up 20% to 30% of the body's total energy expenditure. You have already learned the positive effects of physical activity, one of which is to burn calories and maintain a healthy weight.

### Calories

The third, and last, factor included in how your body expends energy is known as the *thermic effect*, or the amount of energy required to digest specific foods. The energy used by the body can be measured in calories, and four different sources contribute calories to a person's diet. These sources include carbohydrates, fats, proteins, and alcohol.

Together, the three factors (BMR, level of physical activity, and the thermic effect of food) determine how many calories your body needs each day. If you take in fewer calories than you need, you lose weight. If you take in more calories than you need, you gain weight. The combination of these three components can be calculated as follows:

- For those who are not physically active: weight (lbs) × 14 = estimated calories/day
- For those who are moderately active: weight (lbs) × 17 = estimated calories/day
- For active individuals: weight (lbs) × 20 = estimated calories/day

### Body Mass Index

**Body mass index (BMI)** measures an individual's ratio of fat to lean body mass. It can be calculated by using the following formula: [weight (pounds) ÷ height (inches)$^2$] × 703. There are also tables such as the one shown in Figure 16-5 that can be used to calculate the BMI by finding the patient's height in inches on the left hand side of the chart and moving across the chart at the level of the height until you find the approximate weight. At that point on the chart, move upward, noting the BMI and category (normal, overweight, obese, or extremely obese) along the top of the chart.

With the increased incidence of obesity, physicians are turning to using the BMI to assess a patients' risk for obesity. For adults who are 20 years of age or older, the condition of being overweight or obese is based on their BMI level only (i.e., regardless of age or gender). For children and adolescents, however, weight status is

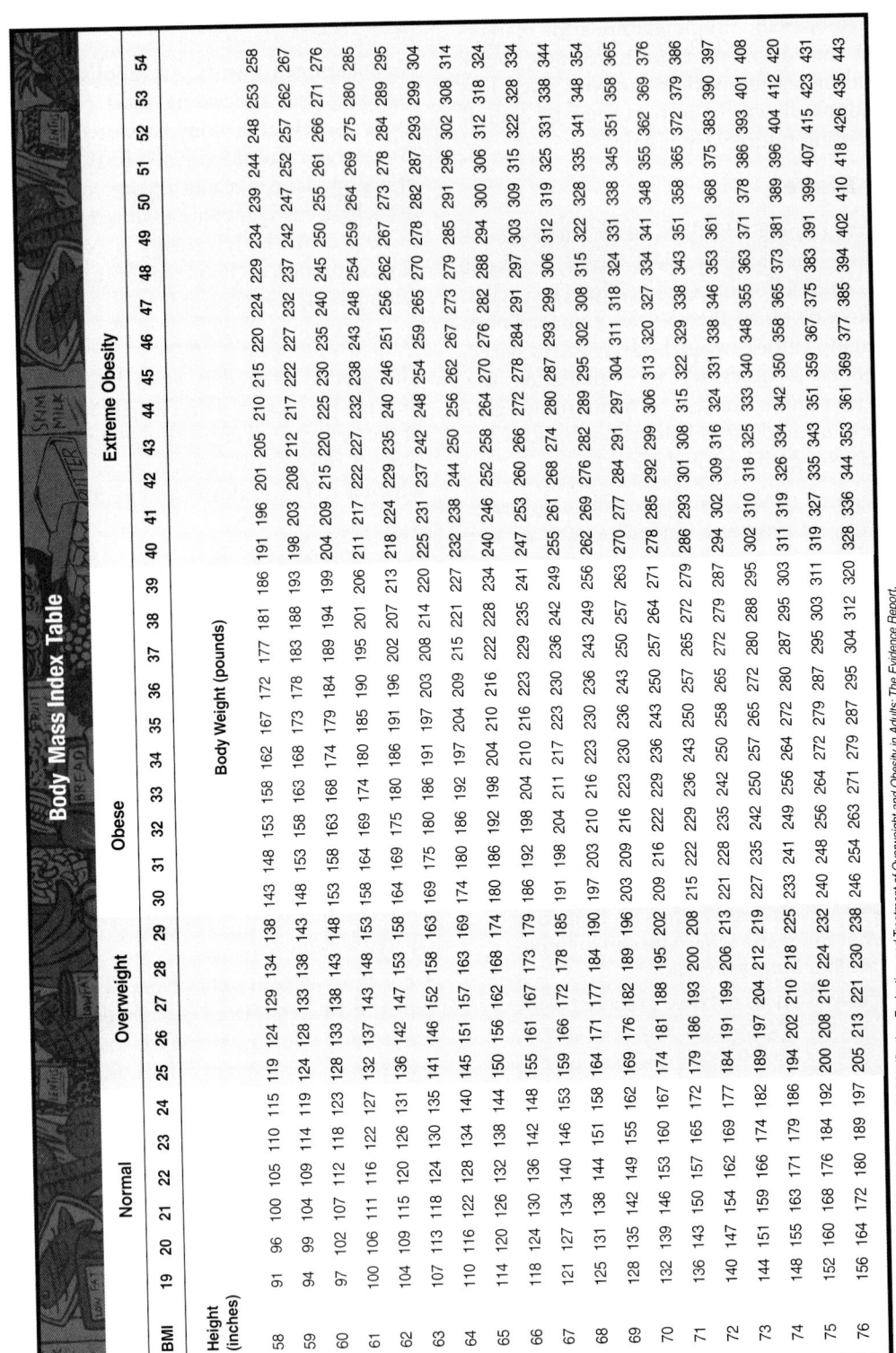

**Figure 16-5 • Body mass index (BMI) table.**

determined by taking into account not only BMI level but also age and gender (Box 16-2).

A BMI over 30 is considered obese. The Centers for Disease Control and Prevention offer a body mass calculator on their Web site. By going to the CDC Web site and searching for the BMI calculator (http://www.cdc.gov/healthyweight/assessing/bmi/), you can enter the patient's requested information and print a BMI graph and information for the patient about their weight and BMI.

## CHECKPOINT QUESTION

7. A patient asks Jack Stone what is meant by BMR and how is this different from the BMI. How should Jack answer this question?

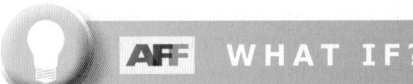

## WHAT IF?

You are assisting your physician-employer in the exam room one afternoon when the two of you see a patient who has gained 30 pounds in a year. She appears depressed and complains of leg pain and increased difficulty getting around. The physician explains that she needs to make some changes in her diet (low calorie, low fat) and asks you to assist the patient in getting started. Where should you begin?

You should refer to the *Dietary Guidelines for Americans, 2010* from the USDA and go over the following points:

- *Monitor calories and nutrients.* Eat foods with more nutrients per calorie, and limit saturated and trans fats, added sugars, cholesterol, sodium, and alcohol.
- *Manage your weight.* To prevent weight gain, slightly decrease calories consumed and increase daily physical activity. To maintain a healthy weight, find a balance between the number of calories consumed each day and an appropriate amount of exercise.
- *Exercise regularly.* To prevent unhealthy weight gain, exercise for 60 minutes (moderate to vigorous activity) most days of the week. Include cardiovascular training, flexibility exercises, and weight training to receive the full benefits of physical fitness.
- *Make healthy food choices.* Eat a variety of fruits and vegetables every day, being sure to consume the recommended amount of servings based on energy needs. When selecting foods from the grains food group, choose whole-grain products. Be sure to include the recommended daily servings of milk or milk products in your diet as well.
- *Limit fats.* Try to consume no more than 20% to 35% of calories from fat each day. Most fats in your diet should come from natural sources, such as nuts, vegetable oils, and fish. Limit other fats by selecting foods that are designated as low-fat, nonfat, or lean, and avoid trans fats.
- *Choose healthy sources of carbohydrates.* Select carbohydrate sources that are also high in fiber, such as fruits, vegetables, and whole-grain products. Avoid foods and beverages that contain added sugars or sweeteners.
- *Monitor sodium and potassium intake.* Limit sodium to less than 2,300 mg per day. Select foods that are high in potassium, such as fruits and vegetables.
- *Limit alcohol consumption.* Consume alcohol in moderation; women should not exceed one drink per day, and men should not exceed two drinks per day. Those who should avoid alcohol include pregnant or lactating women, women who may become pregnant, children, adolescents, individuals taking medication that should not be mixed with alcohol, and people who have certain medical conditions.
- *Prevent food-borne illness.* Wash hands, food preparation surfaces, and fruits and vegetables. Cook foods long enough and at high enough temperatures to kill dangerous microorganisms. Properly store perishable items and avoid unpasteurized milk products, raw eggs, undercooked meat or poultry, and raw sprouts.

*Remember to document all instructions, verbal and written, in the medical record.*

### BOX 16-2   The Body Mass Index (BMI) Measurement

Because BMI takes into account both weight and height, it is a more accurate way to measure body fat than by measuring weight alone. It is important to note, however, that BMI is not the sole method used to determine obesity. It does have limitations; BMI can overestimate body fat in someone who is very muscular or underestimate body fat in an individual with decreased muscle mass. Other factors including age, gender, and ethnicity also cause variations in the relationship between BMI and body fat. Slightly reducing caloric intake for children who are overweight will decrease their body fat. Only the physician can make a diagnosis of obesity after taking all factors including BMI into consideration.

### Sociologic and Psychological Issues

Almost every social event you attend centers around food. Food is a part of many of our traditions, such as birthdays, holidays, and family gatherings for any occasion. Eating has become entertainment for many people in our culture.

In addition to these social events, the consumption of food can also be psychological. Perhaps you remember having snacks prepared by your mother and ready for you after school or a treat such as a lollipop when you scraped your knee. Many people are what researchers call "emotional eaters." Instead of facing the stresses of everyday life, emotional eaters use food to cope. Others eat when they are happy as a form of celebration or as a reward for an accomplishment.

Food is everywhere; it is necessary for life. Experts warn that we must make some major lifestyle changes, make better food choices, and become more active to stop the growing epidemic of obesity. This starts with changing bad habits. Your role as a professional medical assistant begins with examining your own eating habits, making better choices, and becoming an example for patients who want or need to make better choices for a healthier life. Of course, understanding why people eat and how food plays a part in our social and psychological well-being is important to making any changes for better health, both for yourself and your patients.

 **CHECKPOINT QUESTION**

8. What are the ill effects of excess body fat?

## Staying Well

Maintaining the proper body weight and consuming the right nutrients in the right amounts are necessary for good health. But, in our busy world, it is difficult to follow a rigid diet or a confining exercise regimen.

With some planning and determination, though, you can make even subtle changes to improve your health and quality of life. Eating more slowly, sleeping more, and taking the stairs instead of an elevator are just a few of the things that you can do every day to make you feel better. A healthy body has a better immune system.

## Stress

Although a certain amount of good stress is needed to function and thrive in everyday life, too much stress can be harmful. High stress levels are known to cause a long list of health problems. Everything from headaches to leg cramps can be indicators of too much stress. Keep lists of suggestions to manage stress in a central patient education area or waiting area of the office. During waiting times in the examination room, talk to patients about their stress levels. To lessen stress, try using some of the following techniques:

- Think positively. Look for the good in each situation instead of focusing on the bad.
- Devote at least 30 minutes of each day to an activity you truly enjoy, such as spending time with friends, reading, or pursuing a favorite hobby.
- Take a moment to calm your thoughts when faced with a situation that causes you to become angry or agitated.
- Know your limits, and don't take on too many obligations.
- Get a good night's sleep.

Even leisure activity reduces stress by providing a temporary break from the everyday pressures and obligations that can make life stressful. Not only will you be better equipped to handle life's daily challenges, but you will also reduce your physical symptoms of stress. High levels of stress and its effects on the body can contribute to heart disease, ulcers, and other conditions in individuals who are **predisposed**, or genetically programmed, for such problems. Stress can also exacerbate chronic conditions, like diabetes, and have a negative impact on a person's emotional health and interpersonal relationships.

Relaxation exercises can calm you down in times of high stress. Sitting or lying comfortably with your eyes closed while imagining a quiet, peaceful place is a self-relaxation technique called **guided imagery**. Meditation is a relaxation technique that calms the mind and the body, relieving physical and emotional stress.

## Pollution

Air pollution can negatively affect health. Those who live in areas with high levels of pollution might suffer from respiratory problems and general discomfort due to burning eyes or irritated throats. A number of chemicals detected in polluted air have been linked to birth defects, certain cancers, respiratory disorders, and brain damage. Accidental releases of some chemicals have been known to cause serious injury or even death.

The effects of air pollution on the environment are also problematic. Examples of harm to the environment include the destruction of trees and plants, the pollution of water, and the killing of fish and other animals. Environmental changes may result from damage to the ozone layer, increasing instances of skin cancer and eye damage.

The Clean Air Act of 1990 is a federal law that limits the amounts of certain pollutants that may be released into the air in the United States. This act is designed to provide the same basic health and environmental protection to all Americans; however, it is up to the states to regulate these levels. States may set up stricter laws concerning pollution, but they may not adopt weaker pollution controls than the federal law mandates. A federal agency, the Environmental Protection Agency (EPA), is in place to help the states meet federal regulations. The EPA conducts research and provides funding to support state programs designed to reduce air pollution.

To minimize the harmful effects of pollution, experts suggest that you avoid secondhand smoke, areas with heavy traffic, and inhaling highway fumes. When exercising outdoors, try to avoid busy roads or high-pollution areas when smog levels are high. Check air quality levels that are monitored and reported by your local news stations. Shrubbery in your yard is recommended because it protects you from breathing in pollution and dirt from the street.

## Seat Belt Use and Airbags

According to the National Highway Traffic Safety Administration, almost 22,000 people were occupants in passenger vehicles who died in 2012 as a result of automobile accidents. Although seat belt usage was reported as 86% by this agency in 2012, 63% of adults between the ages of 21 to 24 years were not restrained. When the front of a vehicle hits an unmoving object in an automobile accident, the car stops abruptly, but the driver and passengers do not. Momentum keeps moving their bodies forward at the same speed the vehicle was traveling until they are stopped by unmoving objects inside the vehicle, such as the dashboard, steering wheel, or windshield. The impact can cause serious, and sometimes fatal, injuries. However, properly worn seat belts prevent that second crash. Seat belts should fit snugly so the hips and shoulders suffer the greatest impact. These areas of the body can best withstand the impact of a crash. Both the lap belt and shoulder restraint are necessary for the greatest protection. The lap belt keeps the body from moving forward, and the shoulder restraint protects the head and face from coming into contact with the vehicle's dashboard or windshield.

Because a large percentage of motor vehicle deaths result from frontal impact crashes, air bags are engineered to protect passengers and drivers involved in these types of accidents. Although air bags can reduce injuries to the head and chest, they are not intended to replace seat belts. In fact, air bags make seat belts even more effective. When air bags are used in addition to lap belts and shoulder restraints, the risk of injury to the head is greatly reduced.

Distraction on the part of the driver can also be a cause of motor vehicle accidents. According to a U.S. Department of Transportation Web site that focuses on distracted drivers (http://www.distraction.gov), more than 3,000 people were killed in the United States in 2012 due to a distracted driver. Distractions can occur in three forms: visual (taking your eyes off of the road), manual (taking your hands off of the steering wheel), and cognitive (taking your mind off of the task of driving). Sending text messages, for example, is one of the most dangerous activities listed because it involves all three types of distractions. Other activities that can be distracting include talking on a cell phone; eating or drinking; using a PDA (personal digital assistant) or navigation device such as a GPS (global positioning system); watching a video; or changing the radio station, CD, or MP3 player.

## 🔍 CHECKPOINT QUESTION

9. What human health effects are thought to be caused by air pollution?

## Dental Health

Dental health is an important part of a person's overall health. Regular brushing and flossing removes plaque between and around the individual teeth reducing **dental cavities** (decay and holes in the teeth) and promoting healthy gums. Unattended cavities have a profound effect on the gums as well as on the sinuses and the throat. There are many affordable dental products that make dental health simple for patients, including battery-powered toothbrushes, plastic floss holders, and tongue cleaners. Keeping teeth in good repair with regular dental checkups promotes better general health.

## Positive Mental Outlook

Having a positive mental outlook can benefit your health and well-being and possibly even prolong life. Experts say that genetics may play a part in mental attitude, but you also have control over your feelings and emotions. Maybe you cannot control certain events, but you can control your reactions to them or how you let the events affect your daily activities or interactions with others. There have been many instances of terminally ill patients who fared better than expected because they maintained a positive outlook. In almost every situation, you can identify positive and negative aspects. If you pay attention to the positive and downplay the negative, you can train your brain to have a positive attitude.

## Genetics

It is undeniable that genetics determine a great deal in regard to your health. However, even if your parents suffered from ill health, there are ways of reducing your own health risks. Studies have shown that genetics play a large role in what diseases a person contracts, but patients should not use this as an excuse to ignore risk factors. Even if there has been no lung cancer in a family, tobacco use would still increase the risk. In other words, good genes can be negated by bad health habits.

### Infectious Disease Prevention

Fortunately, the body is equipped with a remarkable immune system that protects a healthy person from illness or injury from most germs or pathogens. However, you can control how many of these germs enter the body by taking a few precautions. Proper hand washing is known to be the best defense against illness. Because germs must enter the body to make you sick, the hands are usually the mode of transportation. Wearing personal protective equipment when handling body fluids will protect you in the workplace. As a health care worker, you are trained to stay safe from blood-borne pathogens. These same actions should be taken at home. Using safe practices in the kitchen and bathroom will also reduce the spread of disease. Preventing the spread of infection takes care and attention. Box 16-3 gives some tips for avoiding infectious or contagious diseases.

## Substance Abuse

Substance abuse is characterized by the excessive use of and dependency on drugs. Some abused substances are legal (e.g., alcohol, nicotine), whereas others are illegal (e.g., marijuana, cocaine). Patients with substance abuse problems may seek help from trained specialists or counselors or they may come to the physician office seeking help with their dependency issue. Because substance abuse can be highly detrimental to your patients' health, it is important that you have information available about substance abuse for patients who may have a substance abuse problem. Although many national organizations can provide information, your medical office should also have information available for patients on any local chapters or organizations that may help these patients.

## Alcohol

Alcohol is one of the most commonly abused legal substances. Although there have been studies done that link a daily glass of red wine to a potential reduced risk for heart disease, overconsumption of alcohol can contribute to certain health problems. These problems include high blood pressure, cardiomyopathy, fetal alcohol syndrome, and, in some cases of long-term alcohol abuse, possible liver damage.

## BOX 16-3    Things to do to Prevent Infectious Diseases

1. Keep immunizations up to date:
   • Follow recommended immunizations for children and adults.
   • Immunize your pets.
2. Wash your hands often, especially during cold and flu season. Be sure to wash hands:
   • After using the bathroom
   • Before preparing or eating food
   • After changing a diaper
   • After blowing your nose or sneezing or coughing
   • After caring for a sick person
   • After playing with a pet
3. Prepare and handle food carefully:
   • Keep hot foods hot and cold foods cold until eaten or cooked.
   • Be sure temperature controls in refrigerators and freezers are working properly.
   • Wash counters, cutting boards, and utensils frequently with soap and hot water, especially after preparing poultry and other meats.
   • Wash fresh fruits and vegetables before eating.
   • Cook ground beef until you can no longer see any pink.
4. Use antibiotics only for infections caused by bacteria:
   • Take antibiotics exactly as prescribed, and complete the full course of treatment.
   • Never self-medicate with antibiotics or share them with family or friends.
   • Report to your doctor any quickly worsening infection or any infection that does not get better after you finish a prescribed antibiotic.
5. Avoid insect bites:
   • Use insect repellents on skin and clothing when in areas where ticks or mosquitoes are common.
   • If you have visited wooded or wilderness areas and become sick, tell your doctor all the details in order to help diagnose both rare and common illnesses quickly.
6. Stay alert to disease threats when you travel or visit developing countries:
   • Get all recommended immunizations.
   • Use protective medications for travel, especially to areas with malaria.
   • Do not drink untreated water while hiking or camping.
   • If you become ill when you return home, tell your doctor where you've been.
7. Develop healthy habits:
   • Eat well, get enough sleep, exercise, and avoid tobacco and illegal drug use.
   • When sick, allow yourself time to heal and recover.
   • Be courteous to others: wash your hands frequently, and cover your mouth when you sneeze or cough.

*Source*: Epidemiology and Disease Control and Prevention http://www.edcp.org/factsheets/prevent.cfm

Some people can drink in moderation. Others are prone to addiction, which is an illness and should be treated as such. Because alcohol contains ethanol, it is considered a mind-altering substance. Ethanol works as a depressant within the central nervous system. The effects of alcohol intoxication include a lack of coordination, slurred speech, blurred vision, and impaired brain function. Large quantities of alcohol can have a negative effect on such basic functions as breathing and heart rate. The long-term effects of excessive alcohol use can include cirrhosis of the liver, certain cancers, an increased risk of stroke, and nutritional deficiencies.

## Drugs

Some drugs, like marijuana and hashish, impair short-term memory and comprehension. In addition to altering the user's sense of time and reducing the ability to perform tasks requiring concentration and coordination, these drugs also increase the heart rate and appetite. Long-term users may develop psychological dependence. Because these drugs are inhaled as unfiltered smoke, users take in more cancer-causing agents and do more damage to the respiratory system than with regular filtered tobacco smoke.

Cocaine and crack cocaine are extremely addictive. These illegal drugs stimulate the central nervous system. Crack cocaine is particularly dangerous because this pure form of cocaine is usually smoked and absorbed rapidly in the bloodstream. Use of these drugs can result in psychological and physical dependency and may even cause sudden death. The physical effects of using these substances include dilated pupils, increased pulse rate, elevated blood pressure, insomnia, loss of appetite, paranoia, and seizures. It can also cause death by disrupting the brain's control of the heart and respiration.

Stimulants and amphetamines can have the same effect as cocaine, causing increased heart rate and blood pressure. Symptoms of stimulant use include dizziness, sleeplessness, anxiety, psychosis, hallucinations, paranoia, and even physical collapse. The long-term effects of these substances include hypertension, heart disease, stroke, and renal and liver failure.

Depressants and barbiturates can also cause physical and psychological dependence. Abuse of these drugs can lead to respiratory depression, coma, and death, especially when they are taken with alcohol. Withdrawal can lead to restlessness, insomnia, convulsions, and death.

Hallucinogens, such as lysergic acid diethylamide (LSD), phencyclidine ("angel dust" or PCP), mescaline, and peyote, all interrupt brain messages that control the intellect and keep instincts in check. Large doses can produce seizures, coma, and heart and lung failure. Chronic users complain of persistent memory problems and speech difficulties for up to a year after discontinuing use. Because hallucinogens stop the brain's pain sensors, drug experiences may result in severe self-inflicted injuries.

Narcotics, such as heroin, codeine, morphine, and opium, are addictive drugs. These drugs can produce euphoria, drowsiness, and blood pressure and pulse fluctuations. An overdose can lead to seizures, coma, cardiac arrest, and death.

It is important to teach all pregnant women the damage substance abuse may do to their unborn child and to refer pregnant patients to support services. The most important role of the medical assistant in educating patients about any type of substance abuse is to be supportive and have a list of community resources available to assist patients who need them. Provide positive reinforcements as appropriate and offer services to patients for cessation programs.

## Smoking Cessation

The health risks associated with smoking have been well documented for many years. Nicotine is highly addictive whether ingested by inhaling or chewing. This drug reaches the brain in 6 seconds, damages the blood vessels, decreases heart strength, and is associated with many cancers. The withdrawal symptoms include anxiety, progressive restlessness, irritability, and sleep disturbances. There are numerous methods to try to stop smoking; however, the methods vary greatly. Some programs have the patient gradually stop, while other programs seek a total, abrupt stoppage. There are research data to support both methods.

### PATIENT EDUCATION

**Smoking Cessation Requires Help**

Here are some suggestions to help patients stop smoking:

- Find local smoking cessation support groups. Provide phone numbers and contact names of these groups to your patients.

- If there are no local support groups, the American Heart Association, American Lung Association, or American Cancer Society may help.
- Discuss with the physician the options of prescribing various patches, gums, or other interventions for the patient. Some products have side effects, and the physician may opt not to order them based on the patient's age or other medical illnesses.

### ROLE-PLAYING ACTIVITY

Review the case study found at the beginning of this chapter. Role-play the following scenario assuming you are Jack, the medical assistant at Great Falls Medical Center, and another student is Katie, the mother of a 7-year-old girl named Tabitha. Katie has brought Tabitha in to be seen by the physician because the school sent home a note saying she was "overweight." Tabitha is in the second grade and is 49 inches tall and weighs 75 pounds. Research this weight and/or calculate the BMI for this child. Is she overweight for her age, gender, and height? Her mother insists that she is not overweight and is angry about the school sending home a note "implying" she is a "bad mother" and "does not take care of her children." How should Jack respond to this mother who is angry and defensive? Why would Katie feel like the school is calling her a "bad mother?" When speaking with Katie, Tabitha begins to whine that she "wants to leave" and that her mother promised her a milkshake on the way home. How should Jack respond to Tabitha's request? Explain your response, perhaps having another student role play Tabitha. Your instructor will give you additional information about this activity!

## *español* SPANISH TERMINOLOGY

**Debes llevar una dieta balanceada. Utiliza la pirámide de alimentos como guía para ayudarte a escojer los mejores alimentos.**
You should have a balanced diet. Using the food guide pyramid helps you to choose the right foods.

**En estas fotos, voy a poner un círculo en todos los alimentos que puede comer.**
Using these pictures, I'll circle the foods you can have.

**Estos son los alimentos que debe evitar.**
These are the foods you should avoid.

**Debe hacer ejercicios por lo menos tres veces a la semana.**
You should exercise at least three times a week.

**Su salud oral es muy importante; asegurese de cuidar sus dientes.**
Your oral health is very important; take care of it.

**El Indice de Masa Corporal es un indicador muy importante de su estado de Nutrición y Bienestar.**
BMI is a very important indicator of Nutrition and Wellness.

**Los carbohidratos son communmente conocidos como azucares.**
Carbohydrates are commonly known as sugars.

**Legumbres son una fuente natural de proteínas.**
Legumes are a source of incomplete proteins.

**Los Lipidos son conocidos como las grasas.**
Lipids are also known as fats.

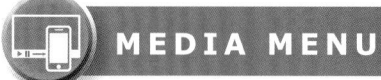

# MEDIA MENU

**Student Resources** on thePoint®

• **CMA/RMA Certification Exam Review**

**Internet Resources**

**Your guide to lowering your cholesterol with TLC**.
NIH Publication No. 06-5235, December 2005
http://www.nhlbi.nih.gov/health/public/heart/chol/chol_tlc.pdf

**The President's Challenge Adult Fitness Test**
http://www.adultfitnesstest.org/

**Health Information for Individuals and Families**
http://www.health.gov/

**Health People government website**
http://www.healthypeople.gov/2020/default.aspx

**Body Mass Index**
http://www.cdc.gov/healthyweight/assessing/bmi/

**Dietary Guidelines**
http://www.health.gov/dietaryguidelines

**U.S. Department of Agriculture's MyPlate Website**
http://www.choosemyplate.gov/

**American Running and Fitness Association**
http://www.americanrunning.org

**President's Council on Fitness, Sports & Nutrition**
http://www.fitness.gov

**American Alliance for Health, Physical Education, Recreation and Dance**
http://www.aahperd.org

**March of Dimes**
http://www.marchofdimes.com

**American Heart Association**
http://www.heart.org/HEARTORG

**American Lung Association**
http://www.lungusa.org

**Information on Alcoholism**
http://www.cdc.gov/alcohol/faqs.htm

## EMR Activity

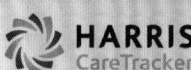

Harris CareTracker is a Web-based electronic medical record (EMR) application that you will use for the EMR activities included in this section at the end of each chapter. This application is actually used in physician offices, but is provided to you through the publisher, Wolters Kluwer Health, to give you hands-on practice working with EMRs. Your instructor will have more information about accessing your username, login, and Quickstart guide.

Prerequisite Activities in Harris CareTracker

*Note*: The Getting Started and Quickstart documents and EMR Activities Step-by-Step Instructions listed below are available at http://thePoint.lww.com/KronenbergerComp5e

Activity Details

Using only legitimate sources, create a healthy eating plan brochure to share with diabetic patients. Use a computer word processing software to create your brochure, cite your sources at the end, and upload it into Harris CareTracker using *Patient Education Upload* under the *Clinical* tab of the *Administration* module.

## Chapter Summary

- Good nutrition and a healthy lifestyle are important to everyone. Knowing the guidelines for a healthy and safe life is important, but practicing those guidelines is essential.
- There is a growing trend in the United States toward obesity, especially among children and young people. The federal government is working to reverse this trend.
- Following the recommendations of the physician will give your patients a better chance at good health and longevity.
- There are ways to stay as safe and healthy, even during daily activities like driving a car. Medical assistants should be prepared to teach these safe and healthy living habits.
- The same safe practices for reducing the spread of disease in the health care workplace, such as hand washing, can be used at home to keep you, your family, and your patients safe from pathogens and infectious diseases.
- To increase chances of good health, patients should be encouraged to limit or avoid harmful substances such as nicotine, alcohol, and drugs. Knowing the benefits of good nutrition, physical fitness, and applying suggestions for staying safe and healthy will give patients a good foundation for making the right choices in life.

## Warm-Ups for Critical Thinking

1. The physician asks you to assist a 65-year-old patient with a low-cholesterol diet. Write a plan for the instruction. Help her plan several sample meals to help get her started. What would you say to her?
2. A 12-year-old boy presents for his routine yearly physical. His current weight is 150 pounds, and his growth chart indicates a steady increase in body weight. Explain the dangers of obesity to the patient's mother. Go to http://www.cdc.gov, search for body mass index, and click on the BMI calculator. Enter the information to complete a BMI chart for the patient with the following measurements: 5 feet, 5 inches tall, 150 pounds, date of birth 5/28/1994.
3. Keep track of all of the food that you consume over a 24-hour period. Calculate your total fat and total carbohydrate intake. Do your meals follow the MyPlate guidelines? If not, what do you need to do to improve your nutritional status? Using pictures from magazines, create well-balanced breakfast, lunch, and dinner plates. Hint: Your plate should be colorful.

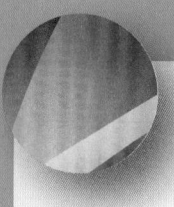

# PSY PROCEDURE 16-1

## Teach a Patient How to Read Food Labels

**Purpose:** To instruct a patient in how to read a food label so that he or she may make better food choices

**Equipment:** Two boxes of the same item, one low calorie or "lite" and the other regular; measuring cup; two bowls; refer to Figure 16-4 for reference

| STEPS | REASONS |
|---|---|
| 1. Identify the patient. | Correctly identifying the patient prevents errors. |
| 2. **AFF** Introduce yourself and explain the procedure including the rationale. | Explaining procedures including the rationale may reduce patient anxiety and improve compliance. |
| 3. Have the patient look at the labels, briefly comparing the two. | Taking an overall look at the label will show the patient the types of items listed. |
| 4. Ask the patient to pour out a normal serving into a bowl. | The patient's perception of a normal serving size may be wrong. |
| 5. Measure the exact serving size printed on the label. Compare the two. Discuss the difference, if any. | Using a measuring cup will show the patient the accuracy of the serving size. Serving sizes noted on package labels are often lesser amounts than what a patient might naturally consume without measuring, which would result in more calories. |
| 6. Explain to the patient each section of the label:<br>a. Serving size and servings per package<br>b. Column for amount in serving<br>c. Column for % daily value (formerly called the *recommended daily allowance [RDA]*) | The patient may be surprised that his or her servings are more or less than on the label, which changes the weights and daily values. |
| 7. Explain calories and calories from fat. Have the patient calculate the percentage of fat calories by multiplying the grams of fat by 9 and dividing that number by the total calories per serving as listed on the label. Multiply the answer by 100. This number is the percentage of calories from fat. | Although manufacturers are required to list this information, patients should know how this is calculated. |
| 8. Read down the label and discuss each nutrient, pointing out the amounts and percentages. | Seeing the labels will help the patient understand. |
| 9. Have the patient compare the two labels and tell you how many total carbohydrates, sugars, and amounts of protein, etc., are on each label. | This will ensure that the patient understands how to determine the types and amounts of ingredients. |
| 10. **AFF** Explain how to respond to a patient who has a religious or personal belief against specific food groups such as meats. | Patients with religious or personal beliefs that eliminate specific foods or food groups may need to be referred to a registered dietician as directed by the physician. Always make sure the physician is aware of any food preferences or allergies. |
| 11. Ask the patient if he or she has any questions. | Having the patient answer your questions and giving him or her an opportunity to ask you questions will ensure the patient's comprehension of the information. |

*(continues on page 400)*

## PROCEDURE 16.1 (continued)

| STEPS | REASONS |
|---|---|
| 12. **AFF** Log into the Electronic Medical Record (EMR) using your username and secure password OR obtain the paper medical record from a secure location and assure it is kept away from public access. | The integrity of the medical record must be maintained at all times to protect patient privacy. |
| 13. Chart the verbal and written instructions given to the patient. When finished, log out of the EMR and/or replace the paper medical record in an appropriate and secure location. | The physician and other workers in the office may need to know what the patient has been taught. Remember, if it's not in the chart, it did not happen. |

---

**Charting Example**

*9/25/15 Pt. given instructions on reading a food label. Pt. verbalized understanding and eagerness to make healthier food choices. Instructed to call the office for any questions or concerns* _____
_____ *C. Parent, CMA(AAMA)*

---

Note: *The medical assistant may sign his/her name in the patient record using only the "CMA" credential if the office has a signature log denoting the entire credential as "CMA(AAMA)."*

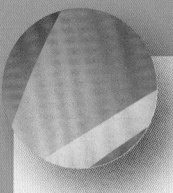

**PSY** PROCEDURE 16-2

## Develop a Meal Plan Utilizing Basic Principles of Nutrition and Instruct a Patient According to Patient's Special Dietary Needs

**Purpose:** To develop a meal plan and instruct a patient so that he or she may achieve better health based on medical needs and physician instructions

**Equipment:** Reference materials related to dietary choices that include nutritional components (i.e., calories and nutrient amounts such as protein, fat, and carbohydrates), a physician order, and the patient medical record

| STEPS | REASONS |
|---|---|
| 1. Review the physician order to determine the specific nutritional information necessary for patient instruction. | Only the physician or other health care professional legally permitted to diagnose and treat patients may prescribe dietary changes. |
| 2. Identify the patient. | Correctly identifying the patient prevents errors. |
| 3. Introduce yourself and explain the procedure including the rationale. | Explaining procedures may reduce patient anxiety and improve compliance. |
| 4. Develop a meal plan based on a regular (i.e., no special dietary needs) 2,000-calorie diet and include information on basic nutrition (nutrients, serving sizes, and calories). Printable materials may be used during instruction from the choosemyplate.gov Web site if approved by the physician. | Never assume the patient has knowledge of basic nutrients. |
| 5. **AFF** Observe the patient during instruction for nonverbal signs such as confusion, interest or disinterest, emotions, etc. | Revising instruction as needed based on the patient responses during instruction may clarify any misperceptions and/or increase compliance with instructions. |
| 6. **AFF** Explain how to respond to a patient who verbalizes concern about the ability to purchase fresh fruits and vegetables due to lack of monetary resources and reliance on public transportation to shop for groceries. | Regardless of a patient's economic status, purchasing fresh fruits or vegetables may be less expensive than canned varieties, which may contain increased sugar or salt. Explain that canned foods may be acceptable, but look for labels that indicate no sugar or salt. Always demonstrate respect for individual patient diversity. |
| 7. Instruct a patient according to one of the following special dietary needs as ordered by the physician:<br>a. Low sodium<br>b. Low fat<br>c. Low carbohydrate<br>d. High protein<br>e. Restricted calorie (i.e., 1,500, 1,800, etc.)<br>f. Lactose free<br>g. Gluten free<br>h. High fiber | Explaining the special dietary needs may increase compliance with the prescribed diet and provide health benefits to the patient. |
| 8. Ask the patient questions during instruction and allow the opportunity for the patient to ask questions during instruction and at the end. | Having the patient answer your questions and giving him or her an opportunity to ask you questions will ensure the patient's comprehension of the information. |

*(continues on page 402)*

## PROCEDURE 16.2 (continued)

| STEPS | REASONS |
|---|---|
| 9. **AFF** Explain how to respond to a patient who has a religious or personal belief against specific food groups such as a vegetarian. | Patients with religious or personal beliefs that eliminate specific foods or food groups may need to be referred to a registered dietician as directed by the physician. Always make sure the physician is aware of any food preferences or allergies. |
| 10. **AFF** Log into the Electronic Medical Record (EMR) using your username and secure password OR obtain the paper medical record from a secure location and assure it is kept away from public access. | The integrity of the medical record must be maintained at all times to protect patient privacy. |
| 11. Chart the verbal and written instructions given to the patient. When finished, log out of the EMR and/or replace the paper medical record in an appropriate and secure location. | The physician and other workers in the office may need to know what the patient has been taught. Remember, if it's not in the chart, it did not happen. |

Charting Example
*04/11/15 Pt. instructed on 2,000-calorie, low-salt diet. Pt. verbalized understanding and was given written information including a sample meal plan. Instructed to call the office for any questions or concerns*
_____ *P. Bratt, RMA*

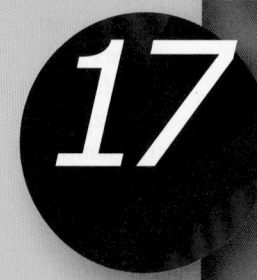

# 17 Medical Asepsis and Infection Control

## Outline

**Microorganisms, Pathogens, and Normal Flora**
Conditions That Favor the Growth of Pathogens
**The Infection Cycle**
Modes of Transmission

**Principles of Infection Control**
Medical Asepsis
Levels of Infection Control
**Infection Control for the Medical Office**
Exposure Risk Factors and the Exposure Control Plan

Standard Precautions
Personal Protective Equipment
Handling Environmental Contamination
Disposing of Infectious Waste
Hepatitis B and Human Immunodeficiency Viruses

## Learning Outcomes

### COG Cognitive Domain*

1. Spell and define key terms
2. *Describe the infection cycle, including the infectious agent, reservoir, susceptible host, means of transmission, portals of entry, and portals of exit*
3. *List major types of infectious agents*
4. *Identify different methods of controlling the growth of microorganisms*
5. Define the following as practiced within an ambulatory care setting: a. medical asepsis b. surgical asepsis
6. *List the various ways microbes are transmitted*
7. *Define the principles of standard precautions*
8. Compare the effectiveness in reducing or destroying microorganisms using the various levels of infection control
9. Identify personal safety precautions as established by the Occupational Safety and Health Administration (OSHA)
10. *Define personal protective equipment (PPE) for the following: a. all body fluids, secretions, and excretions; b. blood; c. nonintact skin; d. mucous membranes*
11. *Identify Center for Disease Control (CDC) regulations that impact health care practices*
12. List the required components of an exposure control plan
13. Explain the facts pertaining to the transmission and prevention of the hepatitis B virus and the human immunodeficiency virus in the medical office

### PSY Psychomotor Domain*

1. *Perform a medical aseptic hand washing procedure (Procedure 17-1)*
2. Select appropriate PPE and remove contaminated gloves (Procedure 17-2)
3. Clean and decontaminate biohazardous spills (Procedure 17-3)
4. Participate in blood-borne pathogen training (Procedure 17-4)

### AFF Affective Domain*

1. *Incorporate critical thinking skills when performing patient care*
2. *Recognize the implications for failure to comply with the Center for Disease Control (CDC) regulations in health care settings*

*Note: AAMA/CAAHEP 2015 Standards are italicized.*

### ABHES Competencies

1. Apply principles of aseptic techniques and infection control
2. Use standard precautions
3. Dispose of biohazardous materials

*(continues on page 404)*

aerobe
anaerobe
asymptomatic
bactericidal
biohazardous
carriers
Centers for Disease
  Control and Prevention
  (CDC) disease
disease

disinfection
exposure control
  plan
exposure risk factor
germicide
immunization
infection
medical asepsis
microorganisms
normal flora

Occupational Safety and
  Health Administration
  (OSHA)
pathogens
personal protective
  equipment (PPE)
postexposure testing
resident flora
resistance
sanitation

sanitization
spores
standard precautions
sterilization
transient flora
vector
viable
virulent

## Case Study

*B*onita Jackson, RMA, is responsible for infection control practices in the urgent care, walk-in clinic at Great Falls Medical Center where she works as a clinical medical assistant. Part of her responsibilities include conducting standard precautions training for all new employees and yearly training for all current employees. Today, she is orienting Robert Townsend, a medical assistant student, to the office. Part of the orientation includes giving him the office policy and procedures manual to review, which includes information about infection control practices and standard precautions. Bonita also shows the student where the hazard communication safety data sheets are located. The student asks whether these are the same as material safety data sheets. He also asks why some trash containers in the examination room have red bags and others have white ones and whether different types of trash should go in each. Finally, he asks why there is an office policy about not putting gauze or adhesive bandages contaminated with blood in the sharps container. How would you answer his questions?

Many patients are seen daily in the medical office for a variety of reasons, including physical examinations for employment, reassurance about a current health problem, and follow-up care for a chronic condition or surgical procedure. In addition, many patients request appointments because of illness. It is important for you to protect patients from each other with regard to contagious diseases and for you to protect yourself from acquiring the many microorganisms with which you will come into contact every day.

To prevent the spread of **disease** in the medical office, medical assistants must meet two goals. First, you must understand and practice **medical asepsis** at all times, using specific practices and procedures to prevent disease transmission. These practices and procedures also allow you to work with ill patients while reducing the chances that you will spread disease to other patients or become infected yourself. Second, you must teach the

patients and their families about techniques to use at home to prevent the transmission of disease. Hand washing, the cornerstone of infection control, is discussed in this chapter and is emphasized in all subsequent chapters wherever contact with infectious material might be expected. In addition, this chapter describes how disease is transmitted and, most important, how to prevent the spread of disease.

## cog MICROORGANISMS, PATHOGENS, AND NORMAL FLORA

**Microorganisms**, living organisms that can be seen only with a microscope, are part of our normal environment. In addition to our physical environment, many microorganisms can be found on your skin and throughout your gastrointestinal, genitourinary, and respiratory systems, and some of these are required for good health. These microorganisms are normal and are referred to as **normal flora** or **resident flora**. Some microorganisms, however, are not part of the normal flora and may cause disease or **infection**. Disease-producing microorganisms are referred to as **pathogens** and are classified as bacteria, viruses, fungi, or protozoa. (Refer to Chapter 44 for a more detailed discussion of microorganisms.)

When normal flora become too many in number or are transmitted to an area of the body in which they are not normally found, they are referred to as **transient flora**, which can become pathogens under the right conditions. For example, *Staphylococcus aureus*, a microorganism commonly found on the skin, may get into underlying tissue if the skin is broken. In this situation, the normal flora of the skin has become transient flora and may cause disease. Decreased **resistance** in the host is one condition that may allow transient flora to become pathogenic. Individuals who are elderly, receiving certain drugs to treat cancer, or under unusual stress may have a lowered resistance and be particularly susceptible to infections.

Although the body is protected by many nonspecific defenses against disease, infection or illness may occur if the natural barriers are overpowered or breached. The following are some of the body's natural defenses that may prevent the invasion of pathogens into various body organs:

- *Skin*. As long as the skin is kept clean and remains intact or unbroken, staphylococcal (Staph) bacteria are not considered dangerous. Washing the skin frequently will flush away many of these bacteria along with any other microorganisms.
- *Eyes*. The eyelashes act as a barrier by trapping dust that may carry microorganisms before they have an opportunity to enter the eye. If any microorganisms do enter the eye, the enzyme lysozyme normally found in tears will destroy some microorganisms, including bacteria.
- *Mouth*. The greatest variety of microorganisms in the body is in the mouth. Saliva is slightly **bactericidal**, and good oral hygiene will remove or prevent the growth of many of the pathogens in the mouth.
- *Gastrointestinal tract*. Hydrochloric acid normally found in the stomach destroys most of the disease-producing pathogens that enter the gastrointestinal system. One bacterium, *Escherichia coli*, is resident flora found in the large intestine and is necessary for digestion. It does not usually cause disease as long it remains within the gastrointestinal tract. *Helicobacter pylori* also resides in the digestive tracts of some individuals and may cause gastric ulcers.
- *Respiratory tract*. Hairs and cilia on the membrane lining of the nostrils are early defenses against airborne microorganisms. If these physical barriers do not stop

an invasion, mucus from the membranes lining the respiratory tract should trap the microorganisms and facilitate their removal from the respiratory system as the person swallows, coughs, or sneezes.
- *Genitourinary tract*. The reproductive and urinary systems provide a less hospitable environment for microorganisms. The slightly acidic environment of these body systems reduces the ability of many microorganisms to survive. In addition, frequent urination flushes the urinary tract and removes many transient microorganisms.

Although these systems have protective mechanisms to prevent infection, any of them may be overpowered by a particularly **virulent** organism. Transient flora is not usually pathogenic unless the person's defenses are compromised by a decrease in resistance.

## CHECKPOINT QUESTION

1. Based on what Bonita learned in her medical assisting program, what are pathogenic microorganisms? How does the body prevent an invasion and subsequent infection naturally?

## Conditions That Favor the Growth of Pathogens

All microorganisms require certain conditions to grow and reproduce. To reduce the number of microorganisms and potential pathogens in a clinical setting, you must eliminate as many of their life requirements as possible. These requirements include the following:

- *Moisture*. Few microorganisms can survive with little water or moisture. However, some microorganisms form **spores** and remain dormant until moisture is available.
- *Nutrients*. Microorganisms depend on their environment for nourishment. Surfaces (tables, counters, equipment, etc.) that are contaminated with organic matter (food products, body fluids, or tissue) promote the growth of microorganisms.
- *Temperature*. Although some microorganisms can survive even in freezing or boiling temperatures, those that thrive at a normal body temperature of 98.6°F are most likely to be pathogenic to humans. Many microorganisms that leave an infected person can survive for a while at room temperature; therefore, surfaces that are contaminated with dried organic material should be considered possibly pathogenic.
- *Darkness*. Many pathogenic bacteria are destroyed by bright light, including sunlight.
- *Neutral pH*. The pH of a solution refers to the measurement of its acid–base balance on a scale of 1 to 14, with 7 being neutral. Many microorganisms are

destroyed in an environment that is not neutral. The pH of blood (7.35 to 7.45) is preferred by microorganisms that thrive in the human body.

• *Oxygen.* Microorganisms that need oxygen to survive are called **aerobes**. A few, however, do not require oxygen; these are called **anaerobes**. Although most pathogens are aerobic, the microbes that cause tetanus and botulism are anaerobic.

If any one of these conditions is altered in any way, the growth and reproduction of the pathogen will be affected. Your role as a professional medical assistant in a medical office includes using this knowledge of microbial growth to inhibit the growth and reproduction of microorganisms in the office.

### 🔍 CHECKPOINT QUESTION

2. Given the six conditions that favor the growth of pathogens, explain how you can alter the growth and reproduction of microorganisms by changing these factors.

### 🎓 THE INFECTION CYCLE

The infection cycle is often thought of as a series of specific links of a chain involving a causative agent or invading microorganism (Fig. 17-1). The first link in the chain is the reservoir host; this is the person who is infected with the microorganism. Although this person may or may not show signs of infection, his or her body

is serving as a source of nutrients and an incubator in which the pathogen can grow and reproduce. These persons are also called **carriers**, or reservoirs, of disease.

The reservoir host may transmit disease only when the pathogen has a means of exit. The second link in the chain is the manner in which the pathogen leaves the reservoir host. Means of exit include the mucous membranes of the nose and mouth, the openings of the gastrointestinal system (mouth or rectum), and an open wound.

In addition to the means of exit, the microbe must have a vehicle in which to leave the host. This next link in the chain, the means of transmission, involves the vehicle that is used by the pathogen when it leaves the reservoir host and spreads through the environment. Vehicles include mucus or air droplets from the oral or nasal cavities and direct contact between an unclean hand and another person or object. Sneezing and coughing without covering the nose and mouth are excellent methods of transmitting microorganisms into the environment and potential hosts.

The fourth link in the chain of the infectious process cycle is the portal of entry. This is the route by which the pathogen enters the next host. With inhalation of contaminated air droplets, the respiratory system is the portal of entry. Another portal of entry is the gastrointestinal system: the pathogen enters the body in contaminated food or drink. Any break in the skin or mucous membranes can be a portal of entry for pathogenic microorganisms.

The final link in the infectious process cycle is the susceptible host (Box 17-1). This host is one to whom the pathogen is transmitted after leaving the reservoir

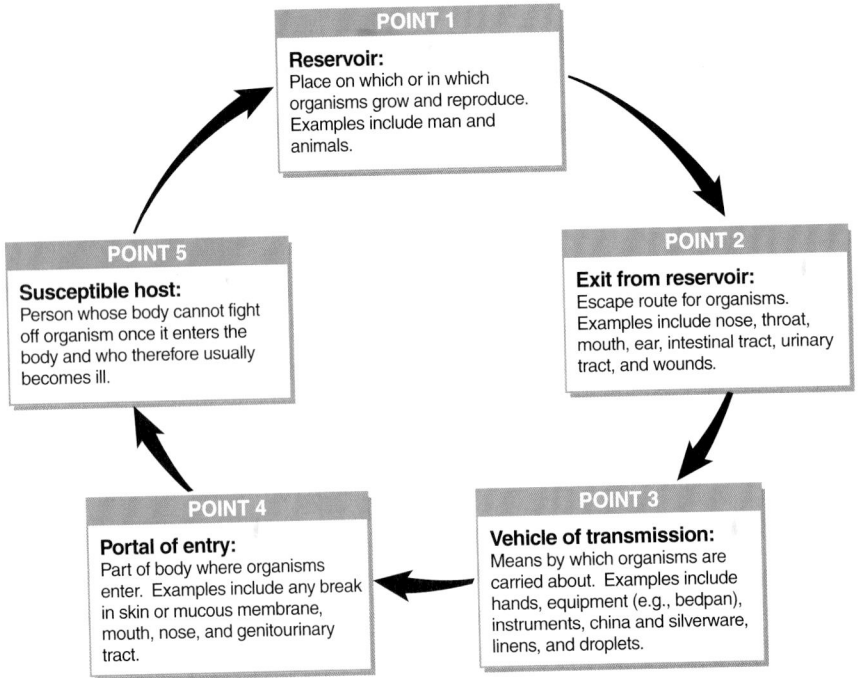

**Figure 17-1 •** The infectious process cycle. Infections and infectious diseases are spread by starting from the reservoir (point 1) and moving in a circle to the susceptible host (point 5). Microorganisms can be controlled by interfering at any point in the cycle.

The susceptible host is unable to resist the invading pathogens for a variety of reasons:

- *Age.* As the body ages, defense mechanisms begin to lose their effectiveness. The immune system is no longer as active or as efficient as in youth. The immune system may also not be fully functional in the very young.
- *Existing disease.* The stress of an existing illness may deplete the immune system and allow microorganisms to cause illness in someone who might otherwise be able to fight it naturally.
- *Poor nutrition.* A diet deficient in nutrients such as proteins, carbohydrates, fats, vitamins, or minerals will not allow cells of the body to repair or reproduce as they are weakened by disease.
- *Poor hygiene.* Although multitudes of microbes exist on our skin, keeping the numbers down by practicing good hygiene will reduce the numbers of pathogens.

host. If the conditions in the susceptible host are conducive to reproduction of the pathogen, the susceptible host becomes a reservoir host and the cycle repeats.

## CHECKPOINT QUESTION

3. Bonita explains how the first and fifth links of the infection cycle are related. In your own words, can you explain how these links are related?

## Modes of Transmission

In the third link of the infectious process cycle, the vehicle that spreads the microorganism is often called the mode of transmission. It is important for you to understand the mode of transmission used by various pathogens so that you can break this link in the infectious cycle and prevent the spread of disease.

### Direct Transmission

Direct contact between the infected reservoir host and the susceptible host produces direct transmission. Direct transmission may occur when one touches contaminated blood or body fluids, shakes hands with someone who has contaminated hands, inhales infected air droplets, or has intimate contact, such as kissing or sexual intercourse, with someone who is contaminated.

### Indirect Transmission

Indirect transmission may occur through contact with a vehicle known as a **vector**. Vectors include contaminated food or water, disease-carrying insects, and inanimate

objects such as soil, drinking glasses, wound drainage, and infected or improperly disinfected medical instruments. While visible blood and body fluids are obvious sources of infection, many infectious organisms remain **viable** for long periods on inanimate surfaces that are not visibly contaminated.

## Sources of Transmission

Most reservoir hosts are humans, animals, and insects. Human hosts include people who are ill with an infectious disease, people who are carriers of an infectious disease, and people who are incubating an infectious disease but are not exhibiting symptoms. This last group can transmit disease even though they are ambulatory and **asymptomatic** (have no symptoms). Animal sources, which are less common, include infected dogs, cats, birds, cattle, rodents, and animals that live in the wild. Diseases that may be transmitted to humans from infected animals include anthrax and rabies.

In addition to flies and roaches, which carry many diseases, other insect sources feed on the blood of an infected reservoir host and then pass the disease to another victim or susceptible host. Ticks and mosquitoes may transmit diseases, including Lyme disease (ticks) and malaria (mosquitoes). Table 17-1 lists some common diseases and their methods of transmission.

## CHECKPOINT QUESTION

4. Great Falls Medical Center has a policy about not opening windows that do not have screens in examination rooms and the reception area. Why do you think this policy is or is not important?

## WHAT IF?

**Many of the symptoms of Ebola virus disease (EVD) are symptoms of other less serious diseases. What if a patient comes into the office where you work and exhibits symptoms of the Ebola virus?**

Ebola, also known as hemorrhagic fever, is caused by a virus originally found in some African countries. While the source of human transmission is not known, infection with the virus typically occurs as a result of direct contact with blood and body fluids or contaminated objects of a person infected with the virus. Generally, the virus is not spread through air, water, or food.

The symptoms of EVD may include fever, severe headache, muscle pain, weakness, diarrhea, nausea and vomiting, abdominal pain, and unexplained bleeding or bruising. The Centers for Disease Control and Prevention (CDC) recommends health care workers respond to possible cases of EVD by utilizing the following steps:

- **Identify**
  - Ask every patient if they have traveled to any high-risk countries (Guinea, Liberia, or Sierra Leone) or if they may have come into contact with anyone infected with EVD.
- **Isolate**
  - If a patient answers "yes" to either of the questions above, immediately isolate the patient by placing them in an exam room by themselves, determine the types of personal protective equipment needed, and have minimal contact with the patient if possible.
- **Inform**
  - Once the patient is isolated, inform the public health department that you may have a patient who has been exposed to the Ebola virus. The public health department officials will assist you in transferring the patient to a facility that can further assess the patient. The patient can only be transferred to a facility that has been approved by the public health department.

*Source*: http://www.cdc.gov/vhf/ebola/index.html

## PRINCIPLES OF INFECTION CONTROL

Most transmission of infectious disease in the medical office can be prevented by strict adherence to guidelines issued by the **Occupational Safety and Health Administration (OSHA)** and the **Centers for Disease Control and Prevention (CDC)**. While most medical assistants take extraordinary precautions when dealing with patients who are known carriers of infectious microorganisms, you may also treat an estimated five unknown carriers for each patient known to be infectious. Therefore, knowledge and use of effective infection control in relation to all patients is essential.

## Medical Asepsis

Medical asepsis does not mean that an object or area is free from all microorganisms. It refers to practices that render an object or area free from pathogenic microorganisms. Commonly known as clean technique, medical asepsis prevents the transmission of microorganisms from one person or area to any other within the medical office (Box 17-2).

Hand washing is the most important medical aseptic technique to prevent the transmission of pathogens. The proper procedure for washing your hands is detailed in Procedure 17-1. Always wash your hands:

- Before and after every patient contact
- After coming into contact with any blood or body fluids
- After coming into contact with contaminated material
- After handling specimens
- After coughing, sneezing, or blowing your nose
- After using the restroom
- Before and after going to lunch, taking breaks, and leaving for the day

Because you should always assume that blood and body fluids are contaminated with pathogens, you should wear gloves when handling any specimens or when contact with contaminated material is anticipated.

## TABLE 17-1  Common Communicable Diseases

| Disease | Method of Transmission |
|---|---|
| AIDS | Contact, or contact with contaminated sharps |
| Chicken pox (varicella) | Direct contact or droplets |
| Cholera | Ingestion of contaminated food or water |
| Diphtheria | Airborne droplets, infected carriers |
| Hepatitis B | Direct contact with infectious body fluid |
| Influenza | Airborne droplets, infected carriers, or direct contact with contaminated articles such as used tissues |
| Measles (rubeola) | Airborne droplets, infected carriers |
| Meningitis | Airborne droplets |
| Mononucleosis | Airborne droplets or contact with infected saliva |
| Mumps | Airborne droplets, infected carriers, or direct contact with materials contaminated with infected saliva |
| Pneumonia | Airborne droplets or direct contact with infected mucus |
| Rabies | Direct contact with saliva of infected animal such as an animal bite |
| Rubella (German measles) | Airborne droplets, infected carriers |
| Tetanus | Direct contact with spores or contaminated animal feces |
| Tuberculosis | Airborne droplets, infected carriers |

## BOX 17-2   Guidelines for Maintaining Medical Asepsis

- Avoid touching your clothing with soiled linen, table paper, supplies, or instruments. Roll used table paper or linens inward with the clean surface outward.
- Always consider the floor to be contaminated. Any item dropped onto the floor must be considered dirty and be discarded or cleaned to its former level of asepsis before being used.
- Clean tables, counters, and other surfaces frequently and immediately after contamination. Clean areas are less likely than dirty ones to harbor microorganisms or encourage their growth.
- Always presume that blood and body fluids from any source are contaminated. Follow the guidelines published by OSHA and the CDC to protect yourself and to prevent the transmission of disease.

However, wearing gloves does not replace hand washing! In fact, your hands should be washed before you apply gloves and after you remove them in all situations to prevent disease transmission.

Other medical aseptic techniques include general cleaning of the office, including the examination and treatment rooms, waiting or reception area, and clinical work areas. Floors are always considered contaminated, and dust and dirt are vehicles for transmission of microorganisms and should be regularly cleaned from all surfaces, including the floor. In addition, you should teach patients and their caregivers proper medical aseptic techniques for use in the home to prevent the spread of disease.

## CHECKPOINT QUESTION

5. Robert is curious about the office policy directing employees to wash their hands after removing examination gloves. Explain why wearing exam gloves does not replace hand washing.

## PATIENT EDUCATION

### Basic Aseptic Technique

While performing procedures, take the opportunity to instruct your patients in basic aseptic techniques they can use at home to reduce the spread of disease.

- *Hand washing.* This routine aseptic technique is particularly important for patients and families in preventing the spread of disease. Instruct patients to wash their hands before and after eating meals; after sneezing, coughing, or blowing the nose; after using the bathroom; before and after changing a dressing; and after changing diapers.

- *Use tissue.* Explain to patients with respiratory symptoms that using a disposable tissue to cover the mouth and nose when coughing and sneezing decreases the potential to transmit the illness throughout the household. In addition, immediate and proper disposal of the used tissue is essential to prevent the spread of infection.
- *Changing bandages.* Patients and family members who change dressings on wounds should be instructed in the proper procedure for using sterile dressings and clean bandages. Always demonstrate the procedure for the patient and have the patient or family member return the demonstration to ensure their understanding.
- *Sanitation.* Explain the proper techniques for disposing of waste from members of the household with communicable diseases. If in doubt, consult the local public health department for guidelines.

## Levels of Infection Control

**Sterilization,** the highest level of infection control, destroys all forms of microorganisms, including spores, on inanimate surfaces. Sterilization methods include exposing the articles to various conditions, including steam under pressure in an autoclave; specific gases, such as ethylene oxide; dry heat ovens; and immersion in an approved chemical sterilizing agent (see Chapter 21 for a more complete discussion of sterilization techniques). Instruments or devices that penetrate the skin or come into contact with areas of the body considered sterile, such as the urinary bladder, must be sterilized using one of these methods. To save time, many medical offices use disposable sterile supplies and equipment to eliminate the need for manual sterilization (Fig. 17-2).

The next highest level of infection control is **disinfection.** Disinfectants or germicides inactivate virtually all recognized pathogenic microorganisms except spores on inanimate objects. There are three levels of disinfection—high, intermediate, and low. Each is described in more detail in the following section.

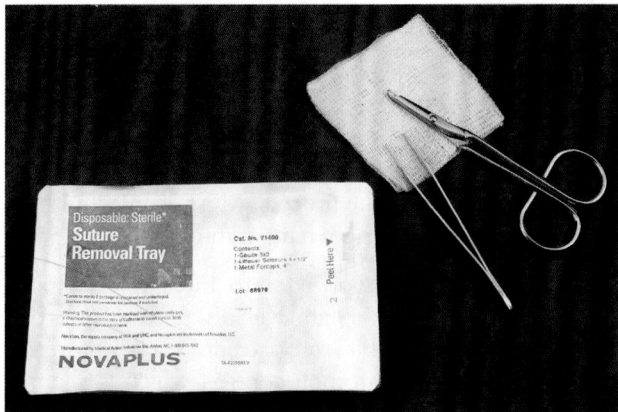

**Figure 17-2 •** Some surgical kits are prepackaged and disposable meant for one-time use only.

The lowest level of infection control is **sanitization,** which is cleaning any visible contaminants from the item using soap or detergent, water, and manual friction. This is the type of infection control used when you manually wash dishes in your kitchen and is usually sufficient to eliminate microorganisms that could cause disease on eating utensils.

## Sanitation

Most instruments, equipment, and supplies used in medical offices must be sanitized regularly according to the recommendations of the manufacturer. **Sanitation** is the maintenance of a healthful, disease-free, and hazard-free environment. Sanitation often involves sanitization procedures that reduce the number of microorganisms on an inanimate object to a safe or relatively safe level. This is accomplished by thoroughly cleaning items such as instruments and equipment with warm, soapy water with mechanical action to remove organic matter and other residue. Cleaning or sanitizing must precede disinfection and/or sterilization in the medical office.

## Disinfection

Disinfectants, or germicides, are chemicals or procedures that inactivate virtually all recognized pathogenic microorganisms but not necessarily all microbial forms, including spores, on inanimate objects. The following factors may affect disinfection:

- Prior cleaning of the object. Equipment and supplies that have been sanitized first are more effectively disinfected.
- The amount of organic material on the object. The more organic matter, such as blood or body tissues, on the item, the more disinfectant agent you must use.
- The type of microbial contamination. All blood and body fluids should be considered contaminated with blood-borne pathogens such as hepatitis B virus (HBV) and human immunodeficiency virus (HIV).
- The concentration of the **germicide** or chemical disinfectant that kills pathogens. Disinfectants diluted with water are relatively ineffective at killing microbes.
- The length of exposure to the germicide. The longer the disinfectant comes into contact with the contaminated object, the more thorough disinfection is likely to be.
- The shape or complexity of the object being disinfected. Objects that have rough edges, corners, or otherwise difficult-to-clean areas may require special techniques to disinfect all surfaces.
- The temperature of the process. Most disinfectants work adequately at room temperature.

Disinfection is categorized into three levels—high, intermediate, and low. High-level disinfection destroys most forms of microbial life except certain bacterial spores. This level of infection control, which is slightly less effective than sterilization, is commonly used to clean reusable instruments that come into contact with mucous membrane–lined body cavities that are not considered sterile, such as the vagina and the rectum. Methods of high-level disinfection include immersion in boiling water for 30 minutes (rarely used in the medical office) and immersion in an approved disinfecting chemical, such as glutaraldehyde or isopropyl alcohol, for 45 minutes or according to the guidelines in the disinfectant label.

Intermediate-level disinfection destroys many viruses, fungi, and some bacteria, including Mycobacterium tuberculosis, the bacterium that causes tuberculosis. However, intermediate disinfection does not kill bacterial spores. Intermediate disinfection is used for surfaces and instruments that come into contact with unbroken skin surfaces, including stethoscopes, blood pressure cuffs, and splints. Commercial chemical germicides that kill *M. tuberculosis* and solutions containing a 1:10 dilution of household bleach (2 oz of chlorine bleach per quart of tap water) are effective intermediate disinfectants.

Low-level disinfection destroys many bacteria and some viruses, but not M. tuberculosis or bacterial spores. This type of disinfection is adequate in the medical office for routine cleaning and removing surface debris when no visible blood or body fluids are on the items being disinfected. Disinfectants without tuberculocidal properties are used for low-level disinfection (Fig. 17-3). Table 17-2 describes disinfection methods, uses, and precautions of various chemicals.

---

### CHECKPOINT QUESTION

6. What level of disinfection would you use to clean a reusable instrument that comes into contact with the vaginal mucosa, such as a vaginal speculum? Why?

---

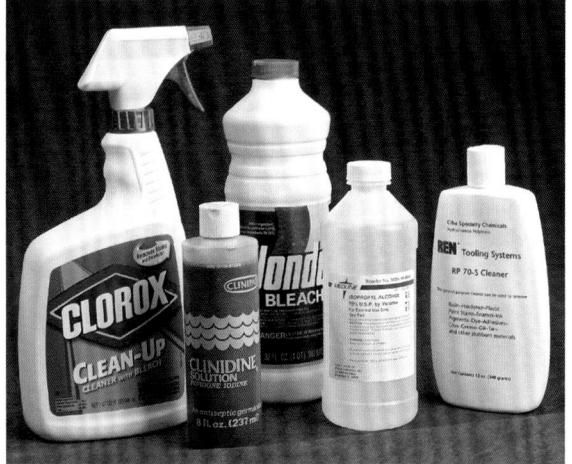

**Figure 17-3 •** These products destroy many pathogenic microorganisms if used correctly.

## INFECTION CONTROL FOR THE MEDICAL OFFICE

OSHA is the federal agency responsible for ensuring the safety of all workers, including those in health care. OSHA promulgates and enforces federal regulations that must be

| TABLE 17-2 | Disinfection Methods |
|---|---|
| **Method** | **Uses and Precautions** |
| Alcohol (70% isopropyl) | Used for noncritical items (countertops, glass thermometers, stethoscopes) |
| | Flammable; damages some rubber, plastic, and lenses |
| Chlorine (sodium hypochlorite or bleach) | Dilute 1:10 (1 part bleach to 10 parts water) |
| | Used for a broad spectrum of microbes |
| | Inexpensive and fast acting |
| | Corrosive, inactivated by organic matter, relatively unstable |
| Formaldehyde | Disinfectant and sterilant |
| | Regulated by OSHA |
| | Warnings must be marked on all containers and storage areas |
| Glutaraldehyde | Alkaline or acid. Effective against bacteria, viruses, fungi, and some spores |
| | OSHA regulated; requires adequate ventilation, covered pans, gloves, and masks; must display biohazard or chemical label |
| Hydrogen peroxide | Stable and effective when used on inanimate objects |
| | Attacks membrane lipids, DNA, and other essential cell components |
| | Can damage plastic, rubber, and some metals |
| Iodine or iodophors | Bacteriostatic agent |
| | Not to be used on instruments |
| | May cause staining |
| Phenols (tuberculocidal) | Used for environmental items and equipment |
| | Requires gloves and eye protection |
| | Can cause skin irritation and burns |

DNA, deoxyribonucleic acid.

followed by all medical offices. The practices of individual offices regarding employees' health and safety must be either put into a policy and procedure manual or compiled separately as an infection control manual. Regardless of where the office policies are kept, however, they must be readily available to both employees of the medical office and OSHA representatives.

## Exposure Risk Factors and the Exposure Control Plan

Medical offices must provide clear instructions in the policy or infection control manual for preventing employee exposure and reducing the danger of exposure to biohazardous materials. The **exposure risk factor** for each worker by job description must be included in the written policy. It is based on the employee's risk of exposure to communicable disease. Administrative medical assistants have a low exposure risk and require only minimal protection to perform the duties associated with that position. However, clinical medical assistants have a higher exposure risk and require access to a variety of **personal protective equipment** (PPE), such as gloves, goggles, and/or face shields depending on the task at hand, and **immunization** against hepatitis B at no charge to the employee. The medical office must provide the appropriate equipment and supplies as outlined in this office policy according to OSHA.

Another written policy required by OSHA for offices with 10 or more employees is the **exposure control plan**. The medical office must have a written plan of action for all employees and visitors who may be exposed to **biohazardous** material despite all precautions. In the event of an exposure, you must first apply the principles of first aid and notify your immediate supervisor, office manager, or the office physician. The physician or supervisor should provide guidance regarding **postexposure testing** and follow-up procedures. Next, you should complete and file an incident report (or exposure report) form explaining the circumstances surrounding the exposure. This report form not only documents the incident but also allows management to establish a policy to prevent this type of exposure in the future. In addition, the employer must record the exposure on an OSHA 300 log (Fig. 17-4) and report the exposure to OSHA if one or more of the following criteria are present:

- The work-related exposure resulted in loss of consciousness or necessitated a transfer to another job.
- The exposure resulted in a recommendation for medical treatment, such as vaccination or medication to prevent complications.
- The exposure resulted in the conversion of a negative blood test for a contagious disease into a positive blood test in the employee who was exposed.

Box 17-3 describes biohazard and safety equipment commonly used in medical offices.

## OSHA's Form 300
# Log of Work-Related Injuries and Illnesses

You must record information about every work-related death and about every work-related injury or illness that involves loss of consciousness, restricted work activity or job transfer, days away from work, or medical treatment beyond first aid. You must also record significant work-related injuries and illnesses that are diagnosed by a physician or licensed health care professional. You must also record work-related injuries and illnesses that meet any of the specific recording criteria listed in 29 CFR Part 1904.8 through 1904.12. Feel free to use two lines for a single case if you need to. You must complete an Injury and Illness Incident Report (OSHA Form 301) or equivalent form for each injury or illness recorded on this form. If you're not sure whether a case is recordable, call your local OSHA office for help.

**Attention:** This form contains information relating to employee health and must be used in a manner that protects the confidentiality of employees to the extent possible while the information is being used for occupational safety and health purposes.

Year 20___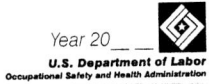

**U.S. Department of Labor**
Occupational Safety and Health Administration

Form approved OMB no. 1218-0176

Establishment name _____

City _____  State _____

Figure 17-4 • The OSHA 300 Log form. (Courtesy of the U.S. Department of Labor.)

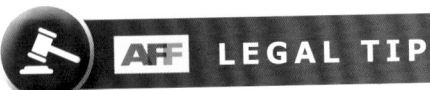

## CHECKPOINT QUESTION

7. How would Bonita explain the difference between exposure risk factors and the exposure control plan to Robert?

**AFF** **LEGAL TIP**

### Blood-Borne Pathogen Standard Training

According to OSHA, health care facilities, including physician offices, must provide training to newly hired employees who will be exposed to blood or other possibly infectious material while caring for patients. This training must be repeated yearly and include any new issues or policies recommended by OSHA, the CDC, the Department of Health and Human Services, or the U.S. Public Health Service. The following items must be included in the training:

- A description of blood-borne diseases, including the transmission and symptoms
- PPE available to the employee and the location of the PPE in the medical office
- Information about the risks of contracting hepatitis B and about the HBV vaccine
- The exposure control plan and postexposure procedures, including follow-up care, in the event of an exposure

## Standard Precautions

**Standard precautions** are a set of procedures recognized by the CDC to reduce the chance of transmitting infectious microorganisms in any health care setting, including medical offices. By presuming that all blood and body fluids, except perspiration, are contaminated and by following these precautions, you can protect yourself and prevent the spread of disease. Specifically, these precautions pertain to contact with blood, all body fluids except sweat, damaged skin, and mucous membranes and require that you do the following:

- Wash your hands with soap and water after touching blood, body fluids, secretions, and other contaminated items, whether you have worn gloves or not.
- Use an alcohol-based hand rub (foam, lotion, or gel) to decontaminate the hands if the hands are not visibly dirty or contaminated.
- Wear clean nonsterile examination gloves when contact with blood, body fluids, secretions, mucous membranes, damaged skin, and contaminated items is anticipated.
- Change gloves between procedures on the same patient after exposure to potentially infective material.
- Wear equipment to protect your eyes, nose, and mouth and avoid soiling your clothes by wearing

---

**BOX 17-3   Biohazard and Safety Equipment in the Medical Office**

- *Hazard communication safety data sheets.* Formerly known as material safety data sheets, these are forms prepared by the manufacturers of all chemical and hazardous substances used in all types of settings including the medical office. In 2012, OSHA revised the standard for these sheets and changed the name to safety data sheets (SDSs). Each sheet describes how to handle and dispose of the chemical and, most important, the health hazards of the chemical and safety equipment needed when using it.
- *Biohazard waste containers.* Only waste contaminated with blood or body fluids or other potentially infectious material (OPIM) should be placed in biohazard waste containers. Sharps containers are used for disposal of items that have the potential to puncture or cut the skin.
- *Personal protective equipment.* Employers are required to provide PPE appropriate to the risk of

exposure. For example, employees who may come into contact with blood, such as the clinical medical assistant giving an injection, need to be protected only by wearing gloves. However, situations that may cause a splash or splatter of blood require full coverage of the skin, eyes, and clothing.
- *Eyewash basin.* Pressing the lever on the basin and turning on the faucets produces a stream of water that forces open the caps of the eyewash basin. To remove contaminants or chemicals from the eyes, lower your face into the stream and continue to wash the area until the eyes are clear or for the amount of time recommended on the safety data sheets (SDSs).
- *Immunization.* Employers are required by OSHA to provide immunization against blood-borne pathogens if vaccines are available.

---

a disposable gown or apron when performing procedures that may splash or spray blood, body fluids, or secretions.
- Dispose of single-use items appropriately; do not disinfect, sterilize, and reuse.
- Take precautions to avoid injuries before, during, and after procedures in which needles, scalpels, or other sharp instruments have been used on a patient.
- Do not recap used needles or otherwise manipulate them by bending or breaking. If recapping is necessary to carry a used needle to a sharps container, use a one-handed scoop technique or a device for holding the needle sheath (see Chapter 24).
- Place used disposable syringes and needles and other sharps in a puncture-resistant container (sharps) as close as possible to the area of use.
- Use barrier devices (e.g., mouthpieces, resuscitation bags) as alternatives to mouth-to-mouth resuscitation (see Chapter 26).
- Do not eat, drink, or put candy, gum, or mints into your mouth while working in the clinical area. Keep your hands away from your face.

## CHECKPOINT QUESTION

8. How will following standard precautions help to protect you against contracting an infection or communicable disease?

## Personal Protective Equipment

In any area of the medical office where exposure to biohazardous materials might occur, PPE must be made available and used by all health care workers, including medical assistants. For instance:

- Gloves must be available and accessible throughout the office. If you or a patient is sensitive to the latex found in regular examination gloves, proper alternatives such as vinyl gloves must be available (Box 17-4).
- Disposable gowns, goggles, and face shields must be available in areas where splattering or splashing of airborne particles may occur (Fig. 17-5).
- You must wear gloves when performing any procedure that carries any risk of exposure, such as surgical procedures or drawing blood specimens, disposing of biohazardous waste, or touching or handling surfaces that have been contaminated with biohazardous materials, or if there is any chance at all, no matter how remote, that you may come into contact with blood or body fluids.

Employers who do not make this equipment available are not in compliance with OSHA regulations and may face significant fines. However, employees are responsible for using the PPE correctly and appropriately and washing their hands frequently throughout the day. Remember, pathogens may be carried home to family members and to other persons who come into contact with you or the patient. When

## BOX 17-4    Latex Allergy and Prevention

The incidence among health care workers of allergic reactions to proteins in latex has increased in recent years. The proteins in latex, a product of the rubber tree that is used to make many products including examination gloves, may cause allergic reactions, especially with repeated exposure. The reactions can be mild (skin redness or rash, itching, or hives) or severe (difficulty breathing, coughing, or wheezing). Respiratory reactions often result when the powder in the gloves becomes airborne and is inhaled as the gloves are removed after use. To protect yourself from exposure and allergy to latex, the following guidelines may be useful:

- Use gloves that are not latex for tasks that do not involve contact or potential contact with blood or body fluids.
- When contact with blood or body fluids is possible, wear powder-free latex gloves. Powder-free gloves contain less protein than the powdered ones, reducing the risk of allergy.
- Avoid wearing oil-based lotions or hand creams before applying latex gloves. The oil in these products can break down the latex, releasing the proteins that cause the allergic reactions.
- Wash your hands thoroughly after removing latex gloves.
- Recognize the symptoms of latex allergy in yourself, your coworkers, and your patients.

removing PPE after a procedure, remove all protective barriers before removing your gloves. Once you have removed all PPE, including your contaminated gloves (Procedure 17-2), always wash your hands (see Procedure 17-1).

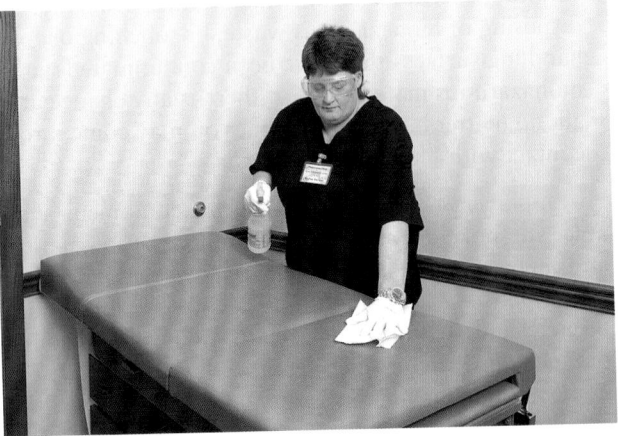

**Figure 17-5** • Personal protective equipment that must be provided for employees who may come into contact with contaminated materials includes gloves, goggles, face shields, and gowns or aprons to protect clothing.

## CHECKPOINT QUESTION

9. The physician asks Bonita to assist with a wound irrigation. What PPE should she wear during this procedure?

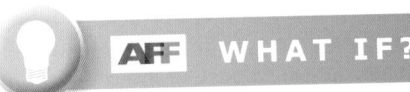

## WHAT IF?

**What if your patient is offended that you are wearing gloves when drawing a blood specimen?**

Sometimes, patients become defensive and make statements to the effect that they are "disease free." If this happens to you, reassure the patient by saying that wearing gloves is a standard practice and is used for the protection of the patient also. Use this occasion to teach the patient about standard precautions and the importance of following these guidelines in preventing the spread of disease.

## Handling Environmental Contamination

Although not all equipment or surfaces in the medical office must be sterile (free from all microorganisms), all equipment and areas must be clean. Sanitization is cleaning or washing equipment or surfaces by removing all visible soil. Any detergent or low-level disinfectant can be used to clean and disinfect areas such as floors, examination tables, cabinets, and countertops. Because you may be expected to perform cleaning tasks routinely or when these surfaces become soiled with visible blood or body fluids, you should understand how these procedures are correctly performed.

Any surface contaminated with biohazardous materials should be promptly cleaned using an approved germicide or a dilute bleach solution. OSHA requires that spill kits or appropriate supplies be available, and commercial kits make cleaning contaminated surfaces relatively safe and easy. Commercial kits include clean gloves, eye protection if there is a risk of splashing, a gel to absorb the biohazardous material, a scoop, towels, and a biohazard waste container to discard all used items (Fig. 17-6). If your office does not purchase commercial kits, you should gather and store the following items together in the event that a biohazardous spill occurs:

- Eye protection, such as goggles
- Clean examination gloves
- Absorbent powder, crystals, or gel
- Paper towels
- A disposable scoop
- At least one biohazard waste bag
- A chemical disinfectant

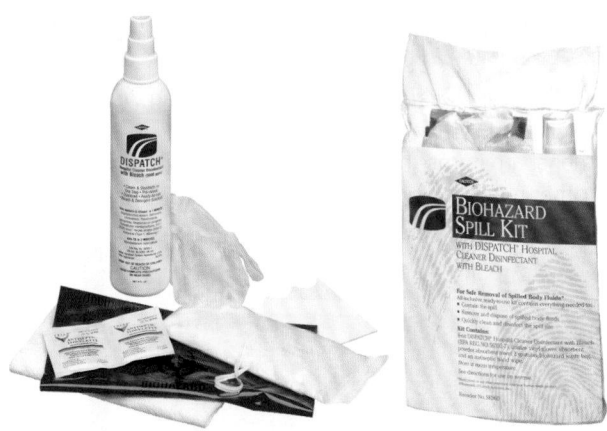

**Figure 17-6 •** A commercially prepared biohazard spill kit contains gloves, absorbent material, eye protection, and a bio-hazard bag for proper disposal. (Courtesy of Caltech Industries, Midland, MI.)

In some cases, you may need a sharps container (Fig. 17-7) and spill control barriers. If there is a large amount of contamination on the floor, you should put on disposable shoe coverings to avoid transmitting microorganisms on your shoes. All gloves, paper towels, eye protection, and shoe coverings should be discarded in the biohazardous waste bags, which must be disposed of properly. Procedure 17-3 outlines the procedure for an area contaminated with blood or body fluids.

Although most medical offices use disposable patient gowns and drapes, some offices continue to use cloth. Hygienic storage of clean linens is recommended, and proper handling of soiled linens, disposable or not, is required. After applying clean examination gloves, handle soiled linen, including examination table paper, as little as possible by folding it carefully so that the most contaminated surface is turned inward to prevent contamination of the air. Contaminated linen should be placed in a biohazard bag in the examination room where the contamination occurred rather than carried through the hallways of the medical office. Some offices using cloth linens contract with an outside company for the laundering. If linen materials are laundered at the office, use normal laundry cycles following the recommendations of the washer, detergent, and fabric.

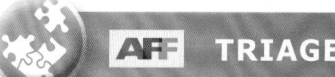

## CHECKPOINT QUESTION

10. While helping Bonita by carrying a urine specimen to the physician laboratory area for testing, Robert accidently spills some of the urine on the floor. How would Bonita explain the cleanup process to Robert who is unsure about how to clean up a spilled urine specimen? Is this a biohazardous situation? Why or why not?

### AFF TRIAGE

The following three situations occur at the same time in the office where you are employed:

A. You have just finished changing the dressing on a wound that is draining a moderate amount of blood. You still have your gloves on, but you need to document the procedure in the patient's medical record and instruct the patient regarding wound care.
B. As you are cleaning up the materials used to irrigate the wound, you spill the basin used to collect the irrigating solution and blood obtained from the procedure.
C. Another staff member knocks on the door of the examination room and informs you that you have a phone call.

**How do you sort these tasks? What do you do first? Second? Third?**

Tell the staff member in situation C that you cannot take a phone call now and ask him or her to take a message or refer the call to another medical assistant. The spill in situation B is a biohazardous spill and should be cleaned up and the area decontaminated immediately. You should be familiar with the policy and procedures of the medical office and clean the spill accordingly. Once the spill is cleaned and decontaminated, remove your gloves and wash your hands. Document the wound irrigation, dressing change, and patient education in situation A only after removing your gloves and washing your hands. To prevent the spread of microorganisms to the medical record, you should never handle the medical record while wearing contaminated gloves.

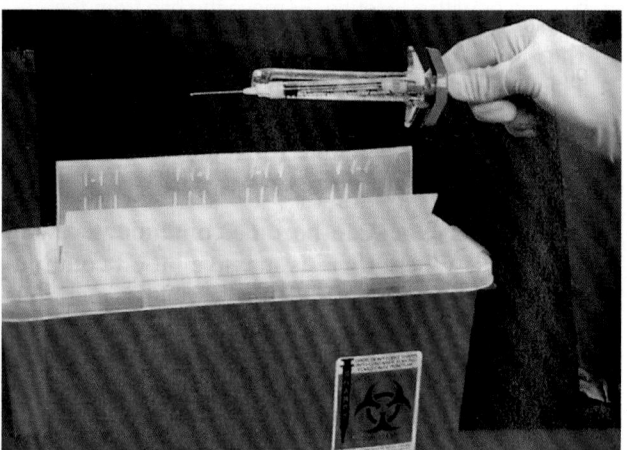

**Figure 17-7 •** All sharps should be disposed of properly by placing them in a plastic puncture-resistant sharps container like the one shown here. Note the biohazard symbol on the sharps container.

## Disposing of Infectious Waste

Federal regulations from the Environmental Protection Agency (EPA) and OSHA set the policies and guidelines for disposing of hazardous materials, but individual states determine policies based on these guidelines. As a result, policies vary widely, and you should review your state and local regulations before making waste disposal decisions. Most medical offices are considered small generators of waste because they produce <50 pounds of waste each month. Facilities such as hospitals and large clinics that generate more than 50 pounds are considered large generators and must obtain a certificate of registration from the EPA and maintain a record of the quantity of waste and disposal procedures.

To remain compliant with any state and federal laws, facilities that are considered large generators of infectious waste and some smaller medical offices use an infectious waste service to dispose of biohazardous waste appropriately and safely. These services supply the office with appropriate waste containers and pick up filled containers regularly (Box 17-5). Once the filled containers are picked up by the waste service, the infectious waste is disposed of according to EPA and OSHA guidelines. The service maintains a tracking record listing the type of waste, its weight in pounds, and the disposal destination. When the waste has been destroyed, a tracking form documenting the disposal is sent to the medical office and should be retained in the office records for 3 years. This documentation must be provided to the EPA should an audit be performed to assess compliance. States impose stiff penalties, including fines and/or imprisonment, for violations of regulations involving biohazardous waste.

Because the fee charged by an infectious waste service is based on the type and amount of waste generated, you should follow these guidelines to help keep the cost down while maintaining safety:

- Use separate containers for each type of waste. Don't put bandages in sharps containers (puncture-resistant containers for needles or other sharp items) or paper towels used for routine hand washing in a biohazard bag.
- Fill sharps containers two-thirds full before disposing of them. Most containers have fill lines that must not be exceeded.
- Use only approved biohazard containers.
- When moving filled biohazard containers, secure the bag or top with a closure for that specific container.
- If the container is contaminated on the outside, wear clean examination gloves, secure it within another approved container, and wash your hands thoroughly afterward.
- Place biohazard waste for pick up by the service in a secure, designated area.

## CHECKPOINT QUESTION

11. After drawing a blood specimen from a patient, you notice that the tube of blood is leaking onto the examination table where you put it while finishing the procedure. How do you clean up the blood spill?

### BOX 17-5   Biohazard Waste Disposal

A biohazard waste container has a red bag with the biohazard symbol on it and should only be used for nonsharp items that are contaminated with blood or other potentially infectious material (OPIM).

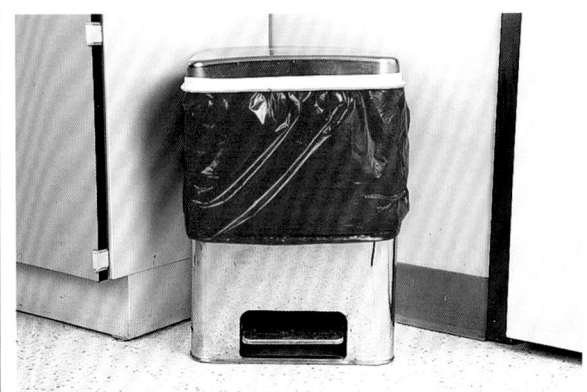

A regular waste container should be used only for disposal of waste that is not biohazardous, such as paper, plastic, disposable tray wrappers, packaging material, unused gauze, and examination table paper. To prevent leakage and mess, nonbiohazardous liquids should be discarded in an acceptable and approved area such as a sink or other washbasin, not in the plastic bag inside the waste can. Biohazard liquid spills (any waste containing blood or other body fluids) should be cleaned according to the office policy using the guidelines noted in Procedure 17-3. **Never discard sharps of any kind in plastic bags; these are not puncture resistant, and injury may result even with careful handling.** Regardless of the type of waste container used (biohazard or nonbiohazard), bags should not be filled to capacity. When the plastic bag is about two-thirds full, it should be removed from the waste can, with the top edges brought together and secured by tying or with a twist tie. Remove the bag from the area and follow the office policy and procedures for disposal. Put a fresh plastic bag into the waste can.

## Hepatitis B and Human Immunodeficiency Viruses

One of the most persistent health care concerns in the medical office is the transmission of HBV and HIV. Although HIV is the most visible public concern, HBV has been an occupational hazard for health care professionals for many years. HBV is more viable than HIV and may survive in a dried state on clinical equipment and counter surfaces at room temperature for more than a week. In this dried state, HBV may be passed through the medical setting by way of contact with contaminated hands, gloves, or other means of direct transmission.

Fortunately, HBV can be contained by the proper use of standard precautions, and it can be killed easily by cleaning with a dilute bleach solution.

HBV and HIV are both transmitted through exposure to contaminated blood and body fluids. Accidental punctures with sharp objects contaminated with blood are one way to become infected, but the viruses may also enter the body through broken skin. Disorders of the skin, including dry cracked skin, dermatitis, eczema, and psoriasis, also allow entrance into the body if contact with contaminated surfaces or equipment occurs.

While there is no vaccine to prevent infection with HIV, employers whose workers, including clinical medical assistants, are at risk for HBV exposure are mandated by OSHA to provide the vaccine to prevent HBV at no cost to the employee. This vaccine is given in a series of three injections that normally produce immunity to the disease. It is recommended that a blood sample be drawn 6 months after the third injection of HBV vaccine to determine whether the person has developed immunity. The blood test can detect the presence, or titer, of antibodies against hepatitis B. The series is repeated if HBV immunity is not found, but the vaccine has been found to be very effective. The immunity may last as long as 10 years. Employees who choose not to receive the vaccine must sign a waiver or release form stating that they are aware of the risks associated with HBV. Individuals who contract hepatitis B may develop cirrhosis (destruction of the cells of the liver) and are at increased risk for developing liver cancer.

In the event of exposure to blood or body fluids infected with HBV, the postexposure plan should include an immediate blood test of the employee. Repeat blood titers should be obtained at specific intervals, usually 6 weeks, 3 months, 6 months, 9 months, and 1 year, as a comparison. If you have been immunized against HBV, usually no further treatment is required. However, if you waive the HBV series, hepatitis B immunoglobulin can be given by injection for immediate short-term protection, and the general series of three immunizations should be started.

The same schedule of evaluation is required after HIV exposure. Again, there is no vaccine to prevent HIV, but other HIV treatments for preventing transmission are being tested (Box 17-6).

## CHECKPOINT QUESTION

12. Robert asks Bonita which virus is more of a threat to the clinical medical assistant: HIV or HBV? How would you answer this question? Why?

## BOX 17-6 HIV Testing

According to the Centers for Disease Control and Prevention (CDC), there are an estimated 1,178,350 Americans who are HIV positive. Unfortunately, 240,000 of those Americans are not aware of their HIV status. What tests are available to detect the presence of the human immunodeficiency virus? This is a question that you may be asked from patients or other curious individuals, and as a professional health care worker, you should be able to answer this question with the most current information available.

Currently, there are three types of tests available to diagnose HIV. The first type, antibody tests, is used to detect the presence of HIV antibodies in blood, oral fluid (not saliva), or urine and includes enzyme immunoassay (EIA) tests. The results from these tests may take up to 2 weeks. Rapid HIV antibody tests are also available, which produce results in 20 to 30 minutes. It is recommended that individuals using an antibody test who test negative get retested at 3 months after the possible exposure because of the possibility of false-negative results if performed too early after the initial infection. It is also recommended that individuals who test positive have a Western blot test performed to confirm the positive result.

The second type of HIV testing includes antigen tests. These tests may diagnose HIV infection 1 to 3 weeks after infection and require only the use of blood samples. These tests require specialized equipment in the laboratory and are not as common as antibody tests.

The third type of HIV testing detects genetic material in the virus 2 to 3 weeks after infection. Technically, these tests are known as PCR or polymerase chain reaction tests. Again, these tests require specialized equipment and specially trained technicians and are not as common as antibody tests at this time.

There are currently 2 FDA-approved home tests on the market to detect HIV. These tests include the Home Access HIV-1 Test System and the OraQuick In-Home HIV test. The Home Access system requires individuals to stick a finger with a lancet that is provided in the kit, collect a blood sample, send the specimen collected to a laboratory, and call for the results after a specified amount of time. The OraQuick test uses oral fluid swabbed from the mouth and allows for testing the specimen at home, getting results in about 20 minutes. Positive results for either of these in-home tests require follow-up with medical care and counseling. Because of the possibility of false-negative results, negative results may need additional testing at a later date.

(http://www.cdc.gov/hiv/testing/lab/hometests.html)

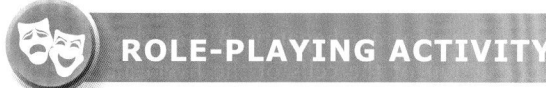

## ROLE-PLAYING ACTIVITY

You are working with Bonita Jackson, the medical assistant found in the case study at the beginning of the chapter. Role-play yourself as Bonita or Janie, a new medical assistant hired to work with another physician in the office. Janie confides in Bonita that she is reluctant to get the hepatitis B vaccine even though the office is providing it free of charge. What issues might be behind Janie's reluctance to get the vaccine? Are there side effects to getting this vaccine and if so, what symptoms or problems could Janie experience? Should Bonita try to talk Janie into getting the vaccine? Role-play this scenario assuming you are Bonita and another student is Janie. Use interpersonal skills and professionalism to discuss this benefits and risks of this vaccine staying within your scope of practice. Switch roles and assume you are Janie. Your instructor will give you additional information about this activity!

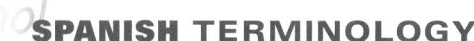

## SPANISH TERMINOLOGY

**Lávese las manos frecuentemente.**
Wash your hands frequently.

**Cúbrase la boca al toser.**
Cover your mouth when coughing.

**¿Es alérgico/alergica al latex?**
Are you allergic to latex?

**¿Tiene fiebre?**
Do you have a fever?

**¿Qué síntomas tiene?**
What symptoms do you have?

**Esta infección se transmite por fluidos corporales.**
This infection is transmitted by body fluids.

**Para minimizar que la infección se expanda, tiene que sanitizar y desinfectar sus articulos personales.**
To minimize the spread of infection, you have to sanitize and disinfect your personal items.

**¿Ya se vacunó?**
Are you vaccinated?

**Hay una epidemia de esta enfermedad en este Estado.**
There is an outbreak of this disease in this state.

**El paciente necesita estar aislado.**
The patient needs to be isolated.

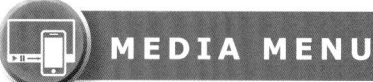

## MEDIA MENU

**Student Resources** on thePoint®
- *Video:* Hand Washing (Procedure 17-1)
- *Video:* Removing Contaminated Gloves (Procedure 17-2)
- CMA/RMA Certification Exam Review

**Internet Resources**
**Occupational Safety and Health Administration:**
http://www.osha.gov
**Latex Allergy Prevention:**
http://www.cdc.gov/niosh/docs/98-113/
**Food and Drug Administration:**
http://www.fda.gov
**Workplace Safety and Health Topics, Health Care Workers:**
http://www.cdc.gov/niosh/topics/healthcare/
**HIV and AIDS:**
http://www.AIDS.gov
**Centers for Diseases Control and Prevention:**
http://www.cdc.gov

## EMR Activity

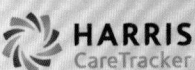

Harris CareTracker is a Web-based electronic medical record (EMR) application that you will use for the EMR activities included in this section at the end of each chapter. This application is actually used in physician offices but is provided to you through the publisher, Wolters Kluwer Health, to give you hands-on practice working with EMRs. Your instructor will have more information about accessing your username, log-in, and Quickstart guide.

### Prerequisite Activities in Harris CareTracker

*Note: The Getting Started and Quickstart documents and EMR Activities Step-by-Step Instructions listed below are available at* http://thePoint.lww.com/KronenbergerComp5e.

### Activity Details

Add an allergy to latex gloves to the *Allergies* section of the EMR for new patient Tom Bankson. He experiences a hives reaction whenever he is touched with latex products of any kind. Make sure to indicate this as a "Pop-Up Alert" in the EMR.

## Chapter Summary

- Following the principles of medical asepsis and infection control helps ensure a safe environment for patients and health care providers in the medical office. If you fail to follow these principles consistently, you will place yourself and others at risk for infection that may impair patients' recovery and affect health care workers' performance.
- Although avoiding contact with microorganisms in the environment is impossible, sanitation and disinfection will reduce the numbers of microorganisms and potential pathogens, making the environment clean and as disease free as possible.
- OSHA and the CDC issue regulations and standards for health care workers who work with blood and body fluids, and you must always follow them, including wearing PPE. In case of exposure, your office must have an exposure control plan and a postexposure plan to assist you in receiving appropriate medical attention and follow-up care.
- *Remember*: Hand washing is the single most effective measure to prevent the spread of infection. Wearing gloves does *not* replace hand washing. Hands must *always* be washed after removing gloves.

## Warm-Ups for Critical Thinking

1. Review Table 17-1 on common communicable diseases. Create a patient education brochure that focuses on the spread of these diseases.
2. A patient who comes into your office has a leg wound that must be cared for at home. When asked about caring for the wound, he tells you that he knows how to do it, but you think he may be confused about the importance of using medical asepsis. How do you handle this situation?
3. On a busy morning in the medical office, you accidently spill a small amount of urine from a specimen container onto the counter. Your coworker needs you to assist with a pediatric injection in the examination room down the hall. Would it be acceptable to clean up the urine spill after you help your coworker? Why or why not?
4. Develop a written policy for new employees regarding disinfecting individual examination rooms in the medical office. Be specific and include issues related to safety.

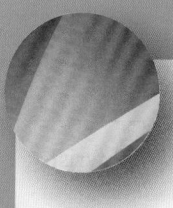

## PROCEDURE 17-1

# Hand Washing for Medical Asepsis

**PSY** Perform hand washing

**Purpose:** To prevent the growth and spread of pathogens

**Equipment:** Liquid soap, disposable paper towels, an orangewood manicure stick, a waste can

**Standard:** This task should take 2 to 3 minutes.

| STEPS | PURPOSE |
|---|---|
| 1. Remove all rings and your wristwatch if it cannot be pushed up onto the forearm. | Rings and watches may harbor pathogens that may not be easily washed away. Ideally, rings should not be worn when working with material that may be infectious. |
| 2. Stand close to the sink without touching it. | The sink is considered contaminated, and standing too close may contaminate your clothing. |
| 3. Turn on the faucet and adjust the temperature of the water to warm. | Water that is too hot or too cold will crack or chap the skin on the hands, which will break the natural protective barrier that prevents infection. |
| 4. Wet your hands and wrists under the warm running water, apply liquid soap, and work the soap into a lather by rubbing your palms together and rubbing the soap between your fingers at least 10 times. | This motion dislodges microorganisms from between the fingers and removes transient and some resident organisms. |

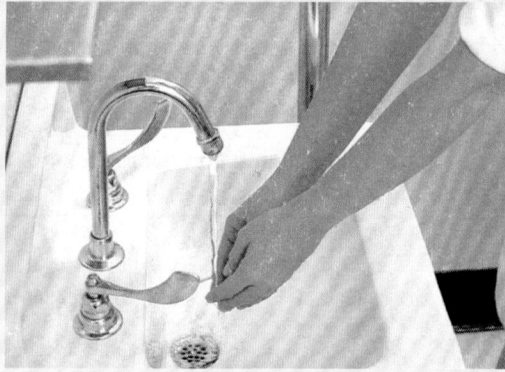

Step 4. Wet hands and wrists.

5. Scrub the palm of one hand with the fingertips of the other hand to work the soap under the nails of that hand; then, reverse the procedure and scrub the other hand. Also scrub each wrist.

Friction helps remove microorganisms.

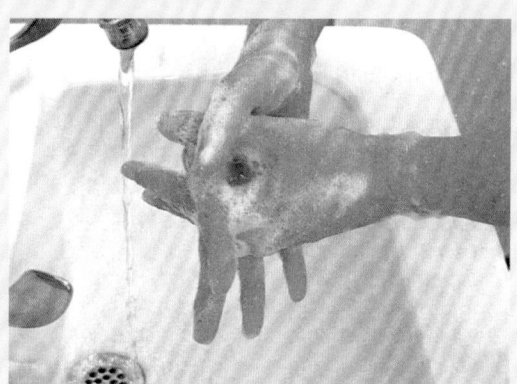

Step 5. Wash hands and wrists with firm rubbing and circular motions.

(continues on page 422)

PROCEDURE 17-1 (continued)

| STEPS | PURPOSE |
|---|---|
| 6. Rinse hands and wrists thoroughly under running warm water, holding hands lower than elbows; do not touch the inside of the sink. | Holding the hands lower than the elbows and wrists allows microorganisms to flow off the hands and fingers rather than back up the arms. |

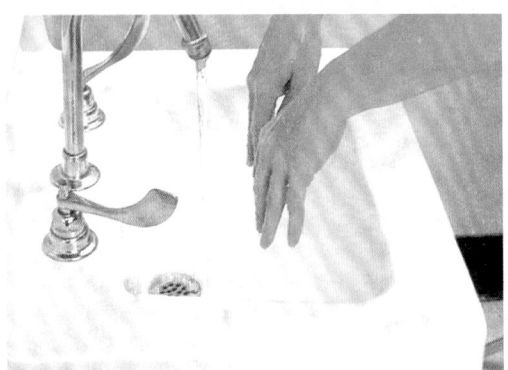

**Step 6.** Rinse hands thoroughly.

7. Clean under the nails by scraping the fingernails of one hand against the soapy palm of the other hand for 10 seconds. Repeat with other hand.

Nails may harbor microorganisms. Do this at the beginning of the day, before leaving for the day, or after coming into contact with potentially infectious material.

8. Reapply liquid soap and rewash hands and wrists.

Rewashing the hands after cleaning the nails washes away any microorganisms that may have been loosened and/or removed.

9. Rinse hands thoroughly again while holding hands lower than wrists and elbows.

10. Gently dry hands with a paper towel. Discard the paper towel and the orangewood stick if used to clean the nails.

Hands must be dried thoroughly and completely to prevent drying and cracking.

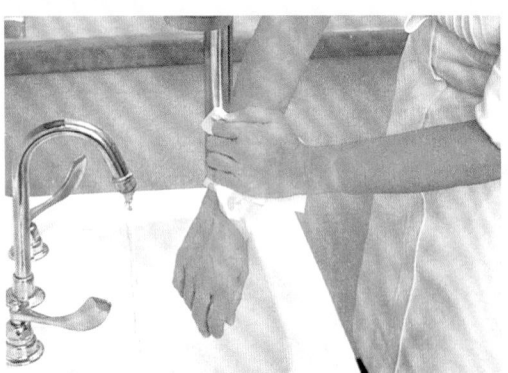

**Step 10.** Dry hands gently with a paper towel.

11. Use a dry paper towel to turn off the faucets, and discard the paper towel.

Your hands are clean and should not touch the contaminated faucet handles.

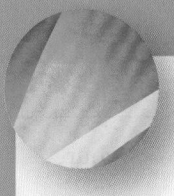

## PROCEDURE 17-2

### Select Appropriate Personal Protective Equipment and Remove Contaminated Gloves

**PSY**  Select appropriate barrier/personal protective equipment (PPE)

**Purpose:** To select appropriate PPE and properly remove contaminated gloves to prevent the spread of pathogenic microorganisms

**Equipment:** PPE (clean examination gloves, goggles or disposable masks with eye/splash guard, disposable masks, disposable gown) and biohazard waste container

**Standard:** This task should take 1 to 2 minutes.

| STEPS | PURPOSE |
|---|---|
| 1. Given a potentially biohazardous situation, choose the correct PPE:<br>a. Cleaning up spilled urine<br>b. Irrigating a wound<br>c. Giving an injection<br>d. Disinfecting examination tables | Gloves should be worn whenever contact with potentially infected blood or body fluids is a possibility. If there may be splashing, eye protection must be worn including either goggles or a mask with an attached face shield to protect the eyes. |
| 2. Apply appropriately chosen PPE. If a gown, mask, and goggles are necessary, apply the gown and mask/goggles first. Choose the appropriate size gloves for your hands and put them on last. | The disposable gown should open in the back, covering all of your clothing. Tie the gown at the neck without making a knot in the strings so that it can be removed easily. Apply the mask with attached face shield or a separate mask and eye goggles next. Clean gloves should be put on last and should fit comfortably, not too loose and not too tight. |
| 3. Make sure clothing is protected if a gown is worn and no skin is showing. | Pull cuff of gloves over end of sleeve of gown on both arms. |
| 4. After the procedure is finished, appropriately remove PPE by removing the gloves first, next the gown, and last the goggles and mask or face shield. | The gloves should be removed first because they are potentially the most contaminated. |
| 5. To remove gloves, grasp the glove of your nondominant hand at the palm and pull the glove away. | To avoid transferring contaminants to the wrist, be sure not to grasp the glove at the wrist. |

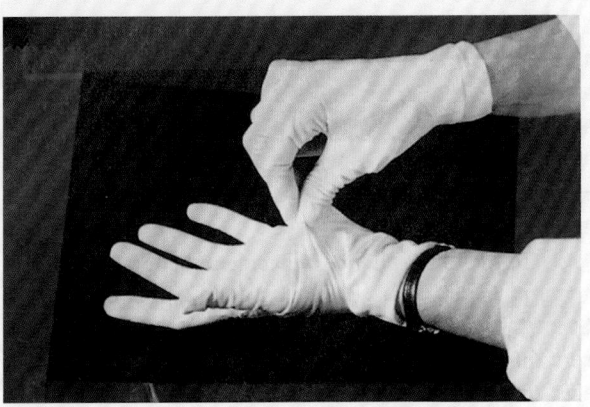

**Step 5.** Grasp the palm of the glove on your nondominant gloved hand.

*(continues on page 424)*

## PROCEDURE 17-2 (continued)

| STEPS | PURPOSE |
|---|---|
| 6. Slide your hand out of the glove, rolling the glove into the palm of the gloved dominant hand. | You should avoid touching either glove with your ungloved hand. |

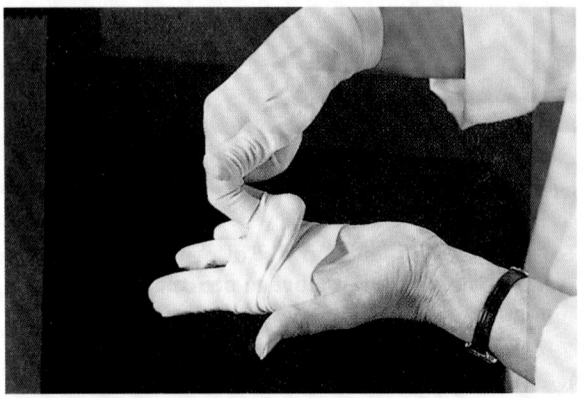

**Step 6A.** Carefully remove the glove and avoid contaminating your bare skin.

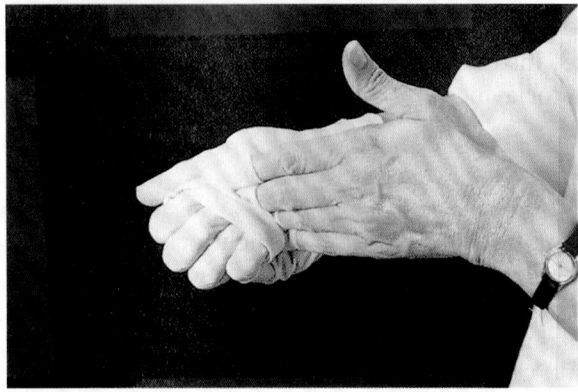

**Step 6B.** Grasp the soiled glove with your gloved dominant hand.

7. Holding the soiled glove in the palm of your gloved hand, slip your ungloved fingers under the cuff of the glove you are still wearing, being careful not to touch the outside of the glove.

Skin should touch skin but never the soiled part of the glove.

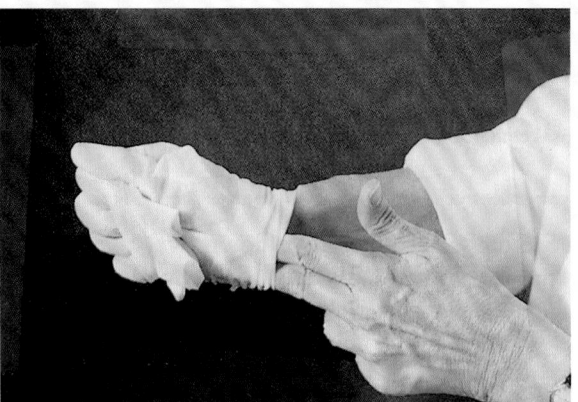

**Step 7.** Slip your free hand under the cuff of the remaining glove.

## PROCEDURE 17-2 (continued)

| STEPS | PURPOSE |
|---|---|
| 8. Stretch the glove of the dominant hand up and away from your hand while turning it inside out, with the already removed glove balled up inside. | Turning it inside out ensures that the soiled surfaces of the gloves are enclosed. |

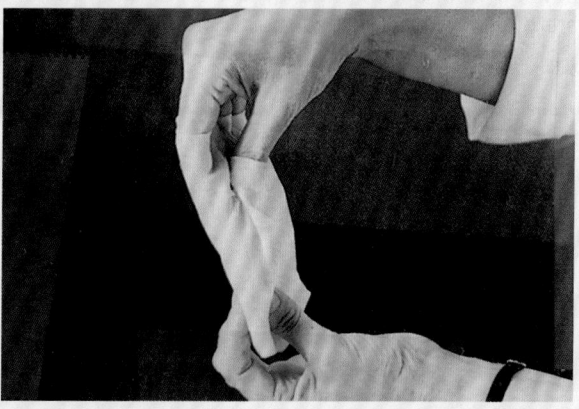

**Step 8.** Remove the glove by turning it inside out over the previously removed glove.

| STEPS | PURPOSE |
|---|---|
| 9. Both gloves should now be removed, with the first glove inside the second glove and the second glove inside out. | |
| 10. Discard both gloves as one unit into a biohazard waste receptacle. | |
| 11. If only gloves were worn as PPE, wash your hands. | Wearing gloves is *not* a substitute for washing your hands! |
| 12. If other PPE were worn (i.e., gown, mask, goggles), remove gloves following the procedure above and untie the gown carefully at the neck. Pull the neck strings of the gown toward the front of the body with the arms straight. Pull each arm out of the sleeve, making the sleeves inside out. Continue removing the gown, rolling it into a ball, touching only the uncontaminated inside of the gown with the hands. Drop the rolled gown in a biohazard waste container. | The contaminated side of the gown will be rolled inside so that your hands are only touching the part of the gown that was next to your clothing. |
| 13. Remove the goggles, face shield, and/or mask. Dispose of any disposable items appropriately. If goggles are nondisposable, place in a designated area for disinfecting. | Carefully remove the goggles and face shield by grasping the sides of goggles or elastic bands of mask. Avoid touching the front of each piece of PPE. |
| 14. Wash your hands. | Always wash hands after removing PPE. |

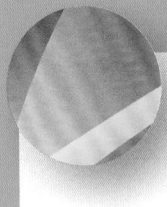

## PROCEDURE 17-3

# Cleaning Biohazardous Spills

**Purpose:** To safely clean contaminated surfaces

**Equipment:** Commercially prepared germicide *or* 1:10 bleach solution, gloves, disposable towels, chemical absorbent, biohazardous waste bag, protective eye wear (goggles or mask and face shield), disposable shoe coverings, disposable gown or apron made of plastic, or other material that is impervious to soaking up contaminated fluids

**Standard:** This task should take 3 to 5 minutes.

| STEPS | PURPOSE |
|---|---|
| 1. Put on gloves. Wear protective eyewear, gown or apron, and shoe coverings if you anticipate any splashing. | A plastic gown or apron will protect your clothing from contaminants. |
| 2. Apply chemical absorbent material to the spill as indicated by office policy. Clean up the spill with disposable paper towels, being careful not to splash. | |

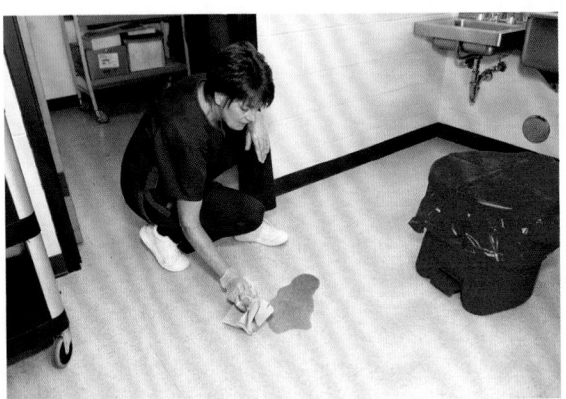

**Step 2.** Wearing PPE, carefully clean up biohazardous spills immediately after they occur.

3. Dispose of paper towels and absorbent material in a biohazard waste bag.

The bag will alert anyone handling the waste that it contains biohazardous material.

4. Spray the area with commercial germicide or bleach solution and wipe with disposable paper towels. Discard towels in a biohazard bag.

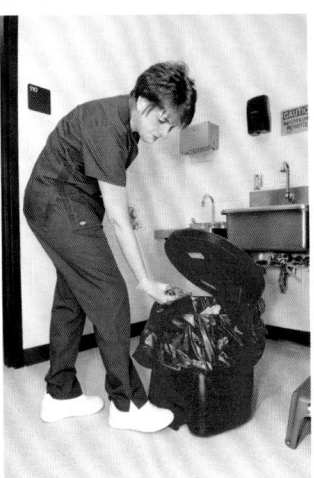

**Step 4.** Place contaminated materials into a biohazard bag.

## PROCEDURE 17-3 (continued)

| STEPS | PURPOSE |
|---|---|
| 5. With your gloves on, remove the protective eyewear and discard or disinfect per office policy. Remove the gown or apron and shoe coverings and put in the biohazard bag if disposable or the biohazard laundry bag for reusable linens. | |
| 6. Place the biohazard bag in an appropriate waste receptacle for removal according to your facility's policy. | |
| 7. Remove your gloves and wash your hands thoroughly. | Wearing gloves does *not* replace proper hand washing. |

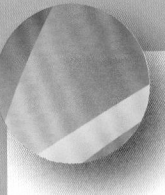

# PROCEDURE 17-4

## Blood-Borne Pathogen Training

**PSY** Participate in Blood-Borne Pathogen Training

**Purpose:** To participate in training about safely working in an environment where exposure to blood-borne pathogens is possible

**Equipment:** A commercial kit that includes presentation materials with current OSHA guidelines regarding blood-borne pathogen training and participation log documenting training including date

**Standard:** This task should take 30 to 45 minutes.

| STEPS | PURPOSE |
|---|---|
| 1. Plan ahead to attend the training as scheduled by your facility. | This training is mandatory for health care workers and must be conducted annually. |
| 2. Come to the training on time and prepared to take notes and ask questions. | Active listening demonstrates participation. Writing may help you remember important information. |
| 3. The training includes information about the following:<br>a. Blood-borne pathogens and diseases<br>b. Exposure control plan<br>c. Engineering and workplace practice controls<br>d. Postexposure evaluation and follow-up procedures | This information may be presented using commercially prepared presentation kits or from individually prepared presentation materials. The exposure control plan must be updated annually according to recent OSHA guidelines. |
| 4. After participating in the training, you should be able to define blood-borne pathogens and the diseases that may affect humans from these pathogens. Procedures to follow in case of an accidental exposure, and engineering and workplace controls to reduce the likelihood of contamination. | Blood-borne pathogens that may cause disease in humans include hepatitis B virus (HBV), hepatitis C virus (HCV), and human immunodeficiency virus (HIV). |
| 5. Sign and date the Blood-Borne Pathogen Training log to document your attendance. | The training is required by your employer each year, and they are required to document that this training was provided to employees. |

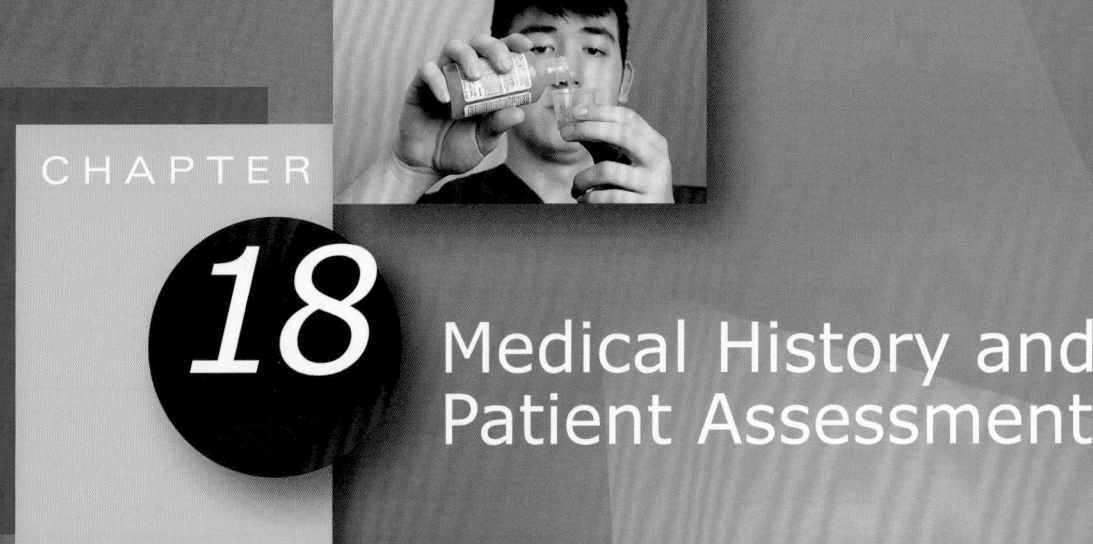

# CHAPTER

# 18 Medical History and Patient Assessment

---

## Outline

**The Medical History**
  Methods of Collecting
    Information
  Elements of the Medical History

**Conducting the Patient Interview**
  Preparing for the Interview
  Introducing Yourself
  Barriers to Communication

**Assessing the Patient**
  Signs and Symptoms
  Chief Complaint and Present Illness

---

## Learning Outcomes

### COG Cognitive Domain*

1. Spell and define key terms
2. *Recognize barriers to communication*
3. *Identify techniques for overcoming communication barriers*
4. Give examples of the type of information included in each section of the patient history
5. Identify guidelines for conducting a patient interview using principles of verbal and nonverbal communication
6. *Differentiate between subjective and objective information*
7. Discuss open-ended and closed-ended questions and explain when to use each type during the patient interview

### PSY Psychomotor Domain*

1. *Use feedback techniques to obtain patient information including the following: (a) reflection, (b) restatement, and (c) clarification*
2. *Use medical terminology correctly and pronounced accurately to communicate information to providers and patients*
3. *Respond to nonverbal communication*

4. Obtain and record a patient history (Procedure 18-1)
5. Accurately document a chief complaint and present illness (Procedure 18-2)

### AFF Affective Domain*

1. Incorporate critical thinking skills when performing patient assessment
2. *Demonstrate (a) empathy, (b) active listening, and (c) nonverbal communication*
3. *Demonstrate sensitivity to patient's rights*
4. *Demonstrate principles of self-boundaries*
5. *Demonstrate respect for individual diversity including (a) gender, (b) race, (c) religion, (d) age, (e) economic status, and (f) appearance*

*\*Note: AAMA/CAAHEP 2015 Standards are italicized.*

### ABHES Competencies

1. Be impartial and show empathy when dealing with patients
2. Interview effectively
3. Recognize and respond to verbal and nonverbal communication
4. Obtain chief complaint, recording patient history

*(continues on page 430)*

| | | | |
|---|---|---|---|
| assessment | hereditary | homeopathic medication | signs |
| chief complaint (CC) | Health Insurance Portability | medical history | symptoms |
| demographic | and Accountability Act | over-the-counter | |
| familial | (HIPAA) | medication | |

## Case Study

*T*he internal medicine clinic at Great Falls Medical Center is busy serving adult patients with many different health issues. Steve Barnett, RMA, works in this clinic and is responsible for checking in new patients and updating information for established patients. This morning, he has checked in four new patients to be seen by the physician. Although all new patients are sent a packet of information and paperwork to be completed and brought to the office at the first visit, only one of the new patients actually had the forms completed correctly. Those who did not have the paperwork completed were asked to fill out the forms while sitting in the waiting room. When he reviewed the paperwork upon calling patients back to the exam room, Steve noticed several blank areas on the forms. Who is responsible for obtaining the information from the patient: the receptionist, the physician, or Steve, the clinical medical assistant? Why is it important to know all details of a family history? One patient, a 53-year-old man, told Steve he was only seeking health care because his wife made the appointment. Would it be appropriate for Steve to discuss the importance of regular checkups with this patient? Why are regular checkups important for adults?

To diagnose a patient's present illness, the physician needs the patient's past and current health information. As a professional medical assistant, you are often responsible for obtaining this information as part of the **medical history** and **assessment**. The medical history is a record containing information about a patient's past and present health status, the health status of related family members, and relevant information about a patient's social habits. Assessment begins with gathering information to determine the patient's problem or reason for seeking medical care. Typically, you ask standard questions and document the patient's responses during the assessment on preprinted forms or in a manner decided by the physician and outlined in the medical office policy and procedure manual.

## THE MEDICAL HISTORY

## Methods of Collecting Information

To complete the patient's medical history, you and the physician work cooperatively with the patient. In some medical practices, medical assistants gather initial patient information by interviewing the patient using a printed list of questions. Other medical offices ask the patient to fill out a standard form before or during the first appointment. Patients who receive the form in the mail are instructed to bring the completed document to the office at the initial visit. In either case, you must check the form for completeness because the physician uses this information as the basis for more extensive questioning during the examination.

In other practices, the physician may prefer to complete the medical history form during the initial patient interview and examination. In this situation, you should be familiar with the form and ready to assist the physician if needed or asked to do so.

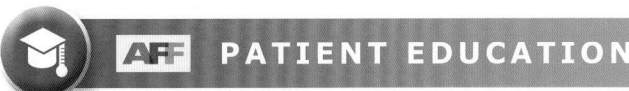

## PATIENT EDUCATION

### General Topics

While assessing a patient, you can also teach. Your teaching may include information about a specific disease or general care. For example, a diabetic patient may need instruction on glucose testing or diet control. General topics for all patients can include the following:

- Blood pressure management
- Stress management
- Diet or weight control tips
- The importance of exercise
- The effects of alcohol and tobacco
- Instructions for conducting breast or testicular self-examinations
- The importance of proper immunizations
- Cancer warning signs and prevention tips

## LEGAL TIP

### Safeguarding Patient Information

You are responsible for ensuring that information in the patient's medical history is kept confidential. Legally and ethically, the patient has a right to privacy concerning his or her medical records, which includes storage in a secure place. Only health care providers directly involved in the patient's care should be allowed access to the records. Although electronic health records makes it easier and more convenient to access patient medical information from a variety of sources, many employers monitor employee access and have policies that require termination of employees who access medical information without having a "need to know" that information, such as information regarding family members, friends, and celebrities.

 ## Elements of the Medical History

The medical history forms used by the office may vary with the practice specialty, but most forms are composed of these common elements: identifying data (database), past history (PH), review of systems (ROS), family history (FH), and social history. Figure 18-1 shows a medical history form. This information is confidential and protected by the **Health Insurance Portability and Accountability Act** (**HIPAA**), a federal law that protects the privacy of health information. No one except those directly involved in the patient's care may have access to it without the patient's permission.

The following are the main elements of the medical history:

- Identifying data (database). The **demographic** information in this section, required for administrative purposes, always includes the patient's name, address, and phone number. It also includes the name, address, and phone number of the patient's employer and insurance carrier and the patient's health insurance policy number, social security number, marital status, gender, and race.
- Past history (PH). This section addresses the patient's prior health status and helps the physician plan appropriate care for any present illness. Information in this section typically includes allergies, immunizations, childhood diseases, current and past medications, and previous illnesses, surgeries, and hospitalizations.
- Review of systems (ROS). A thorough review of each body system may elicit information that the patient forgot to mention earlier or thought was irrelevant. Specific questions, such as symptoms or known diseases, related to each system of the body are included in this section.
- Family history (FH). This section contains the health status of the patient's parents, siblings, and grandparents. This information is important because certain diseases or disorders have **familial** or **hereditary** tendencies. Familial diseases tend to occur often in a particular family, whereas hereditary diseases are transmitted from parent to offspring. If any immediate family member is deceased, the cause of death should be documented.
- Social history. The social history covers the patient's lifestyle, such as marital status, occupation, education, and hobbies. It may also include information about the patient's diet, use of alcohol or tobacco, and sexual history. This information may help the physician understand how present illness, including any treatment, may affect the lifestyle or how the lifestyle may affect the illness. The social history may also provide a guide for patient education, since some behaviors, such as tobacco use or a diet high in fat, may not yet be causing illness but can cause illness in the future.

## CHECKPOINT QUESTION

1. An elderly patient asks Steve what the difference is between the past history and the family history. How would Steve explain the difference?

**Professional Medical Associates – History Form**

NAME: _____ DATE OF BIRTH: _____

What is the main reason for your visit to the doctor? _____

_____

Were you referred? _____ if so, by whom? _____

**PAST MEDICAL HISTORY:**

Are you allergic to any medication? _____

If so, list medications: _____

List current medications, dosage, and how many times a day you take them:

| **Medication** | **Dose** | **Times A Day** |
| --- | --- | --- |
| | | |
| | | |

Alcohol Consumption:    What type? _____ Amount _____ How Often? _____

History of Alcoholism? _____

When was your last TB or Tine test? _____

Have you ever had a positive test for tuberculosis? _____

When was your last Tetanus shot? _____

List all surgeries you have had in the past:

| **Date** | **Type of Surgery** |
| --- | --- |
| | |
| | |

List all past hospitalizations (not involving surgeries above):

| **Date** | **Reason For Hospital Stay** |
| --- | --- |
| | |
| | |

List all past problems with trauma (broken bones, lacerations, etc.):

_____

**REVIEW OF SYSTEMS, PAST MEDICAL PROBLEMS:**
If you have been told you have any of the problems listed below, or are having any of the problems listed below, please CIRCLE:

1. <u>GENERAL:</u> Weight loss, weight gain, fever, chills, night sweats, hot flashes, tire easily, problems with sleep, crying spells, history of cancer.

2. <u>SKIN:</u> Rash, sores that won't heal, moles that are new or changing, history of skin problems.

3. <u>HEENT:</u> Headache, eye problems, hearing problems, sinus problems, hay fever, dizziness, hoarseness, sores in your mouth that won't heal, dental problems.

    Do you chew tobacco or dip snuff? _____

4. <u>METABOLIC/ENDOCRINE:</u> Thyroid problems, diabetes or sugar problems, high cholesterol.

**Figure 18-1** • A sample medical history form, front and back.

5. <u>RESPIRATORY:</u> Cough, wheezing, breathing problems, history of asthma, history of lung problems.

Do you smoke cigarettes or pipe? _____

How much? _____ For how long? _____

6. <u>BREAST (WOMEN):</u> Breast lumps, changes in nipples, nipple discharge, breast problems, family history of breast cancer. When was your last mammogram? _____

7. <u>CARDIOVASCULAR:</u> Heart murmur, rheumatic fever, high blood pressure, angina, heart problems, heart attack, abnormal heart rhythm, chest pain, palpitations, leg swelling, history of phlebitis or blood clots.

8. <u>GI:</u> Problems with appetite, swallowing, heartburn, nausea, vomiting, pain in the abdomen, constipation, diarrhea, blood in stool, history of ulcers, liver problems, hepatitis, jaundice, pancreas problems, gallbladder problems, or colon problems.

9. <u>REPRODUCTIVE (WOMEN):</u> Problems with irregular menstrual cycles, abnormal vaginal bleeding or discharge, history of sexually transmitted diseases, sexual problems.

AGE OF FIRST MENSES (PERIOD) _____ AGE OF MENOPAUSE _____

LAST PAP SMEAR _____ METHOD OF CONTRACEPTION _____

**Obstetric History (Women)**

NUMBER OF PREGNANCIES _____ PLEASE LIST AS FOLLOWS:

Delivery Date      Pregnancy Complications     Type Delivery     Baby's Weight

_____

_____

<u>MEN:</u> Problems with genital discharge, history of venereal diseases, sexual problems, prostate problems.

METHOD OF CONTRACEPTION _____

10. <u>UROLOGIC:</u> Problems with painful urination, urinary frequency, blood in urine, weak urinary stream, history of bladder or kidney infections, or kidney stones.

11. <u>MUSCULOSKELETAL:</u> Arthritis, back pain, cramps in legs.

12. <u>NEUROLOGIC:</u> Seizures, stroke, arm or leg weakness or numbness, black-out spells, memory or thinking problems, depression, anxiety, psychiatric problems.

13. <u>HEMATOLOGIC:</u> Anemia, bleeding problems, enlarged lymph nodes.

HAVE YOU EVER HAD A BLOOD TRANSFUSION? _____ DATE _____

**FAMILY HISTORY:**

List any medical problems that run in your family and which family members have these problems.

_____

_____

**SOCIAL HISTORY:**

MARITAL STATUS: _____

OCCUPATION: _____

EDUCATION: _____

HOBBIES: _____

WHAT DO YOU DO FOR ENJOYMENT? _____

**Figure 18-1** • (*Continued*)

## 🔁 CONDUCTING THE PATIENT INTERVIEW

### Preparing for the Interview

As a medical assistant, your primary goal during a patient interview is to obtain accurate and pertinent information. To do this, you need to understand the basic components of communication and to use active listening skills. You should also use a variety of interviewing techniques, including reflecting, restating or paraphrasing, asking for examples, asking questions, summarizing, and allowing silence (see Chapter 3). Communication also includes observation. Specifically, any objective or observable information concerning the patient's physical or mental status should be noted and documented in the patient's record as appropriate. Examples of observations about a patient's physical status include the general appearance (bruising or injury, pale or flushed skin). The mental or emotional condition of the patient includes observations such as lethargy, crying, tearfulness, and confusion. Judgments made about these observations should not be documented in the patient's record because the terminology used (depressed, abused) may be diagnostic, which is out of the scope of training for the medical assistant. In the case of suspected abuse, you should document the observable information in the medical record and alert the physician regarding your suspicions. Procedure 18-1 outlines the process for conducting a successful patient interview.

Before you start interviewing the patient, make sure you are familiar with the medical history form and any previous medical history provided by the patient. Shuffling papers or looking at a computer or tablet screen while the patient is talking or asking questions out of order may distract the patient and disrupt the flow of the interview. If the patient is new to the medical practice, review the new patient questionnaire before beginning the interview. Review the chart of any established patient, and update information as indicated.

To safeguard confidential patient information and allow for open communication, conduct the interview in a private and comfortable place. Avoid public areas, such as the reception area, where distractions are likely and where others may hear the patient's answers. Interview the patient alone unless he or she wishes to have family members or significant others present (Fig. 18-2).

### PATIENT EDUCATION

#### Genetic Diseases

The patient's family history can provide you with many teaching opportunities. If a patient indicates that previous members of his or her family had certain diseases, then there may be a genetic link. A genetic disease is noted by a mark on the DNA (genetic material) for a specific illness or disease. The patient receives this mark from either or both parents. Some common examples include some forms of high blood pressure, diabetes, heart disease, obesity, and certain cancers. Examples of less common genetic disorders are Tay-Sachs disease, Marfan syndrome, and Huntington disease. Great strides have been made in genetic testing. This allows the patient to have the DNA examined for potential markers of diseases. For example, color blindness is a genetic disorder that can easily be seen on a DNA chain. Patients can have genetic testing done to see whether they carry a particular disease marker. Genetic counseling may also be appropriate depending on the type of genetic disorder. Some insurance plans will pay for genetic testing and counseling. Advise the patient to contact his or her insurance company directly for specific coverage guidelines.

### PATIENT EDUCATION

#### Preventative Medicine

While interviewing the patient about his or her chief complaint, you may have an opportunity to teach the patient about various topics. Emphasize to the patient that illnesses can often be treated easier and quicker if prompt medical attention is received. This is a very important point to stress to older patients with chronic medical problems such as diabetes. For example, a diabetic patient who presents with a small foot ulcer in its early stages may be able to be treated with medicated dressings. However, if the ulcer goes untreated and gets bigger, the patient may need surgery to clean the wound and may even require hospitalization for antibiotics. While interviewing the patient about their chief complaint, take the opportunity to stress the importance of preventative medicine.

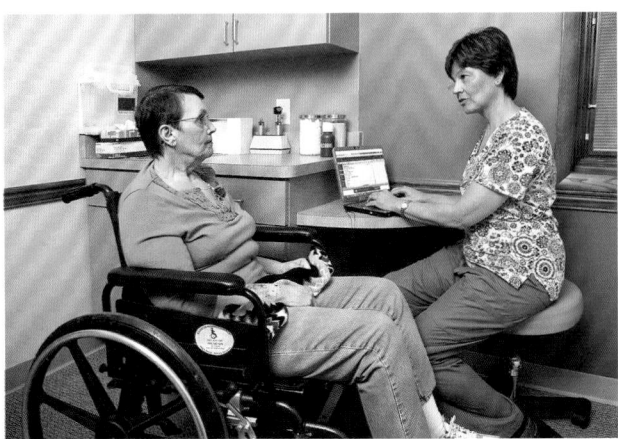

**Figure 18-2 •** Conduct the patient interview in a private office or exam room.

## ▣ Introducing Yourself

Always begin the interview with new or established patients by identifying yourself, your title, and the purpose of the interview. For example, you might say, "Good morning, Mr. Frank. My name is Angela, and I'm Dr. Martin's medical assistant. I would like to ask you a few questions that will help the doctor diagnose and treat you appropriately. Please be assured that your responses will be kept in strict confidence." Under no circumstance should you identify yourself as a nurse because it is unethical and illegal to give the patient a false impression of your credentials.

The initial impression you make will be a lasting one, so be sure that your demeanor and words communicate genuine respect and concern. By developing professional rapport, you will gain the patient's confidence and trust in you, the physician, and the office staff. Some patients may be reluctant to share private information with you until a sense of trust has been established. This makes the professional role of the medical assistant as a caring and empathic health care worker even more important.

## ▣ Barriers to Communication

As you begin speaking with the patient, you must assess any barriers to communication, such as unfamiliarity with English, hearing impairment, or cognitive impairment. Note the patient's verbal and nonverbal behavior during the interview and adjust your questioning if necessary. Avoid using highly technical or medical terminology when conversing with most patients. If the patient has impaired hearing or vision or difficulty understanding or speaking English, adjust your interviewing techniques to fit the patient's needs; however, remember that raising your voice is not necessary and will not improve communication or understanding with these patients. Instead, it is best to face the patient and maintain eye contact when speaking and use physical cues as appropriate (see Chapter 3 for more details about overcoming communication barriers).

### 🔍 CHECKPOINT QUESTION

2. Steve takes a few minutes to look over the medical history form before going into the exam room to interview a new patient. Why is it important to review the medical history form before beginning the interview?

3. Why should you let the patient know that any information shared during the interview will be kept confidential?

## ▣ ASSESSING THE PATIENT

### Signs and Symptoms

During the interview, listen carefully as the patient describes current medical problems to identify **signs** and **symptoms**. Signs are objective information that can be observed or perceived by someone other than the patient. Signs include such things as rash, bleeding, coughing, and vital sign measurements. Signs may also be found during the physician's examination.

Symptoms, or subjective information, are indications of disease or changes in the body as sensed by the patient. Usually, symptoms are not discernible by anyone other than the patient. They include complaints such as leg pain, headache, nausea, and dizziness. Observable signs that may indicate that a patient is having these symptoms include facial expressions, such as wincing during pain, holding onto rails or furniture for balance when walking, and gagging.

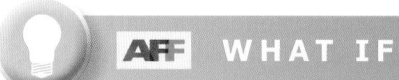

### 💡 AFF   WHAT IF?

**What if the patient appears highly anxious or intimidated about procedures that seem routine?**

You can help put patients at ease by following these steps:

- Treat each patient as an individual with unique needs. Help elderly or disabled patients onto the examination table. If they are unsteady, keep them seated in a regular chair.
- When weighing patients, do not announce their weight aloud, since they may be embarrassed. Instead, ask them in the privacy of the examination room if they want to know their weight.
- Always offer a sheet or blanket to a patient who must change into an examination gown.
- When preparing a patient for a gynecologic examination, have her sit on the examination table until the physician is ready.
- If the physician is delayed, let the patient know. Explain generally the reason for the delay (e.g., an emergency), and let the patient know the approximate length of the delay.

## ▣ Chief Complaint and Present Illness

After recording the patient's medical history and reviewing the information for accuracy and clarity, you must find out exactly why the patient has come to see the physician for this appointment (Procedure 18-2). Ask an open-ended question to encourage the patient to describe the chain of events leading to this visit.

Open-ended questions allow the patient to answer with more than one or two words. For example, you might ask, "What is the reason for your appointment today?" or "Can you describe what has been going on?" Such questions require the patient to explain the visit by giving additional information. In contrast, answers to closed-ended questions usually necessitate only one or two words. Examples of closed-ended questions are "Do you have pain?" and "Are you able to sleep?" These questions can be answered with a simple yes or no and are not going to elicit responses that will be useful to the physician attempting to make a diagnosis.

When open-ended questions are used to determine the reason for the visit, the patient's answer will reveal the **chief complaint** (**CC**). The CC, which is one statement describing the signs and symptoms that led the patient to seek medical care, is documented in the patient's medical record at each visit. Examples of a CC might include "I've had a headache for the past 3 days" or "Yesterday I lifted a heavy crate and hurt my back." You should document the CC on the progress report form in the patient's paper or electronic medical record, using the patient's own words in quotation marks whenever possible. The entry should include the date (day, month, and year) and the time of day.

Once you have obtained the CC, continue to probe for more details to further define the patient's present illness (PI). The PI includes a chronologic order of events, including dates of onset and any home remedies or other self-care activities, including **over-the-counter** and **homeopathic medications**. Over-the-counter medications are those that are available without prescriptions. They include natural drugs, such as herbs, vitamins, and some homeopathic agents. Homeopathic medications include small doses of agents that cause similar symptoms in healthy individuals and are given to a person who is ill to help cure the disease causing the symptoms. The following questions could be used to obtain the PI:

- Chronology. How did this first begin?
- Location. Can you explain or show me exactly where the pain is?
- Severity. Can you describe the pain? Is the pain constant?
- Self-treatment. What medications have you taken for the pain? Do they help?
- Quality. Does anything that you do make the symptoms better or worse?
- Duration. Have you had these symptoms before?

Avoid suggesting answers with questions such as "Is the pain sharp?" or "Is the pain worse when you walk?" Many patients will agree or answer positively because they think this must be the expected answer. In addition, do not coax patients by making suggestions of symptoms you might expect them to have based on the chief complaint. Some patients may agree to have the symptoms you describe if they feel that you are suggesting those that "should" be present.

After asking several open-ended questions, it may be appropriate to ask closed-ended questions to obtain specific data. For example, you might ask the patient, "How long have you had this pain?" This kind of question requires only a short answer, not a lengthy description.

Of course, not all patients visit the doctor because they are ill. Some appointments are for routine examinations or tests. In this case, the CC will include a statement about the reason for the visit (e.g., annual physical examination, employment examination); however, you should obtain any additional PI information as appropriate.

## CHECKPOINT QUESTION

4. Explain the difference between a sign and a symptom, and give one example of each.

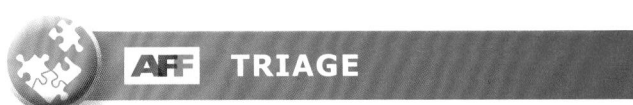

## TRIAGE

While working in the medical office, you begin the day by placing the following three patients into examination rooms:

A. Patient A, a new patient, arrives on time and was given the two-page medical history form to complete.
B. Patient B is an established patient who is scheduled to have his blood pressure checked today because he started a new antihypertensive medication last month.
C. Patient C is a 1-year-old baby who is scheduled to be seen today for a well-child checkup and immunizations.

**How would you sort these patients? Who should be seen first? Second? Third?**

Patient B should be called back first, since he will probably take the least amount of time. Unless this patient's blood pressure is not responding to the antihypertensive medication or he has unanticipated problems, this type of visit is typically conducted in a timely manner as a convenience to the patient. Patient C should be seen next, since infant checkups usually require additional procedures that may require more time from the medical assistant and physician. Patient A should be given an adequate amount of time to complete the medical history forms, since this information will be necessary for the physician to understand the patient's current and future health problems. The patient should not be rushed to complete this paperwork. If necessary, you may call the patient back and assist with completion of the form, especially if the patient is having difficulty due to a physical disability, such as visual impairment, deformity, or trouble holding a pen or pencil because of arthritis.

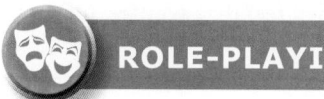

## ROLE-PLAYING ACTIVITY

Find two students to role-play this scenario, taking turns assuming the roles described below. You are either working at the busy internal medicine as a professional medical assistant with Steve Barnett (refer to case study at the beginning of this chapter) or you are a patient/caregiver. As the medical assistant, you are calling patients back from the reception area to an examination room. One of the patients is a 55-year-old man, Russ Smalley, who lives alone since his wife passed away 3 years ago. He has a history of cardiovascular disease and recently had a pacemaker inserted. Using the information on the medical history form, interview the patient to update his information using professionalism and interpersonal skills such as maintaining eye contact. Avoid using medical jargon without being unprofessional or condescending. During the conversation, Russ admits to you that he takes many over-the-counter vitamins and dietary supplements, but he would like more information about a "natural" supplement that improves memory (he cannot remember the name of it and wants you to tell him). He would also like to "get a prescription" for the medication to "help with impotence" because he has recently started dating and is "having problems in that area." Respond to this while staying within your scope of practice and maintaining professionalism. Another patient is an elderly woman, Bertha McIntosh, who is 88 years old and lives with her daughter Mildred who brought her into the office today. Bertha is not sure where she is and seems reluctant to answer questions directly, usually looking to Mildred who is eager to answer all questions for her mother. Again, update the medical history form after calling Ms. McIntosh back to the exam room. Your instructor will give you additional information about this activity!

## *español* SPANISH TERMINOLOGY

**Mi nombre es _____.**
My name is _____.

**¿Cuál es su nombre?**
What is your name?

**¿Dónde nació?**
When were you born?

**¿Dónde vive?**
Where do you live?

**Cuál es su domicilio?**
What is your address?

**¿Usted toma algún medicamento?**
Are you taking any medications?

**¿Le han hecho alguna cirugía?**
Have you had any surgery?

**Fuma usted tabaco o bebe alcohol?**
Do you smoke or drink alcohol?

**Cuantos cigarros al dia?**
How many cigarettes per day?

**Cuantas bebidas alcohólicas y de que tipo usted normalmente bebe?**
How much and what type of alcoholic beverage you usually drink?

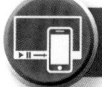

## MEDIA MENU

**Student Resources** on the Point®
• **CMA/RMA Certification Exam Review**

**Internet Resources**
**The Health Insurance Portability and Accountability Act**
http://www.cms.gov/HIPAAGenInfoAmerican

**Autoimmune Related Diseases Association**
http://www.aarda.org

**March of Dimes**
http://www.marchofdimes.com

**Genetic Alliance**
http://www.geneticalliance.org

## EMR Activity

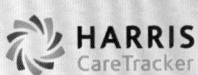

Harris CareTracker is a Web-based electronic medical record (EMR) application that you will use for the EMR activities included in this section at the end of each chapter. This application is actually used in physician offices but is provided to you through the publisher, Wolters Kluwer Health, to give you hands-on practice working with EMRs. Your instructor will have more information about accessing your username, log-in, and Quickstart guide.

### Prerequisite Activities in Harris CareTracker

*Note: The Getting Started and Quickstart documents and EMR Activities Step-by-Step Instructions listed below are available at* http://thePoint.lww.com/KronenbergerComp5e.

### Activity Details

In the *Medical Record* module, *History*, then *General Medical History* section of the *Patient History* screen, click "Yes" on the conditions noted as follows for new patient Penelope Wringer, and save your entries when finished: allergies, pneumonia, anxiety, depression, kidney stones, and hypertension. Click on the *Family History* tab and note "Yes" for the following conditions for her immediate family and save your entries when finished: ovarian CA (mother), osteoporosis (mother), anxiety (mother), diabetes (father), and hypercholesterolemia (father).

# Chapter Summary

- In every medical practice, a history is taken from each patient and updated regularly.
- As a professional medical assistant, you need to know the components of a standard medical history form. You may be required to obtain and document the information on the history form and to interview the patient to elicit the chief complaint and present illness.
- The physician relies on the information that you gather and document for diagnosing and treating patients, so it is essential that you question the patient carefully and document accurately.

# Warm-Ups for Critical Thinking

1. Mrs. Smythe has always been impeccably groomed, articulate, and punctual for her monthly blood pressure checks. Today, she was 15 minutes late, her hair was not combed, she wore no makeup, and her clothes did not match. Are any of these observations worth noting on her chart?

2. After reviewing the following items, determine in which section of the medical history the information should be included and explain why. Identify any items that are irrelevant.
   - Sister died of breast cancer.
   - Son had chicken pox last year.
   - Patient has many allergies.
   - Father died of heart disease.
   - Mother is alive and well.
   - Brother works in real estate.
   - Patient smokes three packs of cigarettes a day.
   - Patient works in a cotton mill.
   - Patient is a runner and teaches aerobics.
   - Patient has recently lost 60 pounds.
   - Patient had an angioplasty last year.

3. Determine which of the following are signs and which are symptoms.
   - Nausea
   - Vomiting
   - Itching
   - Rash
   - Dizziness
   - Abdominal pain
   - Pallor
   - Tingling fingers and toes
   - Ringing in the ears
   - Fever
   - Edema

4. Provide open-ended questions for obtaining additional information from patients with the following complaints:
   - "I am tired; I don't sleep well at night."
   - "I have pain in the bottom of my foot when I walk."
   - "My stomach hurts, and I threw up yesterday."
   - "I have indigestion every day."

5. An elderly patient, Mr. Barnes, comes into the office and is given the medical history form, a pen, and a clipboard. He is unable to hold the pen due to arthritic deformities of his hands. Would it be appropriate to sit with Mr. Barnes in the waiting room and complete the form for him? Why or why not?

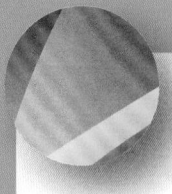

**PSY** PROCEDURE 18-1

## Interviewing the Patient to Obtain a Medical History

**PSY** Use feedback techniques to obtain patient information including the following: (a) reflection, (b) restatement, and (c) clarification.

**Purpose:** Review and complete the various sections of a medical history form while interviewing a patient

**Equipment:** Paper medical history form or questionnaire, black or blue pen

**Standard:** This task should take 10 minutes.

| STEPS | REASONS |
|---|---|
| 1. Gather the supplies. | Make sure you have everything you need before you begin. |
| 2. Review the medical history form. | Be familiar with the order of the questions and the type of information required to allow for smooth communication with the patient. |
| 3. **AFF** Take the patient to a private and comfortable area of the office. | A private place prevents distractions and ensures confidentiality. |
| 4. Sit across from the patient at eye level and maintain frequent eye contact. | Standing above the patient may be perceived as threatening and may result in poor communication. |
| 5. Introduce yourself and explain the purpose of the interview. | This helps to establish a professional rapport with the patient. |
| 6. Using language the patient can understand, ask the appropriate questions, and document the patient's responses. Be sure to determine the patient's CC and PI. | You must obtain accurate and complete data for the physician. |
| 7. Use feedback techniques including the following:<br>**a.** Reflection<br>**b.** Restatement<br>**c.** Clarification | Patients can sense when the interviewer is not listening, so be sure that you show interest in what the patient is saying. To make sure you understand what the patient is communicating, use techniques such as reflection, restatement, and clarification. |
| 8. **AFF** Regardless of the confidences shared by the patient, avoid projecting a judgmental attitude with words or actions. | Maintain professionalism, and ensure the patient's trust. |
| 9. **AFF** Explain how to respond to a patient who has English as a second language. | Solicit assistance from anyone who may be with the patient or a staff member who speaks the patient's native language to interpret if available. If no interpreter is available, use hand gestures or pictures to explain procedure to the patient. |
| 10. **AFF** Explain to the patient what to expect during examinations or procedures at that visit. | Keeping the patient informed about his or her care may decrease anxiety. |

## PROCEDURE 18.1 (continued)

| STEPS | REASONS |
|---|---|
| 11. Review the history form for completion and accuracy. | The patient record is a legal document, and information placed in the record must be accurate. |
| 12. Thank the patient for cooperating during the interview, and offer to answer any questions. | Courtesy encourages the patient to have a positive attitude about the physician's office. |
| 13. Describe examples of applying local, state, and federal health care legislation and regulation in the medical office. | Local regulations include required reporting of communicable diseases or injuries involving violence. State and federal regulations may include issues related to reimbursement, collection of fees, and privacy (HIPAA). |

Charting Example:
10/14/2015 11:00 AM CC: New pt. checkup. Medical hx form complete, pt. indicates no physical or health problems at this time. Family history of colon cancer and hypertension noted _____
E. Parker, CMA(AAMA)

---

Note: *The medical assistant may sign his/her name in the patient record using only the "CMA" credential if the office has a signature log denoting the entire credential as "CMA(AAMA)."*

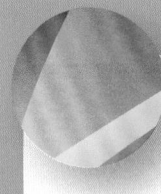

**PSY** PROCEDURE 18-2

# Document a Chief Complaint (CC) and Present Illness (PI)

**PSY** Use medical terminology correctly and pronounced accurately to communicate information to providers and patients.

**PSY** Respond to nonverbal communication.

**PSY** Apply HIPAA rules in regard to release of information.

**Purpose:** Accurately record a CC and PI using open-ended and closed-ended questions while interviewing the patient

**Equipment:** A paper or electronic medical record including a cumulative problem list or progress notes form, black or blue ink pen

**Standard:** This procedure should take 10 minutes or less.

| STEPS | REASONS |
|---|---|
| 1. Gather the supplies, including the medical record containing the cumulative problem list or progress note form. | You should have everything you need before you start. |
| 2. Review new or established patient's medical history form. | Be as familiar as possible with the patient to help you obtain a complete CC and PI. |

---

**Professional Medical Associates – History Form**

NAME: *Fred Smart*                    DATE OF BIRTH: *09-15-1945*

What is the main reason for your visit to the doctor? *Physical Exam*

Were you referred? *No*          if so, by whom? _____

**PAST MEDICAL HISTORY:**

Are you allergic to any medication? *Yes*

If so, list medications: *Penicillin*

List current medications, dosage, and how many times a day you take them:

| **Medication** | **Dose** | **Times A Day** |
|---|---|---|
| *Multivitamin* | *1 tablet* | *every day* |

Alcohol Consumption:    What type? *Beer*      Amount *2-3*      How Often? *Every week*

History of Alcoholism? *No*

When was your last TB or Tine test? *I can't remember*

Have you ever had a positive test for tuberculosis? *No*

When was your last Tetanus shot? *Last year, I cut my finger when fishing.*

List all surgeries you have had in the past:

| **Date** | **Type of Surgery** |
|---|---|
| *1952-childhood?* | *Tonsillectomy* |

List all past hospitalizations (not involving surgeries above):

| **Date** | **Reason For Hospital Stay** |
|---|---|
| *Spring, 1999* | *Pneumonia* |

List all past problems with trauma (broken bones, lacerations, etc.):
*Cut my finger while fishing last year. I had a broken leg from a car accident in 1984.*

**REVIEW OF SYSTEMS, PAST MEDICAL PROBLEMS:**
If you have been told you have any of the problems listed below, or are having any of the problems listed below, please CIRCLE:

1. GENERAL:  Weight loss, weight gain, fever, chills, night sweats, hot flashes, tire easily, problems with sleep, crying spells, history of cancer.

2. SKIN:  Rash, sores that won't heal, moles that are new or changing, history of skin problems.

3. HEENT:  Headache, eye problems, hearing problems, sinus problems, hay fever, dizziness, hoarseness, sores in your mouth that won't heal, dental problems.

    Do you chew tobacco or dip snuff? *No*

4. METABOLIC/ENDOCRINE:  Thyroid problems, diabetes or sugar problems, high cholesterol.

**Step 2A.** Completed medical history form—front

## PROCEDURE 18.2 (continued)

**STEPS**                                                      **REASONS**

5. RESPIRATORY: Cough, wheezing, breathing problems, history of asthma, history of lung problems.

   Do you smoke cigarettes or pipe? *Cigarettes* _____

   How much? *1 pack a day* _____  For how long? *20 years* _____

6. BREAST (WOMEN): Breast lumps, changes in nipples, nipple discharge, breast problems, family history of breast cancer. When was your last mammogram? _____

7. CARDIOVASCULAR: Heart murmur, rheumatic fever, high blood pressure, angina, heart problems, heart attack, abnormal heart rhythm, chest pain, palpitations, leg swelling, history of phlebitis or blood clots.

8. GI: Problems with appetite, swallowing, heartburn, nausea, vomiting, pain in the abdomen, constipation, diarrhea, blood in stool, history of ulcers, liver problems, hepatitis, jaundice, pancreas problems, gallbladder problems, or colon problems.

9. REPRODUCTIVE (WOMEN): Problems with irregular menstrual cycles, abnormal vaginal bleeding or discharge, history of sexually transmitted diseases, sexual problems.

   AGE OF FIRST MENSES (PERIOD) _____  AGE OF MENOPAUSE _____

   LAST PAP SMEAR _____  METHOD OF CONTRACEPTION _____

   **Obstetric History (Women)**

   NUMBER OF PREGNANCIES _____  PLEASE LIST AS FOLLOWS:

   Delivery Date    Pregnancy Complications    Type Delivery    Baby's Weight

   _____

   _____

   MEN: Problems with genital discharge, history of venereal diseases, sexual problems, prostate problems.

   METHOD OF CONTRACEPTION _____

10. UROLOGIC: Problems with painful urination, urinary frequency, blood in urine, weak urinary stream, history of bladder or kidney infections, or kidney stones.

11. MUSCULOSKELETAL: Arthritis, back pain, cramps in legs.

12. NEUROLOGIC: Seizures, stroke, arm or leg weakness or numbness, black-out spells, memory or thinking problems, depression, anxiety, psychiatric problems.

13. HEMATOLOGIC: Anemia, bleeding problems, enlarged lymph nodes.

   HAVE YOU EVER HAD A BLOOD TRANSFUSION? _____  DATE _____

**FAMILY HISTORY:**

List any medical problems that run in your family and which family members have these problems.

*Grandmother had colon cancer; Father has high blood pressure* _____

_____

**SOCIAL HISTORY:**

MARITAL STATUS: *Married for 30 years* _____

OCCUPATION: *Mail Carrier* _____

EDUCATION: *Graduated high school 1963* _____

HOBBIES: *Fishing, camping* _____

WHAT DO YOU DO FOR ENJOYMENT? _____

**Step 2B.** Completed medical history form—back

**Step 2C.** A complete medical record

*(continues on page 444)*

## PROCEDURE 18.2 (continued)

| STEPS | REASONS |
|---|---|
| 3. Greet and identify the patient while escorting him or her to the examination room. | Greeting the patient by name helps develop a professional rapport and eases patient's anxiety. Correctly identifying the patient may help to prevent errors. |

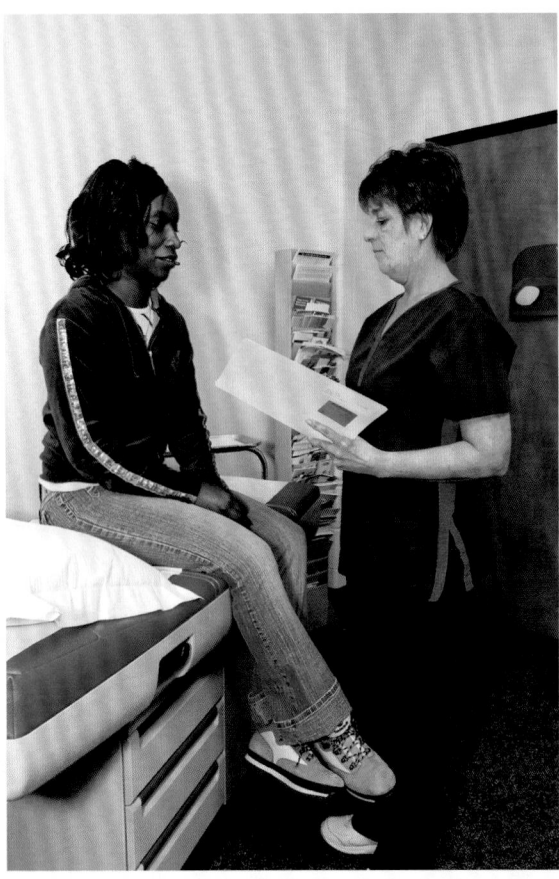

**Step 3.** Always check patient identification information with what is recorded in the medical record.

| STEPS | REASONS |
|---|---|
| 4. **AFF** Using open-ended questions, find out why the patient is seeking medical care; maintain eye contact. | Maintaining eye contact demonstrates that you are actively listening. |
| 5. When reviewing medical history including medications with patient, pronounce all terms and medications accurately. | Correct pronunciation of medical terms and medications improves patient confidence. |
| 6. **AFF** Explain how to respond to a patient who has dementia and whose facial expression shows confusion. | Solicit assistance from caregiver or other staff member to help during the procedure. Give simple directions to the patient about what he/she should do. Speak clearly, not loudly. Nonverbal signs such as a look of confusion should be acknowledged and information clarified if possible. |
| 7. Determine the PI using open-ended and closed-ended questions. | Use closed-ended questions to obtain specific data only after the patient has responded to open-ended questions. |

# PROCEDURE 18.2 (continued)

| STEPS | REASONS |
|---|---|
| 8. Document the CC and PI correctly on the cumulative problem list or progress report form. | Documentation should include the date, time, CC, PI, and your signature (first initial, last name, and title). Use only correct medical terminology and approved abbreviations. |

*09/15/2016*

*9:45 a.m. CC: Pt. c/o headache and nausea x3 days. Has taken ibuprofen for the pain with "some relief." The pain is a "dull ache" in the frontal area of the head and face. Denies emesis. Face flushed, skin warm and dry. T 98.9°F, P88, R24, BP 190/110 (L) sitting.*

*S. Vincer, CMA*

**Step 8.** Sample documentation in the patient record.

| STEPS | REASONS |
|---|---|
| 9. How would you respond to a patient who is moving to another town and asks about having his/her medical records transferred to a physician in another town? | You should be familiar with the office policy regarding release of information, but generally, the patient will need to sign a release form that shows exactly what records or part of the record should be released, a signature line, and a date line. |
| 10. Thank the patient for cooperating, and explain that the physician will soon be in to examine the patient. | Courtesy encourages a positive attitude about the physician's office. If you indicate a time frame in reference to the physician coming into the examination room, be honest. |

**Charting Example:**
09/15/2016 9:45 AM CC: Pt. c/o headache and nausea × 3 days. Has taken ibuprofen for the pain with "some relief." The pain is a "dull ache" in the frontal area of the head and face. Denies emesis. Face flushed, skin warm and dry.
T 98.8°F, P 88, R 24, BP 190/110 (L) sitting_____ S. Vincer, CMA

*Note: The medical assistant may sign his/her name in the patient record using only the "CMA" credential if the office has a signature log denoting the entire credential as "CMA (AAMA)."*

# CHAPTER

# 19

# Anthropometric Measurements and Vital Signs

## Outline

**Anthropometric Measurements**
Weight
Height

**Vital Signs**
Temperature
Pulse

Respiration
Blood Pressure

## Learning Outcomes

### COG Cognitive Domain*

1. Spell and define key terms
2. Explain the procedures for measuring a patient's height and weight
3. Identify and describe the types of thermometers
4. Compare the procedures for measuring a patient's temperature using the oral, rectal, axillary, and tympanic methods
5. List the fever process, including the stages of fever
6. Describe the procedure for measuring a patient's pulse and respiratory rates
7. Identify the various sites on the body used for palpating a pulse
8. Define Korotkoff sounds and the five phases of blood pressure
9. Identify factors that may influence the blood pressure
10. Explain the factors to consider when choosing the correct blood pressure cuff size

### PSY Psychomotor Domain*

1. Measure and record a patient's weight (Procedure 19-1)
2. Measure and record a patient's height (Procedure 19-2)
3. Measure and record a patient's rectal temperature (Procedure 19-3)
4. Measure and record a patient's axillary temperature (Procedure 19-4)
5. Measure and record a patient's temperature using an electronic thermometer (Procedure 19-5)
6. Measure and record a patient's temperature using a tympanic thermometer (Procedure 19-6)
7. Measure and record a patient's temperature using a temporal artery thermometer (Procedure 19-7)

8. Measure and record a patient's radial pulse (Procedure 19-8)
9. Measure and record a patient's respirations (Procedure 19-9)
10. Measure and record a patient's blood pressure (Procedure 19-10)
11. *Instruct and prepare a patient for a procedure or a treatment*
12. *Document patient care accurately in the medical record*
13. *Coach patients appropriately considering cultural diversity, developmental life stage, and communication barriers*

### AFF Affective Domain*

1. *Incorporate critical thinking skills when performing patient assessment*
2. *Demonstrate respect for individual diversity including gender, race, religion, age, economic status, and appearance*
3. *Explain to a patient the rationale for performance of a procedure*
4. *Demonstrate empathy, active listening, and nonverbal communication*
5. *Demonstrate the principles of self-boundaries*
6. *Show awareness of a patient's concerns related to the procedure being performed*

*Note: AAMA/CAAHEP 2015 Standards are italicized.*

### ABHES Competencies

1. Take vital signs
2. Document accurately

afebrile
anthropometric measurements
apnea
baseline data
calibrated
cardiac cycle
cardiac output

cardinal signs
diaphoresis
diastole
dyspnea
febrile
hyperpnea
hyperpyrexia

hypertension
hyperventilation
hypopnea
intermittent fever
orthopnea
palpation
postural hypotension

pyrexia
relapsing fever
remittent fever
sphygmomanometer
sustained fever
systole
tympanic

## Case Study

Yvonne Torres, CMA (AAMA), has worked in a family practice since graduating from her medical assistant education program 5 years ago. There are three physicians and two nurse practitioners in her office. This afternoon, several patients were seen in the office, including a young mother who complains of being "feverish," two high school students who need physical examinations to play sports, an elderly woman with a history of kidney disease who receives dialysis three times a week, and a middle-aged man who has high blood pressure. What would be the best way to obtain a temperature on the young mother, and how would Yvonne know whether she has a fever? Should Yvonne expect a difference in the pulse or respiratory rate between patients based on age? What are some causes of inaccurate blood pressure readings?

Vital signs, also known as **cardinal signs**, are measurements of bodily functions essential to maintaining life processes. Vital signs frequently measured and recorded by the medical assistant include the temperature (T), pulse rate (P), respiratory rate (R), and blood pressure (BP). In addition, medical assistants take **anthropometric measurements**, or the height and weight, of patients and document them in the medical record. This information is essential for the physician to diagnose, treat, and prevent many disorders.

Measurements taken at the first visit are recorded as **baseline data** and are used as reference points for comparison during subsequent visits. After the first office visit, the height is usually not taken; however, the vital signs and weight are taken and recorded for each adult patient at each visit to the medical office.

## ANTHROPOMETRIC MEASUREMENTS

### Weight

An accurate weight is always required for pregnant patients, infants, children, and the elderly. In addition,

weight monitoring may be required if the patient has been prescribed medications that must be carefully calculated according to body weight or for a patient who is attempting to gain or lose weight.

Since most medical practices have only one scale, placement of the scale is important. Many patients are uncomfortable if they are weighed in a place that is not private. Types of scales used to measure weight include balance beam scales, digital scales, and dial scales (Fig. 19-1). Weight may be measured in pounds or kilograms, depending upon the preference of the physician and the type of scale in the medical office. Procedure 19-1 describes how to measure and record a patient's weight.

### Height

Height can be measured using the movable ruler on the back of most balance beam scales. Some offices use a graph ruler mounted on a wall (Fig. 19-2), but more accurate measures can be made with a parallel bar moved down against the top of the patient's head. Height is measured in inches or centimeters, depending upon the physician's preference. Procedure 19-2

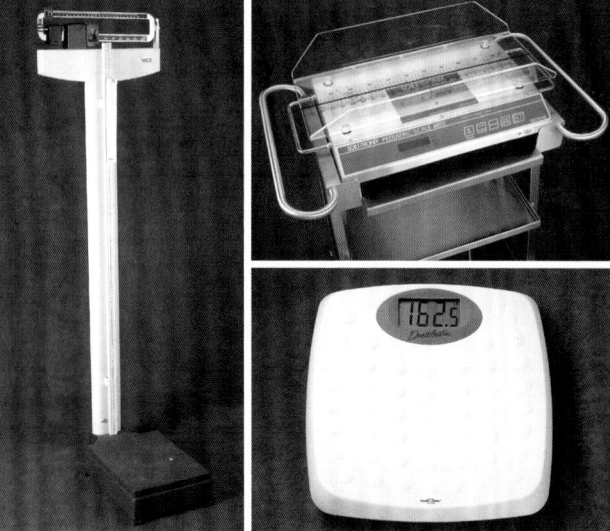

**Figure 19-1** • The three types of scales used in medical offices include the digital, dial, and balance beam scale.

describes how to measure an adult patient's height. Refer to Chapter 38 for the procedure for measuring the height and weight of infants and children.

## CHECKPOINT QUESTION

1. Why is it important for Yvonne to accurately measure vital signs at every patient visit?

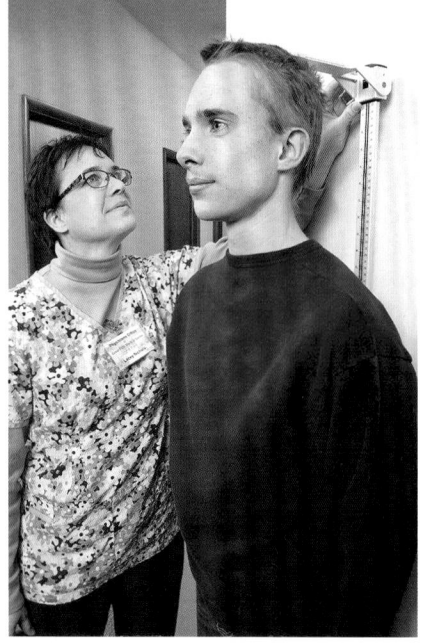

**Figure 19-2** • A wall-mounted device to measure height in the physician office.

## VITAL SIGNS

### Temperature

Body temperature reflects a balance between heat produced and heat lost by the body (Fig. 19-3). Heat is produced during normal internal physical and chemical processes called *metabolism* and through muscle movement. Heat is normally lost through several processes, including respiration, elimination, and conduction through the skin (Table 19-1). Normally, the body maintains a constant internal temperature of around 98.6° Fahrenheit (F) or 37.0° Celsius (C) (centigrade). A patient whose temperature is within normal limits is said to be **afebrile**, whereas a patient with a temperature above normal is considered **febrile** (has a fever).

Thermometers are used to measure body temperature using either the Fahrenheit or Celsius scale. Box 19-1 compares temperatures taken a variety of ways in Celsius and in Fahrenheit. Because thermometers used in the medical office may be in either scale, you should be able to convert from one scale to another (see Appendix G). The patient's temperature can be measured using the oral, rectal, axillary, **tympanic**, or temporal artery methods. The oral method is most commonly used, but use of the tympanic and temporal artery thermometers is also more prevalent, especially in pediatric offices (Fig. 19-4). The tympanic thermometer measures the temperature of blood in the tympanic membrane, while the temporal artery thermometer measures the temperature of the blood within the temporal artery through the skin. If used accurately, both the tympanic thermometer and the temporal artery thermometer give readings that are comparable to the oral temperature.

A reading of 98.6°F orally is considered a normal average for body temperature, with the normal range being 97°F to 99°F. Rectal and axillary readings will vary slightly. Generally, rectal temperatures are 1°F higher than the oral temperatures because of the vascularity

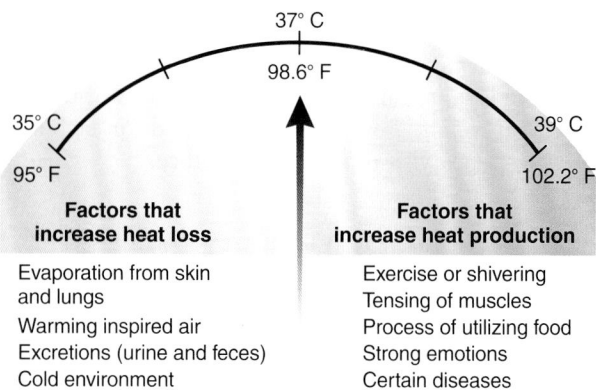

**Figure 19-3** • Factors affecting the balance between heat loss and heat production.

| TABLE 19-1 | Mechanisms of Heat Transfer | |
|---|---|---|
| **Mechanism** | **Definition** | **Example** |
| Radiation | Diffusion or dissemination of heat by electromagnetic waves | The body gives off waves of heat from uncovered surfaces. |
| Convection | Dissemination of heat by motion between areas of unequal density | An oscillating fan blows cool air across the surface of a warm body. |
| Evaporation | Conversion of liquid to vapor | Body fluid (perspiration and insensible loss) evaporates from the skin. |
| Conduction | Transfer of heat during direct contact between two objects. The body gives off waves of heat from uncovered surfaces. | The body transfers heat to an ice pack, melting the ice. |

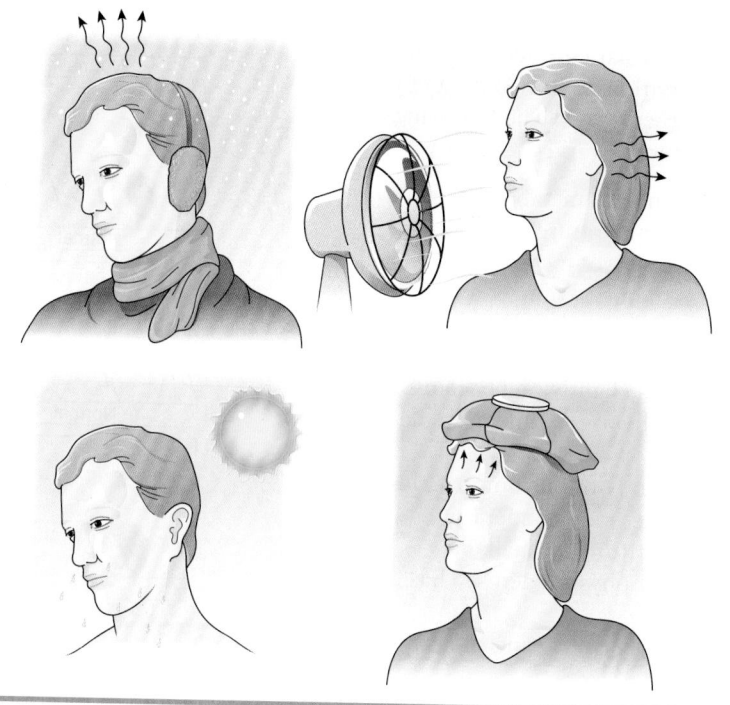

and tightly closed environment of the rectum. Axillary temperatures are usually 1°F lower because of lower vascularity and difficulty in keeping the axilla tightly closed. When recording the body temperature, you must indicate the temperature reading and the method used to obtain it, such as oral, rectal, axillary, tympanic, or temporal artery. A rectal temperature reading of 101°F is equivalent to 100°F orally, and an axillary reading of 101°F is equivalent to 102°F orally.

| BOX 19-1 | Temperature Comparisons | |
|---|---|---|
| | **Fahrenheit** | **Centigrade or Celsius** |
| Oral | 98.6 | 37.0 |
| Rectal | 99.6 | 37.6 |
| Axillary | 97.6 | 36.4 |
| Tympanic or temporal | 98.6 | 37.0 |

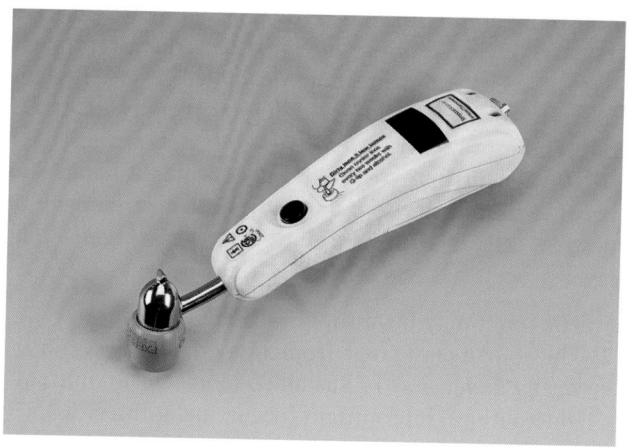

**Figure 19-4 •** A temporal artery scanning thermometer.

## CHECKPOINT QUESTION

2. How does an oral temperature measurement differ from a rectal measurement? Why?

## Fever Processes

Although a patient's temperature is influenced by heat lost or produced by the body, it is regulated by the hypothalamus in the brain. When the hypothalamus senses that the body is too warm, it initiates peripheral vasodilation to carry core heat to the body surface via the blood and increases perspiration to cool the body by evaporation. If the temperature registers too low, vasoconstriction to conserve heat and shivering to generate more heat will usually maintain a fairly normal core temperature. Temperature elevations and variations are often a **sign** of disease but are not diseases in themselves. The following factors may cause the temperature to vary:

- *Age.* Children usually have a higher metabolism and therefore a higher body temperature than do adults. The elderly, who have slower metabolisms, usually have lower readings than do younger adults. Temperatures of both the very young and the elderly are easily affected by the environment.
- *Gender.* Women usually have a slightly higher temperature than do men, especially at the time of ovulation and during pregnancy.
- *Exercise.* Activity causes the body to burn more calories for energy, which raises the body temperature.
- *Time of day.* The body temperature is usually lowest in the early morning before physical activity has begun.
- *Emotions.* Temperature tends to rise during times of stress and fall with depression.
- *Illness.* High or low body temperatures may result from a disease process.

## Stages of Fever

An elevated temperature, or fever, usually results from a disease process, such as a bacterial or viral infection. Body temperature may also rise during intense exercise, anxiety, or dehydration unrelated to a disease process, but these elevations are not considered fevers. **Pyrexia** refers to a fever of 102°F or higher rectally or 101°F or higher orally. An extremely high temperature, 105°F to 106°F, is **hyperpyrexia** and is considered dangerous because the intense internal body heat may damage or destroy cells of the brain and other vital organs. The fever process has several clearly defined stages:

1. The *onset* may be abrupt or gradual.
2. The *course* may range from a day or so to several weeks. Fever may be **sustained** (constant), **remittent** (fluctuating), **intermittent** (occurring at intervals), or **relapsing** (returning after an extended period of normal readings). Table 19-2 describes and illustrates these courses of fever.

| TABLE 19-2 | Variations in Fever Patterns: Temperature Comparisons | |
|---|---|---|
| | **Fahrenheit** | **Celsius** |
| Oral | 98.6 | 37.0 |
| Rectal | 99.6 | 37.6 |
| Axillary | 97.6 | 36.4 |
| Tympanic | 98.6 | 37.0 |

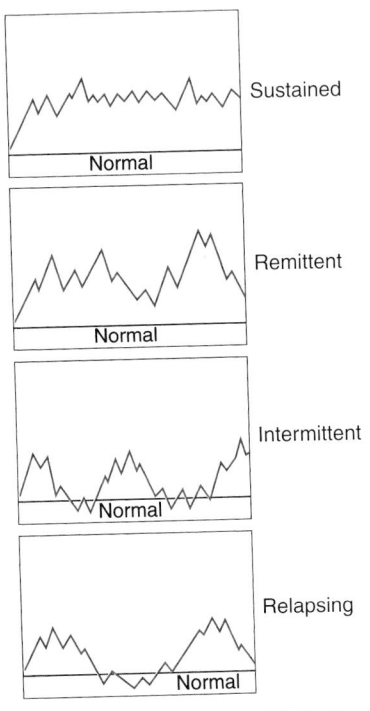

3. The *resolution*, or return to normal, may occur as either a *crisis* (abrupt return to normal) or *lysis* (gradual return to normal).

 **PATIENT EDUCATION**

### Fever

When instructing patients about fever, explain that temperature elevations are usually a natural response to disease and that efforts to bring the temperature back to normal may be counterproductive. However, if the patient is uncomfortable or the temperature is abnormally high, it should be brought down to about 101°F; the body's natural defenses may still be able to destroy the pathogen without extreme discomfort to the patient.

After consulting with the physician, instruct all patients regarding the following comfort measures:

- Consume clear fluids by mouth as tolerated to rehydrate the tissues if nausea and vomiting are not present.

- Keep clothing and bedding clean and dry, especially after **diaphoresis** (sweating).
- Avoid chilling. Chills cause shivering, which raises the body temperature.
- Rest and eat a light diet as tolerated.
- Use antipyretics to keep comfortable, but **do not** give aspirin products to children under 18 years of age. Aspirin has been associated with Reye syndrome, a potentially fatal disorder, following cases of viral illnesses and varicella zoster (chicken pox).

## CHECKPOINT QUESTION

3. How would Yvonne explain why the body temperature of a young child may be different from that of an adult.

## Types of Thermometers

### Glass Thermometers

In the past, oral, rectal, and axillary temperatures have been measured using a mercury glass thermometer. Because mercury is a hazardous chemical if exposure occurs, a mercury spill kit must be available should a mercury thermometer break. The exposed mercury must be cleaned using proper procedures according to the office policy and procedure manual. Never allow anyone to touch or manipulate the mercury from a broken thermometer.

Although most medical offices today do not use mercury-filled glass thermometers, glass thermometers are available that contain a nonmercury substance. Some offices may use these thermometers or have some available for use in the event the electronic thermometers malfunction. These thermometers are similar in appearance to mercury thermometers. Both the mercury and nonmercury glass thermometers consist of a glass tube divided into two major parts. The bulb end is filled with mercury or the nonmercury substance and may have a round or a slender tip. Glass thermometers have different shapes for oral and rectal use. Rectal thermometers have a rounded, or stubbed, end and are usually color-coded red on the opposite flat end of the

thermometer. Thermometers with a long, slender bulb are used for axillary or oral temperatures and are color-coded blue (Fig. 19-5). When the glass thermometer is placed in position for a specified period, body heat expands the chemical in the bulb, which rises up the glass column and remains there until it is physically shaken back into the bulb.

The long stem of the Fahrenheit thermometer is **calibrated** with lines designating temperature in even degrees: 94°F, 96°F, 98°F, 100°F, and so on. Uneven numbers are marked only with a longer line. Between these longer lines, four smaller lines designate temperature in 0.2-degree increments. The thermometer is read by noting the level of the mercury or nonmercury substance in the glass column. For example, if the level of the chemical falls on the second smaller line past the large line marked 100, the reading is 100.4°F. Celsius thermometers are marked for each degree (35°C, 36°C, 37°C, and so on), with 10 markings between the whole numbers (Fig. 19-5). If the mercury falls on the third small line past the line marked 37, the temperature reading is recorded as 37.3°C.

Glass thermometers may be reused if properly disinfected between patients. Also, before using a glass thermometer, place it in a disposable clear plastic sheath. When you take the thermometer from the patient, remove the sheath by pulling the thermometer out, which turns the sheath inside out and traps the saliva inside it. Dispose of the sheath in a biohazard container, sanitize, and disinfect the thermometer according to the office policy. Usually, washing the thermometers with warm—not hot—soapy water and soaking in a solution of 70% isopropyl alcohol is sufficient for disinfection.

The procedures for measuring a rectal or axillary temperature using either the glass thermometer or the electronic thermometer are described in Procedures 19-3 and 19-4.

### Electronic Thermometers

Electronic thermometers are portable battery-operated units with interchangeable probes (Fig. 19-6). The base unit of the thermometer is battery operated, and the interchangeable probes are color-coded blue for oral or axillary and red for rectal. When the probe is properly positioned, the temperature is sensed, and a digital readout shows in the window of the handheld base.

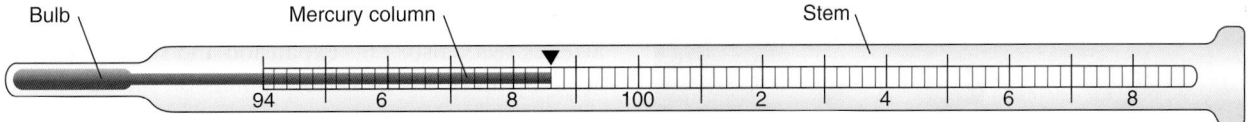

A **Fahrenheit (F°) thermometer** is scaled from 94°F to 108°F. Each long line indicates 1 degree and each short line indicates $^2/_{10}$ (0.2) of a degree. This thermometer is reading 98.6°F.

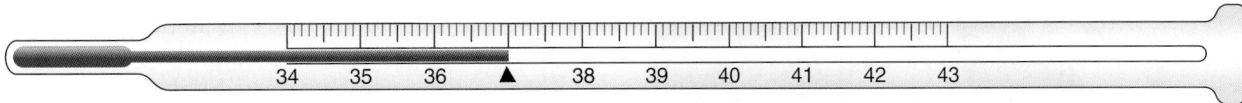

A **Celsius (C°) thermometer** is scaled from 34°C to 43°C. Each long line indicates 1 degree and each short line indicates $^1/_{10}$ (0.1) of a degree. This thermometer is reading 37°C.

**Figure 19-5 •** The two glass thermometers on the top are calibrated in the Celsius (centigrade) scale, and the two on the bottom use the Fahrenheit scale. Note the blunt bulb on the rectal thermometers and the long thin bulb on the oral thermometers.

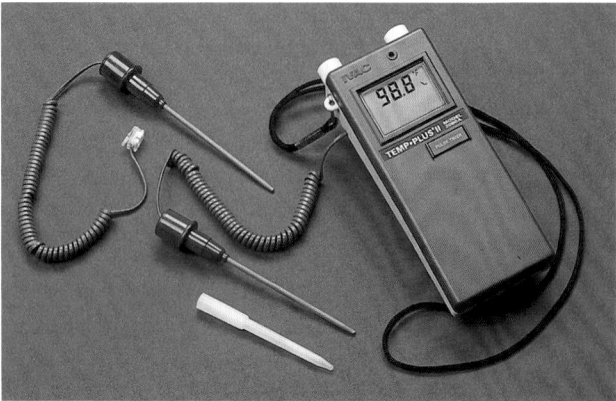

**Figure 19-6** • Two types of electronic thermometers and probes.

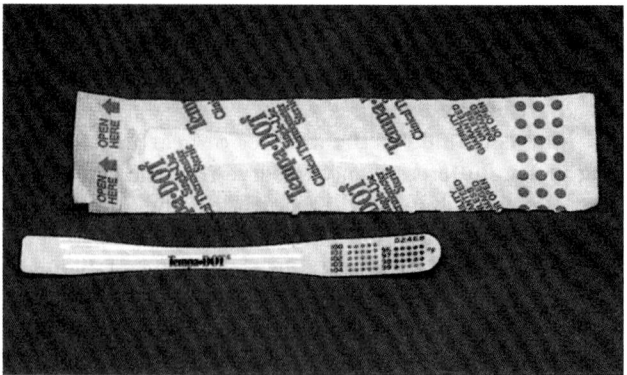

**Figure 19-8** • Disposable paper thermometer. The dots change color to indicate the body temperature.

Electronic thermometers are usually kept in a charging unit between uses to ensure that the batteries are operative at all times. The procedure for taking and recording an oral temperature using an electronic thermometer is described in Procedure 19-5.

### Tympanic Thermometers

Another type of thermometer used in medical offices today is the tympanic, or aural, thermometer. This device is usually battery powered. The end is fitted with a disposable cover that is inserted into the ear much like an otoscope (Fig. 19-7). With the end of the thermometer in place, a button is pressed, and infrared light bounces off the tympanic membrane, or eardrum. When correctly positioned in the ear, the sensor in the thermometer determines the temperature of the blood in the tympanic membrane. The temperature reading is displayed on the unit's digital screen within 2 seconds. This device is considered highly reliable for temperature measurement. Procedure 19-6 describes the complete process for obtaining a body temperature with a tympanic thermometer.

### Temporal Artery Thermometer

The temporal artery thermometer measures actual blood temperature by placing the unit on the front of the forehead, pressing the "on/off" button, and sliding the probe scanner

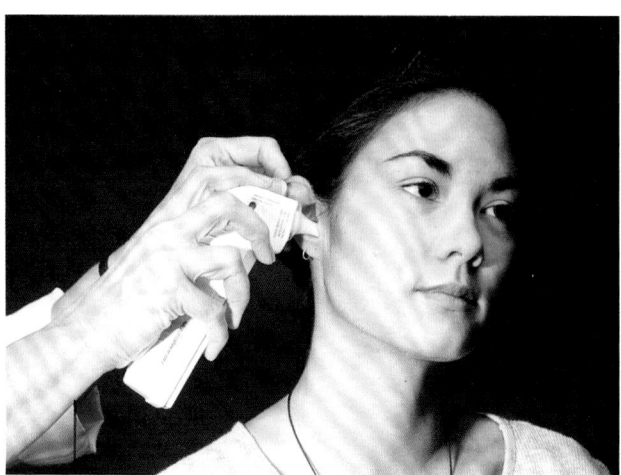

**Figure 19-7** • The tympanic thermometer in use.

over the forehead and down to the temporal artery area of the forehead. Upon releasing the "on/off" button, the temperature is immediately recorded in the digital display box located on the front of the thermometer. Depending on the brand and type of temporal artery thermometer purchased, you should read the manufacturer's instructions carefully for proper use and care of the unit. Procedure 19-7 describes the steps for taking a temperature for taking a temperature using the temporal artery thermometer.

### Disposable Thermometers

Single-use disposable thermometers are fairly accurate but are not considered as reliable as electronic, tympanic, or glass thermometers. These thermometers register quickly by indicating color changes on a strip. They are not reliable for definitive measurement, but they are acceptable for screening in settings such as day care centers and schools (Fig. 19-8). Other disposable thermometers are available for pediatric use in the form of sucking devices, or pacifiers, but these are not used in the medical office setting.

### CHECKPOINT QUESTION

4. How is the reading displayed on an electronic, tympanic, and temporal artery thermometer?

## Pulse

As the heart beats, blood is forced through the arteries, expanding them. With relaxation of the heart, the arteries relax also. This expansion and relaxation of the arteries can be felt at various points on the body where you can press an artery against a bone or other underlying firm surface. These areas are known as pulse points. With **palpation**, each expansion of the artery can be felt and is counted as one heartbeat. A pulse in specific arteries supplying blood to the extremities also indicates that oxygenated blood is flowing to that extremity.

The heartbeat can be palpated (felt) or auscultated (heard) at several pulse points. The arteries most commonly used are the carotid, apical, brachial, radial, femoral, popliteal, posterior tibial, and dorsalis pedis (Fig. 19-9). Palpation of the pulse is performed by

**A** Carotid

**B** Brachial

**C** Radial

**D** Femoral

**E** Popliteal

**F** Dorsalis pedis

**G** Posterior tibial

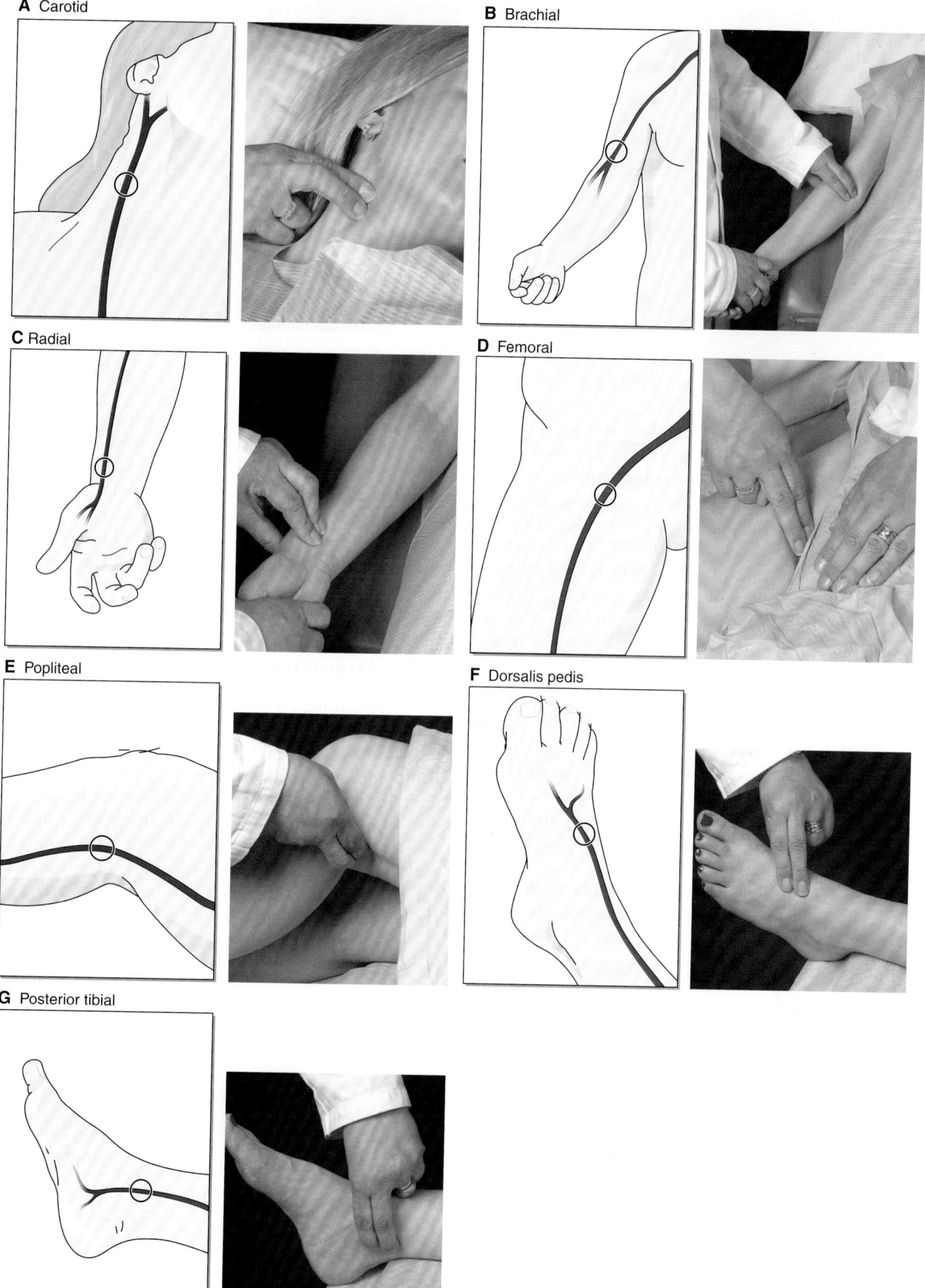

**Figure 19-9** • Sites for palpation of peripheral pulses.

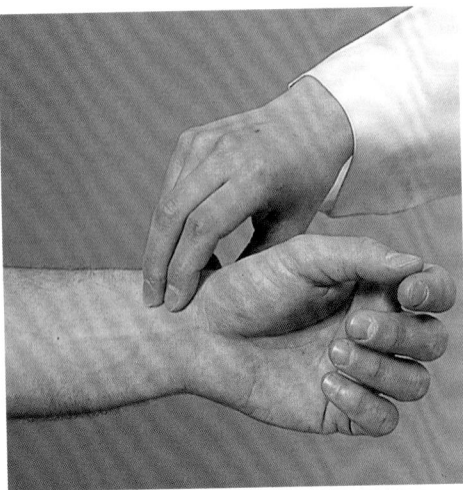

**Figure 19-10 •** Measuring a radial pulse.

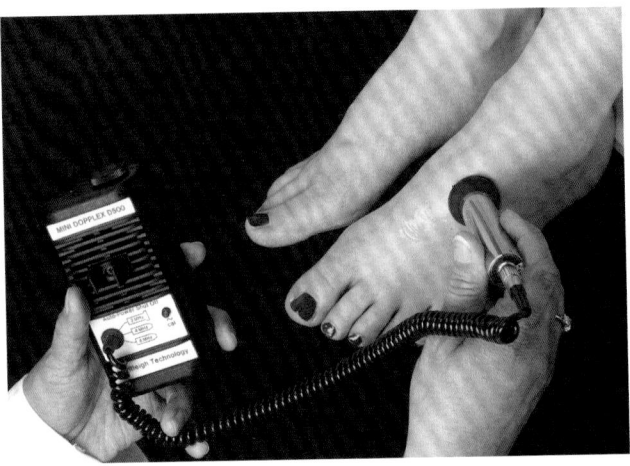

**Figure 19-12 •** The dorsalis pedis pulse being auscultated using a Doppler device.

placing the index and middle fingers, the middle and ring fingers, or all three fingers over a pulse point (Fig. 19-10). The thumb is not used to palpate a pulse. The apical pulse is auscultated using a stethoscope with the bell placed over the apex of the heart (Fig. 19-11). A Doppler unit may be used to amplify the sound of peripheral pulses that are difficult to palpate (Fig. 19-12). This unit is a small battery-powered or electric device that consists of a main box with control switches, a probe, and an earpiece unit that plugs into the main box and resembles the earpieces to a stethoscope. The earpiece may be detached so the sounds can be heard by everyone in the room if desired. Follow the following steps to use a Doppler device:

1. Apply a coupling or transmission gel on the pulse point before placing the end of the probe, or transducer, on the area. This gel creates an airtight seal between the probe and the skin and facilitates transmission of the sound.
2. With the machine on, hold the probe at a 90-degree angle with light pressure to ensure contact. Move

the probe as necessary in small circles in the gel until you hear the pulse. When contact with the artery is made, the Doppler will emit a loud pumping sound with each heartbeat. Adjust the volume control on the Doppler unit as necessary.
3. After assessing the rate and rhythm of the pulse, clean the patient's skin and the probe with a tissue or soft cloth. Do not clean the probe with water or alcohol, as this may damage the transducer.

## Pulse Characteristics

While palpating the pulse, you also assess the rate, rhythm, and volume as the artery wall expands with each heartbeat. The **rate** is the number of heartbeats in 1 minute. This number can be determined by palpating the pulse and counting each heartbeat while watching the second hand of your watch either for 30 seconds and then multiplying that number by 2 or for 1 minute. In healthy adults, the average pulse rate is 60 to 100 beats per minute. At other ages, there is a large variance of pulse rates, as shown in Table 19-3.

The **rhythm** is the interval between each heartbeat or the pattern of beats. Normally, this pattern is regular, with each heartbeat occurring at a regular, consistent rate. An irregular rhythm should be counted for 1 full

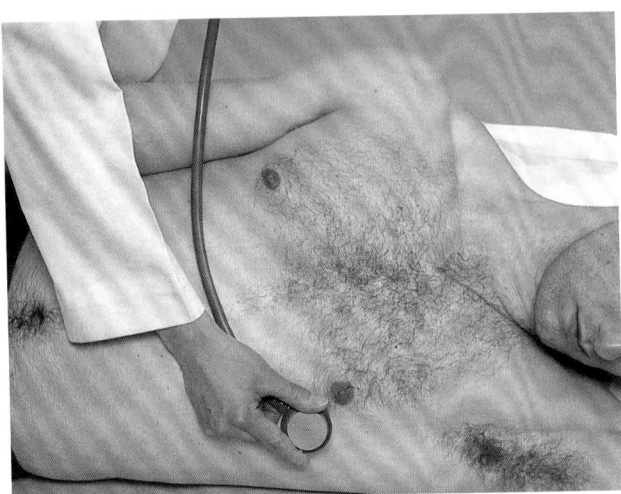

**Figure 19-11 •** Measuring an apical pulse.

| TABLE 19-3 | Variations in Pulse Rate by Age |
|---|---|
| **Age** | **Beats per Minute** |
| Birth to 1 year | 110–170 |
| 1–10 years | 90–110 |
| 10–16 years | 80–95 |
| 16 years to midlife | 70–80 |
| Elderly adult | 55–70 |

minute to determine the rate, and the irregular rhythm should be documented with the pulse rate.

**Volume,** the strength or force of the heartbeat, can be described as soft, bounding, weak, thready, strong, or full. Usually, the volume of the pulse is recorded only if it is weak, thready, or bounding.

### Factors Affecting Pulse Rates

Many factors affect the force, speed, and rhythm of the heart. Young children and infants have a much faster heart rate than do adults. A conditioned athlete may have a normal heart rate below 60 beats per minute. Older adults may have a faster heart rate, as the myocardium compensates for decreased efficiency. Other factors that affect pulse rates are listed in Table 19-4.

The radial artery is most often used to determine pulse rate because it is convenient for both the medical assistant and the patient (Procedure 19-8). If the radial pulse is irregular or hard to palpate, then the apical pulse is the site of choice (Fig. 19-13). To assess the flow of blood into the extremities, you may be asked to palpate peripheral pulses such as the dorsalis pedis. Peripheral pulses that are difficult to palpate may be auscultated with a Doppler unit to check for the presence of blood flow.

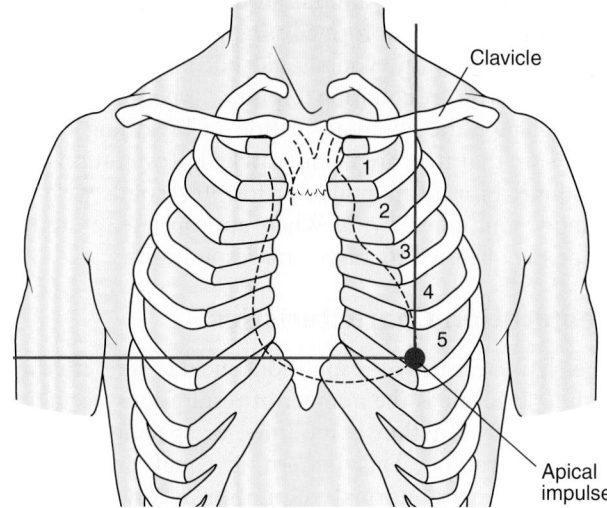

**Figure 19-13** • The apical pulse is found at the 5th intercostal space at the midclavicular line.

### CHECKPOINT QUESTION

5. Yvonne measures vital signs for a variety of patients each day. What characteristics of a patient's pulse should be assessed, and how should they be recorded in the medical record?

## Respiration

Respiration is the exchange of gases between the atmosphere and the blood in the body. With respiration, the body expels carbon dioxide ($CO_2$) and takes in oxygen ($O_2$). External respiration is inhalation and exhalation, during which air travels through the respiratory tract to the alveoli so that oxygen can be absorbed into the bloodstream. Internal respiration is the exchange of gases between the blood and the tissue cells. Respiration is controlled by the respiratory center in the brainstem and by feedback from chemosensors in the carotid arteries that monitor the $CO_2$ content in the blood.

As the patient breathes in (inspiration), oxygen flows into the lungs, and the diaphragm contracts and flattens out, lifting and expanding the rib cage. During expiration, air in the lungs flows out of the chest cavity as the diaphragm relaxes, moves upward into a dome-like shape, and allows the rib cage to contract. Each respiration is counted as one full inspiration and one full expiration.

| TABLE 19-4 | Factors Affecting Pulse Rates |
|---|---|
| **Factor** | **Effect** |
| Time of day | The pulse is usually lower early in the morning than later in the day. |
| Gender | Women have a slightly higher pulse rate than do men. |
| Body type and size | Tall, thin people usually have a lower pulse rate than do shorter, stockier people. |
| Exercise | The heart rate increases with the need for increased **cardiac output** (the amount of blood ejected from either ventricle in 1 minute). |
| Stress or emotions | Anger, fear, excitement, and stress will raise the pulse; depression will lower it. |
| Fever | The increased need for cell metabolism in the presence of fever raises the cardiac output to supply oxygen and nutrients; the pulse may rise as much as 10 beats/minute per degree of fever. |
| Medications | Many medications raise or lower the pulse as a desired effect or as an undesirable side effect. |
| Blood volume | Loss of blood volume to hemorrhage or dehydration will increase the need for cellular metabolism and will increase the cardiac output to supply the need. |

Observing the rise and fall of the chest to count respirations is usually performed as a part of the pulse measurement. Generally, you should not make the patient aware that you are counting respirations because patients often change the voluntary action of breathing if they are aware that they are being watched. Respirations can be counted for a full minute or for 30 seconds with the number multiplied by 2. When appropriate, a stethoscope may be used to auscultate respirations.

## Respiration Characteristics

The characteristics of respirations include rate, rhythm, and depth. **Rate** is the number of respirations occurring in 1 minute. **Rhythm** is the time, or spacing, between each respiration. This pattern is equal and regular in patients with normal respirations. Any abnormal rhythm is described as irregular and recorded as such in the patient's record after the rate.

**Depth** is the volume of air being inhaled and exhaled. When a person is at rest, the depth should be regular and consistent. There are normally no noticeable sounds other than the regular exchange of air. Respirations that are abnormally deep or shallow are documented in addition to the rate. Abnormal sounds during inspiration or expiration are usually a sign of a disease process. These abnormal sounds are usually recorded as crackles (wet or dry sounds) or wheezes (high-pitched sounds) heard during inspiration or expiration.

## Factors Affecting Respiration

In healthy adults, the average respiratory rate is 12 to 20 breaths per minute. Table 19-5 shows the normal variations in respiratory rates according to age. Patients with an elevated body temperature usually also have increased pulse and respiratory rates. A respiratory rate that is much faster than average is called tachypnea, and a respiratory rate that is slower than usual is referred to as bradypnea. Further descriptions of abnormal or unusual respirations include the following:

- **Dyspnea:** difficult or labored breathing
- **Apnea:** no respiration
- **Hyperpnea:** abnormally deep, gasping breaths
- **Hyperventilation:** a respiratory rate that greatly exceeds the body's oxygen demand
- **Hypopnea:** shallow respirations
- **Orthopnea:** inability to breathe lying down; the patient usually has to sit upright to breathe

Procedure 19-9 lists the steps for counting and recording respirations.

## CHECKPOINT QUESTION

6. What happens within the chest cavity when the diaphragm contracts?

## Blood Pressure

Blood pressure is a measurement of the pressure of the blood in an artery as it is forced against the arterial walls. Pressure is measured in the contraction and relaxation phases of the **cardiac cycle**, or heartbeat. When the heart contracts, blood is forced from the atria and ventricles in the phase known as **systole**. This highest pressure level during contraction is recorded as the systolic pressure and is heard as the first sound in taking blood pressure.

As the heart pauses briefly to rest and refill, the arterial pressure drops. This phase is known as **diastole**, and the pressure is recorded as the diastolic pressure. Systolic and diastolic pressure result from the two parts of the cardiac cycle, the period from the beginning of one heartbeat to the beginning of the next. When measured using a stethoscope and **sphygmomanometer**, or blood pressure cuff, these two pressures constitute the blood pressure and are written as a fraction, with the systolic pressure over the diastolic pressure. Table 19-6 describes the classification of blood pressure readings for adults with normal, prehypertension, and hypertension blood pressures. A lower pressure may be normal for athletes with exceptionally well-conditioned cardiovascular systems. Blood pressure that drops suddenly when the patient stands from a sitting or lying position is **postural hypotension**, or *orthostatic hypotension*; it may cause symptoms including vertigo. Some patients with postural hypotension may faint. Extra precautions should be taken when assessing patients going from lying down to sitting or standing.

Two basic types of sphygmomanometers are used to measure blood pressure: the aneroid, which has a circular dial for the readings, and the mercury, which has a mercury-filled glass tube for the readings (Fig. 19-14). Although only one type actually contains mercury, both types are calibrated and measure blood pressure in millimeters of mercury (mm Hg). A blood pressure of 120/80 indicates the force needed to raise a column of mercury to the 120 calibration mark on the glass tube during systole and to 80 during diastole. The elasticity of the person's arterial walls, the strength of the heart muscle, and the quantity and viscosity (thickness) of the blood all affect the blood pressure.

The sphygmomanometer is attached to a cuff by a rubber tube. A second rubber tube is attached to a

| TABLE 19-5 | Variations in Respiration Ranges by Age |
|---|---|
| **Age** | **Respirations per Minute** |
| Infant | 20+ |
| Child | 18–20 |
| Adult | 12–20 |

## TABLE 19-6   Blood Pressure Readings

|  | Systolic BP |  | Diastolic BP |
|---|---|---|---|
| Normal | <120 mm Hg | and | <80 mm Hg |
| Prehypertension | 120–139 mm Hg | or | 80–89 mm Hg |
| Hypertension, stage I | 140–159 mm Hg | or | 90–99 mm Hg |
| Hypertension, stage II | >160 mm Hg | or | >100 mm Hg |

*Source*: U.S. Department of Health and Human Services, National Institutes of Health, National Heart, Lung, and Blood Institute.

hand pump with a screw valve. This device is used to pump air into the rubber bladder in the cuff. When the screw valve is turned clockwise, the bladder in the cuff around the patient's arm is inflated by multiple compressions of the pump. As the bladder inflates, the pressure created against the artery at some point prohibits blood from passing through the vessel. When the screw valve is slowly opened by turning it counterclockwise, the blood pressure can be determined by listening carefully with the stethoscope placed on the artery to the sounds produced as the blood begins to flow through the vessel. Procedure 19-10 describes the steps for correctly obtaining a patient's blood pressure using the radial artery.

### CHECKPOINT QUESTION

7. What is happening to the heart during systole? During diastole?

### Korotkoff Sounds

Korotkoff sounds can be classified into five phases of sounds heard while auscultating the blood pressure as described by the Russian neurologist Nicolai Korotkoff. Only the sounds heard during phase I (represented by the first sound heard) and phase V (represented by the last sound heard) are recorded as blood pressure. You may hear other Korotkoff sounds during the procedure, but it is not necessary to record them. Table 19-7 describes the five phases of Korotkoff sounds that may be heard when auscultating blood pressure.

### WHAT IF?

**What if a patient has a dialysis shunt (a surgically made venous access port that allows a patient with little or no kidney function to be connected to a dialysis machine) in his left arm? Should you use that arm to take his blood pressure?**

*No!* By taking a blood pressure in that arm, you could cause the shunt to be permanently damaged, and the patient would not be able to receive dialysis until another shunt was prepared by a surgeon. The patient's chart should be clearly marked indicating that a shunt is in place and which arm it is located in. Most dialysis patients are keenly aware of the importance of this shunt and will alert you to the location of their shunt. Also, you should not draw blood from this arm.

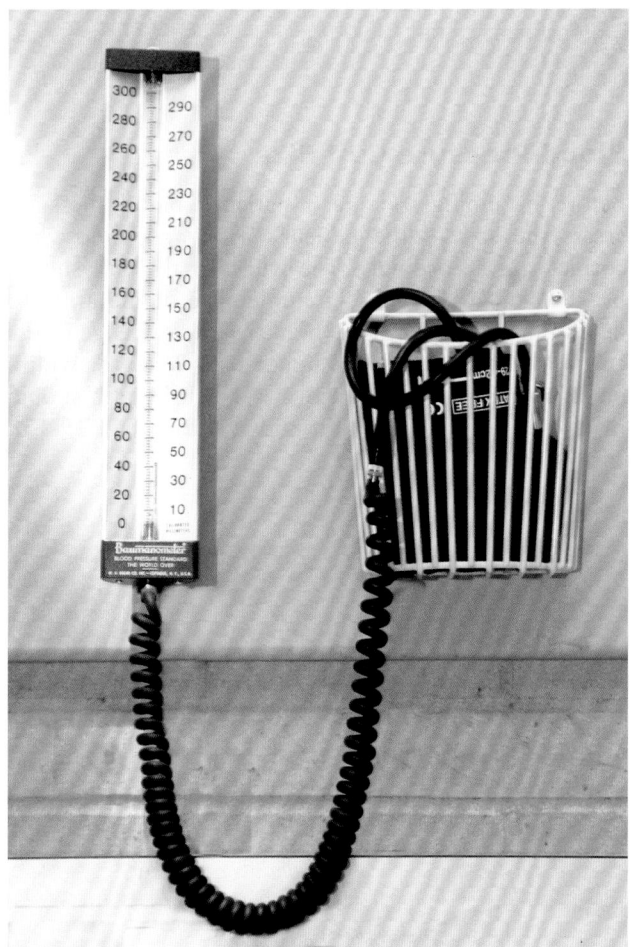

**Figure 19-14** • A mercury column sphygmomanometer.

| TABLE 19-7 | Five Phases of Blood Pressure |
|---|---|
| **Phase** | **Sounds** |
| I | Faint tapping heard as the cuff deflates (systolic blood pressure) |
| II | Soft swishing |
| III | Rhythmic, sharp, distinct tapping |
| IV | Soft tapping that becomes faint |
| V | Last sound (diastolic blood pressure) |

## Pulse Pressure

The difference between the systolic and diastolic readings is known as the pulse pressure. For example, with the average adult blood pressure of 120/80, the difference between the numbers 120 and 80 is 40. The average normal range for pulse pressure is 30 to 50 mm Hg. Generally, the pulse pressure should be no more than one-third of the systolic reading. If the pulse pressure is more or less than these parameters, the physician should be notified.

## Auscultatory Gap

Patients with a history of **hypertension**, or elevated blood pressure, may have an auscultatory gap heard during phase II of the Korotkoff sounds. An auscultatory gap is the loss of any sounds for a drop of up to 30 mm Hg (sometimes more) during the release of air from the blood pressure cuff after the first sound is heard. If the last sound heard at the beginning of the gap is recorded as the diastolic blood pressure, the documented blood pressure is inaccurate and may result in misdiagnosis and treatment of a condition that the patient does not have. As a result, it is important for you to listen and watch carefully as the dial or column of mercury falls until you are certain that you have heard the last sound, or diastolic pressure.

## Factors Influencing Blood Pressure

Atherosclerosis and arteriosclerosis are two disease processes that greatly influence blood pressure. These diseases affect the size and elasticity of the artery lumen. The general health of the patient is also a major factor and includes dietary habits, alcohol and tobacco use, the amount and type of exercise, previous heart conditions such as myocardial infarctions, and family history for cardiac disease. Other factors that may affect blood pressure include the following:

- *Age.* As the body ages, vessels begin to lose elasticity and will require more force to expand the arterial wall. The buildup of atherosclerotic patches inside the artery will also increase the force needed for blood flow.

- *Activity.* Exercise raises the blood pressure temporarily, while inactivity or rest will usually lower the pressure.
- *Stress.* The sympathetic nervous system stimulates the release of the hormone epinephrine, which raises the pressure in response to the fight or flight syndrome.
- *Body Position.* Blood pressure will normally be lower in the supine position.
- *Medications.* Some medications will lower the pressure, while others may cause an elevation.

## PATIENT EDUCATION

### Hypertension

After taking a patient's blood pressure, you should tell the patient what you obtained for the blood pressure reading. Patients with hypertension, or high blood pressure, should be encouraged to keep a personal log of their readings and bring this to each physician office appointment. Because the freestanding blood pressure machines found in pharmacies and supermarkets are not always reliable, you should teach patients with hypertension how to take their blood pressure at home.

## Blood Pressure Cuff Size

Before beginning to take a patient's blood pressure, assess the size of the patient's arm, and choose the correct size accordingly. The width of the cuff should be 40% to 50% of the circumference of the arm. To determine the correct size, hold the narrow edge of the cuff at the midpoint of the upper arm. Wrap the width, not the length, around the arm. The cuff width should reach not quite halfway around the arm (Fig. 19-15).

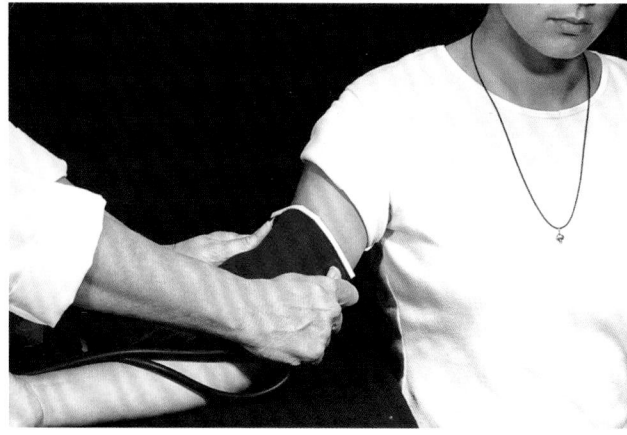

**Figure 19-15 •** Choosing the right blood pressure cuff.

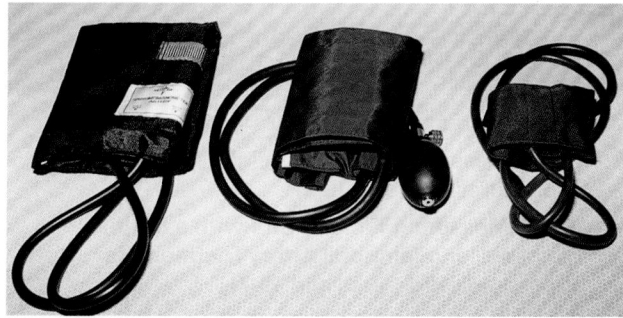

**Figure 19-16** • Three sizes of blood pressure cuffs (from left): a large cuff for obese adults, a normal adult cuff, and a pediatric cuff.

Varying widths of cuffs are available, from about 1 inch for infants to 8 inches for obese adults (Fig. 19-16). The blood pressure measurement may be inaccurate by as much as 30 mm Hg if the cuff size is incorrect. Box 19-2 lists causes of errors in blood pressure readings.

 **CHECKPOINT QUESTION**

8. How are the pulse pressure and the auscultatory gap different?

---

**BOX 19-2 Causes of Errors in Blood Pressure Readings**

- Wrapping the cuff improperly
- Failing to keep the patient's arm at the level of the heart while taking the blood pressure
- Failing to support the patient's arm on a stable surface while taking the blood pressure
- Recording the auscultatory gap for the diastolic pressure
- Failing to maintain the gauge at eye level
- Applying the cuff around the patient's clothing and attempting to listen through the clothing
- Allowing the cuff to deflate too rapidly or too slowly
- Failing to wait 1 to 2 minutes before rechecking using the same arm

---

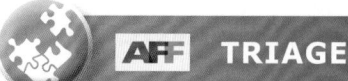 **TRIAGE**

While working in a medical office, you have just taken the following three patients' vital signs:

A. A 52-year-old woman complaining of dyspnea. Her respiratory rate is 38, her pulse is 112 and irregular, and her blood pressure is 150/86.
B. A 43-year-old man with a pulse of 54 and blood pressure of 98/52. He denies any shortness of breath, chest pain, or dizziness.
C. A 65-year-old man who had open-heart surgery 2 weeks ago. He states that yellow drainage is coming from the surgical wound on his chest. His temperature is 101.8°F orally, his blood pressure is 188/62, and his pulse is 118 and regular.

**How do you sort these patients? Who should be seen first? Second? Third?**

Patient A should be seen first. The physician should immediately see any patient complaining of trouble breathing. Her respiratory and pulse rates are faster than normal for an adult. Patient C should be seen second because of his temperature and pulse rate. Patient B should be seen last. A pulse rate of 52 and blood pressure of 98/52 are low, but the patient is not complaining of any symptoms. If he is physically fit, his vital signs may normally be lower than average. If he were complaining of dizziness or feeling faint, he would need to be seen sooner.

---

 **ROLE-PLAYING ACTIVITY**

Assume you are Yvonne Torres, the medical assistant discussed in the case study at the beginning of this chapter. Today, you are working with Dr. Thomas and are checking in a young man, Brett Armstrong, who is being seen for a high school sports physical. Have another student assume the role of Brett, the 16-year-old high school baseball player who cannot understand why he needs his vital signs taken because he is "not sick." Obtain Brett's height, weight, and vital signs, and record these measurements in the medical record. Respond to Brett's analysis that his blood pressure is "not normal" and his anxiety about you recording this on his physical form because this "will keep him off the team." Your instructor will give you additional information about this activity!

## *español* SPANISH TERMINOLOGY

**Voy a tomarle su pulso radial.**
I am going to take your radial pulse.

**Voy a tomarle la presión sanguínea.**
I am going to take your blood pressure.

**Voy a tomarle su temperatura.**
I am going to take your temperature.

**¿Siente que tiene fiebre ó calentura?**
Do you feel feverish?

**Por favor quitese sus zapatos para tener un peso y estatura más correcta.**
Please remove your shoes for more accuracy in your height and weight.

**Voy a tomarle la temperatura en su oído.**
I'm going to measure your temperature in your ear.

**Voy a medir sus respiraciones.**
I'm going to measure your respiratory rate.

**¿Ha comido, tomado alguna bebida ó fumado en los ultimos 15 minutos?**
Have you eaten, drunk, or smoked in the last 15 minutes?

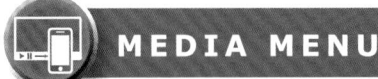

## MEDIA MENU

**Student Resources** on thePoint*

- *Video:* **Measuring an Adult Height and Weight (Procedures 19-1 and 19-2)**
- *Video:* **Measuring Temperature with a Digital, Tympanic, and Temporal Artery Thermometer (Procedures 19-5, 19-6, and 19-7)**
- *Video:* **Measuring a Patient's Pulse and Respirations (Procedures 19-8 and 19-9) Video: Measuring a Patient's Blood Pressure (Procedure 19-10)**
- *Animation:* **Breathing Sounds**
- *Animation:* **Cardiac Cycle**
- *Animation:* **Hypertension**
- **CMA/RMA Certification Exam Review**

**Internet Resources**
**National Reye's Syndrome Foundation**
http://www.reyessyndrome.org

**American Society of Hypertension**
http://www.ash-us.org

**American Lung Association**
http://www.lungusa.org

**National Heart Lung and Blood Institute**
http://www.nhlbi.nih.gov

**American Heart Association**
http://www.heart.org

# EMR Activity

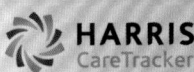

**Harris CareTracker** is a Web-based electronic medical record (EMR) application that you will use for the EMR activities included in this section at the end of each chapter. This application is actually used in physician offices but is provided to you through the publisher, Wolters Kluwer Health, to give you hands-on practice working with EMRs. Your instructor will have more information about accessing your username, log-in, and Quickstart guide.

Prerequisite Activities in Harris CareTracker

*Note: The Getting Started and Quickstart documents and EMR Activities Step-by-Step Instructions listed below are available at* http://thePoint.lww.com/KronenbergerComp5e.

Activity Details

In the *Medical Record* application of the EMR, document vital signs and anthropometric measurements for each of the following patients:

1. Bobby Turner 6 feet, 3 inches, 265 pounds; temperature, 98.8 oral; pulse, 98; respirations, 32; BP, 146/88 (left arm, sitting)
2. Amanda Panci 5 feet 2 inches, 155 pounds; temperature, 100.4 temporal; pulse, 118; respirations, 24; BP, 132/78 (right arm, sitting)
3. Lonnie Taylor, 5 feet, 9 inches, 195 pounds; temperature, 99.2 tympanic; pulse, 72; respirations, 20; BP, 168/90 (right arm, sitting)
4. Sarah Smith, 5 feet, 0 inches, 90 pounds; temperature, 98.6 oral; pulse, 80; respirations, 16; BP, 110/64 (left arm, sitting)

## Chapter Summary

- Anthropometric measurements include height and weight. Vital signs include the following:
  - Temperature (T)
  - Pulse (P)
  - Respirations (R)
  - Blood pressure (BP)
- When a patient first visits the medical office, these measurements are recorded as a baseline and used as a comparison for data collected at subsequent visits. These measurements, which provide important data for the physician to use in diagnosing and treating illnesses, are very frequently performed by medical assistants.

## Warm-Ups for Critical Thinking

1. You are asked to teach a patient, Mr. Stone, how to take his blood pressure at home once in the morning and once at night and record these readings for 1 month. Create a patient education brochure that explains the procedure in understandable terms, and design a sheet that Mr. Stone can easily use to record these readings.
2. Ms. Black arrived at the office late for her appointment; she was frantic and explained that she had experienced car trouble on the way to the office, could not find a parking place, and just locked her keys inside her car. How would you expect these events to affect her vital signs? Explain why.
3. What size of cuff would you choose for Mrs. Cooper, an elderly female patient who is 5 feet 3 inches tall and weighs approximately 90 pounds? Why?
4. How would you respond to a patient who asks you to give advice on what type of thermometer to buy for use at home? Would the age of the patient be relevant with regard to the type of thermometer you might suggest?
5. An elderly male patient tells you that he is considering stopping the blood pressure medication the physician ordered at the previous visit. He further explains that he has "read all about this drug on the Internet," and he informs you that "it has side effects," although he denies experiencing any at this time. Describe how you would handle this situation.

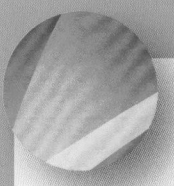

## PSY PROCEDURE 19-1

## Measuring Weight

**PSY** Measure and record weight; instruct and prepare a patient for a procedure or a treatment; document patient care accurately in the medical record.

**Purpose:** Accurately measure and record a patient's weight

**Equipment:** Calibrated balance beam scale, digital scale, or dial scale; paper towel

**Standard:** This procedure should take 5 minutes.

| STEPS | REASONS |
|---|---|
| 1. Wash your hands. | Hand washing before contact with patients aids in infection control. |
| 2. Ensure that the scale is properly balanced at zero. | This helps prevent an error in measurement. |

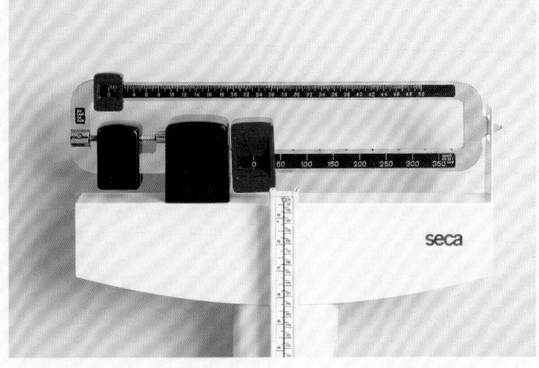

Step 2. A balance beam scale with the weights at zero

| STEPS | REASONS |
|---|---|
| 3. Greet and identify the patient. Explain the procedure. | Identifying the patient prevents errors; explaining the procedure promotes cooperation. |
| 4. Escort the patient to the scale, and place a paper towel on the scale. | Since the patient will be standing in bare feet or stockings, the paper towel minimizes microorganism transmission. |
| 5. Have the patient remove shoes and heavy outerwear and put down purse. | Unnecessary items must be removed to get an accurate reading. |
| 6. Assist the patient onto the scale facing forward and standing on paper towel without touching or holding on to anything if possible, while watching for difficulties with balance. | Some patients may feel unsteady as the plate of the scale settles. |

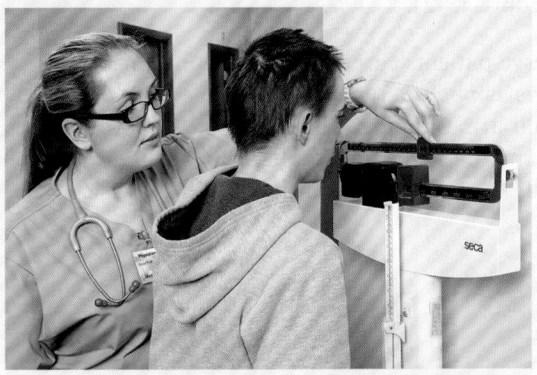

Step 6. The patient should stand erect on the scale.

(continues on page 464)

## PROCEDURE 19-1 (continued)

| STEPS | REASONS |
|---|---|

7. Weigh the patient:

A. Balance beam scale: Slide counterweights on bottom and top bars (start with heavier bars) from zero to approximate weight. Each counterweight should rest securely in the notch with indicator mark at proper calibration. To obtain measurement, the balance bar must hang freely at exact midpoint. To calculate weight, add top reading to bottom one (e.g., if bottom counterweight reads 100 and lighter one reads 16 plus three small lines, record weight as 116 3/4 lb).

B. Digital scale: Read and record weight displayed on digital screen.

C. Dial scale: Indicator arrow rests at patient's weight. Read this number directly above the dial.

> If the counterweight is not resting in the notch, the weight will not be accurate. The weight noted on a digital scale may include decimals such as 155.3 pounds.
>
> Reading at an angle will result in an incorrect measurement.

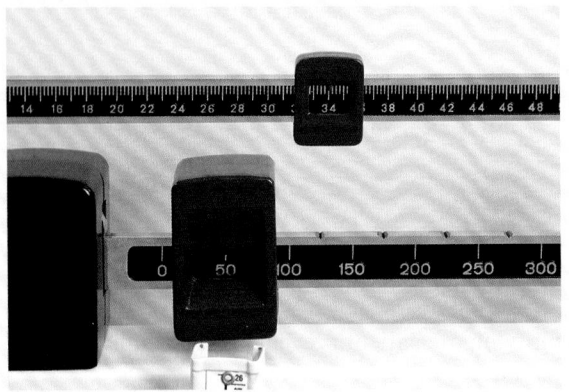

8. Return the bars on the top and bottom to zero.

> **Step 7.** The weight of this patient using the balance beam scale is 175 pounds.
>
> A balance beam scale should be returned to zero after each use.

9. Assist the patient from the scale if necessary, and discard the paper towel.

> Patients may lose balance and fall when stepping down from the scale; they should be observed and assisted as necessary. The paper towel may be left in place on the balance beam scale if the height is going to be obtained using this scale.

10. Record the weight.

> If the weight and height are measured at the same time, they will be recorded together (see example in Procedure 19-2).

11. **AFF** Explain how to respond to a patient who is visually impaired.

> Observe patients carefully to prevent injury and always ask before offering assistance or taking hold of their arm to guide. Make sure the path to the scales is clear from items that could trip or cause the patient to fall. Assist onto the scales and off of the scales as needed.

**PSY** PROCEDURE 19-2

## Measuring Height

**PSY** Measure and record height; instruct and prepare a patient for a procedure or a treatment; document patient care accurately in the medical record.

**Purpose:** Accurately measure and record a patient's height

**Equipment:** A scale with a ruler

**Standard:** This procedure should take less than 5 minutes.

| STEPS | REASONS |
|---|---|
| 1. Wash your hands if this procedure is not done at the same time as the weight. | Typically, height is obtained with weight; your hands are already washed. |
| 2. Have the patient remove shoes and stand straight and erect on the scale, with heels together and eyes straight ahead. (The patient may face the ruler, but a better measurement is made with the patient's back to the ruler.) | The posture of the patient must be erect for an accurate measurement. |
| 3. With the measuring bar perpendicular to the ruler, slowly lower it until it firmly touches the patient's head. Press lightly if the hair is full or high. | Hair that is full should not be included in the height measurement. |

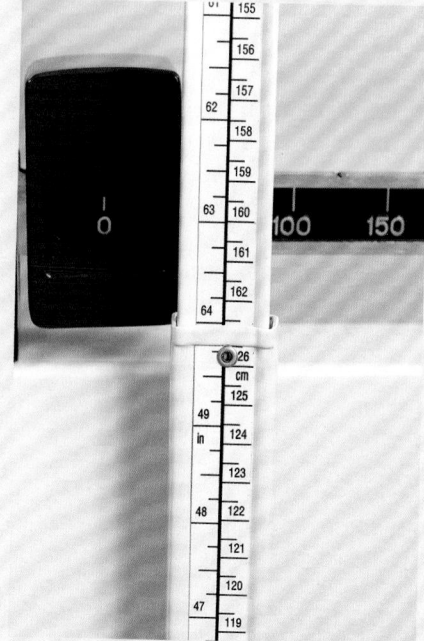

**Step 3.** Measure where the bar slides out of the scale (or point of movement). This measure reads 63 inches, or 5 feet 3 inches.

4. Read the measurement at the point of movement on the ruler. If measurements are in inches, convert to feet and inches (e.g., if the bar reads 65 plus two smaller lines, read it at 65½. Remember that 12 inches equals 1 foot; therefore, the patient is 5 feet, 5½ inches tall).

*(continues on page 466)*

## PROCEDURE 19-2 (continued)

| STEPS | REASONS |
|---|---|
| 5. Assist the patient from the scale if necessary; watch for signs of difficulty with balance. | Elderly or ill patients may be unsteady. |
| 6. Record the weight and height measurements in the medical record. | Procedures not recorded are considered not to have been done. |
| 7. **AFF** Explain how to respond to a patient who has dementia. | Solicit assistance from caregiver or other staff member to help the patient off and on the scale. Give simple directions to the patient about what he or she should do. Speak clearly, not loudly. |

Charting Example:
*10/14/2016 9:15 AM Ht. 5 ft, 5 ½ inches, Wt. 136 ¼ lb* _____ *Y. Torres, CMA*

Note: *The medical assistant may sign his or her name in the patient record using only the "CMA" credential if the office has a signature log denoting the entire credential as "CMA(AAMA)."*

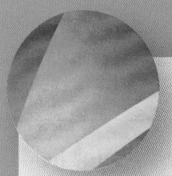

## PSY  PROCEDURE 19-3

# Measuring a Rectal Temperature

**PSY**  Measure and record temperature; instruct and prepare a patient for a procedure or a treatment; document patient care accurately in the medical record.

**Purpose:** Accurately measure and record a rectal temperature using an electronic thermometer with a rectal probe attached

**Equipment:** Electronic thermometer with rectal probe; tissues or cotton balls; disposable plastic sheaths; surgical lubricant; biohazard waste container, gloves

**Standard:** This procedure should take 5 minutes.

| STEPS | REASONS |
|---|---|
| 1. Wash your hands and assemble the necessary supplies. | Hand washing aids infection control. |
| 2. Insert the thermometer into a plastic sheath. | Follow the package instructions for placing the sheath correctly onto the rectal probe that has been correctly inserted into the electronic thermometer base. |

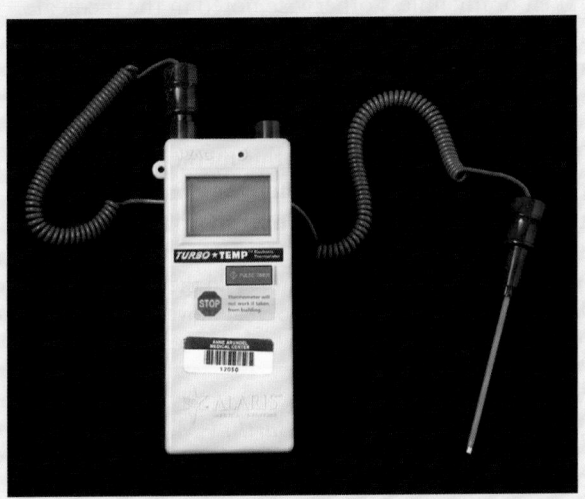

**Step 2.** Rectal thermometers are noted by the color red on the probe.

| STEPS | REASONS |
|---|---|
| 3. Spread lubricant onto a tissue and then from the tissue onto the sheath of the thermometer. | When using a tube of lubricant, avoid cross-contamination by not applying the lubricant directly to the thermometer. A lubricant should always be used for rectal insertion to prevent patient discomfort. |
| 4. Greet and identify the patient and explain the procedure. | |
| 5. Ensure the patient's privacy by placing the patient in a side-lying position facing the examination room door and draping appropriately. | If the examination room door is opened, a patient facing the door is less likely to be exposed. The side-lying position facilitates exposure of the anus. |
| 6. Apply gloves and visualize the anus by lifting the top buttock with your nondominant hand. | Never insert the thermometer without first having a clear view of the anus. |
| 7. Gently insert the thermometer past the sphincter muscle about 1½ inches for an adult, 1 inch for a child, and ½ inch for an infant. | Inserting the thermometer at these depths helps prevent perforating the anal canal. |

*(continues on page 468)*

## PROCEDURE 19-3 (continued)

| STEPS | REASONS |
|---|---|
| 8. Release the upper buttock and hold the thermometer in place with your dominant hand for 3 minutes. Replace the drape without moving the dominant hand. | The thermometer will not stay in place if it is not held. Replacing the drape will ensure the patient's privacy. |
| 9. The electronic thermometer will signal when the reading is obtained. Discard the sheath into an appropriate waste container, and note the reading. | The electronic thermometer will have a digital display of the reading (see Procedure 19-6). |
| 10. Replace the electronic thermometer into the charger as necessary. | Always make sure thermometers are ready for the next patient. |
| 11. Remove your gloves, and wash your hands. | This prevents the spread of microorganisms. |
| 12. Record the procedure and mark the letter R next to the reading, indicating that the temperature was taken rectally. | Temperature readings are presumed to have been taken orally unless otherwise noted in the medical record. The vital signs (temperature, pulse, respirations, and blood pressure) are usually recorded together. |
| 13. **AFF** Explain how to respond to a patient who is developmentally challenged. | To avoid injury, do not use this method to obtain a temperature on an adult when there is the possibility that the patient may not cooperate to avoid injury. |

*Note:* Infants and very small children may be held in the lap or over the knees for this procedure. Hold the thermometer and the buttocks with the dominant hand while securing the child with the nondominant hand. If the child moves, the thermometer and the hand will move together, avoiding injury to the anal canal.

---

Charting Example:
*09/11/2016 8:30 AM T 100.2°F (R)* _____ *J. Barth, CMA*

---

Note: *The medical assistant may sign his or her name in the patient record using only the "CMA" credential if the office has a signature log denoting the entire credential as "CMA(AAMA)."*

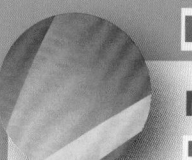

## PSY PROCEDURE 19-4

# Measuring an Axillary Temperature

**PSY** Measure and record temperature; instruct and prepare a patient for a procedure or a treatment; document patient care accurately in the medical record.

**Purpose:** Accurately measure and record an axillary temperature using an electronic thermometer

**Equipment:** Electronic thermometer (oral or rectal); tissues or cotton balls; disposable plastic sheaths; biohazard waste container

**Standard:** This procedure should take 15 minutes.

| STEPS | REASONS |
|---|---|
| 1. Wash your hands and assemble the necessary supplies. | Hand washing aids infection control. |
| 2. Insert the electronic thermometer probe into a plastic sheath. | Follow the package instructions for placing the sheath correctly onto the thermometer. |
| 3. Expose the patient's axilla without exposing more of the chest or upper body than is necessary. | The patient's privacy must be protected at all times. |
| 4. Place the tip of the thermometer deep in the axilla and bring the patient's arm down, crossing the forearm over the chest. Drape the patient as appropriate for privacy. | This position offers the best skin contact with the thermometer and maintains a closed environment. |

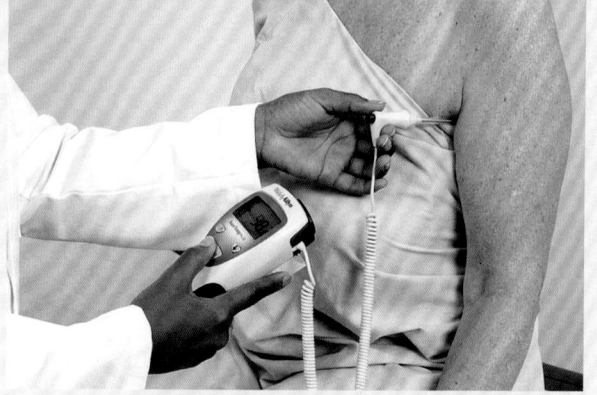

**Step 4.** With the thermometer in the axilla, the arm should be down, and the forearm should be crossed across the chest.

| STEPS | REASONS |
|---|---|
| 5. The electronic thermometer will signal when the reading is obtained. Discard the sheath into an appropriate waste container, and note the reading. | Axillary temperatures using a glass thermometer take longer than do oral or rectal ones. The sheath may obscure the column in a glass thermometer and should be removed before you read the thermometer. The electronic thermometer will have a digital display of the reading (see Procedure 19-5). |
| 6. Replace the electronic thermometer into the charger as necessary. | Always make sure thermometers are ready for the next patient. |
| 7. Wash your hands. | This prevents the spread of microorganisms. |

*(continues on page 470)*

## PROCEDURE 19-4 (continued)

| STEPS | REASONS |
|---|---|
| 8. Record the procedure and mark a letter A next to the reading, indicating that the reading is axillary. | Temperature readings are presumed to have been taken orally unless otherwise noted in the medical record. The vital signs (temperature, pulse, respirations, and blood pressure) are usually recorded together. |
| 9. **AFF** Explain how to respond to a patient who is from a different generation. | Refer to an elderly patient by their correct title (Mr., Mrs., Miss, etc.). Be respectful to the patient by only using the patient's first name after he or she has given you permission to do so and do not assume the patient is hearing or cognitively impaired. |

Charting Example:
*02/01/2016 3:45 PM T 97.8°F (A)* _____ *B. DeMarcus, CMA*

Note: *The medical assistant may sign his or her name in the patient record using only the "CMA" credential if the office has a signature log denoting the entire credential as "CMA(AAMA)."*

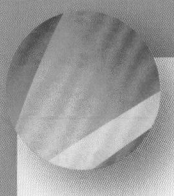

## PSY PROCEDURE 19-5

## Measuring an Oral Temperature Using an Electronic Thermometer

**PSY** Measure and record temperature; instruct and prepare a patient for a procedure or a treatment; document patient care accurately in the medical record.

**Purpose:** Accurately measure and record a patient's temperature using an electronic thermometer

**Equipment:** Electronic thermometer with oral or rectal probe; disposable probe covers; biohazard waste container; gloves for taking a rectal temperature

**Standard:** This task should take 5 minutes.

| STEPS | REASONS |
|---|---|
| 1. Wash your hands and assemble the necessary supplies. | Hand washing aids infection control. |
| 2. Greet and identify the patient and explain the procedure. | Identifying the patient prevents errors. |
| 3. Choose the most appropriate method (oral, axillary, or rectal) and attach the appropriate probe to the battery-powered unit. | Many electronic thermometers come with an oral probe and a rectal probe. |
| 4. Insert the probe into a probe cover. Covers are usually carried with the unit in a specially fitted box attached to the back or top of the unit. | All probes fit into one size probe cover. If using the last probe cover, be sure to attach a new box of covers onto the unit to be ready for the next patient. |
| 5. Position the thermometer appropriately for the method. To take an oral temperature, place the end of the thermometer under the patient's tongue to either side of the frenulum. | This is the area of highest vascularity and will give the most accurate reading. Refer to Procedures 19-3 and 19-4 if taking the temperature using the rectal or axillary methods. |

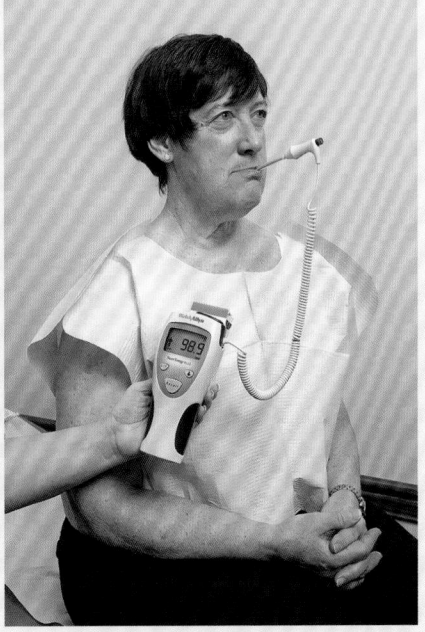

**Step 5.** Place the thermometer to one side of the frenulum.

*(continues on page 472)*

# PROCEDURE 19-5 (continued)

| STEPS | REASONS |
| --- | --- |
| 6. Wait for the electronic thermometer unit to "beep" when it senses no signs of the temperature rising further. This usually occurs within 20–30 seconds. | Removing the thermometer before it signals may result in the recording of an inaccurate temperature. |
| 7. After the beep, remove the probe and note the reading on the digital display screen on the unit before replacing the probe into the unit. | Most units automatically shut off when the probe is reinserted into the unit. |
| 8. Discard the probe cover by pressing a button, usually on the end of the probe, while holding the probe over a biohazard container. After noting the temperature, replace the probe into the unit. | Probe covers should be discarded appropriately. Placing the probe back in the unit often turns the unit off in most models of electronic thermometers. |
| 9. Remove your gloves, if used; wash your hands; and record the procedure. | The vital signs (temperature, pulse, respirations, and blood pressure) are usually recorded together. |
| 10. Return the unit and probe to the charging base. | Although the unit is battery powered, it should be kept in the charging base so that the battery is adequately charged. |
| 11. **AFF** Explain how to respond to a patient who is hearing impaired. | Make sure the patient can see your face as you are speaking. Speak clearly, not loudly. |

---

Charting Example:
*11/28/2016 10:15 AM T 101°F (O)* _____ *D. Shaper, CMA*

---

Note: *The medical assistant may sign his or her name in the patient record using only the "CMA" credential if the office has a signature log denoting the entire credential as "CMA(AAMA)."*

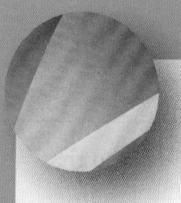

**PSY** PROCEDURE 19-6

# Measuring Temperature Using a Tympanic Thermometer

**PSY** Measure and record temperature; instruct and prepare a patient for a procedure or a treatment; document patient care accurately in the medical record.

**Purpose:** Accurately measure and record a patient's temperature using a tympanic thermometer

**Equipment:** Tympanic thermometer, disposable probe covers, biohazard waste container

**Standard:** This task should take 5 minutes.

| STEPS | REASONS |
|---|---|
| 1. Wash your hands and assemble the necessary supplies. | Hand washing aids infection control. |
| 2. Greet and identify the patient and explain the procedure. | Identifying the patient prevents errors. |
| 3. Insert the ear probe into a probe cover. | Always put a clean probe cover on the ear probe before inserting it. |
| 4. Place the end of the ear probe into the patient's ear canal with your dominant hand while straightening out the ear canal with your nondominant hand. | Straighten the ear canal of most patients by pulling the top, posterior part of the outer ear up and back. For children under 3 years of age, pull the outer ear down and back. |

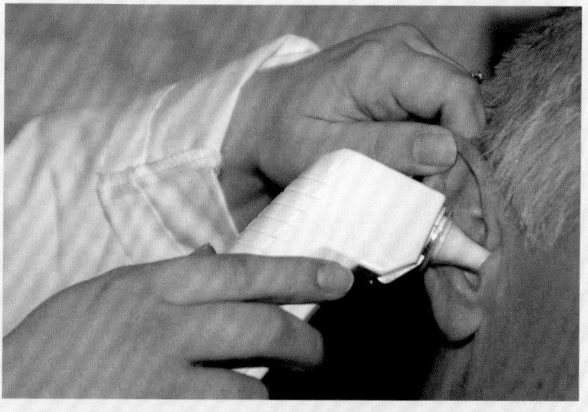

**Step 4.** Place the probe into the ear canal while straightening the ear canal.

| STEPS | REASONS |
|---|---|
| 5. With the ear probe properly placed in the ear canal, press the button on the thermometer. The reading is displayed on the digital display screen in about 2 seconds. | Pressing the button on the thermometer before the probe is properly placed in the ear will result in an inaccurate reading. |
| 6. Remove the probe and note the reading. Discard the probe cover into an appropriate waste container. | The probe covers are for one patient use only. |
| 7. Wash your hands and record the procedure. | Be sure to indicate that the tympanic temperature was taken. The vital signs (temperature, pulse, respirations, and blood pressure) are usually recorded together. |

*(continues on page 474)*

## PROCEDURE 19-6 (continued)

| STEPS | REASONS |
|---|---|
| 8. Return the unit to the charging base. | The unit should be kept in the charging base so that the battery is always adequately charged. |
| 9. **AFF** Explain how to respond to a patient who is deaf. | Solicit assistance from anyone who may be with the patient or a staff member who knows sign language to interpret if available. If no interpreter is available, use hand gestures or pictures to explain procedure to the patient. |

Charting Example:
*04/13/2016 2:00 PM T 99.4°F tympanic_____M. Smythe, CMA*

Note: *The medical assistant may sign his or her name in the patient record using only the "CMA" credential if the office has a signature log denoting the entire credential as "CMA(AAMA)."*

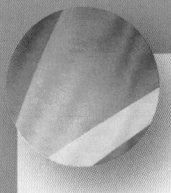

## PSY PROCEDURE 19-7

## Measuring Temperature Using a Temporal Artery Thermometer

**PSY** Measure and record temperature; instruct and prepare a patient for a procedure or a treatment; document patient care accurately in the medical record.

**Purpose:** Accurately measure and record a patient's temperature using a temporal artery thermometer

**Equipment:** Temporal artery thermometer; alcohol wipe

**Standard:** This task should take less than 5 minutes.

| STEPS | REASONS |
|---|---|
| 1. Wash your hands and assemble the necessary supplies. | Hand washing aids infection control. |
| 2. Greet and identify the patient and explain the procedure. | Identifying the patient prevents errors. |
| 3. Place the probe end of the handheld unit on the forehead of the patient. Make sure the patient's skin is dry. | If the patient is diaphoretic, dry the skin with a towel first or take the temperature using another method. |
| 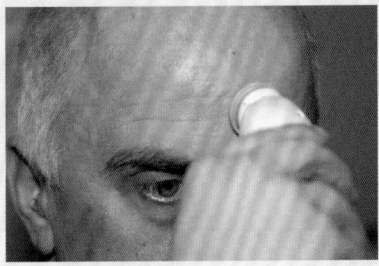 | **Step 3.** The temporal artery thermometer is placed flat against the forehead. |
| 4. With the thermometer against the forehead, depress the on/off button, move the thermometer across and down the forehead, and release the on/off button with the unit over the temporal artery. | Some units may indicate that you should lift the thermometer from the temporal artery and place it behind the ear before releasing the on/off button. |
| 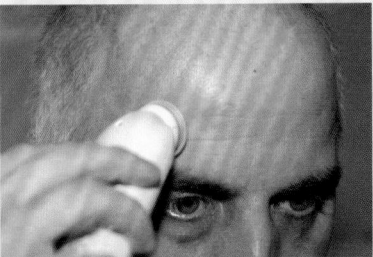<br>A | **Step 4A.** Slide the unit across the forehead. |
| 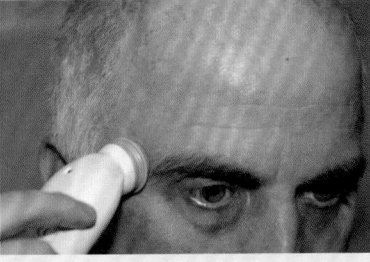<br>B | **Step 4B.** Stop over the temporal artery before releasing the on/off button. |

*(continues on page 476)*

## PROCEDURE 19-7 (continued)

| STEPS | REASONS |
|---|---|
| 5. The reading is displayed on the digital display screen in 1–2 seconds. | |
| 6. Properly disinfect the end of the thermometer according to manufacturer instructions. | Thermometers must be disinfected between patients. |
| 7. Wash your hands and record the procedure. | Be sure to indicate that a temporal artery temperature was taken. The vital signs (temperature, pulse, respirations, and blood pressure) are usually recorded together. |
| 8. Return the unit to the charging base. | The unit should be kept in the charging base so that the battery is always adequately charged. |
| 9. **AFF** Explain how to respond to a patient who is visually impaired. | Observe patients carefully to prevent injury and always ask before offering assistance or taking hold of their arm to guide. Face the patients when speaking and always let them know what you are going to do before touching them. |

Charting Example:
*09/22/2016 9:30 AM T 98.6°F temporal artery* _____ *N. Hoffman, CMA*

Note: *The medical assistant may sign his or her name in the patient record using only the "CMA" credential if the office has a signature log denoting the entire credential as "CMA(AAMA)."*

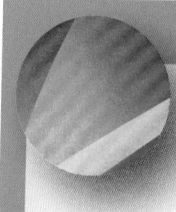

## **PSY** PROCEDURE 19-8

# Measuring the Radial Pulse

**PSY** Measure and record the pulse; instruct and prepare a patient for a procedure or a treatment; document patient care accurately in the medical record.

**Purpose:** Accurately measure and record a patient's radial pulse

**Equipment:** A watch with a sweeping second hand

**Standard:** This procedure should take 3 to 5 minutes.

| STEPS | REASONS |
|---|---|
| 1. Wash your hands. | Hand washing is an infection control technique and should be performed before and after any patient contact. |
| 2. Greet and identify the patient and explain the procedure. | In most cases, the pulse is taken at the same time as the other vital signs. |
| 3. Position the patient with the arm relaxed and supported either on the lap of the patient or on a table. | If the arm is not supported or the patient is uncomfortable, the pulse may be difficult to find, and the count may be affected. |
| 4. With the index, middle, and ring fingers of your dominant hand, press with your fingertips firmly enough to feel the pulse but gently enough not to obliterate it (see Fig. 19-11). | Do not use your thumb; it has a pulse of its own that may be confused as the patient's. You may place your thumb on the opposite side of the patient's wrist to steady your hand. |
| 5. If the pulse is regular, count it for 30 seconds, watching the second hand of your watch. Multiply the number of pulsations by 2 since the pulse is always recorded as beats per minute. If the pulse is irregular, count it for a full 60 seconds. | Counting an irregular pulse for less than 60 seconds will give an inaccurate measurement. |
| 6. Record the rate in the medical record with the other vital signs. Also note the rhythm if irregular and the volume if thready or bounding. | Procedures are considered not to have been done if they are not recorded. The vital signs (temperature, pulse, respirations, and blood pressure) are usually recorded together. |
| 7. **AFF** Explain how to respond to a patient who is developmentally challenged. | To avoid injury to the patient, assess for safety before completing a procedure when there is the possibility that the patient may not cooperate. |

**Charting Example:**
*06/12/2016 11:30 AM Pulse 78 and irregular* _____ *E. Kramer, CMA*

Note: *The medical assistant may sign his or her name in the patient record using only the "CMA" credential if the office has a signature log denoting the entire credential as "CMA(AAMA)."*

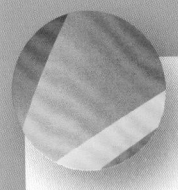

**PSY** PROCEDURE 19-9

## Measuring Respirations

**PSY** Measure and record respirations; instruct and prepare a patient for a procedure or a treatment; document patient care accurately in the medical record.

**Purpose:** Accurately measure and record a patient's respirations

**Equipment:** A watch with a sweeping second hand.

**Standard:** This procedure should take 3 to 5 minutes.

| STEPS | REASONS |
|---|---|
| 1. Wash your hands. | Hand washing aids in infection control. |
| 2. Greet and identify the patient and explain the procedure. | In most cases, the respirations are counted at the same time as the pulse. |
| 3. After counting the radial pulse and still watching your second hand, count a complete rise and fall of the chest as one respiration. Note: Some patients have abdominal movement rather than chest movement during respirations. Observe carefully for the easiest area to assess for the most accurate reading. | A patient who is aware that you are observing respirations may alter the breathing pattern. It is best to begin counting respirations immediately after counting the pulse without informing the patient. |

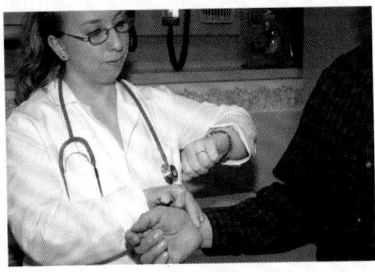

**Step 3.** Continue holding the wrist after taking the pulse and begin counting the respirations.

| STEPS | REASONS |
|---|---|
| 4. If the breathing pattern is regular, count the respiratory rate for 30 seconds and multiply by 2. If the pattern is irregular, count for a full 60 seconds. | Counting an irregular respiratory pattern for <60 seconds may give an inaccurate measurement. |
| 5. Record the respiratory rate in the medical record with the other vital signs. Also, note whether the rhythm is irregular, along with any unusual or abnormal sounds such as wheezing. | Procedures are considered not to have been done if they are not recorded. The vital signs (temperature, pulse, respirations, and blood pressure) are usually recorded together. |
| 6. **AFF** Explain how to respond to a patient who has dementia. | Solicit assistance from caregiver or other staff member to help during the procedure. Give simple directions to the patient about what he or she should do. Speak clearly, not loudly. |

**Charting Example:**
*09/15/2016 8:45 AM Resp 16 _____ J. Thompson, CMA*

Note: *The medical assistant may sign his or her name in the patient record using only the "CMA" credential if the office has a signature log denoting the entire credential as "CMA(AAMA)."*

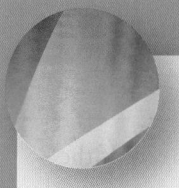

**PSY** PROCEDURE 19-10

## Measuring Blood Pressure

**PSY** Measure and record blood pressure; instruct and prepare a patient for a procedure or a treatment; document patient care accurately in the medical record.

**Purpose:** Accurately measure and record a patient's blood pressure

**Equipment:** Sphygmomanometer; stethoscope

**Standard:** This procedure should take 5 minutes.

| STEPS | REASONS |
|---|---|
| 1. Wash your hands and assemble your equipment. | Hand washing aids infection control. |
| 2. Greet and identify the patient and explain the procedure. | Identifying the patient prevents errors and explaining the procedure eases anxiety. |
| 3. Position the patient with the arm to be used supported with the forearm on the lap or a table and slightly flexed, with the palm upward. The upper arm should be level with the patient's heart. | Positioning the arm with the palm upward facilitates finding and palpating the brachial artery. If the upper arm is higher or lower than the heart, an inaccurate reading may result. |

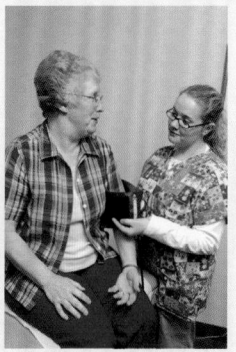

**Step 3.** Support the arm on the patient's lap, slightly flexed with the palm upward.

| STEPS | REASONS |
|---|---|
| 4. Expose the patient's arm. | Any clothing over the area may obscure the sounds. If the sleeve is pulled up, it may become tight and act as a tourniquet, decreasing the flow of blood and causing an inaccurate blood pressure reading. |
| 5. Palpate the brachial pulse in the antecubital area and center the deflated cuff directly over the brachial artery. The lower edge of the cuff should be 1–2 inches above the antecubital area. | If the cuff is placed too low, it may interfere with the placement of the stethoscope and cause noises that obscure the Korotkoff sounds. |

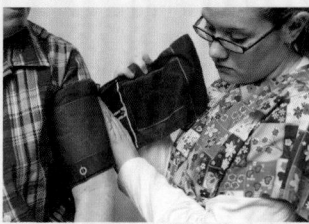

**Steps 5 and 6.** Center the cuff over the brachial artery.

| STEPS | REASONS |
|---|---|
| 6. Wrap the cuff smoothly and snugly around the arm and secure it with the Velcro edges. | If the cuff does not fit smoothly and snugly around the arm, the blood pressure reading may be inaccurate. |

**PROCEDURE 19-10** (continued)

| STEPS | REASONS |
|---|---|
| 7. With the air pump in your dominant hand and the valve between your thumb and the forefinger, turn the screw clockwise to tighten. Do not tighten it to the point that it will be difficult to release. | The cuff will not inflate with the valve open. If the valve is too tightly closed, it will be difficult to loosen with one hand after the cuff is inflated. |

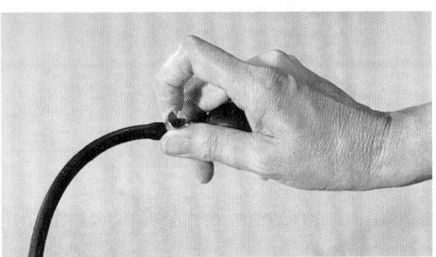

**Step 7.** Holding the bulb and the screw valve properly allows you to inflate and deflate the cuff easily.

| STEPS | REASONS |
|---|---|
| 8. While palpating the brachial pulse with your non-dominant hand, inflate the cuff and note the point or number on the dial or mercury column at which you no longer feel the brachial pulse. | The dial or mercury column should be at eye level. Noting this number gives you a reference point for reinflating the cuff when taking the blood pressure. |

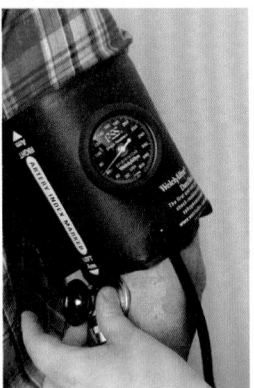

**Step 8.** Palpate the brachial pulse and place the stethoscope diaphragm bell over this artery.

9. Deflate the cuff by turning the valve counterclockwise. Wait at least 30 seconds before reinflating the cuff.

Always wait at least 30 seconds after deflating the cuff to allow circulation to return to the extremity.

10. Place the stethoscope earpieces in your ears with the openings pointed slightly forward. Stand about 3 feet from the manometer with the gauge at eye level. Your stethoscope tubing should hang freely without touching or rubbing against any part of the cuff.

With the earpieces pointing forward in the ear canals, the openings follow the natural opening of the ear canal. The manometer should be at eye level to decrease any chance of error when it is read. If the stethoscope rubs against other objects, environmental sounds may obscure the Korotkoff sounds.

11. Place the diaphragm of the stethoscope against the brachial artery and hold it in place with the non-dominant hand without pressing too hard.

If not pressed firmly enough, you may not hear the sounds. Pressing too firmly may obliterate the pulse.

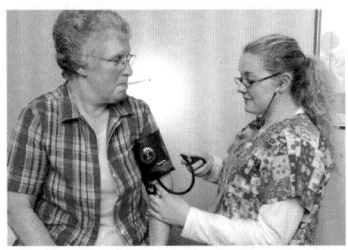

**Step 11.** Hold the stethoscope diaphragm firmly against the brachial artery while taking the blood pressure and listening carefully.

## PROCEDURE 19-10 (continued)

| STEPS | REASONS |
|---|---|
| **12.** With your dominant hand, turn the screw on the valve just enough to close the valve; inflate the cuff. Pump the valve bulb to about 30 mm Hg above the number felt during Step 8. | Inflating more than 30 mm Hg above baseline is uncomfortable for the patient and unnecessary; inflating less may produce an inaccurate systolic reading. |
| **13.** Once the cuff is appropriately inflated, turn the valve counterclockwise to release air at about 2–4 mm Hg per second. | Releasing the air too fast will cause missed beats, and releasing it too slowly will interfere with circulation. |
| **14.** Listening carefully, note the point on the gauge at which you hear the first clear tapping sound. This is the systolic sound, or Korotkoff I. | Aneroid and mercury measurements are always made as even numbers because of the way the manometer is calibrated. |

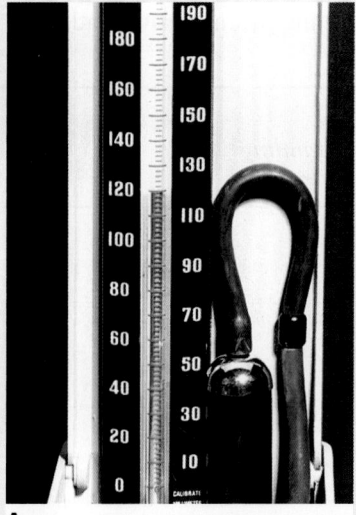

A

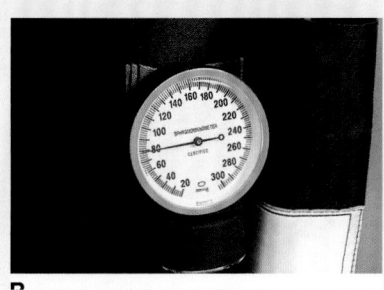

**Step 14A.** The meniscus on the mercury column in this example reads 120 mm Hg.

**Step 14B.** The gauge on the aneroid manometer reads 80 mm Hg.

| STEPS | REASONS |
|---|---|
| **15.** Maintaining control of the valve screw, continue to listen and deflate the cuff. When you hear the last sound, note the reading and quickly deflate the cuff. *Note:* Never immediately reinflate the cuff if you are unsure of the reading. Totally deflate the cuff and wait 1–2 minutes before repeating the procedure. | The last sound heard is Korotkoff V and is recorded as the bottom number or diastolic blood pressure. |
| **16.** Remove the cuff and press the air from the bladder of the cuff. | Removing the remaining air from the bladder of the cuff will allow for better storage. |

*(continues on page 482)*

# PROCEDURE 19-10 (continued)

| STEPS | REASONS |
|---|---|
| 17. If this is the first recording or a new patient, the physician may also want a reading in the other arm or in another position. | Blood pressure varies in some patients between the arms or in different positions such as lying or standing. |
| 18. Put the equipment away and wash your hands. | Hand washing should be done after any patient encounter. |
| 19. Record the reading with the systolic over the diastolic pressure, noting which arm was used (120/80 LA). Also, record the patient's position if other than sitting. | Procedures are considered not done if they are not recorded. The vital signs (temperature, pulse, respirations, and blood pressure) are usually recorded together. |
| 20. **AFF** Explain how to respond to a patient who is from a different culture. | Be respectful of the cultural differences by explaining why procedures are important. Provide additional privacy if necessary. |

Charting Example:
*11/08/2016 3:30 PM T 98.6°F O, P 78, R 16, BP 130/90 LA sitting, 110/78 LA standing*
_____ *Y. Torresnn, CMA*

# CHAPTER

## 20

# Assisting with the Physical Examination

## Learning Outcomes

**COG Cognitive Domain***

1. Spell and define the key terms
2. Identify and state the use of the basic and specialized instruments and supplies used in the physical examination
3. Describe the four methods used to examine the patient
4. State your responsibilities before, during, and after the physical examination
5. List the basic sequence of the physical examination
6. *Describe the normal function of each body system*

**PSY Psychomotor Domain***

1. Assist with the adult physical examination (Procedure 20-1)
2. *Assist provider with a patient exam*
3. *Coach patients appropriately considering cultural diversity, developmental life stages, and communication barriers*
4. *Document accurately in the medical record*

**AFF Affective Domain***

1. *Incorporate critical thinking skills when performing patient assessment*
2. *Show awareness of a patient's concerns related to the procedure being performed*
3. *Explain to a patient the rationale for performance of a procedure*
4. *Demonstrate empathy, active listening, and nonverbal communication*
5. *Demonstrate respect for individual diversity including gender, race, religion, age, economic status, and appearance*
6. *Protect the integrity of the medical record*

**Note: AAMA/CAAHEP 2015 Standards are italicized.*

**ABHES Competencies**

1. Prepare and maintain examination and treatment area
2. Prepare patient for examinations and treatments
3. Assist physician with routine and specialty examinations and treatments

*(continues on page 484)*

# Key Terms

## Case Study

One of the physician offices at Great Falls Medical Center employs several medical assistants including Jackie Bohr, CMA (AAMA). Jackie finished her medical assistant program last year and was placed at this office for her practicum experience. After completing the required number of hours necessary for her program, the practice manager, Julie Smith, hired Jackie to work primarily in the clinical area for Dr. Rowe, a general surgeon. Because Jackie learned the knowledge and skills necessary to work in the front (administrative) and the back (clinical) areas of the medical office, Jackie works with the scheduler and the office biller on days when Dr. Rowe is scheduled to be in surgery. Today, several patients are scheduled for the clinical area including eight postoperative patients, six patients who have been referred to Dr. Rowe for possible surgical procedures, and four patients who need a physical examination before having surgical procedures next week. What is Jackie's role as a medical assistant in the adult physical examination? Are the supplies and equipment used in a physical examination the same for all patients? One patient being seen for a physical examination today is physically disabled. How will Jackie assist Dr. Rowe in examining this patient? An elderly male patient admits to taking ginkgo, a natural dietary supplement that is available over the counter, to "improve his memory." How important is it for Jackie to make sure the physician knows the patient is taking this supplement?

The purpose of the complete physical examination is to assess the patient's general state of health and detect signs and symptoms of disease. New patients usually receive a complete physical examination, which gives the physician baseline information about the patient. This baseline information is valuable for future comparison and can aid the physician in **diagnosis** (identifying a disease or condition). Routine examinations are performed thereafter at regular intervals to help maintain the patient's health and prevent disease.

When a patient comes into the office, the physician can make a **clinical diagnosis** based only on the patient's symptoms. At other times, symptoms are vague and could be caused by one of several diseases. In this situation, a **differential diagnosis** is made by comparing

symptoms of several diseases. To make any diagnosis, the physician will rely on three basic components: the medical history, the physical examination, and any laboratory and diagnostic tests. Once the data from these three components are collected and evaluated, the physician will make a judgment about the patient's condition and devise a plan of care including appropriate treatment. As a medical assistant, you are responsible for assisting with taking the medical history, preparing the patient for the examination, and assisting the physician during the examination so that a clinical or differential diagnosis can be made as accurately as possible. In addition, you may collect specimens for diagnostic testing. During the examination, you must anticipate the needs of the physician and patient and be prepared to assist as necessary.

## 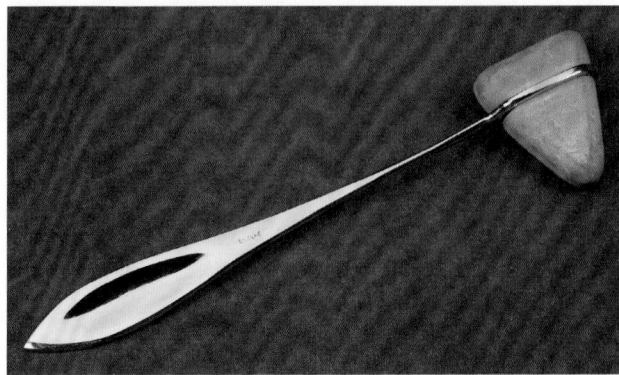 BASIC INSTRUMENTS AND SUPPLIES

Instruments used during the physical examination enable the examiner to see, hear, or feel areas of the body being assessed. In most cases, it is the physician who uses these instruments, but you must be familiar with instruments and supplies. These instruments should be kept in a special tray or drawer in a convenient location in each examination room. The exact equipment used varies among medical offices according to physicians' preferences and the specialty. Supplies that should be available in the examination room include a tape measure, gloves, tongue depressors, and cotton-tipped applicators (Fig. 20-1). The purpose of the most common instruments used in the physical examination is described in the following sections.

### CHECKPOINT QUESTION

1. Jackie works in a general surgery physician office. Instruments and supplies in her office may be different from those found in a pediatric office. Why is there variation in the types of instruments and supplies used in each medical office?

### Percussion Hammer

The percussion hammer is used to test neurologic reflexes. Also called a *reflex hammer*, this instrument has a stainless steel handle and a hard rubber head (Fig. 20-2). The head is used to test reflexes by striking

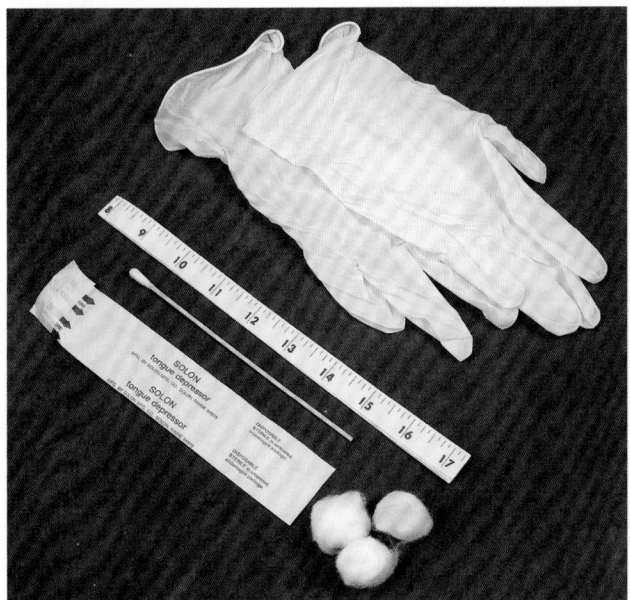

**Figure 20-1** • Common supplies used in the adult physical examination: tape measure, gloves, tongue depressor, and cotton-tipped applicator.

**Figure 20-2** • A reflex hammer.

the tendons of the ankle, knee, wrist, and elbow. The tip of the handle may be used to stroke the sole of the foot to assess the **Babinski reflex** (a reflex noted by extension of the great toe and abduction of the other toes). Some hammers have a brush and needle in the handle specifically used to test sensory perception.

### Tuning Fork

The tuning fork is used to test hearing. It is a stainless steel instrument with a handle at one end and two prongs at the other end (Fig. 20-3). The examiner strikes the prongs against his or her hand, which causes them to vibrate and produce a humming sound. While vibrating, the handle is placed against a bony area of the skull near one of the ears, and the patient is asked to describe what, if anything, is heard in that ear. Depending on the results of this hearing test, the physician may order additional auditory tests.

### Nasal Speculum

The nasal **speculum** is a stainless steel instrument that is inserted into the nostril to assist in the visual inspection of the lining of the nose, nasal membranes, and septum. The tip of the instrument is inserted into the nose, and the handles are squeezed, opening the end and allowing for visualization (Fig. 20-4). Nasal specula are also available in a disposable form.

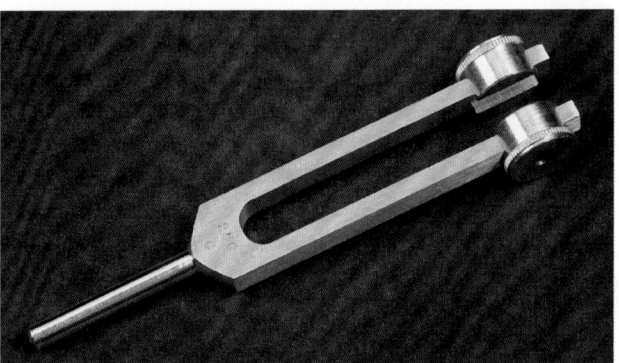

**Figure 20-3** • A tuning fork.

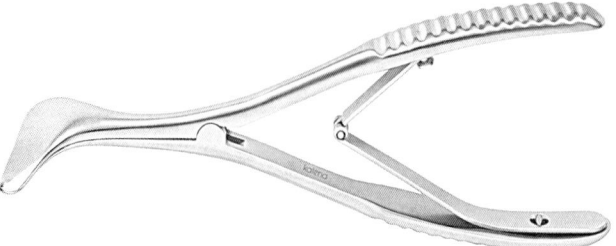

**Figure 20-4** • A nasal speculum.

## Otoscope and Audioscope

The otoscope permits visualization of the ear canal and tympanic membrane. The **tympanic membrane**, or eardrum, is a thin, oval membrane between the outer and middle ear that transmits sound vibrations to the inner ear. The otoscope has a stainless steel handle at one end and a head with a light, a magnifying lens, and a cone-shaped hollow speculum at the other end. A portable otoscope has batteries in the handle to operate the light in the head; other otoscopes are part of a unit attached to the wall and plugged into an electrical outlet (Fig. 20-5A, B). In both types, the hollow speculum is covered with a disposable speculum cover before it is placed in the ear canal. An otoscope with a specialized nasal speculum tip may be used to examine the nose.

The audioscope is used to screen patients for hearing loss. Although it looks like an otoscope, the audioscope's handle has a variety of indicators and selection buttons that can be used to adjust its tones (Fig. 20-6). The examiner places the tip of the audioscope in the patient's ear and asks the patient to respond to each of the tones that is produced. The results are recorded in the patient's medical record.

## Ophthalmoscope

The ophthalmoscope is used to examine the interior structures of the eyes. Like the otoscope, it may have a stainless steel handle that contains batteries or may be mounted on the wall (Fig. 20-7). The head of the ophthalmoscope also has a light source, magnifying lens, and opening through which to view the eye. Portable units may have a common base handle with various otoscope or ophthalmoscope tips that can be attached for different examinations.

## Examination Light and Gooseneck Lamp

Some offices are equipped with an adjustable overhead examination light for better visualization during the examination. The gooseneck lamp is a floor lamp with a movable stand that bends at the neck for use when the overhead lighting is not adequate (Fig. 20-8). You have the responsibility to make sure all examination lights are in proper working order and to direct the light toward the area of the body as indicated by the physician.

## Stethoscope

The stethoscope is used for listening to body sounds. The bell or diaphragm is at one end and is placed on the patient's body. This end is connected to two earpieces by flexible rubber or vinyl tubing (Fig. 20-9). The two earpieces have plastic or rubber tips that must be adjusted and directed outward before being placed in the examiner's ears. The stethoscope is used to listen to the sounds of the heart, lungs, and intestines. It is also used for taking blood pressure.

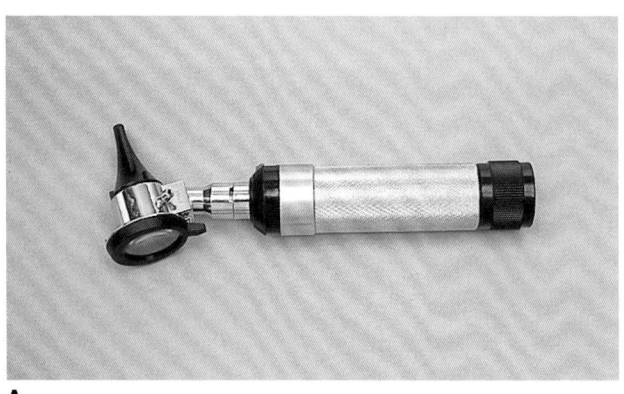

**A**

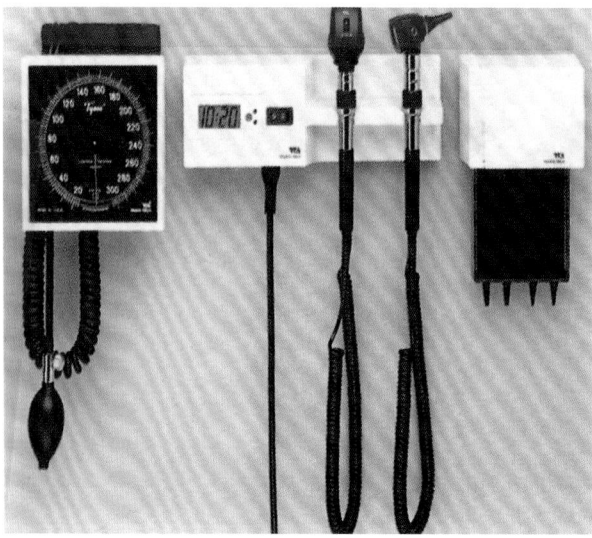

**B**

**Figure 20-5** • **A**: A portable otoscope. **B**: Wall-mounted examination instruments. From left: sphygmomanometer with cuff, ophthalmoscope, otoscope, and dispenser for disposable otoscope speculum covers.

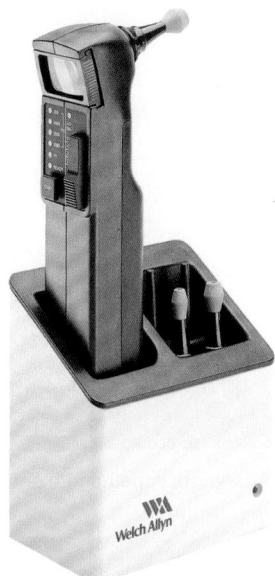

Figure 20-6 • An audioscope.

## Penlight or Flashlight

A penlight or flashlight provides additional light to a specific area during the examination. The penlight is the shape and size of a ballpoint pen and is easily carried in the examiner's pocket (Fig. 20-10). A common flashlight may be used if a penlight is not available. The penlight is often used to examine the eyes, nose, and throat.

### ✎ CHECKPOINT QUESTION

2. Dr. Rowe would like to check the hearing of a preoperative patient. Which instruments should Jackie make available for Dr. Rowe to test the ears and hearing?

## INSTRUMENTS AND SUPPLIES USED IN SPECIALIZED EXAMINATIONS

In addition to the basic instruments described previously, specialized equipment may be used during the physical examination. This chapter introduces the specialized

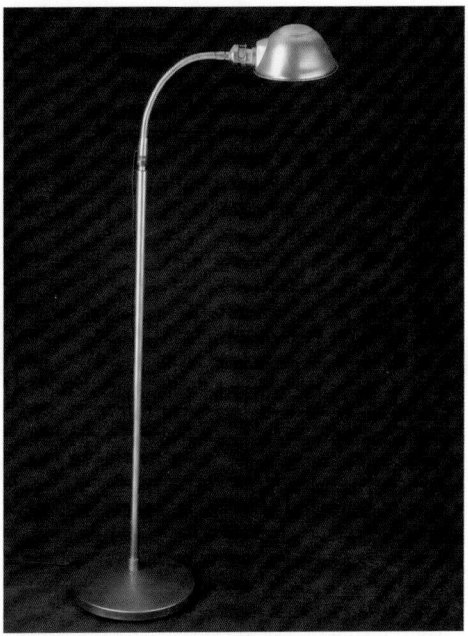

Figure 20-8 • An examination light.

examinations and equipment. A more detailed description of specialty examinations is provided in Unit Five.

## Headlight or Mirror

An ear, nose, and throat specialist (otorhinolaryngologist) may wear a headlight or head mirror during the examination of these structures. This instrument consists of a light or mirror attached to a headband that fits over the examiner's head (Fig. 20-11). A headlight provides direct light on the area being examined; the mirror reflects light from the examination light into the area.

## Laryngeal Mirror and Laryngoscope

The laryngeal mirror is a stainless steel instrument with a long, slender handle and a small, round mirror. It is used to examine areas of the patient's throat and larynx that may not be directly visible.

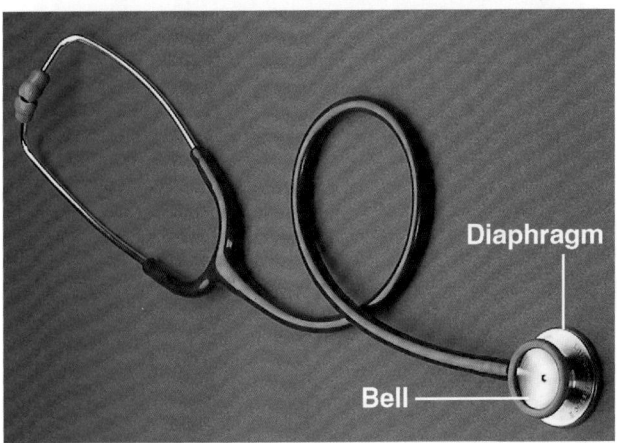

Figure 20-9 • A stethoscope.

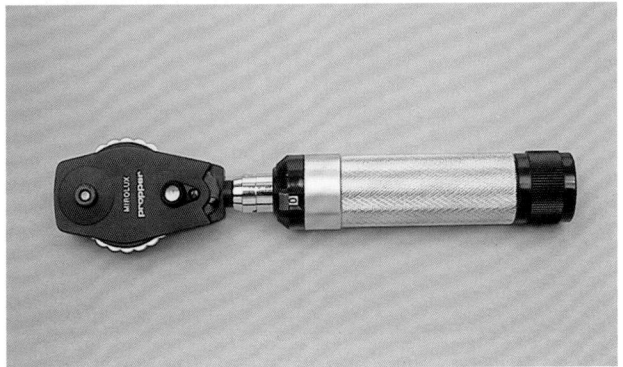

Figure 20-7 • A portable ophthalmoscope.

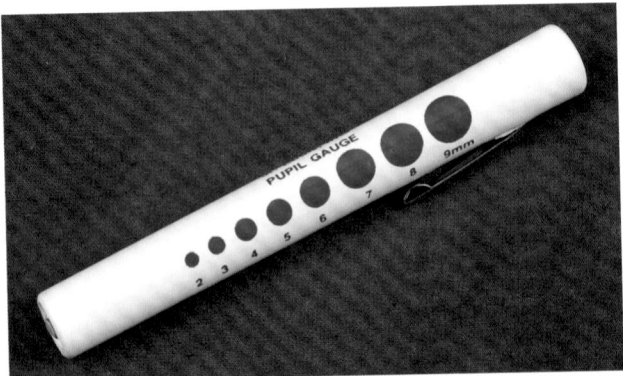

**Figure 20-10** • A penlight.

The laryngoscope handle is similar to the battery handle of a portable otoscope or ophthalmoscope, but the head allows attachment of curved or straight laryngoscope stainless steel blades and a small light source (Fig. 20-12). The examiner places the blade in the patient's throat to visualize the larynx or vocal cords, which cannot be seen by simply looking down the patient's throat.

## Vaginal Speculum

The general physical examination of female patients may include a pelvic examination and **Papanicolaou (Pap) smear**. This is a simple test in which cells obtained from the cervix or vagina are examined microscopically for abnormalities including cancer. To obtain the cells for a Pap smear, or to visually examine internal female reproductive structures, the vaginal speculum is inserted into the vagina to expand the opening (Fig. 20-13). This instrument is made of stainless steel or disposable plastic.

To obtain vaginal or cervical cells, the physician may use the Ayre spatula or cervical scraper (Fig. 20-14). This scraper is about 6 inches long and made of plastic or wood. One tip has an irregular shape that is placed in

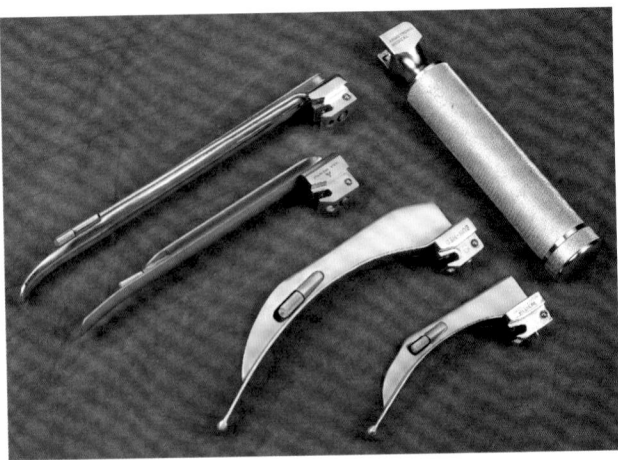

**Figure 20-12** • A laryngoscope handle and blades (straight and curved).

the cervical opening and rotated to collect the specimen; the other end is rounded and may be used to collect cells from the vaginal cul-de-sac. A histobrush may also be used to obtain cells for a Pap smear; it is made of nylon or plastic with soft bristles at one end. The collected cells are transferred to either a glass slide or a liquid preservative and sent to a laboratory for analysis. Chapter 36 has additional information about the gynecologic examination and the role of the medical assistant.

## Lubricant

Lubricant is a water-soluble gel used to reduce friction and provide easy insertion of an instrument in the physical examination. After cells are obtained for a Pap smear, lubricant may also be used for a **bimanual** examination. This examination allows the examiner to palpate internal structures of the pelvic cavity with one hand on the abdomen and with two fingers of the other gloved hand inserted into the vagina. Lubricant may also be used for rectal examinations.

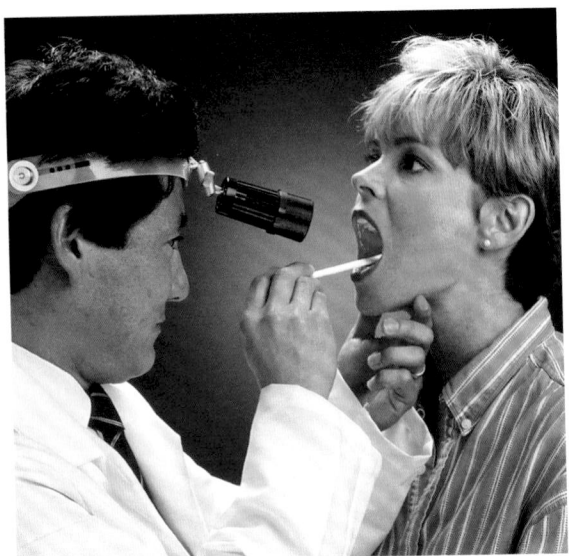

**Figure 20-11** • A headlight.

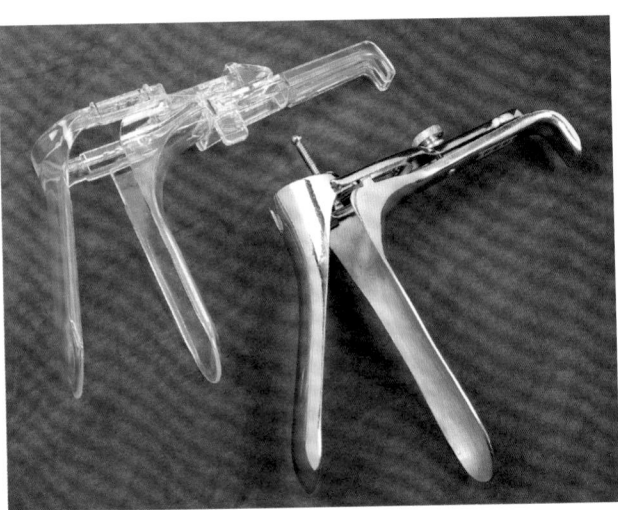

**Figure 20-13** • Vaginal specula.

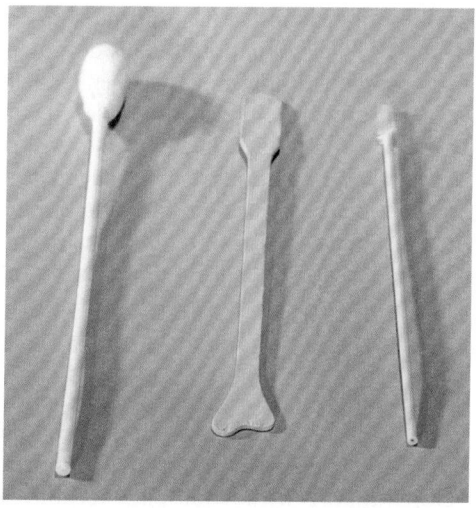

**Figure 20-14** • Cotton-tipped applicator **(left)**, Ayre spatula **(center)**, and histobrush **(right)**. Cotton-tipped applicators of this size are frequently used to remove excess vaginal secretions or to apply medications during the gynecologic examination.

## Anoscope, Proctoscope, and Sigmoidoscope

The instruments used for examination of the rectum and colon vary in length as appropriate for the structure to be examined. The anoscope is a short stainless steel or plastic speculum that is inserted into the rectum to inspect the anal canal. An **obturator** with a rounded tip extends beyond the anoscope to allow the instrument to be easily inserted into the rectum (Fig. 20-15). After the anoscope is inserted, the obturator is removed for visualization of the internal lining of the rectum.

The proctoscope is another type of speculum that is used to visualize the rectum and the anus. It is longer than the anoscope and allows the examiner to inspect more areas of the rectum. While it also consists of an obturator that is removed after the instrument is inserted, a fiberoptic light handle and magnifying lens are attached. The tubular part of the scope is marked in centimeters so that the depth of abnormalities in the anal canal can be noted.

A longer instrument used to visualize the rectum and the sigmoid colon is the sigmoidoscope. This instrument

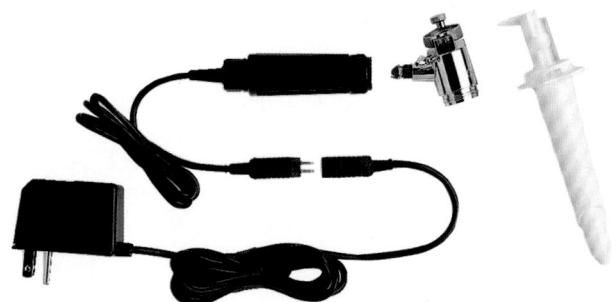

**Figure 20-15** • The anoscope with the obturator.

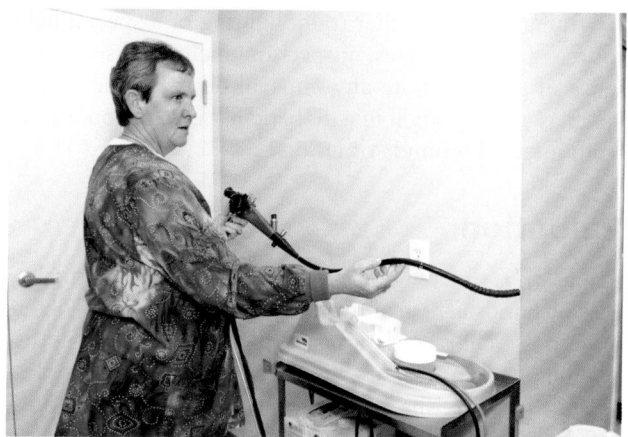

**Figure 20-16** • A flexible sigmoidoscope.

consists of a tube with an obturator, fiberoptic light handle, and magnifying lens (Fig. 20-16). It may be rigid and made of stainless steel, or it may be flexible. The advantages of the flexible sigmoidoscope include a smaller diameter, greater depth during the examination, better visualization of the intestinal mucosa, and less discomfort for the patient.

During all rectal examinations, you need a suction machine, cotton-tipped applicators, glass microscope slides, specimen containers, and laboratory request slips available. Tissue or stool specimens obtained during any rectal procedure must be properly preserved and protected for transport to the laboratory for analysis. More information regarding examinations of the colon is found in Chapter 33.

### CHECKPOINT QUESTION

3. What are the uses of the anoscope, proctoscope, and sigmoidoscope? How would Jackie explain the function of an obturator?

## COG EXAMINATION TECHNIQUES

While performing the physical examination, the physician uses four basic techniques to gather information. These include **inspection, palpation, percussion,** and **auscultation.** Each technique is described in more detail in the following sections.

### Inspection

Inspection is looking at areas of the body to observe physical features. The examiner inspects the patient's general appearance, including movements, skin and membrane color, contour, and **symmetry** or **asymmetry,** which is equality or inequality in size and shape. Inspection is done both with the naked eye and with instruments, using either room lighting or a special light source. In some cases, inspection includes use of the sense of smell to note any unusual odors of the breath (such as a fruity smell in a diabetic patient) or foul odors from infected wounds or lesions.

## Palpation

Palpation is touching or moving body areas with the fingers or hands. The examiner palpates the body to determine pulse characteristics and the presence of growths, swelling, tenderness, or pain. Organs can be palpated to assess their size, shape, and location. Skin temperature, moisture, texture, and elasticity may also be assessed by palpation. Palpation performed with both hands is called bimanual palpation; if the fingers are used, it is called a digital examination. **Manipulation** is the passive movement of the joints to determine the extent of movement or **range of motion (ROM)**.

## Percussion

Percussion is tapping or striking the body with the hand or an instrument to produce sounds. Direct percussion is performed by striking the body with a finger. Indirect percussion is done by placing a finger on the area and then striking this finger with a finger of the other hand while listening to the sounds and feeling the vibrations. This allows the examiner to determine the position, size, and density of air or fluid within a body cavity or organ.

## Auscultation

Auscultation is listening to the sounds of the body. This examination method uses a stethoscope or the ear placed directly on the patient's body. Areas of the body that can be auscultated include the heart, lungs, abdomen, and blood vessels. In the abdominal examination, auscultation is performed before palpation and percussion, which can affect normal bowel sounds.

 **CHECKPOINT QUESTION**

4. Jackie is assisting Dr. Rowe with physical examinations today. Which of the examination techniques used by Dr. Rowe require the use of the hands and fingers to feel organs or structures?

# RESPONSIBILITIES OF THE MEDICAL ASSISTANT

## Room Preparation

Medical assistants are usually responsible for preparing the examination rooms, equipment, and supplies in the clinical area. The examination room should be clean, well

lighted, well ventilated, and at a comfortable temperature for the patient. The examination table is decontaminated with an appropriate disinfectant between patients, and the paper on the table is removed and replaced with clean paper. At the beginning of each day, you are responsible for checking each examination room for adequate supplies and equipment, including the working condition of equipment. Batteries in otoscopes, ophthalmoscopes, and laryngoscopes are to be checked daily and replaced as needed.

## Patient Preparation

Once the examination room is ready, you will call the patient back by name from the waiting room and escort him or her to the treatment room. It is important that you develop rapport with your patients and practice good interpersonal skills. This helps put your patients at ease and increases their confidence in you and the physician. Your goal is to create a positive, supportive, caring, and friendly atmosphere. Treat each patient as an individual, and speak clearly with a confident tone of voice as you explain any procedures.

Before the physician sees the patient, it may be your responsibility to obtain and record the patient's history, chief complaint, and vital signs. If a urine specimen is needed, explain how to obtain the specimen, direct the patient to the bathroom, and explain what to do with the specimen.

Once in the examination room, give the patient instructions for disrobing and putting on the examination gown. Depending on the type of examination to be performed, the patient may wear the gown with the opening in the front or in the back. Leave the room while the patient undresses unless the patient needs help. Then ask the patient to sit on the examination table, helping if

 **PATIENT EDUCATION**

### Vitamins, Herbs, and Natural Remedies

When obtaining the patient's history, it is important to ask about medications and treatments that the patient may be using on a regular basis but may not mention. Many times, patients think that vitamins, herbs, and other over-the-counter products are not medications; however, these should be noted in the medical record because they may interact with prescription drugs that the physician has ordered. In addition, some dietary supplements such as ginkgo purchased over the counter may cause increased bleeding and should be discontinued before any surgical procedure no matter how minor. Although patients may have specific questions about their medications, advise them that the physician will answer specific questions about drug interactions and complications.

needed, and cover the legs with a drape. Place the chart outside the examining room door and notify the physician that the patient is ready.

## CHECKPOINT QUESTION

5. Each morning, Jackie prepares the examination rooms by making sure there are adequate supplies and equipment is ready for use. What would be the advantage of checking the working condition of equipment at the beginning of each work day?

## Assisting the Physician

During the physical examination, you may assist the physician by handing him or her instruments or supplies and directing the light appropriately. Procedure 20-1 describes the steps for assisting the physician with the physical examination.

Depending on the examination and the physical condition of the patient, you may also assist the patient into an appropriate position and adjust the drape to expose only the body area being examined (Fig. 20-17A–K). Be supportive and offer reassurance to the patient during the examination. Always assess the patient's facial

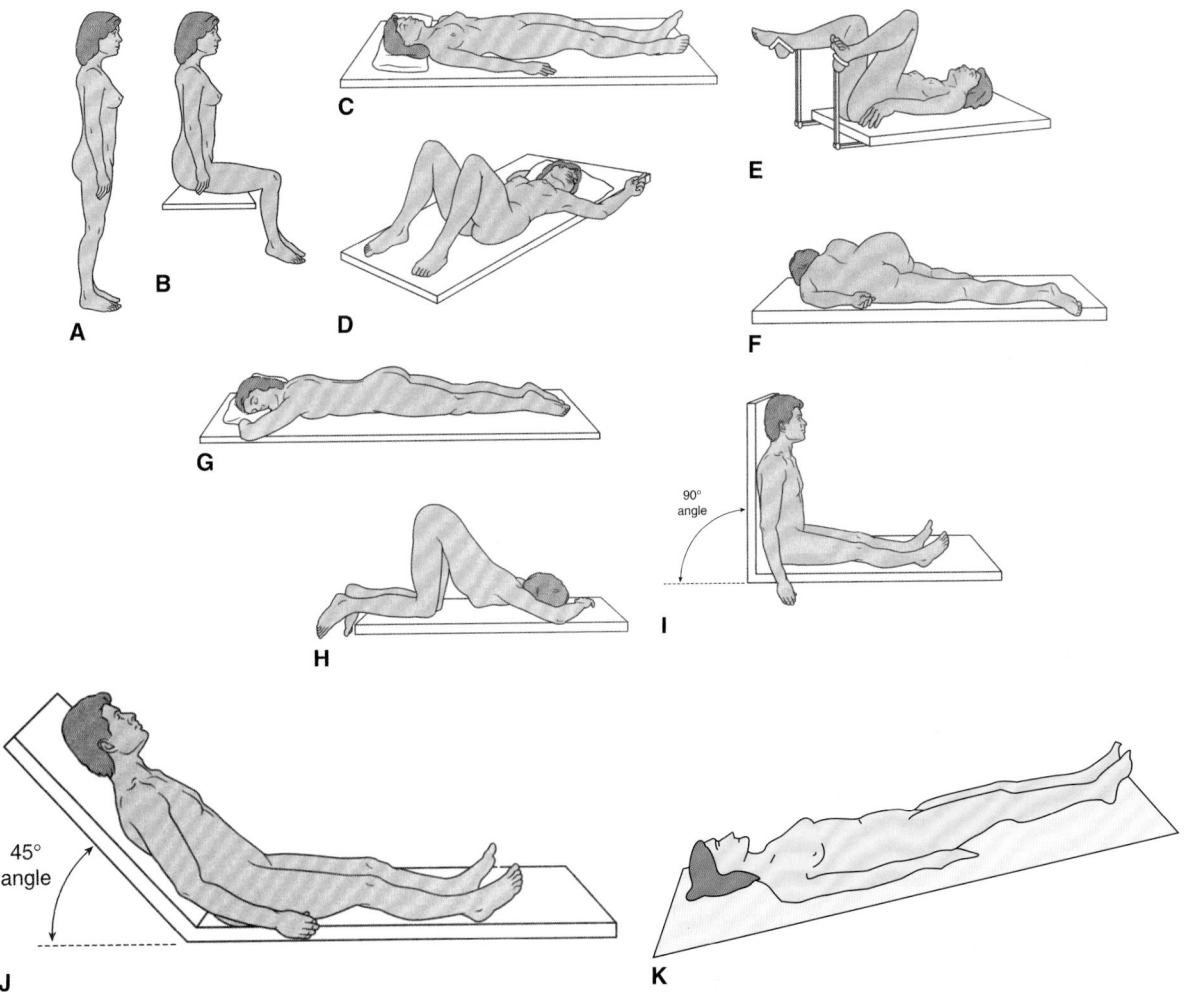

**Figure 20-17** • Patient examination positions. **A:** The erect or standing position. The patient stands erect facing forward with the arms at the sides. **B:** The sitting position. The patient sits erect at the end of the examination table with the feet supported on a footrest or stool. **C:** The supine position. The patient lies on the back with arms at the sides. A pillow may be placed under the head for comfort. **D:** The dorsal recumbent position. The patient is supine with the legs separated, knees bent, and feet flat on the table. **E:** The lithotomy position is similar to the dorsal recumbent position but with the patient's feet in stirrups rather than flat on the table. The stirrups should be level with each other and about 1 foot out from the edge of the table. The patient's feet are moved into or out of the stirrups at the same time to prevent back strain. **F:** The Sims position. The patient lies on the left side with the left arm and shoulder behind the body, right leg and arm sharply flexed on the table, and left knee slightly flexed. **G:** The prone position. The patient lies on the abdomen with the head supported and turned to one side. The arms may be under the head or by the sides, whichever is more comfortable. **H:** Knee–chest position. The patient kneels on the table with the arms and chest on the table, hips in the air, and back straight. **I:** Fowler position. The patient is half-sitting with the head of the examination table elevated 80 to 90 degrees. **J:** Semi-Fowler position. The patient is in a half-sitting position with the head of the table elevated 30 to 45 degrees and the knees slightly bent. **K:** Trendelenburg position. The patient lies on the back with arms straight at either side, and the head of the bed is lowered with the head lower than the hips; the legs are elevated at approximately 45 degrees.

| TABLE 20-1 | **Examination Positions and Their Uses** | |
|---|---|---|
| **Position** | **Body Parts** | **Instruments Needed** |
| Sitting | General appearance | |
| | Head, neck | Stethoscope |
| | Eyes | Ophthalmoscope, penlight |
| | Ears | Otoscope, tuning fork |
| | Nose | Nasal speculum, penlight, substances to smell |
| | Sinuses | Penlight |
| | Mouth | Glove, tongue blade, penlight |
| | Throat | Glove, tongue blade, penlight, laryngeal mirror, laryngoscope |
| | Axilla, arms | |
| | Chest | Stethoscope |
| | Breasts | |
| | Upper back | Stethoscope |
| | Reflexes | Percussion hammer |
| Supine | Chest | Stethoscope |
| | Abdomen | Stethoscope |
| | Breasts | |
| Lithotomy, dorsal recumbent, Sims | Female genitalia and internal organs | Gloves, vaginal speculum, Ayre spatula, histobrush, lubricant |
| Standing, dorsal recumbent, Sims | Male genitalia and hernia | Gloves |
| | Male rectum | Gloves, lubricant, fecal occult blood test |
| | Prostate | Gloves, lubricant |
| | Legs | Percussion hammer |
| | Spine, posture, gait, coordination, balance, strength, flexibility | |
| Prone | Back, spine, legs | |
| Knee–chest | Rectum | Glove, lubricant, anoscope, proctoscope, or sigmoidoscope, fecal occult blood test |
| | Female genitalia | Glove, lubricant, vaginal speculum, Ayre spatula, histobrush |
| | Prostate | Glove, lubricant |
| Fowler | Head, neck, chest | Stethoscope |

expression and level of anxiety by noting verbal and nonverbal behavior during the examination. Table 20-1 lists standard examination positions, the body parts usually examined in these positions, and the instruments needed by the physician for these examinations.

## Postexamination Duties

After the physical examination, you should perform any follow-up treatments and procedures as necessary or as ordered by the physician. Always offer the patient help returning to a sitting position after the examination. Ask the patient to dress, and leave the room unless the patient needs your assistance. Tell the patient what to do after getting dressed. In many offices, the patient gets dressed and remains in the examining room until the medical assistant gives further instructions; in other offices, patients are told to go to the front desk to schedule future appointments or receive further instructions or prescriptions. In either situation, you are responsible for reinforcing any instructions given by the physician and providing appropriate patient education. Unless the patient was advised to wait in the examination room for instructions after dressing, escort the patient to the front desk for scheduling future appointments and addressing billing issues while maintaining confidentiality. Check the medical record to be sure that all data have been accurately documented before releasing the record to the billing department.

Clean all reusable equipment, and properly dispose of any disposable supplies or equipment used during the examination. Cover the examination table with clean paper, and prepare the room for the next patient.

## CHECKPOINT QUESTION

6. When assisting Dr. Rowe with performing physical examinations, what are her four basic responsibilities?

## PHYSICAL EXAMINATION FORMAT

The physical examination of the patient begins with the patient seated on the examining table with a drape sheet over the lap and covering the legs. The physician usually progresses through the examination in an orderly, methodical sequence. The patient's general appearance, behavior, speech, posture, nutritional status, hair distribution, and skin are observed throughout the examination. The next sections describe the areas of the body examined, including normal and abnormal findings.

### Head and Neck

The patient's skull, scalp, hair, and face are inspected and palpated for size, shape, and symmetry. The examiner looks for nodules, masses, and local trauma. The patient may be asked to roll the head in all directions to assess range of motion and to check for any limitations of movement. The trachea and lymph nodes on the anterior neck are palpated for size and symmetry.

The thyroid gland, also on the anterior neck, is palpated for size and symmetry. The patient may be asked to swallow to facilitate palpating this gland. The carotid arteries are palpated and auscultated on both sides of the neck to check for any **bruit** (abnormal sound) caused by abnormal blockage.

### Eyes and Ears

Usually, you perform the visual acuity test before the physician's examination (see Chapter 29). The physician also inspects the **sclera**, or fibrous tissue covering the eye, for normal color. The pupils are inspected with a light to see if they are equal in size, round, and normally reactive to light and accommodation (adjustment). Normal pupil reaction is recorded as **PERRLA**, which means the **p**upils are **e**qual, **r**ound, and **r**eactive to **l**ight and **a**ccommodation. Eye movement is assessed by asking the patient to follow the examiner's fingers. Normal movement may be documented as "EOM intact," which means **extraocular** (outside the eye) movement intact. **Peripheral vision**, or side vision while looking straight ahead, may also be assessed. Using the ophthalmoscope, the physician visualizes the interior of the eye and evaluates the condition of the retina and any pathology of the interlobular blood vessels.

The ears are inspected and palpated for size, symmetry, lesions, and nodules. The otoscope is used to examine the interior of the ear canal, including any **cerumen**, or ear wax. The tympanic membrane is checked for color and intact or broken condition. Normally, the tympanic

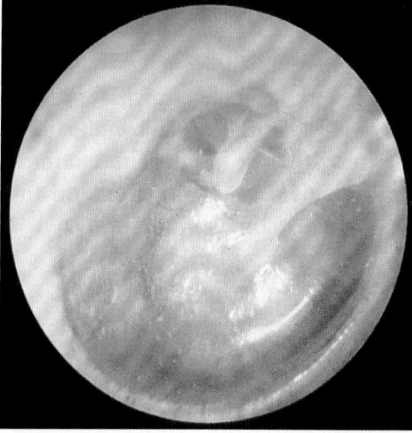

**Figure 20-18 •** A normal tympanic membrane. (Reprinted from Moore KL, Agur AM, Dalley AF. *Essential clinical anatomy* (4th ed.). Baltimore, MD: Lippincott Williams & Wilkins, 2011, with permission.)

membrane is pearly gray and concave (Fig. 20-18). However, infection may cause discoloration, and fluids behind the eardrum may cause the membrane to bulge outward. Auditory acuity is tested with the tuning fork or the audioscope (see Chapter 30).

### Nose and Sinuses

The external nose is palpated for abnormalities and inspected using a nasal speculum and light. The position of the **nasal septum** is noted for any deviation to the right or left. Each nostril is inspected for color of the mucosa, discharge, lesions, obstructions, polyps, swelling, or tenderness. The sense of smell may be assessed by having the patient close the eyes and identify a common substance such as alcohol, lemon, strawberry, or peppermint.

The paranasal sinuses are also inspected and palpated. With the technique of **transillumination** to visualize the sinuses, the room is darkened and a penlight or flashlight is placed against the upper cheek or periorbital ridge.

 **PATIENT EDUCATION**

### The Sense of Taste and Smell

When obtaining the medical history, ask the patient whether he or she has had any problems with tasting or smelling. A sudden loss in the ability to taste or smell can be the result of medication, sinus infection, and certain types of tumor. Lack of taste sensation can be the result of normal aging. Normally, the tongue is covered with small bumps called papillae. Each papilla holds about 100 taste buds that allow sweet, salty, sour, and bitter tastes to be identified. The average adult has about 10,000 taste buds. The cells that make up the taste buds are replaced about every 2 weeks. Scientists estimate that by 80 years of age, most people have lost 60% to 80% of their taste buds, and unfortunately, the remaining taste buds are less sensitive than earlier in life. Sweet and salty taste buds tend to be the most affected.

## Mouth and Throat

The physician inspects the mucous membranes of the mouth, gums, teeth, tongue, tonsils, and throat using clean gloves, a light source, and a tongue blade. A laryngeal mirror may also be used. The examiner assesses general dental hygiene and salivary gland function and looks for any abnormalities in the oral cavity, including color, ulcerations, and nodules.

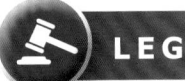

### CHECKPOINT QUESTION

7. What is the tympanic membrane, and how does infection affect its appearance?

## Chest, Breasts, and Abdomen

The anterior chest is examined with the gown removed to the waist. The physician observes the general appearance and symmetry of the chest and breast area, the respiratory rate and pattern, and any obvious masses or swelling. Palpation includes the axillary lymph nodes and the area over the heart. Underlying structures may also be percussed. Using a stethoscope, the examiner auscultates the lungs for abnormal sounds, at which time the patient may be asked to take deep breaths. The heart sounds and apical pulse are also assessed.

Inspection and palpation of the posterior chest include the muscles of the back and spine. This is followed by percussion of the back to assess lung fields. With a stethoscope, the examiner listens to posterior lung sounds, again with the patient asked to take deep breaths.

The breasts may be palpated in both male and female patients. The supine position is preferred for palpation of the breasts because the breast tissue flattens out, making any abnormalities easier to feel. The tissue subject to breast examination includes not only the breast and nipple, but the tissue extending up to the clavicle, under the axilla, and down to the bottom of the rib cage.

After the breasts are examined, the drape is lowered to expose the abdomen to the pubic area. The patient's chest is draped or gowned to just below the breasts. The abdomen is inspected for contour, symmetry, and pulsations from the aorta, a large artery that extends from the heart down the center of the thoracic and abdominal cavities. The examiner uses the stethoscope to auscultate the bowel sounds. Percussion may be used to determine the outlines of the abdominal organs, and palpation is used to assess any organ enlargement, masses, pain, or tenderness.

The lower abdomen and groin are palpated to assess enlargement of **inguinal** lymph nodes and detect any **hernia**. A hernia is protrusion of an organ, such as the intestines, through a weakened muscle wall. The femoral arteries, which pass through each groin, may also be palpated and auscultated.

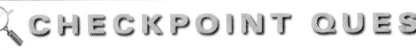

### CHECKPOINT QUESTION

8. Jackie assists a patient into position for a breast examination. Why is the patient supine for palpation of the breasts?

---

### ⚖ LEGAL TIP

#### Assisting During Exams

During the physical examination, it is recommended that you remain in the examination room if the physician is examining a patient of the opposite gender. For example, if a male physician is performing a gynecologic examination, the medical assistant should remain in the room to protect the physician from being accused of inappropriate behavior. A female physician should also ask the medical assistant to remain present during the examination of a male patient for similar reasons. Although physicians perform these examinations routinely and medical assistants are often busy performing many tasks at once, taking the time to be present during these examinations will provide legal protection for the physician should an accusation of impropriety arise at a later date.

## Genitalia and Rectum

The physician puts on clean gloves to examine the external male genitalia and then the rectum. The male genitalia are inspected to note symmetry, lesions, swelling, masses, and hair distribution. The scrotal contents may be visualized using transillumination in a darkened room. In addition, the scrotum is palpated for testicular size, contour, and consistency. The male patient is then asked to stand and bear down as if having a bowel movement while the examiner places a gloved index finger upward along the side of the scrotum in the inguinal ring to assess for a hernia.

The physician asks the patient either to bend over the examination table or to assume the Sims position to inspect the anus for lesions and hemorrhoids. The examiner inserts a gloved and lubricated finger into the rectum to palpate the rectal sphincter muscle and prostate gland for size, consistency, and any masses. An **occult blood** (hidden blood) stool test may be obtained on any stool obtained from the gloved finger. (Chapter 33 describes the procedure for processing the occult blood stool specimen.)

The female genitalia and rectum are usually examined with the patient in the lithotomy position and with one corner of the drape extending over the genitalia and the other corner covering the patient's chest. A gooseneck lamp is adjusted to direct light on the vaginal area, and the external genitalia are inspected for lesions, edema, cysts, discharge, and hair distribution. With clean gloves, the examiner inserts the vaginal speculum and inspects the condition of the vaginal mucosa and cervix. A Pap smear sample from the cervix is obtained, and the speculum is removed. At this time, the examiner performs a bimanual examination to palpate the internal reproductive organs for size, contour, consistency, and any masses. Two fingers of the gloved dominant hand are inserted into the vagina while the gloved nondominant hand is placed on the lower abdomen to compress the internal organs. (See Chapter 36 for a complete description of the procedure for assisting with a gynecologic examination.)

Sometimes, a **rectovaginal** examination is necessary to palpate the posterior uterus and vaginal wall. The examiner places a gloved index finger in the vagina and the middle finger of the same hand in the rectum at the same time. The rectum is usually inspected and palpated for lesions, hemorrhoids, and sphincter tone. A stool specimen may be obtained from the gloved finger to test for occult blood.

## WHAT IF?

**What if you are assisting the physician during a genital and pelvic examination on a disabled female patient who cannot be placed into the lithotomy position?**

Both genital and rectal examinations may be performed with the patient in the dorsal recumbent or Sims position for patients who cannot comfortably assume the usual positions, including the lithotomy position.

## Legs

The legs are inspected and the peripheral pulse sites palpated with the patient supine. The patient stands, with assistance if needed, and the peripheral pulse sites may be palpated again and the legs observed for varicose veins.

## Reflexes

The examiner uses the percussion hammer to test the patient's reflexes by striking the biceps, triceps, patellar, Achilles, and plantar tendons. The patient is usually sitting when these reflexes are checked but may move to supine for checking the plantar reflexes.

## Posture, Gait, Coordination, Balance, and Strength

The general posture of the patient and the spine may be inspected with the patient standing. The patient may be asked to walk and perform other movements so that **gait** and coordination can be observed. A balance test may be done by having the patient stand with the feet together and eyes closed. Range of motion and strength of arms and legs are assessed.

## CHECKPOINT QUESTION

9. Why would Dr. Rowe perform rectovaginal and bimanual pelvic examinations?

## TRIAGE

While working in a family practice office, you have to complete the following three tasks:

A. A patient was just discharged, and the examination room has to be cleaned and restocked.
B. The physician states that she is ready to perform a gynecologic examination and needs your assistance.
C. A suture tray has to be set up for a 3-year-old child with a facial laceration.

**How do you sort these tasks? What do you do first? Second? Third?**

First, assist the physician with the examination. When possible, limit the waiting time for female patients to have their gynecologic examination. Next, set up the suture tray. Third, clean and restock the examination room.

## GENERAL HEALTH GUIDELINES AND CHECKUPS

Physicians vary as to how often they recommend a complete physical examination. For patients aged 20 to 40 years, physical examinations are scheduled about every 1 to 3 years. Annual examinations are typically performed on patients over age 40 unless a medical condition requires more frequent visits.

For women, the American Cancer Society recommends the first Pap smear when sexual activity occurs, but no later than 21 years of age. This test should be done annually for conventional testing or every 2 years if the practitioner uses a liquid-based Pap test. A breast examination by a physician is recommended every 3 years for women aged 20 to 40 to detect lumps and thickenings that could be malignancies, but breast self-examinations (BSEs) should be performed monthly to allow the patient to detect and report any abnormalities in breast tissue between visits to the physician (see Chapter 36). As with most cancers, early detection of breast cancer is the key to survival. A baseline mammogram is recommended for those aged 35 and yearly after 40. If the patient is at risk for developing breast cancer, the physician may recommend mammograms earlier and more often.

The American Cancer Society also recommends that male patients have the prostate-specific antigen (PSA) blood test and digital rectal examination (DRE) yearly beginning at age 50 to detect early signs of prostate cancer. Men who are high risk for developing prostate cancer should have these tests starting at age 45. Risk factors include African-American men and those with close family members (father, brothers, or sons) who were diagnosed with prostate cancer before the age of 65. Again, early detection is important for early treatment, which saves lives.

All patients should have a baseline electrocardiogram (ECG) at age 40 and follow-up ECGs as necessary. In addition, a rectal examination and fecal occult blood test are recommended annually beginning at age 40. At age 50, a proctoscopic examination (colonoscopy) is recommended, and if the results are negative, this exam should be performed every 3 to 5 years thereafter.

The Centers for Disease Control and Prevention recommends the following immunizations for all adults. Adults who may be at a higher risk to serious health problems due to health, job, or lifestyle have additional recommendations in addition to the ones listed here. All adults should consult a health care provider to determine what immunizations are best for their situation.

• Tdap (tetanus, diphtheria, and pertussis) once and a tetanus (Td) booster every 10 years, or sooner if the patient has an open wound.
• Measles, mumps, rubella (MMR) one or two doses between the ages of 19 and 55 years for patients who do not have documentation of having the vaccine or for those who have never had the disease.
• The varicella vaccine (chicken pox) should be given in two doses for adults who do not have documentation of having the vaccine or for those who have never had the disease.
• Seasonal flu (Influenza) is recommended each year for everyone 6 months of age and older including pregnant women.
• One injection of pneumococcal vaccine should be given at age 65 years.
• Some doctors also recommend a series of three hepatitis B injections for any adult patient who has not received this immunization.

You should take every opportunity to educate patients regarding the signs and symptoms that may signal health problems and when to call the physician.

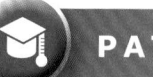

## PATIENT EDUCATION

### The Body's Warning Signals

Teach patients the CAUTION acronym to recognize these early warning signs of cancer:

C     Change in bowel or bladder habits
A     A sore that does not heal
U     Unusual bleeding or discharge
T     Thickening, lumps, or changes in the shape of the breasts or testicles
I     Indigestion or difficulty swallowing
O     Obvious change in a wart or mole
N     Nagging cough or hoarseness of the voice

Frequent, severe headaches and persistent abdominal pain are other signals that should not be ignored. Instruct patients not to overlook the following signs in their children:

• Continual crying for no obvious reason
• Unexplained nausea and vomiting
• General failure to thrive
• Spontaneous bleeding or bleeding that does not stop in the normal amount of time
• Bumps, lumps, masses, or swelling anywhere on the body
• Frequent stumbling for no apparent reason

## CHECKPOINT QUESTION

10. Dr. Rowe asks Jackie to explain the procedure to perform a self-breast examination to a young female patient. Why are monthly breast self-examinations important for women aged 20 to 40 years?

## ROLE-PLAYING ACTIVITY

Working in a general surgery physician office can be a busy but rewarding experience. Choose another student and take turns playing the role of Jackie Bohr, the medical assistant discussed in the case study at the beginning of this chapter, and the patients being seen in the office today. The first patient seen is Becky Trainor, a 36-year-old female who has been referred by her family physician for a suspicious mole removal from her right posterior scapular area. Becky admits to you that she "loves to sunbathe" and has recently joined a tanning salon. How would you respond? After obtaining a chief complaint and present illness, advise Becky on what clothing she will need to remove for Dr. Rowe to examine the area of concern. Record the chief complaint in the medical record. Assuming Dr. Rowe is ready to examine Becky, assist Becky into the most appropriate position for examination. Your instructor will give you additional information about this activity!

## *español* SPANISH TERMINOLOGY

**Voy a examinarlo/la.**
I am going to examine you.

**Voy a examinar sus oídos.**
I am going to check your ears.

**Voy a examinar su nariz.**
I am going to check your nose.

**Por favor saque la lengua.**
Please stick out your tongue.

**Voy a examinar su piel.**
I am going to examine your skin.

**Voy a examinar su abdomen (vientre).**
I am going to examine your abdomen.

**Voy a examinar su espalda.**
I am going to examine your back.

**Por favor pongase esta bata con la apertura para atrás.**
Please wear this gown with the opening to the back.

**Por favor acuéstese con cara para arriba.**
Please lie down face up.

**Por favor acuéstese con la cara para arriba y doble sus rodillas.**
Please lie down face up and bend your knees.

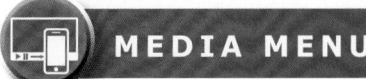

## MEDIA MENU

**Student Resources** on thePoint®

- **CMA/RMA Certification Exam Review**

**Internet Resources**
**American Academy of Family Physicians**
http://www.aafp.org/online/en/home.html

**Family Doctor**
http://www.familydoctor.org/online/famdocen/home.html

**American College of Physicians—Internal Medicine**
http://www.acponline.org

**CDC Screen for Life: National Colorectal Cancer Action Campaign**
http://www.cdc.gov/cancer/colorectal/sfl

**American Cancer Society**
http://www.cancer.org

**National Breast Cancer Foundation**
http://www.nationalbreastcancer.org

## EMR Activity

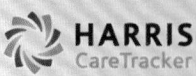

Prerequisite Activities in Harris CareTracker

- *The Getting Started and Quickstart documents and EMR Activities Step-by-Step Instructions are available at* http://thePoint.lww.com/KronenbergerComp5e.
- *Note: You must first enter each patient into the EMR as new patients before completing the following EMR activity as given in the EMR Step-by-Step Instructions.*

Activity Details

In the patient's *Medical Record* application of the EMR, enter the following chief complaints for each patient listed. Also indicate an appropriate present illness for each patient based on the chief complaint and the questions you would ask as determined by the medical history and chief complaint. Although the patient position utilized during the examination is NOT recorded in the medical record, what position would be the most appropriate in order to assist the physician performing the examination?

1. Erica Tomkin: Annual gynecology examination
2. Tammy Leonard: Headaches for 1 week
3. Steve Sutter: Lower back pain after working in yard last weekend
4. Katlyn Bobbitt: Left ear pain and fever
5. Oscar Tinner: Hypertension and right knee pain

## Chapter Summary

- Your role as a medical assistant during the physical examination is to assist both the physician and the patient.
- Efficiency, accuracy, and attention to detail are crucial as you assist the physician and anticipate what will be needed in the examination.
- Assessing the patient's needs, developing a good interpersonal relationship, and providing support to the patient are important to help the patient have a pleasant office visit.

## Warm-Ups for Critical Thinking

1. During the physical examination, the physician asks the patient to walk across the room. What can be determined about the patient's health from observing the patient's gait?
2. After the physical examination, a patient asks you, "Why did the physician hit my chest with his fingers while listening?" How do you explain to the patient what the doctor was doing?
3. Why is it possible for the physician to assess vascular health by checking the interior eye with the ophthalmoscope?
4. How can you anticipate what instruments or supplies the physician may need during the physical examination? Why is this important?
5. When checking the ophthalmoscope for working condition, you discover that it is not working. What do you think might be the problem? How would you handle this situation?

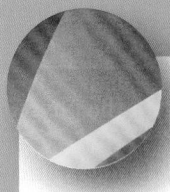

## PSY PROCEDURE 20-1

## Assisting with the Adult Physical Examination

**AFF** Assist provider with patient examination.

**PSY** Instruct and prepare a patient for a procedure or a treatment.

**PSY** Document patient care accurately in the medical record.

**Purpose:** Prepare the room and patient for the general physical examination, assist the physician during the examination, assist the patient as needed after the examination, and clean up the examination room.

**Equipment:** A variety of instruments and supplies, including the stethoscope, ophthalmoscope, otoscope, penlight, tuning fork, nasal speculum, tongue blade, percussion hammer, gloves, water-soluble lubricant, an examinations light, and patient gown and draping supplies

**Standard:** This procedure should take 15 minutes.

| STEPS | REASONS |
| --- | --- |
| 1. Wash your hands. | Handwashing aids infection control. |
| 2. Prepare the examination room and assemble the equipment. | A clean room that is free of contamination prevents transfer of microorganisms. |

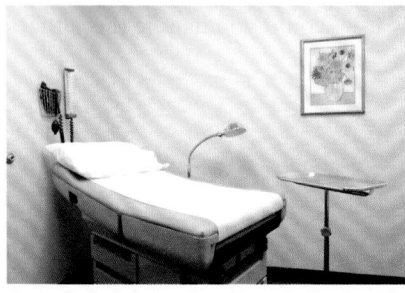

Step 2. The examination room should be clean, neat, and orderly.

| 3. Greet the patient by name and escort him or her to the examining room. | Identifying the patient by name prevents errors. |

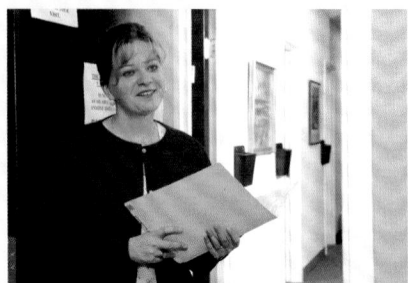

Step 3. Identify the patient and escort him or her to the exam room.

| 4. Explain the procedure. | Explaining the procedure reduces anxiety and may help to ensure compliance. |

# PROCEDURE 20-1 (continued)

| STEPS | REASONS |
|---|---|
| 5. Obtain and record the medical history and chief complaint. | Documenting the chief complaint supports the physician and creates a legal document for the visit. |
| 6. Take and record the vital signs, height, weight, and visual acuity. | The vital signs and other measurements give the physician an overall picture of the patient's health. |

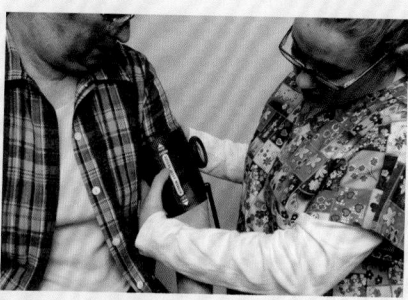

**Step 6.** Taking the patient's vital signs is an important part of the physical exam.

| STEPS | REASONS |
|---|---|
| 7. If the physician requires it, instruct the patient to obtain a urine specimen and escort him or her to the bathroom (refer to Chapter 43 for more information on obtaining a urine specimen). | Even if a urine specimen is not part of the physical examination, an empty bladder makes abdominal and/or pelvic examinations more comfortable. |
| 8. Once inside the examination room, instruct the patient in disrobing including directions on how to put the gown on (open in the front or back). Leave the room unless the patient needs assistance. | The gown must open in the direction that provides accessibility for the examination. Elderly and disabled persons may need help disrobing and putting on the gown. |
| 9. **AFF** Explain how to respond to a patient who has cultural or religious beliefs who may be uncomfortable about disrobing. | Being respectful of the cultural or religious differences by explaining why procedures are needed is important. Provide additional privacy if necessary. |
| 10. Help the patient sit on the edge of the examination table and cover the lap and legs with a drape. | The sitting position is often the first position used by the physician. |

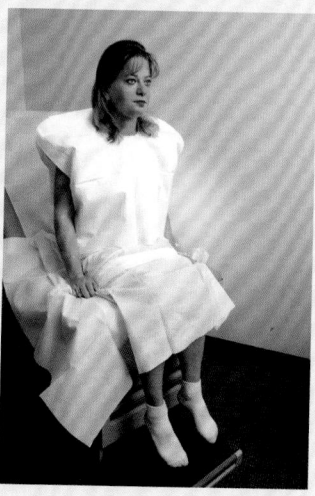

**Step 10.** The patient should be draped appropriately.

*(continues on page 502)*

## PROCEDURE 20-1 (continued)

| STEPS | REASONS |
|---|---|

**11.** **AFF** Place the medical record outside the examination room and notify the physician that the patient is ready. If your office uses an electronic medical record, assure you have entered and updated all information necessary and log off the computer before leaving the room.

Make sure the patient's name on the medical record is facing inward to maintain confidentiality from anyone passing by the room. Alerting the physician helps prevent delays.

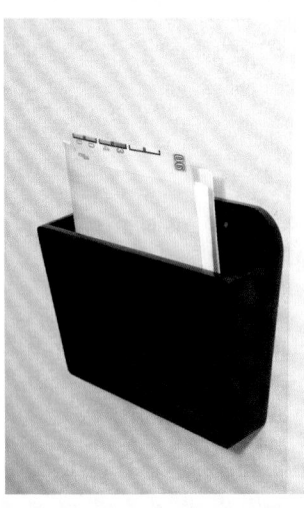

**Step 11.** Place the medical record with identifying information turned away from the hallway.

**12.** Assist the physician by handing him or her the instruments as needed and positioning the patient appropriately.

**A.** Begin by handing the physician the instruments necessary for examining the following:
- Head and neck:    stethoscope
- Eyes:    ophthalmoscope, penlight
- Ears:    otoscope, tuning fork
- Nose:    penlight, nasal speculum
- Sinuses:    penlight
- Mouth:    tongue blade, penlight
Hand the tongue blade to the physician by holding it in the middle. When it is returned to you, grasp it in the middle again so that you do not touch the end that was in the patient's mouth.
- Throat:    glove, tongue blade, laryngeal mirror, penlight

**B.** Help the patient drop the gown to the waist for examination of the chest and upper back. Hand the physician the stethoscope.

**C.** Help the patient pull the gown up and remove the drape from the legs so that the physician can test the reflexes. Hand the physician the percussion hammer.

Anticipating the physician's needs promotes efficiency and saves time. Only the parts of the body being examined should be exposed. Always preserve patients' privacy and keep them covered as much as possible.

## PROCEDURE 20-1 (continued)

| STEPS | REASONS |
|---|---|
| **D.** Help the patient to lie supine, opening the gown at the top to expose the chest again. Place the drape to cover the waist, abdomen, and legs. Hand the physician the stethoscope. | |
| **E.** Cover the patient's chest and lower the drape to expose the abdomen. Hand the physician the stethoscope. | |
| **F.** Assist with the genital and rectal examinations. Hand the patient tissues following these examinations. | Tissues may be used to wipe off excess lubricant. |

For females:
- Assist the patient to the lithotomy position and drape appropriately.
- For examination of the genitalia and internal reproductive organs, provide a glove, lubricant, speculum, microscope slides or liquid prep solution, and Ayres spatula or brush.
- For the rectal examination, provide a glove, lubricant, and fecal occult blood test slide.

For males:
- Help the patient stand and have him bend over the examination table for a rectal and prostate examination.
- For a hernia examination, provide a glove.
- For a rectal examination, provide a glove, lubricant, and fecal occult blood test slide.
- For a prostate examination, provide a glove and lubricant.

**G.** With the patient standing, the physician can assess the legs, gait, coordination, and balance.

| STEPS | REASONS |
|---|---|
| **13.** Help the patient sit at the edge of the examination table. | The physician often discusses findings with the patient at this time and may provide instructions. |
| **14.** Perform any follow-up procedures or treatments. | After the physician examines the patient, there may be additional procedures such as preparing specimens that were obtained. |
| **15.** Leave the room while the patient dresses unless he or she needs assistance. | Leaving the room provides privacy for the patient. |
| **16.** Return to the examination room when the patient has dressed to answer any questions, reinforce physician instructions, and provide patient education. | Compliance depends on full understanding of the treatment plan. Patient education is the responsibility of all health care workers, including the medical assistant. |
| **17.** Escort the patient to the front desk. | You can clarify appointment scheduling or billing issues. |

*(continues on page 504)*

## PROCEDURE 20-1 (continued)

| STEPS | REASONS |
|---|---|
| 18. Properly clean or dispose of all used equipment and supplies. Clean the room with a disinfectant and prepare for the next patient. | All instruments, supplies, and equipment that came into direct contact with the patient must be appropriately decontaminated or disposed of. |
| 19. Wash your hands and record any instructions from the physician. Also note any specimens and indicate the results of the test or the laboratory where the specimens are being sent for testing. | Procedures and instructions are considered not to have been done if they are not recorded. |

Charting Example:
*01/19/2016:30 pm CC: Annual physical exam complete per Dr. Smith. ECG done; results given to Dr. Smith. Blood drawn and sent to Acme lab for CBC, electrolytes, and liver panel. Pt. instructed to return to office in 2 weeks to discuss laboratory results. Pt. given written and verbal instructions for 1,800-calorie, low-sodium diet as ordered. Pt. verbalized understanding* _____ *J. Bohr, CMA*

Note: *The medical assistant may sign his or her name in the patient record using only the "CMA" credential if the office has a signature log denoting the entire credential as "CMA (AAMA)."*

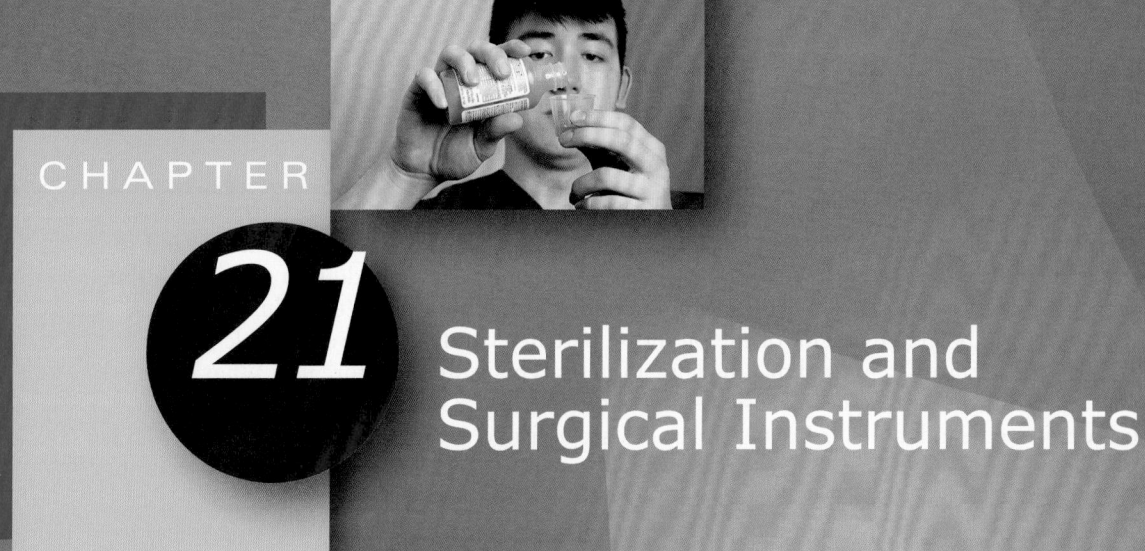

# CHAPTER 21

# Sterilization and Surgical Instruments

## Outline

**Principles and Practices of Surgical Asepsis**
  Sterilization
**Surgical Instruments**
  Forceps

Scissors
Scalpels and Blades
Towel Clamps
Probes and Directors
Retractors

**Care and Handling of Surgical Instruments**
**Storage and Record Keeping**
**Maintaining Surgical Supplies**

## Learning Outcomes

**COG Cognitive Domain***

1. Spell and define the key terms
2. *Define the following as practiced within an ambulatory care setting: surgical asepsis*
3. *Identify quality assurance practices in health care*
4. Describe several methods of sterilization
5. Categorize surgical instruments based on use and identify each by its characteristics
6. Identify surgical instruments specific to designated specialties
7. State the difference between reusable and disposable instruments
8. Explain how to handle and store instruments, equipment, and supplies
9. Describe the necessity and steps for maintaining documents and records of maintenance for instruments and equipment

**PSY Psychomotor Domain***

1. Sanitize equipment and instruments (Procedure 21-1)
2. *Prepare items for autoclaving*
3. Properly wrap instruments for autoclaving (Procedure 21-2)
4. *Perform sterilization procedures*
5. Perform sterilization technique and operate an autoclave (Procedure 21-3).
6. *Perform a quality control measure*

***Note: AAMA/CAAHEP 2015 Standards are italicized.***

**ABHES Competencies**

1. Wrap items for autoclaving.
2. Practice quality control.
3. Use standard precautions.
4. Perform sterilization techniques.

## Key Terms

autoclave
disinfection
ethylene oxide
forceps
hemostat

needle holder
obturator
**Occupational Safety and Health Administration (OSHA)**

ratchet
sanitation
scalpels
scissors
serrations

sound
sterilization

## Case Study

Cindy Tackett, RMA, works in a dermatology office at Great Falls Medical Center and assists the physician with many different types of procedures a day. In addition to assisting the physician, her responsibilities include cleaning nondisposable equipment used during surgical procedures and processing them for use on future patients. Cindy is also responsible for the inventory of sterilized items and making sure all items remain sterile before use. What is the difference, if any, between medical asepsis and surgical asepsis? Once sterilized, are items considered sterile indefinitely? Because microbes are invisible to the naked eye, how does Cindy know items are sterile? This chapter answers these questions and presents various sterilization procedures, including those involving the autoclave. This chapter also covers surgical instruments that may be used in minor office surgical procedures. Although not all medical assistants work in specialties or settings in which surgical procedures are performed, all should have the knowledge and skills necessary to maintain both medical and surgical asepsis.

The goal of surgical asepsis is to free an item or area from all microorganisms, including pathogens and other microorganisms (see Chapter 17). The practice of surgical asepsis, also known as sterile technique, should be used during any office surgical procedure, when handling sterile instruments to be used for incisions and excisions into body tissue, and when changing wound dressings. Surgical asepsis prevents microorganisms from entering the patient's environment; medical asepsis prevents microbes from spreading to or from patients.

In a medical office, your responsibilities may include assisting with minor surgical procedures while maintaining surgical asepsis. To manage this responsibility, you must do the following:

- Become familiar with many types of surgical instruments.
- Understand the principles and practices of surgical asepsis.
- Understand and use **disinfection** and **sterilization** techniques.
- Use equipment designed for sterilization, treatment, and diagnostic purposes.
- Maintain accurate records and inventory of purchases related to surgical equipment and supplies.

The physician expects you to understand sterile technique and to be able to maintain sterility throughout procedures. Any break in sterile technique, no matter how small, can lead to infection the body cannot fight. Even small infections can delay the patient's recovery and are physically, mentally, and financially costly to the patient. Your attention to detail and professional integrity during any surgical aseptic procedure is essential in preventing serious patient complications.

## COG PRINCIPLES AND PRACTICES OF SURGICAL ASEPSIS

As a medical assistant, you are responsible for preventing infection in accordance with the principles and practices of asepsis as it relates to items used during minor office surgical procedures. Surgical asepsis requires the absence of microorganisms, infection, and infectious material on instruments, equipment, and supplies. Disinfection, or medical asepsis, is different from sterilization (Table 21-1). By becoming familiar with the

### TABLE 21-1   Comparison of Medical and Surgical Asepsis

|  | Medical Asepsis | Surgical Asepsis |
|---|---|---|
| Definition | Destroys microorganisms after they leave the body | Destroys microorganisms before they enter the body |
| Purpose | Prevents transmission of microbes from one person to another | Prevents entry of microbes into the body during invasive procedures |
| When used | During contact with a body part that is not normally sterile | During contact with a normally sterile part of the body |
| Differences in hand washing technique | Hands and wrists are washed for 1–2 minutes. | Hands and forearms are washed for 5–10 minutes with a brush. |

manufacturer's recommendations for processing instruments according to the purposes for which the items will be used, you will be able to determine the appropriate level of asepsis.

## Sterilization

While **sanitation** and disinfection are adequate for maintaining medical asepsis in the medical office, these practices are not sufficient to process instruments and equipment used during sterile procedures (see Chapter 17). Objects requiring surgical asepsis must be sanitized first and sterilized by either a physical or chemical process. Procedure 21-1 describes the procedure for sanitizing instruments in preparation for sterilization. Sterilization is the complete elimination or destruction of all forms of microbial life, including spore forms. Steam under pressure, dry heat, ethylene oxide gas, and liquid chemicals are principal sterilizing agents. Although steam under pressure is the most frequently used method of sterilization in the medical office, the method depends on the nature of the material to be sterilized and the type of microorganism to be destroyed. Table 21-2 describes the various methods of sterilization and the temperatures and time of exposure if applicable.

 **CHECKPOINT QUESTION**

1. How would Cindy Tackett explain the difference between sanitization, disinfection, and sterilization to a medical assistant student?

 **LEGAL TIP**

### The Right to Know

**Occupational Safety and Health Administration (OSHA)** and state regulations have defined a specific law to protect you from hazardous materials. The law, The Right to Know, requires that all companies, including medical offices, using hazardous materials have hazard communication safety data sheets (SDS) formerly known as material safety data sheets (MSDS) available to their employees. Safety data sheets (SDS) are prepared by the chemical manufacturer and clearly state how to handle and dispose of the chemical. These forms also include a list of possible health hazards to workers and identify the safety equipment needed for using the chemical. Never handle any type of chemical spill without first reading the safety data sheet. You are required to have a binder available that includes a safety data sheet for all hazardous materials in your office. It may be your responsibility to update the binder and/or add safety data sheets that accompany any supplies or equipment containing hazardous materials. This notebook should be placed in a stationary area where it can be easily consulted in case of an emergency involving hazardous materials.

### Sterilization Equipment

Several types of sterilization equipment are used in clinics and medical offices. As a clinical medical assistant, it is your responsibility to do the following:

- Become familiar with the uses and operation of each piece of equipment.

| TABLE 21-2 Sterilization Methods | |
| --- | --- |
| **Methods** | **Concentration or Level** |
| **Heat** | |
| Moist heat (steam under pressure) | 250°F or 121°C for 30 minutes |
| Boiling | 212°F or 100°C for <30 minutes |
| Dry heat | 340°F or 171°C for 1 hour |
| | 320°F or 160°C for 2 hours |
| **Liquids** | |
| Glutaraldehyde | Follow manufacturer's recommendations or OSHA requirements and guidelines. |
| Formaldehyde | Follow manufacturer's recommendations or OSHA requirements and guidelines. |
| **Gas** | |
| Ethylene oxide | 450–500 mg/L 50°C |

OSHA, Occupational Safety and Health Administration.

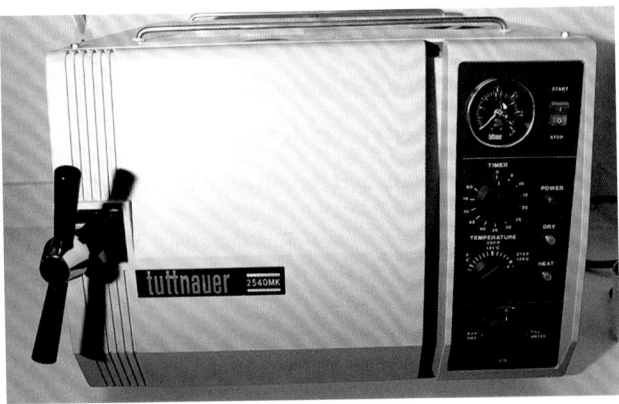
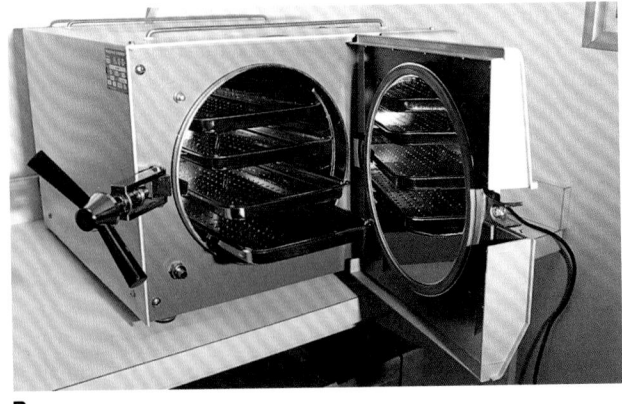

**A**   **B**

Figure 21-1 • **(A)** An autoclave that may be found in the medical office. **(B)** The interior of the autoclave.

- Schedule periodic preventive maintenance or servicing of the equipment.
- Maintain adequate supplies for general operational needs.

## The Autoclave

The most frequently used piece of equipment for sterilizing instruments today is the **autoclave** (Fig. 21-1A, B). The autoclave has two chambers: an outer one where pressure builds and an inner one where the sterilization occurs. Distilled water is added to a reservoir, where it is converted to steam as the preset temperature is reached. The steam is forced into the inner chamber, increasing the pressure and raising the temperature of the steam to 250°F or higher, well above the ordinary boiling temperature of water (212°F or 100°C). The pressure has no effect on sterilization other than to increase the temperature of the steam. The high temperature allows for destruction of all microorganisms, including viruses and spores.

An air exhaust vent on the bottom of the autoclave allows the air in the chamber to be pushed out and replaced by the pressurized steam. When no air is present, the chamber seals and the temperature gauge begins to rise. Most automatic autoclaves can be set to vent, time, turn off, and exhaust at preset times and levels. Older models may require that the steps be advanced manually. All manufacturers provide instructions for operating the machine and recommendations for the times necessary to sterilize different types of loads. These instructions should be posted in a prominent place near the machine.

Sterilization is required for surgical instruments and equipment that will come into contact with internal body tissues or cavities that are considered sterile. The autoclave is commonly used to sterilize minor surgical instruments, surgical storage trays and containers, and some surgical equipment, such as bowls for holding sterile solutions. Instruments or equipment subject to damage by water should not be sterilized in the autoclave. These items can be sterilized with gas. Items that are not subject to water damage but may be destroyed by heat can be cold-sterilized or soaked for a prescribed amount of time in a liquid such as glutaraldehyde or formaldehyde. Always follow the manufacturer's recommendations for sterilizing instruments or equipment and for using any chemical products for sterilization. Procedure 21-2 describes preparation of instruments for sterilization in the autoclave.

## CHECKPOINT QUESTION

2. Why is the properly working autoclave more effective at sterilizing equipment compared to boiling water?

### Sterilization Indicators

Tape applied to the outside of the material used to wrap instruments or supplies for the autoclave indicates that the items have been exposed to steam, but *the tape cannot ensure the sterility of the contents* (Box 21-1). This special tape (Fig. 21-2) is used to close and label the contents of wrapped packages before placing items in the autoclave. The stripes on the tape become dark upon exposure to steam and allow you to easily determine whether or not a pack has been placed in the autoclave.

---

**BOX 21-1   Autoclave Indicator Tape**

Autoclave tape is designed to change color in the presence of heat and steam. In extreme instances, the tape may change appearance when stored too close to heat sources. Most tapes have imprinted lines that darken after exposure, but *sterilization of the package contents is not ensured by a color change on the autoclave tape.* Proper sterilization can be assumed only if accompanying sterilization indicators have registered that all elements of the sterilization process (time and temperature) have been achieved.

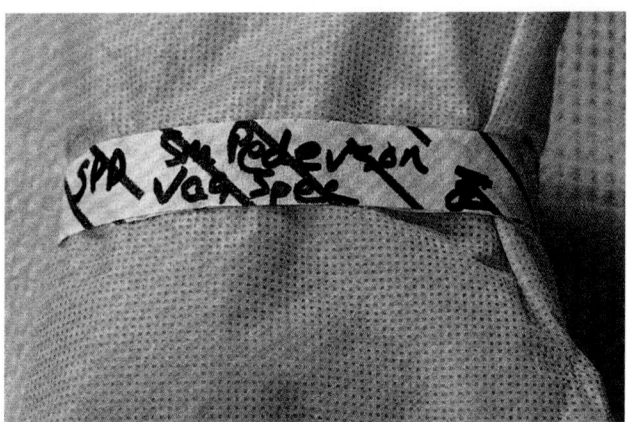

**Figure 21-2** • The stripes on autoclave tape change color, indicating that the pack has been exposed to steam.

Because microorganisms are not visible to the naked eye, sterilization indicators must be placed inside each pack that are designed to register that the proper pressure, temperature, and time were attained in the autoclave to assure destruction of all microbial life (Fig. 21-3). Improper wrapping, loading, or operation of the auto clave may prevent the indicator from registering properly, and the sterility of the contents cannot be assured. Various types of sterilization indicators are available, including those that change colors at high temperatures and those that contain wax pellets, which indicate that the required temperature was reached evidenced by the melted wax. Although most types of sterilization indicators work well, the best method for determining effectiveness of sterilization is the culture test. Strips impregnated with heat-resistant spores are wrapped and placed in the center of the autoclave between the packages in a designated load, such as the first load of the day. The strips are removed from their packets and placed in a broth culture to be incubated according to the instructions of the manufacturer. At the end of the incubation period, the culture is compared to a control to determine that all spores have been killed. If sterilization

was not achieved, the load must be reprocessed before the items put through the sterilization process can be used in surgical procedures.

## CHECKPOINT QUESTION

3. Cindy's responsibilities in the dermatology office include making sure surgical instruments are sterilized and ready for the physician to use. What is the difference between a sterilization indicator and autoclave tape?

### Loading the Autoclave

Improper loading of the autoclave will prevent steam from penetrating the items inside the packs completely, compromising the sterility of the contents. Load the autoclave loosely to allow steam to circulate. Place empty wrapped containers or bowls on their sides with the lids wrapped separately. If containers are upright in the autoclave, air, which is heavier than steam, will settle into the interior of the container and keep steam from circulating to the inner surfaces. Place all packs on their sides to allow for the maximum steam circulation and penetration (Fig. 21-4).

### Operating the Autoclave

All components of autoclaving—temperature, pressure, steam, and time—must be correct for the items to reach sterility. Follow the instruction manual carefully. All machines use the same principles, but operation varies. Become familiar with the function of the machine in your facility. Instructions may be covered in plastic or laminated and posted beside the machine for easy reference.

The autoclave has a reservoir tank that should be filled with distilled water only. Tap water contains chemicals and minerals that would coat the interior chamber, clog the exhaust valves, and hinder the overall operation of the autoclave. When filling the internal chamber of the autoclave with distilled water from the reservoir,

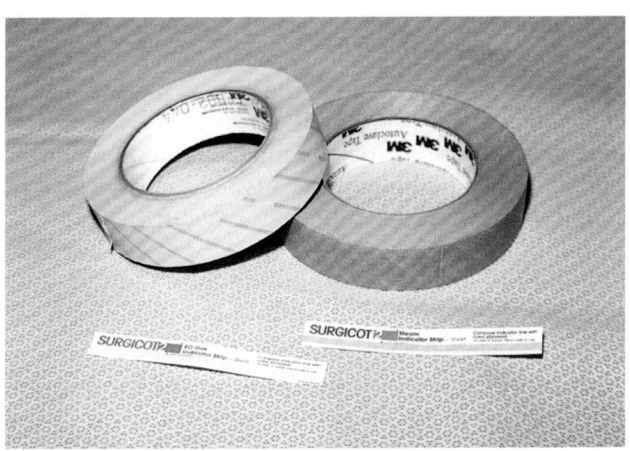

**Figure 21-3** • Autoclave tape (*top*: steam and gas tape) and sterilization indicators (*bottom left and right*).

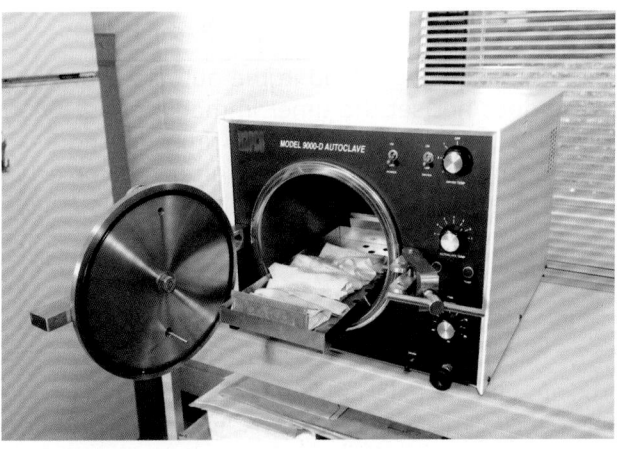

**Figure 21-4** • Properly loaded autoclave.

be sure the water level is at the fill line. If too much water is added to the chamber, the steam will be saturated and may not be efficient, and too little water will not produce the required amount of steam. Procedure 21-3 outlines the general steps for operating an autoclave.

The temperature, pressure, and time required vary with the items being sterilized. In most cases, 250°F at 15 pounds of pressure for 20 to 30 minutes will be sufficient, but you should follow the manufacturer's instructions for the load content. Solid or metal loads take slightly less time than soft, bulky loads. The timer should not be set until the proper temperature has been attained. Some microorganisms, such as spores, are killed only if exposed to high enough temperature for a specific amount of time.

When the items have been in the autoclave at the right temperature for enough time, the timer will sound, indicating that the cycle is finished. Be sure to vent the autoclave to allow the pressure to drop safely. After the pressure has dropped to a safe level, open the door of the autoclave slightly to allow the temperature to drop and the load to cool and dry. Newer autoclaves vent automatically. Do not handle or remove items from the autoclave until they are dry because bacteria from your hands would be drawn through the moist coverings and contaminate the items inside the wrapping. Once the items are dry, remove the packages and store them in a clean, dry, dust-free area. Packs that are sterilized on site in the autoclave are considered sterile for 30 days and must be sterilized again after this period. Always store recently autoclaved items toward the back of the cabinet, rotating the previously autoclaved items to the front. In addition, you are responsible for performing maintenance on the autoclave at regular intervals. Post a schedule for this maintenance near the machine; allow for cleaning the lint trap, washing out the interior of the chamber with a cloth or soft brush, and checking the function of all components. This schedule can remind and document the service with space for initialing or signing after the maintenance has been done.

### CHECKPOINT QUESTION

4. Cindy is running a load in the autoclave but she does not set the timer immediately.
   Why is it important to set the timer on the autoclave during a cycle only after the correct temperature has been reached?

## ⚙ SURGICAL INSTRUMENTS

You must be able to identify surgical instruments according to their design and function. A surgical instrument is a tool or device designed to perform a specific function,

such as cutting, dissecting, grasping, holding, retracting, or suturing. Surgical instruments are designed to perform specific tasks based on their shape; they may be curved, straight, sharp, blunt, serrated, toothed, or smooth. Many are made of stainless steel and are reusable; others are disposable. It is your responsibility to know the proper use and care of the surgical instruments in your clinical setting.

Most instruments used in office procedures can be identified by carefully examining the instrument. The most widely used surgical instruments are **forceps**, **scissors**, **scalpels**, and clamps. Table 21-3 shows the most commonly used instruments and equipment by specialty.

### Forceps

Forceps are surgical instruments used to grasp, handle, compress, pull, or join tissue, equipment, or supplies. The types of forceps include the following:

- **Hemostat**: A surgical instrument with slender jaws used for grasping blood vessels and establishing hemostasis.
- **Kelly clamp**: A curved or straight forceps or hemostat; those with long handles are widely used in gynecologic procedures.
- **Sterilizer forceps**: Used to transfer sterile supplies, equipment, and other surgical instruments to a sterile field. May also be called sterile transfer forceps.
- **Needle holder**: Used to hold and pass a needle through tissue during suturing.
- **Spring or thumb forceps**: Used for grasping tissue for dissection or suturing, such as tissue forceps and splinter forceps.

A variety of forceps can be seen in Figure 21-5A–Q. All forceps are available in many sizes, with or without **serrations** or teeth, with curved or straight blades, and with ring tips, blunt tips, or sharp tips. Many have **ratchets** in the handles to hold the tips tightly together; these are notched mechanisms that click into position to maintain tension. Some have spring handles that are compressed between the thumb and index finger to grasp objects.

Physicians use a variety of forceps. You should study the names and purposes of each type to assist the physician when a specific instrument is requested.

### CHECKPOINT QUESTION

5. The physician Cindy works with in the dermatology office uses a variety of surgical instruments. What are the most common instruments used in a medical office including dermatology?

## TABLE 21-3    Commonly Used Instruments and Equipment by Specialty

|  | Instrument | Use |
|---|---|---|
| **Obstetrics, Gynecology** | Vaginal speculum | Open vagina to view vaginal walls, cervical os; perform procedures; sized; may be reusable metal or disposable plastic |
|  | Tenaculum | Grasping and holding tissue with hooklike tips |
|  | Uterine sound | Assess depth of uterus; graduated in inches or centimeters |
|  | Uterine dilator | Widens cervical os; usually 3–18 mm |
|  | Curet | Blunt or sharp; for scraping endometrium |
|  | Biopsy forceps | Secure pieces of tissue for microscopic study |

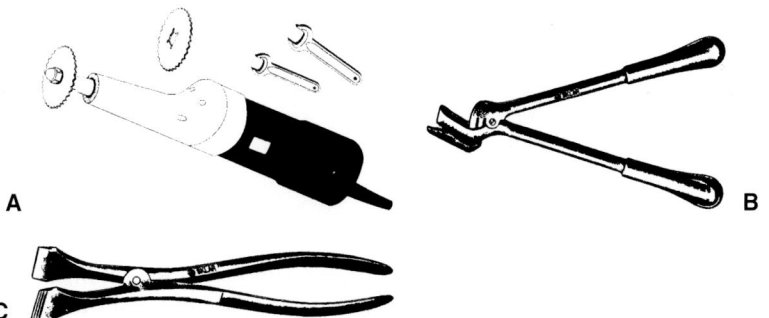

*Gynecology instruments:* **(A)** Graves vaginal speculum. **(B)** Pederson vaginal speculum. **(C)** Duplay tenaculum forceps. **(D)** Schroeder tenaculum forceps. **(E)** Sims uterine sound. **(F)** Simpson uterine sound, malleable. **(G)** Hand uterine dilator. **(H)** Hegar uterine dilator. **(I)** Thomas uterine curets. **(J)** Sims uterine curets

| **Orthopedics** | Cast saw | Remove cast |
|---|---|---|
|  | Cutters or spreaders | Cutters are scissor-like instruments used to cut casting material; spreaders are used to separate the edges of a cast that has been cut. |

*Orthopedic instruments:* **(A)** Oscillating plaster saw. **(B)** Stille plaster shears. **(C)** Henning plaster spreader

(*continued*)

**TABLE 21-3    Commonly Used Instruments and Equipment by Specialty (continued)**

| | Instrument | Use |
|---|---|---|
| **Urology** | Urethral sounds | Explore bladder depth and direction; dilate urethral meatus in stenosis; sized Fr 8–26 |
| | Prostate biopsy | Removes tissue for microscopic study |

*Urology instruments*: **(A)** Otis-Dittel urethral sound. **(B)** Dittel urethral sound

| | Instrument | Use |
|---|---|---|
| **Proctology** | Anoscopes, proctoscopes | Visualize lower intestinal tract. Most have **obturator** for ease of insertion. |
| | Sigmoidoscope | Visualize lower sigmoid colon. Rigid or flexible, with fiberoptic light. Some have suction device. |
| | Punch biopsy | Remove small piece of tissue via small circular hole |
| | Alligator biopsy | Jaws grasp and excise tissue |

*Proctology instruments*: **(A)** Ives rectal speculum (Fansler). **(B)** Pratt rectal speculum. **(C)** Hirschman anoscope

| | Instrument | Use |
|---|---|---|
| **Otology, Rhinology** | Nasal or ear forceps | Insert or remove materials from nose or ear canal |
| | Nasal speculum | Opens, extends nostrils for visualization of nasal passages |
| | Curet | Remove cerumen from deep ear canal |

*Otology and rhinology instruments*: **(A)** Wilde ear forceps. **(B)** Lucae bayonet forceps. **(C)** Buck ear curet. **(D)** Vienna nasal speculum

**TABLE 21-3  Commonly Used Instruments and Equipment by Specialty (continued)**

| | Instrument | Use |
|---|---|---|
| **Ophthalmology** | Eye loop, lid retractor | Hold eyelids open for removal of foreign bodies |
| | Tonometer | Measure intraocular pressure to diagnose glaucoma |

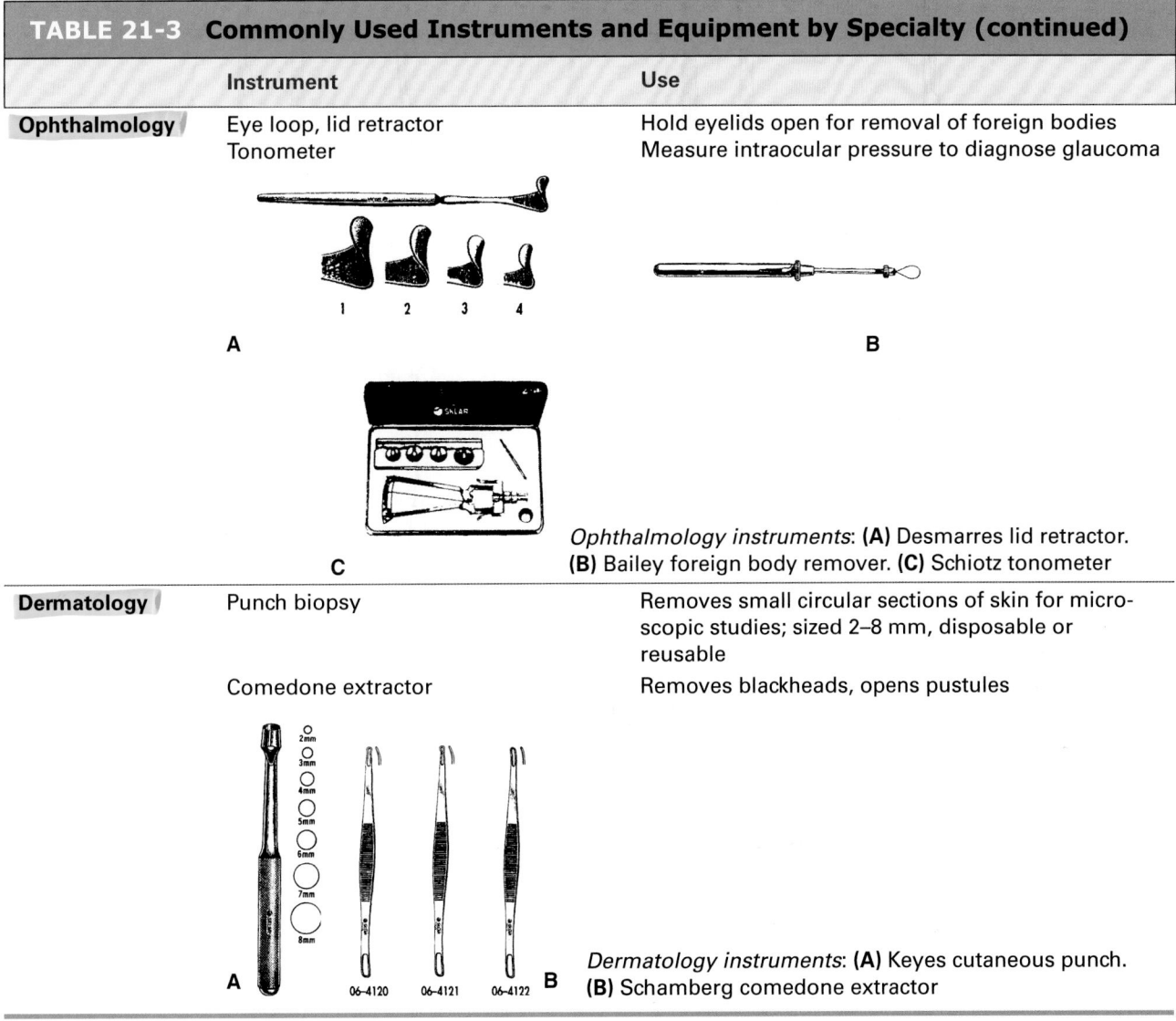

*Ophthalmology instruments*: **(A)** Desmarres lid retractor. **(B)** Bailey foreign body remover. **(C)** Schiotz tonometer

| | Instrument | Use |
|---|---|---|
| **Dermatology** | Punch biopsy | Removes small circular sections of skin for microscopic studies; sized 2–8 mm, disposable or reusable |
| | Comedone extractor | Removes blackheads, opens pustules |

*Dermatology instruments*: **(A)** Keyes cutaneous punch. **(B)** Schamberg comedone extractor

## Scissors

Scissors are sharp instruments composed of two opposing cutting blades held together by a central pin at the pivot. Scissors are used for dissecting superficial, deep, or delicate tissues and for cutting sutures and bandages. Scissors have blade points that are blunt, sharp, or both, depending on the use of the instrument. The types of scissors include the following:

- Straight scissors cut deep or delicate tissue and sutures.
- Curved scissors dissect superficial and delicate tissues.
- Suture scissors cut sutures; they have straight top blades and curved-out, or hooked, blunt bottom blades to fit under, lift, and grasp sutures for snipping.

- Bandage scissors remove bandages; this type has a flattened blunt tip on the bottom longer blade that safely fits under bandages; most common type is the Lister bandage scissors.

Figure 21-6A–C shows various types of scissors.

## Scalpels and Blades

A scalpel is a small surgical knife with a straight handle and a straight or curved blade. A reusable steel scalpel handle can hold different blades for different surgical procedures. Straight or pointed blades are used for incision and drainage procedures, while curved blades are used to excise tissue. Reusable handles are used only with disposable blades. Many offices use disposable handles and blades packaged as one sterile unit. Figure 21-7A–C shows various scalpels and blades.

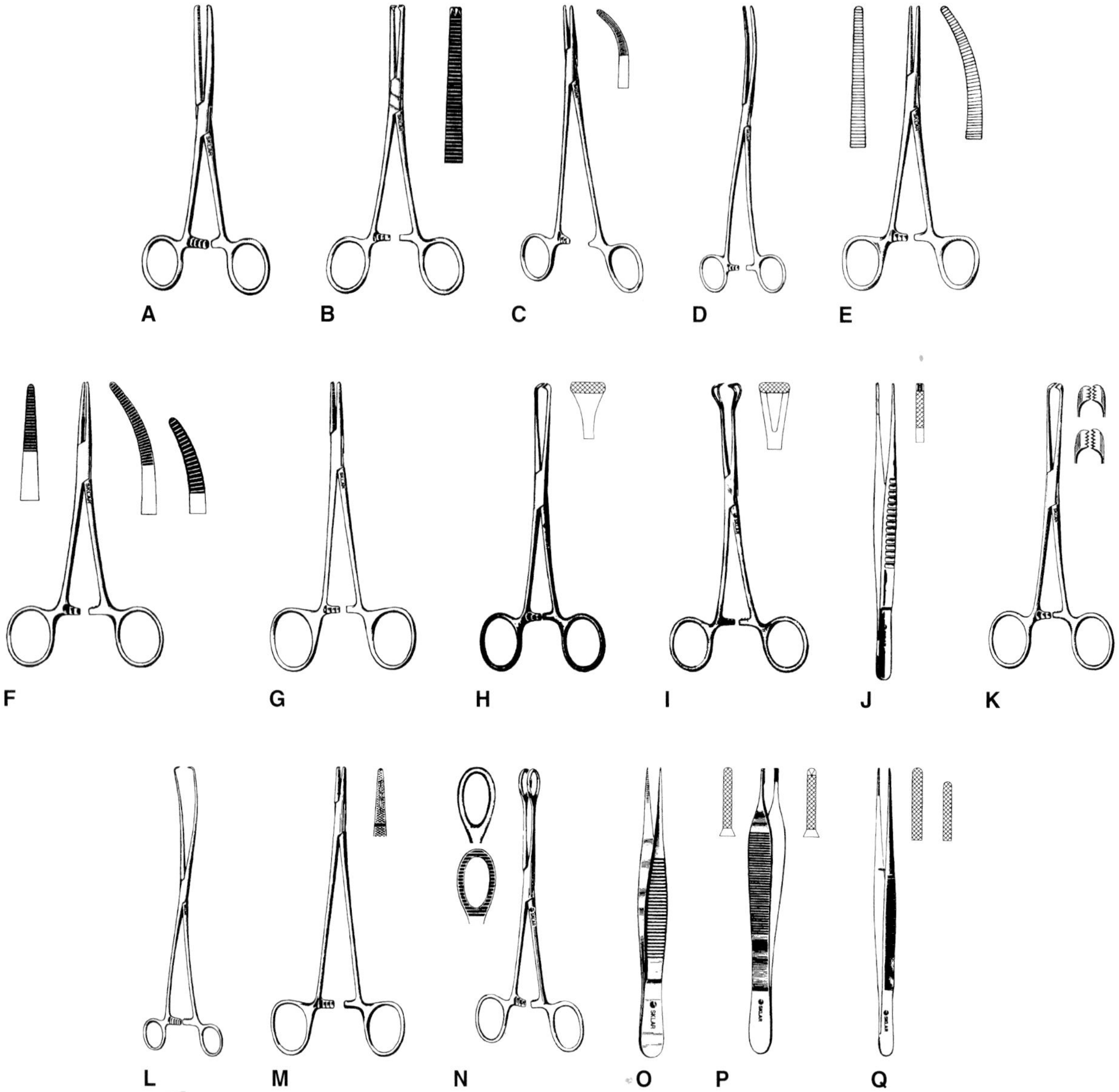

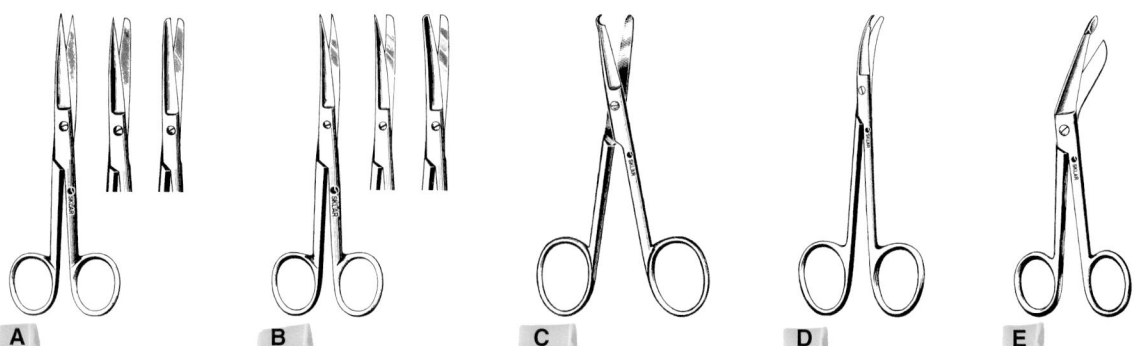

**Figure 21-5** • Forceps: **(A)** Rochester-Pean forceps. **(B)** Rochester-Ochsner forceps. **(C)** Adson forceps. **(D)** Bozeman forceps. **(E)** Crile hemostat. **(F)** Kelly hemostat. **(G)** Halsted mosquito hemostat. **(H)** Allis forceps. **(I)** Babcock forceps. **(J)** DeBakey forceps. **(K)** Allis tissue forceps. **(L)** Duplay tenaculum forceps. **(M)** Crile-Wood needle holder. **(N)** Ballenger sponge forceps. **(O)** Fine-point splinter forceps. **(P)** Adson dressing forceps. **(Q)** Potts-Smith dressing forceps. (Courtesy of Sklar Instruments, West Chester, PA.)

**Figure 21-6** • Scissors: **(A)** Straight blade operating scissors. *Left to right:* S/S, S/B, B/B. **(B)** Curved blade operating scissors. *Left to right:* S/S, S/B, B/B. **(C)** Spencer stitch scissors. **(D)** Suture scissors. **(E)** Lister bandage scissors. S/S, sharp/sharp; S/B, sharp/blunt; B/B, blunt/blunt. (Courtesy of Sklar Instruments, West Chester, PA.)

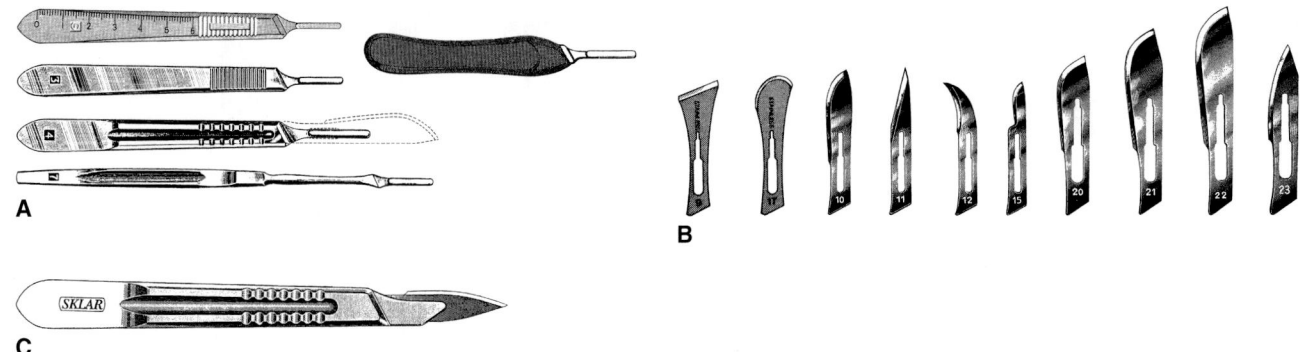

**Figure 21-7 •** Scalpels: **(A)** Scalpel handles. **(B)** Surgical blades. **(C)** Complete sterile disposable scalpel. (Courtesy of Sklar Instruments, West Chester, PA.)

## Towel Clamps

Towel clamps are used to maintain the integrity of the sterile field by holding the sterile drapes in place, allowing exposure of the operative site (Fig. 21-8A, B). A sterile field is a specific area that is considered free of all microorganisms.

## Probes and Directors

Before entering a cavity or site for a procedure, the physician may first probe the depth and direction of the operative area. A probe shows the angle and depth of the operative area, and a director guides the knife or instrument once the procedure has begun (Fig. 21-9A–C).

## Retractors

Retractors hold open layers of tissue, exposing the areas beneath. They may be plain or toothed; the toothed retractor may be sharp or blunt. Retractors may be designed to be held by an assistant or screwed open to be self-retaining. Figure 21-10A–C shows several types of retractors.

### CHECKPOINT QUESTION

6. What types of instruments are used to remove tissue during a biopsy?

## CARE AND HANDLING OF SURGICAL INSTRUMENTS

To ensure that surgical instruments always function properly, follow these guidelines:

1. Do not toss or drop instruments into a basin or sink. Surgical instruments are delicate, and the blade or tip is easily damaged by improper handling. Should you drop an instrument accidentally, carefully inspect it for damage. Damaged instruments can usually be repaired and should not be discarded unless repair is not feasible.
2. Avoid stacking instruments in a pile. They may tangle and be damaged when separated.

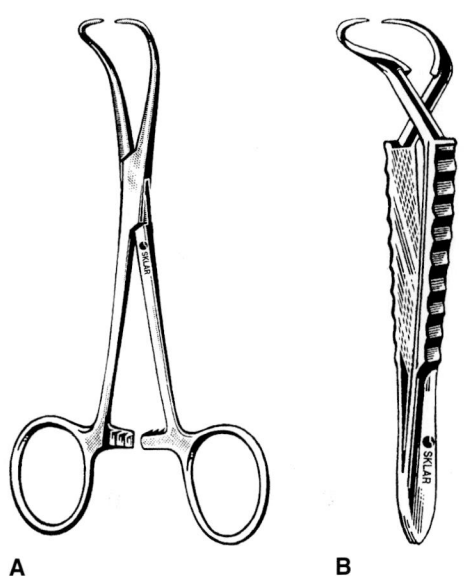

**Figure 21-8 •** Towel clamps: **(A)** Backhaus towel clamp. **(B)** Jones cross-action towel clamp. (Courtesy of Sklar Instruments, West Chester, PA.)

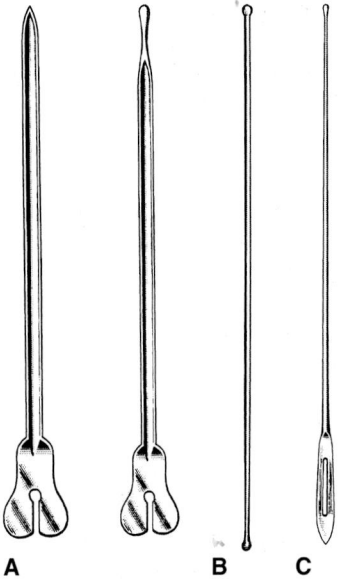

**Figure 21-9 •** Probes: **(A)** Director and tongue tie. **(B)** Double-ended probe. **(C)** Probe with eye. (Courtesy of Sklar Instruments, West Chester, PA.)

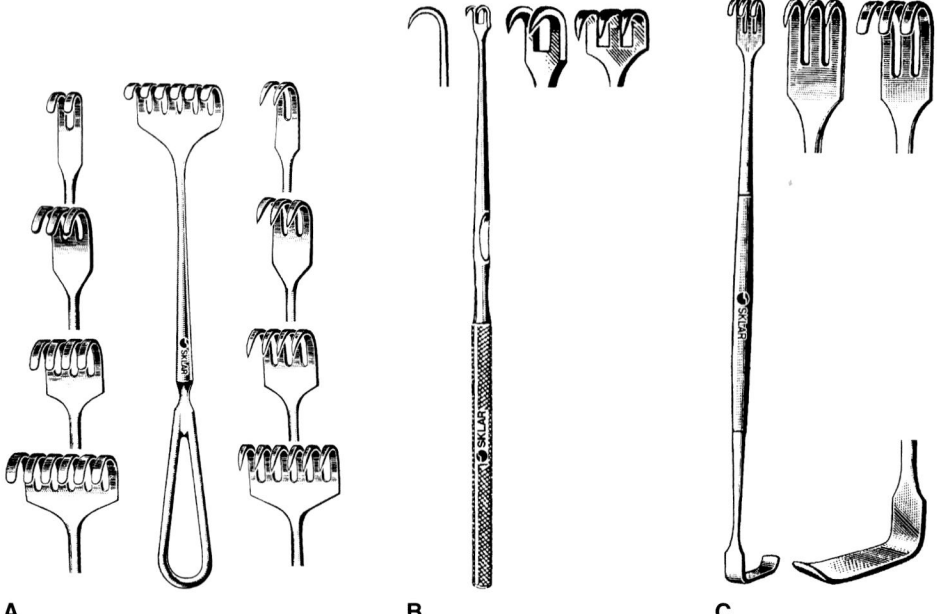

**Figure 21-10 •** Retractors: **(A)** Volkman retractor. **(B)** Lahey retractor. **(C)** Senn retractor. (Courtesy of Sklar Instruments, West Chester, PA.)

3. Always store sharp instruments separately to prevent dulling or damaging the sharp edges and to prevent accidental injury. Disposable scalpel blades should be removed from reusable handles and placed in puncture-proof sharps biohazard containers. If a disposable scalpel is used, the whole unit is discarded into the sharps container. Syringes with needles attached and suture needles should also be discarded in a sharps container and never in the trash or with other instruments for processing. Delicate instruments, such as scissors or tissue forceps or those with lenses, are kept separate to be sanitized and sterilized appropriately.

4. Keep ratcheted instruments open when not in use to avoid damage to the ratchet mechanism.

5. Rinse gross contamination from instruments as soon as possible to prevent drying and hardening, which makes cleaning more difficult. Always wear gloves and follow OSHA standards to prevent contact with possibly infected blood or body fluids.

6. Check instruments before sterilization to ensure that they are in good working order, and identify instruments in need of repair.
   A. Blades or points should be free of bends and nicks.
   B. Tips should close evenly and tightly.
   C. Instruments with box locks should move freely but should not be too loose.
   D. Instruments with spring handles should have enough tension to grasp objects tightly.
   E. Scissors should close in a smooth, even manner with no nicks or snags. (Scissors may be checked by cutting through gauze or cotton to be sure there are no rough areas).
   F. Screws should be flushed with the instrument surface. They should be freely workable but not loose.

7. Use instruments only for the purpose for which they were designed. For instance, never use surgical scissors to cut paper or open packages, because this may damage the cutting edges.

8. Sanitize instruments before they are sterilized so that sterilization will work effectively.

## CHECKPOINT QUESTION

7. While assisting the physician during a minor office surgical procedure, Cindy drops a hemostat on the exam table. What should you do if you drop a surgical instrument accidentally?

## STORAGE AND RECORD KEEPING

When using and maintaining sterile instruments, equipment, and supplies, staff are responsible for correctly storing these items, keeping accurate records of warranties and maintenance agreements, and keeping reordering information on hand. You should be familiar with the manufacturer's recommendations for each instrument or piece of equipment. Most offices have specific storage or supply areas for keeping sterile and other instruments and equipment. This area should be kept clean and dust-free and should be close to the area of need. Clean and sterile supplies and equipment must be separated from soiled items and waste.

Medical assistants are also responsible for keeping accurate records of sterilized items and equipment. Information that must be recorded includes maintenance records and load or sterilization records. These records should include the following:

- Date and time of the sterilization cycle
- General description of the load
- Exposure time and temperature
- Name or initials of the operator
- Results of the sterilization indicator
- Expiration date of the load (usually 30 days)

The maintenance records include service provided by the manufacturer's representative and daily or recommended maintenance to keep the equipment in optimum working condition.

### CHECKPOINT QUESTION

8. When updating a sterilization record, what six items should Cindy include on the document?

## MAINTAINING SURGICAL SUPPLIES

As a clinical medical assistant, you should keep an up-to-date master list of all supplies, including purchases and replacements. Generally, one person is responsible for maintaining inventory, keeping maintenance schedules, and placing orders. If too many staff are involved, these tasks may be overlooked, or efforts may be duplicated. Instruction manuals for all equipment should be kept on file and consulted when ordering supplies for replacement or maintenance. Equipment records for each item should include the following:

- Date of purchase
- Model and serial numbers of the equipment
- Time of recommended service
- Date service was requested
- Name of the person requesting the service
- Reason for the service request
- Description of the service performed and any parts replaced
- Name of the person performing the service and the date the work was completed
- Signature and title of the person who acknowledged completion of the work

Warranties and guarantees should be kept with the equipment records, along with the name of the manufacturer's contact person. A file should be kept to remind the staff of the need for manufacturer service and concurrent or periodic maintenance by the staff.

Parts and supplies for items that are vital to the operation of the facility should always be kept on hand. The shelf life of the item, the storage space available, and the time required to order and receive an item should be considered when deciding what items to keep in inventory. If a piece of equipment cannot function without all of its components or if some of those components have a short

life, replacements must be readily available. For example, an ophthalmoscope without a light is virtually useless.

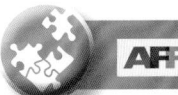

### AFF TRIAGE

While you are working in a medical office, the following three situations arise:

A. You need to wrap instruments for the autoclave that were sanitized earlier in the day.
B. A 45-year-old woman who just had a mole removed needs postoperative instructions before discharge, and the treatment room where the procedure was done is in need of cleaning for the next patient.
C. A load in the autoclave that ran earlier is finished. The sterilized packs have to be put away.

**How do you sort these tasks? What do you do first? Second? Third?**

The patient in situation B should be taken care of first. You should take time to explain any postoperative instructions and follow-up care clearly as indicated by the physician. Once the patient is discharged, the treatment room should be cleaned, and any used surgical equipment should be discarded appropriately or prepared for sanitation according to appropriate standard precautions. The next task includes wrapping the sanitized instruments in preparation for the autoclave. After unloading the autoclave and putting the sterilized packs away, the clean wrapped instruments can be placed in the autoclave for sterilization.

### WHAT IF?

**Your medical office has one designated room for minor office surgical procedures, and two physicians in your office have scheduled minor office procedures for the same day and time. What should you do?**

It is your responsibility to anticipate what the physician needs and address any concerns immediately. Upon discovering that two patients are scheduled for procedures on the same day and time, you should advise both physicians of the situation immediately. In some cases, the patient may have been told not to eat or drink anything (NPO, or nil per os, which is Latin for "nothing by mouth") on the morning of the procedure, and if this is the case and it is agreeable with both physicians, it would be most appropriate to schedule the patient who is NPO earliest in the day. Once the physicians determine who should use the room first, you should then call the patient who will need to be scheduled at a later time, using this opportunity to remind them of any preoperative orders if necessary. Always allow plenty of time between procedures for disinfecting the room, restocking the room with equipment and supplies, and sanitizing and sterilizing any equipment that was used and may be needed for the following procedure.

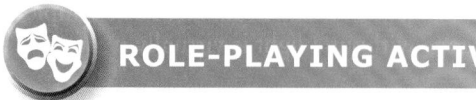

## ROLE-PLAYING ACTIVITY

A professional medical assistant must often communicate "bad" news to the physician and/or practice manager. For example, Cindy Tackett, the medical assistant referred to in the case study at the beginning of this chapter, is responsible for inspecting equipment such as surgical instruments for good working order during the sanitizing and sterilization process. Items that are broken must be repaired or replaced and this can be costly! Not only is surgical equipment expensive to fix or replace, but if there is only one item for use in the office, this could mean patient procedures have to be cancelled and rescheduled.

Role-playing as Cindy, communicate information about a broken surgical instrument professionally to another student who is acting as the physician. The student playing the role of the physician should keep in mind the cost to replace or repair the item while also acknowledging the effect on patient care in the office. Switch roles, perhaps taking on different personalities that are unique to different physicians and employees including medical assistants.

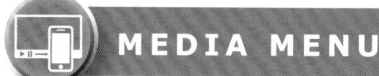

## MEDIA MENU

**Student Resources** on thePoint®

• **CMA/RMA Certification Exam Review**

**Internet Resources**
Medical Resources New and Reconditioned Equipment: Midmark and Ritter Autoclaves
http://www.medicalresources.com

**Amsco Autoclaves and Sterilizers: Alfa Medical**
http://www.sterilizers.com

**Sklar Surgical Instruments**
http://www.sklarcorp.com

**Glutaraldehyde Guidelines for Safe Use and Handling in Health Care Facilities**
http://www.nj.gov/health/surv/documents/glutar.pdf

**Occupational Safety and Health Administration**
http://www.osha.gov

## español SPANISH TERMINOLOGY

**Por favor no toque esta bandeja.**
Please do not touch this tray.

**El doctor estará con usted pronto.**
The doctor will be in shortly.

**¿Tiene usted alguna pregunta?**
Do you have any questions?

**Voy a quitarle el vendaje en estos momentos.**
I will take off the bandage now.

**¿Está cómodo/cómoda?**
Are you comfortable?

**Usted necesita un procedimiento quirúrgico menor.**
You need a minor surgical procedure.

**Su procedimiento será sencillo con anestesia local.**
Your procedure will be simple with local anesthesia.

## EMR Activity

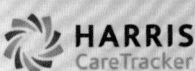

Harris CareTracker is a Web-based electronic medical record (EMR) application that you will use for the EMR activities included in this section at the end of each chapter. This application is actually used in physician offices but is provided to you through the publisher, Wolters Kluwer Health, to give you hands-on practice working with EMRs. Your instructor will have more information about accessing your username, log-in, and Quickstart guide.

Prerequisite Activities in Harris CareTracker

• *The Getting Started and Quickstart documents and EMR Activities Step-by-Step Instructions are available at* http://thePoint.lww.com/KronenbergerComp5e.

Activity Details

Equipment necessary for scheduled procedures in the office must be available and ready for use at the time of the patient's scheduled procedure appointment. Medical assistants are responsible for making sure the equipment is in working order and sterilized before the appointment and must have a system in place to ensure there are no unnecessary delays because the medical equipment is not ready.

In the *Custom Resources* section under the *Setup* tab in the *Administration* module of the EMR, indicate that the equipment necessary for Dr. Jim Schroeder's scheduled balloon sinuplasty is now sterilized and available.

## Chapter Summary

- Most areas of the medical office require medical asepsis to maintain cleanliness and prevent the spread of infection to the patients and staff.
- When body tissues need repair or must be opened surgically, sterile technique or surgical asepsis is required.
- You are responsible for maintaining surgical asepsis, which necessitates that you understand the principles and practices of medical and surgical asepsis.
- You will need to know disinfection and sterilization techniques commonly used in the medical office including the equipment used to sterilize and disinfect items.
- It will be your responsibility to keep accurate records and adequate supplies on hand.
- In addition, your responsibilities include being familiar with instruments used in office surgical procedures, which is the content of the next chapter.

## Warm-Ups for Critical Thinking

1. As the clinical medical assistant at Dr. Will's office, you have been asked to orient new employees to various aspects of the practice and develop an orientation booklet for all staff members. Design a booklet that contains the following information:
   - A basic explanation of the surgical equipment commonly used in the practice
   - The procedures for sanitizing, disinfecting, and sterilizing instruments
   - The operating instructions for the autoclave
   - Create a record that can be used to document sterilization using the autoclave.
2. Research the various types of commercial cold chemical sterilization solutions. Design a step-by-step procedure for using the solution to disinfect and sterilize. Note any hazards or safety precautions that should be followed when working with the chemical.
3. The physician is scheduled to perform a minor office surgical procedure this afternoon, and you realize the instrument she needs for the procedure is broken. How would you handle this situation? What can you do to prevent this situation in the future?
4. When checking the biological sterilization indicator as required to be done weekly by your office policy, you discover that the autoclave has not been reaching the appropriate temperature sufficient to kill all microorganisms and their spores. The logbook indicated that the check last week found the autoclave to be in good working order. Can you be sure that all items autoclaved this past week are sterilized? What would you do?

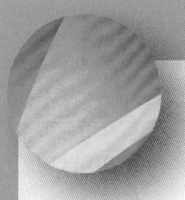

## PSY PROCEDURE 21-1

## Sanitizing Equipment for Disinfection or Sterilization

**PSY** Prepare items for autoclaving.

**Purpose:** Properly sanitize instruments in preparation for disinfection or sterilization

**Equipment:** Instruments or equipment to be sanitized, gloves, eye protection, impervious gown, soap and water, and small handheld scrub brush

| STEPS | REASONS |
|---|---|
| 1. Put on gloves, gown, and eye protection. | These devices protect against splattering and prevent contamination of your clothes. |

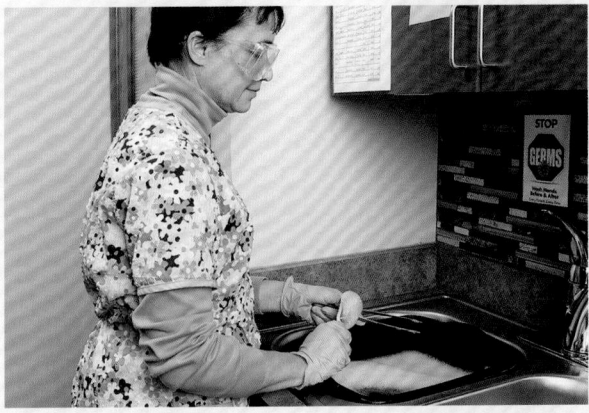

**Step 1.** Always wear personal protective equipment when a splash may occur.

2. Take any removable sections apart. If cleaning is not possible immediately, soak the instrument or equipment to prevent the parts from sticking together.

3. Check for operation and integrity of the equipment. Defective equipment should be repaired or discarded appropriately according to office policy.

4. Rinse the instrument with cool water.    Hot water cooks proteins on, making the contaminants more difficult to remove.

5. After the initial rinse, force streams of soapy water through any tubular or grooved instruments to clean the inside as well as the outside.

6. Use a hot, soapy solution to dissolve fats or lubricants on the surface. Use the soaking solution indicated by office policy.

*(continues on page 522)*

## PROCEDURE 21-1 (continued)

| STEPS | REASONS |
|---|---|
| **7.** After soaking for 5–10 minutes, use friction with a soft brush or gauze to wipe down the instrument and loosen transient microorganisms. Abrasive materials should not be used on delicate instruments and equipment. Brushes work well on grooves and joints. Open and close the jaws of scissors or forceps several times to ensure that all material has been removed. | These devices protect against splattering and prevent contamination of your clothes. |

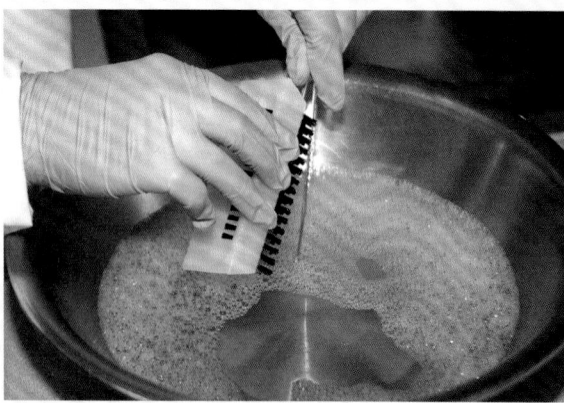

**Step 7.** Use a brush to loosen microorganisms on instruments.

| STEPS | REASONS |
|---|---|
| **8.** Rinse well. | Proper rinsing removes soap or detergent residue and any remaining microorganisms. |
| **9.** Dry well before autoclaving or soaking in disinfectant. | Excess moisture decreases the effectiveness of the autoclave by delaying drying, and it dilutes the disinfectant. |
| **10.** Any items (brushes, gauze, solution) used in sanitation are considered grossly contaminated and must be properly disinfected or discarded. | |

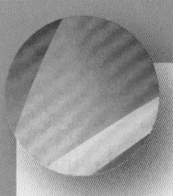

**PSY  PROCEDURE 21-2**

# Wrapping Instruments for Sterilization in an Autoclave

**PSY**  Prepare items for autoclaving; perform a quality control measure.

**Purpose:** Properly prepare and wrap instruments for sterilization in the autoclave

**Equipment:** Instruments or equipment to be sterilized, wrapping material, autoclave tape, sterilization indicator, and black or blue ink pen

| STEPS | REASONS |
|---|---|
| 1. Assemble the equipment and supplies. Check the instruments being wrapped for working order. | Any instruments found to be defective, broken, or otherwise needing repair should not be wrapped or autoclaved. |
| 2. Be sure that the wrapping material has these properties:<br>• Permeable to steam but not contaminants<br>• Resists tearing and puncturing during normal handling<br>• Allows for easy opening to prevent contamination of the contents<br>• Maintains sterility of the contents during storage | The wrap may be double layers of cotton muslin, special paper, or appropriately sized instrument pouches. |

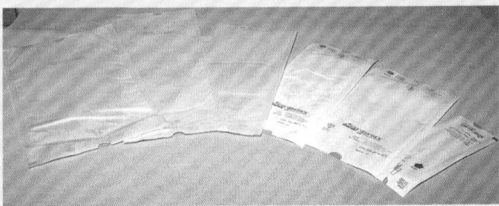

A

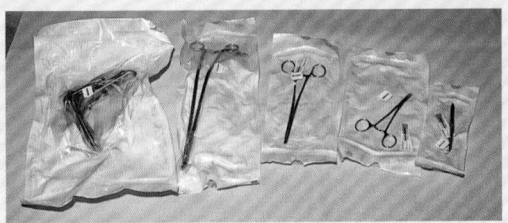

B

| STEPS | REASONS |
|---|---|
| | **Step 2.** (A and B) Autoclave pouches are convenient and come in a variety of sizes. |
| 3. Tear off one or two pieces of autoclave tape. On one piece, indicate in ink the contents of the pack or the name of the instrument that will be wrapped, the date, and your initials. | After the item is wrapped, the contents cannot be seen. Also, dating the package allows the user to determine the quality of the contents based on the amount of time (usually 30 days) that sterilized contents are considered sterile. |

*(continues on page 524)*

## PROCEDURE 21-2 (continued)

| STEPS | REASONS |
|---|---|

4. When using autoclave wrapping material made of cotton muslin or special paper, begin by laying the material diagonally on a flat, clean, dry surface.

   Place the instrument in the center of the wrapping material with the ratchets or handles open. Include a sterilization indicator.

The ratchets should be left open during autoclaving to allow steam to penetrate and sterilize all surfaces.

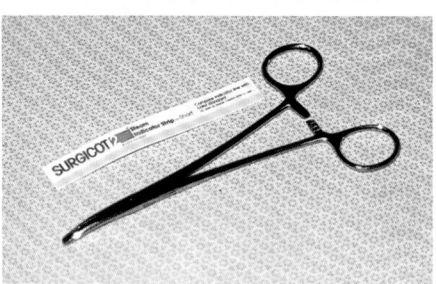

**Step 4.** The ratchets are open.

5. Fold the first flap at the bottom of the diagonal wrap up and fold back the corner, making a tab.

Making a tab allows for easier opening of the pack without contaminating the contents.

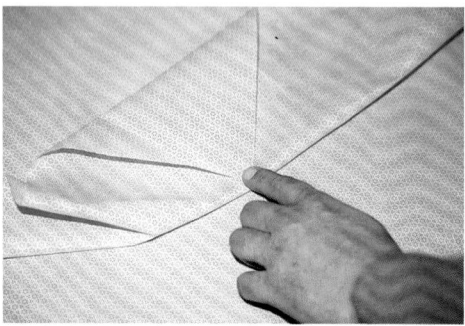

**Step 5.** Make a tab with the corner.

6. Fold the left corner of the wrap and then the right corner, each making a tab for opening the package. Secure the package with autoclave tape.

If the package is not secured with autoclave tape, the contents could become contaminated.

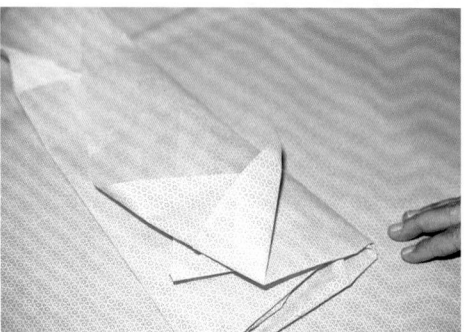

**Step 6.** The bottom, left, and right corners of the wrap are folded.

## PROCEDURE 21-2 (continued)

| STEPS | REASONS |
|---|---|
| 7. Fold the top corner down, making the tab tucked under the material. | Tucking the tab prevents the material from coming loose and contaminating the contents. |

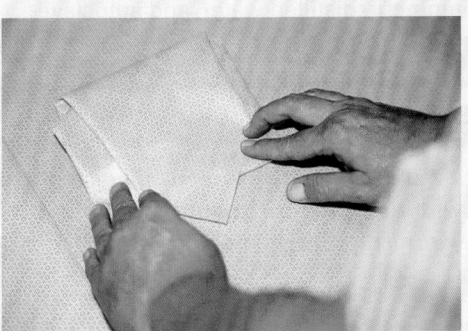

**A**

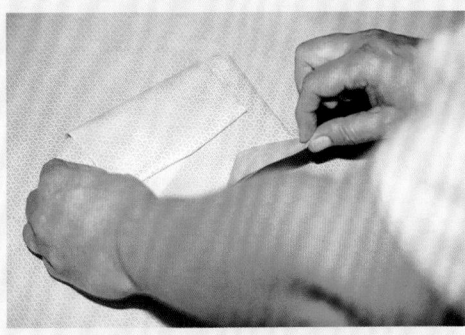

**B**

**Step 7.** (**A**) The top corner is folded down. (**B**) Secure the wrapped instrument package with autoclave tape.

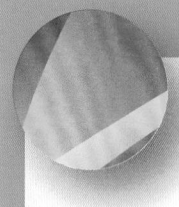

**PSY** PROCEDURE 21-3

## Operating an Autoclave

**PSY** Perform sterilization procedure.

**Purpose:** Safely sterilize instruments or equipment using an autoclave

**Equipment:** Sanitized and wrapped instruments or equipment, distilled water, and autoclave operating manual

| STEPS | REASONS |
|---|---|
| **1.** Assemble the equipment, including the wrapped articles with a sterilization indicator in each package according to office policy. | Some offices want a separately wrapped indicator autoclaved with the load for checking that the procedure was performed properly without opening a pack. |

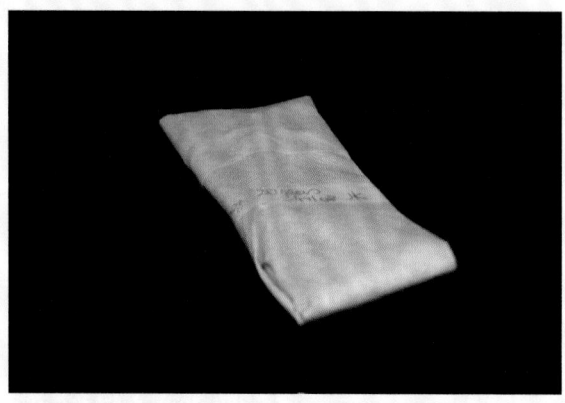

**Step 1.** Properly wrapped items.

| | |
|---|---|
| **2.** Check the water level of the autoclave reservoir and add more if needed. | Use only distilled water in the reservoir tank. |
| **3.** Add water to the internal chamber of the autoclave to the fill line. | The ratchets should be left open during autoclaving to allow steam to penetrate and sterilize all surfaces. |
| **4.** Load the autoclave:<br>**A.** Place trays and packs on their sides 1–3 inches apart.<br>**B.** Put containers on their side with the lid off.<br>**C.** In mixed loads, place hard objects on the bottom shelf and softer packs on the top racks. | Air circulation is not possible if items are tightly packed. Vertical placement forces out heavier air rather than pooling in the containers.<br>Air can circulate in containers on their side with the lid off.<br>Hard objects may form condensation that will drip onto softer items and wet them. |
| **5.** Read the instructions and close the machine. Most machines follow the same protocol:<br>**A.** Close the door and secure or lock it.<br>**B.** Turn the machine on.<br>**C.** When the temperature gauge reaches the point required for the contents of the load (usually 250°F), set the timer. Many autoclaves can be programmed for the required time.<br>**D.** When the timer indicates that the cycle is over, vent the chamber.<br>**E.** After releasing the pressure to a safe level, crack the door of the autoclave to allow additional drying. Most loads dry in 5–20 minutes. Hard items dry faster than soft ones. | You should be familiar with the autoclave and how to operate it safely. |

## PROCEDURE 21-3 (continued)

| STEPS | REASONS |
|---|---|
| 6. When the load has cooled, remove the items. | When the load is finished, the contents will be hot to touch. |
| 7. Check the separately wrapped sterilization indicator, if used, for proper sterilization. | If the indicator registers that the load was properly processed, the items in the additional packs are considered sterile; if not, the items should be considered not sterile, and the load must be reprocessed. |
| 8. Store the items in a clean, dry, dust-free area for 30 days. | After 30 days, reprocessing is necessary. The pack need not be rewrapped, but the autoclave tape should be replaced with new tape with the current date. |
| 9. Clean the autoclave per manufacturer's suggestions, usually by scrubbing the interior chamber with a mild detergent and a soft brush. Attention to the exhaust valve will prevent lint from occluding the outlet. Rinse the machine thoroughly and allow it to dry. | Always follow the manufacturer's recommendations for cleaning the autoclave. |

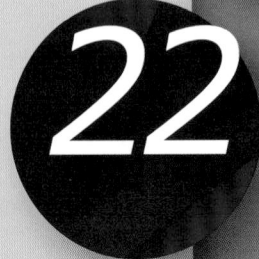

# 22 Assisting with Minor Office Surgery

## Learning Outcomes

### COG Cognitive Domain*

1. Spell and define key terms
2. List your responsibilities before, during, and after minor office surgery
3. Identify the guidelines for preparing and maintaining sterility of the field and surgical equipment during a minor office procedure
4. State your responsibility in relation to informed consent and patient preparation
5. Explain the purpose of local anesthetics and list three commonly used in the medical office
6. Describe the types of needles and sutures and the uses of each
7. Describe the various methods of skin closure used in the medical office
8. Explain your responsibility during surgical specimen collection
9. List the types of laser surgery and electrosurgery used in the medical office and explain the precautions for each
10. Describe the guidelines for applying a sterile dressing

### PSY Psychomotor Domain*

1. Open sterile surgical packs (Procedure 22-1)
  a. *Prepare a sterile field*
2. Use sterile transfer forceps (Procedure 22-2)
3. Add sterile solution to a sterile field (Procedure 22-3)
  a. *Prepare a sterile field*
  b. *Perform within a sterile field*
4. Perform skin preparation and hair removal (Procedure 22-4)
  a. *Instruct and prepare a patient for a procedure or a treatment*
5. Apply sterile gloves (Procedure 22-5)
6. Apply a sterile dressing (Procedure 22-6)
  a. *Instruct and prepare a patient for a procedure or a treatment*
  b. *Prepare a sterile field*
  c. *Perform within a sterile field*
  d. *Perform wound care*
  e. *Demonstrate proper disposal of biohazardous material: sharps and regulated waste*
  f. *Coach patients appropriately considering cultural diversity, developmental life stage, and communication barriers*
  g. *Document patient care accurately in the medical record*

7. Change an existing sterile dressing (Procedure 22-7)
   a. *Instruct and prepare a patient for a procedure or a treatment*
   b. *Prepare a sterile field*
   c. *Perform within a sterile field*
   d. *Perform wound care*
   e. *Demonstrate proper disposal of biohazardous material: sharps and regulated waste*
   f. *Coach patients appropriately considering cultural diversity, developmental life stage, and communication barriers*
   g. *Document patient care accurately in the medical record*
8. Assist with excisional surgery (Procedure 22-8)
   a. *Instruct and prepare a patient for a procedure or a treatment*
   b. *Prepare a sterile field*
   c. *Perform within a sterile field*
   d. *Perform wound care*
   e. *Demonstrate proper disposal of biohazardous material: sharps and regulated waste*
   f. *Coach patients appropriately considering cultural diversity, developmental life stage, and communication barriers*
   g. *Document patient care accurately in the medical record*
9. Assist with incision and drainage (Procedure 22-9)
   a. *Instruct and prepare a patient for a procedure or a treatment*
   b. *Prepare a sterile field*
   c. *Perform within a sterile field*
   d. *Perform wound care*
   e. *Demonstrate proper disposal of biohazardous material: sharps and regulated waste*
   f. *Coach patients appropriately considering cultural diversity, developmental life stage, and communication barriers*
   g. *Document patient care accurately in the medical record*

10. Remove sutures (Procedure 22-10)
    a. *Instruct and prepare a patient for a procedure or a treatment*
    b. *Demonstrate proper disposal of biohazardous material: sharps and regulated waste*
    c. *Coach patients appropriately considering cultural diversity, developmental life stage, and communication barriers*
    d. *Document patient care accurately in the medical record*
11. Remove staples (Procedure 22-11)
    a. *Instruct and prepare a patient for a procedure or a treatment*
    b. *Demonstrate proper disposal of biohazardous material: sharps and regulated waste*
    c. *Coach patients appropriately considering cultural diversity, developmental life stage, and communication barriers*
    d. *Document patient care accurately in the medical record*

### AFF Affective Domain*

1. *Incorporate critical thinking skills when performing patient care*
2. *Demonstrate empathy, active listening, and nonverbal communication*
3. *Explain to a patient the rationale for performance of a procedure*
4. *Show awareness of a patient's concerns related to the procedure being performed*
5. *Protect the integrity of the medical record*

*Note: AAMA/CAAHEP 2015 Standards are italicized.*

### ABHES Competencies

1. Prepare patients for examinations and treatments.
2. Assist physician with minor office surgical procedures.
3. Dispose of biohazardous materials.
4. Use standard precautions.
5. Document accurately.

## Key Terms

| | | | |
|---|---|---|---|
| **Approximate** | **Coagulate** | **Electrode** | **Preservative** |
| **Atraumatic** | **Cryosurgery** | **Fulguration** | **Purulent** |
| **Bandage** | **Dehiscence** | **Keratosis** | **Swaged needle** |
| **Cautery** | **Dressing** | **Lentigines** | **Traumatic** |

## Case Study

$R$ob Long, CMA, has worked in an urgent care center for 6 years and often prepares patients for minor surgical procedures. Today, a 42-year-old male has come into the clinic with a large sebaceous cyst on his back. The physician assistant Barbara Lambert has decided to excise the lesion and has asked Rob to prepare for the procedure. In addition to preparing the patient for a surgical procedure, he must also set up a sterile field, making sure all the necessary supplies and equipment are ready before the procedure is started. Rob must have not only the knowledge and skills to assist with surgical procedures but also the interpersonal skills to win the patient's trust. Rob must use verbal and nonverbal skills to communicate with the patient to prepare for the procedure, relieve anxiety during the procedure, and assure understanding of postoperative instructions after the procedure. Rob must also maintain clear communication with Barbara, who trusts him to prepare the patient, set up the sterile field, and assist during the procedure. Often, Rob is expected to anticipate what the patient and Barbara may need, relying on experience, education and training, and general "people" skills, also known as professionalism.

As a clinical medical assistant, you will have many responsibilities when minor surgery is performed in the physician's office. These include the following:

1. Reinforcing the physician's instructions to the patient regarding preparation for surgery, including at-home skin preparation as directed, fasting from food or fluids, bowel preparation, and other preparations that may be ordered
2. Identifying the patient and gathering the proper equipment and supplies before the physician is ready to do the procedure
3. Obtaining and witnessing the informed consent document if instructed to do so by the physician
4. Preparing the treatment room, instruments, supplies, and equipment
5. Assisting the physician during the procedure
6. Applying a dressing and bandage to the surgical wound
7. Instructing the patient about postoperative wound care, including observing the wound for changes that indicate infection or problems with healing
8. Assisting the patient as needed before, during, and after the procedure
9. Assisting with postoperative instructions such as prescriptions, medications, and scheduling return visits
10. Removing and caring for instruments, equipment, and supplies, including properly disposing of disposable items, sharps, and contaminated or unused supplies
11. Preparing the room for the next patient

Although the types of surgery performed in the medical office vary with the type of medical specialty, the procedure for preparing the patient and setting up the supplies and equipment will require the same process, known as sterile technique. Procedures performed in many general practice offices include suture insertion and removal, incision and drainage, and sebaceous cystectomy. Some gynecologic procedures and urinary procedures also require sterile technique.

## COG PREPARING AND MAINTAINING A STERILE FIELD

Minor office surgery involves procedures that penetrate the body's normally intact surface. Whenever a patient has an open wound, surgical asepsis must be maintained to prevent pathogens from entering the body tissues and causing an infection. Follow the following guidelines to maintain sterility before and during a sterile procedure:

1. Do not let sterile packages get damp or wet. Microorganisms can be drawn into the package by wicking or absorption of the liquid along with the pathogens in it. If a package sterilized in the medical office gets moist, it must be repackaged in a clean, dry wrapper and sterilized again. Damp or wet disposable packages must be discarded.
2. Always face a sterile field to ensure that the area has not been contaminated. If you must leave the area or work with your back to the sterile field, the field must be covered with a sterile drape using sterile technique.
3. Hold all sterile items above waist level. When sterile items are not in your field of vision, you must presume that they have become contaminated.
4. Place sterile items in the middle of the sterile field. A 1-inch border around the field is considered contaminated.
5. Do not spill any liquids, even sterile liquids, onto the sterile field. Remember, the surface below the field is not sterile, and moisture will allow microorganisms to be wicked up into the surgical field.

6. Do not cough, sneeze, or talk over the sterile field. Microorganisms from the respiratory tract can contaminate the field.
7. Never reach over the sterile field. Dust or lint from clothing can contaminate the sterile field.
8. Do not pass soiled supplies, such as gauze or instruments, over the sterile field.
9. If you know or suspect that the sterile field has been contaminated, alert the physician. Sterility must be re-established before the procedure can continue.

## Sterile Surgical Packs

Preparing the treatment or examination room for a surgical procedure is usually the responsibility of the medical assistant. Many medical offices keep a box with index cards or a loose-leaf binder listing the surgical procedures that are commonly performed in the office, including the items needed for setup. Some medical offices prepackage sterile setups in a suitable wrapper and prepare them in the office by autoclave sterilization (Fig. 22-1). These setups are labeled according to the type of procedure (e.g., lesion removal, suture setup) and contain the general instruments for that procedure. Some basic supplies (e.g., gauze sponges, cotton balls, and towels) may also be included before autoclaving.

To reduce the time and effort of sterilizing packs on site, many offices use commercially packaged disposable surgical packs. Disposable surgical packs have become increasingly popular because they are convenient and come with an almost infinite variety of contents. They may contain one sterile article (such as a 4 × 4 sterile dressing) or a complete sterile surgical setup. Many of the supplies are packaged in peel-apart wrappers with two loose flaps that can be pulled apart, and the sterile items can be dropped carefully onto the operative field. The insides of the wrappers may be opened out and used as a sterile field. Some packages are enclosed in plastic and wrapped inside a barrier material that can be used as a sterile field.

Directions for opening are clearly marked on the outside of sterile packs and should be read carefully before opening. If the surgical pack is opened improperly, the contents will be contaminated and cannot be used. Commercially prepared sterile packs are generally more expensive than packages prepared at the medical office, so care must be taken to avoid waste. Labels on commercially prepared packs list the contents in the pack item by item; site-prepared packs usually only state the type of setup. You should check the expiration date on the package; if the pack has expired, it must not be used because sterility is in question. Procedure 22-1 describes the steps for opening sterile surgical packs.

As discussed in Chapter 21, a sterilization indicator should be put inside each surgical package to show that it has been properly sterilized. Tapes, strips, and packaging with indicator stripes or dots on the outside of the packs do not guarantee sterility. In the autoclave, sterility is achieved only by the right combination of temperature, pressure, steam, and time. In addition, improperly packing the autoclave can impede steam penetration to the articles. Therefore, sterilization indicators should be packaged within each pack and must be checked before beginning the surgical procedure. When you open a package of sterile objects, the procedure is the same whether the items are sterilized at the office or commercially prepared. For all sterile packs or supplies, keep the following in mind:

1. Clean hands are used to open the sterile items or packages. The unsterile area is the outside surface of the outside wrapper.
2. The sterile area includes the inside surface of the outside wrapper, the inside wrapper if any, and the contents of the package. These areas or items must not come into contact with any surface, including the hands, or they are considered contaminated and must be replaced.
3. Items are considered contaminated and should be repackaged and sterilized again:
   A. When moisture is present on the pack
   B. If the items are dropped outside the sterile field
   C. If the date on the outside of the package is beyond 30 days for site-prepared packages or it is past the posted expiration date on commercially prepared packages
   D. If the sterilization indicator inside the pack has not changed color
   E. If the wrapper is torn, damaged, or wet
   F. When any area is known or thought to have been touched by a contaminated item

### CHECKPOINT QUESTION

1. What are the nine guidelines that Rob must follow to maintain a sterile field?

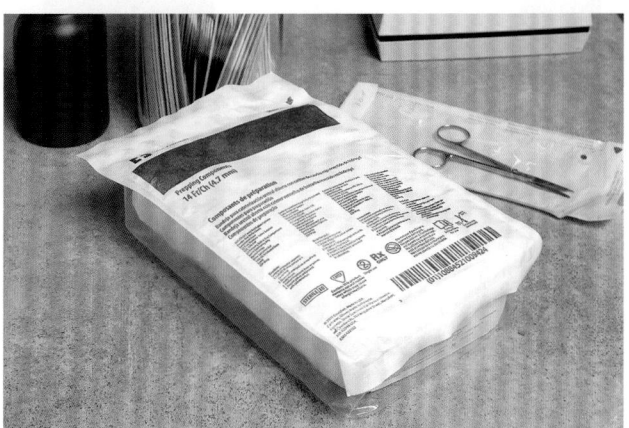

**Figure 22-1** • A wrapped sterile surgical package.

## Sterile Transfer Forceps

Setting up the sterile field requires clean hands and careful technique to avoid contaminating the contents inside the sterile area or field. In the event that sterile items must be manipulated or placed on the sterile field, sterile transfer

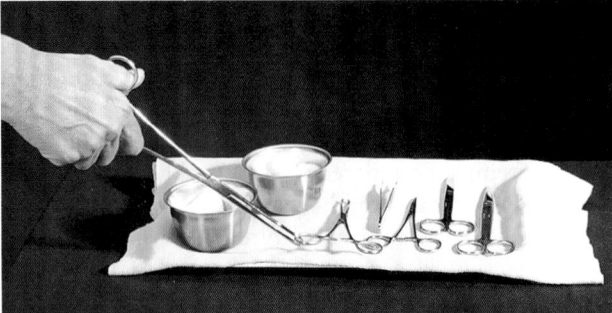

**Figure 22-2 •** Sterile transfer forceps may be used to add or move items on the sterile field.

## Adding Peel-Back Packages and Pouring Sterile Solutions

Procedure packages are frequently prepared with supplies (e.g., cotton balls and gauze squares) to eliminate the need to add more at the time of setup. However, patient assessment at the time of surgery may suggest the need for additional items. These small supplies are usually provided commercially in peel-apart packages. These packages may contain small or single items to be added to the surgical field. The package has an upper edge with two flaps that are used to open the package in a manner that maintains the sterility of the contents. To properly open a package, use both hands with the thumbs just inside the tops of the edges. Separate the flaps using a slow, outward motion of the thumbs and flaps (Fig. 22-3A, B>). Keep in mind that the inside of the sealed package and the contents are sterile but will be contaminated if touched by anything that is not sterile, such as your fingers, or if talking, coughing, or sneezing occurs as you open the package. There are three ways to add the contents of peel-back packages to the sterile field:

forceps or sterile gloved hands must be used, since the hands can never be sterilized. The tips of the forceps and the articles being transferred must both remain sterile (Fig. 22-2). The handles, however, are considered medically aseptic, not sterile, because these are touched by the bare hands of the person using them. Sterile transfer forceps are stored in a dry sterile container, in a wrapped sterile package, or in a sterile solution in a closed container system, such as the Bard Parker, which helps protect the tips of the forceps from contamination. In a closed dry container system, the forceps and container must be sanitized and autoclaved daily. In a closed sterile solution system, the forceps and the container are sterilized at least every day, and fresh sterilization solution is added daily. Only one forceps should be stored in a container to decrease the chance of contamination. After using the sterile transfer forceps without contaminating, place the forceps back in the container for use throughout the procedure or in other procedures scheduled that day. Follow office policy for sterilizing the forceps. Proper use of sterile transfer forceps requires that certain guidelines be followed (Procedure 22-2).

1. *Sterile transfer forceps.* Peel the edges apart with a rolling motion as described earlier. Holding down the two edges, lift the contents up and away with the forceps (Fig. 22-4).
2. *Sterile gloved hand.* This method requires two persons, usually the medical assistant, who opens the package, and the physician, who removes the contents with a sterile gloved hand. You must carefully hold the edges to avoid contaminating the physician's gloves (Fig. 22-5).
3. *Flip off the contents onto a sterile field.* To do this, you step back from the sterile field to prevent your hands and the outer wrapper, which is not sterile, from crossing it. Pull the edges down and away

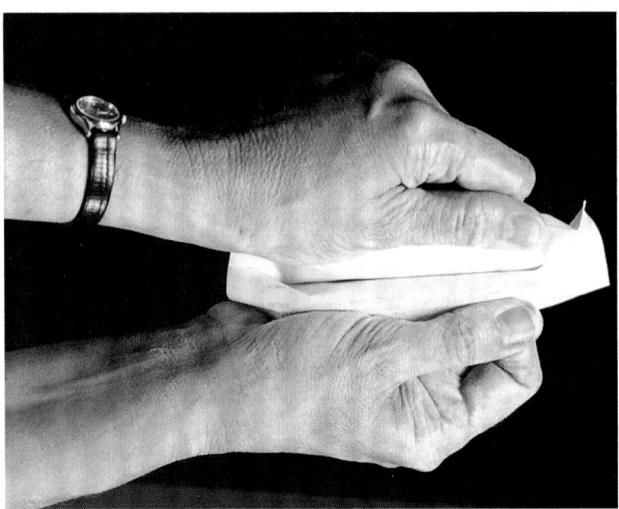

**A**

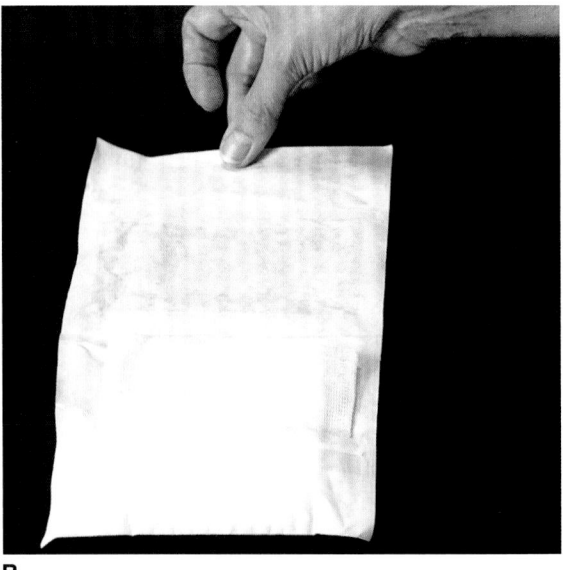

**B**

**Figure 22-3 •** **(A)** Open sterile packets by grasping the edges and rolling the thumbs outward. **(B)** Opening the packet properly forms a sterile field.

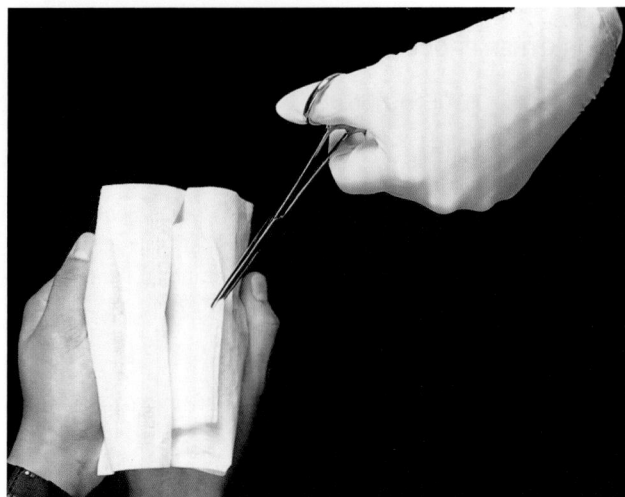

**Figure 22-4** • The physician may use sterile forceps to remove small supplies from peel-back packages.

from the package contents and carefully toss or flip the item onto the middle of the sterile field without touching the 1-inch border around the sterile field. This 1-inch area is considered not sterile.

In most cases, items in presterilized peel-back envelopes cannot be sterilized after being opened and must be discarded even if not used. Because such items are relatively expensive, they should not be opened unnecessarily. A supply of items that might be needed during the procedure should be placed conveniently close to the area and added only if needed.

Whether site prepared or commercially prepared, trays are not processed or stored with liquids in open containers. Solutions must be added as needed at the time of setup. Some procedures require sterile water or saline, while others require an antiseptic solution, such as Betadine. These will be poured into sterile containers added to the sterile field with sterile transfer forceps (Procedure 22-3).

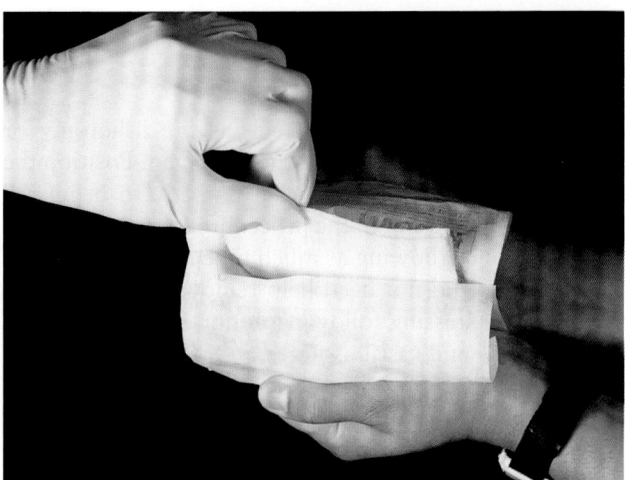

**Figure 22-5** • Sterile gloved hands may be used to remove sterile items.

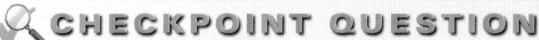

## CHECKPOINT QUESTION

2. What are three ways that Rob can add contents of peel-back packages to the sterile field?

## OG PREPARING THE PATIENT FOR MINOR OFFICE SURGERY

### Patient Instructions and Consent

Many of the minor surgical procedures that are performed in the medical office require a full explanation of the procedure and informed consent (Fig. 22-6). Either the patient agrees and the procedure is performed or the patient refuses and the procedure is not done. The informed consent document must state the procedure and its purpose and expected results along with possible side effects, risks, and complications. Although the physician is responsible for informing the patient of the details of the procedure and any risks involved, the patient may ask questions, including how long the procedure will last, what preparations will be needed, or whether fasting will be necessary. You may answer these questions after verifying the information with the physician.

It is always a good practice to give specific written instructions to the patient for any preparations to be made before arriving at the office so that the procedure can be done on schedule and with no preventable risk to the patient. The physician may prescribe medication for the patient to take at home before the procedure. As with any patient instructions, you should notify the physician if the patient seems confused or does not understand the instructions. Encourage the patient to call the office if questions arise later. Of course, the instructions should be documented in the medical record.

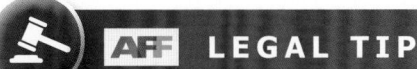

### AFF  LEGAL TIP

#### Informed Consent

In today's litigious society, physicians routinely obtain signed informed consent forms even for minor office procedures. Printed forms are available, or the office may have its own form. Such forms may be used for procedures requiring legal witnessed signatures. Other more generic ones have blank spaces to add information relevant to the procedure to be performed. All forms should have spaces for the date and signatures of the patient, physician, and witness or witnesses. The medical assistant is *not* responsible for informing the patient but often witnesses the signing of the document by the patient. It is the physician's legal responsibility to inform the patient before the consent form is signed by the patient or legal guardian.

SPECIAL CONSENT TO OPERATION OR OTHER PROCEDURE(S)

PATIENT _____    PATIENT NUMBER _____

DATE _____    TIME _____

1.  I HEREBY AUTHORIZE DOCTOR _____ AND/OR SUCH ASSIS-
    TANTS AS MAY BE SELECTED BY HIM, TO PERFORM THE FOLLOWING PROCEDURE(S):

    _____

    ON _____
         (NAME OF PATIENT OR MYSELF)

2.  THE PROCEDURE(S) LISTED ABOVE HAVE BEEN EXPLAINED TO ME BY DR. _____
    AND I UNDERSTAND THE NATURE AND THE CONSEQUENCES OF THE PROCEDURE(S).

3.  I RECOGNIZE THAT, DURING THE COURSE OF THE OPERATION, UNFORESEEN CONDI-
    TIONS MAY NECESSITATE ADDITIONAL OR DIFFERENT PROCEDURES THAN THOSE SET
    FORTH. I FURTHER AUTHORIZE AND REQUEST THAT THE ABOVE NAMED SURGEON, HIS
    ASSISTANTS, OR HIS DESIGNEES PERFORM SUCH PROCEDURES AS ARE IN HIS PRO-
    FESSIONAL JUDGMENT NECESSARY AND DESIRABLE, INCLUDING, BUT NOT LIMITED TO,
    PROCEDURES INVOLVING PATHOLOGY AND RADIOLOGY. THE AUTHORITY GRANTED
    UNDER THIS PARAGRAPH SHALL EXTEND TO REMEDYING CONDITIONS NOT KNOWN TO
    DR. _____ AT THE TIME THE OPERATION IS COMMENCED.

4.  I AM AWARE THAT THE PRACTICE OF MEDICINE AND SURGERY IS NOT AN EXACT SCI-
    ENCE AND I ACKNOWLEDGE THAT NO GUARANTEES HAVE BEEN MADE TO ME AS TO THE
    RESULTS OF THE OPERATION OR PROCEDURE.

5.  TISSUE REMOVED DURING SURGERY SHALL BE SENT TO PATHOLOGY TO BE EXAMINED
    AND DISPOSED OF IN ACCORDANCE WITH THE RULES AND REGULATIONS OF THE MED-
    ICAL STAFF OF THE SURGERY CENTER.

_____    _____
Procedure has been discussed with patient. (Surgeon's Signature)        SIGNATURE OF PATIENT

PATIENT IS UNABLE TO SIGN BECAUSE    ❑  HE (SHE) IS A MINOR _____ YEARS OF AGE

                                     ❑  OTHER (SPECIFY) _____

_____            _____
         WITNESS                             PERSON AUTHORIZED TO SIGN FOR PATIENT

                                             _____
                                             RELATIONSHIP OF ABOVE TO PATIENT

**Figure 22-6 •** Sample consent form.

## Positioning and Draping

Before positioning the patient for a minor surgical procedure, ask the patient to void; this helps prevent discomfort during the procedure. Offer to help the patient remove whatever clothing is necessary to expose the operative site. Expose only the area necessary for the procedure to ensure the patient's privacy. An air-conditioned office may be uncomfortably cool for patients. You may provide additional sheets or a blanket for comfort.

Assist the patient to assume a comfortable position on the examining table that offers exposure of and access to the operative site. Provide pillows for comfort and support. Do not make the patient maintain an uncomfortable position, such as the lithotomy or knee–chest, while waiting for the physician. Position the patient only when the physician is ready to begin the procedure. At the end of the procedure, assist the patient from the table, allowing as much time as needed. Often, patients who did not need help removing clothing will require help dressing following minor office surgery. Be aware of this and assist as necessary.

The type of procedure and the patient's position determine the type of drapes used to expose the operative site and cover the patient. Disposable paper drapes are most commonly used in the medical office. They come in many sizes and shapes, each suited for specific uses. Paper drapes can be used alone, in combination,

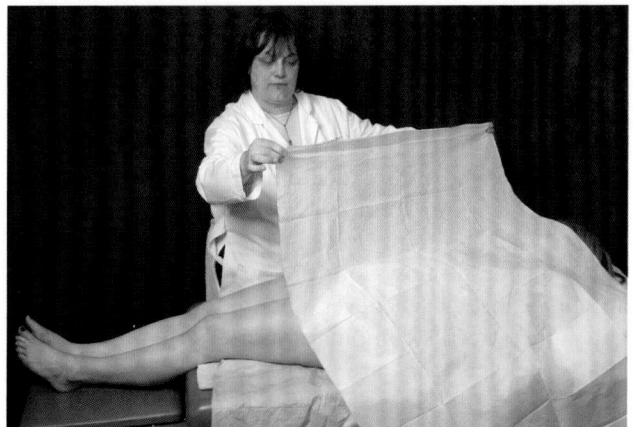

**Figure 22-7 •** Applying a sterile drape.

or with separate drape sheets and towels. Fenestrated drapes have an opening to expose the operative site while covering adjacent areas. Fenestrated drapes may be small, such as those used for suture insertion, or large, such as those used to cover the legs and lower abdomen but expose the perineal area. Some sterile drapes are combined with adhesive-backed clear plastic, which sticks to the patient's skin and eliminates the need for towel clamps. Sterile drapes are applied by picking up the drape on the 1-inch border (no gloves needed), lifting over the surgical area without contaminating the drape, and laying the drape on the patient from farthest away to closest (Fig. 22-7). This ensures that you do not reach over the drape after it is placed on the patient.

When removing contaminated drapes from the patient following a procedure, put on clean examination gloves and carefully roll the items away from the body, keeping the contaminated areas innermost, preventing contamination. This helps to surround the dirtier areas of the sheet with the cleaner area and helps prevent contaminating your clothing. Because the sheets, towels, or drapes may be contaminated with blood or other body fluids, follow standard precautions (see Chapter 17).

## Preparing the Patient's Skin

The goal of preoperative skin preparation is to remove as many microorganisms as possible from the skin to decrease the chance of wound contamination. Skin preparation may be simply applying an antiseptic solution to the area or may include removing gross contaminants and hair from the operative area. Hair can be removed with depilatory creams but often requires shaving the skin (Procedure 22-4).

### CHECKPOINT QUESTION

3. Barbara asks Rob for a fenestrated drape for the sebaceous cyst excision she is going to perform. What is a fenestrated drape?

## ASSISTING THE PHYSICIAN

### Local Anesthetics

When office surgery of any kind is performed, the site is first anesthetized (numbed) with a local anesthetic to minimize the pain and discomfort felt by the patient. Occasionally, when a wound contains embedded debris that must be removed prior to repair, the local anesthetic will be injected before preparing the wound site to facilitate wound cleaning. Lidocaine and lidocaine with epinephrine (0.5% to 2%) are two of the many local anesthetics commonly used in medical offices. Others are mepivacaine (Carbocaine™) and bupivacaine (Marcaine™). Epinephrine is added to local anesthetics to cause vasoconstriction and to slow absorption by the body and lengthen the anesthetic's effectiveness. It may be used when the physician anticipates a long procedure, but anesthesia with epinephrine should never be used on the tips of the fingers, toes, nose, or penis, since the vasoconstriction may cause death of tissue in these distal areas.

One of two methods may be used to administer local anesthesia. In one method, you draw the anesthetic for the physician into a syringe, keeping the vial beside the syringe for the physician's approval. In this case, the anesthetic is usually given to the patient before the physician puts on sterile gloves because the outside of the syringe and needle unit is not sterile.

The second method is used if the physician puts on sterile gloves before administering the anesthetic. In this case, a sterile syringe and needle are included on the sterile field setup. When the physician is ready to administer the anesthetic, you show the physician the label on the vial, clean the rubber stopper of the vial with an alcohol swab, and hold the vial while the physician draws the required amount into the syringe. There are many methods of holding the vial securely while the physician withdraws the medication; however, the most common way is for you to hold the vial with one hand while supporting your wrist with the other hand (Fig. 22-8). You and the physician together develop a method to maintain surgical asepsis.

### Wound Closure

Many types of wounds require closure to ensure rapid healing with minimal scarring. This is accomplished by bringing the edges of the wound as close together as possible in their original position (approximation). Sutures are used to close wounds and incisions and to bring tissue layers into close approximation. Skin closures are performed after cyst or tissue sample removal, to close lacerations, or any time skin surfaces require assistance for healing. Supplies used to suture skin include needles and suture material. Skin staples are sometimes used to close large incisions over areas where **dehiscence** can occur, such as the knee, hip, or abdomen, but these are not usually inserted in the medical office.

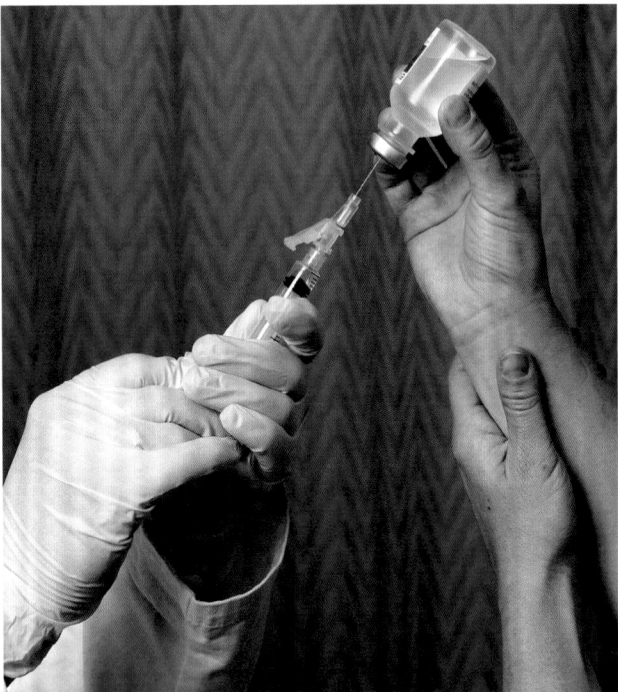

**Figure 22-8** • Hold the vial containing the anesthetic downward, supporting that wrist with the other hand.

## Needles and Sutures

Needles used in minor office surgery are chosen for the type of surgery to be performed. Needles are classified as follows:

- By shape: curved or straight
- By point: tapered or cutting
- By eye: **atraumatic** (swaged) or **traumatic** (with an eye)

Round straight needles are called *domestic needles*, and straight cutting needles are called *Keith needles*. Curved needles used in surgical procedures are usually clamped in a needle holder before being handed to or used by the physician. Straight needles are not clamped in a needle holder but are handed to the physician with the point up. Straight needles are rarely used in medical offices.

Cutting needles are used on tough tissues, such as skin. Round or tapered (noncutting) needles are used on subcutaneous tissue, peritoneum, and muscle. Atraumatic needles, or **swaged needles**, have suture material that has been mechanically attached to the needle by the manufacturer and do not require threading. These are called atraumatic because they cause less trauma than threaded needles as they pass through the tissues. Unlike atraumatic or swaged needles, threaded needles have an eye with a double thickness of suture that must be pulled through tissues. The double thickness of this suture makes a larger and therefore more traumatic opening in the tissues than a swaged suture.

In medical offices, curved swaged needles are used far more often than any other type. Swaged needles are selected for a procedure according to the size and length of the suture material and the attached needle gauge clearly marked on the packaging material. When a suture must be threaded through an eyed needle, both needle gauge and suture size must be selected. The physician usually selects the suture and needle, but you should know your physician's preferences and anticipate needs whenever possible. Sutures, needles, and suture–needle combinations are contained in peel-apart packages that are sterile on the inside so that they can be added to the sterile field (Fig. 22-9). This may be done by sterile transfer forceps, by a sterile gloved hand, or by carefully flipping them onto the sterile field.

Sutures come in various gauges (diameters) and lengths. Very thick sutures are numbered 1 to 5, with 5 being the thickest. Sutures smaller than size 1 are expressed with added zeros. Small sutures, which become progressively smaller, range from 1-0 to 10-0 or smaller (i.e., 1-0, 2-0, 3-0, and so forth). A very fine 10-0 suture, which is about the diameter of a human hair, is generally used in microsurgery. When a fine suture is needed, such as on the face and neck, 23-0 and 24-0 sutures are commonly used. A very fine suture decreases scarring and gives a better cosmetic result.

Sutures also come in absorbable and nonabsorbable forms. Absorbable sutures, or catgut (made from the intestines of sheep or cattle), are readily broken down in the body and usually do not have to be removed. The two forms of absorbable gut suture are chromic, which is chemically treated to delay absorption for several days, and plain, which is not treated and is more quickly absorbed. Absorbable sutures are used most frequently in hospitals during surgery on deep tissues.

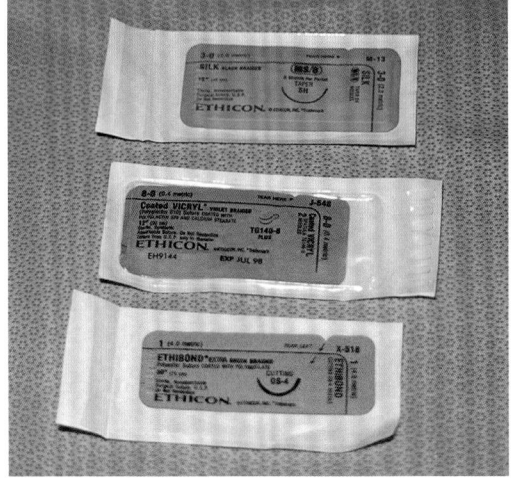

**Figure 22-9** • Suture material and needles are supplied in see-through packages with the size of the suture material and the type of needle listed on the packet. The inside of the packet is sterile.

Nonabsorbable sutures are available in a great variety of brands, sizes, lengths, and swaged needles; they are the most versatile. Nonabsorbable sutures either remain in the body permanently or are removed after healing. Nonabsorbable sutures are used on the skin, intestines, or bone, to ligate larger vessels, and to attach heart valves and various artificial and natural grafts. Nonabsorbable sutures are made of fibers such as silk, nylon, Dacron, or cotton or stainless steel wire.

## Skin Staples

Another form of nonabsorbable suture is the metal skin clip or staple. These are commonly made of stainless steel, but some very specialized types are made of sterling silver for use in neurosurgery and other procedures. When nonabsorbable sutures or staples are used to close skin wounds, they must be removed when the wound has healed completely. Depending on the location of the skin wound, nonabsorbable sutures or staples remain in place for varying lengths of time; the head and neck may require 3 to 5 days due to increased blood supply to these areas. Sutures in the arms and legs may require 7 to 10 days.

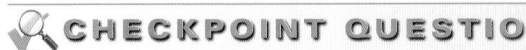

### CHECKPOINT QUESTION

4. How do swaged needles differ from threaded ones?

## Adhesive Skin Closures

Adhesive skin closures are used to **approximate** the edges of a small wound if sutures are not needed. They are appropriate where there is little tension on the skin edges. The strips are placed transversely across the line of the wound to bring the wound edges in close approximation (Fig. 22-10A, B). In most instances, the strips are left in place until they fall off. However, in some cases, the physician may want them removed or replaced if soiled with drainage. When removing these strips, carefully lift the edges distal to the wound and pull gently toward the wound. Never pull the strips away from the wound because tension on the wound site may disrupt the healing process.

## Specimen Collection

Many minor office surgical procedures yield specimens that must be sent to a laboratory to be examined by a pathologist. Specimens include samples of tissue, wound exudate, foreign bodies, and so on. The medical assistant must choose the proper container with the appropriate **preservative** (substance that delays decomposition) for the type of procedure being performed. The laboratory where the specimen is sent usually provides the appropriate containers with preservative, and you should have a stock of them on hand. Hold the open container steady to avoid touching the sides as the physician drops the specimen into the preservative (Fig. 22-11).

You are responsible for attaching a label to the specimen container with the patient's name and the date written clearly on the label, and you must complete a laboratory request form to send with the specimen. These forms require information such as the patient's name, age, sex, and identification number or social security number, date, type of specimen, type of examination, and the physician's name or laboratory contact number. Specimens obtained during a minor surgical procedure must be transported to the pathology laboratory as quickly as possible.

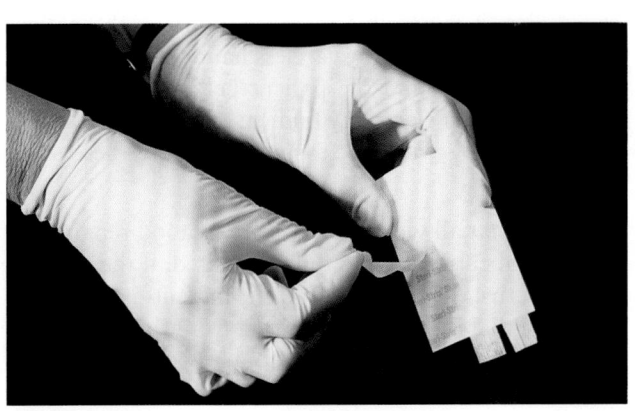
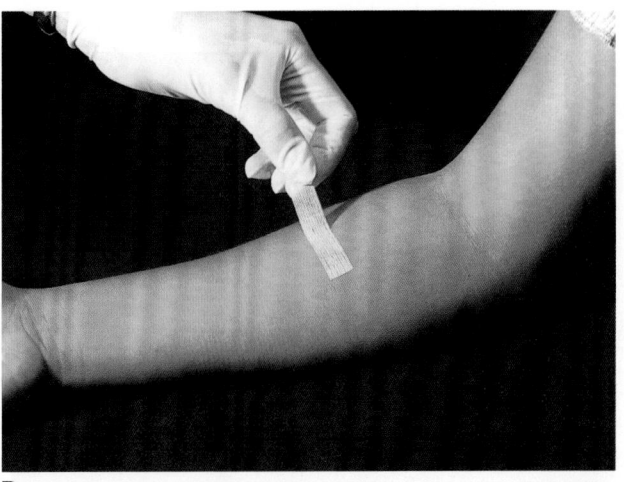

**A**   **B**

**Figure 22-10** • Adhesive skin closures. **(A)** These lightweight lengths of porous tape are used for closing small wounds. **(B)** Strips are placed transversely across a wound.

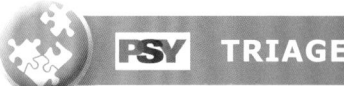

## TRIAGE

The physician has just performed a needle biopsy for a lesion on Mr. Smith's lower back. You have to do the following three tasks:

A. Label the specimen and complete the laboratory requisition form.
B. Apply a dressing to Mr. Smith's lower back.
C. Help Mr. Smith get dressed and into a wheelchair.

**How do you sort these tasks? What do you do first? Second? Third?**

The correct order is A, B, C. All specimens must be immediately labeled. Incorrectly labeled specimens or poorly completed requisition forms may result in the laboratory not being able to test the specimen. It is appropriate to apply a dressing to the wound and then assist the patient to get dressed and into a wheelchair.

## Electrosurgery

Electrosurgery uses high-frequency alternating electric current to destroy or cut and remove tissue. It is used to **coagulate**, or clot, small bleeding vessels. Electrosurgery is considered an alternative to traditional office surgery and is rapidly gaining favor for many procedures. An advantage of electrical surgery is the **cautery** produced by the electricity that seals small bleeding vessels and coagulates nearby cells to reduce bleeding and loss of cell fluid. Electrosurgical units use disposable **electrodes** with tips of various sizes and shapes to deliver the desired amount of electric current to the tissues (Fig. 22-12). The following procedures are considered electrosurgery:

- **Fulguration** destroys tissue with controlled electric sparks. As the physician holds the electrode tip 1 to 2 mm from the site, a series of sparks destroys the superficial cells at the site.

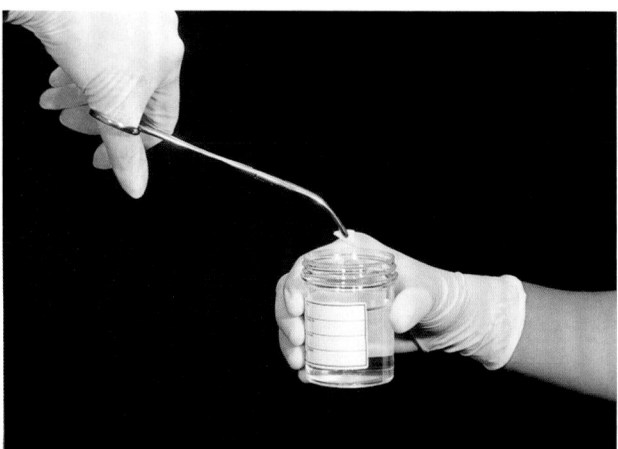

**Figure 22-11 •** Tissue samples are placed in the preservative by the physician.

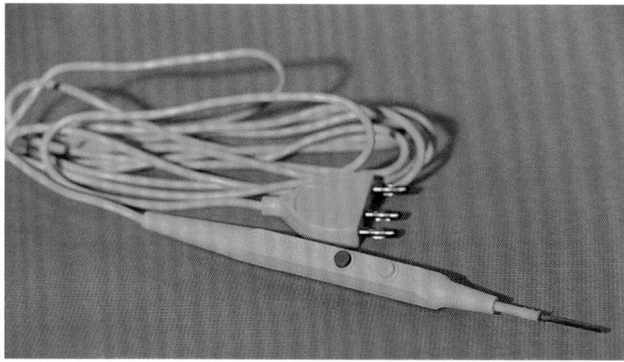

**Figure 22-12 •** A disposable electrosurgical unit. The blade is designed either to cut or to cauterize.

- *Electrodesiccation* dries and separates tissue with an electric current. The electrode is placed directly on the site.
- *Electrocautery* causes quick coagulation of small blood vessels with the heat created by the electric current. Electrocautery is commonly referred to as electrocoagulation.
- *Electrosection* is used for incision or excision of tissue. Bleeding is minimal with this type of procedure, but more damage can occur to surrounding tissues.

Medical offices frequently use electrosurgery to remove moles, cysts, warts, and certain types of skin and cervical cancers. Electrosurgical equipment includes various electrode tips, such as blades, needles, loops, and balls, each with specific uses.

During electrosurgery, your responsibilities are to ensure the safety and comfort of the patient and to pass the electrode to the physician as needed. As with all instruments, the electrode must be passed in its functional position. The electrode is handed to the physician with the tip down.

Because electric current is delivered to the tip by the electrosurgical machine, great care should be exercised to prevent injuries. Although the physician activates the device, it is possible to cause injury to the patient, physician, or yourself by careless handling of the device. Take care to ground the patient before electrosurgery. Metal conducts electricity and can cause serious burns. When assisting with electrosurgery, follow these safety measures:

- Ensure that all working parts are in good repair. The electrical current is carefully regulated; if the machine is defective, serious injury to the patient may occur.
- Ensure that all metal is removed from the patient. The patient must be asked about any metal implants or a cardiac pacemaker. Metal conducts electricity and can cause burns. Metal implants may become very hot, and pacemakers may malfunction during the procedure.

- Ensure that the patient is grounded with a pad supplied by the manufacturer. Attach it to the patient at a site recommended by the manufacturer (some recommend placing the pad far from the operative site; others suggest placing it near the site). Improper placement can result in injury.
- Place the grounding pad firmly and completely against the patient's skin. Apply a conducting gel to the pad and to the patient's skin, or use an adhesive-backed pad to facilitate conduction through the grounding pad. Areas of skin against the pad that are not well connected will result in hot spots and may burn the patient.

Although disposable tips are usually used today, reusable tips may still be used in some medical offices. Reusable tips are disinfected and processed in the autoclave according to the manufacturer's directions. Reusable tips may be polished with steel wool if they become dull. Disposable tips should be discarded after use. Electrosurgical machines should be inspected periodically to ensure proper working order. The operating manual states the periodic maintenance to be performed by office staff and routine inspections to be performed by trained technicians. Surfaces should be kept clean and dry; machines should be kept covered when not in use.

## CHECKPOINT QUESTION

5. Which type of electrosurgery is used for incision or excision of tissue?

## Laser Surgery

Lasers are devices that focus high-intensity light in a narrow beam to create extreme heat and energy. In medicine, lasers can be used to cut tissue and coagulate small bleeding vessels. There are many types of lasers, each with fairly specific applications in medicine. The following are the most common types of lasers encountered in the medical office:

- Argon laser: used for coagulation
- Carbon dioxide laser: used for cutting tissue
- Nd:YAG laser: used for coagulation and to separate warts and moles from surrounding tissues

Light from the laser is not usually visible. Colored filters are used to illuminate the laser's target, enabling the physician to direct the laser beam to the affected area. As with other electronic devices, attention to care and handling of the laser helps ensure that it is in good working order when it is needed. It is important to read and follow the manufacturer's recommended maintenance procedures as described in the instruction manual.

Everyone who is in the room, including the patient, during the laser procedure is required to wear goggles for eye protection. Health care workers are recommended to complete a training program before assisting with laser procedures to ensure that safety precautions are followed.

## CHECKPOINT QUESTION

6. What is one important safety feature worth noting when assisting with a laser procedure?

## PATIENT EDUCATION

### Postoperative Instructions

After any surgical procedure, the patient should receive written and verbal discharge instructions, including how to care for the postoperative wound, taking prescribed medications correctly, and returning to the office for follow-up visits, dressing changes, and suture removal as ordered by the physician. The patient should be informed of the signs and symptoms of infection and should be instructed to report the following conditions:

- Excessive bleeding from the wound (additional teaching should include how to stop any excessive bleeding by applying direct pressure or elevating the body area)
- Redness, red streaks, or excessive swelling around the surgical site
- Fever

Tell the patient to call the office if these symptoms arise. In addition, you will tell the patient the following:

- When to return to the office to have the dressing or bandage changed or how and when to change the bandage or dressing at home.
- The need for follow-up visits. Have the patient schedule the appointment or appointments before leaving and provide an appointment card for each appointment.
- After speaking with the physician, tell the patient when he or she can take a shower or bath and whether the surgical wound can get wet. (Whether the wound may get wet depends on location and depth of the wound and the surgeon's preference.)
- If a specimen was taken for a pathology test, tell the patient when the results will be available.
- Answer any questions about postoperative experience and always encourage patients to call the office at any time if a problem or concern arises.

# POSTSURGICAL PROCEDURES

## Sterile Dressings

Sterile dressings are items such as 4- × 4-inch absorbent gauze sponges and nonadhering dressings that have been processed for use on open wounds. Sterile dressings are generally prepackaged in small numbers but may come in bulk containers. They are manufactured in various sizes and shapes, each for a specific use and chosen according to the size of the wound and the amount of drainage. Dressings should be handled with sterile technique. A sterile dressing may be secured by various bandages (sling, cravat, roller, tubular gauze) to hold the dressing in place, protect the injured part, or restrict movement. Chapter 28 describes bandaging techniques. Procedure 22-5 describes putting on sterile gloves, Procedure 22-6 describes applying a sterile dressing to a surgical wound, and Procedure 22-7 describes changing an existing dressing on a wound.

A sterile dressing is considered contaminated if it is damp or outdated, if its wrapper is damaged, or if it is improperly removed from its wrapper. Sterile dressings are used directly over a wound for the following reasons:

1. To cover and protect from contamination
2. To absorb drainage such as blood, serum, or pus
3. To exert pressure on an open wound to control bleeding
4. To hide disfigurement during healing
5. To hold medications against a wound to facilitate healing

When you remove a dressing, always wear clean examination gloves and carefully observe the wound

for any drainage or exudates, noting this in the patient's chart. The terminology for describing wound drainage is outlined in Box 22-1. Immediately following the closure of a wound, it is normal to see serous or serosanguineous drainage in scant or moderate amounts, depending on the extent of the wound or incision. **Purulent** drainage, or drainage with color other than pink, is a sign of infection. Notify the physician when the wound is uncovered so that it can be examined and a decision can be made regarding how well healing is progressing. Box 22-2 describes the types and phases of wound healing.

---

**BOX 22-1 Wound Drainage**

When observing wound drainage, be sure to note:

**Color**
- Serous (clear)
- Sanguineous (blood tinged)
- Serosanguineous (pinkish or clear and red mixed)
- Purulent (white, green, or yellow-tinged drainage; usually accompanied by an unpleasant odor characteristic of infection)

**Amount**
- Copious (large amount)
- Medium (moderate amount)
- Scant (small amount)

The amount can also be quantified by indicating the size of the drainage (e.g., 2 inch diameter, entire 4 × 4 dressing saturated) or the size of the dressing.

---

**BOX 22-2 The Healing Process**

*Healing by Primary Intention:* This simplest form of healing occurs in wounds whose edges are closely approximated, allowing the entrance of little or no bacteria to complicate the process. The edges of the wound lie closely together, new cells form quickly to bind the site, and capillaries expand themselves across the tissue break to restore circulation to the tissues. Scarring is usually minimal.

*Healing by Secondary Intention:* Granulation of tissue is present in the wound, and the edges of the wound join indirectly. Because the skin edges are not closely approximated, additional new cells are required to fill spaces in the lesion. Capillaries may

not be able to reach across the gap to restore full circulation. Nerves may not rejoin, which results in diminished nerve stimulus through the area. A large scab forms to protect the area while healing goes on below it. Scarring is more severe than with primary intention healing.

*Healing by Tertiary Intention:* The wound initially is left open if there is the possibility that the wound may already be contaminated with microorganisms and closing it would only trap the microorganisms, increasing the potential for an infection. The wound is left open to fill in with granular tissue. There is considerable scar formation.

## BOX 22-2  The Healing Process (continued)

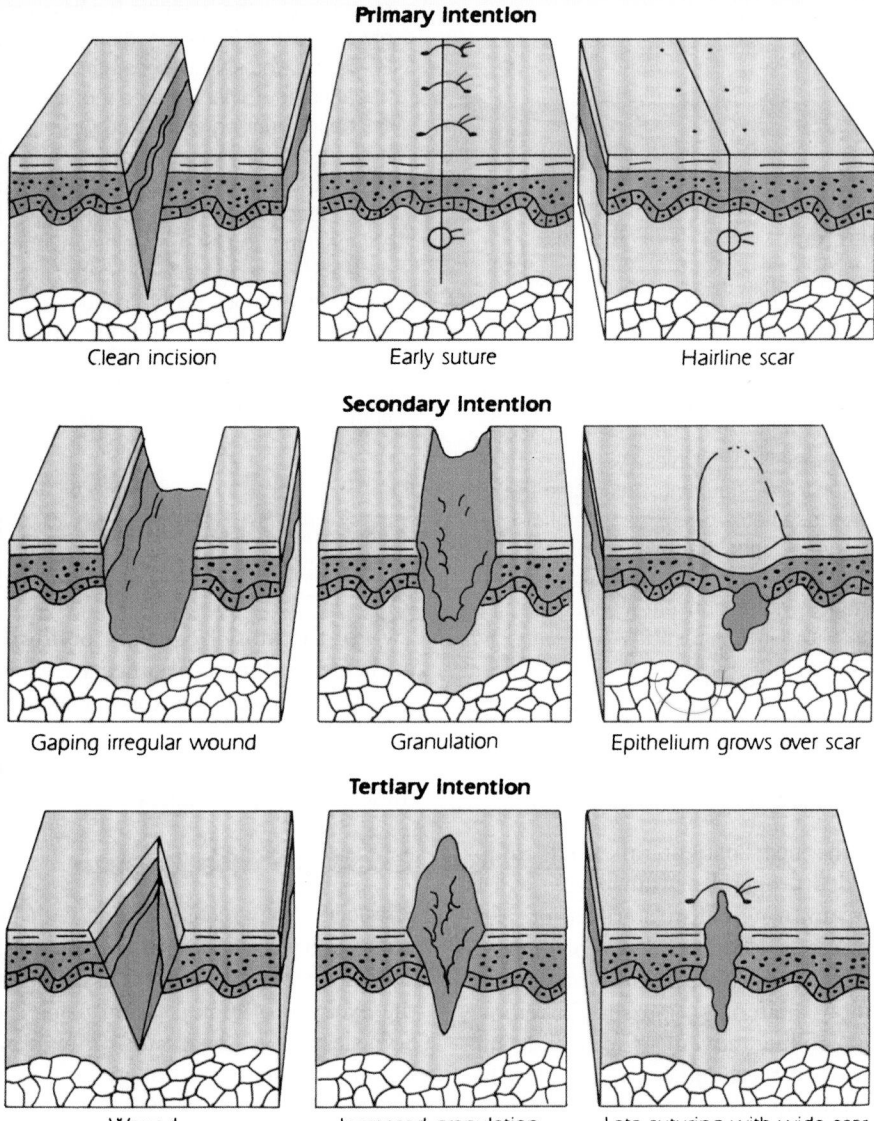

**Primary Intention**
*Left to right:* Clean incision — Early suture — Hairline scar

**Secondary Intention**
*Left to right:* Gaping irregular wound — Granulation — Epithelium grows over scar

**Tertiary Intention**
*Left to right:* Wound — Increased granulation — Late suturing with wide scar

Types of wound healing. (*Top*) Primary intention. *Left to right:* Clean incision, early suture, hairline scar. (*Center*) Secondary intention. *Left to right:* Gaping irregular wound, granulation, epithelium grows over scar. (*Bottom*) Tertiary intention. *Left to right:* Wound, increased granulation, late suturing with wide scar.

### Phases of Wound Healing

*Phase I (inflammatory, lag, or exudative phase):* This phase usually lasts from 1 to 4 days. The body attempts to heal itself by increasing the circulation to the part and by beginning to reroute or repair the supplying vessels. The increased circulation brings with it more white blood cells to mount a defense against pathogens. Serum and red blood cells brought by the additional blood form a glue-like fibrin to plug the wound. As the fibrin dries, it pulls the edges of the wound closer together and forms a scab. Signs that this phase is working are edema from the tissue fluid, warmth from the extra blood, redness from the vasodilation, and pain from the pressure on the nerve endings caused by the edema.

*Phase II (proliferative, healing, or granulation phase):* This phase may last from several days to several weeks. The vessels continue to repair themselves and may reroute if damage is severe. The scab from phase I continues to dry and to pull the edges of the wound as closely together as possible.

*Phase III (remodeling, maturation, or scarring phase):* This phase may take from weeks to years, depending upon the severity of the wound. Fibroblasts build scar tissue to guard the area.

7. How would Rob explain the difference between a dressing and a bandage?

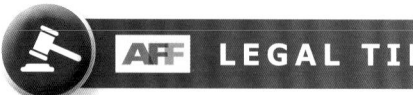

### Protected Health Information

Often, patients who are seen in the medical office for minor surgical procedures must have a note from the physician in order to return back to work or to school. Some offices have a standard form that can be filled out and signed by the physician indicating very generally that the patient has had a procedure and should return back to school or work on a specific day. Unless you have the patient's written consent, you should never indicate the type of procedure on these notes or answer specific questions via the telephone should employers or school personnel call the office for information. Giving information without the patient's written consent would be a violation of the privacy laws included in HIPAA (Health Insurance and Portability Act of 1996).

## Cleaning the Examination Table and Operative Area

In preparation for the next patient, all used equipment must be discarded properly or transported to the equipment room for sanitizing before sterilization. The examination room must be cleaned as part of the procedure using standard precautions. Because of the possibility of biohazardous materials, you should remove papers and sheets in a rolling movement so outside surfaces cover the interior of the bundle. Do not let table covers and sheets come into contact with your clothing. Discard the sheets and covers appropriately. After applying gloves, wipe down the examination table, surgical stand, sink, counter, and other surfaces used during the procedure with an approved disinfectant or dilute bleach solution and allow them to dry. Replace the table sheet paper for the next patient.

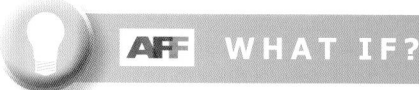

**What if you accidentally cut your finger while cleaning up after a minor office surgical procedure?**

Remove your gloves and immediately wash your hands with an antiseptic solution. Then, have the physician evaluate the wound. The physician will suggest that you wash the wound by performing a hand washing procedure, and antibiotics may be prescribed. The patient should be asked for permission to take a blood sample to test for hepatitis B, hepatitis C, and HIV. State laws vary regarding the legality of health care workers demanding a blood sample for testing. After blood from the patient is examined for the hepatitis B surface antigen, you may be given hepatitis B immunoglobulin (HBIG) and/or hepatitis B vaccine. You should consider obtaining the vaccine for hepatitis now. Many states require that health care workers be immunized at their employer's expense. Finally, be sure to notify your supervisor of any work-related injury so that it may be appropriately documented. The Needlestick Safety and Prevention Act requires that a sharps injury log be maintained and that it include the type and brand of device involved in the incident, the area in which the incident occurred, and a description of the incident. The name of the employee should not be recorded in the injury log. Preventing accidental exposure to contaminated blood or body fluids requires being alert and working without distractions.

## COMMONLY PERFORMED OFFICE SURGICAL PROCEDURES

Two of the most frequently performed minor surgeries in the general medical office are excision of skin lesions (moles, **lentigines, keratoses,** and skin tags) and incision and drainage of abscesses. Always use sterile technique and follow standard precautions when assisting with these surgical procedures.

### Excision of a Lesion

Physicians may excise lesions with electrocautery, laser, **cryosurgery,** or standard surgical equipment. Procedure 22-8 describes the steps for assisting the physician during the excision of a skin lesion using standard equipment. Some lesions are desiccated or fulgurated; however, many lesions are sent to pathology for diagnosis after excision.

### Incision and Drainage

An abscess is a local collection of pus in a cavity surrounded by inflamed tissue. It results from the body's response to an infectious process when pathogens have entered through a break in the skin. Abscesses may be referred to as boils, furuncles (one lesion), or carbuncles (several lesions grouped closely together) and are very painful. The site must be incised and the infected material drained before healing can take place (Procedure 22-9).

## ASSISTING WITH SUTURE AND STAPLE REMOVAL

In many instances, you will be required to remove sutures from a wound. Patients should understand that they might feel a pulling sensation during suture removal but should not feel pain. First, cleanse the area with an antiseptic solution. Either wearing sterile gloves or using

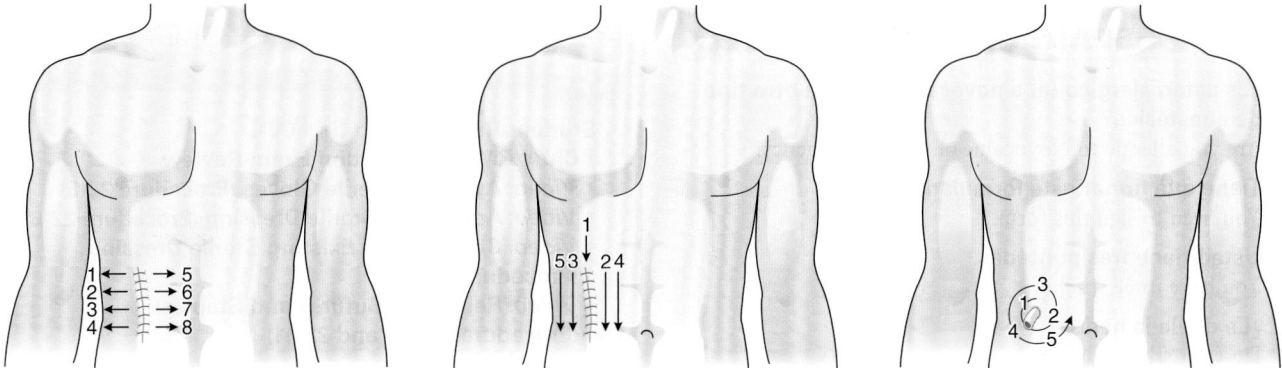

**Figure 22-13** • Clean a wound outward from the site following any of the numbered patterns shown here.

sterile transfer forceps with clean hands, clean the area in a circular motion away from the wound or in straight wipes away from the suture line (Fig. 22-13). The wipe is discarded after each sweep, and a new one is used for the next sweep across the area. Either a sterile disposable suture removal kit, which contains all of the equipment needed for suture removal (Fig. 22-14), or sterile reusable equipment may be used (Procedure 22-10).

Following hospital surgery, some incisions are closed with metal staples rather than sutures. Patients often leave the hospital before the staples can be removed safely and return later to the physician's office to have them removed. Frequently, it will be your responsibility to remove the staples. Most offices use staple removal kits similar to the kits supplied for suture removal. Included in the staple removal kit is a special instrument for removing the staples instead of suture scissors. Procedure 22-11 describes the process for removing staples.

## CHECKPOINT QUESTION

8. What methods may be used to excise lesions in the medical office?

## ROLE-PLAYING ACTIVITY

Role-play the following scenario with another student, alternating the role of patient and physician using different verbal and nonverbal language. Call the "patient" to the exam room, and after verifying their identity, reinforce the reason for the visit today as having an incision and drainage of a lesion on the right posterior thigh area. The patient has never had any type of surgery before today and is very nervous about having this done. The "patient" should express this anxiety using verbal and nonverbal communication. The "medical assistant" should offer explanations using calm and reassuring verbal and nonverbal communication, avoiding giving false hope or advice that could be perceived as practicing medicine. Switch roles and assume the same scenario, perhaps with different personalities. Debrief after role-playing to discuss any concerns or suggestions. Your instructor will give you additional information about this activity!

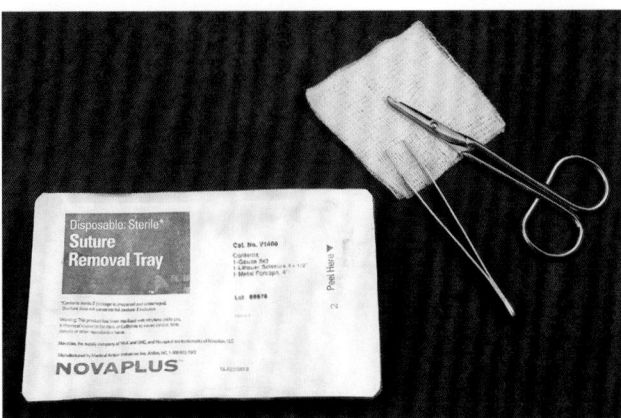

**Figure 22-14** • A disposable suture removal kit.

## *español* SPANISH TERMINOLOGY

**¿Es usted alérgico (a) a novocaína o algún otro tipo de anestésico?**
Are you allergic to Novocaine or other anesthetics?

**Tiene que firmar este formulario.**
You need to sign this form.

**Usted tiene tres puntadas.**
You have three stitches.

**¿Le duele la herida?**
Do your stitches hurt?

**Regrese a la oficina el lunes.**
Return to the office on Monday.

**El doctor usó un material que se deshace solo.**
The doctor used absorbable suture; it will dissolve.

**¿Es usted alérgico (a) to Iodo?**
Are you allergic to iodine?

**Su vendaje necesita estar seco por tres días, si se baña debe protejerlo.**
The dressing needs to be dry for three days; if you shower, you must protect it.

**Si usted nota que la herida está muy irritada, le duele y nota secreción, tiene que llamarnos.**
You have to call us if the wound looks very red, is painful, and has discharge.

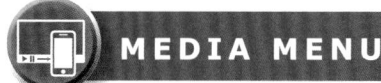

## MEDIA MENU

**Student Resources** on thePoint®
- **CMA/RMA Certification Exam Review**
- *Video:* **Applying Sterile Gloves (Procedure 22-5)**
- *Video:* **Applying a Sterile Dressing (Procedure 22-6)**
- *Video:* **Changing an Existing Sterile Dressing (Procedure 22-7)**
- *Video:* **Removing Sutures and Staples (Procedures 22-10 and 22-11)**

**Internet Resources**
**American Society of Plastic Surgeons**
http://www.plasticsurgery.org
**American Society for Dermatologic Surgery**
http://www.asds.net
**Center for Laser Surgery**
http://www.lasersurgery.com
**The Association for the Advancement of Wound Care**
http://www.aawconline.org

## EMR Activity

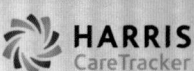

Harris CareTracker is a Web-based electronic medical record (EMR) application that you will use for the EMR activities included in this section at the end of each chapter. This application is actually used in physician offices but is provided to you through the publisher, Wolters Kluwer Health, to give you hands-on practice working with EMRs. Your instructor will have more information about accessing your username, log-in, and Quickstart guide.

Prerequisite Activities in Harris CareTracker

- *The Getting Started and Quickstart documents and EMR Activities Step-by-Step Instructions are available at* http://thePoint.lww.com/KronenbergerComp5e.
- *Note: You must first enter the patient into the EMR as a new patient before completing the following EMR activity as given in the EMR Step-by-Step Instructions.*

Activity Details

Accurately document a follow-up about today's visit in the *Medical Record* module, *Progress Notes* application of the EMR for new patient Lawrence Black, who recently had a sebaceous cyst removed from his back. The patient c/o feeling achy with particular soreness at the surgical site. You note the incision edges are well approximated but appear to be red and slightly swollen.

## Chapter Summary

- With the spiraling costs of health care, many procedures that were once performed only in hospitals are now being performed in medical offices.
- As a medical assistant, you will be required to become more proficient in minor surgical procedures as offices change to meet the needs of the patients. Continuing education, research, and on-the-job training will keep you current on the changes in the field of surgery and in the new equipment that is used during minor office surgical procedures.
- No matter how technical or sophisticated the surgical procedure or equipment, you must not forget the feelings of apprehension many patients have. Although it is your responsibility to prepare the treatment room and assist the physician, you are also obligated to instruct the patient accurately on any presurgical preparations, obtain third-party authorization if necessary, reassure the patient during the procedure, and give the patient accurate information about postsurgical care as ordered by the physician.
- After the procedure, you must disinfect the examination room and prepare it for future patients.

## Warm-Ups for Critical Thinking

1. Dr. Brown has just informed Mrs. Levine that she should return tomorrow for office surgery. While you are alone with the patient, Mrs. Levine begins to cry and expresses great concern about the procedure. What should you do?
2. Refer to an anatomy book and review the anatomy of a hair follicle. Why are skin nicks more likely if the hair is shaved in the opposite direction of its natural growth?
3. Why is it preferable for infected wounds to heal with delayed or unclosed surface edges?
4. Prepare a patient education sheet outlining postoperative wound care.
5. This morning, you are assisting Dr. Patrick with an ingrown toenail removal. When the patient arrives, you notice that the consent form has not been signed. The patient agrees to sign the consent form but indicates that he has some questions about the risks involved. Should you let him sign the consent? Why or why not? What would you do?

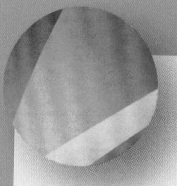

## **PSY** PROCEDURE 22-1

# Opening Sterile Surgical Packs

**PSY** Prepare a sterile field.

**Purpose:** Open sterile packages without contaminating the contents

**Equipment:** Surgical pack and surgical or Mayo stand

| STEPS | REASONS |
|---|---|
| 1. Wash your hands. | Hand washing aids in infection control. Your hands should be clean for this procedure. |
| 2. Verify the procedure to be performed and remove the appropriate tray or item from the storage area. Check the label for contents and expiration date. Check the package for tears and moisture. | Packages that have passed the expiration date should not be used. Moist or torn areas contaminate the contents of the package. |
| 3. Place the package, with the label facing up, on a clean, dry, flat surface such as a Mayo or surgical stand. | Although the field will be protected by a barrier undersurface, microorganisms must be kept at a minimum by using an area as free of pathogens as possible. The surgical stand makes it easy to move the field for the physician's convenience. |
| 4. Without tearing the wrapper, carefully remove the sealing tape. With commercial packages, carefully remove the outer protective wrapper. | Many disposable packages are wrapped in clear plastic film that will become the sterile field when properly opened. Packages prepared in the office are sealed with autoclave tape, which should clearly indicate that the package has been through the autoclave. |
| 5. Loosen the first flap of the folded wrapper by pulling it up, out, and away; let it fall over the far side of the table or stand. | This prevents you from having to reach across the sterile field again. |

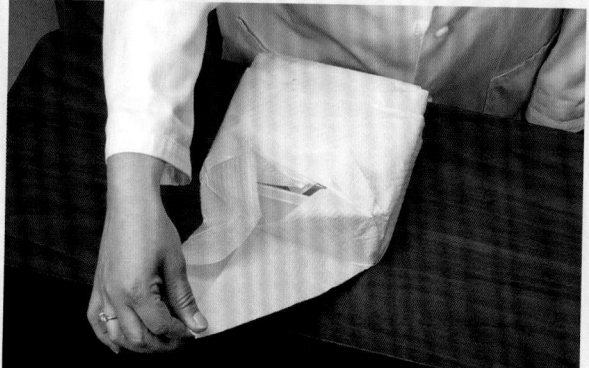

Step 5. Open the first flap away from you.

*(continues on page 548)*

## PROCEDURE 22-1 (continued)

| STEPS | REASONS |
|---|---|

6. Open the side flaps in a similar manner, using your left hand for the left flap and your right hand for the right flap. Touch only the unsterile outer surface; do not touch the sterile inner surface.

This method minimizes your movement over the sterile areas of the package.

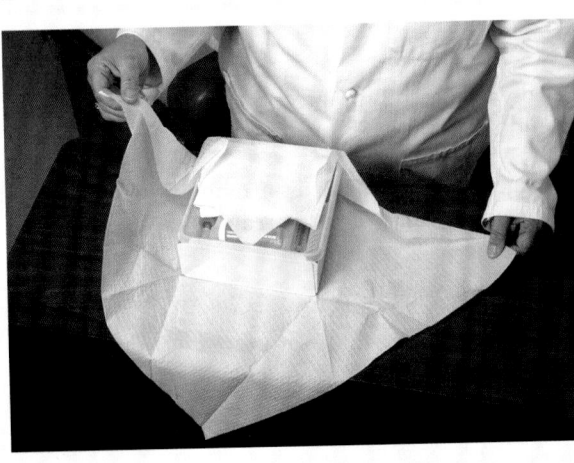

**Step 6.** Open the side flaps.

7. Pull the remaining flap down and toward you by grasping the outside surface only. The outer surface of the wrapper is now against the surgical stand; the sterile inside of the wrapper forms the sterile field.

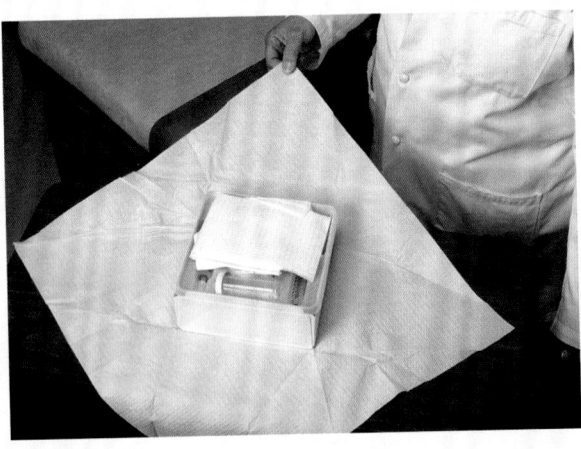

**Step 7.** Pull the remaining flap down and toward you.

8. Repeat Steps 5 to 7 for packages with a second or inside wrapper. This wrapper also provides a sterile field upon which to work. The field is now ready for the procedure to begin.

## PROCEDURE 22-1 (continued)

| STEPS | REASONS |
|---|---|
| 9. If you must leave the area after opening the field, cover the tray and its contents with a sterile drape. Without leaving or turning your back on the sterile setup area, open the sterile drape and carefully lift it out of the package by the edges without contaminating it. Carefully lay the drape over the sterile field, working from your body out so that your arms do not cross the uncovered sterile field but do cross the drape that has been placed over the tray. | Leaving or turning your back on a sterile field makes the sterile field contaminated. |

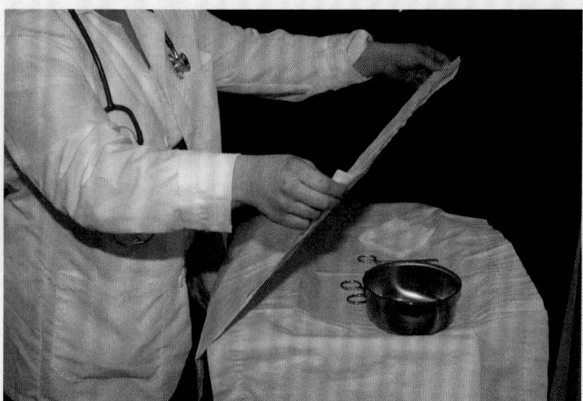

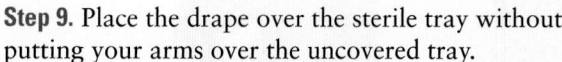

**Step 9.** Place the drape over the sterile tray without putting your arms over the uncovered tray.

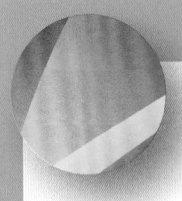

## PSY PROCEDURE 22-2

# Using Sterile Transfer Forceps

**Purpose:** Use sterile transfer forceps without contamination during a sterile setup

**Equipment:** Sterile transfer forceps in a container with sterilization solution, a sterile field, and sterile items to be transferred

| STEPS | REASONS |
|---|---|
| 1. Slowly lift the forceps straight up and out of the container without touching the outside of the container or its inside above the level of the solution. | The area above the soaking solution and the rim are considered not sterile. |
| 2. Hold the forceps with the tips down at all times. | This prevents the solution from running toward the unsterile handles and then back to the grasping blades and tips, which would contaminate them. |

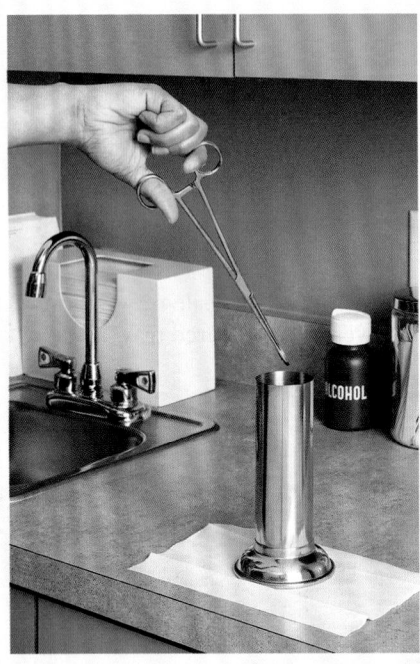

**Step 2.** The tips of the forceps should be held in a downward position.

| STEPS | REASONS |
|---|---|
| 3. Keep the forceps above waist level. | This prevents accidental and unnoticed contamination. |
| 4. With the forceps, pick up the articles to be transferred and drop them onto the sterile field, but do not let the forceps come into contact with the sterile field. | The forceps may be moist from the soaking solution, which may wick microorganisms from the surface below onto the sterile field. Note: Transfer forceps that have been wrapped and autoclaved may be placed with tips on the sterile field and handles extending beyond the 1-inch border that is considered contaminated. Doing this allows you to move objects around the field for the physician's convenience. |

# PROCEDURE 22-2 (continued)

| STEPS | REASONS |
|---|---|
| 5. Carefully place the forceps back in the sterilization solution. | The sterilization solution in the forceps container keeps the tips of the forceps sterile for future use. The solution should be changed at least daily or according to office policy. |

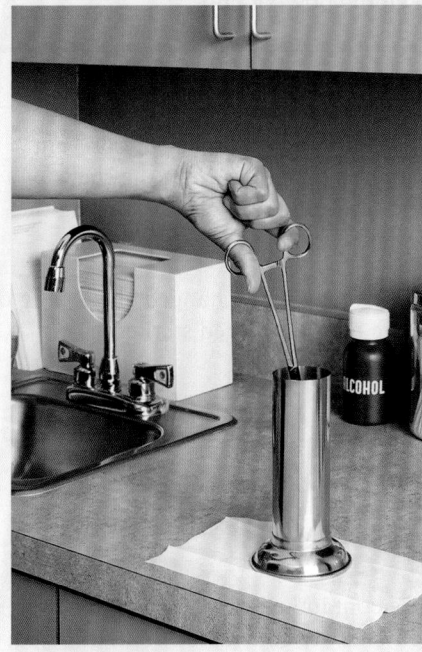

**Step 5.** Put the forceps into the container without contaminating them.

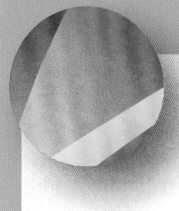

## PSY PROCEDURE 22-3

# Adding Sterile Solution to a Sterile Field

**PSY** Prepare a sterile field; perform within a sterile field.

**Purpose:** Pour a sterile solution into a container on the sterile field without contamination

**Equipment:** Sterile setup, container of sterile solution, and sterile bowl or cup

| STEPS | REASONS |
|---|---|
| 1. As with any drug or medication, identify the correct solution by carefully reading the label. If necessary, use the sterile transfer forceps and place the sterile bowl or cup on the sterile field. | The label should be checked three times to prevent errors: when taking the container from the shelf, before pouring the solution, and when returning the container to the shelf. |
| 2. Check the expiration date on the label; do not use the solution if it is out of date, if the label cannot be read, or if the solution appears abnormal. Sterile water and saline bottles must be dated when opened and must be discarded if not used within 48 hours. | Out-of-date solutions may have changed chemically or deteriorated and are not considered sterile. |
| 3. If you are adding medication, such as lidocaine, to the solution, show the medication label to the physician now. | This allows for verification of the contents. |
| 4. Remove the cap or stopper. Hold the cap with your fingertips, with the cap opening down to prevent contamination of the inside of the cap. If you must put the cap down, place it on a side table (not the sterile field) with the open end up. If you are pouring the entire contents onto the sterile field, discard the cap. Retain the bottle to keep track of the amount added to the field and for charting later. It can then be discarded. | If the cap becomes contaminated and is returned to the bottle, the contents are considered contaminated. Placing the cap on a surface with the opening up prevents contamination of the interior of the cap. |

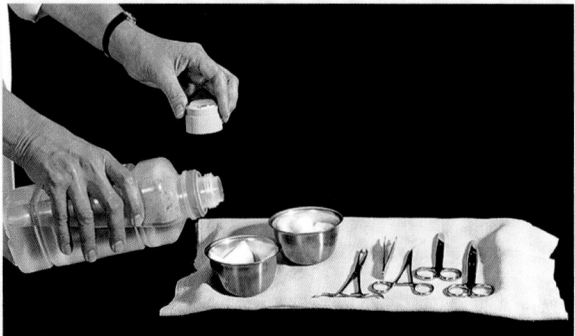

**Step 4.** Hold the cap facing downward to prevent contamination of the inside.

## PROCEDURE 22-3 (continued)

| STEPS | REASONS |
|---|---|
| **5.** Grasp the container with the label against the palm of your hand (known as palming the label). | If solution runs down the side of the bottle in this position, it will not obscure the label. |

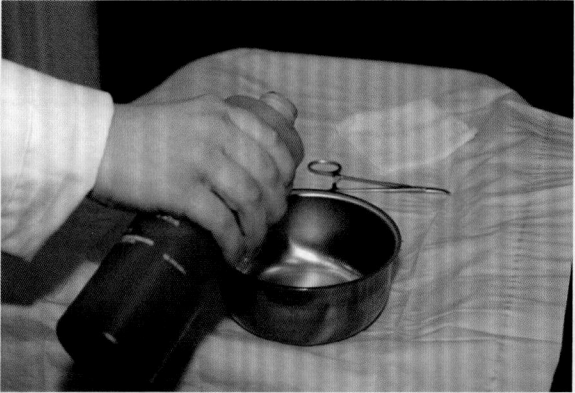

**Step 5.** Hold the bottle of sterile solution with the label in your palm.

| STEPS | REASONS |
|---|---|
| **6.** Pour a small amount of the solution into a separate container or waste receptacle. | The lip of the bottle is considered contaminated; pouring off this small amount cleanses the lip. |
| **7.** Without reaching across the sterile field, carefully and slowly pour the desired amount of solution into the sterile container from not less than 4 and not more than 6 inches above the container. The bottle of solution should never touch the sterile container or tray, as this will cause contamination. | Pouring the solution slowly reduces the chance of splashing and overfilling. Solution poured too fast or from an improper height may splash. Touching the container to objects on the sterile field contaminates the field. If the solution splashes onto the field, wicking will cause contamination from the surface below. |
| **8.** After pouring the desired amount of solution into the sterile container, recheck the label for the contents and expiration date and replace the cap carefully, without touching the bottle rim with any unsterile surface of the cap. | This ensures accuracy. Careful replacement of the cap ensures that the contents remain sterile. |
| **9.** Return the solution to its proper storage area or discard the container after checking the label again. | You will have checked the solution label a total of three times to avoid errors. |

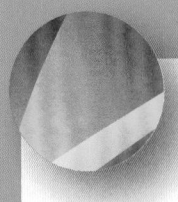

## **PSY** PROCEDURE 22-4

# Performing Hair Removal and Skin Preparation

**PSY** Instruct and prepare a patient for a procedure or a treatment.

**Purpose:** Prepare the skin by removing any hair and applying an antiseptic solution before a surgical procedure

**Equipment:** Nonsterile gloves; shave cream, lotion, or soap; new disposable razor; gauze or cotton balls; warm water; antiseptic; and sponge forceps

| STEPS | REASONS |
|---|---|
| 1. Wash your hands. | Hand washing aids infection control. |
| 2. Assemble the equipment. | This ensures that all supplies are available. A new razor must be used for each patient to prevent the transmission of pathogens and to ensure the closest possible shave. |
| 3. Greet and identify the patient. Explain the procedure and answer any questions. | This prevents errors in treatment, helps gain compliance, and eases anxiety. |
| 4. Put on gloves and prepare the patient's skin: <br> **A.** For shaving, apply shaving cream or soapy lather to the area. Pull the skin taut and shave by pulling the razor across the skin in the direction of hair growth. Repeat this procedure until all hair is removed from the operative area. Rinse and thoroughly pat the shaved area dry with a gauze square. <br> **B.** If the patient's skin is not to be shaved, wash and rinse the skin with soap and water and dry the skin thoroughly. | Gloves must be worn when contact with blood or body fluids is possible. Shaving cream or soapy lather on the skin reduces friction and helps prevent scratching. Shaving in the direction of hair growth gives the closest shave while reducing the chance of nicking the skin. Rinsing removes soap residue and hair from the shaved area. Pat dry rather than rub to prevent abrasions. Using gauze squares for drying picks up stray hairs that might have been left behind during rinsing. |
| 5. Apply antiseptic solution of the physician's choice to the skin surrounding the operative area using sterile gauze sponges, sterile cotton balls, or antiseptic wipes. Holding the gauze or cotton ball in the sterile sponge forceps, wipe the skin in circular motions starting at the operative site and working outward. Discard each sponge after a complete sweep has been made. If the area is large or circles are not appropriate, the sponge may be wiped straight outward from the operative site, then discarded, and the procedure repeated until the entire area has been thoroughly cleaned. At no time should a wipe that has passed over the skin be returned to the cleaned area or to the antiseptic solution. | Discarding sponges after each stroke prevents contamination of the wound by microorganisms brought back to the area from the surrounding skin. |
| 6. Holding dry sterile gauze sponges in the sponge forceps, thoroughly pat the area dry. In some instances, the area may be allowed to air-dry. | Moist skin may moisten the sterile drapes, causing wicking and contaminating the site. |
| 7. Instruct the patient not to touch or cover the prepared area. | This avoids contaminating the operative site, which would require repeating the procedure. |

## PROCEDURE 22-4 (continued)

| STEPS | REASONS |
|---|---|
| 8. **AFF** Explain how to respond to a patient who is developmentally challenged. | To avoid injury to the patient, assess for safety before completing a procedure when there is the possibility that the patient may not cooperate. |
| 9. Inform the physician that the patient is ready for the procedure. Drape the prepared area with a sterile drape if the physician will be delayed for more than 10 or 15 minutes or if the sterile tray will be unattended for any length of time. | |

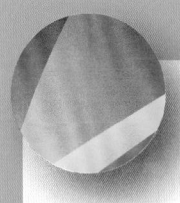

**PSY** PROCEDURE 22-5

## Applying Sterile Gloves

**Purpose:** Apply prepackaged sterile gloves without contamination
**Equipment:** One package of sterile gloves in the appropriate size

| STEPS | REASONS |
|---|---|
| 1. Remove rings and other jewelry. | Rings may pierce the gloves and contaminate the procedure. |
| 2. Wash your hands. | Wearing gloves is not a substitute for hand washing but must be done in addition to it. |
| 3. Place the prepackaged gloves on a clean, dry, flat, surface with the cuffed end toward you. | Sterile gloves are packaged for ease of application in this fashion. |

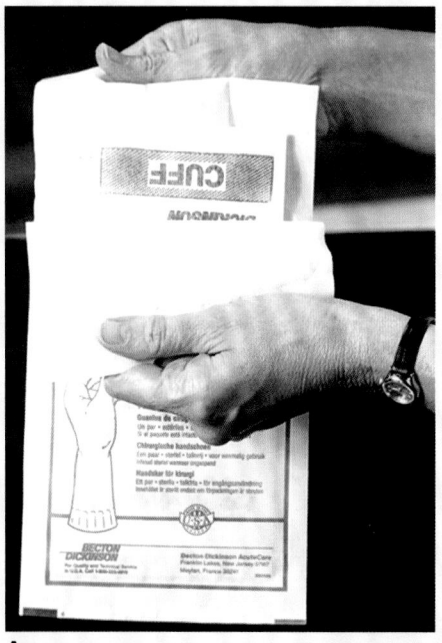

A

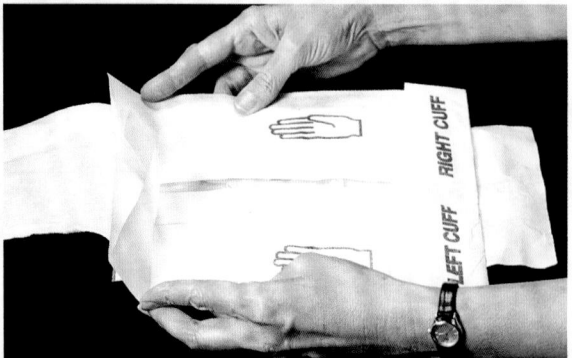

B

Step 3. (**A**) Pull the outer wrapping apart to expose the sterile inner wrap. (**B**) With the cuffs toward you, fold back the inner wrap to expose the gloves.

## PROCEDURE 22-5 (continued)

| STEPS | REASONS |
|---|---|
| **4.** Grasping the edges of the outer paper, open the package out to its fullest. | The inner surface of the package is a sterile field. |

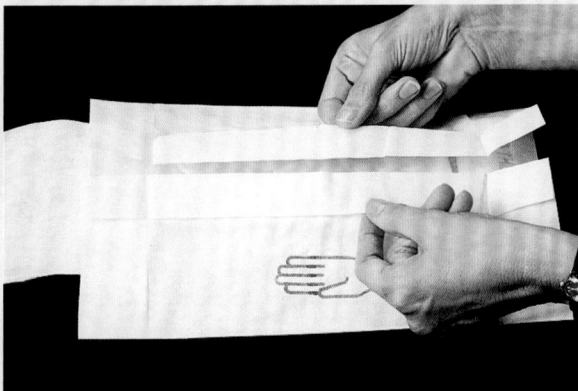

**A**

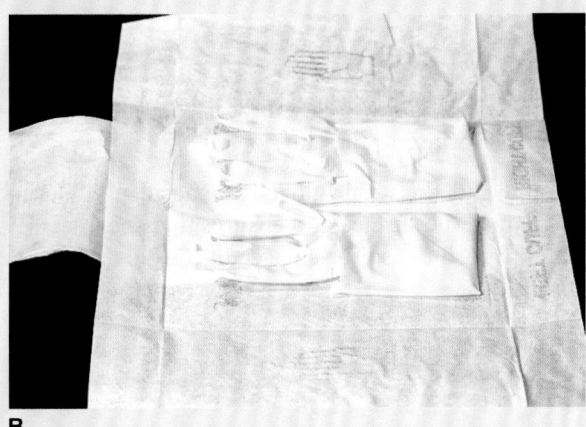

**B**

**Step 4. (A and B)** Grasp the edges and open the packages.

| | |
|---|---|
| **5.** Using your nondominant hand, pick up the dominant hand glove by grasping the folded edge of the cuff and lifting it up and away from the paper. The folded edge of the cuff is contaminated as soon as it is touched with the ungloved hand. Be very careful not to touch the outside surface of the sterile glove with your ungloved hand. | Lift it up and away to avoid letting the fingers of the glove brush an unsterile surface. |

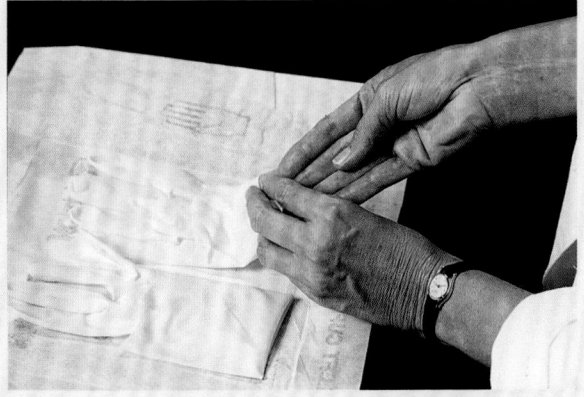

**Step 5.** Using your nondominant hand, lift the cuff of the glove for the dominant hand, touching only the inner surface of the cuff. Curl your thumb inward as you insert your hand.

*(continues on page 558)*

## PROCEDURE 22-5 (continued)

| STEPS | REASONS |
|---|---|
| 6. Curl your fingers and thumb together and insert them into the glove. Then, straighten your fingers and pull the glove on with your nondominant hand still grasping the cuff. | This prevents accidental touching of the outside surface of the glove. |
| 7. Unfold the cuff by pinching the inside surface that will be against your wrist and pulling it toward the wrist. | This ensures that only the unsterile portions are touched by the hands. |

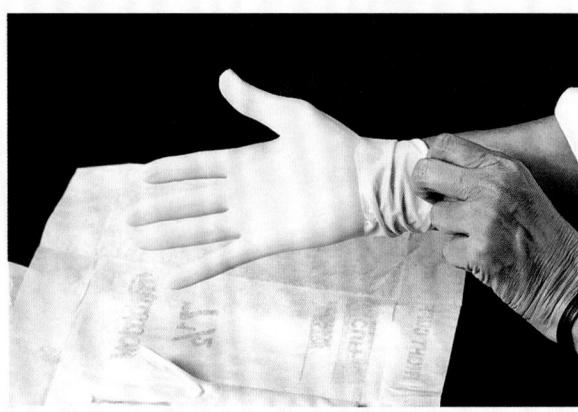

**Step 7.** Pull the glove snugly into place, touching only the inside surface of the cuff.

8. Place the fingers of your gloved hand under the cuff of the remaining glove, lift the glove up and away from the wrapper, and slide your ungloved hand carefully into the glove with your fingers and thumb curled together.

This prevents the sterile glove from accidentally touching an unsterile surface and ensures that the fingers will not brush the sterile surface of the glove.

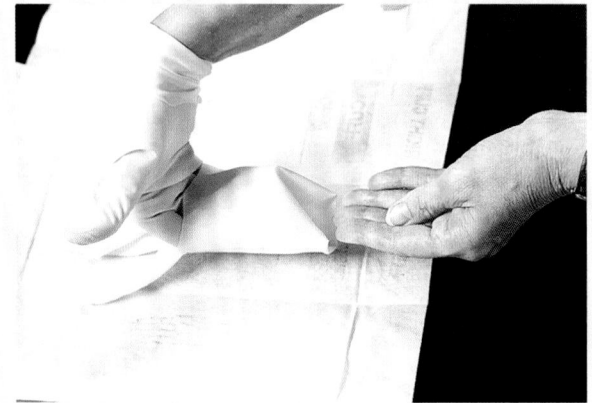

**Step 8.** With your thumb curled, slip the gloved dominant hand into the cuff of the remaining glove.

## PROCEDURE 22-5 (continued)

| STEPS | REASONS |
|---|---|
| 9. Straighten your fingers and pull the glove up and over your wrist by carefully unfolding the cuff. | At all times, sterile must touch sterile only. Folding the cuffs out to their fullest allows the greatest area of sterility. |

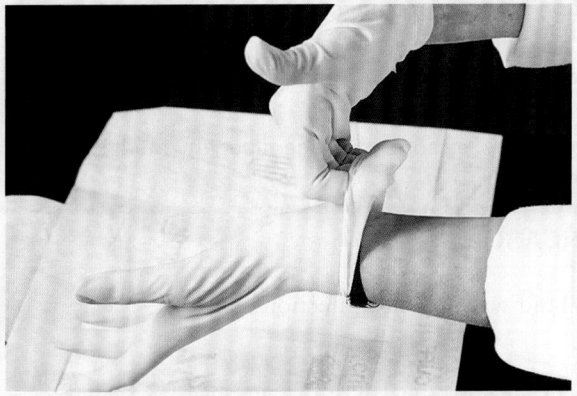

**Step 9.** Unfold the cuff and pull the glove on snugly.

| STEPS | REASONS |
|---|---|
| 10. Settle the gloves comfortably onto your fingers by lacing your fingers together and adjusting the tension over your hands. | The gloves should fit snugly without wrinkles or areas that bind the fingers. |

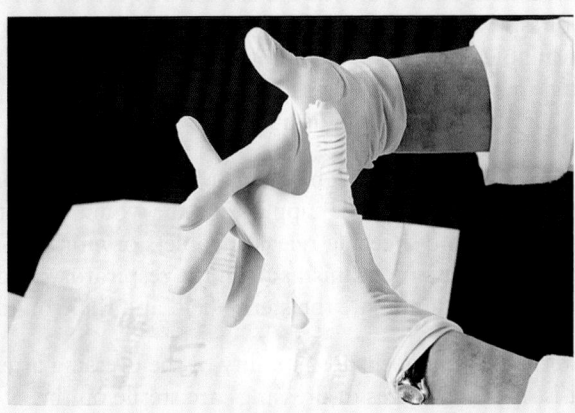

**Step 10.** Adjust the fingers for a comfortable fit.

| STEPS | REASONS |
|---|---|
| 11. Remove contaminated sterile gloves exactly as you would remove contaminated nonsterile gloves and discard them appropriately. | If removed correctly, one glove will be balled into the other with no opportunity to touch the soiled area of either glove. |

*(continues on page 560)*

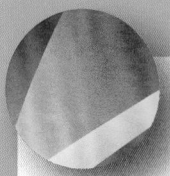

**PSY** Procedure 22-6

## Applying a Sterile Dressing

**PSY** Instruct and prepare a patient for a procedure or a treatment; prepare a sterile field; perform within a sterile field; perform wound care; demonstrate proper disposal of biohazardous material, sharps and regulated waste; coach patients appropriately considering cultural diversity, developmental life stage, and communication barriers; document patient care accurately in the medical record.

**Purpose:** Using sterile dressings and sterile technique, apply a sterile dressing to a surgical wound without contamination

**Equipment:** Sterile gloves, sterile gauze dressings, scissors, bandage tape, any medication to be applied to the wound if ordered by the physician

| STEPS | REASONS |
|---|---|
| 1. Wash your hands and assemble the necessary supplies. | Hand washing aids infection control. |
| 2. Assemble the equipment and supplies. | This ensures that all of the supplies are available before beginning the procedure. |
| 3. Greet and identify the patient. Ask about any allergies before selecting tape. With the size of the dressing in mind, cut or tear lengths off to secure the dressing. Set the tape aside in a convenient place. | Patients must be identified to prevent errors in tape treatment. Some patients are sensitive to certain tape adhesives. Many types of hypoallergenic tape are available. Having tape cut and prepared saves time and may prevent the dressing from slipping while tape is cut after the dressing is applied. |
| 4. Explain the procedure and instruct the patient to remain still during the procedure and to avoid coughing, sneezing, and talking until the procedure is complete. | Unexpected movements by the patient may result in contamination of the sterile supplies and the wound. Talking, coughing, and sneezing release droplets of moisture-containing microorganisms from the respiratory tract that may contaminate the sterile field and the wound. |
| 5. Open the dressing pack to create a sterile field, leaving the sterile dressing on the inside of the opened package. Observe the principles of surgical asepsis. Many packets are designed to be peeled apart. | Sterile technique ensures sterility of the dressing after it is open. Packages of dressings are sterile on the inside; if opened properly, the inner surface may be used as a sterile field. |

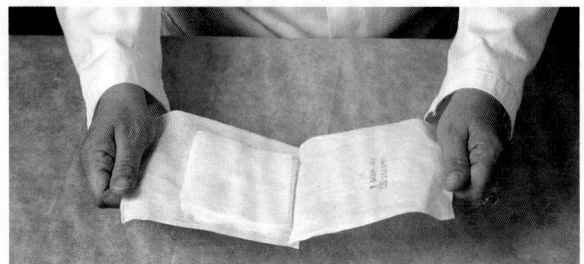

**Step 5.** Open the sterile dressing pack or packs.

6. To maintain sterility:
   **A.** If sterile gloves are to be used, open the appropriate package of gloves. Using sterile technique, put on the gloves before touching any sterile items.
   **B.** If using sterile transfer forceps to apply the dressing (the no-touch method), use sterile technique to arrange the dressing on the wound, and do not touch the dressing or the site with the hands.

Sterile items may only be touched with sterile gloves *or* sterile transfer forceps.

**PROCEDURE 22-6** (continued)

| STEPS | REASONS |
|---|---|

**7.** If ordered by the physician, apply topical medication to the sterile dressing that will directly cover the wound, being careful not to touch the end of the medication bottle or tube to the dressing.

The outside end of the medication bottle or tube may not be sterile.

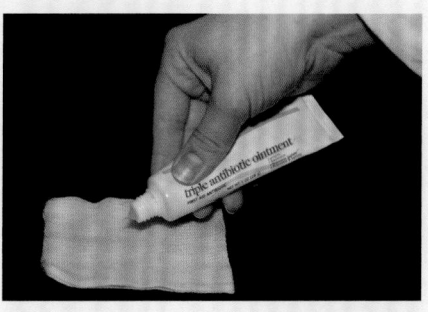

**Step 7.** Apply medication if ordered without touching the end of the container to the dressing.

**8.** Using the already opened sterile dressings and sterile technique, apply the number of dressings necessary to cover and protect the wound. Sterile dressings must be carefully placed on the wound and not allowed to drag over the skin.

If the dressing is dragged over the skin, it will be contaminated by microorganisms from the surrounding skin and may cause infection.

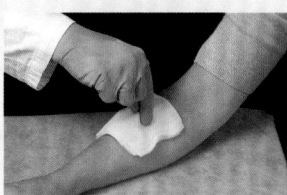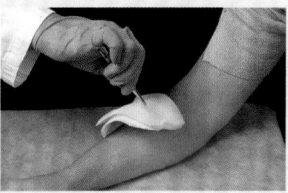

**Step 8.** Using sterile gloves (*left*). Using sterile forceps (*right*).

**9.** Apply the previously cut lengths of tape over the dressing to secure it, but avoid overuse of tape. When the wound is completely covered, you may remove your gloves or keep them on while you tape the dressing. Discard the gloves in the proper receptacle.

Tape is used only to keep the dressing in place. It should allow observation of any bleeding or drainage. Too much tape can cause perspiration that will dampen the dressing and compromise sterility. Tape should not obstruct blood circulation. Excessive tape also must later be removed, which may hurt.
A bandage may be applied over the dressing to hold it in place, add support, or immobilize the area.

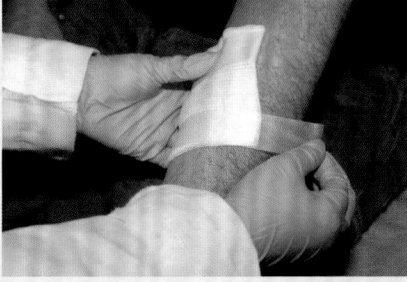

**A**

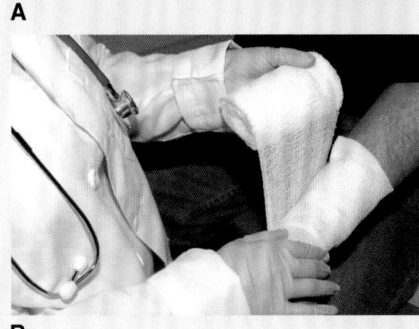

**B**

**Step 9.** (**A**) Securing a dressing with tape. (**B**) Securing a dressing with a bandage.

*(continues on page 562)*

## PROCEDURE 22-6 (continued)

| STEPS | REASONS |
|---|---|
| **10.** When the patient is to change dressings at home, provide appropriate instructions. Dressings should be kept clean and dry and changed when wet or soiled. Otherwise, dressings should be changed as instructed by the physician. Make sure patients understand the signs of infection, such as redness, swelling, pain, or undue warmth at the site, and instruct them to call the office at once if these appear. Also say what to do in case of excessive bleeding or drainage and how to manage any drains. | Microorganisms may be transported to the wound by capillary action if the dressing is wet or soiled. |
| **11.** **AFF** Explain how to respond to a patient who is visually impaired. | Face the patient when speaking and always let him or her know what you are going to do before touching him or her. Give the patient written and oral instructions. Confirm instructions with caregiver. |
| **12.** Wearing clean examination gloves, properly dispose of or care for equipment and supplies. Disposable articles contaminated with wound drainage or blood go into a biohazard container. Clean the work area, remove your gloves, and wash your hands. | Follow standard precautions. |
| **13.** Return reusable supplies (unopened sterile gloves or dressings, tape) to their appropriate storage areas; all others should be discarded correctly. | Unopened supplies should be returned to the appropriate storage areas for reuse. Discarding uncontaminated reusables is wasteful. |
| **14.** Record the procedure. | Procedures are considered not to have been done if they are not recorded in the patient's medical record. |

---

**Charting Example:**
*10/14/2016 4:45 PM DSD applied to surgical wound (L) anterior forearm. No bleeding from incision, edges well approximated with 4 sutures intact. Pt. given verbal and written instructions on dressing change and wound care at home. To RTO in 5 days for suture removal* _____ R. Long, CMA

---

**Note:** *The medical assistant may sign his or her name in the patient record using only the "CMA" credential if the office has a signature log denoting the entire credential as "CMA(AAMA)."*

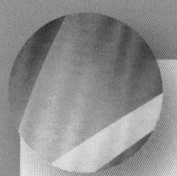

**PSY** PROCEDURE 22-7

# Changing an Existing Sterile Dressing

**PSY** Instruct and prepare a patient for a procedure or a treatment; prepare a sterile field; perform within a sterile field; perform wound care; perform a dressing change; demonstrate proper disposal of biohazardous material, sharps and regulated waste; coach patients appropriately considering cultural diversity, developmental life stage, and communication barriers; document patient care accurately in the medical record.

**Purpose:** Carefully remove an existing dressing from a wound and cover it with a sterile dressing using sterile technique

**Equipment:** Sterile gloves, nonsterile gloves, sterile dressing, prepackaged skin antiseptic swabs or sterile antiseptic solution in a sterile basin and sterile cotton balls or gauze, tape, and approved biohazard container

| STEPS | REASONS |
|---|---|
| 1. Wash your hands and assemble the necessary supplies. | Hand washing aids infection control. |
| 2. Assemble the equipment and supplies. | This ensures that all supplies are available before you begin the procedure. |
| 3. Greet and identify the patient. Explain the procedure and answer any questions. | This prevents errors in treatment, helps gain compliance, and eases anxiety. |
| 4. Prepare a sterile field, including opening sterile dressings. If using a sterile container and solution, open the package containing the sterile basin and use the inside of the wrapper as the sterile field for the basin. Flip the sterile gauze or cotton balls into the basin and appropriately pour in the antiseptic solution. If using prepackaged antiseptic swabs, carefully open an adequate number for the size of the wound and set them aside without contaminating them. | Opening sterile supplies after applying sterile gloves will cause contamination of your gloves and your supplies. |
| 5. Instruct the patient not to talk, cough, sneeze, laugh, or move during the procedure. | Respiratory droplets may contaminate the sterile field. Movement may cause accidental contamination of the field. |
| 6. Wearing clean gloves, carefully remove the tape from the wound dressing by pulling it toward the wound. Remove the old dressing. Note: If the dressing is difficult to remove because of dried blood, it may be soaked with sterile water or saline for a few minutes to loosen it. Gently pull the edges of the dressing toward the center. Never pull on a dressing that does not come off easily. If this procedure does not sufficiently loosen the dressing or causes undue discomfort to the patient, immediately notify the physician. | Tape pulled away from the direction of the wound may pull the healing edges of the wound apart. |

*(continues on page 564)*

## PROCEDURE 22-7 (continued)

**STEPS**

**REASONS**

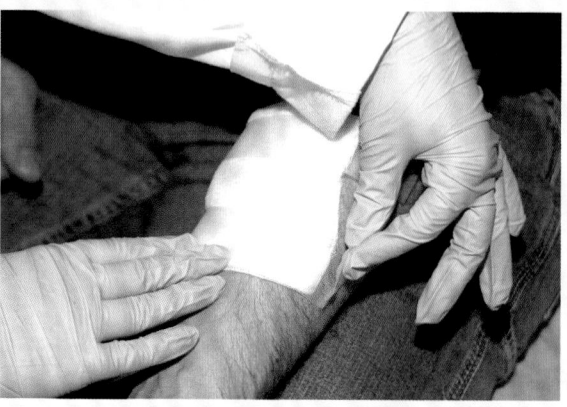

7. Discard the soiled dressing into a biohazard container. Do not pass it over the sterile field.

8. Inspect the wound for degree of healing, amount and type of drainage, appearance of wound edges, and so on.

9. Observing medical asepsis, remove and discard your gloves. The physician may want to inspect the wound before you remove exudate or drainage to determine whether healing is proceeding as expected. If a culture is ordered, the specimen must be taken before the wound is cleaned to ensure the most reliable findings.

10. Using proper technique, put on sterile gloves. Clean the wound with the antiseptic solution ordered by the physician. Clean in a straight motion with the cotton or gauze or the prepackaged antiseptic swab. Discard the wipe (cotton ball, swab) after each stroke and use a fresh sterile one to continue. Never return the wipe to the antiseptic solution or to the skin after one sweep across the area.

11. Remove your gloves and wash your hands.

12. Change the dressing using the procedure for sterile dressing application and using sterile gloves or sterile transfer forceps (Procedure 22-6).

13. **AFF** Explain how to respond to a patient who has dementia.

**Step 6.** Pull the tape toward the wound.

The dressing will be soiled with blood and body fluids and must be considered hazardous. Dressings passed over the sterile field will shed microorganisms and contaminate the area.

The wound is inspected now because wound cleaning removes most exudate. Make a mental note for charting when the procedure is complete.

The wound must be cleaned before fresh dressings are applied. Returning the wipe to the wound area or solution brings microorganisms from the surrounding skin to the open lesion.

Your hands must be washed before you apply the sterile dressing with sterile gloves or sterile forceps.

The old dressing is removed with clean gloves but sterile technique must be used when applying a new sterile dressing.

Solicit assistance from a caregiver or other staff member to help during the procedure. Give simple directions to the patient about what he or she should do. Speak clearly, not loudly.

## PROCEDURE 22-7 (continued)

| STEPS | REASONS |
|---|---|
| **14.** Record the procedure. | Procedures are considered not to have been done if they are not recorded. |

---

Charting Example:

*11/23/2016 11:30 AM Dressing to (R) lower leg changed, small amount of yellow purulent drainage noted____*
*Dr. Blake aware. Wound culture for C&S obtained and sent to Acme laboratory. Wound cleansed with Betadine*
*as ordered; DSD reapplied. Moderate amount of redness and swelling at wound site; edges well approximated.*
*Instructed to RTO in 2 days for C&S results and dressing change _____*
*R. Long, CMA*

---

Note: *The medical assistant may sign his or her name in the patient record using only the "CMA" credential if the office has a signature log denoting the entire credential as "CMA(AAMA)."*

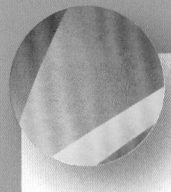

**PSY** PROCEDURE 22-8

## Assisting with Excisional Surgery

**PSY** Instruct and prepare a patient for a procedure or a treatment; prepare a sterile field; perform within a sterile field; perform wound care; demonstrate proper disposal of biohazardous material, sharps and regulated waste; coach patients appropriately considering cultural diversity, developmental life stage, and communication barriers; document patient care accurately in the medical record.

**Purpose:** Prepare for and assist with excisional surgery while maintaining sterile technique

**Equipment:** At the side, sterile gloves, local anesthetic, antiseptic wipes, adhesive tape, and specimen container with completed laboratory request. On the field, basin for solutions, gauze sponges and cotton balls, antiseptic solution, sterile drape, dissecting scissors, disposable scalpel, blade of physician's choice, mosquito forceps, tissue forceps, needle holder, and suture and needle of physician's choice.

| STEPS | REASONS |
|---|---|
| 1. Wash your hands and assemble the necessary supplies. | Hand washing aids infection control. |
| 2. Assemble the equipment. | This ensures that all supplies are available. |
| 3. Greet and identify the patient. Explain the procedure and answer any questions. | This prevents errors in treatment, helps gain compliance, and eases anxiety. |
| 4. Set up a sterile field on a surgical stand with the at-the-side equipment close at hand. Cover the field with a sterile drape until the physician arrives. | Covering the sterile field with a sterile drape will prevent the sterile field from becoming contaminated. |
| 5. Position the patient appropriately. | The required position depends on the location of the lesion. |
| 6. Put on sterile gloves or use sterile transfer forceps and cleanse the patient's skin as described in Procedure 24-4. Some physicians prefer to do this themselves after gloving, using supplies on the field. The physician's preference always takes precedence over any outlined procedure. | The antiseptic discourages the entrance of microorganisms into the wound. After cleansing the skin, remove the gloves, if used, and wash your hands. |
| 7. The physician will perform the procedure; you may be asked to assist. This usually involves adding supplies as needed, watching closely for opportunities to assist the physician, and comforting the patient. | It is not necessary for you to wear sterile gloves during the procedure unless the physician requires you to handle sterile instruments or supplies. |
| 8. If the lesion is to be referred to pathology for analysis, you will be required to assist with collecting the specimen in an appropriate container. | Always follow standard precautions, wearing examination gloves when handling specimens. Have the container ready to receive the specimen. |
| 9. At the end of the procedure, wash your hands and dress the wound using sterile technique (Procedure 22-6). | The wound must be covered to protect the incision from contamination. |
| 10. **AFF** Explain how to respond to a patient who is hearing impaired. | Make sure the patient can see your face as you are speaking. Speak clearly, not loudly. |

## PROCEDURE 22-8 (continued)

| STEPS | REASONS |
|---|---|
| 11. Thank the patient and give appropriate instructions for care of the operative site, changing the dressing, postoperative medications, and follow-up visits as ordered by the physician. | Courtesy encourages the patient to have a positive attitude about the physician's office. |
| 12. Wearing gloves, clean the examining room in preparation for the next patient. Discard all used disposables in appropriate biohazard containers. Return unused items to their proper places. Remove your gloves and wash your hands. | Standard precautions must be followed. |

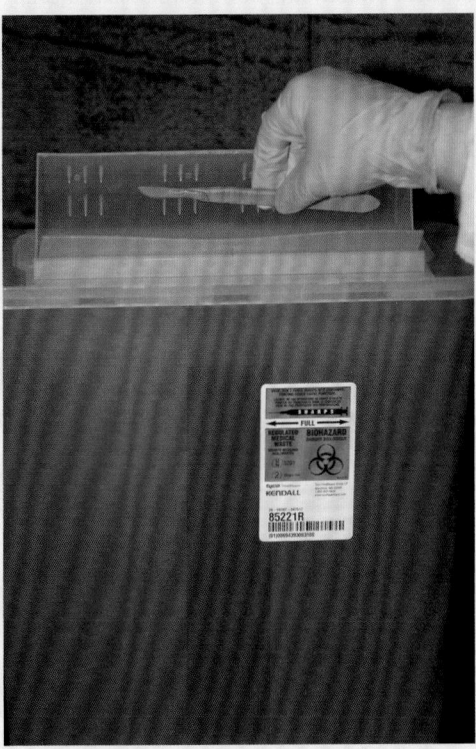

**Step 11.** Discard any disposable sharp items, such as a scalpel, into the appropriate biohazard container.

| | |
|---|---|
| 13. Record the procedure. | Procedures not recorded in the patient record are not considered to have been done. |

Charting Example:
*09/19/2016 8:45 AM Mole to posterior (L) shoulder removed per Dr. Snider. Specimen sent to Acme lab. T 98.4 (O), P 96, R 20, BP 134/78 (R) sitting. 4 × 4 DSD applied to surgical incision; minimal sanguineous drainage noted. Pt. given verbal and written instructions on wound care, postop antibiotics, pain medication, and follow-up visits. Verbalized understanding. To RTO × 2 days for drsg change* _____
*R. Long, CMA*

Note: *The medical assistant may sign his or her name in the patient record using only the "CMA" credential if the office has a signature log denoting the entire credential as "CMA(AAMA)."*

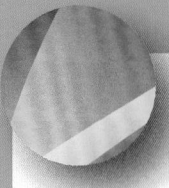

## PSY PROCEDURE 22-9

### Assisting with Incision and Drainage (I&D)

**PSY** Instruct and prepare a patient for a procedure or a treatment; prepare a sterile field; perform within a sterile field; perform wound care; demonstrate proper disposal of biohazardous material, sharps and regulated waste; coach patients appropriately considering cultural diversity, developmental life stage, and communication barriers; document patient care accurately in the medical record.

**Purpose:** Prepare for and assist with an incision and drainage procedure while maintaining sterile technique

**Equipment:** At the side, sterile gloves, local anesthetic, needle and syringe if not placed on sterile field, antiseptic wipes, adhesive tape, sterile dressings, packing gauze, and culture tube if the wound may be cultured. On the field, basin for solutions, gauze sponges and cotton balls, antiseptic solution, sterile drape, syringes and needles for local anesthetic, commercial I&D sterile setup or scalpel, dissecting scissors, hemostats, tissue forceps, sterile 4 × 4 gauze sponges, and sterile probe (optional)

## STEPS

The steps for this procedure are similar to those in procedure 22-8. Specifically, you are expected to prepare the surgical field and the patient's surgical area as instructed or preferred by the physician. After the procedure, the wound must be covered to avoid further contamination and to absorb drainage. The exudate is a hazardous body fluid requiring standard precautions. Although a culture and sensitivity may be ordered on the drainage from the infected area, no other specimen is usually collected.

> Charting Example:
> *04/15/2012 11:30 AM Postop VS T 100.4 (O), P 88, R 24, BP 128/88 (R) sitting. 4 × 4 DSD applied to surgical wound on (L) posterior neck. Given verbal and written instructions on wound care, dressing changes, and follow-up. Verbalized understanding* ———————————————————— *R. Long, CMA*

> Note: *The medical assistant may sign his or her name in the patient record using only the "CMA" credential if the office has a signature log denoting the entire credential as "CMA(AAMA)."*

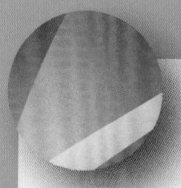

## PSY  PROCEDURE 22-10

# Removing Sutures

**PSY** Instruct and prepare a patient for a procedure or a treatment; prepare a sterile field; perform within a sterile field; perform wound care; demonstrate proper disposal of biohazardous material, sharps and regulated waste; coach patients appropriately considering cultural diversity, developmental life stage, and communication barriers; document patient care accurately in the medical record.

**Purpose:** Using aseptic technique, remove sutures from a wound

**Equipment:** Skin antiseptic, clean exam gloves, sterile gloves, and prepackaged suture removal kit *or* thumb forceps, suture scissors, and 2 × 2 gauze

| STEPS | REASONS |
|---|---|
| 1. Wash your hands and apply clean examination gloves. | Hand washing aids infection control. |
| 2. Assemble the equipment. | This ensures that all supplies are available. |
| 3. Greet and identify the patient. Explain the procedure and answer any questions. | This prevents errors in treatment, helps gain compliance, and eases anxiety. |
| 4. If dressings have not been removed, remove them and properly dispose of them in the biohazard container. Remove your gloves and wash your hands if a soiled dressing was removed. | Always wash your hands after removing gloves. |
| 5. Put on clean examination gloves and cleanse the wound with an antiseptic, such as Betadine, using a new antiseptic gauze for each swipe down the wound and removing any old drainage or blood. | The wound must be as free of pathogens as possible before removal of the sutures to prevent contamination of the wound. |
| 6. Open the suture removal packet using sterile asepsis or set up a field for on-site sterile equipment. Put on sterile gloves. | Suture removal is a sterile procedure. |
| 7. The knots will be tied so that one tail of the knot is very close to the surface of the skin; the other will be closer to the area of suture that is looped over the incision. | |

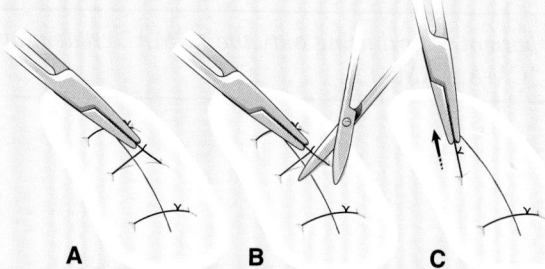

A    B    C

**Step 7. (A)** With the hemostat or thumb forceps, lift the stitch up and away from the skin. **(B)** Cut the stitch near the skin. **(C)** Using the forceps, pull the freed stitch up and out.

*(continues on page 570)*

## PROCEDURE 22-10 (continued)

| STEPS | REASONS |
|---|---|
| **A.** With the thumb forceps, grasp the end of the knot closest to the skin and lift it slightly and gently up from the skin. | |
| **B.** Cut the suture below the knot as close to the skin as possible. | **B.** Cutting below the knot and close to the skin frees the knot at an area that has not been exposed to the outside surface of the body. The only part of the suture that will pull through the tissues will be the suture that was under the skin surface. |
| **C.** Use the thumb forceps to pull the suture out of the skin with a smooth, continuous motion, at a slight angle in the direction of the wound. | C. This prevents tension on the healing tissue. |
| **8.** Place the suture on the gauze sponge. Repeat the procedure for each suture to be removed. | This helps in counting the number removed; if six sutures were inserted and are now to be removed, there should be six sutures on the gauze sponge at the end of the procedure. |
| **9.** Clean the site with an antiseptic solution, and if the physician has so indicated, cover it with a sterile dressing. | Some wounds still need to be protected; some have healed well enough to be left uncovered. |
| **10.** **AFF** Explain how to respond to a patient who is developmentally challenged. | To avoid injury to the patient, assess for safety before completing a procedure when there is the possibility that the patient may not cooperate. |
| **11.** Thank the patient and properly dispose of the equipment and supplies. Clean the work area, remove your gloves, and wash your hands. | Standard precautions must be followed. Courtesy encourages a positive attitude about the physician's office. |
| **12.** Record the procedure, including the time, location of sutures, number removed, and condition of the wound. | Procedures are considered not to have been done if they are not recorded. |

---

**Charting Example:**
*06/26/2012 3:30 PM × 6 sutures removed from (L) ring finger. Wound well approximated, no drainage*
*_____R. Long, RMA*

---

**Note:** *The medical assistant may sign his or her name in the patient record using only the "CMA" credential if the office has a signature log denoting the entire credential as "CMA(AAMA)."*

**PSY** PROCEDURE 22-11

## Removing Staples

**PSY** Instruct and prepare a patient for a procedure or a treatment; demonstrate proper disposal of biohazardous material, sharps and regulated waste; coach patients appropriately considering cultural diversity, developmental life stage, and communication barriers; document patient care accurately in the medical record.

**Purpose:** Using aseptic technique, remove staples from a wound

**Equipment:** Antiseptic solution or wipes, gauze squares, sponge forceps, prepackaged sterile staple removal instrument, examination gloves, and sterile gloves

| STEPS | REASONS |
|-------|---------|
| 1. Wash your hands. | Hand washing aids infection control. |
| 2. Assemble the equipment. | This ensures that all supplies are available. |
| 3. Greet and identify the patient. Explain the procedure and answer any questions. | This prevents errors in treatment, helps gain compliance, and eases anxiety. |
| 4. If the dressing is still in place, put on clean examination gloves and remove it. Dispose of the dressing in a biohazard container. | The dressing is contaminated and must be handled with standard precautions. Remove gloves and wash your hands. |
| 5. Clean the incision with antiseptic solution. Pat dry with sterile gauze sponges. | The incision must be cleaned before removing the staples to avoid infection. If exudate is present, the staples may not be easy to see. |
| 6. Put on sterile gloves. | Staple removal is a sterile procedure. |
| 7. Gently slide the end of the staple remover under each staple to be removed. Press the handles together to lift the ends of the staple out of the skin. | The remover is designed to open the staple so that the ends will lift free and minimize discomfort. |

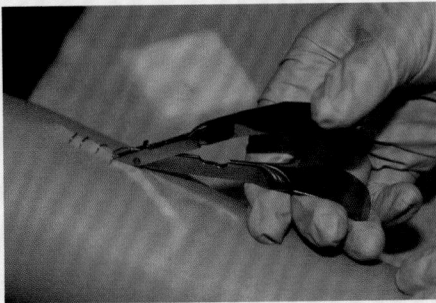

**Step 7.** Slide the end of the staple remover under each staple. Press the handles together to lift the ends of the staple out of the skin.

| | |
|-------|---------|
| 8. Place each staple on a gauze square as it is removed. | This helps in counting the staples at the end of the procedure. |
| 9. When all staples are removed, gently clean the incision as instructed for all procedures. Pat dry and dress the site if ordered to do so by the physician. | The area should be cleaned and dried before any new dressing is applied to avoid wicking microorganisms. Healing may be far enough along to allow the wound to remain uncovered. |
| 10. **AFF** Explain how to respond to a patient who is visually impaired. | Face the patient when speaking and always let him or her know what you are going to do before touching him or her. |

*(continues on page 572)*

## PROCEDURE 22-11 (continued)

| STEPS | REASONS |
| --- | --- |
| 11. Thank the patient and properly care for or dispose of all equipment and supplies. Clean the work area, remove your gloves, and wash your hands. | Standard precautions must be followed. |
| 12. Record the procedure. | Procedures are not considered to have been done if they are not recorded. |

Charting Example:

*3/17/2016 10:30 AM × 15 staples removed from (L) knee incision; edges well approximated, no redness or drainage noted. Wound left open to air as ordered by Dr. Perez* _____
*R. Long, CMA*

Note: *The medical assistant may sign his or her name in the patient record using only the "CMA" credential if the office has a signature log denoting the entire credential as "CMA(AAMA)."*

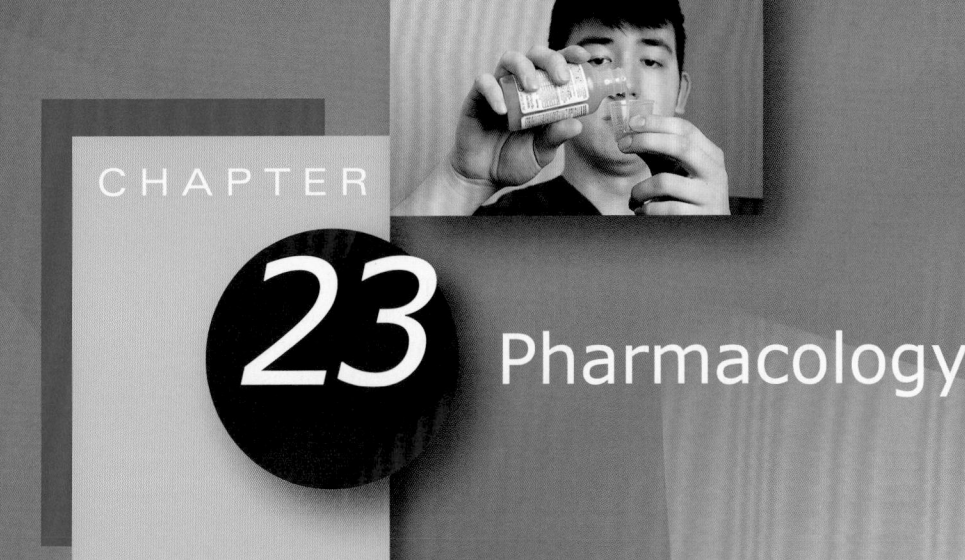

# 23 Pharmacology

## Outline

**Medication Names**
**Legal Regulations**
  Food and Drug Administration
  Drug Enforcement Administration
  Inventory, Storage, Dispensation, and
    Disposal of Medications

**Sources of Drugs**
**Drug Actions and Interactions**
  Pharmacodynamics
  Pharmacokinetics
  Drug Interactions
  Side Effects and Allergies

**Sources of Information**
**Prescriptions**
  Refilling Prescriptions

## Learning Outcomes

**COG Cognitive Domain***

1. Spell and define key terms
2. Describe the relationship between anatomy and physiology of all body systems and medications used for treatment in each
3. Identify chemical, trade, and generic drug names
4. Discuss all levels of governmental legislation and regulation as they apply to medical assisting practice, including FDA and DEA regulations
5. Explain the various drug actions and interactions including pharmacodynamics and pharmacokinetics
6. *Identify the classifications of medications, including indications for use, desired effects, side effects, and adverse reactions*

7. Name the sources for locating information on pharmacology

*\*Note: AAMA/CAAHEP 2015 Standards are italicized.*

**ABHES Competencies**

1. Properly utilize PDR, drug handbook, and other drug references to identify a drug's classification, usual dosage, usual side effects, and contradictions
2. Identify and define common abbreviations that are accepted in prescription writing
3. Understand legal aspects of writing prescriptions, including federal and state laws

## Key Terms

| | | | |
|---|---|---|---|
| allergy | contraindications | pharmacodynamics | side effect |
| anaphylaxis | drug | pharmacokinetics | synergism |
| antagonism | generic name | pharmacology | trade name |
| chemical name | interactions | potentiation | |

## Case Study

*E*laine Black, RMA, is employed in a clinic at Great Falls Medical Center where many patients seek treatment for chronic pain management. There are three physicians in this practice as well as two nurse practitioners, and Elaine rotates between each provider depending on the day of the week and the personal schedules of the providers. Although many of the patients seen at this clinic are established and are seen regularly to treat pain associated with back and neck injuries, car accidents, and osteoarthritis, some are also treated by other physicians for chronic health problems such as hypertension, diabetes, and emphysema. New patients also come into the clinic seeking pain medication, and the clinic management has had to write office policies to address the national problem of substance abuse and patients who are addicted and may be obtaining pain medications from multiple sources. Why is it important for Elaine to ask established and new patients about other medications they may be taking to treat non–pain-related issues? Should Elaine ask patients about the use of vitamins, dietary supplements, and over-the-counter medications? Why or why not? How should Elaine deal with patients suspected of abusing or selling pain medications, but seeking treatment for pain? This chapter addresses the topic of pharmacology and the issues surrounding working with medications as a health care professional.

As a clinical medical assistant, you may be responsible for administering medications under the supervision of the physician. It is important that you acquire knowledge of medications, their uses and potential abuses, range of dosages, methods of administration, and adverse effects. **Pharmacology** is the term given to the study of drugs and their actions, dosages, and side effects. A **drug** is a chemical substance that affects body function or functions. Medications are available in many forms and are administered in various ways to produce therapeutic effects.

## **MEDICATION NAMES**

Most medications have a **chemical name**, a **generic name**, and a **trade name** (Box 23-1). The chemical name is the first name given to any medication. It identifies the chemical components of the drug. The generic name is assigned to the medication during research and development. When the drug is available for commercial use and distribution by the original manufacturer, it is given a brand, or trade, name. The trade name is registered

by the U.S. Patent Office and has the official trademark symbol (™) after its name. After the patent expires, any other company that manufactures the medication may assign its own trade name to the generic equivalent. The first letter of a trade name is always capitalized; generic names begin with lowercase letters.

Drugs can be classified according to their actions and effects on the body. Table 23-1 lists some commonly used drugs, prescription and nonprescription, and their classifications.

### CHECKPOINT QUESTION

1. What is the difference between a drug's chemical name and trade name?

## **LEGAL REGULATIONS**

### Food and Drug Administration

Consumers in the United States are protected by federal regulations regarding the production, prescribing, or dispensing of medications. In 1906, the Pure Food and Drug Act was passed. After being amended in 1938, it required that the safety of a drug be proved before distribution to the public. The amended law was renamed the Federal Food, Drug, and Cosmetic Act. In 1952, the Durham-Humphrey Amendment banned many drugs from being dispensed without a prescription. The Kefauver-Harris Amendment of 1962 required testing of prescription and nonprescription medications for effectiveness before their release for sale. The U.S. Food and Drug Administration (FDA)

| BOX 23-1 | Drug Names |
|---|---|
| Chemical Name | 7-chloro-1,3-dihydro-1-methyl-5-phenyl-2H-1,4-benzodiaxepin-2-one |
| Trade Name | Valium™ |
| Generic Name | Diazepam |

## TABLE 23-1   Classifications of Drugs

| Therapeutic Classification | Effect or Action/Uses | Common Examples |
|---|---|---|
| Adrenergic blocking agents | Affect the alpha receptors of adrenergic nerves | Metoprolol tartrate (Lopressor™), propranolol hydrochloride (Inderal™) |
| Adrenergics | Mimic the activity of the sympathetic nervous system | Epinephrine (Adrenaline™), ephedrine sulfate |
| Analgesics | Used to relieve pain | Aspirin, acetaminophen (Tylenol™), codeine |
| Antacids | Neutralize or reduce the acidity of the stomach | Magnesium (Milk of Magnesia™), calcium carbonate (Tums™) |
| Anthelmintics | Kills parasitic worms | Piperazine citrate, mebendazole (Vermox™) |
| Antianginal agents | Promote vasodilation hydrochloride | Nitroglycerin, diltiazem (Cardizem™) |
| Antianxiety agents | Act on subcortical areas of the brain to relieve symptoms of anxiety | Alprazolam (Xanax™), chlordiazepoxide (Librium™), diazepam (Valium™) |
| Antiarrhythmics | Various actions and effects | Disopyramide (Norpace™), procainamide hydrochloride (Pronestyl™), esmolol (Brevibloc™) |
| Antibiotics | Destroy, interrupt, or interfere with the growth of microorganisms | Penicillin, ampicillin, cefaclor, tetracycline |
| Anticoagulants and thrombolytics | Used to prevent the formation of blood clots or dissolve blood clots | Heparin sodium, streptokinase (Streptase™) |
| Anticonvulsants | Reduce the excitability of the brain | Phenobarbital, phenytoin (Dilantin™) |
| Antidepressants | Various actions | Amitriptyline hydrochloride (Elavil™), fluoxetine hydrochloride (Prozac™) |
| Antidiarrheals | Decrease intestinal peristalsis | Loperamide hydrochloride (Imodium A-D™) |
| Antiemetic agents | Prevents nausea and vomiting | Dimenhydrinate (Dramamine™), promethazine hydrochloride (Phenergan™) |
| Antifungals | Destroy or retard the growth of fungi | Ketoconazole (Nizoral™), miconazole nitrate (Monistat 3™ or 7™) |
| Antihistamines | Counteracts the effects of histamine on body organs and structures | Chlorpheniramine maleate (Chlor-Trimeton™), diphenhydramine hydrochloride (Benadryl™) |
| Antihypertensives | Increase the size of arterial blood vessels | Methyldopa (Aldomet™), prazosin (Minipress™) |
| Anti-inflammatory agents | Reduce irritation and swelling of tissues | Aspirin, ibuprofen (Motrin™), naproxen (Naprosyn™) |
| Antineoplastic agents | Slow the rate of tumor growth | Cyclophosphamide (Cytoxan™) |
| Antipsychotics | Exact mechanism not understood; used to treat psychoses | Thorazine, Haldol |
| Antipyretics | Decrease body temperature | Aspirin, acetaminophen (Tylenol™) |
| Antitussives, mucolytics, and expectorants | Relieve coughing, loosen respiratory secretions, or aid in the removal of thick secretions | Codeine sulfate, Benylin, Entex |
| Antivirals | Inhibit viral replication | Acyclovir (Zovirax™), AZT |
| Bronchodilators | Dilate the bronchi | Albuterol sulfate (Ventolin™), metaproterenol (Alupent™) |
| Cardiotonics | Increase the force of the myocardium | Digoxin (Lanoxin™), milrinone (Primacor™) |
| Cholinergic blocking agents | Affect the autonomic nervous system | Atropine sulfate, scopolamine hydrobromide |
| Cholinergics | Mimic the activity of the parasympathetic nervous system | Neostigmine (Prostigmin™), pilocarpine hydrochloride |

(continues on page 576)

| TABLE 23-1 | Classifications of Drugs (continued) | |
|---|---|---|
| Therapeutic Classification | Effect or Action/Uses | Common Examples |
| Decongestants | Reduce swelling of nasal passages | Pseudoephedrine hydrochloride (Sudafed™) |
| Diuretics | Increase the secretion of urine by the kidneys | Furosemide (Lasix™), chlorothiazide (Diuril™) |
| Emetics | Promote vomiting | Ipecac syrup |
| Histamine H₂ antagonists | Inhibit the action of histamine at the H₂ receptor cells of the stomach | Cimetidine (Tagamet™), ranitidine (Zantac™) |
| Hormones, female | Used to prevent symptoms of menopause | Estradiol (Estraderm™), medroxyprogesterone acetate (Provera™) |
| Hormones, male | Androgen therapy to treat testosterone deficiency | Fluoxymesterone (Halotestin™) |
| Immunologic agents (vaccines) | Stimulate the immune response to create protection against disease | Pneumococcal vaccine, influenza virus vaccine, diphtheria and tetanus toxoid |
| Insulin and oral hypoglycemics | Used to control diabetes | NPH and ultralente insulin, tolbutamide (Orinase™), glipizide (Glucotrol™) |
| Sedatives and hypnotics | Sedatives relax and calm; hypnotics induce sleep | Butabarbital sodium, temazepam (Restoril™) |
| Stimulants | Increase activity of the central nervous system | Doxapram hydrochloride (Dopram™), amphetamine sulfate |
| Thyroid and antithyroid agents | Used to increase or decrease the amount of thyroid hormone produced | Levothyroxine sodium (T₄; Levothroid™) |

Summarized from Scherer JC, Roach SS. *Introductory Clinical Pharmacology*, 5th ed. Philadelphia, PA: Lippincott-Raven Publishers; 1996.

was established to regulate the manufacture and distribution of drugs and food products and to ensure accuracy in the ingredients listed on the labels of food and drug products.

## Drug Enforcement Administration

In 1970, the Controlled Substances Act was passed to regulate the manufacture and distribution of drugs whose use may result in dependency or abuse. . This act also requires that anyone who manufactures, prescribes, administers, or dispenses controlled substances register with the United States Attorney General under the Bureau of Narcotics and Dangerous Drugs (BNDD). The Drug Enforcement Administration (DEA) is a branch of the Department of Justice (DOJ) and is designated to exercise strong regulatory control over all drugs listed by the BNDD. This authority extends to prescribing, refilling, and storing controlled substances in the medical office. The DEA is concerned with controlled substances only; medications not subject to abuse are not regulated by this agency.

As a medical assistant, you may be responsible for maintaining or reminding the physician about professional records and licensure, including registration with the DEA. When the physician registers with the U.S.

Attorney General under the BNDD, a registration number (DEA number) is issued. Physicians are registered for 3 years after application and acceptance. The DEA does not take responsibility if the physician's registration expires. The registration retires with the physician; it does not stay with the medical office.

The DEA is also responsible for revising the list of drugs in the Schedule of Controlled Substances (Table 23-2). These substances have been identified as having a potential for abuse and dependency. Drug dependence, sometimes referred to as addiction, can be psychological, physical, or both. A patient who has developed physical dependence on a drug will have mild to severe physiologic symptoms that gradually decrease in intensity after the drug is stopped. Patients who are psychologically dependent have acquired a need for the feeling brought on by the drug. Patients who are prescribed controlled substances must be monitored closely for signs of physical or psychological dependence.

Controlled substances in Schedule II are received from suppliers using a Federal Triplicate Order Form DEA 222. Schedules III, IV, and V do not require triplicate forms, but invoices for receipts of the substances must be maintained for 2 years. Box 23-2 describes how to handle inventory of controlled substances.

## TABLE 23-2   Controlled Substances

| Schedule | Description | Examples |
|---|---|---|
| I | These drugs have the highest potential for abuse and have no currently accepted medicinal use in the U.S. There are no accepted safety standards for use of these drugs or substances even under medical supervision, although some are used experimentally in carefully controlled research projects. | *Opium, marijuana, lysergic acid diethylamide (LSD), peyote, mescaline* |
| II | These drugs have a high potential for abuse. They have a current accepted medicinal use in the U.S., but with severe restrictions. Abuse of these drugs can lead to dependence, either psychological or physiologic. Schedule II drugs require a written prescription and cannot be refilled or called into the pharmacy by the medical office. Only in extreme emergencies may the physician call in the prescription. A handwritten prescription must be presented to the pharmacist within 72 h. | *Morphine, codeine, cocaine, Seconal™, amphetamines, Dilaudid™, Ritalin™* |
| III | These drugs have a limited potential for psychological or physiologic dependence. The prescription may be called in to the pharmacist by the physician and refilled up to five times in a 6-month period. | *Paregoric, Tylenol with codeine™, Fiorinal™* |
| IV | These drugs have a lower potential for abuse than do those in Schedules II and III. They can be called into the pharmacist by a medical office employee and may be filled up to five times in a 6-month period. | *Librium™, Valium™, phenobarbital* |
| V | These drugs have a lower potential for abuse than do those in schedules I, II, III, and IV. | *Lomotil™, Dimetane™, Expectorant DC™, Robitussin-DAC™* |

Five schedules, or categories, of controlled substances were established by the Bureau of Narcotics and Dangerous Drugs. Medications in the five schedules may be revised periodically after review.

---

### BOX 23-2   Handling Inventory of Controlled Substances

1. When you receive controlled substances, make sure that both you and a second employee sign the receipt.
2. List all controlled substances on the appropriate inventory form (see Fig. 23-1).
3. When a controlled substance leaves the medical office inventory, record the following information: drug name, patient, dose, date, ordering physician, and employee who handled the procedure.
4. Keep all controlled substance inventory forms for 2 years.
5. Ensure that controlled substances are kept in a locked safe or in a secure locked box.
6. Notify the local law enforcement agency immediately if these drugs are lost or stolen.

---

If controlled substances are prescribed and not administered at the office, some states require only that the information be recorded in the patient's chart; others require a separate file of prescription copies of controlled substances. Law enforcement officials recommend that the DEA number not be preprinted on the prescription. Officials at regional DEA offices are available to answer any questions regarding the drugs under its control. As a medical assistant, you should make sure the physician's office is on the DEA's periodic mailing list to keep abreast of changes.

### CHECKPOINT QUESTION

2. After a controlled substance is administered, what information should Elaine document and where should this information be recorded?

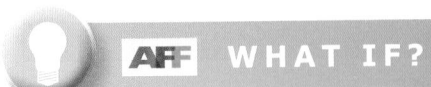

## WHAT IF?

**Bob Sandler, a 38-year-old accountant, was first seen in the office 2 weeks ago for a back injury that occurred after doing some home repair work the previous weekend. At the initial visit, the physician prescribed an opioid pain medication and a muscle relaxant. Today, Mr. Sandler tells you that his medications were stolen, and he would like a refill for both. What if both drugs had a high potential for abuse and were often purchased illegally on the street? Would you suspect that the patient was selling his medication? How could you be sure that this was not occurring?**

Although the medical assistant must be an advocate for the patient, he or she must also be vigilant about the possibility of drug abuse in the patient population and the community at large. It is imperative that the medical assistant gather as much information as possible about "lost" or "stolen" medications and report any illegal activities to the proper authorities. Patients who have had medications stolen that have a high abuse potential will want to report the theft to the police. Some physicians want to see a police report before issuing another prescription.

## Inventory, Storage, Dispensation, and Disposal of Medications

Most medical offices store medications in the office for use during office hours or to give to patients for use at home. Often, pharmaceutical company sales representatives will leave medication samples specifically for you to dispense at the direction of the physician. In either situation, it will be your responsibility to maintain an inventory of these medications, including the amount of each drug being stored and a written record of medications taken for administration in the office or dispensed to the patient for use at home (Fig. 23-1). Medications kept in the medical office should be stored away from patients or other visitors who may come to the office. Ideally, the medication area should be locked and accessible only by authorized clinical staff. It will be your responsibility to keep this medication area clean, neat, and organized.

When disposing of medications other than controlled substances, you should follow the office policy and procedure manual. In some cases, the appropriate pharmaceutical representative may need to be notified and may advise you to place any expired medications into a container to be picked up and disposed of by the company. Never dispose of expired medications in regular trash containers. For controlled substances that need to be disposed, a witness should watch the disposal, and both parties will be required to sign appropriate DEA forms noting the name of the drug and the amount disposed.

| Controlled Substance: | | Meperidine (Demerol) 50 mg Injection | | | | |
|---|---|---|---|---|---|---|
| Amount Ordered: | | 50 mg vials/ampules | | | Date: | |

| Date | Patient Name | Ordering Physician | Dose Given | Amount Discarded | Employee Signature |
|---|---|---|---|---|---|
| | | | | | |
| | | | | | |
| | | | | | |
| | | | | | |
| | | | | | |
| | | | | | |
| | | | | | |
| | | | | | |
| | | | | | |
| | | | | | |

**Figure 23-1** • Controlled substance inventory form.

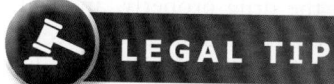

## LEGAL TIP

### Reporting Suspected Abuse of Controlled Substances in the Medical Office

If you suspect that a physician or any other health care professional is illegally diverting controlled substances, you have a legal and ethical responsibility to report this suspicion. Gather and document evidence and the reasons you suspect diversion of substances. You should have a clear and compelling case to present to the proper authorities, usually the local police. In addition, if a physician is involved, report this evidence to the Drug Enforcement Agency and the American Medical Association (AMA). You should also notify the state medical society. If the suspected health care worker is not a physician, report it to the appropriate supervisor or superior. Most states have programs to assist health care professionals in obtaining appropriate psychological help to deal with addiction or dependency issues. In most instances, you will remain anonymous.

## SOURCES OF DRUGS

Drugs are available from numerous natural sources, such as plants, minerals, and animals. They may also be synthetic (prepared in the laboratory by artificial means). Table 23-3 lists a number of commonly prescribed drugs and their sources.

## DRUG ACTIONS AND INTERACTIONS

### Pharmacodynamics

Pharmacodynamics is the study of the ways drugs act on the body, including the actions on specific cells, tissues, and organs. All drugs cause cellular change (drug action) and some degree of physiologic change (drug effect). An action of a local drug, such as an ointment or lotion applied to the skin, is limited to the area where it is administered. A drug administered for a systemic effect is absorbed into the blood and carried to the organ or

### TABLE 23-3 Common Drugs and Their Sources

| Source | Drug | Use |
|---|---|---|
| *Plants* | | |
| Cinchona bark | Quinidine | Antiarrhythmic |
| Purple foxglove | Digitalis | Cardiotonic |
| Opium poppy | Paregoric | Antidiarrheal |
| | Morphine | Analgesic |
| | Codeine | Antitussive, analgesic |
| *Minerals* | | |
| Magnesium | Milk of magnesia | Antacid, laxative |
| Silver | Silver nitrate | Placed in eyes of newborns to kill *Neisseria gonorrhoeae;* chemical cautery of lesions |
| Gold | Solganal™ | Arthritis treatment |
| *Animal Proteins* | | |
| Porcine or bovine | Insulin | Antidiabetic hormone pancreas |
| Porcine or bovine stomach acids | Pepsin | Digestive hormone |
| Animal thyroid glands | Thyroid, USP | Hypothyroidism |
| *Synthetics* | | |
| | Demerol™ | Analgesic |
| | Lomotil™ | Antidiarrheal |
| | Gantrisin™ | Sulfonamide |
| *Semisynthetic* | | |
| *Escherichia coli* bacteria and altered DNA molecules | Humulin™ | Antidiabetic hormone |

tissue on which it will act. An example of this is antibiotic therapy for a urinary tract infection. The antibiotic tablets are taken orally, but once they are absorbed, the action takes place in the urinary bladder, where the drug destroys any microorganisms. A systemic effect can be produced by administering drugs orally (by mouth), sublingually (under the tongue), rectally, by injection, transdermally (through the skin), or by inhalation (through the lungs). A number of factors can influence a drug's action in the body including the following:

- *Age*: Elderly people have slower metabolic processes. Age-related kidney and liver dysfunctions also extend the breakdown and excretion times in these patients, so it is necessary to monitor the cumulative effects of drugs in the elderly. Children may have a more immediate response to drugs and, therefore, must be assessed frequently.
- *Weight*: Many drug dosages are calculated and administered according to the patient's weight. As a general rule, the larger the patient, the greater the dose; however, individual sensitivity to the effects of drugs should be taken into consideration.
- *Sex*: Women may react differently to certain drugs than do men because of the ratio of fat to body mass or fluctuating hormone levels.
- *Existing pathology*: If the body is compromised by a disease process, absorption, distribution, metabolism, and excretion may be altered.
- *Tolerance*: Some medications given over a long period of time may cause the body to become resistant to their effects, requiring larger doses to achieve the desired response.

Medical assistants should always administer medications under the direct order of a physician. Under no circumstance should the dosage be adjusted or altered unless they are specifically instructed to do so by the physician. In most states, medical assistants can also administer medications upon the order of a physician assistant; however, state laws vary regarding the delegation of medication administration by an advanced practice nurse or nurse practitioner. You must be familiar with the state laws in which you are employed.

## Pharmacokinetics

**Pharmacokinetics** is the study of the action of drugs within the body based on the route of administration, rate of absorption, duration of action, and elimination from the body. Specifically, the processes included in pharmacokinetics include absorption (getting the drug into the bloodstream), distribution (movement of the drug from the bloodstream into the cells and tissues), metabolism (the physical and chemical breakdown of drugs by the body, including the liver), and excretion (byproducts sent to the kidneys to be removed from the body). In the presence of hepatic disease, the liver may

not be able to break down the drug properly, and the patient may undergo toxic effects caused by an accumulation of the drug in the liver or the bloodstream. In this situation, the drug may be noted as contraindicated by the manufacturer, or not recommended for use, in patients with a history of liver disease. Some drugs reach the kidneys relatively unchanged; these drugs can be detected in the urine during excretion, when the waste products of drug metabolism are eliminated from the body. However, if the kidneys are compromised by disease, medication may not be properly eliminated, adding to the danger of a cumulative, or building, effect and possible toxicity or poisoning.

 **CHECKPOINT QUESTION**

3. Why should pharmacokinetics be taken into consideration before administering medications?

 **PATIENT EDUCATION**

### Food–Drug Interaction

Many medications interact with food. Some medications are best absorbed when taken on an empty stomach. Two such medications are the antibiotics ampicillin and nafcillin (Unipen™). Other medications should be taken with food to decrease the potential for stomach upset. These include ibuprofen (Motrin™), an analgesic and anti-inflammatory; amoxicillin, an antibiotic; and verapamil (Calan™), a heart medication. Certain medications interact with specific types of food. For example, green leafy vegetables can interact with Coumadin, an anticoagulant, and make the patient's bleeding time increase. Also, grapefruit juice interacts with atorvastatin (Lipitor™), a medication used to lower blood cholesterol levels, to reduce its efficacy. It is important for patients to know about any food–drug interaction that may affect them. Information about food and drug interactions can be found in most pharmacology books. You will need to learn as much as you can about the medications that are commonly prescribed by the physician with whom you are working.

## Drug Interactions

When two or more drugs are taken simultaneously, one drug may increase, decrease, or cancel the effects of the other. These **interactions** may occur with prescribed drugs, over-the-counter medications, herbal or other natural supplements, and alcohol consumption. These interactions must always be taken into account when prescribing medications, administering medications, obtaining a medication history, or educating a

| TABLE 23-4 | Drug-Related Terms to Know |
|---|---|
| **Term** | **Meaning** |
| Therapeutic classification | States purpose for the drug's use (e.g., cardiotonic, anti-infective, antiarrhythmic). |
| Teratogenic category | Relates the level of risk to fetal or maternal health. These rank from Category A through D, with increasing danger at each level. Category X indicates that the particular drug should never be given during pregnancy. |
| Indications | Gives diseases for which the particular drug would be prescribed. |
| Contraindications | Indicates conditions or instances for which the particular drug should not be used. |
| Adverse reactions | Refers to undesirable side effects of a particular drug. |
| Hypersensitivity | Refers to an excessive reaction to a particular drug; also known as a drug allergy. The body must build this response; the first exposures may or may not indicate that a problem is developing. |
| Idiosyncratic reaction | Refers to an abnormal or unexpected reaction to a drug peculiar to the individual patient; not technically an allergy. |

patient about taking medications. Types of interactions include **synergism** (two drugs working together), **antagonism** (an effect in which one drug decreases the effect of another), and **potentiation** (occurs when one drug prolongs or multiplies the effect of another drug). Physicians prescribing two or more drugs may be using these drug interactions to cause a desired effect, or the patient may not realize these interactions exist and cause problems by taking them together. An example of two drugs working together is the use of a muscle relaxant and a pain medication to reduce the pain associated with an injury to a muscle or muscle group (synergism). However, some drug interactions produce undesirable effects. For example, antacids taken to relieve symptoms of indigestion may prevent absorption of antibiotics, such as tetracycline (antagonism). Potentiation occurs when sedatives and barbiturates are taken together, resulting in increased central nervous system depression or when a physician used lidocaine with epinephrine during a surgical procedure. The epinephrine in the lidocaine solution results extends the effects of the numbing medication (i.e. lidocaine), resulting in less pain over a longer period of time after the procedure. Table 23-4 lists other important drug-related terms you should know.

## Side Effects and Allergies

When gathering a patient's medical history, you must always ask about allergies of any sort, particularly allergies to medications. A drug **allergy** is a reaction such as hives, dyspnea, or wheezing. In addition, the allergic reaction **anaphylaxis** can be life threatening. Allergic reactions can be immediate or delayed 2 hours or longer, depending on the route of administration; however, many allergic reactions occur within minutes if the medication is administered by injection. The medical

assistant must interview the patient carefully about symptoms of allergies and note in the medical record the names of any medications that produce true allergic symptoms. Drug allergies should always be noted prominently on the front of the patient's medical record and on each page of the medication record. Because of the possibility of an anaphylactic reaction, patients should never be given medications that they have had an allergic reaction to in the past. You should always check the chart and ask the patient before administering any medications in the medical office as an additional safety measure.

Many patients state that they have an allergy to certain medications when in fact the reaction was a **side effect**. Side effects are reactions to medications that are predictable (as noted by the manufacturer of the medication) and that occur in some patients who take the medication. For example, some medications may cause nausea unless taken with food, and in this case, nausea may be listed by the manufacturer as a side effect. Other medications may cause drowsiness or dryness of the mouth. While side effects are often annoying, they are not life threatening and should not be noted on the patient's allergy list.

If a patient is receiving allergy medications or any medication that has a high incidence of allergic reactions (e.g., penicillin), the patient should wait for 20 to 30 minutes and be rechecked before leaving the office. Some offices require all patients receiving injections to wait for a specific amount of time (15 to 20 minutes) before leaving the office. Always follow the policies of the medical office with regard to administering medications.

## CHECKPOINT QUESTION

4. How does synergism differ from antagonism?

# ☰ SOURCES OF INFORMATION

The *Physician's Desk Reference* (PDR) is widely used as a reference for drugs in current use. It is intended for physicians, but since the medical assistant must know about various medications administered in the office, the PDR is a valuable resource for anyone, including the medical assistant, to use before administering medications (Fig. 23-2). This resource is clearly written to identify a drug's chemical name, brand name or names, and generic name. It also lists the properties, indications, side effects, **contraindications**, dosages, and so on. One section of the PDR contains pictures of various medications. This book is sometimes distributed to physicians free of charge; however, it is also available for use in libraries and for purchase in bookstores.

The *United States Pharmacopeia Dispensing Information* (USPDI) consists of two paperback volumes providing drug information for the health care provider. It defines drug sources, chemistry, physical properties, tests for identity, storage, and dosage. The USPDI does not contain photographs of the medications and must be purchased by the physician.

The *American Hospital Formulary Service* (AHFS), which is distributed to practicing physicians, contains concise information arranged according to drug classifications. The *Compendium of Drug Therapy* is published annually and is also distributed to physicians. It includes photographs of the drugs and phone numbers of major pharmaceutical companies and poison control centers.

# ☰ PRESCRIPTIONS

Medications may be administered (given in the office), dispensed (a supply given for later use), or prescribed (a written order to be filled by a pharmacist). You may be

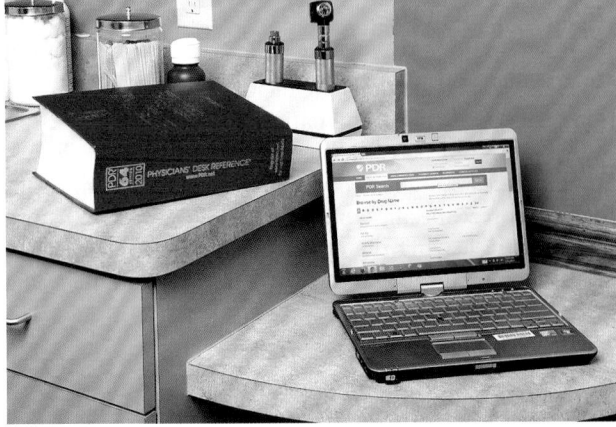

**Figure 23-2 •** The PDR.

permitted to complete the prescription form and obtain the physician's signature if directed to do so by the physician. An established protocol and traditional form must be followed when filling out prescriptions:

Line 1. *Date*. Prescriptions must be filled within 6 months of the date of issuance.

Line 2. *Patient's name and address*. The pharmacist needs this information to fill the prescription.

Line 3. *Superscription*. The symbol $R_x$ is found at the top left of the blank prescription pad. Literally it means recipe, or "take thou."

Line 4. *Inscription*. This includes the name of the medication, the desired form (e.g., liquid, tablet, capsule), and the strength (e.g., 250 mg, 500 mL).

Line 5. *Subscription*. This states the amount to be dispensed (e.g., 60 tablets, 120 mL).

Line 6. *Signature*. This section notes any instructions for taking the medication (e.g., with meals, three times a day, four times a day).

Line 7. *Refills*. The number of times a prescription can be refilled should be indicated on the prescription and is generally no more than five times within 6 months. If no refills are indicated, the word none should be circled, or 0 should be written in.

Line 8. *Physician's signature*. The physician is responsible for prescriptions written in his or her office and should check and sign all prescriptions.

Line 9. *Generic*. Some physicians and insurance companies allow generic substitutes for some medications but not others. Note on the prescription whether generic substitutions can be made. If the physician does not want a specific medication substituted with a generic drug, "DAW" can be written on the prescription, which means "dispense as written."

All prescribed medications must be documented in full in the patient's record (Fig. 23-3). Prescriptions that are called or faxed to the pharmacist must also be documented. The chart is a legal document and may be called into court in the event of legal action. If the medication order is not recorded, it will be presumed that the medication was never ordered. Figure 23-4 shows a sample prescription form.

## Refilling Prescriptions

In most situations, a patient needing one or more prescriptions refilled will be required to make an appointment to see the physician, especially if the medications are controlled substances. Occasionally, a patient may phone the office requesting an emergency refill for a medication that is prescribed to be taken daily but has no additional refills noted on the bottle by the pharmacist. You should pull the patient's chart and check with the physician before calling any

| DATE | TIME | ORDERS |
|------|------|--------|
| 7/5/XX | 1000 | Prescription for ampicillin 250 mg, p.o., qid X7 days as ordered by Dr. Smith |
| | | *Sally Smith, CMA* |
| | | |
| | | |
| | | |
| | | |

**Figure 23-3** • Documentation of a prescribed medication in a patient record.

prescriptions into the pharmacy. This is also true if the pharmacist calls the medical office requesting the refill for the patient. Always check with the physician before authorizing the refill of any medication.

Some drugs, such as digoxin, have a cumulative effect and may become toxic if blood levels are not monitored closely. For this reason, it is important that you be familiar with the medications prescribed by the physician and promptly schedule any laboratory tests ordered by the physician. In addition, you should be vigilant about notifying the physician with the results of any patient laboratory blood tests that may be ordered to monitor the effects of medications. Patients who

request phone refills for medications that need blood monitoring should be encouraged to comply with the physician's recommendations for such laboratory tests. It will be your responsibility to help patients understand the importance of maintaining therapeutic blood levels of these medications.

**CHECKPOINT QUESTION**

5. What does the superscription on the prescription indicate, and how does it differ from the subscription?

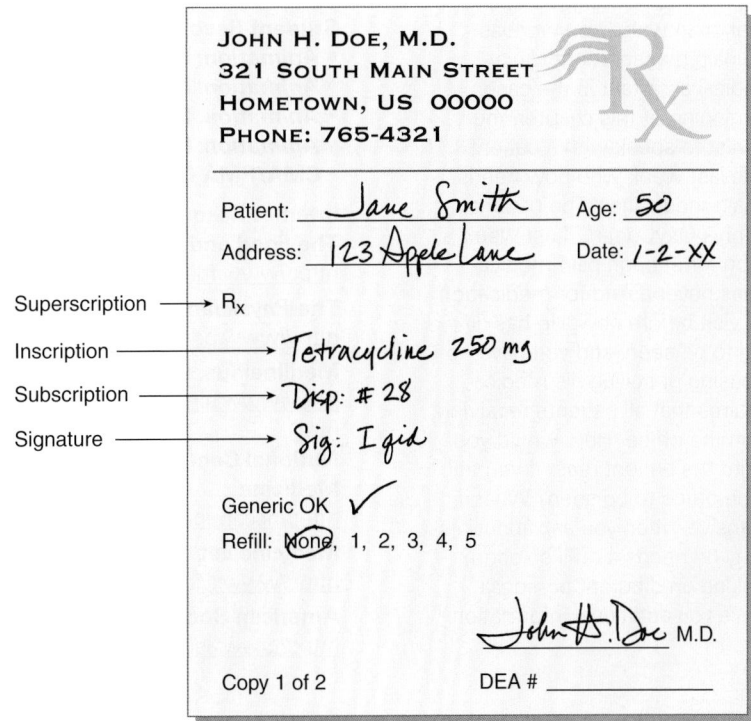

**Figure 23-4** • Prescription form.

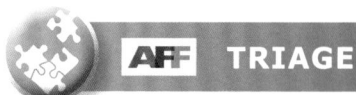

## TRIAGE

**Three patients have called the office asking you for prescription refills. It is 10 AM. What is the correct priority order for looking at the patient's medical record and calling the pharmacy for a refill?**

A. A 52-year-old patient says she went to take her methyldopa (Aldomet™) this morning but was out of it. She takes it every morning at 9:00 for her blood pressure.

B. A mother says her 3-year-old son spilled the bottle of ampicillin on the floor. The next dose is due at 2:00 this afternoon.

C. A 66-year-old patient says she is out of her sleeping pills. She wants a refill for temazepam (Restoril™).

**How do you sort these patients? Which prescription should be called in to the pharmacy first? Second? Third?**

Important: Before calling any medication refill into the pharmacy, you must look at the patient's medical record and be sure there are refill orders on the chart. Also, you must follow your office's policy on prescription refills.

Patient A should be done first; it is important that blood pressure medications be taken at the same time every day. Patient B is next so that the 2:00 PM dose is not missed. Patient C's prescription should be handled last.

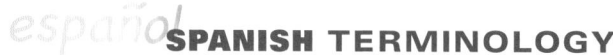

## *español* SPANISH TERMINOLOGY

**Por favor tome este medicamento tres veces al dia ó cada ocho horas.**
Please take this medicine three times a day or every 8 hours.

**Debe ir a la farmacia para conseguir este medicamento.**
Please go to the pharmacy to pick up this medicine.

**¿Ha tomado algun medicamento o remedio para aliviar su malestar?**
Have you taken any medications or remedies for this (illness)?

**Esta medicina puede provocarle cansancio.**
This medicine may make you tired.

**No maneje si está tomando este medicamento.**
Do not drive while taking this medicine.

**Por favor tome este medicamento con alimentos.**
Please take this medicine with food.

**Por favor tome este medicamento con el estómago vacio.**
Please take this medicine with an empty stomach.

**El engargado de la farmacia le va a imprimir una explicación detallada de las propiedades y efectos secundarios de esta medicina.**
The pharmacist will give you a printout to explain the properties and side effects of this drug.

## ROLE-PLAYING ACTIVITY

After choosing another student or as assigned by your instructor, role-play a situation in which you work as a medical assistant in the pain management clinic with Elaine Black, the medical assistant in the case study described at the beginning of this chapter. You are asked by the receptionist to speak with a patient who was seen in the clinic last week who now needs another prescription for pain medication. The patient tells you that he "is out of his OxyContin." Last week, he was given a prescription for enough pain medication for 1 month and he has never asked for medication before his monthly office visit before now. He has difficulty getting to the clinic to be seen, and you have no reason to believe he is abusing or selling his medication. The office policy requires that all patients receiving pain medication be seen in the office. How would you handle this call? How might the patient react if you tell him he must come into the office to be seen? What if the patient becomes defensive when you ask about his recent medication and why he needs a refill so soon? Reverse roles, perhaps taking on different personalities. Your instructor will give you additional information about this activity!

## MEDIA MENU

**Student Resources** on thePoint*
- *Animation:* **Drug Absorption**
- *Animation:* **Drug Distribution**
- *Animation:* **Drug Binding**
- *Animation:* **Drug Excretion**
- **CMA/RMA Certification Exam Review**

**Internet Resources**
**The Food and Drug Administration**
http://www.fda.gov/medwatch
**The *Physician's Desk Reference***
http://www.pdr.net
**MedlinePlus, National Institutes of Health**
http://www.nlm.nih.gov/medlineplus/druginformation.html
**National Center of Complementary and Alternative Medicine**
http://nccam.nih.gov
**MedicineNet**
http://www.MedicineNet.com
**American Society of Health-System Pharmacists**
http://www.ashp.org

## EMR Activity

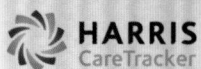

Harris CareTracker is a web-based electronic medical record (EMR) application that you will use for the EMR activities included in this section at the end of each chapter. This application is actually used in physician offices, but is provided to you through the publisher, Wolters Kluwer Health, to give you hands-on practice working with EMRs. Your instructor will have more information about accessing your username, log-in, and Quickstart guide.

Prerequisite Activities in Harris CareTracker

- *The Getting Started and Quickstart documents and EMR Activities Step-by-Step Instructions are available at* http://thePoint.lww.com/KronenbergerComp5e
- *Note: You must first enter the patients into the EMR as new patients before completing the following EMR activity as given in the EMR Step-by-Step Instructions*

Activity Details

Most electronic medical record software programs allow for e-prescriptions where the provider electronically writes the order for the medication to be taken by the patient and sends it immediately to the pharmacy to be filled and picked up by the patient after the office visit. Document the following new or refill prescriptions in the *Medical Record* module, *Medications* application of the EMR as ordered for the following patients for Dr. Christy Boling. Keep in mind that you may have to add medications by using the *Medication Search* dialog box.

1. Thomas Barter: Tylenol No. 3, 2 tablets every 4 to 6 hours as needed for knee pain.
2. Sue Tamrick: tramadol hydrochloride 50 mg by mouth every 4 to 6 hours as needed for back pain.
3. Justin Jones: cephalexin 250 mg by mouth four times a day for 7 days
4. Kathy Newman: refill for Synthroid 150 mcg by mouth 1 tablet daily, 12 refills

## Chapter Summary

- Medications are administered, dispensed, or prescribed to patients to produce therapeutic effects. They are available in many forms and can be administered in various ways.
- Some medications, called controlled substances, may result in dependency and abuse. These drugs are strictly regulated by the federal government.
- As a medical assistant, you will need to keep current on the legal regulations concerning the manufacture, sale, and prescribing of medications. You must also understand the actions, effects, and interactions of drugs to carry out a physician's medication orders.
- Whether administering medications in the office or refilling a prescription order to a pharmacy over the phone, you must always have a physician order. Never recommend any medication, even an over-the-counter remedy, to a patient.

## Warm-Ups for Critical Thinking

1. What type of information regarding medications do patients need to know? Is there anything they do not need to know?
2. Using a drug reference book such as the PDR, look up a medication that you have taken. What are the medication's trade and generic names? Are there any side effects or contraindications? Explain what you learned about this medication that you did not already know.
3. How would you interact with a patient who insists that he/she should leave immediately after receiving an injection when the office policy states that patients should remain in the office for 15 minutes after receiving an injection?
4. Describe how you could keep prescription pads secure during the typical day working in the medical office.

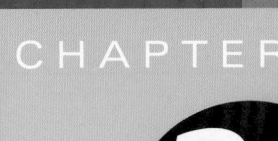

# CHAPTER

## 24

# Preparing and Administering Medications

## Outline

**Medication Administration Basics**
Safety Guidelines
Seven Rights for Correct Medication Administration
Systems of Measurement

**Routes of Medication Administration**
Oral, Sublingual, and Buccal Routes
Parenteral Administration
Other Medication Routes

**Principles of Intravenous Therapy**
Intravenous Equipment
Troubleshooting Problems

## Learning Outcomes

### COG Cognitive Domain*

1. Spell and define the key terms
2. *Demonstrate knowledge of basic math computations*
3. *Apply mathematical computations to solve equations*
4. *Define basic units of measurement in metric and household systems*
5. *Convert among measurement systems*
6. *Identify abbreviations and symbols used in calculating medication dosages*
7. List the safety guidelines for medication administration
8. Explain the differences between various parenteral and nonparenteral routes of medication administration
9. Describe the parts of a syringe and needle and name those parts that must be kept sterile
10. List the various needle lengths, gauges, and preferred site for each type of injection
11. Compare the types of injections and locate the sites where each may be administered safely
12. Describe principles of intravenous therapy

### PSY Psychomotor Domain*

1. Administer oral medications (Procedure 24-1).
   a. *Verify rules of medication administration (right patient, medication, dose, route, time, documentation)*
   b. *Administer oral medications*
   c. *Document patient care accurately in the medical record*
2. Prepare injections (Procedure 24-2)

3. Administer an intradermal injection (Procedure 24-3)
   a. *Verify rules of medication administration (right patient, medication, dose, route, time, documentation)*
   b. *Select proper sites for administration of parenteral medication*
   c. *Instruct and prepare a patient for a procedure or treatment*
   d. *Calculate proper dosages of medication for administration*
   e. *Administer parenteral (excluding IV) medications*
   f. *Demonstrate proper disposal of biohazard material, sharps, and regulated waste*
   g. *Document patient care accurately in the medical record*
4. Administer a subcutaneous injection (Procedure 24-4)
   a. *Verify rules of medication administration (right patient, medication, dose, route, time, documentation)*
   b. *Select proper sites for administration of parenteral medication*
   c. *Instruct and prepare a patient for a procedure or treatment*
   d. *Calculate proper dosages of medication for administration*
   e. *Administer parenteral (excluding IV) medications*
   f. *Demonstrate proper disposal of biohazard material, sharps, and regulated waste*
   g. *Document patient care accurately in the medical record*

*(continues on page 588)*

5. Administer an intramuscular injection (Procedure 24-5)
   a. *Verify rules of medication administration (right patient, medication, dose, route, time, documentation)*
   b. *Select proper sites for administration of parenteral medication*
   c. *Instruct and prepare a patient for a procedure or treatment*
   d. *Calculate proper dosages of medication for administration*
   e. *Administer parenteral (excluding IV) medications*
   f. *Demonstrate proper disposal of biohazard material, sharps, and regulated waste*
   g. *Document patient care accurately in the medical record*
6. Administer an intramuscular injection using the Z-track method (Procedure 24-6)
   a. *Verify rules of medication administration (right patient, medication, dose, route, time, documentation)*
   b. *Select proper sites for administration of parenteral medication*
   c. *Instruct and prepare a patient for a procedure or treatment*
   d. *Calculate proper dosages of medication for administration*
   e. *Administer parenteral (excluding IV) medications*
   f. *Demonstrate proper disposal of biohazard material, sharps, and regulated waste*
   g. *Document patient care accurately in the medical record*
7. Apply transdermal medications (Procedure 24-7)
8. *Complete an incident report related to an error in patient care* (Procedure 24-8)

**AFF Affective Domain***

1. *Incorporate critical thinking skills when performing patient care*
2. *Verify ordered doses/dosages prior to administration*
3. *Show awareness of the patient's concerns related to the procedure being performed*
4. *Demonstrate empathy, active listening, and nonverbal communication*
5. *Demonstrate respect for individual diversity including gender, race, religion, age, economic status, and appearance*
6. *Explain to a patient the rationale for performance of a procedure*
7. *Protect the integrity of the medical record*

***Note: AAMA/CAAHEP 2015 Standards are italicized***

**ABHES Competencies**

1. Demonstrate accurate occupational math and metric conversions for proper medication administration
2. Apply principles of aseptic techniques and infection control
3. Maintain medication and immunization records
4. Use standard precautions
5. Prepare and administer oral and parenteral medications as directed by physician
6. Document accurately
7. Dispose of biohazardous materials

## Key Terms

| | | | |
|---|---|---|---|
| ampule | induration | ophthalmic | vial |
| apothecary system | infiltration | otic | Z-track method |
| buccal | Mantoux test | parenteral | |
| diluent | metric system | sublingual | |
| gauge | nebulizer | topical | |

## Case Study

*P*am King, CMA (AAMA), works in a busy family practice office at Great Falls Medical Center. Her responsibilities at the office include assisting with all aspects of patient care including obtaining vital signs, assisting the physician with examinations, and administering medications. Today, the office has scheduled several pediatric patients for immunizations in the morning and sick patients for the afternoon. Another employee has drawn up a medication to be given and has asked Pam to administer the injection to a patient in an examination room. Pam is not familiar with this patient and is reluctant to give a medication that she has not drawn up herself. However, she knows the employee who did prepare the medication and feels that she is trustworthy. How should Pam handle this situation? Who should document the medication administered: Pam, the other employee, or the physician who ordered the medication? All aspects of medication administration are addressed in this chapter, including the role of the professional medical assistant.

Administering medications in most physician offices may be an important part of the clinical duties assigned to medical assistants. Become familiar with the laws in the state where you live—some states do not allow medical assistants to administer medications. However, there are many states that do permit medical assistants to administer medications. Medical assistants living in those states have a responsibility to perform these skills with accuracy and competence. This chapter gives detailed information about the preparation and administration of medications in the medical office.

## COG MEDICATION ADMINISTRATION BASICS

Before administering any medications in the medical office, you should be familiar with the medication ordered by the physician and the procedures necessary to administer the drug accurately and safely. As a clinical medical assistant, you must look up any drugs you are not familiar with to determine the drug classification, the usual dosage, and the route of administration. In addition, you should be thoroughly familiar with the terminology, abbreviations, symbols, and signs used in prescribing, administering, and documenting medications. The abbreviations listed in Table 24-1 are most commonly used and should be memorized. Although most physician offices are not accredited by The Joint Commission, the abbreviations listed in red have been identified as potentially dangerous to use by The Joint Commission and may result in medication errors. These abbreviations are not permitted in facilities that are accredited by The Joint Commission; however, they are frequently used in physician offices.

### Safety Guidelines

To ensure safety when administering medications, follow these guidelines:

1. Know the policies of your office regarding the administration of medications.
2. Give only the medications that the physician has ordered in writing. Do not accept verbal orders.
3. Check with the physician if you have any doubt about a medication or an order.
4. Avoid conversation and other distractions while preparing and administering medications. It is important to remain attentive during this task.
5. Work in a quiet, well-lighted area.
6. Check the label when taking the medication from the shelf, when preparing it, and when replacing it on the shelf or disposing of the empty container. This is known as the three checks for safe administration.
7. Place the order and the medication side by side to compare for accuracy.
8. Check the strength of the medication (e.g., 250 mg vs. 500 mg) and the route of administration.
9. Read labels carefully. Do not scan labels or medication orders.
10. Check the patient's medical record for allergies to the actual medication or its components before administering.
11. Check the medication's expiration date. Outdated medications should be discarded according to office policy and should never be administered to a patient.
12. Be alert for color changes, precipitation, odor, or any indication that the medication's properties have changed. If the medication has changed in consistency, color, or odor, discard it appropriately.
13. Measure exactly. There should be no bubbles in liquid medication.
14. Have sharps containers as close to the area of use as possible.
15. Put on gloves for all procedures that might result in contact with blood or body fluids.
16. Stay with the patient while he or she takes oral medication. Watch for any reaction and record the patient's response.
17. Never return a medication to the container after it is poured or removed.
18. Never recap, bend, or break a used needle.
19. Never give a medication poured or drawn up by someone else.
20. Never leave the medication cabinet unlocked when not in use.
21. Never give keys for the medication cabinet to an unauthorized person. Limit access to the medication cabinet by limiting access to the cabinet keys.
22. Never document medication given by someone else, and do not ask someone else to document medication that you have administered.

When the physician writes a prescription for a medication, you will often be the health care provider who gives this prescription to the patient and records that this medication was ordered on the medication record in the patient health record (see Legal Tip box). In some cases, the physician may ask you to dispense a sample of the prescribed medication provided by the pharmaceutical representative to the patient until the prescription can be filled later at the pharmacy. Once the patient takes the prescription to the pharmacy, the pharmacy will fill the prescription according to the physician orders. In addition, the pharmacist will give the patient written information about taking the medication and any side effects that might be encountered. Also, the pharmacist will note any specific instructions and warnings on the medication container. Patients should always be encouraged to contact the office for any questions or problems concerning medications ordered by the physician.

## TABLE 24-1 Abbreviations

The abbreviations in red have been identified as potentially dangerous to use by The Joint Commission and may result in medication errors. However, most physician offices are not accredited by The Joint Commission and may use these abbreviations.

| Abbreviation | Meaning | Abbreviation | Meaning |
| --- | --- | --- | --- |
| ac | Before meals | NS | Normal saline |
| ad lib | As desired | OD | Right eye |
| AM, am, A.M. | Morning | OS | Left eye |
| amp | Ampule | OU | Both eyes |
| amt | Amount | oz | Ounce |
| **AD** | **Right ear** | p | After |
| **AS** | **Left ear** | pc | After meals |
| **AU** | **Both ears** | PM, pm, P.M. | Afternoon or evening |
| aq | Aqueous | po, PO | By mouth |
| bid | Twice a day | prn, PRN | Whenever necessary |
| ⁻c | With | q | Every |
| cap | Capsule | **qd** | **Every day** |
| **cc** | **Cubic centimeter** | qh | Every hour |
| **DC, disc, d/c** | **Discontinue** | q2h | Every 2 hours |
| disp | Dispense | q3h | Every 3 hours |
| dl, dL | Deciliter | qid | Four times a day |
| elix | Elixir | **qod** | **Every other day** |
| et | And | qs | Quantity sufficient |
| ext | Extract | qt | Quart |
| fl, fld | Fluid | R | Right, rectal |
| g, gm | Gram | Rx | Take, prescribe |
| **gr** | **Grain** | ⁻s | Without |
| gt(t) | Drop(s) | SC, subcu, S/Q, SQ | Subcutaneously |
| h, hr | Hour | Sig | Label |
| hs, HS | Hour of sleep | SL | Sublingual |
| Id, ID | Intradermal | ss | One-half |
| IM | Intramuscular | stat, STAT | Immediately |
| IV | Intravenous | supp | Suppository |
| Kg | Kilogram | syr | Syrup |
| L, l | Liter | tab | Tablet |
| lb | Pound | T, tb, tbs, tbsp | Tablespoon |
| **mcg, μg** | **Microgram** | t, tsp | Teaspoon |
| mEq | Milliequivalent | tid | Three times a day |
| ml, mL | Milliliter | tinc | Tincture |
| NaCl | Sodium chloride | **u** | **Units** |
| NKA | No known allergies | ung | Ointment |
| NPO | Nothing by mouth | | |

## CHECKPOINT QUESTION

1. When are the "three checks" for safe medication administration that should be performed by Pam before administering any medication in the physician office?

## Seven Rights for Correct Medication Administration

Medication errors should not occur during careful preparation or administration. By observing the seven rights during medication administration, you will eliminate the potential for many errors. The seven rights are as follows:

1. Right patient. Ask the patient to state his or her name. Some patients will answer to any name, so simply saying the name is not assurance that you have the correct patient.
2. Right time. Most medications ordered to be given in the office are to be given before the patient leaves. Some patients may have to be told when the next dose is due.
3. Right dose. Check doses carefully. Many medications come in various strengths.
4. Right route. Some medications are prepared for administration by a variety of routes. Is it oral, **parenteral, otic, ophthalmic,** or **topical?**
5. Right drug. Many medication names are very much alike; for instance, Orinase and Ornade™ may be confused if you are not careful. Always look up unfamiliar medications in a drug reference book such as the *Physician's Desk Reference* (PDR).
6. Right technique. Check how the medication is to be given, such as orally and with or without food. Intramuscular, subcutaneous, and intradermal injections should be given only after carefully choosing a site and with the correct procedure.
7. Right documentation. The medical record is a legal document. Make sure that the medication is documented after it is administered (not before) and that you have documented it in the correct medical record. All medications given in the medical office must be documented immediately with the name of the medication, the dose, the route, and the site (if injected), and the documentation must be signed by the medical assistant. The patient's response should be charted as well, when appropriate.

## CHECKPOINT QUESTION

2. After administering a medication, what information should Pam record in the patient's medical record?

## LEGAL TIP

### Medication Errors

Even if you are extremely careful, you may make an error when administering a medication. It is imperative that you report the error to the physician and that intervention measures start immediately. The error and all corrective actions must be documented thoroughly in the patient's medical record. An incident report should be completed for the error and filed in the medical office as verification that all possible precautions were taken for the patient.

## Systems of Measurement

The most common system of measurement used in the medical office is the **metric system;** however, the **apothecary system** of measurement may still used by some physicians. The household system of measurement is most often used by patients (Box 24-1). Both the apothecary and the household systems of measurement should be avoided in the medical setting, since the measurements are not as accurate as in the metric system. While working in the clinical setting, you may find it necessary to convert from one system to another. In addition, you may be required to calculate a dose in one system of measurement using mathematical equations. It is necessary to master the elements of the systems of measurement before attempting to calculate dosages.

### Metric, Household, and Apothecary

The metric system is used in the United States and throughout the world. Because the metric system is based on multiples of 10, decimals, not fractions, are used in calculating and recording dosages. In the metric system, the base unit of *length* is the *meter* (m). The base unit of *weight* is the *gram* (g or gm), and the liter

---

### BOX 24-1 Household Measures

Household measurements include cups, medicine droppers, teaspoons, and tablespoons. Some of the approximate equivalents to household measurements are as follows:

   1 teaspoon = 1 fluid dram = 5 mL
   1 tablespoon = 1/2 fluid ounce = 4 fluid drams = 15 mL
   2 tablespoons = 1 fluid ounce = 30 mL

   Caution patients who will be using household measurements to avoid using table flatware and regular cups. Standard measuring spoons and cups are more accurate.

(L or l) is used to measure fluid and gas volume. Prefixes used in the metric system show a fraction or multiple of the base. The following prefixes are often used:

- Micro- (0.000001)
- Milli- (0.001)
- Centi- (0.01)
- Deci- (0.1)
- Kilo- (1,000.0)

For example, using the base unit of a gram, fractional measurements are as follows:

- Microgram (mcg, μg), one-millionth of a gram (×0.000001)
- Milligram (mg), one-thousandth of a gram (×0.001)
- Kilogram (kg), 1,000 grams (×1,000.0)

Decagrams and centigrams are not used in medication administration.

With the base unit of a liter (1 L = approximately 1.06 quarts), fractional measurements in milliliters (ml, mL) are commonly used in medication administration. Also, 1 cubic centimeter (cc) is equivalent to 1 mL, and therefore, the measures are used interchangeably at times.

The apothecary system is used less frequently now than in the past and is gradually being replaced by the metric system. In the apothecary system, liquid measurements include drop (gt) or drops (gtt), minim (min, m), fluid dram (fl dr), fluid ounce (fl oz), pint (pt), quart (qt), and gallon (gal). Measurements for solid weights include grain (gr), dram (dr), ounce (oz), and pound (lb). Roman numerals are used for smaller numbers, and fractions may be used when necessary. Decimals are never used in the apothecary system.

The household system of measurement includes measures such as the teaspoon (tsp), tablespoon (tbsp), ounce (oz), cup (c), pint (pt), quart (qt), and pound (lb). While this system is not used in the medical office for calculating doses, patients may need to be instructed on the proper household measurement for taking medications ordered in the metric system (e.g., 5 mL is equivalent to 1 tsp). Table 24-2 lists commonly used equivalents in the metric, apothecary, and household systems of measurement.

 **CHECKPOINT QUESTION**

3. What are three systems of measurement? Which is the most commonly used in the medical office?

## Converting Between Systems of Measurement

### Apothecary or Household to Metric

To convert from one system to another system, use the following rules:

- To change grains (apothecary system) to grams (metric system), divide the number of grains ordered by 15. Example: gr 30 ÷ 15 = 2 g.

| TABLE 24-2 | Most Commonly Used Approximate Equivalents | |
|---|---|---|
| **Metric** | **Apothecary** | **Household** |
| 60 mg | gr i | |
| 0.06 mL | Minim i | 1 drop |
| 1.0 g | gr xv | |
| 1.0 mL | Minim xv | 1/5 tsp |
| 5.0 mL | 1 dram | 1 tsp |
| 15 mL | 1/2 oz | 1 tbsp |
| 30 mL | 1 oz | 2 tbsp |
| 500 mL | 6 oz | 1 pint |
| 1,000 mL | 2 oz | 1 quart |

There are many discrepancies among these approximate equivalents. For example, 30 mL is the accepted equivalent for 1 oz, but 29.57 mL is the exact equivalent. Such discrepancies are inevitable when equivalencies between the two systems are not exact. The discrepancies are within a 10% margin of error, which usually is acceptable in pharmacology.

Reprinted from Taylor C, Lillis C, Le Mone P. *Fundamentals of Nursing: The Art and Science of Nursing Care*, 2nd ed. Philadelphia, PA: Lippincott Williams & Wilkins, 1993:1347, with permission.

- To change grains (apothecary system) to milligrams (metric system), multiply the grains by 60. Use this rule with less than 1 grain. Example: gr 1/4 × 60 = 15 mg.
- To change ounces (household) to milliliters (metric system), multiply the ounces by 30. Example: 4 oz × 30 = 120 mL.
- To change milliliters (metric system) to fluid ounces (household system), divide the milliliters by 30. Example: 150 mL ÷ 30 = 50 oz.
- To change kilograms (metric system) to pounds (household system), multiply the kilograms by 2.2. Example: 50 kg × 2.2 = 110.0 lb.
- To change pounds to kilograms (metric system), divide the pounds (household system) by 2.2. Example: 44 lb ÷ 2.2 = 20 kg.

### Metric to Metric

In the metric system, it is sometimes necessary to convert measurements using the same unit of measure. For example, the physician may order 0.5 g of medication, and the medication label reads 500 mg. To convert within the metric system, use the following rules:

- To change grams to milligrams, multiply grams by 1,000 or move the decimal point three places to the right. Example: 0.5 g × 1,000 = 500 mg.
- To change milligrams to grams, divide the milligrams by 1,000 or move the decimal point three places to the left. Example: 500 mg ÷ 1,000 = 0.5 g.
- To change milligrams to micrograms, multiply the milligrams by 1,000 or move the decimal point three places to the right. Example: 5 mg × 1,000 = 5,000 μg.

- To change micrograms to milligrams, divide the micrograms by 1,000 or move the decimal point three places to the left. Example: 500 µg ÷ 1,000 = 0.5 mg.
- To change liters to milliliters, multiply the liters by 1,000 or move the decimal point three places to the right. Example: 0.01 L × 1,000 = 10 mL.
- To change milliliters to liters, divide the milliliters by 1,000 or move the decimal point three places to the left. Example: 100 mL ÷ 1,000 = 0.1 L.

There is no conversion necessary when changing cubic centimeters to milliliters; they are approximately the same.

## Calculating Adult Dosages

Administration of medication is an exact science; errors in calculation can kill the patient. Although the physician will order the dose of medication to be administered to the patient, you may have to calculate the amount of medication to withdraw into a syringe or pour into a medicine cup. In addition to the physician's order, you must also be aware of the label on the medication container (Fig. 24-1) since both the physician's order and the information on the medication label are used to calculate the amount given. There are two methods by which doses are most frequently calculated for adults: the ratio method and the formula method. Measurements must be in the same system (preferably metric) and unit before a calculation can be made. For example, if the medication is ordered in the apothecary or household system but is packaged in the metric system, you must first convert the order (apothecary or household) to the metric system. If the medication is ordered in grams but is packaged in milligrams, the ordered dose must be converted to milligrams before any calculations can be made. When using the metric system, be careful to keep the decimal point in the correct place during calculations and be sure to convert fractions to decimals.

### Ratio and Proportion

When using the ratio method to calculate doses, you must use the amount of medication ordered and the information on the medication label to create a ratio. Once the ratio has been determined, the proportion, or relationship between the two ratios, can be calculated to give you the amount of medication to administer. To calculate a dose using the ratio and proportion method, set up the problem as follows:

Dose on hand: Known quantity = Dose desired: Unknown quantity

**Example 1.** The physician orders erythromycin 250 mg. The label on the package reads erythromycin 100 mg/mL. The equation can be written as follows:

$$100 \text{ mg} : 1 \text{ mL} = 250 \text{ mg} : X$$

Multiply the extremes (first and fourth terms) = 100X

Multiply the means (second and third terms) = 250

Write the proportion as follows : 100X = 250

Divide both sides of the equal sign by 100 to solve for X.

$$250 \div 100 = 2.5$$

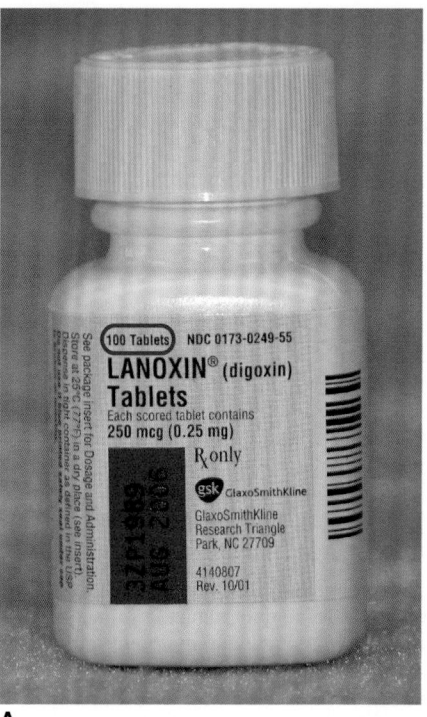
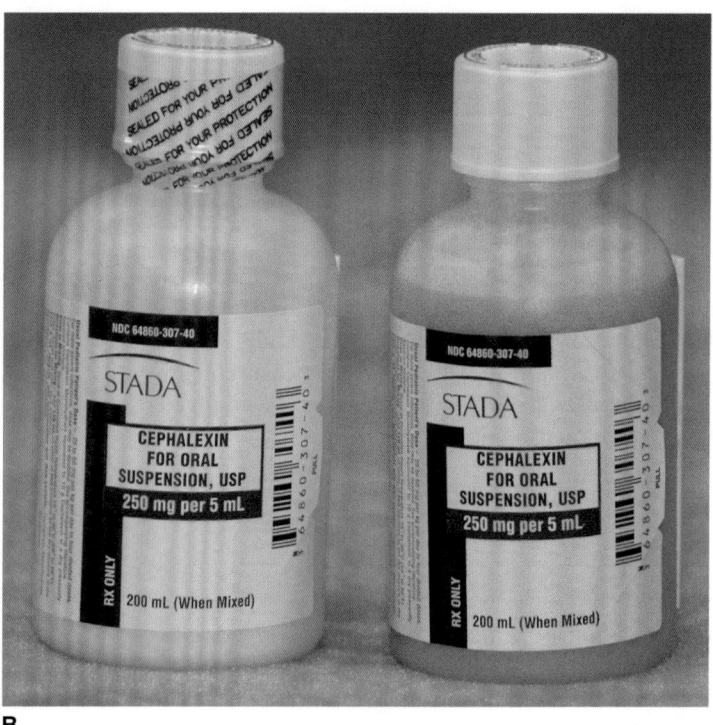

**A**    **B**

**Figure 24-1 •** Medication labels include the name of the medication and the dose per unit such as **(A)** 0.25 mg per tablet or **(B)** 250 mg per 5 mL.

Therefore, you administer 2.5 mL of erythromycin for the patient to receive the 250 mg ordered by the physician. *Note*: When you document the medication after administration, the amount given is the amount ordered by the physician in milligrams, not the amount in milliliters administered.

**Example 2.** The physician orders phenobarbital 25 mg. On hand are 12.5-mg tablets. State the equation as follows:

$$12.5 \text{ mg} : 1 \text{ tablet} = 25 \text{ mg} : X$$

$$\text{Multiply the extremes} = 12.5X$$

$$\text{Multiply the means} = 25 \text{ mg}$$

$$25 = 12.5X$$

$$\text{Divide both sides by } 12.5$$

$$25 \div 12.5 = 2 \text{ tablets}$$

In this example, you administer two tablets of phenobarbital to the patient and record that 25 mg was given.

### The Formula Method

The formula method is written as follows:

$$(\text{Desired} \div \text{On hand}) \times \text{Quantity} = \text{Dose}$$

**Example 1.** The physician orders ampicillin 0.5 g. On hand, you have ampicillin 250-mg capsules. How much ampicillin should be administered? Remember, both doses must be in the same unit of measure. Convert grams in the physician's order to milligrams by multiplying the grams by 1,000 (or move the decimal point three places to the right). The answer is 0.5 g equals 500 mg. With this information, you may set up your problem:

$$500 \text{ mg (desired)} \div 250 \text{ mg (on hand)} \times 1 \text{ (quantity)}$$
$$= 2 \times 1 = 2$$

In this example, the quantity (one capsule) is how the medication (ampicillin 250 mg) comes supplied. You administer two capsules and chart that 0.5 g or 500 mg was given to the patient.

**Example 2.** The physician orders 0.35 g of a medication, and you have on hand a liquid form of the medication that is labeled 700 mg/mL. How many milliliters do you prepare to administer? Remember, measurements must be in equivalent units, so 0.35 g must be changed to 350 mg before setting up the formula.

$$(350 \text{ mg} \div 700 \text{ mg}) \div 1 \text{ mL} = 0.5 \text{ mL} = 0.5 \text{ mL}$$

### 🔍 CHECKPOINT QUESTION

4. Before calculating a dose, what must be done with the measurements if the physician orders the medication in milligrams and the medication is supplied in grams?

## Calculating Pediatric Dosages

Although several formulas may be used to calculate children's doses, one method uses the body surface area (BSA) and is considered to be the most accurate method for children up to 12 years of age or adults who are below normal percentiles for body weight. A scale known as a nomogram (Fig. 24-2) is used to estimate the BSA in square meters according to the patient's height and weight. A straight line is drawn from the patient's height in inches or centimeters in column 1 to the patient's weight in kilograms or pounds in column 3 (Fig. 24-3). The line intersects on the BSA column (column 2) to give the BSA of the child. Once the BSA is determined, the following formula is used to calculate the medication dosage:

$$(\text{BSA} \times \text{Adult dose}) \div 1.7 = \text{Child's dose}$$

Other rules for calculating pediatric doses include Young's rule, Clark's rule, and Fried's rule. Young's rule is used to calculate doses for children aged 12 months to 12 years. This method requires that you determine

| Height | | Surface Area | Weight | |
|---|---|---|---|---|
| Feet | Centimeters | Square Meters | Pounds | Kilograms |

**Figure 24-2 •** Nomogram for estimating surface area of infants and young children. To determine the surface area of the patient, draw a straight line between the point representing the height on the left vertical scale and the point representing the weight on the right vertical scale. The point at which this line intersects the middle vertical scale represents the patient's surface area in square meters.

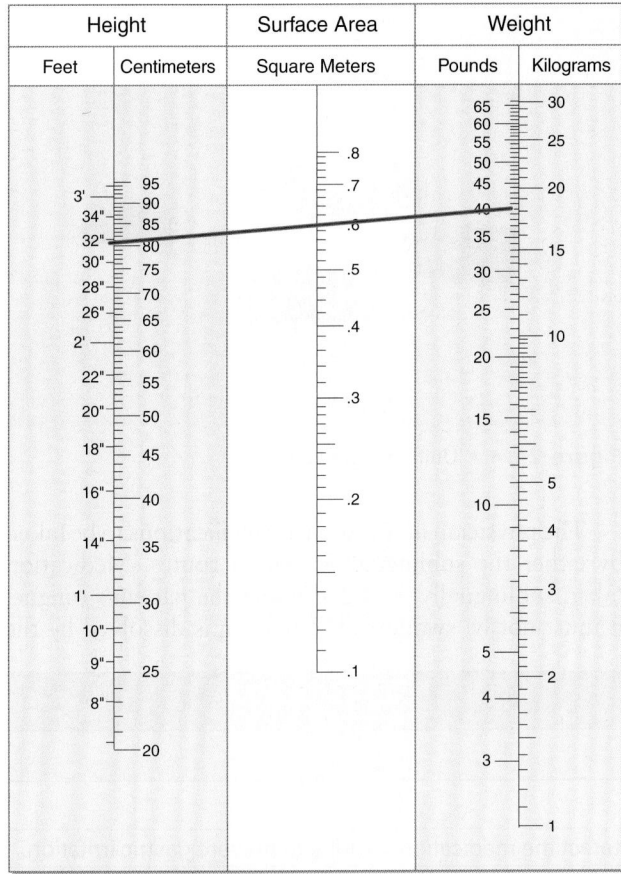

| Height | | Surface Area | Weight | |
|---|---|---|---|---|
| Feet | Centimeters | Square Meters | Pounds | Kilograms |

**Figure 24-3** • Using the nomogram, the child who is 32 inches tall and weighs 40 pounds has a BSA of 0.6 m².

the age of the child in years and divide by the age of the child in years plus 12. This number is multiplied by the adult dose.

Pediatric dose = ×Adult dose

Clark's rule is more accurate than Young's rule because it allows for variations in body size and weight for different ages. Using Clark's rule, the weight of the child is divided by 150 (presumed weight of average adult) and multiplied by the average adult dose to determine the pediatric dose.

Pediatric dose = ×Adult dose

Fried's rule, which is used for calculating doses for infants less than 2 years of age, bases the dose on the age of the child in months. In this case, 150 used in calculations is the age in months of a 12.5-year-old child, presuming that a child of that age would be eligible for an adult dose. Using Fried's rule, the child's age in months is divided by 150 and then multiplied by the average adult dose.

Pediatric dose = ×Adult dose

Some medications that require careful calibration are dosed per kilogram of body weight. Instructions for

calculation are included in the package insert that comes with the medication or in the *Physician's Desk Reference.* For instance, the insert may state to give adults and children over 25 kg (55 lb) 500 mg of a particular medication and use the formula 25 mg/kg for children who weigh less than 25 kg. If the child weighs 20 lb, this weight must be converted to kilograms before any calculations are made. Since 1 kg is equal to 2.2 lb, the child who weighs 20 lb also weighs 9 kg. The equation for calculating the child's dosage would be set up as follows:

$$25 \text{ mg} \times 9 \text{ kg} = 225 \text{ mg}$$

Therefore, the physician will use this calculation to determine how much medication (225 mg) is appropriate for the child who weighs 20 lb (9 kg).

## CHECKPOINT QUESTION

5. When the physician is calculating how much medication to prescribe for an infant or child, which method for calculating pediatric dosages is most often used?

## WHAT IF?

**A child is brought to the medical office having difficulty breathing and needing emergency medications? How does the physician have time to calculate the dose for the child's body weight?**

In such a situation, the physician does not have the time to perform the calculations and instead may rely on a printed graph that lists precalculated emergency drug doses or on medication reference books. There is also computer software that is available that will automatically calculate and print a list of pediatric emergency medications and their doses. In this situation, it is important to remain calm and notify emergency services as directed by the physician since these trained professionals will have the knowledge and equipment required to resuscitate a child should the emergency situation deteriorate.

## ROUTES OF MEDICATION ADMINISTRATION

Medication can be administered in many ways and is chosen by the physician after considering many factors. Sometimes, the route is chosen because of cost, safety, or the speed by which the drug will be absorbed into the body. Certain drugs may be administered by only one route, while others may be administered in a variety of ways. Some drugs may be toxic if given by a certain route, some may be effective only if given by a specific route, and sometimes absorption will occur only through one particular route.

## 💿 Oral, Sublingual, and Buccal Routes

Of all of the medication routes, the oral route is most preferred by patients and is the easiest to administer. However, medications taken orally, or by mouth, are usually slow to take effect, and this route cannot be used for unconscious patients, those with nausea and vomiting, or those who are ordered to take nothing by mouth. Drugs given orally may be administered as tablets, capsules, pills, or liquids (Procedure 24-1). Most are absorbed through the walls of the gastrointestinal tract. Drugs given orally in the medical office usually come in unit dose packs that contain the amount of the drug for a single dose (Fig. 24-4). These may be left by pharmaceutical sales representatives to be given as samples to patients. Unit dose packages are labeled with the trade name, generic name, precautions, instructions for storage, and an expiration date. Table 24-3 lists common solid and liquid forms of oral medications.

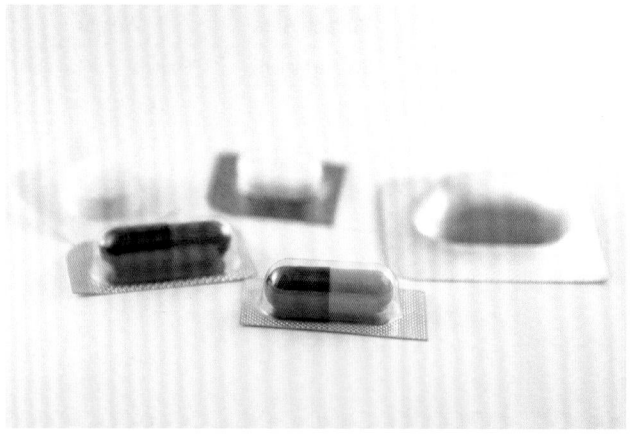

**Figure 24-4** • Unit-dose packages.

The physician may also order medications to be taken by either the **sublingual** or **buccal** routes. Medication taken sublingually is placed under the patient's tongue; it must not be swallowed. The drug is dissolved by the

| TABLE 24-3 | Forms of Oral Medications |
|---|---|
| **Form** | **Description** |
| *Solids* | |
| Buffered caplet | Agents are added to decrease or counteract the medication's acidity to prevent gastric irritation. |
| Capsule | Powdered or granulated medication is enclosed in a gelatin capsule designed to dissolve in gastric enzymes or high in the small intestines. |
| Enteric coated tablet | A compressed dry form of a medication coated to withstand the gastric acidity and dissolve in the intestines. These may be medications that would be destroyed by the gastric enzymes or might be damaging to the gastric mucosa. Never crush or break enteric coated tablets. |
| Gelcap | An oil-based medication enclosed in a soft gelatin capsule. |
| Lozenge | A firm, compressed form of medication, usually for a local effect in the mouth or throat. Caution patients to let lozenges dissolve slowly and avoid drinking any fluids for a period of time after using the lozenge. |
| Powder | A finely ground form of medication; may be difficult for some patients to swallow |
| Spansule or time-release capsule | Gelatin capsules are filled with forms of the medication that will dissolve over a period of time rather than all at once. Never open spansules unless this is recommended by the manufacturer. |
| Tablet | Medication is formed into many shapes and colors for easy identification. Tablets usually dissolve high in the gastrointestinal tract. These may be broken into halves only if they have been scored for that purpose. |
| *Liquids* | |
| Elixir | Medication is dissolved in alcohol, and flavoring is added. These are less sweet than syrups and are usually preferred by adults. They should not be used with alcoholics or diabetics. |
| Emulsion | Medication is combined with water and oil. Emulsions must be thoroughly shaken to disperse the medication evenly. |
| Extract | This is a very concentrated form of medication made by evaporating volatile plant oils. Extracts may be administered as drops and are usually given in a liquid to disguise their strong taste. |
| Gel | Medication is suspended in a thin gelatin or paste base. |
| Suspension | Particles are dissolved in a liquid that must be shaken well before administered. |
| Syrup | This very sweet form of medication is used frequently for children's medications and is usually flavored in addition to having a high sugar content. |

saliva in the mouth and is absorbed directly into the bloodstream through the oral mucosa covering the sublingual vessels. Caution the patient not to eat or drink until the medication has totally dissolved.

Medication given by the buccal route is placed in the pouch between the cheek and gum at the side of the mouth. Buccal absorption of medication occurs through the vascular oral mucosa. Although few medications are manufactured for this route, the patient must not eat or drink until the medication is completely absorbed if this method is used to administer medications.

 **CHECKPOINT QUESTION**

6. Pam is instructed by the physician to administer a medication orally. What are the disadvantages of the oral route for medication administration?

## Parenteral Administration

If a patient cannot take medications orally, if the drug cannot be absorbed through the gastrointestinal system, or if rapid absorption of the drug is desired, the parenteral route is used. Parenteral administration refers not only to injections but to all ways drugs are administered other than via the gastrointestinal tract. Administration by injection is the most efficient method of parenteral drug administration, but it can also be the most hazardous. While the effects may be quite rapid, the medication cannot be retrieved once injected, and because the skin is broken, it is possible for infection to develop if strict aseptic technique is not followed (Box 24-2).

 **Equipment for Injections**

*Ampules, Vials, Cartridges*

Medications used for injections are supplied in **ampules**, **vials**, and cartridges (Fig. 24-5). Ampules are small glass containers that must be broken at the neck so that the solution can be aspirated into the syringe. When the ampule is opened, all medication in it must be either used or discarded. It must not be saved for later use because once the ampule is broken, sterility cannot be maintained.

---

**BOX 24-2** **Injections: Maintaining Sterility**

The following parts of a hypodermic setup must be kept sterile:

- Syringe tip
- Inside of barrel
- Shaft of plunger
- Needle

---

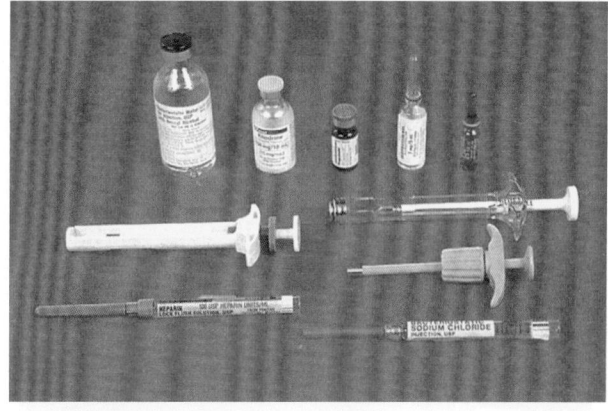

**Figure 24-5 •** Ampules, vials, prefilled cartridges, and holders.

Vials are glass or plastic containers sealed at the top by a rubber stopper. They may be single-dose or multiple-dose containers. The contents of vials may be in solution or in powder, which requires reconstitution with a specific amount and type of **diluent** (diluting agent), usually sterile water or saline. Certain drugs, such as phenytoin (Dilantin), require a special diluent supplied by the manufacturer. When a powdered drug is reconstituted in a multiple-dose vial, the following must be written on the label:

1. Date of reconstitution
2. Initials of the person who reconstituted the drug
3. Diluent used

To reconstitute dry medication, withdraw the diluent using aseptic technique, add the diluent to the vial containing the powder, and roll the bottle between your palms to dissolve the medication completely. Shaking the vial may cause unnecessary bubbles. When the powder has completely dissolved, calculate the dose based on the amount of diluent added to the powder. The instructions from the manufacturer of the drug usually indicate how much diluent to add to the powder and the resulting concentration of the mixture necessary for calculating dosages. You should always check the vial label or manufacturer's instructions before adding the diluent to determine the resulting dosage.

Vials intended for multiple doses may hold up to 50 mL and may be used repeatedly by inserting a needle through the self-sealing rubber stopper to remove a portion of the solution. Unit dose vials usually contain 1 to 2 mL, and all of the solution is removed for a single injection.

Prefilled syringes contain a premeasured amount of medication in a disposable cartridge with a needle attached. The prefilled cartridge and needle are placed in a holder for administration (Fig. 24-6). Examples of prefilled cartridges and holders are the Tubex™ and the Carpuject™. After a prefilled cartridge and holder are used, only the used cartridge should be discarded in a sharps biohazard container. The holder is reusable.

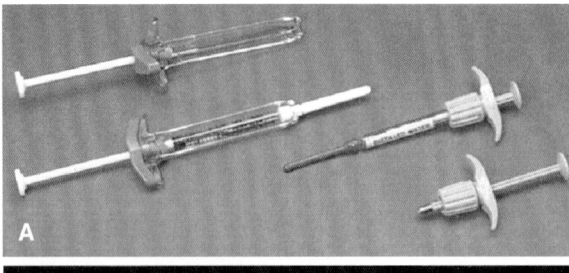

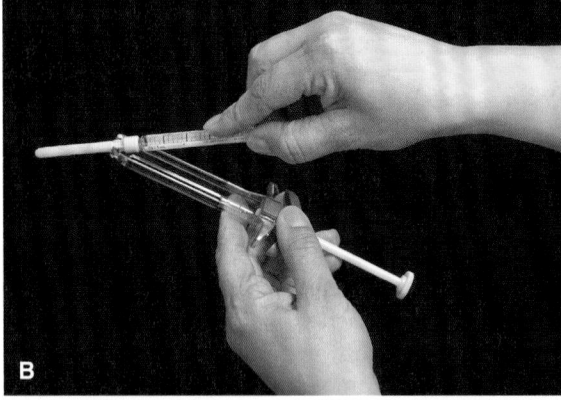

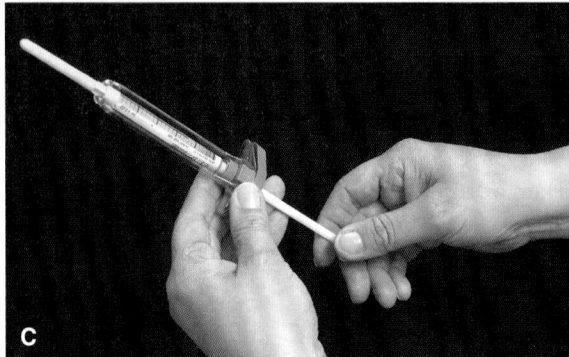

**Figure 24-6 •** Prefilled syringes. **(A)** Prefilled medication cartridges and injector devices. **(B)** Inserting the cartridge into the injector device. **(C)** Ready for injection.

## Needles and Syringes

The choice of needle and syringe used for an injection depends on the type of injection and the size of the patient. The 1-mL and 3-mL hypodermic syringe are the sizes most commonly used for injections. In the medical office, syringes designed to hold 5 mL or more are usually used for irrigation only, not for injections. All syringes consist of a plunger, body or barrel, flange, and tip (Fig. 24-7). Types of syringes used for parenteral administration include tuberculin, or 1-mL, syringes, 3-mL syringes, and insulin syringes that are calibrated in units and are used for insulin only (Fig. 24-8).

Needle lengths vary from 3/8 inch to 1 1/2 inch for standard injections. Gauge refers to the diameter of the needle lumen. Needle gauge varies from 18 (large) to 30 (small); the higher the number, the smaller the gauge. Medical supply companies package hypodermic needles separately in color-coded packages (Fig. 24-9) or in color-coded envelopes with the syringe attached. The sizes are also written on the package. Choose the

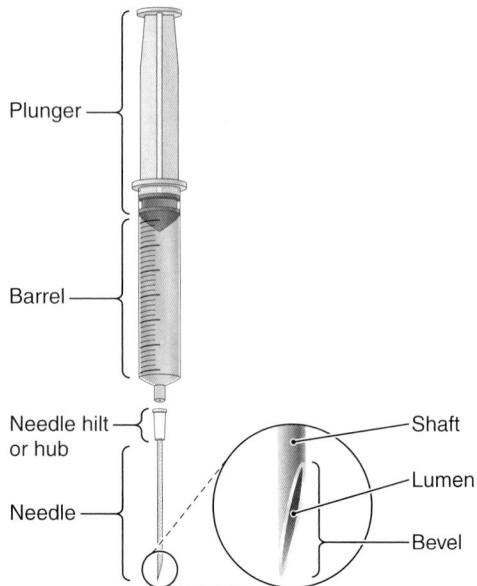

**Figure 24-7 •** Parts of a syringe and needle. (Reprinted from Cohen BJ. *Medical terminology: An illustrated guide,* 6th ed. Philadelphia, PA: Lippincott Williams & Wilkins, 2011, with permission.)

package with a needle length and gauge appropriate for the route of the injection. For example, an intramuscular injection for an adult requires a needle length of 1 to 1 1/2 inches, depending on the size of the patient and the fat to muscle ratio. The needle gauge varies from 20 to 25 depending on the thickness of the medication to be administered. Thick medications, such as penicillin and hormones, are difficult to draw into a syringe using a small-gauge needle, such as a 25 or 27, and equally difficult to inject into the patient. Subcutaneous injections are generally given using a short, small-gauge needle: 23 to 25 gauge, 5/8 inch to 1/2 inch.

All hypodermic syringes are marked with 10 calibrations per milliliter on one side of the syringe. Each small line represents 0.1 mL. The other side of the syringe may

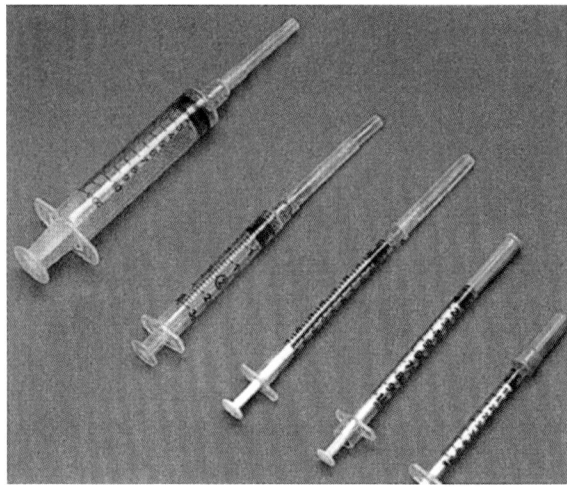

**Figure 24-8 •** Syringes (*from top to bottom*): 10 mL, 3 mL, tuberculin or 1 mL, insulin, and low-dose insulin.

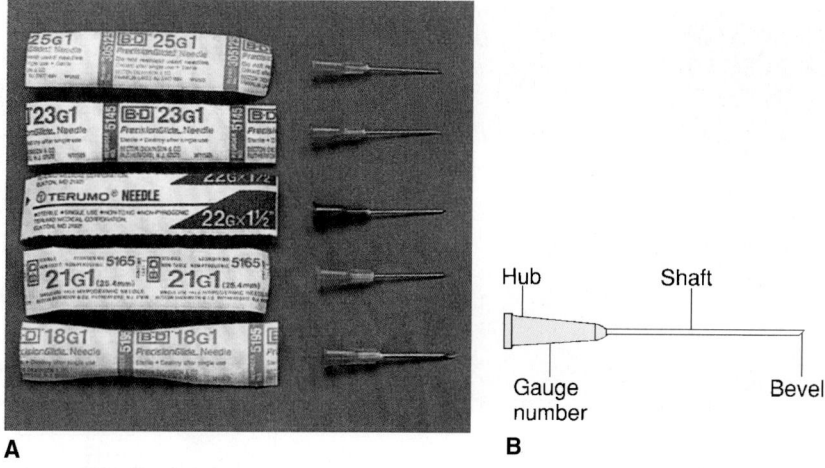

**Figure 24-9** • Needles. **(A)** Different gauges and lengths. **(B)** Parts of a needle.

be marked in minims (m), which are rarely used today. The tuberculin (TB) syringe is narrow and has a total capacity of 1 mL. There are 100 calibration lines marking the TB 1-mL syringe, with each line representing 0.01 mL. Every tenth line is longer than the others to indicate 0.1 mL. TB syringes are used for newborn and pediatric doses, for intradermal skin tests, and any time small amounts of medication (<1 mL) are to be given. The needle size for intradermal injections using a TB syringe is 25 to 27 gauge, 3/8 to 5/8 inch.

The insulin syringe is used strictly for administering insulin subcutaneously to diabetic patients and has an orange cap. It has a total capacity of 1 mL; however, the 1-mL volume is marked as 100 units (U) to represent the strength of 100 U insulin per milliliter when full. Each group of 10 U is divided by five small lines, and each line represents 2 U. Most of the insulin used today is U-100, which means that it has 100 U of insulin in each milliliter. The insulin syringe must be marked U-100 to match the insulin used.

Procedure 24-2 describes the steps required for preparing an injection.

### CHECKPOINT QUESTION

7. What are ampules and vials, and how do they differ?

## Types of Injections

 Intradermal Injections

Intradermal medications are administered into the dermal layer of the skin by inserting the needle at a 10 to 15 degree angle, almost parallel to the skin surface (Fig. 24-10). When an intradermal injection is administered correctly, the needle tip and lumen are slightly visible under the skin, and a small bubble, known as a wheal, is raised in the skin. Recommended sites for intradermal injections include the anterior forearm

and the back. Intradermal injections are used exclusively to administer skin tests for tuberculosis screening, the **Mantoux test**, and allergy testing. Procedure 24-3 describes the steps for giving an intradermal injection.

The tine test is another skin test used for routine screening of tuberculosis, but it is not considered as diagnostic as the Mantoux test. Both methods use purified protein derivative (PPD) from a live tuberculin bacillus culture to test for the presence of tuberculin antibodies. The tine applicator contains small tines impregnated with PPD. After cleansing the forearm, press the tine applicator firmly into the intradermal

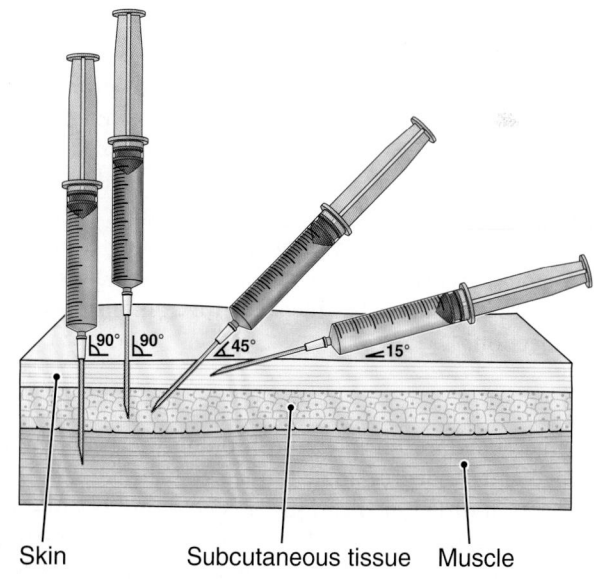

**Figure 24-10** • Comparison of the angles of insertion for intramuscular, subcutaneous, and intradermal injections. (Reprinted from Cohen BJ. *Medical terminology: An illustrated guide,* 6th ed. Philadelphia, PA: Lippincott Williams & Wilkins, 2011, with permission.)

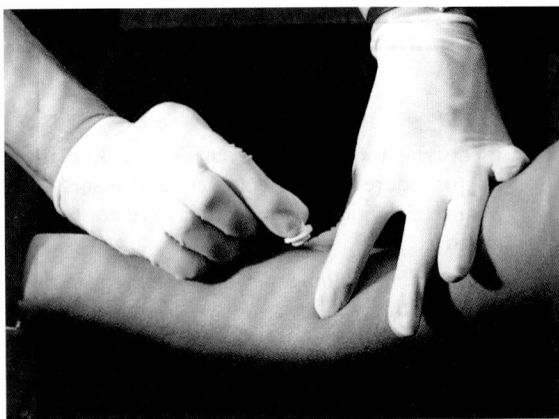

**Figure 24-11** • Administering the tine test for tuberculosis screening.

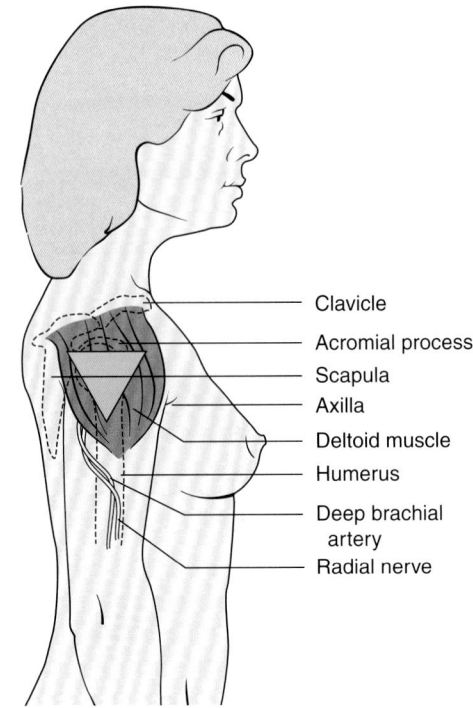

**Figure 24-12** • The deltoid muscle site for intramuscular injection is located by palpating the lower edge of the acromial process. At the midpoint, in line with the axilla on the lateral aspect of the upper arm, a triangle is formed. Medications are administered within this triangle.

layer of the skin (Fig. 24-11). A positive tine test is usually followed by a Mantoux test. Both the tine test and the Mantoux test must be read within 48 to 72 hours. A positive Mantoux reaction has induration, a hard raised area over the injection site, larger than 10 mm. This positive reaction indicates the possibility of exposure to tuberculosis; however, it does not indicate that the patient has active tuberculosis (see Chapter 31). A complete medical history and further testing by sputum culture and radiography are required for a definitive diagnosis. Redness over the intradermal injection site should not be considered induration. An induration of less than 10 mm in a patient with no known risk factors, such as previous tuberculosis or HIV infection, is considered negative.

 ## Subcutaneous Injections

Subcutaneous (SQ or SC) injections are given into the fatty layer of tissue below the skin by positioning the needle and syringe at a 45 degree angle to the skin (see Fig. 24-10). The SQ route is chosen for drugs that should not be absorbed as rapidly as through the intramuscular (IM) or intravenous (IV) route. Common sites include the upper arm, thigh, back, and abdomen. Procedure 24-4 describes the steps for administering an SQ injection.

 ## Intramuscular Injections

IM injections are given by positioning the needle and syringe at a 90 degree angle to the skin (see Fig. 24-10). Absorption of IM medications is fairly rapid because of the rich vascularity of muscle. If slower absorption is desired, the medication is mixed with an oil base rather than saline or water to prolong absorption time. A 1-inch to 1 1/2–inch needle is required to administer an intramuscular injection to an adult. The length of the needle depends on the muscle chosen for injection and the size of the patient.

Recommended muscles used for IM injections include the deltoid (Fig. 24-12), dorsogluteal (Fig. 24-13), ventrogluteal (Fig. 24-14), and vastus lateralis (Fig. 24-15).

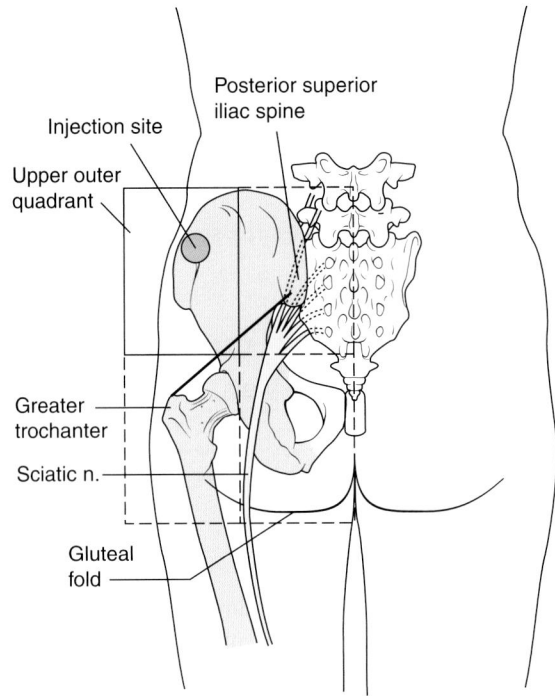

**Figure 24-13** • The dorsogluteal site for administering an IM injection is lateral and slightly superior to the midpoint of a line drawn from the trochanter to the posterior superior iliac spine. Correct identification of this site minimizes the possibility of accidentally damaging the sciatic nerve.

The rectus femoris (Fig. 24-16) can also be used when the other sites are contraindicated. It is recommended that no more than 1 mL be injected into the deltoid muscle and no more than 3 mL be injected into the other muscles in an adult. Children younger than 2 years of age should never receive injections in the gluteal muscle, since this muscle is not well developed until the child is walking. The muscle chosen for the injection depends on the preference of the medical assistant, the patient, and the amount of medication to be administered. Also, some pharmaceutical companies recommend specific sites for medications to be injected intramuscularly, and the medical assistant should use these sites as indicated. Gold sodium thiomalate, a medication used to treat arthritis, and some vaccines are examples of medications that have specific guidelines for administration set forth by the manufacturer. Procedure 24-5 describes the steps for administering an intramuscular injection.

### Z-Track Method of Intramuscular Injections

The Z-track method is used for IM administration of medications that may irritate or damage the tissues if allowed to leak back along the line of injection. An example of a medication that should be administered using this technique is iron dextran, which is used to treat iron deficiency anemia. The Z-track method prevents leakage by sealing off the layers of skin along the route of the needle (Fig. 24-17). If the medication is extremely caustic, directions may include changing the needle after drawing up the solution. An additional precaution may include drawing up to 0.5 mL of air into the syringe after the medication has been aspirated into the syringe. When the medication is injected

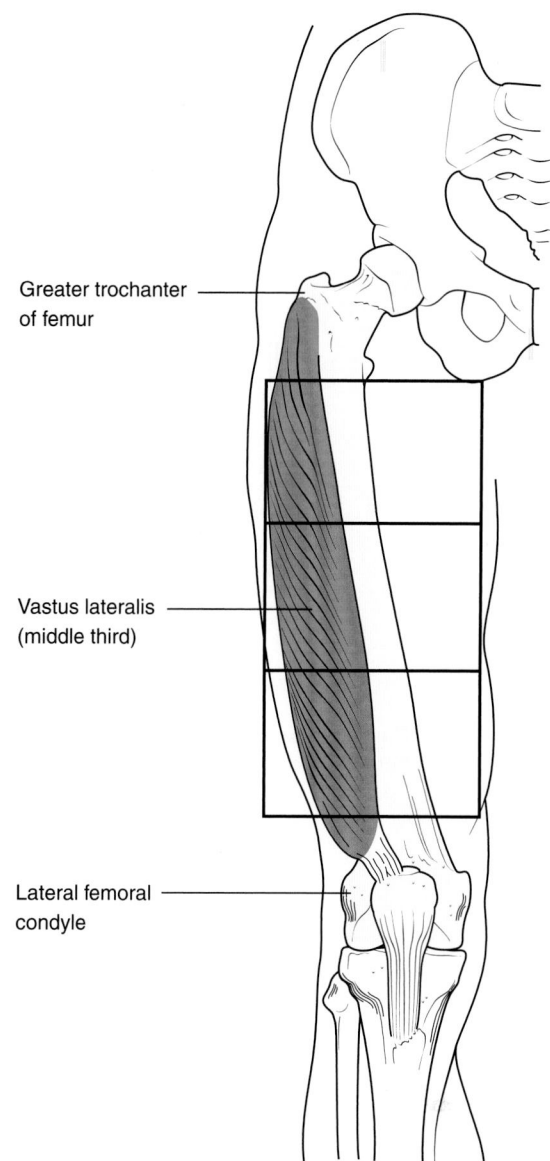

**Figure 24-15** • The vastus lateralis site for IM injections is identified by dividing the thigh into thirds horizontally and vertically. The injection is given in the outer middle third.

Greater trochanter of femur

Vastus lateralis (middle third)

Lateral femoral condyle

at a 90 degree angle, the additional air rises to the top of the syringe and is injected after the medication. This clears the needle and the path of the injection (Fig. 24-18). Procedure 24-6 describes the steps for administering an intramuscular injection using the Z-track method.

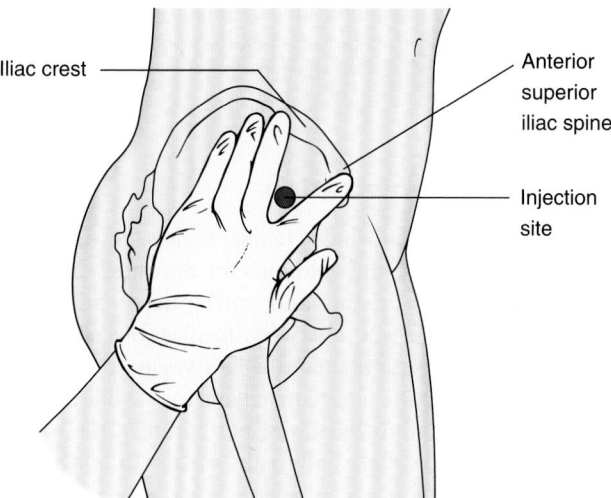

Iliac crest

Anterior superior iliac spine

Injection site

**Figure 24-14** • The ventrogluteal site is located by placing the palm on the greater trochanter and the index finger toward the anterior superior iliac spine. The middle finger is then spread posteriorly away from the index finger as far as possible. A "V" or triangle is formed by this maneuver. The injection is made in the middle of the triangle.

### 🔍 CHECKPOINT QUESTION

8. Pam attended an accredited medical assisting program and was taught to administer a variety of injection methods. Name the types of injections and the possible sites for each type.

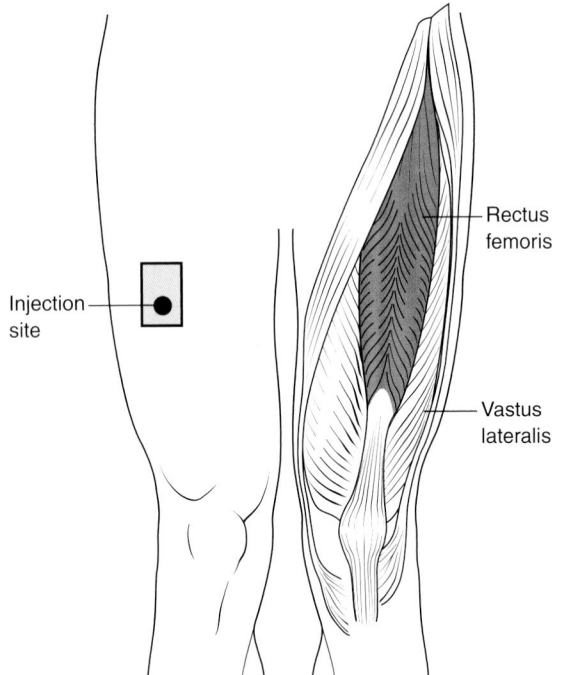

**Figure 24-16** • The rectus femoris site for IM injections is used only when other sites are contraindicated.

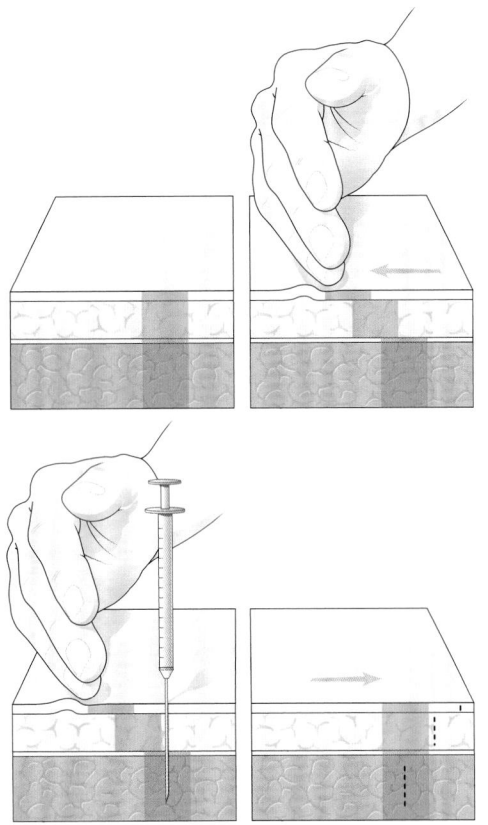

**Figure 24-17** • The Z-track technique is used to administer medications that are irritating to SQ tissue. The skin is pulled to one side, the needle is inserted, and the solution is injected after careful aspiration. When the needle is withdrawn and the displaced tissue is allowed to return to its normal position, the solution is prevented from escaping from the muscle tissue.

# Other Medication Routes

## Rectal Administration

Rectal medications are packaged in the form of suppositories or liquids administered as a retention enema (Fig. 24-19). They can provide a local effect or be absorbed through the rectal mucosa for a systemic effect. Rectal medications may be used for patients who are NPO (allowed nothing by mouth) or who have nausea and vomiting, but they are never used for patients who have diarrhea. Suppositories have a cocoa butter or glycerin base that melts at body temperature. They should be stored in the refrigerator to prevent melting. Rectal medications are rarely administered in the medical office, but you may be required to instruct the patient the proper technique for administration at home. Both retention enemas and rectal suppositories should be retained by the patient for about 20 to 30 minutes before elimination.

 **PATIENT EDUCATION**

### Administering Rectal Medications at Home

Some medications have to be administered rectally. You should teach the patient or family member to perform this procedure if the medication is to be taken at home. Here are some key points to discuss:

- Gloves should be worn.
- A small amount of a lubricant should be added to the suppository for easy insertion. The lubricant may be supplied with the suppository, or it can be purchased separately at the pharmacy.
- Advise the patient to remain lying on the bed for about 15 minutes after the suppository is inserted.
- The suppository should be inserted past the anal sphincter.

## Vaginal Administration

Vaginal medications include creams, tablets, cocoa butter-based suppositories, and solutions for douches. Examples include hormonal creams and antibiotic or antifungal preparations (Fig. 24-20). Very few medications other than those for local effects are prescribed for vaginal administration. Instruct the patient to remain lying for a while after the insertion of vaginal medications. For comfort, the patient may have to wear a light pad to absorb any drainage.

 ## Transdermal Administration

Dermal medications, which are applied to the skin, include topical creams, lotions, ointments, and transdermal medications. Topical medications (creams, ointments, sprays, and lotions) produce local effects, while

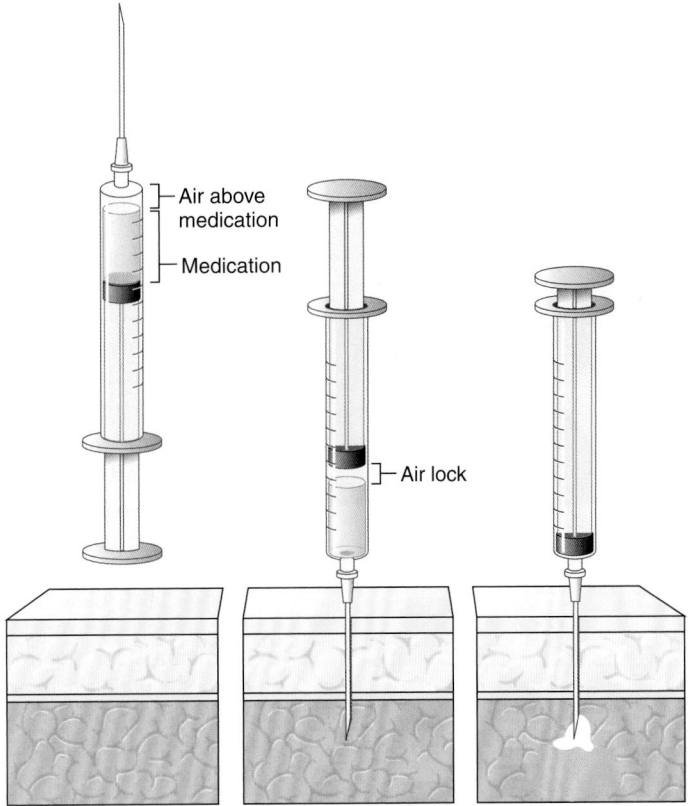

**Figure 24-18 •** An air bubble added to the syringe after the medication has been accurately measured helps to expel solution that is trapped in the shaft of the needle when the injection is given. It also helps to trap the injected solution in the IM tissue.

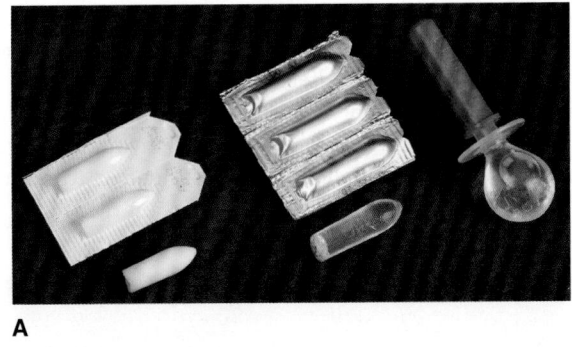

transdermal medications produce systemic effects. Medication administered transdermally is delivered to the body by absorption through the skin. Delivery is slow and maintains a steady, stable level of medication. You should never cut a transdermal patch, since doing so alters the rate of absorption. Dermal patches are placed on the skin, usually on the chest or back, upper arm, or behind the ear (for medications that prevent motion sickness). Procedure 24-7 describes the steps for applying transdermal medications.

## Inhalation

Inhalation is administration of medication, water vapor, or gas by inspiration of the substance into the lungs. Medication administered by inhalation is absorbed quickly through the alveolar walls into the capillaries, but a disease condition may make absorption difficult to predict. Patients with chronic pulmonary disease or disorder may self-administer certain medications with a handheld **nebulizer** or inhaler, both producing a fine spray of medicated mist that is inhaled directly into the lungs (see Chapter 31).

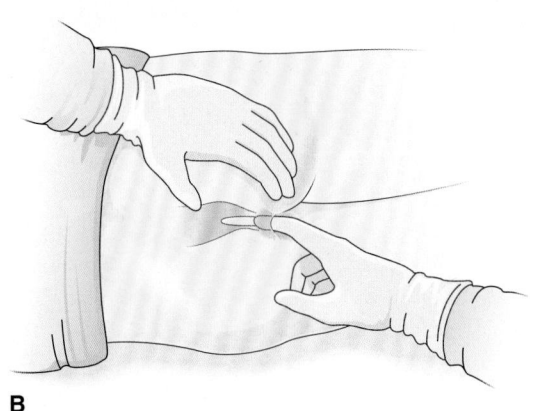

**B**

**Figure 24-19 •** **(A)** These are examples of suppositories. **(B)** Rectal suppositories should be introduced into the anus well beyond the internal sphincter.

### CHECKPOINT QUESTION

9. How are medications given by the inhalation route absorbed?

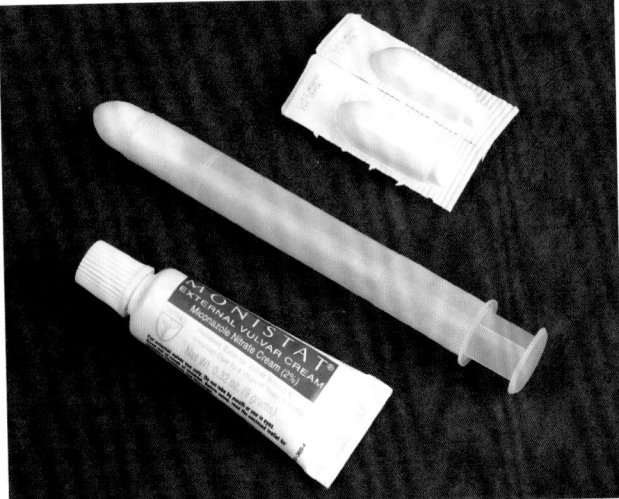

**A**

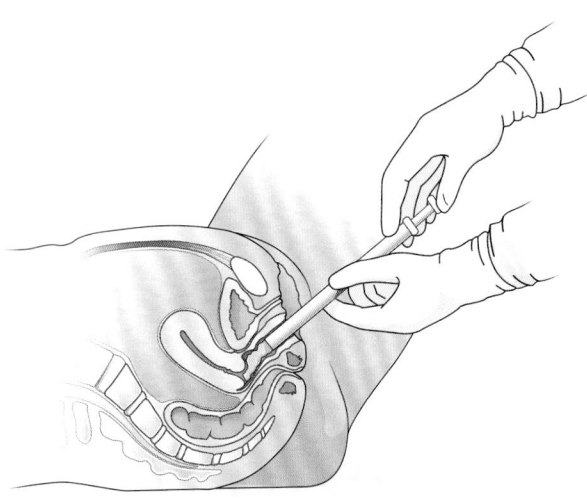

**B**

**Figure 24-20 • (A)** Vaginal suppository and applicator. **(B)** Insertion of vaginal cream using applicator.

# PRINCIPLES OF INTRAVENOUS THERAPY

With the IV route, a sterile solution of a drug is injected through a catheter or needle that has been inserted into a vein by a procedure known as *venipuncture* (refer to Chapter 41). IV medication has the quickest action because it enters the bloodstream immediately. In most cases, the physician administers IV medications, but some ambulatory care centers expect medical assistants to be proficient at setting up the equipment and fluids for an IV, performing the venipuncture, and regulating the IV fluids as directed by the physician. Some states may have laws that prohibit a medical assistant from starting an IV line or administering IV medications. Only drugs intended for IV administration should be given by this route.

## AFF  TRIAGE

While you are working in a medical office setting, the following three situations arise:

A. A 50-year-old man is complaining of dyspnea, and the doctor has ordered a nebulizer treatment.
B. A 65-year-old woman needs her first dose of an antibiotic.
C. A 47-year-old woman slipped on the ice in the parking lot and is having moderate pain in the right ankle. The doctor has ordered a pain medication injection.

**How do you sort these patients? Who do you see first? Second? Third?**

Patient A should be treated first; any patient with chest pain or shortness of breath should be treated as a number 1 priority. Patient C should be medicated for pain control. Last, patient B should be given the antibiotic. Remember, you must closely monitor this patient for 30 minutes for signs of an allergic reaction. All three of these patients need to be closely evaluated after receiving their medications. Ask yourself, is the patient breathing better? Is the pain better? Communicate your findings with the physician.

## Intravenous Equipment

The equipment necessary for starting an IV includes the fluids (determined by the physician), the IV catheter (angiocatheter), and the tubing and valve that connect the IV fluids to the catheter and regulate the flow of fluids into the patient (Fig. 24-21). Once the IV line is started, the fluids are administered through the vein either to replace fluids lost by the patient or to administer medications through special ports on the tubing.

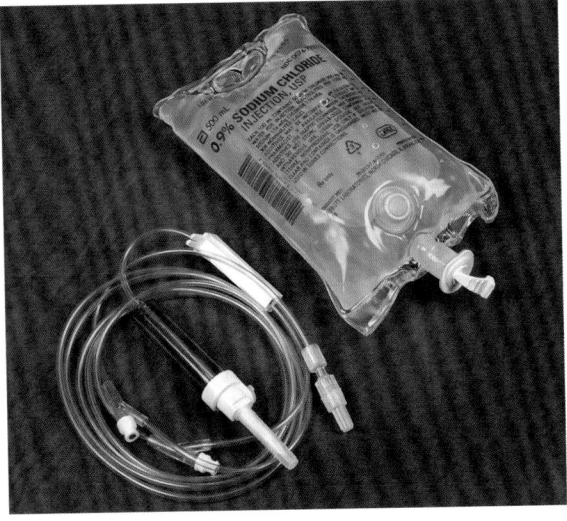

**Figure 24-21 •** IV equipment including the fluid and tubing.

Examples of fluids that come prepackaged for use in IV therapy are Ringer's lactate (RL), dextrose 5% and water (D5W), 0.9% normal saline, 0.45% normal saline, or a combination (D5NS, D5RL). The physician chooses the type and amount of fluid to be administered. An administration set (tubing) is used, with one end (the end with the drip chamber) inserted into the IV fluid bag and the other end inserted into the IV catheter after it is in the vein. After securing the IV catheter and attaching the administration set tubing, adjust the flow of fluids by adjusting the roller clamp and carefully watching the fluids drip into the drip chamber. Carefully count the drops per minute so you can adjust the flow of fluids to the exact rate desired. The amount of fluid to be administered is ordered by the physician in terms of milliliters per hour (e.g., 125 mL/hour). Using this physician order, determine how fast to run the solution following this procedure:

- Determine the drop factor (number of drops needed to deliver 1 mL of fluid) as noted on the administration set tubing package (macrodrip systems deliver 10 or 20 drops per milliliter, and microdrip systems deliver 60 drops per milliliter.)
- The physician order will include the type of fluid (e.g., RL, $D_5W$), the amount (e.g., 125 mL), and the time frame (e.g., per hour).
- Use the following formula to calculate the number of drops per minute necessary to deliver the amount of fluid:

$$(\text{Volume in milliliters} \times \text{Time in minutes})$$
$$\times \text{Drop factor (gtt / min)}$$
$$= \text{Drops per minute}$$

For example, if the physician orders an IV of RL at 100 mL/hour and the administration set delivers 10 gtt/mL, the formula would be set up as follows:

$$(100 \text{ mL} \div 60 \text{ minutes}) = 1.67$$
$$1.67 \times 10 \text{ gtt / mL} = 17 \text{ gtt / min } (16.7 \text{ rounded up to nearest tenth} = 17)$$

In this situation, you would regulate the roller clamp so that 17 drops per minute flow into the drip chamber to deliver 100 mL/hour as ordered by the physician. If the physician would like the patient to have an IV line available, but not necessarily for administering fluids, a to-keep-open (TKO) or keep-vein-open (KVO) rate will be ordered. The flow of fluids into the vein to prevent clotting may be 15 to 30 mL/hour as determined by the physician. The same formula is used to calculate this rate: (rate = volume ÷ time ÷ drop factor).

## Troubleshooting Problems

The medical assistant must be vigilant about watching the IV fluids and the site of venipuncture. **Infiltration** occurs when IV fluid infuses into the tissues surrounding the vein, usually because the catheter has been dislodged. Carefully securing the IV catheter and the administration tubing usually prevents infiltration. In case of infiltration, stop the flow of fluids, remove the catheter, and notify the physician. Infiltration is characterized by the following:

- Swelling and pain at the IV site
- A slow or absent flow rate into the drip chamber of the administration set with the roller clamp open
- No blood return or backup into the tubing when the fluid bag is below the level of the heart

Phlebitis may occur when the IV catheter has caused inflammation in the vein or when there is an infection present. Often, the irritation or infection occurs at the insertion site and is characterized by redness, swelling, and tenderness. There may also be a red streak starting at the insertion site and following the vein upward on the extremity. Although the IV may be flowing without difficulty, signs of infection or inflammation indicate that the IV line should be removed and reinserted as ordered by the physician. Regardless of the reason for reinserting an IV, you must use either the other arm or a site above the level of infiltration or infection.

### CHECKPOINT QUESTION

10. How would you explain an IV that is not flowing even with the roller clamp open?

### ROLE-PLAYING ACTIVITY

Review the case study found at the beginning of this chapter. Role-play the scenario, assuming the role of Pam King, the medical assistant asked to give an injection drawn up by another employee. Another classmate can assume the role of the other employee. How would you respond? Would your response be different if the medication was drawn up and you were asked to administer it by someone in the office you did not know or trust? Role-play this scenario, perhaps switching roles so that you are the other employee and your classmate is Pam King. Your instructor will give you additional information about this activity!

## *español* SPANISH TERMINOLOGY

**¿Es alérgico/alérgica a algo?**
Do you have any allergies?

**Tome tres cucharaditas cuatro veces al dia ó cada seis horas.**
Take three teaspoons 4 times a day or every 6 hours.

**Tengo que ponerle una inyección.**
I need to give you an injection.

**No mastique este medicamento.**
Please do not masticate/chew this medication

**¿Quiere un poco de agua?**
Would you like some water?

**¿Hay algo que lo/la ayude a aliviar el dolor?**
Does anything help the pain?

**En una escala de 1 al 10, siendo el 10 el máximo, que numero le daría al suyo.**
On a pain scale of 1 to 10, with 10 being the highest, how would you grade yours?

**Este es un medicamento que va debajo de la lengua, no lo mastique ó trague.**
This is a sublingual medication; do not swallow or chew it.

**La medicina está en el parche, su piel la va a absorver.**
The medicine is in the patch; your skin will absorb it.

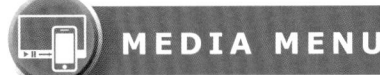

## MEDIA MENU

**Student Resources** on thePoint®

- *Animation:* Intramuscular Injection
- *Animation:* Intravenous Injection
- CMA/RMA Certification Exam Review
- *Video:* Administering Oral Medications (Procedure 24-1)
- *Video:* Preparing Injections (Procedure 24-2)
- *Video:* Administering an Intradermal Injection (Procedure 24-3)
- *Video:* Administering a Subcutaneous Injection (Procedure 24-4)
- *Video:* Administering an Intramuscular Injection and the Z-Track Method (Procedures 24-5 and 24-6)
- *Video:* Applying Transdermal Medications (Procedure 24-7)

**Internet Resources**
**Medwatch**
http://www.fda.gov/medwatch

**Physician's Desk Reference**
http://www.pdr.net/Default.aspx

**FDA Medication Guides**
http://www.fda.gov/Drugs/DrugSafety/ucm085729.htm

**National Center for Complimentary and Alternative Medicine**
http://nccam.nih.gov

**Institute for Healthcare Improvement**
http://www.ihi.org/IHI

**Patient Safety and Quality Healthcare**
http://www.psqh.com/index.html

## EMR Activity

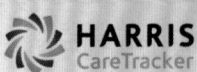

Harris CareTracker is a Web-based electronic medical record (EMR) application that you will use for the EMR activities included in this section at the end of each chapter. This application is actually used in physician offices but is provided to you through the publisher, Wolters Kluwer Health, to give you hands-on practice working with EMRs. Your instructor will have more information about accessing your username, log-in, and Quickstart guide.

Prerequisite Activities in Harris CareTracker

• *The Getting Started and Quickstart documents and EMR Activities Step-by-Step Instructions are available at* http://thePoint.lww.com/KronenbergerComp5e.

Activity Details

In the *Medical Record* module, *Progress Note* application, accurately document the following medications ordered by Dr. Kyle Dunn and administered by you in the medical office today for the following patients:

1. Erica Tompkin Rocephin 1 gram IM right dorsogluteal muscle
2. Sarah Banks Tripedia 0.5cc IM right vastus lateralis muscle
3. Lawrence Black Depo-Testosterone 200mg IM left dorsogluteal muscle

## Chapter Summary

- The administration of medication is one of the most challenging and exacting procedures performed in the medical office.
- Few other procedures require such intense concentration and attention to detail or include such potential for danger to the patient.
- You will be asked to practice interpersonal skills, such as tact and diplomacy, to make these procedures acceptable to the patient and to allay the anxiety felt by almost all patients during the administration of medications.
- It is also your responsibility to be familiar with and follow the laws in your state regarding the administration of medications.

## Warm-Ups for Critical Thinking

1. Design a patient education brochure that will teach patients about administering rectal medications at home.
2. After inserting the needle while giving an IM injection, you aspirate by pulling back slightly on the plunger. As you do this, blood appears in the syringe. What has happened? What should you do?
3. Another coworker has just given an oral medication to a patient in the office. She asks you to document the procedure. How would you handle this situation?
4. When preparing a medication for injection, you become distracted and forget how much medication you need to draw up into the syringe. What should you do?

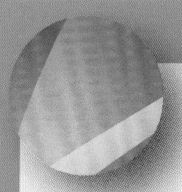 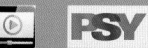 PROCEDURE 24-1

## Administering Oral Medications

**PSY** Verify rules of medication administration; administer oral medications; document patient care accurately in the medical record.

**Purpose:** Accurately administer oral medications

**Equipment:** Physician's order, oral medication, disposable calibrated cup, glass of water, and patient medical record

| STEPS | REASONS |
|---|---|
| 1. Wash your hands. | Handwashing aids infection control. |
| 2. Review the physician's medication order and select the correct medication. Compare the label to the physician's instructions. Note the expiration date. Check the label three times: when taking it from the shelf, while pouring, and when returning it to the shelf. | Carefully dispensing medications helps prevent errors. Outdated medication should not be administered but should be discarded appropriately. |
| 3. Calculate the correct dosage to be given if necessary. | Some medications, such as vaccines, are given in specific milliliters and do not need to have a dosage calculated. |
| 4. If using a multidose container, remove the cap from the container, touching only the outside of the lid. Single-dose, or unit-dose, medications come individually wrapped in packages that may be opened by pushing the medication through the foil backing or peeling back a tab on one corner. | The inside of the lid of a multidose bottle will be contaminated if touched. |
| 5. According to your calculations and the label, remove the correct dose of medication.<br>  A. For solid medications:<br>    (1) Pour the capsule or tablet into the bottle cap to prevent contamination. | The amount the physician orders is in milligrams. You will need to calculate the amount of milliliters to administer to deliver the milligrams ordered. |

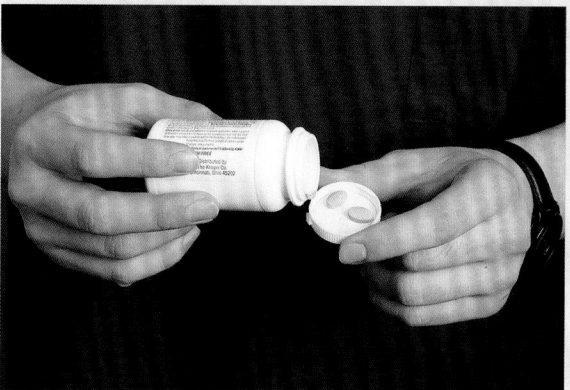

**Step 5A (1).** Pour the tablet into the bottle cap.

*(continues on page 610)*

# PROCEDURE 24-1 (continued)

| STEPS | REASONS |
|---|---|

**(2)** Transfer the medication to a disposable cup.

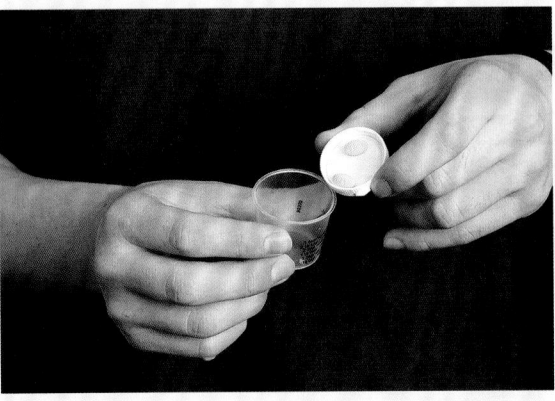

**Step 5A (2).** Transfer the medication into a disposable cup.

**B.** For liquid medications:
  **(1)** Open the bottle and place the lid on a flat surface with the open end up to prevent contamination of the inside of the cap.
  **(2)** Palm the label to prevent liquids from dripping onto the label and possibly damaging it or making it illegible.

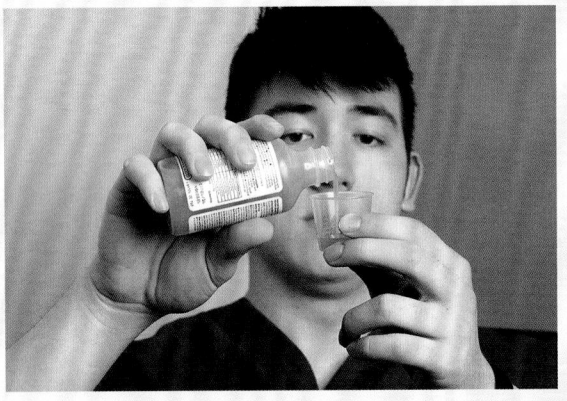

**Step 5B (2).** Palm the label of the container when pouring liquids.

  **(3)** With the opposite hand, place your thumbnail at the correct calibration on the cup. Holding the cup at eye level, pour the proper amount of medication into the cup, using your thumbnail as a guide.

**6.** Greet and identify the patient. Explain the procedure. Ask the patient about medication allergies that might not be noted on the chart.

Identifying the patient prevents errors. Explaining the procedure helps ease anxiety and may improve compliance. The medical record should be checked for allergies, but the patient should also be asked, since allergies may not have been noted.

**7.** Give the patient a glass of water to wash down the medication unless contraindicated and administer the medication by handing the patient the disposable cup containing the medication.

Water helps the patient swallow the medication, but water is contraindicated for medications intended for a local effect (such as cough syrup or lozenges) and for buccal or sublingual medications.

## PROCEDURE 24-1 (continued)

| STEPS | REASONS |
|---|---|
| 8. Remain with the patient to be sure that all of the medication is swallowed. Observe any unusual reactions, report them to the physician, and enter them in the medical record. | You cannot assume that the patient swallowed the medication unless you observe it. |
| 9. **AFF** Explain how to respond to a patient who is hearing impaired. | Make sure the patient can see your face as you are speaking. Speak clearly, not loudly. |
| 10. Thank the patient and give any appropriate instructions. | |
| 11. Wash your hands. | Always wash your hands after a patient encounter. |
| 12. **PSY** Log into the electronic medical record (EMR) using your username and secure password OR obtain the paper medical record from a secure location and assure it is kept away from public access. Record the procedure noting the date, time, name of medication, dose administered, route of administration, and your name. | The integrity of the medical record must be maintained at all times to protect patient privacy. |
| 13. When finished, log out of the EMR and/or replace the paper medical record in an appropriate and secure location. | The physician and other workers in the office may need to know what the patient has been taught. Remember, if it's not in the chart, it did not happen. |

Charting Example:

*12/14/2016 8:45 AM Ampicillin 125 mg PO given to pt. NKA* _____ *P. King, CMA*

Note: *The medical assistant may sign his or her name in the patient record using only the "CMA" credential if the office has a signature log denoting the entire credential as "CMA(AAMA)."*

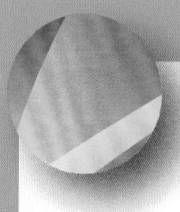 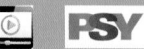

## PSY PROCEDURE 24-2

### Preparing Injections

**Purpose:** Accurately prepare a medication by injection

**Equipment:** Physician's order, medication for injection (ampule or vial), antiseptic wipes, needle and syringe of appropriate size, small gauze pad, biohazard sharps container, patient's and medical record

| STEPS | REASONS |
|---|---|
| 1. Wash your hands. | Handwashing aids infection control. |
| 2. Review the medication order and select the correct medication. Compare the label to the physician's instructions. Note the expiration date. Check the label three times: when taking it from the shelf, while drawing it up into the syringe, and when returning it to the shelf. | Carefully dispensing medications helps prevent errors. Outdated medication should not be administered to a patient but should be discarded appropriately. |
| 3. Calculate the correct dosage to be given if necessary. | |
| 4. Choose the needle and syringe according to the route of administration, type of medication, and size of the patient. | A shorter needle is used for SQ medications, whereas a larger gauge may be necessary for thick medications. |
| 5. Open the needle and syringe package. Assemble if necessary. Make sure the needle is firmly attached to the syringe by grasping the needle at the hub and turning it clockwise onto the syringe. | Needles and syringes often are preassembled, or they may be purchased separately. A needle that is not firmly attached may be detached during the procedure. |

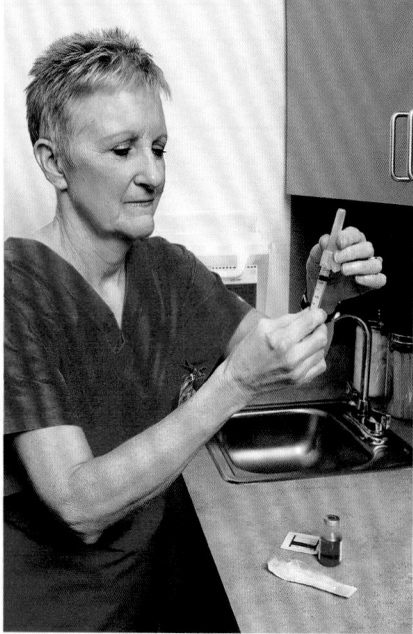

**Step 5.** Grasp the needle at the hub and turn it clockwise.

| STEPS | REASONS |
|---|---|
| 6. Withdraw the correct amount of medication:<br>**A.** From an ampule:<br>(1) With the fingertips of one hand, tap the stem of the ampule lightly to remove any medication in or above the narrow neck. | Administering an incorrect amount of medication will result in the patient getting too little or too much of a medication. |

## PROCEDURE 24-2 (continued)

**STEPS**

**REASONS**

(2) Wrap a piece of gauze around the ampule neck to protect your fingers from broken glass. Grasp the gauze and ampule firmly with the fingers. Snap the stem off the ampule with a quick downward movement of the gauze. Be sure to aim the break away from your face. Dispose of the ampule top in a biohazard sharps container to prevent injury.

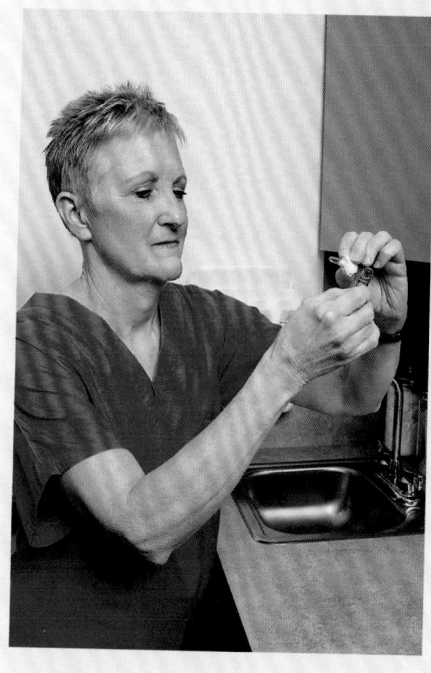

**Step 6A (2).** Grasp the gauze and ampule firmly.

(3) After removing the needle guard, insert the needle lumen below the level of the medication. Withdraw the medication by pulling back on the plunger of the syringe without letting the needle touch the contaminated edge of the broken ampule. Withdraw the desired amount of medication and dispose of the ampule in a biohazard sharps container.

(4) Remove any air bubbles by holding the syringe with the needle up and gently tapping the barrel of the syringe until the air bubbles rise to the top. Draw back on the plunger to add a small amount of air, then gently push the plunger forward to eject the air out of the syringe. Be careful not to eject any medication if the required dosage has been drawn up.

*(continues on page 614)*

## PROCEDURE 24-2 (continued)

| STEPS | REASONS |
|---|---|

**B.** From a vial:

(1) Using the antiseptic wipe, cleanse the rubber stopper of the vial to avoid introducing bacteria into the medication.

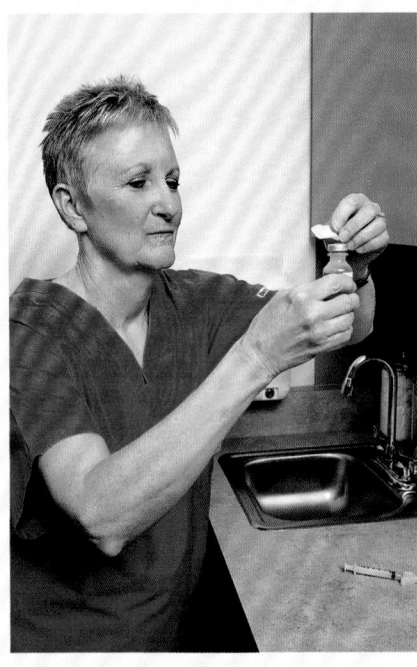

**Step 6B (1).** Clean the rubber stopper with an antiseptic wipe.

(2) Remove the needle guard and pull back on the plunger to fill the syringe with an amount of air equal to the amount of medication to be removed from the vial.

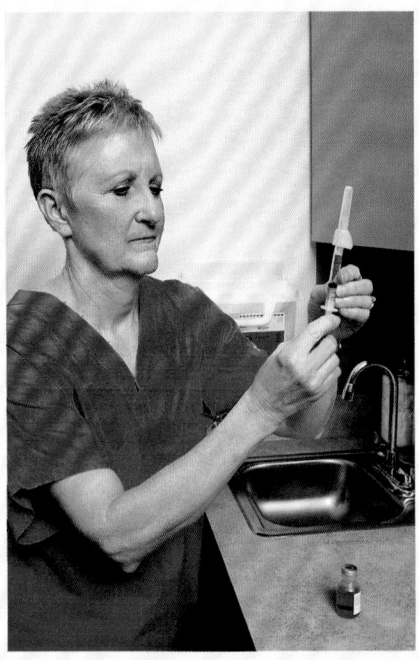

**Step 6B (2).** Pull back on the plunger, sucking air into the syringe.

## PROCEDURE 24-2 (continued)

| STEPS | REASONS |
|---|---|
| (3) Insert the needle into the vial through the center of the cleansed vial top. Inject the air from the syringe into the vial above the level of the medication to avoid producing foam or bubbles in the medication. | |

(3) Insert the needle into the vial through the center of the cleansed vial top. Inject the air from the syringe into the vial above the level of the medication to avoid producing foam or bubbles in the medication.
Injecting an equal amount of air into the vial will prevent a vacuum from forming in the vial, which would make withdrawal of the medication difficult.

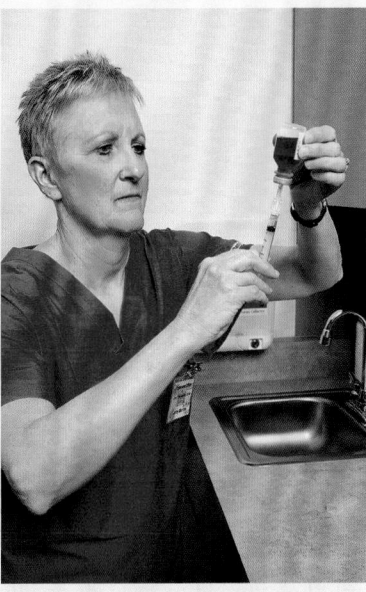

Step 6B (3). Insert the needle through the rubber stopper.

(4) With the needle inside the vial, invert the vial, holding the syringe at eye level. Aspirate, or withdraw, the desired amount of medication into the syringe.

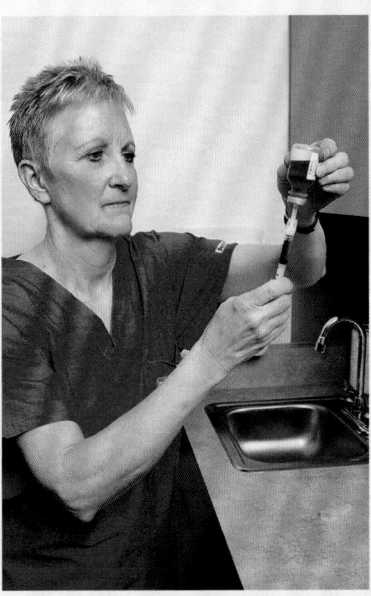

Step 6B (4). Invert the vial.

(continues on page 616)

## PROCEDURE 24-2 (continued)

**STEPS**                                           **REASONS**

(5) Displace any air bubbles in the syringe by
gently tapping the barrel of the syringe with
the fingertips. Remove the air by pushing the
plunger slowly and forcing the air into the vial.

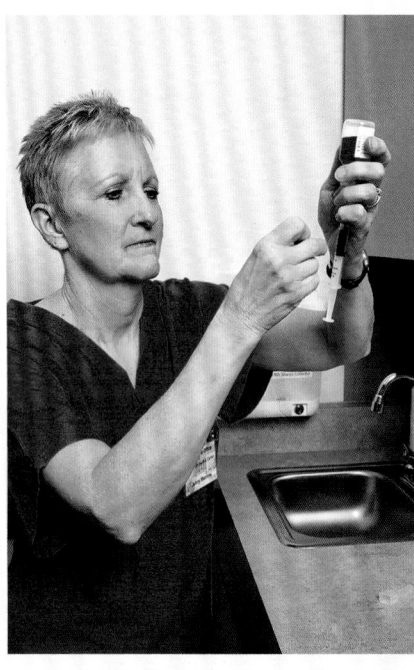

**Step 6B (5).** Tap the barrel gently to remove air bubbles
from the medication.

7. Carefully recap the needle by placing the needle
guard on a hard, flat surface, and without contaminating the needle, insert the needle into the
cap and scoop up the cap with one hand.

Recapping the needle protects the sterility of the needle
until the medication can be administered. Recapping
with two hands should be avoided to prevent needle
sticks, especially after giving an injection.

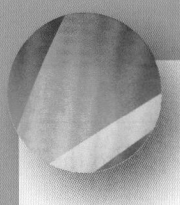 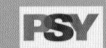 PROCEDURE 24-3

## Administering an Intradermal Injection

**PSY** Verify rules of medication administration; select proper sites for administering parenteral medication; instruct and prepare a patient for a procedure or treatment; calculate proper dosages of medication for administration; administer parenteral (excluding IV) medication; demonstrate proper disposal of biohazard material, sharps, and regulated waste; document patient care accurately in the medical record.

**Purpose**: Accurately prepare and administer a medication by intradermal injection

**Equipment**: Physician's order, medication for injection (ampule or vial), antiseptic wipes, needle and syringe of appropriate size, small gauze pad, biohazard sharps container, clean exam gloves, and patient's medical record

| STEPS | REASONS |
|---|---|
| 1. Wash your hands. | Handwashing aids infection control. |
| 2. Review the order and select the correct medication. Compare the label to the physician's instructions. Note the expiration date. Check the label three times: when taking it from the shelf, while drawing it up into the syringe, and when returning it to the shelf or discarding the unit dose vial or ampule. | Carefully dispensing medications helps prevent errors. Outdated medication should not be administered to a patient but should be discarded appropriately. |
| 3. Prepare the injection according to the steps in Procedure 24-2. | Regardless of the type of injection, the preparation is the same. |
| 4. Greet and identify the patient. Explain the procedure and ask the patient about medication allergies that might not be noted on the medical record. | Correctly identifying the patient prevents errors. |
| 5. Select the appropriate site for the injection. Recommended sites are the anterior forearm and the middle of the back. | The anterior forearm is used for tuberculosis testing, whereas the back is often used for allergy testing. |
| 6. Prepare the site by cleansing with an antiseptic wipe using a circular motion starting at the anticipated injection site and working toward the outside. Do not touch the site after cleaning. | The site must be prepared by first removing microorganisms from the area. Wiping in a circular motion will carry the microorganisms away from the site. |
| 7. Put on gloves. | Standard precautions must be followed for protection against potential exposure to blood. |
| 8. Remove the needle guard. Using your nondominant hand, pull the patient's skin taut. | Stretching the skin allows the needle to enter the skin with less resistance and secures the patient against movement. |

*(continues on page 618)*

## PROCEDURE 24-3 (continued)

| STEPS | REASONS |
|---|---|

**9.** With the bevel of the needle facing upward, insert the needle at a 10 to 15 degree angle into the upper layer of the skin. When the bevel of the needle is under the skin, stop inserting the needle. The needle will be slightly visible below the surface of the skin. It is not necessary to aspirate when performing an intradermal injection.

The needle should be inserted almost parallel to the skin to ensure that penetration occurs within the dermal layer. The bevel of the needle facing up will allow the wheal to form. If the bevel faces downward, no wheal will be formed.

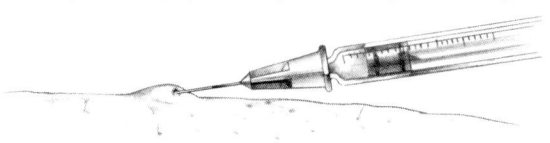

**Step 9.** Insert the needle at a 10 to 15 degree angle.

**10.** Inject the medication slowly by depressing the plunger. A wheal will form as the medication enters the dermal layer of the skin. Hold the syringe steady for proper administration.

Moving the needle once it has penetrated the skin will cause discomfort to the patient.

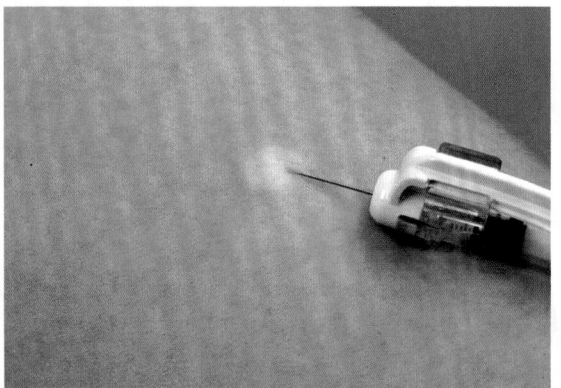

**Step 10.** A wheal is formed when the medication is injected under the skin in an intradermal injection.

**11.** Remove the needle from the skin at the angle of insertion. Do not use an antiseptic wipe or gauze pad when withdrawing the needle. Do not press or massage the site. Do not apply an adhesive bandage.

Pressure on the wheal may press the medication into the tissues or out of the injection site. Any redness or swelling produced by applying an adhesive bandage could result in an inaccurate reading of the test.

**12.** **AFF** Explain how to respond to a patient who has dementia.

Solicit assistance from a caregiver or other staff member to help during the procedure. Give simple directions to the patient about what he or she should do. Speak clearly, not loudly.

**13.** Do not recap the needle. Dispose of the needle and syringe in an approved biohazard sharps container. The sharps container should be placed where you have easy access to it after the injection is given.

Discarding the needle and syringe without recapping helps reduce the risk of an accidental needle stick.

**14.** Remove your gloves and wash your hands.

## PROCEDURE 24-3 (continued)

| STEPS | REASONS |
|---|---|
| 15. Depending upon the type of skin test administered, the length of time required for the body tissues to react, and the policies of the medical office, perform one of the following:<br>A. Read the test results. Inspect and palpate the site for the presence and amount of induration.<br>B. Tell the patient when to return (date and time) to the office to have the results read.<br>C. Instruct the patient to read the results at home. Make sure the patient understands the instructions. Have the patient repeat the instructions if necessary. | To make sure the results are accurate and that the patient does not have a serious reaction, you must be familiar with the skin test given and follow all procedures accordingly. |
| 16. **AFF** Log into the electronic medical record (EMR) using your username and secure password OR obtain the paper medical record from a secure location and assure it is kept away from public access. Record the procedure noting the date, time, name of medication, dose administered, route of administration, and your name. | The integrity of the medical record must be maintained at all times to protect patient privacy. |
| 17. When finished, log out of the EMR and/or replace the paper medical record in an appropriate and secure location. | The physician and other workers in the office may need to know what the patient has been taught. Remember, if it's not in the chart, it did not happen. |

Charting Example:
05/04/2016 10:35 AM *Mantoux test, 0.1 mL PPD ID, (L) anterior forearm. Pt. given verbal and written instructions to RTO in 48 to 72 hours to have results read. Pt. verbalized understanding*
——————————————————————— *P. King, CMA*

Note: *The medical assistant may sign his or her name in the patient record using only the "CMA" credential if the office has a signature log denoting the entire credential as "CMA(AAMA)."*

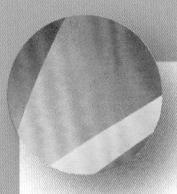
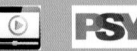

## PROCEDURE 24-4

### Administering a Subcutaneous Injection

**PSY** Verify rules of medication administration; select proper sites for administering parenteral medication; instruct and prepare a patient for a procedure or treatment; calculate proper dosages of medication for administration; administer parenteral (excluding IV) medication; demonstrate proper disposal of biohazard material, sharps, and regulated waste; document patient care accurately in the medical record.

**Purpose:** Accurately prepare and administer a medication by SQ injection

**Equipment:** Physician's order, medication for injection (ampule or vial), antiseptic wipes, needle and syringe of appropriate size, small gauze pad, biohazard sharps container, clean exam gloves, adhesive bandage, and patient's medical record

| STEPS | REASONS |
|---|---|
| 1. Wash your hands. | Handwashing aids infection control. |
| 2. Review the medication order and select the correct medication. Compare the label to the physician's instructions. Note the expiration date. Check the label three times: when taking it from the shelf, while drawing it up into the syringe, and when returning it to the shelf. | Carefully dispensing medications helps prevent errors. Outdated medication should not be administered to a patient but should be discarded appropriately. |
| 3. Prepare the injection according to the steps in Procedure 24-2. | Regardless of the type of injection, the preparation is the same. |
| 4. Greet and identify the patient. Explain the procedure and ask the patient about medication allergies that may not be noted on the medical record. | Correctly identifying the patient prevents errors. |
| 5. Select the appropriate site for the injection. Recommended sites include the upper arm, thigh, back, and abdomen. | These areas of the body usually have additional adipose tissue. |
| 6. Prepare the site by cleansing with an antiseptic wipe using a circular motion starting at the anticipated injection site and working toward the outside. Do not touch the site after cleaning. | The site must be prepared by first removing microorganisms from the area. Wiping in a circular motion will carry the microorganisms away from the site. |
| 7. Put on gloves. | Standard precautions must be followed for protection against exposure to blood. |
| 8. Remove the needle guard. Using your nondominant hand, hold the skin surrounding the injection site in a cushion fashion. | Holding the skin up and away from the underlying muscle will ensure entrance into the SQ tissues. Proper technique will help ensure that the SQ tissue, not the muscle, is entered. |

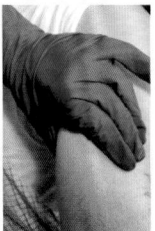

**Step 8.** Cushion the tissue between your fingers for the SQ injection.

## PROCEDURE 24-4 (continued)

| STEPS | REASONS |
|---|---|
| 9. With a firm motion, insert the needle into the tissue at a 45 degree angle to the skin surface. Hold the barrel between the thumb and the index finger of the dominant hand and insert the needle completely to the hub. | A quick, firm motion is less painful to the patient. Full insertion ensures that the medication is inserted into the proper tissue. |

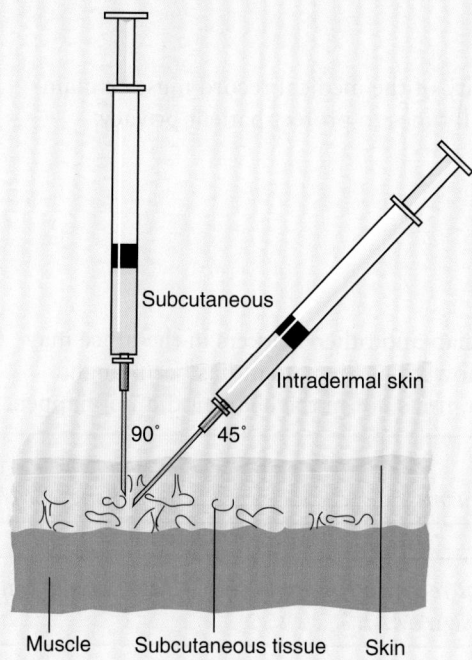

Subcutaneous

Intradermal skin

90°     45°

Muscle     Subcutaneous tissue     Skin

**Step 9.** Insert the needle at a 45 degree angle for an SQ injection.

| STEPS | REASONS |
|---|---|
| 10. Remove your nondominant hand from the skin. | Your nondominant hand will be used to pull back on the plunger in the next step. |
| 11. Holding the syringe steady, pull back on the syringe gently. If blood appears in the hub or the syringe, a blood vessel has been entered. If this occurs, do not inject the medication. Remove the needle and prepare a new injection. | If medication intended for SQ administration is administered into a blood vessel, the medication can be absorbed too quickly, producing undesirable results. |
| 12. Inject the medication slowly by depressing the plunger. | If medication is injected too rapidly, pressure is created, which will cause patient discomfort and may cause tissue damage. |
| 13. Place a gauze pad over the injection site and remove the needle at the angle at which it was inserted. Gently massage the injection site with the gauze pad with one hand while discarding the needle and syringe into the sharps container with the other hand. Do not recap the used needle. Apply an adhesive bandage if needed. | Discarding the needle and syringe without recapping helps reduce the risk of an accidental stick. Massaging helps to distribute the medication so that it can be more completely absorbed. |
| 14. **AFF**  Explain how to respond to a patient who is deaf, hearing impaired, visually impaired, or does not speak English. | Solicit assistance from anyone who may be with the patient or a staff member who speaks his or her native language to interpret if available. If no interpreter is available, use hand gestures or pictures to explain procedure to the patient. |

*(continues on page 622)*

## PROCEDURE 24-4 (continued)

| STEPS | REASONS |
|---|---|
| 15. Remove your gloves and wash your hands. | |
| 16. An injection given for allergy desensitization requires that the patient remain in the office for at least 30 minutes for observation of any reaction. If the patient experiences any unusual reaction after any injection, notify the physician immediately. | An unusual reaction after an allergy injection could be fatal. |
| 17. **AFF**   Log into the electronic medical record (EMR) using your username and secure password OR obtain the paper medical record from a secure location and assure it is kept away from public access. Record the procedure noting the date, time, name of medication, dose administered, route of administration, and your name. | The integrity of the medical record must be maintained at all times to protect patient privacy. |
| 18. When finished, log out of the EMR and/or replace the paper medical record in an appropriate and secure location. | The physician and other workers in the office may need to know what the patient has been taught. Remember, if it's not in the chart, it did not happen. |

Charting Example:
*03/04/2016 9:30 AM Regular insulin 5 units SQ (R) posterior upper arm* _____ *P. King, CMA*

Note: *The medical assistant may sign his or her name in the patient record using only the "CMA" credential if the office has a signature log denoting the entire credential as "CMA(AAMA)."*

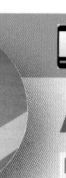  PROCEDURE 24-5

## Administering an Intramuscular Injection

**PSY** Verify rules of medication administration; select proper sites for administering parenteral medication; instruct and prepare a patient for a procedure or treatment; calculate proper dosages of medication for administration; administer parenteral (excluding IV) medication; demonstrate proper disposal of biohazard material, sharps, and regulated waste; Document patient care accurately in the medical record.

**Purpose:** Accurately prepare and administer a medication by IM injection

**Equipment:** Physician's order, medication for injection (ampule or vial), antiseptic wipes, needle and syringe of appropriate size, small gauze pad, biohazard sharps container, clean exam gloves, adhesive bandage, and patient's medical record

| STEPS | REASONS |
|---|---|
| 1. Wash your hands. | Handwashing aids infection control. |
| 2. Review the order and select the correct medication. Compare the label to the physician's instructions. Check the label three times: when taking it from the shelf, while drawing it up into the syringe, and when returning it to the shelf. | Carefully dispensing medications helps prevent errors. Outdated medication should not be administered to a patient but should be discarded appropriately. |
| 3. Prepare the injection according to the steps in Procedure 24-2. | Regardless of the type of injection, the preparation is the same. |
| 4. Greet and identify the patient. Explain the procedure and ask the patient about medication allergies that might not be noted on the medical record. | Correctly identifying the patient prevents errors. |
| 5. Select the appropriate site for the injection. Recommended sites include the deltoid, vastus lateralis, dorsogluteal, and ventrogluteal areas; however, the site should be chosen based on the medication and age and size of the patient. | Skill and accuracy are crucial when locating IM injection sites since major blood vessels and nerves may lie near the muscles. |
| 6. Prepare the site by cleansing with an antiseptic wipe using a circular motion starting at the anticipated injection site and working toward the outside. Do not touch the site after cleaning. | The site must be prepared by first removing microorganisms from the area. Wiping in a circular motion will carry the microorganisms away from the site. |
| 7. Put on gloves. | Standard precautions must be followed for protection against potential exposure to blood. |

*(continues on page 624)*

## PROCEDURE 24-5 (continued)

| STEPS | REASONS |
|---|---|
| 8. Remove the needle guard. Using your nondominant hand, hold the skin surrounding the injection site taut with the thumb and index fingers or grasp the muscle in a small person with little body fat. | Holding the skin taut in an average or overweight person will allow for easier insertion of the needle. Bunching the muscle produces a deeper muscle mass in a very thin person. |

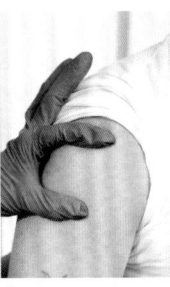

**A**

**Step 8 (A).** Hold the skin taut for an average size person.

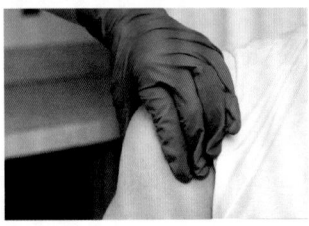

**B**

**Step 8 (B).** Bunch the muscle in a thin person.

9. While holding the syringe like a dart, use a quick, firm motion to insert the needle into the tissue at a 90 degree angle to the surface. Hold the barrel between the thumb and the index finger of the dominant hand and insert the needle completely to the hub.

A quick, firm motion is less painful to the patient. Full insertion at 90 degree ensures that the medication is inserted into the proper muscle tissue.

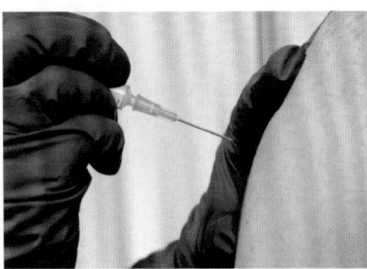

**Step 9.** Insert the needle at a 90 degree angle to the hub.

10. Remove your nondominant hand from the skin and gently pull back on the plunger while holding the syringe steady. If blood appears in the hub or the syringe, a blood vessel has been entered. If this occurs, do not inject the medication. Remove the needle and prepare a new injection.

If medication intended for IM administration is administered into a blood vessel, the medication can be absorbed too quickly, producing undesirable results.

11. Inject the medication slowly by depressing the plunger.

If medication is injected too rapidly, pressure is created, which will cause patient discomfort and may cause tissue damage.

## PROCEDURE 24-5 (continued)

| STEPS | REASONS |
|---|---|
| 12. Place a gauze pad over the injection site and remove the needle at the same angle at which it was inserted. Gently massage the injection site with the gauze pad with one hand while discarding the needle and syringe into the sharps container with the other hand. Do not recap the used needle. Apply an adhesive bandage if needed. | Discarding the needle and syringe without recapping helps reduce the risk of an accidental needle stick. Massaging helps to distribute the medication into the tissues so that it can be more completely absorbed. |
| 13. **AFF** Explain how to respond to a patient who is visually impaired. | Face the patient when speaking and always let him or her know what you are going to do before touching him or her. |
| 14. Remove your gloves and wash your hands. | |
| 15. Observe the patient for any unusual reactions. If the patient experiences any unusual reaction after any injection, notify the physician immediately. | Unusual reactions after administering injections may be the beginning of a life-threatening emergency. |
| 16. **AFF** Log into the electronic medical record (EMR) using your username and secure password OR obtain the paper medical record from a secure location and assure it is kept away from public access. Record the procedure noting the date, time, name of medication, dose administered, route of administration, and your name. | The integrity of the medical record must be maintained at all times to protect patient privacy. |
| 17. When finished, log out of the EMR and/or replace the paper medical record in an appropriate and secure location.<br><br>Document the procedure, the site, results, and instructions if given. | The physician and other workers in the office may need to know what the patient has been taught. Remember, if it's not in the chart, it did not happen. |

**Charting Example:**
*05/06/2012 2:00 PM Solu-Medrol 20 mg IM (L) DG* _____ *P. King, CMA*

Note: *The medical assistant may sign his or her name in the patient record using only the "CMA" credential if the office has a signature log denoting the entire credential as "CMA(AAMA)."*

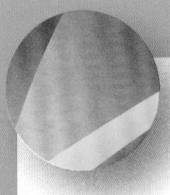

**PSY** PROCEDURE 24-6

## Administering an Intramuscular Injection Using the Z-Track Method

**PSY** Verify rules of medication administration; select proper sites for administering parenteral medication; instruct and prepare a patient for a procedure or treatment; calculate proper dosages of medication for administration; administer parenteral (excluding IV) medication; demonstrate proper disposal of biohazard material, sharps, and regulated waste; Document patient care accurately in the medical record.

**Purpose:** Accurately prepare and administer a medication by Z-track IM injection

**Equipment:** Physician's order, medication for injection (ampule or vial), antiseptic wipes, needle and syringe of appropriate size, small gauze pad, biohazard sharps container, clean exam gloves, adhesive bandage, and patient's medical record

| STEPS | REASONS |
|---|---|
| 1. Follow steps 1 through 7 as described in Procedure 24-5 (Administering an Intramuscular Injection). *Note*: The ventrogluteal, vastus lateralis, and dorsogluteal sites work well for the Z-track method; the deltoid does not. | |
| 2. Remove the needle guard. Rather than pulling the skin taut or grasping the tissue as you would for an IM injection, pull the top layer of skin to the side and hold it with the nondominant hand throughout the injection. | The skin pulled to the side will eventually be released after the medication is administered and will act as a barrier to prevent the medication from leaving the injection site in the muscle. |

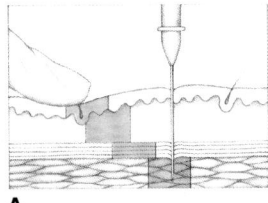

**A**

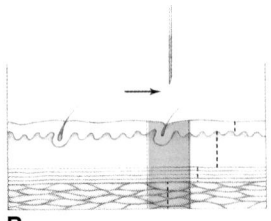

**B**

**Step 2.** Pull the top layer of skin to one side using the edge of your nondominant hand.

| STEPS | REASONS |
|---|---|
| 3. While holding the syringe like a dart, use a quick, firm motion to insert the needle into the tissue at a 90 degree angle to the skin surface. Hold the barrel between the thumb and the index finger of the dominant hand and insert the needle completely to the hub. Continue to hold the skin to one side with the nondominant hand. | A quick, firm motion is less painful to the patient. Full insertion at 90 degree ensures that the medication is inserted into the proper muscle tissue. |
| 4. Aspirate by withdrawing the plunger slightly. If no blood appears, push the plunger in slowly and steadily. Count to 10 before withdrawing the needle. | If medication intended for IM administration is administered into a blood vessel, the medication can be absorbed too quickly, producing undesirable results. Counting to 10 before removing the needle allows time for the tissues to begin absorbing the medication. |

## PROCEDURE 24-6 (continued)

| STEPS | REASONS |
|---|---|
| 5. Remove the needle at the same angle at which it was inserted while releasing the skin. Do not massage the area. Discard the needle and syringe into the sharps container. Apply an adhesive bandage if needed. | Discarding the needle and syringe without recapping helps reduce the risk of an accidental needle stick. |
| 6. Remove your gloves and wash your hands. | |
| 7. Observe the patient for any unusual reactions. If the patient experiences any unusual reaction after any injection, notify the physician immediately. | An unusual reaction may be the start of a life-threatening emergency. |
| 8. **AFF** Log into the electronic medical record (EMR) using your username and secure password OR obtain the paper medical record from a secure location and assure it is kept away from public access. Record the procedure noting the date, time, name of medication, dose administered, route of administration, and your name. | The integrity of the medical record must be maintained at all times to protect patient privacy. |
| 9. When finished, log out of the EMR and/or replace the paper medical record in an appropriate and secure location. | The physician and other workers in the office may need to know what the patient has been taught. Remember, if it's not in the chart, it did not happen. |

Charting Example:
*07/11/2016 3:30 PM Imferon 25 mg IM Z-track (R) DG* _____ *P. King, CMA*

Note: *The medical assistant may sign his or her name in the patient record using only the "CMA" credential if the office has a signature log denoting the entire credential as "CMA(AAMA)."*

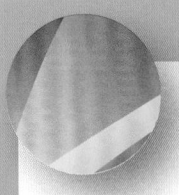 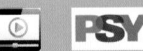 **PROCEDURE 24-7**

## Applying Transdermal Medications

**PSY** Verify rules of medication administration; select proper sites for administering parenteral medication; instruct and prepare a patient for a procedure or treatment; calculate proper dosages of medication for administration; administer parenteral (excluding IV) medication; demonstrate proper disposal of biohazard material, sharps, and regulated waste; document patient care accurately in the medical record.

**Purpose**: Accurately prepare and administer a transdermal medication

**Equipment**: Physician's order, medication, clean exam gloves, and patient's medical record

| STEPS | REASONS |
|---|---|
| 1. Wash your hands. | Handwashing aids infection control. |
| 2. Review the order and select the correct medication. Compare the label to the physician's instructions. Note the expiration date. Check the label three times: when taking it from the shelf, before taking it into the patient exam room, and before applying it to the patient's skin. | Carefully dispensing medications helps prevents errors. Outdated medications should not be administered to a patient but should be discarded appropriately. |
| 3. Greet and identify the patient. Explain the procedure and ask the patient about medication allergies that might not be noted on the medical record. | Correctly identifying the patient prevents errors. |
| 4. Select the appropriate site and perform any necessary skin preparation. The sites are usually the upper arm, the chest or back surface, or behind the ear. These sites should be rotated. Ensure that the skin is clean, dry, and free from any irritation. Do not shave areas with excessive hair; trim the hair closely with scissors | Shaving may abrade the skin and cause the medication to be absorbed too rapidly. |
| 5. If there is a transdermal patch already in place, remove it carefully while wearing gloves. Discard the patch in the trash container. Inspect the site for irritation. | Touching the medication with bare hands may cause it to be absorbed into your skin, causing undesirable reactions. |
| 6. Open the medication package by pulling the two sides apart. Do not touch the area of medication. | Touching the area of medication will remove some and prevent the patient from getting the prescribed amount. |

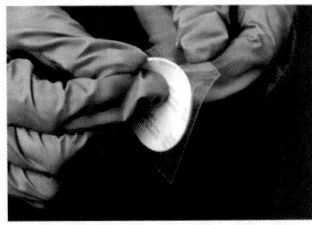

**Step 6**. Open the transdermal medication by pulling the wrapper apart.

| | |
|---|---|
| 7. Apply the medicated patch to the patient's skin following the manufacturer's directions. Press the adhesive edges down firmly all around, starting at the center and pressing outward. If the edges do not stick, fasten with tape. | Starting at the center eliminates air spaces that may prevent contact with the skin. |

## PROCEDURE 24-7 (continued)

| STEPS | REASONS |
|---|---|
| 8. **AFF** Explain how to respond to a patient who is uncomfortable exposing skin on areas such as the chest or arms due to cultural or religious beliefs. | Be respectful of cultural differences by explaining why procedures are important. Provide additional privacy measures if necessary. |
| 9. Wash your hands. | Always wash your hands after a patient encounter. |
| 10. **AFF** Log into the electronic medical record (EMR) using your username and secure password OR obtain the paper medical record from a secure location and assure it is kept away from public access. Record the procedure noting the date, time, name of medication, dose administered, route of administration, site of the new patch, and your name. | The integrity of the medical record must be maintained at all times to protect patient privacy. |
| 11. When finished, log out of the EMR and/or replace the paper medical record in an appropriate and secure location. | The physician and other workers in the office may need to know what the patient has been taught. Remember, if it's not in the chart, it did not happen. |

**Charting Example:**
09/06/2016 8:30 AM *Transdermal nitroglycerin 0.2 mg/h patch to (L) anterior chest* _____
*P. King, CMA*

Note: *The medical assistant may sign his or her name in the patient record using only the "CMA" credential if the office has a signature log denoting the entire credential as "CMA(AAMA)."*

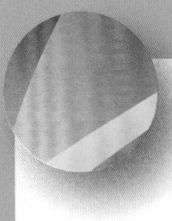

**PSY** PROCEDURE 24-8

# Complete an Incident Report

**PSY** Complete an incident report related to an error in patient care.

**Purpose**: Recognize a medication error has occurred and complete the documentation required as a result of this error

**Scenario**: After administering medication, you realize the wrong dose was given.

**Equipment**: An incident form

| STEPS | REASONS |
|---|---|
| 1. Recognize the error in patient care (i.e., medication administration) and notify the physician immediately after assessing the patient and providing emergency procedures if appropriate. | Ethically, you must acknowledge the error and let the physician know so that steps can be taken to protect the patient if necessary. |
| 2. Once the patient is assessed and necessary interventions taken as per physician instructions, complete an incident report form. | Because this incident was not part of the "normal" routine, it should be documented according to office policy and procedure. |
| 3. Sign and date the incident report form and file with the office or practice manager. | The incident report form should not be placed into the patient's medical record. |
| 4. **AFF** Advise the patient on any follow-up procedures as instructed by the physician. | The patient must be made aware of the error and given any treatment or follow-up procedures as necessary. |

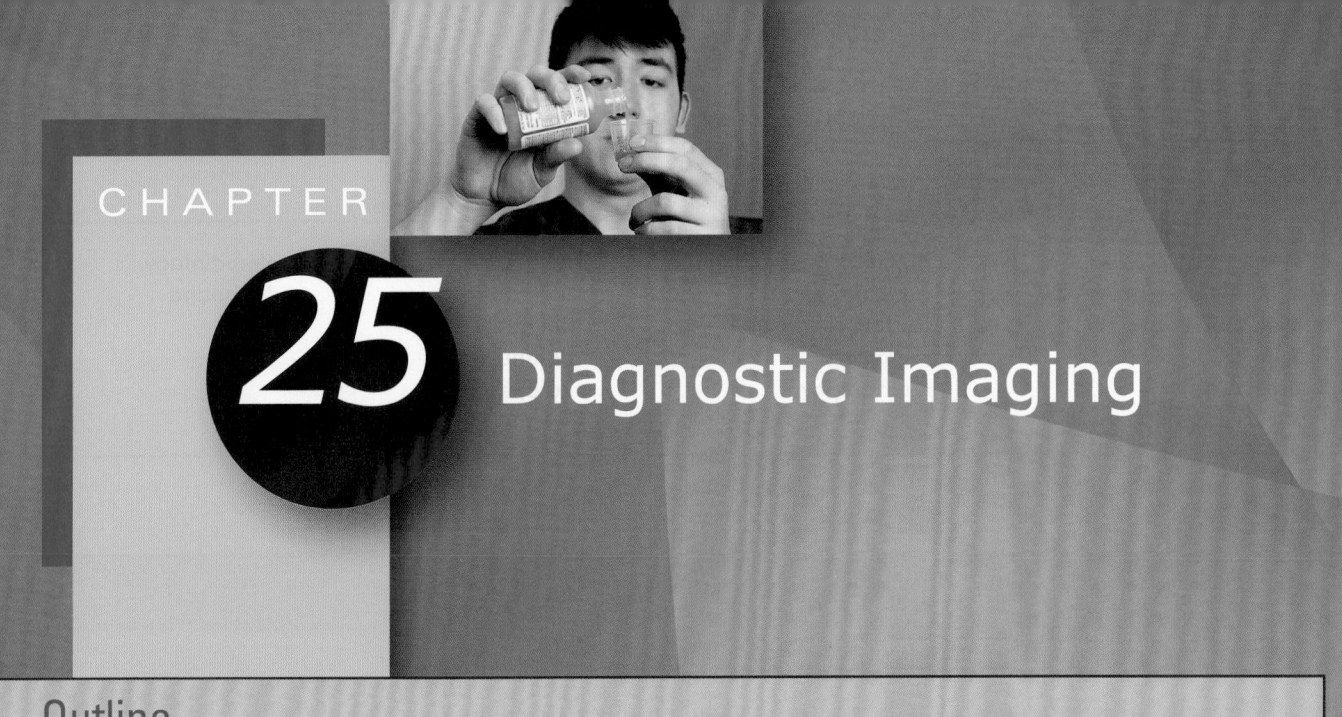

## Outline

## Learning Outcomes

### COG Cognitive Domain*

1. Spell and define the key terms
2. Explain the theory and function of x-rays and x-ray machines
3. State the principles of radiology
4. Describe routine and contrast media, fluoroscopy, computed tomography, sonography, magnetic resonance imaging, nuclear medicine, and mammographic examinations
5. Explain the role of the medical assistant in radiologic procedures
6. *Describe body planes, directional terms, quadrants, and cavities*
7. *Identify critical information required for scheduling patient procedures*

### PSY Psychomotor Domain*

1. Assist with x-ray procedures (Procedure 25-1)
  a. *Instruct and prepare a patient for a procedure or treatment*
  b. *Respond to nonverbal communication*
  c. *Coach patients appropriately considering cultural diversity, developmental life stage, and/or communication barriers*
  d. *Document patient care accurately in the medical record*

### AFF Affective Domain*

1. *Incorporate critical thinking skills when performing patient care*
2. *Show awareness of a patient's concerns related to the procedure being performed*
3. *Demonstrate respect for individual diversity including gender, race, religion, age, economic status, and appearance*
4. *Explain to a patient the rationale for performance of a procedure*
5. Demonstrate empathy, *active listening, and nonverbal communication*
6. *Protect the integrity of the medical record*

*\*Note: AAMA/CAAHEP 2015 Standards are italicized.*

### ABHES Competencies

1. Assist the physician with the regimen of diagnostic and treatment modalities as they relate to each body system
2. Comply with federal, state, and local health laws and regulations
3. Communicate on the recipient's level of comprehension
4. Serve as a liaison between the physician and others
5. Show *empathy and impartiality when dealing with patients*

cassette
computed tomography (CT)
contrast medium
film
fluoroscopy

magnetic resonance
  imaging (MRI)
nuclear medicine
radiograph
radiography

radiologist
radiology
radiolucent
radionuclides
radiopaque

teleradiology
ultrasound
x-rays

## Case Study

$M$ary Smalley, CMA (AAMA), works in an internal medicine office that is part of Great Falls Medical Center. All of the patients seen in this office are adults and most of them are over the age of 55 years. It is common for the physicians to order diagnostic imaging procedures to determine the cause of patient symptoms or screen for possible diseases that would be best treated if diagnosed at an early stage. Although the diagnostic imaging procedures ordered by the physician are not actually performed in the internal medicine office, Mary must schedule these procedures and give patients instructions about preparing for them as necessary. What types of diagnostic imaging procedures might require patient preparation? How should Mary respond to a patient who calls the office the day of the procedure and says he is not adequately prepared for the procedure? Is it Mary's responsibility to provide information about diagnostic imaging procedures or is this the responsibility of the imaging facility? The answers to these questions are found in this chapter on diagnostic imaging procedures and the role of the medical assistant.

The discovery of **x-rays** in the late 19th century forever changed the practice of medicine. Routine x-ray imaging, **computed tomography (CT)**, sonography, **magnetic resonance imaging (MRI)**, and **nuclear medicine** are now commonly used diagnostic and therapeutic procedures. Advances in radiation therapy continue to be at the forefront of the treatment for cancer.

## PRINCIPLES OF RADIOLOGY

**Radiology** continues to evolve through technologic changes that provide ever-increasing diagnostic information to physicians. As the technology advances, the need to teach patients becomes even more important. Medical assistants are often directly involved in preparing patients for outpatient radiographic procedures, performing basic radiographic procedures in the medical office, and assisting in the general educational process.

## X-Rays and X-Ray Machines

X-rays are high-energy waves that cannot be seen, heard, felt, tasted, or smelled and that can penetrate fairly dense objects, such as the human body. This penetrating ability is what allows x-rays to be powerful diagnostic and therapeutic tools. Diagnostically, these penetrating waves create two-dimensional shadowlike images on **film** that is similar to photographic film. Unprocessed film must be protected from light and kept in a special holder called a **cassette** before use. Once the film inside the cassette has been exposed to x-rays, the cassette is placed in a special machine that removes the film and processes it. The processed film containing a visible image is called a **radiograph** (Fig. 25-1). The process by which these films are produced is called **radiography**.

Electricity of extremely high voltage in the x-ray tube produces x-rays. The x-rays leave the tube in one primary direction as a beam, through a device used to control the size of the beam. The light that shines on the patient is not part of the beam but is a positioning aid that illuminates the area covered by the beam. A patient may hear noises

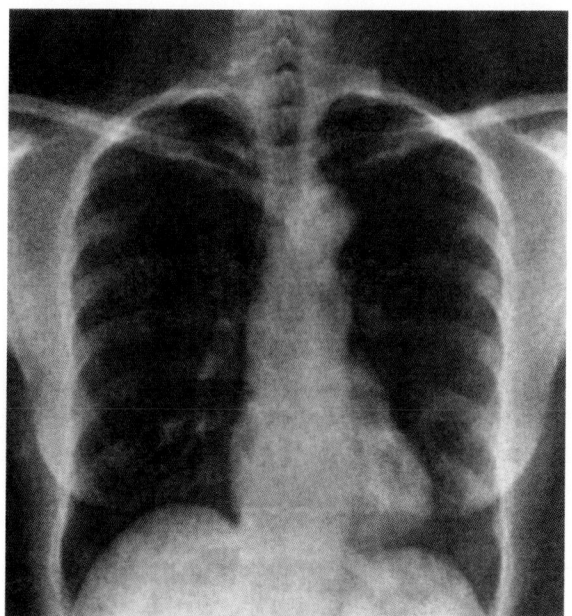

**Figure 25-1** • Radiograph of chest.

coming from the tube area during an exposure, but these are made by the equipment, not the x-rays.

Today, x-ray machines are sophisticated and technologically advanced. Many are designed to work with computers to produce digital images of the body (Fig. 25-2). Fluoroscopic units can reveal motion within the body. Most permanently installed radiographic units include a special table, some of which can be electronically rotated from the horizontal to the vertical. In this situation, the radiographic film is placed in a cassette that slides into a slot or opening on the table.

Images are formed on the x-ray film as the rays either pass through or are absorbed by the tissues of the body. **Radiolucent** tissues, such as air in the lungs, permit the passage of x-rays, while **radiopaque** tissues, such as bone, do not permit the passage of x-rays. Because bone is dense and absorbs much of the radiation beam, these structures appear white on a radiograph. Air is not dense and does not absorb much radiation. Therefore, air in a structure shows up dark

on a radiograph. Other body tissues, such as muscle, fat, and fluid, show as varying shades of gray because of the way each tissue absorbs the x-rays. Physicians who specialize in interpreting the images on the processed film are **radiologists**.

## Outpatient X-Rays

The medical community is making a conscious effort to have as much treatment as possible done on an outpatient basis, and thus, some medical offices have on-site x-ray equipment. Outpatient diagnostic imaging centers have also been created to offer these services. Some companies specialize in providing minimal x-ray services to patients in long-term care facilities or the patients' homes.

In some states, you may be permitted to take and process simple images such as bone or chest radiographs as permitted by state law. The training for medical assistants varies, but some programs include a formal course in the theory of radiography and a written examination offered by the state radiographic association for the general operator. In other states, only licensed radiographers may take and process radiographs. You should be familiar with your state laws and comply with any regulations.

### ✎ CHECKPOINT QUESTION

1. A patient asks Mary about x-rays and if these are harmful to the body. How would Mary describe x-rays to a patient including the harmful effects?

## Patient Positioning

The x-ray exposure on film is a two-dimensional image. Because the human body is a three-dimensional structure, x-ray examinations usually require a minimum of two exposures taken at 90 degree to each other. For instance, a chest radiographic examination requires one exposure from the back and another from the side (Fig. 25-3). Other examinations necessitate three or more exposures at different angles. These different angles of exposure are the basis for standard positioning for x-ray examinations (Box 25-1).

## Examination Sequencing

Most radiographic procedures can be performed in any order of convenience, but certain procedures must follow certain sequences in specific situations. For example, patients with gallbladder symptoms may go through a series of procedures, progressing from the simple noninvasive oral cholecystogram (an x-ray of the gallbladder after the ingestion of a **contrast medium** orally) to the more complex operative cholangiogram (x-ray of the

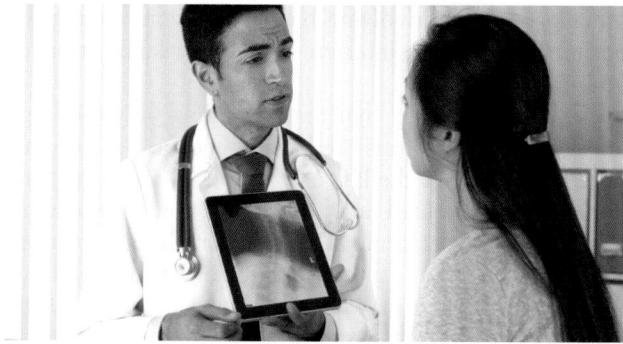

**Figure 25-2** • Digital radiographic image.

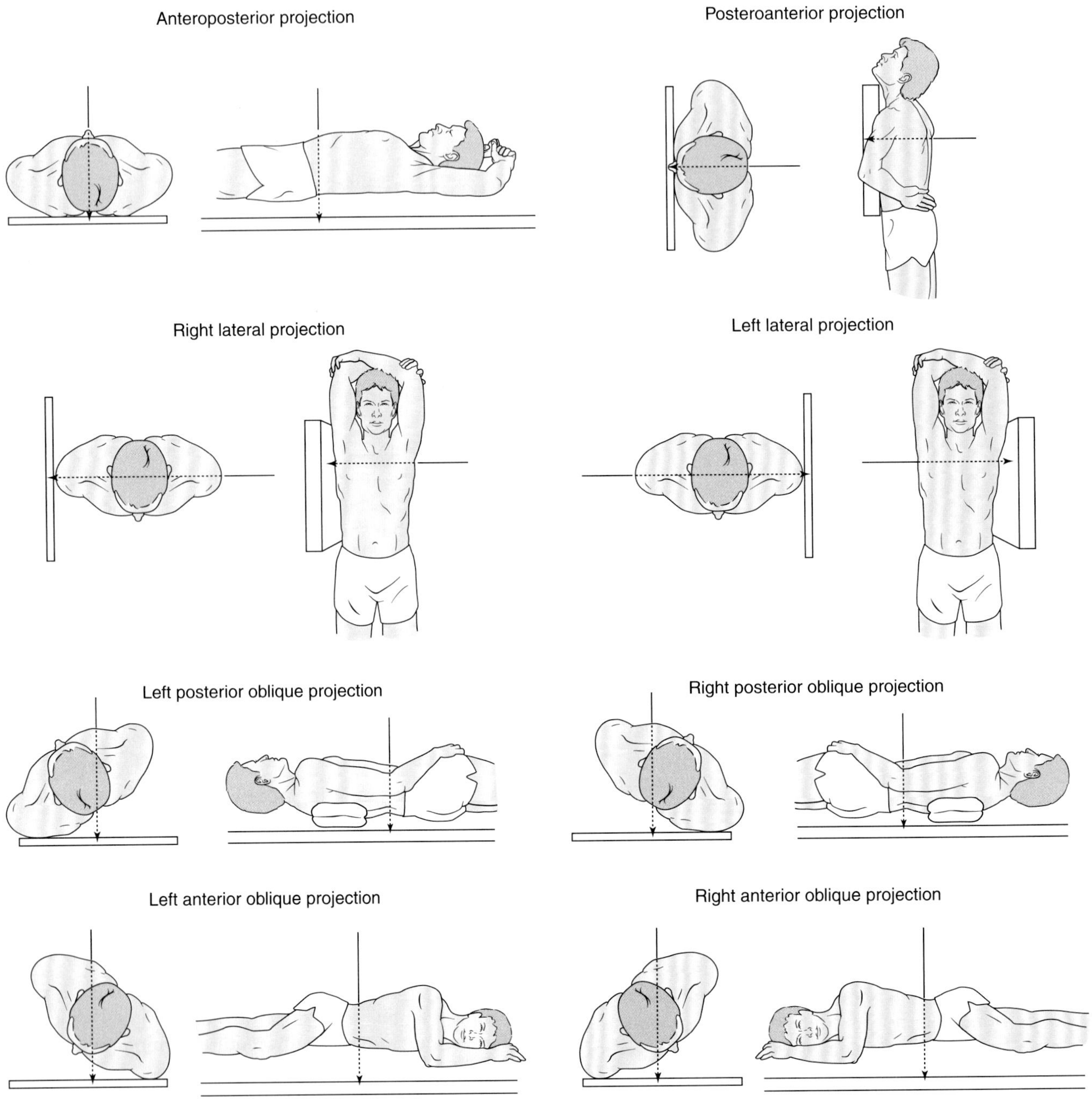

Anteroposterior projection

Posteroanterior projection

Right lateral projection

Left lateral projection

Left posterior oblique projection

Right posterior oblique projection

Left anterior oblique projection

Right anterior oblique projection

**Figure 25-3** • Standard positions.

bile ducts after injection with a contrast medium during a surgical procedure).

Another example is barium studies, the name given to examinations performed after administration of barium sulfate. A patient with gastrointestinal (GI) symptoms may undergo a series of barium studies to assist the physician in diagnosis. Because of the nature of the barium studies and the length of time required to eliminate the barium from the digestive tract, barium enemas are usually scheduled before upper GI examinations. If an endoscopic study, such as an esophagogastroscopy, is

ordered, it is imperative that these be scheduled before other procedures involving barium to avoid having the barium obstruct or interfere with the visualization of internal structures.

The barium study that requires filling only the large intestine with barium is the barium enema. Because this procedure involves the last part of the GI tract, this barium can be eliminated fairly quickly so that other examinations can be performed. If an upper GI examination, commonly referred to as an upper GI or barium swallow, is performed first, it may be several days before all of the barium is out of the patient's system. Any residual barium in the GI tract can obscure vital structures in subsequent procedures, preventing them from contributing diagnostic information. The proper sequencing of scheduling the barium enema first and the upper GI last will usually provide diagnostic information in a shorter time.

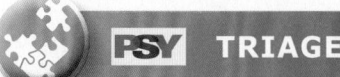

## TRIAGE

While working in a medical office setting, the physician has asked you to call the hospital and schedule Mrs. Roberts for the following three tests:

**A.** An esophagogastroduodenoscopy (EGD)
**B.** Barium enema
**C.** Barium swallow

**What is the correct order for scheduling these tests to be performed?**

The correct order is the EGD, the barium enema, and finally the upper GI series or barium swallow. It is important that these procedures be scheduled in this order to ensure optimal results.

---

## CHECKPOINT QUESTION

2. Why would Mary schedule a barium enema before an upper GI or barium swallow?

---

## BOX 25-1 Standard Terminology for Positioning and Projection

**Radiographic View**
Describes the body part as seen by an x-ray film or other recording medium, such as a fluoroscopic screen. Restricted to the discussion of a *radiograph* or *image*.

**Radiographic Position**
Refers to a specific body position, such as supine, prone, recumbent, erect, or Trendelenburg. Restricted to the discussion of the *patient's physical position.*

**Radiographic Projection**
Restricted to the discussion of the *path of the central ray.*

**Positioning Terminology**
Lying Down

1. *Supine,* lying on the back
2. *Prone,* lying face downward
3. *Decubitus,* lying down with a horizontal x-ray beam
4. *Recumbent,* lying down in any position

Erect or Upright

1. *Anterior position,* facing the film
2. *Posterior position,* facing the radiographic tube
3. *Oblique position,* erect or lying down
   A. Anterior, facing the film
      i. *Left anterior oblique,* body rotated with the left anterior portion closest to the film
      ii. *Right anterior oblique,* body rotated with the right anterior portion closest to the film
   B. *Posterior,* facing the radiographic tube
      i. *Left posterior oblique,* body rotated with the left posterior portion closest to the film
      ii. *Right posterior oblique,* body rotated with the right posterior portion closest to the film

From The American Registry of Radiologic Technologists® "Content Specifications for The Examination in Radiography." Publication date: July 2004.

## Radiation Safety

Of primary concern to all radiation workers and patients is the proper and safe use of radiant energy. The hazards of radiation have been known for many decades, and warnings about x-ray radiation are usually posted in appropriate areas (Fig. 25-4). X-rays have the potential to cause cellular or genetic damage to the body, and the results of this damage may not manifest for several years after exposure. The adverse effects are most extreme for rapidly reproducing cells. Pregnant women, children, and reproductive organs of adults are at the highest risk because of their rapid cell division and growth.

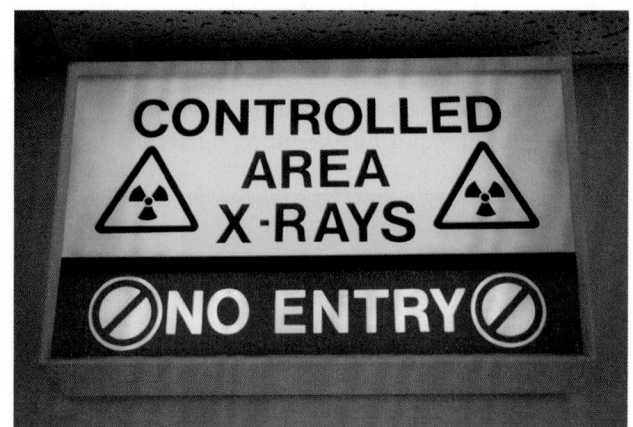

**Figure 25-4 •** X-ray warning sign.

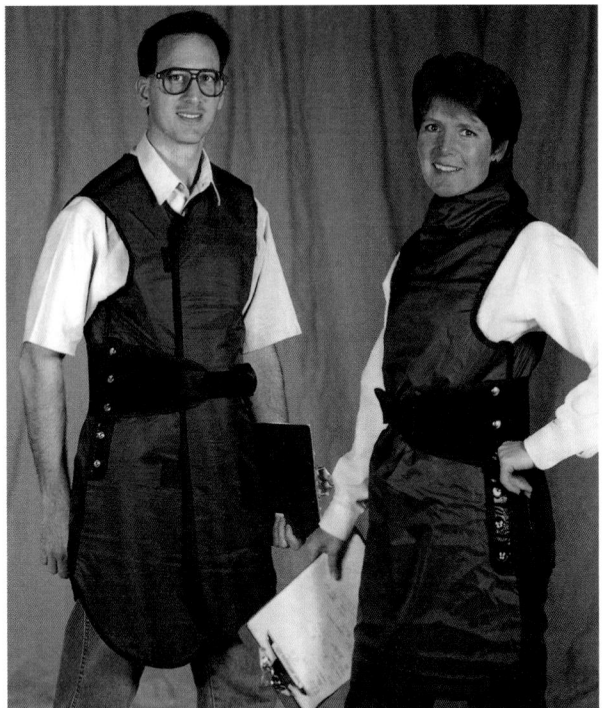

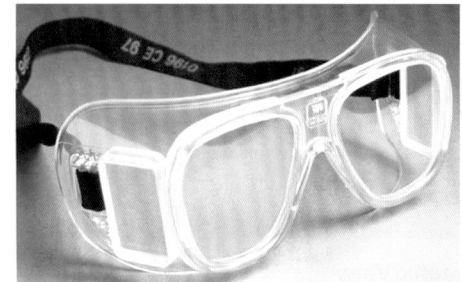

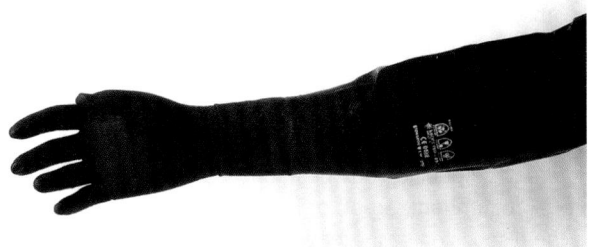

**Figure 25-5** • X-ray protection equipment.

Radiation safety procedures for patients include the following:

1. Minimizing exposure amounts
2. Avoiding unnecessary examinations
3. Limiting the area of the body exposed
4. Shielding sensitive body parts, such as the gonads and the thyroid gland
5. Evaluating the pregnancy status of female patients before performing examinations

Safety procedures for clinical staff working around x-ray equipment include the following:

1. Limiting the amount of time exposed to x-rays
2. Staying as far away from the x-rays as possible during exposure, preferably standing behind a barrier such as a wall lined with lead
3. Using available shielding for protection, such as lead aprons and gloves (Fig. 25-5)
4. Avoiding holding patients during exposures. For children requiring assistance, a parent

wearing a lead apron may be recruited during the procedure.

5. Wearing individual dosimeters, which are small devices that contain radiographic film clipped to the outside of the uniform, to record the amount of radiation, if any, to which the worker has been exposed (Fig. 25-6). These badges are provided by the employer and are obtained from companies that specifically monitor any radiation exposure of individual health care providers.
6. Ensuring proper working condition of the equipment by scheduling routine maintenance

For both patients and medical assistants working around radiation, these concerns can be summed up in what is called the ALARA concept: doing whatever is necessary to keep radiation exposure as low as reasonably achievable.

## DIAGNOSTIC PROCEDURES

Routine radiographic examinations require little or no preparation of the patient and are the most commonly performed examinations. These procedures are most readily accepted by the patient and are named for the part of the body involved in the radiographic procedure (Table 25-1). These studies are performed for viewing primarily bone structure or abnormalities.

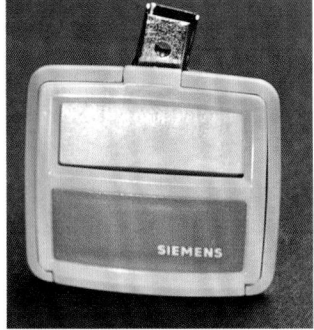

**Figure 25-6** • Dosimeter badge.

### CHECKPOINT QUESTION

3. How does the dosimeter protect you from radiation?

| TABLE 25-1 | Routine Radiographic Examinations by Body Region |
|------------|---------------------------------------------------|
| **Region** | **Patient Preparation** |
| Trunk | Disrobing of the area: chest, ribs, sternum, shoulder, scapula, clavicle, abdomen, hip, pelvis, sternoclavicular, acromioclavicular, sacroiliac joints |
| Extremities | Removing jewelry or clothing that might obscure parts of interest: fingers, thumb, hand, wrist, forearm, elbow, humerus, toes, foot, os calcis, ankle, lower leg, knee, patella, femur |
| Spine | Disrobing of the appropriate area: cervical, thoracic, or lumbar spine; sacrum; coccyx |
| Head | Removing eyewear, false eyes, false teeth, earrings, hairpins, and hairpieces: skull, sinuses, nasal bones, facial bones and orbits, optic foramen, mandible, temporomandibular joints, mastoid and petrous portion, zygomatic arch |

## Mammography

Mammography, an x-ray examination of the breast, is used as a screening tool for breast cancer (Box 25-2). Each breast is compressed in a specialized device to even the thickness, allowing for an optimal diagnostic image. Needle localization studies using the information gained from the mammogram allow the physician to withdraw small amounts of cells from suspicious areas in a minimally invasive procedure. Mammography has become a vital adjunct to biopsy (Fig. 25-7).

## Contrast Medium Examinations

Within the abdomen, many structures having similar radiation absorption rates are superimposed on each other. This makes differentiating structures difficult.

The use of a radiopaque contrast medium helps differentiate between body structures by artificially changing the absorption rate of a particular structure. For example, barium sulfate absorbs radiation and shows white on a radiograph (Fig. 25-8). There are many contrast media for various applications. Iodinated compounds are used in many areas of the body, including the kidneys and blood vessels, and in some CT scans. Patients who may have an intestinal perforation may be given an iodinated contrast medium instead of barium because that material spilling into the peritoneum is much less troublesome to the patient than barium.

Radiographic examinations using contrast media are performed to evaluate not only a structure but also its function. For example, patients having excretory urography have a contrast medium injected, and the anatomic structure of each kidney is evaluated as the medium passes through the urinary tract. Contrast media may be introduced into the body in several ways, including by mouth, intravenously, or through a catheter, depending on the material and area of the body being examined. It is important that you ask the patient about allergies, especially shellfish allergies. Usually, patients allergic to shellfish are actually allergic to the high iodine content

### BOX 25-2 American Cancer Society (ACS) Guidelines for Breast Cancer Screening

The ACS recommends mammography for women yearly starting at the age of 40. However, women with known risk factors such as a family history of breast cancer may have mammography screenings earlier than the age of 40 years. The following breast cancer screenings are recommended:

- Mammography over the age of 40 every year as long as the woman is in good health
- Clinical breast exam or breast exam by a physician or nurse about every 3 years for women in their 20s and 30s and every year starting at the age of 40 years
- Women should be familiar with how their breasts normally look and feel. Breast self-exam (BSE) may be an option monthly starting in the 20s to check for the presence of lumps, changes in the size or shape of the breast, or any other changes in the breasts or underarm. Any changes should be reported promptly to the health care provider.
- A mammography and MRI of the breasts yearly for women at high risk for developing breast cancer

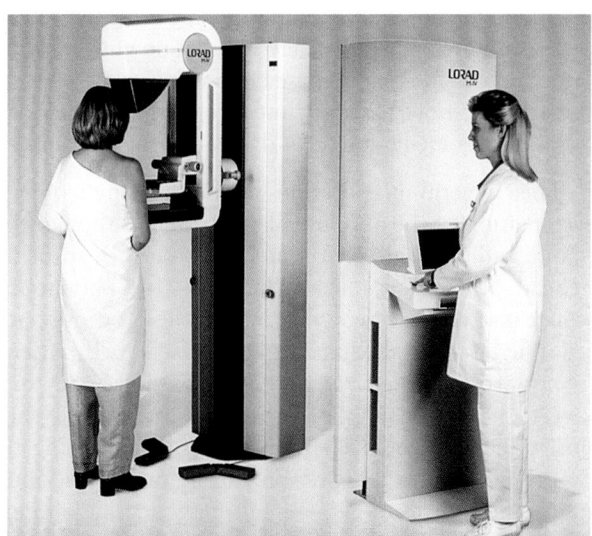

**Figure 25-7 •** Mammography machine.

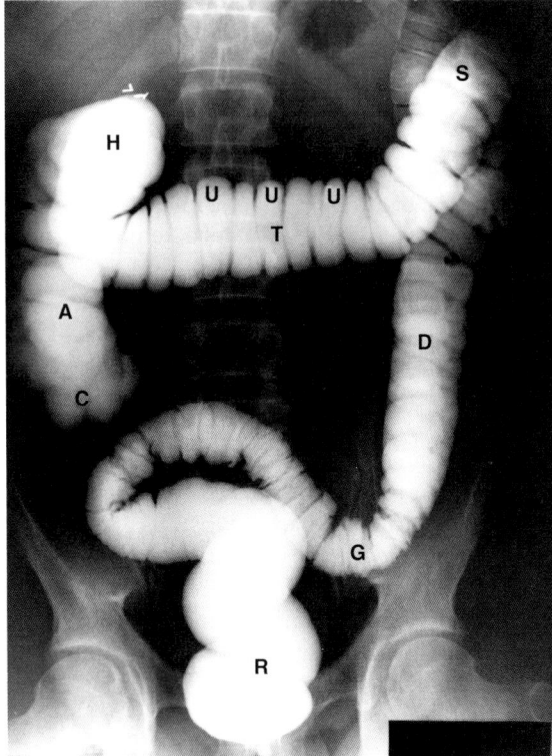

**Figure 25-8** • Barium-filled large intestine.

of the shellfish, and because injectable contrast media are iodine based, this information needs to be relayed to the radiology center before the patient is scheduled. Another concern for patients undergoing radiographic procedures requiring contrast media is the preparation that they must undergo before some of these procedures, especially barium studies. Preparation of the patient for a barium study might include the following:

- Liquid diet only for the evening meal on the day before the examination
- Laxatives the day preceding the examination to help clean the intestinal tract
- Nothing by mouth (NPO) after midnight the day before the examination. This usually includes no gum chewing or cigarette smoking because both activities increase gastric secretions that may interfere with the ability of the contrast medium to coat the wall of the intestine.

This general preparation applies to any contrast examination of the abdominal structures. Although this type of radiographic procedure is not performed in the medical office, you must ensure that the patient has proper instructions for preparing for the procedure and is notified of the scheduled time and facility. If patients are not properly prepared for contrast studies, they may have to be rescheduled for another time and day and must undertake the preparations again. Explaining the importance of the preparation can be one of the most important contributions you can make to the patient's care in contrast examinations.

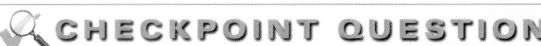

**CHECKPOINT QUESTION**

4. How would Mary explain the purpose of contrast media aid in differentiating between body structures?

## Fluoroscopy

**Fluoroscopy**, or fluoro studies, uses x-rays to observe movement within the body. The movement of a contrast medium in the body could include barium sulfate through the digestive tract or iodinated compounds in the blood as it flows through the heart or blood vessels. Fluoroscopy is also used as an aid to other types of treatments, such as reducing fractures and implanting devices such as pacemakers.

## Computed Tomography

CT is a procedure in which the x-ray tube and film move in relation to one another during the exposure, blurring out all structures except those in the focal plane. CT uses a combination of x-rays from a tube circling the patient and computers that analyze the x-rays to create cross-sectional images of the body. CT may be done with or without contrast medium. In addition, some CT units can create three-dimensional images so that organs can be viewed from all angles (Fig. 25-9).

**CHECKPOINT QUESTION**

5. What procedures would require the use of fluoroscopy?

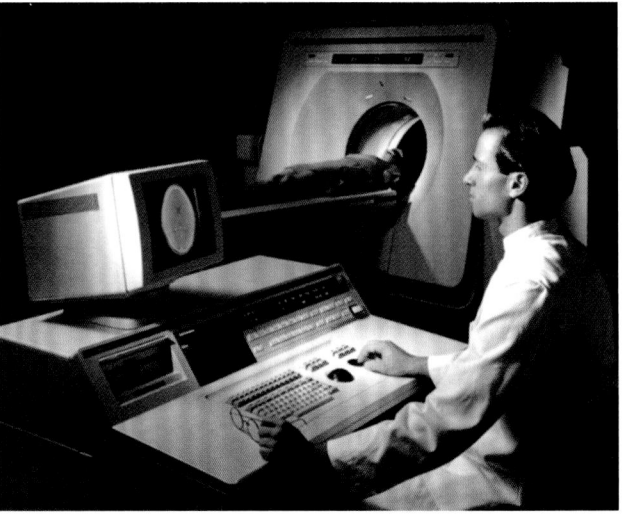

**Figure 25-9** • A CT scanner.

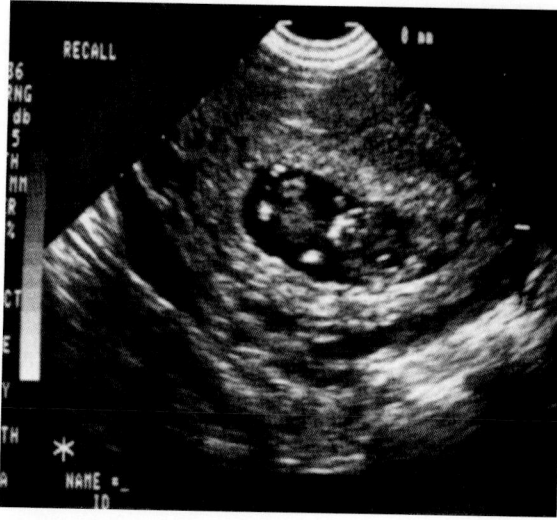

**Figure 25-10** • A sonogram.

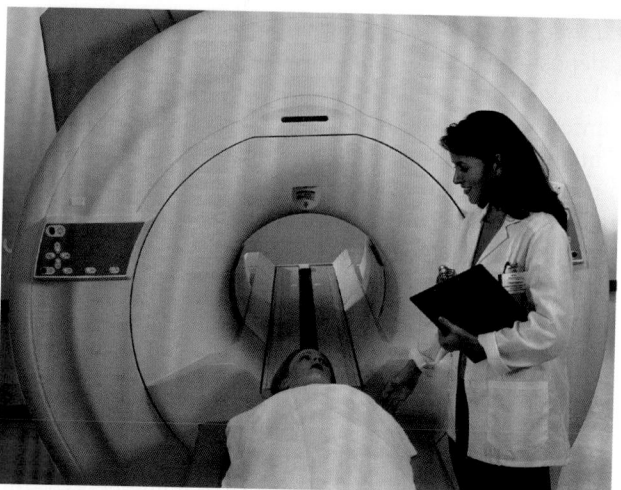

**Figure 25-11** • An open MRI.

## Sonography

**Ultrasound**, or sonography, uses high-frequency sound waves, not x-rays, to create cross-sectional still or real-time (motion) images of the body, usually with the help of a computer. This application is often used to demonstrate heart function or abdominal or pelvic structures. It is commonly used in prenatal testing to visualize the developing fetus. Many obstetricians routinely schedule at least one sonogram before the 4th month of pregnancy (Fig. 25-10).

## Magnetic Resonance Imaging

MRI uses a combination of high-intensity magnetic fields, radio waves, and computer analysis to create cross-sectional images of the body. MRI does not use x-rays. The image depends on the chemical makeup of the body. MRI is commonly used for a variety of studies, including the central nervous system and joint structure. Some MRI studies are performed with contrast. Typically, the patient must be prepared for a long procedure snugly enclosed in a machine that makes numerous knocking and whirring noises. Some facilities use open MRI, which does not make a patient feel as claustrophobic as the closed MRI (Fig. 25-11). Patients with a fear of enclosed places may require a mild sedative before closed MRI.

## Nuclear Medicine

Nuclear medicine entails the injection of small amounts of **radionuclides**, which are radioactive materials with short life spans, designed to concentrate in specific areas of the body. Sophisticated computer cameras detect the radiation and create an image. This technique is commonly used to study the thyroid, brain, lungs, liver, spleen, kidney, bone, and breast. These examinations are commonly called scans.

A sophisticated nuclear medicine study, *positron emission tomography* (PET), uses specialized equipment to produce detailed sectional images of the body's physiologic processes. Another procedure, *single photon emission computed tomography* (SPECT), is a nuclear study that produces sectional images of the body as detectors move around the patient. Both of these procedures are useful in the early diagnosis of physiologic and cellular abnormalities, such as those associated with cancerous tumors.

###  CHECKPOINT QUESTION

6. Which diagnostic imaging technique would most likely be ordered for diagnosing cancer in the early stages?

## **COG** INTERVENTIONAL RADIOLOGIC PROCEDURES

Interventional radiologic techniques are designed to treat specific disease conditions. For some patients, these therapeutic techniques are so effective that there is no need for surgery. Some interventional procedures may be life-saving. The following are some types of techniques:

- *Percutaneous transluminal coronary angioplasty* (PTCA), also known as *balloon angioplasty*, is used to enlarge the lumen of a coronary artery with a balloon-tipped catheter. Using fluoroscopy, the catheter is placed at a point of partial occlusion or stenosis. The balloon is then briefly inflated, compressing the plaque against the sides of the vessel. After the balloon is deflated, the catheter is removed, and the lumen of the vessel remains larger, allowing for improved blood flow through the blood vessel. Balloon angioplasties may be performed in almost any blood vessel.

- *Laser angioplasties* use laser beams to remove deposits in vessels using fluoroscopy.
- *Vascular stents* (plastic or wire tubes) may be inserted into the stenosed, or constricted, area of a vessel to maintain its patency. Fluoroscopy is used to guide placement of the stent.
- *Embolizations* artificially stop active bleeding from a blood vessel or reduce blood flow to a diseased area of an organ.

## RADIATION THERAPY

A major force in the fight against cancer for many years has been radiation therapy. The use of high-energy radiation to destroy cancer cells may not only prolong the lives of many patients but also saves lives. Used in conjunction with surgery, chemotherapy, or both, radiation is possibly the best-known treatment for cancer. Because the radiation is intense enough to destroy cancer cells, it may also damage adjacent normal cells. Therefore, treatments must be planned carefully and precisely by a radiologist, a physician who specializes in radiology.

Treatment consists of a precise, carefully planned regimen of therapy, including the frequency and amount of radiation to be used and the number of exposures during a given period. The area of the body to be exposed must be defined exactly so that each treatment is identical. The therapy consists of placing the patient in a position described by the treatment plan and having the exact amount of radiation administered by a radiology technician. Usually, the patient has little to do but lie still.

The patient's prognosis varies with the situation. Most patients have some side effects, which may include hair loss, weight loss, loss of appetite, skin changes, and digestive system disturbances. Once the treatment plan is carried out, most of the side effects disappear.

### CHECKPOINT QUESTION

7. What type of health care practitioner is responsible for prescribing and monitoring the effects of radiation therapy for the treatment of cancer?

## THE MEDICAL ASSISTANT'S ROLE IN RADIOLOGIC PROCEDURES

Because professional medical assistants have a variety of responsibilities in patient care, they often are in an ideal position to help alleviate patients' anxiety regarding radiology. Patient anxiety may be relieved by giving

patients information about examinations that they do not understand, by making patients feel comfortable enough to ask questions, and by answering questions in terms that the patient can understand.

## Calming the Patient's Fears

Some patients who have experience with the medical system have learned to overcome their anxieties and to find answers to their questions. No matter how much they have been through before, however, there is always something new or something they do not understand that may make them feel as if they have lost control of their situation. Being sensitive to patients' feelings is one of the greatest talents anyone in medicine can possess and should be an important part of your training and personality.

Unfortunately, many patients must undergo procedures they do not understand and do not know enough about to be able to ask relevant questions. Many feel like spectators rather than participants in their own care. Medical assistants can affect a patient's emotional response to a radiologic procedure by explaining what to expect in simple, everyday language, not technical medical terms. The technical aspects of radiology make it difficult for patients to understand. The key to success in explaining radiology procedures to patients is simplicity, leaving the details to the physician.

As noted earlier, explaining the preparations for examinations and their importance is vital to the success of many procedures. Equally important may be an explanation of what to do after the procedure. A barium enema, for instance, can lead to constipation if the patient does not drink enough fluids after the examination. This simple direction can save the patient much distress.

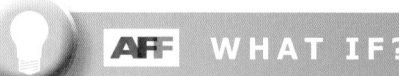 **WHAT IF?**

**A patient has been scheduled for a barium study at a local outpatient facility but calls your office to ask what to do if he ate breakfast this morning. What should you do?**

As a medical assistant, you must understand the reason for fasting before certain diagnostic procedures. In this situation, the patient should be instructed to call the diagnostic facility for further instructions, which will include rescheduling the procedure. Emphasize to the patient the importance of following all instructions carefully since not doing so will interfere with the procedure and/or the results. Not following instructions will result in further inconvenience of the patient and delay of a possible diagnose, further delaying treatment and outcomes for the patient.

## Assisting with Examinations

As a medical assistant, you may be expected to assist with radiologic examinations in the following ways:

- Tell the patient what clothing to remove or assist with clothing removal as needed.
- Help the patient take the position for the procedure, emphasizing the importance of remaining still and following breathing directions.
- Perform specific radiologic procedures, such as bone or chest radiography, as permitted by your state's laws and your education and training.
- Place film in an automatic processor and reload new film into the cassette.
- Distribute or file radiographs and reports appropriately.
- Procedure 25-1 details the procedure for assisting with x-ray procedures.

## Handling and Storing Radiographic Films

Advancing technology and the need for quality control have led to automated processing and developing of film to eliminate human error. Automated processing machines produce a film usually in less than 2 minutes. Because processors vary by manufacturer, you need to be proficient in the operation of your particular facility's equipment.

Unexposed film must be protected from moisture, heat, and light by storage in a cool, dry place, preferably in a lead-lined box. Film packets, exposed or unexposed, must be opened in a darkroom using only the darkroom light for illumination. The film is placed in a cassette for use in any area outside the darkroom. Intensifying screens in the cassette are used to reduce the amount of exposure required. Special sleeves or envelopes of various sizes are available for storing the film that has been labeled with the name of the patient (Fig. 25-12). Film must be protected and stored in a cool, dry area.

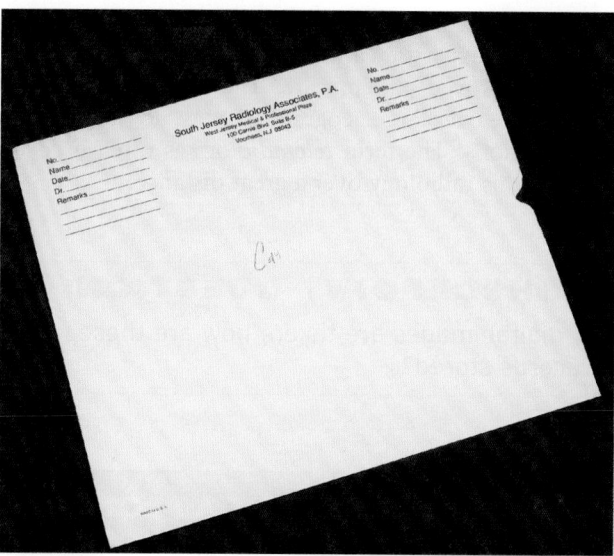

**Figure 25-12** • An x-ray envelope.

the examination to the referring physician. You may need the patient's permission to have the summary of findings sent to the office physician.

With a short-term referral, the examining physician usually returns the films to the referring physician. Patients who have ongoing concerns or who change physicians may request the information contained in their records after submitting written consent. In addition, the patient may obtain copies of the original radiographs if necessary.

### CHECKPOINT QUESTION

8. How can a medical assistant such as Mary help with radiologic examinations?

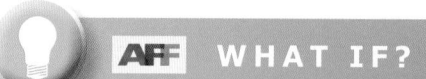

### WHAT IF?

**What if your patient asks you to give him the results of a recently taken chest x-ray?**

Many patients are anxious to find out test results including the results of radiology procedures. Often, these patients will ask you for the results before the physician has had an opportunity to read any radiology reports or to look at the actual radiograph. You should tell this patient that the physician would prefer to talk to him about the results and any questions can be answered at that time by the physician. Although you may have access to radiology reports, it is not appropriate to discuss the results with the patient unless the physician has given you permission to do so.

## TRANSFER OF RADIOGRAPHIC INFORMATION

Radiographic images obtained on site for use by the physician remain part of the patient's permanent record. Digital images can be saved on a computer diskette or compact disk. In many cases, however, radiographic studies are performed at one site for consultation or referral at another site. X-ray films belong to the site where the study was performed. The examining physician or radiologist generally writes a summary of

## Teleradiology

The use of computed imaging and information systems, **teleradiology**, is providing new benefits in medicine. Many institutions use a picture archiving and communication system (PACS) in which computers store and transmit images. Digital images from CT, for instance, can be transmitted via telephone lines to distant locations. This allows consultation with experts on a difficult case within a matter of minutes. Previously unavailable expertise can be brought to rural areas for greatly improved patient care. The result is improved patient care over large geographic areas, not just in specific locations. The term *teleradiology* is often used to describe this radiology over a great distance.

## CHECKPOINT QUESTION

9. If digital images are taken, how are these records stored?

## PATIENT EDUCATION

### Advances in Surgical Procedures

Today, many surgeries that once required large abdominal incisions and extended hospital stays are performed in outpatient ambulatory surgical centers through small incisions and a laparoscope. For example, gallstones are removed with a laparoscope guided by an interventional radiologist, and the patient returns home the same day of surgery. Abdominal aortic aneurysms are treated with a similar procedure, resulting in shorter hospital admissions and less pain. You need to stay current regarding new procedures and surgical techniques so that you can be informed and reassure patients and their families who may not be as aware of the advances made in health care.

## ROLE-PLAYING ACTIVITY

You are a practicum student at the internal medicine physician office with Mary Smalley, CMA (refer to the case study at the beginning of the chapter). Unless roles are assigned by your instructor, ask another student to assume the role of the following patients.

1. Madge Blankenship (age 72 years). Madge is being seen today for pain in her lower back and right leg. She is normally very active and has continued to drive even though she has increased pain upon "pushing the gas pedal." The physician suspects a herniated disk and has ordered a CT scan of her lower back, and this must be scheduled at the local radiology center. Madge does not want to rely on others for assistance and is cooperative with the physician, but irritable with you when you go to speak with her about the CT scan. She is concerned that she will not be "able to find" the radiology center.

2. George Temple (age 60 years). George is being seen today for abdominal pain after eating. The physician suspects gallbladder disease and orders an ultrasound of the gallbladder to be scheduled at the local radiology center. George explains to you that he "cannot miss work" because he had to take most of his vacation time this year to care for his wife who had a stroke. He is also concerned that this "test" will be painful.

How would you relate to each of these patients? Is their age a factor? Why or why not? Your instructor will give you additional information about this activity!

## *español* SPANISH TERMINOLOGY

**Tiene que estar en ayunas antes de la prueba.**
You must be fasting before the test.

**Puede tomar una comida ligera la noche antes de la prueba.**
You may eat a light supper the night before the test.

**Debe seguir estas instrucciónes al pie de la letra.**
You must follow these directions exactly.

**Tengo que tomarle una placa de rayos x.**
I have to take an x-ray.

**Por favor quítese todos los metales que traiga, collares, reloj, anillos, aretes, etc.**
Please remove all metals from your body: necklaces, rings, watch, etc.

**¿Se practicó el enema?**
Did you have the enema?

**¿Está usted embarazada?**
Are you pregnant?

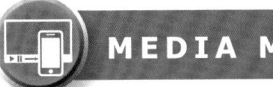

## MEDIA MENU

**Student Resources** on thePoint®
• **CMA/RMA Certification Exam Review**

**Internet Resources**
**Radiology Info**
http://www.radiologyinfo.org

**Virtual Hospital**
http://www.vh.org

**American Society of Radiologic Technologists**
http://www.asrt.org

**Access Excellence Resource Center: The Living Skeleton**
http://www.accessexcellence.org/RC/VL/xrays/index.php

**Medline Plus: X-Rays**
http://www.nlm.nih.gov/medlineplus/xrays.html

**The Registry of Radiologic Technologists**
http://www.arrt.org

## EMR Activity

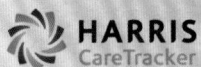

Harris CareTracker is a Web-based electronic medical record (EMR) application that you will use for the EMR activities included in this section at the end of each chapter. This application is actually used in physician offices but is provided to you through the publisher, Wolters Kluwer Health, to give you hands-on practice working with EMRs. Your instructor will have more information about accessing your username, log-in, and Quickstart guide.

Prerequisite Activities in Harris CareTracker

- *The Getting Started and Quickstart documents and EMR Activities Step-by-Step Instructions are available at* http://thePoint.lww.com/KronenbergerComp5e.

Activity Details

Preauthorization for diagnostic procedures has been requested from the insurance companies for the following patients. Using the *ToDo* application in each patient's EMR, send a note to yourself to check the status of the preauthorization in 3 days at 3:00 PM.

1. Tom Bankston, preauthorization requested for MRI of the cervical spine
2. Lawrence Black, preauthorization requested for MRI of the left ankle and foot

## Chapter Summary

- Radiology is continually evolving as a tool to diagnose and treat disease. As a medical assistant:
  - You must understand the common types of diagnostic and therapeutic radiologic procedures that may be ordered by the physician.
  - You may also be responsible for teaching patients about these procedures in general and about any particular preparations required.
  - When assisting the physician, you must always follow radiation safety precautions carefully for the protection of yourself and your patient.

## Warm-Ups for Critical Thinking

1. While preparing a female patient for an x-ray procedure, she explains to you that she might be pregnant. How would you handle this situation?
2. Create a poster for your office summarizing the key points of radiation safety.
3. Constipation is a common problem among patients who have barium studies. How can patient education diminish this problem?
4. An elderly woman is concerned about having an ultrasound of her gallbladder and states that she does not want to have any more x-rays. Based on what you know about sonography, how would you respond to this patient?
5. Explain the importance of patient privacy laws (Health Insurance Portability and Accountability Act of 1996 [HIPAA]) and teleradiology. What is your role in maintaining privacy in using teleradiology?

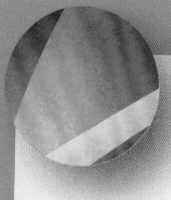

**PSY PROCEDURE 25-1**

# Assist with X-Ray Procedures

**PSY** Instruct and prepare a patient for a procedure or treatment; respond to nonverbal communication; coach patients appropriately considering cultural diversity, developmental life stage, and/or communication barriers; document patient care accurately in the medical record.

**Purpose:** Prepare the patient for general x-ray procedure

**Equipment:** Patient gown and drape

**Standard:** This procedure should take 5 minutes.

| STEPS | REASONS |
|---|---|
| 1. Wash your hands. | Handwashing aids infection control. |
| 2. Greet the patient by name, introduce yourself, and escort him or her to the room where the x-ray equipment is maintained. | Identifying the patient prevents errors. |
| 3. **AFF** Explain how to respond to a patient who speaks English as a second language (ESL). | With the patient's permission, have an interpreter in the room to assist with translation. Arrange this before the patient comes into the office if possible. If one is not available, utilize a picture chart or nonverbal gestures to help the patient understand. |
| 4. Ask female patients about the possibility of pregnancy. If the patient is unsure or indicates pregnancy in any trimester, consult with the physician before proceeding with the x-ray procedure. | Fetal exposure to x-rays may be damaging to developing organs and tissues. |
| 5. After explaining what clothing should be removed, if any, give the patient a gown and provide privacy. | For a chest x-ray, you will have the patient remove all clothing from the waist up. Jewelry such as necklaces may also have to be removed because these will show up on the x-ray and may obscure the images the physician needs to view for diagnosis. |
| 6. Notify the x-ray technician or physician that the patient is ready for the x-ray procedure. Stay behind the lead-lined wall during the x-ray procedure to avoid exposure to x-rays during the procedure. | Depending on state law, you may or may not be trained to perform x-ray procedures. |
| 7. After the x-ray, ask the patient to remain in the room until the film has been developed and checked for accuracy and readability. | On occasion, the x-ray will need to be repeated for clarity or adjusted patient position. |
| 8. Once you have determined that the exposed film is adequate for the physician to view for diagnosis, have the patient get dressed and escort him or her to the front desk. | At that time, you can explain any further physician instructions or billing procedures. |
| 9. **AFF** Log into the electronic medical record (EMR) using your username and secure password OR obtain the paper medical record from a secure location and assure it is kept away from public access. | |

## PROCEDURE 25-1 (continued)

| STEPS | REASONS |
|---|---|
| 10. Document the procedure in the medical record. | Procedures are considered not to have been done if they are not recorded. |
| 11. When finished, log out of the EMR and/or replace the paper medical record in an appropriate and secure location. | The integrity of the medical record must be maintained at all times to protect patient privacy. |

---

Charting Example:

*10/19/2016 AP Chest x-ray obtained per x-ray tech. Radiograph placed on viewbox—Dr. Jones notified*

*———————————————————————————————————— M. Smalley, CMA*

---

Note: *The medical assistant may sign his or her name in the patient record using only the "CMA" credential if the office has a signature log denoting the entire credential as "CMA (AAMA)."*

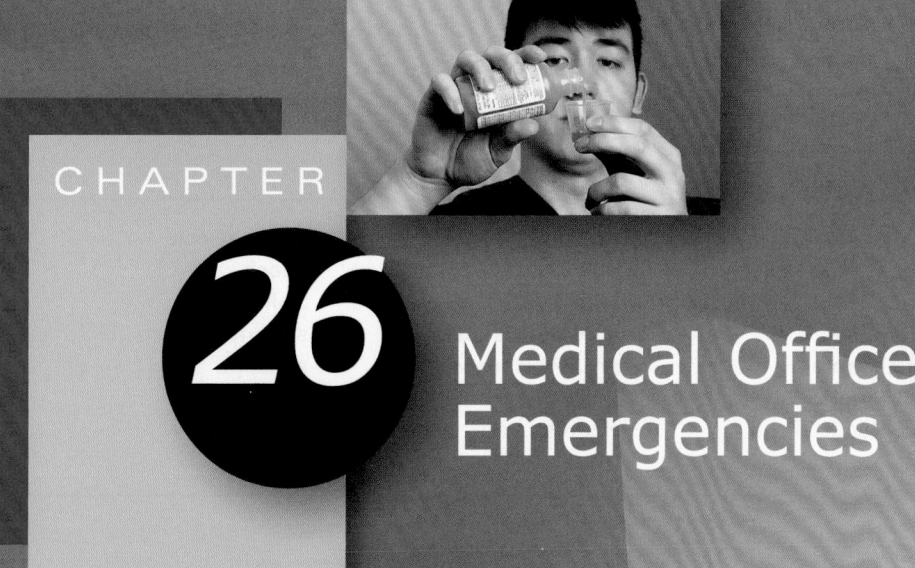

# CHAPTER 26

# Medical Office Emergencies

## Outline

**Medical Office Emergency Procedures**
Preparation for an Emergency
Patient Assessment

## Learning Outcomes

### COG Cognitive Domain*

1. Spell and define key terms
2. *List principles and steps of professional/provider CPR*
3. *Describe basic principles of first aid as they pertain to the ambulatory health care setting*
4. Identify the five types of shock and the management of each
5. Describe how burns are classified and managed
6. Explain the management of allergic reactions
7. Describe the management of poisoning and the role of the poison control center
8. List the three types of hyperthermic emergencies and the treatment for each type
9. Discuss the treatment of hypothermia
10. Describe the role of the medical assistant in managing psychiatric emergencies

### PSY Psychomotor Domain*

1. Administer oxygen (Procedure 26-1)
2. Perform cardiopulmonary resuscitation (Procedure 26-2)
   a. *Produce up-to-date documentation of provider/ professional level CPR*
3. Use an automatic external defibrillator (Procedure 26-3)
4. Manage a foreign body airway obstruction (Procedure 26-4)
5. Control bleeding (Procedure 26-5)
   a. *Perform first aid procedures for bleeding*
6. Respond to medical emergencies other than bleeding, cardiac/respiratory arrest, or foreign body airway obstruction (Procedure 26-6)
   a. *Perform first aid procedures for fractures, seizure, shock, and syncope*
7. *Document patient care accurately in the medical record*

### AFF Affective Domain*

1. *Incorporate critical thinking skills in performing patient assessment*
2. *Incorporate critical thinking skills in performing patient care*
3. *Show awareness of patients' concerns related to the procedure being performed*
4. *Demonstrate empathy, active listening, nonverbal communication*
5. *Demonstrate respect for individual diversity including gender, race, religion, age, economic status, and appearance*
6. *Explain to a patient the rationale for performance of a procedure*
7. Protect the integrity of the medical record
8. Demonstrate self-awareness in responding to an emergency situation

*\*Note: AAMA/CAAHEP 2015 Standards are italicized.*

### ABHES Competencies

1. Document accurately
2. Recognize and respond to verbal and nonverbal communication
3. Adapt to individualized needs
4. Apply principles of aseptic techniques and infection control
5. Recognize emergencies and treatments and minor office surgical procedures
6. Use standard precautions
7. Perform first aid and CPR
8. Demonstrate professionalism by exhibiting a positive attitude and sense of responsibility

| | | | |
|---|---|---|---|
| allergen | heat cramps | infarction | septic shock |
| anaphylactic shock | heat exhaustion | ischemia | shock |
| cardiogenic shock | heat stroke | melena | Splint |
| contusions | hematomas | neurogenic shock | superficial burn |
| ecchymosis | hyperthermia | partial-thickness | syncope |
| full-thickness burn | hypothermia | burn | |
| frostbite | hypovolemic shock | seizures | |

## Case Study

$B$etsy Reynolds, CMA (AAMA), recently transferred from an orthopedic physician's office to the urgent care center in the Great Falls Medical Center. Her experience working with patients who had bone, joint and soft tissue injuries was a favorable quality to the office manager and physician who interviewed and ultimately hired her for the current position. Betsy works the afternoon and evening shift and is responsible for assessing patients who come into the center. She must also determine the urgency of the situation and what immediate action should be taken, if any. In addition to her training in emergency office procedures, Betsy may draw on the urgent care center's extensive policy and procedure manual, which covers in detail the various types of medical emergencies that may be seen in the center and the role of the medical assistant in addressing them. There are two physicians and one physician assistant available at all times. Today, Betsy has taken care of five adult patients and three children brought in by caregivers. The illnesses and injuries have included a sore throat and fever, a sprained ankle, a second-degree burn on the forearm, and a lacerated thumb that required suturing. This chapter includes some of the medical office emergencies seen in Betsy's clinic today and the role of the medical assistant.

Emergency medical care is the immediate care given to sick or injured persons. When properly performed, it can mean the difference between life or death, rapid recovery or long hospitalization, and temporary or permanent disability. Emergency care in the medical office entails identifying the emergency, delivering basic first aid, and furnishing temporary assistance or basic life support until a rescue squad and advanced life support can be obtained.

## ☯ MEDICAL OFFICE EMERGENCY PROCEDURES

An emergency can occur anywhere, to anyone, at any time. For example, a patient who is being seen for a routine examination may have a heart attack, collapse, and require immediate cardiopulmonary resuscitation (CPR). A diabetic patient or coworker may lapse into a diabetic coma (see Chapter 37 for diabetic emergency procedures). A patient may fall down a flight of stairs and receive trauma to the head or limbs. In a life-threatening situation, the well-prepared medical assistant can obtain important information and perform lifesaving procedures before the ambulance or rescue squad arrives, increasing the patient's chance for survival. Medical assistants should be certified in CPR, using the automatic external defibrillator (AED) and removing foreign body airway obstructions. Although the American Association of Medical Assistants (AAMA) required certified medical assistants (CMAs) to demonstrate proof of CPR certification to recertify their credential several years ago, proof of CPR certification is no longer required. However, accredited education programs for medical assistants must require students to obtain documentation of provider/professional level CPR. This training may be provided by the American Red Cross, American Heart Association, American Safety and Health Institute, or National Safety Council. You should contact one of these agencies for specific information regarding training and certification. This chapter is not meant to provide a comprehensive study of all aspects of emergency care; instead, it briefly reviews the information in such a training course.

## Preparation for an Emergency

Every medical office should have an emergency action plan, including the following:

- The local emergency rescue service telephone number (usually 911)
- Location of the nearest hospital emergency department
- Telephone number of the local or regional poison control center
- Procedures for various emergencies
- List of office personnel who are trained in CPR
- Location and list of contents of the emergency medical kit or crash cart

Whether confronted with a cardiac emergency or psychiatric crisis, medical assistants must be able to coordinate multiple ongoing events while rendering patient care. Contributing to the complexity of a medical emergency are such factors as panicky family members, the arrival of emergency personnel, and possibly language barriers. You must be able to remain calm in these situations while reacting competently and professionally.

### Emergency Medical Kit

Proper equipment and supplies should be readily available in a medical emergency. Although the office's equipment and supplies vary with the medical specialty, emergency equipment and supplies are fairly standard. This equipment should be kept in a designated location that is accessible to all staff. Standard supplies for a medical emergency kit are listed in Box 26-1. Although items used during an emergency should be replaced as soon as possible, a medical assistant or other staff member should check the contents of the emergency kit or crash cart regularly, perhaps weekly, to verify that contents are available and that no item has gone beyond the expiration date. If so, the expired items should be replaced immediately.

### The Emergency Medical Services System

The initial element of any emergency medical services (EMS) system is citizen access. The availability of rapid, systematic intervention by personnel specifically trained in providing emergency care is an integral part of the EMS system. Most communities have a 911 system to report emergencies and summon help by telephone. The communications operator at the local EMS station will answer the call, take the information, and alert the EMS, fire, or police department as needed. In communities

---

**BOX 26-1** Emergency Medical Kit and Equipment

The following are standard supplies that can be used to make up an emergency medical kit:

- Acetic acid solution (4% to 6%) or vinegar
- Activated charcoal
- Adhesive strip bandages, assorted sizes
- Adhesive tape, 1- and 2-inch rolls
- Alcohol (70%)
- Alcohol wipes
- Antimicrobial skin ointment
- Chemical ice pack
- Cotton balls
- Cotton swabs
- Disposable gloves
- Elastic bandages, 2- and 3-inch widths
- Gauze pads, 2 × 2– and 4 × 4–inch widths
- Roller, self-adhesive gauze, 2- and 4-inch widths
- Safety pins, various sizes
- Scissors
- Spray bottle for cool water
- Syrup of ipecac
- Thermometer
- Tweezers

In addition to these contents, the following equipment should be available:

- Blood pressure cuff (pediatric and adult)
- Stethoscope
- Bag–valve–mask device with assorted size masks
- Flashlight or penlight
- Portable oxygen tank with regulator
- Oxygen masks
- Suction unit and catheters

Additional equipment that may be available includes the following:

- Various sizes of endotracheal tubes
- Laryngoscope handle and various sizes of blades
- AED
- IV supplies (catheters, administration set tubing, assorted solutions)
- Emergency drugs including atropine, epinephrine, and sodium bicarbonate

---

without a 911 system, emergency calls are usually made directly to the local ambulance, fire, or police department. You should know the emergency system used in your community. Emergency phone numbers should be prominently displayed by all telephones in the medical office.

Some communities have an enhanced 911 system that automatically identifies the caller's telephone number and location. If the telephone is disconnected or the caller loses consciousness, the communications operator can still send emergency personnel to the scene. In the medical office, an emergency requiring notification of the EMS includes situations that are life threatening or have the potential to become life threatening, such as the symptoms of a heart attack, shock, or severe breathing difficulties. In each of these cases, the medical assistant provides immediate care to the patient, including CPR if necessary, while directing another staff member to notify the physician. During assessment of the emergency by the physician, the medical assistant should continue to provide first aid or be prepared to assist the physician in administering first aid while another staff member notifies the EMS. The staff member who calls EMS should be able to describe the emergency to the communications operator. The operator will then know what level of emergency personnel and rescue equipment to send. Excellent communication skills and cooperation between health care team members are essential during a medical office emergency.

Documentation in the medical record is an important responsibility in all patient care, including emergency care. EMS personnel depend on accurate and complete information regarding the patient's symptoms, the nature of the emergency, and any treatment performed prior to their arrival. This information should be placed in the patient's record in chronological order as events occurred or treatments were performed. Any vital signs taken during the emergency should also be recorded. Emergencies that involve visitors or staff must also be documented, and in this case, a blank paper or progress note page will be sufficient to record the details and outline the care provided. Information should include but not be limited to the following:

1. Basic identification, including name, age, address, and location of the patient's emergency contact if known
2. The chief complaint if known
3. Times of events, beginning with recognition of the emergency, management techniques, and changes in patient's condition
4. The patient's vital signs
5. Specific emergency management rendered in the office, such as CPR, bandaging, splinting, and medications administered before and after the emergency
6. Observations of the patient's condition, including any slurred speech, lethargy, confusion, and so on
7. Any medical history, allergies, or current medications if known

When the EMS personnel arrive, assist them as necessary. Let them examine the patient and take over the emergency care. You can also help by removing any obstacles to removal of the patient by stretcher and keeping family members in the reception area or a private room.

## CHECKPOINT QUESTION

1. Betsy was ordered by the physician to notify emergency medical services for a patient who needed to be transported to an acute care facility or hospital. What should Betsy document before the ambulance arrives in an emergency?

## Patient Assessment

The two primary objectives in assessment of the patient are to identify and correct any life-threatening problems and provide necessary care. Each step of the assessment must be managed effectively before proceeding to the next. For example, airway, breathing, and circulation must be intact before you take a history. In addition, survey the scene quickly to identify hazards or clues to the patient's condition. For example, an elderly person found at the bottom of a stairway will likely have head or neck injuries and should be treated in such a way as to avoid moving the head, neck, or spinal column. Emesis found near a person that resembles coffee grounds may be a clue to bleeding in the gastrointestinal system that may result from peptic ulcer disease and hemorrhage.

### Recognizing the Emergency

When providing emergency care, do not assume that the obvious injuries are the only ones. Less noticeable or internal injuries may also have occurred during an accident. You should look for the causes of the injury, which may provide a clue to the extent of physical damage. For example, the elderly patient who fell down the stairs may have a noticeable bump on the forehead; this is obvious, but perhaps the patient has an injury in the cervical spine that is not as readily noticeable. In the case of an injury to the head or back when spinal fracture is possible, be especially careful not to move the victim any more than necessary and avoid rough handling.

### The Primary Assessment

Once you are at the victim's side, an initial survey of the patient is the first step in emergency care. This is a rapid evaluation, usually done in less than 45 seconds. The purpose of the primary assessment is to identify and correct any life-threatening problems. Quickly assess the following aspects of the patient:

- Responsiveness
- Circulation
- Airway
- Breathing

Checking for responsiveness means noting whether the patient is conscious or unconscious. If the patient is unconscious, attempt to awaken the patient by speaking and touching the shoulder. If no response occurs, check

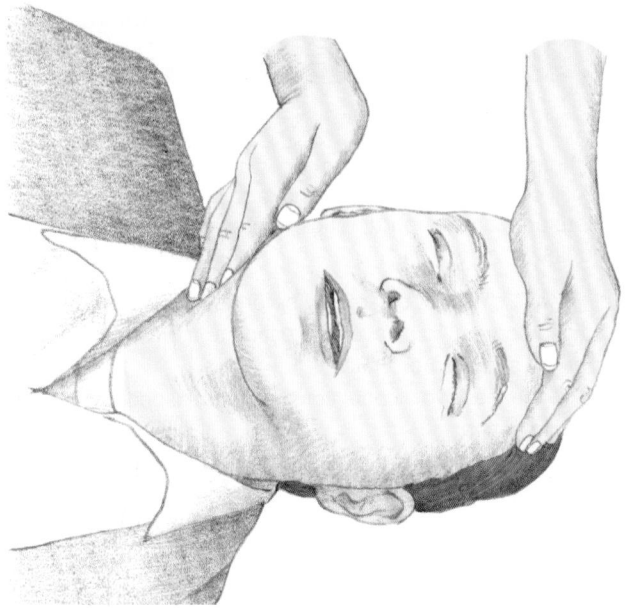

**FIGURE 26-1** • Check for circulation by palpating the carotid pulse. (From *Nursing Procedures*, 4th ed. Ambler, PA: Lippincott Williams & Wilkins, 2004.)

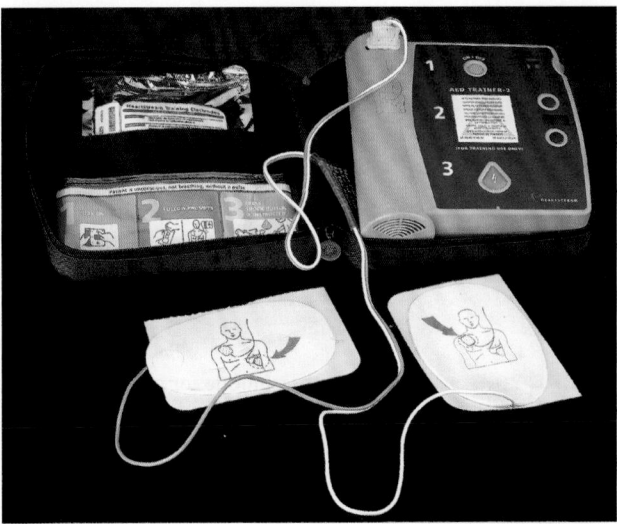

**FIGURE 26-3** • The AED can be used to defibrillate a life-threatening heart rhythm.

for circulation. Evaluate circulation in adults and children by checking the carotid pulse (Fig. 26-1). The brachial pulse is used to evaluate circulation in infants. If no pulse is found, begin CPR chest compressions immediately (Fig. 26-2). Some medical offices may have an AED as part of the emergency medical kit (Fig. 26-3). Training to use the AED is included in most CPR classes. Many public places such as airports and shopping malls have AED units available for use by those individuals trained appropriately. If no pulse present, begin chest compressions.

After 30 compressions, assess the patient's airway by using the head tilt–chin lift method (Fig. 26-4). Patients who may have neck injuries should have the airway opened using the jaw thrust method to avoid further injury to the spinal cord (Fig. 26-5). An unconscious patient who is supine is likely to have a partial or total

airway obstruction caused by the tongue falling back into the oropharynx, producing snoring respirations or total airway obstruction. Opening the patient's airway may be necessary to allow adequate respirations. In the event of a foreign body airway obstruction, it will be necessary to clear the airway to perform effective rescue breathing.

Once the airway is open, evaluate the patient's breathing by watching for movement of the chest up or down while listening and feeling over the mouth and nose for signs of adequate ventilation. If the patient is not breathing, rescue breathing must be started immediately. A face mask with a one-way valve or a bag–valve–mask device is required when performing rescue breathing

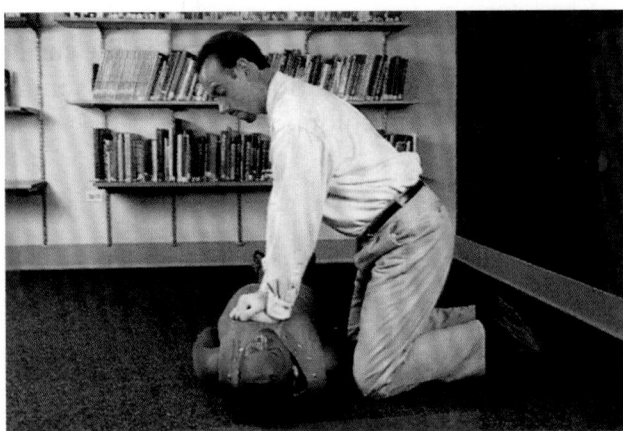

**FIGURE 26-2** • Chest compressions should be started if no signs of circulation, including a pulse, are present.

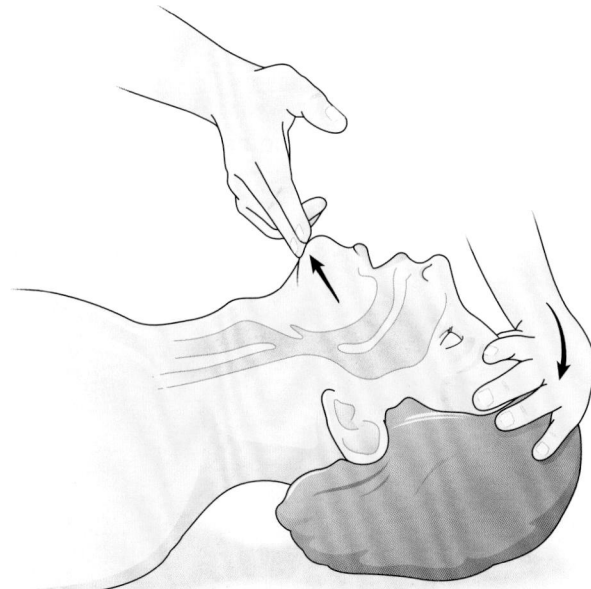

**FIGURE 26-4** • The head tilt–chin lift technique for opening the airway. The head is tilted backward with one hand (*down arrow*) while the fingers of the other hand lift the chin forward (*up arrow*).

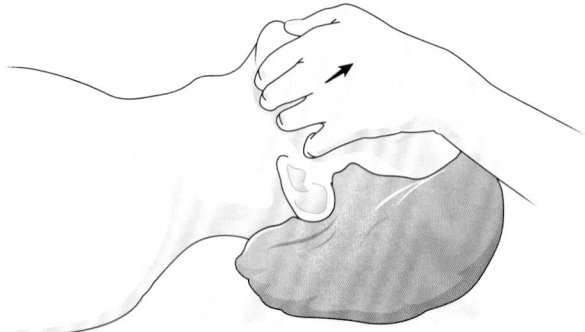

**FIGURE 26-5** • The jaw thrust technique for opening the airway. The hands are placed on either side of the head. The fingers of both hands grasp behind the angle of the jaw, bringing it up (*arrow*).

(Fig. 26-6). Respirations that are too fast, too slow, or irregular also require medical intervention. Immediate intervention for these conditions may include breathing into a mask or paper bag for respirations that are too fast (hyperventilation) or administering oxygen as directed by the physician. Any obvious noises, such as stridor or wheezes, are noted and reported to the physician (see Chapter 31). Continue cardiopulmonary procedures until relieved by another health care staff member or EMS personnel arrive and take over. Procedure 26-1 describes the procedure for administering oxygen in the medical office, while Procedures 26-2, 26-3, and 26-4 explain CPR, the use of the AED, and managing a patient with a foreign body airway obstruction.

During the primary assessment, also check for any hemorrhage, and if found, control the bleeding quickly (Procedure 26-5). Evaluate perfusion, or blood flow through the tissues, by checking the temperature and moisture of the skin.

### CHECKPOINT QUESTION

2. What is the purpose of the primary assessment?

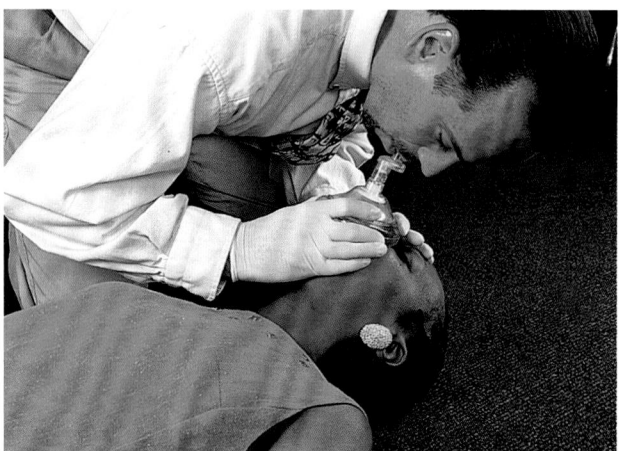

**FIGURE 26-6** • Using a mask with a one-way valve, begin rescue breathing if no breathing is noted in the primary survey.

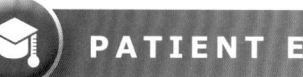

## PATIENT EDUCATION

### Choking

Although the danger of choking is always present with small children, many adults choke to death each year. Here are some important tips to prevent choking in adults:

- Always chew food carefully before swallowing. Focus on eating by avoiding eating and driving a car at the same time.
- Avoid excessive alcohol consumption, especially while eating.
- Laughter and talking increase your chance of choking. Do not talk with food in your mouth.
- Older adults who wear dentures should go for an annual dental evaluation to make sure dentures fit snugly.
- With age, saliva production decreases, making it more difficult to swallow. Encourage older patients to take smaller bites and chew food longer, sipping liquids as needed.

## The Secondary Assessment

After conducting a primary assessment and assessing that the patient's airway, breathing, and circulation are adequate, a secondary assessment can be performed. The secondary assessment includes asking the patient questions to obtain additional information and performing a more thorough physical evaluation to find less obvious problems than those noted in the primary assessment. To gain an accurate impression during the secondary assessment, the following four areas are assessed:

1. *General appearance.* The patient's skin color and moisture, facial expression, posture, motor activity, speech, and state of alertness provide important clues about the mental and physical condition. Check for a medical bracelet or necklace. Medicine bottles in a pocket or purse can also be helpful.
2. *Level of consciousness.* By the time you have completed the primary survey and noted the patient's general appearance, the level of consciousness may be apparent. A decrease in oxygen to the cells of the brain, neurologic damage from a cerebrovascular accident (stroke), and intracranial swelling are just some of the conditions that may alter a patient's level of consciousness. The AVPU system uses a common language to describe the patient's level of consciousness:
   - A, **A**wake and alert
   - V, responds to **V**oice
   - P, responds only to **P**ain
   - U, **U**nresponsive or unconscious

3. *Vital signs.* After noting the general appearance and determining the level of consciousness, assess the vital signs, including the pulse and respiratory rates and blood pressure. Assessment of temperature is important for patients who have altered skin temperature or have been exposed to environmental temperature extremes. Patients with a history of infection, chills, or fever and children with **seizures** should always have their temperature taken.

4. *Skin.* An initial evaluation of the temperature and moisture of skin should have been noted during the primary survey. A more thorough look should now be taken. Skin is normally dry and somewhat warm. Moist, cool skin may indicate poor blood flow to the tissues and possibly shock. The color of the skin should be noted as an indication of the circulation near the surface of the body and oxygenation of the tissues.

## WHAT IF?

**What if your patient has a cervical fracture?**

Fractures to the cervical spine can be life threatening or seriously disabling. There are seven cervical vertebrae in the neck, and fractures to the first cervical vertebra (C1), the most superior vertebra, tend to be fatal unless immediately and aggressively treated by emergency services personnel before transport to a trauma center. Fractures to the second and third cervical vertebrae (C2 and C3) often result in permanent or long-term respiratory dependency on a mechanical ventilator since the involuntary respiratory center of the brain is affected. Vertebrae fractures of the fourth to seventh cervical vertebrae (C4 to C7) will result in various levels of paralysis and motor impairment. If you suspect a patient has a cervical fracture or other vertebral fracture, keep the head and neck of the patient still and call for emergency personnel. Never move the patient unless the patient is in immediate danger. The emergency medical technicians will properly immobilize the head and neck of the patient for transport to the hospital, where radiographic tests will diagnose the extent of the injury.

## The Physical Examination

A head-to-toe survey that includes examination of the head and neck, chest and back, abdomen, and extremities in this sequence should be done only after completing the primary and secondary surveys. Although the physician usually performs this examination, you must be prepared to assist as needed while continuing to reassure the patient.

### Head and Neck

If a cervical spine injury is suspected, immediately immobilize the spine and avoid manipulating the neck during examination of the head. Inspect the face for edema, bruising, bleeding, and drainage from the nose or ears. Examine the mouth for loose teeth and dentures. The condition and severity of a neurologic injury or patient with altered consciousness can be assessed by checking the pupils with a flashlight or penlight. The pupils should be checked for several characteristics:

- Equality in size
- Dilation bilaterally in darkness or dim light
- Rapid constriction to light in both eyes
- Equal reaction to light

To evaluate the pupils for these qualities, shade both eyes from the light and use a flashlight or small penlight at an angle 6 to 8 inches from each eye. The conscious patient should not look directly into the light. Report the findings to the physician.

### Chest and Back

The anterior chest is evaluated to some degree when the patient's respiratory status is evaluated. A further inspection of the chest should be done after removing clothing from a patient with trauma or abnormal vital signs. Patients with cardiac or respiratory complaints should also have their chest more thoroughly evaluated. Palpation of the chest and back may reveal the possibility of rib fractures.

### Abdomen

The abdomen of all patients is evaluated, but it is particularly important for those with GI symptoms or suspicion of blood or fluid loss as seen in vaginal bleeding, vomiting, or melena (blood in the stool). The abdomen is inspected for scars, bruises, and masses. A distended abdomen may indicate hemorrhage in the abdominal cavity.

### Arms and Legs

An examination of the arms and legs is the last step of the head-to-toe survey. Inspect the arms and legs for swelling, deformity, and tenderness. Also note any tremors in the hands. To determine the neurologic status of the arms and legs, assess strength, movement, range of motion, and sensation, including comparing one side of the body with the other. Muscle strength in the upper extremities is checked by having the patient squeeze both of your hands at the same time. Leg strength may be determined by having the patient push each foot against your hand, again at the same time, while noting any weakness in one side or the other. Assess sensation by using a safety pin or other tool to determine the patient's response to pain. Throughout the examination, you must note the comparison of both sides, including any weakness or decreased sensation in one side or the other. Again, the physician will most likely be performing this examination, but you must be prepared to assist as needed.

## CHECKPOINT QUESTION

3. What diagnostic signs would Betsy evaluate in the secondary assessment?

# Types of Emergencies

## Shock

**Shock** is lack of oxygen to the individual cells of the body, including the brain, as a result of a decrease in blood pressure. Although the cause of the low blood pressure varies, the body initially adjusts for any type of shock by increasing the strength of the heart contractions and the heart rate while constricting the blood vessels throughout the body. As shock progresses, the body has more difficulty trying to adjust, and eventually, tissues and body organs have such severe damage that the shock becomes irreversible and death ensues. The signs and symptoms of shock include the following:

- Low blood pressure
- Restlessness or signs of fear
- Thirst
- Nausea
- Cool, clammy skin
- Pale skin with cyanosis (bluish color) at the lips and earlobes
- Rapid and weak pulse

## Types of Shock

**Hypovolemic shock** is caused by loss of blood or other body fluids. If the cause is blood loss, it is hemorrhagic shock. Dehydration caused by diarrhea, vomiting, or profuse sweating can also lead to hypovolemic shock. **Cardiogenic shock** is an extreme form of heart failure that occurs when the function of the left ventricle is so compromised that the heart can no longer adequately pump blood to body tissues. This type of shock may follow death of cardiac tissue during a myocardial infarction (heart attack). **Neurogenic shock** is caused by a dysfunction of the nervous system following a spinal cord injury. Normally, the diameter of all blood vessels is controlled by the involuntary nervous system and smooth muscles surrounding the vessels. After a spinal cord injury, the nervous system loses control of the diameter of the blood vessels, and vasodilation ensues. Once the blood vessels are dilated, there is not enough blood in the general circulation, so that blood pressure falls and shock ensues. **Anaphylactic shock** is an acute general allergic reaction within minutes to hours after the body has been exposed to an offending foreign substance. You must carefully observe patients for this type of shock after giving medications and during allergy testing (see later section on anaphylaxis). **Septic shock** is caused by a general infection of the bloodstream in which the patient appears seriously ill. It may be associated with an infection such as pneumonia or meningitis, or it may occur without an apparent source of infection, especially in infants and children. Initially, a fever is present, but the body temperature falls, a clinical sign suggestive of sepsis.

## Management of the Patient in Shock

Because shock can result from many types of medical situations or trauma, you should always be prepared to treat the patient for shock in any emergency situation that occurs in the medical office. After performing the primary and secondary assessments, the following list of general guidelines for managing a patient in shock should be observed:

1. Observe the patient for and maintain an open airway and adequate breathing.
2. Control bleeding.
3. Administer oxygen as directed by the physician.
4. Immobilize the patient if spinal injuries may be present.
5. Splint fractures.
6. Prevent loss of body heat by covering the patient with a blanket, especially if the patient is cold.
7. Assist the physician with starting an intravenous (IV) line as ordered (see Chapter 24).
8. Elevate the feet and legs of a patient with low systemic blood pressure.
9. Transport the patient to the closest hospital as soon as possible by notifying the EMS as directed by the physician.

## CHECKPOINT QUESTION

4. What does it mean when a patient is in shock?

# Bleeding

Soft tissue injuries involve damage to the skin and/or underlying musculature. When a blunt object strikes the body, it may crush the tissue beneath the skin. Although the skin does not always break, severe damage to tissue and blood vessels may cause bleeding within a confined area. This is called a closed wound. Types of closed wounds include **contusions**, **hematomas**, and crush injuries. A contusion is a bruise or collection of blood under the skin or in damaged tissue (Fig. 26-7). The site may swell immediately or 24 to 48 hours later. As blood accumulates in the area, a characteristic black and blue mark, called **ecchymosis**, is seen.

A blood clot that forms at the injury site, generally when large areas of tissue are damaged, is a hematoma. As much as a liter of blood can be lost in the soft tissue when a large bone is fractured. Crush injuries are usually caused by extreme external forces that crush both tissue and bone. Even though the skin remains intact, underlying organs may be severely damaged. Regardless of the type of swelling in a closed wound, the treatment includes the application of ice to reduce and prevent additional swelling to the area (see Procedure 29-2 in Chapter 29).

In an open wound, the skin is broken, and the patient is susceptible to external hemorrhage and wound

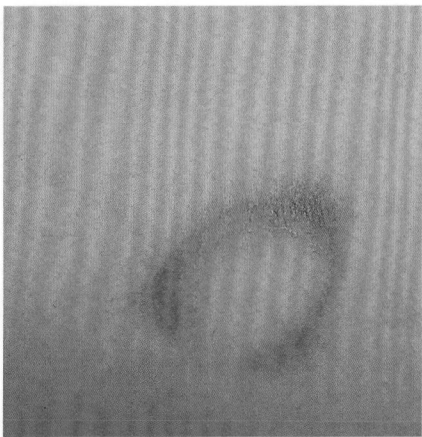

**FIGURE 26-7** • A closed wound; contusion.

- *Abrasion*, the least serious type of open wound, is little more than a scratch on the surface of the skin. All abrasions, regardless of size, are painful because of the nerve endings involved.
- *Laceration* results from snagging or tearing of tissues that leaves a freely bleeding jagged wound. Skin may be partly or completely torn away, and the laceration may contain foreign matter that can lead to infection. A wound caused by a broken bottle or a piece of jagged metal is a laceration.
- *Major arterial laceration* can cause significant bleeding if the sharp or jagged instrument cuts the wall of a blood vessel, especially an artery. Uncontrolled major arterial bleeding can result in shock and death.
- *Puncture wounds* can result from sharp, narrow objects like knives, nails, and ice picks. Punctures also can be caused by high-velocity penetrating objects, such as bullets. A special case of the puncture wound is the *impaled object wound*, in which the instrument that caused the injury remains in the wound. The object can be anything—a stick, arrow, piece of glass, knife, or steel rod—that penetrates any part of the body.
- *Avulsion* is a flap of skin torn loose; it may either remain hanging or tear off altogether. Avulsions usually bleed profusely. Most patients who present with an avulsion work with machinery. Home accidents with lawn mowers and power tools are common causes of avulsion.
- *Amputation* is caused by the ripping, tearing force of industrial and automobile accidents, often great enough to tear away or crush limbs from the body.

contamination. An open wound may be the only surface evidence of a more serious injury, such as a fracture. Open wounds include abrasions, lacerations, major arterial lacerations, puncture wounds, avulsions, amputations, and impalements (Fig. 26-8). When managing any patient with an open wound, follow standard precautions to protect yourself against disease transmission and to protect the patient from further contamination. An open injury to these tissues is a wound. Box 26-2 describes common soft tissue injuries and wounds.

### Management of Bleeding and Soft Tissue Injuries

Management of open soft tissue injuries includes controlling bleeding by applying direct pressure (Procedure 26-5). Sterile gauze should be used to cover the wound if possible to avoid introducing microorganisms into the wound. Management of an amputated body part includes controlling the bleeding but also preserving the severed part for possible reattachment later. To preserve the severed body part:

- Place the severed part in a plastic bag.
- Place this bag in a second plastic bag. This second bag will provide added protection against moisture loss.
- Place both sealed bags in a container of ice or ice water, but do not use dry ice.

An impaled object should not be removed but requires careful immobilization of the patient and the injured area of the body (Fig. 26-9). Because any motion of the impaled object can cause additional damage to the surface wound and underlying tissue, you must stabilize the object without removing it by placing gauze pads around the object and securing with tape. The immobilized impaled object can be carefully removed after transportation to the hospital.

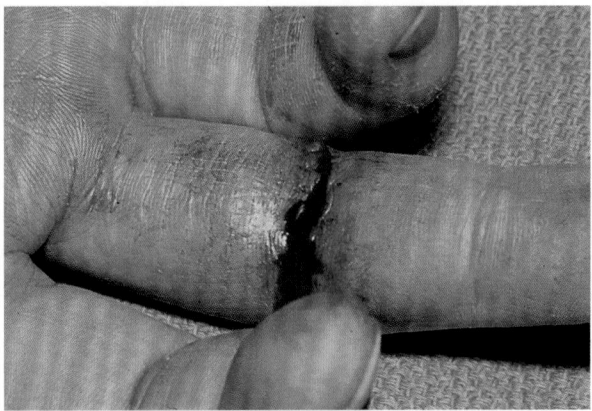

**FIGURE 26-8** • An open wound; laceration.

### CHECKPOINT QUESTION

5. A patient presents into the urgent care clinic with a lacerated thumb. How should Betsy treat an open wound that is bleeding?

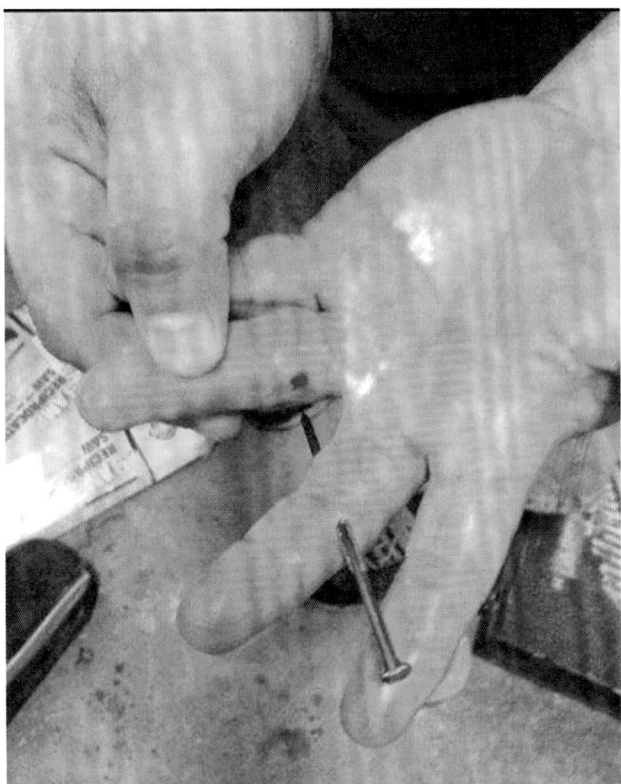

**FIGURE 26-9** • An impaled object.

## Burns

The four major sources of burn injury are thermal, electrical, chemical, and radiation. *Thermal burns*, also called heat burns, result from contact with hot liquids, solids, superheated gases, or flame. *Electrical burns* are caused by contact with low- or high-voltage electricity. Lightning injuries are also considered electrical burns. *Chemical burns* result when wet or dry corrosive substances come into contact with the skin or mucous membranes. The amount of injury with a chemical burn depends on the concentration and quantity of the chemical agent and the length of time it is in contact with the skin. *Radiation burns* are similar to thermal burns and can occur from overexposure to ultraviolet light or from any extreme exposure to radiation.

### Classification of Burn Injuries

Classification of burn injuries depends on the depth or tissue layers involved. Factors that determine the depth of the burn include the agent causing the burn, the temperature, and the length of time exposed. Burns are classified according to the depth of injury: **superficial** (first-degree), **partial-thickness** (second-degree), or **full-thickness** (third-degree) **burns** (Fig. 26-10).

### Calculation of Body Surface Area Burned

The extent of body surface area (BSA) injured by the burn is most commonly estimated by a method called the rule of nines. This method calculates the percentage of

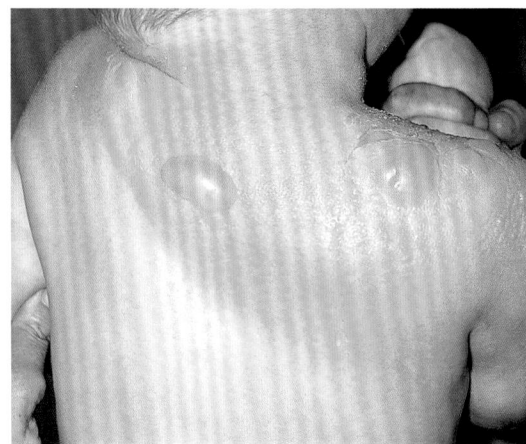

**FIGURE 26-10** • Second-degree sunburn. (From Fleisher GR, Ludwig S, Baskin MN. *Atlas of Pediatric Emergency Medicine.* Philadelphia, PA: Lippincott Williams & Wilkins, 2004.)

total body surface of individual sections of the body. With the rule of nines for an adult, 9% of the skin is estimated to cover the head and another 9% for each arm, including front and back (Fig. 26-11). Twice as much, or 18%, of the total skin area covers the front of the trunk, another 18% covers the back of the trunk, and 18% covers each lower extremity. The area around the genitals is the additional 1% of the BSA. In infants and children, the percentages are the same except that the head is 18% and each lower extremity is 13.5% of the total BSA. Usually, the emergency

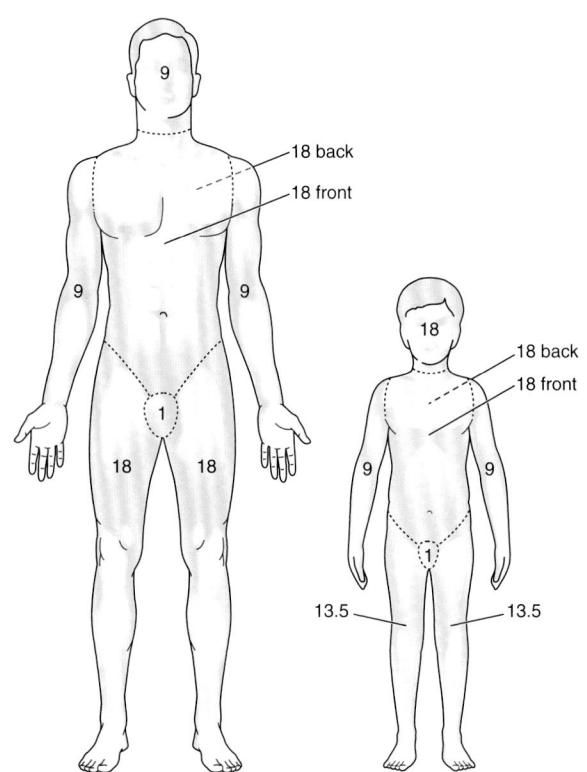

**FIGURE 26-11** • The rule of nines.

room physician determines the percentage of body burned using this rule, not the medical assistant.

## Management of the Burn Victim

Follow these guidelines for managing burn patients in the medical office:

1. Eliminate the source of the burn, if necessary, by washing the area with cool water.
2. Have someone notify the physician, and take the patient immediately to an examination or treatment room.
3. Continually assess the patient's airway, breathing, and circulation. Begin CPR if necessary.
4. Remove all jewelry and clothing as necessary to evaluate the extent of the burn.
5. Administer oxygen as instructed by the physician.
6. Treat the patient for shock and accompanying low blood pressure.
7. Notify the EMS as directed by the physician.
8. Document the time and type of treatments given.
9. Assist with the necessary procedures for transporting the patient to the hospital.

## CHECKPOINT QUESTION

7. What are the four major sources of burn injuries?

## Musculoskeletal Injuries

Injuries to muscles, bones, and joints are some of the most common problems encountered in providing emergency care. The seriousness varies widely, from simple injuries, such as a fractured finger, to major or life-threatening conditions, such as open fracture to the femur, which can cause severe bleeding. Injuries to muscles, tendons, and ligaments occur when a joint or muscle is torn or stretched beyond its normal limits. Fractures and dislocations are usually associated with external forces, although some arise from disease, such as bone degeneration.

## Management of Musculoskeletal Injuries

It is often difficult to distinguish between strains, sprains, fractures, and dislocations in an emergency. Therefore, in most cases, assume the area is fractured and immobilize it accordingly. Proper splinting includes immobilizing the joint above and below the fracture site. Splinting helps prevent further injury to soft tissues, blood vessels, and nerves from sharp bone fragments and relieves pain by stopping motion at the fracture site. As soon as possible, apply ice to the injured area to reduce the swelling that commonly occurs with this type of injury, but never attempt to reduce, or put back into place, a dislocated area. For injuries to the upper extremities, an arm sling may be ordered (Procedure 29-1 in Chapter 29 describes how to apply an arm sling).

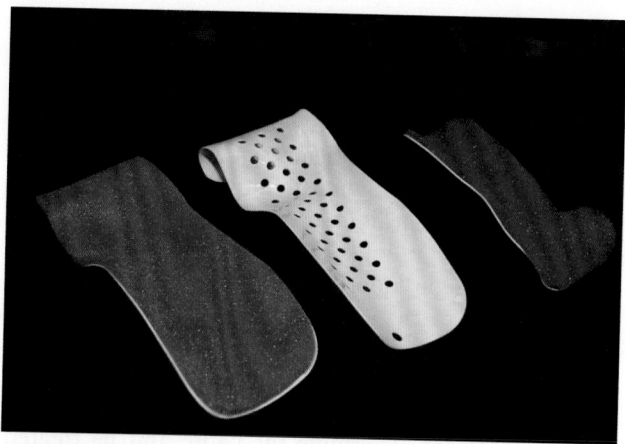

**FIGURE 26-12 •** Types of splints.

## Types of Splints

Any device used to immobilize a sprain, strain, fracture, or dislocated limb is a **splint**. Splinting material may be soft or rigid and can be improvised from almost any object that can provide stability. Commercial types include traction, air, wire ladder, and padded board splints (Fig. 26-12). Regardless of the type of splint, once applied, you must examine the extremity for signs of impaired circulation. To check the circulation of an extremity:

• Observe the skin color and nail beds of the affected extremity. A pale or cyanotic color indicates that the circulation is impeded.
• Locate a pulse in the artery distal to the affected extremity. A weak or absent pulse also indicates that circulation is decreased to the area.
• Watch for increased swelling of the extremity. Although this may not indicate that the circulation is impaired, the swelling itself can reduce circulation.

If the circulation is impaired with the splint in place, it must be removed or loosened immediately to provide for adequate blood flow, or tissue **ischemia** (decrease in oxygen) and **infarction** (death) may occur.

## CHECKPOINT QUESTION

6. The physician asks Betsy to splint the arm of a patient who may have a fractured bone in her lower arm. What is the purpose of applying a splint?

## Cardiovascular Emergencies

According to the American Heart Association, cardiovascular disease is the leading cause of death in adults aged 75 and older and second for adults 45 to 74 years of age. The most common problem is coronary artery disease. Approximately two-thirds of sudden deaths from coronary artery disease occur out of the hospital, and most occur within 2 hours of the onset of symptoms. As coronary artery disease progresses, less and less oxygen can get to the cardiac muscle, which leads to tissue ischemia and eventual infarction of the cardiac tissue. Patients who experience **syncope**, a brief loss of consciousness also known as fainting, should be evaluated to rule out cardiovascular conditions. There are many causes for fainting, but the underlying reason is a sudden decrease in blood flow to the brain. Conditions that may cause syncope include anemia, stress, and dehydration; however, more serious conditions such as a stroke or heart attack may also be the root cause of syncope. A thorough medical examination by a health care provider can determine the cause and be treated accordingly.

The early symptoms of a myocardial infarction (heart attack) include the following:

- Chest pain not relieved by rest
- A complaint of pressure in the chest or upper back
- Nausea or indigestion
- Chest pain that radiates up into the neck and jaw or down one arm
- Anxiety

Early treatment, including basic life support, early defibrillation, and advanced life support can prevent many of these deaths. If CPR is initiated promptly and the patient is rapidly and successfully defibrillated, the patient's survival chances improve. As noted earlier, an AED may be available in your medical office and should be used as soon as possible after it is determined that the victim does not have a pulse. When applied to the patient's chest, the AED will analyze the rhythm and advise the operator to shock, or defibrillate, the patient by simply pressing a button.

## Neurologic Emergencies

A seizure is caused by an abnormal discharge of electrical activity in the brain. During a seizure, erratic muscle movements, strange sensations, and a complete loss of consciousness can occur. A seizure is not a disease but a manifestation or symptom of an underlying disorder. Epilepsy, head injury, and drug toxicity can cause seizures in adults. Children may also have seizures due to an elevated body temperature. A thorough patient history is important when assessing these patients. It should include the following:

- Information about previous seizure disorders
- Frequency of seizures if recurrent
- Prescribed medications
- Any history of head trauma
- Alcohol or drug abuse
- Recent fever
- Stiff neck (as seen in meningitis)
- A history of heart disease, diabetes, or stroke

In managing a patient having a seizure, you must give priority to assessing the patient's responsiveness,

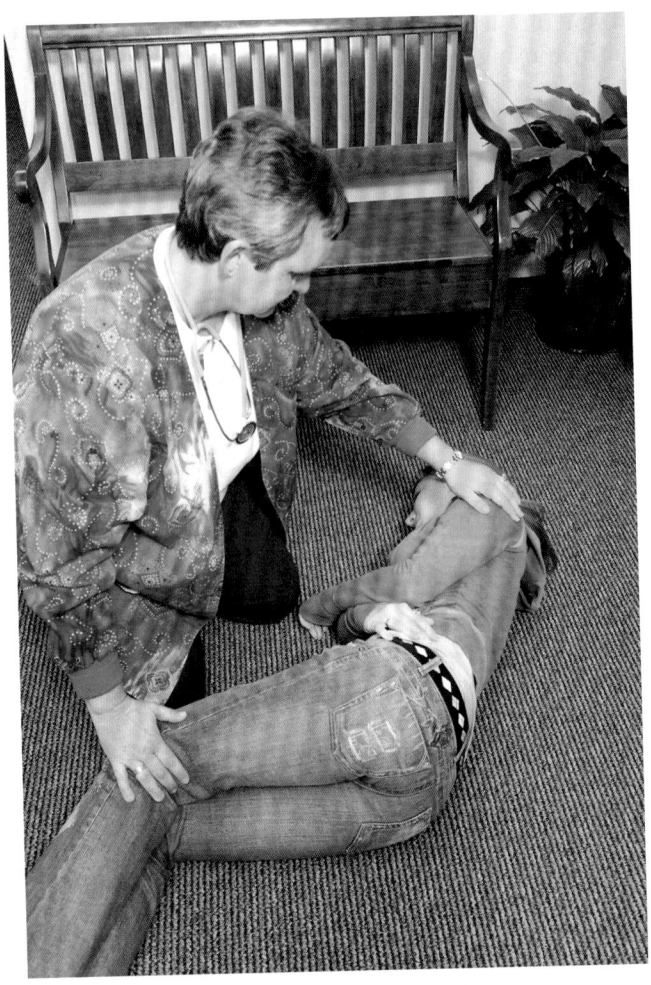

**FIGURE 26-13** • Patient in recovery position.

airway, breathing, and circulation. In certain types of seizures, the patient loses consciousness and, therefore, cannot protect the airway. During the seizure, the muscles of the body, including those of the face, will contract tightly. If you attempt to force an object between the teeth to prevent the patient from biting the tongue, the result will most likely be injury to you or the patient. Frequently, a patient may vomit during the seizure and lose bowel or bladder control. Particular attention and care are necessary to clear and maintain the airway without causing injury to yourself or the patient. Assisting the patient into the recovery position (on one side) will help secretions such as blood or vomit drain from the mouth (Fig. 26-13). Secretions may be removed from the mouth using a suction machine if available. It is helpful to also note how long the seizure lasted including the time between seizures if the patient experiences multiple seizures. Be sure to report this information to the physician and the emergency services personnel.

The most important thing you can do for a patient during a seizure is protect the patient from injury. If the patient lost consciousness and fell at the beginning of the seizure, care will be necessary to protect the neck and cervical spine until immobilization can occur.

## CHECKPOINT QUESTION

8. What are some causes of seizure activity in a patient?

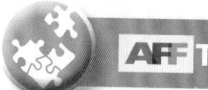 **TRIAGE**

While working in a busy medical urgent care center, the following three patients arrive at the same time:

A. A 4-year-old child arrives, carried in by his mother who states that he has had vomiting and diarrhea for approximately 2 days but has recently become "sleepy and hard to arouse."

B. A 36-year-old female presents in complaining of pain in her hand after spilling a cup of hot coffee on it. You notice that the palm of her left hand is red and has several small blisters on it.

C. A 40-year-old man had cut his thumb while using a box cutter at work. He has a towel on it and notes that the bleeding has "stopped," but he still would like to have it evaluated by the physician.

**How do you sort these patients? Who do you see first? Second? Third?**

Anytime there is change in anyone's mental status, it should be treated as a priority. See patient A first since he may be dehydrated and headed for hypovolemic shock. Patient B should be seen next. She has a first- and second-degree burn, and although these may be painful, she is not in immediate danger of shock. Patient C should be seen last. The patient is capable of holding pressure to the site to control bleeding, but he may need sutures to close the wound as well as a tetanus injection.

## Allergic and Anaphylactic Reactions

A severe allergic reaction called anaphylaxis causes most emergency department visits related to allergies. An allergic reaction is a generalized reaction that can occur within minutes to hours after the body has been exposed to a substance recognized by the immune system as foreign and to which it is oversensitive. The systemic signs and symptoms of anaphylaxis are more severe compared to a simple allergic reaction, but repeated exposure to a substance that produces allergic reactions may ultimately lead to an anaphylactic reaction and should be avoided.

### Common Allergens

An **allergen** is a substance that gives rise to hypersensitivity or allergy. The allergen may be a drug, insect venom, food, or pollen and may be injected, ingested, inhaled, or absorbed through the skin or mucous membranes. A person may have symptoms within seconds after exposure to an allergen, or the reaction may be delayed for several hours. You must ask every patient about allergies at every visit and note these on the front of the patient's chart and the medication record. Check the patient's medical record and ask about allergies *before* administering any medications in the office; this is essential to prevent allergic reactions or anaphylaxis in patients with known hypersensitivity.

Although the exact incidence of anaphylactic reactions is difficult to pinpoint, it is estimated that 1% to 2% of patients who receive penicillin in the United States have some form of allergy to the drug and that one in 50,000 injections of penicillin results in death from anaphylaxis. However, you must be alert to the signs and symptoms of allergic reactions after administering any medication, not just penicillin. Patients with moderate to severe allergy symptoms often receive frequent injections of specific allergens to reduce the symptoms associated with allergies. These patients should be monitored closely for anaphylaxis, and they should not be permitted to leave the office for a prescribed amount of time, often 20 to 30 minutes after the injection. When documenting that an injection was given, you should also note the condition of the patient upon discharge.

### Signs and Symptoms

The initial signs and symptoms of an allergic reaction may include severe itching, a feeling of warmth, tightness in the throat or chest, or a rash. The primary rule for any exposure is that the sooner the symptoms occur after the exposure, the more severe the reaction is likely to be. Be observant and ready to treat any patient who has these symptoms. Airway obstruction, cardiovascular collapse, and shock can occur if the situation worsens. Because the primary cause of death in an anaphylactic reaction is swelling of the tissues in the airway causing airway obstruction, observe the patient closely for signs of airway involvement, including wheezing, shortness of breath, and coughing. Choking or tightness in the neck and throat may signal this danger. Tachycardia, hypotension, pale skin, dryness of the mouth, diaphoresis (profuse sweating), and other signs of shock may also be present.

### Management of Allergic and Anaphylactic Reactions

The patient having a severe allergic reaction will often be anxious. Some allergic reactions are mild, without respiratory problems or signs of shock. These simple reactions can be managed by administering oxygen or medications such as antihistamines to relieve symptoms as directed by the physician. If respiratory involvement occurs without signs of shock, the physician may order that epinephrine (1:1,000) be given subcutaneously. The patient with a severe anaphylactic reaction who is in shock needs more aggressive therapy, including additional medications, an IV line, and monitoring of the cardiac rhythm. The primary goal when treating a patient having an anaphylactic reaction is restoring respiratory and circulatory function. The following steps are required for managing allergic reactions, including anaphylaxis:

- Do not leave the patient, but have another staff member request that the physician immediately evaluate the patient and bring the emergency kit or cart, including oxygen.
- Assist the patient to a supine position.
- Assess the patient's respiratory and circulatory status by obtaining the blood pressure, pulse, and respiratory rates.
- Observe the skin color and warmth.
- If the patient complains of being cold or is shivering, cover him or her with a blanket.
- Upon the direction of the physician, start an IV line (see Chapter 24) and administer oxygen.
- As ordered by the physician, administer medications such as epinephrine as ordered.
- Document vital signs and any medications and treatments given, noting the time each set of vital signs is taken or medications are administered.
- Communicate relevant information to the EMS personnel, including copies of the progress notes or medication record as needed.

### ✎ CHECKPOINT QUESTION

9. What is the primary cause of death in anaphylaxis?

## Poisoning

The likelihood that one will be exposed to toxins in the home or workplace is increasing. In addition to over-the-counter and prescription medications often found in the home, household chemicals are an additional hazard and are often designed to have a pleasant odor and color. Industrial chemicals offer another possibility of poisoning. These chemicals may affect a single victim or many victims in the event of a hazardous materials incident. Most toxic exposures occur in the home and almost 50% occur in children aged 1 to 3 years (Fig. 26-14). Although about 90% of reported poisonings are accidental, intentional exposures usually affect adolescents and adults, and they tend to have a higher death rate. Fortunately, deaths from drug overdoses and poisoning are rare, but you must know how to respond if a patient comes to the office or telephones with a possible poisoning.

### Poison Control Center

The American Association of Poison Control Centers (AAPCC) has established standards and regional poison control centers throughout the country. These centers

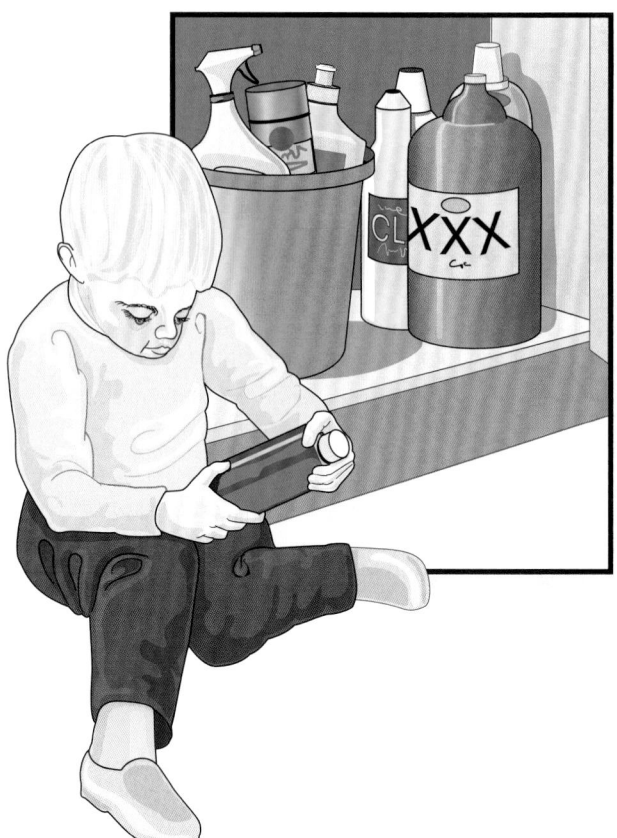

**FIGURE 26-14 •** Advise adults to store cleaning products out of the reach of small children.

are staffed by physicians, nurses, and pharmacists. When information about a poisoning or drug overdose is not readily available, the poison control center is a valuable resource, and the phone number should be posted near all phones in the medical office. The professionals at the poison control center can usually evaluate a potential or known toxic exposure, instruct the caller in the use of syrup of ipecac to induce vomiting if indicated, and check on the patient's progress by follow-up telephone calls.

### Management of Poisoning Emergencies

Exactly how and when a poison control center is consulted should be part of the medical office's protocol. Few toxic substances have specific antidotes, so the management of the poisoning is aimed at treating the signs and symptoms and assessing the involved organ systems. The patient may go to the medical office after the poisoning, or more commonly, the patient or caregiver telephones the office requesting information. In either situation, you must obtain the following information *before* making the call to poison control:

- The nature of the poisoning (ingested, inhaled, skin exposure)
- The age and weight of the victim
- The name of the substance

- An estimate of the amount of poison
- When the exposure occurred
- The patient's present signs and symptoms

Once the poison control center has been notified and instructions given, you must be prepared to treat the patient as directed and notify the EMS to transport the patient to the hospital. Never give a patient syrup of ipecac or otherwise induce vomiting unless directed to do so by the professionals at the poison control center.

## CHECKPOINT QUESTION

10. Why is it important to have the phone number of the poison control center near the telephone in the medical office?

## Heat- and Cold-Related Emergencies

Environmental temperature is one of the many variables to which the body normally adjusts, maintaining equilibrium. Human beings depend on the ability to control core body temperature within a range of several degrees. Measured rectally, this core temperature is 37.6°C (99.6°F). The peripheral temperature is usually lower (98.6°F orally). Several conditions can disrupt the normal heat-regulating mechanisms of the body. These are divided into two main categories: **hyperthermia** and **hypothermia**.

### Hyperthermia

Hyperthermia is the general condition of excessive body heat. Correct management depends on assessment of the underlying cause. The first type of hyperthermia and the least severe includes **heat cramps**, which is muscle cramping that follows a period of heavy exertion and profuse sweating in a hot environment. While sweat is primarily water, it also contains the electrolyte sodium, which is needed for muscle function. Heavy sweating, which is a normal compensatory mechanism to cool the body, will result in a sodium deficit, which compromises muscle function and produces muscle cramps. A patient with heat cramps often complains of cramping in the calves of the legs and in the abdomen. Cramping may also occur in the hands, arms, and feet. Mental status and blood pressure usually remain normal, although an increased pulse rate is common.

Heat cramps signal the need for cooling and rest. In uncomplicated cases, the patient is encouraged to take fluids by mouth, but nausea may make IV infusion necessary. If the patient is able to take fluids by mouth, give a commercial electrolyte solution, or salt can be added to water or fruit juice at 1 teaspoon per pint. Cramps can sometimes be prevented entirely with similar oral intake before physical exertion and every 20 minutes during exercise. Salt tablets are not recommended because they may cause nausea.

**Heat exhaustion** results most often from physical exertion in a hot environment without adequate fluid replacement and may follow heat cramps that are not treated. Body temperature usually remains normal or slightly above normal. Patients have central nervous system symptoms such as headache, fatigue, dizziness, or syncope (fainting). Although the skin is typically moist and the pulse rate is high, skin color, blood pressure, and respiratory rate vary with the degree to which the body is able to hold off the distress. Patients in late stages of heat exhaustion have pale skin, low blood pressure, and rapid respiration. Treatment includes having the patient lie down in a cool room, removing clothing, and spraying the patient a cool water spray. The patient should also be encouraged to drink cool fluids including water or a commercial electrolyte solution as with heat cramps.

**Heat stroke** is a true emergency and is the most serious of the heat-related emergencies. The body is no longer able to compensate for the rapid rise in body temperature (past 105°F), and the patient may undergo brain damage or death. Heat stroke victims can deteriorate quickly to coma, and many patients have seizures. The skin is classically hot, flushed, and dry. Vital signs are elevated initially but may drop, with ensuing cardiopulmonary arrest. Heat stroke demands rapid cooling of the body by immersing the patient in cold water up to the chin or wrapping the body in sheets or towels that have been soaked in cold water. This patient will need to be transported to the hospital immediately and you may be required to activate the EMS and communicate appropriately and clearly.

For any heat-related emergency, you should alert the physician and follow office policy for the management of hyperthermia including these basic steps:

- Move the patient to a cool area.
- Remove clothing that may be holding in the heat.
- Place cool, wet clothes or a wet sheet on the core surface areas of the body where the ability to cool the central blood is the greatest: the scalp, neck, axilla, and groin.
- Administer oxygen as directed by the physician and apply a cardiac monitor.
- Notify the EMS for transportation to the hospital as directed by the physician.

### Hypothermia

The body's core temperature can drop several degrees without loss of normal body function. The body usually tolerates a 3°F to 4°F drop in temperature without symptoms; hypothermia is an abnormally low body temperature, below 35°C (95°F). Internal metabolic factors and significant heat loss to the external environment can lead to hypothermia. Very cold air and immersion in cold water can cause a rapid drop in core temperature. The following are the signs and symptoms of hypothermia:

- Cool, pale skin
- Lethargy and mental confusion
- Shallow, slow respirations
- Slow, faint pulse rate

Basic management of hypothermia includes handling the patient gently, removing wet clothing, and covering the patient to prevent further cooling. If there is evidence of rewarming (skin warm, respirations approaching normal, no shivering) and the patient is alert and able to swallow, give warm fluids by mouth. Avoid drinks that constrict peripheral blood vessels, such as those that contain caffeine (coffee and tea). Fluids that cause dilation of the blood vessels, such as alcohol, should also be avoided. Warm beverages with sugar, such as hot chocolate, can be given to begin replacement of the fuel that the body needs to restore normal heat production. No fluids should be given by mouth to patients who have a diminished or changing level of consciousness.

### Frostbite

Windy subfreezing weather creates the greatest risk for **frostbite**. Small body parts with a high ratio of surface area to tissue mass (fingers, toes, ears, and nose) are most vulnerable to frostbite, although larger areas of the extremities are also vulnerable during profound cooling. Exposure to cold can cause tissues to freeze, and the frozen cells will die.

The type and duration of contact are the two most important factors in determining the extent of frostbite injury. Touching cold fabric, for example, is not nearly as dangerous as coming into direct contact with cold metal, particularly if the skin is wet or even damp. The combination of wind and cold is dangerous. *Superficial frostbite* appears as firm and waxy gray or yellow skin in an area that loses sensation after hurting or tingling. Prolonged exposure can lead to blistering and eventually *deep frostbite*, which most often affects the hands and feet. No warning symptoms appear after the initial loss of feeling. Freezing progresses painlessly once the nerve endings are numb. Skin becomes inelastic and the entire area feels hard to the touch. Deep frostbite results in tissue death, and the affected tissue must be removed surgically or amputated.

Superficial frostbite can be managed by warming the affected part with another body surface, for example, placing an ungloved hand over the nose or ears. Management for more than superficial frostbite is rapid rewarming after any system-wide hypothermia has been corrected. Deep frostbite should be managed only in the hospital to prevent further damage to the tissue. You may be asked to do the following as directed by the physician:

- Immerse the frozen tissue in lukewarm water (41°C, 105°F) until the area becomes pliable and the color and sensation return.
- Do not apply dry heat.
- Do not massage the area; massage may cause further tissue damage.
- Avoid breaking any blisters that may form.
- Upon the direction of the physician, notify the EMS for transportation to a hospital.

If rewarming is not attempted, bandage the frostbitten part with dry sterile dressings. Frostbitten tissue is similar to burned tissue in that it is vulnerable to infection. Take care to keep the affected part as clean as possible. All frostbite victims should be assessed for hypothermia. Clothing offers good protection against weather only if it is loose enough to avoid restricting circulation. Tight gloves, cuffs, boots, and straps add to the danger.

### CHECKPOINT QUESTION

11. How would Betsy explain the difference between heat exhaustion and heat stroke to a student she is working with at the urgent care today?

## Behavioral and Psychiatric Emergencies

Psychological distress may be mild, moderate, or severe. The degree of intensity determines the type and amount of intervention necessary. A psychiatric emergency is different from an emotional crisis, and you must know how to differentiate between the two. A psychiatric emergency is any situation in which the patient's moods, thoughts, or actions are so disordered or disturbed that harm or death may result for the patient or others if no intervention occurs. An emotional crisis, on the other hand, is a situation with much less intensity. While it may be distressing to the patient, in most cases, it is not likely to end in danger, harm, or death without immediate intervention. However, if neglected entirely, an emotional crisis may escalate to a full psychiatric emergency.

A true behavioral emergency, like a medical emergency, carries a serious threat. Urgent behavioral situations usually require some form of professional psychological evaluation and intervention and require transportation to the hospital. The following guidelines are useful for handling a psychiatric emergency:

- Notify the physician and EMS as directed.
- Offer reassurance and general support to the patient and any caregivers or family members who may be present.
- Accurately document information including vital signs and the patient's behavior.

## ROLE-PLAYING ACTIVITY

With four other students, role-play the following situation as if you are working in the urgent care with Betsy Reynolds, the medical assistant described in the case study at the beginning of this chapter. Take turns being the medical assistant and the patients:

Four patients come into the urgent care at the same time.

Patient #1: A 36-year-old male who is complaining of severe indigestion. His color is pink, but he is holding his chest and says he is having "trouble" breathing.

Patient #2: A 7-year-old boy is with his mother who says he was stung by a bee in the bottom of his left foot earlier this afternoon, but the area has become more swollen and he is complaining of severe pain. He is seated in a chair in the waiting area playing a handheld video game.

Patient #3: An elderly man is holding a towel to his forehead and says he received a cut while working in his garage. His color is pale and he is shaking but walked in with his wife who drove him to the clinic.

Patient #4: A 22-year-old college student complains of a sore throat and fever since yesterday that has gotten "worse" today. His skin is flushed and hot.

Which of these patients should be taken to an exam room first in your opinion? How would you respond if the wife of the elderly man fainted in the waiting room? Your instructor will give you additional information about this activity!

## SPANISH TERMINOLOGY

*español*

**¿Le duele algo?**
Are you in pain?

**¿Tiene dificultad para respirar?**
Are you having any problem breathing?

**¿Cuándo ocurrió el accidente?**
When did the accident happen?

**Calmese, por favor. La ambulancia está de camino.**
Calm down, please. The ambulance is on the way.

**¡Por favor llame al 911 y trae el desfibrilador!**
Please call 911 and bring the AED!

**¡Por favor llame inmediatamente al Centro de Envenenamiento!**
Please call Poison Control immediately!

**¡Todo va a estar bien!, ya avisamos a su familia, tranquilícese.**
Everything will be all right! We already notified your family, relax!

**¡Tráiganme la Epinefrina!**
Bring me the EpiPen!

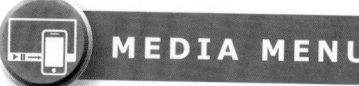

## MEDIA MENU

**Student Resources** on **thePoint®**

• **CMA/RMA Certification Exam Review**

• *Video:* **Administering Oxygen (Procedure 26–1)**

**Internet Resources**
**American Association of Poison Control Centers**
http://www.aapcc.org

**American Heart Association**
http://www.heart.org/HEARTORG/

**American Red Cross**
http://www.redcross.org

**Safety and Health Institute**
http://www.hsi.com

**National Safety Council**
http://www.nsc.org/pages/home.aspx

**Occupational Health and Safety Administration**
http://www.osha.gov

# EMR Activity

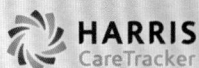

Harris CareTracker is a Web-based electronic medical record (EMR) application that you will use for the EMR activities included in this section at the end of each chapter. This application is actually used in physician offices but is provided to you through the publisher, Wolters Kluwer Health, to give you hands-on practice working with EMRs. Your instructor will have more information about accessing your username, log-in, and Quickstart guide.

Prerequisite Activities in Harris CareTracker

- *The Getting Started and Quickstart documents and EMR Activities Step-by-Step Instructions are available at* http://thePoint.lww.com/KronenbergerComp5e.
- *Note: You must first enter the patients into the EMR as new patients before completing the following EMR activity as given in the EMR Step-by-Step Instructions.*

Activity Details

Enter the following encounter information into the *Medical Record* application of the EMR for the following patient using today's date:

1. Patient: Linda Bankston came to the urgent care clinic today for a laceration on her left thumb. After controlling the bleeding and applying a sterile gauze pad, you took her vital signs (temperature 98.6 degrees Fahrenheit orally, pulse 110 and regular, respirations 24, and blood pressure 124/88 right arm sitting). Her skin is pink, warm, and dry.

## Chapter Summary

Dealing with a medical emergency will require you to:

- Communicate clearly and calmly.
- Recognize the need for immediate medical intervention.
- Perform emergency procedures immediately and competently.
- Provide first aid and life support measures that can mean the difference between life and death.
- Reassure the patient and family members.
- Work with the physician and other health care team members efficiently and with confidence.

## Warm-Ups for Critical Thinking

1. When an emergency occurs, the patient's family members may become anxious and emotionally distraught. How can you help to calm an anxious family member?
2. Investigate the Good Samaritan law in your state. Prepare a poster describing the laws in your state.
3. While obtaining a chief complaint, your patient complains of shortness of breath. His respiratory rate is 36, and his skin is cool and clammy. What should be your next steps? Why?
4. The mother of a 15-year-old boy calls the office and tells you that her son has just been stung by a bee. She says he has never been stung before, and she is concerned about the amount of swelling around the site of the sting on his arm. However, you hear him coughing in the background. Are there any questions that you might want to ask the mother? How would you handle this call?
5. On a hot summer day, the mail carrier comes into your office to deliver the mail and collapses on the floor in the reception area. You notice that his skin is flushed and hot to touch. Should you move this person to an exam room? What could be the possible cause for his symptoms? How would you treat this patient?

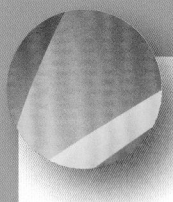

## PSY PROCEDURE 26-1

## Administer Oxygen

**Purpose:** Administer oxygen according to the physician's order

**Equipment:** Oxygen tank with regulator and oxygen delivery system (nasal cannula, mask)

| STEPS | REASONS |
|---|---|
| 1. Wash your hands. | Handwashing aids infection control. |
| 2. Check the physician order for the amount of oxygen and the delivery method (nasal cannula, mask). | |
| 3. Assemble the equipment. | |
| 4. Greet and identify the patient. Explain the procedure. | Identifying the patient prevents errors. Explaining the procedure helps ease anxiety and may improve compliance. |
| 5. **AFF** Explain how to respond to a patient who has dementia. | Solicit assistance from caregiver or other staff member to help during the procedure. Give simple directions to the patient about what he/she should do. Speak clearly, not loudly. |
| 6. Connect the distal end of the tubing on the oxygen delivery method (nasal cannula or mask) to the adapter on the regulator, which is connected to the oxygen tank. | The oxygen tank must have a regulator attached that allows the nasal cannula or mask tubing to be connected. The tubing cannot be connected with a regulator on the oxygen tank. |

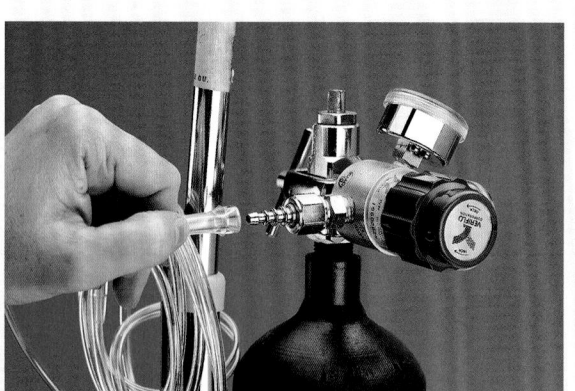

**Step 6.** Connect the distal end of the oxygen tubing to the regulator on the oxygen tank.

## PROCEDURE 26-1 (continued)

| STEPS | REASONS |
|---|---|
| 7. Place the oxygen delivery system (nasal cannula or mask) on the patient. | |

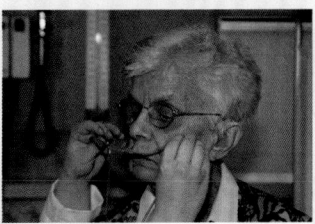

**A**

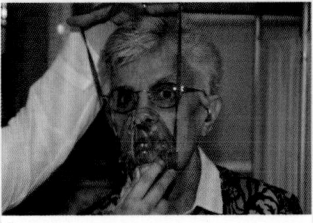

**B**

**Step 7.** Step 7A: Place the nasal cannula into the patient's nares. Step 7B: Secure the mask over the nose and mouth.

8. Turn the regulator dial to the appropriate number of liters per minute as ordered by the physician.

Oxygen is considered a medication and must be ordered by a physician.

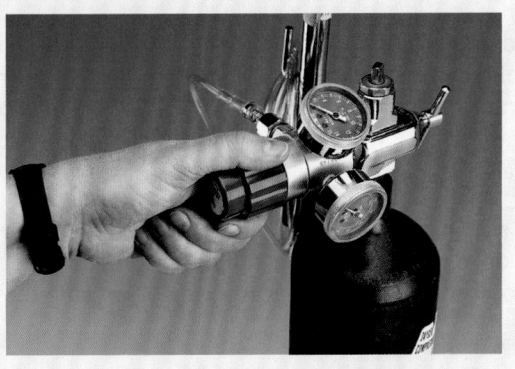

**Step 8.** Turn on the oxygen by rotating the dial on the oxygen tank regulator.

9. **AFF** Log into the electronic medical record (EMR) using your username and secure password OR obtain the paper medical record from a secure location and assure it is kept away from public access.

10. Record the procedure in the patient's medical record.

Procedures are considered not to have been done if they are not recorded.

11. When finished, log out of the EMR and/or replace the medical record in an appropriate and secure location to protect patient privacy.

The integrity of the medical record must be maintained at all times.

---

Charting Example:
*12/23/2016 2:15 PM Oxygen applied per nasal cannula at 4 L/min as ordered* _____
*B. Reynolds, CMA.*

---

Note: *The medical assistant may sign his or her name in the patient record using only the "CMA" credential if the office has a signature log denoting the entire credential as "CMA (AAMA)."*

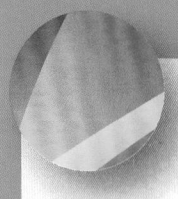

**PSY** PROCEDURE 26-2

## Perform CPR (Adult)

**PSY** Produce up-to-date documentation of provider/professional level CPR.

**Purpose:** Perform rescue breathing and chest compressions (cardiopulmonary resuscitation) on an adult

**Equipment:** CPR mannequin for practice, mouth-to-mask barrier device, and gloves

*Note:* Demonstration of competency depends upon the individual student and the most current structured educational protocol by certified trainers for the American Heart Association, American Red Cross, or the National Safety Council.

| STEPS | REASONS |
|---|---|
| 1. Determine unresponsiveness by shaking the patient and shouting "Are you okay?" Instruct another staff member to get the physician, emergency cart/supplies, and AED. If gloves are easily accessible, put clean gloves on both hands. Otherwise, put them on when the emergency medical cart arrives. | Establishing unresponsiveness prevents rescue measures being taken for a patient who does not need them. High-quality CPR and early defibrillation will improve survival from sudden cardiac arrest. |
| 2. If the patient does not respond, assess for cardiac function by feeling for a pulse using the carotid artery on the side of the patient's neck. | The most current guidelines require rescuers to check for a pulse *before* checking the airway or breathing. |
| 3. If no pulse is present, follow the protocol for chest compressions according to the standards of the training provided by the American Heart Association, the American Red Cross, or the National Safety Council. | Instead of using the acronym "ABC," use "CAB" (circulation, airway, breathing). The physician will probably want EMS notified at this point since quick access to advanced care will increase the patient's chance for survival. |
| 4. After 30 compressions, check for airway patency and respiratory effort using the head tilt–chin lift maneuver with the patient in a supine position. | If you suspect a neck injury, use the jaw thrust maneuver to open the airway after rolling the patient carefully to his/her back without twisting or moving the neck. |
| 5. After opening the airway, begin rescue breathing by placing a mask over the patient's mouth and nose and giving two slow breaths, causing the chest to rise without overfilling the lungs. | Giving slow breaths will provide oxygen without overfilling the lungs. Overfilling the lungs with air may cause gastric distention and vomiting. |
| 6. Continue chest compressions and rescue breathing at a ratio of 30:1 until relieved by another health care provider or EMS arrives. | If an AED is available, follow the recommended guidelines for using this device. |

| STEPS | REASONS |
|---|---|
| 7. Utilize the recovery position if the patient regains consciousness or a pulse and adequate breathing. | The recovery position includes the patient lying on his/her side, which facilitates respirations and prevents aspiration of emesis in the event that the patient vomits. |

*Note:* In the clinical situation, respiratory barrier devices and gloves will be available to protect you from the patient's oral secretions and should be used appropriately.

All health care professionals should receive training for proficiency in CPR in an approved program. The procedure described here is not intended to substitute for proficiency training with a mannequin and a structured protocol.

---

Charting Example:

*10/14/ 2016 10:30 AM Pt c/o chest pain. Skin diaphoretic, color pale. Pulse 125 and regular, BP 88/54 (L). Collapsed in exam room, Dr. Barton notified. Pulse and respirations absent, CPR started. EMS notified per Dr. Barton _____ S. Pencil, CMA*

---

*10/14/2016 10:40 AM CPR continued per EMS, pt. unresponsive. Transported to General Hospital. Patient's wife, Helen, notified of transport _____ S. Pencil, CMA*

---

Note: *The medical assistant may sign his or her name in the patient record using only the "CMA" credential if the office has a signature log denoting the entire credential as "CMA (AAMA)."*

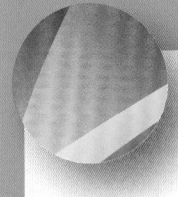

**PSY** PROCEDURE 26-3

## Use an AED (Adult)

**Purpose:** Correctly apply and use an AED on an adult patient

**Equipment:** Practice AED, chest pads with connection cables appropriate for the AED machine, scissors, dry gauze pads, gloves, and mannequin

| STEPS | REASONS |
|---|---|
| 1. Determine unresponsiveness by shaking the patient and shouting, "Are you okay?" | Establishing unresponsiveness prevents rescue measures being taken for a patient who does not need them. |
| 2. Have another staff member get the physician, medical emergency cart or bag, and AED. Follow the procedure for CPR procedures according the most recent guidelines (see Procedure 26-2). | High-quality CPR and early defibrillation will improve survival from sudden cardiac arrest. |
| 3. When the AED is available, continue CPR while a second rescuer removes the patient's shirt and prepares the chest for the AED electrodes. This second rescuer will be in control of operating the AED. | If the patient's skin is wet, use a dry towel or cloth to dry the chest. If the patient is wearing a transdermal medication patch on the chest, remove the patch and wipe any excess medication off of the chest. If there is excessive hair on the patient's chest, use a disposable razor to remove any hair over where the chest electrode pads will be placed. |
| 4. After removing the sticky paper backing on the AED electrode pads, apply the chest electrodes onto the patient's chest, one on the upper right chest and the other on the lower left chest. | Placing the electrodes on the chest as directed will allow the best conduction of electricity to the heart muscle. |

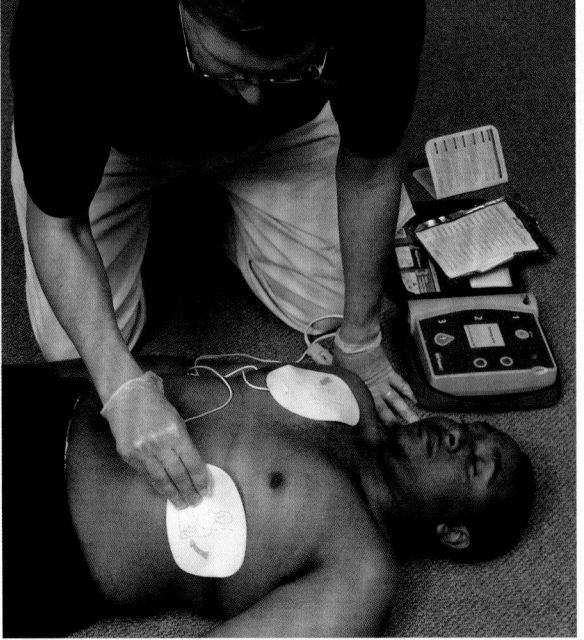

**Step 4.** Place the AED pads on the upper right chest and the lower right chest.

## PROCEDURE 26-3 (continued)

| STEPS | REASONS |
|---|---|
| **5.** Once the electrodes are in place, connect the wire from the electrodes to the AED unit and turn the AED on. | Although AED machines vary, most ask you to place the electrodes on the patient before connecting the wires to the AED machine. |

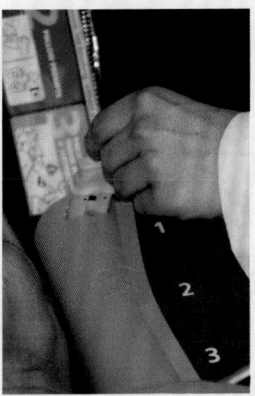

**Step 5.** Connect the AED electrode wires to the AED machine.

**6.** Follow the instructions given by the AED as the heart rhythm is being analyzed. Do not touch the patient during the analysis, including doing CPR. If no shock is necessary, the AED will indicate this and instruct you to resume CPR.

The AED will verbally tell you what to do. Listen to all instructions and follow the directions given by the machine.

**7.** If the AED instructs you that an electrical shock is necessary, the second rescuer will operate the machine, making sure that no person is touching the patient or the exam table (if the patient is on a table) before pressing the appropriate button on the AED to deliver the electrical shock.

If another person is touching the patient or the exam table when an electrical shock is delivered, the shock will be given to that person as well as the patient.

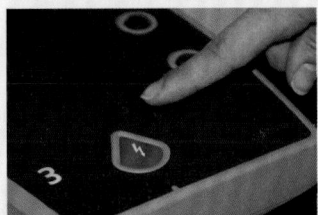

**Step 7.** The second rescuer delivers the electrical shock if indicated.

**8.** After delivering the shock, the AED will again analyze the patient's heart rhythm. The patient must not be touched during this process.

If a shock is not advised and CPR is resumed, the AED will ask you to stop CPR periodically to reanalyze the rhythm. Do not touch the patient while the AED is analyzing the heart rhythm.

*(continues on page 672)*

## PROCEDURE 26-3 (continued)

| STEPS | REASONS |
|---|---|
| 9. Continue to follow the instructions given by the AED, which will include either reshocking the patient or resuming CPR. | Continue this pattern until EMS arrives and takes over the emergency procedures. |

*Note:* All health care professionals should take an approved training course in CPR and use of an AED. This procedure is not intended to substitute for proficiency training with a mannequin in a structured educational protocol.

---

Charting Example:
*11/15/2016 3:15 PM Pt. became unresponsive while waiting in reception area; no pulse or respiratory effort. Dr. Barton notified, CPR started* _____ *J. Crete, CMA*

---

*11/15/2016 3:18 PM AED applied, 2 electrical shocks delivered, pulse returned, no respiratory effort. Rescue breathing resumed* _____ *J. Crete, CMA*

---

*11/15/2016 3:25 PM EMS here. Pt. transported to General Hospital* _____ *J. Crete, CMA*

---

Note: *The medical assistant may sign his or her name in the patient record using only the "CMA" credential if the office has a signature log denoting the entire credential as "CMA (AAMA)."*

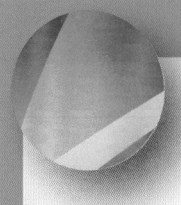

## **PSY** PROCEDURE 26-4

# Manage a Foreign Body Airway Obstruction (Adult)

**Purpose:** Respond appropriately to an adult (conscious and unconscious) with a foreign body airway obstruction

**Equipment:** Mouth to mask with barrier device, gloves, and CPR mannequin

| STEPS | REASONS |
|---|---|
| 1. For a conscious patient, ask, "Are you choking?" If the patient can speak or cough, the obstruction is not complete. Observe the patient for increased distress and assist as needed, but do not perform abdominal thrusts. | The patient who is coughing or speaking can breathe and may be able to remove the obstruction without assistance. Performing abdominal thrusts on a patient who is not in need of assistance may cause injury. |
| 2. If the patient cannot speak or cough and is displaying the universal sign of distress (grasping the throat with both hands), follow these steps to perform abdominal thrusts and have a coworker notify the physician:<br>**A.** Stand behind the patient and wrap your arms around his or her waist.<br>**B.** Make a fist with your nondominant hand, with the thumb side against the patient's abdomen between the navel and the xiphoid process. | Excess pressure on the xiphoid process may cause it to break off. Applying pressure at or below the navel may not produce enough force on the diaphragm to expel the foreign object. |
| 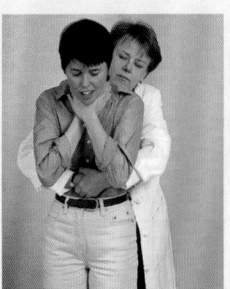<br>**C.** Grasp your fist with your dominant hand and give quick upward thrusts. Completely relax your arms between each thrust and make each thrust forceful enough to dislodge the obstruction in the airway. | **Step 2B.** Make a fist, with the thumb side against the abdomen. |
| 3. Repeat the thrusts until the object is expelled and the patient can breathe or the patient becomes unconscious. | Several thrusts may be necessary to expel the object. |
| 4. If the patient is unconscious OR becomes unconscious, perform a tongue–jaw lift followed by a finger sweep to remove the object if possible. | Before performing the tongue–jaw lift and finger sweep, apply clean examination gloves to avoid contact with the patient's oral secretions. |
| 5. Open the airway and try to give the patient two rescue breaths. | Repositioning the patient's head ensures that the airway obstruction is not caused by improper head position. |

*(continues on page 674)*

## PROCEDURE 26-4 (continued)

| STEPS | REASONS |
|---|---|
| **6.** If rescue breaths are obstructed, begin abdominal thrusts:<br>   **A.** Straddle the patient's hips.<br>   **B.** Place the palm of one hand between the patient's navel and the xiphoid process.<br>   **C.** Lace your fingers with the other hand against the back of the properly positioned hand. | |
| **7.** Give five abdominal thrusts, and then repeat the tongue–jaw lift and finger sweep maneuver. Attempt to give rescue breaths. If rescue breaths adequately ventilate the patient, continue rescue breaths until the patient resumes breathing or EMS arrives, as indicated by the physician. While you are performing rescue breathing, periodically check for a carotid pulse and be prepared to start chest compressions if necessary. | A patient with a foreign object may not be able to breathe; however, cardiac function may continue. |
| **8.** If no object is removed after the finger sweep or the lungs cannot be inflated during the attempted rescue breaths, continue the cycle of abdominal thrusts, tongue–jaw lift, finger sweep, and rescue breaths until EMS arrives. | |

*Note:* Obese or pregnant patients require chest thrusts rather than abdominal thrusts. Children over the age of 8 years are considered to be adults for the purpose of foreign body airway obstruction.

All health care professionals should take an approved training course in CPR, use of an AED, and managing a foreign body airway obstruction in an approved program. This procedure is not intended to substitute for proficiency training with a mannequin in a structured educational protocol.

---

**Charting Example:**
*07/09/2016 2:15 PM Pt. choked on a throat lozenge in the examination room. Abdominal thrusts x6 administered; lozenge removed. Dr. Kramer notified. Pulse 104, respirations 26, BP 160/98 (R)*
———————————————————————— *R. Lent, CMA*

---

Note: *The medical assistant may sign his or her name in the patient record using only the "CMA" credential if the office has a signature log denoting the entire credential as "CMA (AAMA)."*

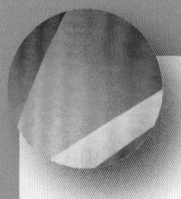

## **PSY** PROCEDURE 26-5

### Control Bleeding

**PSY** Perform first aid procedures for bleeding; document patient care accurately in the medical record.

**Purpose:** Adequately control external bleeding to prevent further hemorrhage and shock

**Equipment:** Gloves and sterile gauze pads

| STEPS | REASONS |
|---|---|
| 1. Identify the patient and determine, if possible, what type of accident caused the external bleeding. Immediately escort the patient to an examination room and have someone notify the physician. | Injuries that are due to the use of a weapon will require reporting to the local law enforcement authorities. |
| 2. Obtain clean examination gloves and an adequate supply of sterile gauze pads, preferably 4 × 4–size pads. | The gloves will protect you from the patient's blood, whereas the sterile gauze pads will prevent microorganisms from entering the open wound. If sterile gauze pads are not immediately available, the use of nonsterile gauze pads to control bleeding is appropriate until sterile pads can be obtained. |
| 3. Apply the exam gloves and quickly open two to three packages of gauze pads. Instruct the patient to lie down on the exam table if he or she has not already done so. | Having the patient lie down reduces the risk of fainting and falling. |
| 4. Using the sterile gauze pads, apply direct pressure to the wound. Maintain pressure until the bleeding stops. Hold pressure for at least 20 minutes without removing the gauze to check for bleeding. | Lifting the gauze to check for continued bleeding may remove any clots that are beginning to form, causing the bleeding to resume or worsen. |

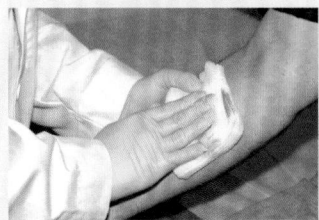

**Step 4.** Apply direct pressure to the wound.

| | |
|---|---|
| 5. If the bleeding continues or seeps through the gauze, do not remove it. Apply additional gauze on top of the saturated gauze while continuing to apply direct pressure. | Removing the saturated gauze may dislodge a blood clot that is trying to form, causing an increase in bleeding. |
| 6. As directed by the physician, apply direct pressure to the artery delivering blood to the area while continuing to apply direct pressure to the wound. | Pressure points include the brachial artery, the radial artery, the femoral artery, and the popliteal artery. |

*(continues on page 676)*

## PROCEDURE 26-5 (continued)

| STEPS | REASONS |
|---|---|
| 7. Once the bleeding is controlled, be prepared to assist the physician with a minor office surgical procedure to close the wound *or* notify EMS for transport to the hospital as directed by the physician. | Always monitor the patient for signs of shock and treat the patient appropriately. |

Charting Example:
*01/20/2016 1:45 PM Pt. presented with laceration to left hand due to hand saw accident at home. Wound approximately 4 inches across palm of hand and bleeding profusely. Direct pressure applied. Dr. Smith notified* _____ S. Jones, CMA

*01/20/2016 1:50 PM Bleeding controlled after direct pressure to brachial artery per Dr. Smith. Wound bandaged, pt. transported to General Hospital emergency room per EMS* _____ S. Jones, CMA

Note: *The medical assistant may sign his or her name in the patient record using only the "CMA" credential if the office has a signature log denoting the entire credential as "CMA (AAMA)."*

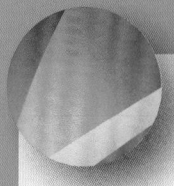

## PSY PROCEDURE 26-6

# Respond to Medical Emergencies Other Than Bleeding, Cardiac/Respiratory Arrest, or Foreign Body Airway Obstruction

**PSY** Perform first aid procedures for fracture, seizure, shock, and syncope; document patient care accurately in the medical record.

**Purpose:** Adequately respond to a variety of medical emergencies.

**Equipment:** A medical emergency kit that contains a minimum of personal protective equipment including gloves, low-dose aspirin tablets, 2 × 2 and 4 × 4 sterile gauze pads, vinegar or acetic acid solution, blood pressure cuff and stethoscope, sterile water or saline for irrigation, ice bags, and towel or rolled gauze bandage material

| STEPS | REASONS |
|---|---|
| 1. Identify the patient and determine, if possible, what type of medical emergency is involved. Immediately escort the patient to an examination room. | Injuries that are due to the use of a weapon will require reporting to the local law enforcement authorities. |
| 2. Have another staff member get the physician, medical emergency cart or bag, and AED. | High-quality CPR and early defibrillation will improve survival from sudden cardiac arrest should the medical emergency progress to cardiac or respiratory arrest. |
| 3. Apply clean examination gloves and other personal protective equipment as appropriate. | The gloves will protect you from the patient's blood or body fluids. |
| 4. Assist the patient to the exam table and have him or her lie down if he/she has not already done so. | Having the patient lie down reduces the risk of fainting and falling. |
| 5. Treat the patient according to the physician instructions and the most current guidelines for first aid procedures: | |
| A. Chest pain: Activate EMS and have patient chew one (1) adult non–enteric-coated aspirin or two (2) low-dose aspirin tablets unless contraindicated. | Patients who have a history of aspirin allergy or recent gastrointestinal bleeding should not be given aspirin. |
| B. Snakebite: Apply pressure bandage to *all* venomous snakebites. A blood pressure cuff may be used to apply pressure. 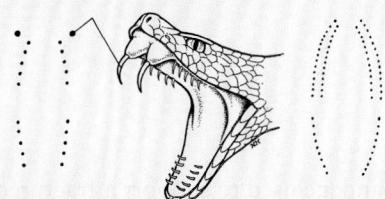 | Applying pressure will slow the lymph flow and reduce the absorption of the venom. Use the following mmHg guidelines if a blood pressure cuff is used to apply pressure: Upper extremity: greater than 40 mm Hg and less than 70 mm Hg Lower extremity: greater than 55 mm Hg and less than 70 mm Hg **Step 5B.** Teeth marks of a poisonous snake (**A**) as compared with that of (**B**) a nonpoisonous snake. (From Neil O. Hardy, Westpoint, CT.) |

*(continues on page 678)*

## PROCEDURE 26-6 (continued)

| STEPS | REASONS |
|---|---|
| **C.** Jellyfish sting: Wash the area for at least 30 seconds with acetic solution, such as vinegar or a 4%–6% acetic acid solution. | Washing with acetic solution will deactivate the venom. |
| Remove nematocysts and apply or immerse the area in hot water for 20 minutes. | Removing the nematocysts and applying hot water will reduce the pain. |

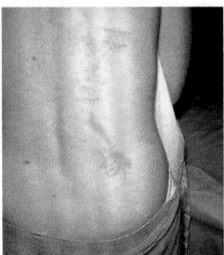

**Step 5C**. Jellyfish sting. Note the whiplike shape of the lesions. (From Goodheart HP. *Goodheart's Photoguide of Common Skin Disorders*, 2nd ed. Philadelphia, PA: Lippincott Williams & Wilkins, 2003.)

| STEPS | REASONS |
|---|---|
| **D.** Dental injuries: | |
| *Chipped tooth:* Patient should follow up with a dentist. | A chipped tooth may not be painful but may require repair to prevent further problems or for cosmetic reasons. |
| *Cracked or broken tooth:* Patient should follow up with a dentist as soon as possible to prevent further damage. | A root canal or tooth extraction may be necessary. Patient may experience pain and sensitivity to hot/cold and air. |
| *Tooth removed:* Rinse tooth with water but do not scrub the tooth or remove any attached tissue. Do not allow the tooth to dry. Attempt to reinsert the tooth into the socket or store it in a container of milk. The patient should see a dentist immediately. | Rinsing removes any debris. The tooth should be reimplanted by a dentist within 30 minutes for the best success with reimplantation; however, there may be success for up to 2 hours. |
| *Broken jaw:* Secure the jaw with a towel tied around the jaw over the top of the head. Depending on the assessment of the physician, the patient may need to be transported to the hospital emergency room or a dentist or oral surgeon may be consulted. | The physician will determine the extent of the injury and if additional treatment is warranted. |

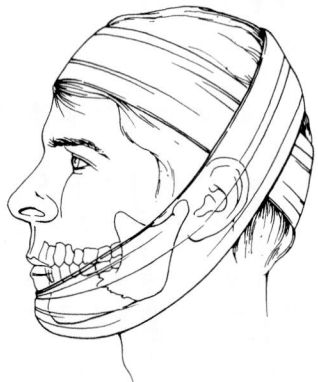

**Step 5D**. Barton bandage used to support a fractured mandible. (From Harwood-Nuss A, Wolfson AB, et al. *The Clinical Practice of Emergency Medicine*, 3rd ed. Philadelphia, PA: Lippincott Williams & Wilkins, 2001.)

## PROCEDURE 26-6 (continued)

| STEPS | REASONS |
|---|---|
| E. Fracture injuries: Apply ice and splint the limb or area appropriately. Remove rings and other jewelry on the affected extremity before swelling increases; these items restrict circulation. Watch the extremity for signs of impaired circulation (refer to Chapter 29, Orthopedics, for more information on fractures). | Do not apply an ice or cold pack directly to the skin. Place a towel or other material between the ice bag/cold pack and the skin to prevent damage to the skin. Signs of impaired circulation include pale or cyanotic color of the skin or nailbeds, increased swelling, and a decrease or absent pulse distal to the injury. |
| F. Seizure: Prevent injury by moving furniture and other objects out of the way in the event the patient becomes unconscious during the seizure. Assess breathing during the seizure but do NOT attempt to insert anything between the teeth. Note the duration of the seizure and report this to the physician and/or EMS personnel. | If the patient may have injured his/her neck or back when falling during the seizure, protect the cervical spine by not twisting the patient or allowing them to sit up or move after the seizure. |
| G. Shock: For a patient exhibiting signs of shock, lie the patient down and elevate the feet if possible. Cover the patient with a blanket or other material and monitor vital signs. Do not give the patient anything to eat or drink. | A patient in shock will have a low blood pressure and weak, thread, fast heart rate. Elevating the feet will keep blood in the trunk and head, oxygenating vital organs such as the kidneys and brain. Covering the patient with a blanket or other material will prevent the patient from shivering. Giving the patient who may be in shock food or drink may result in vomiting. |
| H. Syncope: Any patient who complains of dizziness or lightheadedness should be assisted to a supine position immediately as these symptoms may lead to loss of consciousness or fainting. After lying the patient down, take the blood pressure and obtain a heart rate. If the patient loses consciousness, prevent injury if possible by moving objects out of the way. If there is a possibility the patient injured his/her neck or back during the fall, avoid twisting movements or allowing the patient to sit up or move when awake. | There are usually underlying medical issues associated with syncope. Obtain as much history from the patient as possible before any loss of consciousness or upon awakening. Report any medical conditions to the physician. |
| 6. If the patient develops cardiac or respiratory arrest, follow the procedure for CPR according to the most recent guidelines (see Procedures 26-2 and 26-3). | High-quality CPR and early defibrillation will improve survival from sudden cardiac arrest. |

---

Charting Example:
*01/20/2016 1:45 PM Pt. presented with complaint of snakebite to right anterior forearm. No identification of snake determined, forearm shows 2 small pinpoint wounds with increased redness and swelling. Dr. Jones notified. Sterile gauze placed over wound and pressure applied via a blood pressure cuff at 50 mmHg. EMS notified as ordered. Pt. anxious, pulse 122, respirations 32, nonlabored. _____*
*B. Reynolds, CMA*

---

Note: *The medical assistant may sign his or her name in the patient record using only the "CMA" credential if the office has a signature log denoting the entire credential as "CMA (AAMA)."*

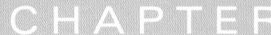

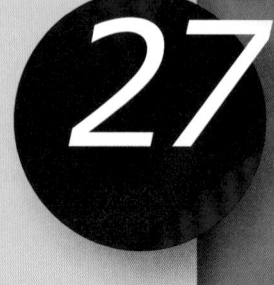

# 27 Disaster Preparedness and the Medical Assistant

## Outline

**Emergency Preparedness**
Emergency Medical Kit
Emergency Action Plan
Central Operation Centers
**Examples of Disasters: One Natural and One Man-Made**
Epidemics and Pandemics

Bioterrorism
**Emergency Preparedness Plans in Your Community**
Your Role in Emergency Preparedness
Environmental Safety Plan
Conducting a Mock Environmental Exposure Drill

**Effects of Stress and Emergencies**
**Principles for Evacuation During an Emergency**
Evacuation Plan for the Physician Office

## Learning Outcomes

**COG Cognitive Domain***

1. Spell and define the key terms
2. Describe what is meant by a disaster and disaster preparedness
3. List several types of disasters
4. *Identify critical elements of an emergency plan for response to a natural disaster or other emergency*
5. *Describe fundamental principles for evacuation of a health care setting*
6. Identify emergency preparedness plans in your community
7. Discuss potential role(s) of the medical assistant in emergency preparedness

**PSY Psychomotor Domain***

1. Respond to a simulated disaster (Procedure 27-1)
    a. *Participate in a mock exposure event with documentation of specific steps*
    b. *Report relevant information concisely and accurately*

2. Maintain a list of community resources for emergency preparedness (Procedure 27-2)
3. Develop a personal safety plan (Procedure 27-3)

**AFF Affective Domain***

1. *Recognize the physical and emotional effects on persons involved in an emergency situation*
2. *Demonstrate self-awareness in responding to an emergency situation*
3. Apply active listening skills
4. Use appropriate body language and other nonverbal skills in communicating with patients, family, and staff

*Note: AAMA/CAAHEP 2015 Standards are italicized.*

**ABHES Competencies**

1. Serve as liaison between physician and others
2. Perform risk-management procedures

## Key Terms

bioterrorism          disaster          epidemic          pandemic

## Case Study

*T*aylor Tonninger, RMA, works for Great Falls Medical Center physician offices as the practice manager for a busy multiphysician ear, nose, and throat group located downtown in a large city. Within a twenty-mile radius of the practice, there are many manufacturing companies, four hospitals, three public high schools, two colleges, and one university. The city has an efficient public transportation system, and most employees, including Taylor, use this as their primary means of getting into the city to work each day. Taylor shares an apartment with another medical assistant, Sarah White, RMA, who works for a smaller, private physician office in a neighboring quiet town. Sarah and Taylor are happy in their current employment and would not trade places despite Taylor's longer commute each day and Sarah's limited access to shopping and food during the day. Of the two offices, which is more likely to experience a disaster and therefore should be ready to respond? If both offices have an emergency disaster plan, should they include the same information? What types of disasters would be likely for Taylor's office? What types of disasters would be likely for Sarah's office?

The answers to these questions are found in this chapter.

A successful and safe medical practice needs an effective medical office process or plan to respond to **disasters**, which are unplanned events that may cause damage to property or life. This process or plan must be a team effort among the physicians, practice managers, and the office staff members. Because disasters occur when least expected and may be caused by accidents or nature, emergency preparedness has become a way of life in the United States. All medical assistants must be able to recognize and respond to many types of emergencies including disasters. The medical assistant must be able to communicate with patients, other staff members, and emergency personnel calmly in the event of a disaster and possible evacuation of the medical office.

## COG EMERGENCY PREPAREDNESS

Disasters, whether arising from natural or man-made circumstances, usually strike without warning and could occur during a typical workday in any type of medical office. During a crisis, you should be prepared to assist not only patients and coworkers but the community at large. In fact, your medical training will cause many people including patients to look to you for guidance and reassurance during an emergency (Fig. 27-1). In some cases, emergency medical personnel may be unable to respond immediately, and part of your job will be to respond appropriately to keep everyone safe while maintaining a calm demeanor.

Natural disasters are outside of human control and can occur forcefully and abruptly or slowly over a period of time. Some examples of natural disasters include the following:

- Drought
- Earthquake
- Epidemics
- Flood
- Hurricane
- Tornado
- Snowstorm
- Storms
- Volcanic eruption
- Tidal wave (tsunami)
- Mudslide
- Avalanche
- Famine

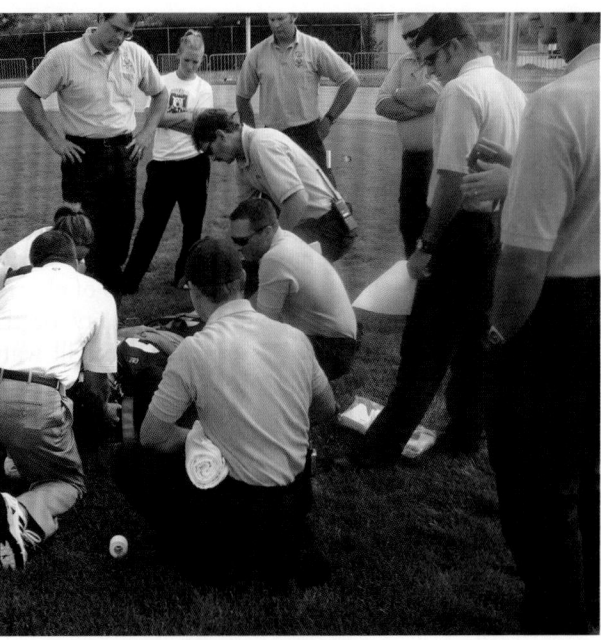

**Figure 27-1 •** A trained medical assistant is prepared to assist in a disaster or emergency.

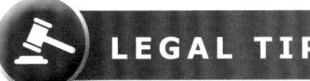

## LEGAL TIP

### Flood Insurance and the Medical Office

Individuals and businesses may be affected by damages incurred as a result of flooding. In some cases, flooding is a result of plumbing issues such as clogged toilets, septic tanks, or roots from trees or large shrubs that damage underground pipes. Flooding may also result from natural disasters such as tornadoes, hurricanes, or earthquakes. In either case, property damage that results from flooding is often not part of a standard homeowner, renter, or business owner property or mortgage insurance policy.

In 1968, the National Flood Insurance Program (NFIP) was created to and passed into law to financially protect homeowners, renters, and businesses in the event of property damage as a result of flooding. Specifically, this program offered flood insurance to those individuals or businesses if their community agreed to participate in the program. To participate, communities agreed to adopt and enforce ordinances that reduced the risk of flooding. Although the Federal Emergency Management Agency (FEMA) was not created until 1979, NIFP has been reformed several times since 1968 and now requires participating communities to adopt and enforce ordinances that meet or exceed FEMA requirements to reduce the risk of flooding. The most recent law passed in March 2014 to reform NFIP was the Homeowner Flood Insurance Affordability Act (HFIAA). This reform, like others before it, strengthens NFIP and offers resources to individuals and businesses who would like more information about flood insurance or who need assistance after a flood.

*Source:* http://www.fema.gov/national-flood-insurance-program

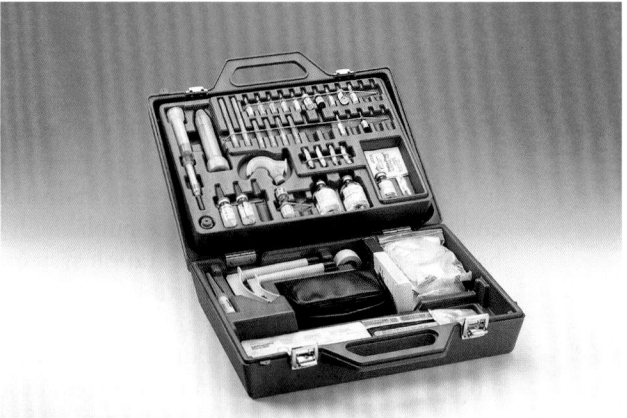

**Figure 27-2** • The medical emergency supply kit should be easily accessible.

supplies are fairly standard (see Chapter 26, Medical Office Emergencies). This equipment should be kept in a designated location that is accessible to all staff (Fig. 27-2). Standard supplies for a medical emergency kit are listed in Box 26-1 (Chapter 26). Although items used during an emergency should be replaced as soon as possible, a medical assistant or other staff member should check the contents of the emergency kit or crash cart regularly, perhaps weekly, to verify that contents are available and that no item has gone beyond the expiration date. If so, the expired items should be replaced immediately. Knowing where this kit is kept and assurance that it is complete and contains up-to-date supplies are essential in the event of a disaster and possible medical emergency!

## Emergency Action Plan

It is important for every medical office to develop a plan jointly or in consultation with the local Office of Emergency Services, Emergency Medical Services, Department of Health Services, hospital planners, and/or neighboring clinics.

Every medical office should have an emergency action plan, including the following information in a binder or other notebook:

- The local emergency rescue service telephone number (usually 911)
- Location of the nearest hospital emergency department
- Telephone number of the local or regional poison control center
- Procedures for various emergencies
- List of office personnel who are trained in CPR
- Location and list of contents of the emergency medical kit or crash cart

Whether confronted with a cardiac emergency, a natural disaster event, or another unexpected crisis, medical assistants must be able to coordinate multiple ongoing

Other emergencies may be caused by or controlled by humans. These include accidents involving multiple vehicles, plane crashes, or train derailments. Disasters involving biohazardous materials may be natural or man-made. Although you cannot anticipate all disasters, being prepared for those that are likely and having a plan to deal with problems such as loss of electric power are essential to maintaining continuity of the office and providing focused assistance. You will want to remain calm and as in control as possible should you or your community have an unplanned event requiring an immediate response.

## Emergency Medical Kit

Proper equipment and supplies should be readily available for any disaster that could include a medical emergency. Although the office's equipment and supplies vary with the medical specialty, emergency equipment and

events while rendering patient care. Contributing to the complexity of a medical emergency are such factors as panicky family members, the arrival of emergency personnel, and possibly language barriers. In the event of a disaster, details specific to the type of event will also add to the complexity and chaos. The key to being prepared is having and being familiar with a well-written plan that is functional, flexible, and easy to implement. It is important to test the plan during nonpeak hours when facilities lack optimum leadership and staff, because disasters can occur at any time. Testing should include observers to report the strengths and weaknesses of the plan and the need for training in specific areas. The plan should be modified to eliminate or minimize any vulnerability revealed during testing. In some communities, coordinating the testing of your disaster plan may be done with professional emergency services personnel who can give feedback and suggestions for making the plan work smoothly in case of an actual disaster. In addition, many communities have resources available to assist with developing a disaster plan.

## Central Operation Centers

Before a disaster occurs, a location in or near the medical office should be identified that can become a central operation center to coordinate activities. The development of a central operation center is vital to successful disaster and emergency response operations (Fig. 27-3). Although this center provides coordination of all activities, it should be located in an area that is away from the center of activities. An alternate site may also be

established should the primary site become inoperable or contaminated.

The site should be equipped with adequate administrative supplies including frequently used telephone numbers, maps and marking pens, paper, floor plans of the facility (including utility shut-off valves), and locations of fire extinguishers and emergency exits. The emergency operation center should also be supplied with adequate emergency supplies including water, food, a portable radio, a first aid kit, a flashlight and batteries, and backup power.

Another important aspect of the response is to be able to adequately perform triage on a scalable basis. Preassembled paper medical records should be available to quickly process a rapid influx of patients. Additional forms may also be necessary and should be available in a folder labeled accordingly.

## WHAT IF?

**What happens now?**

It is difficult to think about, but the possibility of a major disaster involving an entire community is a reality. How does a medical office come back from a catastrophe? Recovery operations often take longer than the emergency itself. All health care facilities, including medical offices, must attempt to resume business after a damaging emergency. Documentation is crucial for reimbursement of damages and costs associated with response and recovery. You should assume that typical computer function may be inoperable and, therefore, backup paper billing systems should be planned for in advance of a disaster. During a recovery period, it is critical for staff members to attend to the psychosocial trauma of disaster. Staff members should be encouraged to debrief often, but this should not be forced.

## CHECKPOINT QUESTION

1. Taylor has been asked to develop a disaster plan for the office. What is the purpose of a central operations center?

## COG EXAMPLES OF DISASTERS: ONE NATURAL AND ONE MAN-MADE

### Epidemics and Pandemics

Each year, the virus that causes influenza causes illness in many individuals and, in some cases, death. Fortunately, a vaccine is developed every year to protect

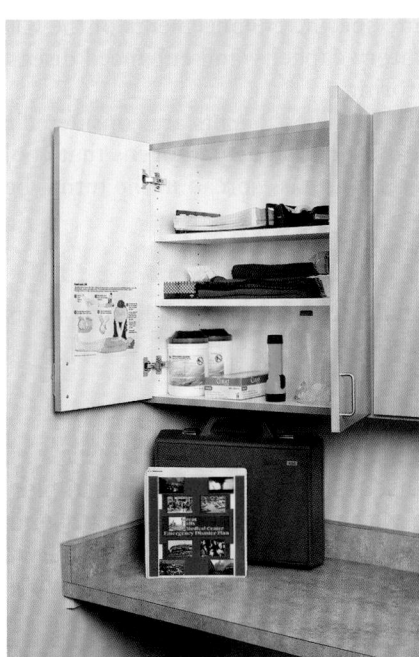

**Figure 27-3 •** A central location to meet and store essential supplies is part of the disaster plan.

those who get the immunization against the specific virus for that year. You will come into contact with many patients who suffer from "cold-like" symptoms in the winter months, and it will be in your best interest to get this vaccine during the fall months to protect yourself.

When a disease affects numerous people within a specific geographical area, it is known as an **epidemic**. However, when a disease affects numerous people in many areas of the world at the same time, it is known as a **pandemic**. One of the oldest examples of an epidemic that became a pandemic is the bubonic plague. According to the Centers for Disease Control and Prevention (CDC), approximately 25% of the world's population died from the plague known as "Black Death" from 1345 to 1360. This disease originated in central Asia and was carried to other countries and continents by rodents who, in turn, carried infected fleas. This disease has never been eradicated, and India reported several cases in the 1990s that resulted in heightened awareness and alerts for travelers to and from that country. Fortunately, this did not result in a global pandemic, but the ease with which people travel around the world raises concerns for all health care professionals who must plan for the possibility of an epidemic or pandemic. The CDC provides a guide for medical offices to develop a plan of action before an epidemic or pandemic occurs. This guide is called "Abbreviated Pandemic Influenza Plan

Template for Primary Care Provider Offices: Guidance from Stakeholders" and can be found on the following Web site: http://www.cdc.gov/h1n1flu/guidance/pdf/abb_pandemic_influenza_plan.pdf

## Bioterrorism

**Bioterrorism** refers to the purposeful infliction of an agent (e.g., bacteria, virus, radiation, etc.) into a populated area with the intent to cause destruction of the environment, people, or animals living in the area. Bioterrorism is a very serious man-made threat that can trigger a large-scale emergency. The CDC classifies a biologic agent as a weapon when it is easy to disseminate, has a high potential for mortality, can cause a public panic or social disruption, and requires public health preparedness. There are many government Web sites available that provide information about various agents of bioterrorism, and they may be classified into three major categories according to the CDC:

1. Category A—These include organisms or toxins that pose the highest risk to the public and national security. Specifically, these agents have the potential to:
   - Spread easily from person to person
   - Result in high death rates
   - Cause public panic and social disruption
   - Require special action for public health preparedness
2. Category B—These agents have the potential to:
   - Spread moderately easy
   - Result in moderate illness rates and low death rates
   - Require specific enhancements of the CDC's laboratory capacity and enhanced disease monitoring
3. Category C—These agents are considered emerging threats and include pathogens that could be engineered for mass spread in the future because they are
   - Easily available
   - Easily produced and spread
   - Potentially lethal with possible high morbidity and mortality rates

## PATIENT EDUCATION

### Better Safe Than Sorry

Although we can protect ourselves from certain disease-causing microorganisms like the virus that causes the flu, there is always the possibility that unexpected microorganisms will cause disease in an area or, worse yet, the world. In April of 2009, the first cases of the H1N1 virus were documented in the United States, and by June of that same year, the World Health Organization (WHO) declared a global pandemic. By the fall of 2009, the worst of the pandemic of H1N1 was over for people living in the United States, partly due to the response of the CDC education efforts and the development and availability of a vaccine to immunize against this specific influenza.

We should encourage our patients to get immunized as directed by the physician each year for all types of influenza for which there are available vaccines, especially the elderly and those with chronic diseases such as asthma or chronic obstructive pulmonary disease.

 **CHECKPOINT QUESTION**

2. When discussing her medical office plan for dealing with a pandemic, Taylor's friend Sarah asks her to explain the difference between an epidemic and a pandemic. How would she explain the difference?

## PATIENT EDUCATION

### Preparing for a Bioterrorist Attack

The CDC and the American Red Cross have a guide for anyone who would like more information on preparing for a bioterrorist attack (http://www.bt.cdc.gov/preparedness). Share the following information with patients who are concerned and would like more information about preparing for such an attack:

- Maintain a supply of food, water, and other items for your family. Although a 3-day supply of items for each member of the family is a good start, having enough clean water and supplies for up to 2 weeks is best.
- Develop a family emergency preparedness plan. Everyone in the family should know the plan and how to respond in the event of an attack.
- Be informed and stay informed. Pay attention to the local news and follow any advice given.

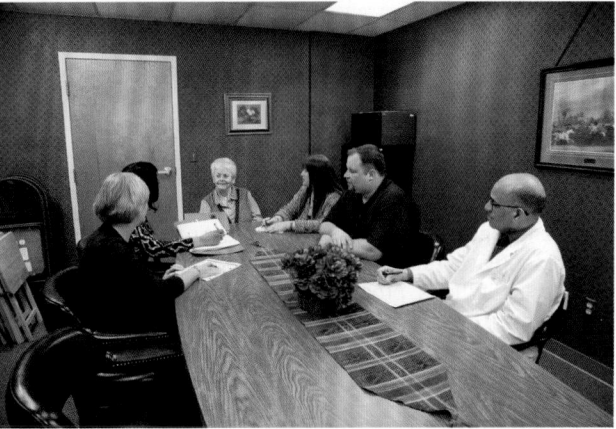

**Figure 27-4** • Many types of health care professionals including medical assistants should be part of a community medical disaster planning committee.

A good place to start is with your community's online Web site. Many towns and cities post their emergency preparedness plans on their Web sites. If you cannot find the plan online, call the police or fire departments or the public safety officer in your town or city. Staff there can often direct you to the right person or, even better, send you a copy of the emergency plan for the community. You can utilize this plan to develop a personal plan and a plan for the physician office.

## EMERGENCY PREPAREDNESS PLANS IN YOUR COMMUNITY

In addition to the medical emergencies that may confront you in a medical setting, you also need to be prepared for emergencies that affect an entire community and you personally. Unfortunately, the Department of Homeland Security (DHS) reports that even people who think they are prepared for disasters often aren't as prepared as they think. In a national survey, the DHS found that 40% of respondents did not have household plans, 80% had not conducted home evacuation drills, and nearly 60% did not know their community's evacuation routes.

Technically, all emergencies are local when they affect you, your family and friends, or your workplace. Although federal and state governments can and will step in to help in the event of a major emergency, response and recovery begins and ends with local governments. The success of those actions depends on the level of planning governments have already completed. Such plans typically reside within the public services departments, such as police, fire, and emergency services. However, you should not leave all the planning and implementation up to public service professionals. You, a member of the medical community, also have an important role to play. It is extremely important that you learn about your community's emergency plans and your role in those plans.

### Your Role in Emergency Preparedness

The professional medical assistant can provide significant administrative and clinical contributions during an emergency. When it comes to planning, make sure that you represent the professional medical assistant on planning committees at the community, hospital, and office levels (Fig. 27-4). Your role in an emergency could include the following:

- Organizing, stocking, and managing on-site medical clinics
- Performing first-aid and CPR
- Serving as a liaison between the physician and others
- Interviewing patients and family members to collect pertinent personal and medical information
- Creating and maintaining medical records during and after an emergency
- Taking and recording vital signs
- Assisting physicians with examinations, procedures, and treatments
- Transferring and transporting patients as needed
- Preparing and administering medications as directed by the physician

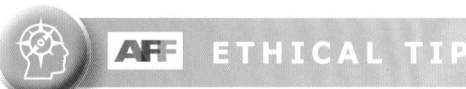

### Disaster Assistance and Ethical Dilemmas

Education and training for medical assistants includes the knowledge and skills taught, practiced, and assessed according to standards approved by educational institutions, program accreditation agencies, and competent instructors or educators. In the classroom and eventually the medical office, you will have access to supplies and equipment that are disinfected, in good working order, and/or sterilized according to standard procedures. Medications and other supplies are kept in secure locations including refrigeration when required.

Unfortunately, the supplies or equipment you have available may be less than desired during or immediately after a disaster. Even a fully stocked emergency supply kit will run out of supplies eventually! How would you handle a situation in which you need medical supplies, but the ones left are questionable with regard to sterility, or you have to improvise and use something else in place of an item that would be optimum? An example would be having sterile gauze to put on an open wound versus using another clean cloth to control bleeding or cover a wound should a sterile gauze pad not be available. What about using medications such as vaccines that have not been refrigerated due to a loss of power? If a patient has been injured and the physician orders you to give a tetanus injection, how would you feel about giving a vaccine that may or may not prevent a disease because it has not been properly stored according to the manufacturer's instructions?

While it is the hope of everyone involved that you do not ever have to encounter these situations, providing medical care involves actions that a *reasonable person* would do in the same or a similar situation. These scenarios are real possibilities during and after a disaster, but thinking about these or other ethical dilemmas may help in coping with your actions after the fact.

## Environmental Safety Plan

If you work in a medical office that has a laboratory that uses potentially dangerous chemicals, you should have an environmental safety plan. This is a written document that outlines how your office will implement and maintain environmental safety procedures. It should include the following:

- A plan for handling and disposing of hazardous waste
- A commitment and plan to train employees on environmental safety guidelines
- Procedures to notify staff and patients in the event of an environmental emergency
- Procedures to notify fire and police of the environmental emergency

- Communication procedures
- A plan to prevent pollution in the laboratory and/or office
- Opportunities to reduce wasted resources such as energy and water
- Emergency responses to fires, spills, and similar events in the facility
- A list of safety equipment available to all personnel including fire extinguishers, safety showers, eyewash stations, spill kits, gloves, and eye protection
- A schedule of self-inspections and annual audits for the medical office
- A policy for chemical storage

### CHECKPOINT QUESTION

3. Why is it important to involve the community in disaster preparedness?

## Conducting a Mock Environmental Exposure Drill

Having a written plan outlining what to do in the event of an environmental threat is a major step in being prepared (Fig. 27-5). However, practicing the plan will give everyone in your office an opportunity to practice putting the plan into action. Conducting regular mock emergency drills will assure that everyone is prepared in the event a real disaster strikes. A drill can be as simple as "walking through" the evacuation of the office or as elaborate as a community-wide disaster drill involving the police, fire department, and hospitals. In addition to the "professionals" who will be directly involved in helping during the disaster, volunteer victims are assigned roles in the drill. The "victim" in Figure 27-6 is playing the part of a tornado survivor injured by flying debris.

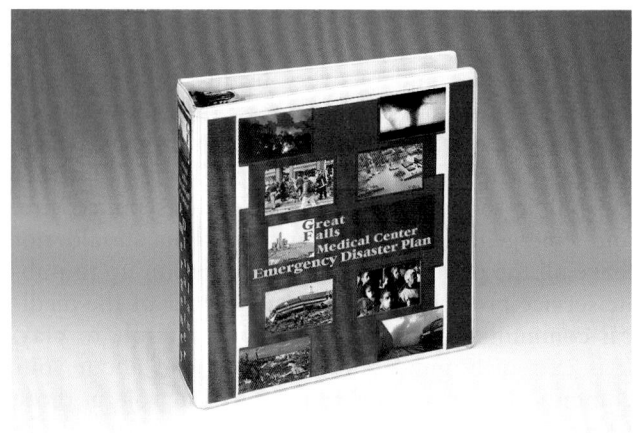

**Figure 27-5 •** A medical office disaster plan.

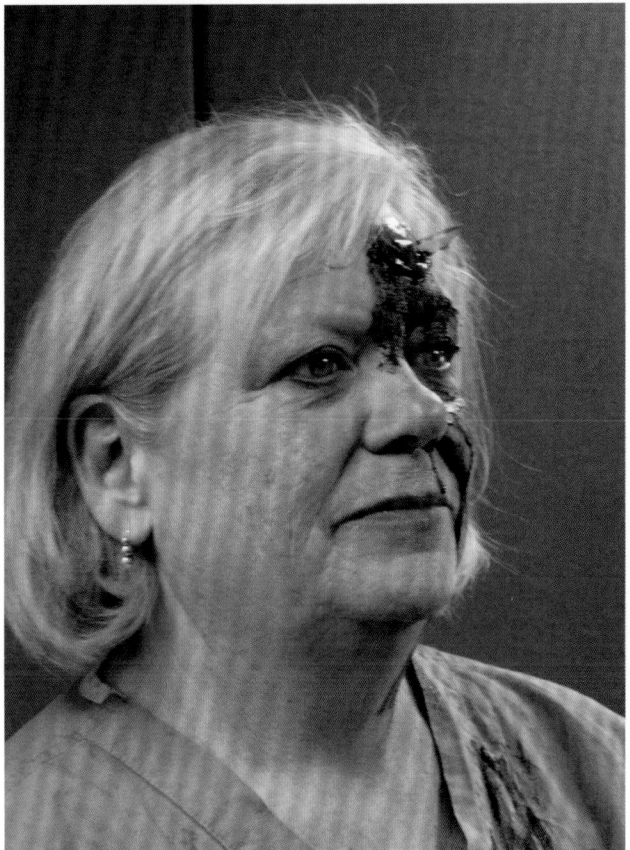

**Figure 27-6** • A volunteer victim in a mock disaster drill is prepared by a make-up artist to portray a tornado survivor injured by flying debris.

Box 27-1 details important parts to include when planning a mock emergency drill.

After conducting a mock emergency drill, don't forget to plan for a "postmortem" meeting, often the next day following the mock incident. This will help you identify what worked and what did not work before, during, and after the drill. The results of this analysis should be used to revise your office environmental safety plan

---

**BOX 27-1   Mock Emergency Drill Planning**

The following factors must be considered when planning a mock emergency drill:

• When and how the drill will occur
• The type of environmental exposure that will occur in the drill
• How the initial alarm will be sounded
• The type of damage and/or injuries that will result
• Individuals who should be notified of the drill
• The roles that people will play in the drill including what they should say and how they should behave
• Any special effects, clothing, or equipment required to make the drill as realistic as possible

---

# EFFECTS OF STRESS AND EMERGENCIES

Although this chapter has described the importance of dealing with safety and emergencies in the medical office, significant consideration must be given to the psychological effects of dealing with such emergencies. Often, the psychological component of a disaster is overshadowed by the acute needs of the physical casualty. Experts estimate that for every 1 physical casualty of a disaster, there are 20 psychological victims. Dealing with disasters and emergencies causes stress over a broad spectrum of individuals depending on the proximity to the disaster and the experience of the disaster on the individual. There are six categories of experience that may describe an individual exposed to a disaster:

• Primary victims: Individuals who experience maximum exposure to the disaster
• Secondary victims: Relatives and friends of the primary victims
• Third-level victims: First responders and health care personnel who participate in rescue and recovery activities
• Fourth-level victims: The community, including those who can converge, who altruistically offer help, who share the grief and loss, or are involved in some way
• Fifth-level victims: Individuals who are upset or psychologically distressed but not directly involved in the disaster
• Sixth-level victims: Those individuals indirectly or vicariously affected by the disaster

The process of coping with the disaster experience begins with feelings of disbelief, bewilderment, and difficulty concentrating. Denial is used as the primary defense. Anxiety and fear represent the next phase and are followed by varying degrees of sadness and depression.

Most victims of stress will recover using their own coping mechanisms without any residual effects. However, some individuals may be affected by acute traumatic stress or posttraumatic stress disorder (PTSD). Acute traumatic stress usually resolves within 2 to 4 weeks of the disaster event. However, posttraumatic stress disorder (PTSD) may be delayed in onset up to 4 weeks and typically lasts for 4 weeks or more. Box 27-2 identifies some characteristics of individuals who may be suffering from acute traumatic stress or posttraumatic stress disorder.

Of greatest concern is the risk that people exposed to trauma from natural or man-made disasters are at risk for the development of a major psychiatric disorder. The effects of stress associated with the disaster may include aggravation or exacerbation of any preexisting mental health condition, such as depression, generalized anxiety disorder, panic disorder, or PTSD (Fig. 27-7).

> **BOX 27-2    Characteristics of Acute Traumatic Stress or Posttraumatic Stress Disorder (PTSD)**
>
> 1. Reliving the traumatic event through intrusive thoughts or images, nightmares, or flashbacks
> 2. Avoidance of associations of the traumatic event and feelings of numbness and detachment
> 3. Increased arousal as evidenced by being jumpy, nervous, or defensive much of the time
> 4. Difficulty sleeping and an inability to concentrate

Factors that may contribute to severe psychological reactions after an event include lack of family and social support, personal loss, adverse reactions from others, and survivor guilt. Psychological first aid for anyone suffering from a stress disorder includes the following:

- Immediate physical care and medical attention
- Appropriate comforting and consolation
- Protection from further threat and distress
- Facilitating some sense of being in control
- Allowing for sharing of experience, but not forcing it
- Provision of culturally appropriate ways of grieving
- Normalization of activity and routine as possible
- Facilitating links with private or community resources

Disaster responders, including medical personnel, are at high risk for developing trauma-related disorders. If possible, take regular rest periods during a disaster response and encourage coworkers to do the same. Seek psychological care including counseling if symptoms of stress persist after the disaster including sleep disorders, excessive fatigue, mood changes, anxiety, and developing problems with relationships.

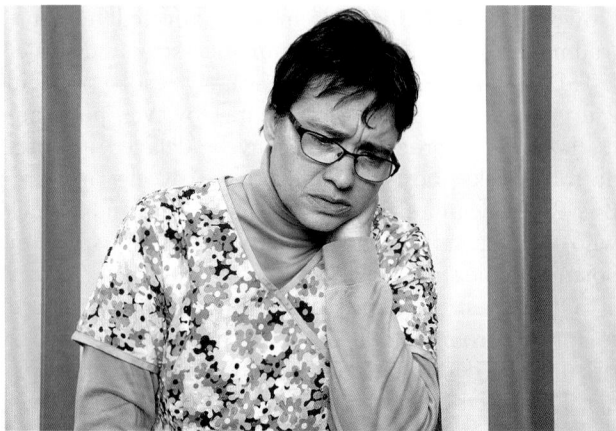

**Figure 27-7 •** There may be psychological effects on health care workers including medical assistants after a disaster or emergency.

> **⚲ CHECKPOINT QUESTION**
>
> 4. What psychological first aid may be helpful for anyone experiencing the effects of stress after an emergency or disaster?

# PRINCIPLES FOR EVACUATION DURING AN EMERGENCY

During an emergency or natural disaster, it may be necessary to evacuate the medical office. Ideally, your facility will have an evacuation plan and will train all employees in its implementation. Because your reactions may determine how other employees and patients respond, it is important that you remain calm during an evacuation. Encourage an orderly evacuation by walking swiftly, but not running. Do not use elevators during an emergency, and, depending on the urgency of the situation, do not worry about personal belongings. You may need to close windows and lock doors as well as forward the phones or implement the answering service if there is time to do so. Again, this is something that should be determined during the planning process. Principles to consider in any evacuation plan include the following:

- Identify the person responsible for ordering the evacuation.
- Determine the facility or location that you will evacuate to. Choose a backup site, if available, just in case the planned location or facility is not available.
- Identify evacuation routes.
- Define individual staff responsibilities. Plan for the likelihood that not all staff will be available.
- Identify what critical supplies or equipment will need to be transported and who will be responsible for transporting them.
- Determine how individuals will be accounted for during and after the evacuation.
- Develop a procedure to handle patient/staff illness or death during the evacuation.
- Develop a medical office reentry plan. Who will authorize reentry after the emergency? How will the medical office be inspected to determine safety after returning?

## Evacuation Plan for the Physician Office

Although it is not as involved as the scene in a hospital or nursing home, evacuating a physician office still requires planning and practice. It is important that you be familiar with the key elements of such an evacuation plan because you will, by necessity, play an important role in any emergency evacuation.

The first step is to know what constitutes an emergency requiring evacuation. This could be a fire, a chemical spill, impending weather-related emergencies, a threat of violence, or even a highly infectious patient. You should discuss the specific situations that might trigger an evacuation order in your office with your physician, office manager, and other staff and develop a policy to guide the process.

In addition to the key elements already mentioned, other items to be considered for a physician office include the following:

- Communicating the evacuation. This may be done verbally, through an e-mail or text message, or with an alarm. Include how patients will be notified of the evacuation before, during, and after the event.
- Determining who is responsible for giving the evacuation order. This will most likely be a physician or the office manager.
- Identifying specific staff responsibilities including who will be in charge of evacuating patients currently in the office, both those patients who are well-bodied and those who need assistance.
- Determining how patient records will be protected and/or transported.
- Identifying available transportation for the evacuation.
- Determining a meeting place for all employees once the evacuation is complete.
- Identifying at least two exit routes from your work area.
- Identifying any employees with disabilities who may require special attention during an evacuation. It should be clarified how these individuals will be assisted.
- Determining how the office will be secured during and after the evacuation.
- Identifying what, if anything, should be taken from the office and who should be responsible for seeing that the item(s) are removed and secure.
- Identifying who will communicate with emergency personnel.

- Determining if any personnel should remain behind after the primary evacuation.
- Identifying a way to account for employees during and after the evacuation.
- Identifying the person who will be responsible for notifying the public utilities (electricity, telephone, water, gas, etc.) that the building or office has been evacuated.
- Identifying and obtaining any special equipment that may be required for evacuation such as safety goggles, masks, gloves, etc.

## ROLE-PLAYING ACTIVITY

Role-play a scenario with your classmates or as assigned by your instructor where you are employed as a medical assistant in the ENT office where Taylor Tonninger, RMA works (refer to the case study at the beginning of this chapter for more information). One day while you both are working, a strong smell of gas overwhelms the inside of the office and before Taylor can call the utility department, an explosion is heard outside the building. Several patients and visitors in the office complain of nausea from the odor, and two elderly patients are light-headed and pale in color. Four people run into the office with blood running down their faces and asking for help. You look out the window and see that the street is covered with debris, which will make it difficult for emergency equipment to reach the office. The emergency management system was notified and you were told that it would be at least 4 hours before anyone the street could be cleared enough for help to arrive. Role-play this situation using 4 to 6 students as "patients" and "victims" from the explosion who are not regular patients but are seeking help from your office. You and another student are Taylor and the other medical assistant working that day. Your instructor will give you additional information about this activity!

## español SPANISH TERMINOLOGY

**Necesitamos irnos de este lugar.**
We need to evacuate this place.

**¿Esta lastimado? ¿Tiene alguna herida?**
Do you have any injuries?

**¿Puede caminar?**
Are you able to walk?

**Ya llamamos a la policia y a los bomberos.**
We have called the police and fire department.

**Por favor cálmese y sígame.**
Remain calm and follow me.

**¿Quiere que le hable a alguién?**
Is there someone I can call for you?

**Usted necesita un Botiquín de Primeros Auxilios.**
You need a First Aid Kit.

**Fuego en el edificio!**
Fire in the building!

**Terremoto! Tirese, Cúbrase y Agárrese!**
Earthquake! Drop, cover, and hold on!

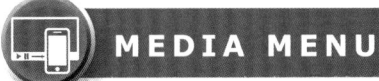

## MEDIA MENU

**Student Resources** on the Point®

• **CMA/RMA Certification Exam Review**

**Internet Resources**
**Occupational Safety and Health Administration**
http://www.osha.gov

**American Red Cross**
http://www.redcross.org

**American Safety and Health Institute**
http://www.hsi.com/

**National Safety Council**
http://www.nsc.org/Pages/Home.aspx

**Federal Emergency Management Agency**
http://www.fema.gov/

**Disaster Assistance**
http://www.disasterassistance.gov/

**Ready.gov**
http://www.ready.gov/

**U.S. Department of Homeland Security**
http://www.dhs.gov/

**Disaster Distress Helpline**
http://disasterdistress.samhsa.gov/disasters/

## EMR Activity

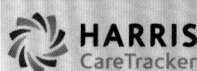

Harris CareTracker is a web-based electronic medical record (EMR) application that you will use for the EMR activities included in this section at the end of each chapter. This application is actually used in physician offices, but is provided to you through the publisher, Wolters Kluwer Health, to give you hands-on practice working with EMRs. Your instructor will have more information about accessing your username, login, and Quickstart guide.

Prerequisite Activities in Harris CareTracker

• *The Getting Started and Quickstart documents and EMR Activities Step-by-Step Instructions are available at* http://thePoint.lww.com/KronenbergerComp5e

Activity Details

Send an e-mail to your instructor from *New Mail* dialog box in the *Messages* tab of the *Home* module advising that the annual inspection of all fire extinguishers was done yesterday and that everything has been approved for 1 year. The new inspection certificate is in the equipment log book.

## Chapter Summary

- Dealing with a disaster or medical emergency in the office or community will require you to communicate clearly and calmly and work effectively as a team member with other employees and emergency personnel or law enforcement.
- You may be involved with developing a disaster plan jointly or in consultation with local or community agencies.
- Adequately prepare for several types of disasters including those that are natural or man-made.
- Participate in mock disaster drills, and provide constructive input regarding any strengths or weaknesses in the disaster plan.
- Recognize the effects of trauma from disasters on the psychological well-being of individuals involved directly in the disaster.

## Warm-Ups for Critical Thinking

1. Plan a mock disaster drill for a medical office: assign employees to certain tasks including "victims," and design a form to document the drill and the postdrill discussion.
2. It is 7:30 AM, and you are preparing the office for the busy day ahead. The first patient is scheduled for 8:00 AM, and when you check the voicemail messages, you realize all but one employee, the medical billing specialist, has called in sick due to flu-like symptoms. Would this situation be appropriate for the medical office emergency disaster plan? What steps should be taken initially to deal with this situation?
3. Research the resources in your community that could assist in providing information or materials for preparing a disaster plan or binder.

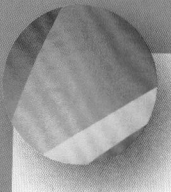

**PSY** PROCEDURE 27-1

# Respond to a Simulated Disaster

**PSY** Participate in a mock exposure event with documentation of specific steps; Report relevant information concisely and accurately.

**Purpose:** Respond appropriately to a given a simulated disaster scenario

**Equipment:** Phone, disaster drill manual for a medical office, paper medical record forms and folders, pen, portable emergency kit.

| STEPS | REASONS |
|---|---|
| 1. Develop and/or review an emergency/disaster procedure manual. | Being familiar with what to do before an emergency or disaster occurs is essential to remaining calm and responding appropriately. |
| 2. As assigned by your instructor, assume the role of an employee, patient, or visitor in a medical office. | By assuming different roles, you will experience the actual feelings and behaviors of various people who may be in a medical office during a disaster or emergency. |
| 3. During a "normal" workday, a disaster occurs unexpectedly. Your instructor will give you more information as the disaster unfolds. | Disasters are often unplanned events that can occur during any workday. Some events can be predicted (i.e. hurricane or tornado), but most are not. Anticipating a disaster and having a plan to follow may decrease loss of life and property during an actual event. |
| 4. At the conclusion of the mock disaster event, discuss the event including the strengths and weaknesses of the emergency plan. | Part of any disaster drill should include a reflection on how a plan worked or did not work. This allows the plan to be revised and improved should a "real" disaster occur. |
| 5. **AFF** Complete a reflection paper about the mock disaster as assigned by your instructor. | Responding to an emergency and disaster may have long-term unintended effects on the individuals involved in the event. This assignment will encourage self-awareness of you as a responder and help you to recognize the possible physical and emotional effects of being involved in a disaster. |

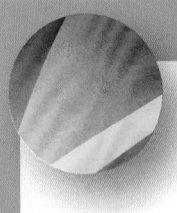

**PSY** PROCEDURE 27-2

## Maintain a List of Community Resources for Emergency Preparedness

**Purpose:** Research and document community resources that are available to prepare and respond to potential disasters.

**Equipment:** Phone, computer with Internet access, paper and pen, binder.

| STEPS | REASONS |
|---|---|
| 1. Determine the geographical area of your community including the city or town, county, and surrounding counties or towns as appropriate. | Identifying the components of your community will help your research of possible resources. |
| 2. Complete an Internet search of the possible resources that make up your community, beginning with the local resources. | Depending on the size and local economy and the nature of the emergency or disaster, you may need to expand your search for resources beyond your local area. |
| 3. Create a list of resources including the name of the agency, resources available, phone numbers, addresses, and Web address if available. | If a local agency has limited information on the Internet, you may have to contact the agency by phone. When speaking with representatives from various agencies, always explain the purpose of your research. Some agencies may provide additional information or resources if you explain that you are pursuing a health care career. |
| 4. Organize the resources you find in a binder or other notebook for easy reference. | Your instructor may want you to submit your binder or notebook for a grade. In the medical office, this binder should be accessible to all employees. |

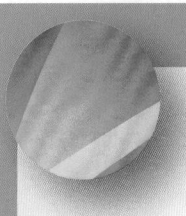

## PSY   PROCEDURE 27-3

### Develop a Personal Safety Plan

**Purpose:** Create a plan for maintaining personal safety in the event of a local or community disaster.

**Equipment:** Phone, computer with Internet access, paper and pen, binder.

| STEPS | REASONS |
|---|---|
| 1. Download an electronic version of a family or personal safety plan template from a reputable Web site such as Ready.gov: http://www.ready.gov/sites/default/files/documents/files/RRToolkit.pdf | Using a template to create a personal or family safety plan may save time and prevent you from forgetting essential information. |
| 2. Gather information needed for inclusion in the safety plan such as important names and addresses, pharmacy information, insurance information (health, home, car, etc.), medications and/or prescription numbers, veterinarian and other pet information (kennels, etc.), and other information that may be needed during or after a disaster event. | Include any information that may be needed should you or your family have to evacuate your home without access to this information. |
| 3. Speak with family members and decide how you will contact each other in the event of a disaster. Also discuss where family members will go and/or meet if a disaster occurs when everyone is not together. | Your skills as a professional medical assistant will be invaluable to the community in the event of a disaster. Preparing yourself and your family before a disaster happens will allow you to focus on providing care to others in the community instead of focusing on personal and family safety. |
| 4. Once the personal or family plan is developed, keep a copy in the emergency supply kit or another safe place. | All members of the family should know where the emergency supply kit and plan are located. |

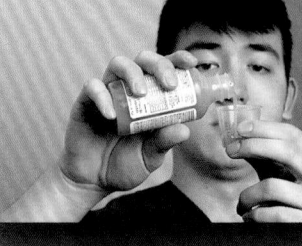

CHAPTER

# 28 Dermatology

## Outline

## Learning Outcomes

**OG Cognitive Domain***

1. Spell key terms
2. *Define medical terms and abbreviations related to all body systems*
3. *Describe structural organization of the human body*
4. *List major organs in each body system*
5. *Identify the anatomical location of major organs in each body system*
6. *Describe the normal function of each body system*
7. *Identify common pathology related to each body system including signs, symptoms, and etiology*
   a. Describe common skin disorders
8. Explain the difference between bandages and dressings and give the purpose of each
9. Identify the guidelines for applying bandages

**PSY Psychomotor Domain***

1. Apply a warm or cold compress (Procedure 28-1)
   a. *Instruct and prepare a patient for a procedure or treatment*
   b. *Coach patients appropriately considering cultural diversity, developmental life stage, and communication barriers*
   c. *Coach patients regarding disease prevention and treatment plans*
   d. *Document patient care accurately in the medical record*
2. Assist with therapeutic soaks (Procedure 28-2)
   a. *Instruct and prepare a patient for a procedure or treatment*
   b. *Coach patients appropriately considering cultural diversity, developmental life stage, and communication barriers*
   c. *Coach patients regarding disease prevention and treatment plans*
   d. *Document patient care accurately in the medical record*
3. Apply a tubular gauze bandage (Procedure 28-3)
   a. *Instruct and prepare a patient for a procedure or treatment*
   b. *Coach patients appropriately considering cultural diversity, developmental life stage, and communication barriers*
   c. *Coach patients regarding disease prevention and treatment plans*
   d. *Document patient care accurately in the medical record*

**AFF Affective Domain***

1. Incorporate critical thinking skills when performing patient assessment
2. Incorporate critical thinking skills when performing patient care
3. Show awareness of a patient's concerns related to the procedure being performed
4. Demonstrate empathy, active listening, and nonverbal communication
5. Demonstrate respect for individual diversity including gender, race, religion, age, economic status, and appearance
6. Explain to a patient the rationale for performance of a procedure

7. Demonstrate sensitivity to patient rights
8. Protect the integrity of the medical record

***Note: AAMA/CAAHEP 2015 Standards are italicized.**

### ABHES Competencies

1. Assist the physician with the regimen of diagnostic and treatment modalities as they relate to each body system
2. Comply with federal, state, and local health laws and regulations
3. Communicate on the recipient's level of comprehension
4. Serve as a liaison between the physician and others
5. Show empathy and impartiality when dealing with patients

## Key Terms

| | | | |
|---|---|---|---|
| alopecia | erythema | intertrigo | pustule |
| bulla | folliculitis | macule | seborrhea |
| carbuncle | furuncle | neoplasm | urticaria |
| cellulitis | herpes simplex | pediculosis | verruca |
| dermatophytosis | herpes zoster | pruritus | vesicle |
| eczema | impetigo | psoriasis | vitiligo |

## Case Study

$A$lthough patients with skin disorders are seen in many types of medical offices every day, those who need specialized care may be referred to a dermatologist. Great Falls Medical Center physician offices include a dermatology office with one physician, two physician assistants, and one advanced practice nurse. Barry Barth, CMA (AAMA), has worked in this office for 5 years and has recently assisted the office in transitioning from a paper medical records system to an electronic medical record (EMR) system. He says that although using the EMR requires spending more time with the patients at each visit, the system allows for a more thorough and systematic questioning and is getting easier and quicker to navigate. Today, Barry is assisting the physician assistants in the morning with several established patients, including six adolescent patients being treated for acne vulgaris, follow-up visits with four patients who had skin lesions removed last week, and eight new patients referred to the office from their primary care physicians for various reasons. This afternoon, Barry is assisting the physician with four minor office surgery procedures. What specialized skills would be essential for Barry to have to work efficiently and competently in this dermatology office? Is Barry at a higher risk for contracting communicable diseases compared to medical assistants working in another office such as family practice? What types of skin disorders are commonly seen in a dermatology office? These questions and others are addressed in this chapter.

The skin, or integument, is the largest organ of the body. Clear skin glowing with health indicates a good general state of wellness; pallor, cyanosis, or dry, scaly skin indicates poor general health. Although it has many functions, including maintaining homeostasis, one of the most important functions of the integumentary system is to protect the underlying tissues and organs from the external environment. Figure 28-1 shows a cross section of the normal anatomy of the skin and accessory structures. Unbroken skin provides a protective barrier that prevents the entrance of microorganisms and is the body's first line of defense against infection. In addition, the skin protects the body from mechanical injury, damaging substances, and the ultraviolet rays of the sun. The study of the skin is dermatology, and a physician who specializes in disorders of the skin is a dermatologist. The general practice physician may diagnose diseases of the integumentary system or may refer patients to the dermatologist.

### ✎ CHECKPOINT QUESTION

1. How would Barry explain how the skin prevents infectious microorganisms from entering the body?

## ⬡ COMMON DISORDERS OF THE INTEGUMENTARY SYSTEM

### Skin Infections

Many integumentary disorders are manifested by lesions or abnormalities in skin tissue (Fig. 28-2A–P). These lesions may be primary or secondary to primary lesions. When working with a patient who may have a skin infection, you should always wear protective equipment, such as examination gloves, since the drainage from any lesions may be infective.

### Bacterial Infections

#### Impetigo

**Impetigo** is a contagious bacterial infection of the skin that is common in young children. It may be caused by Staphylococcus or Streptococcus microorganisms. Lesions appear on exposed areas, such as the face and neck. Terms used to describe many skin lesions, not

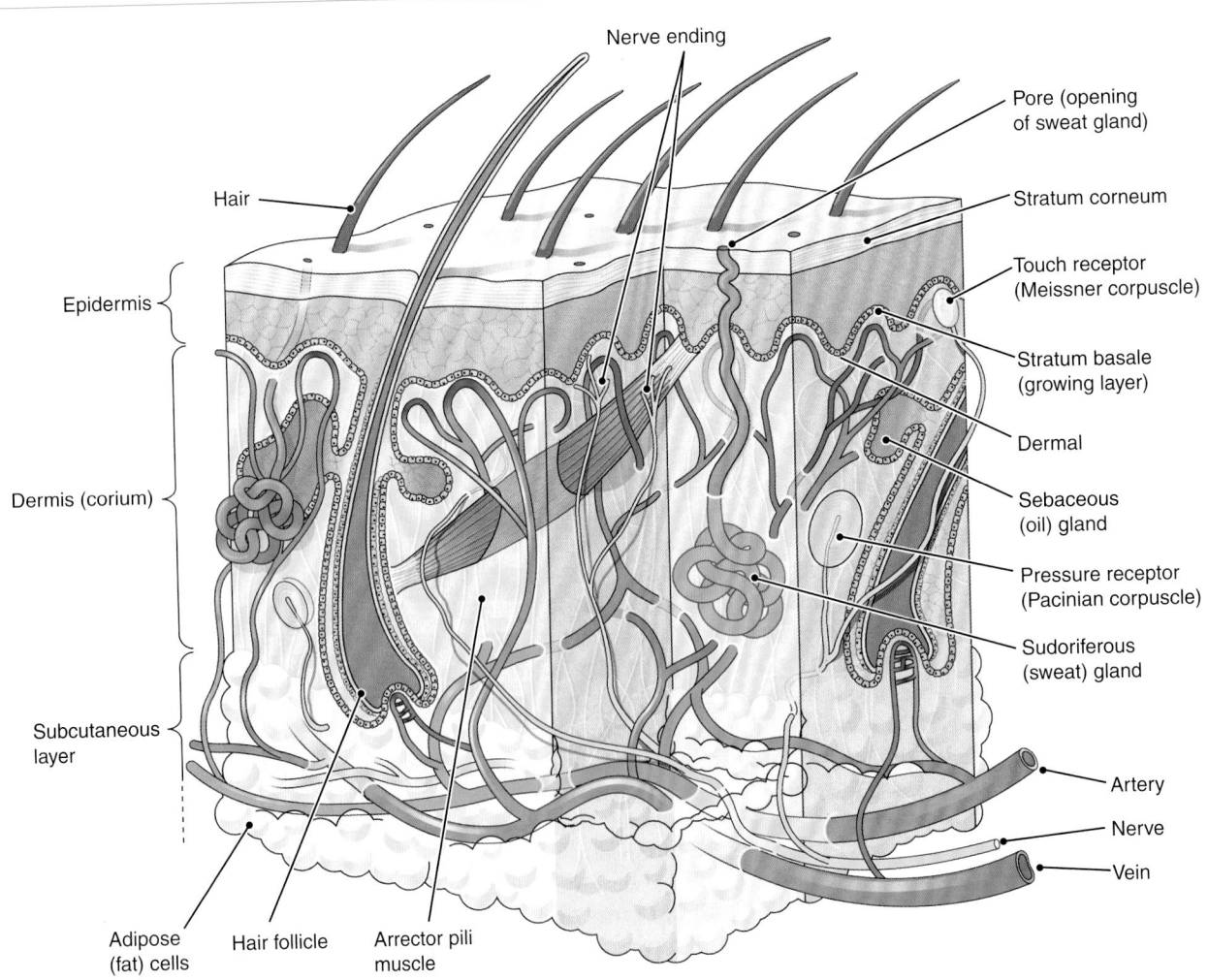

**FIGURE 28-1** • Cross-section of the skin. (Reprinted from Cohen BJ. *Memmler's The Human Body in Health and Disease*, 11th ed. Philadelphia, PA: Lippincott Williams & Wilkins, 2009, with permission.)

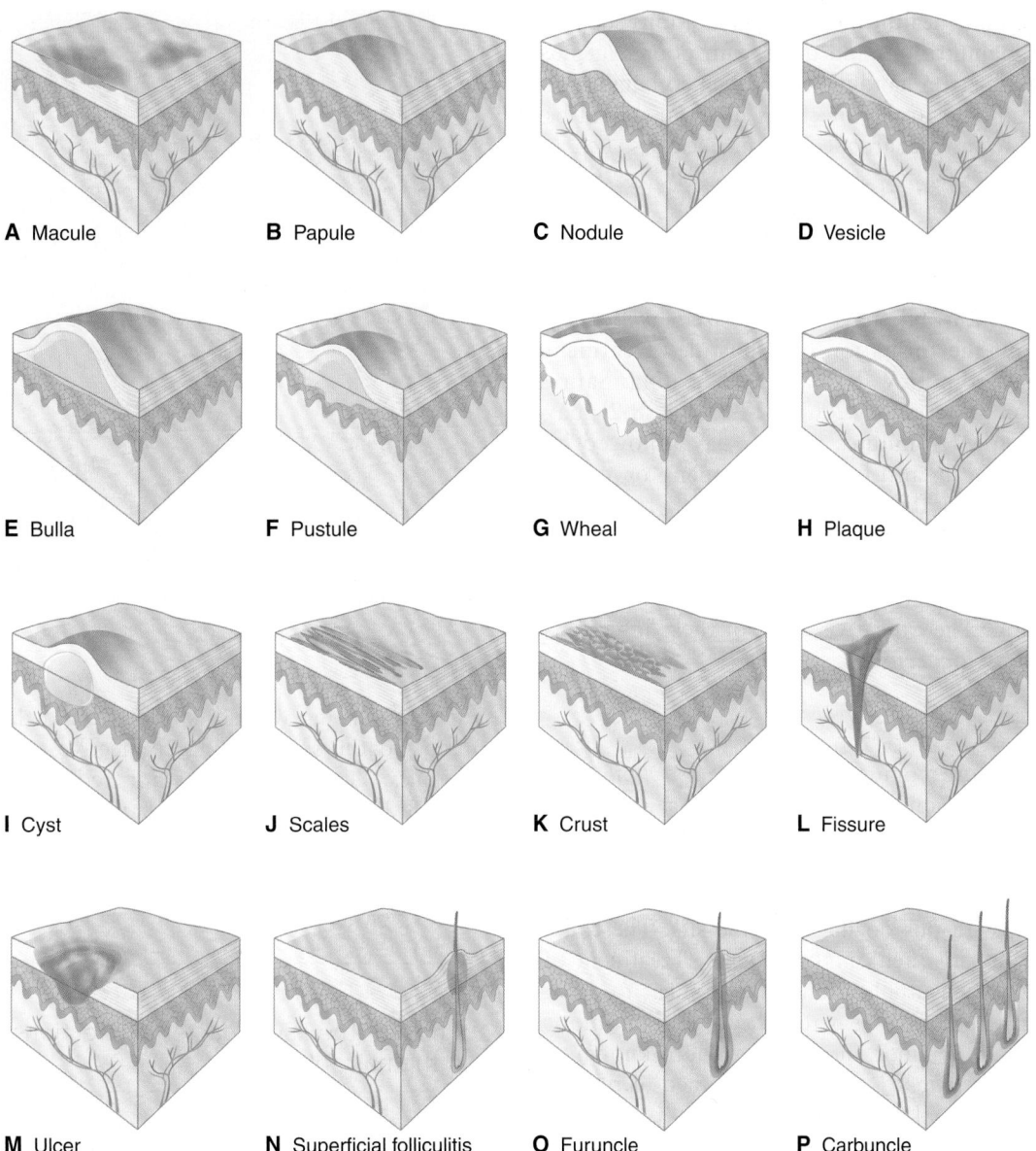

**FIGURE 28-2 •** Skin lesions. Primary lesions: **(A)** Macule. Flat, circumscribed discoloration. **(B)** Papule. Palpable elevated solid lesion smaller than 1 cm; colors vary. **(C)** Nodule. Raised solid lesion larger than 1 cm. **(D)** Vesicle. Small elevation filled with clear fluid. **(E)** Bulla. Vesicle or blister larger than 1 cm. **(F)** Pustule. Lesion containing pus. **(G)** Wheal. Transient elevation of the skin caused by edema of the dermis and surrounding capillary dilation. **(H)** Plaque. Elevated solid lesion on skin or mucosa; larger than 1 cm. **(I)** Cyst. Tumor that contains semisolid or liquid material. Secondary lesions: **(J)** Scales. Heaped-up horny layer of dead epidermis. **(K)** Crust. Covering formed from serum, blood, or pus drying on the skin. **(L)** Fissures. Cracks in the skin. **(M)** Ulcer. Lesion formed by local destruction of the epidermis and part of the underlying dermis. Other lesions: **(N)** Superficial folliculitis. Local infection of a hair follicle. **(O)** Furuncle. Acute inflammation deep within hair follicle. **(P)** Carbuncle. Infection involving subcutaneous tissues around several hair follicles.

just those seen in a patient with impetigo, include the following:

**Macule:** small, flat skin discoloration (see Fig. 28-2A)
**Vesicle:** small fluid-filled sac (see Fig. 28-2D)
**Bulla:** large fluid-filled sac (see Fig. 28-2E)
**Pustule:** pus-filled sac (see Fig. 28-2F)

Initially, impetigo may appear as an area of **erythema**; however, patches of vesicles that produce honey-colored drainage and crusts follow the redness (see Fig. 28-2K). These vesicles leave red areas when the crusts are removed. Treatment is washing the area two or three times a day and applying a topical antibiotic as ordered by the physician. Oral antibiotics may also be prescribed for severe cases. Scratching must be discouraged to prevent the spread of the infection, and patients must be instructed to wash towels, washcloths, and bed linens daily. Individuals at risk for developing impetigo are those in poor health, those with conditions such as anemia or malnutrition, and those with poor hygiene; however, any person handling contaminated laundry or otherwise exposed to the infectious material should be encouraged to practice frequent medical asepsis such as handwashing.

## Folliculitis

**Folliculitis** is a superficial infection of a hair follicle (see Fig. 28-2N). It is characterized by itching, burning, and the formation of a pustule. Treatment is aimed at promoting drainage and healing. Saline soaks or compresses (Procedures 28-1 and 28-2) may be ordered for 15 minutes twice a day followed by application of an anti-infective ointment or cream and a dressing to absorb any drainage. If folliculitis is left untreated, it may lead to the formation of an abscess. An abscess is formed when a small sac of pus, or purulent material, accumulates at the site of inflammation. The causative agent of these infections is often *Staphylococcus*.

## Furuncle

A **furuncle**, more commonly known as a *boil*, is a deep-seated infection of a hair follicle or gland (see Fig. 28-2O). Friction and pressure at the site may contribute to its formation. A hard, painful nodule forms (see Fig. 28-2C), enlarges for several days, and then erupts, with pus oozing from the site. The cause of the infection is often *Staphylococcus*. Treatment of a furuncle includes application of moist heat to assist in ripening it, or bringing it to a head, and antibiotic therapy. Often, a minor surgical procedure known as *incision and drainage (I & D)* is performed to remove the purulent material and facilitate healing. (Chapter 22 discusses incision and drainage in detail.)

## Carbuncle

A **carbuncle** consists of infection in an interconnected group of hair follicles or several furuncles joined together in a mass (see Fig. 28-2P). The subcutaneous tissue in the surrounding area is also involved, and *Staphylococcus* is often responsible. Carbuncles are hard, round, extremely painful swellings that enlarge over several days to a week. Eventually, they soften and erupt, discharging pus from several sites. When the skin sloughs away, a scarred cavity remains. The patient often has a fever.

Treatment of a carbuncle is with systemic antibiotics, moist heat (Procedures 28-1 and 28-2), and incision and drainage once the lesion has matured. A topical anti-infective agent and loose bandages are also applied to the area. The site may require a wick, or sterile gauze packing, to remain in the cavity for several days to facilitate healing.

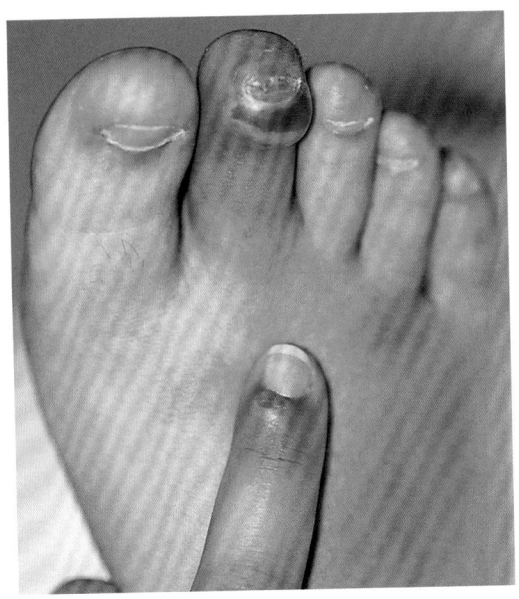

**FIGURE 28-3** • Cellulitis infection.

## Cellulitis

When an existing wound is infected and the infection spreads to the surrounding connective tissue, **cellulitis** results. The skin becomes hot, red, and edematous (Fig. 28-3). If it is not treated, the underlying tissue may be destroyed or develop an abscess. A systemic anti-infective, such as an antibiotic, usually provides rapid and successful treatment.

 **CHECKPOINT QUESTION**

2. Which of the listed bacterial infections develop in the hair follicles?

---

## PATIENT EDUCATION

### MRSA

A strain of *Staphylococcus aureus* bacteria that must be considered as the cause of some skin infections is **methicillin-resistant Staphylococcus aureus** or MRSA (pronounced "mersa"). This microorganism is resistant to many antibiotics used to treat common staphylococcus skin infections. Patients who become infected with MRSA in a health care setting such as a hospital or long-term care facility have health care–associated MRSA (HA-MRSA), while those who become infected in the community have community-associated MRSA (CA-MRSA). In a health care facility, MRSA may be contracted as a result of invasive procedures such as surgeries and intravenous or urinary catheters. In the community, MRSA is contracted through direct contact (skin to skin) with the microorganism. The microorganism may

## PATIENT EDUCATION
### (CONTINUED)

be present on objects or the skin of people who are not infected. Symptoms of CA-MRSA include one or more painful skin boils that eventually drain purulent material. Diagnosis is made by obtaining a culture of the exudates and sending to a lab for evaluation of the causative microbe.

People at risk include those who live in crowded living spaces, child care workers, students who participate in contact sports such as wrestling, and anyone who is immunosuppressed. Treatment includes incision and drainage (I & D) of the abscessed area and the administration of specific antibiotics that are effective at killing the microorganism. Although hospitalized patients are typically placed in isolation to prevent the spread of this microorganism, patients may be seen in the medical office. The following preventative measures should be taken by health care personnel working with patients with skin infections:

- Frequent handwashing. Hand sanitizer may be used when access to soap and water are not possible; however, the product should be at least 60% alcohol.
- Cover wounds. Infected areas should be covered with sterile dressings and bandages until completely healed to prevent infected exudate from coming into contact with other areas of the body, other people, or objects in the environment.
- After each patient encounter, sanitize and disinfect items in the exam room, such as the exam table, that come into contact with patients.

Patient education must include the preventative measures noted above and should also include these:

- Avoid sharing personal items such as towels, sheets, razors, clothing, and athletic equipment. MRSA spreads on contaminated objects as well as through direct contact.
- Personal hygiene should include frequent showers, especially for student athletes after athletic games or practices. Showering should include the use of soap and water.
- Towels and bed linens should be washed frequently in hot water using an appropriate laundry detergent and the addition of bleach if possible. Washed items should be dried in a hot dryer.

Your role may also include educating family and the general community about MRSA including preventative measures. Because of the negative stigma that some patients and their families have about MRSA, education and a nonjudgmental attitude will go a long way toward reducing fear and preventing the spread of this microbe!

# Viral Infections

## Herpes Simplex

**Herpes simplex** infections produce lesions commonly known as *cold sores* or *fever blisters*. The lesions, which appear on the lips, mouth, face, and nose, are small vesicles grouped on a red base. They eventually erupt, leaving a painful ulcer and then a crust. The infection may be precipitated by other infections, such as upper respiratory infections, or by menstruation, fatigue, trauma, stress, or exposure to the sun.

The causative agent is herpes simplex virus I (HSVI). Herpes simplex II is responsible for the sexually transmitted disease known as *genital herpes*. Typically, HSVI infections are recurrent, and no effective treatment eliminates or controls the disease. During an outbreak, the lesions appear and demonstrate the characteristics noted earlier and should be considered infectious. Antiviral drugs, such as valacyclovir or acyclovir, have been shown to decrease the severity of the outbreaks in some people, but they do not offer a cure. Treatment is aimed at relieving discomfort with topical anesthetic ointment to relieve the pain until the lesions heal, usually in 5 to 7 days.

## Herpes Zoster

**Herpes zoster**, or shingles, is caused by the same virus that causes chicken pox. It is believed that after an initial infection with the varicella virus, the virus lies dormant in the nervous system for years. Herpes zoster usually occurs in adults and may become active in times of physical or emotional stress or immunosuppression. When reactivated, the virus spreads down a nerve to the skin, causing redness, swelling, and pain. After about 48 hours, a band of lesions develops (Fig. 28-4).

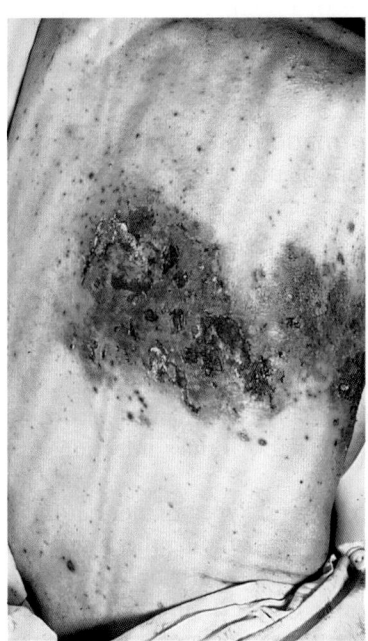

**FIGURE 28-4** • Herpes zoster (shingles).

They begin as papules, which are small, red solid elevations on the skin (see Fig. 28-2B). Shingles commonly appear on the face, back, and chest and are frequently unilateral. These lesions progress to vesicles and pustules and then dry crusts and may last for 2 to 5 weeks. Scarring and alterations in pigmentation are common. Pain often remains after the lesions have disappeared, in some cases for several months.

The treatment of a herpes zoster breakout includes an opioid analgesic for the discomfort or nerve block for severe pain. Locally, calamine lotion may be used for itching. The area must be protected from air and the irritation of clothing. Antiviral medications such as acyclovir or Valtrex may be prescribed to alleviate the severity of the disease. A vaccine for shingles is available, and although it may not prevent an outbreak, it may decrease the course and duration of the disease.

## Verruca

A **verruca** is a wart, or squamous cell papilloma (benign skin tumor), that appears as a rough, raised lesion with a pitted surface. Verruca may occur singly or in groups and may be found anywhere on the skin or mucous membranes. They commonly appear on the fingers, hands, or feet and may vary in size, shape, and appearance. The causative agents include papilloma viruses, and the treatment is removal. Removing a wart may be achieved with keratolytic agents, which cause softening and shedding of the skin; liquid nitrogen, which freezes and destroys the affected tissue; podophyllum resin, a caustic agent found in many over-the-counter wart medications; laser therapy, which removes the affected tissue using radiation of the visible infrared spectrum of light; or surgical excision. They may also disappear spontaneously.

 **CHECKPOINT QUESTION**

3. What information could Barry use to inform patients about preventing viral skin infections?

## Fungal Infections

Fungal infection of the skin (**dermatophytosis**) is caused by a group of molds called *dermatophytes*. The group of fungal diseases called tinea is collectively known as *ringworm*; its members are named according to the area of the body infected. All tinea infections are considered contagious.

There are several types of dermatophytes, but the treatment is similar, including the application of topical antifungal powders, creams, or shampoos. Antifungal medications such as griseofulvin may be prescribed orally for severe cases. Inflamed lesions may be treated with wet compresses or soaks.

## Tinea Capitis

Tinea capitis affects the scalp. It is contagious and appears most frequently in children. It is characterized by round gray scaly patches (dried skin flakes) and areas of **alopecia** (baldness). There are usually no symptoms except light itching.

## Tinea Corporis

Tinea corporis (also known as tinea circinata) manifests on hairless portions of the body. It is characterized by itchy red rings that are clear in the center with a scaly border (see Fig. 28-2J). It is frequently found on the face and arms but may also be found on the trunk (Fig. 28-5).

## Tinea Cruris

Tinea cruris, known in lay terms as jock itch, is found on the skin in the groin area and the gluteal folds. The lesions, which cause marked itching, are red macules with clear centers and scaly borders.

## Tinea Pedis

Tinea pedis, or athlete's foot, is characterized by itching, burning, and stinging between the toes and on the soles of the feet. The lesions may appear as red, weepy vesicles, as chronic dry scales, or as fissures (crack-like lesions) between the toes (see Fig. 28-2L).

## Tinea Unguium

Also known as onychomycosis, tinea unguium causes thickening, discoloration, and crumbling of the nails, most often the toenails. It is difficult to cure and often requires months of local antifungal preparations. In severe cases, an oral antifungal medication, griseofulvin, is prescribed.

## Tinea Versicolor

Tinea versicolor, also known as pityriasis versicolor, is a fungal infection; however, it is not caused by dermatophytes. It is not known exactly what sort of

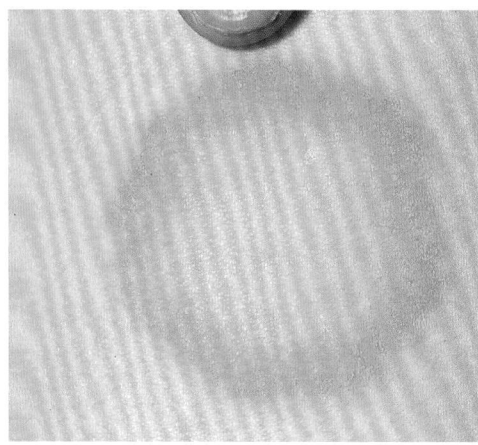

**FIGURE 28-5** • Tinea corporis (ringworm) fungal infection.

fungus is the causative agent. The disease causes a multicolor rash, generally over the upper trunk. It is most common in young people during warm weather, and it is chronic. Its lesions vary from macular to raised, round, or oval, vary from darkly pigmented to depigmented, and are slightly scaly. There are usually no symptoms. Diagnosis of tinea versicolor is determined with a Wood light, an ultraviolet light used in a darkened room to show abnormalities in the skin as fluorescent. Treatment includes the use of selenium sulfide for 7 days along with topical antifungal cream or lotion.

 **CHECKPOINT QUESTION**

4. A new patient has a skin lesion and asks Barry to "touch it." Why should Barry avoid direct contact with skin lesions?

 **AFF  PATIENT EDUCATION**

### Preventing Fungal Infections

Because fungi thrive in moist conditions, a general measure for treating fungal infections and preventing the spread of infection is to keep the infected area clean and dry. Instruct patients diagnosed with fungal infections to wear loose-fitting clothing and launder clothing daily. Socks and underclothing should be changed frequently, and clothing should not be shared with others. Shower shoes should be worn in public showers and pools since these areas are usually wet, providing an optimum environment for the fungus to grow on floors and be transmitted directly to the feet.

## Parasitic Infections

### Scabies

Scabies is a contagious skin disorder caused by the itch mite *Sarcoptes scabiei*. It is spread by direct contact and produces small vesicles or pustules between the fingers and at the inner wrist, elbows, axillae, waist, and groin. The itching caused by the mite is worst at night, when the female burrows under the epidermis to lay her eggs.

Treatment for scabies is aimed at disinfestation. For adults, an antiparasitic such as 1% lindane cream is applied from the neck down at bedtime. One application of 5% permethrin, or Elimite, cream is effective and is the drug of choice for children. All bedding and clothing for the entire family should be laundered daily until the infestation is resolved.

### Pediculosis

**Pediculosis** is an infestation of the skin with a parasite known commonly as *lice*. Three types of the louse *Pediculus humanus* infest the body: *P. humanis* var. *capitis* infests the scalp (pediculosis capitis) and the eyelashes or eyelids (pediculosis palpebrarum); and *P. humanis* var. *corporis* or var. *vestimenti* is found on the body (pediculosis corporis) and the pubic hairs (pediculosis pubis). Wherever they are found, itching is intense, and the skin often becomes secondarily infected from scratching. Lice feed on human blood and lay eggs (nits) on body hair or clothing fibers. Nits may be seen on hair shafts close to the skin or in seams of clothing.

Pediculosis is common among populations with overcrowding, such as head lice in schools, and poor hygiene. The infestation is transmitted through physical contact with an infested person, by sitting on an infested toilet seat, or by sharing a comb, brush, clothing, or bedding that is infested. Benzene hexachloride creams, lotions, or shampoos are used for all types of pediculosis. All clothing and linen must be dry cleaned or washed in hot water and ironed. Sealing items in plastic bags for 30 days or heating them to 140°F will kill lice on items that cannot be laundered.

 **CHECKPOINT QUESTION**

5. How are parasitic skin infections spread?

## Inflammatory Reactions

### Eczema

**Eczema** is an inflammatory skin disorder usually involving only the epidermal layer of the skin. It is more common in children than adults and is characterized by itching and lesions that generally begin as red patches, proceed to weepy vesicles, and end up as dry scaly crusts (Fig. 28-6). They appear on the face, neck, bends of the knees and elbows, and the upper trunk. It is not clear why some patients develop this disorder, which is chronic and may have periods of remission and exacerbation. Possible causes of eczema depend on the individual and may include the following:

- Food allergies to fish, eggs, and milk products
- Medication or chemical allergies

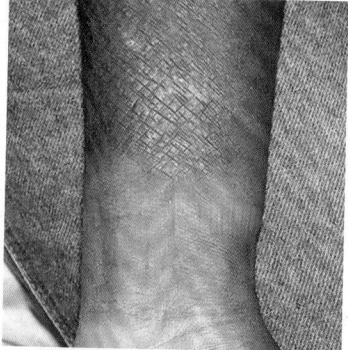

**FIGURE 28-6 •** Eczema.

- Sensitivity to irritating soaps, household cleaning products, deodorants, and perfumes
- Inhalants such as pollen, dust, or animal dander
- Poor circulation to a body part
- Ultraviolet rays

Treatment is removing the cause and promoting healing of the lesions. The causative agent should be avoided if it is known. The patient should maintain good hydration and keep the skin well moistened with emollients. A humid environment is recommended. Warm, not hot, baths should be taken daily with a nondrying soap. The skin should be dried immediately, and scratchy clothing should be avoided.

Exudative lesions are treated with soaks, baths, or wet dressings for 10 to 30 minutes three or four times daily. Domeboro™, Aveeno™, or bicarbonate is good for these purposes. In addition, the physician may order the following treatments:

- Topical corticosteroid lotion, cream, or ointment to be used twice a day.
- Bandages at night to protect against scratching.
- Antihistamines for severe **pruritus** (itching).
- For scales, a topical steroid ointment. Systemic corticosteroids, such as prednisone, may be ordered in severe cases.

## Seborrheic Dermatitis

Seborrheic dermatitis (skin inflammation), also known as **seborrhea**, is an overproduction of sebum. It is a chronic disorder resulting in greasy yellow scales primarily on the scalp, where it is called *seborrheic dandruff*. Underlying redness and pruritus may be present. The eyelids, face, chest, back, umbilicus, and body folds may also be affected. It is thought that seborrhea is caused by a genetic predisposition and a combination of hormones, nutrition, infection, or stress. It is treated with shampoo and topical corticosteroid lotion.

## Urticaria

**Urticaria**, or hives, is an acute inflammatory reaction of the dermis. It begins with itching, followed by erythema and swelling. The wheals (see Fig. 28-2G) have a pale center with a red edge. They resemble a mosquito bite and appear in clusters anywhere on the body. Hives are self-limiting, lasting from a few days to a few weeks. The most common causes include contact with these substances:

- Foods, including shellfish, strawberries, tomatoes, citrus fruits, eggs, and chocolate
- Inhalants, including feathers or animal dander
- Chemicals, cosmetics, and medications
- Sunlight
- Insect bites or stings
- Heat, cold, or pressure on the skin
- Infection
- Stress

Treatment of urticaria is reduction of the inflammatory response. The cause should be avoided if known. Antihistamines are usually given to reduce itching and swelling, and a short course of prednisone is sometimes ordered. Starch or Aveeno baths twice a day may be ordered to make the patient more comfortable. Epinephrine is given if the symptoms of urticaria develop rapidly and are associated with dyspnea. These symptoms are indicative of anaphylaxis, a severe life-threatening emergency (see Chapter 26).

## Acne Vulgaris

Acne vulgaris is an inflammatory disease of the sebaceous glands. Its cause is not known in all cases, and although it may occur in any adult, it more commonly occurs during adolescence as a result of the increase in hormone production. It is characterized by pimples, comedones (blackheads), cysts (fluid-filled sacs beneath the skin) (see Fig. 28-2I), and scarring. The lesions may occur on the face, neck, upper chest, back, and shoulders. Overactive sebaceous glands produce excessive sebum that gets trapped in a follicle, producing a dark substance that results in a blackhead. Leukocytes accumulate, producing pus.

Treatment for acne includes a regimen of tretinoin (Retin-A™), benzoyl peroxide, and tetracycline. Sunlamp treatments are sometimes used to dry the lesions.

## Psoriasis

**Psoriasis** is a chronic inflammatory skin disorder characterized by bright red plaques (see Fig. 28-2H) covered with dry, silvery scales. Although the cause is unknown, it is a chronic disorder and often difficult to treat. Psoriasis is usually found on the scalp, elbows, knees, base of the spine, palms, soles, and around the nails (Fig. 28-7). There are usually no vesicles, and itching varies from mild to severe. Exacerbations are common during cold weather, stress, and pregnancy. Treatment includes tar preparations and topical steroid cream or ointment. Exposure to ultraviolet light three times a week may also be prescribed.

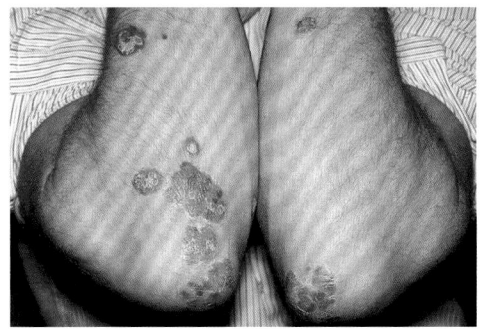

**FIGURE 28-7 •** Psoriasis.

## CHECKPOINT QUESTION

6. A patient asks Barry about the differences between eczema and psoriasis. How would Barry answer this question?

## Disorders of Wound Healing

### Keloids

Keloids, an overproduction of scar tissue, occur as a complication of wound healing. The scar tissue forms as a result of excessive collagen accumulation. A raised nodule forms and does not resolve with time. The cause is unknown. It occurs most frequently in young women, especially during pregnancy, and is particularly common in African Americans. The most common sites are the neck and shoulders. Injections of cortisone are sometimes effective in treating keloids.

## Disorders Caused by Pressure

### Callus and Corn

A callus, sometimes called a callosity, is a raised painless thickening of the epidermis. It is caused by pressure or friction on the hands and feet. A corn is a hard, raised thickening of the stratum corneum on the toes. It results from chronic friction and pressure, especially from poorly fitting shoes. The pressure compresses the dermis, making it thin and tender and causing pain and inflammation. Soft corns can form between the toes.

The treatment for calluses and corns begins with relieving the pressure. Shoes should be made of soft leather and fit properly. Liners may be inserted in shoes to relieve pressure. Bandages and corn pads also help correct the problem. In some cases, the physician recommends surgical intervention or use of a keratolytic agent to cause chemical peeling.

### Decubitus Ulcers

Decubitus ulcers are also called *pressure sores* and are caused by prolonged pressure to an area of the body, usually over a bony prominence (see Fig. 28-2M). The pressure impairs blood supply, oxygen, and nutrition to the area, which results in an ulcerative lesion and eventual tissue death. The most common sites are over the sacrum and hips, but these ulcers may also occur on the back of the head, ears, elbows, heels, and ankles (Fig 28-8). They are most common in aged, debilitated, and immobilized patients. Bedridden and wheelchair-bound patients are at risk for developing decubiti unless they are repositioned frequently, every 2 hours, to relieve pressure. Special mattresses, pads, and pillows are useful in preventing pressure sores.

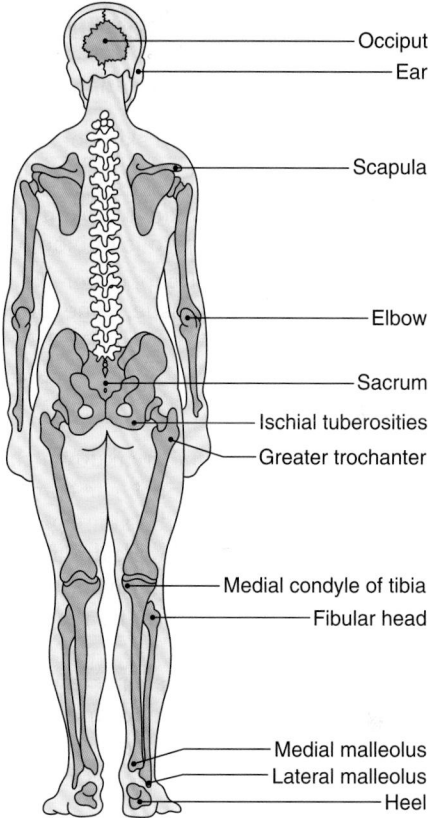

Occiput
Ear
Scapula
Elbow
Sacrum
Ischial tuberosities
Greater trochanter
Medial condyle of tibia
Fibular head
Medial malleolus
Lateral malleolus
Heel

**FIGURE 28-8** • Areas susceptible to pressure sores. (From Nettina SM. *The Lippincott Manual of Nursing Practice*, 7th ed. Philadelphia, PA: Lippincott Williams & Wilkins, 2001.)

Decubitus ulcers are graded, or staged, according to the degree of tissue involvement (Table 28-1). Treatment consists of topical antibiotic powder and adhesive absorbent bandages and dressings. Deep infections may require systemic antibiotics and possibly surgical débridement.

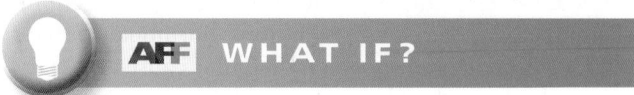

**AFF** WHAT IF?

**An elderly patient comes into the office with multiple decubitus ulcers. What should you do?**

Older adults are always at risk for developing skin ulcerations; however, the physician must assess the situation to determine whether the patient is receiving adequate care at home. Patients who arrive in the medical office with multiple ulcers in different stages of healing may be abused or neglected. Elder abuse is less often identified, but some experts believe it is as common as child abuse. If you suspect elder abuse, contact your local department of social services. The investigation may substantiate the abuse (requiring referral to law enforcement) or may identify ways to alleviate the situation (caregiver education, respite care) without removing the patient from home. In some states, the law requires reporting elder abuse. The physician who fails to do so can be fined or be subject to other penalties.

| TABLE 28-1 | Staging or Grading for Decubitus Ulcers |
|---|---|
| **Stage** | **Description** |
| I | Red skin does not return to normal when massaged or when pressure is relieved. |
| II | Skin is blistered, peeling, or cracked superficially. |
| III | Skin is broken, with loss of full thickness; subcutaneous tissue may be damaged; serous or bloody drainage may be present. |
| IV | Deep, crater-like ulcer shows destruction of subcutaneous tissue; fascia, connective tissue, bone, or muscle may be exposed and may be damaged. |

## Intertrigo

**Intertrigo** is a disorder of skin breakdown that occurs in the body folds of obese persons. The combination of heat, moisture, and friction of the skin against itself in these areas causes the skin to break down. Humid climates and poor hygiene often aggravate the condition. Erythema and skin fissures result, and the affected area itches, stings, and burns.

Treatment for intertrigo is proper hygiene and an attempt to keep the area clean and dry. Talcum powder or cornstarch is often recommended. Antibacterial or antifungal lotion or powder is necessary if secondary infection is present.

 **CHECKPOINT QUESTION**

7. What patients are most at risk for developing decubitus ulcers?

## Alopecia

Alopecia, or baldness, may be the result of physical trauma, systemic disease, bacteria or fungal infection, chemotherapy, excessive radiation, hormonal imbalance, or genetic predisposition. Baldness caused by scarring and inherited male pattern baldness are permanent and cannot be reversed; however, the drug minoxidil may be recommended by the physician to stimulate hair growth in male pattern baldness. For other causes of baldness, treatment of the underlying disorder often results in new hair growth.

## Disorders of Pigmentation

### Albinism

Albinism is a genetically determined condition of partial or total absence of the pigment melanin in the skin, hair, and eyes. The skin is pale, the hair is white, and the irises of the eyes appear pink (Fig. 28-9). The skin will not tan and is prone to sunburn. Because no pigment is present to protect the underlying eye structures from the ultraviolet rays of the sun, eye problems may develop as a result of this disorder. Albinism has no treatment.

## Vitiligo

**Vitiligo** is a progressive chronic destruction of melanocytes, which are cells in the epidermis that produce melanin, a skin pigment. This disorder is thought to be an autoimmune disorder in patients with an inherited predisposition. The depigmented areas occur as white patches that sometimes have a hyperpigmented border. It usually occurs in exposed areas of the skin.

There is no effective treatment for vitiligo. Patients are advised to protect the areas from the sun because they are prone to sunburn in the absence of melanin. Waterproof cosmetics may be used to cover the area.

## Leukoderma

Leukoderma is a permanent local loss of skin pigment that results from damage caused by skin trauma. It is particularly common in African Americans. Causes of

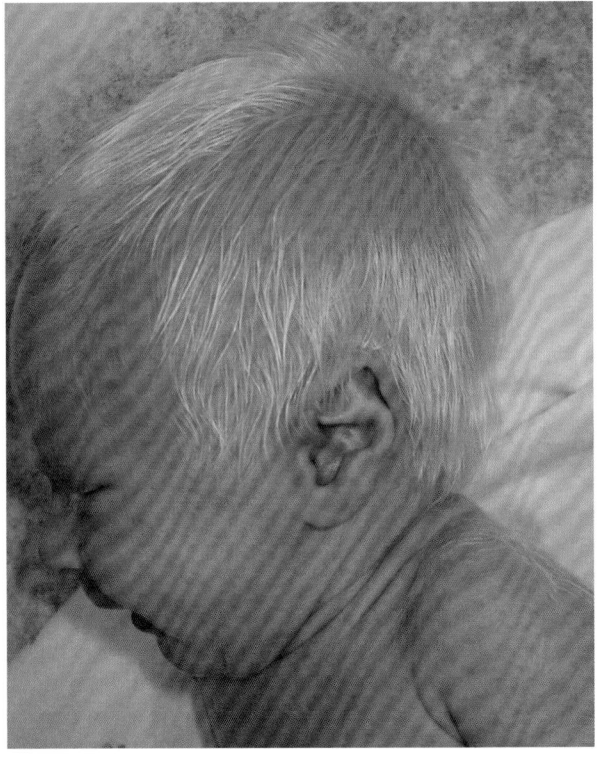

**FIGURE 28-9 •** Albinism.

**When Is a Skin Lesion Abnormal?**

Most melanomas, a type of skin cancer, are pigmented, elevated skin lesions that frequently develop from a new or existing mole. The key to treatment of this potentially deadly cancer is early detection of changes in size, color, shape, elevation, texture, or consistency of any pigmented area, old or new, or of any spot or bump. Being familiar with what is normal for you will help you notice what is abnormal.

The eventual outcome of melanoma is governed by how deeply it has invaded the skin, which also determines how aggressively the cancer will be treated. Because many skin cancers develop from overexposure to the sun, a cancer prevention message first used in Australia and currently being promoted in the United States is "Slip! Slop! Slap! Wrap!" This may help individuals to remember how to protect the skin: slip on a shirt, slop on sunscreen, slap on a hat, and put on wraparound sunglasses to protect your eyes and the skin around them.

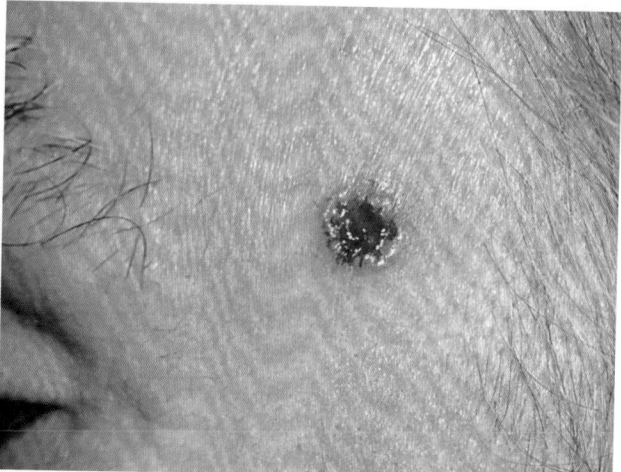

**FIGURE 28-10** • Basal cell carcinoma. (Reprinted from Goodheart HP. *Goodheart's Photoguide of Common Skin Disorders*. Philadelphia, PA: Lippincott Williams & Wilkins, 2003, with permission).

leukoderma include contact with caustic chemicals and the sequela of burns or infection.

## Nevus

A nevus, also known as a *birthmark* or *mole*, is a congenital pigmented skin blemish. It is usually circumscribed and may involve the epidermis, connective tissue, nerves, or blood vessels. Nevi are usually benign, not cancerous, but may become malignant (cancerous). Patients should be cautioned to watch for changes in the color, size, and texture of any nevus. Bleeding and itching should also be reported (Box 28-1).

### CHECKPOINT QUESTION

8. Which of the disorders of pigmentation are inherited?

## Skin Cancers

### Basal Cell Carcinoma

Basal cell carcinoma is a slow-growing cancer that appears most commonly on exposed areas of the body, usually the face, but may also occur on the shoulders or chest. The lesion has a waxy appearance with a depressed center and a rolled edge where blood vessels may be apparent. Metastasis (spreading to other areas of the body) almost never occurs, but if left untreated, the lesions will grow locally and may ulcerate and damage surrounding tissues (Fig. 28-10). The most common treatment for basal cell carcinoma is surgical removal, and this may be done in

the physician's or dermatologist's office. Radiation therapy and cryosurgery, or removal using a cold agent such as liquid nitrogen, are alternative treatments.

### Squamous Cell Carcinoma

Squamous cell carcinoma is slightly less common than basal cell carcinoma and occurs in any squamous (scaly) epithelial area of the body, such as the lungs, cervix, or anus, but is most frequently found on the skin (Fig. 28-11). This type of skin cancer is a slow-growing, malignant **neoplasm** (tumor). The lesions are firm, red, horny or prickly, and painless, and they range widely in size. Those on exposed areas are thought to result from exposure to the sun. Other areas not normally exposed, such as mucous membranes, are thought to be affected as the result of frequent irritation. Treatment is the same as for basal cell carcinoma. Although basal cell carcinoma is not generally metastatic, squamous cell carcinoma will spread readily through underlying and surrounding tissues.

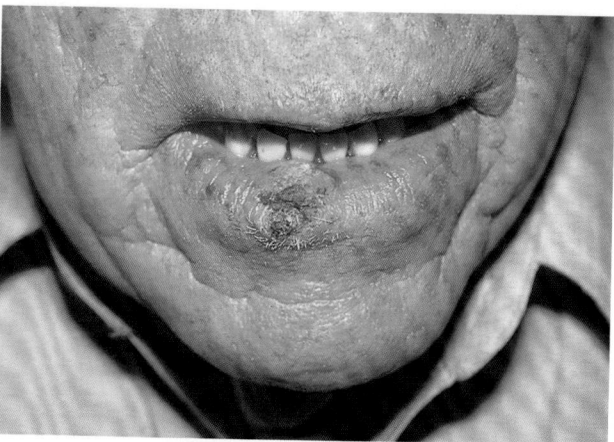

**FIGURE 28-11** • Squamous cell carcinoma. (Reprinted from Goodheart HP. Goodheart's Photoguide of Common Skin Disorders. Philadelphia, PA: Lippincott Williams & Wilkins, 2003, with permission.)

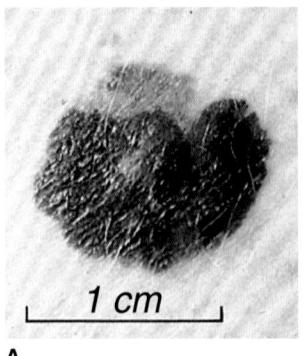 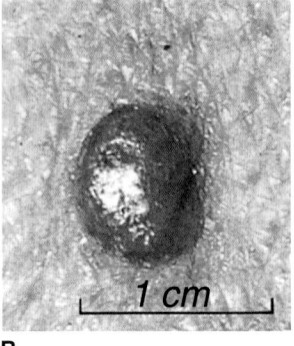

**A**    **B**

**FIGURE 28-12** • Malignant melanoma. **(A)** Superficial melanoma. **(B)** Nodular melanoma.

## Malignant Melanoma

Malignant melanoma is a cancer of the skin that forms from melanocytes. Lesions vary from macules to nodules and often have an irregular border and a variety of colors (Fig. 28-12). Mixtures of white, blue, purple, and red are the most common. The tumor grows both in radius and in depth into the dermis. The American Cancer Society notes that melanoma is primarily a disease of whites, who are 10 times more likely to have a melanoma compared to African Americans. The rates for men getting this type of cancer are 50% higher than for women.

Risk factors for developing malignant melanoma include a personal or family history of melanoma and the presence of multiple moles. In some cases, skin cancer grows in a pre-existing nevus, so patients should be encouraged to have new, unusual, or changing skin lesions evaluated by the physician. Other risk factors include those for all types of skin cancer: sensitivity to the sun (e.g., fair skin, blond or red hair) and a history of sunburns, tanning, pre-existing immunosuppressive diseases, and a past history of basal or squamous cell skin cancers (Box 28-2).

Treatment of malignant melanoma is surgical removal after a biopsy, possibly including removal of

---

### BOX 28-2    Effects of Sunlight on the Skin

In addition to sunburn and premature aging, exposure to the sun's ultraviolet rays is the major cause of skin cancers. Primary prevention of skin cancer consists of limiting exposure to ultraviolet light by wearing proper clothing and using sunscreen. Exposure to the sun is not recommended during the 5 peak hours of the day: 10:00 AM to 3:00 PM A sunscreen with at least a 15 SPF (sun protective factor) is considered good protection in blocking ultraviolet rays. Although many sunscreens contain PABA (aminobenzoic acid), which may cause allergy in some people, a number of PABA-free sunscreens are available. Exposure to ultraviolet rays through the use of sunlamps and tanning beds should also be discouraged.

---

lymph tissue. The patient's prognosis depends on the depth of the tumor. Tumors over 1.5 mm often metastasize to the lymph nodes, liver, lungs, and brain and are often fatal.

### CHECKPOINT QUESTION

9. Which is more likely to metastasize, basal cell or squamous cell carcinoma?

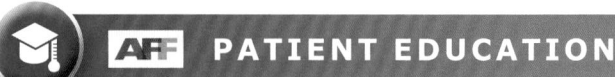

### PATIENT EDUCATION

#### Playing It Safe in the Sun

During the summertime, many teenagers enjoy lying on the beach and acquiring a tan, while others are exposed to the sun by working outdoors in jobs such as lifeguarding. These two habits can lead to long-term skin problems. As a medical assistant, you can help educate teenagers about these risks. The following patient education tips are useful reminders for any patient who is exposed to excessive sunlight:

- The powerful rays of the sun can injure your eyes. Always wear sunglasses.
- Even one sunburn can increase your potential for developing skin cancer.
- A hat can prevent sunburn on the scalp. Also, a hat can help keep the sun away from the face.
- Use the highest level of sun block that is available. Apply it frequently.
- Do not apply oil to the skin to tan faster.
- Avoid lying on the beach during peak sun hours. Enjoy beach activities during the early morning or late afternoon.

## DIAGNOSTIC PROCEDURES

### Physical Examination of the Skin

Examination of the skin is performed primarily by inspection. Many lesions can be diagnosed by the characteristic size, shape, and distribution on the skin; however, laboratory studies may be necessary to confirm a diagnosis. As the medical assistant, you may assemble the equipment as directed by the physician, verify that an informed consent has been obtained for surgical procedures, and properly direct specimens to the appropriate laboratories. Observe standard precautions when handling any specimens, including those obtained from the skin.

Before the examination, prepare the examination room and the patient. Use a gown and draping appropriate to the patient's symptoms and area to be examined. During the examination, aid the physician by ensuring that the lighting is adequate and directed properly, assisting in obtaining wound cultures, maintaining asepsis, and applying topical medications, sterile dressings, and bandages. Protect skin lesions from further infection by using medical or surgical asepsis as indicated.

After the dermatologic examination, reinforce the physician instructions about caring for the skin condition at home, including the following:

- Keeping bandages clean and dry
- Returning to the office to have sutures or staples removed
- How long to avoid getting the area wet
- Applying topical medications

When the patient has left the office, clean and disinfect the examination room according to the office policy.

## Wound Cultures

Obtain a wound culture by getting a sample of wound exudate (drainage) using a sterile swab, applying the specimen to a growth medium, and allowing the microorganisms to grow. A sample of the culture is typically collected by the medical assistant and sent to an outside laboratory. At the laboratory, the specimen is placed on a slide and observed under a microscope to diagnose the type of the bacterial or fungal infection. Chapter 44 describes the specific procedure for collecting a wound specimen and preparing the specimen for transport to an outside laboratory.

### CHECKPOINT QUESTION

10. What are the responsibilities of Barry as a professional medical assistant with regard to diagnosing skin lesions?

## Skin Biopsy

The purpose of a skin biopsy is to remove a small piece of tissue from a lesion so that it may be examined under a microscope to determine whether it is a benign or malignant growth. A local anesthetic is injected by the physician, and sterile asepsis is used throughout the procedure (see Chapter 22). The three types of skin biopsy performed by the physician are excision, punch, and shave. In an excision biopsy, the entire lesion is removed for evaluation. When a punch biopsy is done, a small section is removed from the center of the lesion. A shave biopsy cuts the lesion off just above the skin line. Regardless of the method used to obtain the skin biopsy, samples of tissue are sent to the laboratory for analysis.

## Urine Melanin

Melanin is not normally present in the urine unless the patient has malignant melanoma. A urine test to detect the presence of melanin is done with a random sample

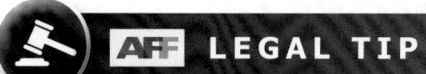

### LEGAL TIP

## Informed Consent

Some dermatology procedures, such as biopsies, are invasive and require a sample of tissue for analysis. Although some office procedures may be considered "minor," patients must always be informed of the actual procedure and the potential risks involved. It is in the best interest of the medical office to have consent forms signed no matter how minor the surgical procedure.

Although the physician is responsible for informing the patient about the procedure, including the benefits and risks, it is the responsibility of the medical assistant to make sure the consent form is signed and in the medical record before the procedure is started. In some cases, you may be asked to obtain the signature of the patient on the consent form. This is acceptable; however, if the patient has specific questions about the procedure or feels unsure if this is the right decision, always let the physician know before the patient signs the form so that questions and concerns can be addressed. It is always better to err on the side of caution than proceed without a signed consent form or with a signed form when the patient was not truly informed.

of urine from the patient. The specimen is sent to the laboratory, allowed to sit for 24 hours, and then examined under a microscope for the presence of melanin. Chapter 45 describes the procedure for instructing a patient on collecting a urine sample and transporting the sample to the laboratory.

## Wood Light Analysis

Wood light is a dark, ultraviolet light that is used to primarily detect a fungal infection. However, alterations in pigment, scabies, and other types of infections may also be detected with a Wood light. Normally, the skin does not appear fluorescent when exposed to this type of ultraviolet light. Any areas that appear fluorescent when exposed to a Wood light are considered abnormal and can be diagnosed by the physician and treated accordingly. This procedure is not invasive and requires no preparation by the patient or the medical assistant; however, any creams or ointments may need to be removed before using the Wood light on the skin.

### CHECKPOINT QUESTION

11. A patient in the dermatology office is concerned about having a skin biopsy. Why are skin biopsies performed?

## ᴄᴏɢ  BANDAGING

Bandages are strips of woven materials, typically absorbent, that are used for many purposes, such as

1. Applying pressure to control bleeding
2. Holding a dressing in place
3. Protecting dressings and wounds from contamination
4. Immobilizing an injured part of the body
5. Supporting an injured part of the body

### Types of Bandages

• *Roller bandages* are soft woven materials packaged in a roll. Roller bandages are available in various lengths and widths from 1 inch to 6 or more inches (Fig. 28-13). The bandage size used depends on the part being bandaged and the desired thickness of the completed bandage. Most bandages are made of a porous, lightweight material and may be either sterile or clean. Gauze bandages conform easily to angular surfaces of the body. A crepe-like stretchy gauze is made to adjust to various body contours and resists unrolling much better than plain roller gauze. Kling and Conform are two frequently used brands.

• *Elastic bandages*, such as the Ace brand, are special bandage rolls with elastic woven throughout the fabric (Fig. 28-14). They are generally brownish tan. Unlike other types of roller gauze, elastic bandages can be given to the patient to take home to be washed and reused many times. Because of the elastic fibers, great care must be exercised when applying the bandage to prevent compromising circulation and still provide support to the injured part. Elastic bandages should be applied without wrinkling in concentric or overlapping layers.

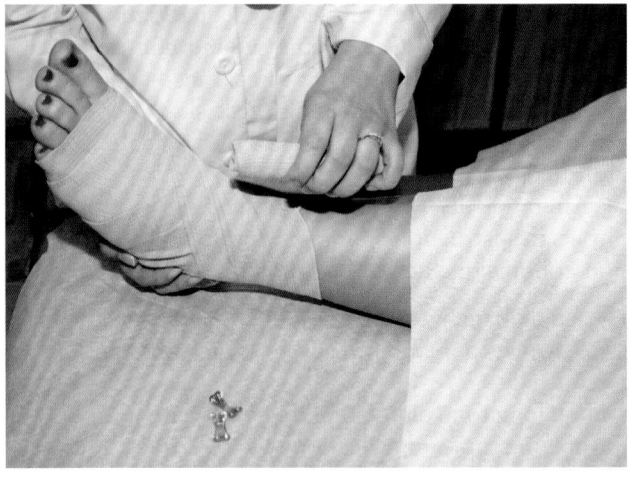

**FIGURE 28-14** • An elastic bandage.

Bandages should fit snugly but not too tightly. Adjust the bandage if it seems too loose or if the patient says it is uncomfortable or tight. Some elastic bandages have an adhesive backing, which helps keep the layers in place and provides a secure, snug, and comfortable fit. To avoid applying it too tightly, never stretch or pull on the elastic bandage during application. Ask the patient how tight the bandage feels as it is being applied, and instruct the patient on signs of impaired circulation by checking the extremity distal to the bandage for the following indications:

• Increased swelling or pain
• Pale skin
• Cool skin compared to the other extremity

• *Tubular gauze bandages* are used to enclose rounded body parts. The bandage resembles a hollow tube and is very stretchy (Fig. 28-15). It is used to enclose fingers, toes, arms, and legs and even the head and trunk. Tubular gauze bandages are available in various widths to fit any part of the body from 1/2 inch to 7 inches. Tubular gauze is

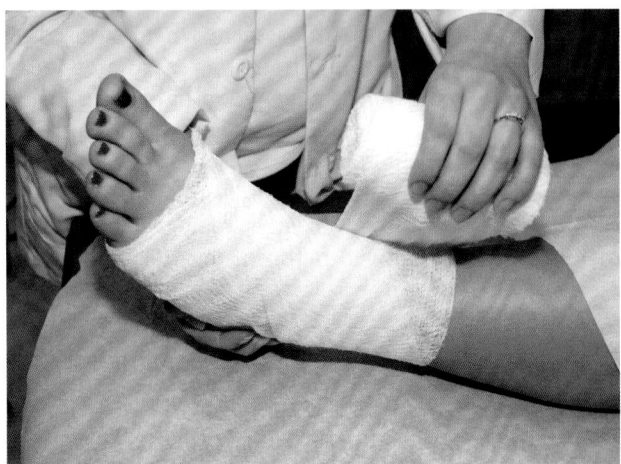

**FIGURE 28-13** • Gauze roller bandage.

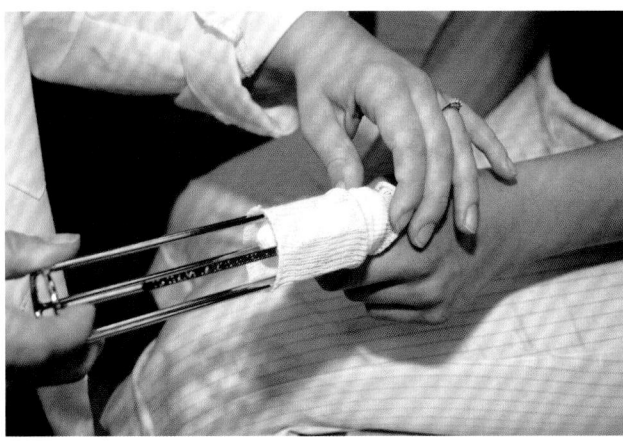

**FIGURE 28-15** • A tubular bandage.

applied using a metal or plastic tubular frame-like applicator. The applicator is available in various sizes and should be slightly larger than the body part to be covered. This enables the gauze to slide easily over the body part. Applicators are marked according to a size number that corresponds to different sizes of tubular gauze. Procedure 28-3 describes the specific steps for applying a tubular gauze bandage.

## Bandage Application Guidelines

When properly applied, bandages should feel comfortably snug and should be fastened securely enough to remain in place until removed. Bandages can be fastened with safety pins, adhesive tape, or clips. You gain the patient's confidence when you apply a bandage that is comfortable and neat looking and that stays in place. Patients become understandably upset when bandages fall off during normal activities. The following are general guidelines for applying bandages:

1. Observe the principles of medical asepsis, including handwashing, to prevent the transfer of pathogens. Surgical asepsis is not necessary. The bandage may be used to cover a sterile dressing or may be used alone if there is no open wound.
2. Keep the area to be bandaged and the bandage itself dry and clean because moisture may wick bacteria into the wound. A moist bandage encourages the growth of pathogens and is uncomfortable for the patient.
3. Never place a bandage directly over an open wound. Apply a sterile dressing first, and cover it with a bandage for protection. The bandage should extend approximately 1 to 2 inches beyond the edge of the dressing.
4. Never allow skin surfaces of two body parts to touch each other under a bandage. Wound healing may cause opposing surfaces to adhere and result in scar tissue formation. For example, burned fingers must be dressed separately but may be bandaged together.
5. Pad joints and any bony prominence to help prevent skin irritation caused by the bandage rubbing against the skin over a bony area.
6. Bandage the affected part in the normal position: joints should be slightly flexed to avoid muscle strain, discomfort, and pain. Muscle spasms may occur if the part is made to assume an unnatural position.
7. Apply bandages beginning at the distal part and extending to the proximal part of the body. Bandage turns that extend distal to proximal aid in return

of venous blood to the heart and help make the bandage more secure.
8. Always talk with the patient during the bandaging. If the patient complains that it is too tight or too loose, adjust the bandage. Instruct the patient to do the same at home. The bandage should fit snugly, but if it is too tight, it may impair circulation. If it is too loose, it may fall off.
9. When bandaging hands and feet, leave the fingers and toes exposed whenever possible to make it easier to check for circulatory impairment. If the skin feels cold or looks pale, the nail beds look cyanotic, or the patient complains of swelling, numbness, or tingling of the toes or fingers, remove the bandage immediately and reapply it correctly.

Figure 28-16A–F illustrates various techniques for wrapping bandages.

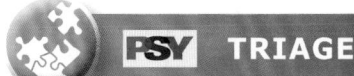

## PSY TRIAGE

While working in a medical office setting, the following three situations occur:

A. The physician has asked you to apply a new dressing to a 24-year-old man who lacerated his finger today and just had four sutures inserted by the physician.
B. The receptionist informs you that a patient has arrived and signed in but is complaining of a rash that is "itching." The receptionist is concerned that the scratching patient may be contagious, and she would like him put into an examination room right away.
C. A 32-year-old woman is waiting in the procedure room to have a suspicious mole removed from her back. You need to set up the sterile tray for this minor office surgical procedure.

**How do you sort these patients? Who do you see first? Second? Third?**

Patient B should be taken directly to an examination room since the cause for the patient's symptom (itching) is not known. If you will be expected to assist the physician with the minor surgical procedure, it would be best to take care of patient A because applying a dressing should take only a few minutes. After applying the dressing and discharging the patient, then you can set up for the surgical procedure and assist the physician. However, if your physician does not usually require you to assist during minor procedures, it might be more logical to set up for the procedure then apply the dressing to patient A, allowing plenty of time for wound care instructions if necessary.

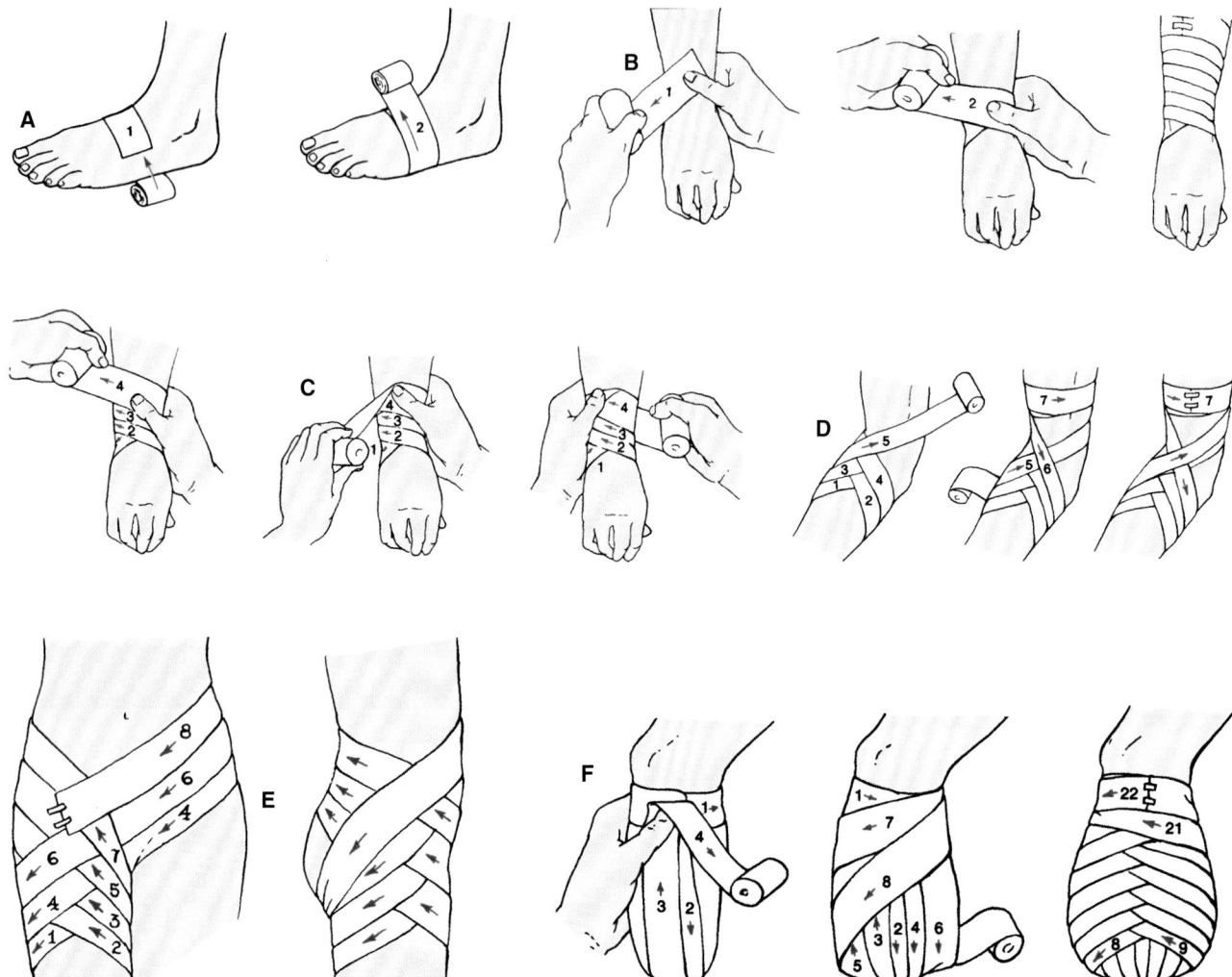

**FIGURE 28-16** • The six basic techniques for wrapping a roller bandage. **(A)** A *circular turn* is used to anchor and secure a bandage when it is started and ended. Hold the free end of the rolled material in one hand and wrap it about the area and back to the starting point. **(B)** A *spiral turn* partly overlaps a previous turn. The overlapping varies from half to three-fourths of the width of the bandage. Spiral turns are used to wrap a cylindrical part of the body like the arms and legs. **(C)** A *spiral reverse turn* is a modification of a spiral turn. The roll is reversed halfway through the turn. This works well on tapered body parts, such as the forearm and wrist. **(D)** A *figure-of-eight turn* is best used when an area spanning a joint, like the elbow or knee, requires bandaging. It is made by making oblique turns that alternately ascend and descend, simulating the number 8. **(E)** A *spica turn* is a variation of the figure-of-eight turn. It differs in that the wrap includes a portion of the trunk or chest. **(F)** The *recurrent turn* is made by passing the roll back and forth over the tip of a body part. Once several recurrent turns have been made, the bandage is anchored by completing the application with another basic turn like the figure of eight. A recurrent turn is especially beneficial when wrapping the stump of an amputated limb.

## Commonly Prescribed Dermatology Medications

**Note:** *The generic name of the drug is listed first and is written in all lower case letters. Brand names are in parentheses and the first letter is capitalized.*

| | | |
|---|---|---|
| Acyclovir (Zovirax) | Capsules: 200 mg<br>Injection: 500 mg/vial, 1 g/vial<br>Suspension: 200 mg/5 mL<br>Tablets: 400 mg, 800 mg | Antiviral |
| Crotamiton (Eurax) | Cream: 10%<br>Lotion: 10% | Scabicide |
| Diphenhydramine hydrochloride (Benadryl) | Capsules: 25 mg, 50 mg<br>Injection: 50 mg/mL (IM)<br>Tablets: 25 mg, 50 mg | Antihistamine |
| Epinephrine (adrenaline) (EpiPen) | Injection (IM or SC):<br>0.1 mg/mL (1:10,000)<br>0.5 mg/mL (1:2,000)<br>1 mg/mL (1:1,000) | Bronchodilator |
| Famciclovir (Famvir) | Tablets: 125 mg, 250 mg, 500 mg | Antiviral |
| Hydrocortisone (Cortizone 5, 10; Scalpicin; Dermolate) | Cream: 0.5%, 1%, 2.5%<br>Topical solution: 1%, 2.5% | |
| Isotretinoin (Accutane) | Capsules: 10 mg, 20 mg, 30 mg, 40 mg | Retinoic acid derivative |
| Itraconazole (Sporanox) | Capsules: 100 mg<br>Oral solution: 10 mg/mL | Antifungal |
| Ketoconazole (Nizoral) | Tablets: 200 mg | Antifungal |
| Lindane (Hexit) | Cream: 1%<br>Lotion: 1%<br>Shampoo: 1% | Pediculicide; scabicide |
| Linezolid (Zyvox) | Tablets: 600 mg | Antibiotic |
| Minoxidil (Rogaine) | Topical foam: 5% | |
| Topical solution: 2%, 5% | Vasodilator | |
| Permethrin (Acticin, Elimite, Nix) | Cream: 5%<br>Lotion: 1%<br>Topical liquid (cream rinse): 1% | Pediculicide |
| Pyrethrins and piperonyl butoxide (RID, A-200, Pronto) | Lotion: 0.3% and 2%<br>Mousse: 0.33% and 4%<br>Shampoo: 0.33% and 4%<br>Topical gel: 0.3% and 3% | Pediculicide |
| Terbinafine hydrochloride (Lamisil) | Oral granules (packets): 125 mg, 187.5 mg<br>Tablets: 250 mg | Antifungal |
| Tetracycline hydrochloride (Sumycin) | Capsules: 250 mg, 500 mg<br>Oral suspension: 125 mg/5 mL | Antibiotic |
| Tretinoin (Retin-A; Atralin) | Cream: 0.02%, 0.025%, 0.05% 0.1%<br>Gel: 0.05%, 0.01%, 0.025%<br>Microsphere gel: 0.04%, 0.1% | Retinoid |
| Triamcinolone acetonide (Kenalog, Triderm) | Cream: 0.025%. 0.1%, 0.5%<br>Lotion: 0.025%, 0.1%<br>Ointment: 0.025%, 0.1%, 0.5% | Corticosteroid |
| Vancomycin hydrochloride (Vancocin) | Capsules: 125 mg, 250 mg<br>Powder for injection (IV): 500 mg vial, 1 g vial | Antibiotic |
| Zoster vaccine, live (Zostavax) | Injection: single dose (SC) | Vaccine |

 ## ROLE-PLAYING ACTIVITY

With cooperation from classmates or as assigned by your instructor, role-play a situation in which an elderly patient is referred to the Great Falls Medical Center dermatology office and diagnosed with a scabies infection on both arms and his back. You must explain the infection to the patient and the treatment ordered by the physician's assistant (lindane cream 1%) to be applied in a thin layer every 12 hours. The patient is having difficulty understanding why he can't just "get a shot" and is not sure how he will apply it to his back (he lives alone). How would you respond? What advice could you give him about applying the cream to his back? Switch roles and role-play a scenario in which an adolescent patient is diagnosed by the physician's assistant with severe acne vulgaris. He does not seem to be compliant with the previous physician orders with regard to cleansing his face and back and taking the prescribed medication (oral tetracycline hydrochloride 500 mg every day and Atralin gel applied daily in the evening). What issues might be preventing the patient from being noncompliant? How would you encourage compliance? Your instructor will give you additional information about this activity!

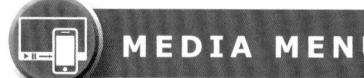 ## MEDIA MENU

**Student Resources** on thePoint®
- *Animation:* Acute Inflammation
- *Animation:* Wound Healing
- *Video:* Applying A Tubular Gauze Bandage (Procedure 28-3)
- **CMA/RMA Certification Exam Review**

**Internet Resources**

**American Cancer Society**
http://www.cancer.org

**American Academy of Dermatology**
http://www.aad.org

**American Board of Dermatology**
http://www.abderm.org

**American Society of Dermatology**
http://www.asd.org

## español SPANISH TERMINOLOGY

**¿Desde hace cuánto tiene usted ese lunar?**
How long have you had that mole?

**He tenido este lunar desde hace cinco (5) años.**
I have had this mole for 5 years.

**Esta ampolla es dolorosa.**
This blister is painful.

**¿Tiene comezón?**
Do you feel itchy?

**¿Cual loción ó jabón está usando?**
What kind of lotion/soap are you using?

**Por favor pare de usar esa loción/jabón inmediatamente.**
Please stop using that lotion/soap immediately.

**¿Ha estado usted en contacto con una substancia química desconocida?**
Have you been in contact with an unknown chemical, food, shampoo, soap, etc.?

## EMR Activity

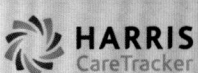

Harris CareTracker is a Web-based electronic medical record (EMR) application that you will use for the EMR activities included in this section at the end of each chapter. This application is actually used in physician offices but is provided to you through the publisher, Wolters Kluwer Health, to give you hands-on practice working with EMRs. Your instructor will have more information about accessing your username, log-in, and Quickstart guide.

Prerequisite Activities in Harris CareTracker

• *The Getting Started and Quickstart documents and EMR Activities Step-by-Step Instructions are available at* http://thePoint.lww.com/KronenbergerComp5e.

Activity Details

Accurately document the following treatments ordered by dermatologist, Dr. Schroeder.

1. Patient: Tammy Leonard; treatment, cool compress applied to rash on posterior lower leg for 10 minutes
2. Patient: Steve Sutter; treatment, Triderm cream 0.025% applied to left thumb after wart removed and a dry sterile dressing applied followed by a tubular gauze bandage

## Chapter Summary

- The skin and its accessories make up the largest and most visible organ of the body.
- Assessment of the integument offers the first glimpse into a person's total state of health.
- The medical physician who treats disorders of the skin is called a *dermatologist*; however, the medical assistant working in other offices will also be exposed to various types of integumentary system disorders.
- A responsibility of the medical assistant includes assisting the physician in correctly identifying and treating various forms of skin lesions.
- Typically, the medical assistant will be responsible for applying sterile dressings directly over a skin lesion or wound and should always remember to follow sterile technique.
- Always provide patient instruction during and after bandaging, alerting the patient to the signs and symptoms of impaired circulation.
- Bacterial skin infections may be contagious, and you should follow standard precautions, including good handwashing, after being with any patient with a skin disorder that may be infectious.

## Warm-Ups for Critical Thinking

1. Sunlight or ultraviolet rays are needed to convert vitamin D, which is necessary for calcium and phosphorous absorption. Why is it important that children be exposed to sunlight regularly during their growing years?
2. After considering the factors needed for any microorganism to thrive, explain why molds and fungi thrive in a public shower or pool.
3. Create a patient information sheet describing the difference between eczema and psoriasis.
4. Using a drug reference book, research the usual dosage, side effects, and contraindications of the drug minoxidil, which is used to treat alopecia.
5. How would you respond to a patient who complains that his friend has recently been diagnosed with vitiligo and he is worried that he might also get this disease?

## PSY PROCEDURE 28-1

## Applying a Warm or Cold Compress

**PSY** Instruct and prepare a patient for a procedure or treatment; coach patients regarding disease prevention and treatment plans; coach patients appropriately considering cultural diversity, developmental life stage, and communication barriers; document patient care accurately in the medical record.

**Purpose:** Apply warm or cold compresses according to a physician's order

**Equipment:** Warm compresses, appropriate solution (water with possible antiseptic if ordered) warmed to 110°F or recommended temperature, bath thermometer, absorbent material (cloth, gauze), waterproof barriers, hot water bottle (optional), clean or sterile basin, and gloves; cold compresses, appropriate solution, ice bag or cold pack, absorbent material (cloth, gauze), waterproof barriers, and gloves

| STEPS | REASONS |
|---|---|
| 1. Wash your hands. | Handwashing aids in infection control. |
| 2. Check the physician's order and assemble the equipment and supplies. | Hot and cold compresses must be ordered by the physician. |
| 3. Pour the appropriate solution into the basin. For hot compresses, check the temperature of the warmed solution. 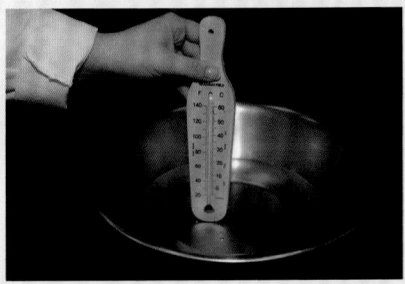 | The solution must not be hot enough to injure the patient.<br><br><br><br><br>**Step 3.** Check hot solution with a bath thermometer if available. |
| 4. Greet and identify the patient. Identify yourself including your title. Explain the procedure. | Identifying the patient prevents errors in treatment. Explaining the procedure helps ease anxiety and ensure compliance. |
| 5. Ask patient to remove clothing as appropriate and to put on a gown. Drape as appropriate. | Privacy must always be provided. |
| 6. **AFF** Explain how to respond to a patient who is hearing impaired. | Solicit assistance from anyone who may be with the patient or a staff member who knows sign language to interpret if available. If no interpreter is available, use hand gestures or pictures to explain the procedure to the patient. |
| 7. Protect the examination table with a waterproof barrier. | Wet surfaces are uncomfortable for the patient and may cause chilling. |
| 8. Place absorbent material or gauze in the prepared solution. Wring out excess moisture. | Compresses should be moist but not dripping; avoid wetting the patient. |
| 9. Lightly place the compress on the patient's skin and ask about the temperature for comfort. Observe the skin for changes in color. | Always ask the patient whether the temperature of the compress is causing pain or discomfort. |

*(continues on page 718)*

## PROCEDURE 28-1 (continued)

| STEPS | REASONS |
|---|---|
| 10. Gently arrange the compress over the area and contour the material to the area. Insulate the compress with plastic or other waterproof barrier. 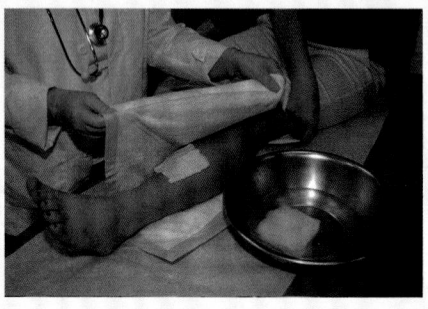 | Unless the material is against the skin, temperature will not be transferred to the area of concern. Insulating the area with the waterproof barrier will retard temperature loss and avoid getting the rest of the patient wet.<br><br>**Step 10.** Place a waterproof barrier over the compress material. |
| 11. Check the compress frequently for moisture and temperature. Hot water bottles or ice packs may be used to maintain the temperature. Rewet absorbent material as needed. | The temperature should stay fairly constant. If the material dries, benefits will be lost. |
| 12. After the prescribed amount of time, usually 20 to 30 minutes, remove the compress, discard disposable materials, and disinfect reusable equipment. | Equipment should be available for the next use. Cross-contamination must be avoided. |
| 13. Remove your gloves and wash your hands. | |
| 14. **AFF** Log into the electronic medical record (EMR) using your username and secure password OR obtain the paper medical record from a secure location and assure it is kept away from public access. Record the procedure, including the duration of the treatment, type of solution, temperature of the solution if a warm compress is used, skin color after the treatment, assessment of the area, and the patient's response. Your entry must include the date, time, and your name/credentials. | The integrity of the medical record must be maintained at all times to protect patient privacy. Procedures are considered not to have been done if they are not recorded. |
| 15. When finished, log out of the EMR and/or replace the paper medical record in an appropriate and secure location. | |

*Note:* If the compress is being applied to an area with an open lesion, sterile technique is required.
Warm compresses will speed suppuration to increase healing. Cold compresses will slow bleeding and decrease inflammation.

---

**Charting Example:**
*10/16/2016 10:45 AM Hot compress applied to the left ankle ×20 min. Skin pink after treatment; no broken areas or blisters noted on the skin _____ B. Barth, CMA*

---

Note: *The medical assistant may sign his or her name in the patient record using only the "CMA" credential if the office has a signature log denoting the entire credential as "CMA (AAMA)."*

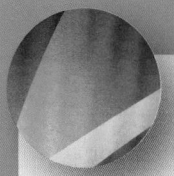

**PSY** PROCEDURE 28-2

## Assisting with Therapeutic Soaks

**PSY** Instruct and prepare a patient for a procedure or treatment; coach patients regarding disease prevention and treatment plans; coach patients appropriately considering cultural diversity, developmental life stage, and communication barriers; document patient care accurately in the medical record.

**Purpose:** Perform a therapeutic soak as directed by the physician

**Equipment:** Clean or sterile basin or container in which to place the body part comfortably, solution and/or medication, dry towels, bath thermometer, and gloves

| STEPS | REASONS |
|---|---|
| 1. Wash your hands. | Handwashing aids in infection control. |
| 2. Assemble the equipment and supplies, including a basin or container of the appropriate size. | If the container is uncomfortably small, soaking the body area will be difficult and may cause muscle spasms. Surfaces should be padded for comfort. |
| 3. Fill the container with solution and check the temperature with a bath thermometer. The temperature should be below 110°F to avoid blood pressure changes caused by vasodilation. | Assessing the temperature will prevent burning or injuring tissues. |
| 4. Greet and identify the patient. Identify yourself including your credentials. Explain the procedure. | Identifying the patient prevents errors in treatment. Explaining the procedure helps ease anxiety and ensure compliance. |
| 5. Slowly lower the area to be soaked into the container and check the patient's reaction. Arrange the part comfortably. Check for pressure areas and pad the edges as needed for comfort. | Immersing the part too quickly can shock the patient. If the patient is not comfortable, muscle spasms or strain may result. |

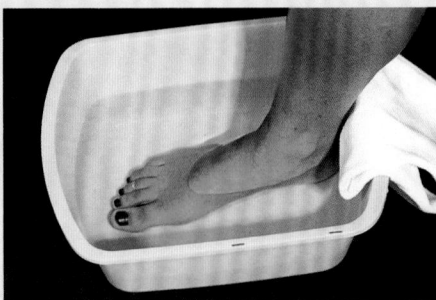

**Step 5.** The basin should be large enough to immerse the entire body area.

| | |
|---|---|
| 6. **AFF** Explain how to respond to a patient who has dementia. | Solicit assistance from a caregiver who may have accompanied patient to the office visit or ask another staff member to help during the procedure if necessary. Give simple directions to the patient about what he or she should do. Speak clearly, not loudly. |

*(continues on page 720)*

## PROCEDURE 28-2 (continued)

| STEPS | REASONS |
|---|---|
| 7. While soaking, check the temperature of the solution every 5 to 10 minutes. If additional water or solution must be added to maintain the temperature, remove some of the solution and then add warmed solution while holding your hand between the patient and the stream of the solution being poured. Mix or swirl the soak to ensure constant, even temperature. | The proper temperature must be maintained for maximum benefit. Avoid pouring the solution or water directly against the patient's skin. |

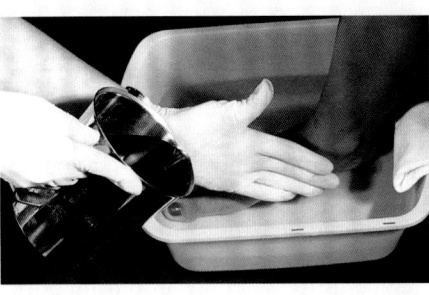

**Step 7.** Shield the patient's skin when adding warm solution to the soak.

| | |
|---|---|
| 8. Soak for the prescribed amount of time, usually 15 to 20 minutes. Remove the part from the solution and carefully dry the area with a towel. | The area may be sensitive to brisk rubbing but must be dried to prevent chilling the patient or causing discomfort. |
| 9. Properly care for the equipment; appropriately dispose of single-use supplies and wash your hands. | |
| 10. **AFF** Log into the electronic medical record (EMR) using your username and secure password OR obtain the paper medical record from a secure location and assure it is kept away from public access. Record the procedure, including duration of treatment; type and temperature of solution; skin color after treatment; assessment of the area; including the condition of any lesions; and the patient's response. Your entry must include the date, time, and your name/credentials. | The integrity of the medical record must be maintained at all times to protect patient privacy. Procedures are considered not to have been done if they are not recorded. |
| 11. When finished, log out of the EMR and/or replace the paper medical record in an appropriate and secure location. | |

---

Charting Example:

4/19/2016 12:20 PM *Left great toe soaked in Betadine solution × 15 min. Mod. amount of tan drainage from edges of toenail noted after soak _____ J. Brighton, RMA*

---

Note: *The medical assistant may sign his or her name in the patient record using only the "CMA" credential if the office has a signature log denoting the entire credential as "CMA (AAMA)."*

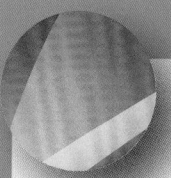

## PSY  PROCEDURE 28-3

### Applying A Tubular Gauze Bandage

**PSY** Instruct and prepare a patient for a procedure or treatment; coach patients regarding disease prevention and treatment plans; coach patients appropriately considering cultural diversity, developmental life stage, and communication barriers; document patient care accurately in the medical record.

**Purpose:** Apply tubular gauze bandage to a digit or extremity

**Equipment:** Tubular gauze, applicator, tape, and scissors

| STEPS | REASONS |
|---|---|
| 1. Wash your hands. | Handwashing aids in infection control. |
| 2. Greet and identify the patient. Explain the procedure. | This prevents error in treatment, helps gain the patient's compliance, and eases anxiety. |
| 3. **AFF** Explain how to respond to a patient who is visually impaired. | Face the patient when speaking and always let him or her know what you are going to do before touching him or her. |
| 4. Choose the appropriate size tubular gauze applicator and gauze width according to the size of the area to be covered. Manufacturers of tubular gauze supply charts with suggestions for the appropriate size for various body parts. | The applicator and gauze should slip easily over the body part. Choose an applicator slightly larger than the part to be covered. The gauze designed to fit the chosen applicator will provide a secure fit. |
| 5. Select and cut or tear adhesive tape in lengths to secure the gauze ends. | Tape ensures that the gauze will not slip off. Having it at hand before beginning the procedure saves time and effort. |
| 6. Place the gauze bandage on the applicator in the following manner:<br>A. Be sure the applicator is upright (open end up) and placed on a flat surface.<br>B. Pull a sufficient length of gauze from the stock box; do not cut it yet.<br>C. Open the end of the length of gauze and slide it over the upper end of the applicator; estimate and push the amount of gauze that will be needed for this procedure onto the applicator. | |

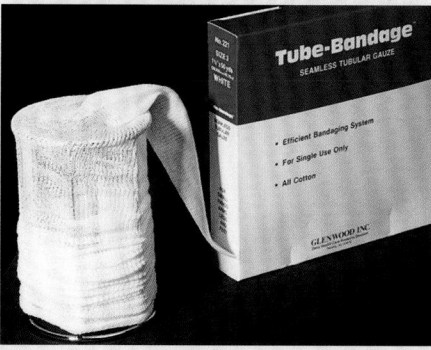

**Step 6C.** Place the applicator upright and slide the end of the gauze over the applicator.

D. Cut the gauze when the required amount of gauze has been transferred to the applicator.

*(continues on page 722)*

## PROCEDURE 28-3 (continued)

| STEPS | REASONS |
|---|---|
| **7.** Place the applicator over the distal end of the affected part (finger, hand, toe, leg) and begin to apply the gauze by pulling it over the applicator onto the skin. Hold it in place as you move to Step 8. | The applicator should begin distally and work proximally. |
| **8.** Slide the applicator up to the proximal end of the affected part. Holding the gauze at the proximal end of the affected part, pull the applicator and gauze toward the distal end.<br><br>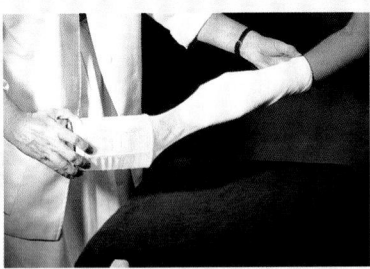 | This keeps the bandage from slipping. If the bandage is not held in place at the early stages of application, it may not completely cover the part.<br><br><br>**Step 8.** Hold the gauze at the proximal end of the affected part and pull the applicator toward the distal end. |
| **9.** Continue to hold the gauze in place at the proximal end. Pull the applicator 1 to 2 inches past the end of the affected part if the part is to be completely covered. Sometimes, the gauze need not extend beyond a limb but covers only the area of the wound.<br><br>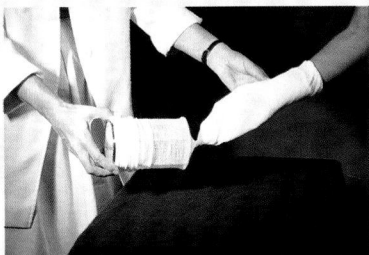 | The bandage will be secured at the distal end if the part is to be completely covered. If the distal portion of the limb is not to be covered, the bandage must extend at least 1 inch beyond the wound site to ensure adequate coverage. |
| **10.** Turn the applicator one full turn to anchor the bandage. | **Step 9.** Pull the applicator 1 to 2 inches past the affected area.<br><br>The bandage will be securely held in place by the twist. |
| **11.** Move the applicator toward the proximal part as before.<br><br>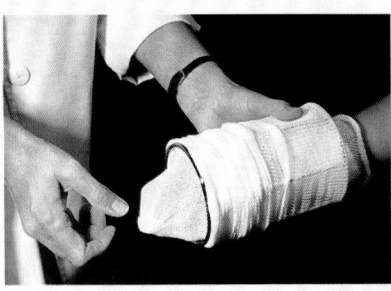 | Moving the applicator and gauze up and down over the affected body part creates a layer of bandage material, adding additional protection to the wound.<br><br><br><br>**Step 11.** Move the applicator toward the proximal part. |

# PROCEDURE 28-3 (continued)

| STEPS | REASONS |
|---|---|
| **12.** Move the applicator forward about 1 inch beyond the original point. Anchor the bandage again by turning it as before. 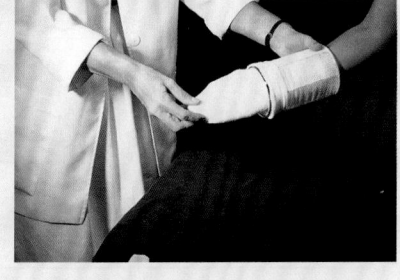 | Anchoring provides a secure fit. |
| | **Step 12.** Move the applicator forward about 1 inch beyond the starting point. |
| **13.** Repeat the procedure until the desired coverage is obtained. The final layer should end at the proximal part of the affected area. Any extra length of gauze can be cut from the applicator. Remove the applicator. | The part should be adequately covered to protect the wound. |
| **14.** Secure the bandage in place with adhesive tape, or cut the gauze into two tails and tie them at the base of the tear. Tie the two tails around the closest proximal joint. Use the adhesive tape sparingly to secure the end if not using a tie. 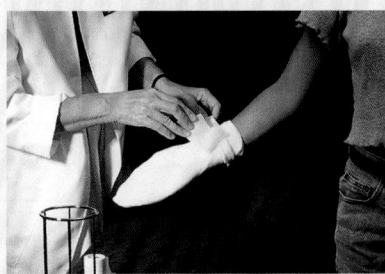 | The bandage must be securely fastened to keep it in place until it is changed. |
| | **Step 14.** Secure the bandage with adhesive tape. |
| **15.** Properly care for or dispose of equipment and supplies. Clean the work area. Wash your hands. | Standard precautions must be followed. |
| **16.** **AFF** Log into the electronic medical record (EMR) using your username and secure password OR obtain the paper medical record from a secure location and assure it is kept away from public access. Record the procedure and the patient's response. Your entry must include the date, time, and your name/credentials. | The integrity of the medical record must be maintained at all times to protect patient privacy. Procedures are considered not to have been done if they are not recorded. |
| **17.** When finished, log out of the EMR and/or replace the paper medical record in an appropriate and secure location. | |

**Charting Example:**
*02/08/2016 9:15 AM Sterile dressing change to right index finger, tubular bandage applied and secured over dressing _____ T. Matthews, CMA*

Note: *The medical assistant may sign his or her name in the patient record using only the "CMA" credential if the office has a signature log denoting the entire credential as "CMA (AAMA)."*

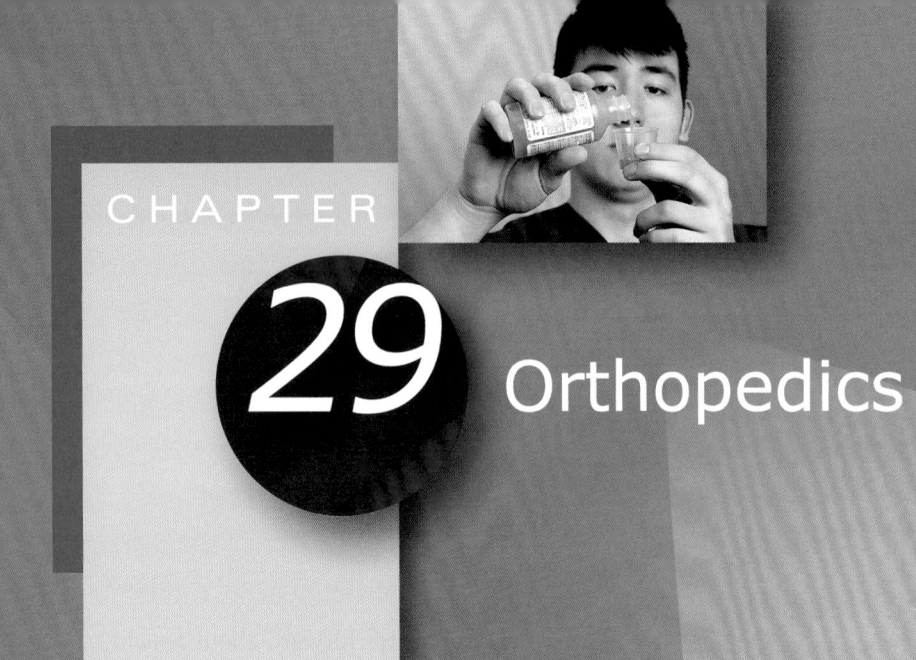

# CHAPTER 29 Orthopedics

## Learning Outcomes

**COG Cognitive Domain***

1. Spell key terms
2. Define medical terms and abbreviations related to all body systems
3. Describe structural organization of the human body
4. List major organs in each body system
5. Identify the anatomical location of major organs in each body system
6. Describe the normal function of each body system
7. Identify common pathology related to each body system including signs, symptoms, and etiology
   a. Describe common disorders of the musculoskeletal system
   b. Compare the different types of fractures
   c. Identify and explain diagnostic procedures of the musculoskeletal system
8. Discuss the role of the medical assistant in caring for the patient with a musculoskeletal system disorder
9. Describe the various types of ambulatory aids

**PSY Psychomotor Domain***

1. Apply an arm sling (Procedure 29-1)
   a. Instruct and prepare a patient for a procedure or treatment

   b. Coach patients appropriately considering cultural diversity, developmental life stage, and communication barriers
   c. Coach patients regarding disease prevention and treatment plans
   d. Document patient care accurately in the medical record
2. Apply cold packs (Procedure 29-2)
   a. Instruct and prepare a patient for a procedure or treatment
   b. Coach patients appropriately considering cultural diversity, developmental life stage, and communication barriers
   c. Coach patients regarding disease prevention and treatment plans
   d. Document patient care accurately in the medical record
3. Use a hot water bottle or commercial hot pack (Procedure 29-3)
   a. Instruct and prepare a patient for a procedure or treatment
   b. Coach patients appropriately considering cultural diversity, developmental life stage, and communication barriers
   c. Coach patients regarding disease prevention and treatment plans
   d. Document patient care accurately in the medical record

4. Measure a patient for axillary crutches (Procedure 29-4)
   a. *Instruct and prepare a patient for a procedure or treatment*
   b. *Coach patients appropriately considering cultural diversity, developmental life stage, and communication barriers*
   c. *Coach patients regarding disease prevention and treatment plans*
   d. *Document patient care accurately in the medical record*
5. Instruct a patient in various crutch gaits (Procedure 29-5)
   a. *Instruct and prepare a patient for a procedure or treatment*
   b. *Coach patients appropriately considering cultural diversity, developmental life stage, and communication barriers*
   c. *Coach patients regarding disease prevention and treatment plans*
   d. *Document patient care accurately in the medical record*

### AFF  Affective Domain*

1. *Incorporate critical thinking skills when performing patient assessment*
2. *Incorporate critical thinking skills when performing patient care*

3. *Show awareness of a patient's concerns related to the procedure being performed*
4. *Demonstrate empathy, active listening, and nonverbal communication*
5. *Demonstrate respect for individual diversity including gender, race, religion, age, economic status, and appearance*
6. *Explain to a patient the rationale for performance of a procedure*
7. *Demonstrate sensitivity to patient rights*
8. *Protect the integrity of the medical record*

***Note: AAMA/CAAHEP 2015 Standards are italicized.***

### ABHES Competencies

1. Assist the physician with the regimen of diagnostic and treatment modalities as they relate to each body system
2. Comply with federal, state, and local health laws and regulations
3. Communicate on the recipient's level of comprehension
4. Serve as a liaison between the physician and others
5. Show empathy and impartiality when dealing with patients
6. Document accurately

## Key Terms

| | | | |
|---|---|---|---|
| ankylosing spondylitis | callus | goniometer | phonophoresis |
| arthrograms | contracture | iontophoresis | prosthesis |
| arthroplasty | contusions | kyphosis | reduction |
| arthroscopy | electromyography | lordosis | scoliosis |
| bursae | embolus | Paget disease | |

## Case Study

*T*onya Burton, RMA, works in the orthopedic practice that is part of the Great Falls Medical Center Corporation. The office has eight orthopedic physicians and four physician assistants. In addition to the five medical assistants who work at the front desk, each physician and physician assistant has an assigned medical assistant in the clinical area. The orthopedic physician Tonya works for specializes in disorders of the knees and hips. Although patients with sports injuries are commonly seen in the office, many patients are referred to this office for back pain and follow-up care after receiving care from the local hospital for fractures. Many of the patients seen by Tonya and the physician she works with are elderly and require surgery to replace joints (knee or hip replacements) after injury. Why are the elderly more likely to break bones of the hip during a fall compared to younger patients? What are the differences in the way bones heal depending on age? With the approval of the physician, how can Tonya educate patients about avoiding back injuries? These questions and others are addressed in this chapter.

Muscles allow movement of the body through contraction and relaxation. Bones support the body and respond to the contractions and relaxations (Fig. 29-1). Because the two systems depend on each other to function, they are often referred to as a single system—the musculoskeletal system. Within this system are joints, areas where two or more bones are held together by connective tissue and cartilage. The integrity of the entire system is required for normal body support and movement (Fig. 29-2).

# THE MUSCULOSKELETAL SYSTEM AND COMMON DISORDERS

When there is a problem with the musculoskeletal system, orthopedists and physical therapists often provide appropriate treatment and rehabilitation. However, medical assistants working in other specialties, such as family practice or urgent care centers, also care for patients with musculoskeletal disorders. The most common disorders of the musculoskeletal system are sprains, dislocations, fractures, joint disruptions, and degeneration. The musculoskeletal system reacts to injury or disease with pain, swelling, inflammation, deformity, and/or limitation of range and function (Box 29-1).

## Sprains and Strains

Injury to a joint capsule and its supporting ligaments is called a **sprain**, and injury to a muscle and its supporting tendons is called a **strain**. Damage to a muscle, ligament, or tendon may result in joint instability. If the ligament is completely torn, it cannot efficiently stabilize the joint. Common symptoms are inflammation and pain. Applying ice at the time of injury helps reduce swelling and pain. For mild sprains, treatment includes exercise to prevent joint stiffness and muscle atrophy. Therapeutic devices and compression wraps reduce swelling. Moderate sprains must be treated with care to prevent further injury because the ligaments are weakened and healing may take 6 to 8 weeks. Severe sprains often require surgery, and the recovery may take longer than 8 weeks.

In the spine, a sprain to the facet joint (the area between vertebrae) can cause pain not only at the point of difficulty but also radiating into an extremity (radicular pain) as a result of impingement on the nerve root that passes close to the joint. For example, an injury to the facet joint between vertebrae of the lower back often causes pain in the back that radiates down one leg or the other. An injury to the anterior cruciate ligament in the knee greatly compromises the joint's stability. The knee becomes swollen, painful, and unstable and has limited motion. Complete tears in the ligaments of the knee require surgery and extensive rehabilitation.

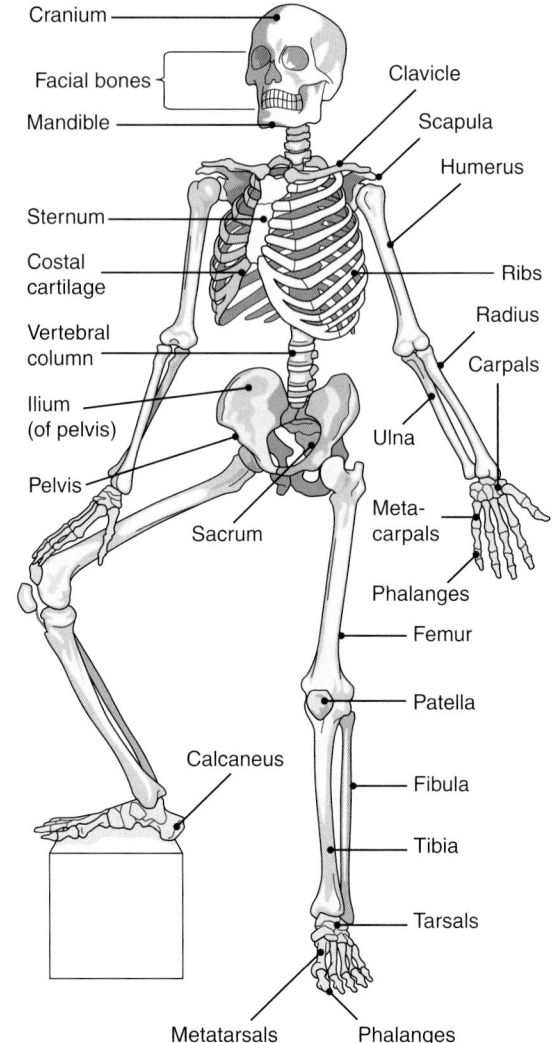

**Figure 29-1 •** The axial skeleton is shown in yellow; the appendicular skeleton is shown in blue. (Reprinted from Cohen BJ. *Memmler's The Human Body in Health and Disease*, 11th ed. Philadelphia, PA: Lippincott Williams & Wilkins, 2009, with permission.)

An injury to the Achilles tendon in the lower posterior leg is extremely painful and limits the ability to walk. A tear in this tendon requires surgery followed by immobilization.

## Dislocations

Dislocation of a joint, also called a **luxation**, occurs when the end of the bone is displaced from its articular surface. It can be caused by trauma or disease, or it may be congenital. Common sites of dislocations include the shoulders, elbows, fingers, hips, and ankles. A *subluxation* is a partial dislocation in which the bone is pulled out of the socket but all joint structures maintain their proper relationships. Partial dislocations can result from weakness, decreased muscle tone, gravity, or neurologic deficit. The muscles bear most of the responsibility for preventing subluxation. Common symptoms of dislocations include pain, pressure, limited movement, and

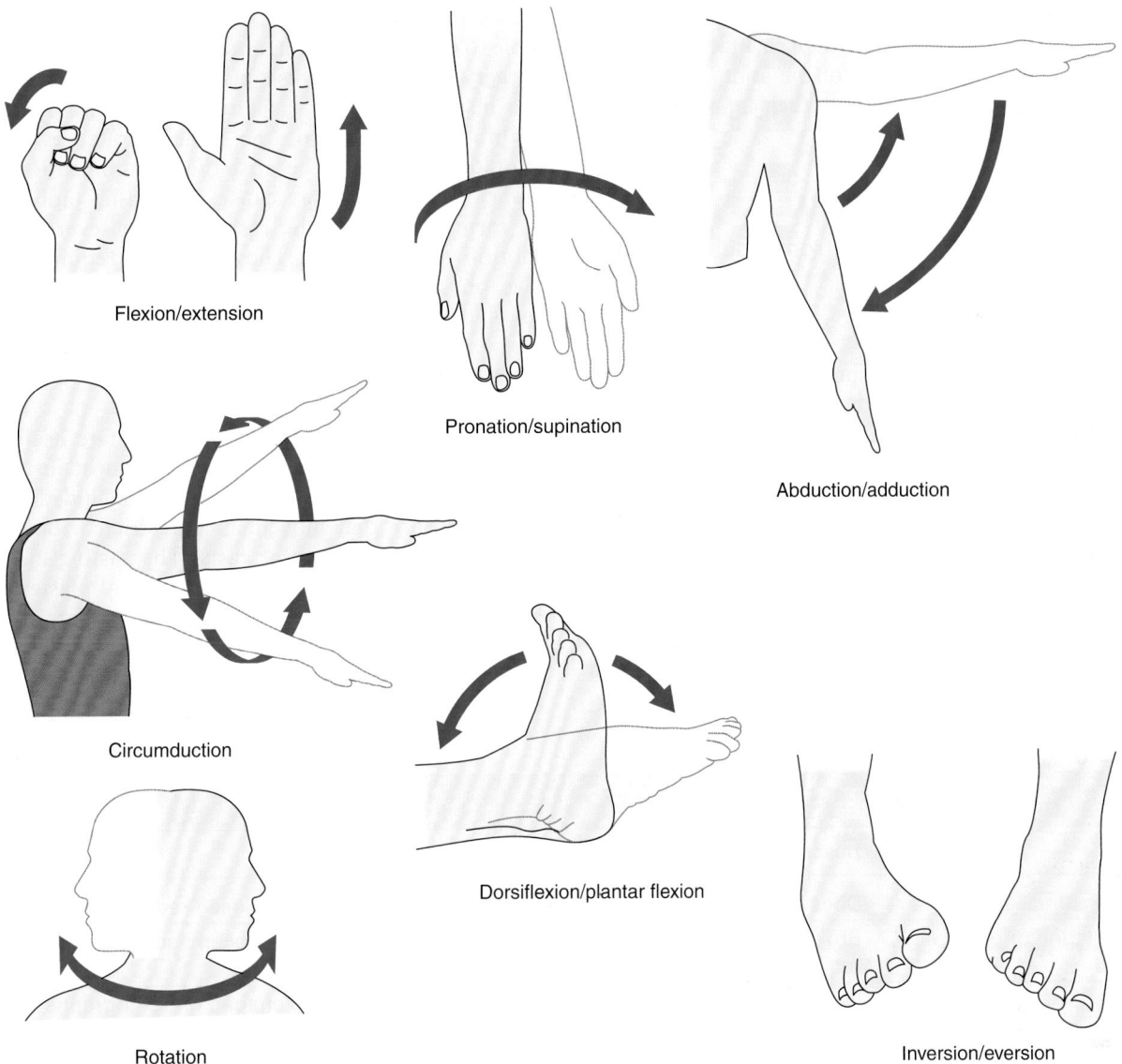

Flexion/extension

Pronation/supination

Abduction/adduction

Circumduction

Dorsiflexion/plantar flexion

Rotation

Inversion/eversion

**Figure 29-2** • Normal range of motion of selected joints: flexion/extension; pronation/supination; abduction/adduction; circumduction; dorsiflexion/plantar flexion; inversion/eversion; and rotation. (Reprinted from Cohen BJ. *Memmler's The Human Body in Health and Disease*, 11th ed. Philadelphia, PA: Lippincott Williams & Wilkins, 2009, with permission.)

## BOX 29-1 Musculoskeletal Pain

Rest, immobilization, or both may be needed to relieve pain in acute soft tissue strains, sprains, and inflammations. Because painful movement may cause further damage to the injured tissue, restriction of movement may also be required. This can be accomplished by rest and by the use of a cast, brace, sling, splint, collar, elastic wrap, or corset. If weight bearing is painful or inadvisable because of fracture or musculoskeletal pathology, an ambulatory aid (e.g., cane, walker, or crutches) may be used.

The use of hot moist packs, a heating pad, or warm baths can help increase circulation, relax spasms, and ease sore muscles. Ice packs help prevent swelling, decrease inflammation, and reduce contusions, which may follow a direct blow on a muscle.

With contusions, the capillaries (small blood vessels) rupture and bleed into the tissue. Swelling and inflammation may result. Reduction of the bleeding is crucial; it is accomplished by applying cold packs and a pressure bandage. Immobilization to prevent further injury is also important. Within a few days, pain-free exercises and heat applications should be introduced to begin healing.

Generally, movement should begin as soon as possible after a soft tissue injury to maintain a healthy joint and resilient muscles. Gentle active or passive movement in the pain-free range, mild joint immobilization, traction, or exercise can be effective in maintaining normal range, function, and strength.

deformity. Numbness and loss of a pulse in the affected extremity can also occur. Treatment includes realigning the bones and immobilization of the joint. The patient may have to do exercises to strengthen supporting muscles to avoid recurrences.

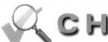

## CHECKPOINT QUESTION

1. How does a luxation differ from a subluxation?

## Fractures

A fracture is a break or disruption in a bone caused by falls, other trauma, disease, tumors, or unusual stress. There are many types of fractures, each with its own set of problems (Table 29-1). However, all fractures have one symptom in common: pain. Other manifestations may include swelling, hemorrhage, lack of movement or unusual movement, **contusions**, and deformity of the body part involved.

Treatment of a fracture is known as a **reduction** (realigning the bones) by placing the broken ends into proper alignment. Casting, splinting, wrapping, and taping are means of maintaining and immobilizing a

closed reduction while the bone heals. If it is not possible to obtain proper alignment by a closed reduction, surgery is required; this open reduction may require the insertion of pins, a plate, or other hardware to maintain alignment of the bones. Fractures in the shoulder are serious because the immobilization necessary for healing may cause scar tissue (adhesions) to form in the capsule, resulting in a severe loss of motion and function. These patients require extensive physical therapy to regain complete use of the involved arm.

## Casts

Fractures must be immobilized to facilitate healing of the bone in the proper alignment. In most instances, both proximal and distal joints are included in the cast to ensure that movement is restricted. Box 29-2 describes various types of casts. The casting material is either plaster or fiberglass. Traditional plaster casts are bandages impregnated with calcium sulfate crystals and are supplied as rolls of material in widths appropriate to a variety of sites. After water is added to the dry rolls of bandage and the wet material is applied to

| TABLE 29-1 | Types of Fractures |
|---|---|
| **Type** | **Description** |
| Simple or closed | Does not protrude through the skin; usually treated with a closed reduction |
| Compound or open | Broken end protrudes through the skin; infection a major concern; surgery often required |
| Spiral | Occurs with torsion or twisting injuries; appears to be S shaped on radiographs |
| Impacted | One bone segment driven into another |
| Greenstick | Common injury in children; partial or incomplete break in which only one side of a bone is broken, like a green stick |
| Transverse | At right angles to axis of bone; generally caused by excessive bending force or direct hit on bone |
| Oblique | Slanted across axis of bone |
| Comminuted | Bone is fragmented, usually by much direct force; difficult to reduce because many pieces of bone must be held in proper alignment; more complicated to treat if articular surface is involved, so surgery usually required; severe soft tissue damage common because of the force necessary to cause the fracture |
| Compression | Damage from application of strong force against both ends, such as a fall; vertebrae susceptible to compression fractures, especially in older adults |
| Depressed | Fracture of flat bones (usually skull), causing fragment to be driven below the surface of the bone |
| Avulsion | Caused by strong force applied to the bone by sharp twisting, pulling motion of attached ligaments or tendons resulting in a tearing away of bone fragments |
| Pathologic | Usually result of disease process such as osteoporosis (brittle bones), **Paget disease** (a chronic skeletal disease in older adults with bowing of the long bones), bone cysts, tumors, or cancers |

| TABLE 29-1 | Types of Fractures (Continued) |
|---|---|
| Type | Description |

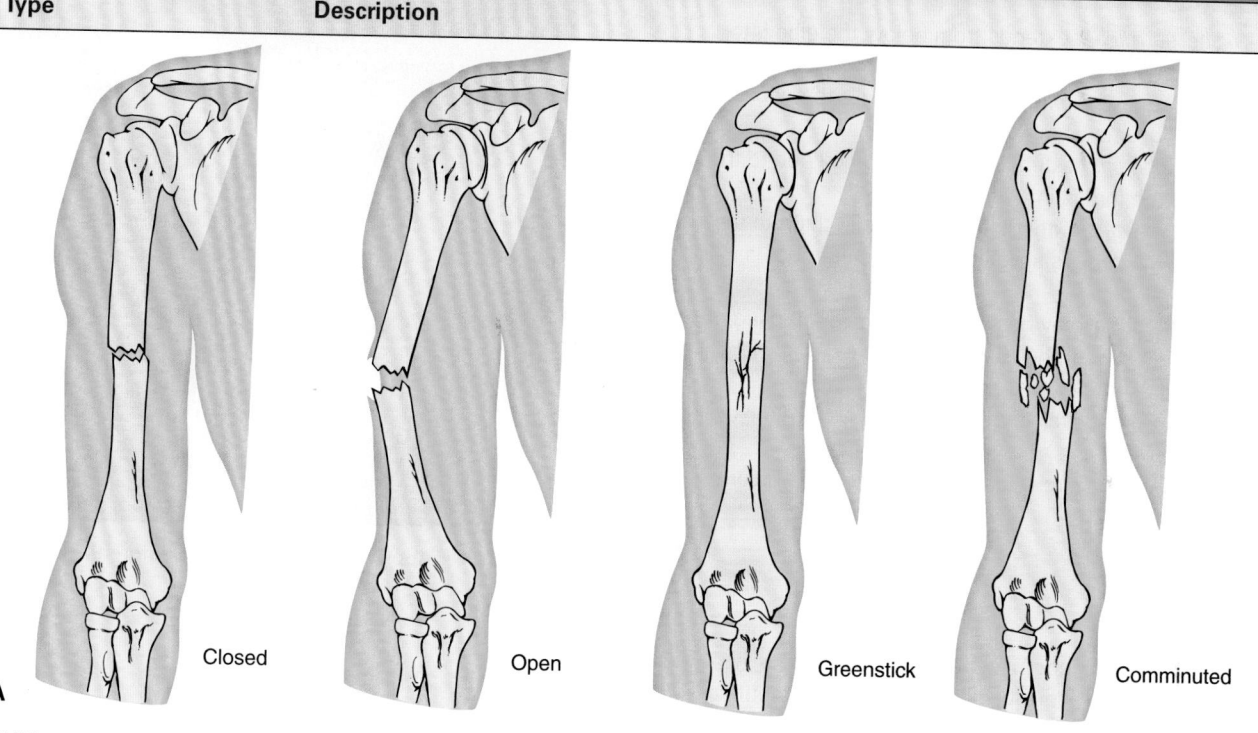

**(A)** Types of fractures: closed, open, greenstick, comminuted.

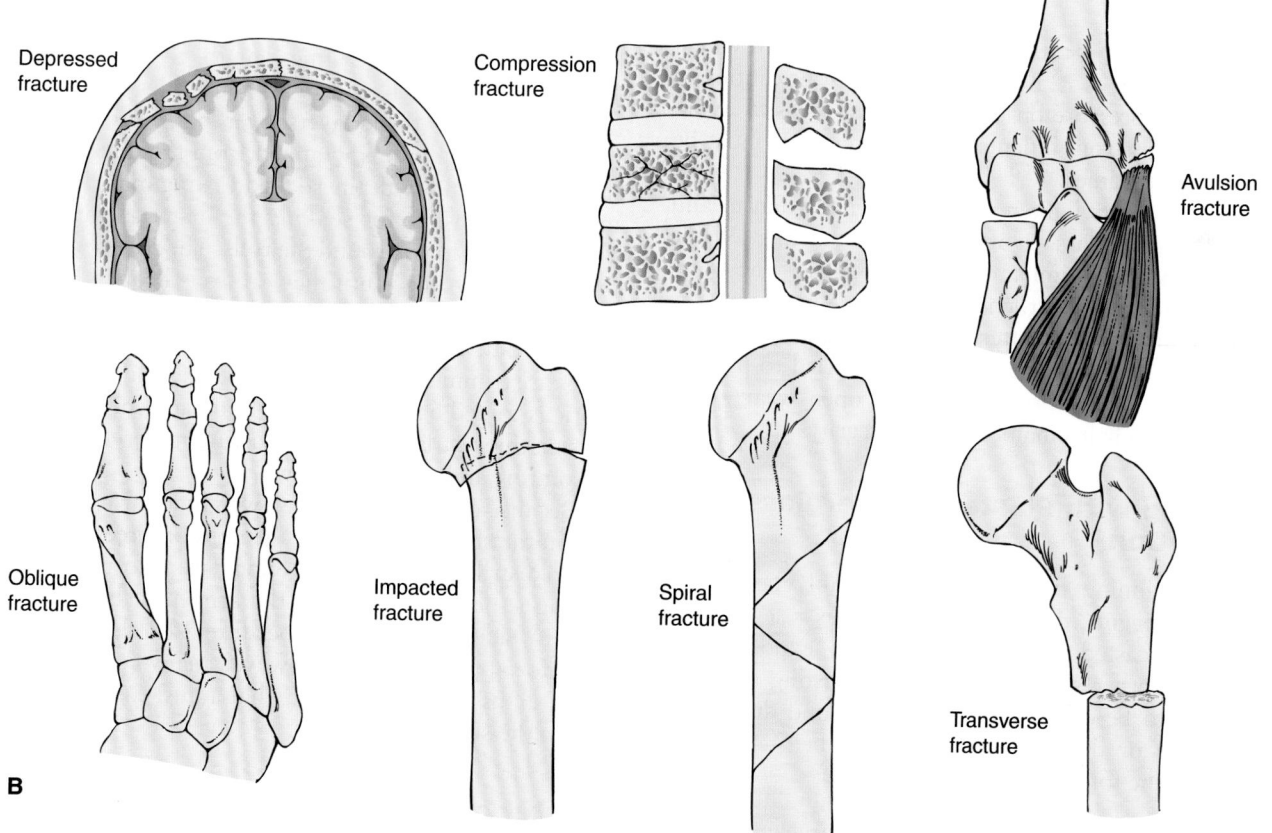

**(B)** Types of fractures: depressed fracture, compressed fracture, avulsion fracture, oblique fracture, impacted fracture, spiral fracture, transverse fracture.

## BOX 29-2    Types of Casts

- *Short arm cast* extends from below the elbow to midpalm.
- *Long arm cast* extends from the axilla to midpalm. The elbow is usually at a 90° angle.
- *Short leg cast* extends from below the knee to the toes; the foot is in a natural position.
- *Long leg cast* extends from the upper thigh to the toes; the knee is slightly flexed, and the foot is in a natural position.
- *Walking cast* may be either short leg or long leg; the cast is extra strong to bear weight and may include a walking heel.
- *Body cast* encircles the trunk, usually from the axilla to the hip.
- *Spica cast* encircles part of the trunk and one or two extremities.

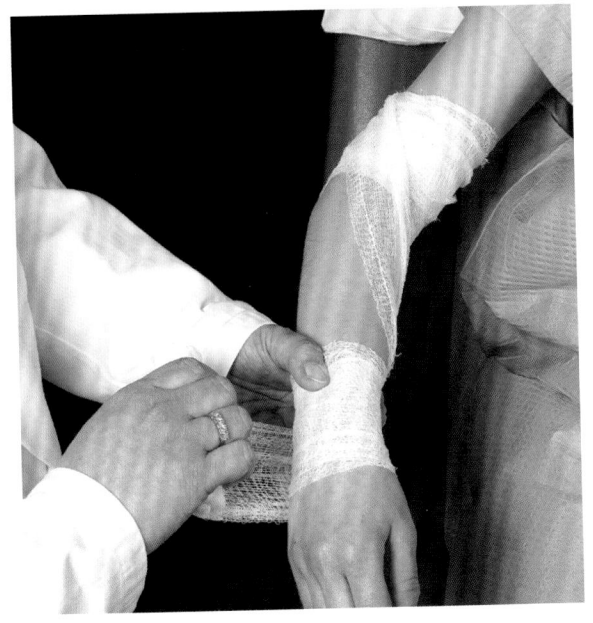

**Figure 29-3** • Applying a roller bandage before the casting material.

the extremity, a chemical reaction generates heat that may be uncomfortable to the patient for a short time, usually less than 30 minutes. This chemical reaction is necessary to produce a rigid dressing when dry. The bandage will mold smoothly to the casting site as it is applied.

A plaster cast is rather soft until it is fully dry, which can take as long as 72 hours. Patients must be cautioned not to exert pressure on the drying cast so as to avoid pressure sores from indentations. Plaster casts must be kept dry at all times.

Because of its lighter weight, water resistance, and durability, fiberglass is often used for casting. While the application is similar to the plaster cast, the polyurethane additives harden in minutes, eliminating the extended drying time. After the cast has set, the material will not soften when wet but must be dried to prevent skin lesions. The fabric has a more open weave than plaster, which helps maintain skin integrity.

### Assisting with Plaster or Fiberglass Cast Application

After positioning the patient comfortably before the procedure begins, drape the patient to expose only the part to be casted, avoiding unnecessary exposure and protecting other skin areas from the casting material. The part to be casted should be clean and dry; apply a bandage or dressing to any lesions before casting. Assemble the following items:

- Tubular soft fabric stocking material large enough to encircle the limb
- Roller padding, also called *sheet wadding*
- Casting material

- Bucket of cool or tepid water
- Plaster or cast knife
- Utility gloves

The limb is covered first with the soft knitted tubular material with extra fabric above and below the projected casting length to allow for a padded fold at each end. The soft roller padding is applied in fairly thick layers over bony prominences (Fig. 29-3). The limb is wrapped from the distal end to the proximal end with the soaked casting material. You may be responsible for soaking the material until bubbles no longer form around the rolls. The rolls should be pressed, not wrung, until they are wet through but not dripping. Wear utility gloves to protect your hands from the material. When the site is adequately covered, rough edges are trimmed with the plaster knife, and the knitted fabric is folded back to form cuffs at each end. The skin outside the cast is cleansed of casting material to avoid discomfort and skin breakdown.

Because of the unsupported weight an arm cast may put on the shoulder muscles, a sling is ordered to relieve and redistribute the weight. Slings are also used when casting is not necessary, but the arm must be immobilized to facilitate healing. Procedure 29-1 describes the steps for applying a sling; however, many commercially made slings are now available that adjust easily depending on the size of the patient.

### Plaster or Fiberglass Cast Removal

To remove a plaster or fiberglass cast, cuts are made in the cast through its length on opposite sides, dividing it into halves. An electric oscillating circular saw known as

## PATIENT EDUCATION

### Cast Care

Instruct patients with casts to do the following:

- Be aware of the initial warmth of the drying cast; this will diminish in 20 to 30 minutes.
- Keep a plaster cast dry.
- Avoid indentations by allowing the cast to dry completely before handling or propping it on a hard surface.
- Note that the fingers and toes are left uncovered to check for color, swelling, numbness, and temperature; report any impairment to the physician immediately.
- Report odors, staining, or undue warmth of the cast.
- Prevent swelling by elevating the limb for at least 24 hours after casting and as often as possible after that time.
- Never insert any object under the cast to scratch beneath it. Breaks in the skin may become infected and require that the cast be removed prematurely.

a *cast cutter* is used (Fig. 29-4). Assure the patient that this will not cut the skin. Wear safety goggles to protect your eyes from flying particles and caution the patient also. The cast will be split apart with a cast spreader, and the padding will be cut with utility scissors. The patient should be warned that the skin will be pale and dry and the muscle will be weak and shrunken from disuse. Also, explain that the skin may be sensitive to touch and temperature. Creams and lotions help alleviate the dryness, and physical therapy and exercise will restore the muscle tone.

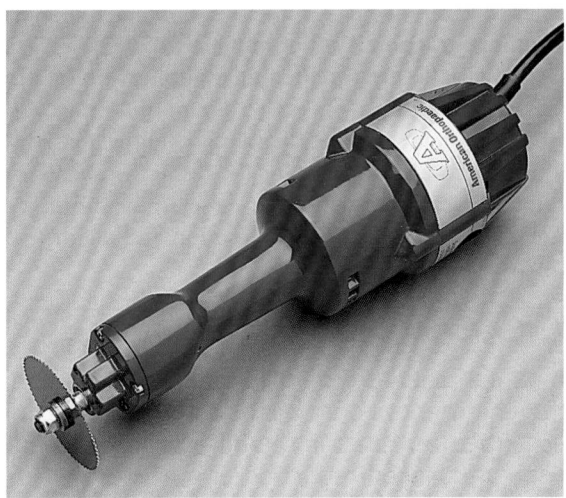

**Figure 29-4** • A cast cutter and saw. (Courtesy of M-PACT Worldwide, Eudora, KS.)

## CHECKPOINT QUESTION

2. After applying a plaster cast, Tonya tells the patient she should avoid touching it until it is completely dry. Why is it important to not touch plaster casts until completely dry?

## LEGAL TIP

### Assessing Circulation after a Cast Application

A cast that is applied improperly can lead to nerve and vascular damage, resulting in permanent loss of function to the extremity. In extreme situations, a surgical amputation may be required. To ensure proper care and to avoid lawsuits, it is essential that distal extremity circulation be assessed and documented before and after reductions and casting. Also, the patient should be taught to watch for and report signs of impaired circulation.

### Healing of Fractures

The most important criterion for successful healing of a fracture is an adequate blood supply. In dermatology, the term "callus" describes a raised painless thickening of the epidermis. However, the blood secretes an important glue-like substance also known as **callus**, which is deposited around a break in any bone. Callus holds the ends of the bones together; with time, the callus turns to bone. The bone cells mold the callus and smooth the fracture site to close to its original size. Immobilization of the fracture site allows successful molding and reshaping. Older adults may heal slowly, and prosthetic joint replacement may be necessary if bone restructuring is inadequate (Box 29-3).

### BOX 29-3 Bone Healing in Older Adults

A fractured femur in older adults raises special concerns. Bone-repairing osteoblasts are less able to use calcium to restructure bone tissue at any site in older adults, but the neck of the femur, the most common fracture site, is especially vulnerable to delayed or imperfect healing because the blood supply is poor. Fractures through this area, involving the femoral head or neck or just inferior to the greater trochanter, may require hip arthroplasty or total hip replacement.

Most hip joint replacement prostheses are metal or polyethylene molded to conform to the joints they

## BOX 29-3    Bone Healing in Older Adults (Continued)

are designed to replace. Total hip replacement, usually used for degenerative joint disease or rheumatoid arthritis, replaces the head and neck of the femur and the acetabular surface. Knee replacement replaces both the head of the tibia and the distal epiphysis of the femur.

Early repair and return to mobility prevent contractures and atrophy of the supporting muscles. Postoperative walking prevents many of the complications associated with prolonged confinement in older adults, such as pathologic fractures, static pneumonia, and renal calculi.

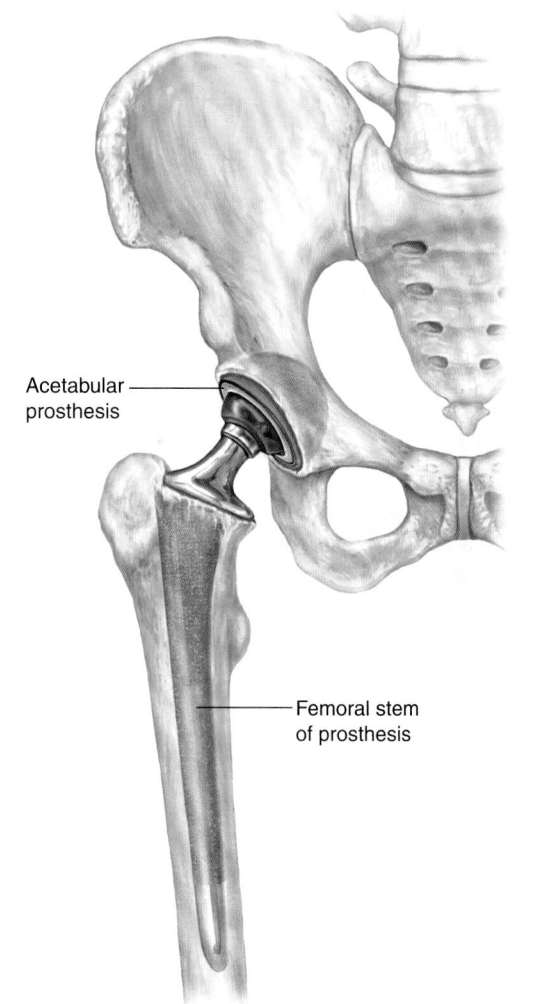

Acetabular prosthesis

Femoral stem of prosthesis

Hip and knee replacement: acetabular (pelvic) component; femoral (proximal) component; femoral (distal) component; and tibial component. (Asset provided by Anatomical Chart Co.)

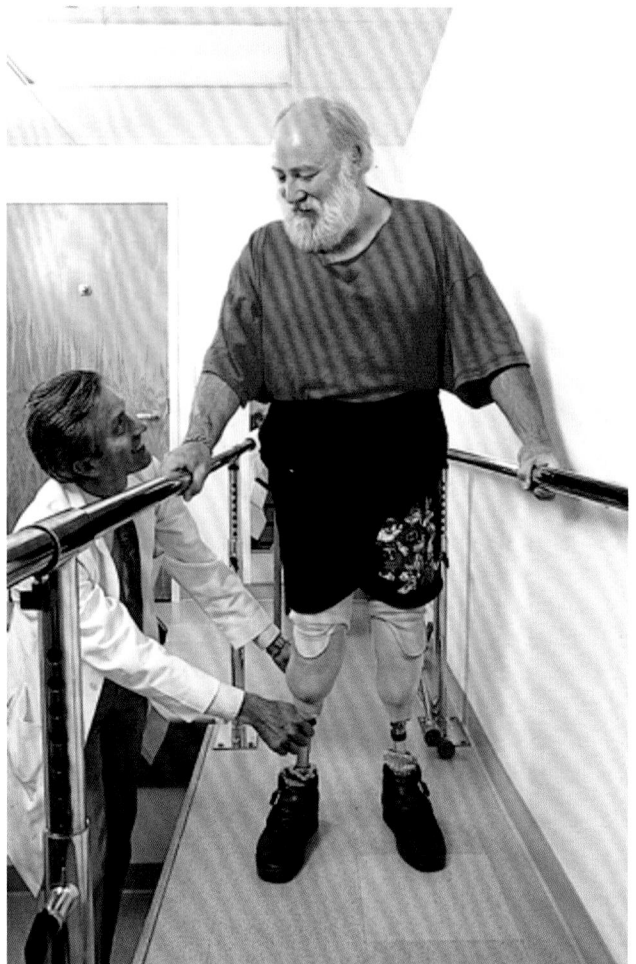

**Figure 29-5** • A patient with a prosthetic device.

If the blood supply is inadequate to the healing bone or tissue, union may be delayed or absent. If damage is sufficient or if severe trauma, disease, tumor, or complications are involved, amputation may be necessary. Amputation is a drastic measure that is performed only when all other avenues are exhausted. A **prosthesis** enables the amputee to resume functional activities such as walking, grasping, and holding (Fig. 29-5).

A potentially life-threatening complication of a fracture is a fat **embolus**. This type of embolus results from the release of fat droplets from the yellow marrow of the long bones. If the embolus lodges in the coronary or pulmonary vessels or in a large vessel in the brain, it can block the vessel, causing an infraction and death.

## 🔍 CHECKPOINT QUESTION

3. A patient seen by the orthopedic physician in the emergency room needs an open reduction of a fracture. What is the difference between an open and closed reduction of a fracture?

## Helping Elderly Patients Avoid Hip Fractures

Older patients are particularly likely to fall and fracture bones, and when this happens, one of the most common bones broken is the head of the femur. These fractures take a long time to heal and often result in the patient being admitted to a skilled nursing facility for rehabilitation. Therefore, it is important for you to teach older patients fall prevention techniques. Here are some important tips:

- Always wear shoes with good, solid tie strings.
- Be sure that lighting is adequate, both inside and outside the home.
- Remove scatter rugs inside the home.
- Place grab bars throughout the home where extra assistance may be needed in getting out of chairs or off of the toilet.

Advise the patient that one-floor living is best, and teach the patient ways to reorganize the home to avoid climbing stairs.

## Bursitis

**Bursae,** small pad-like sacs filled with a clear synovial fluid, surround some joints in areas of excessive friction, such as under tendons and over bony prominences. Their primary purposes are to reduce friction between moving parts and to prevent damage. The subdeltoid bursa in the shoulder between the deltoid muscle and the joint capsule is the most common site of bursitis, an inflammation of the bursa. Other frequent sites include the olecranon process at the elbow, the trochanter at the hip, the prepatellar bursae at the knee, and the heel.

The most common symptom of bursitis is pain during range-of-motion movement (see Fig. 29-2). In subdeltoid bursitis, pain occurs in the midrange of abduction but not at the beginning or end of the range. Pain occurs in the shoulder and arm when the inflamed bursa is pinched between the head of the humerus and the clavicle during abduction.

Treatment for bursitis usually consists of anti-inflammatory medications, rest, heat or cold applications, ultrasound to promote healing, and activities within the pain-free range. Physical therapy for range-of-motion exercises may also be ordered by the physician.

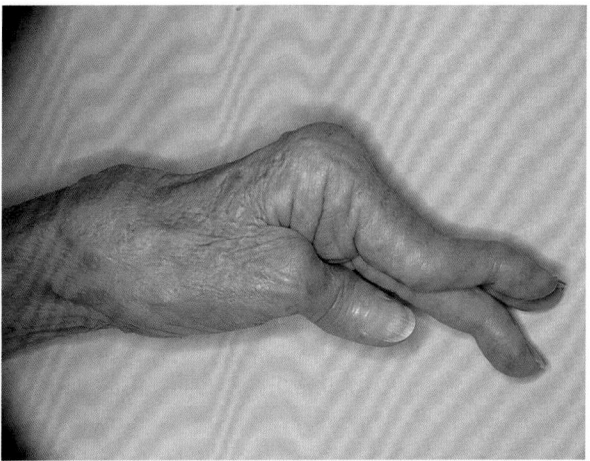

**Figure 29-6 •** Hand of a patient with rheumatoid arthritis. (From Strickland JW, Graham TJ. *Master Techniques in Orthopaedic Surgery: The Hand,* 2nd ed. Philadelphia, PA: Lippincott Williams & Wilkins, 2005.)

## Arthritis

Osteoarthritis, or degenerative joint disease, is caused by wear and tear on the weight-bearing joints. As the articular cartilage degenerates, the ends of the bones enlarge, causing an intrusion of bone into the joint cavity. The patient has pain and restricted movement in the affected joint. Treatment of osteoarthritis includes administration of anti-inflammatory medications and intra-articular corticosteroid injections to control the pain and inflammation. Patients may also require the use of an ambulatory aid such as a cane, walker, or crutches to decrease joint stress.

Rheumatoid arthritis is a systemic autoimmune disease that attacks the synovial membrane lining of the joint. Ultimately, it leads to inflammation, pain, stiffness, and crippling deformities (Fig. 29-6). It usually begins in non–weight-bearing joints such as the fingers but eventually may affect many joints, including the hands, wrists, elbows, feet, ankles, knees, and neck.

Marie-Strumpell disease, or **ankylosing spondylitis,** is rheumatoid arthritis of the spine. It is characterized by extreme forward flexion of the spine and tightness in the hip flexors. Rheumatoid arthritis in children is known as *Still disease.*

The treatment for rheumatoid arthritis is similar to the treatment for osteoarthritis: anti-inflammatory medications orally and corticosteroid or gold injections into the affected joint, heat and cold applications, and protection of painful joints with splints or braces. In severe cases, the joint may be surgically replaced with an artificial one.

### CHECKPOINT QUESTION

5. A patient asks Tonya to explain the difference between osteo- and rheumatoid arthritis. How does osteoarthritis differ from rheumatoid arthritis?

### CHECKPOINT QUESTION

4. What is the most common site of bursitis?

## Tendonitis

Muscles are attached to bones by tendons, which aid the body's mobility and stability. Tendonitis is inflammation of these structures. This disorder usually occurs after strains, sprains, overuse, or overstretching of the tissue. Although pain does not occur with passive movement, active movement is painful, and resistance to movement is intensely painful because the tissue must contract during active and resisted movement. Local tenderness is usual. The most common site of tendonitis is at the supraspinatus tendon in the shoulder, one of the rotator cuff muscles. Palpation over the tendon will elicit extreme pain. Sometimes, tendonitis is caused by calcium deposits, and this type is called *calcific tendonitis*.

The treatment for tendonitis consists of oral anti-inflammatory medications, rest, heat or cold applications, ultrasound, **iontophoresis** (electrical transfer of ions), massage, and transverse friction massage (deep massage across the fibers of the tendons). Usually, the patient is referred to a licensed massage therapist for the massage or transverse friction massage.

## Fibromyalgia

Fibromyalgia causes multiple and often nonspecific symptoms including widespread pain in specific body areas, muscular stiffness, fatigue, and difficulty sleeping. This disorder varies from person to person, and the symptoms can be intermittent, making diagnosis difficult. Although the exact cause of this disorder is not known, some evidence suggests abnormalities in the immune system, perhaps resulting from a viral infection. Although it does not lead to other serious diseases, fibromyalgia tends to be chronic and is diagnosed by ruling out all other diseases and disorders with similar symptoms.

Treatment for fibromyalgia is based on relieving the symptoms with nonsteroidal anti-inflammatory medications, exercise, rest, and personal counseling, as indicated for the clinical depression that often accompanies this disorder because it is chronic.

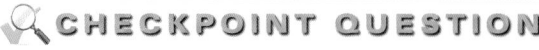

### ⚲ CHECKPOINT QUESTION

6. What is the usual cause of tendonitis?

## Gout

Gout, a metabolic disease of overproduction of uric acid, is a form of arthritis caused by the deposit of uric acid crystals into a joint, usually in the great toe. Although the cause of gout is unknown, the patient may have a history of injury to the joint, obesity, and a high-protein diet, especially a diet high in purines (alcoholic beverages, turkey, sardines, trout, bacon, and organ meats). The patient with gout complains of a painful, hot, inflamed joint; symptoms worsen unless treated (Fig. 29-7). Periods of

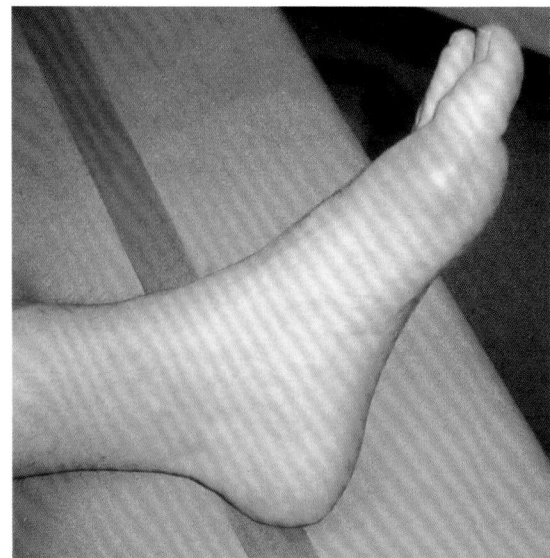

**Figure 29-7** • Tenderness and erythema on the medial aspect of the first metatarsophalangeal joint caused by gout. (From Berg D, Worzala K. *Atlas of Adult Physical Diagnosis.* Philadelphia, PA: Lippincott Williams & Wilkins, 2006.)

remission and exacerbation may occur. Gout may become chronic and can lead to multiple joint involvement with chronic pain, degeneration, and deformity. Symptoms are relieved by taking nonsteroidal anti-inflammatory medications and by avoidance of purine-rich foods and alcohol. Medication to prevent uric acid formation or foster its excretion from the body may also be prescribed.

### ⚲ CHECKPOINT QUESTION

7. The physician asks Tonya to educate a patient with gout about their diet. What foods should be avoided in the patient with gout?

## Muscular Dystrophy

The congenital disorders collectively known as *muscular dystrophy* are characterized by varying degrees of progressive wasting of skeletal muscles. There is no neurologic involvement, but the skeletal muscles waste and weaken. Some forms of the disease affect the heart and other organs. The most common type of muscular dystrophy, Duchenne, is apparent in males in early childhood and is usually fatal by young adulthood as respiratory and cardiac muscles fail. Several forms, such as facioscapulohumeral and limb girdle dystrophy, progress slowly from a childhood onset and result in varying degrees of disability. Duchenne, facioscapulohumeral, and limb girdle dystrophies are genetically transmitted.

Diagnosis of muscular dystrophy is based on family and patient history. The characteristic signs are frequently the most obvious diagnostic indicators of the disease. They include muscle weakness, clumsiness, frequent falling, and muscle spasms. **Electromyography**

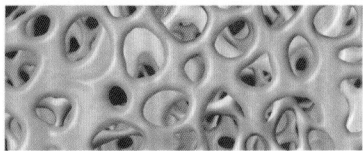

Healthy bone

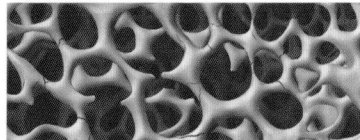

Bone with osteoporosis

**Figure 29-8** • Healthy bone versus bone with osteoporosis.

and muscle biopsy are used to rule out nervous system involvement. There is no known cure for any form of muscular dystrophy; however, exercise, physical therapy, and the use of splints or braces can relieve the symptoms. As mobility decreases, the use of a cane, walker, or wheelchair may be useful in maintaining independence.

## Osteoporosis

Porous bones, or osteoporosis, is a condition in which the bones are deficient in calcium and phosphorus, making them brittle and vulnerable to fractures (Fig. 29-8). The cause may be dietary, with general deficiencies in calcium, vitamin D, or phosphorus, or it may be primary progressive inability to metabolize calcium brought on by estrogen deficiency in elderly women or sedentary lifestyle, alcoholism, liver disorder, or rheumatoid arthritis.

There are few signs of osteoporosis other than a gradual loss of stature or height, progressive kyphosis (or dowager's hump), and spontaneous, nontraumatic fractures (Fig. 29-9). Diagnosis includes bone scan, densitometry (a test that measures the density of the bones), thyroid and parathyroid studies, and serum calcium and

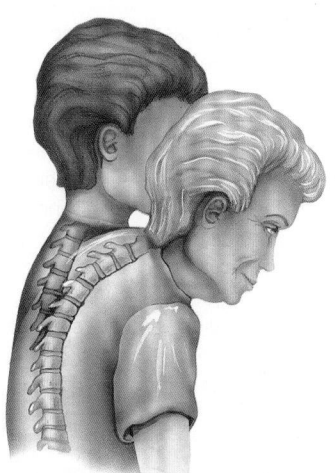

**Figure 29-9** • The progression of kyphosis in osteoporosis.

phosphorus determinations. Treatment is preventing fractures by increasing appropriate levels of exercise to strengthen the bones. Hormone therapy with estrogen or a combination of estrogen and progesterone may be prescribed for postmenopausal women to prevent loss of minerals from the bones that occurs with the natural decrease in these hormones during menopause. Calcium and vitamin D supplements are beneficial to arrest the progression but will not cure the underlying degenerative factors once osteoporosis has begun.

## Bone Tumors

Bone tissue is rarely the primary site for malignancies but is frequently a site of metastasis. Primary osteosarcomas occur most often in young men, although they may occur at any age in either sex. Osteogenic sarcomas originate in the bony tissue, while nonosseous tumors seed to the bones from other sites. Ewing sarcoma, originating in the marrow and invading the shaft of the long bones, is common in young adults, especially adolescent boys.

There is no known cause of malignant skeletal tumors, but one hypothesis is that rapid development of bone tissue during growth spurts is a predisposing factor. Bone pain is the most common early sign. The pain is most intense at night, is usually dull and centered at the site, and is not relieved by resting the body part. Depending on the site, the mass may be palpable through the skin and muscles. Biopsy is the definitive diagnostic test after a bone scan suggests the need. Surgical treatment includes excision of the tumor, including a large margin of surrounding bone structure and nearby lymph nodes, or amputation if the tumor is in an extremity. Chemotherapy and radiation are usually indicated also.

### CHECKPOINT QUESTION

8. Why is exercise used to treat or prevent osteoporosis?

## Spine Disorders

The vertebral column (Fig. 29-10) is made up of 33 vertebrae and numerous joints. The cervical, thoracic, and lumbar vertebrae are separated from each other by 23 intervertebral discs; the vertebrae of the sacrum and coccyx are fused, with no discs separating the bones. These vertebrae and their discs absorb and transmit the shock of running, walking, and jumping and keep the spine flexible for a high degree of mobility. Many strong ligaments and structures support and protect the spine, including the anterior and posterior longitudinal ligaments and the four natural curves in the spine. However, back injuries are common and are a leading cause of work-related injury among health care professionals. Box 29-4 offers some suggestions for avoiding back strain, and patients can use these general guidelines as well.

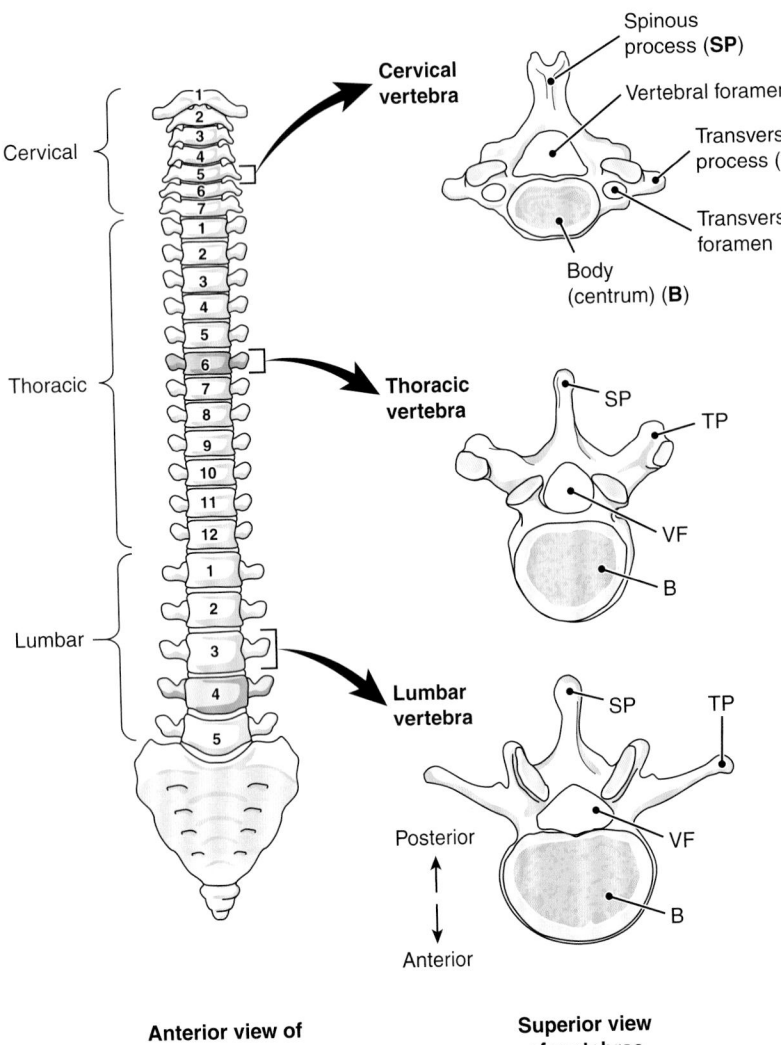

Spinous
process (**SP**)

Cervical
vertebra

Vertebral foramen (**VF**)

Transverse
process (**TP**)

Transverse
foramen

Body
(centrum) (**B**)

Cervical

Thoracic

Thoracic
vertebra

SP

TP

VF

B

Lumbar

Lumbar
vertebra

SP    TP

Posterior

VF

B

Anterior

Anterior view of
vertebral column

Superior view
of vertebrae

**Figure 29-10 •** (**Left**) Front view of
the vertebral column. (**Right**) Vertebrae
from above. (Reprinted from Cohen BJ.
*Memmler's The Human Body in Health
and Disease*, 11th ed. Philadelphia, PA:
Lippincott Williams & Wilkins, 2009, with
permission.)

## BOX 29-4   Avoiding Back Strain

You can prevent back strain by using good body
mechanics:

- When lifting a heavy object, keep the object close
  to your body. Never lift an object with extended
  arms.
- Never lift and twist at the same time. Lift the object,
  and then reposition your feet by pivoting or taking
  two steps to turn.
- Bend your knees, not your back, when lifting.
- Ask for assistance from coworkers when you must
  lift or move obese patients or heavy objects.
- Maintain proper posture at all times; slouching
  causes muscle strain.
- If you do sustain an injury at work, inform your
  supervisor immediately and document what happened. Complete an incident report in accordance
  with the facility's policy.

## PATIENT EDUCATION

### Posture and Back Pain

Although there are many reasons for poor posture including the aging process, the result of poor posture includes
back pain, which often results in more pain and poor
posture. In patients with poor posture, the bones are not
aligned properly, and the muscles, joints, and ligaments
become strained and stressed. As the discs between the
vertebra become less resilient, there is increased pressure from forces such as gravity and body weight, which
results in the loss of flexibility in the muscles of the back
and spine and spine degeneration. Weak, tight, and inflex-
ible muscles cannot support the back's natural curves.

The most common posture faults are the forward
head posture and rounded shoulders. Maintaining good
posture—or correcting poor posture—can help reduce
a bulging disc or relieve the biomechanical stress
caused by poor skeletal alignment, greatly aiding musculoskeletal system functioning.

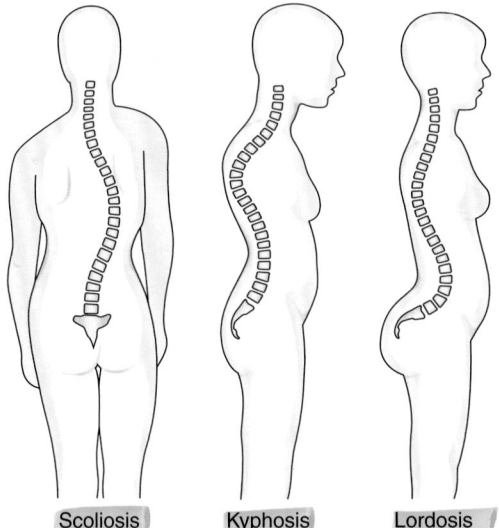

**Figure 29-11 •** Abnormalities of the spinal curves. (Reprinted from Cohen BJ. *Memmler's The Human Body in Health and Disease*, 11th ed. Philadelphia, PA: Lippincott Williams & Wilkins, 2009, with permission.)

## Abnormal Spine Curvatures

Exaggerated or abnormal curvatures of the spine affect the posture and the alignment of the shoulders and hips. An abnormally deep lumbar curve is **lordosis**, or swayback. Abnormal thoracic curvature, particularly of the upper portion, is called **kyphosis**, or hunchback. A side-to-side or lateral curvature is called **scoliosis;** it is commonly screened for in school children, especially girls, and if severe enough, it is surgically corrected during adolescence (Fig. 29-11).

Treatment of abnormal spinal curvatures entails the use of bracing to straighten the curve to a normal position. Transcutaneous muscle stimulation devices cause the muscles on one side to contract and draw the spine into its proper position. When necessary, orthopedic surgery is performed to straighten the spinal column.

## Herniated Intervertebral Disc

The lumbar spine is one of the most frequently injured parts of the body because it absorbs the body's full weight and the weight of anything that is carried. Because most of the movement in the lumbar spine occurs at the L4 to L5 and L5 to S1 segments, most herniated discs are seen at these levels, but injury can occur in any disc in the spine (Fig. 29-12).

A disc herniates when its soft center, known as the nucleus, ruptures through its tough outer layer to protrude into the spinal canal, sometimes pressing on the spinal cord. It is usually caused by severe trauma, degenerative change, or strenuous strain. Common symptoms include severe back pain, numbness in one or both extremities, spasms, weakness, and limitation of movement. Flexion radiates pain into the extremities, and exten-

SAGITTAL VIEW OF LOWER SPINE

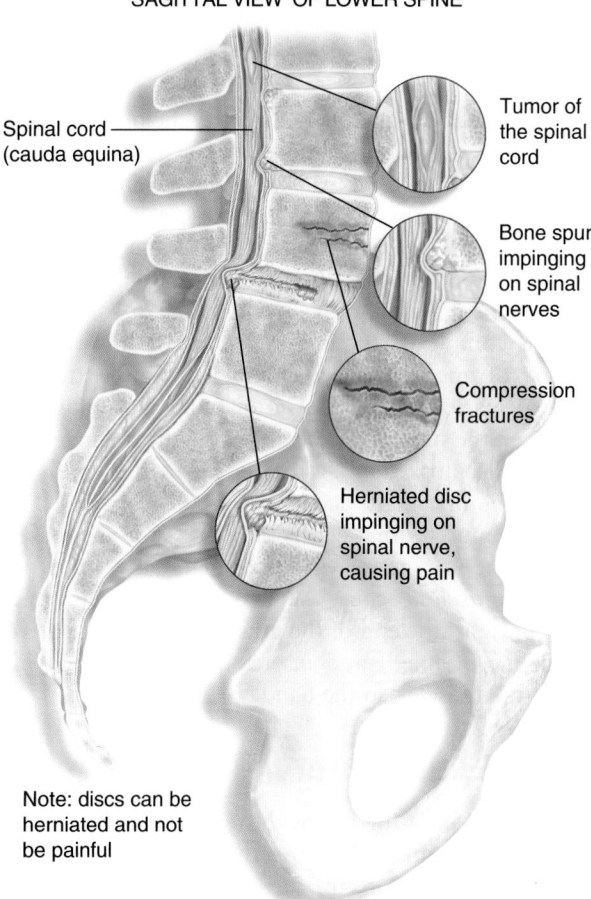

**Figure 29-12 •** Causes of low back pain.

sion is restricted and causes pain at the spinal segment. Having the patient raise one leg from the supine position (known as the *straight leg raise test*) indicates whether the back pain is from a disc. A positive sign includes back pain with the leg at 45 to 60 degrees. A flattened lumbar curve and a lateral shift of the spine are fairly common. Radiography may show a narrowed disc space.

Because bone strength throughout the body is diminished during confinement or inactivity, total bed rest is no longer a common treatment for most musculoskeletal disorders, including herniated discs, although pain limits activity. The treatment for herniated discs may include physical therapy for traction, massage, and mild extension exercises. While most disc herniations and bulges can be treated successfully without surgery, severe, unremitting pain, numbness, and progressive weakness of an extremity are indications for surgery to remove the injured disc.

### CHECKPOINT QUESTION

9. Tonya has a medical assistant student working with her today. How would she explain the three abnormal curvatures of the spine?

# ☼ DISORDERS OF THE UPPER EXTREMITIES

The structures of the upper extremity include the shoulder, elbow, wrist, and hand. Movement of the shoulder occurs in a ball-and-socket joint, which is the most mobile joint in the body. The elbow, a hinge joint, is made up of the articulation of the humerus with the radius (lateral) and the ulna (medial) and allows movement in one direction only.

The complex structure of the wrist allows for a variety of movements, including flexion, extension, ulnar deviation, radial deviation, and circumduction. However, the most intricate and specialized movements of the musculoskeletal system occur in the hand. The thumb, the first digit, accounts for 50% of hand function. The muscles that control the precision movements and fine motor activities of the hand are known as *intrinsic muscles* because they have both of their attachments, origin (the end of the muscle that stays relatively stationary or fixed) and insertion (the more movable end of the muscle), in the hand.

## Rotator Cuff Injury

The rotator cuff is formed by the tendons of four muscles that hold the joint surfaces together during joint motion. Injury to the rotator cuff muscles in the shoulder can cause severe pain, weakness, and loss of function (Fig. 29-13). Surgical intervention for rotator cuff injury is often necessary because the tendons do not heal quickly on their own. An extended period of postoperative rehabilitation and physical therapy is usually needed to increase range of motion and strength and to regain the use of the shoulder. Professional athletes, particularly baseball pitchers, are prone to rotator cuff injuries.

## Adhesive Capsulitis, or Frozen Shoulder

Frozen shoulder, a shortening of the muscles and joint structures known as a **contracture**, affects the entire shoulder joint and its capsule. It usually results from a fracture or disease process that prevents movement; however, anything that causes pain or restricts motion (e.g., tendonitis, bursitis, nerve damage, stroke, sprain, or strain) can lead to a frozen shoulder.

Contractures develop when the joint is immobilized, allowing the collagen fibers to stick to each other and thereby limit the movement in the joint. Adhesions and additional collagen are produced in response to injury, which results in a painful, tight, and constricted capsule. The shoulder movements most restricted are abduction and external rotation. Because full active range of motion is not possible, weakness and atrophy ensue.

Treatment consists of administration of anti-inflammatory medications and heat or cold applications. The physician may also prescribe physical therapy to include ultrasound, mobilization or manipulation, and stretching exercises. Recovery is slow and typically painful. Contractures in the joints are often preventable with proper management and by moving the joint through a full range of motion each day.

## Lateral Epicondylitis, or Tennis Elbow

Lateral epicondylitis, often called *tennis elbow*, is a common elbow injury involving a sprain or strain of the tendons of origin of the wrist and finger extensor muscles. Symptoms include extreme pain with extension of the wrist, such as when trying to lift a cup or glass. Resistance to wrist extension and supination are the diagnostic tests for tennis elbow because both movements greatly increase the pain.

Treatment consists of ice applications, **phonophoresis** (ultrasound with cortisone) or iontophoresis, avoiding movements that cause the pain, use of a forearm strap just distal to the elbow to take the pressure off the tendon, transverse friction massage, and gentle passive exercise to maintain mobility. In prolonged, extreme cases, surgery may be indicated.

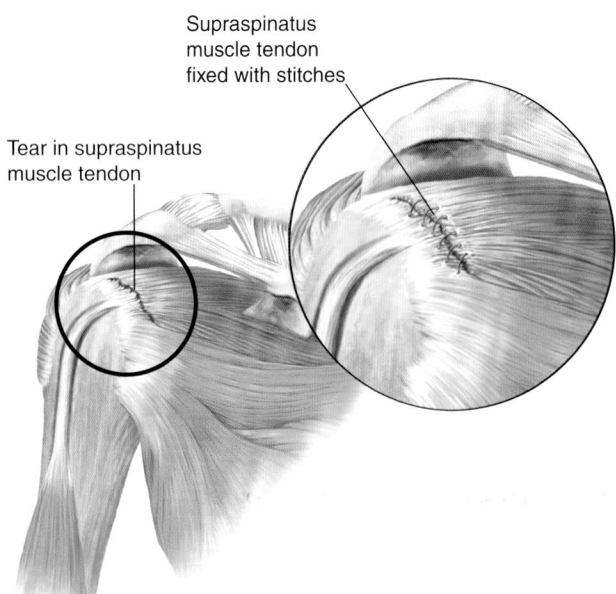

Supraspinatus muscle tendon fixed with stitches

Tear in supraspinatus muscle tendon

**Figure 29-13 •** Rotator cuff tear.

## 🔍 CHECKPOINT QUESTION

10. Which of the disorders of the upper extremities may result from decreasing movement of the arm and shoulder?

## Carpal Tunnel Syndrome

A repetitive motion injury, carpal tunnel syndrome occurs when the carpal bones and transverse carpal ligaments compress the median nerve at the wrist. Symptoms include numbness in the thumb and index and middle fingers and pain and weakness in the affected hand and wrist. Often, pain awakens the patient at night.

Diagnostic tests for carpal tunnel syndrome include the Phalen test, in which holding the wrist in flexion reproduces the symptoms; Tinel test, in which the wrist is held in hyperextension and the transverse carpal ligament is thumped, causing tingling in the hand and fingers; and nerve conduction tests.

Treatment of carpal tunnel syndrome can be conservative, with anti-inflammatory medications and immobilization of the wrist with a brace or splint. If surgical intervention is necessary, it consists of release of the transverse carpal ligament.

### PATIENT EDUCATION

#### Living with Carpal Tunnel Syndrome

Patients with carpal tunnel syndrome should be questioned regarding their work environment. This syndrome is common among typists, computer operators, assembly line workers, and other professions that demand frequent grasping, twisting, and flexion of the wrist. Caution a patient who does a lot of word processing or typing to maintain good body alignment at all times in a properly proportioned and well-constructed chair. Palm supports for computer keyboards decrease the degree of wrist flexion. Advise the patient to take breaks and, if possible, to alternate computer work with other tasks. A physical therapist may offer range-of-motion exercises that the patient can do throughout the day to alleviate wrist tension. An occupational therapist can evaluate the work area and make suggestions for changes. Always consult the physician before making referrals.

## Dupuytren Contracture

Dupuytren contracture results in flexion deformities of the fingers, most often the ring and little fingers. It is caused by contractures of the fascia in the palm of the hand due to the proliferation or overgrowth of fibrous tissue (Fig. 29-14). As the fibrous tissue grows thicker, function is lost because the fingers cannot be straightened. Dupuytren contracture is easily diagnosed by inspection and palpation. Surgery is often required to release the contractures. Although no medications are

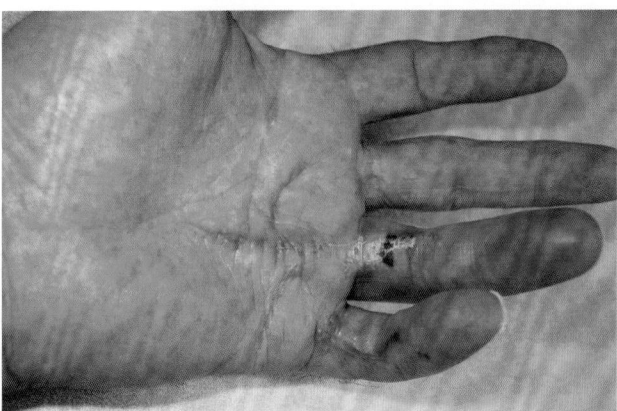

**Figure 29-14 •** A Dupuytren contracture.

available to treat this disorder, corticosteroid injections may temporarily improve function in the hand. Stretching of the tight structures in the early stages may slow the progression.

### CHECKPOINT QUESTION

11. A patient is diagnosed with carpal tunnel syndrome in Tonya's office today. What treatment might be ordered by the physician for carpal tunnel syndrome?

## DISORDERS OF THE LOWER EXTREMITIES

The musculoskeletal structures of the lower extremities include the hip, knee, ankle, and feet. The hip, a ball-and-socket joint, is important for weight bearing and walking. The acetabulum, the socket of the hip joint, is deep enough to hold most of the femoral head and is surrounded by three strong ligaments.

The largest joint in the body, however, is the knee. Locking the knee into extension allows one to stand for long periods without using the muscles. An integral part of the knee is the patella, which lies inside the quadriceps tendon and protects the hinge joint. Two important sets of ligaments, the collateral and cruciate ligaments, stabilize the knee. The knee is often injured because it is supported entirely by muscles and ligaments and because it is one of the most stressed joints, lying as it does between the two longest bones in the body.

## Chondromalacia Patellae

Chondromalacia patellae is a degenerative disorder affecting the cartilage that covers the back of the patella, or kneecap. It usually occurs in young women and in athletes who perform activities that stress the knee,

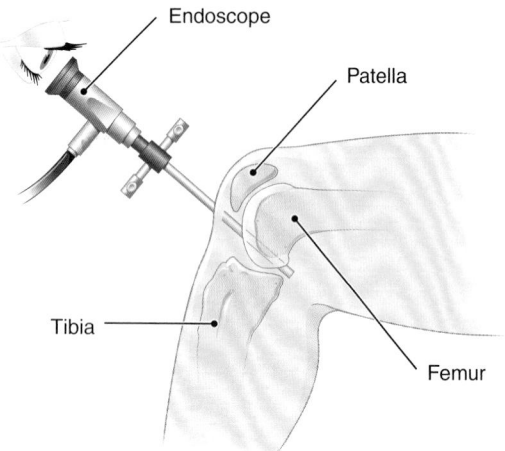

**Figure 29-15** • An arthroscopic examination of the knee. (Reprinted from Cohen BJ. *Medical Terminology: An Illustrated Guide*, 6th ed. Philadelphia, PA: Lippincott Williams & Wilkins, 2011, with permission.)

such as running, jumping, and bicycling. A common complaint is pain when walking downstairs or getting out of a chair. Rest, physical therapy, bracing or taping the knee, anti-inflammatory medications, ice therapy, and exercises to strengthen the quadriceps muscles can help to relieve the symptoms. If these treatments are not effective, an endoscope may be used to examine the joint and surrounding tissue for further problems (**arthroscopy**) (Fig. 29-15). In severe and chronic cases, a surgical procedure, **arthroplasty**, may be performed to repair or remove damaged cartilage.

## Plantar Fasciitis

Plantar fasciitis, inflammation of the plantar fascia ligament that stretches across the bottom of the foot, is the most frequent cause of pain in the bottom of the foot. Although the cause of plantar fasciitis is not always known, repetitive activities that stress the plantar fascia ligament, such as running and walking for extended periods on hard surfaces, may cause it. Factors that may aggravate it include wearing improperly fitted shoes and being overweight. Diagnosis includes a history of pain in the foot and heel when getting out of bed or after sitting for long periods. Deep palpation over the plantar (sole) surface of the heel bone will elicit pain. Radiography of the foot may be ordered to identify stress fractures, bone cysts, or heel spurs; however, ligaments do not show up clearly on radiographs, which are not routinely ordered to diagnose plantar fasciitis.

The treatment of choice for plantar fasciitis is a foot orthotic device (splint or heel pad) to support the arch and distribute the weight evenly. Physical therapy to stretch the ligament, ice therapy, massage, ultrasound,

and nonsteroidal anti-inflammatory medications may also relieve the pain. Chronic planter fasciitis may necessitate wearing a night splint, which holds the affected foot at a 90° angle, preventing shortening and tightening of the plantar fascia during the night. Surgery is rarely done because of the high incidence of recurrence.

## COG COMMON DIAGNOSTIC PROCEDURES

### Physical Examination

The physician's evaluation of the musculoskeletal system usually includes an assessment of structure and function, movement, and pain. An important part of the evaluation is the history, which includes the patient's description of the events and circumstances that led to the decision to seek medical help.

The physician observes the patient's overall physical state by noting how the patient walks, sits, stands, and moves. Concentrating on the area of concern, the physician evaluates the problem by visual inspection, palpation, and diagnostic tests. Pain and limited or compromised functions are warning signals. Strength also affects function and is a part of any musculoskeletal evaluation. Other important considerations are skin color, temperature, tone, and tenderness; abnormal findings may indicate underlying disease.

### Diagnostic Studies

The most frequently used tools for detecting disorders of the musculoskeletal system are radiology and diagnostic imaging, which are used to diagnose fractures, dislocations, and degeneration or diseases of the bones and joints. Other radiographic studies include **arthrograms**, x-ray studies of the joints that may show joint disease, and **myelograms**, which help detect intervertebral disc conditions. A bone scan analyzes bone growth, density, tumors, and other pathology.

Computed tomography (CT) and magnetic resonance imaging (MRI) may reveal soft tissue disease, such as tumor, metastatic lesions, and ruptured or bulging discs. Electromyography and nerve conduction velocity tests measure the health and fitness of the nerves as they relate to conduction of nerve impulses and muscle function.

Goniometry is measurement of the amount of movement available in a joint by a protractor-like device called a **goniometer** (Fig. 29-16). A bone or muscle biopsy is also a valuable diagnostic tool. It allows intense examination of the tissue under a microscope to determine cell damage, neoplasms (tumor or growth), or other types of diseases.

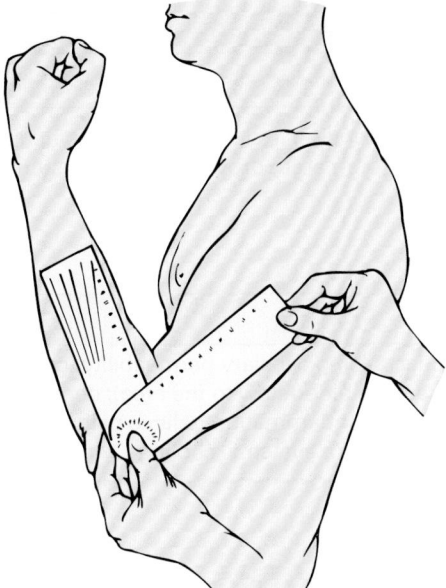

**Figure 29-16** • A goniometer. (Reprinted from Weber J, Kelley J. *Health Assessment in Nursing.* Philadelphia, PA: Lippincott Williams & Wilkins, 2003, with permission.)

---

### CHECKPOINT QUESTION

12. What procedures can be used to diagnose musculoskeletal disorders?

---

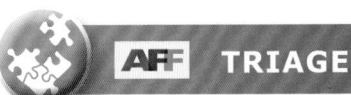 **TRIAGE**

While working in a medical office setting, the following three situations occur:

A. You need to teach a 78-year-old patient how to use a walker.

B. A 47-year-old woman just arrived in the office complaining of pain in her left wrist. She fell in the parking lot. You have been instructed to apply a cold pack to her wrist.

C. A 12-year-old patient needs a sling applied to her right arm.

**How do you sort these patients? Who do you see first? Second? Third?**

Patient B should be attended first. A cold pack should be applied to the injured wrist as soon as possible to help control the swelling and decrease the pain. Patient C should be seen next. Applying a sling will take less time than teaching patient A how to use the walker. Teaching an older patient may take extra time, skill demonstration, and return demonstration. In addition, a detailed patient education instruction pamphlet about the use of the walker should be given to the patient and explained in detail.

##  THE ROLE OF THE MEDICAL ASSISTANT

### Warm and Cold Applications

Because of the time necessary for warm or cold applications, these procedures are not often done in the office. However, your responsibility may include instructing the patient in administering the treatments at home. Patients should understand the purpose of the procedure, how to perform it, the expected results, and any precautions or danger signs. Table 29-2 discusses the types of heat and cold applications and the purposes of each. Procedure 28-2 describes the steps for applying a cold pack, and Procedure 29-3 describes a hot pack application.

### PATIENT EDUCATION

#### Heating Pads

Heating pads are not often used in the office, but a heating pad may be ordered by the physician for the patient to use at home. The patient must be aware of the potential for injury if strict guidelines are not followed. Share these safety tips with your patient:

1. Most heating pads are equipped with a cover to ensure comfort and safety. If one is not provided, wrap the pad in a soft cover before applying to the skin.
2. Do not fold or bend the pad; wires may break and form an electrical short if not kept in alignment.
3. Do not use safety pins on the heating pad. Pins may cause malfunction if they come into contact with the wiring inside the pad.
4. Never place heating pads under the body; heat may build up as it is reflected from the surface below and cause burns.
5. Set the temperature to be comfortably warm at first touch (usually the low or medium setting); do not turn the temperature up to high as the body adjusts to the temperature.
6. Keep to the recommended time for heat treatments and allow circulation to return to normal at intervals.

### Precautions

When exposed to cool or warm temperatures, the body quickly adapts. For example, the water in a swimming pool feels cool at first, but after a short while, the body becomes used to the temperature, and it no longer feels cool. The body has adapted. Using this reasoning, patients should be instructed that the benefits of heat or cold therapy are continuing even though they may not be able to feel the initial temperature change.

The body responds to extremes of temperature for extended periods by exerting an opposite effect called the *rebound phenomenon.* For example, heat applied to

| TABLE 29-2 | **Heat and Cold Treatments: Types and Purposes** | |
|---|---|---|
| **Dry Heat** | **Moist Heat** | **Purposes** |
| Hot water bottle<br>Heating pad<br>Thermal pad<br>Disposable heat pack<br>Heat lamp | Compresses<br>Warm soaks | Relieve muscle spasms or tension; relieve pain; hasten healing by increasing blood flow to an area; provide local or systemic warming |
| **Dry Cold** | **Moist Cold** | **Purposes** |
| Ice bag<br>Ice collar<br>Disposable ice pack | Compresses<br>Cold soaks | Limit initial edema by decreasing capillary permeability (caution: cold retards edema by decreasing blood flow to the area); decrease bleeding or hemorrhage; decrease inflammation; relieve pain by numbing nerve pathways; provide local or systemic cooling |

an area will cause dilation of the blood vessels, or vaso-dilation. However, if heat is applied beyond 30 minutes, vasoconstriction will occur as the body attempts to compensate for the heat. Therefore, applications left on longer than recommended by the physician will have an opposite effect to the one intended.

Some areas of the body with thin skin and few nerve receptors, such as the abdomen, are more sensitive to heat than areas such as the palms of the hands. When applying heat, remember that the very young, older adults, the confused or disoriented patient, and patients with circulatory disorders or diabetes are particularly subject to burns.

Generally, the temperature of heat and cold therapy should be kept within the following guidelines:

- Warm: tepid, 95°F to 98°F, to very warm, 115°F
- Cold: neutral, 93°F to 95°F, to very cold, 50°F

After checking with the physician, you should caution patients as follows:

Do not use heat:

- Within 24 hours after an injury, because it may increase bleeding
- For noninflammatory edema, because increased capillary permeability will allow additional tissue fluid to build up
- In cases of acute inflammation, because increased blood supply will increase the inflammatory process
- In the presence of malignancies, because cell metabolism will be enhanced
- Over the pregnant uterus
- On areas of erythema or vesicles, because it will compound the existing problem
- Over metallic implants, because it will cause discomfort

Do not use cold:

- On open wounds, because decreased blood supply will delay healing
- In the presence of already-impaired circulation, because it will further impair circulation

## CHECKPOINT QUESTION

13. How does the body respond to prolonged exposure to temperature extremes?

## Ambulatory Assist Devices

Patients may lose their ability to move normally because of an accident or injury, disease process, neurologic or muscular defect, or degeneration. Patients who require assistance to maintain mobility may use crutches, a cane, a walker, or a wheelchair. Medical assistants often are responsible for teaching patients how to use these ambulatory aids safely. Remind the patient to

- Check the rubber tips frequently and replace worn tips immediately. (Most ambulatory aids require rubber tips, although some walkers have rollers.)
- Check screws and bolts frequently; tighten as needed.
- Remove scatter rugs and small pieces of furniture that may cause falls.
- Use caution on wet surfaces to avoid falling.
- To avoid damage to the axillary nerve, do not place the axillary bars against the axilla.
- Avoid back and neck strain by standing straight and looking ahead.

### Crutches

Crutches may be made of wood or tubular aluminum and may be ordered for short-term use or when the patient will need assistance long term for several months or years. Axillary crutches are the most common form and extend from just under the patient's axillae to the floor with hand grips to distribute weight to the palms. These crutches are typically prescribed for short-term conditions when the patient cannot bear weight on one extremity. The Lofstrand, or Canadian, crutch is usually aluminum and reaches just to the forearms, with a metal cuff to maintain its position on the arms and a covered hand grip to distribute the weight (Fig. 29-17A, B). Lofstrand crutches allow the patient to release and use the hands without losing the crutches. These work well for patients who will need crutches for a long period or for those who have poor coordination. Procedure 29-4 explains the steps necessary for measuring and fitting a patient with axillary crutches, and Procedure 29-5 explains how to teach a patient the proper gait techniques.

## PATIENT EDUCATION

### Tips for Crutch Walking

**To go up stairs**:

- Stand close to the bottom step.
- With the body's weight supported on the hands, step up on the first step with the unaffected leg.
- Bring the affected side and the crutches up to the step at the same time.
- Resume balance before proceeding to the next step.
- *Remember*: The good side goes up first!

**To go down stairs**:

- Stand close to the edge of the top step.
- Bend from the hips and knees to adjust to the height of the lower step. Do not lean forward (leaning forward may cause a fall).
- Carefully lower the crutches and the affected leg to the next step before moving the other extremity.
- Next, lower the unaffected leg to the lower step and regain balance.
- *Remember*: The affected foot goes down first!

**To sit**:

- Back up to the chair until you feel its edge on the back of your legs.
- Move both crutches to the hand on the affected side and reach back for the chair with the hand on the unaffected side.
- Lower yourself slowly into the chair.

## Canes

A cane is used when the patient needs extra support and stability but requires only a small measure of assistance with weight bearing. The standard cane may be used when the patient needs very slight assistance. The tripod (three legs) or quad cane (four legs) is useful when the patient needs greater stability (Fig. 29-18A–C). Tripod and quad canes can stand alone when patients need to use their hands or have other support. They tend to be bulkier and heavier than standard canes, but

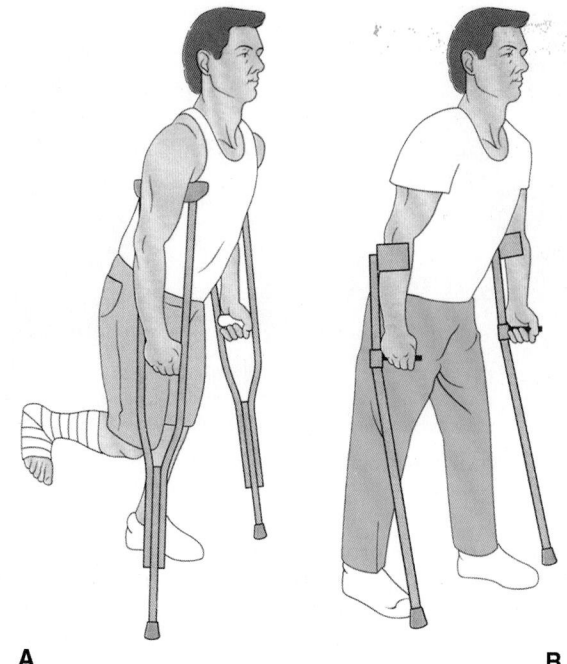

**A**                                    **B**

**Figure 29-17** • Types of crutches. **(A)** Axillary crutches. **(B)** Lofstrand crutches (also known as *Canadian* or *forearm crutches*).

because they offer greater stability and safety, they are good for patients who need more support than the standard cane affords.

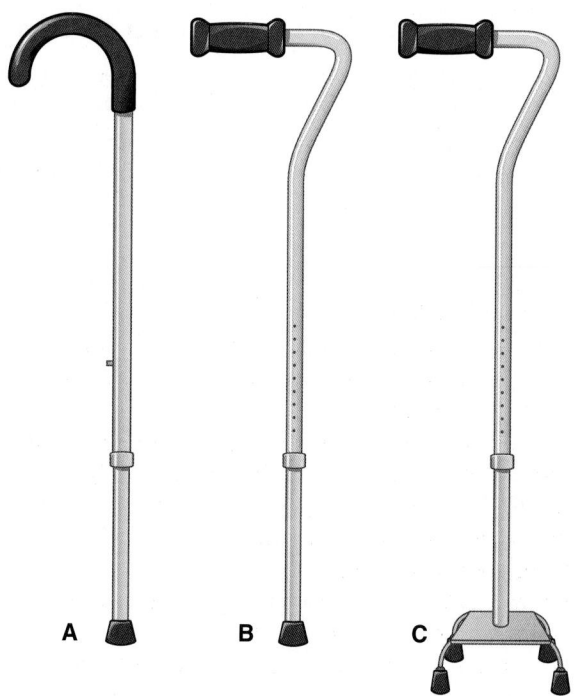

**A**          **B**          **C**

**Figure 29-18** • Three types of canes. **(A)** Single-ended canes with half-circle handles are recommended for patients requiring minimal support. **(B)** Single-ended canes with straight handles are recommended for patients with hand weakness. **(C)** Three- or four-prong canes are recommended for patients with poor balance.

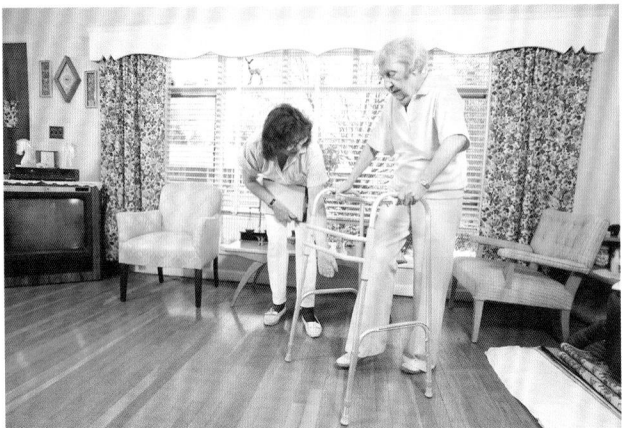

**Figure 29-19 •** A properly adjusted walker.

To measure for proper cane length, have the patient stand erect. The cane should be level with the patient's greater trochanter, and the patient's elbow should be bent at a 30 degree angle. To walk with a cane, the patient should

1. Position the cane on the unaffected side about 4 to 6 inches to the side and about 2 inches ahead of the foot.
2. Advance the cane and the affected leg together.

3. Bring the unaffected leg forward to a position just ahead of the cane.
4. Repeat the steps.

### Walkers

A walker is a comfortable aid for older adults and others with conditions that cause weakness or poor coordination. A walker is a lightweight aluminum frame-shaped–like three sides of a rectangle; however, because walkers are somewhat bulky, maneuvering in close quarters can be difficult. The walker frame should be level with the patient's hip, and the patient's elbow should be bent at about a 30-degree angle (Fig. 29-19). To use a walker

1. Stand erect and move the walker ahead about 6 inches.
2. Using an easy walking gait with hands on the walker grips, step into the walker.
3. Move the walker ahead again.
4. Repeat the steps.

### CHECKPOINT QUESTION

14. When instructing a patient on using a cane, on which side of the body should Tonya explain the cane positioned?

## MEDICATION BOX

### Commonly Prescribed Orthopedic Medications

**Note:** *The generic name of the drug is listed first and is written in all lower case letters. Brand names are in parentheses and the first letter is capitalized.*

| | | |
|---|---|---|
| Acetylsalicylic acid (aspirin) (Bayer, Ecotrin) | Tablets: 325 mg, 500 mg | Analgesic |
| Acetaminophen and codeine (Tylenol #3) | Tablets: 300 mg acetaminophen and codeine 30 mg | Analgesic |
| Adalimumab (Humira) | Injection: 40 mg/0.8 mL prefilled syringe | Antirheumatic |
| Alendronate sodium (Fosamax) | Tablets: 5 mg, 10 mg, 35 mg, 40 mg, 70 mg | Antiresorptive |
| Allopurinol (Lopurin, Zyloprim) | Tablets: 100 mg, 300 mg | Antigout |
| Calcium citrate (Citracal) | Tablets: 250 mg, 950 mg | Calcium |
| Carisoprodol (Soma) | Tablets: 250 mg, 350 mg | Muscle relaxant |
| Celecoxib (Celebrex) 200 mg, 400 mg | Capsules: 50 mg, 100 mg, NSAID | |
| Colchicines (Colcrys) | Tablets: 0.6 mg | Antigout |
| Cyclobenzaprine (Flexeril, Amrix) | Capsules: 15 mg, 30 mg | Muscle relaxant |
| Gold sodium thiomalate (Aurolate, Myochrysine) | Injection: 50 mg/mL (IM) | Antirheumatic |
| Hydrocodone and acetaminophen (Vicodin, Lortab) | Tablets: 500 mg acetaminophen and 5 mg hydrocodone | Analgesic |
| Ibandronate sodium (Boniva) | Tablets: 2.5 mg, 150 mg Injection: 3 mg/3 mL prefilled syringe (IV) | Antiresorptive |
| Ibuprofen (Motrin, Advil) | Capsules: 200 mg Tablets: 100 mg, 200 mg, 400 mg, 800 mg | NSAID |

## MEDICATION BOX (continued)

| | | |
|---|---|---|
| Indomethacin (Indocin) | Capsules: 25 mg, 50 mg Oral suspension: 25 mg/5 mL | NSAID |
| Meperidine hydrochloride (Demerol) | Tablets: 50 mg, 100 mg<br>Injection (IM): 25 mg/mL, 50 mg/mL, 75 mg/mL | Analgesic |
| Morphine sulfate (Duramorph, Kadian, Roxanol) | Tablets: 15 mg, 30 mg<br>Capsules: 30 mg to 120 mg<br>Oral solution: 10 mg/5 mL | Analgesic |
| Naproxen (Naprosyn) | Tablets: 200 mg, 250 mg, 375 mg, 500 mg | NSAID |
| Oxycodone (OxyContin, Roxicodone) | Capsules: 5 mg<br>Oral solution: 5 mg/5 mL<br>Tablets: 5 mg, 10 mg, 15 mg, 20 mg, 30 mg | Analgesic |
| Tramadol hydrochloride (Ultram) | Tablets: 50 mg | Analgesic |

## ROLE-PLAYING ACTIVITY

With cooperation from classmates or as assigned by your instructor, role-play interaction in the orthopedic office in which you are a medical assistant working with Tonya Barton (refer to the case study at the beginning of the chapter). An older teenager comes into the office with a below-the-knee cast on his leg that was applied 3 weeks ago for a broken tibia. His mother says he has been complaining of "severe itching" underneath the cast for about one week. You notice a scratch on the skin where the cast stops on the front of the leg. There is also an odor coming from the cast. What would you say to this patient? What questions would you ask about the care of the cast? In another situation, a patient comes into the office complaining of chronic back pain since he "fell" at work a year ago. He says his previous doctor said his back "could not be fixed" and gave him pain medications, but now, the doctor has retired and the patient would like more pain medication. Do you have any concerns or judgments about this patient or his request? How would you respond? Your instructor will give you additional information about this activity!

## español SPANISH TERMINOLOGY

**Voy a ponerle una tabilla en la pierna.**
I am going to put a splint on the leg.

**Voy a examinarle la pierna.**
I am going to examine your leg.

**Doble las rodillas, no la espalda.**
Bend your knees, not your back.

**¿Tiene dolor en sus articulaciones ó coyonturas?**
Do you feel pain in your joints?

**¿Tiene dolor en sus musculos?**
Do you feel pain in your muscles?

**Usted tiene un desgarro muscular.**
You have a strained muscle.

**Usted tiene un desgarre en un ligamento.**
You have a sprained ligament.

**Usted tiene que hacer estiramiento por lo menos diez minutos antes de hacer ejercicio.**
You need to stretch for at least ten minutes before exercising.

**R.I.C.E significa reposo, hielo, compresión y elevación**
R.I.C.E. means rest, ice, compression, and elevation.

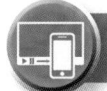

## MEDIA MENU

**Student Resources** on thePoint®
* *Animation:* Muscle Contraction
* *Video:* Measure a Patient for Axillary Crutches and Instruct in Various Gaits (Procedures 29-4 and 29-5)
* CMA/RMA Certification Exam Review

**Internet Resources**
**Arthritis Foundation**
http://www.arthritis.org
**Muscular Dystrophy Association**
http://www.mdausa.org
**About.com: What you need to know about orthopedics**
http://orthopedics.about.com
**American Association of Neurological Surgeons**
http://www.aans.org/Patient%20Information.aspx

# EMR Activity

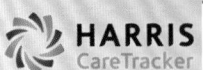
**HARRIS**
CareTracker

Harris CareTracker is a Web-based electronic medical record (EMR) application that you will use for the EMR activities included in this section at the end of each chapter. This application is actually used in physician offices, but is provided to you through the publisher, Wolters Kluwer Health, to give you hands-on practice working with EMRs. Your instructor will have more information about accessing your username, login, and Quickstart guide.

Prerequisite Activities in Harris CareTracker

*Note: The Getting Started and Quickstart documents and EMR Activities Step-by-Step Instructions are available at* http://thePoint.lww.com/KronenbergerComp5e

Activity Details

Document a note in each patient's EMR for an outgoing referral to the physical therapist's office noting insurance authorization for 10 physical therapy sessions starting today and good for 90 days.

1. Patient: Bobby Turner: Referral from Dr. Kyle Dunn to Rahim Patel, PT; insurance authorization PT9877611
2. Patient: Tammy Leonard: Referral from Dr. Kyle Dunn to Rahim Patel, PT; insurance authorization PT82259

## Chapter Summary

- The musculoskeletal system has many functions including the following:
  - Providing support and protection for vital organs
  - Allowing movement and mobility
  - Providing a frame (the skeleton) on which muscles are attached and the bones are held together at the joints
  - Providing stability and flexibility of the body

- Although the orthopedic physician specializes in the diagnosis and treatment of these conditions, you should expect to see patients with disorders of the musculoskeletal system in various medical offices, including pediatrics and family practice. In this chapter, you learned the following:
  - Common disorders of the musculoskeletal system including the upper and lower extremities
  - Diagnostic procedures including x-ray procedures that may be ordered by the physician to assist in diagnosing disorders of the musculoskeletal system
  - Various types of ambulatory assist devices that may be necessary for patients who have mobility problems related to disorders of the musculoskeletal system including canes and crutches
  - Your role in working with patients in the medical office who may have disorders of the musculoskeletal system

## Warm-Ups for Critical Thinking

1. Create a patient education brochure for the use of ambulatory aids. Be sure to include a brief description of the purpose of each aid along with the procedure steps.
2. The youth baseball league playoffs are coming to your town, and you are asked to staff the first aid station. What kinds of orthopedic injuries do you expect to see, and why? Develop a list of the first aid supplies that you want to have available and explain the reasons for your selections.
3. How would you respond to a patient with impaired circulation who tells you that he often uses a heating pad to relieve the pain in his legs although the physician has warned him not to do so?
4. Your patient with plantar fasciitis asks you why the pain is worse in the morning when first getting out of bed. Describe how you could explain this condition to a patient with limited understanding of human anatomy.
5. Using a drug reference book, look up several anti-inflammatory medications (naproxen sodium, ibuprofen). What gastrointestinal disorders may result from taking these medications, and how can these side effects be avoided?

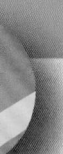

## **PSY** PROCEDURE 29-1

### Apply an Arm Sling

**PSY** Instruct and prepare a patient for a procedure or treatment; coach patients regarding disease prevention and treatment plans; coach patients appropriately considering cultural diversity, developmental life stage, and communication barriers; and document patient care accurately in the medical record.

**Purpose:** Correctly apply an arm sling

**Equipment:** A canvas arm sling with adjustable straps

| STEPS | PURPOSE |
|---|---|
| 1. Wash your hands. | Hand washing aids infection control. |
| 2. Assemble the equipment and supplies. | Be prepared before beginning any procedure. |
| 3. Greet and identify the patient and explain the procedure. Identify yourself including your credentials. | Identifying the patient prevents errors in the treatment. Explaining the procedure helps ease anxiety and ensure compliance. |
| 4. **AFF** Explain how to respond to a patient who does not speak English or speaks English as a second language (ESL). | Solicit assistance from anyone who may be with the patient or get another staff member who speaks his or her native language to interpret if available. If no interpreter is available, use hand gestures or pictures to explain the procedure to the patient. |
| 5. Position the affected limb with the hand at slightly less than a 90° angle so that the fingers are a bit higher than the elbow. | This position helps reduce swelling of the hand and fingers. |
| 6. Insert the arm into the pouch end of the sling with the elbow fitting into the pocket corner. | The elbow should fit snugly into the sling. |

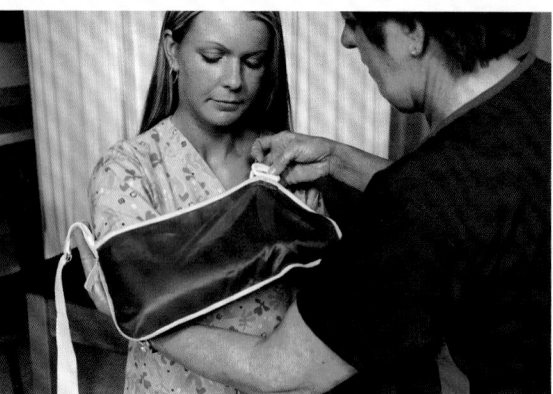

**Step 6.** Insert elbow into the pocket of sling.

## PROCEDURE 29-1 (continued)

| STEPS | PURPOSE |
|---|---|
| **7.** Bring the strap across the back and over the opposite shoulder to the front of the patient. | The back and unaffected shoulder will support the weight of the affected arm. |

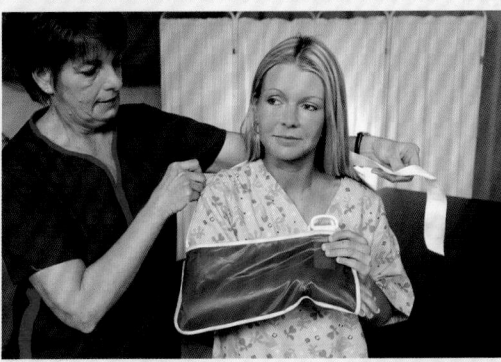

**8.** Secure the Velcro end of the strap by inserting the end of it under the loop on the sling. Pull the strap through the loop an adequate amount so that the arm and hand inside the sling continue to be slightly elevated at a 90 degree angle.

**Step 7.** Bring strap across back and to front of the patient.

The arm and hand should be at 90° to prevent swelling of the hand and fingers.

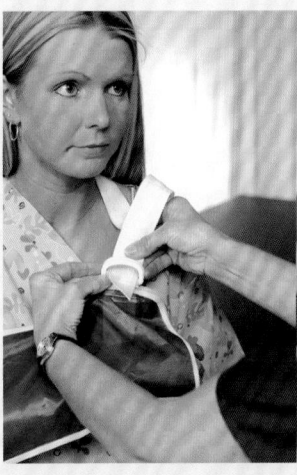

**9.** Press the Velcro ends together and check the patient's comfort and distal extremity circulation.

**Step 8.** Bring strap through loop.

Check circulation by palpating a radial pulse.

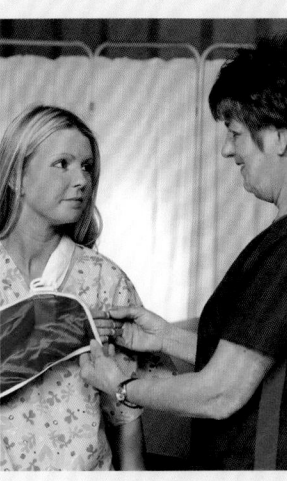

**Step 9.** Check circulation.

(continues on page 750)

## PROCEDURE 29-1 (continued)

| STEPS | PURPOSE |
|---|---|
| 10. Wash your hands. | |
| 11. **AFF** Log into the electronic medical record (EMR) using your username and secure password OR obtain the paper medical record from a secure location and assure it is kept away from public access. Record the application of the sling. Your entry must include the date, time, and your name/credentials. | The integrity of the medical record must be maintained at all times to protect patient privacy. Procedures are considered not to have been done if they are not recorded. |
| 12. When finished, log out of the EMR and/or replace the paper medical record in an appropriate and secure location. | |

Charting Example:
*10/28/2016 11:15 AM Arm sling applied to (R) arm as ordered. Fingers to (R) hand warm and pink, no swelling. To RTO in 4 days _____ T. Burton, RMA*

Note: *The medical assistant may sign his or her name in the patient record using only the "CMA" credential if the office has a signature log denoting the entire credential as "CMA(AAMA)."*

**PSY** PROCEDURE 29-2

## Apply Cold Packs

**PSY** Instruct and prepare a patient for a procedure or treatment; coach patients regarding disease prevention and treatment plans; coach patients appropriately considering cultural diversity, developmental life stage, and communication barriers; and document patient care accurately in the medical record.

**Purpose:** Apply a cold pack appropriately according to the physician's order

**Equipment:** Ice bag and ice chips or small cubes or a disposable cold pack, small towel or cover for the ice pack, and gauze or tape

| STEPS | PURPOSE |
|---|---|
| 1. Wash your hands. | Hand washing aids infection control. |
| 2. Assemble the equipment and supplies, checking the ice bag for leaks. If using a commercial cold pack, read the manufacturer's directions. | Avoid wetting and chilling the patient. Small bits of ice help the bag to conform to the patient's contours better than large pieces. |
| 3. Fill a reusable ice bag about two-thirds full. Press it flat on a surface to express air from the bag. Seal the container. | If the bag is too full of ice or air, it will not conform easily to the patient's contours. |
| 4. If using a commercial chemical ice pack, activate it according to the manufacturer's instructions. | Commercially prepared chemical ice packs contain chemicals that must be mixed before the pack will become cold. |
| 5. Cover the bag in a towel or other suitable cover. | The cover will absorb condensation and make the procedure more comfortable for the patient. |

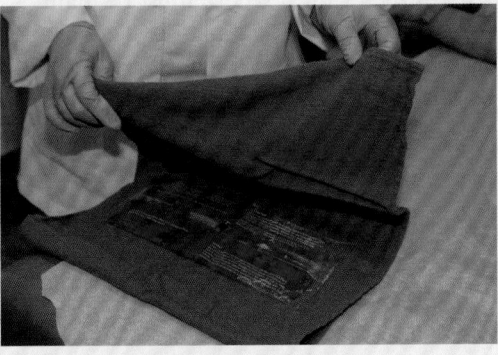

**Step 5.** Place the ice pack in a protective cover.

| STEPS | PURPOSE |
|---|---|
| 6. Greet and identify the patient. Identify yourself including your credentials. Explain the procedure. | Identifying the patient prevents errors in the treatment. Explaining the procedure helps ease anxiety and ensures compliance. |
| 7. **AFF** Explain how to respond to a patient who has cultural or religious beliefs that prohibit disrobing. | Be respectful of the cultural differences by explaining why procedures are important. Provide additional privacy if necessary. |
| 8. After assessing the skin for color and warmth, place the covered ice pack on the area. | The area must be assessed for the documentation before treatment begins. The cold pack should not come into direct contact with the skin. |

# PROCEDURE 29-2 (continued)

| STEPS | PURPOSE |
|---|---|
| 9. Secure the ice pack with gauze or tape. | The ice pack should lie securely against the patient's skin for the greatest benefit. Pins may puncture the ice bag. |

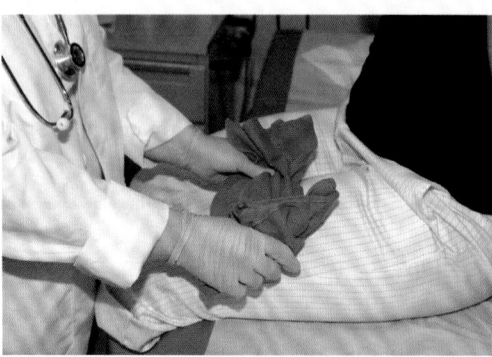

**Step 9.** Secure the ice pack with gauze or tape.

| STEPS | PURPOSE |
|---|---|
| 10. Apply the treatment for the prescribed amount of time and no longer than 30 minutes. | Longer than the prescribed time or 30 minutes may cause an adverse rebound effect, causing increased blood flow and swelling. |
| 11. During the treatment, assess the skin under the pack frequently for mottling, pallor, or redness. Remove the ice pack at once if these appear. | These signs indicate an adverse reaction and should be reported to the physician immediately after removing the ice pack. |
| 12. Properly care for or dispose of equipment and supplies. Wash your hands. | If the equipment is reusable, it should be prepared for the next patient by disinfecting according to office policy. If it is disposable, discard it appropriately. |
| 13. **AFF** Log into the electronic medical record (EMR) using your username and secure password OR obtain the paper medical record from a secure location and assure it is kept away from public access. Record the procedure, site of the application, results including the condition of the skin after the treatment, and the patient's response. Your entry must include the date, time, and your name/credentials. | The integrity of the medical record must be maintained at all times to protect patient privacy. Procedures are considered not to have been done if they are not recorded. |
| 14. When finished, log out of the EMR and/or replace the paper medical record in an appropriate and secure location. | |

---

Charting Example
*11/22/2016 10:45 AM Ice bag applied to (L) anterior thigh as ordered × 20 minutes. Skin before treatment swollen, with large contusion noted, no break in skin. After treatment, area pale and cool to touch, swelling decreased. Verbal and written instructions given for application qid at home; pt. verbalized understanding*
_____ *B. Barry, CMA*

---

Note: *The medical assistant may sign his or her name in the patient record using only the "CMA" credential if the office has a signature log denoting the entire credential as "CMA(AAMA)."*

**PSY** PROCEDURE 29-3

## Apply a Hot Water Bottle or Commercial Hot Pack

**PSY**  Instruct and prepare a patient for a procedure or treatment; coach patients regarding disease prevention and treatment plans; coach patients appropriately considering cultural diversity, developmental life stage, and communication barriers; and document patient care accurately in the medical record.

**Purpose**: Apply a hot pack appropriately according to the physician's order

**Equipment**: A hot water bottle or commercial hot pack and towel or other suitable covering for the hot pack

| STEPS | PURPOSE |
|---|---|
| 1. Wash your hands. | Hand washing aids infection control. |
| 2. Assemble equipment and supplies, checking the hot water bottle for leaks. | Checking for leaks avoids wetting the patient. |
| 3. Fill the hot water bottle about two-thirds full with warm (110°F) water; place the bottle on a flat surface with the opening up and press out the excess air. | Excess air will prevent the bottle from conforming to the patient's contours. |

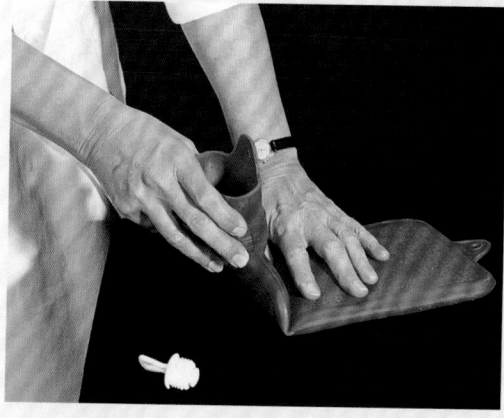

**Step 3.** Express air from the bottle before capping.

| | |
|---|---|
| 4. If using a commercial hot pack, follow the manufacturer's directions for activating it. | Commercially prepared chemical hot packs contain chemicals that must be mixed before the pack will become hot. |
| 5. Wrap and secure the pack or bottle before placing it on the patient's skin. | Covering the bag will increase the patient's comfort and prevent burning the skin. |

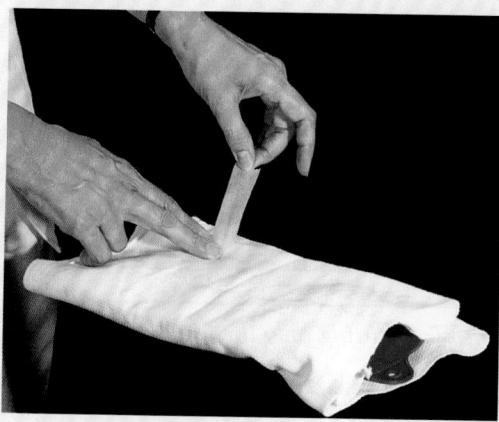

**Step .5** Wrap and secure the bag before placing on the patient's skin.

## PROCEDURE 29.3 (continued)

| STEPS | PURPOSE |
|---|---|
| **6.** Greet and identify the patient. Explain the procedure. | Identifying the patient prevents errors in the treatment. |
| **7.** After assessing the color of the skin where the treatment is to be applied, place the covered hot pack on the area. | The area must be assessed for documentation before the treatment begins. The hot pack should not touch the skin. Heat therapy should be used cautiously in patients with circulatory disorders, diabetics, and older adults. |
| **8.** **AFF** Explain how to respond to a patient who is from a different generation than you. | Refer to an elderly patient by his or her correct title (Mr., Mrs., Miss, etc.). Be respectful to the patient by only using his or her first name after they have given you permission to do so. Do not assume the patient is hearing or cognitively impaired because of his or her age. |
| **9.** Secure the hot pack with gauze or tape. | It should be securely against the patient's skin for the greatest benefit. Pins may puncture the hot pack. |
| **10.** Apply the treatment for the prescribed amount of time but for no longer than 30 minutes. | Longer than the prescribed time or 30 minutes may cause an adverse rebound effect and decreased blood flow to the area. |
| **11.** During the treatment, assess the skin every 10 minutes for pallor (rebound), excessive redness (pack too hot), and swelling (tissue damage). If you see any of these signs, immediately remove the hot pack. | These signs indicate an adverse reaction and should be reported to the physician immediately after you remove the hot pack. |
| **12.** Properly care for or dispose of equipment and supplies. Wash your hands. | Reusable equipment should be disinfected for the next patient. Disposables should be discarded appropriately. |
| **13.** **AFF** Log into the electronic medical record (EMR) using your username and secure password *or* obtain the paper medical record from a secure location and assure it is kept away from public access. Record the procedure, site of the application, results including the condition of the skin after the treatment, and the patient's response. Your entry must include the date, time, and your name/credentials. | The integrity of the medical record must be maintained at all times to protect patient privacy. Procedures are considered not to have been done if they are not recorded. |
| **14.** When finished, log out of the EMR and/or replace the paper medical record in an appropriate and secure location. | |

---

Charting Example:
*7/11/2016 3:00 PM Hot pack to (L) shoulder × 30 minutes as ordered. Skin pink before treatment, slightly reddened after treatment. Pt. stated pain in upper back and shoulder relieved. Oral and written instructions given for applications at home qid, Pt. verbalized understanding* _____ *S. Rose, CMA*

---

Note: *The medical assistant may sign his or her name in the patient record using only the "CMA" credential if the office has a signature log denoting the entire credential as "CMA(AAMA)."*

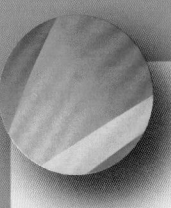

## PSY   PROCEDURE 29-4

# Measure a Patient for Axillary Crutches

**PSY** Instruct and prepare a patient for a procedure or treatment; coach patients regarding disease prevention and treatment plans; coach patients appropriately considering cultural diversity, developmental life stage, and communication barriers; and document patient care accurately in the medical record.

**Purpose**: Accurately measure a patient for axillary crutches

**Equipment**: Axillary crutches with tips, pads for the axilla, and hand rests as needed

| STEPS | PURPOSE |
|---|---|
| 1. Wash your hands. | Hand washing aids infection control. |
| 2. Assemble the equipment, including crutches' correct size. | Axillary crutches must always be fitted to the height of the patient. |
| 3. Greet and identify the patient. Identify yourself including your credentials. | This helps avoid errors in treatment. |
| 4. Ensure that the patient is wearing low-heeled shoes with safety soles. | Low-heeled shoes with good soles assist with adjusting the crutches to the patient's height and help prevent falls. While using the crutches, patients should wear shoes with the same heel height to avoid an improper crutch fit. |
| 5. Have the patient stand erect. Support the patient as needed. | Standing will allow you to adjust the crutches to the correct height. |
| 6. **AFF** Explain how to respond to a patient who is hearing impaired. | Make sure the patient can see your face as you are speaking. Speak clearly, not loudly. |
| 7. While standing erect, have the patient hold the crutches naturally with the tips about 2 inches in front of and 4 to 6 inches to the sides of the feet. This is called the *tripod position*, and all crutch gaits start from this position. | This is the *tripod position*, and all crutch gaits start from this position. |
| 8. Adjust the central support in the base so that the axillary bar is about two fingerbreadths below the patient's axillae. Tighten the bolts for safety at the proper height. | If the axillary bar presses on the axillae, nerve damage may occur. If it is too low, the crutches will be difficult to manage and will cause poor posture and back strain. |

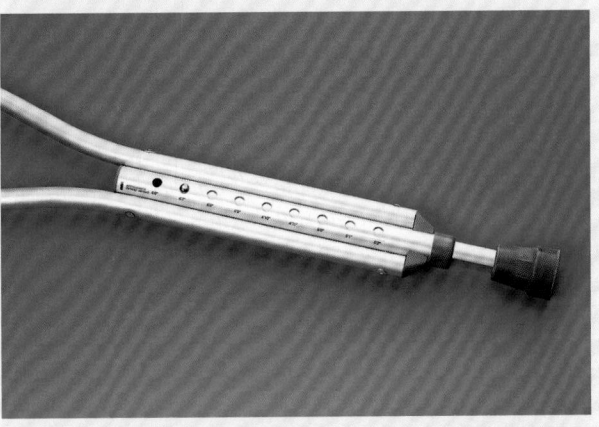

**Step 8.** (**A**) Adjust the crutches to the patient's height by removing the wing nut and bolt and moving the extension. (**B**) Tighten the bolt securely.

| STEPS | PURPOSE |
|---|---|
| 9. Adjust the hand grips by raising or lowering the bar so that the patient's elbow is at a 30° angle when the bar is gripped. Tighten bolts for safety. | Hand grips that are too high or too low will compromise safety and may cause nerve pressure. |

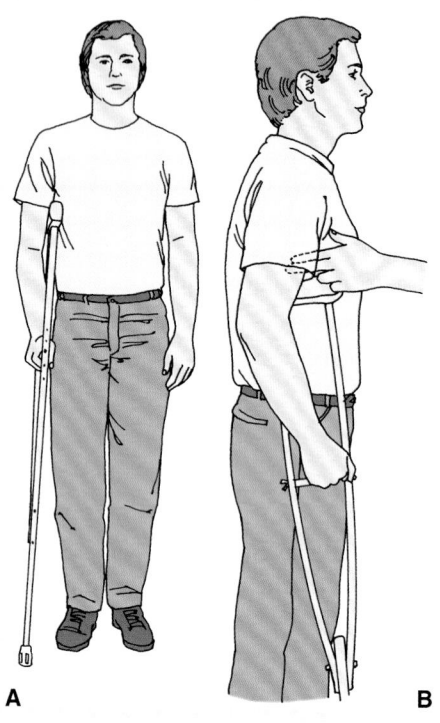

**A**      **B**

**Step 9.** (**A**) Adjust the hand grips by raising or lowering along the shaft of the crutch. (**B**) Crutches are properly adjusted when the patient's elbow is at a 30 degree angle and two fingers can be inserted under the axilla on top of the crutch axillary bar.

| STEPS | PURPOSE |
|---|---|
| 10. If needed, pad axillary bars and hand grips with soft material, such as large gauze pads or small towels, and secure with tape to prevent friction. | If padding is used on the axillary bars, make sure the padding is not touching the axilla; this is to avoid pressure and damage to the axillary nerve. |
| 11. Wash your hands. | |
| 12. **AFF** Log into the electronic medical record (EMR) using your username and secure password OR obtain the paper medical record from a secure location and assure it is kept away from public access. Record the procedure, site of the application, results including the condition of the skin after the treatment, and the patient's response. Your entry must include the date, time, and your name/credentials. | The integrity of the medical record must be maintained at all times to protect patient privacy. Procedures are considered not to have been done if they are not recorded. |
| 13. When finished, log out of the EMR and/or replace the paper medical record in an appropriate and secure location. | |

---

Charting Example:

*3/17/2016 4:40 PM Pt. measured for axillary crutches as ordered; no pressure to axilla, elbows at a 30° angle. Given oral and written instructions for crutch safety and the 3-point and swing-through gaits. Demonstrated both gaits without difficulty. Verbalized understanding of instructions. Reinforced physician order for no weight bearing on (L) leg × 3 days, to return to office in 4 days* _____ *B. Daye, RMA*

---

Note: *The medical assistant may sign his or her name in the patient record using only the "CMA" credential if the office has a signature log denoting the entire credential as "CMA(AAMA)."*

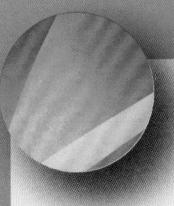

PROCEDURE 29-5

# Instruct a Patient in Various Crutch Gaits

**PSY** Instruct and prepare a patient for a procedure or treatment; coach patients regarding disease prevention and treatment plans; coach patients appropriately considering cultural diversity, developmental life stage, and communication barriers; and document patient care accurately in the medical record.

**Purpose**: Properly instruct a patient in various gaits using axillary crutches

**Equipment**: Axillary crutches measured appropriately for a patient

| STEPS | PURPOSE |
|---|---|
| 1. Wash your hands. | Hand washing aids infection control. |
| 2. Have the patient stand up from a chair, holding both crutches on the affected side, then sliding to the edge of the chair. The patient pushes down on the chair arm on the unaffected side, then pushes to stand. With one crutch in each hand, he or she rests on the crutches until balance is restored. | Encourage the patient to use the large leg and arm muscles to stand instead of back muscles to avoid straining the back. |
| 3. **AFF** Explain how to respond to a patient who is visually impaired. | Observe patients carefully to prevent injury. Face the patient when speaking, and always let him or her know what you are going to do before touching him or her. |
| 4. Assist the patient to the tripod position. | To ensure safety and proper balance, crutches should be in this position before proceeding with any gait. |
| 5. Depending on the patient's weight-bearing ability, coordination, and general state of health, instruct the patient in one or more of the following gaits: | Most patients will use one or two gaits and should be taught how to use those gaits safely. |

5. A. Three-point gait, most commonly used for crutch training. For use when only one leg can bear weight or only partial weight bearing is allowed on the affected leg. Used by amputees, those with injury to one leg, and leg or foot surgery patients. Requires coordination and upper body strength
   (1) Move both crutches forward with the unaffected leg bearing weight
   (2) Supporting weight on hand grips, bring unaffected leg past crutches
   (3) Repeat.

B. Two-point gait requires partial weight bearing and good coordination. Two points are raised, and two points are always on the floor.
   (1) Move right crutch and left foot forward.
   (2) As these points rest, move right foot and left crutch forward.
   (3) Repeat.

C. Four-point gait, slowest and safest of the gaits. At least three points are on the ground at all times. The affected leg must bear partial weight. Used by patients with degenerative diseases, spasticity, or poor coordination
   (1) Move right crutch forward.
   (2) Move left foot just ahead of left crutch.

*(continues on page 758)*

# PROCEDURE 29-5 (continued)

| STEPS | PURPOSE |
|---|---|

**(3)** Move left crutch forward.
**(4)** Move right foot just ahead of right crutch.
**(5)** Repeat.
D. Swing-through gait
　**(1)** Move both crutches forward.
　**(2)** With weight on hands, swing body ahead of crutches, with both legs leaving the floor together.
　**(3)** Move crutches ahead.
　**(4)** Repeat.
E. Swing-to gait
　**(1)** Move both crutches forward.
　**(2)** With weight on hands, swing body even with crutches, with both legs leaving the floor.
　**(3)** Move crutches ahead.
　**(4)** Repeat.

| 4 POINT GAIT | 2 POINT GAIT | 3 POINT GAIT | SWING TO | SWING THROUGH |
|---|---|---|---|---|
| • Partial weight bearing both feet<br>• Maximal support provided<br>• Requires constant shift of weight | • Partial weight bearing both feet<br>• Provides less support than 4 point gait<br>• Faster than a 4 point gait | • Non weight bearing<br>• Requires good balance<br>• Requires arm strength<br>• Faster gait<br>• Can use with walker | • Weight bearing both feet<br>• Provides stability<br>• Requires arm strength<br>• Can use with walker | • Weight bearing<br>• Requires arm strength<br>• Requires coordination/balance<br>• Most advanced gait |
| 4. Advance right foot | 4. Advance right foot and left crutch | 4. Advance right foot | 4. Lift both feet/swing forward/land feet next to crutches | 4. Lift both feet/swing forward/land feet in front of crutches |
| 3. Advance left crutch | 3. Advance left foot and right crutch | 3. Advance left foot and both crutches | 3. Advance both crutches | 3. Advance both crutches |
| 2. Advance left foot | 2. Advance right foot and left crutch | 2. Advance right foot | 2. Lift both feet/swing forward/land feet next to crutches | 2. Lift both feet/swing forward/land feet in front of crutches |
| 1. Advance right crutch | 1. Advance left foot and right crutch | 1. Advance left foot and both crutches | 1. Advance both crutches | 1. Advance both crutches |
| Beginning stance | Beginning stance | Beginning stance | Beginning stance | Beginning stance |

**Step 5.** Crutch gaits.

## PROCEDURE 29-5 (continued)

| STEPS | PURPOSE |
|---|---|
| 6. Wash your hands. | |
| 7. **AFF** Log into the electronic medical record (EMR) using your username and secure password OR obtain the paper medical record from a secure location and assure it is kept away from public access. Record the patient education and instructions. Your entry must include the date, time, and your name/credentials. | The integrity of the medical record must be maintained at all times to protect patient privacy. Procedures are considered not to have been done if they are not recorded. |
| 8. When finished, log out of the EMR and/or replace the paper medical record in an appropriate and secure location. | |

Charting Example:
*See Charting Example for Procedure 29-4.*

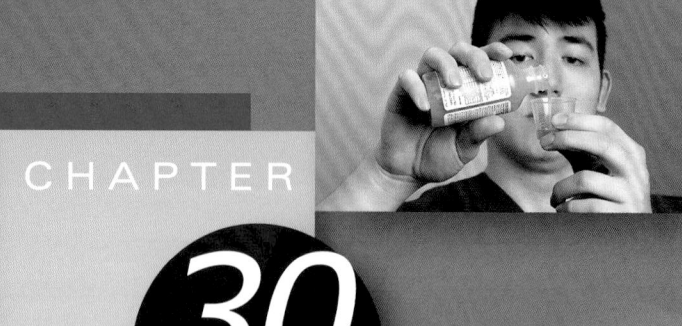

# CHAPTER

# 30

# Ophthalmology and Otolaryngology

## Outline

**Common Disorders of the Eye**
Cataract
**Stye or Hordeolum**
Conjunctivitis
Corneal Ulcer
Retinopathy
Glaucoma
Refractive Errors
Strabismus
Color Deficit
**Diagnostic Studies of the Eye**
Visual Acuity Testing
Color Deficit Testing
Tonometry and Gonioscopy
**Therapeutic Procedures for the Eye**
Instilling Eye Medications

**Common Disorders of the Ear**
Ceruminosis
Conductive and Perceptual Hearing Loss
Ménière Disease
Otitis Externa
Otitis Media
Otosclerosis
**Diagnostic Studies of the Ear**
Visual Examination
Audiometry and Tympanometry
Tuning Fork Tests
**Therapeutic Procedures for the Ear**
Irrigations and Instillations

**Common Disorders of the Nose and Throat**
Allergic Rhinitis
Epistaxis
Nasal Polyps
Sinusitis
Pharyngitis and Tonsillitis
Laryngitis
**Diagnostic Studies of the Nose and Throat**
Visual Inspection
**Therapeutic Procedures for the Nose and Throat**
Throat Culture

## Learning Outcomes

### COG Cognitive Domain*

1. Spell key terms
2. *Define medical terms and abbreviations related to all body systems*
3. *Describe structural organization of the human body*
4. *List major organs in each body system*
5. *Identify the anatomical location of major organs in each body system*
6. *Describe the normal function of each body system*
7. *Identify common pathology related to each body system including signs, symptoms, and etiology*
   a. Describe common eye, ear, nose, and throat disorders
   b. Identify and explain diagnostic eye, ear, nose, and throat procedures
8. Describe patient education procedures associated with the eye, ear, nose, and throat

### PSY Psychomotor Domain*

1. Measure distance visual acuity with a Snellen chart (Procedure 30-1)
   a. *Instruct and prepare a patient for a procedure or treatment*
   b. *Coach patients appropriately considering cultural diversity, developmental life stage, and communication barriers*
2. *Document patient care accurately in the medical record.* Measure color perception with an Ishihara color plate book (Procedure 30-2)
   a. *Instruct and prepare a patient for a procedure or treatment*
   b. *Coach patients appropriately considering cultural diversity, developmental life stage, and communication barriers*
   c. *Document patient care accurately in the medical record*

3. Instill eye medication (Procedure 30-3)
   a. *Instruct and prepare a patient for a procedure or treatment*
   b. *Coach patients appropriately considering cultural diversity, developmental life stage, and communication barriers*
   c. *Document patient care accurately in the medical record*
4. Irrigate the eye (Procedure 30-4)
   a. *Instruct and prepare a patient for a procedure or treatment*
   b. *Coach patients appropriately considering cultural diversity, developmental life stage, and communication barriers*
   c. *Document patient care accurately in the medical record*
5. Irrigate the ear (Procedure 30-5)
   a. *Instruct and prepare a patient for a procedure or treatment*
   b. *Coach patients appropriately considering cultural diversity, developmental life stage, and communication barriers*
   c. *Document patient care accurately in the medical record*
6. Administer an audiometric hearing test (Procedure 30-6)
   a. *Instruct and prepare a patient for a procedure or treatment*
   b. *Coach patients appropriately considering cultural diversity, developmental life stage, and communication barriers*
   c. *Document patient care accurately in the medical record*
7. Instill ear medication (Procedure 30-7)
   a. *Instruct and prepare a patient for a procedure or treatment*
   b. *Coach patients appropriately considering cultural diversity, developmental life stage, and communication barriers*
   c. *Document patient care accurately in the medical record*
8. Instill nasal medication (Procedure 30-8)
   a. *Instruct and prepare a patient for a procedure or treatment*
   b. *Coach patients appropriately considering cultural diversity, developmental life stage, and communication barriers*
   c. *Document patient care accurately in the medical record*

### AFF Affective Domain*

1. *Incorporate critical thinking skills when performing patient assessment*
2. *Incorporate critical thinking skills when performing patient care*
3. *Show awareness of a patient's concerns related to the procedure being performed*
4. *Demonstrate empathy, active listening, and nonverbal communication*
5. *Demonstrate respect for individual diversity including gender, race, religion, age, economic status, and appearance*
6. *Explain to a patient the rationale for performance of a procedure*
7. *Demonstrate sensitivity to patient rights*
8. *Protect the integrity of the medical record*

*Note: AAMA/CAAHEP 2015 Standards are italicized.*

### ABHES Competencies

1. Assist the physician with the regimen of diagnostic and treatment modalities as they relate to each body system
2. Comply with federal, state, and local health laws and regulations
3. Communicate on the recipient's level of comprehension
4. Serve as a liaison between the physician and others
5. Show empathy and impartiality when dealing with patients
6. Document accurately

# Key Terms

| | | | |
|---|---|---|---|
| astigmatism | intraocular pressure | optometrist | retinal degeneration |
| cerumen | myopia | otolaryngologist | strabismus |
| decibel (db) | myringotomy | otoscope | tinnitus |
| fluorescein angiography | ophthalmologist | presbycusis | tonometry |
| hordeolum | ophthalmoscope | presbyopia | |
| hyperopia | optician | refraction | |

## Case Study

Charlene Mayers, CMA (AAMA), is a new medical assistant who works in the Great Falls Medical Center Ear, Nose, and Throat Office. Before moving to this office, Charlene worked in a family practice office for 5 years, a pediatric office for 2 years, and an urgent care office for 4 years. In all these settings, she worked with patients with eye and ear problems. She learned of an opening in this specialty office through a local chapter meeting for professional medical assistants and decided to apply for the position after speaking with several medical assistants employed at the office. The office staff include two physicians, a nurse practitioner, an audiologist, four certified medical assistants, a receptionist, and a scheduler who works with the hospital to schedule patients for inpatient and outpatient procedures. Today, a 62-year-old patient is seen in the office with complaints of "hearing problems" and difficulty breathing due to a "stuffy nose." He believes the symptoms are related and has many questions about getting hearing aids and allergy shots. When Charlene asked for his arm to take his blood pressure, he said he had "not had blood taken in a while" and he did not answer and continued to read a pamphlet he picked up on hearing loss when Charlene asked him if he snores during sleep. How should Charlene or any medical assistant communicate with a patient who has known or suspected hearing loss? Should Charlene advise him that he probably has allergies because many people do and that he may benefit from allergy shots? Why or why not? These and other questions related to the eyes and ears are addressed in this chapter.

Medical assistants working for **ophthalmologists**, who specialize in disorders of the eyes, or **otolaryngologists**, who specialize in disorders of the ears, nose, and throat (also known as *ENT physicians*), are expected to perform basic procedures associated with these body systems. Medical assistants working in general family practice and pediatric offices also encounter patients with eye or ear disorders and are expected to perform basic procedures associated with the eyes, ears, nose, and throat in these settings as well. This chapter describes the various disorders, diagnostic tests, and treatment modalities that are included in the eye, ear, nose, or throat examination.

## COMMON DISORDERS OF THE EYE

Light waves are reflected off of all objects and are transmitted through various structures of the eye including the cornea, lens, and retina (Fig. 30-1). These impulses are transmitted via the optic nerve to the occipital lobe of the cerebral cortex in the brain. When the rays of light are bent, or refracted, by the curvature of the cornea and lens, the occiput recognizes whether the objects are in or out of focus. If the objects are out of focus to the occiput, impulses are sent to change the shape of the lens or the position of the extrinsic muscles to sharpen the image.

While the eye is a complex, highly developed organ, any of its many components may malfunction or become infected or diseased. The most common eye disorders that you may encounter in a medical office are described in the following sections. In addition, Box 30-1 describes guidelines for assisting sight-impaired patients in a medical office.

## Cataract

A cataract is an opacity, or clouding, of the lens that leads to decreased visual acuity. Most commonly, cataracts are bilateral and seen in older adults. A rare condition in infancy can result from maternal exposure to the rubella virus. This condition is known as *congenital cataracts*. Occasionally, trauma to the lens or chemical toxicity causes clouding of the lens.

The symptoms include gradual blurring and loss of vision over months as the clouding of the lens slowly progresses. The observer may see a milky opacity at the pupil rather than the normal black opening (Fig. 30-2). An examination with an **ophthalmoscope** reveals the white area behind the pupil if the cataract has not advanced to the point where it can be seen unassisted.

The treatment for cataracts is surgical removal of the opaque lens. This surgery is beneficial in 95% of patients and is usually an outpatient procedure. After the cloudy lens has been removed, an intraocular lens is implanted, or the patient's vision is corrected by contact lenses or special glasses.

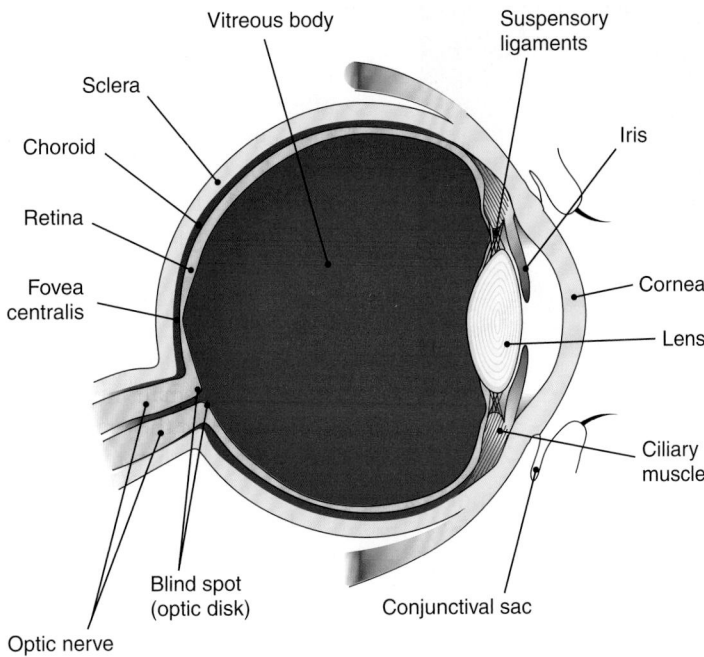

**FIGURE 30-1** • The eye. (Reprinted from Cohen BJ. *Memmler's The Human Body in Health and Disease*, 11th ed. Philadelphia, PA: Lippincott Williams & Wilkins, 2009, with permission.)

# STYE OR HORDEOLUM

A stye, or hordeolum, is an infection of any of the lacrimal glands of the eyelids, causing redness, swelling, and pain. The causative infectious organism is often *Staphylococcus aureus*, a microorganism commonly found on the skin. Warm compresses will hasten suppuration of the infection, and topical antibiotic drops or ointments attack the microorganism. You may be responsible for teaching the patient the procedure for applying warm compresses and instilling ophthalmic drops or ointment.

## CHECKPOINT QUESTION

1. What are the symptoms of a cataract?

## Conjunctivitis

Conjunctivitis, an infection of the mucous membrane covering the sclera and cornea (conjunctiva) of the eye, is caused by several species of bacteria or viruses. Additional causes of conjunctivitis include allergens or irritants without an infectious process. Many pathogens cause unilateral conjunctivitis, but allergic conjunctivitis is almost always bilateral.

---

**BOX 10-1   Assisting Sight-Impaired Patients**

Follow these tips to assist a sight-impaired patient:

• Ask patients how you can help, and follow their requests and suggestions. Many sight-impaired patients know best what they need.

• When escorting the patient, offer your arm. Tell the patient the approximate length of the hallway and advise the patient of any turns, such as "It should be about 20 steps and then we'll take a right." Avoid stairs if possible, but if you must assist a sight-impaired patient up or down stairs, advise the person of the number of steps. Many patients prefer to hold the railings for balance.

• If the patient has a guide dog, do not approach the dog without first speaking to the patient and receiving approval.

• If the patient needs extensive teaching on a particular subject, suggest using a tape recorder to record the instructions.

---

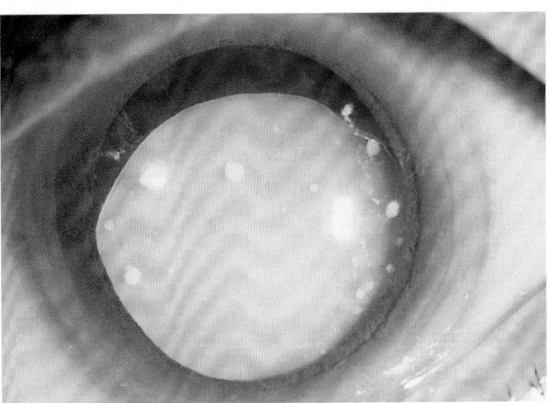

**FIGURE 30-2** • An eye with a cataract.

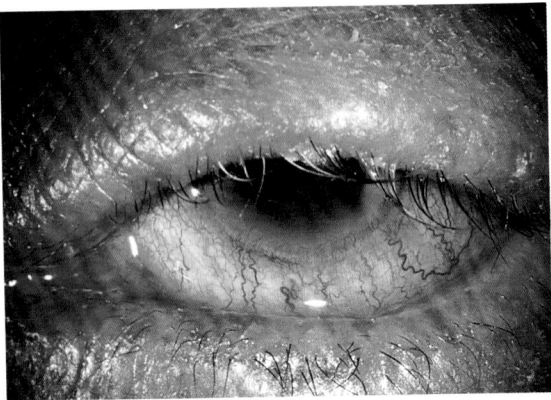

**FIGURE 30-3** • Conjunctivitis.

Signs and symptoms of conjunctivitis include tearing and occasionally exudates and pain (Fig. 30-3). Bacterial and viral conjunctivitis, or pink eye, is highly contagious and can rapidly spread through schools and day care centers. It is spread by contact; for example, an infectious child rubs the eyes, handles objects such as toys or books, and spreads the infection to the next child who comes into contact with the contaminated object. The infected child should not go to school or day care until the infection is treated and has been resolved. Good hygiene, including hand washing, helps prevent the spread of infectious conjunctivitis. Antibiotic ophthalmic drops or ointment are prescribed by the physician if the cause of the conjunctivitis is bacterial. To prevent the spread of conjunctivitis, you should instruct the patient to do the following:

- Avoid rubbing the eyes to prevent spreading the infection to the other eye or to other people.
- Discard all eye makeup that may be infectious.
- Wash all towels, washcloths, and pillowcases after use.

## Corneal Ulcer

A corneal ulcer is erosion of the surface of the cornea, leaving scar tissue that may lead to visual disturbances or blindness. Corneal ulcers are caused by several types of bacteria, fungi, viruses, and protozoa or by trauma, allergen, or toxin. Signs and symptoms include tearing, pain on blinking, and sensitivity to light. A visual examination with a penlight shows an irregular corneal surface. A fluorescein dye is administered by placing a strip gently in the sulcus of the eye; this stains the perimeter of the ulcer to confirm the diagnosis. Treatment includes rest and antibiotic therapy.

### CHECKPOINT QUESTION

2. Explain the difference between a stye and conjunctivitis.

## Retinopathy

Retinopathy is a general term for disease or disorder affecting the retina. A decrease in the blood supply to the highly vascular retina will cause **retinal degeneration**, pathologic changes in cell structure that impair or destroy the retina's function. The causes include atherosclerosis that impedes blood flow to the retina, the microcirculatory changes associated with diabetes (diabetic retinopathy), and vascular changes resulting from long-term hypertension. Depending on the cause, the patient's loss of vision may be sudden or gradual. Loss of vision may be preceded by small intraocular hemorrhages, night blindness, or loss of the central visual field. If small vessels rupture and scar, they may pull against the retina and cause retinal detachment that results in blindness.

Diagnosis of retinopathy is made by a thorough eye examination and **fluorescein angiography**. This procedure involves injection of fluorescent dye into one of the veins of the arms and photographing the blood vessels of the eye as the dye moves through it. The treatment of retinopathy is based on treating the underlying cause. Although some forms of retinopathy respond well to treatment, others progress to full blindness.

## Glaucoma

Glaucoma describes a group of disorders that result in increased **intraocular pressure**, or pressure within the eye. As aqueous humor is formed in the posterior chamber just in front of the lens, it flows through the pupil to the anterior chamber just behind the cornea. It eventually filters into the canal of Schlemm. Any pathology that impedes the outflow of aqueous humor (genetics, vasoconstriction) will increase the pressure, either very gradually or quite suddenly. The gradual form of glaucoma (open-angle glaucoma) may present with mild or no pain, visualizing halos around lights, and loss of peripheral vision. Most adult glaucoma patients have this type of glaucoma. Angle-closure glaucoma, an acute and sudden blockage, is characterized by severe eye pain, blurred vision, headache, nausea, and vomiting. Blindness may result within days of the onset of acute glaucoma unless the condition is diagnosed and treated quickly.

Treatment for chronic glaucoma includes medication, often a diuretic, to decrease intraocular pressure by slowing the formation of aqueous humor within the eyes or by improving the flow. Acute glaucoma may necessitate an iridectomy, or removal of part of the iris, to increase the outflow of the humor. Frequent eye examinations, including **tonometry**, may detect glaucoma and facilitate treatment before visual deficiencies and blindness result.

## Refractive Errors

Errors of **refraction** are the most common of all eye problems. The primary types of refractive errors are **hyperopia**, **myopia**, **astigmatism**, and **presbyopia** (Fig. 30-4A, B).

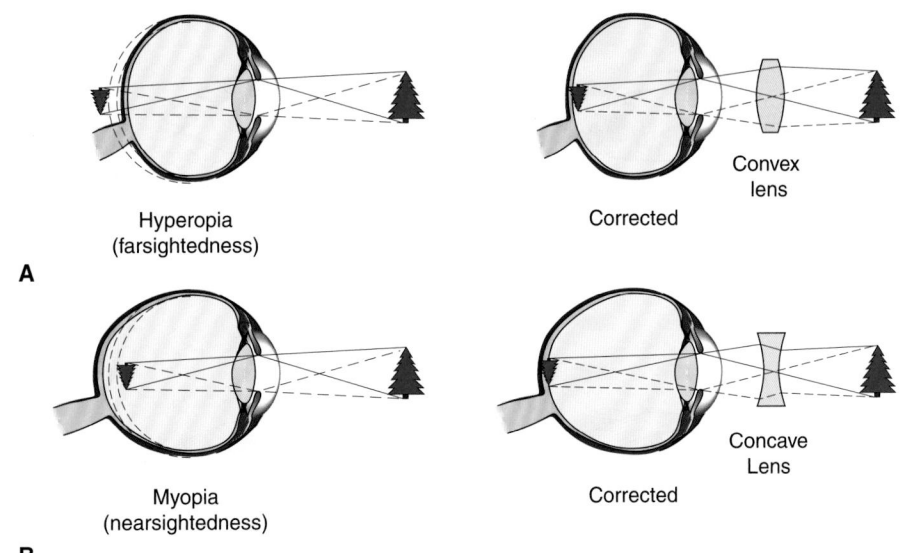

**FIGURE 30-4** • Errors of refraction. **(A)** The hypertrophic eye with convex corrective lens. **(B)** The myopic eye with concave corrective lens. (Reprinted from Cohen BJ. *Memmler's The Human Body in Health and Disease*, 11th ed. Philadelphia, PA: Lippincott Williams & Wilkins, 2009, with permission.)

Hyperopia, also known as farsightedness, occurs in an eyeball that is too short from front to back to allow the lines of vision to reflect distinctly on the fovea centralis. The person with hyperopia cannot focus on objects near the face.

Myopia, also known as nearsightedness, results when the eyeball is too long. The lines of vision converge before they reach the fovea centralis and begin to diverge again at the fovea. Objects must be near the face for the image to be focused far back on the retina.

Astigmatism is unfocused refraction of light rays on the retina resulting from lens or corneal irregularities. If the cornea is not smooth, images refracted through it will not project sharply onto the retina; the effect is much like peering through wavy glass.

Presbyopia is vision change resulting from loss of lens elasticity with age. The lens normally adjusts to refract light from near or far. As a person ages, the ciliary bodies that hold and adjust the lens and the lens itself lose elasticity and no longer accommodate near vision; far vision may be unaffected. Symptoms usually begin gradually around age 40 years. Most adults are affected to some degree by age 50 years.

All refractive errors are treated with either corrective lenses or reshaping the lens with laser surgery (Box 30-2). An **optometrist** is a trained specialist who measures errors of refraction and prescribes lenses. An **optician** is a trained specialist who grinds lenses to fulfill corrective prescriptions written by either an optometrist or an ophthalmologist, a medical doctor who treats eye disorders or performs surgical corrections.

## CHECKPOINT QUESTION

3. What are the four common refractive errors? Briefly explain each.

## Strabismus

Strabismus is a misalignment of eye movements, usually caused by muscle incoordination. Although most newborns are born with some degree of strabismus, coordination improves as the infant grows and the eye muscles strengthen. However, the strabismus does not resolve in

---

**BOX 10-2   Laser Surgery to Correct Errors of Refraction**

A procedure that is popular among patients to correct myopia, hyperopia, and astigmatism is a surgical procedure called *LASIK*, which stands for laser in situ keratomileusis. An ophthalmologist uses a laser to reshape the cornea, allowing the light to properly focus on the retina and correcting these errors of refraction. Advantages of this procedure include the following:

• It is an outpatient procedure that takes very little time to perform.
• The vision of most people is corrected within 24 hours.
• There is a quick recovery time with very little pain.
• There is no need for glasses or contacts in most patients after the procedure.

Disadvantages include the following:

• The procedure is expensive.
• Changes made to the cornea cannot be reversed.
• Some side effects, such as dry eyes, may be experienced by some patients.

Patients wanting to know more about this procedure should be referred to an ophthalmologist.

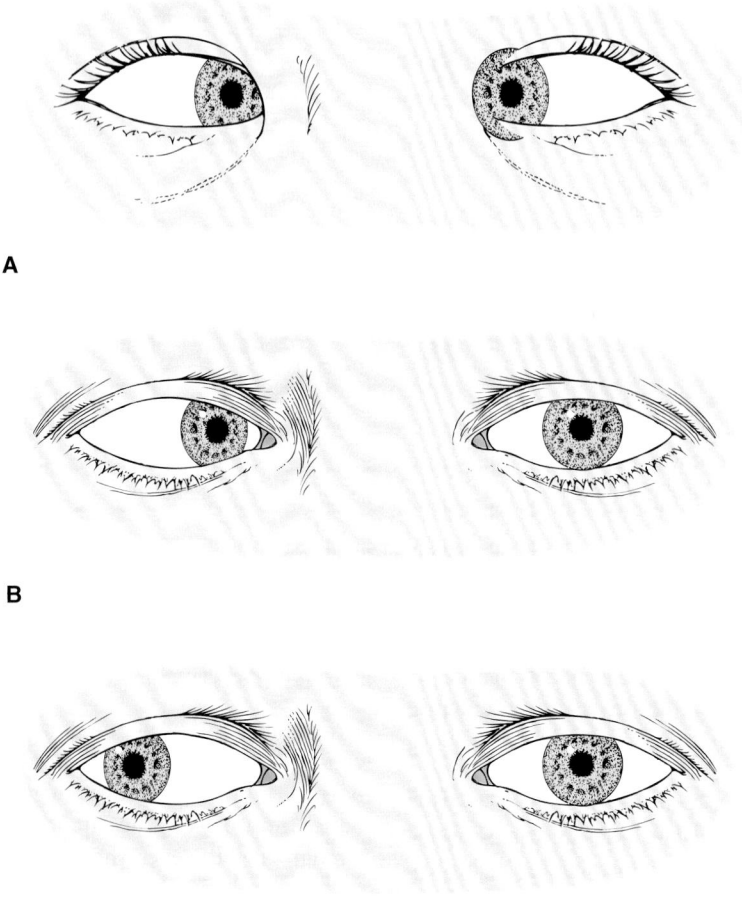

**FIGURE 30-5** • Forms of strabismus. **(A)** Esotropic. **(B)** Exotropic. **(C)** Hypotrophic. (From Weber J, Kelley J. *Health Assessment in Nursing.* 2nd ed. Philadelphia: Lippincott Williams & Wilkins; 2003.)

some cases and requires medical intervention. Strabismus may take any of the following forms (Fig. 30-5A–C):

- Esotropic, also known as *cross eyes* or *convergent eyes*
- Exotropic, also known as *wall eyes* or *divergent eyes*
- Hypotrophic, deviation downward
- Hypertrophic, deviation upward
- Concomitant, with both eyes moving together
- Nonconcomitant, with the two eyes moving independently

Treatment may require only patching, or covering, the unaffected eye to force the affected eye's muscles to strengthen. In some cases, surgery is required to correct the deviant muscle or muscles.

## Color Deficit

Color deficit is an absence of or a defect in color perception. Red, green, or blue perception may be impaired or absent. The term "color deficient" or "color deficit" is commonly used rather than referring to the disorder as *color blindness.*

This disorder is usually inherited on the X chromosome and affects more men than women. Occasionally, color deficit results from damage to the cones by medications or other substances that are toxic to the color-receptive nerve cells. Color deficit has no cure or correction.

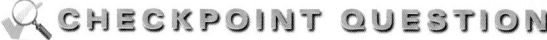

**CHECKPOINT QUESTION**

4. How is strabismus corrected?

## DIAGNOSTIC STUDIES OF THE EYE

In most medical offices, the basic examination equipment includes the ophthalmoscope, the lighted instrument used to examine the inner surfaces of the eye (Fig. 30-6). In many instances, visually examining the interior structures of the eyes can alert the physician to a number of vascular and hypertensive conditions because the blood vessels of the eye and the inner structures, such as the retina, are easily viewed.

Normal vision (20/20) means the patient can see at 20 feet what the normal eye sees at 20 feet. The figures on the charts—letters, numbers, a series of E's, or common symbols—become progressively smaller to test levels of perception (Fig. 30-7). For patients who cannot read or who do not speak English, the E chart may be used. A patient who can see only the line (letters or E's) on the chart at the 20/40 level has visual acuity at 20 feet equivalent to what a person with normal vision can see at 40 feet. The patient should wear any corrective lenses for the test unless the physician requests that the examination be done without them. Each eye is tested separately, with the opposite eye covered but not closed.

The picture chart is used for children. If a child is to be tested, first spend a few moments familiarizing the child with the objects on the chart. For example, if the picture is of a dog and the child has never seen one, the illustration may not be recognized as a dog. If necessary, enlist a parent or coworker to help with the eye cover.

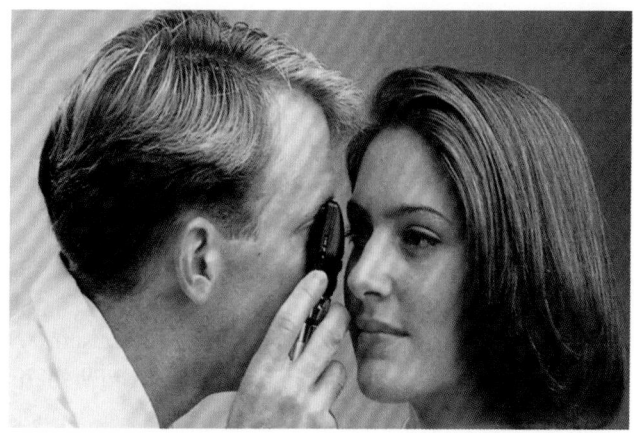

**FIGURE 30-6** • Examination of the eye with an ophthalmoscope. (Reprinted from Willis MC. *Medical Terminology: A Programmed Learning Approach to the Language of Health Care*. Baltimore, MD: Lippincott Williams & Wilkins, 2002, with permission.)

## Visual Acuity Testing

Visual acuity, or clearness, is commonly assessed in the medical office using the Snellen eye chart. These charts are hung 20 feet from the patient at eye level in an area with good lighting and few distractions (Procedure 30-1).

## CHECKPOINT QUESTION

5. When is the E chart used to test visual acuity?

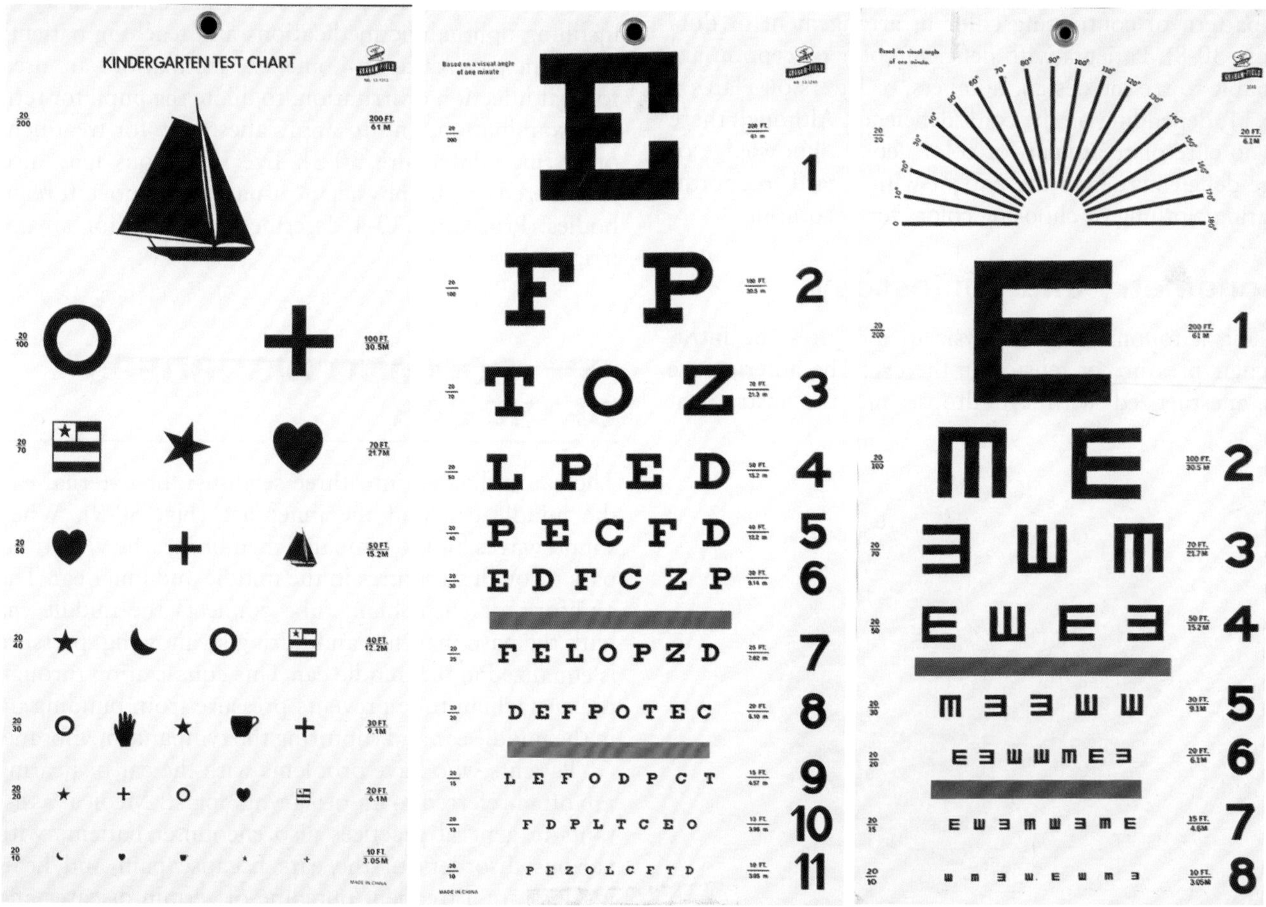

**FIGURE 30-7** • Snellen charts used to assess distant vision. The charts on the left and right are used for young children and illiterate adults.

## PATIENT EDUCATION

### Preventative Eye Care

Preventive care of the eye is a vital component of patient education. Regular eye checkups, proper care of contact lenses, control of diabetes and hypertension, annual tonometer checks for glaucoma yearly after age 40 years, and proper attention to eye injuries are important aspects of eye health maintenance.

Advise patients to wear sunglasses with ultraviolet protection during any sun exposure to avoid damage to the eyes. Children should also be fitted for sunglasses to protect their eyes against sun damage.

Advise patients not to rub their eyes. This can spread infection from person to person and can damage the cornea if a small foreign object is in the eye. Wearing goggles or safety glasses at appropriate times can prevent disease transmission and injury caused by foreign bodies.

## Color Deficit Testing

The Ishihara method is used to test for color deficits (Procedure 30-2). It consists of 14 color plates with many four-colored dots forming a number, a letter, or a pattern of contrasting color in arrangement of dots (Fig. 30-8). Patients with deficient color perception are unable to see the design, numbers, or letters on Plates 1 to 11, depending on the color deficiency. Although there is no cure or treatment for color deficits, knowledge of the deficit may help the patient with regard to coordinating clothing or choosing colors for decorating.

## Tonometry and Gonioscopy

Using a tonometer, the physician measures the intraocular pressure or tension in the eye. The anterior eye is anesthetized with eye drops, and the instrument

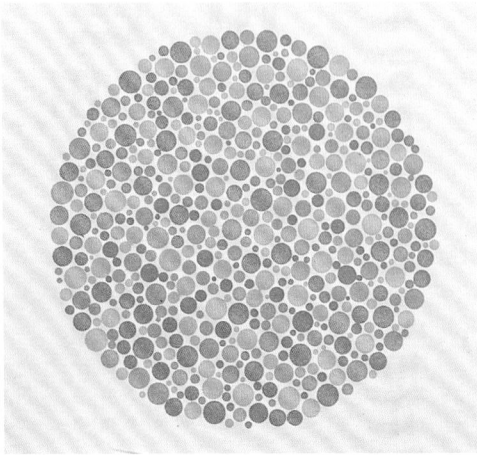

**FIGURE 30-8 •** Ishihara color plate. (Courtesy of B. Proud. Copyright.)

is moved against the cornea to measure the pressure required to produce an indentation or to flatten a small area of the cornea. This test is an important part of the eye examination to diagnose glaucoma. Although it is not routinely performed at the general practice medical office, tonometry is painless and done regularly at the ophthalmologist's or optometrist's office.

Gonioscopy, also performed at the ophthalmologist's or optometrist's office, is the use of a special instrument (gonioscope) to measure the angle of the anterior chamber between the iris and the cornea. This test is useful to the physician in determining the cause of the increased intraocular pressure.

 **CHECKPOINT QUESTION**

6. Why is it important to have the pressure of the eye measured with a tonometer?

## **COG** THERAPEUTIC PROCEDURES FOR THE EYE

### Instilling Eye Medications

Medical assistants frequently have the responsibility of instilling ophthalmic medications and teaching patients about the procedure for home use. Instillations are used to treat infection or irritation, to dilate the pupil for retinal examination, and to apply anesthetic for treatment or testing (Procedure 30-3). Eye irrigations may also be ordered by the physician, usually to remove foreign bodies. Procedure 30-4 describes the steps for an eye irrigation.

## **COG** COMMON DISORDERS OF THE EAR

The ear is divided into three sections: the external ear, the middle ear, and the inner ear (Fig. 30-9). When sound waves hit the tympanic membrane, the vibrations pass through structures in the middle and inner ear. The auditory, or eustachian, tube connects the middle ear with the nasopharynx, and during swallowing, pressure is equalized in the middle ear. This equalization through the eustachian tube prevents pressure from building up in the middle ear and rupturing the tympanic membrane.

Patients who have problems with the ear or hearing are often referred to an otolaryngologist. Medical assistants in general practices also encounter patients with various disorders of the ears because pain and hearing loss are a frequent outcome of certain diseases and can occur at any age. Box 30-3 describes guidelines for assisting hearing-impaired patients in a medical office.

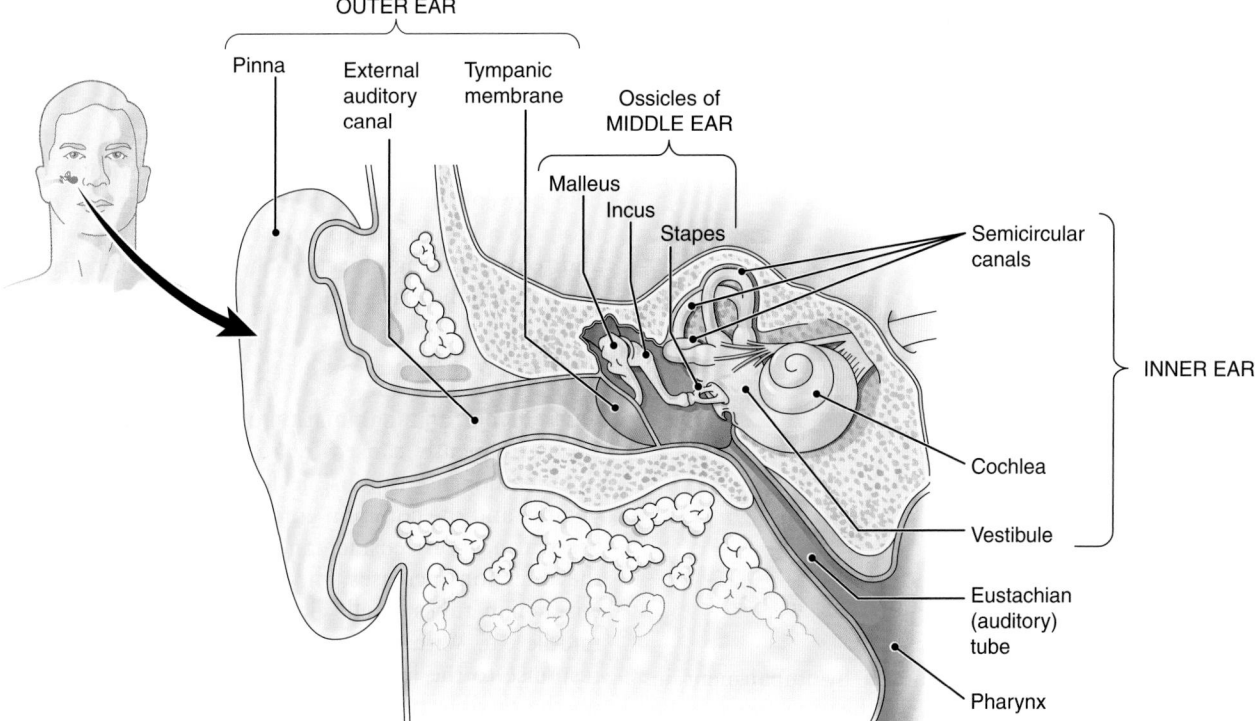

**FIGURE 30-9 •** The ear, showing the outer, middle, and inner subdivisions. (Reprinted from Cohen BJ. *Memmler's The Human Body in Health and Disease*, 11th ed. Philadelphia, PA: Lippincott Williams & Wilkins, 2009, with permission.)

## Ceruminosis

Ceruminosis, or impacted earwax, is a frequent reason for diminished hearing. **Cerumen** is usually soft and moist and leaks out in such small amounts that it is unnoticed. Occasionally, the cerumen becomes hard and dry or excessive hair in the ear holds the wax in the ear canal, causing it to build up against the tympanic membrane.

The presenting symptoms may be a gradual hearing loss or **tinnitus**, an extraneous noise heard in one or both ears. An examination of the ear canal with an **otoscope** shows the obvious reason. The wax may be softened by warm ear drops or hydrogen peroxide and removed by an ear curet or by gently washing with an irrigating device using water at room temperature (Procedure 30-5).

## Conductive and Perceptual Hearing Loss

Conductive and perceptual hearing loss are the two categories of hearing impairment. In conductive loss, sound waves are not appropriately transmitted to the level of the cochlea. In perceptual, or sensorineural, loss, transmission from the oval window to the receptors in the brain is impaired. Many patients present with both, a condition called *mixed deafness*.

Causes of hearing loss include heredity, infection, trauma, ototoxic drugs, some neurologic diseases, exposure to loud noises, and **presbycusis**. Presbycusis usually results from a hardening of the joints between the ossicles (three small bones in the middle ear), which occurs with aging.

Diagnosis of hearing loss of any type is done by testing the hearing using an audiometer (Fig. 30-10) in the medical office. Procedure 30-6 describes the steps for performing a hearing test using the audiometer. Treatment is aimed at addressing the underlying cause of the hearing loss if possible. A stapedectomy may be performed for otosclerosis, with a replacement for the impaired joint. Cochlear implants are gaining favor for

### BOX 10-3  Assisting Hearing-Impaired Patients

Follow these tips to assist a hearing-impaired patient:

- Speak normally; do not yell or raise your voice. Doing so will not facilitate the hearing capabilities of the patient.
- Get the patient's attention before speaking and make sure he or she can see your lips while you talk.
- Speak clearly, but remember that the patient is hearing impaired, not mentally challenged.
- If the patient is deaf and requires an interpreter, speak to the patient, not the interpreter.

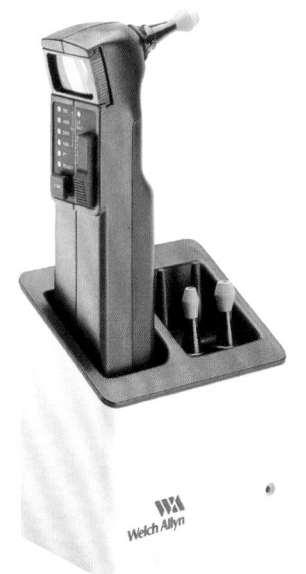

**FIGURE 30-10** • The audiometer.

those whose hearing loss is caused by impairment in the cochlear receptors. Conductive hearing loss can be treated successfully in most instances with hearing aids; perceptual loss is far more difficult to correct.

## CHECKPOINT QUESTION

7. How would Charlene explain the difference between conductive and perceptual hearing loss?

## Ménière Disease

Ménière disease, a degenerative condition of unknown cause, affects the inner ear and upsets the body's ability to maintain equilibrium in addition to causing loss of hearing. The symptoms include vertigo, sensorineural hearing loss, and tinnitus. Severe symptoms may lead to nausea and vomiting. Periods of remission are followed by exacerbation. Although there is no cure, many of the symptoms can be treated with palliative medication. If the symptoms persist or increase and become incapacitating, it may be necessary to destroy the organs of the inner ear. The result of this drastic measure is immediate relief of symptoms, but the patient is irreversibly deaf.

## Otitis Externa

Also known as swimmer's ear, otitis externa is an inflammation or infection of the external ear. It is common in the summer and is caused by any number of pathogens that grow in the warm, moist ear canal. The presenting symptoms include pain on movement of any adjoining structures around the ear, jaw, and auricle. Otoscopy reveals a red, swollen ear canal

(Fig. 30-11). Although the physician may order that debris (pus or excessive cerumen) be gently washed from the area, otitis externa is best treated by an antibiotic, either topical (Procedure 30-7) or systemic, warm compresses, and medication to relieve pain.

Applying an alcohol solution after swimming can help prevent this problem. Encourage patients who are prone to otitis externa to wear earplugs while swimming and to avoid using objects such as swabs or hairpins to clean inside the ear canal.

## Otitis Media

Otitis media, an inflammation or infection of the middle ear, is frequently caused by an upper respiratory infection. Pathogens responsible for pharyngitis, nasopharyngitis, and the common cold frequently travel through the warm, moist eustachian tube to the middle ear. As the infection increases, the mucous membranes of the eustachian tubes swell, closing off the opening to the middle ear. With no way to drain, fluid builds up as a response to the infection and causes pain and pressure on the flexible tympanic membrane. If pressure is sufficient, the membrane may tear or perforate spontaneously to relieve the pressure.

This disorder is common in infants and children because of the relatively horizontal position of the eustachian tube between the nasopharynx and middle ear. Children have very short, almost horizontal, eustachian tubes, which can be problematic if microorganisms from the nasopharynx are forced into the middle ear by coughing. The problem is compounded for children who are put to bed with a bottle of milk or formula. The milk acts as a hospitable medium for bacteria.

Symptoms include severe pain, fever of varying degrees, and mild to moderate hearing loss. Infants may be fussy and tug at their ears. Any elevation in a child's temperature should be a warning to check for otitis media. Diagnosis is usually made by otoscopy, which may reveal a reddened, bulging tympanic membrane (Fig. 30-12). Bubbles can sometimes be seen behind the thin membrane. Treatment is an antibiotic for bacterial infection and an analgesic for

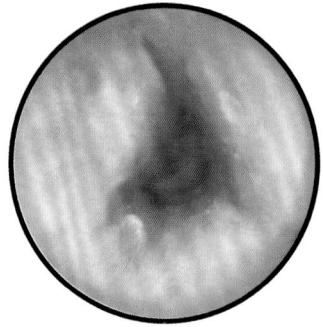

**FIGURE 30-11** • The red, swollen ear canal of a patient with otitis externa. (From Bickley LS, Szilagyi P. *Bates' Guide to Physical Examination and History Taking.* 8th ed. Philadelphia: Lippincott Williams & Wilkins; 2003.)

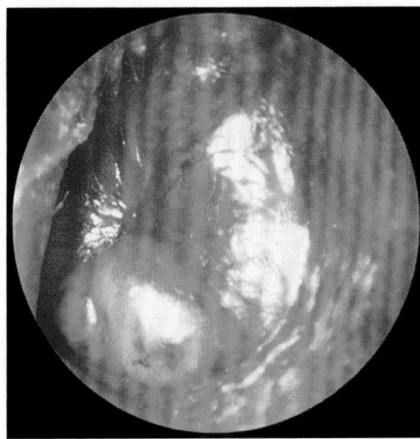

**Otitis media**

**FIGURE 30-12** • A bulging tympanic membrane of a patient with otitis media. (From Moore KL, Dalley AF II. *Clinical Oriented Anatomy.* 4th ed. Baltimore: Lippincott Williams & Wilkins; 1999.)

pain relief. A decongestant may reduce some of the swelling. In severe chronic cases, a **myringotomy** (surgical incision into the tympanic membrane) may be performed to relieve pressure. Tubes may be inserted through the tympanic membrane and remain for several months to equalize the pressure if the problem persists.

 **CHECKPOINT QUESTION**

8. A mother brings her 9-month-old infant into the ENT office after getting a referral from the pediatrician for recurrent otitis media infections. What are the symptoms of otitis media in an infant?

## PATIENT EDUCATION

### Otologic Disorders

Teach patients to recognize symptoms of otologic disorders (hearing loss, pain, drainage) and to report them promptly to the physician. Proper attention at the early stage of an infection or injury can often prevent serious or irreversible damage.

Instruct patients that it is acceptable to clean the external ear with a cotton-tipped applicator but that they should not put the applicator inside the ear canal. This drives cerumen deeper into the ear and creates more impaction than may already be present.

Tell children not to put small objects such as beans, peas, or small parts of toys in their ears because they may become lodged and removal may require surgery. Caution parents to complete all antibiotic treatment for children's ear infections even though the symptoms subside. The infection may linger after the patient is asymptomatic. Ear recheck appointments should be kept as scheduled to ensure that the child is free of infection.

## Otosclerosis

Otosclerosis is a disorder of the ossicles of the middle ear, especially the stapes bone. This disorder, thought to be hereditary, results from ossification or hardening of the bones causing loss of hearing of low tones. The treatment for otosclerosis is hearing aids or microsurgical implantation of a stapedial prosthesis to replace the sclerotic joint and allow movement of the bones.

## COG DIAGNOSTIC STUDIES OF THE EAR

### Visual Examination

Using an otoscope, the physician can view the auditory canal and eardrum (Fig. 30-13). Disposable otoscopes are available; reusable otoscopes use disposable speculum covers that are changed between patients. Some reusable otoscopes use the same base as an ophthalmoscope.

### Audiometry and Tympanometry

An audiometer can be used to detect hearing loss (Procedure 30-6). Audiometers produce pure tones of various **decibel (dB)** levels and frequencies heard through earphones or an instrument that resembles an otoscope. The decibel is a unit for measuring the intensity of sound. Speech audiometry uses voice tones rather than pure tones to assess hearing.

Impedance audiometry evaluates tympanic membrane and ossicle mobility. A probe is inserted into the auditory meatus and emits tones of various intensity levels that bounce back to the probe receiver. If the tympanic membrane and ossicles are normal, the movement is transmitted and rebound is picked up by the receiver to produce a curve on the graph. If the tympanic

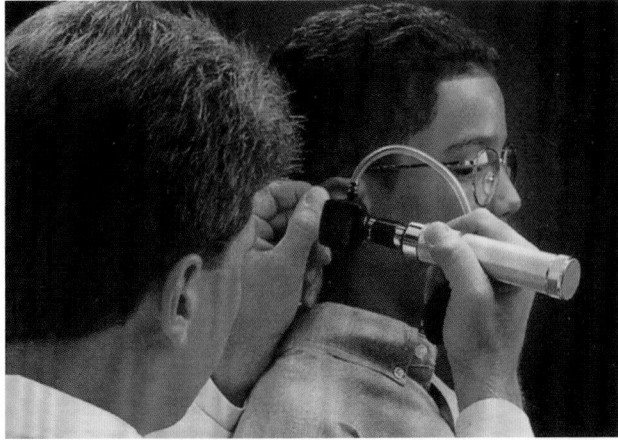

**FIGURE 30-13** • Examination of the ear with an otoscope. (Reprinted from Willis MC. *Medical Terminology: A Programmed Learning Approach to the Language of Health Care.* Baltimore, MD: Lippincott Williams & Wilkins, 2002, with permission.)

membrane and ossicles are less mobile than normal, much of the sound transmitted bounces back and is reflected to the instrument to produce a distinct curve on the graph. Tympanometry works like the audiometer but uses air pressure rather than tones to produce the graph.

## CHECKPOINT QUESTION

9. The ENT physician wants to visualize the ear canal and tympanic membrane. Which of the instruments described allows the physician to visualize the ear canal and tympanic membrane?

## Tuning Fork Tests

Two tests that may be performed using the tuning fork are the Rinne test and the Weber test. The Rinne test entails lightly tapping the tuning fork, placing the end of it on the mastoid bone, and then moving it to the external auditory meatus to determine conductive hearing loss. In normal hearing, the sound is louder through the external auditory meatus than the bone. The Weber test entails gently tapping the tuning fork and placing it on the midline of the forehead to differentiate between conductive and sensorineural hearing loss. In conductive loss, the sound is louder in the affected ear; in sensorineural loss, the sound is louder in the unaffected ear. Although the physician most likely is the one who performs the tuning fork tests, you should ensure that the tuning fork is available and assist as needed.

## WHAT IF?

**What if your patient asks you if a hearing aid could help her?**

Hearing aids help many people, but they do not fully restore the ability to hear. The purpose of the aid is to amplify sound waves. Not all patients with hearing loss are good candidates for hearing aids. For example, patients who have permanent nerve damage generally do not have significant improvement with standard hearing aids.

The two basic types of aids are bone conduction receivers, which sit behind the ear and press against the skull, and air conduction receivers, which fit into the auditory canal. The size and type of hearing aid depends on the patient's specific condition and need. Binaural (both ears) aids are available and often can be fitted into eyeglasses for inconspicuous appearance.

Patients must understand that a hearing aid will improve their hearing, not correct it. Teach patients about maintenance requirements so they can keep the device in good working condition, and explain how to adjust the volume control. Have the patient speak to the physician regarding any concerns about purchasing and using a hearing aid.

## THERAPEUTIC PROCEDURES FOR THE EAR

### Irrigations and Instillations

Ear irrigations are performed to relieve pain, to remove debris or foreign objects, or to apply medication solutions. Ear instillations may include a local anesthetic for the relief of pain associated with otitis externa or otitis media or a topical antibiotic for otitis externa. These medications include the words "for otic use" on the label. For medication irrigations and instillations, observe the principles of medication administration, including checking the medication label for the expiration date.

## COMMON DISORDERS OF THE NOSE AND THROAT

### Allergic Rhinitis

Allergic rhinitis is inflammation of the mucous membranes of the nasal passages usually resulting from exposure to an allergen. Symptomatic treatment with antihistamine medication is usually offered to relieve the symptoms. It is also known as *hay fever* or *seasonal allergic rhinitis* when it appears in response to seasonal plant pollens. If the symptoms are present year round, it is perennial allergic rhinitis and is usually a reaction to household irritants, such as dust mites and pet dander. The signs are obvious, with paroxysmal sneezing, intense rhinorrhea (nasal drainage), congestion, and watery reddened eyes.

Diagnosis usually entails history and differential diagnosis. Mucous secretions may reveal an increase in immunoglobulin E in response to the allergens. An allergist may isolate the offending protein by skin testing. Allergy treatment entails exposure to the allergen in minute doses to desensitize the immune reaction.

### Epistaxis

Commonly known as nosebleed, epistaxis generally occurs from trauma to the nasal membranes, but it may be secondary to another disorder, such as hypertension, malignancy, polyps, or the fragile capillaries associated with pregnancy. Diagnosis necessitates a history and inspection of the nasal mucosa with a nasal speculum (Fig. 30-14). The initial therapy for simple epistaxis is having the patient sit upright with the head slightly forward to avoid postnasal drainage that may lead to nausea. Compress the nares against the septum for 5 to 10 minutes with either ice or a cold, wet compress. Advise the patient to remain still and not to blow the nose until the physician concludes that all danger is past.

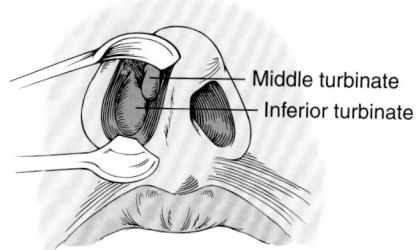

— Middle turbinate
— Inferior turbinate

**FIGURE 30-14** • Physical examination of the nose with a nasal speculum. (Reprinted from Nettina SM. *The Lippincott Manual of Nursing Practice*. Philadelphia, PA: Lippincott Williams & Wilkins, 2001, with permission.)

Bleeding that continues more than 10 minutes after treatment begins is considered severe. For severe epistaxis, the physician may insert nasal packing or a balloon catheter that may remain in place several hours to several days. For secondary bleeding, treatment of the underlying cause may be indicated. Cautery to an exposed blood vessel helps if that is the only cause.

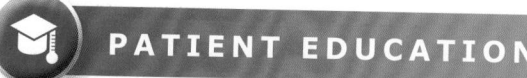

### CHECKPOINT QUESTION

10. A patient complains to Charlene that he has frequent nosebleeds. What factors may contribute to epistaxis?

## Nasal Polyps

Nasal polyps are small pendulous tissues that obstruct breathing. Polyps usually occur in the mucous membranes of the nasal passages as a response to long-term allergies. Symptoms include a feeling of fullness or congestion and occasionally a nasal discharge. Diagnosis requires direct examination with a nasal speculum or radiography of the nasal structures. Treatment may be corticosteroids applied either topically or by injection directly into the polyps. The underlying allergy must be treated to prevent recurrence of polyps. If conservative treatment is not effective, conventional or laser surgery is required.

## Sinusitis

Sinusitis, or inflammation of one or more of the sinus cavities, can be either acute or chronic. Acute sinusitis is usually the result of an upper respiratory infection and is fairly easily resolved. Chronic sinusitis is more persistent and more difficult to control. Either form is particularly common when microorganisms are forced into the moist sinus cavities during hard nose blowing.

Symptoms of sinusitis include the obvious signs of an upper respiratory infection, with the addition of a purulent nasal discharge and facial pain over the sinus areas. Diagnosis requires direct visualization using a nasal speculum, radiography of the sinuses, needle puncture of the sinuses to withdraw a specimen for culture, and ultrasound.

Serious complications in the brain and middle ear may occur if sinusitis is not treated promptly with antihistamines or ephedrine nose drops to shrink mucosal tissue and relieve pressure. Steroidal nasal sprays may also be prescribed. Procedure 29-8 describes the steps for instilling nasal medication. If the cause of the sinusitis is a bacterial infection, antibiotics are prescribed by the physician and effectively relieve symptoms within 7 to 10 days. Chronic sinusitis may require treatment for 4 to 6 weeks. Total blockage of the sinus cavity may result if the disorder is not treated; this may require surgery to puncture the wall between the nose and the involved sinus cavity to allow drainage.

### CHECKPOINT QUESTION

11. What is the usual cause of a sinus infection?

### 🎓 PATIENT EDUCATION

#### Nasal Disorders

Patients need to be alert for any changes in their breathing pattern. The early symptoms of any nasal disorder must be treated as soon as possible to prevent complications. Instruct children not to put small pieces of food or toys in the nose.

Instruct patients about the rebound phenomena of nasal sprays and drops. If used without the advice of a physician, these medications may become addictive. After frequent use, the nasal mucosa responds to withdrawal of the medication with congestion. Nasal preparations should never be used more than four times a day for 3 days unless specified by the physician.

## Pharyngitis and Tonsillitis

Inflammation of the epithelial tissues of the throat and of the tonsils produces similar symptoms of sore throat and difficulty swallowing. Examination of the throat reveals red, swollen tissues and possibly pustules on the tonsils or in the throat (Fig. 30-15). You may be asked to obtain a throat specimen from these patients for transportation to an outside laboratory for a culture, or you may be

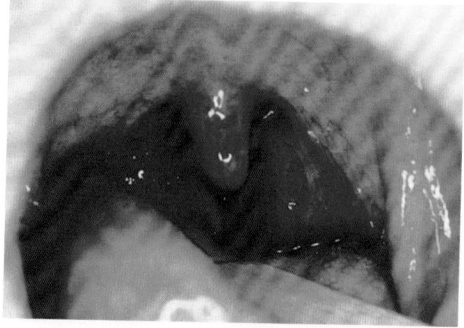

**FIGURE 30-15** • Pharyngitis with swollen tonsils. (From The Wellcome Trust. *National Medical Slide Bank*. London, UK.)

required to perform a rapid strep test on the specimen in the office. (Chapter 44 describes the steps for collecting throat specimens.) Treatment of a sore throat may include gargles, an analgesic, and an antibiotic, especially if the throat culture reveals a bacterial infection. Tonsillitis may be treated with an antibiotic, or if the problem is chronic, the tonsils may be surgically removed—a tonsillectomy. This procedure usually includes removal of both pharyngeal tonsils (adenoids) and palatine tonsils.

## LEGAL TIP

A patient calls the office at 4:45 pm complaining of a sore throat. Scheduled appointments are running 1 to 2 hours behind. Because it is the middle of flu season, you think it is safe to tell the patient that he has a virus and can be seen in the morning. During the night, the patient's throat closes because of the infection and obstructs his airway. The patient dies, and the autopsy report shows a tonsillar abscess. Could the patient's family sue you? Yes! As a medical assistant, you cannot presume to diagnose medical conditions. You made a medical decision and diagnosed the patient when you decided that the symptoms indicated a virus. Only the physician can make a diagnosis. Always follow office policy regarding telephone advice, and document all phone conversations after bringing them to the physician's attention.

## Laryngitis

Inflammation of the larynx can result from an infection, irritation, or overuse of the voice. The result is hoarseness, cough, and difficulty speaking. Diagnosis is made after a thorough history and visual inspection of the pharynx for redness and signs of infection. Laryngitis may be treated with an antibiotic if it is thought to be caused by a bacterial infection, but more often, it is left to resolve on its own. The patient is told to rest the voice and speak as little as possible. A cool-mist humidifier may be helpful in soothing the throat.

## CHECKPOINT QUESTION

12. A patient seen in the ENT office is diagnosed with laryngitis. Describe the symptoms of a patient with laryngitis.

## COG DIAGNOSTIC STUDIES OF THE NOSE AND THROAT

### Visual Inspection

Examination of the nose and throat entails visually inspecting the nose using a nasal speculum or viewing the throat using a penlight and tongue depressor. The physician may order radiography and culture to identify infectious

microorganisms. The physician may also palpate the lymph nodes in the neck and other neck structures related to the upper airway. You may be responsible for preparing the patient and assisting during the examination.

##  COG THERAPEUTIC PROCEDURES FOR THE NOSE AND THROAT

### Throat Culture

A throat culture in cases of suspected pharyngitis or tonsillitis can help determine what microorganism is causing the problem. The patient's throat is gently swabbed with a sterile culture swab to obtain the specimen. A sterile swab is necessary to avoid culturing microorganisms not in the throat. After the specimen is obtained, it is either processed in the office with a commercially prepared test kit such as those that check for streptococcal bacteria or sent to a laboratory for analysis. If the specimen is sent to the laboratory, it must be placed in a culture medium, labeled, and sent in a biohazard bag with the appropriate laboratory request. (Chapter 44 describes the steps for collecting throat specimens.)

## CHECKPOINT QUESTION

13. The physician orders a throat culture, and when gathering the equipment, Charlene obtains a sterile swab. Why is it necessary to use a sterile swab to obtain the throat culture specimen?

## 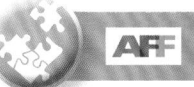 AFF TRIAGE

You have the following three tasks:

1. Patient A is on the phone asking for advice on pain and blurred vision in his left eye after wearing his contact lens through the night.
2. Patient B is waiting in an examination room for you to complete a visual acuity and Ishihara test required for a pre-employment physical exam.
3. A pharmacist telephones with a question about a patient's prescription for glaucoma medication.

**How do you sort these tasks? What do you do first? Second? Third?**

After asking the receptionist to take a message from the pharmacist calling regarding patient C, address patient A since he will need an appointment to be seen right away. Wearing contact lenses longer than prescribed can scratch the cornea, and the patient should be seen as soon as possible to avoid further damage. Next, complete and record the eye examinations for patient B's physical examination. Once these situations are resolved, call the pharmacist and answer any questions, clarify concerns, or refer the matter to the physician.

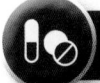

# MEDICATION BOX

## Commonly Prescribed Otic and Ophthalmic Medications

**Note:** *The generic name of the drug is listed first and is written in all lower case letters. Brand names are in parentheses and the first letter is capitalized.*

| | | |
|---|---|---|
| Amoxicillin and clavulanate (Augmentin) | Tablets: 250 mg, 500 mg<br>Oral Suspension: 125 mg/5 mL | Antibiotic |
| Amoxicillin trihydrate (Amoxil) | Capsules: 250 mg, 500 mg<br>Tablets: 500 mg, 875 mg<br>Oral suspension: 50 mg/mL | Antibiotic |
| Atropine sulfate (Isopto Atropine) | Ophthalmic solution: 0.5%, 1%, 2% | Antimuscarinic |
| Azithromycin (Zithromax) | Tablets: 250 mg, 500 mg, 600 mg | Antibiotic |
| Betaxolol hydrochloride (Betoptic) | Ophthalmic solution: 0.5%<br>Ophthalmic suspension: 0.25% | Antiglaucoma |
| Bimatoprost (Latisse) | Ophthalmic solution: 0.03% | Antiglaucoma |
| Brimonidine tartrate (Alphagan-P) | Ophthalmic solution: 0.1%, 0.15%, 0.2% | Antiglaucoma |
| Ceftriaxone sodium (Rocephin) | Injection (IM): 250 mg, 500 mg, 1 g, 2 g | Antibiotic |
| Dexamethasone (Maxidex) | Ophthalmic solution: 0.1%<br>Ophthalmic suspension: 0.1% | Corticosteroid |
| Gentamicin sulfate (Genoptic) | Ophthalmic ointment: 0.3%<br>Ophthalmic solution: 0.3% | Anti-infective |
| Latanoprost (Xalatan) | Ophthalmic solution: 0.005% | Antiglaucoma |
| Loratadine (Claritin, Alavert) | Capsules: 10 mg<br>Syrup: 1 mg/mL<br>Tablets: 10 mg | Antihistamine |
| Tobramycin (Tobrex) | Ophthalmic ointment: 0.3%<br>Ophthalmic solution: 0.3% | Anti-infective |

## ROLE-PLAYING ACTIVITY

With cooperation from classmates or as assigned by your instructor, role-play the scenarios in the ENT office where you are working as a medical assistant with Charlene Mayers (refer to the case study at the beginning of the chapter). A middle-aged patient comes into the office explaining that she made an appointment to see an ENT physician because she "knows" she has a sinus infection but her physician will not prescribe antibiotics. In addition, she asks you to give her some samples of a "nose spray" she got from her family doctor last year for "allergies," and although she cannot remember the name of the spray, she said it helped, was in a "green bottle," and may have been a steroid. Another patient came in to have his hearing evaluated and asks about a cochlear implant. He wants to know what you know about these devices and if there is "any danger of brain cancer" after getting one (he read this on the Internet). Do you have any concerns or judgments about these patients or their requests? How would you respond? Your instructor will give you additional information about this activity!

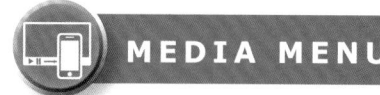

## MEDIA MENU

**Student Resources** on thePoint®
- **CMA/RMA Certification Exam Review**

**Internet Resources**
**American Academy of Otolaryngology-Head and Neck Surgery**
http://www.entnet.org
**Journal of Pediatric Ophthalmology and Strabismus**
http://www.slackjournals.com/jpos
**American Foundation for the Blind**
http://www.afb.org
**Foundation Fighting Blindness**
http://www.blindness.org
**Prevent Blindness America**
http://www.preventblindness.org
**American Optometric Association**
http://www.aoa.org
**Hearing Loss Association of America**
http://www.shhh.org

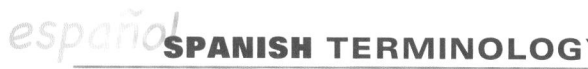

## SPANISH TERMINOLOGY

**El ojo**
The eye

**Los oídos**
(inner) ears

**Las orejas**
(outer) ears

**La nariz**
The nose

**La garganta**
The throat

**¿Cuándo fue la ultima vez que se hizo un examen de la vista?**
When was the last time you had a vision test?

**¿Padece de dolor de oído?**
Do you have earaches?

**El nombre correcto de ojo irritado es conjuntivitis.**
The correct name for pink eye is conjunctivitis.

**Su diagnóstico es Glaucoma, una elevación de la presión dentro de sus ojos.**
Your diagnosis is glaucoma, an elevation of the pressure inside your eyes.

**La membrana de su timpano está rota.**
Your tympanic membrane is ruptured.

**Usted necesita un exámen auditivo con el audiólogo.**
You need a formal hearing screening with the audiologist.

**Usted no puede escuchar correctamente porque tiene un tapón de cerilla ó cerumen.**
Your cannot hear properly because you have a plug of earwax.

## EMR Activity

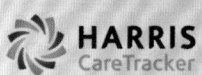

Harris CareTracker is a Web-based electronic medical record (EMR) application that you will use for the EMR activities included in this section at the end of each chapter. This application is actually used in physician offices, but is provided to you through the publisher, Wolters Kluwer Health, to give you hands-on practice working with EMRs. Your instructor will have more information about accessing your username, login, and Quickstart guide.

Prerequisite Activities in Harris CareTracker

- *The Getting Started and Quickstart documents and EMR Activities Step-by-Step Instructions are available at* http://thePoint.lww.com/KronenbergerComp5e

Activity Details

Document the following treatments ordered by Dr. Singer and performed by you today in the ENT:

1. Patient: Kathy Newman; right ear irrigated with 500-cc sterile water for ear wax; return clear with several small pieces of brown wax and one large piece.
2. Patient: Steve Sutter; Omnaris, 2 sprays in both nares and repeat every day as needed.

# Chapter Summary

Although not all patients who have disorders of the eyes or ears need a referral to an ophthalmologist or otolaryngologist, you will routinely encounter patients who need to have these conditions properly diagnosed and treated. Keep in mind that

- Disorders of the eyes, ears, nose, and throat may affect any patient at any age.
- Severe complications, such as an infection of the brain or hearing loss, can result in patients who are not receiving adequate attention or not following the physician's instructions for treatment.
- You will play a vital role by assisting with ear, nose, and throat examinations and educating patients regarding their treatment.

# Warm-Ups for Critical Thinking

1. The mother of a 10-month-old boy explains to you that the baby has had a runny nose and has been fussy for the past 2 days. You notice that he is pulling at his right ear. What equipment do you anticipate that the physician will need for examining the child?
2. A 16-year-old girl complains of a sore throat. Her vital signs are T 102.8 (O), P 112, R 24, and BP 112/84. The physician examines her and tells you to obtain a throat specimen for a rapid strep test to determine whether the pharyngitis is due to an infection with streptococcal bacteria. The patient is reluctant to let you obtain a throat culture, saying it will make her gag and vomit. How do you handle this situation?
3. The school nurse at the local high school phones your office asking for information about a student who has been out of school the past 3 days with conjunctivitis. Specifically, she wants to know whether this student has been diagnosed with this condition or is simply truant. How do you handle this phone call?
4. An elderly patient is having difficulty hearing and would like you to explain why the physician wants you to irrigate his ears for ceruminosis. He is concerned that the procedure will be uncomfortable. What could you say to the patient to ease his anxiety?
5. You notice that another medical assistant working in the office is getting frustrated with an adult male during a visual acuity test using the Snellen eye chart. The patient doesn't seem to know the letters of the alphabet and you suspect that he is illiterate, but may have been embarrassed to tell the other MA before the examination started. Would you intervene? What would you say?

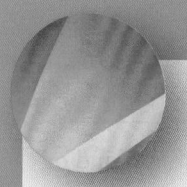

## PSY PROCEDURE 30-1

# Measuring Distance Visual Acuity

**PSY** Instruct and prepare a patient for a procedure or treatment; coach patients regarding disease prevention and treatment plans; coach patients appropriately considering cultural diversity, developmental life stage, and communication barriers; and document patient care accurately in the medical record.

**Purpose:** To assess and document the distance visual acuity of a patient in both eyes, with or without corrective lenses

**Equipment:** Snellen eye chart, paper cup, or eye paddle

| STEPS | PURPOSE |
|---|---|
| 1. Wash your hands. | Hand washing aids infection control. |
| 2. Prepare the examination area. Make sure the area is well lighted, a distance marker is placed exactly 20 feet from the chart, and the chart is at eye level. | All distance visual acuity testing is done at 20 feet for consistency of results. |
| 3. Greet and identify the patient. Identify yourself and your title. Explain the procedure. | Patients who understand the procedure are likely to be compliant and produce an accurate test result. |
| 4. **AFF** Explain how to respond to a patient who is hearing impaired. | Speak clearly, not loudly, and face the patient. |
| 5. Position the patient at the 20-foot marker. | The patient may stand or sit as long as the chart is at eye level and the patient is 20 feet from it. |
| 6. Observe whether the patient is wearing glasses. If not, ask the patient about contact lenses and mark the results of the test accordingly. | The visual acuity examination is usually performed with patients wearing their corrective lenses, if they have them. If the patient wears his or her corrective lenses, then the record must indicate that the lenses were worn for the test. |
| 7. Have the patient cover the right eye with the cup or the eye paddle. Instruct the patient to keep both eyes open. Also, tell him or her to not lean forward and to avoid squinting during the test. | The test starts with the right eye covered for paper consistency. The hand should not be used to cover the eye, since pressure against the eye or peeking through the fingers affects the results. Closing one eye will cause squinting of the other, which changes the vision and skews the findings. |

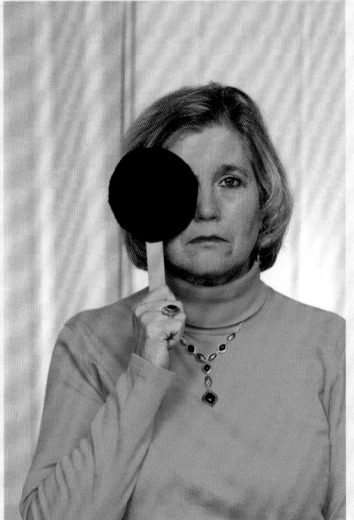

**Step 7.** Have the patient cover the right eye.

## PROCEDURE 30-1 (continued)

| STEPS | PURPOSE |
|---|---|
| 8. Stand beside the chart and point to each row as the patient reads aloud the indicated lines, starting with the 20/200 line. This number is on the right side of the chart next to each line. | It is generally best to start at about the second or third row to judge the patient's response. If these lines are read easily, move down to smaller figures. If the patient has difficulty reading the larger lines, notify the physician. |
| 9. Record the smallest line that the patient can read with two errors or less according to office policy. If the patient reads line 5 with one error with the left eye, it will be recorded as OS (ocularis sinistra) 20/40–1. If that same line is read with two mistakes, it is recorded as OS 20/40–2. If no errors are read at the 20/40 line, it is recorded as OS 20/40. Your physician may prefer that only lines read without any error be counted as correct. | Many offices will consider up to two mistakes acceptable when recording visual acuity. |
| 10. Repeat the procedure with the left eye covered and record as in Step 9, using OD (ocularis dexter). | |
| 11. Wash your hands. | |
| 12. **AFF** Log into the electronic medical record (EMR) using your username and secure password OR obtain the paper medical record from a secure location and assure it is kept away from public access. Record the procedure. Your entry must include the date, time, and your name/credentials. | The integrity of the medical record must be maintained at all times to protect patient privacy. Procedures are considered not to have been done if they are not recorded. |
| 13. When finished, log out of the EMR and/or replace the paper medical record in an appropriate and secure location. | |

Charting Example:
*01/16/2016 4:30 pm Visual acuity OD 20/40–1 OS 20/20 with correction. Dr. Smart aware*
_____ *C. Mayers, CMA*

Note: *The medical assistant may sign his or her name in the patient record using only the "CMA" credential if the office has a signature log denoting the entire credential as "CMA(AAMA)."*

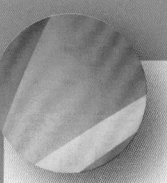

## PSY PROCEDURE 30-2

# Measuring Color Perception

**PSY**  Instruct and prepare a patient for a procedure or treatment; coach patients regarding disease prevention and treatment plans; coach patients appropriately considering cultural diversity, developmental life stage, and communication barriers; and document patient care accurately in the medical record.

**Purpose:** To assess and document color perception

**Equipment:** Ishihara color plates and gloves

| STEPS | PURPOSE |
|---|---|
| 1. Wash your hands, put on gloves, and get the Ishihara color plate book. | Hand washing aids infection control. Gloves in this case are used to protect the plates, not the patient or health care worker. Oils from the hands can alter the colors and interfere with the test results. |
| 2. Greet and identify the patient and yourself including your title. Explain the procedure. | Greeting the patient establishes rapport, and identifying the patient ensures you have the correct patient. |
| 3. Ensure that the patient is seated comfortably in a quiet, well-lighted room. Indirect sunlight is best. (Sunlight should not shine directly on the plates; the colors fade with exposure to bright lights.) Patients who wear glasses or contact lenses should keep them on. | The Ishihara tests color perception, not visual acuity. Corrective lenses do not interfere with accurate test results. |
| 4. **AFF**  Explain how to respond to a patient who is developmentally challenged. | Depending on the level of impairment, speak to the patient accordingly. Explain the procedure using words the patient can understand. Solicit assistance from the caregiver who may be with the patient. |
| 5. After opening the book, hold the first plate in the book about 30 inches from the patient and ask if he or she can see the number in the dots on the plate. | The first plate should be obvious to all patients and serves as an example. |

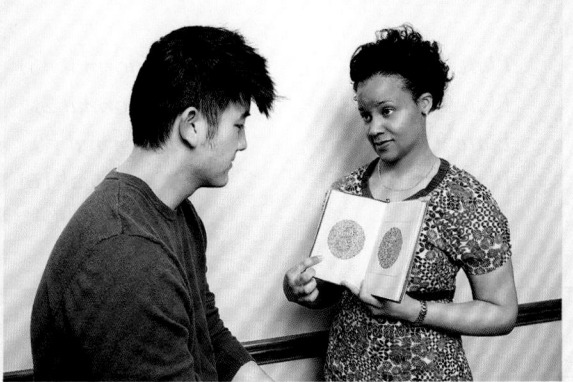

**Step 5.** Hold the first plate about 30 inches from the patient.

## PROCEDURE 30-2 (continued)

| STEPS | PURPOSE |
|---|---|
| 6. Record the results of the test by noting the number or figure the patient reports on each plate, using the plate number followed by the response. If the patient cannot distinguish the pattern, record as the plate number followed by the letter X. The patient should not take more than 3 seconds to read the plates and should not squint or guess. These indicate that the patient was unsure and are recorded as X. | Procedures not recorded in the medical record are considered not to have been done. |
| 7. Record the results for Plates 1 to 10. Plate 11 requires the patient to trace the winding bluish-green line between the two x's. Patients with a color deficit will not be able to trace the line. | If 10 or more of the first 11 plates are read correctly without difficulty, the patient does not have a color deficit. Plates 12, 13, and 14 are usually used to detect the degree of deficiency in patients with red–green color deficiencies. Procedures are considered not to have been done if they are not recorded. |
| 8. Store the book in a closed, protected area away from light. | Storing the book in a dark cabinet will safeguard the integrity of the colors. |
| 9. Remove your gloves and wash your hands. | Wash your hands after any patient contact. |
| 10. **AFF** Log into the electronic medical record (EMR) using your username and secure password OR obtain the paper medical record from a secure location and assure it is kept away from public access. Record the procedure. Your entry must include the date, time, and your name/credentials. | The integrity of the medical record must be maintained at all times to protect patient privacy. Procedures are considered not to have been done if they are not recorded. |
| 11. When finished, log out of the EMR and/or replace the paper medical record in an appropriate and secure location. | |

Charting Example:

12/22/2016 10:30 am Ishihara color deficit testing performed:

| | | | |
|---|---|---|---|
| Plate 1 | 12 | Plate 7 | X (normal 45) |
| Plate 2 | 8 | Plate 8 | X (normal 2) |
| Plate 3 | 5 (normal 2) | Plate 9 | 2 (normal X) |
| Plate 4 | X | Plate 10 | X (normal 16) |
| Plate 5 | 21 (normal 74) | Plate 11 | X (traceable) |
| Plate 6 | X (normal 7) | | |

_____ B. Cotton, CMA

Note: *The medical assistant may sign his or her name in the patient record using only the "CMA" credential if the office has a signature log denoting the entire credential as "CMA(AAMA)."*

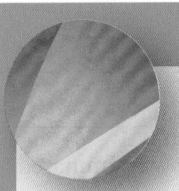

## PSY PROCEDURE 30-3

### Instilling Eye Medications

**PSY** Instruct and prepare a patient for a procedure or treatment; coach patients regarding disease prevention and treatment plans; coach patients appropriately considering cultural diversity, developmental life stage, and communication barriers; and document patient care accurately in the medical record.

**Purpose**: Instill and document ophthalmic medications as ordered by the physician

**Equipment**: Physician's order and patient record, ophthalmic medication, sterile gauze, tissues, and gloves

| STEPS | PURPOSE |
|---|---|
| 1. Wash your hands. | Hand washing aids infection control. |
| 2. Obtain the patient's medical record, including the physician's order, correct medication, sterile gauze, and tissues. | The medication must specify ophthalmic use. Check the label three times before administering the ophthalmic solution or ointment. Medications formulated for other uses may be harmful if used in the eyes. |
| 3. Greet and identify the patient. Identify yourself including your title. Explain the procedure. Ask the patient about any allergies not recorded in the chart. | Identifying the patient prevents errors in treatment. |
| 4. **AFF** Explain how to respond to a patient who does not speak English or who speaks English as a second language (ESL). | Solicit assistance from anyone who may be with the patient or a staff member who speaks the patient's native language to interpret if available. If no interpreter is available, use hand gestures or pictures to explain the procedure to the patient. |
| 5. Position the patient comfortably. | The patient may lie or sit with the head tilted slightly back and the affected eye slightly lower to avoid the medication running into the unaffected eye. |
| 6. Put on gloves and pull down the lower eyelid with sterile gauze while asking the patient to look up. | Since there is potential for contact with secretions from the eye, you must wear gloves. Pulling down the lower lid exposes the conjunctival sac to receive the medication. If the patient is looking up and away from the medication, the blink reflex may not be triggered. |

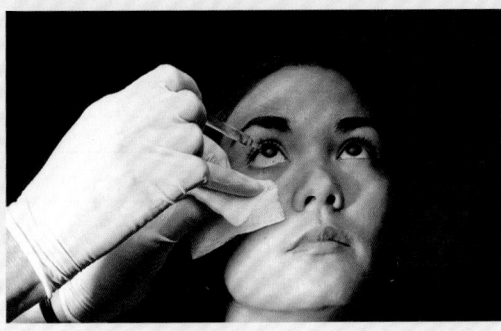

**Step 6.** Pull the lower eyelid down and ask the patient to look up.

## PROCEDURE 30-3 (continued)

| STEPS | PURPOSE |
|---|---|
| 7. Instill the medication: A. Ointment: Discard the first bead of ointment from the container onto a tissue without touching the end of the medication tube to the tissue. Place a thin line of ointment across the inside of the lower eyelid, moving from the inner canthus outward. Release the ointment by twisting the tube slightly. Do not touch the tube to the eye. B. Drops: Hold the dropper close to the conjunctival sac (about half an inch away) but do not touch the patient. Release the proper number of drops into the sac. Discard any medication left in the dropper. | The first bead of ointment is considered contaminated. Placing the ointment in the sac avoids touching the eye with the tip of the ointment tube. Twisting the tube releases the ointment. Discarding the remaining medication prevents contaminating the remainder of a multiple dose container. |
| 8. Release the lower lid and have the patient gently close the eye and roll it to disperse the medication. | Closing the eye will prevent the medication from leaking out. Rolling the eye around will distribute the medication. |
| 9. Wipe off any excess medication with the tissue. Instruct the patient to apply light pressure to the puncta lacrimalis for several minutes. | Pressing the puncta prevents the medication from running into the nasolacrimal sac and duct. |
| 10. Properly care for or dispose of equipment and supplies. Clean the work area and wash your hands. | Always clean up after procedures as soon as possible. Wash your hands after any patient contact. |
| 11. **AFF** Log into the electronic medical record (EMR) using your username and secure password OR obtain the paper medical record from a secure location and assure it is kept away from public access. Record the procedure including the name of the medication, which eye was medicated, and the patient's response. Your entry must include the date, time, and your name/credentials. | The integrity of the medical record must be maintained at all times to protect patient privacy. Procedures are considered not to have been done if they are not recorded. |
| 12. When finished, log out of the EMR and/or replace the paper medical record in an appropriate and secure location. | |

Charting Example:
*10/14/2016 8:45 am Garamycin ophthalmologic ointment applied to OS _____*
*B. Marker, CMA*

Note: *The medical assistant may sign his or her name in the patient record using only the "CMA" credential if the office has a signature log denoting the entire credential as "CMA(AAMA)."*

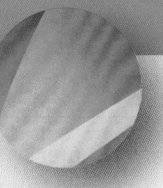

## PSY PROCEDURE 30-4

# Irrigating the Eye

**PSY** Instruct and prepare a patient for a procedure or treatment; coach patients regarding disease prevention and treatment plans; coach patients appropriately considering cultural diversity, developmental life stage, and communication barriers; and document patient care accurately in the medical record.

**Purpose:** Irrigate the eye as ordered by the physician and document the procedure

**Equipment:** Physician's order and patient record, small sterile basin if sterile solution is used, irrigating solution (water) and medication (if ordered), protective barrier or towels, emesis basin, sterile bulb syringe, tissues, and gloves

| STEPS | PURPOSE |
|---|---|
| 1. Wash your hands and put on gloves. | Hand washing aids infection control. You must wear gloves when you are exposed to body fluids. |
| 2. Assemble the equipment, supplies, and medication if ordered. Check the label three times as recommended for medication administration, and make sure the label indicates ophthalmic use. Note: If both eyes are to be treated, use separate equipment (solution and bulb syringe) to avoid cross-contamination. | Unless water is ordered for the eye irrigation, solutions for the eye must be sterile and must be formulated for ophthalmic use. |
| 3. Greet and identify the patient. Identify yourself and your title. Explain the procedure. | Identifying the patient prevents errors in treatment. Patients who understand the procedure are generally cooperative and compliant. |
| 4. **AFF** Explain how to respond to a patient who is hard of hearing. | Make sure the patient can see your face as you speak. Speak clearly, not loudly. |
| 5. Position the patient comfortably, either with the head tilted and the affected eye lower or lying with the affected eye down. | With the affected eye down, there is little chance of contamination running into the unaffected eye. |
| 6. Drape the patient with the protective barrier or towel. | A protective barrier will prevent wetting the patient's clothing. |
| 7. Place the emesis basin against the upper cheek near the eye with the towel under the basin. With clean gauze, wipe the eye from the inner canthus outward to remove debris from the lashes. | Debris from the lashes may be washed into the eye. |
| 8. Separate the lids with the thumb and forefinger of your nondominant hand. To steady your hand, you may lightly support your dominant hand, holding the syringe with solution on the bridge of the patient's nose parallel to the eye. | Because of the natural reflex to close the eye, you must use your nondominant hand to physically separate the eyelids. |

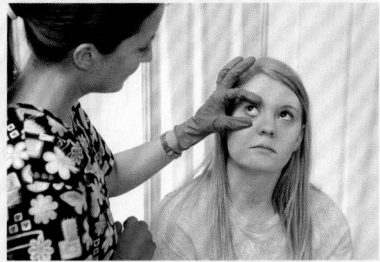

**Step 8.** Separate the eyelids with the thumb and forefinger.

## PROCEDURE 30-4 (continued)

| STEPS | PURPOSE |
|---|---|
| 9. Gently irrigate from the inner to the outer canthus, holding the syringe 1 inch above the eye. Use gentle pressure and do not touch the eye. The physician will order the time or amount of solution to be used. Debris from the lashes may be washed into the eye. | The solution must flow from the inner to the outer canthus to avoid washing pathogens into the punctum. With the syringe 1 inch above the eye, there is little chance of touching the eye and causing discomfort. |

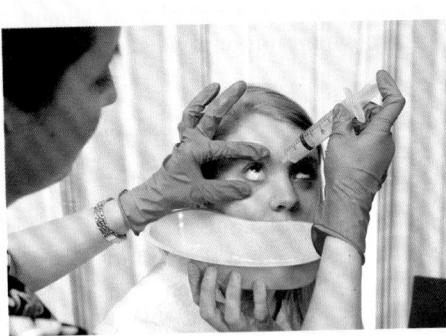

**Step 9.** Hold the syringe 1 inch above the eye.

| STEPS | PURPOSE |
|---|---|
| 10. Use tissues to wipe any excess solution from the patient's face. | This prevents the spread of microorganisms. |
| 11. Properly dispose of equipment or sanitize as recommended and remove your gloves. Wash your hands. | Always clean up as soon as possible after completing procedures. Hands should be washed after patient contact to prevent the spread of disease. |
| 12. **AFF** Log into the electronic medical record (EMR) using your username and secure password OR obtain the paper medical record from a secure location and assure it is kept away from public access. Record the procedure including the amount, type, and strength of the solution; which eye was irrigated; and any observations. Your entry must include the date, time, and your name/credentials. | The integrity of the medical record must be maintained at all times to protect patient privacy. Procedures are considered not to have been done if they are not recorded. |
| 13. When finished, log out of the EMR and/or replace the paper medical record in an appropriate and secure location. | |

Charting Example:
04/16/2016 11:30 am OD irrigated with 500 mL sterile NS, return clear _____
J. Penta, CMA

Note: *The medical assistant may sign his or her name in the patient record using only the "CMA" credential if the office has a signature log denoting the entire credential as "CMA(AAMA)."*

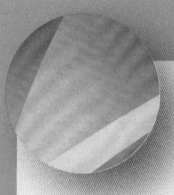

## Procedure 30-5

# Irrigating the Ear

**PSY** Instruct and prepare a patient for a procedure or treatment; coach patients regarding disease prevention and treatment plans; coach patients appropriately considering cultural diversity, developmental life stage, and communication barriers; and document patient care accurately in the medical record.

**Purpose:** Irrigate the ear as ordered and document the procedure

**Equipment:** Physician's order and patient's record, emesis or ear basin, waterproof barrier or towels, otoscope, irrigating solution (water), bowl for solution, and gauze

| STEPS | PURPOSE |
|---|---|
| 1. Wash your hands. | Hand washing aids infection control. |
| 2. Assemble the equipment and supplies. | Ear irrigation is not a sterile procedure. |
| 3. Greet and identify the patient. Identify yourself including your title. Explain the procedure. | Identifying the patient prevents errors in the treatment. Ear irrigations are not usually painful, but the flow of the solution may be uncomfortable. The patient may be more cooperative if this is understood. |
| 4. **AFF** Explain how to respond to a patient who has dementia. | Solicit assistance from a caregiver or other staff member to help during the procedure as needed. Give simple directions to the patient about what he or she should do. Speak clearly, not loudly. |
| 5. Position the patient comfortably erect. | The patient who is comfortably seated may be more cooperative during the procedure. |
| 6. View the affected ear with an otoscope to locate the foreign matter or cerumen. | The area of treatment must be visualized before irrigation begins. If debris from the external auricle is not removed, it may be washed into the canal. |

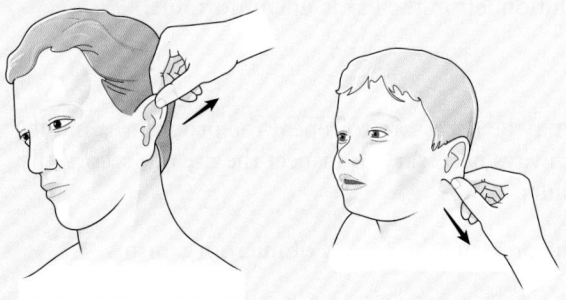

**Step 6.** The shape of the ear canal changes with growth. To allow good inspection, position the ear as illustrated.

| | |
|---|---|
| A. Adults: Gently pull ear up and back to straighten the auditory canal. <br> B. Children: Gently pull ear slightly down and back to straighten the auditory canal. | |
| 7. Drape the patient with a waterproof barrier or towel. | Wet clothing would be uncomfortable for the patient. |
| 8. Tilt the patient's head toward the affected side. | Tilting the head will facilitate the flow of solution. |

*(continues on page 788)*

## PROCEDURE 30-5 (continued)

| STEPS | PURPOSE |
|---|---|

9. Place the drainage basin under the affected ear.

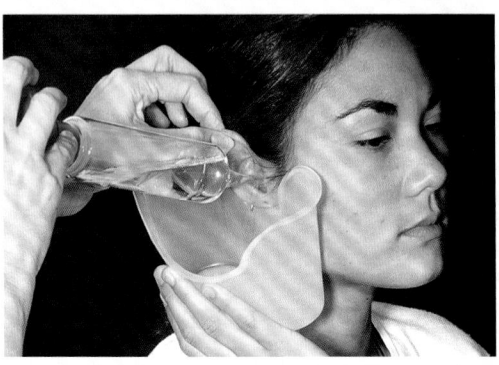

Step 9. Place the basin under the ear.

10. Fill the irrigating syringe or turn on the irrigating device.

Some offices have special systems for irrigating ears, whereas others may have you use a 20-mL or bulb syringe.

11. Gently position the auricle as described, using your nondominant hand.

The canal must be straight for visualization and treatment.

12. With your dominant hand, place the tip of the syringe in the auditory meatus and direct the flow of the solution gently up toward the roof of the canal.

Directing the flow against the upper surface prevents pressure against the tympanic membrane and facilitates the outflow of solution.

13. Continue irrigating for the prescribed period or until the desired result (cerumen removal) is obtained.

If the patient complains of pain or discomfort, stop the irrigation and notify the physician.

14. Dry the patient's external ear with gauze. Have the patient sit for awhile with the affected ear down to drain the solution.

Solution left in the ear is uncomfortable.

15. Inspect the ear with the otoscope to determine the results.

It may be necessary to repeat the procedure, and it is always necessary to inspect the area to record the results.

16. Properly care for or dispose of equipment and supplies. Clean the work area. Wash your hands.

This prevents the spread of microorganisms.

17. **AFF** Log into the electronic medical record (EMR) using your username and secure password OR obtain the paper medical record from a secure location and assure it is kept away from public access. Record the procedure including the amount, type, and strength of the solution; which ear was irrigated; and any observations. Your entry must include the date, time, and your name/credentials.

The integrity of the medical record must be maintained at all times to protect patient privacy. Procedures are considered not to have been done if they are not recorded.

## PROCEDURE 30-5 (continued)

| STEPS | PURPOSE |
|---|---|
| 18. When finished, log out of the EMR and/or replace the paper medical record in an appropriate and secure location. | |

*Note:* If the tympanic membrane appears to be perforated, do not irrigate without checking with the physician; solution may be forced into the middle ear through the perforation. Remove any obvious debris at the entrance of the canal before beginning the irrigation.

---

Charting Example:

*03/17/2016 3:30 pm AD irrigated with 500 mL sterile water; return clear with 2 large pieces of yellow-brown cerumen noted _____ S. Stark, CMA*

---

Note: *The medical assistant may sign his or her name in the patient record using only the "CMA" credential if the office has a signature log denoting the entire credential as "CMA(AAMA)."*

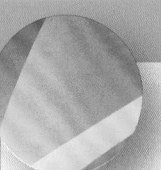

## PSY PROCEDURE 30-6

# Perform Audiometric Hearing Test

**PSY** Instruct and prepare a patient for a procedure or treatment; coach patients regarding disease prevention and treatment plans; coach patients appropriately considering cultural diversity, developmental life stage, and communication barriers; and document patient care accurately in the medical record.

**Purpose:** To accurately assess and document a hearing test using audiometry

**Equipment:** Audiometer and otoscope

| STEPS | PURPOSE |
|---|---|
| 1. Wash your hands. | Hand washing aids infection control. |
| 2. Greet and identify the patient. Identify yourself and your title. Explain the procedure. Take the patient to a quiet area or room for testing. | Patients who understand the procedure are likely to be compliant, producing accurate results. A quiet room allows for accurate results without distraction. Determine the signal (raising the hand, saying yes) to indicate that the tones are heard. |
| 3. **AFF** Explain how to respond to a patient who is visually impaired. | Face the patient when speaking and always let him or her know what you are going to do before touching him or her. |
| 4. Using an otoscope or audioscope with a light source, visually inspect the ear canal and tympanic membrane before the examination. | Looking into the ear canal verifies that there are no obstructions, such as cerumen, to interfere with the test. If you see an obstruction, notify the physician. |
| 5. Choose the correct size tip for the end of the audiometer. Attach a speculum to fit the patient's external auditory meatus, making sure the ear canal is occluded with the speculum in place. | The design of the tip or speculum obviates bulky ear phones. The tip should block any environmental noise during the test. |
| 6. With the speculum in the ear canal, retract the pinna: up and back for adults, down and back for children. | Pulling the pinna up and back for adults and down and back for children straightens the ear canal. |

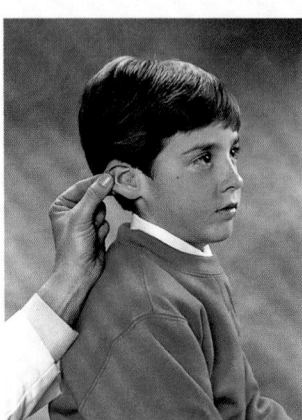

**Step 6.** Pull the pinna down and back for children. (Courtesy of Welch-Allyn.)

## PROCEDURE 30-6 (continued)

| STEPS | PURPOSE |
|---|---|
| **7.** Turn the instrument on and select the screening level. There is a pretest tone for practice if necessary. Press the start button and observe the tone indicators and the patient's responses. | The signal (raising the hand, saying yes) was determined before you began the test. The audiometer will proceed down each tone with a light indicator. |

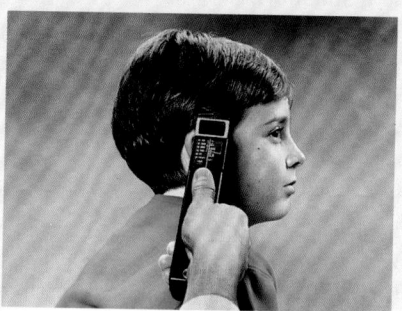

**A**

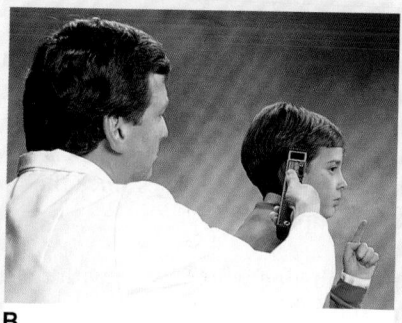

**B**

**Step 7. (A)** Place the audiometer tip in the patient's ear. **(B)** The patient should give a signal when each tone is heard. (Courtesy of Welch-Allyn.)

| STEPS | PURPOSE |
|---|---|
| **8.** Screen the other ear. | Each ear is screened separately. |
| **9.** If the patient fails to respond at any frequency, rescreening is required. | If the patient does not hear a specific tone, a second opportunity should be given. |
| **10.** If the patient fails rescreening, notify the physician. | A patient who fails to hear one or more tones may be referred to an audiologist. |
| **11.** **AFF** Log into the electronic medical record (EMR) using your username and secure password OR obtain the paper medical record from a secure location and assure it is kept away from public access. Record the procedure. Your entry must include the date, time, and your name/credentials. | The integrity of the medical record must be maintained at all times to protect patient privacy. Procedures are considered not to have been done if they are not recorded. |
| **12.** When finished, log out of the EMR and/or replace the paper medical record in an appropriate and secure location. | |

Charting Example:
*02/14/2016 9:00 am Audiometry testing performed AU, results in chart* _____ *S. Smythe, RMA*

Note: *The medical assistant may sign his or her name in the patient record using only the "CMA" credential if the office has a signature log denoting the entire credential as "CMA(AAMA)."*

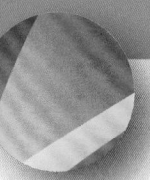

**PSY** PROCEDURE 30-7

# Instilling Ear Medication

**PSY** Instruct and prepare a patient for a procedure or treatment; coach patients regarding disease prevention and treatment plans; coach patients appropriately considering cultural diversity, developmental life stage, and communication barriers; and document patient care accurately in the medical record.

**Purpose:** Instill otic medication as ordered and document the instillation

**Equipment:** Physician's order and patient's record, otic medication with dropper, and cotton balls

**Standard:** This procedure should take 5 minutes.

| STEPS | PURPOSE |
|---|---|
| 1. Wash your hands. | Hand washing aids infection control. |
| 2. Check the medication label three times as specified for medication administration. The label should specify otic preparation. | Medication for otic instillation is formulated for that purpose. |
| 3. Greet and identify the patient. Identify yourself including your title. Explain the procedure. | Identifying the patient prevents errors in the treatment. Patients who understand the procedure are generally compliant. |
| 4. Ask the patient about any allergies not documented in the medical record. | The patient may have developed allergies since the medical record was last updated. |
| 5. **AFF** Explain how to respond to a patient who does not speak English or who speaks English as a second language (ESL). | Solicit assistance from anyone who may be with the patient or a staff member who speaks the patient's native language to interpret if available. If no interpreter is available, use hand gestures or pictures to explain the procedure. |
| 6. Have the patient seated with the affected ear tilted upward. | The medication must be allowed to flow through the canal to the tympanic membrane. |
| 7. Draw up the ordered amount of medication. | Only administer the amount prescribed. |
| 8. Straighten the canal.<br>   **A.** Adults: Pull the auricle slightly up and back.<br>   **B.** Children: Pull the auricle slightly down and back. | Straightening the ear canal will prevent the medication from pooling in the ear canal. |

# PROCEDURE 30-7 (continued)

| STEPS | PURPOSE |
|---|---|
| 9. Insert the tip of the dropper without touching the patient's skin and let the medication flow along the side of the canal. | Touching the patient will contaminate the dropper. The medication should flow gently to avoid discomfort. |

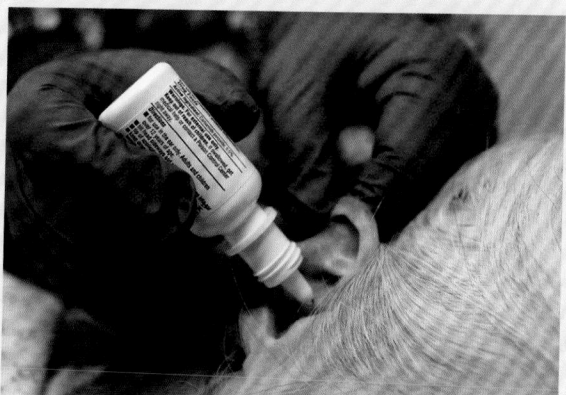

Step 9. Insert the tip of the dropper without touching the ear.

| STEPS | PURPOSE |
|---|---|
| 10. Have the patient sit or lie with the affected ear up for about 5 minutes after the instillation. | The medication should rest against the tympanic membrane for as long as possible. |
| 11. If the medication is to be retained in the ear canal, insert a moist cotton ball into the external auditory meatus without force. | A slightly moist cotton ball will keep the medication in the canal and not wick it out. Forcing the cotton ball into the ear canal could be painful to the patient. |
| 12. Properly care for or dispose of equipment and supplies. Clean the work area. Wash your hands. | This prevents the spread of microorganisms. |
| 13. AFF Log into the electronic medical record (EMR) using your username and secure password OR obtain the paper medical record from a secure location and assure it is kept away from public access. Record the procedure including the name of the medication, which ear was medicated, and the patient's response. Your entry must include the date, time, and your name/credentials. | The integrity of the medical record must be maintained at all times to protect patient privacy. Procedures are considered not to have been done if they are not recorded. |
| 14. When finished, log out of the EMR and/or replace the paper medical record in an appropriate and secure location. | |

Charting Example:
*06/15/2016 12:30 pm Neosporin otic solution, 2 gtt instilled into AS as ordered*
*—————————————————————————————— D. Barth, CMA*

Note: *The medical assistant may sign his or her name in the patient record using only the "CMA" credential if the office has a signature log denoting the entire credential as "CMA(AAMA)."*

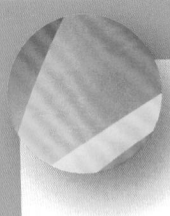

## Procedure 30-8

# Instilling Nasal Medication

**PSY** Instruct and prepare a patient for a procedure or treatment; coach patients regarding disease prevention and treatment plans; coach patients appropriately considering cultural diversity, developmental life stage, and communication barriers; and document patient care accurately in the medical record.

**Purpose:** Instill nasal medication as ordered and document the instillation

**Equipment:** Physician's order and patient's record, nasal medication, drops or spray, tissues, and gloves

| STEPS | PURPOSE |
|-------|---------|
| 1. Wash your hands. | Hand washing aids infection control. |
| 2. Assemble the equipment and supplies. Check the medication label three times. | Medications for use in the nasal passages must be formulated for these surfaces. |
| 3. Greet and identify the patient. Explain the procedure and ask the patient about any allergies not documented. | Identifying the patient prevents errors in the treatment. Nasal instillations are uncomfortable but should not be painful; patients will be more cooperative if they understand the procedure. |
| 4. **AFF** Explain how to respond to a patient who has dementia. | Solicit assistance from the caregiver or another staff member to help during the procedure. Give simple directions to the patient about what he or she should do. Speak clearly, not loudly. |
| 5. Position the patient comfortably recumbent. Extend the patient's head beyond the edge of the examination table or place a pillow under the shoulders. Support the patient's neck to avoid strain as the head tilts back. | The patient must be properly positioned if the medication is to reach the upper nasal passages. |

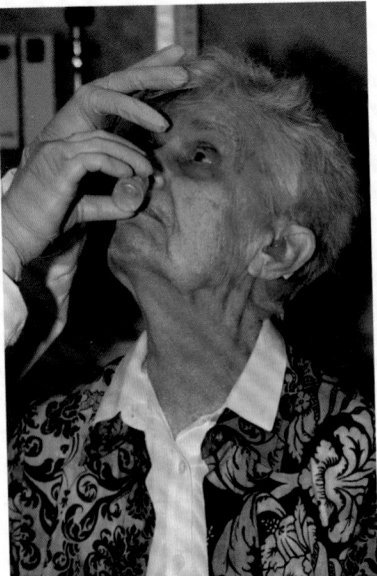

Step 5. Tilt the patient's head back.

## PROCEDURE 30-8 (continued)

| STEPS | PURPOSE |
|---|---|
| 6. Administer the medication. A. Hold the dropper upright just above each nostril and dispense one drop at a time without touching the nares. Keep the patient recumbent for 5 minutes. B. Place the tip of the bottle at the naris opening without touching the patient's skin or nasal tissues and spray as the patient takes a deep breath. | Touching the dropper to the nostril would contaminate the dropper. For effective treatment, the patient must allow the medication to reach the upper nasal passages. The medication must reach the upper passages; if the patient breathes out while the medication is being sprayed, the medication is exhaled and does not reach the nasal passages. |
| 7. Wipe any excess medication from the patient's skin with tissues. | Excess medication around the nares is uncomfortable. |
| 8. Properly care for or dispose of equipment and supplies. Clean the work area. Remove your gloves and wash your hands. | This prevents the spread of microorganisms. |
| 9. **AFF** Log into the electronic medical record (EMR) using your username and secure password OR obtain the paper medical record from a secure location and assure it is kept away from public access. Record the procedure including the name of the medication and the patient's response. Your entry must include the date, time, and your name/credentials. | The integrity of the medical record must be maintained at all times to protect patient privacy.<br><br>Procedures are considered not to have been done if they are not recorded. |
| 10. When finished, log out of the EMR and/or replace the paper medical record in an appropriate and secure location. | |

Charting Example:
*06/15/2016 12:00 pm Oxymetazoline hydrochloride 0.05% nasal spray, 2 sprays to each nostril as ordered per Dr. Greene _____ D. Pratt, CMA*

Note: *The medical assistant may sign his or her name in the patient record using only the "CMA" credential if the office has a signature log denoting the entire credential as "CMA(AAMA)."*

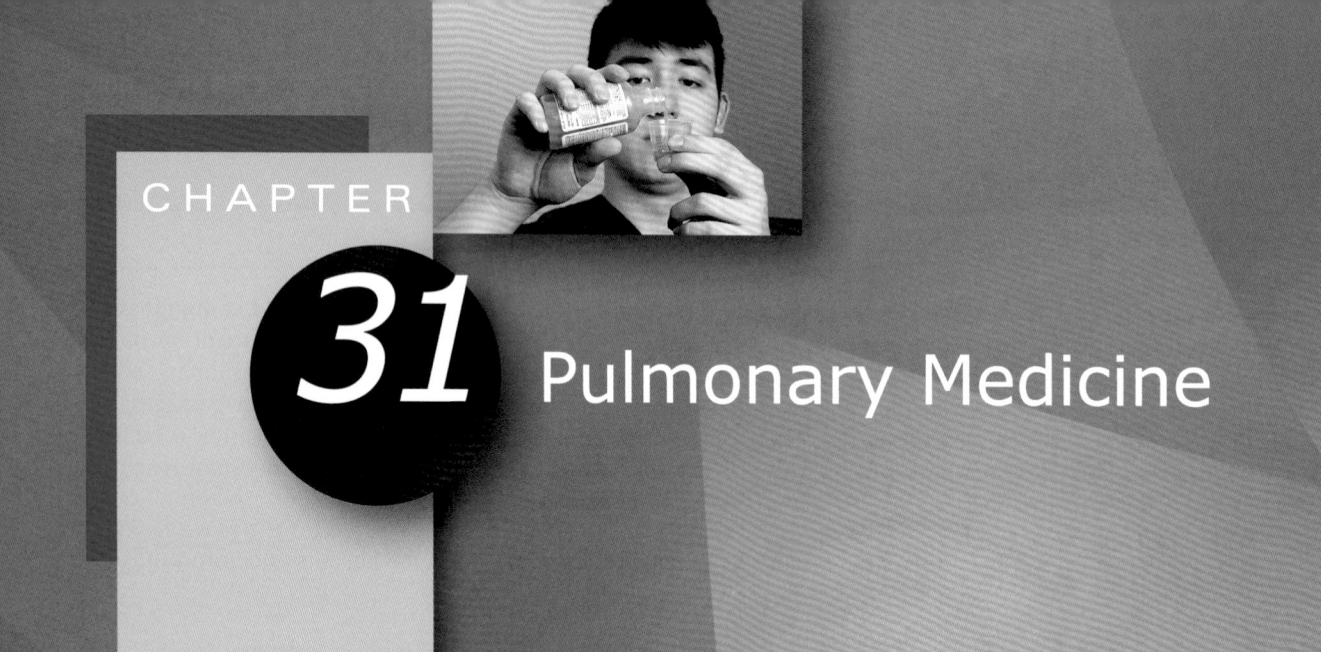

# CHAPTER

# *31* Pulmonary Medicine

## Learning Outcomes

**COG Cognitive Domain\***

1. Spell key terms
2. *Define medical terms and abbreviations related to all body systems*
3. *Describe structural organization of the human body*
4. *List major organs in each body system*
5. *Identify the anatomical location of major organs in each body system*
6. *Describe the normal function of each body system*
7. *Identify common pathology related to each body system including signs, symptoms, and etiology*
   a. Identify the primary defense mechanisms of the respiratory system
   b. Identify and explain diagnostic procedures of the respiratory system
   c. Describe the physician's examination of the respiratory system
8. Discuss the role of the medical assistant with regard to various diagnostic and therapeutic procedures

**PSY Psychomotor Domain\***

1. Instruct a patient in the use of the peak flowmeter (Procedure 31-2)
   a. *Instruct and prepare a patient for a procedure or treatment*
   b. *Coach patients appropriately considering cultural diversity, developmental life stage, and communication barriers*
   c. *Coach patients regarding disease prevention and treatment plans*
   d. *Document patient care accurately in the medical record.*
2. Administer a nebulized breathing treatment (Procedure 31-2)
   a. *Instruct and prepare a patient for a procedure or treatment*
   b. *Coach patients appropriately considering cultural diversity, developmental life stage, and communication barriers*
   c. *Coach patients regarding disease prevention and treatment plans*
   d. *Document patient care accurately in the medical record*
3. Collecting a sputum specimen (Procedure 31-3)
   a. *Instruct and prepare a patient for a procedure or treatment*
   b. *Coach patients appropriately considering cultural diversity, developmental life stage, and communication barriers*
   c. *Coach patients regarding disease prevention and treatment plans*
   d. *Document patient care accurately in the medical record*
4. Perform a pulmonary function test (Procedure 31-4)
   a. *Instruct and prepare a patient for a procedure or treatment*
   b. *Coach patients appropriately considering cultural diversity, developmental life stage, and communication barriers*
   c. *Coach patients regarding disease prevention and treatment plans*
   d. *Document patient care accurately in the medical record*

### AFF Affective Domain*

1. *Incorporate critical thinking skills when performing patient assessment*
2. *Incorporate critical thinking skills when performing patient care*
3. *Show awareness of a patient's concerns related to the procedure being performed*
4. *Demonstrate empathy, active listening, and nonverbal communication*
5. *Demonstrate respect for individual diversity including gender, race, religion, age, economic status, and appearance*
6. *Explain to a patient the rationale for performance of a procedure*

7. *Demonstrate sensitivity to patient rights*
8. *Protect the integrity of the medical record.*

*\*Note: AAMA/CAAHEP 2015 Standards are italicized.*

### ABHES Competencies

1. Assist the physician with the regimen of diagnostic and treatment modalities as they relate to each body system
2. Comply with federal, state, and local health laws and regulations
3. Communicate on the recipient's level of comprehension
4. Serve as a liaison between the physician and others
5. Show empathy and impartiality when dealing with patients
6. Document accurately

## Key Terms

| | | | |
|---|---|---|---|
| atelectasis | dyspnea | laryngectomy | thoracentesis |
| chronic obstructive pulmonary disease (COPD) | forced expiratory volume | palliative | tidal volume |
| | hemoptysis | status asthmaticus | tracheostomy |

## Case Study

*E*llen Barker, CMA (AAMA), finished a 2-year associate degree medical assistant program 2 years ago. The first year after graduating, she worked in a busy urgent care center in the suburb where she grew up. She heard through a friend that the corporate office for Great Falls Medical Center was looking for a credentialed medical assistant to work in the pulmonary medicine office last year, so she applied, interviewed, and was hired after meeting with the physicians in the practice. There are five pulmonary physicians in the practice, and each has his or her own medical assistant. She works for Dr. Richards, one of the younger physicians in the office, who came to the practice 2 years ago. Although Dr. Richards sees some pediatric patients, most of his patients are adults who have chronic respiratory diseases such as asthma and emphysema. Several of the adult patients have a history of smoking cigarettes, and some of those have not quit despite their respiratory difficulties. It is well known that smoking causes lung disease, but what are the specific effects on the lungs that cause patients to have respiratory issues? Will smoking long term cause conditions such as pulmonary fibrosis? Is emphysema reversible? These and other questions are answered in this chapter.

The respiratory system provides the body with the oxygen that all cells need to perform their functions (Fig. 31-1). It also eliminates carbon dioxide, a waste product, and water from the body. The respiratory system works closely with the cardiovascular system to deliver oxygen to every cell in the body. When a cell is too long deprived of oxygen, the cell dies, and when many cells die, so does the tissue.

The upper airways, tracheobronchial tree, and alveoli come into contact with air from the atmosphere or environment, which can contain dust, pathogenic microorganisms, and other irritants. In healthy

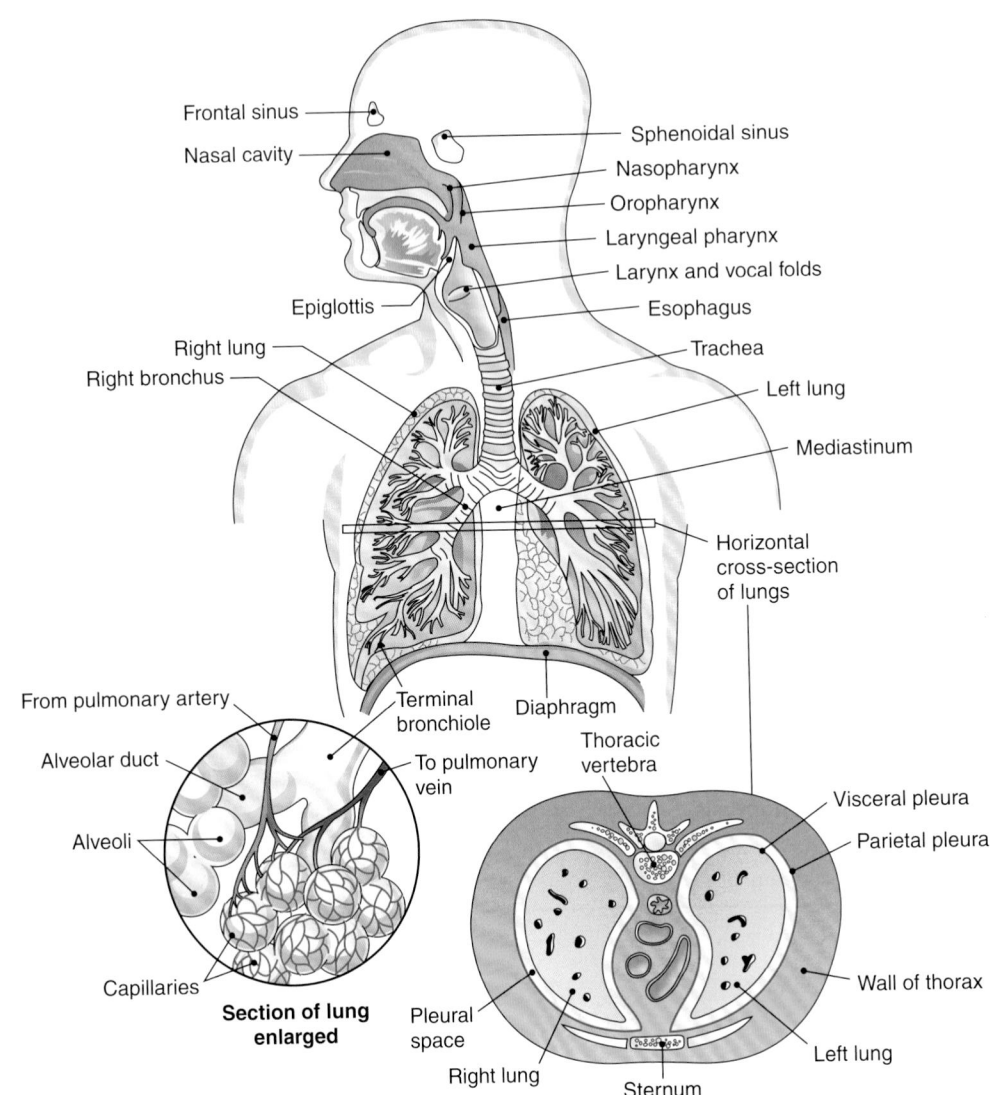

**Figure 31-1 •** The respiratory system. (Reprinted from Cohen BJ. *Memmler's The Human Body in Health and Disease*, 11th ed. Philadelphia, PA: Lippincott Williams & Wilkins, 2009, with permission.)

individuals, defense mechanisms in the respiratory system help to protect the body from disease and illness caused by these environmental contaminants. Table 31-1 summarizes the major defense mechanisms of the respiratory system. Disease can occur, however, when these defenses are overwhelmed by cigarette smoke, air pollution, infectious organisms, or other irritants.

| TABLE 31-1 | Defenses of the Respiratory System |
|---|---|
| **Defense** | **Function** |
| Nasal hairs | Filter large dust particles from the air |
| Mucous membranes | Trap dust and other particles, add moisture |
| Turbinates in the nose | Whirl air around to increase warming, humidifying, filtering |
| Epiglottis | Closes over trachea to prevent aspiration during swallowing |
| Airway reflexes | Trigger cough to clear irritants in pharynx, larynx, trachea |
| Airway smooth muscles | Constrict when irritation occurs to prevent entry of foreign substances |
| Macrophage in alveoli | Phagocytize ("eat") bacteria, other foreign cells, debris |
| Tonsils | Filter air moving through passageways to protect against bacterial invasion; aid in formation of white blood cells |

**COMMON RESPIRATORY DISORDERS**

## Upper Respiratory Disorders

The most common problems of the upper respiratory tract are caused by infectious microorganisms and by allergic reactions that produce inflammation. Acute rhinitis, sinusitis, pharyngitis, tonsillitis, and laryngitis are described in Chapter 30; these are also considered upper respiratory disorders.

## Lower Respiratory Disorders

Diseases of the lower respiratory tract may be acute (sudden in onset with relatively short duration) or chronic (progressing over time or recurring frequently). Acute diseases of the lower respiratory tract include bronchitis and pneumonia. Chronic diseases include asthma, chronic bronchitis, and emphysema. The last two diseases are usually grouped as chronic obstructive pulmonary disease because most patients have elements of both emphysema and chronic bronchitis.

---

### PATIENT EDUCATION

#### Effects of Smoking on the Airways

Cigarette smoking has many harmful effects on the body. Smoke from a cigarette irritates the airways and causes the membrane to produce more mucus. This increased production of mucus, along with the increase in dust and debris that collects in the mucus, slows down the body's normal clearing processes. The smoke anesthetizes the cilia lining the respiratory tract so they stop waving the debris away. Over time, large amounts of thick, sticky mucus are retained in the lungs, blackening the lung tissue and sealing the alveolar sacs. This thick, tarry mucus causes the patient to cough frequently, especially in the mornings, and to be prone to bronchitis, both acute and chronic, as a result of the destruction of the protective mechanisms of the airway from the heat and tar inhaled in the smoke.

---

## Bronchitis

Bronchitis is an inflammation of the mucous membranes of the bronchi caused by infection or irritation that induces increased production of mucus in the trachea, bronchi, and bronchioles. The most prominent symptom of bronchitis is a productive cough. If a bacterial or viral infection is present, the sputum may change color from the normal white or clear to yellow, green, gray, or tan. If an infection is suspected, you may be asked to obtain a sputum specimen for culture and sensitivity to determine the causative microorganism and appropriate antibiotic therapy. (Chapter 44 outlines the procedure for collecting a sputum specimen.) In many cases, the physician bases a diagnosis of bronchitis on the history and symptoms of the patient without ordering a sputum culture.

The treatment of bronchitis generally includes an antibiotic for bacterial infection, smoking cessation, rest, and increased fluid intake. A cough suppressant may be prescribed, especially for use at night, but this is controversial because of the body's need to clear secretions from the airways. Retained secretions can become infected and lead to pneumonia.

## Pneumonia

Pneumonia is a bacterial or viral infection in the alveoli, or tiny air sacs that are the site of gas exchange in the lungs. The buildup of fluid and congestion in the alveoli prevents effective gas exchange. Diagnostic testing usually includes analysis of a sputum specimen and chest radiography. Bacterial pneumonias tend to be sudden and severe in onset, causing a fever, cough, chills, and **dyspnea**. Infections caused by bacteria also tend to be local to one lobe or area of the lung. Treatment of bacterial pneumonia primarily includes an appropriate antibiotic, bed rest, and medication to relieve symptoms. Pneumonia caused by bacteria often requires hospitalization for administration of intravenous antibiotics and oxygen, especially in the elderly or debilitated patients.

Viral pneumonia is usually more gradual in onset but can be just as serious. Antibiotics are ineffective in treating viral pneumonia; however, the physician may order an antibiotic to prevent a secondary bacterial infection. Viral pneumonia tends to spread throughout the lung fields and often is marked by a fever and productive cough. Treatment may include bed rest or hospitalization.

---

### PATIENT EDUCATION

#### Pulmonary Fibrosis

Pulmonary fibrosis is a lung disease that occurs due to damage and scarring of the lung tissue. As more scarring develops, the lungs become stiff and the ability of the alveoli to exchange oxygen and carbon dioxide is decreased. Symptoms of pulmonary fibrosis include dyspnea, a dry cough, fatigue, and weight loss. In some patients, the disease may develop quickly and be severe, while other patients are diagnosed and the disease progresses more slowly, perhaps over months or years. As the disease progresses, the patient will become more short of breath with exertion.

The cause of this disease is often unknown (idiopathic pulmonary fibrosis); however, some patients have developed this disease due to the following:

- Long-term exposure to occupational or environmental pollutants such as asbestos, grain dust, or bird droppings
- Medications such as those used for chemotherapy and cardiac arrhythmias and some antibiotics may damage the lungs and result in pulmonary fibrosis months or years after taking the drug.
- Underlying medical conditions including tuberculosis, pneumonia, rheumatoid arthritis, and systemic lupus erythematosus may cause lung damage that results in pulmonary fibrosis.

Although there is no cure for pulmonary fibrosis, some patients may have significant lung damage and may receive a lung transplant. Most patient care is aimed at education and support including the following:

- Corticosteroids such as prednisone and/or drugs that suppress the immune system.
- Oxygen therapy may be ordered by the physician to decrease symptoms associated with decreased blood oxygen levels.
- A referral for pulmonary rehabilitation may be prescribed by the physician to provide patients with exercises to improve endurance, breathing techniques to improve lung efficiency, emotional support, and nutritional counseling.

Encourage patients who are diagnosed with this disease to do the following:

- Participate in treatment as much as possible.
- Stop smoking and avoid environments where cigarette or cigar smoke is in the air.
- Maintain nutritional status by increasing calories and frequency of meals.
- Receive vaccines as ordered by the physician to avoid respiratory infections.

As the patient's disease progresses, support to both the family and the caregivers will be essential. Discussions for end-of-life care should be directed to the physician and any decisions made respected by the health care team working with the patient and family.

##  CHECKPOINT QUESTION

1. A patient in Ellen Michael's office has been diagnosed with viral pneumonia. What are the characteristics of bacterial and viral pneumonia?

## Asthma

Asthma is a reversible inflammatory process involving primarily the small airways such as the bronchi and bronchioles. Asthma manifests as constriction of the smooth muscle lining the airways, spasms of the bronchi and bronchioles (bronchospasm), swelling of the mucous membranes of the airways, and increased mucus production with productive coughing. All three of these manifestations narrow the airways, making it difficult for the patient to move air into and out of the lungs.

The patient having an asthma attack may have dyspnea, coughing, wheezing, and, in severe cases, cyanosis. Patients with asthma usually have exacerbations, which are periods of frequent attacks, and remissions, which are periods when they are relatively symptom free. Attacks may be triggered by exposure to allergens, such as mold or dust; inhaled irritants, such as cigarette smoke; upper respiratory infections; psychological stress; cold air; or exercise. In some instances, the immediate cause of the asthma attack is unknown. While asthma is considered a chronic disorder that occurs in children or adults, many children with asthma outgrow it by adulthood.

Many medications are available to prevent or control the symptoms of asthma, but it is important that they be used properly. On days that the patient has no symptoms of asthma, he or she should use a device called a peak flowmeter (Fig. 31-2) to determine the amount of air moving into and out of the lungs (Procedure 31-1). Instruct the patient to use the peak flowmeter correctly, and record the results on a chart or diary provided by the medical office. This record, known as the patient's personal best, assists the physician in establishing and maintaining a medication protocol.

Patients with symptoms of asthma, including wheezing and difficulty breathing, may be prescribed a bronchodilator, or medication to dilate the bronchi, such as albuterol (Procedure 31-2). This medication may be administered by way of an inhaler or as a nebulized breathing treatment. The inhaler requires the patient to put the mouthpiece into the mouth and press down on the top of the canister while inhaling through the mouth, administering the medication directly into the lungs. Taken during episodes of wheezing such as an asthma attack, this inhaler may be referred to as a

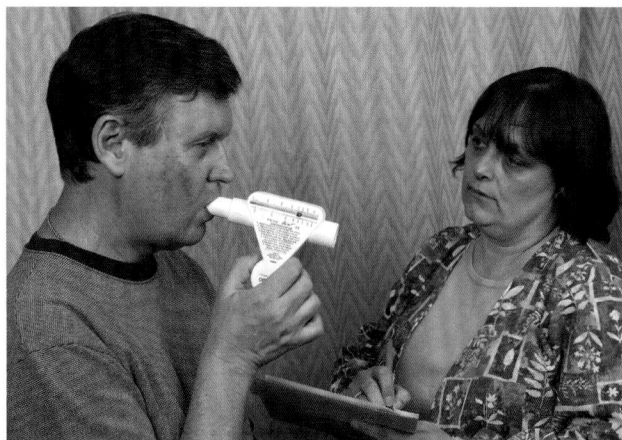

**Figure 31-2** • The peak flowmeter.

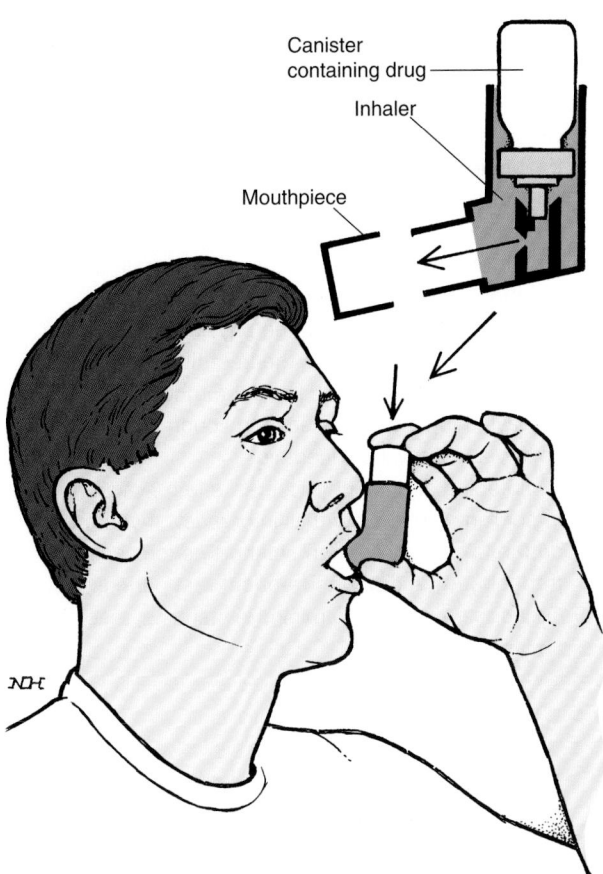

Canister containing drug

Inhaler

Mouthpiece

**Figure 31-3** • An inhaler may be used to administer some medications directly to the lungs.

"rescue inhaler" because it is used during actual bronchoconstriction, not to prevent bronchoconstriction (Fig. 31-3). Children who are prescribed to use inhalers may also attach a device called a "spacer," which is placed between the mouth and the inhaler device (Fig. 31-4). The patient puts the mouthpiece or mask end of the spacer into place and presses the end of the inhaler canister, dispensing the medication into the spacer. Inside the spacer, the medication is trapped while the patient breathes normally through the mouthpiece or mask.

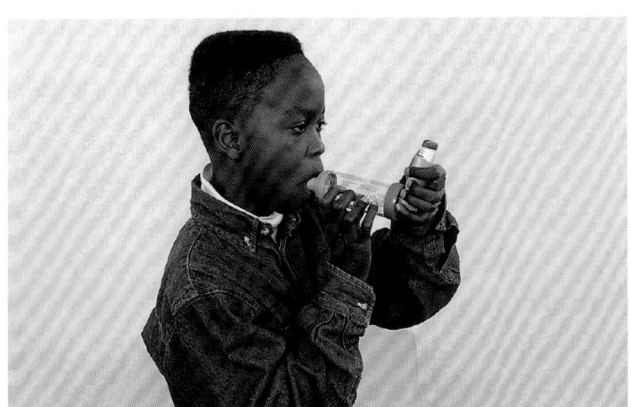

**Figure 31-4** • Pediatric patient using an inhaler with a spacer.

This device prevents medication from the depressed canister from being wasted by not inhaling all of it at one time. Although adults may use a spacer, it is especially useful for small children who must use an inhaler, but may not understand the procedure entirely for inhaling all of the medication with each "puff" or compression of the canister of medication.

Administering a bronchodilator such as albuterol through a nebulized breathing treatment is also an option to deliver medication directly to the lungs. The medication is supplied in a 2-mL or 3-mL solution and requires a nebulizer machine, which is essentially an air compressor that turns the liquid medication into a fine mist for inhalation. After the bronchodilator is in the nebulizer administration setup, the machine is turned on and causes the liquid medication to break apart into a fine spray that is inhaled by the patient through a mouthpiece or mask. Because bronchodilator medications cause an increase in the heart rate, you should monitor the patient's pulse before, during, and after the treatment. If the patient becomes lightheaded, discontinue the treatment, have the patient lie down, obtain the vital signs, and notify the physician.

An asthma attack that does not respond to medication is an emergency known as **status asthmaticus**. Because such attacks can be fatal, the patient needs immediate emergency medical services and hospitalization.

 **CHECKPOINT QUESTION**

2. When discussing asthma with a patient, what factors would she mention that may trigger an asthma attack?

## 🎓 PATIENT EDUCATION

### Using More Than One Inhaler for Asthma

Asthmatics may use more than one inhaler. One medication is usually a bronchodilator to open the bronchioles and control bronchospasms. Another type of inhaler is a corticosteroid. Steroids help to control inflammation in the bronchioles and generally are prescribed only during a respiratory illness. Teach the patient to use the bronchodilator first, wait 5 minutes, and then use the steroid. Using the steroid inhaler after the bronchodilator allows for more steroid medication to enter the lung tissue, making it more effective.

Some patients are prescribed two inhaled bronchodilators. One type is used daily to prevent asthma attacks, and the other is used as a rescue inhaler. The rescue inhaler should be used only when the asthma cannot be controlled with the daily regimen. Before teaching a patient about the correct pattern for using the inhalers, clarify the information with the physician. Each asthmatic responds differently and requires an individualized approach to care.

## Chronic Obstructive Pulmonary Disease

Chronic bronchitis and emphysema are most commonly caused by cigarette smoking. As a result, patients who have smoked over a long period often exhibit signs and symptoms of both of these disorders. Chronic bronchitis is a chronic inflammation and swelling of the airways with excessive mucus production, obstruction of the bronchi, and trapping of air behind mucus plugs. The trapping of this air overinflates the alveoli. Chronic bronchitis is not usually an infectious process but, instead, is produced by chronic irritation of the airways by cigarette smoke or other pollutants. However, because of the increase in sputum and the difficulty these patients have in clearing their sputum, they are prone to develop respiratory infections.

Emphysema is a disease process in which the walls of the damaged alveoli stretch and break down after repeated exposure to irritants such as cigarette smoke and air pollution. The pulmonary capillaries also break down, and the tiny airways leading to each alveolus weaken and collapse. The end result is a sharp reduction in surface area for gas exchange, and once again, air is trapped in the enlarged air sacs that were once clusters of tiny alveoli.

The combination of these diseases, together called **chronic obstructive pulmonary disease (COPD)**, produces characteristic symptoms. COPD is a likely cause of shortness of breath, chronic cough, sputum production, and wheezing in the patient with a history of smoking. The onset of these symptoms is usually slow and gradual over years, and the patient may go a long time without realizing that he or she has signs and symptoms of a disease. Many people with COPD have some of the signs and symptoms of asthma, and many of these patients take asthma medications.

Once a patient is diagnosed with COPD, the disease process is not usually reversible. Many patients have a hard time accepting that fact and insist that their physician provide a cure or restore the lungs to normal function. Although the disease is not curable, the progression of COPD can be slowed and the quality of life improved significantly through education about the disease, a prescribed exercise regimen, proper use of medications, good nutrition, and home oxygen therapy.

### PATIENT EDUCATION

#### Living with COPD

To improve the quality of life, encourage a patient diagnosed with COPD to follow these suggestions:

1. Quit smoking if you haven't already done so! Even though the lungs have been permanently damaged, further deterioration will be reduced if you stop smoking now.

2. Get a flu vaccination each fall and make sure you have had the pneumonia vaccine.
3. Avoid crowds, especially in the winter, when the viruses that cause colds and influenza are prevalent.
4. If pollution is high, stay indoors with the air conditioning on if possible.
5. Use your abdominal muscles instead of your shoulder and neck muscles to avoid strain and fatigue in these muscles.
6. Drink lots of fluids unless the physician has limited your fluid intake. Water is the best fluid. Good fluid intake is the best way to keep the mucus in your airways thin so that it is easy to cough up.
7. Follow a healthy, balanced diet.
8. Avoid doing difficult physical tasks (e.g., vacuuming or mowing the lawn) all in one day. If you must do these chores, do them in short periods spaced throughout the day with frequent rest periods.
9. Organize your home to minimize standing, reaching, and lifting.

### WHAT IF?

#### What if a patient requires home oxygen therapy?

Many patients with severe COPD or end-stage lung cancer are discharged from the hospital with oxygen to use at home. Most surgical supply companies and pharmacies can arrange to have oxygen therapy equipment delivered to the home. The oxygen is usually supplied by a machine called a concentrator that runs on electricity. The concentrator separates oxygen out of room air and concentrates it for delivery to the patient. Attached to the cylinder is a flowmeter, or regulator, that indicates the amount of oxygen being delivered. The patient should be instructed to leave the oxygen at the setting prescribed by the physician. Too much oxygen can be toxic for some patients, such as those with emphysema. A cannula (plastic tube with pronged openings that fit into the nares) is attached to the flowmeter and delivers oxygen to the patient's airways. The company supplying the oxygen should instruct the patient regarding safe home oxygen administration. Since oxygen is highly flammable, you should reinforce safety precautions during oxygen use, including avoiding open flames and sparks. In addition, the supplier should be available 24 hours a day for emergency oxygen maintenance.

## Tuberculosis

Tuberculosis is an infectious disease spread by respiratory droplets from a person infected with Mycobacterium tuberculosis. The patient with active tuberculosis has signs and symptoms such as a productive cough, night sweats, and malaise. Although no tuberculosis vaccine is available, a screening test can be administered to detect a previous infection. However, a patient with a positive screening test for tuberculosis does not necessarily have active disease and therefore may not be contagious. The procedure for administering and reading the results of the screening tests (Mantoux and tine tests) for tuberculosis is described in Chapter 24. Patients with symptoms of tuberculosis should be treated as contagious and encouraged to wear a protective mask over the nose and mouth to prevent spreading the disease through infected droplets released into the air during speaking and coughing. In addition, you are required to report any diagnosis of tuberculosis to the local public health department. The treatment for tuberculosis includes a regimen of antibiotic therapy that lasts for months. You should provide emotional support for these patients, since the treatment lasts up to a year, and encourage compliance with the prescribed regimen at each office visit.

## LEGAL TIP

### Words Have Meaning!

Patients with chronic and irreversible diseases, such as COPD, must never be led to believe that the doctor can cure the disease. Avoid making statements such as "Everything will be okay" or "The doctor can help you," and also be careful not to indicate that the patient will return to normal function. Legally, the doctor is responsible for your actions, including promises, even if they are innocent and were said only to make the patient feel better. These statements may be taken as a guarantee, and if the results are not achieved, the patient may file a lawsuit on the grounds that a contract was broken and the promised results were not delivered.

 CHECKPOINT QUESTION

3. What two disease processes are present in a patient with COPD?

## COMMON CANCERS OF THE RESPIRATORY SYSTEM

### Laryngeal Cancer

Cancer of the larynx is seen most commonly in heavy smokers and alcoholics. The presenting symptoms are usually hoarseness that lasts longer than 3 weeks, a feeling of a lump in the throat, or pain and burning in the throat when drinking citrus juice or hot liquids. A patient with laryngeal cancer may be treated with radiation, surgery, or both. Surgery usually is a laryn-

gectomy, or removal of the larynx, and formation of a permanent **tracheostomy** stoma (Fig. 31-5). Patients who have had a laryngectomy are unable to speak normally but can be trained to use esophageal speech or a prosthetic speech device.

## Lung Cancer

Lung cancer is one of the most common causes of death in both men and women. Cigarette smoking is believed to be the most common cause; 80% of lung cancer patients are smokers. Prognosis is generally poor for patients with lung cancer, with only 8% of men and 12% of women surviving for 5 years. One of the reasons is that symptoms tend to present rather late in the disease, when it has already had a chance to metastasize, or spread to other organs. Also, many of the symptoms are nonspecific and are seen in most heavy smokers. These symptoms include chronic cough, wheezing, dyspnea, **hemoptysis**, and chest pain.

Diagnosis of lung cancer is made by chest radiography, sputum cytology, bronchoscopy, biopsy, or **thoracentesis**. Treatment is generally **palliative**, giving relief but not a cure, and usually includes surgery, radiation, and chemotherapy. These treatments may improve the patient's prognosis and prolong survival.

 CHECKPOINT QUESTION

4. What factor appears to contribute to both laryngeal cancer and lung cancer?

## COMMON DIAGNOSTIC AND THERAPEUTIC PROCEDURES

### Physical Examination of the Respiratory System

The traditional examination of the chest consists of four parts: inspection, palpation, percussion, and auscultation. Each is briefly described in the following sections. For the physician to perform this examination efficiently, the patient should be sitting up, and all clothing should be removed from the waist up. The patient should be given a gown and draped appropriately (see Chapter 20).

### Inspection

Inspection consists of a visual examination of the chest and the patient's respiratory pattern (Table 31-2). During inspection, the physician looks for abnormal shape of the thorax, use of accessory muscles to breathe, surgical scars, cyanosis, and any other visible signs of previous or current respiratory disease.

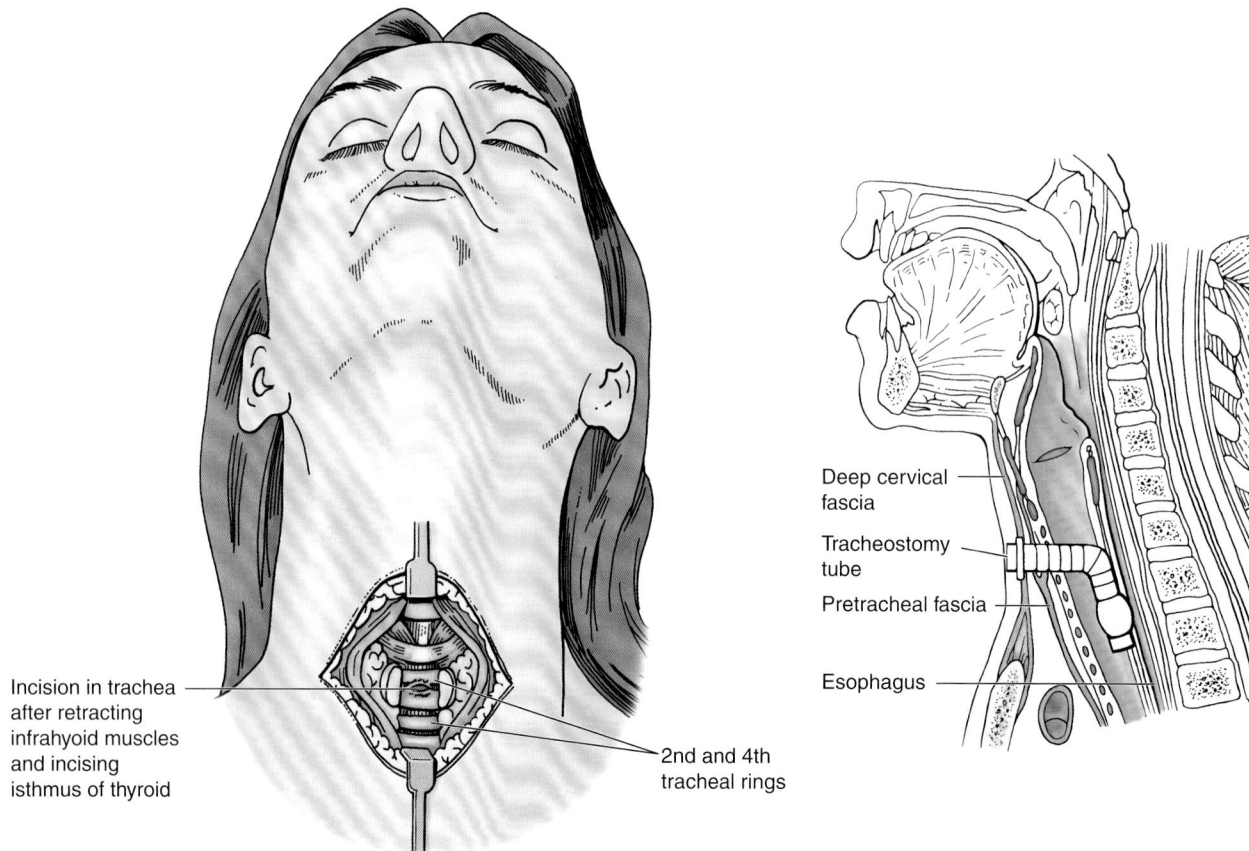

Incision in trachea after retracting infrahyoid muscles and incising isthmus of thyroid

2nd and 4th tracheal rings

Deep cervical fascia

Tracheostomy tube

Pretracheal fascia

Esophagus

**Figure 31-5** • The patient with a tracheostomy. (From Moore KL, Dalley AF II. *Clinical Oriented Anatomy*, 4th ed. Baltimore, MD: Lippincott Williams & Wilkins, 1999.)

## Palpation

In palpation, the physician uses his or her hands to feel the patient's throat for lumps, areas of tenderness, and location of the trachea, which may be displaced by a tumor. The patient may be asked to say "99" while the physician feels the chest wall in different places to assess the vibrations produced. Solid masses (such as tumors) or fluids (as in pneumonia) increase vibrations, whereas increased air (as seen in emphysema) reduces the vibrations.

## Percussion

Percussion is placing a finger (or fingers) on the chest and striking it with the fingers of the other hand. The physician listens for the sound to determine whether it is normal (resonant), like the sound produced by a drum. Dull or flat sounds are heard in patients with consolidation of pulmonary tissue, such as **atelectasis**, pneumonia, or a tumor. A hyperresonant sound is hollow and is heard in patients with emphysema. Children with cystic fibrosis (see Chapter 38) often require chest percussion to loosen the thick respiratory secretions throughout the day.

## Auscultation

Auscultation is listening to the patient's lungs and airway passages with a stethoscope. The physician systematically listens to each side of the chest in each area to compare the sounds bilaterally. The patient should breathe deeply, with an open mouth and the head turned away from the physician's face. The patient is encouraged not to breathe too rapidly to avoid hyperventilation, which

| TABLE 31-2 | **Abnormal Respiratory Patterns** |
|---|---|
| **Pattern** | **Description** |
| Apnea | No respirations |
| Bradypnea | Slow respirations |
| Cheyne-Stokes | Rhythmic cycles of dyspnea or hyperpnea subsiding gradually into brief apnea |
| Dyspnea | Difficult or labored respirations |
| Hypopnea | Shallow respirations |
| Hyperpnea | Deep respirations |
| Kussmaul | Fast and deep respirations |
| Orthopnea | Inability to breathe except while sitting or standing |
| Tachypnea | Fast respirations |

| TABLE 31-3 | Abnormal Breath Sounds |
|---|---|
| **Breath Sound** | **Description** |
| Bubbling | Gurgling sounds as air passes through moist secretions in airways |
| Crackles (rales) | Crackling sound, usually inspiratory, as air passes through moist secretions in airways. Fine to medium crackles indicate secretions in small airways and alveoli. Medium to coarse crackles indicate secretions in larger airways. |
| Friction rub | Dry, rubbing, or grating sound |
| Rhonchi | Low-pitched, continuous sound as air moves past thick mucus or narrowed air passages |
| Stertor | Snoring sound on inspiration or expiration; indicates a partial airway obstruction |
| Stridor | Shrill, harsh inspiratory sound; indicates laryngeal obstruction |
| Wheeze | High-pitched musical sound, either inspiratory or expiratory; indicates partial airway obstruction |

can cause dizziness. During auscultation, the physician listens for abnormal or adventitious sounds, such as crackles and wheezes, which may also indicate a disease process (Table 31-3).

 **CHECKPOINT QUESTION**

5. What are the four methods used to examine the respiratory system?

## Sputum Culture and Cytology

Sputum cultures are obtained to aid with diagnosis and treatment decisions in patients with suspected pneumonia, tuberculosis, or other infectious diseases of the lower airway. A microbiology laboratory will culture and incubate the specimen to identify any pathogenic microorganisms. Sputum specimens obtained for cytology are analyzed in the laboratory for abnormal cells that may indicate precancerous or cancerous conditions of the lung or airway. In all cases, it is important to obtain a specimen that the patient has coughed up and expectorated from the lower airways, with minimal contamination by oral and pharyngeal secretions. The patient is asked to cough deeply and collect the specimen in a sterile container (Procedure 31-3). After instructing the patient on coughing and collecting the specimen, you process the specimen and prepare the laboratory request for transportation to the laboratory for analysis.

Sputum collection for suspected cancer or for tuberculosis may be required over three consecutive mornings. The specimens should be brought into the office as soon as possible to avoid deterioration of the specimen. Most diagnostic specimens are obtained early in the morning, when the greatest volume of secretion has accumulated. If this is not possible, a specimen may also be collected after a nebulized breathing treatment with a bronchodilator. The patient may be weak from illness, thick mucus may be difficult to bring up, and coughing may exhaust the patient. A cool mist humidifier may be ordered for use at home to help loosen thick secretions. It is vitally important that the patient understand that the specimen must be collected from the lung fields and not from the mouth. The difference between saliva and sputum should be explained to the patient at his or her level of understanding.

## Chest Radiography

Chest radiography can help in the diagnosis of a large variety of pulmonary problems, including pneumonia, lung cancer, emphysema, tuberculosis, and pulmonary edema. Often, the physician orders two views: a posteroanterior (PA) view and a lateral view. This gives the physician a three-dimensional view. If the procedure is performed at the hospital or other outpatient facility, you may have to schedule it and request the results after the radiographs are interpreted by the radiologist.

 **CHECKPOINT QUESTION**

6. Dr. Richards has ordered a sputum specimen, and Ellen must instruct the patient on obtaining this specimen. What is being analyzed in a sputum specimen?

## Bronchoscopy

Bronchoscopy is an endoscopic procedure in which a lighted scope is inserted into the trachea and bronchi for direct visualization. This procedure is considered invasive and requires the patient's written consent. It is usually performed in an outpatient surgical setting, and you may have to schedule it. Bronchoscopy can be used for many diagnostic purposes, such as obtaining sputum specimens, obtaining tissue for biopsy, and visually assessing airway changes caused by chronic pulmonary diseases such as COPD or asthma. It can also be used therapeutically, for example, to clear out mucus plugs or to remove a foreign body.

##  Pulmonary Function Tests

Pulmonary function tests are performed with a spirometer that measures the amount of air a patient can

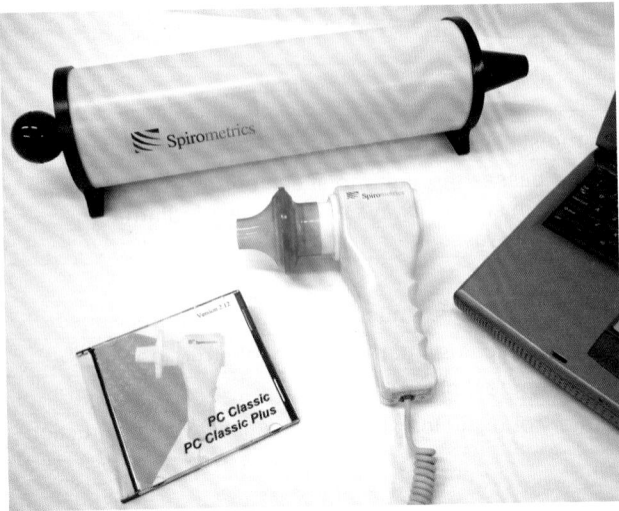

**Figure 31-6** • A pulmonary function testing machine. (Courtesy of Spirometrics.)

move in and out of the lungs (Fig. 31-6). The patient breathes into a mouthpiece and performs several breathing maneuvers that you explain during the test. By measuring the patient's airflow and comparing the results with predicted values for the patient's height, weight, gender, age, and race, the physician gains valuable information concerning whether the patient has mild, moderate, or severe obstructive or restrictive disease. The patient's **tidal volume** and **forced expiratory volume** are two measurements that can be obtained during the pulmonary function test. Procedure 31-4 describes the steps for performing the pulmonary function test.

treatment. Place patient B in an examination room and tell her that you will start the test within 10 minutes or advise her that she can reschedule the test for later this week. Inform patient C that you will schedule her procedure and notify her by phone of the exact date and time. Patients often become anxious about impending tests and can easily become upset with delays. Offer reassurance to the patient as needed.

## Arterial Blood Gases

Arterial blood gas (ABG) determinations measure the pH and pressures of oxygen and carbon dioxide in arterial blood. The results can indicate whether the patient's lungs are adequately exchanging gases. ABGs can also give information about metabolic acid–base problems, such as diabetic ketoacidosis. Drawing blood from an artery takes special training and is not routinely done in the medical office. However, you may be required to schedule a patient for an arterial puncture at a laboratory or hospital and record the results, which are usually phoned to the office.

## Pulse Oximetry

Many medical offices have a pulse oximeter, which quickly and painlessly determines the percentage of oxygen saturation on a patient's capillary blood cells (Fig. 31-7). The pulse oximeter is small, fitting into the palm of the hand, and includes a digital display that notes

### AFF    TRIAGE

While working in a medical office, the following three situations occur this afternoon:

A. Patient A is an elderly male with emphysema who is wheezing. The doctor has ordered a nebulized treatment with a bronchodilator.
B. Patient B is a 34-year-old woman who is scheduled to have a pulmonary function test today as part of a preemployment physical. She is anxious about getting the test "over with" so that she can pick up her children from school.
C. Patient C has been seen and discharged by the doctor but is waiting for you to schedule a bronchoscopy that the physician has ordered to be done later this week.

**How do you sort these patients? Who do you see first? Second? Third?**

Patient A should be seen first. Anyone who has trouble breathing or a respiratory problem must be treated as a priority. It is important to monitor this patient closely for any changes in condition before, during, and after

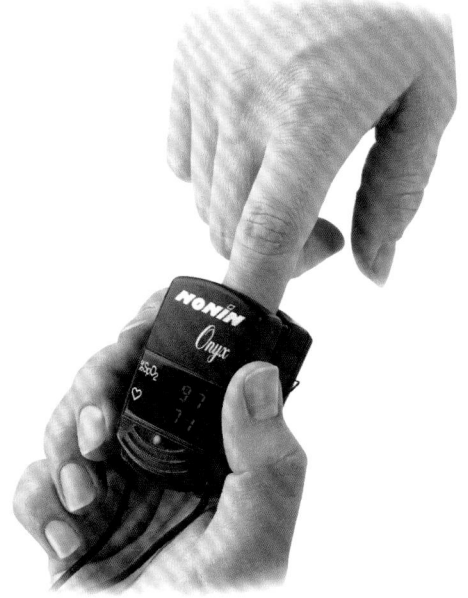

**Figure 31-7** • Pulse oximetry is used to measure oxygen saturation of arterial blood. (Reprinted from Cohen BJ. *Medical Terminology: An Illustrated Guide.* Philadelphia, PA: Lippincott Williams & Wilkins, 2003, with permission.)

the patient's pulse rate and oxygen saturation when a sensor cable is attached to the nail bed of the patient's index finger. Pulse oximeter readings should be obtained as a baseline for patients with chronic respiratory conditions and for patients with respiratory signs and symptoms, such as complaints of dyspnea or wheezing. The results should be recorded as a percentage; readings above 95% are considered normal. Although patients with chronic conditions such as emphysema may have readings of 90% or higher, readings below 90% should be reported to the physician immediately.

 **CHECKPOINT QUESTION**

7. What are the ways the physician can obtain information to help diagnose respiratory disorders?

---

**MEDICATION BOX**

## Commonly Prescribed Respiratory System Medications

**Note:** *The generic name of the drug is listed first and is written in all lower case letters. Brand names are in parentheses and the first letter is capitalized.*

| | | |
|---|---|---|
| albuterol sulfate (Proventil, Ventolin) | Inhalation aerosol: 90 mcg/metered spray<br>Solution for inhalation: 0.083%, 0.5%, 0.42%<br>Tablets: 2 mg, 4 mg | Bronchodilator |
| benzonatate (Tessalon) | Capsules: 100 mg, 200 mg | Local anesthetic |
| budesonide (Pulmicort Respules) | Powder: 90 mcg/dose<br>Inhalation suspension: 0.25 mg, 0.5 mg, 1 mg | Corticosteroid |
| cefdinir (Omnicef) | Capsules: 300 mg<br>Suspension: 125 mg/5 mL, 250 mg/5 mL | Antibiotic |
| cephalexin (Keflex) | Capsules: 250 mg, 333 mg, 500 mg, 750 mg<br>Oral suspension: 125 mg/5 mL | Antibiotic |
| cetirizine hydrochloride (Zyrtec) | Tablets: 5 mg, 10 mg<br>Oral solution: 5 mg/5 mL | Antihistamine |
| dextromethorphan hydrobromide (Delsym, Robitussin, Triaminic) | Gel caps: 15 mg, 30 mg<br>Solution: 3.5 mg/5 mL, 5 mg/5 mL | Cough suppressant |
| fexofenadine hydrochloride (Allegra) | Tablets: 30 mg, 60 mg, 180 mg<br>Oral suspension: 30 mg/5 mL | Antihistamine |
| fluticasone propionate (Flonase) | Nasal spray: 50 mcg/metered spray | Corticosteroid |
| guaifenesin (Mucinex, Robitussin) | Syrup: 100 mg/5 mL<br>Capsules: 200 mg<br>Tablets: 100 mg, 200 mg, 400 mg | Mucolytic (expectorant) |
| influenza virus vaccine, live intranasal (FluMist) | Intranasal spray: 0.2 mL | Vaccine |
| ipratropium bromide (Atrovent) | Inhaler: 17 mcg/metered dose | Bronchodilator |
| ipratropium bromide and albuterol (Combivent) | Inhaler: 18 mcg ipratropium and 90 mcg albuterol/metered dose | Bronchodilator |
| isoniazid (INH) | Injection: 100 mg/mL (IM)<br>Tablets: 100 mg, 300 mg<br>Oral solution: 50 mg/5 mL | Antibiotic |
| levalbuterol (Xopenex) | Inhalation aerosol: 3 mL vials: 45 mcg<br>Solution for inhalation: 0.31 mg, 0.63%, 1.25 mg; 5 mL vials: 1.25 mg | |
| levofloxacin (Levaquin) | Tablets: 250 mg, 500 mg, 750 mg<br>Oral solution: 25 mg/mL | Antibiotic |

*(continues on page 808)*

## MEDICATION BOX (continued)

| loratadine (Claritin, Alavert) | Capsules: 10 mg<br>Syrup: 1 mg/mL<br>Tablets: 10 mg | Antihistamine |
|---|---|---|
| oseltamivir phosphate (Tamiflu) | Capsules: 30 mg, 45 mg, 75 mg<br>Oral suspension: 12 mg/mL | Antiviral |
| pirbuterol acetate (Maxair) | Inhaler: 0.2 mg/metered dose | Bronchodilator |
| rifampin (Rifadin, Rimactane) | Capsules: 150 mg, 300 mg | Antibiotic |
| theophylline (Theochron, Theo-24) | Tablets (Theochron): 100 mg to 600 mg<br>Capsules (Theo-24): 100 mg to 400 mg | Bronchodilator |
| zanamivir (Relenza) | Powder for inhalation: 5 mg/blister | Antiviral |

 **ROLE-PLAYING ACTIVITY**

With cooperation from classmates or as assigned by your instructor, role-play the scenarios as if you are working with Ellen Michael in the pulmonary medicine office (refer to the case study at the beginning of the chapter). A 45-year-old patient is seen in the office today for symptoms of bronchitis and possible emphysema. He has been a smoker for 20 years, and you were instructed by the physician to discuss smoking cessation with him. The patient is tired of being "out of breath" but is not sure he can quit because everyone in his family including his wife smokes. He has not been successful in the past when he has tried to quit. He also tells you that his grandfather starting smoking as a child and lived to be 92 years old. What would you say to this comment? Is there any information you can give to this patient to encourage better choices instead of smoking? How should he deal with secondhand smoke? Do you have any concerns or judgments about this patient? How would you respond? Your instructor will give you additional information about this activity!

### español SPANISH TERMINOLOGY

**¿Tose con flema?**
Do you cough up any phlegm?

**¿De qué color es la flema?**
What color is it?

**Transparente**
Clear

**Blanca**
White

**Amarilla**
Yellow

**Verde**
Green

**Oscura**
Dark

**Necesito que tome una respiración profunda y sople lo más fuerte que pueda.**
I need you to take a deep breath and blow out as hard as you can.

**Sostenga su respiración.**
Hold your breath.

**¿Es su tos seca?**
Is your cough dry?

**¿Siente que le falta el aire? ¿Que no puede respirar?**
Do you feel a shortness of breath?

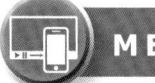 **MEDIA MENU**

**Student Resources** on thePoint®
- *Animation:* **Asthma**
- *Animation:* **Breathing Sounds**
- *Animation:* **Oxygen Transport**
- *Video:* **Administering a Nebulized Breathing Treatment (Procedure 31-2)**
- *Video:* **Perform a Pulmonary Function Test (Procedure 31-4)**
- **CMA/RMA Certification Exam Review**

**Internet Resources**
**Centers for Disease Control and Prevention**
http://www.cdc.gov
**American Lung Association**
http://www.lungusa.org
**American Association of Respiratory Care**
http://www.acr.org
**American Thoracic Society**
http://www.thoracic.org
**American Cancer Society**
http://www.cancer.org

## EMR Activity

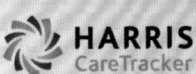

Harris CareTracker is a Web-based electronic medical record (EMR) application that you will use for the EMR activities included in this section at the end of each chapter. This application is actually used in physician offices, but is provided to you through the publisher, Wolters Kluwer Health, to give you hands-on practice working with EMRs. Your instructor will have more information about accessing your username, log-in, and Quickstart guide.

Prerequisite Activities in Harris CareTracker

- *The Getting Started and Quickstart documents and EMR Activities Step-by-Step Instructions listed below are available at* http://thePoint.lww.com/KronenbergerComp5e

Activity Details

Document the following treatments ordered by Dr. Hageman and performed by you today in the pulmonary medicine office

1. Patient: Lonnie Taylor; pulmonary function tests performed
2. Patient: Lawrence Black; patient taught how to use peak flowmeter, albuterol inhaler 2 puffs administered in office

## Chapter Summary

You can play an important role in helping the patient to maintain healthy lungs and in assisting the physician to diagnose and treat respiratory disease. It is important that you remember that:

- Because the air that we breathe is open to the atmosphere, the respiratory system is susceptible to infection and irritant injury.
- Disorders of the respiratory system can affect either the upper respiratory system or the lower respiratory system.
- Chronic disorders of the respiratory system include emphysema and asthma, while acute disorders include sinusitis and the common cold.
- The peak flowmeter is used by patients at home to assess breathing, while a pulmonary function test is done in the office and gives the physician more information about the health of the lungs.
- Diagnosis of infectious respiratory infections can be done through the sputum culture.

## Warm-Ups for Critical Thinking

1. Why do you think it is better to inhale through the nose than through the mouth?
2. Mr. Gardner, age 55 years, has been diagnosed with COPD and has many questions about his condition. Identify the characteristics of COPD. How do you explain this disease to Mr. Gardner?
3. Your patient has recently had an upper respiratory infection and was seen today for bronchitis. Why would the physician tell the patient to take the cough suppressant only at night? Use a drug reference book and look up some possible cough suppressants that might be ordered by the physician. Are there any precautions that the patient should be made aware of before taking these medications?
4. The mother of an 8-year-old child with asthma tells you that the child has tested positive for an allergy to cats. Unfortunately, their family owns two cats. The mother tells you that she is reluctant to give the cats away since her son will "probably outgrow his asthma" according to a family friend whose daughter also has asthma. How would you respond? Could the allergy to cats trigger an asthma attack?
5. Develop a patient brochure on the effects of smoking. Investigate the products available for smoking cessation and include these in your brochure.

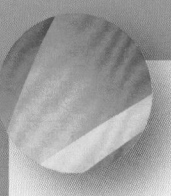

## PSY PROCEDURE 31-1

# Instructing a Patient on Using the Peak Flowmeter

**PSY** Instruct and prepare a patient for a procedure or treatment; coach patients regarding disease prevention and treatment plans; coach patients appropriately considering cultural diversity, developmental life stage, and communication barriers; and document patient care accurately in the medical record.

**Purpose:** Instruct the patient on the correct procedure for using and recording measurements using the peak flowmeter

**Equipment:** Peak flowmeter, recording documentation form

| STEPS | REASONS |
|---|---|
| 1. Wash your hands. | Hand washing aids infection control. |
| 2. Assemble the peak flowmeter, disposable mouthpiece, and patient documentation form. | The flowmeter is used to instruct patients in performing a peak flow reading. A disposable mouthpiece should be used. In some offices, the patient is instructed in using a peak flowmeter that is given to him or her to take home and use. In this case, no disposable mouthpiece is necessary. |
| 3. Greet and identify the patient. Identify yourself including your title and explain the procedure. | Identifying the patient prevents errors. |
| 4. **AFF** Explain how to respond to a patient who is developmentally challenged. | Always explain procedures to the caregiver who accompanies the patient. |
| 5. Holding the peak flowmeter upright, explain how to read and reset the gauge after each reading. | In the upright position, the meter is calibrated with numbers and contains a sliding gauge that should move freely up and down the meter next to the numbers. |

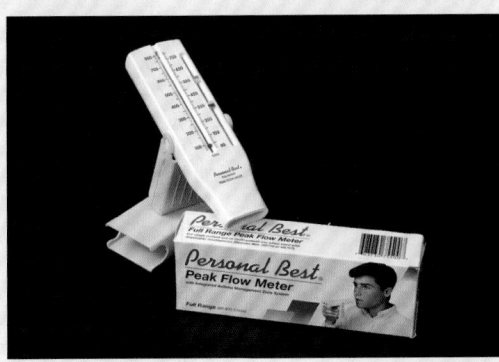

**Step 5.** The peak flowmeter and sliding gauge.

| STEPS | REASONS |
|---|---|
| 6. Instruct the patient to put the peak flowmeter mouthpiece in the mouth, forming a tight seal with the lips. After taking a deep breath, the patient should blow hard into the mouthpiece without blocking the back of the flowmeter. | The patient should close the lips around the mouthpiece without biting down. Blocking the back of the flowmeter will interfere with the movement of the gauge. |
| 7. Note the number on the flowmeter corresponding to the level at which the sliding gauge stopped after the patient blew hard into the mouthpiece. Reset the gauge to zero. | A normal range provided with the flowmeter is based on the patient's age, height, and weight. Ideally, the patient's readings should be within this range. |

*(continues on page 812)*

## PROCEDURE 31-1 (continued)

| STEPS | REASONS |
|---|---|

**8.** Instruct the patient to perform this procedure three times consecutively, in the morning and at night, and to record the highest reading on form.

The highest reading is the patient's best reading. Recording the readings on the form allows the patient to follow his or her progress based on the medication therapy or exposure to allergens.

**Peakflow Meter Daily Record**

Name: Jane Doe

| Date: | 3/05 | 3/06 | 3/07 | | | | | | |
|---|---|---|---|---|---|---|---|---|---|
| Time: | 8am | 8:30 | 8:15 | | | | | | |
| 750 | | | | | | | | | |
| 650 | | | | | | | | | |
| 550 | | ● | | | | | | | |
| 450 | ● | | | | | | | | |
| 350 | | ● | | | | | | | |
| 250 | | | | | | | | | |
| 150 | | | | | | | | | |

**Step 8.** A peak flowmeter documentation form.

**9.** Explain to the patient the procedure for cleaning the mouthpiece by washing with soapy water and rinsing without immersing the flowmeter in water.

Cleaning the mouthpiece is sanitary and prevents the spread of microorganisms.

**10.** **AFF** Log into the electronic medical record (EMR) using your username and secure password OR obtain the paper medical record from a secure location and assure it is kept away from public access. Record the procedure including the name of the medication and the patient's response. Your entry must include the date, time, and your name/credentials.

The integrity of the medical record must be maintained at all times to protect patient privacy. Procedures are considered not to have been done if they are not recorded.

**11.** When finished, log out of the EMR and/or replace the paper medical record in an appropriate and secure location.

Charting Example:

*12/11/2016 3:30 PM Pt. instructed on using a flowmeter—return demonstration without difficulty, verbalized understanding. Given patient documentation form, instructed to record readings in morning and evening. Today's reading 400 LPM. No dyspnea, c/o wheezing or SOB _____ E. Michael, CMA*

Note: *The medical assistant may sign his or her name in the patient record using only the "CMA" credential if the office has a signature log denoting the entire credential as "CMA (AAMA)."*

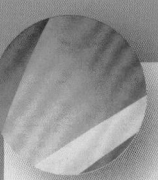

## PSY PROCEDURE 31-2

# Performing a Nebulized Breathing Treatment

**PSY** Instruct and prepare a patient for a procedure or treatment; coach patients regarding disease prevention and treatment plans; coach patients appropriately considering cultural diversity, developmental life stage, and communication barriers; and document patient care accurately in the medical record.

**Purpose:** Set up and administer a nebulized breathing treatment in the medical office

**Equipment:** Physician order, patient's medical record, inhalation medication, nebulizer disposable setup, nebulizer

| STEPS | REASONS |
|---|---|
| 1. Wash your hands. | Hand washing aids infection control. |
| 2. Assemble the equipment and medication; check the medication label three times, as when administering any medications. | Checking the medication label three times prevents errors. |
| 3. Greet and identify the patient. Identify yourself including your title and explain the procedure. | Properly identifying the patient will avoid errors. Explaining the procedure promotes understanding and compliance. |
| 4. **AFF** Explain how to respond to a patient who does not speak English or who speaks English as a second language (ESL). | Solicit assistance from anyone who may be with the patient or a staff member if available who speaks the patient's language. If no interpreter is available, use hand gestures or pictures to explain the procedure to the patient. |
| 5. Remove the nebulizer treatment cup from the setup and add the exact amount of medication ordered by the physician. | The physician bases the amount of bronchodilator on the age and weight of the patient. |

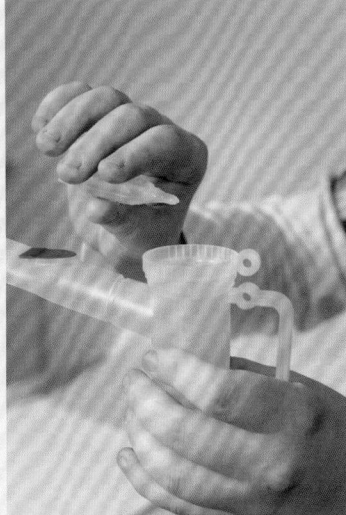

**Step 5.** The nebulizer medication cup.

*(continues on page 814)*

## PROCEDURE 31-2 (continued)

| STEPS | REASONS |
|---|---|
| 6. Place the top on the cup securely, attach the T piece to the top of the cup, and position the mouthpiece firmly on one end of the T piece. | The top of the mouthpiece usually screws onto the bottom of the cup, providing a reservoir for the medication and saline. |

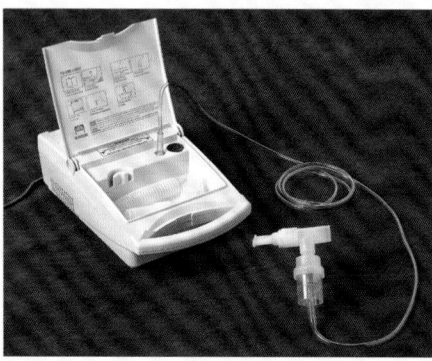

**Step 6.** A nebulizer machine and disposable setup with mouthpiece.

| STEPS | REASONS |
|---|---|
| 7. Attach one end of the tubing securely to the connector on the cup and the other end to the connector on the nebulizer machine. | |
| 8. Ask the patient to put the mouthpiece in the mouth and make a seal with the lips without biting the mouthpiece. Instruct the patient to breathe normally during the treatment, occasionally taking a deep breath. | The patient may have difficulty breathing or be wheezing but should be encouraged to breathe as normally as possible. Breathing too rapidly may cause hyperventilation. Occasionally taking a deep breath will allow medication to be administered to deeper lung tissues. |

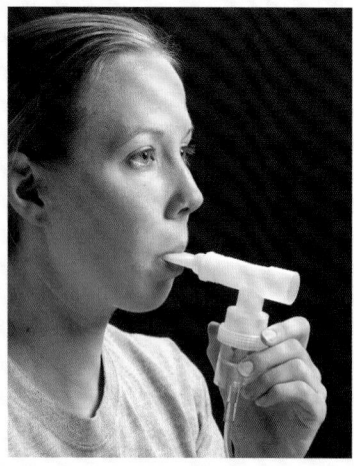

**Step 8.** The T piece and medication cup.

| STEPS | REASONS |
|---|---|
| 9. Turn the machine on. The medication in the reservoir cup will become a fine mist to be inhaled by the patient. | A fine mist will come from the opposite end of the T piece when the patient exhales. |
| 10. Before, during, and after the breathing treatment, take and record the patient's pulse. | Most bronchodilators cause a slight increase in the heart rate. Notify the physician if the increase is significant or if the patient has symptoms such as dizziness. |
| 11. When the treatment is over and the medication cup is empty, turn the machine off and have the patient remove the mouthpiece. | The treatment typically takes about 15 minutes. |

## PROCEDURE 31-2 (continued)

| STEPS | REASONS |
|---|---|
| 12. Disconnect the disposable treatment setup and dispose of all parts in a biohazard container. Properly put away the machine. | The setup equipment, including the mouthpiece, may be contaminated with hazardous microorganisms and should be handled and disposed of properly. |
| 13. Wash your hands | |
| 14. **AFF** Log into the electronic medical record (EMR) using your username and secure password OR obtain the paper medical record from a secure location and assure it is kept away from public access. Record the procedure including the name of the medication and the patient's pulse before, during, and after the treatment. Your entry must include the date, time, and your name/credentials. | Procedures are considered not to have been done if they are not recorded. The bronchodilator used for nebulized treatments may cause the heart rate to increase, and the pulse should be noted and recorded during and after the treatment. The integrity of the medical record must be maintained at all times to protect patient privacy. |
| 15. When finished, log out of the EMR and/or replace the paper medical record in an appropriate and secure location. | |

---

**Charting Example:**

*11/26/2016 9:15 AM Pt. given nebulized breathing treatment with albuterol 2 mg for inhalation—pulse before treatment 88, during treatment 100, and after treatment 110. Pt. states she is "breathing easier" after treatment, skin warm and dry, color pink ———————————————————————————————— J. Barker, CMA*

---

Note: *The medical assistant may sign his or her name in the patient record using only the "CMA" credential if the office has a signature log denoting the entire credential as "CMA (AAMA)."*

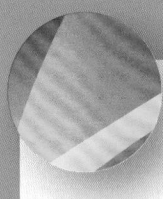

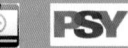 PROCEDURE 31-3

## Collect a Sputum Specimen

**PSY** Instruct and prepare a patient for a procedure or treatment; coach patients regarding disease prevention and treatment plans; coach patients appropriately considering cultural diversity, developmental life stage, and communication barriers; and document patient care accurately in the medical record.

**Purpose:** Instruct a patient on collecting a sputum specimen for culture and sensitivity or cytology and record the procedure

**Equipment:** Physician order, patient's medical record, sterile specimen container, gloves, biohazard transport bag, laboratory request

| STEPS | REASONS |
|---|---|
| 1. Wash your hands. | Hand washing aids infection control. |
| 2. Assemble the equipment. | Having all the necessary equipment and supplies saves time when the patient is ready to undergo the procedures. |
| 3. Greet and identify the patient. Identify yourself including your title and explain the procedure. | Identifying the patient prevents errors, and explaining the procedure promotes compliance. |
| 4. **AFF** Explain how to respond to a patient whose first language is not English. | If a translator is available, speak to the patient while the translator interprets for the patient. The translator may be a family member or friend. If a translator is not available, look at the patient, and use gestures and/or pictures to explain. |
| 5. Provide the patient with a cup of water and instruct him/her to rinse the mouth with water. | Rinsing the mouth reduces contamination of the specimen with microorganisms normally found in the mouth. |
| 6. Ask the patient to cough deeply, using the abdominal muscles as well as the accessory muscles to bring secretions from the lungs and not just the upper airway. | The desired specimen should contain microorganisms and epithelial cells from the lining of the lower respiratory tract. |
| 7. Instruct the patient to expectorate the specimen directly into the container without touching the inside of the container with the lips or tongue and without getting the specimen on the outside of the container. | Approximately 5–10 mL is sufficient for most sputum studies. Touching the inside of the container will contaminate the container and specimen. Sputum on the outside of the container will contaminate the container during handling. |
| 8. When the specimen is in the container, apply gloves, and after taking the container from the patient, cap the container immediately and place into a biohazard bag for transport to the laboratory with a laboratory requisition (see Chapter 40). | The specimen is a biohazardous body fluid and should be handled wearing appropriate PPE. Capping the container immediately eliminates the danger of spreading microorganisms or contaminating the specimen with outside microorganisms. |
| 9. Once the specimen has been routed to the laboratory, remove your gloves and wash your hands. | Hand washing prevents the spread of microorganisms. |

## PROCEDURE 31-3 (continued)

| STEPS | REASONS |
|---|---|
| 10. **AFF** Log into the electronic medical record (EMR) using your username and secure password OR obtain the paper medical record from a secure location and assure it is kept away from public access. Record the procedure including the patient's response. Your entry must include the date, time, and your name/credentials. | The integrity of the medical record must be maintained at all times to protect patient privacy. Procedures are considered not to have been done if they are not recorded. |
| 11. Place the printed results in the medical record or scan into the electronic medical record if appropriate. | |
| 12. When finished, log out of the EMR and/or replace the paper medical record in an appropriate and secure location. | |

**Charting Example:**

*06/12/2016 3:00 PM Moderate amount thick yellow sputum collected and sent to GFMC laboratory for cytology*
*———————————————————————————————————————— J. Barker, CMA*

Note: *The medical assistant may sign his or her name in the patient record using only the "CMA" credential if the office has a signature log denoting the entire credential as "CMA (AAMA)."*

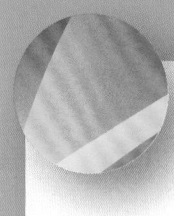

## ▶ **PSY** PROCEDURE 31-4

### Perform a Pulmonary Function Test

**PSY** Instruct and prepare a patient for a procedure or treatment; coach patients regarding disease prevention and treatment plans; coach patients appropriately considering cultural diversity, developmental life stage, and communication barriers; and document patient care accurately in the medical record.

**Purpose:** Perform a pulmonary function test and record the procedure

**Equipment:** Physician order, patient's medical record, spirometer and appropriate cables, calibration syringe and log book, disposable mouthpiece, printer, nose clip

| STEPS | REASONS |
|---|---|
| 1. Wash your hands. | Hand washing aids infection control. |
| 2. Assemble the equipment. | Having all the necessary equipment and supplies saves time when the patient is ready to undergo the procedures. |
| 3. Greet and identify the patient. Identify yourself including your title and explain the procedure. | Identifying the patient prevents errors, and explaining the procedure promotes compliance. |
| 4. **AFF** Explain how to respond to a patient who is visually impaired. | Observe patients carefully to prevent injury and ask before offering assistance or taking hold of their arms to guide. Face the patient when speaking and always let him or her know what you are going to do before touching him or her. |
| 5. Turn the spirometer on, and, if it has not been calibrated according to office policy, calibrate it using the calibration syringe according to the manufacturer's instructions. Record the calibration in the appropriate log book. | The spirometer must be calibrated daily to ensure accurate results. |

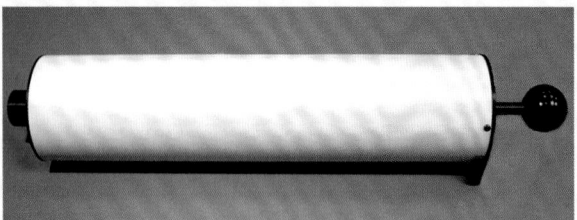

**Step 5.** The calibration syringe used for checking the spirometer.

| STEPS | REASONS |
|---|---|
| 6. With the machine on and calibrated, attach the appropriate cable, tubing, and mouthpiece according to the type of machine being used. | One cable is plugged into an electrical outlet, and another cable or tube is connected to the spirometer and the patient's mouthpiece. |
| 7. Using the keyboard on the machine, enter the patient's name or identification number, age, weight, height, sex, race, and smoking history. | The spirometer automatically takes these parameters into consideration when providing the results. |
| 8. Ask the patient to remove any restrictive clothing, such as a necktie, and show the patient how to apply the nose clip. | Restrictive clothing can stop the chest from fully expanding, causing an inaccurate result. The nose clip stops air from being expelled from the nose during the test. |

## PROCEDURE 31-4 (continued)

| STEPS | REASONS |
|---|---|
| 9. Ask the patient to stand, breathe in deeply, and blow into the mouthpiece as hard as possible. The patient should continue to blow into the mouthpiece until the machine indicates that it is appropriate to stop blowing. A chair should be available in case the patient becomes dizzy or light-headed. | Some machines signal to stop blowing with a buzz or beep; however, you may have to instruct the patient if the machine gives only a visual signal. Some patients become light-headed during this procedure and should be observed closely for signs of difficulty or imbalance. |

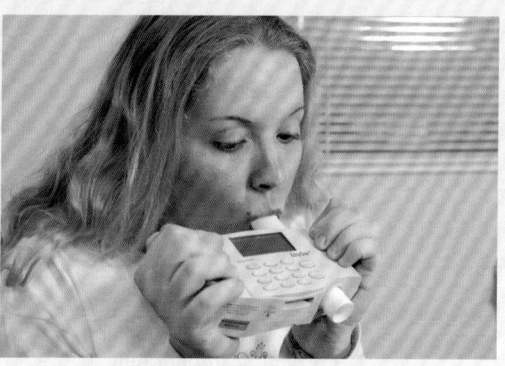

**Step 9.** The patient should blow into the mouthpiece as instructed.

| STEPS | REASONS |
|---|---|
| 10. During the procedure, coach the patient as necessary to obtain an adequate reading. | Many patients feel that they have exhaled all air from the lungs when the machine is instructing them to continue. All air must be exhaled to obtain accurate results. The machine will indicate whether the reading or maneuver is adequate. |
| 11. Continue the procedure until three adequate readings, or maneuvers, are performed. | Three maneuvers are usually required to obtain the patient's best result. The patient may rest between readings if necessary. |
| 12. After printing the results, properly care for the equipment and dispose of the mouthpiece into the biohazard container. Wash your hands. | The mouthpiece may be contaminated and must be handled and discarded properly. |
| 13. **AFF** Log into the electronic medical record (EMR) using your username and secure password OR obtain the paper medical record from a secure location and assure it is kept away from public access. Record the procedure including the patient's response. Your entry must include the date, time, and your name/credentials. | The integrity of the medical record must be maintained at all times to protect patient privacy. Procedures are considered not to have been done if they are not recorded. |
| 14. Place the printed results in the medical record or scan into the electronic medical record if appropriate. | The three maneuvers will be recorded on one printout. |
| 15. When finished, log out of the EMR and/or replace the paper medical record in an appropriate and secure location. | |

Charting Example:
*06/12/2016 3:00 PM PFT performed for employment physical as ordered by Dr. John. ×3 maneuvers obtained without difficulty. Dr. John notified of results in chart _____ J. Barker, CMA*

Note: *The medical assistant may sign his or her name in the patient record using only the "CMA" credential if the office has a signature log denoting the entire credential as "CMA (AAMA)."*

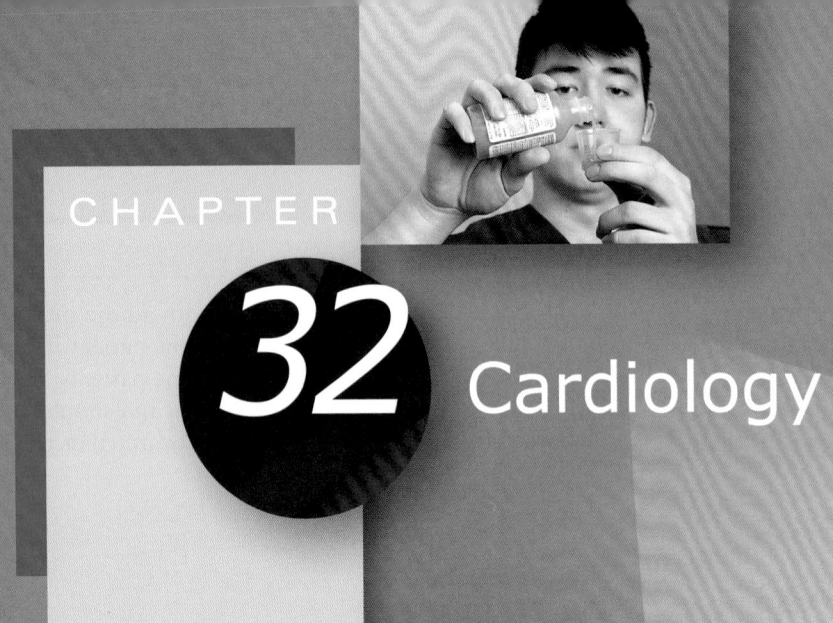

# CHAPTER 32 Cardiology

## Learning Outcomes

**COG Cognitive Domain***

1. Spell key terms
2. *Define medical terms and abbreviations related to all body systems*
3. *Describe structural organization of the human body*
4. *List major organs in each body system*
5. *Identify the anatomical location of major organs in each body system*
6. *Describe the normal function of each body system*
7. *Identify common pathology related to each body system including signs, symptoms, and etiology*
   a. List and describe common cardiovascular disorders
   b. Identify and explain common cardiovascular procedures and tests
8. Describe the roles and responsibilities of the medical assistant during cardiovascular examinations and procedures
9. Discuss the information recorded on a basic 12-lead electrocardiogram
10. Explain the purpose of a Holter monitor

**PSY Psychomotor Domain***

1. Perform electrocardiography (Procedure 32-1)
   a. Instruct and prepare a patient for a procedure or treatment
   b. Coach patients appropriately considering cultural diversity, developmental life stage, and communication barriers

c. Coach patients regarding disease prevention and treatment plans
d. Document patient care accurately in the medical record
2. Apply a Holter monitor for a 24-hour test (Procedure 32-2)
   a. Instruct and prepare a patient for a procedure or treatment
   b. Coach patients appropriately considering cultural diversity, developmental life stage, and communication barriers
   c. Coach patients regarding disease prevention and treatment plans
   d. Document patient care accurately in the medical record

**AFF Affective Domain***

1. *Incorporate critical thinking skills when performing patient assessment*
2. *Incorporate critical thinking skills when performing patient care*
3. *Show awareness of a patient's concerns related to the procedure being performed*
4. *Demonstrate empathy, active listening, and nonverbal communication*
5. *Demonstrate respect for individual diversity including gender, race, religion, age, economic status, and appearance*
6. *Explain to a patient the rationale for performance of a procedure*

**7.** *Demonstrate sensitivity to patient rights*
**8.** *Protect the integrity of the medical record*

***Note: AAMA/CAAHEP 2015 Standards are italicized.***

### ABHES Competencies

**1.** Assist the physician with the regimen of diagnostic and treatment modalities as they relate to each body system
**2.** Perform electrocardiograms

**3.** Comply with federal, state, and local health laws and regulations
**4.** Communicate on the recipient's level of comprehension
**5.** Serve as a liaison between the physician and others
**6.** Show empathy and impartiality when dealing with patients
**7.** Document accurately

## Key Terms

| | | | |
|---|---|---|---|
| aneurysm | cerebrovascular accident (CVA) | lead | pericarditis |
| angina pectoris | | myocardial infarction (MI) | tachycardia |
| artifacts | congestive heart failure | myocarditis | transient ischemic attack (TIA) |
| atherosclerosis | coronary artery bypass graft (CABG) | palpitations | |
| bradycardia | | percutaneous | |
| cardiomegaly | electrocardiography (ECG) | transluminal coronary angioplasty (PTCA) | |
| cardiomyopathy | endocarditis | | |

## Case Study

$A$bby Perez, CMA (AAMA), works in a busy cardiology office at Great Falls Medical Center. This office has many established patients who have chronic heart conditions that must be monitored regularly by a cardiologist. One of the patients seen in the office today is concerned about her "blood being too thin" because she started taking a "blood thinner" last month for atrial fibrillation. What is a blood thinner, and are the patient's concerns warranted? Why would a patient with a heart condition such as atrial fibrillation be prescribed a "blood thinner?" These and other questions related to the heart and blood vessels will be addressed in this chapter.

Cardiovascular disease is a major cause of illness and death. The cardiologist is a physician who specializes in disorders of the heart, and many patients with chronic cardiac conditions are referred to the cardiology office for treatment and follow-up. However, many of these patients are seen in internal medicine or family practice medical offices also. Because medical assistants see patients who have cardiovascular disorders regardless of the medical specialty, you must understand the cardiovascular system, associated disorders, and common tests and procedures that are ordered for diagnosis and treatment.

## COG COMMON DISORDERS OF THE CARDIOVASCULAR SYSTEM

The cardiovascular system consists of the heart (Fig. 32-1) and blood vessels, including the arteries, capillaries, and veins. The rhythmic contractions of the heart pump oxygen-rich blood from the lungs throughout the body to oxygenate and nourish the tissues and remove wastes for elimination. Although the heart and blood vessels

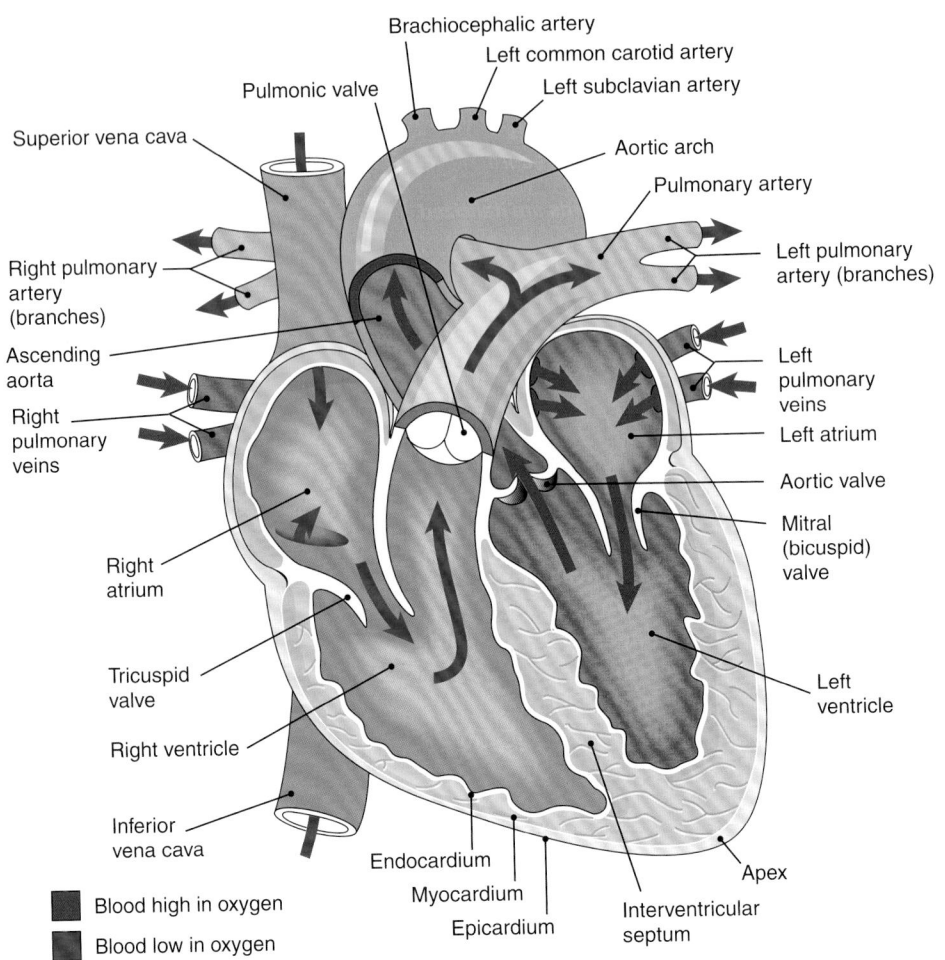

**Figure 32-1** • The heart and great vessels. (Reprinted from Cohen BJ. *Memmler's The Human Body in Health and Disease*, 11th ed. Philadelphia, PA: Lippincott Williams & Wilkins, 2009, with permission.)

are a closed system for the flow of blood (Fig. 32-2), disorders anywhere in this system may adversely affect other body systems that depend on the cardiovascular system for delivery of oxygen and nutrients. Depending on the body system affected by the lack of oxygen and nutrients being delivered, the following can be symptoms of various heart disorders:

- Chest pain
- Dyspnea
- Fatigue
- Diaphoresis
- Nausea and vomiting
- Irregular heartbeat
- Changes in peripheral circulation
- Edema
- Skin ulcers that do not heal
- Pain that increases with walking and decreases with rest
- Changes in skin color

Although some of these symptoms can indicate disorders not related to the heart or blood vessels, you should obtain an accurate history and chief complaint and communicate any finding to the physician through complete documentation.

## Disorders of the Heart

### Carditis

Cardiac inflammation, or carditis, may affect any of the layers of the heart muscle, and, although other factors may be involved, it is usually the result of a systemic infection. **Pericarditis,** an inflammation of the sac that covers the outside of the heart, may be acute or chronic. It is caused by a pathogen, neoplasm, or autoimmune disorder, such as systemic lupus erythematosus or rheumatoid arthritis. Other causes of pericarditis include certain chemicals, radiation, and uremia in patients with kidney failure. Signs and symptoms include a sharp pain in the same locations as with a **myocardial infarction (MI)**, except that pain increases on inspiration and on lying down but decreases on sitting up and leaning forward. Dyspnea, tachycardia, neck venous distention, pallor, and hypertension are warning signs that serous fluid is compressing the heart and interfering with cardiac function. Treatment is relieving the symptoms and, if possible, correcting the underlying cause, including administering an antibiotic for bacterial infection.

**Myocarditis** may be diffused through the heart muscle or may be local to a focal point. Causes include radiation, chemicals, and bacterial, viral, or parasitic infection. Signs and symptoms of early acute episodes are usually

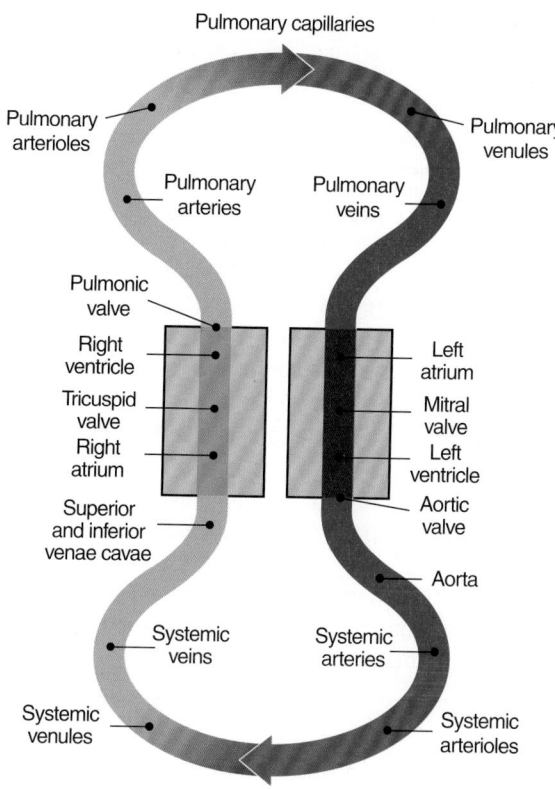

Pulmonary capillaries

Pulmonary arterioles

Pulmonary arteries

Pulmonary venules

Pulmonary veins

Pulmonic valve

Right ventricle

Tricuspid valve

Right atrium

Superior and inferior venae cavae

Left atrium

Mitral valve

Left ventricle

Aortic valve

Aorta

Systemic veins

Systemic arteries

Systemic venules

Systemic arterioles

Systemic capillaries

**Figure 32-2** • Blood vessels form a closed system for the flow of blood. Blood high in oxygen (oxygenated) is shown in red; blood low in oxygen (deoxygenated) is shown in blue. Changes in oxygen content occur as blood flows through capillaries. (Reprinted from Cohen BJ. *Memmler's The Human Body in Health and Disease*, 11th ed. Philadelphia, PA: Lippincott Williams & Wilkins, 2009, with permission.)

nonspecific, such as fatigue, fever, and mild chest pain. Chronic cases may lead to heart failure with **cardiomegaly** (an enlarged heart muscle), arrhythmias, and valvulitis. Treatment is supportive care and medication as ordered by the physician to kill the responsible pathogen.

Chronic or acute **endocarditis** is infection or inflammation of the inner lining of the heart, the endocardium. The lining of the heart and its valves may gather clusters of platelets, fibrin, and white blood cells to trap the pathogens. These clusters, called *vegetations*, may break away to become emboli that travel to the spleen, kidneys, lungs, or nervous system. These formations may also scar the valves and erode the chordae tendineae, small tendons that attach the heart valves to the ventricles. The destruction of these structures may result in reflux, or backflow, of the valves or blood. Diagnosis of endocarditis requires a blood culture to identify the causative agent. Treatment is directed at eliminating the infecting organism.

## CHECKPOINT QUESTION

1. How would Abby describe the difference in pain due to pericarditis from the pain of myocardial infarction?

## Congestive Heart Failure

**Congestive heart failure** (CHF) is a condition in which the heart cannot pump effectively. Failure of the right ventricle causes congestion of the peripheral extremities, while failure of the left ventricle leads to pulmonary congestion. Many patients have failure of both sides of the heart; their signs and symptoms include edema of the lower extremities and dyspnea. As blood flow to organs such as the brain and kidneys decreases, patients may also have complaints related to the organs involved. Progressive heart failure results in damage to vital organs and death.

The causes of CHF include coronary artery disease, myocardial disease, valvular heart disease, and hypertension. While there is no cure for it, treatment is aimed at relieving symptoms and preventing permanent damage to vital organs. Medications given to CHF patients include drugs to increase cardiac function and decrease edema.

## Myocardial Infarction

Death of any part of the heart muscle, called **myocardial infarction**, occurs when one or more of the coronary arteries becomes totally occluded, usually by atherosclerotic plaques or by an embolism. An MI may occur suddenly without prior symptoms or in patients with diagnosed atherosclerotic coronary artery disease. Symptoms of myocardial infarction may be similar to those felt during **angina pectoris** in patients with ischemic heart disease, but this disorder is distinguished by pain that lasts longer than 20 to 30 minutes and is unrelieved by rest. Box 32-1 describes criteria that the physician will use to distinguish the chest pain of angina pectoris from the chest pain of MI. Other symptoms include nausea, diaphoresis, weakness, vomiting, and abdominal cramps. The patient may complain of feeling a viselike grip around the chest cavity. The skin may become cool, clammy, and pale, and the patient may feel anxiety or impending doom. Some patients have nonspecific symptoms such as indigestion and therefore do not seek medical attention. In 20% of patients, the MI may be silent, diagnosed only by routine **electrocardiography** (ECG). It is imperative not to ignore or dismiss complaints by patients with symptoms of MI or to accept the patient's own diagnosis that "It's only indigestion." Although the death of myocardial tissue that occurs during an MI cannot be reversed, early medical intervention may reduce the amount of tissue that dies and increase the patient's chances of survival. Procedures such as **percutaneous transluminal coronary angioplasty** (PTCA) and **coronary artery bypass graft** (CABG) are performed to increase blood flow to the cardiac muscle (Box 32-2).

## CHECKPOINT QUESTION

2. Why is it important to treat a patient with myocardial infarction as early as possible?

**BOX 32-1  Is It Angina or Myocardial Infarction?**

The pain felt with angina and MI is brought about by myocardial anoxia, or an increased need for oxygen to the heart muscle because of exertion, stress, or extremes of heat or cold. Typically, angina is relieved by rest or nitroglycerin, a vasodilator. However, pain from an MI is not relieved by these measures. The following is a brief comparison of these two disorders:

|  | **Angina** | **Myocardial Infarction** |
| --- | --- | --- |
| Description | Moderate pressure deep in the chest; squeezing, suffocating feeling | Severe deep pressure not relieved by reducing stressors; crushing pressure |
| Onset | Pain gradual or sudden; subsides quickly, usually in less than 30 minutes; can be relieved by nitroglycerin, rest, or reducing stressors | Pain sudden; remains after stressors reduced or relieved; not relieved by nitroglycerin |
| Location | Midanterior chest, usually diffuse, radiates to back, neck, arms, jaw, and epigastric area | Midanterior chest with same radiating patterns |
| Signs and symptoms | Dyspnea, nausea, signs of indigestion, profuse sweating | Nausea, vomiting, fear, diaphoresis, pounding heart, palpitations |

Any patient who calls the medical office complaining of chest pain must be examined immediately. The office should have an established protocol for handling these calls. The physician must be consulted to decide whether the patient should be directed to the nearest emergency department or come directly to the office.

## Cardiac Arrhythmia

When the electrical conduction system of the heart is not functioning normally, cardiac arrhythmias may develop and can be detected on the electrocardiography. Cardiac arrhythmia or dysrhythmia is an abnormal heart rhythm that may occur as a primary disorder or as a response to a systemic problem. Arrhythmia may also be a reaction to a drug toxicity or an electrolyte imbalance. Normally, the sinoatrial (SA) node is the pacemaker of the heart (Fig. 32-3), initiating an electrical impulse in the adult at rest 60 to 100 times a minute. This is sinus rhythm. Arrhythmia may occur if the SA node initiates electrical impulses too fast or too slowly. If the SA node is damaged or the conduction pathway is blocked, the heart will beat too slowly to meet the body's demands. This type of arrhythmia, called **bradycardia**, is characterized by a heart rate less than 60 beats per minute. If the SA node initiates an electrical impulse faster than 100 times per minute, the arrhythmia is called **tachycardia**.

More serious arrhythmias occur when the ventricles beat too fast, a condition known as **ventricular tachycardia (VT)**. This condition occurs when some of the electrical signals originate in the ventricles rather than in the SA node. Once the ventricles begin to beat at a very rapid rate, less blood is pumped out of the heart with each contraction, since the heart's chambers do not have time to fill with blood before the next contraction begins. As less blood is pumped into circulation, less oxygen is carried to the tissues. This lack of adequate blood and oxygen may cause dizziness, unconsciousness, or cardiac arrest.

Another arrhythmia is ventricular fibrillation. Ventricular fibrillation is a medical emergency that occurs when the heart is quivering rather than contracting in an organized fashion. In this condition, very little blood is pumped out of the heart, and the patient will fall unconscious and die very quickly unless a shock with a cardiac defibrillator is administered immediately to restore normal cardiac electrical activity. Automatic external defibrillators (AED) are now available in many medical offices and public places, such as airports and shopping malls. All professional medical assistants should receive certification in cardiopulmonary resuscitation (CPR) and use of the AED, which is relatively easy to operate (Box 32-3). Patients who require frequent defibrillation may benefit from the insertion of an implantable cardiac defibrillator that will automatically deliver an electrical shock to restore normal cardiac conduction. These devices should not be confused with cardiac pacemakers, which help to regulate the normal rhythm of the heart.

## Artificial Pacemakers

When a patient's heart conduction system cannot maintain normal sinus rhythm without assistance, an electrical source can be implanted to assist or replace the sinoatrial node. The permanent or temporary artificial pacemaker is surgically implanted either between the chest wall and the rib cage or within the chest cavity (Fig. 32-4). The pacemaker may be programmed to fire, or initiate an electrical charge, continuously at a predetermined rate or on demand, only when the patient's normal heart rate falls below a preset number.

Pacemaker programming initially occurs when the pacemaker is inserted in an outpatient or inpatient surgical facility. If additional programming or assessment is necessary, the pacemaker may be evaluated by telephone monitoring: the patient uses the telephone

## BOX 32-2   Corrective Cardiac Surgery

The least traumatic form of cardiac surgery is the *PTCA*. A double-lumen catheter with a balloon surrounding the upper portion is inserted into a vessel in the groin or axilla. This catheter is threaded into the coronary vessels, with the surgeon watching a fluoroscopic screen while performing the procedure. When the occlusion is found, the balloon is inflated to press the atherosclerotic plaque against the arterial walls and relieve the occlusion. A laser may be used to remove the plaque. A spring or mesh (called a *stent*) may be inserted and left in place within the vessel to maintain patency. This procedure is less invasive than bypass surgery, but occasionally, the artery rebuilds plaque at the site, or the stent may fill with plaque and the artery may occlude again.

 *CABG* is performed by grafting a piece of vessel from another part of the body to the area beyond the occlusion and to the ascending aorta, providing a patent passage for the blood. The surgery requires a still field of surgery, so the heart must be stopped and the patient supported by a cardiopulmonary bypass machine for the length of the operation. The saphenous vein may be used for multiple bypasses; the internal mammary artery is used if the surgery is not extensive. Hospitalization may be as long as 5 to 7 days, and 20% of patients develop a repeat thrombus within 1 year.

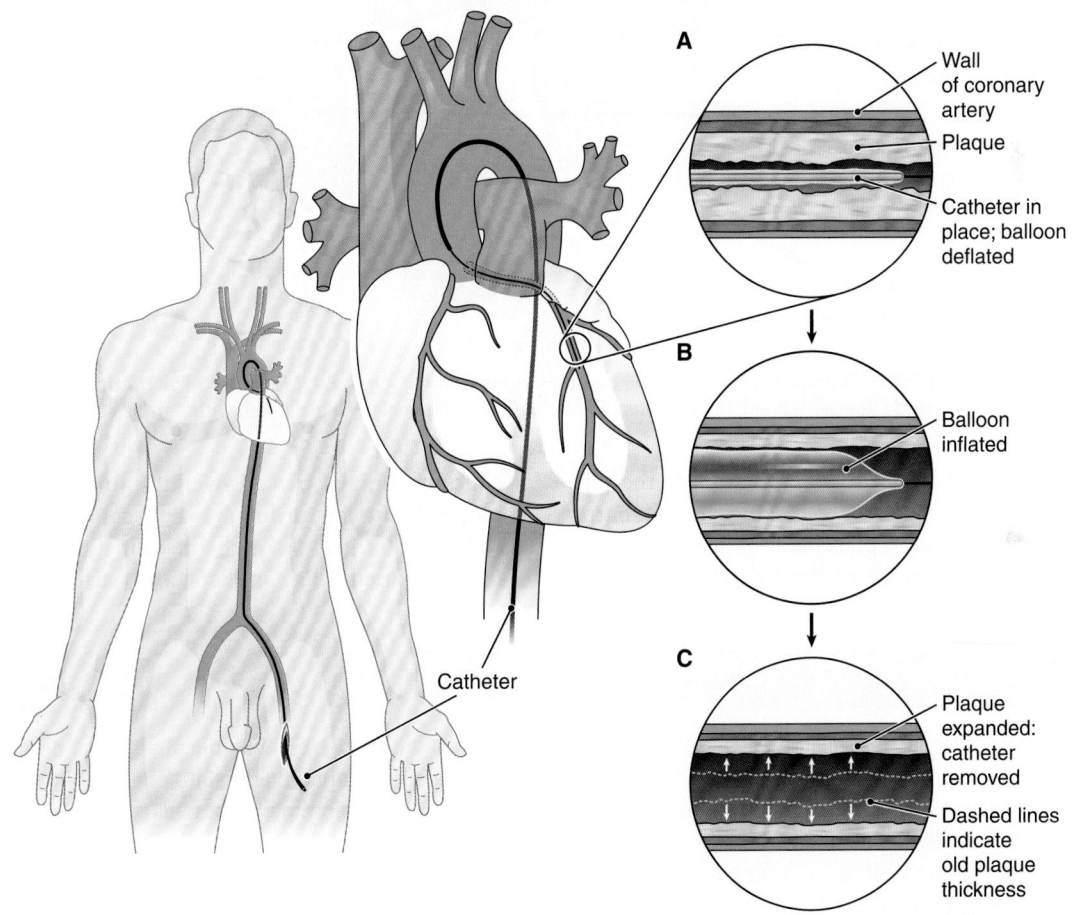

Percutaneous transluminal coronary angioplasty (PTCA). **(A)** A guide is threaded into the coronary artery. **(B)** A balloon catheter is inserted through the occlusion. **(C)** The balloon is inflated and deflated until plaque is flattened and the vessel is opened.

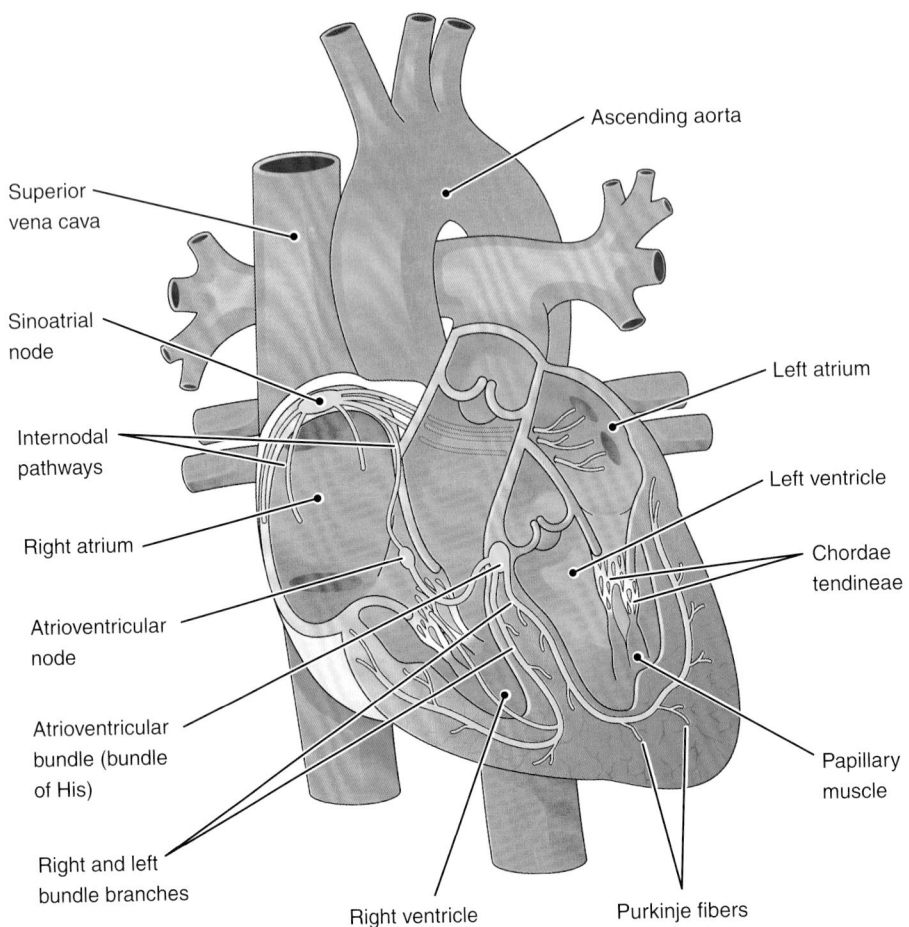

Ascending aorta

Superior vena cava

Sinoatrial node

Internodal pathways

Right atrium

Atrioventricular node

Atrioventricular bundle (bundle of His)

Right and left bundle branches

Right ventricle

Left atrium

Left ventricle

Chordae tendineae

Papillary muscle

Purkinje fibers

**Figure 32-3 •** Conduction system of the heart. (Reprinted from Cohen BJ. *Memmler's The Human Body in Health and Disease*, 11th ed. Philadelphia, PA: Lippincott Williams & Wilkins, 2009, with permission.)

receiver to transmit the rate and function of the pacemaker to a physician at the receiving site. If battery function is failing and replacement is not possible or advisable, batteries can be recharged transdermally. A charging unit is placed over the implantation site and plugged into an ordinary electrical outlet. The power cell is recharged through the skin with no discomfort to the patient. Pacemakers are battery operated and

---

### BOX 32-3   The Automatic External Defibrillator

The automatic external defibrillator (AED) is becoming more widely supplied in public places and medical offices because of the minimal training required and potential to save the life of a patient with sudden cardiac arrest without waiting for emergency medical services or transportation to a hospital.

The device is a small defibrillator in a zippered bag that is usually orange or red with the acronym *AED* written clearly on the front. Inside the bag are also disposable chest pads connected to a cord that is inserted into the connection on the AED. A small washcloth for drying the skin before placing the chest pads if necessary, disposable razor to shave excess chest hair, and examination gloves in the event of possible exposure to blood or other body fluids during the procedure may be added to the AED bag because these items may be necessary to ensure adequate contact between the patient's skin and the chest pads.

In the event that an unconscious patient or victim is found with no pulse (refer to cardiopulmonary resuscitation criteria), the rescuer should apply the chest pads as trained, and using the pictures provided on the pads as a guide, connect the cable to the machine and turn the machine on. The machine has verbal commands to guide the user through the steps necessary to provide an electrical shock if necessary. Do not touch or move the patient while the machine is analyzing the patient's cardiac rhythm or when the machine determines that an electrical shock is necessary.

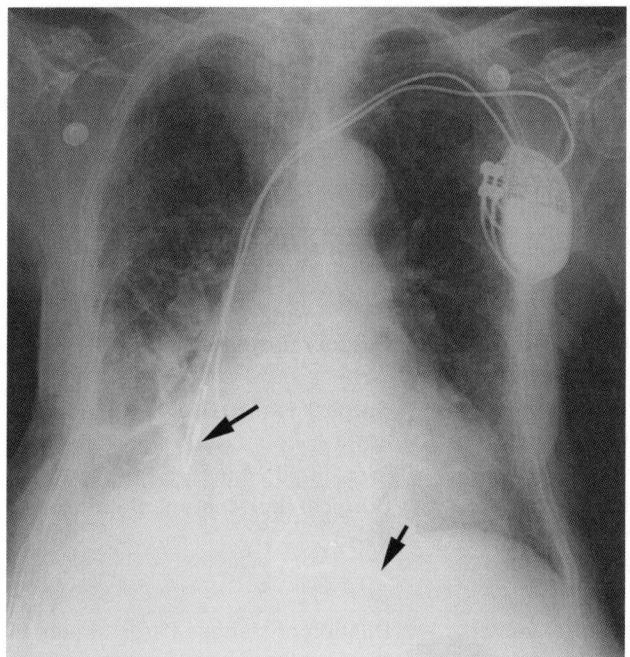

**Figure 32-4 •** Chest x-ray of an intracardiac pacemaker showing the leads (*arrows*) in the right atrium and right ventricle. (From Daffner RH. *Clinical Radiology the Essentials*, 3rd ed. Philadelphia, PA: Lippincott Williams & Wilkins, 2007.)

usually are manufactured to retain their charge for up to 20 years. Recharging or changing the battery in an implanted pacemaker usually requires an outpatient surgical procedure under a local anesthetic.

 **CHECKPOINT QUESTION**

3. Which two cardiac arrhythmias should Abby look for that are emergencies requiring immediate intervention?

 **PATIENT EDUCATION**

### Nitroglycerin

A medication commonly prescribed to increase blood flow to the cardiac muscle is nitroglycerin, a vasodilator. Vasodilators open the lumen of vessels, increasing blood supply to the heart muscle. Patient education should include the following instructions:

- Keep the medication in the dark bottle supplied by the pharmacy because nitroglycerin can be deactivated if exposed to light.
- Be alert for any side effects, such as light-headedness, syncope, and hypotension. Caution patients not to drive or operate other machinery until these symptoms have passed.

- Be aware that nitroglycerin may be prescribed and dispensed as either tablets or a spray to be used as needed, or it may be ordered as a transdermal patch worn constantly to maintain vasodilation. The usual administration guidelines are for three doses at 5-minute intervals. If pain persists, the patient should be advised to call for emergency medical services.
- Patients with arthritis or visual impairment should use nitroglycerin spray. These patients may find the spray easier to use than tablets, since the tablets are very small.
- Check the expiration date of the medication frequently, and always have an adequate supply available at home and when traveling.
- Encourage patients prescribed nitroglycerin to obtain and wear a Medic Alert bracelet or necklace. In the event of an emergency, first responders can assist with administering this medication if necessary.
- Ensure that the medication is kept out of the reach of children.

## Congenital and Valvular Heart Disease

Valvular disease is an acquired or congenital abnormality of any of the four cardiac valves. Valvular heart disease is characterized by stenosis and obstructed blood flow or by valvular degeneration and backflow of the blood against the course of the circulatory pathway. The valves in the left side of the heart are most often affected. The most common congenital valve diseases include atrial septal defect (ASD), ventricular septal defect (VSD), patent ductus arteriosus (PDA), coarctation of the aorta, aortic or pulmonic stenosis, bicuspid aortic valve, mitral valve prolapse, and tetralogy of Fallot (Table 32-1).

Rheumatic heart disease, an acquired valvular disease, presents clinically as a generalized inflammatory disease occurring 10 to 21 days after an upper respiratory infection caused by group A beta hemolytic streptococci. It is characterized by inflammatory lesions of the connective tissues, particularly in the heart, joints, and subcutaneous tissues. The heart valves are damaged by an abnormal response of the immune system caused by the turbulence of the infected blood. This damage results in a systolic murmur. Although it usually attacks children aged 5 to 15, rheumatic heart disease has declined significantly since the 1940s.

Mitral valve stenosis, a condition that occurs when the leaflet cusps of the mitral valve fuse and thicken, may result from rheumatic heart disease. When the valve cusps thicken and fuse, the result is an abnormally narrow valve; hence, mitral regurgitation, or backflow, of blood from the left ventricle into the left atrium occurs. Patients

| **TABLE 32-1** | **Diseases of the Cardiac Valves and Congenital Cardiac Defects** | |
|---|---|---|
| Disorder | Description | Treatment |
| ASD | Abnormal opening between atria, allowing unoxygenated blood in right atrium to mix with oxygenated blood in left atrium; congenital | Surgery to close |
| VSD | Abnormal opening between ventricles, allowing unoxygenated blood in right ventricle to mix with oxygenated blood in left ventricle; congenital | Surgery to close |
| PDA | Abnormal opening between pulmonary artery and aorta; congenital | Surgery to close |
| Coarctation of the aorta | Narrowing of the aorta resulting in high blood pressure in upper extremities and low blood pressure in lower extremities; congenital | Surgery to increase diameter of aorta |
| Bicuspid aortic valve | Aortic valve having two cusps instead of three, resulting in incomplete closure between aorta and left ventricle during systole and diastole; congenital | Surgical replacement of aortic valve |
| Aortic or pulmonic stenosis | Narrowing of aortic or pulmonary artery valve leaflets, causing overwork of cardiac muscle and hypertrophy of ventricles; as stenosis increases, valve becomes less flexible | Dilation of stenosed area or surgical replacement of valve |
| MVP | Drooping of one or both cusps of mitral (bicuspid) valve into left ventricle during systole, resulting in incomplete closure of valve and backflow of blood from left ventricle into left atrium | Usually benign. Treatment is alleviating any symptoms (palpations, chest pain). Prophylactic antibiotic may be ordered before dental procedures |
| Tetralogy of Fallot | Four defects: pulmonary stenosis, dextroposition of aorta, ventricular septal defect, and hypertrophy of right ventricle; congenital | Surgery to correct |

with mitral stenosis often have dyspnea, or shortness of breath, and their ability to exert themselves physically may be limited. Pulmonary edema may also develop and cause symptoms such as dyspnea and a productive cough.

Treatment of valvular disease depends on the type and severity of the abnormality. Severe cases may require medication, low-sodium diet, and prophylactic antibiotic before surgery or dental work. If medication is not successful, surgical replacement of the involved valves may be necessary.

 **CHECKPOINT QUESTION**

4. What microorganism may be responsible for rheumatic heart disease and cardiac valvular damage?

## Disorders of the Blood Vessels

### Atherosclerosis

Diseases of blood vessels—arteries or veins—often begin with collection of fatty plaques made of calcium and cholesterol inside the walls of the vessels. These plaques narrow the lumen, or opening, of the blood vessels and impede blood flow. This condition, which is known as **atherosclerosis**, is problematic in arteries because oxygen and nutrients are prevented from reaching various tissues of the body. In addition to the occlusion that occurs with atherosclerosis, the plaques are rougher than the walls of a normal artery and may remain stationary as a thrombus or break away from the wall of the artery as an embolus (Fig. 32-5). Signs and symptoms of atherosclerosis usually result from ischemia to a body part and may include pain or numbness, loss of normal blood flow, or loss of a palpable pulse to the affected body area.

If the coronary arteries are involved, the condition is coronary artery disease (CAD), the most common type of heart disease and the leading cause of death in men and women in the United States. Patients with CAD may have the following symptoms:

- Angina pectoris (pain radiating to the arm, jaw, shoulder, back, or neck, usually felt on exertion and relieved by rest)
- Pressure or fullness in the chest, felt most severely during exertion and relieved by rest

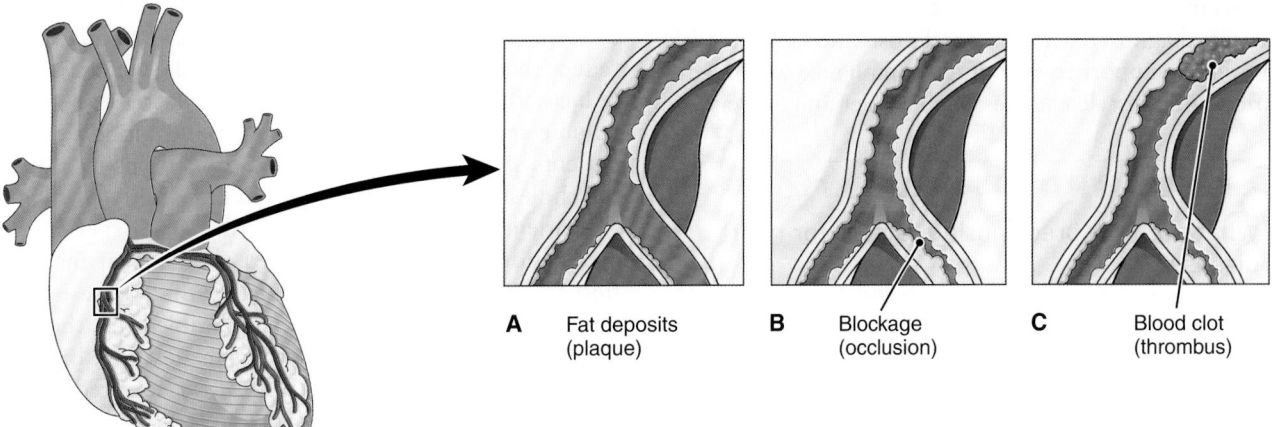

**Figure 32-5** • Coronary atherosclerosis. **(A)** Fat deposits narrow an artery, leading to ischemia. **(B)** Blockage of the coronary artery. **(C)** Formation of a blood clot (thrombus), leading to MI. (Reprinted from Cohen BJ. *Memmler's The Human Body in Health and Disease*, 11th ed. Philadelphia, PA: Lippincott Williams & Wilkins, 2009, with permission.)

- Syncope (fainting)
- Edema of the extremities, especially the legs
- Unexplained cough, generally without respiratory symptoms
- Excessive fatigue
- Dyspnea

Predisposing conditions for atherosclerosis and coronary artery disease (CAD) include a diet high in saturated fats and a family history of hypercholesterolemia. Other risk factors include cigarette smoking, diabetes mellitus, and hypertension. Consuming a diet low in cholesterol and saturated fats, participating in a moderate exercise program, maintaining normal body weight and blood pressure, and not smoking may minimize the chances for developing atherosclerosis and CAD or reduce the progression if a diagnosis has been made. If necessary, the physician may order lipid-lowering medication for patients whose blood cholesterol and triglyceride levels are not affected by dietary or other behavioral changes.

Diagnosis of atherosclerosis is often made by angiography to locate the occlusion and evaluate the degree of obstruction (Fig. 32-6). In this procedure, a catheter is inserted into the blood vessel, and radiographic images are taken as a contrast medium is injected into the vessel. The radiographs are evaluated for the presence and amount of plaque buildup or the presence of a thrombus. Doppler ultrasonography, a test that uses sound waves to produce an image of the blood vessel, may also be ordered to detect atherosclerosis. Doppler ultrasonography, or echocardiography, can be used to determine the ability of the heart to fill and pump blood. This noninvasive test uses sound waves to produce a picture of the heart on a video monitor to detect areas of poor blood flow or damaged muscle.

A relatively new noninvasive test for CAD is cardiac calcium scoring using electron beam computed tomography (CT). In this procedure, CT of the coronary arteries using an electron beam identifies the amount of fat and calcium buildup within the coronary arteries. An elevated score indicates an increased risk for developing CAD, especially if other risk factors are present.

The treatment for atherosclerosis often includes lifestyle changes, as described earlier, to reverse or prevent further atherosclerotic formations. If the condition is severe, lipid-lowering medication may be prescribed. Surgery to remove the plaque or improve blood flow through an artery may also be indicated for some patients. Your responsibilities will include coordinating diagnostic procedures based on the physician's orders and insurance requirements and teaching patients about

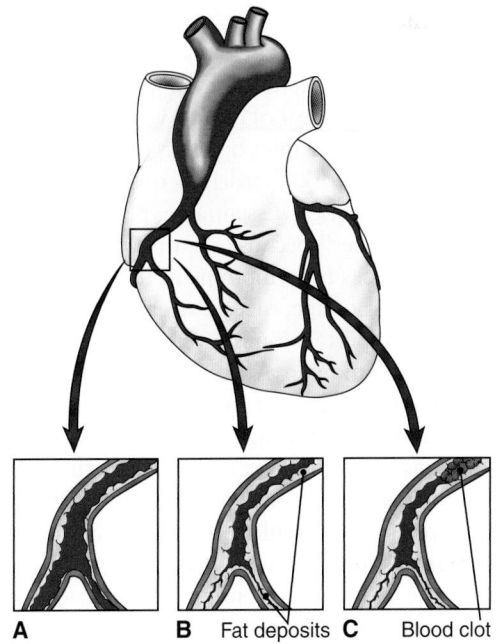

**Figure 32-6** • Atherosclerotic coronary occlusion. (Reprinted from Rubin E, Farber JL. *Pathology*. Philadelphia, PA: Lippincott Williams & Wilkins, 2005, with permission.)

behaviors that can prevent atherosclerosis and CAD. Patients diagnosed with atherosclerosis and CAD require emotional support to encourage compliance with medication and lifestyle changes, such as diet and exercise.

### CHECKPOINT QUESTION

5. What are four predisposing factors for heart disease?

## Hypertension

Patients with a resting systolic blood pressure above 140 mm Hg and a diastolic pressure above 90 mm Hg are said to be hypertensive. Hypertension cannot be diagnosed on the basis of one blood pressure measurement, since other factors, such as emotional upset or anxiety, may cause a temporary increase in blood pressure. Since many factors may affect the blood pressure, the physician often requires several blood pressure readings before making the diagnosis of hypertension. Once a diagnosis of hypertension is made, you may play a major role in assisting with the control of this condition by regularly monitoring the patient's blood pressure and medication prescriptions; teaching the patient about dietary and lifestyle changes, such as smoking cessation and weight loss; and recording complete and accurate information regarding the medical history each time the patient visits the office. Refer to Table 19-6 in Chapter 19 for more information regarding blood pressure readings and what constitutes normal, prehypertension, and hypertension I and II.

One type of hypertension, essential hypertension, is a major cause of stroke and renal failure and is a major consequence of atherosclerosis anywhere in the circulatory system. The long-term effects of essential hypertension may include weakening of the arteries throughout the body and enlargement of the left ventricle of the heart. Left ventricular hypertrophy, or enlargement, occurs gradually as the heart works harder to overcome the higher pressure in the arteries. Essential hypertension is often called a "silent killer" because the disease is gradual and frequently produces no symptoms in the patient, striking anyone regardless of age, race, sex, or ethnic origin.

Malignant hypertension is severe and sudden in onset and is most common in African American men under age 40 years regardless of other risk factors. Patients with malignant hypertension have signs and symptoms including diastolic blood pressure greater than 120 mm Hg and blurred vision, headache, and possibly confusion. The physician should be notified immediately if these symptoms are present.

While the cause of essential hypertension may be unknown, its correlation with an elevated serum cholesterol level has been shown. After diagnosis, some patients can control the high blood pressure with a low-sodium, low-fat diet, an exercise program, weight reduction if needed, and antihypertensive and lipid-reducing medications. Diuretic medication may be prescribed to reduce the amount of sodium in the body, which in turn reduces the total fluid volume. The decrease in fluid volume reduces strain on the heart and blood vessels. Patients should also be informed of methods to reduce the cholesterol and triglycerides in their diet.

Patients who have been prescribed antihypertensive medications should be instructed to take that medication as prescribed. Many patients feel that because their blood pressure has reached a manageable level, they do not need to continue the prescribed medication. Explain that the medication is the cause of the lowered blood pressure and that discontinuing the treatment without consulting the physician may jeopardize their recovery.

### CHECKPOINT QUESTION

6. Several patients in the Great Falls Medical Center cardiology office are being seen for hypertension. What two disorders may result from untreated hypertension?

## Varicose Veins

Varicosities, the most common circulatory disease of the lower extremities, occur when the superficial veins of the legs swell and distend (Fig. 32-7). Eventually, the valves in the veins fail to close properly, allowing blood to pool and stretch the walls of the veins. People who sit or stand for long periods without moving or contracting their leg

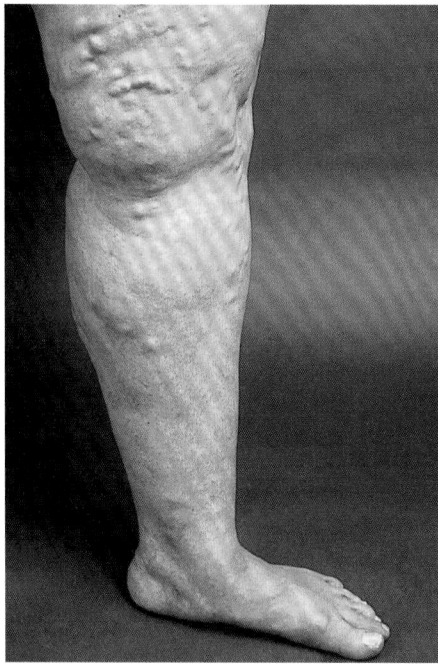

**Figure 32-7 •** Varicose veins of the lower extremities. (Reprinted from Bickley LS, Szilagy PG. *Bates' Guide to Physical Examination and History Taking.* Philadelphia, PA: Lippincott Williams & Wilkins, 2003, with permission.)

muscles are predisposed to varicose veins. A hereditary weakness in the vein walls is also a predisposing factor. Varicosities may also be secondary to deep vein thrombosis. Signs and symptoms of varicose veins are swelling, aching, and a feeling of heaviness in the legs. Varicosities may also be asymptomatic. Many patients consider varicose veins unattractive and seek treatment even without symptoms.

Treatment of varicose veins is usually conservative, with instructions to avoid standing or sitting for long periods to reduce symptoms and prevent the development of further varicosities. Other helpful measures that may be ordered by the physician include wearing elastic support stockings or wrapping the legs with elastic bandages and elevating the legs for specified periods. Surgery to remove the veins is usually the last approach. Another treatment technique is injection of a sclerosing agent into small varicose vein segments, but this is not suggested for large areas.

## Venous Thrombosis and Pulmonary Embolism

Thrombi, or blood clots, in the peripheral or pulmonary veins commonly affect patients with underlying cardiovascular disease. Risk factors for developing thrombi may be either primary (inherited) or secondary (acquired). Primary causes include hemolytic anemia and sickle cell disease, and secondary factors include long-term immobility, chronic pulmonary disease, thrombophlebitis, varicosities, and defibrillation after cardiac arrest. Chemical contraceptives for women have also been implicated in a higher risk of developing thrombi in young women who have none of the usual predisposing factors. The risk increases in women who smoke. A thrombus in the peripheral venous circulatory system may dislodge and become an embolus. This embolus is dangerous to the patient, since the blood clot can lodge in the pulmonary circulation (causing a pulmonary embolism), the cardiac circulation (causing MI), or the cerebral circulation (causing a **cerebrovascular accident [CVA]**).

Peripheral vascular occlusion may also lead to stasis ulcers, which are caused by breakdown of the skin and underlying tissue due to inadequate circulation to the area. These ulcers develop as deep red discolorations, itching, edema, and large areas of scaling skin leading to fissures and ulcers (Fig. 32-8). Increasing circulation to the lower extremities with use of support stockings, weight reduction, and elevating the limbs may prevent formation of these ulcers.

A blood clot lodged in the pulmonary circulation is a pulmonary embolism. Signs and symptoms of a pulmonary embolism include dyspnea, syncope, and severe pleuritic chest pain with respiration. Diagnosis may include chest radiography, an electrocardiogram, a lung scan, or a pulmonary arteriogram. Doppler studies are used to diagnose deep vein thrombosis. Depending on the severity, treatment may include bed rest with elevation of the affected extremity, anticoagulant medication such as Coumadin, or surgery.

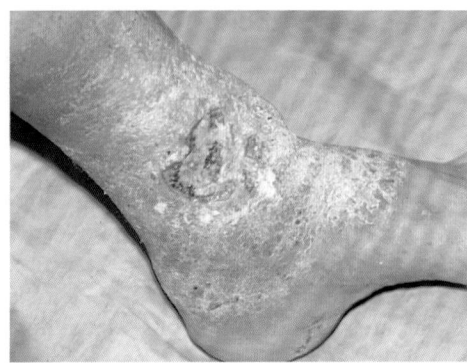

**Figure 32-8** • Stasis dermatitis with venous stasis ulcer. (From Goodheart HP. *Goodheart's Photoguide of Common Skin Disorders*, 2nd ed. Philadelphia, PA: Lippincott Williams & Wilkins, 2003.)

 **CHECKPOINT QUESTION**

7. What disease occurs when the superficial veins in the legs become swollen and distended?

 **PATIENT EDUCATION**

### Anticoagulant Therapy

Patients with certain types of cardiac problems are prescribed anticoagulant medications, commonly called *blood thinners*, which are used to decrease the risk of a thrombus or embolus developing. Coumadin is a common oral anticoagulant. Lovenox™, another anticoagulant, is given as an injection. Teach patients who are prescribed anticoagulants as follows:

- Monitor the mouth, urine, and stool for any signs of bleeding.
- Use a soft-bristle toothbrush.
- Call the office if any signs of bleeding occur.
- Avoid injuries and falls while taking anticoagulant medications.
- Be aware that needlesticks from injections or venipuncture require prolonged application of pressure afterwards to control bleeding and bruising.
- Comply with orders for blood work. Anticoagulant medications necessitate frequent tests for blood counts and bleeding times.
- Limit the intake of foods high in vitamin K (asparagus, cabbage, fish, broccoli, cheese, pork, spinach, cauliflower, and rice). These patients should be given a printed flyer on dietary restrictions.
- Avoid taking over-the-counter (OTC) medications containing aspirin or ibuprofen without consulting the physician. These drugs may cause an increase in bleeding times, interfering with the actions of the anticoagulant.
- Take the medication at the same time every day. If a dose is missed, take it as soon as it is remembered that day but do not take a double dose.

## Cerebrovascular Accident

CVA, sometimes called stroke, results suddenly when damage to the blood vessels in the brain occurs. The damage blocks the circulation, resulting in ischemia, or lack of oxygen, to that part of the brain. Brain tissue dies without adequate oxygen. A common cause of CVA is blockage of the cerebral artery by thrombus or embolus. Hemorrhage, atherosclerotic heart disease, and hypertension are additional causes of CVAs. Unfortunately, CVAs are the most common nervous system disorder in the elderly and one of the leading causes of death in the United States.

Patients who have CVAs usually have varying degrees of weakness or paralysis of one side of the body, with possible involvement of language and comprehension. Symptoms vary according to which artery and which part of the brain is affected. CVAs are fatal when vital centers of the brain are damaged. Once the brain tissue is damaged by a CVA, treatment is aimed at reducing further death of cerebrovascular tissue and assisting the patient to regain any affected function. Patients who have CVAs need many months of rehabilitation, including physical therapy, occupational therapy, and speech therapy. You must remember that, although these patients may not be able to communicate effectively with you, they are capable of understanding and should be treated with respect, dignity, and compassion.

Ischemia to small areas of the brain over short periods is known as **transient ischemic attack (TIA)**. TIA, or ministroke, should be considered a warning sign for a possible impending cerebrovascular accident. TIAs may be caused by atherosclerotic plaques narrowing the arteries supplying blood to the brain, a small embolus that reduces the flow of blood to an area, or spasms of the blood vessels. The symptoms vary according to the arteries affected but usually include the following:

- Mild numbness or tingling in the face or a limb
- Difficulty swallowing
- Coughing and choking
- Slurred speech
- Unilateral visual disturbance
- Dizziness

As many as 50% to 80% of patients who exhibit symptoms of TIAs progress to a stroke. The signs of a major stroke may begin as a TIA and progress to loss of consciousness, hyperpnea (deep, gasping breaths), anisocoria (unequal pupils), and hemiplegia (unilateral paralysis). Any patient who has the signs and symptoms of a TIA or a CVA should be sent to the emergency room following all physician instructions and office policies.

## Aneurysm

Weakened blood vessel walls are predisposed to abnormal dilation. Dilation in the form of an **aneurysm** may occur in any vessel, but arteries are most often affected (Fig. 32-9).

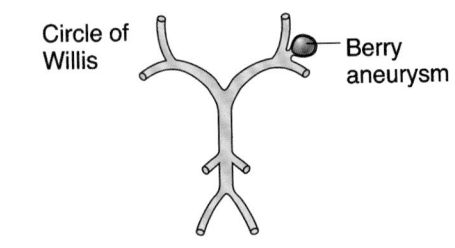

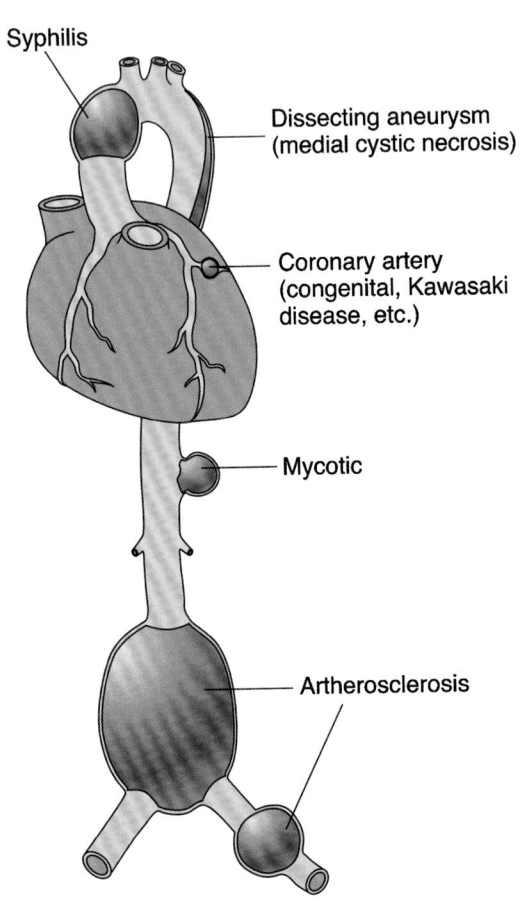

**Figure 32-9** • The locations of aneurysms. (Reprinted from Rubin E. *Pathology: Clinicopathologic Foundations of Medicine.* Philadelphia, PA: Lippincott Williams & Wilkins, 2005, with permission.)

Because of the high pressure so close to the heart, the aorta is the most common site. The normally elastic vessel wall develops a ballooning effect in one or many forms, all of them dangerous:

- A *dissecting aneurysm* tears the inner walls of the artery and allows blood to leak into the lining of the vessel; the wall will eventually die and tear open.
- A *sacculated aneurysm* balloons from the arterial wall into a sac, which may burst.
- A *berry aneurysm* is usually a congenital defect in a cerebral artery.

Causes of aneurysms include trauma, hypertension, atherosclerosis, certain fungal infections, syphilis, and congenital defects. Symptoms include pain or pressure at the site. Death may occur quickly if the tear is not repaired. Diagnosis is based on a thorough history and examination, an arteriogram or aortogram, computed tomography, or magnetic resonance imaging. Surgical resection is the only option.

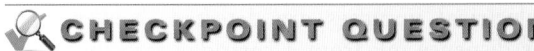

## CHECKPOINT QUESTION

8. What is the physiologic reason for a stroke?

### Anemia

Deficiencies in hemoglobin or in the numbers of red blood cells result in anemia. Anemia is not considered a disease but is a symptom of an underlying disorder. Anemia can result from any of the following:

- Blood loss due to hemorrhage or slow internal bleeding
- A diet low in iron or a malabsorption condition (nutritional anemia)
- Suppressed (by chemotherapeutic medication) or diseased bone marrow, resulting in decreased blood cell formation (aplastic anemia)
- Vitamin $B_{12}$ deficiency due to a lack of intrinsic factor (pernicious anemia)
- Genetic abnormality (sickle cell anemia, thalassemia)
- Destruction of functioning red blood cells by various means, such as liver or spleen dysfunction or toxins (hemolytic anemia)

Symptoms of anemia may include cardiovascular alterations such as tachycardia and pallor, anorexia and weight loss, dyspnea on exertion, and fatigue. Treatment of anemia must address the cause; it can include increasing dietary iron, blood transfusions, and injection of vitamin $B_{12}$ (cyanocobalamin) on a regular basis. Aplastic anemia may require a bone marrow transplantation. Unfortunately, genetic abnormalities, such as sickle cell anemia and thalassemia, cannot be corrected at this time.

## COG COMMON DIAGNOSTIC AND THERAPEUTIC PROCEDURES

Testing for cardiovascular disorders may be either invasive or noninvasive. Invasive techniques require entering the body by the use of a tube, needle, or other device. Noninvasive techniques do not require entering the body or puncturing the skin. Depending on the patient's symptoms, testing may be basic and can be done easily during the general physical examination by auscultating the heart and chest cavity. Additional tests the physician may order that you perform in the medical office can include chest radiography or 12-lead ECG. Sometimes, initial findings indicate the need for a more sophisticated procedure, such as cardiac catheterization, which is performed at an outpatient surgical center or hospital.

## Physical Examination of the Cardiovascular System

The cardiovascular examination is the most basic noninvasive procedure used to assess the heart and blood vessels. When preparing a patient for a cardiovascular examination, you will obtain vital information, including accurate determination of weight, blood pressure, heart and respiratory rates, body temperature, and cardiovascular history. It is also important to obtain a complete list of the patient's medications and current dosages, including any herbal and vitamin supplements and OTC medications. A brief social and family history should include lifestyle and familial risk factors for cardiovascular disorders. The patient should be questioned regarding a history of smoking tobacco, alcohol intake, family history of heart disease, hypercholesterolemia, diet, and exercise. Specifically, you should ask the following questions to elicit important information from a patient with cardiovascular problems:

- Why are you seeing the cardiologist or physician today?
- What symptoms have you been having?
- How long have you had the pain, discomfort, distress, or unusual sensations? (Patients may not think of chest discomfort as a cardiac symptom.)
- Where is the pain or discomfort? Does it stay in one place or radiate in any direction?
- Is the pain associated with any other symptoms, such as shortness of breath, nausea, weakness, sweating, or dizziness?
- If you have been short of breath, does it restrict any of your activities or require you to sleep on additional pillows at night?
- Are you a smoker?
- Do you drink alcoholic beverages?

As you proceed with the interview, keep in mind that patients with cardiovascular problems are usually understandably anxious and concerned. They may bring with them family members who are also concerned or anxious. It is your responsibility to help ease apprehension and to offer reassurance and support when appropriate.

The physician or cardiologist usually begins the examination with a review of the patient's history and reason for the office visit. The physician also reviews the patient's vital signs and medications, noting any allergies to medications and other substances. The physician inspects the patient to evaluate the general appearance, noting the circulation and any swelling of the extremities, color of the skin, and jugular vein distention. Palpation is used to evaluate the efficiency of the circulatory pathways and peripheral pulses. Using auscultation with a stethoscope, the physician can evaluate the sounds made as blood flows through the heart and the valves open and close. Abnormal heart sounds, such as bruits and murmurs, may be detected (Box 32-4).

## BOX 32-4    Abnormal Heart Sounds

Abnormal heart sounds, called *murmurs*, are sounds the blood makes as it courses through the heart valves. The sounds vary with the severity and location of the abnormality. For instance, they may blow, rasp, rub, bubble, whistle, whoosh, and/or click. A murmur is not a disease, but it may indicate organic heart disease.

Functional murmurs may only occur during elevations in body temperature or during times of physical stress and are not usually a cause for concern. *Organic murmurs* indicate structural abnormalities of varying degrees and are always present. A cardiologist evaluates the murmur by noting its location in the heart, when it occurs in the cardiac cycle, how long it lasts, and its characteristic sound.

In addition to obtaining important information and data before the physician examines the patient, you must also provide instructions and materials for proper gown wearing and draping. After the examination, the physician may order an ECG, which you will perform and give to the physician for diagnosis.

## CHECKPOINT QUESTION

9. The cardiologist tells a patient he has a heart murmur. How would Abby explain a heart murmur to a patient?

## Electrocardiogram

One of the most valuable diagnostic tools for evaluating the electrical pathway through the heart is the electrocardiogram, known by the acronym ECG or EKG. The ECG is the graphic record of the electrical current as it progresses through the heart. It can be performed as part of a routine physical examination or as needed for a patient with chest pain, discomfort, or other signs and symptoms of possible cardiac problems. During the ECG, you are responsible for explaining the procedure to the patient and applying combinations of electrodes, called **leads**, on the patient's limbs and precordial area (anterior chest). ECGs are used to assist in diagnosing ischemia, delays in impulse conduction, hypertrophy of the cardiac chambers, and arrhythmias. They are not used to detect anatomic disorders, such as heart murmurs.

The ECG tracing is printed on graph paper that is either blue or black with a heat-labile white coating. Graph lines are printed over the white coating, appearing as small blocks with thicker lines outlining every five small blocks. On standard ECG paper, each small block is 1 mm². The large blocks are 5 mm² (Fig. 32-10A). Some older ECG machines contain a stylus that heats and melts the white coating, exposing the dark background beneath to record the movement of the stylus as the electrical impulses are detected. Newer ECG machines dispense ink from a cartridge into the stylus to mark the ECG tracing paper. The ECG paper may be affected by pressure as well as heat and should be handled carefully to prevent extraneous markings. Each small horizontal block represents time (0.04 seconds), and the vertical small blocks represent voltage (0.1 millivolts). After the heart's electrical markings are traced on the paper, the heart rate and time required for the electrical impulses to spread through the heart can be determined (Fig. 32-10B).

### ECG Leads

Over the years, a standard system of electrode placement has evolved, and nomenclature has been developed for the recordings from different electrode combinations. Each lead records the electrical impulse through the heart from a different angle. Viewing the conduction of the electrical impulses in these various angles gives the physician a fairly complete view of the entire heart. The standard ECG has 12 leads that produce a three-dimensional record of the impulse wave. Four wires are labeled and color coded for the limb that the wire should be connected to, and six wires are labeled for connection to electrodes placed on the anterior chest (Box 32-5). The four limb electrodes should be positioned away from bony areas and on muscular areas, such as the calves, outer thighs, and above the elbow. Adjustments may be necessary for patients with amputations, surgery to the extremity, or trauma to the arms or legs.

The right leg (RL) electrode, the grounding lead, helps reduce alternating current (AC) interference and keeps the average voltage of the patient the same as that of the recording instrument. The other three limb leads attached to electrodes on the patient's left leg and arms make up the combinations necessary for the first six views of the heart in the 12-lead ECG. The first three combinations, which are standard bipolar leads also known as *Einthoven leads*, allow frontal visualization of the heart's electrical activity from side to side. Each lead provides specific measurements:

- Lead I measures the difference in electrical potential between the right arm (RA) and the left arm (LA).
- Lead II measures the difference in electrical potential between the right arm (RA) and the left leg (LL).
- Lead III measures the difference in electrical potential between the left arm (LA) and the left leg (LL).

The same limb electrodes provide measurement of the signal between one electrode and the average of the remaining two. These second three combinations,

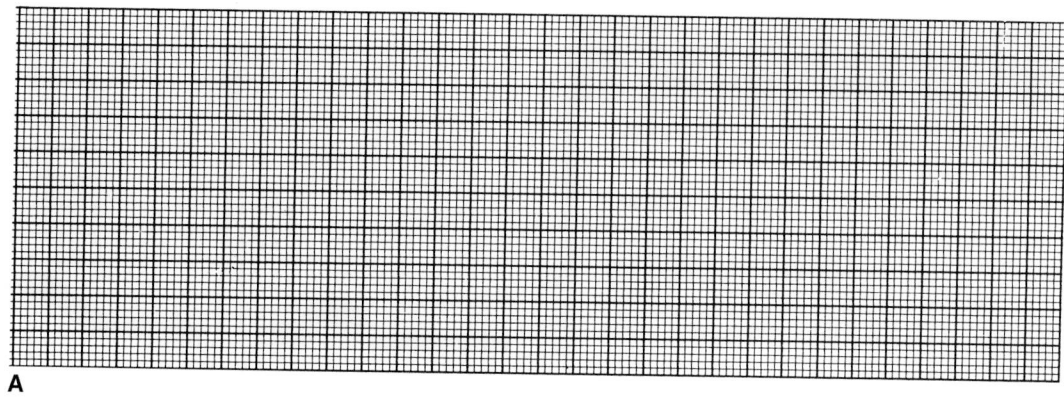

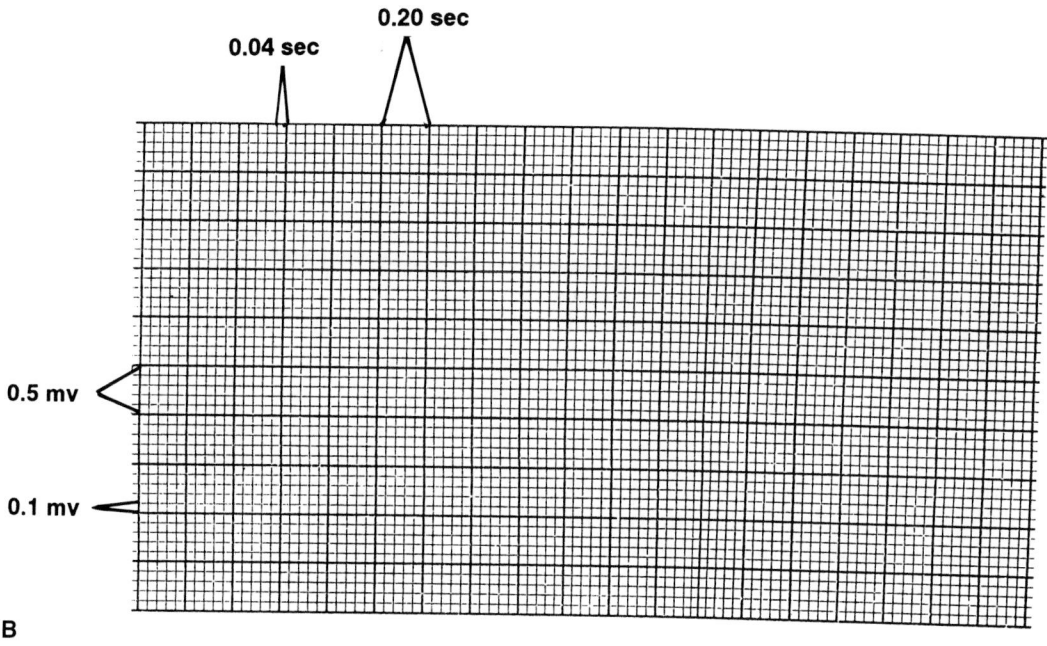

**Figure 32-10 •** ECG graph paper. **(A)** Each small square is 1 mm x 1 mm. Each fifth line is marked darker to make a cube of 5 mm x 5 mm (actual size). **(B)** Horizontally, the graph paper represents time in seconds. Each small square represents 0.04 seconds, and each large square represents 0.2 seconds. Five large squares = 1 second (5 x 0.2).

the augmented unipolar limb leads, allow visualization from a frontal view top to bottom:

• Lead aVR (LL 1 LA) to RA measures the potential at the right arm.

• Lead aVL (LL 1 RA) to LA measures the potential at the left arm.

• Lead aVF (RA 1 LA) to LL measures the potential at the left foot.

For a closer look at the electrical conduction through the heart, electrodes are placed directly on the anterior chest wall, but the limb electrodes must remain attached to the patient. The positioning of the chest electrodes must be precise for accuracy. These leads, the unipolar precordial (chest) leads, show the comparison of the chest electrode potential to the average of the three limb electrodes (Box 32-6). All electrodes must connect to the wires of the ECG machine. Each lead is clearly marked on the ECG paper as it is printed, or specific codes may be printed on the paper to denote each lead (Table 32-2). The recording of the ECG on paper varies from one machine to another, but the principles and techniques are universal (Procedure 32-1).

---

**BOX 32-5    Abbreviations Used in Performing ECGs**

RA—right arm
LA—left arm
LL—left leg
RL—right leg
$V_1$–$V_6$—chest leads
aVR—augmented voltage right arm
aVL—augmented voltage left arm
aVF—augmented voltage left foot or leg

- $LV_1 = (RA + LA + LL)$ to $V_1$: Fourth intercostal space at right margin of sternum
- $LV_2 = (RA + LA + LL)$ to $V_2$: Fourth intercostal space at left margin of sternum
- $LV_3 = (RA + LA + LL)$ to $V_3$: Midway between $V_2$ and $V_4$
- $LV_4 = (RA + LA + LL)$ to $V_4$: Fifth intercostal space at junction of midclavicular line
- $LV_5 = (RA + LA + LL)$ to $V_5$: Horizontal level of $V_4$ at left anterior axillary line
- $LV_6 = (RA + LA + LL)$ to $V_6$: Horizontal level of $V_4$ and $V_5$ at midaxillary line

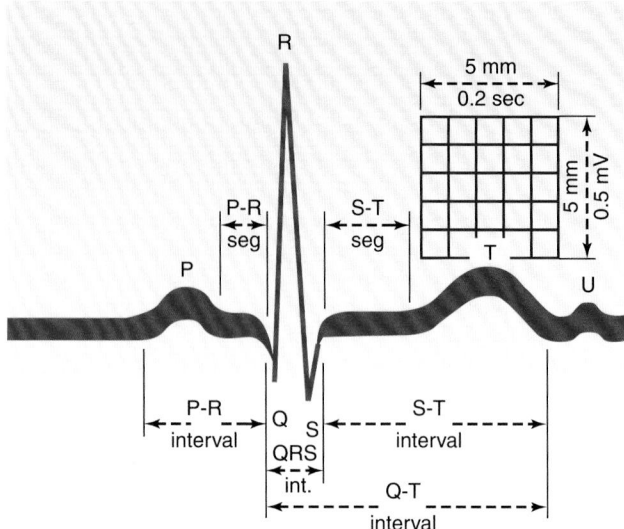

**Figure 32-11** • The cardiac cycle waves, segments, and intervals. (Reprinted from Cohen BJ. *Medical Terminology: An Illustrated Guide*. Philadelphia, PA: Lippincott Williams & Wilkins, 2009, with permission.)

## ECG Interpretation

The physician's interpretation of the standard 12-lead ECG includes an examination of various waveforms associated with the cardiac cycle (Fig. 32-11). Commonly measured components of an ECG tracing are discussed in the following sections.

### PR Interval

The time from the beginning of the P wave to the beginning of the QRS complex is called the *PR interval*. This time interval represents depolarization of the atria and the spread of the depolarization wave up to and including the atrioventricular node.

### PR Segment

The PR segment represents the period between the P wave and QRS complex.

### ST Segment

The distance between the QRS complex and the T wave from the point where the QRS complex ends (J-point) to the onset of the ascending limb of the T wave is called the *ST segment*. On the ECG, this segment is a sensitive indicator of myocardial ischemia or injury.

### Ventricular Activation Time

The time from the beginning of the QRS complex to the peak of the R wave, the *ventricular activation time*, represents the time necessary for the depolarization wave to travel from the inner surface of the heart (endocardium) to the outer surface of the heart (epicardium).

During the ECG, the paper speed on the machine should be set at 25 mm per second, which allows the electrical impulses (seen as waves) on the ECG to be measured using the blocks on the ECG paper as a reference (each small horizontal block is 0.04 seconds). Movement of the electricity through the atria is noted and measured on the ECG tracing as the PR interval (the normal PR interval is 0.12 to 0.20 seconds). Electrical movement through the ventricles is measured and noted on the ECG as the QRS complex, which is normally less than 0.12 seconds. The following elements are taken into consideration:

- Rate: how fast the heart is beating
- Rhythm: regularity of cardiac cycles and intervals
- Axis: position of the heart and direction of depolarization, or electrical movement, through the heart
- Hypertrophy: size of the heart
- Ischemia: decrease in blood supply to an area of the heart
- Infarction: death of heart muscle resulting in loss of function

Under usual diagnostic conditions, the 12-lead ECG provides sufficient data. As the medical assistant, you are responsible for obtaining a good-quality ECG

| TABLE 32-2 | Coding ECG Leads | | |
|------|------|------|------|
| Lead | Code | Lead | Code |
| I | . | V1 | -. |
| II | .. | V2 | -.. |
| III | ... | V3 | -... |
| aVR | - | V4 | -.... |
| aVL | — | V5 | -..... |
| aVF | —- | V6 | -...... |

## TABLE 32-3 Types of Artifacts

**WANDERING BASELINE**

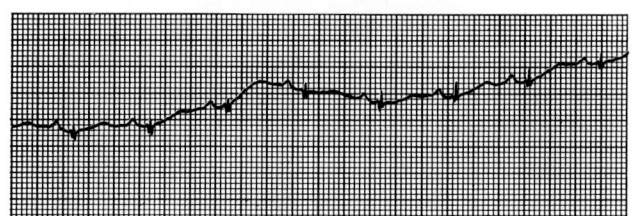

**SOMATIC MUSCLE TREMOR**

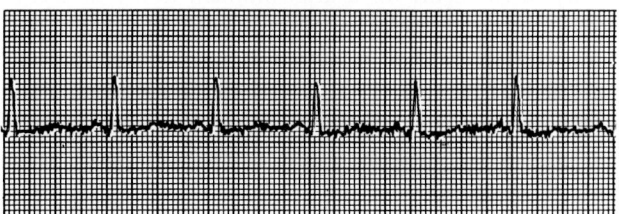

**AC INTERFERENCE**

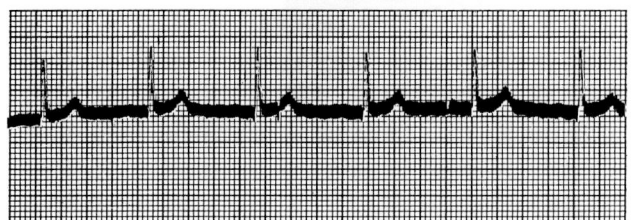

| Artifact | Possible Cause | How to Prevent Problems |
|---|---|---|
| Wandering baseline | Electrodes too tight or too loose; electrolyte gel dried out; skin has oil, lotion, or excessive hair | Apply electrodes properly; apply new electrodes; prepare skin before applying electrodes |
| Muscle or somatic artifact | Patient cannot remain still because of tremors or fear | Reassure patient; explain procedure and stress the need to keep still; patients with disease may be unable to stay motionless |
| Alternating artifact | Improperly grounded ECG machine | Check cables to ensure properly current-grounded machine before beginning test |
| | Electrical interference in room in immediate area | Move patient or unplug appliances |
| | Dangling lead wires | Arrange wires along contours of patient's body |

without avoidable **artifacts**. An artifact is an abnormal signal that does not reflect electrical activity of the heart during the cardiac cycle. Artifacts can be due to movement by the patient, mechanical problems with the ECG machine, or improper technique. Table 32-3 describes three types of artifacts and how to prevent them.

Sometimes, the physician requests a rhythm strip along with the ECG. A rhythm strip is a long strip of a certain lead or a combination of leads. It may be used to define certain cardiac arrhythmias. While most ECG machines have a button that automatically records the 12 views in the 12-lead ECG, a rhythm strip must be obtained using the manual mode on the ECG machine.

 **WHAT IF**

**What if the physician asks you to perform an ECG on a child?**

Although pediatric cardiac problems may not be encountered daily in the medical office, obesity, elevated cholesterol and triglyceride blood levels, and type 2 diabetes are conditions that are seen increasingly frequently in pediatric and family practice offices, and these conditions may require intervention, including electrocardiography. Although the placement of the electrodes is similar to that for an adult, smaller electrodes for use on the smaller patient allow for easier placement. A standard ECG can be done on children over 8 or 9 years of age; however, for younger children, the sensitivity, or gain, on the machine should be changed according to the physician's orders or office policy and procedure manual. If the sensitivity or gain is changed, this must be noted on the ECG before it goes into the medical record.

 **CHECKPOINT QUESTION**

10. Which three waves represent a cardiac cycle on an ECG?

## Holter Monitor

In many instances, an ECG that records the electrical activity of the heart for a brief moment in the medical office does not reveal cardiac problems. For diagnosis of intermittent cardiac arrhythmias and dysfunctions, a monitor that records for at least 24 hours is used. The Holter monitor is small and portable and can be worn comfortably for long periods without interfering with daily activities (Fig. 32-12). It may be set to record continuously or only when the patient presses a record button when feeling symptoms. This record button is also known as an "incident" or "event" button. When applying the Holter monitor, you must instruct the patient to keep a diary of daily activities. The physician will interpret the ECG tracing recorded by the Holter monitor and compare these findings with activities recorded in the diary to get an accurate view of what activities, if any, precipitate cardiac arrhythmias. Procedure 32-2 describes the steps for applying a Holter monitor.

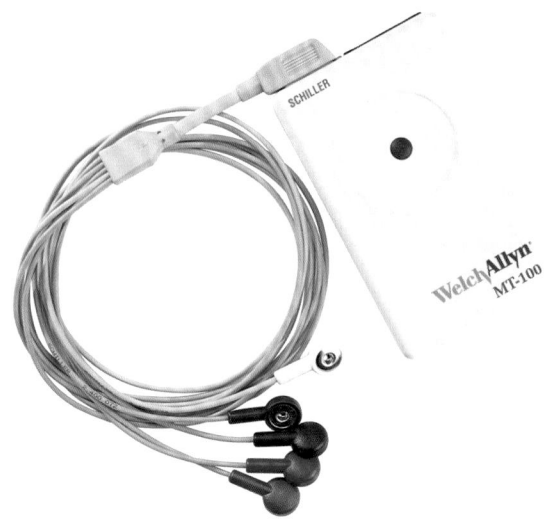

Figure 32-12 • A Holter Monitor. (Courtesy of Welch Allyn.)

### PATIENT EDUCATION

#### The Holter Monitor Patient Diary

A patient with a Holter monitor must keep a diary of daily activities. When the patient has symptoms, he or she depresses an incident (or event) button on the machine and then records in the diary the activity that caused the incident, including the symptoms. At intervals, the patient also records daily activities such as working quietly at a desk, driving a car, eating a meal, watching television, and sleeping. All activities must be noted, including elimination, sexual intercourse, anger, laughter, and so on. Some monitors are equipped with small tape recorders so the patient can keep an audio diary instead of a written one.

## Chest Radiography

Chest radiography provides valuable basic information about the anatomic location and gross structures of the heart, great vessels, and lungs. It also aids in the evaluation of such disorders as CHF and pericardial effusions. Many patients with CHF have an enlarged heart, especially the ventricles, and pericardial effusions appear as white markings around the heart on the film. Many patients with chronic cardiac conditions also have pulmonary problems, and the chest film can be used to assess the lungs. Any abnormal swelling or growth of the heart or great vessels (aorta, inferior vena cava, superior vena cava, pulmonary arteries) can also be assessed.

## Cardiac Stress Test

To measure the response of the cardiac muscle to increased demands of oxygen, the physician may request a cardiac stress test. The heart is usually tested with the patient walking on a treadmill (Fig. 32-13) with periodic increases in the rate or angle of the walk or run, but it may also be done on a stationary bicycle. The patient is attached to an ECG monitor for constant tracing during the test, and the blood pressure is monitored before, during, and after the test. The test is performed according to the physician's orders, and the ECG is interpreted by the physician, but you may be responsible for attaching the electrodes, monitoring and recording the blood pressure, and assisting the physician in watching

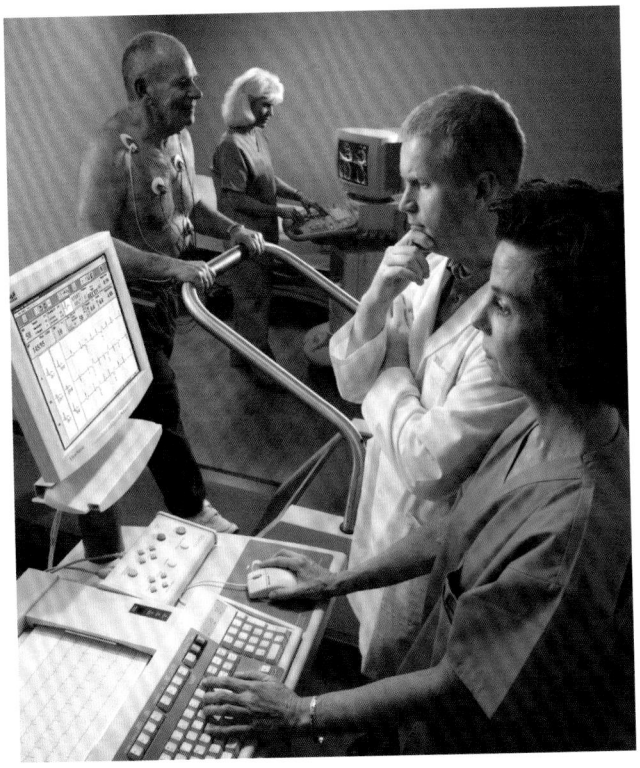

Figure 32-13 • Walking on a treadmill while monitoring the heart's activity with an ECG machine is one way to determine the ability of the heart to adapt to increased work during exercise. (Courtesy of Borgess Medical Center, Kalamazoo, MI.)

the patient for signs of light-headedness. Emergency resuscitation equipment should be available in case of cardiac or respiratory difficulties. This test may indicate the need for further cardiac testing. The cardiac stress test may be done as part of a routine physical examination in adults without symptoms or as a diagnostic tool for patients who have intermittent periods of angina pectoris or **palpitations**.

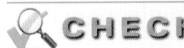

## CHECKPOINT QUESTION

11. What is the purpose of a cardiac stress test?

## Echocardiography

An echocardiogram, or echo, uses sound waves generated by a small device called a transducer. These waves travel through the cardiac chambers, walls, and valves and are transmitted back to a screen, where they can be viewed and interpreted. Echocardiograms help the physician to diagnose suspected or known valvular disease in adults and children. Echocardiograms also aid in diagnosing the severity of heart failure and **cardiomyopathy**. In addition, this test can be used to detect injuries to the heart in patients with trauma. Only the most specialized cardiac medical offices have the equipment and personnel (ultrasonographers) to obtain echocardiographs. In most instances, your role is to schedule the outpatient procedure and give the patient any instructions required by the facility. Usually, no patient preparations are required for echocardiography.

 **COG** TRIAGE

While working in a medical office, the following three situations occur:

A. A 29-year-old woman has been seen by the physician, who orders application of a Holter monitor. She also needs instruction on the importance of completing the diary.

B. A 62-year-old woman needs an ECG. She is complaining of heaviness in her chest.

C. A 17-year-old patient and his mother have just arrived in the office with written orders from an orthopedic surgeon that he needs a "stat preop" ECG. The patient is scheduled for knee surgery in the morning.

**How do you sort these patients? Who do you see first? Second? Third?**

Do the ECG for patient B first. Her chest heaviness may be due to a cardiac problem, and the physician should assess this ECG immediately. See patient A next, since she has been waiting. After applying the Holter monitor and explaining the diary, do the ECG for patient C. Every surgeon has standard orders for various tests he or she wants completed before doing surgery. ECGs are commonly ordered and read by a cardiologist or internist before a surgical procedure. Although the written order is written as stat, the test can be done as soon as possible and convenient.

## Cardiac Catheterization and Coronary Arteriography

Cardiac catheterization is a common invasive procedure used to help diagnose or treat conditions affecting the coronary arterial circulation. It may be performed on patients with shortness of breath, angina, dizziness, palpitations, fluttering in the chest, rapid heartbeat, and other cardiovascular symptoms to determine the severity or cause of the problem. It is often indicated after a cardiac stress test or echocardiogram reveals an abnormality. This procedure is not done in the medical office, but the medical assistant may be responsible for scheduling diagnostic cardiac catheterizations at a local outpatient facility or hospital and giving the patient any instructions required by the outpatient facility. If the procedure is for treatment, it must be done at an inpatient facility that has immediate access to open heart surgical equipment and personnel in the event of an emergency.

During the catheterization, the physician, usually a cardiologist, inserts a flexible tube into a blood vessel in either the arm or the groin and gently guides it toward the heart. When the catheter is in place, coronary arteriography is performed by injecting contrast medium, revealing the heart's chambers, valves, great vessels, and coronary arteries on a monitor. If atherosclerotic plaques are found, an angioplasty may be performed or scheduled for later (see Box 32-2).

## CHECKPOINT QUESTION

12. How is the echocardiography obtained?

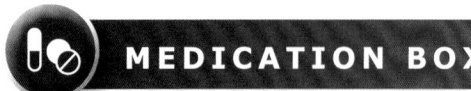

## MEDICATION BOX

### Commonly Prescribed Cardiovascular System Medications

*Note: The generic name of the drug is listed first and is written in all lowercase letters. Brand names are in parentheses, and the first letter is capitalized.*

| | | |
|---|---|---|
| amlodipine (Norvasc) | Tablets: 2.5 mg, 5 mg, 10 mg | Antianginal; antihypertensive |
| atenolol (Tenormin) | Tablets: 25 mg to 100 mg | Antihypertensive |
| carvedilol (Coreg) | Tablets: 3.125 mg to 25 mg | Antihypertensive |
| digoxin (Lanoxin) | Tablets: 0.125 mg, 0.25 mg | Inotropic |
| diltiazem hydrochloride (Cardizem) | Capsules (extended release): 60 mg to 420 mg<br>Tablets: 30 mg to 120 mg | Antianginal; antihypertensive |
| enalapril (Vasotec) | Tablets: 2.5 mg to 20 mg | Antihypertensive |
| ezetimibe (Zetia) | Tablets: 10 mg | Antilipemic |
| furosemide (Lasix) | Tablets: 20 mg to 80 mg | Diuretic; antihypertensive |
| gemfibrozil (Lopid) | Tablets: 600 mg | Antilipemic |
| hydrochlorothiazide (Microzide) | Tablets: 12.5 mg to 100 mg<br>Capsules: 12.5 mg | Diuretic |
| lisinopril (Prinivil; Zestril) | Tablets: 2.5 mg to 40 mg | Antihypertensive |
| metoprolol succinate (Toprol XL) | Tablets: 25 mg to 200 mg | Antihypertensive |
| metoprolol tartrate (Lopressor) | Tablets: 25 mg to 100 mg | Antihypertensive |
| nadolol (Corgard) | Tablets: 20 mg to 160 mg | Antianginal; antihypertensive |
| nitroglycerin (Nitrostat, Nitro-Dur, Nitrolingual) | Capsules: 2.5 mg, 6.5 mg, 9 mg<br>Tablets (sublingual): 0.3 mg, 0.4 mg, 0.6 mg<br>Transdermal: 0.1 mg/hour to 0.8 mg/hour | Antianginal |
| pravastatin sodium (Pravachol) | Tablets: 10 mg to 80 mg | Antilipemic |
| propranolol (Inderal) | Tablets: 10 mg to 80 mg<br>Capsules (extended release): 60 mg to 160 mg | Antianginal; antihypertensive |
| ramipril (Altace) | Capsules: 1.25 mg to 10 mg | Antihypertensive |
| simvastatin (Zocor) | Tablets: 1.25 mg to 10 mg<br>Tablets: 5 mg to 80 mg | Antilipemic |
| verapamil hydrochloride (Calan; Isoptin SR) | Capsules (extended release): 100 mg to 300 mg<br>Tablets: 40 mg to 120 mg | Antianginal; antihypertensive |

 **ROLE-PLAYING ACTIVITY**

With cooperation from classmates or as assigned by your instructor, role-play the scenarios as if you are working with Abby Perez in the cardiology office (refer to the case study at the beginning of the chapter). A 19-year-old patient is seen in the office today for complaints of an "irregular" heart rate. He was referred to the office by his family practice physician who noticed this at his last physical examination appointment. The patient is an athlete and continues to run 5 miles every day after graduating from high school. He is anxious and asking many questions during the 12-lead ECG the physician has asked you to perform. His questions include why is his heartbeat irregular, is this dangerous, is he going to be able to continue running, and will this condition cause him to die suddenly. He has been researching "his condition" on the Internet. What would you say to these questions? Is there anything you can say or do to relieve his anxiety? Your instructor will give you additional information about this activity!

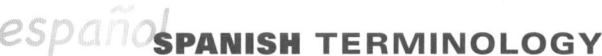 *español* **SPANISH TERMINOLOGY**

**¿Padece de presión alta?**
Do you have high blood pressure?

**¿Tiene dolor de pecho?**
Do you have chest pain?

**¿Ha sentido dolor en el brazo izquierdo?**
Have you ever had pain in the left arm?

**¿Se marea?**
Do you have dizzy spells?

**¿Siente palpitaciones?**
Is your heart pounding?

**¿Siente que se va a desmayar?**
Do you feel like you are going to pass out?

**¿Tiene historia familiar de enfermedades del corazón?**
Do you have family history of cardiac disease?

**Usted necesita un ecocardiograma, es como una fotografía del corazón y no duele nada.**
You need an echocardiogram, which is a picture of your heart and is painless.

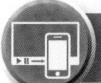 **MEDIA MENU**

**Student Resources on thePoint**
- **Animation:** Cardiac Cycle
- **Animation:** Congestive Heart Failure
- **Animation:** Hypertension
- **Animation:** Myocardial Blood Flow
- **Animation:** Stroke
- **Video:** Perform a Basic 12-Lead Electrocardiogram (Procedure 32-1)
- **Video:** Applying a Holter Monitor (Procedure 32-2)
- **CMA/RMA Certification Exam Review**

**Internet Resources**
**American Heart Association**
http://www.heart.org
**American Red Cross**
http://www.redcross.org
**National Safety Council**
http://www.nsc.org
**American College of Cardiology**
http://www.cardiosource.org/acc
**American Society of Hypertension, Inc.**
http://www.ash-us.org
**American Medical Association**
http://www.ama-assn.org

## EMR Activity

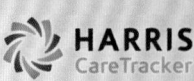

**Harris CareTracker** is a Web-based electronic medical record (EMR) application that you will use for the EMR activities included in this section at the end of each chapter. This application is actually used in physician offices but is provided to you through the publisher, Wolters Kluwer Health, to give you hands-on practice working with EMRs. Your instructor will have more information about accessing your username, log-in, and Quickstart guide.

Prerequisite Activities in Harris CareTracker

• The Getting Started and Quickstart documents and EMR Activities Step-by-Step Instructions are available at http://thePoint.lww.com/KronenbergerComp5e.

Activity Details

Document the following treatments ordered by Dr. White and performed by you today in the cardiology office:

1. Patient: Bobby Turner; 12-lead ECG performed
2. Patient: Sue Tamrick; Holter monitor applied

## Chapter Summary

- The circulatory system is a closed transport system kept in motion by the force of the beating heart.
- Nutrients are delivered to cells, cellular wastes are picked up, hormones are directed to target cells, and disease-fighting mechanisms are transported to areas of concern.
- The patient with undiagnosed cardiac disease may complain of lethargy, shortness of breath, or swelling of the extremities.
- Your responsibility includes:
  - Obtaining a complete cardiac history from all patients.
  - Assisting with the physical examination.
  - Performing or assisting with diagnostic testing.
  - Scheduling any cardiac procedures that are not performed in your medical office.
  - Obtaining necessary referrals from third-party payers when the physician concludes that the patient should be evaluated by a cardiologist.
  - Educating patients at every opportunity to prevent cardiac disease and offering support once a cardiac diagnosis has been made by the physician.

## Warm-Ups for Critical Thinking

1. Draw a diagram of the heart and a cardiac cycle as seen on the ECG. How would you explain an ECG to a patient? How would you assist the patient in relaxing for this procedure?
2. Compare and contrast the signs and symptoms of a CVA and a TIA. What kind of help does a patient need at home after a stroke? What language barriers might you encounter with the patient who has had a stroke, and how could you overcome these barriers?
3. Explain anemia and identify its symptoms. Why does anemia cause these symptoms? What dietary instructions should be given to a patient with iron deficiency anemia?
4. Prepare a patient education brochure that describes hypertension and its causes, symptoms, and possible treatments. In this brochure, explain why hypertension is often referred to as the silent killer.
5. Using a drug reference book, look up nitroglycerin. What is the usual dosage? How often can this drug be taken for the pain of angina?
6. Research the reason for why many patients with mitral valve disease are prescribed prophylactic antibiotics before dental procedures. What would you say to a patient who does not want to take these antibiotics before a dental procedure?

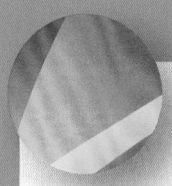

## PSY PROCEDURE 32-1

### Performing a 12-Lead Electrocardiogram

**PSY** Instruct and prepare a patient for a procedure or treatment; coach patients regarding disease prevention and treatment plans; coach patients appropriately considering cultural diversity, developmental life stage, and communication barriers; document patient care accurately in the medical record.

**Purpose:** Prepare a patient and obtain a 12-lead ECG that is free from artifacts

**Equipment:** Physician's order, patient record, ECG machine with cable and lead wires, ECG paper, disposable electrodes that contain coupling gel, gown and drape, skin preparation materials including a razor and antiseptic wipes

| STEPS | REASONS |
|---|---|
| 1. Wash your hands. | Hand washing aids infection control. |
| 2. Assemble the equipment. | Obtain all necessary equipment and supplies before beginning the procedure. |

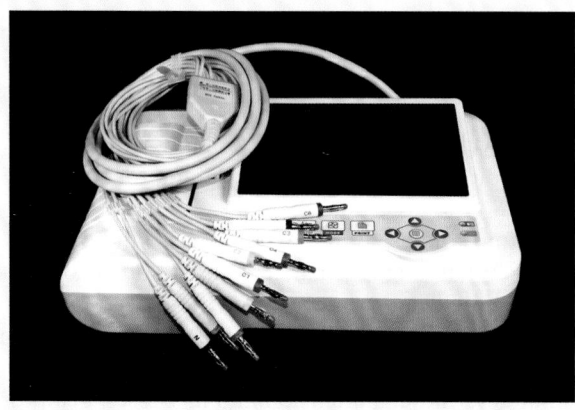

**Step 2.** The ECG machine.

| STEPS | REASONS |
|---|---|
| 3. Greet and identify the patient. Explain the procedure. | This avoids errors in treatment and helps gain compliance. |
| 4. Turn the machine on and enter appropriate data, including the patient's name and/or identification number, age, sex, height, weight, blood pressure, and medications. | This information will assist the physician in determining a proper diagnosis. |
| 5. Instruct the patient to disrobe above the waist, and provide a gown for privacy. Female patients should also be instructed to remove any nylons or tights. | Clothing may interfere with proper placement of the leads. Patients wearing pants do not have to remove them if they can be pulled up to expose the lower legs. |
| 6. Position the patient comfortably supine with pillows as needed for comfort. Drape the patient for warmth and privacy. | If the patient is uncomfortable, too cool, or improperly draped, movement is likely, which will result in artifacts on the ECG tracing. |
| 7. Prepare the skin as needed by wiping away skin oil and lotions with the antiseptic wipes or shaving any hair that will interfere with good contact between the skin and the electrodes. | Skin preparation ensures properly attached leads and helps avoid improper readings and lost time repeating the test. |

## PROCEDURE 32-1 (continued)

| STEPS | REASONS |
|---|---|
| **8.** Apply the electrodes snugly against the fleshy, muscular parts of the upper arms and lower legs according to the manufacturer's directions. Apply chest electrodes, $V_1$–$V_6$. | Electrodes that are not snug against the skin or are on bony prominences may cause improper reading and artifact. In case of an amputation or the otherwise inaccessible limb, place the electrode on the uppermost part of the existing extremity or on the anterior shoulder (upper extremity) and groin (lower extremity). |

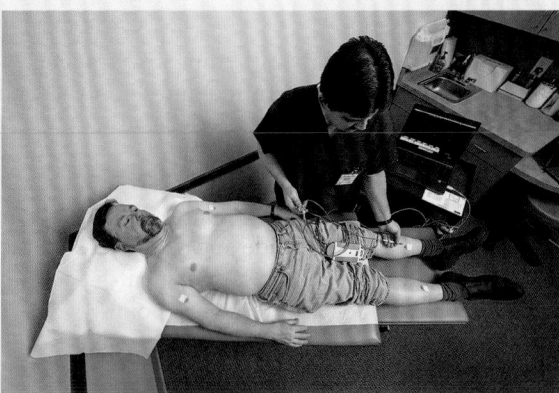

**A**

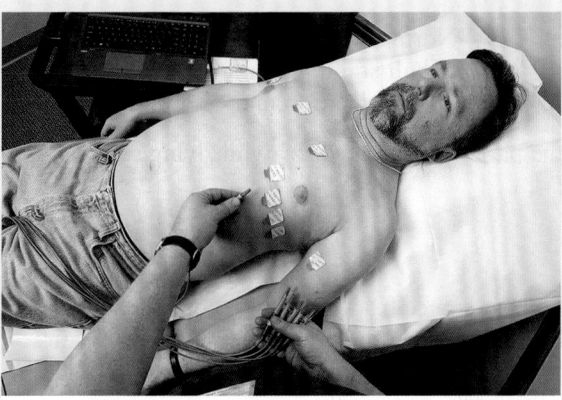

**B**

**Step 8.** (**A**) Applying limb electrodes. (**B**) Applying chest electrodes.

| STEPS | REASONS |
|---|---|
| **9.** Connect the lead wires securely according to the color-coded notations on the connectors (RA, LA, RL, LL, V1–V6). Untangle the wires before applying them to prevent electrical artifacts. Each lead must lie unencumbered along the contours of the patient's body to decrease the likelihood of artifacts. Double-check the placement. | Improperly placed leads will result in both time lost to an inaccurate reading and retesting. |

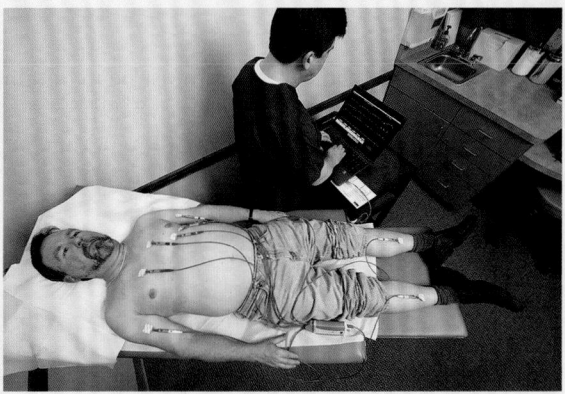

**Step 9.** The wires should lie along the contours of the patient's body.

(continues on page 846)

## PROCEDURE 32-1 (continued)

| STEPS | REASONS |
|---|---|
| 10. Determine the sensitivity, or gain, and paper speed settings on the ECG machine before running the test. Set sensitivity or gain on 1 and paper speed on 25 mm/second. | A sensitivity setting of 1 and a paper speed of 25 mm/second are necessary to obtain an accurate ECG. These settings should not be changed without a direct order from the physician and the changes noted on the final ECG tracing. |
| 11. Depress the automatic button on the ECG machine to obtain the 12-lead tracing. The machine will automatically move from one lead to the next without your intervention. | If the physician wants only a rhythm strip tracing, use the manual mode of operation and select the lead manually. |
| 12. When the tracing is complete and printed, check the ECG for artifacts and a standardization mark. | With sensitivity set on 1, the standardization mark should be 2 small squares wide and 10 small squares high. The standardization mark documents accuracy of operation and provides a reference point. |

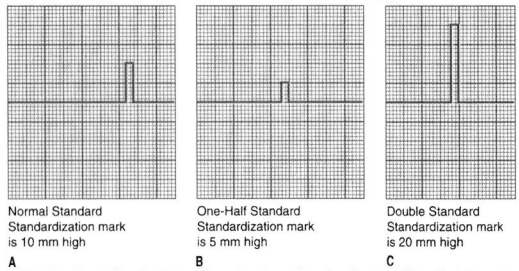

Normal Standard Standardization mark is 10 mm high
A

One-Half Standard Standardization mark is 5 mm high
B

Double Standard Standardization mark is 20 mm high
C

**Step 12.** (**A**) Normal standardization mark is 10 mm high. (**B**) One-half standardization mark is 5 mm high. (**C**) Double standardization mark is 20 mm high.

| STEPS | REASONS |
|---|---|
| 13. If the tracing is adequate, turn off the machine and remove and discard the electrodes. Assist the patient to a sitting position and help with dressing if needed. | Some patients become dizzy while lying supine. |
| 14. **AFF** Explain how to respond to a patient with dementia. | Solicit assistance from a caregiver or other staff member to help during the procedure. Give simple directions to the patient about what he or she should do. Speak clearly, not loudly. |
| 15. If a single-channel machine was used (each lead produced on a roll of paper, one lead at a time), carefully roll the ECG strip without using clips to secure the roll. This ECG must be mounted on 8- × 11-inch paper or a form before going into the medical record according to the office policy and procedure. | Folding the ECG tracing or applying clips may make marks on the surface, obscuring the reading. Special forms may be purchased specifically for mounting a single-channel ECG strip and placing it in the medical record. |
| 16. Wash your hands. | |
| 17. **AFF** Log into the electronic medical record (EMR) using your username and secure password OR obtain the paper medical record from a secure location and assure it is kept away from public access. Record the procedure. Your entry must include the date, time, and your name/credentials. | The integrity of the medical record must be maintained at all times to protect patient privacy. Procedures are considered not to have been done if they are not recorded. |

## PROCEDURE 32-1 (continued)

| STEPS | REASONS |
|---|---|
| 18. Place the printed results in the medical record or scan into the electronic medical record if appropriate. | |
| 19. Let the physician know that the ECG has been completed and is ready for review. | |

**Charting Example:**

*12/02/2016 9:45 AM Pre-employment 12-lead ECG obtained and placed in chart* _____
*A. Perez, CMA*

---

Note: *The medical assistant may sign his or her name in the patient record using only the "CMA" credential if the office has a signature log denoting the entire credential as "CMA(AAMA)."*

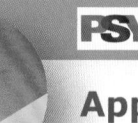

## PSY PROCEDURE 32-2

# Applying a Holter Monitor

**PSY** Instruct and prepare a patient for a procedure or treatment; coach patients regarding disease prevention and treatment plans; coach patients appropriately considering cultural diversity, developmental life stage, and communication barriers; document patient care accurately in the medical record.

**Purpose:** Prepare and instruct a patient on wearing a Holter monitor for continuous cardiac monitoring

**Equipment:** Physician's order, patient record, Holter monitor with appropriate lead wires, fresh batteries, carrying case with strap, disposable electrodes with coupling gel, adhesive tape, gown and drape, skin preparation materials including a razor and antiseptic wipes, diary

**Standard:** This procedure should take 10 minutes.

| STEPS | REASONS |
|---|---|
| 1. Wash your hands. | Hand washing aids infection control. |
| 2. Assemble the equipment. | Obtain all necessary equipment and supplies before beginning the procedure. |
| 3. Greet and identify the patient. Explain the procedure, reminding the patient that it is important to carry out all normal activities for the duration of the test. | Identifying the patient and explaining the procedure avoid errors in treatment and help gain compliance. A normal routine is essential to allow the physician to identify areas of concern. |
| 4. Explain the purpose of the incident diary, emphasizing the need to carry it at all times during the test. Ask the patient to remove all clothing from the waist up and put on the gown, and drape appropriately for privacy. | The chest must be exposed for proper placement of the electrodes. |
| 5. With the patient seated, prepare the skin for electrode attachment. Provide privacy. Shave the skin if necessary and cleanse with antiseptic wipes. | Shaving and cleansing the skin will improve adherence of the adhesive on the electrodes. |
| 6. Expose the adhesive backing of the electrodes and follow the manufacturer's instructions to attach each firmly. Apply the electrodes at the specified sites:<br>**A.** Right manubrium border<br>**B.** Left manubrium border<br>**C.** Right sternal border at the fifth rib<br>**D.** Fifth rib at the anterior axillary line<br>**E.** Right lower rib cage over the cartilage as a ground lead | The electrodes will be worn by the patient for up to 24 hours and must be secure. |

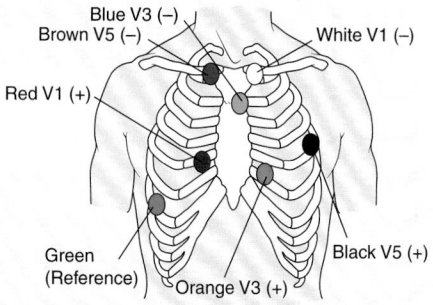

**Step 6.** (A) Sites for Holter electrodes. (B) Place the Holter electrodes as directed by the manufacturer.

## PROCEDURE 32-2 (continued)

| STEPS | REASONS |
|---|---|
| 7. Check the security of the attachments. | Electrodes that are not securely attached will result in poor tracings. |
| 8. Position electrode connectors down toward the patient's feet. Attach the lead wires and secure with adhesive tape. | Application of adhesive tape over the connections will help ensure that the leads do not work loose during the day.

**Step 8.** Securely tape each electrode. Tape the lead wires to the patient's body. |
| 9. Connect the cable and run a baseline ECG by hooking the Holter to the ECG machine with the cable hookup. | Check for accurate function of the Holter before the patient leaves. |
| 10. Assist the patient to dress carefully with the cable extending through the garment opening. Clothing that buttons down the front is convenient. | This prevents pulling and strain on the leads. |
| 11. Plug the cable into the recorder and mark the diary. If needed, explain the purpose of the diary to the patient again. Give instructions for a return appointment to evaluate the recording and the diary. | Keeping the diary is an important part of wearing the Holter monitor and will assist the physician in an accurate diagnosis. |
| 12. Wash your hands. | |
| 13. **AFF** Log into the electronic medical record (EMR) using your username and secure password OR obtain the paper medical record from a secure location and assure it is kept away from public access. Record the procedure. Your entry must include the date, time, patient education given, and your name/credentials. | The integrity of the medical record must be maintained at all times to protect patient privacy.

Procedures are considered not to have been done if they are not recorded. |

**Charting Example:**
*11/28/2016 1:00 PM Holter monitor ordered and applied; baseline ECG done. Oral and written instructions given regarding care and use of monitor. Instructions for completion of diary also given. Pt. verbalized understanding of use of monitor and completion of diary. To RTO tomorrow PM for removal of the monitor*
——————————————————————————————————— *R. Steele, CMA*

**Note:** *The medical assistant may sign his or her name in the patient record using only the "CMA" credential if the office has a signature log denoting the entire credential as "CMA(AAMA)."*

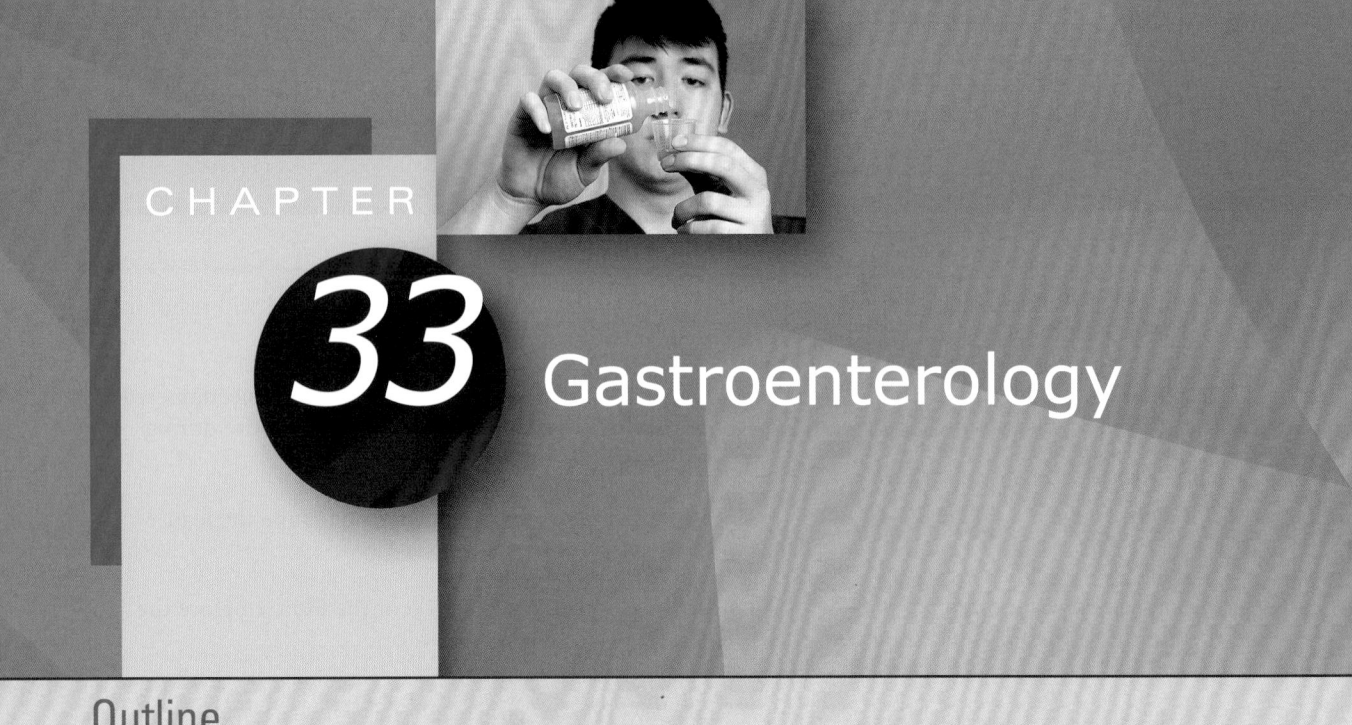

# 33 Gastroenterology

## Outline

## Learning Outcomes

### COG Cognitive Domain*

1. Spell key terms
2. Define medical terms and abbreviations related to all body systems
3. Describe structural organization of the human body
4. List major organs in each body system
5. Identify the anatomical location of major organs in each body system
6. Describe the normal function of each body system
7. Identify common pathology related to each body system including signs, symptoms, and etiology
   a. List and describe common disorders of the alimentary canal and accessory organs
   b. Identify and explain the purpose of common procedures and tests associated with the gastrointestinal system
8. Describe the roles and responsibilities of the medical assistant in diagnosing and treating disorders of the gastrointestinal system

### PSY Psychomotor Domain*

1. Assist with colon procedures (Procedure 33-1)
   a. Instruct and prepare a patient for a procedure or treatment

b. Coach patients appropriately considering cultural diversity, developmental life stage, and communication barriers
   c. Coach patients regarding disease prevention and treatment plans
   d. Document patient care accurately in the medical record
2. Test stool specimen for occult blood: Guaiac method (Procedure 33-2)
   a. Obtain specimens and perform CLIA-waived microbiology tests
   b. Differentiate between normal and abnormal results
   c. Document patient care accurately in the medical record

### AFF Affective Domain*

1. Incorporate critical thinking skills when performing patient assessment
2. Incorporate critical thinking skills when performing patient care
3. Show awareness of a patient's concerns related to the procedure being performed
4. Demonstrate empathy, active listening, and nonverbal communication
5. Demonstrate respect for individual diversity including gender, race, religion, age, economic status, and appearance

6. *Explain to a patient the rationale for performance of a procedure*
7. *Demonstrate sensitivity to patient rights*
8. *Protect the integrity of the medical record*

*Note: AAMA/CAAHEP 2015 Standards are italicized.*

### ABHES Competencies

1. Assist the physician with the regimen of diagnostic and treatment modalities as they relate to each body system

2. Prepare the patient for examinations and treatments
3. Recognize and understand various treatment protocols
4. Comply with federal, state, and local health laws and regulations
5. Communicate on the recipient's level of comprehension
6. Serve as a liaison between the physician and others
7. Show empathy and impartiality when dealing with patients
8. Document accurately

## Key Terms

| | | | |
|---|---|---|---|
| anorexia | hepatomegaly | melena | stomatitis |
| ascites | hepatotoxins | metabolism | turgor |
| dysphagia | insufflator | obturator | |
| guaiac | leukoplakia | peristalsis | |
| hematemesis | malocclusion | sclerotherapy | |

## Case Study

*S*haron Clay, CMA (AAMA), works at the gastroenterology specialty office at Great Falls Medical Center. There are three physicians in this specialty office, and Sharon works for Dr. Damien White. Today, Dr. White is seeing several patients who have been diagnosed with chronic conditions such as gastroesophageal reflux disease (GERD), ulcerative colitis, and Crohn disease. Several patients to be seen today are morbidly obese and are going to be having weight-loss surgery. What is GERD, and what are the signs and symptoms of this disorder? How are ulcerative colitis and Crohn disease different? What surgical procedures are performed to assist with weight loss in a patient who is obese? These and other questions regarding disorders of the gastrointestinal system are addressed in this chapter.

The gastrointestinal (GI) system, or tract, is responsible for the ingestion, digestion, transportation, and elimination of the food we eat (Fig. 33-1). Nutrients are broken down by the action of digestive enzymes into units that can be absorbed through the walls of the GI system into the circulatory and lymphatic systems. This process starts when something is put into the mouth, chewed, and mixed with the enzymes in saliva. Through **peristalsis**, food is pushed along the GI tract, further breaking it down into segments and mixing it with enzymes to hasten the breakdown into nutrients. **Metabolism** is the breakdown of food into usable units through these

physical and chemical changes. Any unused food material is eliminated as waste from the GI system as feces.

Disorders of the GI system may affect the alimentary canal, also called the GI tract, or accessory organs such as the liver, gallbladder, and pancreas. This chapter describes common disorders of the GI system and the accessory organs, diagnostic procedures, and your role as a medical assistant working with patients with GI disorders. Although the physician who specializes in disorders of the GI system is the gastroenterologist, medical assistants working in other offices, such as family practice and internal medicine, often encounter patients with disorders of this body system.

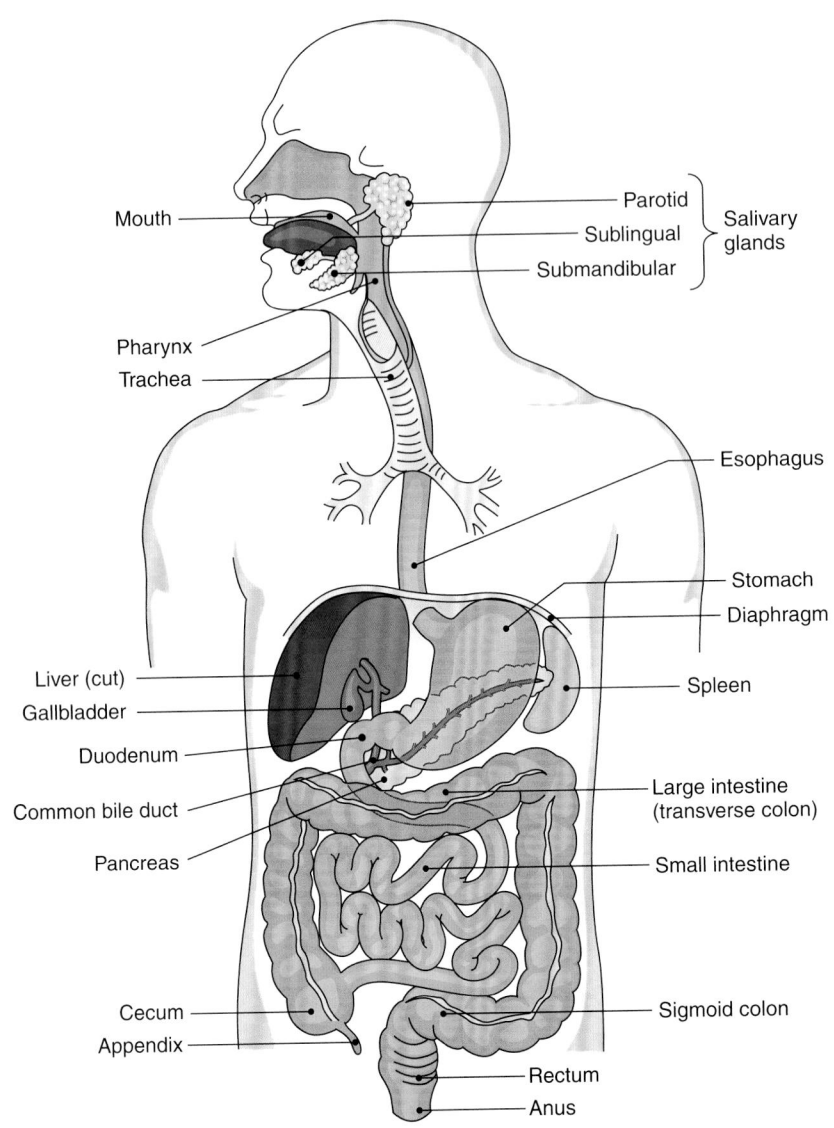

**Figure 33-1** • The digestive system. (Reprinted from Cohen BJ. *Memmler's The Human Body in Health and Disease*, 11th ed. Philadelphia, PA: Lippincott Williams & Wilkins, 2009, with permission.)

# COMMON GASTROINTESTINAL DISORDERS

## Mouth Disorders

Although disorders of the teeth, gums, and oral cavity are typically diagnosed and treated by the dentist, patients requiring a referral to a dentist or oral surgeon may be seen first in the medical office. Physicians and other health care professionals should be aware of these disorders and their importance to the nutrition, digestion, and overall health status of the patient. Your role includes taking an accurate medical history, including inquiring about the condition of the oral cavity and teeth, making referrals as ordered by the physician, and educating patients about the care of the gums and teeth to prevent health problems and loss of teeth.

## Caries

Dental caries (tooth decay) is the most widespread disease of the oral cavity. Bacteria allowed to remain on the teeth erode the enamel and allow infection to reach the inner portions of the tooth. Factors that may contribute to the development of dental caries include a poor diet, inadequate dental hygiene, and **malocclusion**, which is abnormal contact between the upper teeth and the lower teeth. Prevention of dental caries includes consuming a balanced diet low in sugars, good oral hygiene as prescribed by the dentist, and frequent professional dental care. Treatment may include drilling the dental caries and replacing the space with a filling or extraction of the affected teeth. Because dental caries can cause discomfort with chewing or biting, they may affect nutrition and ultimately digestion and the overall health of the patient.

# Stomatitis

**Stomatitis,** an inflammation of the oral mucosa, may be caused by a virus, bacteria, or fungus. The two most common forms are herpetic stomatitis, caused by the herpes simplex virus, and candidiasis, caused by the fungus **Candida albicans.**

Herpes simplex is usually self-limiting after the initial exposure to the virus. The virus is usually transmitted hand to mouth, mouth to mouth, or by vector (e.g., shared drinking glasses or eating utensils). The infection presents as a painful sore on the mucosa of the mouth (commonly called a *canker sore*) or on the lips (commonly called a *fever blister* or *cold sore*). After the initial infection, the virus lies dormant for long periods, with exacerbations during illness, stress, overexposure to the sun, or other trigger. Although there is no cure for herpes simplex, palliative measures such as ointments or creams may be purchased over the counter to relieve the discomfort.

**C. albicans,** formerly called **Monilia albicans,** is an opportunistic yeast or fungus. This organism is always present in the mouth but is kept in check by other normal microorganisms found in the mouth including bacteria. When the normal bacterial balance in the mouth is altered, *C. albicans* microorganisms multiply, causing an infection that appears as a white substance covering the oral cavity and tongue. Factors that can upset the balance of these microorganisms in the mouth include the use of broad-spectrum antibiotics that kill many bacteria throughout the body, including the mouth, allowing the opportunistic organisms to grow without control. In babies, the disease is called *thrush* and commonly is caused by a favorable environment for the growth of *C. albicans*, as milk changes the pH of the mouth. In adults or infants, treatment with an antifungal agent usually cures the disorder and restores the balance of microbes in the mouth.

 **CHECKPOINT QUESTION**

1. A patient seen in the gastroenterology office today has been diagnosed with stomatitis. Sharon Clay, the medical assistant in this office, knows that there are two common causes for this disorder. What are the two most common causes of stomatitis?

# Gingivitis

Gingivitis is an inflammation of the gingiva, or gums. It may lead to periodontitis, or inflammation, and possible destruction of the supporting structures of the teeth, including the gingiva, periodontal ligament, and mandibular or maxillary bone. In Americans, more teeth are lost to gum disease than to tooth decay. Good oral hygiene and frequent dental care help prevent premature loss of teeth. Once diagnosed, gingivitis is usually treated with an antibiotic.

# Oral Cancers

Cancers of the oral cavity are common, especially among individuals who use tobacco products. The constant irritation of the tobacco causes white spots or patches, called **leukoplakia,** to form on the oral mucosa, particularly the lips and tongue. These lesions have clearly defined borders and frequently become malignant. Treatment includes surgery or chemical agents such as radiation or chemotherapy. Although cancer of the lips usually responds well to radiation or surgery, cancers of the margins of the tongue metastasize quickly and are commonly difficult to treat effectively.

 **CHECKPOINT QUESTION**

2. When discussing gingivitis with a patient, how would Sharon explain the way gingivitis can be prevented?

# Esophageal Disorders

## Hiatal Hernia

Hiatal hernia, or diaphragmatic hernia, occurs when the stomach protrudes up into the diaphragm through a weakened or enlarged cardiac sphincter at the bottom of the esophagus, allowing a portion of the stomach to slide up into the chest cavity. This type of hernia is a common condition that frequently affects people over age 40 years. Weight gain, either recent or prolonged, can be a contributing factor. Normally, the cardiac sphincter, a muscle that separates the end of the esophagus from the beginning of the stomach, prevents gastroesophageal reflux, or backflow of gastric acids from the stomach into the esophagus. The presence of a hiatal hernia enables the stomach acid to backflow into the esophagus, causing considerable discomfort, including indigestion and epigastric pain in the upper abdomen (Fig. 33-2).

The symptoms of a hiatal hernia include abdominal pain and indigestion, especially after eating. Diagnosis is made by taking a careful medical history, chest radiographs, barium swallow, or endoscopy. Medical treatment is usually preferred to surgical intervention because surgically corrected hiatal hernias frequently recur. Medical interventions include diet modifications such as small, frequent meals with no food for at least 2 hours before bedtime. In addition, the physician may order antacids, weight loss, elevating the head of the bed when sleeping, and drug therapy to increase the tone of the cardiac sphincter.

Constant exposure to gastric acid from gastroesophageal reflux can lead to esophagitis, a condition that resembles abraded tissue along the lining of the esophagus. Constant irritation of the lining of the esophagus, also known as *Barrett esophagus*, may lead to malignancy. Patients with Barrett esophagus have a 30% to 40%

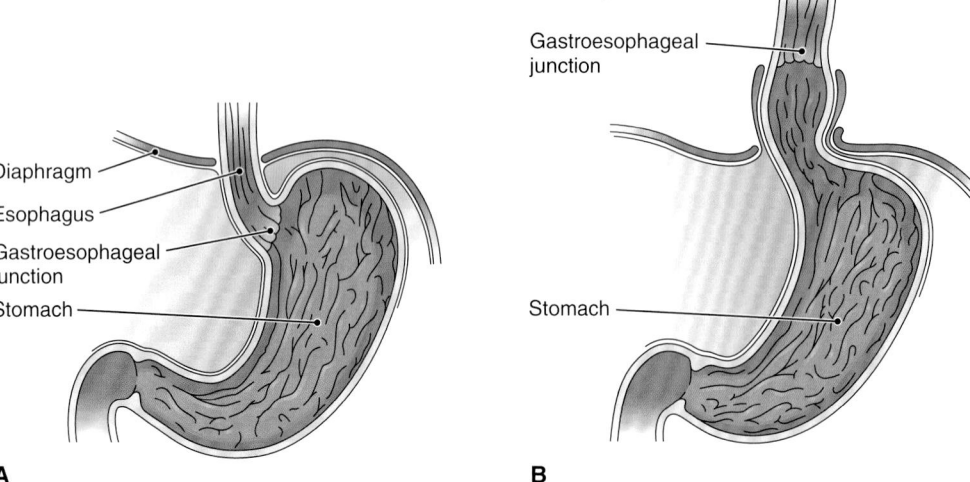

**Figure 33-2** • **(A)** Normal. **(B)** Hiatal hernia. The stomach protrudes through the diaphragm into the thoracic cavity, raising the level of the junction between the esophagus and the stomach. (Reprinted from Cohen BJ, Wood DL. *Memmler's The Human Body in Health and Disease*, 11th ed. Philadelphia, PA: Lippincott Williams & Wilkins, 2009, with permission.)

chance of developing adenocarcinoma. If the source of irritation is gastroesophageal reflux, it will be diagnosed and treated much the same as a hiatal hernia.

## Gastroesophageal Reflux Disease

Patients who complain of any type of chest pain, including heartburn, should be assessed immediately because the chest pain of gastroesophageal reflux disease (GERD) may be similar to the chest pain of a patient having cardiac problems. In addition to the chest pain, signs and symptoms of myocardial involvement can include the following:

- Shortness of breath
- Nausea or vomiting
- Pain that spreads from the chest to the jaw, back, or arms

Chest pain that is not cardiac may be diagnosed by the physician as GERD, a chronic disorder characterized by discomfort in the chest (heartburn) due to the backflow of gastric contents into the esophagus. This disorder is caused by a weak lower esophageal sphincter that normally closes after food is swallowed, keeping the material in the stomach. The symptoms of GERD include the following:

- Frequent heartburn or indigestion relieved by antacids
- Hoarseness or laryngitis
- Sore throat
- A feeling of a lump in the throat
- Chronic cough

A thorough examination by the physician plus endoscopic and radiologic procedures is usually necessary to diagnose GERD. Once diagnosed, this disorder can be treated with appropriate medications. Untreated, GERD can lead to erosion of the esophagus and complications such as esophageal bleeding. GERD may also be the cause of esophageal cancers in some patients.

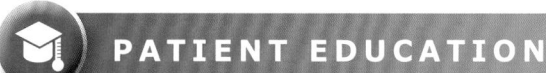

### PATIENT EDUCATION

## Preventing Gastric Reflux

- Avoid spicy foods and chocolate, especially in the evening.
- Limit caffeine.
- Maintain optimum weight.
- Avoid overeating.
- Wait 1 hour after eating before exercising.
- Do not eat just before going to bed.
- Do not lie down just after eating.
- Stop smoking.
- Place blocks, bricks, or a stack of books under the legs of the bed to elevate the head, chest, and abdomen approximately 12 inches.
- See the physician if symptoms persist.

## Esophageal Varices

Varicose veins (varices) of the esophagus result from pressure within the esophageal veins. This condition is commonly seen in patients diagnosed with cirrhosis of the liver. Since drainage from the portal vein is impaired by the liver damage, the veins of the esophagus become distended, resulting in varices. The most common and dangerous problem that results from esophageal varices is hemorrhaging if the distended veins rupture. Before a rupture occurs, the treatment of choice is **sclerotherapy**, which uses a chemical agent to cause fibrosing (hardening) of the area around the varices, preventing hemorrhaging. In the event of esophageal hemorrhage, the patient should be transported immediately to the emergency room, where pressure tubes can be applied directly to the varices to control the bleeding.

## Esophageal Cancer

Cancer of the esophagus is most common among older men and is usually fatal. Predisposing factors for this type of cancer include chronic gastroesophageal reflux, smoking, and drinking alcohol. The malignancy narrows the lumen of the esophagus and causes **dysphagia** (difficulty swallowing). As the mass enlarges, swallowing solid food may become extremely painful. Vomiting and weight loss occur as the symptoms progress. A barium swallow with fluoroscopy outlines the lesion, and esophagoscopy with biopsy confirms the diagnosis. If the disease is local, surgical resection, chemotherapy, and radiation are the therapies of choice. No treatment has proven satisfactory, however, and the survival rates are very low.

 **CHECKPOINT QUESTION**

3. What is a hiatal hernia, and how can it affect the esophagus?

# Stomach Disorders

## Gastritis

Gastritis, an inflammation of the lining of the stomach, can be acute or chronic. The most common causes include irritants such as alcohol and certain drugs, including aspirin and nonsteroidal anti-inflammatory medications (NSAIDs). The bacterium *Helicobacter pylori*, also often implicated, is presumed to enter the body through food contaminated with infected fecal material (fecal–oral route) or from eating or drinking from a utensil also used by someone who is infected with the bacteria (oral–oral route). It resides in the mucous lining of the stomach and secretes enzymes that attack the mucous membrane.

Gastritis can cause significant oozing of blood and may result in a positive test for occult (hidden) blood in the stool. In elderly patients, sufficient blood loss can result in anemia. Signs and symptoms of gastritis include evidence of GI bleeding, epigastric discomfort, nausea, and vomiting. Diagnosis is usually made by obtaining a careful and complete history and direct visualization of the gastric mucosa through an endoscopic procedure known as a gastroscopy. Treatment usually involves eliminating the irritant, restoring the proper gastric acidity, and administering antibiotics as prescribed by the physician.

## Peptic Ulcers

Ulcers in the GI tract are erosions or sores left by sloughed tissues. These erosions can expose small blood vessels and produce bleeding and pain. Peptic ulcers occur from the exposure of the lining of the stomach and first part of the small intestine (duodenum) to hydrochloric acid (HCl), a caustic chemical produced and secreted by the lining of the stomach that may cause erosion if too much is excreted. As the mucosa erodes, the patient has abdominal pain that intensifies during peristalsis, especially after eating. As the erosions and mucosa become more irritated, the ulcers bleed. The bleeding may range from slight oozing to life-threatening hemorrhage. Heavy bleeding will lead to **melena** (black tarry stools) or **hematemesis** (vomiting blood). Ulcers in the upper GI tract may perforate into the abdominal cavity with life-threatening consequences such as hypovolemic shock and peritonitis (Box 33-1). Chronic ulcerative conditions may also progress to malignancies.

The causes of peptic or gastric ulcers may include the use of chemicals that irritate the gastric mucosa, including aspirin, NSAIDs, and alcohol. Many gastric ulcers are also caused by an infection with **H. pylori**, which can be treated effectively with an antibiotic. Overproduction of gastric HCl also irritates the gastric mucosa and may produce erosions. Gastric acid production is under nerve and hormonal control and increases during times of emotional stress. Diagnosis of an ulcer is similar to the diagnosis of gastritis, including a thorough history and possibly endoscopic examination. The prescribed treatment for ulcers is avoiding the irritants causing the erosion, limiting the production of hydrogen by the gastric cells to neutralize the acid in the stomach, and an antibiotic as prescribed. Surgery to cut or disconnect the vagus nerve (vagotomy), which also reduces the secretion of HCl, may be performed if methods to decrease production of gastric acid are ineffective in treating the ulcer.

---

**BOX 33-1 Peritonitis**

Peritonitis, an infection of the lining of the abdominal cavity, is a serious complication of several GI disorders that may occur if contents of the intestines or other organs leak into the abdominal cavity. The patient will be acutely ill and will have a fever and elevated white blood cell count. In addition, the patient will be complaining of severe abdominal pain. Treatment of peritonitis requires hospitalization with intravenous antibiotics and continuous monitoring of the patient for signs of septic shock. This condition can quickly become fatal if not treated appropriately and aggressively.

## Gastric Cancer

Gastric cancer has no known cause, although smoking, excessive alcohol intake, ingesting foods high in preservatives, and genetic predisposition may contribute. Gastric cancer spreads rapidly to adjacent organs (the liver and pancreas) and throughout the peritoneal cavity. Signs and symptoms include chronic indigestion, weight loss, **anorexia**, anemia, and fatigue. The patient may have hematemesis with bright blood or coffee ground vomitus with dark blood. There may also be dark, bloody stools.

Diagnosis of gastric cancer requires an upper GI series with fluoroscopy, fiberoptic gastroscopy, and biopsy of the lesion or tumor. The extent of the disease can be determined by computed tomography (CT) and biopsy of the suspected metastatic sites, including adjacent organs. Surgery to remove the lesion may range from a subtotal gastric resection (removal of part of the stomach) to a total gastrectomy (removal of the entire stomach). If the cancer has metastasized, other organs may be removed, and radiation and chemotherapy may be necessary.

 **CHECKPOINT QUESTION**

4. What microorganism is found to be the cause of peptic ulcers in some patients?

# Intestinal Disorders

## Gastroenteritis

Gastroenteritis is general inflammation of the stomach, small intestine, and/or colon. This condition is caused by ingesting food or water that contains bacteria, viruses, parasites, or irritating agents such as spices. Food allergies and reactions to certain medications, such as antibiotics, may also inflame these organs. Symptoms include abdominal pain and cramping, nausea, vomiting, diarrhea, and fever.

The symptoms of gastroenteritis are self-limiting in most adults, usually lasting a few hours to a couple of days. However, because of the dehydration that can accompany the diarrhea and vomiting, gastroenteritis may be life threatening in the elderly, young children, and persons with diabetes mellitus. Treatment is palliative; it includes reducing the work of the GI tract by limiting food intake; treating the nausea, vomiting, and diarrhea; and maintaining the fluid balance by hydrating the body as needed. In severe cases, intravenous fluids must be administered to prevent dehydration and death, especially in the young and the elderly. If the cause of the inflammation is a bacterial or parasitic infection, an antibiotic or antiparasitic medication may be prescribed once the causative microorganism has been identified through a stool culture and analysis.

## Duodenal Ulcers

Ulcerative lesions in the duodenum are often caused by exposure to highly corrosive gastric acid that is secreted by the stomach or other irritants that pass through the pylorus to the small intestine. Unlike the stomach, the duodenum has a normally alkaline pH, and the mucosa is not as well protected as the gastric mucosa. When food material passes through the pylorus and brings excessive acid or other irritants with it, an ulcer may form in the duodenum. As with the peptic ulcer, an overproduction of gastric acid may arise from ingestion of highly spicy foods or from overproduction of stress hormones, which also increases production of gastric acid. Treatment for duodenal ulcers is limiting or avoiding the irritating factors and reducing gastric acidity. If these measures are not successful, surgery may be an option. Ulcers in the duodenum left untreated may perforate the lining of the small intestine or may progress to cancerous lesions.

## Malabsorption Syndromes

Malabsorption syndromes prevent the normal absorption of certain nutrients through the walls of the small intestines. Commonly, fat is not absorbed. A sign that a patient has a problem with malabsorption of fats includes stools that are frothy and pale. Because fat is necessary for the metabolism of vitamins A, D, E, and K, patients with this disorder require supplemental vitamin therapy.

Celiac sprue is a malabsorption syndrome marked by intolerance to gluten, a protein found in wheat and wheat by-products. Celiac sprue can develop at any stage of life and often causes diarrhea high in fat. The cause of celiac sprue is not known, but it runs in families, suggesting a genetic factor.

Regardless of the nutrient involved in a patient with malabsorption syndrome, the patient is typically treated by addressing the suspected causes and avoiding or replacing the malabsorbed substances.

 **CHECKPOINT QUESTION**

5. How are peptic and duodenal ulcers different?

 **PATIENT EDUCATION**

### Bariatric Surgery to Treat Obesity

Bariatrics is the study of morbid obesity. A popular surgical procedure to treat obesity is gastric bypass. Here are a few facts about this procedure:

• According to the American Society for Metabolic and Bariatric Surgery (http://www.asmbs.org), candidates for the surgery must be severely obese and have failed to lose weight with other methods.

- Candidates for gastric bypass surgery must have either a body mass index greater than 40 (approximately 80 to 100 pounds over the ideal weight for height) or significant medical problems associated with being overweight.
- The abdomen is incised, and the stomach is reduced to about the size of a thumb. The large remainder of the stomach is bypassed, and the new, smaller stomach is attached directly to the small intestine.
- The surgery comes with risks and requires lifestyle changes. Anemia and nutritional deficiencies are long-term risks that must be monitored and prevented or corrected.
- Since weight reduction after this procedure is often quick and dramatic, patients should be encouraged to begin an exercise program following the surgery as indicated by the surgeon.

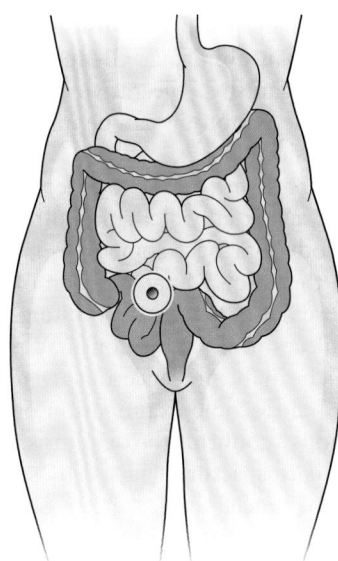

**Figure 33-3** • An ileostomy. The shaded portion indicates the section of the bowel that has been removed or is inactive. (Modified from Cohen BJ. *Medical Terminology: An Illustrated Guide*, Philadelphia, PA: Lippincott Williams & Wilkins, 2003, with permission.)

## Crohn Disease

Crohn disease, also known as **regional enteritis**, is an inflammation of the deep lining of the bowel ranging from very mild to severe and debilitating. The cause of Crohn disease is unclear, but it is thought to be an autoimmune disorder with a possible genetic link. Crohn disease can affect the small bowel and the colon but is more common in the area of the ileocecal valve. The bowel walls become inflamed, and the lymph nodes enlarge, leading to edema of the bowel wall. When the lining of the bowel is swollen, the fluid from the intestinal contents cannot be absorbed, causing diarrhea and cramping, which may lead to more irritation and bleeding. Patients may also have periods of constipation, anorexia, and fever.

Although Crohn disease is a chronic disorder, each episode of inflammation causes scarring. The scarring may lead to narrowing of the colon, obstructing the bowel. Bowel obstruction can be life threatening and is a medical emergency. Diagnosis of Crohn disease necessitates a thorough history and analysis of the blood, which shows an increase in white blood cells and the erythrocyte sedimentation rate. A barium enema, or lower GI radiographic examination, if ordered by the physician, shows strictures alternating with normal bowel. Sigmoidoscopy and colonoscopy show patchy areas of inflammation within the bowel.

The treatment of Crohn disease is symptomatic; it includes restoration of fluids and electrolytes, administering corticosteroids to reduce inflammation, rest, and a low-fiber diet. Surgery is performed in cases of perforation or hemorrhage. If the situation is severe, a colectomy with an ileostomy may be performed (Fig. 33-3).

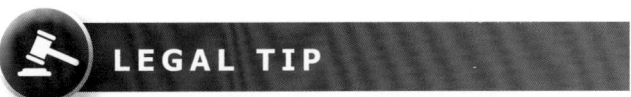

### LEGAL TIP

#### Reminder: Confidentiality and Privacy

Patients with any chronic disease process, such as Crohn disease, often have concerned family members who may call or contact the office for information regarding the health of the patient. It is important to include family members in the care of the patient with a disorder such as this; however, information about the patient or their condition cannot be released without written permission of the patient no matter how well-meaning the requests or questions appear. Many offices have all patients sign a statement annually giving permission as to what family members, if any, can get information about the patient including leaving messages on answering machines about lab or test results. Always check the medical record for signed consents regarding private information, and if no consent is available, do not share any information about the patient.

## Ulcerative Colitis

Like Crohn disease, ulcerative colitis is an inflammatory bowel disease affecting the lining of the colon. It occurs most often in young women but may occur at any age and may affect men also. The cause is not known but is thought to be an abnormal GI immune reaction to foods or microorganisms. Ulcerative colitis is a chronic condition, and the symptoms can be mild or severe with periods of remission.

The tissue that lines the colon becomes congested and edematous, eventually sloughing off and leading to ulcers and bloody diarrhea. Sometimes, pus and mucus are present in the stool. Malabsorption of fluids causes weakness, anorexia, nausea, and vomiting. Scarring can occur as the ulcers heal. The colon may produce pseudopolyps, which can be precancerous. Diagnosis may be determined by endoscopic examination or by a barium enema, and biopsy confirms the diagnosis. Colonoscopy is used to evaluate strictures caused by scarring and to assess the risk of cancer.

Treatment of ulcerative colitis requires controlling the inflammation and preventing the loss of fluids and nutrients during periods of exacerbation. If the disease is severe, a corticosteroid is prescribed to relieve the inflammation. Surgery is a last resort and usually involves a proctocolectomy with an ileostomy.

## CHECKPOINT QUESTION

6. Which of the inflammatory bowel diseases can lead to life-threatening bowel obstruction? How?

## Irritable Bowel Syndrome

Patients with irritable bowel syndrome frequently complain of bouts of constipation alternating with diarrhea. Although the patient may have signs and symptoms resembling those of Crohn disease or ulcerative colitis, irritable bowel syndrome usually does not result in weight loss, and the prognosis is good. However, this disorder can be debilitating because there is no warning for the bouts of diarrhea caused by the spastic colon. Women are more likely than men to have this chronic disorder, whose symptoms may range from mild to severe even though endoscopic examination shows no signs of disease. The origin of irritable bowel syndrome is thought to be psychogenic, a reaction to stress and emotions and the actions of the autonomic nervous system, which partly controls the colon. The consumption of specific food irritants may also precipitate an attack; however, the particular food item that triggers symptoms varies from person to person. Diagnosis requires a careful history, both physical and emotional. Other diseases are ruled out by testing. Treatment is stress management and identifying the offending food irritants. For severe flare-ups, the physician may order corticosteroids and antibiotics.

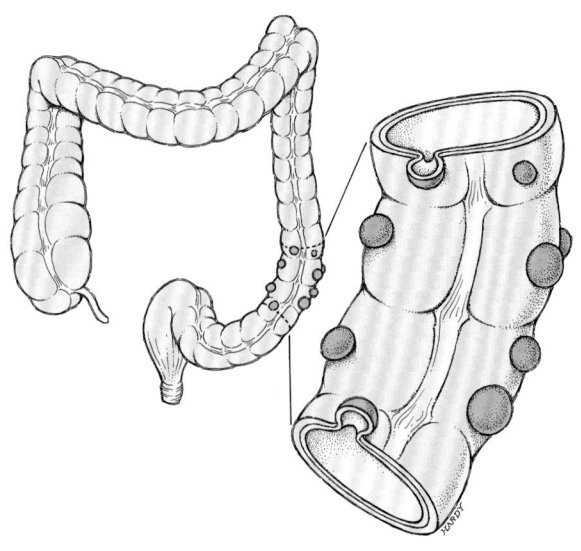

**Figure 33-4 •** Diverticulosis of the sigmoid colon. (Reprinted from Neil Hardy, Westpoint, CT, with permission.)

## Diverticulosis

Diverticulosis is a chronic condition of thinning of the bowel wall, causing small outpouches in the lining of the intestinal wall (Fig. 33-4). This disorder usually occurs in the sigmoid colon but may occur anywhere in the GI tract. The cause has been attributed to a diet deficient in roughage. While many people have diverticulosis without symptoms, the condition becomes more serious when the bowel wall becomes so thin that veins and arteries are exposed. Bleeding can occur when the wall is nicked by a piece of stool and may be severe enough to require surgery to stop the hemorrhage. A diet high in fiber and use of stool softeners may be ordered by the physician to prevent the signs and symptoms of this disorder.

Diverticulosis may progress to diverticulitis or inflammation of these areas of weakness in the bowel wall. The inflammation is usually caused by fecal material becoming lodged in the thin pockets. The symptoms are fever and abdominal pain. As the bowel becomes swollen and distended, the diseased areas may rupture, exposing the peritoneum to fecal material and resulting in peritonitis. The pouches are visualized on films produced from a barium enema or directly through endoscopic studies. During the acute phase, treatment includes a bland diet and stool softeners until the inflammation has subsided.

The frequency of bowel elimination is an individual characteristic. If stools are passed only several times a week but are soft, formed, and passed with little effort, there should be no concern about constipation. However, constipation may be a problem if stools are passed daily but are hard, dry, and difficult to pass.

## PATIENT EDUCATION

### Maintaining Good Bowel Habits

By following these guidelines, patients can prevent common problems of elimination:

- Eat a variety of foods, especially fresh fruits, vegetables, and whole grains. Limit the intake of highly processed foods.
- Drink eight glasses of water a day to keep the stools moist and easy to pass and to hydrate the tissues.
- Get some form of exercise daily. Even a walk around the block will aid muscle tone and help prevent sluggish metabolism.
- Make time for bowel movements when the stimulus is felt. Avoiding or delaying defecation results in loss of moisture from the stool and may make the bowel insensitive to the stimulus.
- Do not use laxatives or enemas. Frequent use may result in a lazy bowel that responds only to these chemical and physical stimuli.

## Polyps

Colon polyps are masses of benign mucous membrane lining the large intestine that are usually slow growing but may become cancerous. Polyps are usually discovered by a barium enema or during a colonoscopy. If the polyps are discovered at an early stage and removed, cancer of the colon may be prevented. Cancer of the colon may invade the muscle of the bowel and metastasize through the lymph system to other organs.

## Hernias

The anterior abdominal wall is covered with various muscles that assist with movement and support and protect the internal structures of the abdomen. When these muscles weaken, the underlying organs or intestines may protrude through the weakened muscle wall, resulting in a hernia. Factors that may increase the risk for developing a hernia include a genetic predisposition to muscular weakness, lifting heavy objects, obesity, and pregnancy. The signs and symptoms of abdominal hernia include a protrusion or bulge over the area of the hernia. Specific types of abdominal hernias are named according to the area of the abdomen: the inguinal hernia occurs in right or left inguinal (groin) areas; the ventral hernia occurs in the front of the abdomen; and the umbilical hernia occurs over the umbilicus. The treatment for abdominal hernias includes surgically repairing the weakened muscle (herniorrhaphy) using grafting material as necessary. To prevent abdominal hernias, encourage the use of abdominal support and good body mechanics when lifting and weight reduction as prescribed by the physician.

## CHECKPOINT QUESTION

7. What has generally been noted as the cause of diverticulosis?

## Appendicitis

The vermiform appendix, a small pouch of tissue protruding from the cecum or first part of the large intestine, is approximately 4 inches long. Although the function of this tissue is not clear, there is no direct involvement with the process of digestion. Appendicitis occurs when the vermiform appendix becomes infected and fills with bacteria, pus, and blood. Adolescents and young adult men are most commonly affected by this condition, but women and young children can also develop appendicitis. The symptoms include severe abdominal pain with tenderness over the right lower quadrant, vomiting, a fever, and an elevated white blood count. A thorough history should be obtained from any patient with these symptoms, and once the physician determines the diagnosis of appendicitis, it is necessary to make arrangements for immediate surgical removal of the infected appendix. If a diagnosis is not made quickly or the appendectomy is delayed, perforation of the appendix and peritonitis can result and make recovery more difficult for the patient (see Box 33-1).

## Hemorrhoids

Hemorrhoids are external or internal dilated veins (varicosities) in the rectum. Internal hemorrhoids may enlarge and may bleed during defecation. A patient with external hemorrhoids may complain of rectal pain and itching and bleeding with bowel movements. Poor abdominal and pelvic floor muscle tone, poor dietary habits including a diet low in fiber, and chronic constipation may cause hemorrhoids. The diagnosis of external hemorrhoids is made by visual inspection, while internal hemorrhoids are diagnosed by anoscopy or proctoscopy. Treatment involves regulating the diet to control constipation, providing local pain relief, using a stool softener, and surgical ligation (hemorrhoidectomy) using standard surgical techniques, laser, or cryosurgery (freezing).

## Colorectal Cancers

Cancer of the colon and rectum is often fatal, but the patient's chances for survival are better with early diagnosis and treatment. Although the cause of colorectal cancer is unknown, it has been linked to diets high in animal fats and low in fiber. It is commonly seen in patients with a history of ulcerative colitis or colorectal

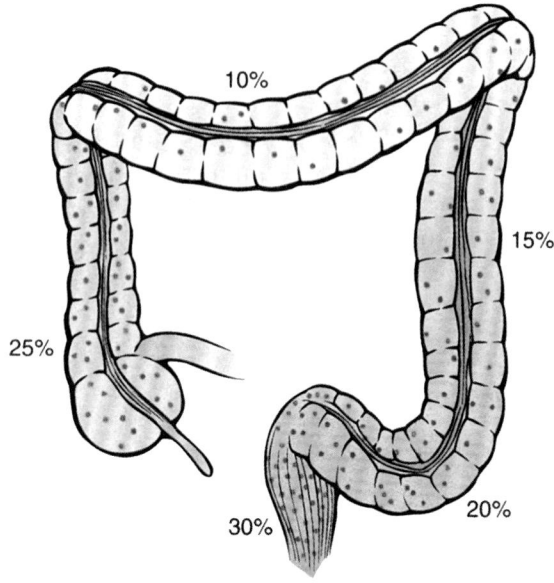

**Figure 33-5 •** Percent distribution of cancer sites in the colon and rectum.

polyps and affects the first and last parts of the colon more often than other areas (Fig. 33-5). Early signs of colorectal cancer are vague abdominal pains with occasional bloody stools. Later signs depend on the section and amount of the colon involved and the degree of metastasis to other organs and tissues.

Many rectal cancers are discovered by a digital examination or an anoscopy, but sigmoidoscopy or colonoscopy is used to determine the extent of involvement. A barium enema with contrast air aids in the diagnosis. Laboratory tests include **guaiac** tests, such as the Hemoccult™, which test for occult (hidden) blood in the stool. Surgical removal of the affected area, usually followed by chemotherapy and radiation, is the treatment of choice.

### Functional Disorders

Functional disorders of the GI tract include the common disorders of constipation, diarrhea, and intestinal gas. Normally, peristalsis causes the products of digestion to move at a constant rate, not too slowly and not too quickly. Constipation occurs when the lower colon retains fecal material too long so that too much moisture is absorbed, making the stool hard and dry. Most constipation is caused by poor bowel habits (avoiding defecation and overusing laxatives), low-fiber diet, and inadequate fluid intake. The quality of the stool is more important than the quantity. To avoid constipation, patients should be encouraged to increase oral fluid intake; eat foods high in fiber, such as raw vegetables and fruit; and maintain regular bowel habits. The physician may also prescribe a stool softener and an over-the-counter fiber product as needed.

When the fluid contents of the bowel are rushed through, as in diarrhea, the water and minerals are not reabsorbed into the system, and the stool is loose and watery. Bacterial or viral infection or a GI irritant causes the smooth muscles and mucous membranes to work to flush out the bowel as quickly as possible. The treatment for diarrhea includes medication to slow peristalsis, a bland diet, and increasing oral fluids to replace fluids and electrolytes lost in the stool.

Intestinal gas, produced by bacterial decomposition of proteins in the digestive tract, can lead to abdominal discomfort. Gas in the intestinal tract causes a feeling of fullness. The gas may be expelled from the stomach through the mouth (eructation, or belching) or from the intestines through the rectum (flatulence). The production of intestinal gas is due to intolerance of milk products, swallowing air through excessive talking or gum chewing, consuming gas-producing spicy or fatty foods, or slow emptying of the stomach and bowels. The problem can usually be relieved by avoiding the offending foods or behaviors. Various over-the-counter preparations and prescription medications can be used if the problem persists.

### CHECKPOINT QUESTION

8. What causes hemorrhoids?

## Liver Disorders

Liver disorders are assessed by observing the cardinal signs of liver dysfunction: jaundice, **ascites** (fluid accumulation in the peritoneal cavity), and **hepatomegaly** (enlargement of the liver). It is vital to obtain a complete medical history from patients with a suspected liver disorder. Particular concern focuses on jaundice, anemia, splenectomy, alcohol use, travel to developing countries, blood transfusions, use of **hepatotoxins** (drugs that are damaging to the liver), and abuse of controlled substances. Diagnostic tests for liver disorders include the following:

• Liver function tests, including prothrombin time and levels of bilirubin, alkaline phosphatase, albumin, and cholesterol
• Radiography and barium study
• Radioisotope liver scan
• Percutaneous peritoneoscopy and biopsy
• Surgical laparotomy and liver biopsy

### Hepatitis

Hepatitis is an inflammation or infection of the liver that may lead to liver destruction and necrosis of hepatic cells. The five types of viral hepatitis are summarized in Table 33-1 and listed here:

• *Hepatitis A (HAV)*, the most common type of viral hepatitis, is also known as infectious hepatitis. HAV spreads in food and water contaminated with fecal

## TABLE 33-1 Types of Viral Hepatitis

| Virus | Transmission | Precautions |
| --- | --- | --- |
| HAV | Fecal–oral route | Hand washing; HAV vaccine |
| HBV | Sera and body fluids | Standard precautions; HBV vaccine |
| HCV | Blood transfusions Percutaneous contamination | Standard precautions |
| HDV | Coinfection with HBV | Standard precautions; HBV vaccine |
| HEV | Fecal–oral route | Hand washing; standard precautions |

material or seafood high in coliform bacteria. It is highly contagious, but the prognosis for recovery after an infection with hepatitis A is good.

- *Hepatitis B (HBV)*, also known as *serum hepatitis*, can be transmitted by contaminated blood and other body fluids. HBV may be so severe that death results, but the use of standard precautions will prevent spread. Fortunately, there is a vaccine to protect against HBV, and it is recommended for all health care workers.
- *Hepatitis C (HCV)*, also known as *non-A, non-B hepatitis*, can be transmitted via blood transfusion or percutaneous contamination. After the initial infection, HCV frequently progresses to chronic hepatitis that may be asymptomatic but is communicable. As with HBV, the use of standard precautions prevents spread.
- *Hepatitis D (HDV)* occurs only in patients who have had HBV; it cannot survive without HBV.
- *Hepatitis E (HEV)* spreads in food or water contaminated with fecal material and ingested by the unsuspecting individual.

While the viruses responsible for the individual types of viral hepatitis are physically different, the symptoms of all types are similar. They may include fatigue, joint pain, flulike symptoms with fever, jaundice, dark urine, and light stools. Complications of hepatitis include long-term impaired liver function, chronic hepatitis, liver cancer, and death.

Diagnosis of the various types of viral hepatitis is made by obtaining a complete medical history, blood analysis for hepatitis antibodies, and liver function studies. There is no cure once infection occurs, but the patient is encouraged to rest and take in a supportive diet. Interferon-α is given to some patients to assist the immune system in responding to viral hepatitis. Standard precautions must be observed to protect caregivers and health care workers from contracting hepatitis.

Another cause of hepatitis, toxic hepatitis, is exposure to chemical toxicants or hepatotoxic substances, including certain medications and alcohol. If the offending toxicant is eliminated early enough, the prognosis for recovery is good. The symptoms of toxic hepatitis resemble viral hepatitis, and the diagnosis is similar. A liver biopsy may identify the underlying pathology.

## Cirrhosis or Fibrosis

Cirrhosis is a chronic disease characterized by destruction of liver cells and the formation of scar tissue or fibers throughout the liver, altering its function and efficiency. The causes of cirrhosis include a history of exposure to hepatotoxins, alcoholism, prolonged biliary obstruction, and a history of hepatitis. In the early stages, symptoms include vague GI discomfort. In the late stages, respiratory efficiency decreases because of ascites that forces the abdominal contents against the diaphragm. Bleeding tendencies result from the loss of clotting factors formed in the liver. Dermal pruritus (itching), jaundice, and hepatomegaly are usually present. Diagnosis is made by liver biopsy, liver scan, and blood work. Treatment includes avoiding the hepatotoxins or abstinence from alcohol to prevent further death of hepatic cells, a good diet, vitamin supplements, and supportive care. In cases of liver failure that accompanies increased destruction of liver tissue, the physician may recommend a liver transplantation.

### CHECKPOINT QUESTION

9. How does the cause of viral hepatitis differ from that of toxic hepatitis?

## Liver Cancer

The liver is rarely a primary site for cancer but is frequently a target site of metastasis. This type of cancer is more common in men than in women and is rapidly fatal. There is no known cause, but primary liver cancers are thought to be due to exposure to carcinogenic chemicals, including hepatotoxins. Patients who have cirrhosis or hepatitis B are more likely than the general population to develop liver cancer.

In the early stages of the disease, patients usually complain of weight loss, weakness, and right upper quadrant pain. Jaundice may be present and will definitely develop as the disease progresses (Fig. 33-6). Diagnosis is

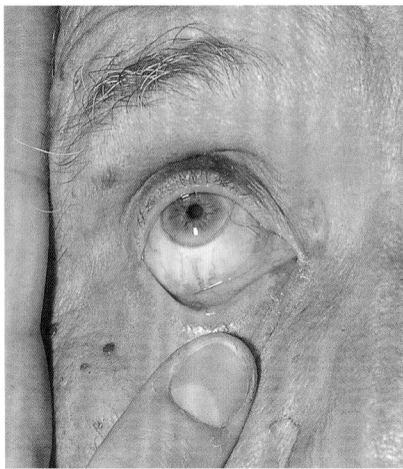

**Figure 33-6** • A patient with jaundice. (From Bickley LS, Szilagyi P. *Bates' Guide to Physical Examination and History Taking*, 8th ed. Philadelphia, PA: Lippincott Williams & Wilkins, 2003.)

confirmed by biopsy, liver function tests, and computed tomography (CT) or magnetic resonance imaging (MRI). If the lesion is small and local, resection is possible. Chemotherapy may be used in some instances. If there is no metastasis, a liver transplantation may be possible.

## Gallbladder Disorders

### Cholelithiasis and Cholecystitis

Cholelithiasis is the formation of gallstones made of cholesterol and bilirubin (Fig. 33-7). When the peristaltic action of the gallbladder is sluggish and bile pools in

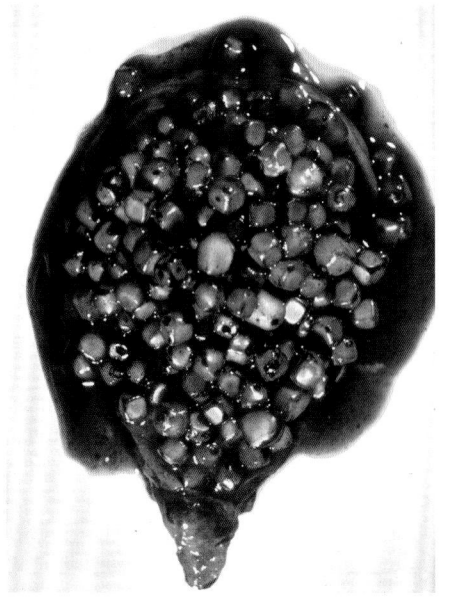

**Figure 33-7** • Cholelithiasis. The gallbladder has been opened to reveal numerous yellow cholesterol gallstones. (Reprinted from Rubin E, Gorstein F, Rubin R, Schwarting R, Strayer D. *Rubin's Pathology: Clinicopathologic Foundations of Medicine*. Philadelphia, PA: Lippincott Williams & Wilkins, 2005, with permission.)

the sac, fluid is absorbed, leaving the solids to concentrate and solidify into stones. Cholecystitis is an acute or chronic inflammation of the gallbladder, usually resulting from an impacted stone in the duct. Cholecystitis or cholelithiasis usually causes pain as peristalsis presses bile against the blockage, especially after a fatty meal.

Signs and symptoms of any gallbladder disorder include acute right upper abdominal quadrant pain that may radiate to the shoulders, back, or chest; indigestion; nausea; and intolerance of fatty foods. Later in the illness, jaundice may appear as the ducts to the liver become blocked. Tests to determine the cause of the symptoms include cholecystography after the ingestion of a radiopaque dye, percutaneous transhepatic cholangiography, endoscopic retrograde cholangiopancreatography (ECRP), and duodenal endoscopy. Noninvasive procedures include ultrasound and CT. Flat plate radiographs are not especially accurate for evaluating gallbladder disorders. The treatment may be supportive or palliative, including pain medication and avoiding fatty foods; however, surgical removal of the stones (cholecystectomy) may be necessary, usually through endoscopic laparotomy. Lithotripsy (crushing the gallstones using sound waves) may also be used to break the stones into small pieces that can pass easily through the bile ducts and into the digestive system for elimination.

### Gallbladder Cancer

Cancer of the gallbladder is rare and difficult to diagnose. Since the symptoms are similar to those of cholecystitis, this cancer is usually discovered during routine gallbladder tests performed to diagnose general gallbladder disease. The signs and symptoms include right upper quadrant pain, nausea and vomiting, weight loss, and anorexia. However, cholecystitis pain is usually sporadic, whereas pain due to malignancy is usually chronic and severe. The gallbladder may be palpable, and jaundice may be present. It is most common in older women and is rapidly fatal. The cause is not known, but theory suggests that cholelithiasis is a predisposing factor. Diagnosis includes liver function tests, CT, MRI, and cholecystography. Surgical cholecystectomy is the primary treatment, but survival rates are low.

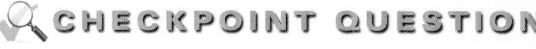

**CHECKPOINT QUESTION**

10. How are cholelithiasis and cholecystitis different?

## Pancreatic Disorders

### Pancreatitis

Pancreatitis is an inflammation of the pancreas that may be related to alcoholism, trauma, gastric ulcer, or biliary tract disease. Signs and symptoms include vomiting and steady epigastric pain radiating to the spine. Signs of progressive disease include abdominal rigidity and decreased bowel activity. Complications include diabetes mellitus, hemorrhage, shock, coma, and death as the digestive enzymes cause the organ to digest itself. Diagnostic blood tests show an increase in serum amylase and glucose levels. Ultrasound and CT are useful for diagnosis. Treatment includes pain relief and medication to reduce pancreatic secretions while the organ recovers. Prognosis depends on the extent and severity of damage to the pancreas.

### Pancreatic Cancer

One of the deadliest malignancies is pancreatic cancer, which kills most patients within a year of diagnosis. There is no definitive cause of pancreatic cancer, but it occurs most often in middle-aged African American men who smoke, who have a diet high in fats and proteins, or who are exposed to industrial chemicals for long periods.

Patients complain of weight loss, back and abdominal pain, and diarrhea. Commonly, they are jaundiced. Diagnosis is made by laparoscopic biopsy, CT, MRI, endoscopic retrograde cholangiopancreatography (ERCP), and pancreatic enzyme studies. Surgical removal of the pancreas (pancreatotomy), chemotherapy, and radiation therapy are used to treat pancreatic cancer, but the survival rate is very low.

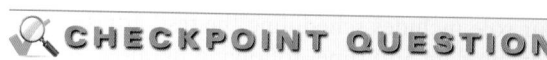

### CHECKPOINT QUESTION

11. What are some complications of pancreatitis?

## COMMON DIAGNOSTIC AND THERAPEUTIC PROCEDURES

### History and Physical Examination of the GI System

Before beginning any patient's care, an adequate history must be obtained. The patient presenting with GI concerns will be assessed for signs (e.g., vomiting) and symptoms (e.g., nausea). From that base, the physician will determine the direction of the diagnostic testing to rule out or to confirm possible diagnosis. The history must include occupation, family history, recent travel to developing countries, and current medications. Patients should also be required to complete a checklist of concerns, which may include heartburn, GI bleeding, weight gain or loss, history of alcohol use, and laxative and enema use.

The physician will assess skin **turgor** (elasticity), jaundice, edema, bruising, breath odor, size and shape of the abdomen, and presence and quality of bowel sounds. The physician will also palpate abdominal contents.

## Blood Tests

Blood work ordered by the physician may include white and red blood cell counts. The red blood cells, hemoglobin, and hematocrit are used to assess possible anemia as the result of GI bleeding. White blood cell counts can help to detect infection, while the erythrocyte sedimentation rate is used to assess inflammatory processes, including inflammation of the GI system.

Blood may also be drawn and sent to the laboratory to determine liver function. Specifically, alkaline phosphatase, serum bilirubin, prothrombin time, and serum glutamic pyruvic transaminase (SGPT) levels are determined in a test collectively known as a **liver panel**. Pancreatic enzyme studies include evaluation of blood for levels of enzymes normally released by the pancreas, including trypsin, chymotrypsin, steapsin, and amylopsin. Results that fall outside of the normal ranges for these substances indicate pathology and necessitate further testing as determined by the physician.

## Radiology Studies

Flat plate radiographs of the abdomen may be ordered for diagnosing GI problems, but without contrast medium, these radiographs are not so useful as contrast radiographs. Radiology studies of the stomach and intestines consist of instilling barium, a radiopaque liquid, into the GI tract orally or rectally to outline the organs and identify abnormalities. The radiographs include standard pictures taken at various intervals after the barium is administered by mouth or by enema. If a fluoroscope (special type of radiographic equipment) is used, movement of the chalky liquid barium is viewed while it fills the esophagus or colon, giving additional diagnostic information.

The barium swallow (also called an *upper GI* or *UGI*) series can reveal abnormal constrictions, masses, and obstruction in the esophagus, stomach, and duodenum. This examination requires that the patient have nothing by mouth (NPO) after midnight the night before the test. A small bowel series is an extension of the UGI that visualizes the barium flowing through the small intestine to diagnose abnormalities of the first part of the small intestine.

A barium enema, or lower GI study, provides an outline of the colon. It can reveal a blockage, cancerous growths, polyps, and diverticula. Since the lower GI study requires that the colon be empty of stool, the patient must be given specific instructions to follow before the examination. Box 33-2 outlines the standard preparation for a barium enema, which should be orally explained to the patient and given in written form.

Cholecystography is radiography of the gallbladder after the patient takes oral tablets containing a contrast material 12 hours prior to the procedure. The contrast medium is excreted from the liver into

## BOX 33-2   Patient Preparation for Bowel Studies

Many bowel studies, such as barium enema and flexible sigmoidoscopy, require that the bowel be completely clear of fecal matter. With minor variations as directed by the physician, the bowel preparation usually includes the following:

- Liquid diet without dairy products for the full day before the procedure or a clear liquid evening meal
- A laxative or enema the evening preceding the procedure
- Nothing by mouth after midnight except water
- Rectal suppository, Fleet's enema, or cleansing enema the morning of the procedure

If inflammatory processes or ulcerations are suspected inside the bowel, only gentle cleansing will be used to avoid undue discomfort or possible perforation of lesions.

the gallbladder, and any abnormalities are viewed on the radiogram. After the initial films are taken, the patient is given a fatty meal that stimulates the contraction of the gallbladder to release bile and contrast medium into the bile ducts. Additional films may be taken to view any obstruction of these ducts by stones. The bile ducts may also be examined using percutaneous transhepatic cholangiography, a test that entails injection of contrast material through a needle inserted through the skin into the hepatic duct. Once the dye is injected, radiography is performed for diagnosis by the physician.

The role of the medical assistant in radiographic procedures includes determining third-party payer (insurance) requirements for referrals or preauthorization, scheduling the procedure in an outpatient facility, and explaining to the patient the preparations for the examination as necessary. When the test is complete, the radiologist will submit a written report to the referring physician. Follow office policy and procedure for routing the report to the physician for review and advising the patient of the examination results.

### CHECKPOINT QUESTION

12. Why are contrast media used in radiography of the GI organs?

## Nuclear Imaging

Radionuclides, or radioactive elements, are often used in the diagnosis of disorders of the liver. After the

elements are injected into the body, images are taken using a nuclear scanning device, and abnormalities can be detected and evaluated by the radiologist. The injected radionuclide remains radioactive for a short specific period, and there is usually very little, if any, patient preparation required for this test. The role of the medical assistant includes coordinating any third-party payer requirements such as preauthorization, scheduling the test at a nuclear imaging center or hospital, and following up with the patient when the results are returned to the medical office as indicated in the policy and procedure manual. Test results indicating abnormalities necessitate additional evaluation and testing as determined by the physician.

## Ultrasonography

The use of high-frequency sound waves to diagnose disorders of internal structures is used in many specialties, including gastroenterology. Abnormalities in the structure of various digestive accessory organs, such as the liver and gallbladder, can be easily viewed using ultrasonography and require very little if any preparation by the patient. As with other diagnostic tests ordered by the physician, your role includes verifying third-party payer guidelines and obtaining preauthorization if needed. Although ultrasound does not use radiation or radiography, ultrasounds are scheduled in the imaging department of many outpatient or inpatient facilities. Your role includes scheduling the test, advising the patient of the date and time, following up after the test to obtain results if necessary, ensuring that the physician is aware of the results, and notifying the patient with any findings or additional instructions as ordered by the physician.

## Endoscopic Studies

Fiberoptic technology has enabled physicians to pass soft, flexible tubes down the esophagus into the stomach and small intestine or up into the colon for direct visualization of these organs. Supplemental laboratory specimens, including tissue biopsy samples; samples of secretions for gastric analysis, including pH; culture sample to check for bacteria; bile for crystals that may lead to the formation of stones; and cells for cytology, including cancerous or otherwise abnormal cells, can be obtained. Endoscopic examinations are also used to diagnose biliary disorders.

Endoscopic retrograde cholangiopancreatography (ERCP) is used to visualize the esophagus, stomach, proximal duodenum, and pancreas with a flexible endoscope. When the endoscope is in place, dye is injected directly into the ducts of the gallbladder and pancreas, and radiographs are taken to determine patency and function of these structures and the biliary ducts (Fig. 33-8). This procedure is usually performed in an outpatient surgical

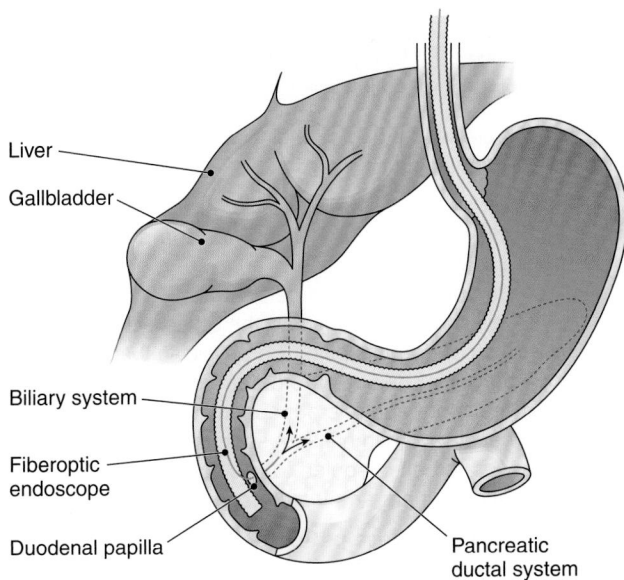

Figure 33-8 • The ducts of the gallbladder and pancreas can be easily visualized during an ERCP. (From Cohen BJ. *Medical Terminology*, 4th ed. Philadelphia, PA: Lippincott Williams & Wilkins, 2003.)

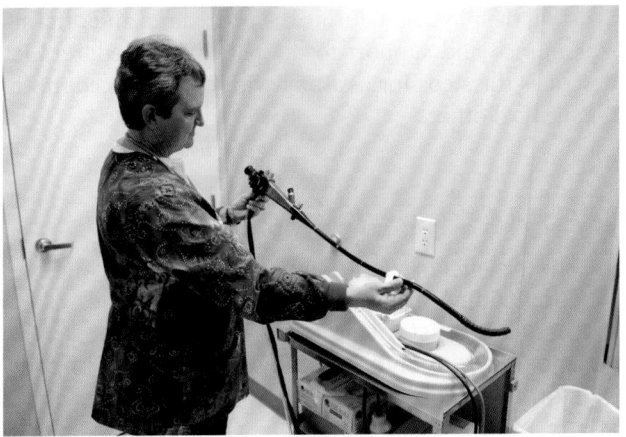

**Figure 33-9** • A flexible sigmoidoscope.

center under anesthesia. Your role includes scheduling the procedure, advising the patient on any instructions prior to the test, and follow-up when the written report is sent by the gastroenterologist or radiologist.

Anoscopy, which may be performed in the medical office, is insertion of a metal or plastic anoscope into the rectal canal for visual inspection of the anus and rectum and to swab for cultures. The sigmoidoscopy examination provides a visual examination of the sigmoid colon using either a rigid sigmoidoscope or the more widely accepted flexible fiberoptic sigmoidoscope. The rigid sigmoidoscope is about 25 cm (10 inches) long. This instrument is supplied as reusable metal or disposable plastic and is calibrated in centimeters. An **obturator** in the lumen allows the instrument to be inserted with minimal discomfort and can be removed after insertion allowing for better visualization and obtaining specimens. The lens at the end magnifies the view for closer observation of the intestinal mucosa and can be moved aside to allow the physician to swab, suction, or sample the mucosa for biopsy. The handle contains the light source. The scope may be equipped with a hand bulb **insufflator**, a device for blowing air into the colon to expand the walls for easier visualization.

The flexible fiberoptic sigmoidoscope is more popular because it offers better visualization and is less uncomfortable for the patient (Fig. 33-9). The scope is very thin, can bend and maneuver curves, and can be inserted much farther than the rigid scope (Fig. 33-10). The instrument is 35 cm (about 14 inches) or 65 cm (about 26 inches). It usually includes an insufflator and suction in addition to the light source. Although smaller

in diameter than the rigid scope, it can also be used to obtain samples and cultures.

Some physicians prefer that the bowel be as free of feces as possible and may order a light, low-residue meal the evening before the endoscopic examination. An evening laxative may also be ordered to be followed by a cleansing enema on the morning of the procedure. A light breakfast may be allowed but only if ordered by the physician. Other physicians prefer to view the mucosa as it normally appears, without preparation. Most medical offices note the preferred preparation in the policy and procedure manual. Your role includes informing the patient of the preferred preparation for the procedure,

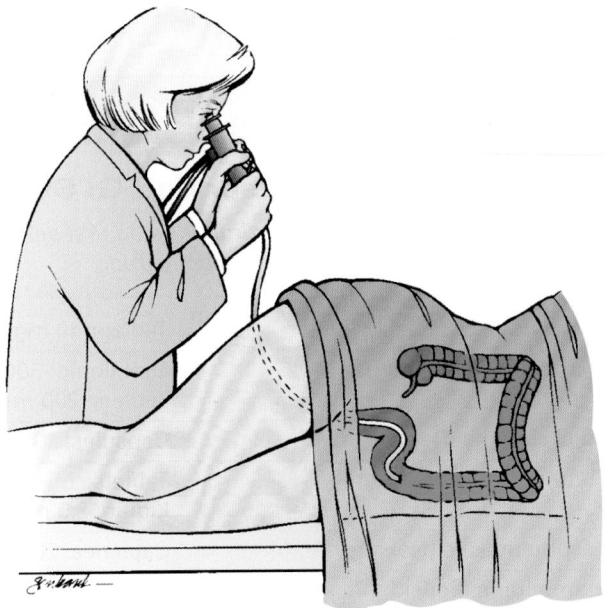

**Figure 33-10** • Sigmoidoscopy. The flexible scope is advanced past the proximal sigmoid colon and into the descending colon. (Reprinted from Cohen BJ. *Medical Terminology: An Illustrated Guide*. Philadelphia, PA: Lippincott Williams & Wilkins, 2003, with permission.)

assisting the physician during the procedure, and offering reassurance and support to the patient. Procedure 33-1 describes the steps for assisting with colon procedures in the medical office.

 CHECKPOINT QUESTION

13. The physician would like to perform an anoscopy today in the office and Sharon, the medical assistant, is assisting. What does anoscopy involve, and how does it differ from sigmoidoscopy?

## Fecal Tests

As part of the routine examination for adult patients, many physicians recommend testing a stool specimen for the presence of occult, or hidden, blood. A stool specimen may also be ordered to test for ova (eggs) and parasites if the physician suspects the patient has a parasite infection. You may be responsible for instructing the patient in the procedure for collecting these specimens, and in some cases, such as in testing the stool for occult blood, you may be responsible for testing the stool specimen after the patient returns it to the office. Procedure 33-2 describes the procedure to test a stool specimen for the presence of occult blood using the guaiac method. Chapter 44 discusses the procedure for instructing a patient to collect a stool specimen for ova and parasites.

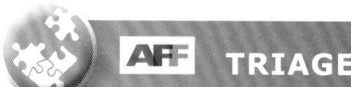 TRIAGE

While you are working in a medical office, the following three situations occur:

A. A 44-year-old man is scheduled for a routine physical. However, he arrives in the office complaining of "heartburn" and is taken to an exam room where the physician has ordered an ECG.

B. An 18-year-old boy comes into the office with lower right abdominal pain. The physician wants blood drawn immediately to determine a white blood cell count and rule out appendicitis.

C. A 52-year-old woman has just seen the physician and needs to be scheduled for a colonoscopy at the local outpatient ambulatory surgical center.

**How do you sort these patients? Who do you see first? Second? Third?**

First, you should do the ECG on patient A. A feeling of indigestion or epigastric discomfort can be a sign of cardiac disease. Next, draw patient B's blood, since an elevation in the white blood cell count indicates the need for additional tests and/or surgery for appendicitis. Finally, schedule the outpatient procedure for patient C after checking for appropriate insurance referrals.

*Note:* This sequence is the accepted triage standard; however, the physician may opt for the blood work to be done first if he or she considers that patient A's discomfort is probably due to gastric difficulties and has ordered the ECG as a prophylactic measure. This decision is based on the physical examinations of both patients. You and the physician must work as a team to achieve the best outcomes.

 MEDICATION BOX

### Commonly Prescribed GI System Medications

*Note: The generic name of the drug is listed first and is written in all lowercase letters. Brand names are in parentheses, and the first letter is capitalized.*

| | | |
|---|---|---|
| bisacodyl (Dulcolax) | Tablets: 10 mg | Laxative |
| cimetidine (Tagamet) | Oral liquid: 300 mg/5 mL<br>Tablets: 200 mg to 800 mg | Antiulcerative |
| dicyclomine (Bentyl) | Capsules: 10 mg, 20 mg | Anticholinergic |
| diphenoxylate (Lomotil) | Tablets: 2.5 mg<br>Liquid: 2.5 mg/5 mL | Antidiarrheal |
| esomeprazole (Nexium) | Capsules: 20 mg to 40 mg | Antiulcerative |
| famotidine (Pepcid) | Gelcaps: 10 mg<br>Tablets: 10 mg to 40 mg | Antiulcerative |
| hepatitis A vaccine, inactivated (Havrix, Vaqta) | Injection: 25 units/0.5 mL (intramuscular) | Vaccine |

## MEDICATION BOX (continued)

| | | |
|---|---|---|
| hepatitis B vaccine, recombinant (Engerix-B, Recombivax HB) | Injection: adults (20 year and older) First dose: 20 mcg intramuscular initially Second dose: 20 mcg after 30 days Third dose: 20 mcg 6 months after second dose | Vaccine |
| infliximab (Remicade) | 100-mg vial (intravenous) | Immunosuppressant |
| lansoprazole (Prevacid) | Capsules: 15 mg and 30 mg Oral suspension: 15 or 30 mg/packet | Antiulcerative |
| metoclopramide (Reglan) | Tablets: 5 mg, 10 mg Intramuscular injection: 5 mg/mL | Antiemetic |
| omeprazole (Prilosec) | Capsules: 10 mg to 40 mg | Antiulcerative |
| ondansetron (Zofran) | Tablets: 4 mg, 8 mg, 24 mg | Antiemetic |
| pantoprazole (Protonix) | Tablet: 20 mg, 40 mg | Antiulcerative |
| phentermine (Adipex-P) | Capsules: 18.75 mg, 30 mg, 37.5 mg Tablets: 37.5 mg | Appetite suppressant |
| polyethylene glycol (MiraLax) | Powder: single-dose (17 g) 16 oz, 24 oz | Laxative |
| rabeprazole (Aciphex) | Tablets: 20 mg | Antiulcerative |
| ranitidine (Zantac) | Tablets: 75 mg | Antiulcerative |
| scopolamine (Scopace; Transderm-Scop) | Tablets: 0.4 mg Transdermal patch: 1.5 mg/2.5 cm$^2$ | Antiemetic |
| sibutramine (Meridia) | Capsules: 5 mg, 10 mg, 15 mg | Appetite suppressant |

 **ROLE-PLAYING ACTIVITY**

With cooperation from classmates or as assigned by your instructor, role-play the scenarios as if you are working with Sharon Clay in the gastroenterology office (refer to the case study at the beginning of the chapter). A patient, Karen Clark, seen today was referred to your office for a bariatric surgery consultation. Karen is 44 years old and she is 5 feet and 4 inches tall, weighing 475 pounds, with a BMI of 81, giving her a diagnosis of morbid obesity. She says she has "tried" all diets and "nothing works," and her family physician has recommended possible surgery for weight loss. She has high blood pressure and diabetes and shows signs of congestive heart failure. Her physician warned her that if she does not lose weight, she may die before she turns 50 years of age. What are your feelings and/or opinions of someone who is overweight? How would you respond to this patient or any patient who is morbidly obese? She tells you that while she is willing to have surgery to lose weight, she is not going to change her eating habits. What would you say to her? Your instructor will give you additional information about this activity!

## *español* SPANISH TERMINOLOGY

**¿Tiene indigestión?**
Do you have indigestion?

**¿Esta estreñido ó constipado?**
Are you constipated?

**¿Tiene diarreas?**
Do you have diarrhea?

**¿Ha notado sangre ó mucosidad en la excreta ó excremento?**
Have you noticed any blood or mucus in the stool?

**¿Cuántas veces ha evacuado hoy?**
How many times have you had bowel movements today?

**¿Puede apuntar con un dedo donde exactamente le duele?**
Can you point with a finger to where the pain is exactly?

**¿Siente que su vientre esta distendido?**
Do you feel bloated?

**Necesita masticar más despacio.**
You need to masticate/chew slowly.

**Las hemorroides son venas que sangran frecuentemente.**
Hemorrhoids are dilated veins that bleed frequently.

**Necesita incluir más fibra en su alimentación.**
You need to include more fiber in your diet.

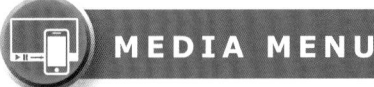

## MEDIA MENU

**Student Resources** on thePoint®
- *Animation:* Cirrhosis
- *Animation:* General Digestion
- CMA/RMA Certification Exam Review

**Internet Resources**
**The American College of Gastroenterology**
http://www.acg.gi.org

**Centers for Disease Control and Prevention**
http://www.cdc.gov/hepatitis

**National Digestive Diseases Information Clearinghouse**
http://digestive.niddk.nih.gov/ddiseases/pubs/cirrhosis

## EMR Activity

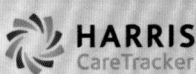

**Harris CareTracker** is a Web-based electronic medical record (EMR) application that you will use for the EMR activities included in this section at the end of each chapter. This application is actually used in physician offices but is provided to you through the publisher, Wolters Kluwer Health, to give you hands-on practice working with EMRs. Your instructor will have more information about accessing your username, log-in, and Quickstart guide.

### Prerequisite Activities in Harris CareTracker

- *The Getting Started and Quickstart documents and EMR Activities Step-by-Step Instructions are available at* http://thePoint.lww.com/KronenbergerComp5e.

### Activity Details

Using only legitimate sources, create a brochure explaining how patients should prepare for a colonoscopy procedure. Use a computer word processing software to create your brochure, cite your sources at the end, and upload it into the EMR using the *Patient Education Upload* feature in the *Clinical* tab of the *Administration* module.

## Chapter Summary

Information regarding the care of a patient with GI disorders requires knowledge of the following:

- Any disruption of the processes of ingestion, absorption, or elimination is pathologic not only to the gastric system, but to other body systems and cells as well.
- Although the medical assistant working in the office of the gastroenterologist encounters many patients with disorders of the GI system, patients with gastric disorders are commonly seen in other offices, including family practice, internal medicine, and pediatrics.
- A thorough history is essential for an accurate diagnosis of any GI disorder.
- Assisting with various diagnostic procedures, such as colon examinations and stool testing, can also help the physician detect abnormalities in GI function.
- Patient education regarding diet and prevention of various gastric disorders is a critical aspect of the professional medical assistant's role and should be considered an ongoing process.

## Warm-Ups for Critical Thinking

1. Review the preparation of the patient for an upper GI series and a barium enema. Create two handouts that include the following:
   - A description of each procedure
   - A list of reasons for the procedure
   - Preparations required to ensure reliable test results
2. Many endoscopic examinations require the patient to be in an uncomfortable and embarrassing position. How can you help alleviate the stress and anxiety?
3. Mrs. Barnes, a 43-year-old patient, was scheduled for a cholecystography at 11:00 AM today and was given all instructions and the oral contrast medium to take the morning of the examination. She calls the office at 10:30 AM and tells you that she forgot to take the dye tablets and wants to know whether she should take them now and go in for her test at the appointed time. What do you tell Mrs. Barnes?
4. Research the various surgeries used to treat obesity. In addition to the risks involved with having abdominal surgery, are there any side effects or risks with each procedure that may further affect the GI system or other body systems?
5. Explain how a patient with gallstones can develop pancreatitis.

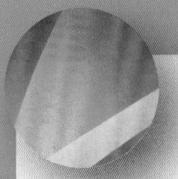

## PSY PROCEDURE 33-1

## Assisting with Colon Procedures

**PSY** Instruct and prepare a patient for a procedure or treatment; coach patients regarding disease prevention and treatment plans; coach patients appropriately considering cultural diversity, developmental life stage, and communication barriers; and document patient care accurately in the medical record.

**Purpose:** To prepare the patient and assist with endoscopic colon procedures

**Equipment:** Appropriate instrument (flexible or rigid sigmoidoscope, anoscope, or proctoscope), water-soluble lubricant, gown and drape, cotton swabs, suction (if not part of the scope), biopsy forceps, specimen container with preservative, completed laboratory requisition form, personal wipes or tissues, equipment for assessing vital signs, examination gloves

| STEPS | REASONS |
|---|---|
| 1. Wash your hands. | Hand washing aids infection control. |
| 2. Assemble the equipment and supplies. Write the name of the patient on the label of the specimen container and complete the laboratory requisition. | The name of the patient must be clearly marked on the container and the laboratory requisition form must be complete for accurate identification and processing of any specimens taken. |
| 3. Check the light source if a flexible sigmoidoscope is being used. Turn off the power after checking for working order to avoid a buildup of heat in the instrument. | If heat is permitted to build up in the scope, the patient may be burned. If the rigid sigmoidoscope, anoscope, or proctoscope is being used, check the examination light for working order. |

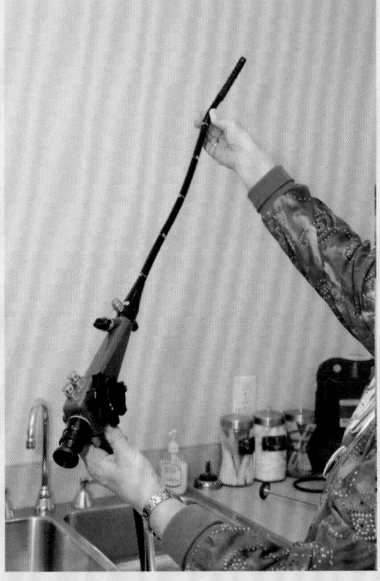

**Step 3.** Make sure the equipment, such as the sigmoidoscope, is in good working order.

4. Greet and identify the patient and explain the procedure. Identify yourself including your title. Inform the patient that a sensation of pressure or the need to defecate may be felt during the procedure and that the pressure is from the instrument and will ease. The patient may also feel gas pressure when air is insufflated during sigmoidoscopy. *Note:* The patient may have been ordered to take a mild sedative before the procedure.

Identifying the patient prevents errors in treatment. Explaining the procedure helps ease anxiety and ensure compliance.

(continues on page 872)

## PROCEDURE 33-1 (continued)

| STEPS | REASONS |
|---|---|
| 5. Instruct the patient to empty the urinary bladder. | Pressure from the instrument may injure a full bladder. Urine in the bladder may increase discomfort. |
| 6. Assess the vital signs and record them in the medical record. | Colon examination procedures may cause cardiac arrhythmias and a change in blood pressure in some patients. Baseline vital signs will allow you to detect variations from the patient's normal vital signs. |
| 7. Have the patient undress completely from the waist down and put on a gown. Drape appropriately. | Drapes will provide privacy and warmth. |
| 8. Assist the patient onto the examination table. If the instrument is an anoscope or a fiberoptic device, Sims position or a side-lying position is most comfortable. If a rigid instrument is used, the patient will assume a knee–chest position or be placed on a proctology table that supports the patient in a knee–chest position. *Note:* Do not ask the patient to assume the knee–chest position until the physician is ready to begin. The position is difficult to maintain. Drape the patient appropriately. | These positions facilitate the procedure by moving the abdominal organs up into the abdominal cavity rather than the pelvis. |

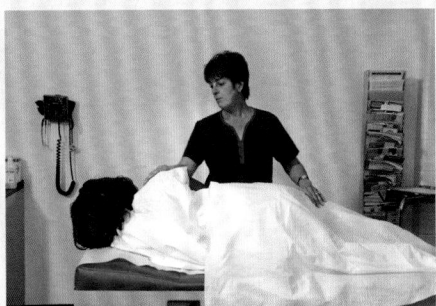

**Step 8.** This patient is in the Sims position.

| STEPS | REASONS |
|---|---|
| 9. **AFF** Explain how to respond to a patient who is visually impaired. | Observe patients carefully to prevent injury and always ask before offering assistance. Face the patient when speaking and always let him or her know what you are going to do before touching him or her. |
| 10. Assist the physician as needed with lubricant, instruments, power, swabs, suction, and specimen containers. | Anticipating what the physician needs and being ready to hand items to the physician will provide for a smooth and quick procedure. |
| 11. During the procedure, monitor the patient's response and offer reassurance. Instruct the patient to breathe slowly through pursed lips. | Reminding the patient how to breathe will aid in relaxation during the procedure. |
| 12. When the physician is finished, assist the patient into a comfortable position and allow a rest period. Offer personal cleaning wipes or tissues. Take the vital signs before allowing the patient to stand, and assist the patient from the table and with dressing as needed. Give the patient any instructions regarding care after the procedure and follow-up ordered by the physician. | A drop in blood pressure on standing is common after lying in any of these positions for an extended period. If the patient complains of dizziness or light-headedness after sitting up, have him or her lie down. If any biopsy samples were taken, the patient may have slight rectal bleeding. |

## PROCEDURE 33-1 (continued)

| STEPS | REASONS |
|---|---|
| 13. Clean the room and route the specimen to the laboratory with the requisition. Disinfect or dispose of the supplies and equipment as appropriate and wash your hands. | Follow standard precautions throughout the procedure. |
| 14. **AFF** Log into the electronic medical record (EMR) using your username and secure password OR obtain the paper medical record from a secure location and assure it is kept away from public access. Because you did not perform the procedure, you do not need to document the colon procedure. However, you are required to document your part in preparing specimens obtained and patient instructions after the procedure. Your entry must include the date, time, and your name/credentials. | Procedures are considered not to have been done if they are not recorded. |
| 15. When finished, log out of the EMR and/or replace the paper medical record in an appropriate and secure location. | |

**Charting Example:**
*05/31/2016 12:45 PM T 98.6 (O), P 100, R 20, BP 144/86 (L). Sigmoidoscopy performed by Dr. Jacobs and specimen obtained—pt. tolerated well. Specimen to Acme Lab, VS after procedure P 112, R 24, BP 146/86 (L). Pt. denied dizziness after procedure. Discharged per Dr. Jacobs _____ . S. Clay, CMA*

Note: *The medical assistant may sign his or her name in the patient record using only the "CMA" credential if the office has a signature log denoting the entire credential as "CMA (AAMA)."*

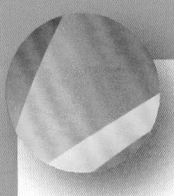

## PSY  PROCEDURE 33-2

# Test stool specimen for occult blood: Guaiac method.

**PSY**  Obtain specimens and perform CLIA-waived microbiology tests; differentiate between normal and abnormal results; document patient care accurately in the medical record.

**Purpose:** To test stool for occult blood from a sample collected by the patient using a test kit and either brought back to the office or mailed into the office per office policy and procedure

**Equipment:** Gloves, labeled specimen pack or packs (the patient may bring in up to 3 samples per the office policy), test developer or reagent drops, biohazardous waste container

| STEPS | REASONS |
|---|---|
| 1. Wash your hands. | Hand washing aids in infection control. |
| 2. Verify the stool sample collected by the patient appropriately labeled and that the physician has ordered a stool for occult blood. Assemble the equipment and supplies and put on gloves. | The physician must order a stool for occult blood. |
| 3. Check the expiration date on the developer or reagent solution. | Solution that has expired may yield inaccurate results. |
| 4. Open the test window on the back of each test pack. Apply one drop of the developer solution to each window according to the manufacturer's instructions. | Following the manufacturer's instructions ensures accurate test results. |
| 5. Read the color change within the specified time period, usually 60 seconds. | The test results must be read within the appropriate time for accurate results. |
| 6. Apply one drop of developer as directed on the control section or window of each test pack. Note whether the control results are positive or negative. If the control results are acceptable, the patient results may be reported. | Patient test results cannot be reported if quality control (QC) results are not acceptable. If control results are not acceptable, do not record the patient results as they may not be accurate. Notify the physician that the test pack did not meet quality control standards. |
| 7. Properly dispose of the test pack or packs and your gloves in a biohazardous waste container. Wash your hands. | The test packs and your gloves are contaminated and must be disposed of properly to prevent the spread of disease. Washing your hands aids in preventing the spread of disease. |
| 8. **AFF**  Log into the electronic medical record (EMR) using your username and secure password OR obtain the paper medical record from a secure location and assure it is kept away from public access. Document the results of the test noting the results as "positive" or "negative" for occult blood. Your entry must include the date, time, and your name/credentials. | Procedures are considered not to have been done if they are not recorded. |

## PROCEDURE 33-2 (continued)

| STEPS | REASONS |
|---|---|
| **9.** When finished, log out of the EMR and/or replace the paper medical record in an appropriate and secure location. | |

**Charting Example:**
*05/31/2016 4:45 PM Occult blood slides x3 returned to office via mail. X3 test packs negative for occult blood*
_____ *S. Clay, CMA*

**Note:** *The medical assistant may sign his or her name in the patient record using only the "CMA" credential if the office has a signature log denoting the entire credential as "CMA (AAMA)."*

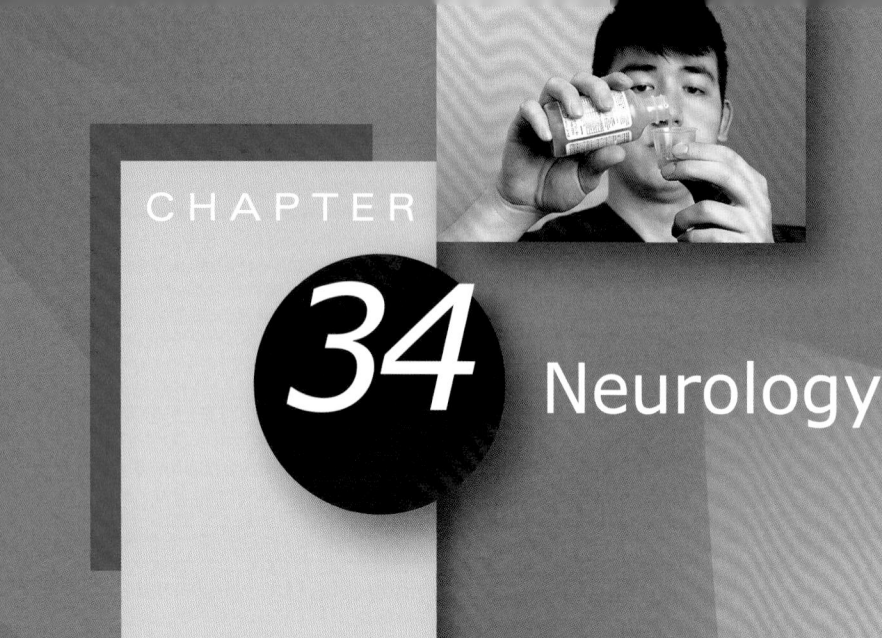

CHAPTER

# *34* Neurology

## Learning Outcomes

### COG Cognitive Domain*

1. Spell key terms
2. *Define medical terms and abbreviations related to all body systems*
3. *Describe structural organization of the human body*
4. *List major organs in each body system*
5. *Identify the anatomical location of major organs in each body system*
6. *Describe the normal function of each body system*
7. *Identify common pathology related to each body system including signs, symptoms, and etiology*
  a. List and describe common diseases of the nervous system
  b. Describe the physical and emotional effects of degenerative nervous system disorders
  c. List potential complications of a spinal cord injury
  d. Name and describe the common procedures for diagnosing nervous system disorders

### PSY Psychomotor Domain*

1. Assist with a lumbar puncture (Procedure 34-1)
  a. *Instruct and prepare a patient for a procedure or treatment*
  b. *Coach patients appropriately considering cultural diversity, developmental life stage, and communication barriers*
  c. *Coach patients regarding disease prevention and treatment plans*
  d. *Document patient care accurately in the medical record*

### AFF Affective Domain*

1. Incorporate critical thinking skills when performing patient assessment
2. Incorporate critical thinking skills when performing patient care
3. Show awareness of a patient's concerns related to the procedure being performed
4. Demonstrate empathy, active listening, and nonverbal communication
5. Demonstrate respect for individual diversity including gender, race, religion, age, economic status, and appearance
6. Explain to a patient the rationale for performance of a procedure
7. Demonstrate sensitivity to patient rights
8. Protect the integrity of the medical record

*Note: AAMA/CAAHEP 2015 Standards are italicized.*

### ABHES Competencies

1. Assist the physician with the regimen of diagnostic and treatment modalities as they relate to each body system
2. Comply with federal, state, and local health laws and regulations
3. Communicate on the recipient's level of comprehension
4. Serve as a liaison between the physician and others
5. Show empathy and impartiality when dealing with patients
6. Document accurately

## Key Terms

## Case Study

*A*lthough patients with disorders of the nervous system may be seen in many types of physician offices, some may be referred to neurologists. The neurology office at Great Falls Medical Center employs two physicians, one physician assistant, and two medical assistants. Brenda Ryan, CMA (AAMA), is one of the medical assistants employed at this office. Today, several patients with seizure disorders are scheduled to be seen and one patient, a 22-year-old college student, has been referred to the neurologist for symptoms consistent with multiple sclerosis. What tests might the physician perform for patients with seizure disorders? What is Brenda's role in assisting the neurologist with examination of the nervous system? These and other questions about the specialty of neurology will be answered in this chapter.

The nervous system is the chief communication and command center for all parts of the body. The nervous system has two divisions: the central nervous system (CNS) and the peripheral nervous system (PNS). The CNS includes the brain and spinal cord (Fig. 34-1), and the PNS contains the nerves that transmit impulses. Nerves are found throughout the body and in the brain. The autonomic nervous system (ANS), a division of the PNS, functions without voluntary action. Together, these divisions of the nervous system allow skeletal movement, maintain vital homeostatic functions such as breathing and heart rate, and promote thought processes including memory and logic. The complexity of the nervous system and its connections with the muscular system make it subject to many disorders that can be difficult to diagnose and treat effectively.

Neurology deals with study of the nervous system and its disorders, and the physician who specializes in this area is a neurologist. The medical assistant who works in a neurology office has many interesting and challenging patients. Also, the medical assistant who works in other medical specialties may also have patients with diseases or disorders of the nervous system. This chapter focuses on some of the common disorders of the nervous system and the role of the medical assistant who works with these patients.

## COG COMMON NERVOUS SYSTEM DISORDERS

### Infectious Disorders

Disorders of the nervous system range from minor inconveniences to lethal diseases. The following sections discuss the disorders in groups: infectious, degenerative, convulsive (**seizures**), developmental, traumatic, neoplastic (tumors), and headache.

### Meningitis

Meningitis is characterized by inflammation of the meninges covering the spinal cord and the brain. The inflammation can result from either bacterial or viral infection. Viral meningitis is usually not life threatening and is often short-lived, but bacterial meningitis is often severe and may be fatal. The infection is usually precipitated by an upper respiratory, sinus, or ear infection. Children are the age group most likely to develop meningitis. Meningitis can also result from head trauma when an open wound allows organisms to enter the cranium and nervous system.

Patients with meningitis have a variety of signs and symptoms, including nausea, vomiting, fever, headache,

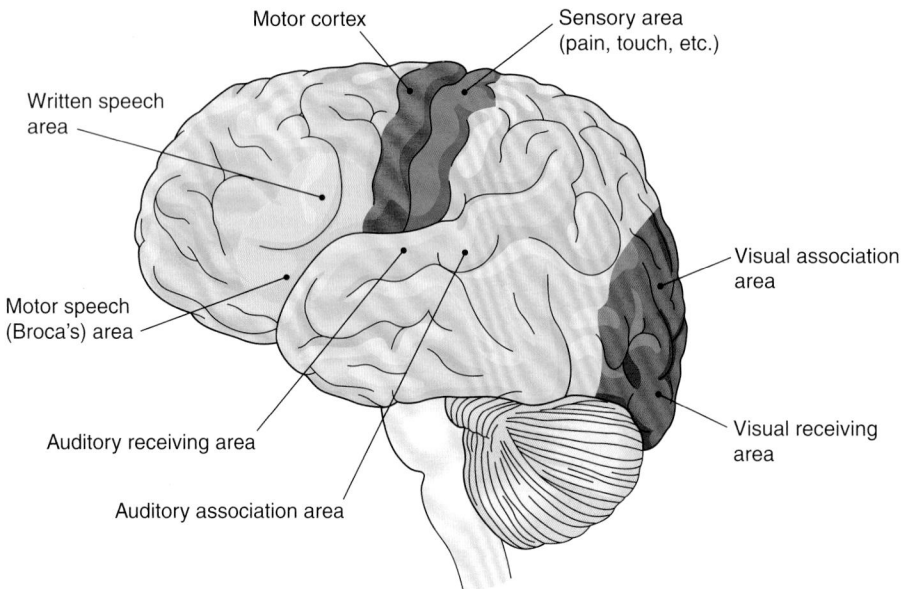

**Figure 34-1** • Functional areas of the cerebral cortex. (Reprinted with permission from Cohen BJ. *Memmler's The Human Body in Health and Disease.* 11th ed. Philadelphia: Lippincott Williams & Wilkins, 2009.)

and a stiff neck. Patients may also complain of photophobia, or intolerance to light. A rash with small, reddish purple dots may appear on the body, and as patients become sicker, they may slip into a coma and have seizures.

To diagnose meningitis, the physician usually orders a complete blood count. If the white blood cell count is high, a lumbar puncture is performed, and cerebrospinal fluid (CSF) is sent to the laboratory for analysis to determine the infectious organism. The treatment of meningitis depends on the organism causing the infection. The treatment for viral meningitis includes fluids and bed rest, and bacterial meningitis is treated with antibiotics and generally requires hospitalization. The local health department must be notified of the diagnosis, and some states require that an infectious disease form be filed. Check your office policy and procedure manual to determine who is responsible for obtaining, completing, and submitting these reports, keeping in mind that, in many offices, it is the medical assistant's responsibility. Depending on the type of meningitis, individuals (family, friends, coworkers, classmates) who have had contact with the patient may require prophylactic treatment.

## Encephalitis

Encephalitis is an inflammation of the brain that frequently results from a viral infection following a varicella (chicken pox), measles, or mumps infection. A strain of the virus is transmitted by mosquitoes. This type is primarily seen on the East and Gulf coasts. Symptoms of all forms include drowsiness, headache, and fever. Seizures and coma may occur in later stages. Diagnosis is made via lumbar puncture and analysis of CSF.

Treatment of encephalitis requires hospitalization for intravenous fluid therapy and supportive care.

The prognosis is usually good if the diagnosis is made early and treatment begins quickly. As with meningitis, the local health department should be notified to identify those who may have been exposed to the disease.

### CHECKPOINT QUESTION

1. How does the treatment of viral meningitis differ from that of bacterial meningitis?

## Herpes Zoster

**Herpes zoster,** or *shingles,* is caused by the virus that causes chickenpox and occurs only in those who have had a varicella infection (see Chapter 28). Herpes zoster usually occurs in adults, often in times of physical or emotional stress. The virus, which lies dormant after the initial infection, becomes reactivated and spreads down the length of a nerve, causing redness, swelling, and pain (Fig. 34-2). After about 48 hours, a band of papules develops on the skin following the nerve pathway. These lesions commonly appear on the face, back, and chest and progress to vesicles, pustules, and then dry crusts similar to chickenpox lesions. The lesions may last for 2 to 5 weeks, and the patient may have pain after the lesions disappear.

The treatment of a herpes zoster breakout includes an analgesic or nerve block for pain. Calamine lotion may be applied to the skin to reduce itching. Antiviral medication, such as acyclovir, may be prescribed to alleviate the severity of the disease.

## Poliomyelitis

Commonly called polio, this highly contagious and resistant virus affects the brain and spinal cord. The virus

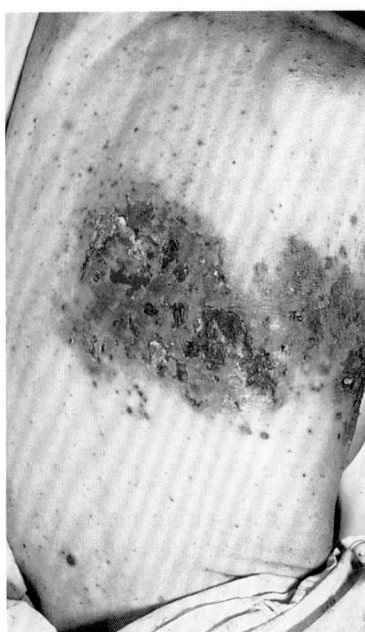

**Figure 34-2** • Primary skin lesions. Herpes zoster (shingles) is an acute, inflammatory, infectious skin disease caused by a herpes virus. (From Weber J, Kelley J. *Health Assessment in Nursing*. 2nd ed. Philadelphia: Lippincott Williams & Wilkins, 2003.)

can live outside the body for several months, making it almost impossible to eliminate once it has appeared in a community. It is transmitted by direct contact, usually through the mouth. In the United States, its incidence has been greatly reduced by aggressive immunization programs. However, because not all children have received the proper schedule of immunizations and because some adults have not been immunized at all, concern about the disease still exists.

In the acute phase, the patient may complain of a stiff neck, fever, headaches, and a sore throat. Nausea, vomiting, and diarrhea may also occur. As the disease progresses, paralysis may develop. Muscle atrophy leads to eventual deformities (Fig. 34-3). If the respiratory muscles are affected, the patient cannot breathe without artificial assistance.

A new dimension of the disease, postpoliomyelitis muscular atrophy (PPMA) syndrome, has been documented in some individuals who had polio as children. Many of these patients have signs and symptoms similar to those that signaled the onset of the original disease. They usually complain of muscle weakness and a lack of coordination. Typically, patients with PPMA are treated on an outpatient basis with supportive care. No cure is available.

During the acute stage of polio, treatment is palliative and supportive. After this acute stage has resolved, treatment of the patient is rehabilitation of the weakened extremities with a strong emphasis on physical and occupational therapy. To increase mobility, patients are fitted with mechanical supports such as braces and splints. Some patients must wear these devices indefinitely. Emotional support is important for these patients,

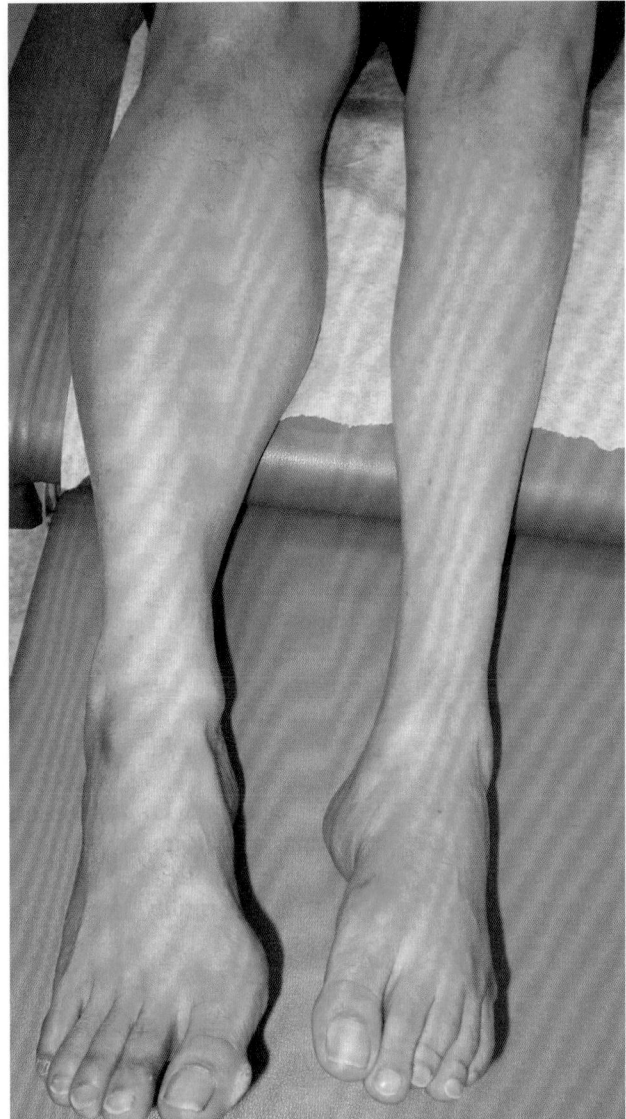

**Figure 34-3** • Muscle atrophy in the left leg due to polio. (Image provided by Stedman's.)

particularly those with PPMA. Many need counseling to reconcile themselves to body image changes caused by the deformities and to allay fear of dependency.

Activities aimed at preventing polio are essential. You may be responsible for patient education regarding immunizations. The previously used oral polio vaccine contained a weakened form of the polio virus, but today's newer injectable form does not contain a live or weakened form of the virus. In the oral form, the virus could be shed in the stool of the immunized child, and caretakers who were not immunized could contract the disease. This is not possible with the newer form of the vaccine.

## Tetanus

Tetanus, commonly called *lockjaw*, is an infection of nervous tissue caused by the tetanus bacillus, *Clostridium tetani*, which lives in the intestinal tract of animals and is excreted in their feces. The microorganism is also found in almost all soil. An infection occurs after the microbe enters the body through an open wound in the skin, often a puncture wound. Wounds caused by farm equipment involving manure are especially susceptible to a tetanus infection. All deep, dirty wounds should be treated as high risk for tetanus.

Tetanus has a slow incubation period. It may inhabit the body for up to 14 weeks before signs and symptoms appear. Initial symptoms include spasms of the voluntary muscles, restlessness, and stiff neck. As the disease progresses, seizures and **dysphagia** (difficulty swallowing) develop. The facial and oral muscles contract, leaving the mouth sealed with the teeth clenched tightly. Untreated, the respiratory muscles become paralyzed, and the disease is typically fatal.

Prevention is the best defense against tetanus. Wounds should be properly cleaned immediately. Dead tissue around the wound must be removed, and an antibiotic should be given if the wound appears infected. To obtain immunity early in life, immunizations are administered to infants and children on a schedule determined by the American Academy of Pediatrics and the Centers for Disease Control and Prevention. After the initial immunization schedule is complete, the vaccine must be given every 10 years for life. Patients who develop an infection with the tetanus microbe require immediate hospitalization and aggressive antibiotic therapy. The prognosis is guarded when tetanus has fully developed.

---

 **CHECKPOINT QUESTION**

2. Although Brenda has never seen a patient with tetanus, what are the initial signs of a tetanus infection?

---

## Rabies

Rabies is caused by a virus that is commonly transmitted by animal saliva through a bite wound from an infected animal and spreads to the organs of the central nervous system. Animals that commonly transmit rabies are skunks, squirrels, raccoons, bats, dogs, cats, coyotes, and foxes. Children are at highest risk for rabies because they are most likely to be bitten by such animals.

The incubation period for rabies ranges from 10 days to many months, depending on the location of the bite. Initial symptoms include fever, general malaise, and body aches. As the disease progresses, mental derangement, paralysis, and photophobia develop. The patient's saliva becomes extremely profuse and sticky, and the throat muscles begin to spasm, making swallowing difficult or impossible, which causes profuse drooling. Muscle spasms of the throat occur at the sight of water or when attempting to drink water, resulting in hydrophobia. The progressive involvement of the tissues of the brain is often fatal.

Immediate treatment of a wound caused by an animal must be the first priority. After the wound is cleansed, the patient should receive an antibiotic and prophylactic vaccine therapy consisting of the human diploid cell vaccine and a rabies immune globulin vaccine. All animal bites must be reported to the city or county animal control center, and you may be responsible for completing and submitting the report. If possible, the animal should be quarantined and evaluated for behavioral changes. If the animal is domestic, a complete veterinary history must be obtained. A copy of the animal's rabies tag and certificate, if available, should be placed in the patient's chart.

## Reye Syndrome

Reye syndrome, a devastating nervous system illness, typically occurs in children after a viral illness, commonly varicella (chickenpox). Studies have found that the use of aspirin in the presence of a viral illness increases the risk of developing Reye syndrome. No other antipyretic agents have been implicated in this disorder. Reye syndrome is not contagious.

While this disorder can affect all organs of the body, it most often affects the liver and the brain. Initial symptoms include vomiting and lethargy, and as the brain swelling continues, confusion, seizures, and coma may develop quickly. The signs and symptoms of Reye syndrome should be treated as a medical emergency because early diagnosis and treatment increase the chances of recovering. The prognosis depends on the amount and severity of cerebral edema. Diagnosis is made by obtaining blood samples to determine liver function, including ammonia, aspartate aminotransferase, and alanine aminotransferase levels. Patients with Reye syndrome require rapid hospitalization, aggressive antibiotic therapy to prevent secondary bacterial infection, and supportive care.

# Degenerative Disorders
## Multiple Sclerosis

The cause of multiple sclerosis (MS) is unknown, but possible origins include a viral infection, autoimmunity, immunologic response, and genetic predisposition. In MS, the myelin sheaths covering many neurons in the body degenerate and are replaced with plaque, which impairs nerve impulse conduction (Fig. 34-4). Multiple sclerosis most commonly occurs in women aged 20 to 40 years and is characterized by remissions and exacerbations. Although there is no cure, the rate and severity of progression vary greatly among patients.

Typically, patients complain initially of progressive loss of muscle control. They may also complain of loss of balance, shaking tremors, and poor muscle coordination. Tingling and numbness can also be the first signs of the disease. **Dysphasia** (difficulty speaking) may be

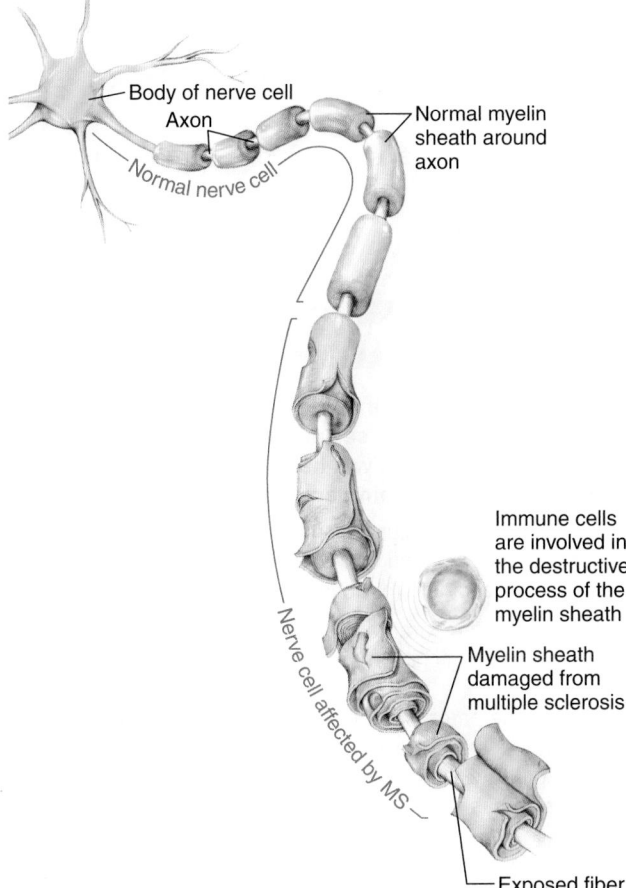

**Figure 34-4 •** Nerve cell in multiple sclerosis.

*Labels on figure:*
Body of nerve cell
Axon
Normal nerve cell
Normal myelin sheath around axon
Immune cells are involved in the destructive process of the myelin sheath
Myelin sheath damaged from multiple sclerosis
Nerve cell affected by MS
Exposed fiber

another sign. As the disease progresses, bladder dysfunction and complaints of visual disturbances are common. Patients may also develop nystagmus (involuntary rapid movement of the eyeball in all directions).

Treatment of MS is palliative. Physical therapy is critical to limit the extent of muscle deterioration and to maintain existing muscle strength. As the disease progresses, the patient is often fitted for prosthetic appliances such as crutches to assist with mobility. Drug therapy includes muscle relaxants and steroids. Because this disease affects persons in the prime of life, patients with MS and their families require psychological support from all of their regular health care providers. Many support groups and counselors specialize in providing therapy for persons with debilitating diseases, including MS, and this information should be shared with patients and families as appropriate.

## Amyotrophic Lateral Sclerosis

Commonly known as Lou Gehrig disease, amyotrophic lateral sclerosis (ALS) causes a progressive loss of motor neurons. ALS is a terminal disease with no known cause, but a strong familial connection has been observed. It occurs most often in middle-aged

men. It begins with loss of muscle mobility in the forearms, hands, and legs and then progresses to the facial muscles, causing dysphasia and dysphagia that worsen over time. Death usually occurs 3 to 5 years after the onset of symptoms.

Treatment of ALS consists of keeping the patient comfortable and educating the family. As the disease progresses, it becomes increasingly difficult for the patient to maintain an unobstructed airway. The family must be taught to prevent and manage choking. Often, the physician discusses advance directives, or end-of-life requests, with the family and the patient. Ideally, the medical assistant will be present for these discussions to provide emotional support.

## Parkinson Disease

This disease is most often seen in older adults; however, it may begin in middle adulthood. Because the disease is a neurologic disorder affecting specific neurotransmitters, or chemicals, in the brain, the symptoms appear gradually and cause a decrease in muscle control. Common symptoms of this disease include rigid muscles, involuntary tremors, and difficulty walking. For more information about Parkinson disease, refer to Chapter 39.

---

### CHECKPOINT QUESTION

3. A patient is seen in the neurology office with a diagnosis of multiple sclerosis. Should health care professionals such as Brenda worry that multiple sclerosis is contagious?

---

## Seizure Disorders

Seizures, commonly called **convulsions,** are involuntary contractions of voluntary muscles caused by a rapid succession of electrical impulses through the brain. Seizures have many causes, including chemical imbalance, trauma, pregnancy-induced hypertension, tumor, and withdrawal from drugs or alcohol. However, many seizures are idiopathic (have no known cause).

Epilepsy is the most common form of seizure disorder. Epilepsy may appear in early childhood or at any life stage. Diagnosis is made through **electroencephalogram (EEG)** studies, blood tests, and radiologic tests. Epileptic seizures are characterized as either petit mal or grand mal. Petit mal seizures, also called *absence seizures* or *partial seizures,* are briefer than grand mal seizures and usually occur only in childhood. The child may appear to fall asleep or drift away momentarily. Some muscle twitching may occur. Then, the child awakes and continues the interrupted activity. Petit mal seizures may go undetected for many years.

Grand mal seizures, also called *tonic–clonic seizures*, are more involved than petit mal seizures. Generally, the patient will go through three phases:

1. The first phase is an **aura**, or warning that a seizure is impending. The aura may include tingling in the extremities, visual signs (such as flashing lights), or perception of a particular taste or odor. Not all patients have auras, but those who do usually perceive the same aural phenomena each time.
2. The second phase is complete loss of consciousness with extensive muscle twitching or contractions, which may be violent. The patient falls and usually loses control of bladder and bowel functions.
3. The third phase is the postictal phase. The patient slowly regains consciousness but remains drowsy for an extended time.

The primary treatment during the actual seizure is preventing injury to the patient (see Chapter 26). Epilepsy is treated with various pharmacologic agents that must be taken by the patient regularly to prevent seizure activity. Instruct patients to take their medication every day as prescribed by the physician, never missing a dose. Many epileptic patients who become stabilized and seizure free on medication decide they no longer need the medication. Remind these patients that stopping the medication may lead to the recurrence of seizures.

A patient who has seizures is usually permitted to have a driver's license, but each state has specific regulations requiring that patients be seizure free for a particular length of time. The patient may ask the physician to complete paperwork from the state issuing the driver's license, and you may be asked to assist with completion of these forms.

## Febrile Seizures

Febrile (fever) seizures occur in a small number of children, most commonly aged 6 months to 3 years, with an elevated body temperature. Children with febrile seizures must have a complete physical and neurologic examination to rule out the possibility of organic origin of the seizures. Typically, children generally outgrow febrile seizures by age 6 or 7 years and have no further seizure activity.

Treatment is gently returning the child's body temperature to a more manageable level. Cool compresses are preferable to ice baths or alcohol sponge baths, which may cause hypothermia. Because of the danger of Reye syndrome, these children should not be given salicylates, or products containing aspirin, to reduce the temperature.

## Focal Seizures

A focal, or *jacksonian*, seizure begins as a small local seizure that spreads to adjacent areas. For instance, the small seizure may begin in the fingers and spread to the hand and arm. The cause of focal seizures must be researched to prevent the progression to general seizures.

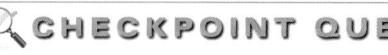

### CHECKPOINT QUESTION

4. How do petit mal seizures differ from grand mal seizures?

### WHAT IF

**What if the mother of a 2-year-old child who recently had a febrile seizure tells you that she is scared that the child will have another seizure and that it will cause brain damage?**

Because febrile seizures can be very scary for parents of small children, you can help them cope with these measures by doing the following:

- Reassure the parents that febrile seizures are common in young children and that they generally are not chronic.
- Allow the parents to be involved in the care of the child. If a seizure occurs in the medical office, urge the parents to hold and comfort the child after the seizure has subsided and the physician has evaluated the child.
- Provide easy-to-understand explanations for all procedures.
- Encourage parents to talk about their fears.
- Remain calm and demonstrate confidence in handling the situation.

## Developmental Disorders
### Neural Tube Defects

Many abnormalities may occur during the embryonic and fetal stages of development. As the embryo develops, the tissue over the neural tube (a tubelike section of the developing embryo) closes and evolves into the components of the CNS. If a developmental failure occurs on the proximal (upper) portion, anencephaly, or the absence of a brain, may result. An abnormality in development in the distal, or caudal, end of the neural tube results in spina bifida. **Spina bifida occulta** is the most benign form. In this condition, the posterior laminae of the vertebrae fail to close, typically at L5 or S1. There are usually no external signs of deformity, although there may be a skin dimple or dark tufts of hair over this area on the lower back. A **meningocele** occurs when the meninges protrude through the spina bifida. In spina bifida with **myelomeningocele**, the most severe form, the spinal cord and meninges protrude externally (Fig. 34-5A–D). The main treatment is surgical intervention; prognosis is based on the extent of spinal cord involvement.

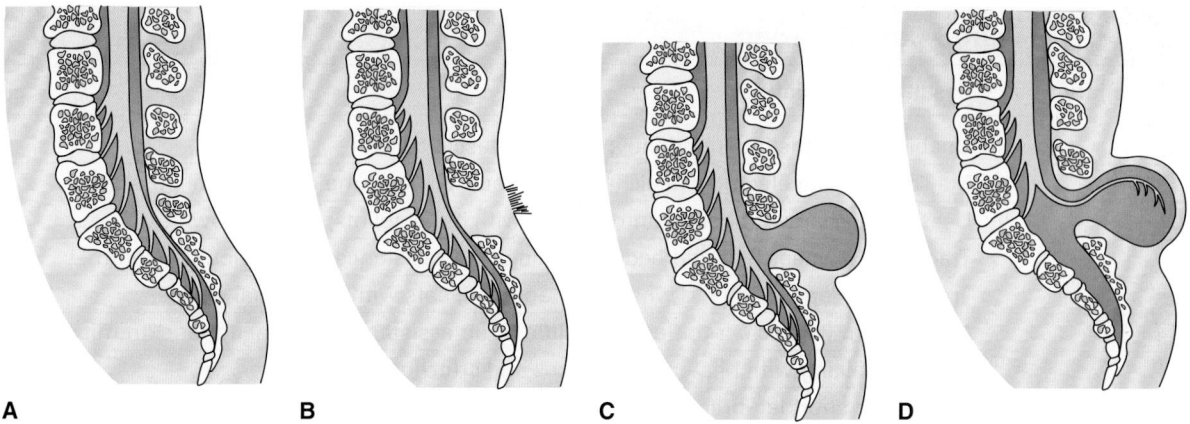

**Figure 34-5 •** Spinal defects. **(A)** Normal spinal cord. **(B)** Spina bifida occulta. **(C)** Meningocele. **(D)** Meningomyelocele. (Reprinted with permission from Pillitteri A. *Maternal and Child Health Nursing: Care of the Childbearing and Childrearing Family.* 5th ed. Philadelphia: Lippincott Williams & Wilkins, 2007.)

 **PATIENT EDUCATION**

### Alpha-Fetoprotein

This blood test is routinely performed during the second trimester (weeks 16 to 18) of pregnancy to check for maternal serum levels of alpha-fetoprotein and screen the fetus for defects in the neural tube. If this protein is found to be high, there may be nervous system disorders in the fetus, such as spina bifida, whereas low levels may indicate trisomy 13 or Down syndrome. Because abnormal results may occur due to more than one fetus or incorrect due dates, high or low results indicate the need for further studies such as sonography or amniocentesis before a definitive diagnosis is made.

## Hydrocephalus

Hydrocephalus occurs when the arachnoid and ventricular spaces of the brain contain excessive CSF. Although it occurs most commonly in infants and children as the result of a defect in CSF production or absorption, hydrocephalus sometimes occurs in adults as a result of tumor or trauma. Treatment is surgical insertion of a shunt, which reroutes the excessive CSF from the brain to the right atrium of the heart or the peritoneal cavity. The prognosis is usually good if hydrocephalus is treated aggressively in the early stages, before CNS damage.

## Cerebral Palsy

Cerebral palsy describes a group of neuromuscular disorders that result from CNS damage during the prenatal, neonatal, or postnatal period. Although cerebral palsy is not progressive, the damage may become more obvious as developmental delays are discovered. Impairment may range from slight motor dysfunction to catastrophic physical and mental disabilities. Prognosis varies with

the site of the damage and its severity. Treatment is supportive and rehabilitative. No cure exists.

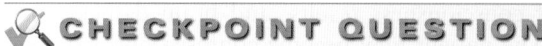 **CHECKPOINT QUESTION**

5. What is spina bifida, and how does it develop?

## Trauma

Traumatic injuries are the most common causes of neurologic disorders and the leading killer of individuals ages 1 to 24 years. The trauma often is a preventable injury to the head that causes edema in the brain tissue or blows to the posterior neck and back, injuring the spinal cord. You can help prevent these types of injuries and the lifelong impairments that accompany permanent damage to the CNS by encouraging parents to require their children to wear a helmet when bicycle riding, skating, skateboarding, and riding in a motor vehicle. Head trauma sustained in a motor vehicle accident often results from the passengers being tossed around the interior of the car or, worse yet, ejected from the vehicle. Inexperienced teenage drivers should also be asked about the use of seat belts not just for themselves but for their passengers as well.

### Traumatic Brain Injuries

Children are at particularly high risk for head trauma. A child's head is large in proportion to the rest of the body; therefore, when children fall (as they frequently do), they often fall head first. Children are also prone to traumatic injuries because their reflex systems are immature. Traumatic injuries to the brain include **concussion**, **contusion**, and intracranial hemorrhage. A concussion is a nonlethal brain injury that results from blunt trauma. The patient may momentarily lose consciousness but promptly return to an awake and alert state. The treatment for concussion is rest and observation for signs of

| TABLE 34-1 | Spinal Cord Injuries |
|---|---|
| **Level of Injury** | **Resulting Disabilities** |
| C1, C2 | Unable to breathe independently; no neck muscle control |
| C3, C4 | May manipulate electric wheelchair with mouthpiece; some neck control possible |
| C5 | Uses wheelchair with hand controls; eats with hand splints; good elbow flexion |
| C6 | Transfers to wheelchair and bed with little or no assistance; good shoulder control |
| C7 | Transfers independently to wheelchair and bed; eats with no special devices |
| T1, T4 | Moves from wheelchair to floor with little or no assistance; normal upper extremity function |
| T5, L2 | Limited walking with bilateral leg braces and crutches |
| L3, L4 | Walks with short leg braces with or without crutches |
| L5, S3 | Walks independently with no equipment if foot strength is good |

C, cervical; L, lumbar; S, sacral; T, thoracic.

a more serious injury, contusion. A contusion is a focal alteration of cerebral circulation. Hemorrhages and extravasation, or pooling, of blood and fluid can result. Loss of consciousness results, and brain damage may occur. The patient may become confused and lethargic and have nausea and vomiting as the intracranial bleeding increases, causing pressure on the brain. Intracranial hemorrhage is bleeding of a vessel inside the skull due to trauma, congenital abnormality, or aneurysm.

Traumatic brain injuries are diagnosed with radiographic studies. Treatment for contusions and hemorrhages can be surgery, drug therapy, and supportive care. The prognosis for all brain injuries depends on the extent of damage and the location of the injury.

## Spinal Cord Injuries

Spinal cord injuries are most common among individuals aged 15 to 35 years. Most spinal cord injuries are due to trauma from a motor vehicle accident, diving accident, or fall. A complete spinal cord injury is one in which the cord is transected and no neurologic abilities remain below the point of injury. An incomplete spinal cord injury is one in which the cord is injured or partially severed, causing minor to severe disability below the point of injury (Table 34-1). The higher in the spinal cord the injury is, the more serious the complications and paralysis for the patient. Table 34-2 describes the types of paralysis that a patient may have and the typical causes of each type.

In caring for patients who may have a spinal cord injury, the initial consideration is to prevent further damage. Accident victims with suspected spinal cord injuries must be kept immobile until proper emergency medical service personnel are present. Treatment in the emergency department is focused on stabilization, and patients usually require an extended hospitalization and rehabilitation, depending on the extent of the damage to the spinal cord.

In the physician's office, recovering trauma patients may receive follow-up treatment and evaluation. These patients are monitored for changes in their reflexes and evaluated for physical therapy and occupational therapy. The goal of long-term care is to prevent complications, which can include skin ulcerations (pressure ulcers), hypostatic pneumonia, bladder infection, muscle contractures, and psychological depression. Most of the physical complications are treated with physical therapy and good care either in the home or in the long-term rehabilitation facility. The mental and emotional complications require intensive therapy by counselors who specialize in treating patients with debilitating disorders.

| TABLE 34-2 | Types of Paralysis | |
|---|---|---|
| **Type** | **Causes** | **Result** |
| Hemiplegia | Cerebrovascular accident; trauma to one side of the brain; tumors | Paralysis on one side of the body, opposite the side of involvement |
| Paraplegia | Spinal cord trauma; spinal tumors | Paralysis of any part of the body below the point of involvement |
| Quadriplegia | Spinal cord trauma; spinal tumors | Paralysis of all limbs (usually cervical or high thoracic vertebra involvement) |

**CHECKPOINT QUESTION**

6. How does a complete spinal cord injury differ from an incomplete one?

## PATIENT EDUCATION

### Spinal Cord and Traumatic Brain Injuries

Spinal cord and traumatic brain injuries are common in young people. Both types of injuries can produce serious, and even fatal, results. As a medical assistant, you must take an active role in educating your community, patients, and friends about prevention of these injuries:

- Use seat belts in automobiles for all passengers.
- Secure infants and young children in approved car seats.
- Avoid alcohol when participating in sporting activities and driving.
- Obey traffic signs and speed limits.
- Avoid illicit drug use and any medication that impairs awareness.
- Wear a helmet while bicycling and riding a motorcycle.
- Never dive head first into water that is shallow or not clear.

## Brain Tumors

A brain tumor may be either malignant or benign and may be a secondary or metastatic site. If the brain tumor is the primary site, it is named for the site of origin (e.g., glioma, meningioma, medulloblastoma). Both malignant and benign tumors can produce serious complications for the patient because of the limited space inside the cranium. Generally, the patient has vague complaints of headaches, blurred vision, personality changes, or memory loss. In more advanced cases, seizures, blindness, and dysphagia may be evident. The type of tumor and its location affect the presenting symptoms, their severity and onset, and the prognosis.

Diagnosis is made primarily with radiologic studies. The treatment can include surgery, radiation therapy, chemotherapy, or a combination of radiation and chemotherapy.

## Headaches

It is estimated that 70% of the population has **cephalalgia**, or headaches. Headaches have a variety of origins, including stress, trauma, bone pathology, infection (e.g., sinus), or vascular disturbance. In many instances, the cause is never known.

**Migraine** headaches are one of the most common types. Migraines can be triggered by stress, high altitude, smoking, certain smells, or ingested chemicals (e.g., caffeine, alcohol, and certain food additives), but in many situations, the cause is unknown. Many patients who have migraines have an aura, or sensory perception such as flashing lights or wavy lines, before onset. Once the migraine headache begins, the symptoms usually include a unilateral temporal headache, photophobia, diplopia (double vision), and nausea. Generally, these headaches are treated with an analgesic, and the patient may be instructed to rest in a dark, quiet room. The physician may also prescribe medication to arrest the headache and symptoms when the migraine begins. These medications, sometimes called *abortive headache medications*, include the triptans (sumatriptan succinate [Imitrex™], naratriptan hydrochloride [Amerge™], and eletriptan hydrobromide [Relpax™]).

Other common types of headaches include the following:

- *Tension headaches* are associated with contraction of the muscles of the neck and scalp due to stress. The treatment is a muscle relaxant, analgesic, and reversing the precipitating factors. Biofeedback techniques may also be useful to assist with coping with stress that cannot be avoided.
- *Cluster headaches* are similar to migraine headaches but typically occur at night. They are usually short lasting but may recur as often as 4 or 5 times a night for several weeks and then not again for weeks or months. Treatment is a muscle relaxant, analgesic, and stress relief techniques.

**CHECKPOINT QUESTION**

7. When obtaining a chief complaint from a patient with migraine headaches, Brenda asked about triggers. What are some triggers for migraine headaches?

## LEGAL TIP

### Risk Management

Risk management includes those activities performed in the medical office that may help reduce or eliminate litigation or lawsuits. A professional medical assistant can practice risk management by

- Documenting concisely and accurately immediately following any patient encounter, either in person or on the telephone
- Being familiar with the office policy and procedure manual and following the guidelines as written
- Communicating clearly with patients and other health care providers while observing the laws regarding confidentiality
- Maintaining compliance with state and federal laws with regard to filing insurance claims and billing procedures
- Practicing within his or her scope of education and training

## ⚙ COMMON DIAGNOSTIC TESTS FOR DISORDERS OF THE NERVOUS SYSTEM

The physician may perform a variety of tests to evaluate a patient's neurologic status. These tests may be invasive or noninvasive and may include radiologic and electrical tests along with physical examination.

### Physical Examination

The physical examination, a key component of diagnosis of nervous system disorders, includes the following evaluations:

- Mental status and orientation
- Cranial nerve assessment
- Sensory and motor functions
- Reflex assessment

The patient's mental status is evaluated by routine questioning to establish mental alertness and orientation. For example, the examiner may ask the patient to count to 10 and to state the president's name and the year.

Cranial nerves are assessed according to the methods described in Table 34-3. Visual acuity may be tested on a chart such as the Snellen eye chart, and the results can indicate a refractive error or a more serious neurologic disorder. Sensory function is tested with the pin versus soft brush method for spinal nerves and cranial nerves. The instrument commonly used is the Buck neurologic hammer (Fig. 34-6). With the patient's eyes closed, the physician uses the pin and brush to determine the patient's ability to distinguish between sensations. The physician evaluates sensory reception and determines whether there is a reception difference on either side of the body.

Motor functioning is tested by watching the patient walk. Many disorders can be detected by observing a patient's gait. Part of this assessment includes the

| **TABLE 34-3** | **Cranial Nerves and Assessment** | | |
| --- | --- | --- | --- |
| Nerve (Number) | Type | Functions | Examination Methods |
| Olfactory (I) | Sensory | Smell | Test each nostril for smell reception, interpretation |
| Optic (II) | Sensory | Vision | Test vision for acuity, visual fields |
| Oculomotor (III) | Motor | Pupil constriction, raise eyelids | Test papillary reaction to light, ability to open and close eyes |
| Trochlear (IV) | Motor | Downward, inward eye movement | Test for downward, inward eye movement |
| Trigeminal (V) | Motor | Jaw movements, chewing, mastication | Ask patient to open and clench jaws while palpating the jaw muscles |
| | Sensory | Sensation on face, neck | Test face and neck for pain sensations, light touch, temperature |
| Abducens (VI) | Motor | Lateral movement of eyes | Test ocular movement in all directions |
| Facial (VII) | Motor | Muscles of face | Ask the patient to raise the eyebrows, smile, show the teeth, puff out the cheeks |
| | Sensory | Sense of taste on anterior two thirds of tongue | Test for taste sensation with various agents |
| Acoustic (VIII) | Sensory | Hearing | Test hearing ability |
| Glossopharyngeal (IX) | Motor | Pharyngeal movement and swallowing | Ask the patient to say "ah," yawn to observe upward movement of soft palate; elicit gag response; note ability to swallow |
| | Sensory | Taste on lower third of tongue | Test for taste with various agents |
| Vagus (X) | Motor | Swallowing, speaking | Ask the patient to swallow, speak; note hoarseness |
| Accessory (XI) | Motor | Movement of shoulder muscles | Ask the patient to shrug against resistance |
| Hypoglossal (XII) | Motor | Movement, strength of tongue against cheek | Ask the patient to protrude the tongue, push the tongue |

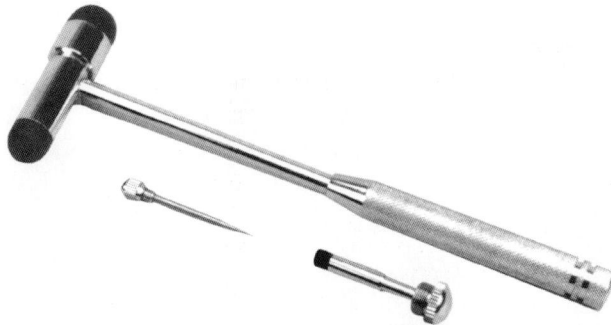

**Figure 34-6 •** The Buck neurologic hammer.

**Romberg test.** The patient is asked to stand with feet together and with the eyes closed. A positive Romberg sign is noted if the patient sways or is unsteady.

The last part of the examination is reflex testing (Table 34-4). Figure 34-7A–D depicts the correct method for tendon reflex testing. Reflexes are scored on the following scale:

0 = No response
1+ = Diminished response
2+ = Normal
3+ = Brisker than normal
4+ = Hyperactive with clonus, which is the repetitive jerking of a muscle and indicates a neurologic disorder

Patients with weak or slow responses to stimuli applied during reflex testing may require additional testing to determine the source of the problem. Since the muscles require electrical impulses from the nervous system to contract, the physician must determine whether the problem is with the muscles or if there is a disorder of the nervous system.

## Radiologic Tests

The most common noninvasive radiologic tests include computed tomography (CT) and magnetic resonance imaging (MRI). These tests may be done with a contrast medium or dye. The contrast medium helps differentiate between the soft tissue areas of the nervous system and the tumors, lesions, or hemorrhages that may blend in with their supporting tissues.

A **myelogram** is an invasive radiologic test in which dye is injected into the CSF. After the dye is injected, the spinal cord is filmed, and any abnormalities, such as tumors or damage from injury, can be detected. The blood vessels of the brain can be visualized on radiographic film by injecting dye through a femoral artery catheter threaded up to the carotid artery in a test called *cerebral angiogram.*

Radiography of the skull may be used to rule out many possible disorders and is diagnostic for fractures.

## Electrical Tests

Electroencephalography (EEG) is a noninvasive test that records electrical impulses in the brain. A variety of electrodes are placed on the patient's scalp, and tracings of brain wave activity are recorded. Typically, the patient is given a mild sedative to induce a quiet state. This test is used to assess hyperactive electrical responses in the brain as seen in patients with seizure disorders. In the inpatient acute care setting, EEG is used to determine brain activity in patients who are on life support but who may be brain dead and have no chance for recovery.

### CHECKPOINT QUESTION
8. What are the differences between a myelogram and an EEG?

## Lumbar Puncture

A lumbar puncture is used to diagnose infectious inflammatory or bleeding disorders affecting the brain

| TABLE 34-4 | Reflex Testing | | |
|---|---|---|---|
| Reflex | Method of Testing | Expected Response | Location |
| Brachioradialis | Tap styloid process of radius | Flexion of elbow | C5, C6 |
| Biceps | Tap biceps tendon | Flexion of elbow | C5, C6 |
| Triceps | Tap triceps | Extension of elbow | C7 |
| Patellar | Tap patellar tendon | Extension of leg | L2, L4 |
| Achilles | Tap Achilles tendon | Plantar flexion of foot | S1 |
| Corneal | Light touch on corneoscleral corner | Closure of eyelid | CN V, VII |

C, cervical; L, lumbar; S, sacral; CN, cranial nerve.

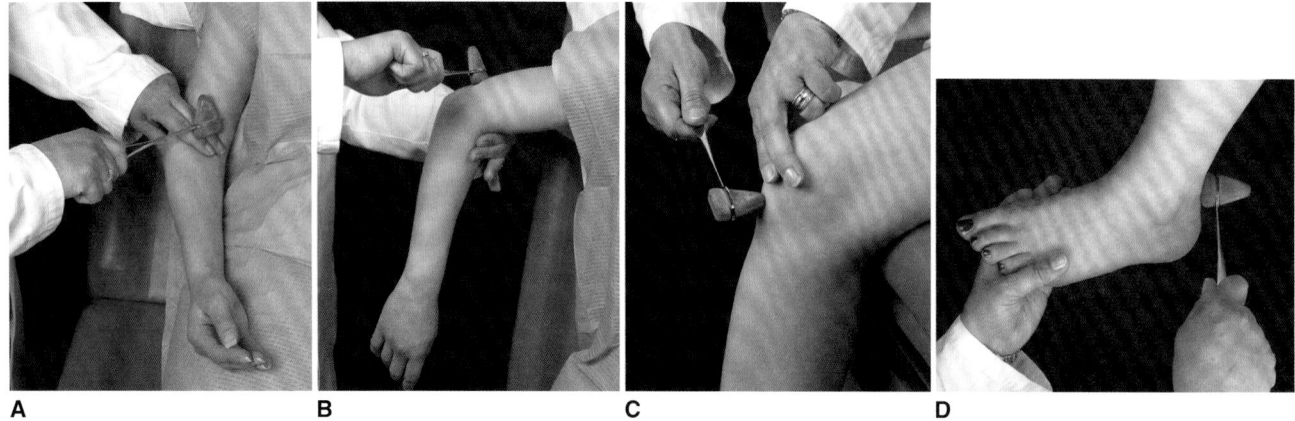

**Figure 34-7** • Techniques for eliciting major tendon reflexes. **(A)** Biceps reflex. **(B)** Triceps reflex. **(C)** Patellar reflex. **(D)** Ankle or Achilles reflex.

and spinal cord or as a means of injecting pain control medication into the spinal column near the nerves producing the pain. A needle is inserted into the subarachnoid space at L4 to L5, below the level of the spinal cord (Fig. 34-8). If CSF is removed and sent to the laboratory, it may be tested for glucose, protein, bacteria, cell counts, and red blood cells, which indicate intracranial bleeding. It may also be performed to evaluate intracranial pressure. An obstruction to CSF flow can be determined with the **Queckenstedt test**. For this test, you will be directed to press against the patient's jugular veins in the neck (right, left, or both) while the physician monitors the pressure of CSF. If CSF pressure increases when the jugular vein is compressed, the finding is normal. If no increase in pressure occurs, the flow of CSF is blocked.

If a lumbar puncture is performed in the medical office, your responsibility includes assisting the patient into a side-lying curled position or a supported forward-bending sitting position and maintaining sterility of the items used during the puncture (see Chapter 22). The physical position is uncomfortable and difficult to maintain, and you should help the patient to relax as much as possible by encouraging slow, deep breathing during the procedure. The steps for assisting the physician with a lumbar puncture are described in Procedure 34-1.

If CSF has been removed, the physician may require that the patient lie flat for 6 to 12 hours to prevent a spinal headache. In addition, the patient may require intravenous fluid and pain medication. For these reasons, the lumbar puncture may be performed in outpatient clinics than in the medical office.

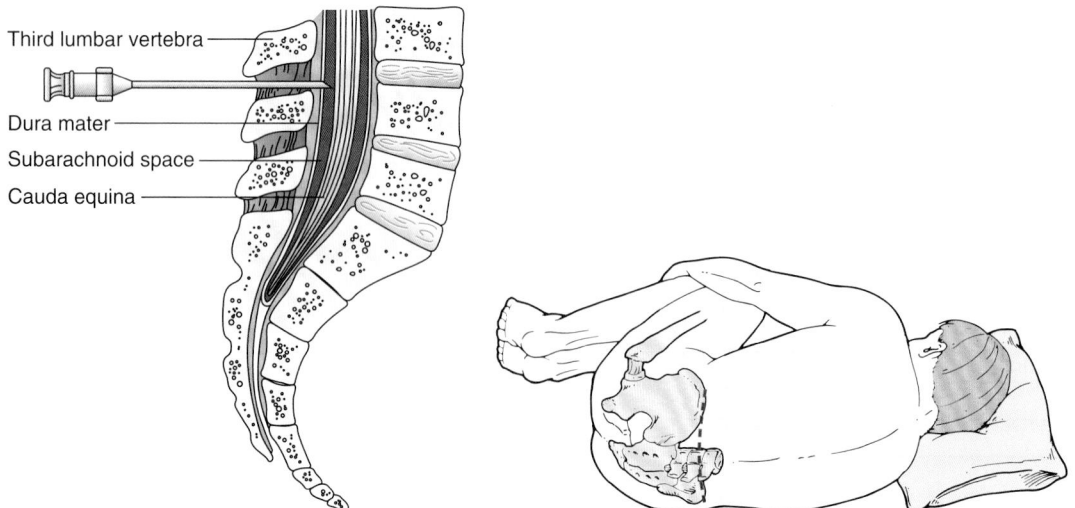

**Figure 34-8** • Technique for lumbar puncture. The L3 to L5 spaces are just below the line connecting the anterior and superior iliac spines. (Taylor C, Lillis CA, LeMone P. *Fundamentals of Nursing.* 2nd ed. Philadelphia: Lippincott Williams & Wilkins, 1993:543.)

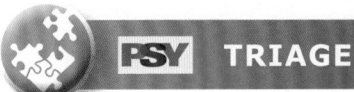

## TRIAGE

While you are working in a medical office, the following three situations occur at the same time:

A. Patient A is a 35-year-old woman who came to the office with a severe migraine. She is sitting in the darkened examination room with an emesis basin because she has been nauseated and vomiting this morning. The physician has ordered an injection of Imitrex™.

B. Patient B is a 46-year-old patient who came to the office for an injection of anesthetic into the spinal column to relieve chronic pain caused by an injury that occurred on the job 2 years ago.

C. Patient C is phoning about a bill received after an office visit last month. The patient is angry and demanding to speak to the physician immediately.

**How do you sort these patients? Who do you see first? Second? Third?**

Patient C should quickly be referred to the office manager or billing supervisor in a calm and professional manner. In most offices, the clinical medical assistant does not have enough information about the patient's account to determine the nature of the problem. Next, patient A should be given the injection and allowed to remain in the examination room until the medication has taken effect or she feels able to leave. While she is resting in the quiet, darkened room after the injection, you can prepare patient B and the treatment room.

## MEDICATION BOX

### Commonly Prescribed Neurology System Medications

**Note:** *The generic name of the drug is listed first and is written in all lowercase letters. Brand names are in parentheses, and the first letter is capitalized.*

| | | |
|---|---|---|
| acetaminophen (Tylenol) | Tablets: 160 mg to 650 mg<br>Caplets: 160 mg, 500 mg<br>Gel caps: 500 mg<br>Oral suspension: 80 mg/0.8 mL<br>Suppositories: 80 mg, 120 mg | Analgesic; antipyretic |
| acyclovir (Zovirax) | Capsules: 200 mg<br>Injection: 500 mg/vial, 1 g/vial (*do not* give intramuscularly or subcutaneously)<br>Tablets: 400 mg, 800 mg | Antiviral |
| carbamazepine (Tegretol) | Capsules: 100 mg, 200 mg, 300 mg<br>Tablets: 200 mg<br>Tablets (chewable): 100 mg | Anticonvulsant |
| cefadroxil (Duricef) | Capsules: 500 mg<br>Oral suspension: 125 mg/5 mL to 500 mg/mL<br>Tablets: 1 g | Antibiotic |
| clonazepam (Klonopin) | Tablets: 0.5 mg, 1 mg, 2 mg<br>Tablets (orally disintegrating): 0.125 mg, 0.25 mg, 0.5 mg, 1 mg, 2 mg | Anticonvulsant |
| eletriptan hydrobromide (Relpax) | Tablets: 20 mg, 40 mg<br>Transdermal: Patches release | Antimigraine |

## MEDICATION BOX (continued)

| | | |
|---|---|---|
| fentanyl transdermal system (Duragesic) | 12.5 mcg, 25 mcg, 50 mcg, 75 mcg, or 100 mcg per hour | Opioid analgesic |
| gabapentin (Neurontin, Gaborone) | Capsules: 100 mg to 400 mg<br>Oral solution: 250 mg/5 mL<br>Tablets: 100 mg to 800 mg | Anticonvulsant |
| ibuprofen (Motrin, Advil, Excedrin IB) | Capsules: 200 mg<br>Oral drops: 40 mg/mL<br>Oral suspension: 100 mg/5 mL<br>Tablets: 100 mg to 800 mg | Analgesic; antipyretic |
| meclizine hydrochloride (Antivert, Dramamine) | Tablets: 12.5 mg, 25 mg, 50 mg | Antiemetic |
| naratriptan (Amerge) | Tablets: 1 mg, 2.5 mg | Antimigraine |
| oxycodone hydrochloride (OxyContin) | Capsules: 5 mg<br>Tablets: 5 mg, 10 mg, 15 mg, 20 mg, 30 mg | Opioid analgesic |
| penicillin G sodium | Injection: (intramuscular or intravenous) 5-million-unit vial | Antibiotic |
| penicillin V potassium (Penicillin VK, Veetids) | Oral suspension: 125 mg/5 mL to 250 mg/mL (after reconstitution)<br>Tablets: 250 mg, 500 mg | Antibiotic |
| phenobarbital (Solfoton) | Elixir: 15 mg/5 mL, 20 mg/5 mL<br>Tablets: 15 mg to 100 mg | Anticonvulsant |
| phenytoin (Dilantin) | Tablets (chewable): 50 mg<br>Oral suspension: 125 mg/5 mL | Anticonvulsant |
| sumatriptan succinate (Imitrex) | Injection: 4 mg/0.5 mL, 6 mg/0.5 mL<br>Tablets: 25 mg, 50 mg<br>Nasal solution: 5 mg/0.1 mL, 20 mg/0.1 mL | Antimigraine |
| tramadol hydrochloride (Ultram) | Tablets: 50 mg | Opioid analgesic |
| valacyclovir (Valtrex) | Tablets: 500 mg, 1,000 mg | Antiviral |

# ROLE-PLAYING ACTIVITY

With cooperation from classmates or as assigned by your instructor, role-play the scenarios as if you are working with Brenda Ryan in the neurology office (refer to the case study at the beginning of the chapter). Haley Brandt, a 22-year-old female, comes into the office today to find out the results of testing she has undergone this past month to determine the cause of general weakness in her arms and tingling in her upper back. You are looking through the medical record and see that the physician has made a diagnosis of multiple sclerosis. The patient is not aware of this diagnosis yet, and after taking her back to the exam room to get her vital signs, she asks you about the results of her tests. She begins to cry and tells you that she is afraid she has something "bad" and is going to "die." What would you say to this patient? How would you respond? Your instructor will give you additional information about this activity!

## *español* SPANISH TERMINOLOGY

**¿Tiene una buena memoria?**
Is your memory good?

**¿Le duele la cabeza?**
Have you any pain in the head?

**¿Se siente mareado?**
Do you feel dizzy?

**¿Se podría voltear por favor para su lado izquierdo/ derecho?**
Can you please turn to your left/right side?

**Por favor cierre sus ojos y toque su nariz con la punta de su dedo.**
Please close your eyes and touch your nose with your pointer finger.

**Usted necesita un electroencefalograma, es un procedimiento sin dolor.**
You need an electroencephalogram; it is a painless procedure.

**Su Sistema Nervioso necesita vitamima B$_{12}$.**
Your nervous system needs vitamin B$_{12}$.

**¿Tiene usted historia familiar de migrañas?**
Do you have family history of migraines?

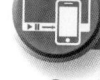

# MEDIA MENU

**Student Resources** on thePoint®
• *Animation:* Nerve Synapse

• **CMA/RMA Certification Exam Review**

**Internet Resources**
**Centers for Disease Control and Prevention**
http://www.cdc.gov/rabies

**National Reye's Syndrome Foundation**
http://www.reyessyndrome.org

**National Institutes of Health**
http://www.nlm.nih.gov/medlineplus/seizures.html;
http://www.nlm.nih.gov/medlineplus/cerebralpalsy.html

**Association for Spina Bifida and Hydrocephalus**
http://www.asbah.org

**Spina Bifida Association of America**
http://www.spinabifidaassociation.org

**National Multiple Sclerosis Society**
http://www.nationalmssociety.org/index.aspx

**Amyotrophic Lateral Sclerosis Association**
http://www.alsa.org

**American Spinal Injury Association**
http://www.asia-spinalinjury.org

## EMR Activity

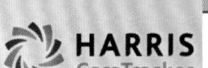

Harris CareTracker is a Web-based electronic medical record (EMR) application that you will use for the EMR activities included in this section at the end of each chapter. This application is actually used in physician offices, but is provided to you through the publisher, Wolters Kluwer Health, to give you hands-on practice working with EMRs. Your instructor will have more information about accessing your username, log-in, and Quickstart guide.

Prerequisite Activities in Harris CareTracker

• *The Getting Started and Quickstart documents and EMR Activities Step-by-Step Instructions are available at* http://thePoint.lww.com/KronenbergerComp5e

Activity Details

Document the vital signs, chief complaint, and present illness in the EMR for each of the following patients seen by Dr. Patel today in the neurology office.

1. Patient: Penelope Wringer: This patient was referred by her family physician, Dr. Kyle Dunn, for complaints of frequent headaches and dizziness for the past month. She tells you she has "a lot of stress" this past month but has continued to work and drive. When asked about her appetite, she says she is sometimes nauseous but has not vomited. Her vital signs are 144/88 (left arm, sitting), radial pulse 76, respirations 16, and temperature using a temporal thermometer 99.0.

2. Patient: Sarah Smith: This patient has a history of epilepsy and is currently taking clonazepam 1.5 mg daily to control her seizures. She says she has not had any seizures in 6 months and is here today for a routine follow-up appointment. Her vital signs are 120/74 (right arm, sitting), radial pulse 72, respirations 20, and temperature 98.4 using the temporal thermometer.

## Chapter Summary

The nervous system is complex and works with both conscious and unconscious functions including providing electrical stimulation to skeletal muscles for movement and psychological processes such as thought and mood. Disorders of the nervous system can be grouped into several types:

- Infectious
- Degenerative
- Convulsive
- Developmental
- Traumatic
- Neoplastic
- Headache

Diagnosing disorders of the nervous system is often complicated and requires many types of tests. Common diagnostic tests include

- Radiologic studies (e.g., CT, MRI)
- EEG
- Physical examination
- Prenatal screening
- Lumbar puncture
- Radiography

Patients with neurological disorders may be seen in any type of medical office; however, some patients may be referred to a neurologist for follow-up or diagnosis. Your responsibilities when working with patients with neurologic disorders may include the following:

- Assisting the physician with the neurologic examination
- Scheduling patients for outpatient procedures
- Providing emotional support to patients and their families or caregivers

## Warm-Ups for Critical Thinking

1. Research and prepare a patient education fact sheet about migraine headaches, including the possible triggers, the causes, and the treatments (include abortive headache medications).
2. A 3-year-old girl comes to the office with varicella zoster (chickenpox). She has a fever, and the physician orders acetaminophen. The child's mother asks, "Why can't she have aspirin instead?" How do you respond?
3. Your patient, a 21-year-old man, was in a motor vehicle accident last year, and a spinal cord injury left him paraplegic. Explain how this injury has most likely affected his life, not just physically but emotionally and psychologically. How do you handle any anger or apathy directed at you or the physician?
4. Prepare a presentation for a preschool class on safety, including riding bicycles or riding other toys outside, wearing helmets, and the importance of being in a booster seat while wearing a seat belt in the car.
5. With cooperation from your instructor, schedule a presentation from a professional at the local health district to discuss communicable diseases such as meningitis and rabies in your community. What questions would you ask about diseases that affect the nervous system?

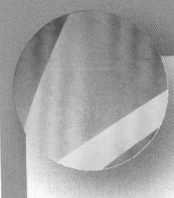

## PSY PROCEDURE 34-1

# Assisting with a Lumbar Puncture

**PSY** Instruct and prepare a patient for a procedure or treatment; coach patients regarding disease prevention and treatment plans; coach patients appropriately considering cultural diversity, developmental life stage, and communication barriers; and document patient care accurately in the medical record.

**Purpose:** To prepare and assist the physician during a lumbar puncture

**Equipment:** Sterile and clean exam gloves, 3- to 5-inch lumbar needle with stylet (physician will specify gauge and length), sterile gauze sponges, sterile specimen container, local anesthetic and syringe, needle, adhesive bandages, fenestrated drape, sterile drape, antiseptic, skin preparation supplies (razor), biohazard sharps container, and biohazard waste container

| STEPS | PURPOSE |
|-------|---------|
| 1. Wash your hands. | Hand washing aids infection control. |
| 2. Assemble the equipment, identify the patient, and explain the procedure. Identify yourself including your title. | Identifying the patient helps prevent errors in treatment. Explaining the procedure helps ease anxiety. |
| 3. Check that the consent form is signed and in the chart. Warn the patient not to move during procedure. Tell the patient that the area will be numb but pressure may still be felt after the local anesthetic is administered. | Because this is an invasive procedure, informed consent should be obtained and the form kept in the chart. Although there is little chance of damage to the spinal cord, movement may injure the patient and will probably contaminate the field. |
| 4. **AFF** Explain how to respond to a patient who has dementia. | Solicit assistance from the caregiver or other staff member to help during the procedure. Give simple directions to the patient about what he or she should do. Speak clearly, not loudly. |
| 5. Have the patient void. Direct the patient to disrobe and put on a gown with the opening at the back. | Emptying the bladder will decrease discomfort during the procedure. The back must be exposed for the procedure. |
| 6. Prepare the skin unless this is to be done with sterile preparation. If the physician prefers to prepare the skin using sterile forceps after gloving, you may have to add sterile solution to the field. Assist as needed with administration of the anesthetic. | Before starting, assess the lumbar region. If the site is hairy, it may be necessary to shave the skin before the procedure. Strict medical and surgical asepsis must be observed to reduce the risk of introducing microorganisms into the nervous system. |
| 7. When the physician is ready, prepare the sterile field and assist with the initial preparations. Assist the patient into the appropriate position.<br>**A.** For the side-lying position, stand in front of the patient and help by holding the patient's knees and top shoulder. Ask the patient to move so the back is close to the edge of the table. | These positions widen the space between the vertebrae to allow entrance of the needle. Your presence will help ensure that the patient does not move. |

# PROCEDURE 34.1 (continued)

| STEPS | PURPOSE |
|---|---|

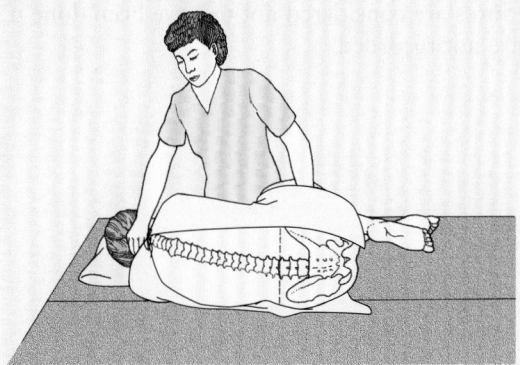

**B.** For the forward-leaning, supported position, stand in front of the patient and rest your hands on the shoulders as a reminder to remain still. Ask the patient to breathe slowly and deeply.

**Step 7.** The patient should be lying on the side with the knees drawn up, the head and neck down, and the back curled as much as possible.

8. Throughout the procedure, observe the patient closely for signs such as dyspnea or cyanosis. Monitor the pulse at intervals and record the vital signs after the procedure. Note the patient's mental alertness and any leakage at the site, nausea, or vomiting. Assess lower limb mobility. Assist the physician as necessary.

When the physician has the needle securely in place, the physician may ask you to help the patient to straighten slightly to ease tension and to allow a normal CSF flow.

9. If specimens are to be taken, put on gloves to receive the potentially hazardous body fluid. Label the tubes in sequence as you receive them. Label them also with the patient's identification and place them in biohazard bags.

Standard precautions must be followed.

10. If the Queckenstedt test is to be performed, you may be required to press against the patient's jugular veins in the neck (right, left, or both) while the physician monitors the pressure of CSF.

Normally, the pressure of CSF will rise and drop rapidly as the veins in the neck are compressed. If an obstruction is present, the rise and return to normal may be slow, or there may be no response to the external application of pressure.

11. At the completion of the procedure, cover the site with an adhesive bandage and assist the patient to a flat position. The physician will determine when the patient is ready to leave the examining room and the office.

Some patients have headache after the procedure and must be monitored carefully during the recovery period.

12. Route the specimens as required. Clean the examination room, and care for or dispose of the equipment as needed. Wash your hands.

Standard precautions must be followed throughout the procedure.

*(continues on page 896)*

## PROCEDURE 34.1 (continued)

| STEPS | PURPOSE |
|---|---|
| 13. **AFF** Log into the electronic medical record (EMR) using your username and secure password OR obtain the paper medical record from a secure location and assure it is kept away from public access. Because you did not perform the procedure, you do not need to document the lumbar puncture procedure. However, you are required to document your part in preparing specimens obtained and patient instructions after the procedure. Your entry must include the date, time, and your name/credentials. | Procedures are considered not to have been done if they are not recorded. |
| 14. When finished, log out of the EMR and/or replace the paper medical record in an appropriate and secure location. | |

Charting Example:
*02/12/16 8:30 AM Pt. positioned and draped for lumbar puncture. VS 120/80 (R), 86, 18. LP per formed by Dr. Alexander* _____ *B. Ryan, CMA*

*9:00 AM LP complete. Pt. tolerated procedure well. CSF specimen to lab. Post LP VS 114/74 (R) 76, 16* _____ *B. Ryan, CMA*

*9:30 AM Pt. denies discomfort. No n/v. No leakage at LP site. Bandage clean and dry. Pt and wife given discharge instructions. Verbalized understanding. Pt d/c per Dr. Alexander* _____ *B Ryan, CMA*

Note: *The medical assistant may sign his or her name in the patient record using only the "CMA" credential if the office has a signature log denoting the entire credential as "CMA(AAMA)."*

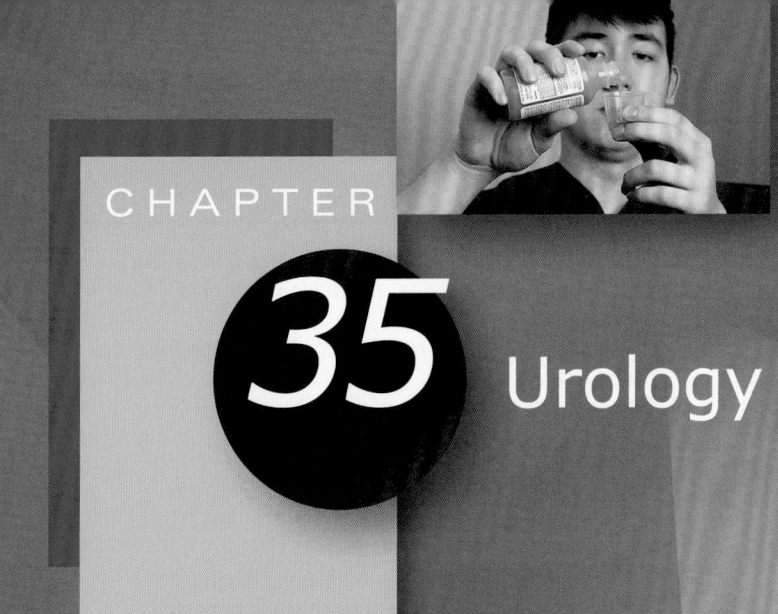

# CHAPTER 35 Urology

## Learning Outcomes

### COG Cognitive Domain*

1. Spell key terms
2. *Define medical terms and abbreviations related to all body systems*
3. *Describe structural organization of the human body*
4. *List major organs in each body system.*
5. *Identify the anatomical location of major organs in each body system*
6. *Describe the normal function of each body system*
7. *Identify common pathology related to each body system including signs, symptoms, and etiology*
   a. List and describe common diseases of the urinary system and the male reproductive system
   b. Describe and explain the purpose of various diagnostic procedures associated with the urinary system
   c. Name and describe the common procedures for diagnosing urinary system disorders
8. Discuss the role of the medical assistant in diagnosing and treating disorders of the urinary system and the male reproductive system

### PSY Psychomotor Domain*

1. Perform a female urinary catheterization (Procedure 35-1)
   a. *Instruct and prepare a patient for a procedure or treatment*
   b. *Coach patients appropriately considering cultural diversity, developmental life stage, and communication barriers*
   c. *Coach patients regarding disease prevention and treatment plans*
   d. *Document patient care accurately in the medical record*
2. Perform a male urinary catheterization (Procedure 35-2)
   a. *Instruct and prepare a patient for a procedure or treatment*
   b. *Coach patients appropriately considering cultural diversity, developmental life stage, and communication barriers*
   c. *Coach patients regarding disease prevention and treatment plans*
   d. *Document patient care accurately in the medical record*

*(continues on page 898)*

## Learning Outcomes (continued)

3. Instruct a male patient on the testicular self-examination (Procedure 35-3)
   a. *Instruct and prepare a patient for a procedure or treatment*
   b. *Coach patients appropriately considering cultural diversity, developmental life stage, and communication barriers*
   c. *Coach patients regarding disease prevention and treatment plans*
   d. *Document patient care accurately in the medical record*

### AFF Affective Domain*

1. *Incorporate critical thinking skills when performing patient assessment*
2. *Incorporate critical thinking skills when performing patient care*
3. *Show awareness of a patient's concerns related to the procedure being performed*
4. *Demonstrate empathy, active listening, and nonverbal communication*

5. *Demonstrate respect for individual diversity including gender, race, religion, age, economic status, and appearance*
6. *Explain to a patient the rationale for the performance of a procedure*
7. *Demonstrate sensitivity to patient rights*
8. *Protect the integrity of the medical record*

*Note: AAMA/CAAHEP 2015 Standards are italicized.*

### ABHES Competencies

1. Assist the physician with the regimen of diagnostic and treatment modalities as they relate to each body system
2. Comply with federal, state, and local health laws and regulations
3. Communicate on the recipient's level of comprehension
4. Serve as a liaison between the physician and others
5. Show empathy and impartiality when dealing with patients
6. Document accurately

## Key Terms

anuria
blood urea nitrogen (BUN)
catheterization
cryptorchidism
cystoscopy
dialysis
dysuria

enuresis
erectile dysfunction
hematuria
hydrocele
incontinence
intravenous pyelogram (IVP)

lithotripsy
nephrostomy
nocturia
oliguria
prostate-specific antigen (PSA)
proteinuria

psychogenic impotence
pyuria
retrograde pyelogram
specific gravity
ureterostomy
urinalysis
urinary frequency

## Case Study

*P*atients with disorders of the urinary system are seen in many types of physician offices, but in some situations, they may be referred to a specialist known as a urologist. Stephanie Strobb, CMA (AAMA), works for a urology group that is part of Great Falls Medical Center. The physicians in this office also see male patients with disorders of the male reproductive system. Today, Dr. O'Brien is seeing several male patients who have symptoms indicative of an enlarged prostate gland. What are the symptoms of an enlarged prostate gland, and how is this disorder treated? What is the difference between a urologist and a nephrologist? These and other questions are addressed in this chapter.

The process of metabolism creates waste products that must be eliminated from the body. Several body systems contribute to preventing a buildup of the end products of metabolism, including the gastrointestinal system, the respiratory system, and the integumentary system. The urinary system also removes waste from the blood while regulating fluid volume, important electrolytes, blood pressure, and pH (acid–base) balance (Fig. 35-1). Disorders of the filters of the urinary system, the kidneys, are diagnosed through various urine and blood tests and radiographs. Patients with kidney problems are typically referred to a nephrologist, a physician who specializes in the physiology of the kidneys. Patients with disorders of the anatomy, or physical characteristics, of the urinary system are referred to another type of specialist, a urologist. Since the male reproductive system is so inextricably linked to the urinary system, disorders of the male reproductive system are also often referred to the urologist. This chapter does not review the anatomy and physiology of the urinary system but, instead, focuses on common disorders, diagnostic procedures, and treatments associated with the urinary and male reproductive systems.

# COMMON URINARY DISORDERS

## Renal Failure

As noted above, patients with disorders affecting the filtration of the kidneys are referred to a nephrologist. However, this disorder will be discussed in this chapter as a disorder of the urinary system. Renal failure is an acute or chronic disorder of kidney function manifested by the inability of the kidney to excrete wastes, concentrate urine, and aid in homeostatic electrolyte conservation. In acute renal failure, the patient has **oliguria** and a corresponding rise in nitrogen-containing wastes in the blood. The causes of acute renal failure include a serious loss of fluid due to severe burn or hemorrhage, trauma, toxic injury to the kidney, and an obstruction beyond the level of the collecting tubules.

Chronic renal failure is a gradual loss of nephrons with corresponding inability of the kidney to perform its functions. It may result from another disease process, such as systemic lupus erythematosus, diabetic neuropathy, radiation, or renal tuberculosis. The patient has general weakness, edema of the lungs and tissues, and neurologic symptoms such as confusion progressing to seizures and coma as the wastes, or toxins, not filtered by the kidneys build up in the blood.

Treatment for both acute and chronic renal failure may involve renal **dialysis** to remove nitrogenous waste products and excess fluid from the body. Dialysis dependence may be short term in an acute illness or long term in end-stage renal disease. Without functional nephrons, wastes must be filtered through membranes other than those in the renal tissues. Two methods are used: hemodialysis and peritoneal dialysis.

With hemodialysis, toxins are removed from the blood by routing the patient's blood through a dialysis machine containing synthetic filters and a dialysate, a substance used to balance the electrolyte concentration in the blood. The machine can be regulated to remove or retain certain substances as needed for the individual patient. This type of dialysis requires that the patient's circulatory system be accessed as often as three times a week for 3 to 4 hours at a time. Therefore, most patients receive a surgical fistula, or graft, between an artery and a vein to make entry with a needle during the procedure easier for the patient (Fig. 35-2). The fistula is often placed in one of the arms, and this arm should not be used for taking blood pressures or for blood draws.

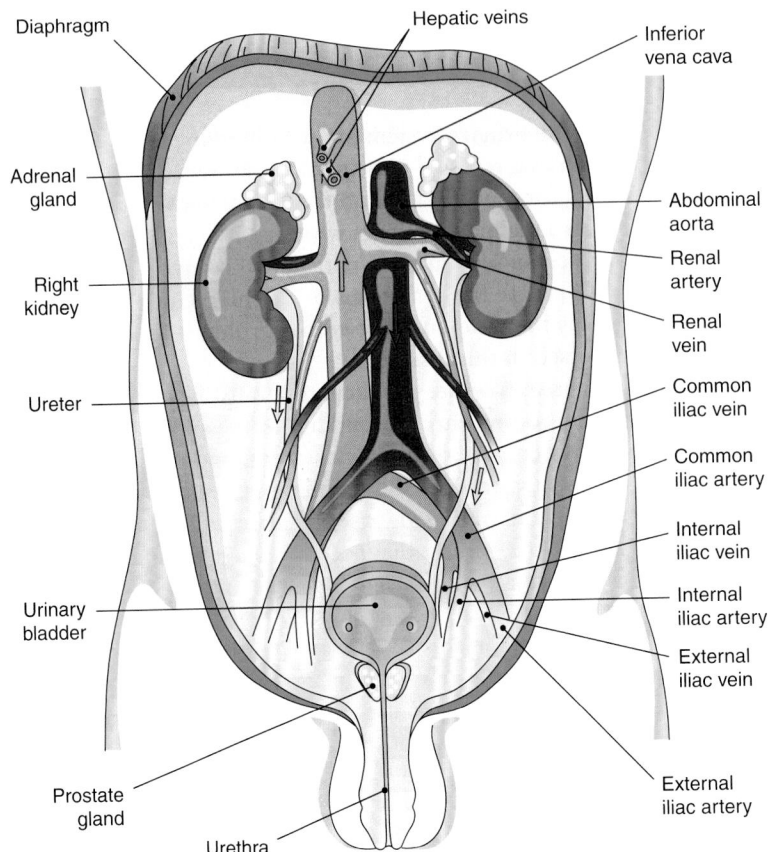

**FIGURE 35-1 •** Urinary system with blood vessels. (Reprinted from Cohen BJ. *Memmler's The Human Body in Health and Disease*, 11th ed. Philadelphia, PA: Lippincott Williams & Wilkins, 2009, with permission.)

Patients receiving peritoneal dialysis often perform the procedure at home. An appropriately balanced dialysate is administered through a catheter into the abdominal cavity, allowed to remain in the abdominal cavity for a specified time, and then drained into a collecting

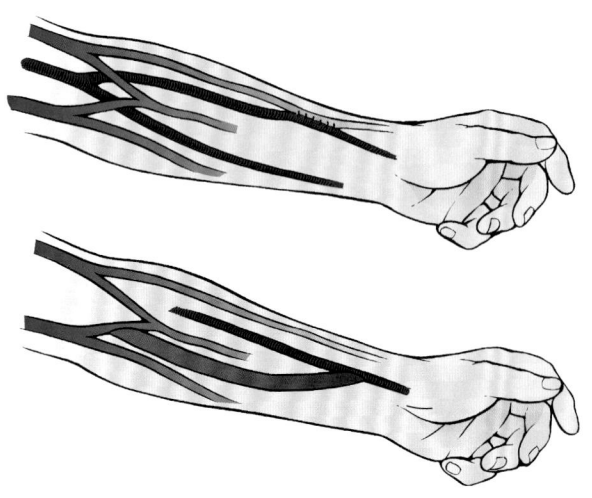

**FIGURE 35-2 •** Hemodialysis access sites. Arteriovenous fistula (**top**). Arteriovenous graft (**bottom**). (Springhouse. *Lippincott's Visual Encyclopedia of Clinical Skills*. Philadelphia, PA: Wolters Kluwer Health, 2009.)

bag. As the dialysate flows from the peritoneal cavity, it brings with it filtered wastes and excess fluid removed from the patient's blood through the blood vessels in the abdominal cavity (Fig. 35-3). Patients who have had extensive abdominal surgery with disruption of the peritoneal membranes are not good candidates for this type of dialysis. Peritoneal dialysis allows the patient the freedom to move about and continue a more normal lifestyle at home than with hemodialysis, which requires that the patient go to an outpatient facility several times a week. However, an abdominal catheter may result in an altered body image and psychological depression. The surgical opening on the abdomen can also become infected, leading to peritonitis, a serious infection in the abdominal cavity.

Neither type of dialysis is a cure for the underlying renal dysfunction, but both can prolong life almost indefinitely. Chronic renal failure frequently involves other systems as well as the urinary system and requires treatment for that involvement.

## 🔍 CHECKPOINT QUESTION

1. Which type of dialysis involves the filtering of wastes from the blood directly?

# PATIENT EDUCATION

## Urinary Tract Health

As the medical assistant, you will teach patients about everyday habits related to good general health. Encourage patients with urinary system symptoms to follow these suggestions to avoid urinary tract infections in the future:

*For All Patients*

- Drink lots of fluids, which help remove waste products from the fluid compartments. We are all generally advised to drink 8 glasses of water a day so that tissues are well hydrated, feces are soft, and infections in the lower urinary system are relatively unlikely.
- Empty your bladder when you feel the need. Urine held beyond comfort causes bladder stress and irritation. Allowing urine to stagnate in the bladder increases the risk of infection.
- Be aware that cranberry juice and vitamin C help acidify the urine and make the urinary system less attractive to bacteria.

*Especially for Women*

- Avoid using perfumed products in the perineal area. The female urinary meatus is very short and prone to irritation. Urethral infections quickly become bladder infections with irritation.
- Avoid tight-fitting lower garments, especially nylon underwear. Loose-fitting cotton underwear absorbs moisture and allows for airflow, making both bladder and vaginal infections less likely.
- Wipe carefully from front to back after using the toilet. Wash with soap and water, and rinse well if infections are a recurrent problem.
- If you are prone to urinary tract infections, void immediately after sexual intercourse to flush the area of bacteria that might have intruded into the urethra.
- Avoid tub baths, particularly bubble baths; showers are less likely to contribute to infections.

## Calculi

Calculi are stone formations that may be found anywhere in the urinary system and may range from granular particles to staghorn structures that fill the renal pelvis. Stones seem most likely to form if the urine is alkaline; the symptoms vary with the size and location of the stone. Hematuria may be present if rough edges of calculi abrade the mucous membrane lining the urinary system. The patient has flank pain if a stone lodges in one of the ureters.

Treatment may not be needed if the stones are small enough to be flushed out with increased fluid intake.

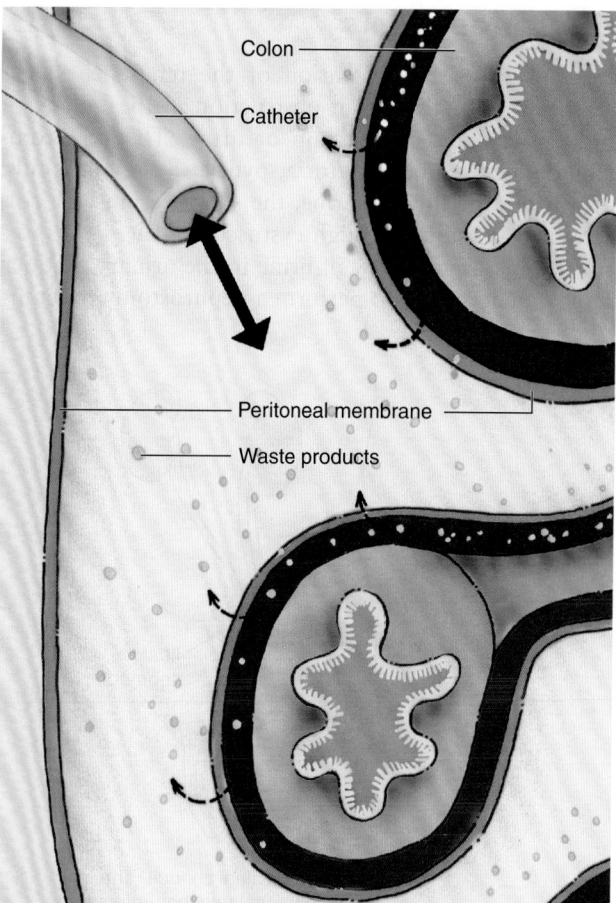

**FIGURE 35-3 •** Continuous ambulatory peritoneal dialysis. Peritoneal dialysis works through a combination of diffusion and osmosis. (Springhouse. *Lippincott's Visual Encyclopedia of Clinical Skills*. Philadelphia, PA: Wolters Kluwer Health, 2009.)

Large stones may require surgery or **lithotripsy**, a procedure in which ultrasound is used to crush the stones. In either case, the chemical makeup of the stones is evaluated for the forming components, and the patient's diet may be adjusted to prevent recurrence.

## Tumors

The urinary system may be a primary or secondary site for tumors. Tumors are more common in the urinary bladder but may also occur in the kidney. Symptoms vary but usually include hematuria and an unexplained abdominal mass. Treatment is based on the extent and type of tumor and may include surgery, chemotherapy, radiation, or a combination.

 **CHECKPOINT QUESTION**

2. A patient seen in the urology office today suspects he has renal calculi, or kidney stones. What are calculi, and when are they more likely to form?

## Hydronephrosis

Hydronephrosis is distention of the renal pelvis and calyces resulting from an obstruction in the kidney or ureter that causes a backup of urine. The symptoms include flank pain, hematuria, pyuria, fever, and chills. To restore the flow of urine, the stricture must be corrected, if possible, through cystoscopy. If it is not possible to restore the flow of urine to the urinary bladder, it may be necessary to perform a **nephrostomy** (opening the kidney and placement of a catheter in the kidney pelvis) or **ureterostomy** (surgical creation of an opening to the outside of the body from the ureter) (Fig. 35-4).

## Urinary System Infections

Glomerulonephritis is the inflammation of the glomerulus, or filtering unit, of the kidney. Symptoms range from very mild edema of the extremities, **proteinuria, hematuria**, and oliguria to complete renal failure. It is occasionally

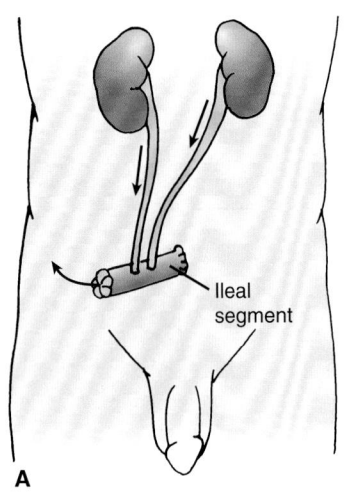

**A**

Conventional ileal conduit. The surgeon transplants the ureters to an isolated section of the terminal ileum (ileal conduit), bringing one end to the abdominal wall. The ureter may also be transplanted into the transverse sigmoid colon (colon conduit) or proximal jejunum (jejunal conduit).

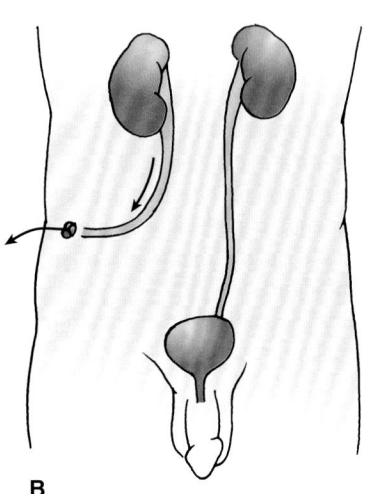

**B**

Cutaneous ureterostomy. The surgeon brings the detached ureter through the abdominal wall and attaches it to an opening in the skin.

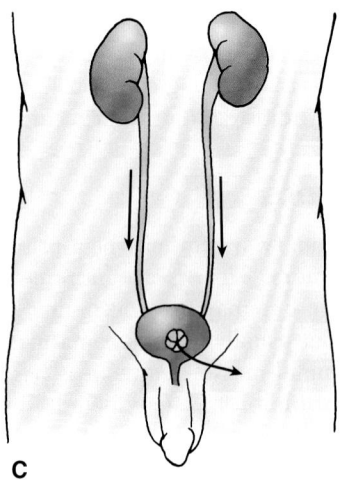

**C**

Vesicostomy. The surgeon sutures the bladder to the abdominal wall and creates an opening (stoma) through the abdominal and bladder walls for urinary drainage.

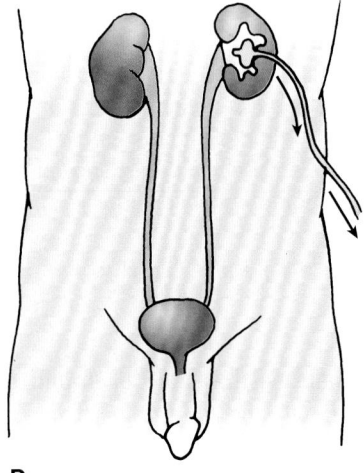

**D**

Nephrostomy. The surgeon inserts a catheter into the renal pelvis via an incision into the flank or, by percutaneous catheter placement, into the kidney.

**FIGURE 35-4 •** A ureterostomy. (Reprinted from Smeltzer SC, Bare BG, Hinkle JL, et al. *Brunner & Suddarth's Textbook of Medical-Surgical Nursing.* Philadelphia, PA: Lippincott Williams & Wilkins, 2008, with permission.)

| TABLE 35-1 | Symptoms of Urinary Tract Disorders and Possible Causes |
|---|---|
| **Symptoms** | **Possible Causes** |
| **Anuria** | Renal failure, acute nephritis, lead or mercury poisoning, complete obstruction of urinary tract |
| Burning during voiding | Urethritis |
| Burning during and after voiding | Cystitis |
| Dysuria | Infection |
| **Enuresis** | Normal to age 3 years |
| Frequency | Infection, diabetes |
| Hematuria | Diseases of glomeruli, trauma, neoplasm, calculi |
| **Incontinence** | Infection, uterine prolapse, nerve damage, neoplasm, senility |
| Nocturia | Infection, prostatic hypertrophy, abdominal pressure (pregnancy), diabetes |
| Oliguria | Acute nephritis, dehydration, fever, urinary obstruction, neoplasm |
| Polyuria | Diabetes mellitus, diabetes insipidus, diuretic use, high fluid intake |
| Proteinuria | Disease of glomeruli or protein metabolism, infection, nephrotic syndrome |
| Pyuria | Infection |
| Renal colic | Calculi |
| Urgency | Infection, disease of the prostate |

seen in children 1 to 4 weeks after a streptococcal infection as the large streptococcal antibodies are trapped in the small capillaries of the glomerulus, causing irritation and inflammation. Glomerulonephritis in adults may be chronic, with scarring and hardening of the glomeruli from repeated episodes of acute glomerulonephritis, and may lead to renal failure. Symptoms of the chronic form include proteinuria, casts in the urine (see Chapter 43), and hematuria. Treatment is usually symptomatic, and if an infection is involved, an antibiotic is prescribed.

Pyelonephritis is inflammation of the renal pelvis and the body of the kidney. It usually results from an ascending infection from the ureters and may be acute or chronic. Symptoms include those of any infection, such as chills and fever, nausea, and vomiting, but also include flank pain and **pyuria** (pus in the urine). Medication to acidify the urine and make the system less hospitable to bacteria may be the treatment of choice for pyelonephritis. In addition, an antibiotic may be prescribed.

Cystitis is an inflammation of the urinary bladder. This condition is far more common in women than in men because a woman's urethra is shorter. Symptoms begin with **urinary frequency**, **dysuria**, and urgency and progress to chills, fever, nausea, vomiting, and flank pain. The causative microorganism is identified with a urine culture, and the treatment usually is an antibiotic once the causative microorganism has been identified.

Urethritis is inflammation of the urethra that may occur before the signs and symptoms of cystitis appear, or it may indicate a sexually transmitted disease, such as gonorrhea or nongonococcal urethritis. The treatment for cystitis is also effective for urethritis. Other signs and symptoms of the urinary system and the possible causes are listed in Table 35-1.

 **CHECKPOINT QUESTION**

3. Why are women more likely than men to have cystitis?

 **WHAT IF?**

**A mother brings her 5-year-old daughter to the office with complaints of burning on urination. What questions do you ask? How do you educate the mother and child?**

First, ask if the child urinates when she feels the urge or if she holds her urine. Some young girls are inclined to hold their urine long past the time to void, setting up a perfect situation for bacterial growth. Caution the child to go to the bathroom when the need arises, making sure to use terms she can understand. Next, ask the mother if she uses bubble bath in the child's bath water. Young girls have a very short urethra and are prone to urethritis if they bathe in water with certain types of bubble bath. Finally, explain that the child must learn to wipe from front to back to avoid urinary tract infections.

# COMMON DISORDERS OF THE MALE REPRODUCTIVE SYSTEM

Male patients with disorders of the reproductive system often have signs and symptoms pertaining to the urinary system. If you work in a family practice or internal medicine office, you may care for male patients with reproductive system disorders, or these patients may be referred to urology for specific treatment or surgery. Common disorders are discussed in the following sections.

## Benign Prostatic Hyperplasia

As most men reach their middle years, the prostate begins to enlarge, or hypertrophy. Benign prostatic hyperplasia is a noncancerous enlargement of the prostate gland that occurs commonly in men over age 40 years. Diagnosis is with a digital rectal examination, which should be performed as part of the routine physical examination in men after age 40 years (Fig. 35-5). Using a gloved hand and water-soluble lubricant, the physician will insert the index finger into the rectum and palpate the prostate for size, shape, and consistency.

As the prostate gland enlarges, it presses on the urethra and urinary bladder, causing urinary symptoms such as frequency and **nocturia**. While this condition is not usually a serious problem, it can be treated medically or surgically by partially or completely removing the prostate gland. The surgical procedure, prostatectomy, can be performed transurethrally or through a surgical opening into the suprapubic area of the lower abdomen. If the prostate is removed transurethrally, the procedure is a transurethral resection of the prostate. Box 35-1 describes the surgical techniques used to treat prostatic hypertrophy in more detail.

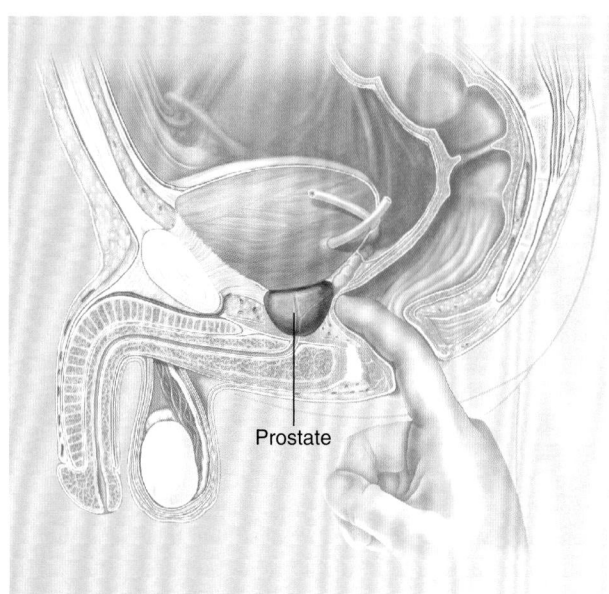

**FIGURE 35-5** • Digital rectal exam (DRE).

---

**BOX 35-1** **Surgical Intervention for Prostatic Hypertrophy**

**Transurethral Resection of the Prostate**
A cystoscope with an electrocautery wire cutting loop, a resectoscope, is inserted through the urethra and rotated through the prostate to remove pieces of the gland. The pieces are washed out with irrigating fluid introduced through the scope. There is no abdominal incision, making this a relatively safe procedure for the high-risk patient. The whole organ is not usually removed for this surgery; therefore, the obstruction frequently returns. This is not a choice for malignancies.

**Suprapubic Prostatectomy**
Performed through the abdominal wall and bladder, suprapubic prostatectomy allows the surgeon to peel out the whole organ through a wide surgical field and to check the bladder for involvement. This approach is the choice for large prostate glands or for malignancies. As in all surgeries, there are postoperative risks, particularly for the elderly. These include pain, hemorrhage, urinary leakage, and prolonged convalescence.

**Perineal Resection**
An incision between the scrotum and the anus is a short, direct route to the prostate without interfering with the bladder and is preferred for some large malignancies. It appears to be relatively nontraumatic for the very old or infirm. Surgeons find that the field offers less room to maneuver than with the suprapubic approach. It is not a good choice for young men because erectile dysfunction and urinary and fecal incontinence are frequent postoperative complications. The proximity of the anal area also increases the risk of infection.

**Retropubic Resection**
A low abdominal incision above the pubis but below the bladder avoids trauma to the bladder and thereby allows a shorter convalescence than with the suprapubic approach. It also provides better removal options than the transurethral approach. It is a good choice if pathology is limited to the prostate, with no bladder involvement.

## Prostate Cancer

Prostate cancer, like most cancers, is best treated when detected early. In the early stages of the disease, many men are asymptomatic. As a result, male patients over age 40 years should be encouraged to have yearly physical examinations that include a digital rectal examination, which often allows the physician to palpate an enlarged gland. If the prostate gland is enlarged, a biopsy of the prostate may be advised to determine the cause of the enlargement.

Another diagnostic test often ordered as part of the routine physical examination is the **prostate-specific antigen**, or **PSA**, blood test. This antigen is normally found in the blood of all men, but its level increases with any inflammation of the prostate, including cancer. While the cause of prostate cancer is not known, it is most common in men over age 50 years, with 75% of diagnoses in men over age 75 years. Treatment depends on the extent of the malignancy and the patient's age and general health status. Prostate cancer is often treated by a combination of surgery, chemotherapy, and radiation.

 **CHECKPOINT QUESTION**

4. Does the patient with benign prostatic hyperplasia have an elevated prostate-specific antigen level? Why or why not?

## Testicular Cancer

Although testicular cancer accounts for only about 1% of all malignancies, the metastatic and mortality rates are high. This type of cancer is most often seen in men ages 15 to 34 years. The cause of testicular cancer is unknown, but predisposing factors may include cryptorchidism, infection, genetic factors, and endocrine abnormalities. The symptoms are gradual and painless and may initially only involve a vague feeling of scrotal heaviness.

Once a diagnosis of testicular cancer has been made, treatment may be orchiectomy, or surgical removal of the testicle. Chemotherapy and radiation may also be used.

## Hydrocele

Hydrocele, a collection of fluid in the scrotum and around the testes, may result from trauma or infection or may simply be due to aging. Diagnosis is based on symptoms and inspection. If the condition is extremely uncomfortable, aspiration of the excessive fluid may be required, and if the condition persists, surgical intervention may be the treatment of choice. In most cases, no treatment is necessary, and the fluid is reabsorbed by the body. Hydrocele is common in male infants but generally subsides without treatment.

## Cryptorchidism

Normally, the testes descend from the abdominal cavity into the scrotal sac in the male fetus by the eighth month of gestation. In a small percentage of male infants, one or both of the testes fail to descend by the time of delivery (Fig. 35-6). **Cryptorchidism** refers to either one or both undescended testes. Surgical correction, known

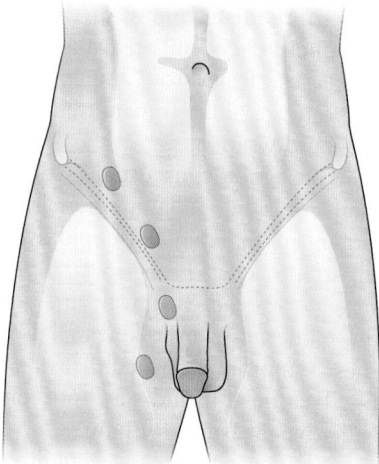

**FIGURE 35-6 •** Possible locations of undescended testicles.

as *orchiopexy*, is usually performed before age 4 years, preferably at age 1 or 2 years. If an undescended testis is not surgically corrected, it results in sterility of the undescended organ and may increase the risk of testicular malignancy later in life.

 **CHECKPOINT QUESTION**

5. A patient in the urology office is diagnosed with a hydrocele. What are the causes of hydrocele?

## Inguinal Hernia

After the testes descend in the male fetus and the inguinal canals close, small rings are left open at the anterior base of the abdominal wall as a passage for the spermatic cord. There is no connection between this area and the abdominal contents, but this area remains a possible site for weakness and protrusion of the intestines with age or exertion. The patient with an inguinal hernia is often asymptomatic unless the intestines protrude through the weakened area, which may result in a noticeable bulge and pain. Diagnosis is made in the early stages by having the patient bear down and cough while the physician inserts a finger into a pouch made by the scrotum up into the external and internal inguinal rings. Pressure against the finger indicates weakness of the muscles in this area.

Treatment of an inguinal hernia depends on the patient's physical condition. Surgical correction of a hernia, called a *herniorrhaphy*, repositions the protruding organ and repairs the opening.

## Infections

Infections of the male urinary tract are likely to spread to the reproductive system because they share many of the same organs. The most common infections of the male reproductive system are epididymitis, orchitis, and prostatitis. Although not all infections result from a sexually transmitted microorganism, many of the infections of the male reproductive system are caused by sexually transmitted diseases. Refer to Chapter 36 for more information about sexually transmitted diseases that affect both men and women.

Infection in the epididymis usually results from an infected prostate or other inflammation in the urinary tract. Microorganisms that may cause epididymitis include staphylococci, streptococci, *Escherichia coli*, chlamydia, and *Neisseria gonorrhoeae*. Symptoms include a swollen scrotum, pain, tenderness, fever, and malaise. Diagnosis is based on these symptoms and a culture of any drainage from the penis. Treatment includes an antibiotic, bed rest, fluids, and palliative measures for pain.

The microorganisms that cause epididymitis often also cause orchitis, and the treatment is virtually the same. Orchitis may also result in hydrocele, which should be treated if it becomes a severe complication.

Chronic prostatitis is common among the elderly and may be confused with prostatic hypertrophy if repeated infections cause the organs to fibrose. The causative agents are much like those of other infections of the male reproductive system, with the leading cause being *E. coli*. It frequently results from catheterization or cystoscopy. Some pathogens reach the prostate by way of the bloodstream of the lymph system. Signs and symptoms may include inguinal pain, fever, low back and joint pain, burning, dysuria, and urethral discharge. Urine specimens contain blood and pus. Diagnosis is based on signs, symptoms, and urinalysis. Antibiotic treatment is required to treat chronic prostatitis.

 **CHECKPOINT QUESTION**

6. What are some microorganisms responsible for causing infections in the male reproductive system?

 **PATIENT EDUCATION**

### HIV/AIDS Prevention

When providing instructions about AIDS prevention, explain to your patient that it is safest, of course, to abstain from sex. Encourage your patients to have sex only with a partner who is known not to be infected, who has sex with no one but the patient, and who does not use needles or syringes. Also, advise the patient to use a latex condom if it is not known whether the sexual partner is infected. Generally, instruct patients to:

- Avoid contact with another person's blood, body fluids, semen, and vaginal secretions.
- Avoid sharing needles, syringes, and any objects that come into contact with blood or body fluids.
- Avoid using alcohol and drugs. Use of these substances can hinder clear thinking and lead to unwise decision making.

## Erectile Dysfunction

**Erectile dysfunction**, also known as *impotence*, is the inability to achieve or maintain an erection; it may be psychological or organic. **Psychogenic impotence** may be caused by something as simple as exhaustion, anxiety, or depression, and in such cases, it usually disappears with resolution of the underlying cause. Organic erectile dysfunction may result from disease in almost any other body system, including endocrine imbalance, cardiovascular problems, nervous system impairment, or urinary disease. Organic erectile dysfunction may also be caused by injury to the pelvic organs or by medication that impairs any of the systems serving the reproductive system.

Diagnosis is based on a detailed medical and sexual history with an analysis of lifestyle and emotional status. Blood studies and measurements of both penile arterial flow and nerve conduction to this area are usually required. Treatment depends on the cause and may include a vacuum tube system that pulls blood into the penis, creating an erection, or vitamin E injections into the penis. Today, many new drugs, such as sildenafil (Viagra™), stimulate erections in the impotent male. If none of these are effective, a penile implant can be inserted surgically.

 **LEGAL TIP**

### Clinical Trials

Physicians who participate in clinical trials using new drugs or procedures have an ethical and legal obligation to follow specific guidelines, including the following:

- Notifying the patient that the drug or procedure is experimental and detailing the risks and benefits of the treatment clearly
- Obtaining an informed written consent before beginning the drug or performing the procedure
- Assuring that the drug or procedure is documented appropriately and reported accurately according to the standards for the research being conducted
- Providing a high standard of care for all patients regardless of whether or not they are participating in a clinical trial

## COMMON DIAGNOSTIC AND THERAPEUTIC PROCEDURES

### Urinalysis

The single most important step in diagnosing urinary diseases is the examination of the patient's urine, or **urinalysis**. Tests should always be performed on a fresh

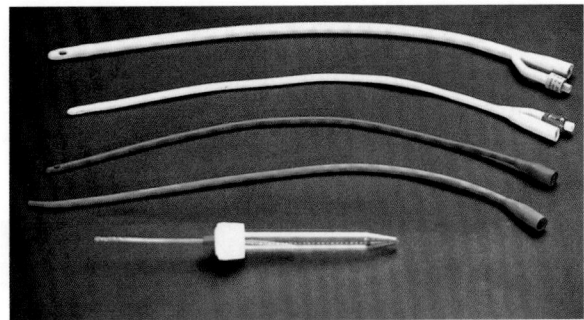

FIGURE 35-7 • Types of catheters. From the *top*: No. 24-French indwelling catheter; No. 16-French indwelling catheter; No. 16-French straight catheter; Coudé catheter; and self-contained catheterization collection unit.

specimen and with the first morning specimen when concentrated urine is needed, such as for pregnancy testing. The urinalysis includes a physical and chemical evaluation, **specific gravity**, and a microscopic examination (see Chapter 45). If an infection is suspected, the physician may also order a urine culture.

The patient may produce the urine specimen by performing a clean-catch midstream procedure after receiving instructions from you on the proper procedure for collecting the specimen. In some cases, the physician may order a urine specimen obtained by **catheterization**, which is the introduction of a sterile flexible tube into the urinary bladder (Fig. 35-7). In the medical office, a straight catheter is used for catheterization and removed once the urine specimen is obtained. Some patients have an indwelling catheter inserted at another facility, such as a hospital. Indwelling catheters are similar to straight catheters, but these types are kept in place by a balloon on the end of the catheter inflated after placement in the bladder (Fig. 35-8). Indwelling catheters are not usually inserted in the medical office.

Catheters are sized 8 to 10 Fr (French) for children and 14 to 20 Fr for adults. (**Note:** French is a unit of measurement to describe the size of the diameter of catheters.) Procedures 35-1 and 35-2 describe the procedure

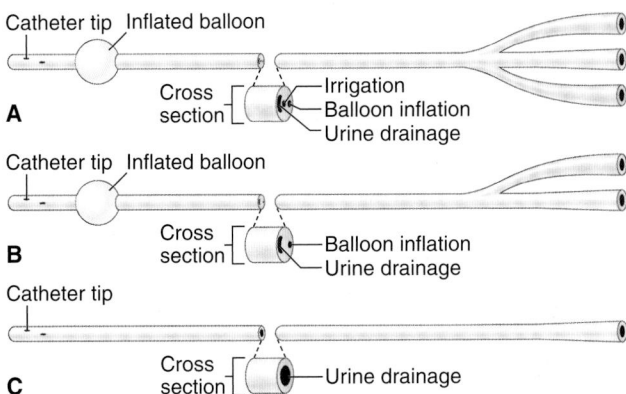

FIGURE 35-8 • Sterile water is inserted into the indicated lumen to inflate the balloon of the indwelling catheter. When the balloon is inflated, the catheter will remain within the bladder.

---

**BOX 34-2  Principles of Catheterization**

Catheterization is usually a last resort for obtaining a urine specimen. Even under the most aseptic conditions, there is a risk of introducing infection into the urinary system. However, some patients require catheterization when there is no other alternative. For example, catheterization is required in the following circumstances:

- It is impossible to obtain a clean-catch midstream specimen for urinalysis.
- The residual urine, or urine left in the bladder after urination, must be measured.
- Medication must be instilled into the bladder to treat an infection.
- The patient has urinary retention or cannot urinate.

Urinary catheter types and sizes vary. They are made of plastic or rubber. If the patient has prostatic hypertrophy, the physician may order a Coudé catheter (see Fig. 34-7), which is slightly curved and a bit stiffer than the other types, so it is easier to advance it beyond the obstructing enlarged prostate gland.

---

for performing a catheterization in females and males, respectively, in the medical office, and Box 35-2 explains some principles of urinary catheterization.

## Blood Tests

Serum levels of uric acid, **blood urea nitrogen (BUN)**, or creatinine may be indicated for the diagnosis of some disease processes of the urinary system. It will likely be your responsibility to draw the patient's blood and process it on-site or direct it to the proper testing facility (see Chapter 41).

## Cystoscopy or Cystourethroscopy

**Cystoscopy** is direct visualization of the bladder and urethra with a lighted instrument called a **cystoscope** (Fig. 35-9). Cystoscopy allows the physician to diagnose many disorders of the lower urinary tract, such as tumors and inflammation. You may be responsible for providing preoperative instructions to the patient as directed by the physician. This procedure is usually done under local anesthesia and may be performed in the urologist's office, but some physicians prefer to have the patient receive a general anesthetic and outpatient hospitalization.

### ⚲ CHECKPOINT QUESTION

7. What is the most common test for disorders of the urinary system performed in the medical office?

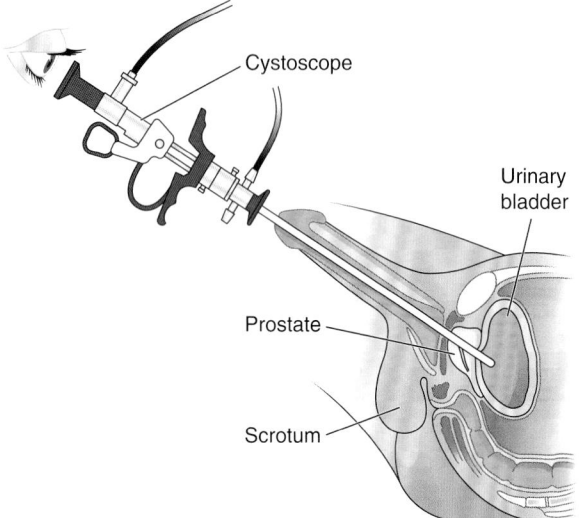

**FIGURE 35-9** • The interior of the urinary bladder as seen through a cystoscope. (Modified from Cohen BJ. *Medical Terminology: An Illustrated Guide*. Philadelphia, PA: Lippincott Williams & Wilkins, 2003, with permission.)

## Intravenous Pyelogram and Retrograde Pyelogram

An **intravenous pyelogram (IVP)** is a radiographic examination of the kidneys and urinary tract using a radiopaque dye injected into the circulatory system. This dye is filtered by the kidneys to serve as a contrast medium and enhance visualization of the renal structures. Although this procedure is not done in the medical office, you will schedule the examination at the appropriate facility and give the patient instructions to be followed before the procedure. Specifically, the patient is required to cleanse the bowels with a laxative the night before the test and to have an enema the morning of the procedure, since feces may prevent adequate visualization of the kidneys. In addition, the patient is asked not to eat or drink anything for at least 8 hours before the dye is injected to increase the blood concentration and visibility of the dye.

You must question the patient carefully about possible iodine allergy, including allergic reactions to seafood, particularly shellfish. Encourage the patient to increase fluid intake after the test to flush out the dye and counteract any dehydration caused by the preliminary cleansing.

A **retrograde pyelogram** is similar to the IVP except that the dye is not injected intravenously but is introduced through a catheter in the ureters through a cystoscope. This test is commonly used when IVP is contraindicated because of poor kidney function. Like IVP, this test is not performed in the medical office, but you may be responsible for making arrangements with the appropriate facility and giving the patient any necessary instructions.

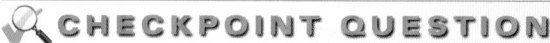

⚲ **CHECKPOINT QUESTION**

8. How does a retrograde pyelogram differ from an intravenous pyelogram?

 **PATIENT EDUCATION**

### Renal Calculi

Clark Watkins, a 45-year-old white man, has severe right flank pain radiating to the suprapubic and inguinal regions of the abdomen. He has a fever of 100.3°F, nausea, and some vomiting. Urinalysis shows gross and microscopic hematuria and calcium crystal casts; it is clear of pyuria and white blood cells. Dr. Brown performs in-office ultrasonography, and the results suggest renal calculi. He orders an IVP, which reveals sand-to-gravel calculi.

Your role is to provide patient education. Demonstrate to Mr. Watkins the procedure for filtering his urine and provide him with the strainer so he can bring in the solid material for analysis. Mr. Watkins's diet will be altered in accordance with the composition of the stones. He may be referred to a dietitian or given a diet list after counseling with Dr. Brown. Encourage Mr. Watkins to increase his fluid intake to flush the stones and to walk frequently to assist peristalsis in the ureters and passing the stones. Urge him to drink fruit juices, especially cranberry juice, in addition to water, and discourage caffeine drinks. He may need an antiemetic if nausea and vomiting interfere with fluid intake. Caution him to watch for signs of infection and obstruction, including cloudy urine, which may contain pus, and fever.

## Ultrasound

Ultrasound is noninvasive use of sound waves to show stones and obstructions in the urinary system and tissues. No special preparation is required other than an explanation of the procedure to the patient. If ordered by the physician, you may be responsible for scheduling this procedure with the appropriate facility.

## Rectal and Scrotal Examinations

For the male patient seen in the physician's or urologist's office, you will assist with examination of the reproductive organs by instructing the patient to disrobe from the waist down and providing him with appropriate draping. The physician will inspect and palpate the scrotum for lumps and inguinal hernia. Using a gloved hand and water-soluble lubricant, the physician will perform a digital rectal examination, inserting the index finger into the rectum and palpating the prostate for size, shape, and consistency.

At home, male patients should perform the testicular self-examination because this is the best method for early detection of testicular cancer. The American Cancer Society recommends that all men perform this examination frequently, possibly weekly, and you are responsible for teaching the patient about this disease and the self-examination. You should explain that the best time for the self-examination is after a warm shower or bath, when the scrotal sac is relaxed (Procedure 34-3). If lumps or thickened areas are palpated during the examination, instruct the patient to notify the physician immediately.

 **CHECKPOINT QUESTION**

9. The medical assistant, Stephanie Strobb, must teach a patient about performing the testicular self-examination. What should she tell the patient is the best time to perform this examination at home?

 **AFF TRIAGE**

While you are working in a medical office, the following three situations occur:

A. Patient A, a 24-year-old patient, has obtained a urine specimen for a work physical.
B. The physician has asked you to teach patient B, a 30-year-old male, to perform the testicular self-examination before discharging him.
C. Patient C is a 67-year-old woman who needs a catheter to relieve bladder distention due to urinary retention.

**How do you sort these patients? Who do you see first? Second? Third?**

First, see patient C, since she has urinary retention and is most likely very uncomfortable. Next, test the urine specimen from patient A. The quality of the urine specimen decreases as the urine specimen sits out, and once it is tested, the results can be given to the physician for diagnosis. Patient B should be addressed last. Patient education should never be rushed, and he should be given an opportunity to ask questions for clarification.

## Vasectomy

A popular form of reproductive control is the vasectomy, or surgical removal of all or a segment of the vas deferens to prevent the passage of sperm from the testes. This procedure is commonly performed in the medical office, and you will assist by instructing the patient on preoperative orders as indicated by the physician. Some physicians order light preoperative sedation and may require that the patient have nothing by mouth after midnight on the day of the procedure.

On the day of the procedure, you should assist the physician by providing the appropriate surgical tray or instruments and assist the disrobed patient into the lithotomy position with appropriate draping materials to provide privacy. The physician will make two small incisions near the scrotal sac, pull each vas deferens (from the right and left testes) through the incision, clamp each vas deferens proximally and distally, and surgically cut and remove a segment of each. The remaining vas deferens ducts are placed back in the scrotal sac after the clamps are removed, and the site is sutured.

Ejaculation and sexual function are not affected by this procedure. The volume of sperm in the ejaculate is so small that it is not noticeable. The sperm produced by the testes after this procedure are absorbed in the testes. Since sterility may not be immediate, the patient should be advised to use another form of birth control, such as a condom, until sperm counts confirm that the ejaculate is free of sperm. You should advise the patient to return to the office for periodic sperm counts until no sperm are found in the ejaculate.

## MEDICATION BOX

### Commonly Prescribed Urinary System Medications

**Note:** The generic name of the drug is listed first and is written in all lowercase letters. Brand names are in parentheses, and the first letter is capitalized.

| | | |
|---|---|---|
| Ciprofloxacin (Cipro) | Oral suspension: 250 mg/mL, 500 mg/mL<br>Tablets: 100 mg, 250 mg, 500 mg, 750 mg | Antibiotic |
| Doxycycline (Oracea) | Capsules: 40 mg | Antibiotic |
| Fesoterodine fumarate (Toviaz) | Tablets: 4 mg, 8 mg | Antimuscarinic |
| Nitrofurantoin (Macrobid, Macrodantin) | Capsules: 25 mg, 50 mg, 100 mg | Antibiotic |

*(continues on page 910)*

| Oxybutynin chloride (Ditropan) | Syrup: 5 mg/5 mL<br>Tablets: 5 mg<br>Transdermal patch: 36 mg patch, delivers 3.9 mg/day | Antimuscarinic |
| --- | --- | --- |
| Phenazopyridine hydrochloride (Pyridium) | Tablets: 95 mg, 97.2 mg, 100 mg, 200 mg | Urinary analgesic |
| Sildenafil citrate (Viagra, Revatio) | Tablets: 20 mg, 25 mg, 50 mg, 100 mg | Erectile dysfunction |
| Sulfamethoxazole (Septra) | Tablets: 400 mg, 800 mg | Anti-infective; sulfonamide |
| Tadalafil (Cialis) | Tablets: 2.5 mg, 5 mg, 10 mg, 20 mg | Erectile dysfunction |
| Tamsulosin hydrochloride (Flomax) | Capsules: 0.4 mg | Benign prostatic hyperplasia |
| Testosterone (Depo-Testosterone, Delatestryl) | Injection: 100 mg/mL<br>200 mg/mL | Androgen hormone |
| Tolterodine tartrate (Detrol, Detrol LA) | Capsules: 2 mg, 4 mg<br>Tablets: 1 mg, 2 mg | Antimuscarinic |

 ## ROLE-PLAYING ACTIVITY

With cooperation from classmates or as assigned by your instructor, role-play the scenarios as if you are working with Stephanie Strobb in the urology office (refer to the case study at the beginning of the chapter). Jason, a 19-year-old male, comes into the office today for a swelling in his scrotum. He is anxious and embarrassed to talk about his symptoms and generally wants to avoid the topic. His mother has come with him to the office and is quiet, but obviously concerned. What would you say to this patient? How would you respond? Your instructor will give you additional information about this activity!

## *español* SPANISH TERMINOLOGY

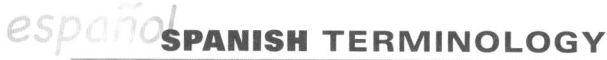

**¿Se orina sin querer?**
Do you pass water involuntarily?

**Necesitamos una muestra de orina.**
We need a urine sample from you.

**Va a ser un poco incómodo.**
It will be a little bit uncomfortable for you.

**¿Tiene dificultades para orinar?**
Do you have any problems when urinating?

**¿Siente que la orina está muy caliente?**
Do you have a burning sensation when urinating?

**¿Tiene que levantarse por la noche a orinar? ¿Cuántas veces?**
Do you have to get up to urinate during the night? How many times?

**¿Tiene usted historia familiar de problemas en la próstata?**
Do you have family history of prostate disease?

**Una dieta alta en sales minerales puede causar piedras en los riñones.**
Consuming an excess of mineral salts can cause kidney stones.

**Necesitamos la primera orina de la mañana.**
We need the first urine of the morning.

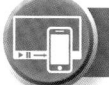 ## MEDIA MENU

**Student Resources** on the Point°
- *Animation:* **Renal Function**
- *Video:* **Performing a Female Urinary Catheterization (Procedure 34-1)**
- **CMA/RMA Certification Exam Review**

**Internet Resources**
**Brady Urological Institute, Johns Hopkins Medical Institutions**
http://urology.jhu.edu
**Urology Channel**
http://www.urologychannel.com
**National Kidney & Urologic Diseases Information Clearinghouse**
http://kidney.niddk.nih.gov
**Prostate Cancer Research Institute**
http://www.prostate-cancer.org/pcricms
**American Cancer Society**
http://www.cancer.org
**National Kidney Foundation**
http://www.kidney.org

## EMR Activity

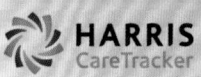
**Harris CareTracker** is a Web-based electronic medical record (EMR) application that you will use for the EMR activities included in this section at the end of each chapter. This application is actually used in physician offices, but is provided to you through the publisher, Wolters Kluwer Health, to give you hands-on practice working with EMRs. Your instructor will have more information about accessing your username, login, and Quickstart guide.

Prerequisite Activities in Harris CareTracker

• *The Getting Started and Quickstart documents and EMR Activities Step-by-Step Instructions are available at* http://thePoint.lww.com/KronenbergerComp5e

Activity Details

Document the chief complaint and present illness for the following patients seen today by Dr. Kyle Dunn.

1. Patient: Sandy Leonard: This patient is an established patient in the urology office for symptoms of recurrent urinary tract infections. The physician asked for a urine specimen via catheterization. You performed the catheterization with a 14-French straight catheter and obtained 350 mL of pale yellow urine. A sterile specimen was sent to Acme Labs for a culture and sensitivity.

2. Patient: Lawrence Black: This patient was referred by his family physician for an elevated PSA found after a routine physical examination. He is a new patient and is worried that he may have "prostate cancer." His vital signs are 148/90 (right arm, sitting), radial pulse 96, respirations 20, and temperature 98.4 using the temporal thermometer.

## Chapter Summary

- The urinary system performs many vital functions to maintain the internal environment of the body. Patients may require an examination of the urinary system for
- Signs and symptoms that indicate disorders of the urinary system, especially infection of the urinary bladder and urethra
- Evaluation during a complete physical examination even if no symptoms are present
- Examination of the male reproductive system, which shares the same organs as the male urinary system, for any disorders of the male reproductive system
- Your role in working with patients with urologic disorders may include
- Assisting the physician as necessary during the physical examination
- Preparing the patient for urologic procedures
- Performing urologic procedures such as urinary catheterization
- Providing patient education as directed by the physician

## Warm-Ups for Critical Thinking

1. Differentiate between peritoneal dialysis and hemodialysis. Why are some patients poor candidates for peritoneal dialysis? What can you ask the patient to determine whether or not the peritoneal catheter is functioning or infected?
2. Research the newest pharmacologic agents used to treat erectile dysfunction and explain the method of action, usual dosages, and side effects.
3. A male patient in your office has just been diagnosed with a low sperm count, and the physician has recommended that he switch from briefs to boxer shorts. How do you think this will affect his sperm count, and why?
4. Create a patient education brochure explaining the procedure for performing the testicular self-examination.
5. Identify the resources in your community for patients diagnosed with renal failure.
6. Elderly patients who experience incontinence may be too embarrassed to discuss this condition with anyone. What interpersonal skills can you use to obtain this information from the patient?

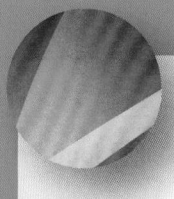

## PSY PROCEDURE 35-1

# Female Urinary Catheterization

**PSY** Instruct and prepare a patient for a procedure or treatment; coach patients appropriately considering cultural diversity, developmental life stage, and communication barriers; and document patient care accurately in the medical record.

**Purpose:** Using sterile aseptic technique, perform a straight catheterization on a female torso model

**Equipment:** Sterile straight catheterization tray with 14- or 16-French catheter, sterile gloves, antiseptic solution, sterile specimen cup with lid, lubricant, sterile drape, examination light, and anatomically correct female torso model

| STEPS | REASONS |
|---|---|
| 1. Wash your hands. | Handwashing aids infection control. |
| 2. Identify yourself, including your title. Also, identify the patient, explain the procedure, and have the patient disrobe completely from the waist down; provide a gown and adequate draping. | Identifying the patient helps prevent errors in the treatment. The privacy of the patient should be maintained at all times. |
| 3. Place the patient in the dorsal recumbent or lithotomy position, draping carefully to prevent unnecessary exposure. Carefully open the tray and place it between the patient's legs. Shine the examination light on the perineum. | The dorsal recumbent or lithotomy position allows the best view of the perineum and urinary meatus. Placing the tray between the legs of the patient allows easy access to the catheter and supplies. Adequate lighting is essential. |
| 4. Remove the sterile glove package and put on the sterile gloves without contaminating them. | Contaminating the gloves will contaminate the supplies and may cause the patient to develop a urinary tract infection after the procedure. |
| 5. Carefully remove the sterile drape and place it under the buttocks of the patient without contaminating your gloves. | If the sterile drape is on top of the tray, it may be carefully lifted out of the tray by the edge with clean hands and carefully placed under the buttocks. This drape is a barrier to protect the examination table from spills. |
| 6. Open the antiseptic swabs and place them upright inside the catheter tray. Open the lubricant and squeeze a generous amount onto the tip of the catheter while it lies in the catheter tray. | The antiseptic swabs should be opened before beginning the actual catheterization. Placing the package upright prevents the antiseptic from spilling. Lubricant applied to the catheter allows for easier insertion. |
| 7. Remove the sterile urine specimen cup and lid and place them to the side of the tray without contaminating your gloves. | Urinary catheterization is a sterile procedure. |
| 8. Using your nondominant hand, carefully expose the urinary meatus by spreading the labia. This hand is now contaminated and must not be moved out of position until the catheter is in the bladder. | Moving this hand during the cleaning process will contaminate the area. |

*(continues on page 914)*

## PROCEDURE 35-1 (continued)

| STEPS | REASONS |
|---|---|
| 9. Cleanse the urinary meatus using the antiseptic swabs by wiping from top to bottom on each side and down the middle of the exposed urinary meatus. Use a separate swab for each side and the middle. | Continue to hold the labia apart with the nondominant hand. |

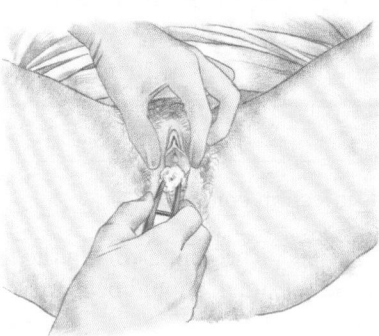

**Step 9.** Expose the urinary meatus and cleanse from top to bottom.

| STEPS | REASONS |
|---|---|
| 10. Using your sterile dominant hand, pick up the catheter and carefully insert the lubricated tip into the urinary meatus approximately 3 inches. The other end of the catheter should be left in the tray, which will collect the urine that drains from the bladder. | The adult female urethra is approximately 2 to 3 inches long. Once urine begins flowing into the catheter tray, the catheter is in far enough. |

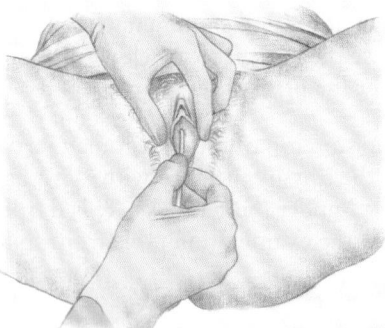

**Step 10.** Insert the catheter approximately 3 inches with the sterile hand, while continuing to hold the labia apart with the nondominant hand.

| STEPS | REASONS |
|---|---|
| 11. Once the urine begins to flow into the catheter tray, hold the catheter in position with your nondominant hand by releasing the labia and moving your fingers down onto the catheter. Use your dominant hand to direct the flow of urine into the specimen cup if a specimen is needed. | Once the catheter is inserted into the bladder, the contaminated hand can hold the external part of the catheter in place while the dominant hand can be used to obtain a specimen. |
| 12. When the urine flow has slowed or stopped *or* 1,000 mL has been obtained, carefully remove the catheter by pulling it straight out. | No more than 1,000 mL of urine should be removed from the bladder, since doing so may cause painful spasms of the bladder. Most patients do not have 1,000 mL. |
| 13. Wipe the perineum carefully with the drape that was under the buttocks. Dispose of the urine appropriately and discard the catheter, tray, and supplies in a biohazard container. | Once the catheter is removed, it is not necessary to keep your dominant hand sterile. |

## PROCEDURE 35-1 (continued)

| STEPS | REASONS |
| --- | --- |
| 14. **AFF** Explain how to respond to a patient who is visually impaired. | Face the patient when speaking to him or her and always let him or her know what you are going to do before touching him or her. |
| 15. If a urine specimen was obtained, properly label the specimen container and complete the laboratory requisition. Process the specimen according to the guidelines of the laboratory. | Specimens obtained to be sent to an outside laboratory should be labeled and accompanied by a completed request form. |
| 16. Remove your gloves and wash your hands. | Standard precautions must be followed throughout the procedure. |
| 17. Instruct the patient to dress and give any follow-up information regarding test results as necessary. | Telling the patient what to do and what to expect will reduce confusion and misunderstanding. |
| 18. **AFF** Log into the electronic medical record (EMR) using your username and secure password OR obtain the paper medical record from a secure location and assure it is kept away from public access. Document the procedure including the size of the catheter used and the amount and quality of the urine obtained. Your entry must include the date, time, and your name/credentials. | Procedures are considered not to have been done if they are not recorded. |
| 19. When finished, log out of the EMR and/or replace the paper medical record in an appropriate and secure location. | The integrity of the medical record must be protected at all times. |

**Charting Example:**
*02/14/2016 9:15 AM Catheterization with a 14-French straight cath, 300 mL dark amber urine obtained, specimen to Acme lab for C & S _____ S. Strobb, CMA.*

Note: *The medical assistant may sign his or her name in the patient record using only the "CMA" credential if the office has a signature log denoting the entire credential as "CMA(AAMA)."*

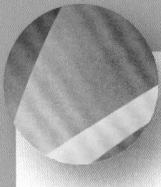

## PSY PROCEDURE 35-2

## Male Urinary Catheterization

**PSY** Instruct and prepare a patient for a procedure or treatment; coach patients appropriately considering cultural diversity, developmental life stage, and communication barriers; and document patient care accurately in the medical record.

**Purpose:** Using sterile aseptic technique, perform a straight catheterization on a male torso model

**Equipment:** Sterile straight catheterization tray with 14- or 16-French catheter, sterile gloves, antiseptic solution, sterile specimen cup with lid, lubricant, sterile drape, examination light, and anatomically correct male torso model

| STEPS | PURPOSE |
|---|---|
| 1. Wash your hands. | Handwashing aids infection control. |
| 2. Identify yourself, including your title. Also, identify the patient, explain the procedure, and have the patient disrobe completely from the waist down while providing a gown and adequate draping. | Identifying the patient helps prevent errors in the treatment. The privacy of the patient should be maintained at all times. |
| 3. Place the patient supine, draping carefully to prevent unnecessary exposure. Carefully open the tray and place it to the side of the patient on the examination table or on top of the patient's thighs. | The male urinary meatus is on the glans penis. Placing the tray on top of the patient's legs allows easy access to the catheter and supplies. |
| 4. Remove the sterile glove package and put on the sterile gloves without contaminating them. | Contaminating the gloves will contaminate the supplies and may cause the patient to develop a urinary tract infection after the procedure. |
| 5. Carefully remove the sterile drape and place it under the glans penis. | If the sterile drape is the top item in the tray, it may be carefully lifted out of the tray by the edge with clean hands and placed under the penis. This drape is a barrier to protect the examination table and patient from any spills. |
| 6. Open the antiseptic swabs and place them upright inside the catheter tray. Open the lubricant and squeeze a generous amount onto the tip of the catheter as it lies in the bottom of the catheter tray. | The antiseptic swabs should be opened before beginning the catheterization. Placing the package upright helps prevent the antiseptic from spilling. Lubricant on the catheter allows for easier insertion. |
| 7. Remove the sterile urine specimen cup and lid and place them to the side of the tray without contaminating your gloves. | Urinary catheterization is a sterile procedure. |
| 8. Using your nondominant hand, carefully pick up the penis, exposing the urinary meatus. This hand is now contaminated and must not be moved out of position until the catheter is inserted into the urinary bladder. | Moving this hand will contaminate the area. |

# PROCEDURE 35-2 (continued)

| STEPS | PURPOSE |
|---|---|
| **9.** Cleanse the urinary meatus using the antiseptic swabs by wiping from top to bottom on each side and down the middle of the exposed urinary meatus. Use a separate swab for each side and the middle. | Continue to hold the penis with the dominant hand. |

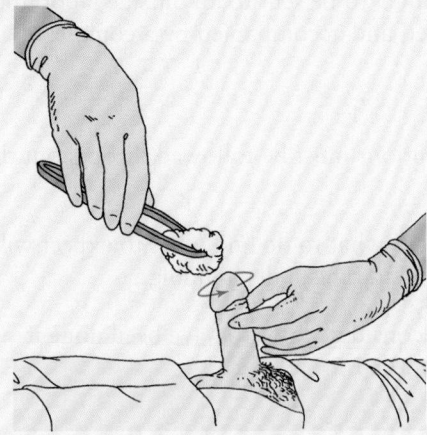

**Step 9.** Expose the urinary meatus and cleanse from top to bottom.

**10.** Using your sterile dominant hand, pick up the catheter and carefully insert the lubricated tip into the urinary meatus approximately 4 to 6 inches. The other end of the catheter should be left in the tray, which will collect the urine that drains from the bladder.

The adult male urethra is approximately 4 to 6 inches long. Once urine begins flowing into the catheter tray, the catheter is in far enough.

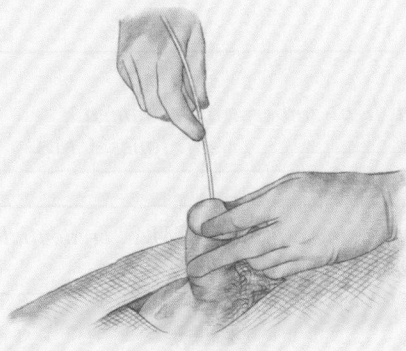

**Step 10.** Carefully insert the catheter into the urethra.

**11.** Once the urine begins to flow, hold the catheter in position with your nondominant hand. Use your dominant hand to direct the flow of urine into the specimen cup if a specimen is needed.

Once the catheter is inserted into the bladder, the contaminated hand can hold the external part of the catheter in place while the dominant hand can be used to obtain a specimen.

**12.** When the urine flow has slowed or stopped *or* 1,000 mL has been obtained, carefully remove the catheter by pulling it straight out.

No more than 1,000 mL of urine should be removed from the bladder, since doing so may cause painful spasms of the bladder.

**13.** Wipe the glans penis carefully with the drape and dispose of the urine, catheter, tray, and supplies appropriately in a biohazard container.

Once the urinary catheter has been removed, it is not necessary to keep the dominant hand sterile.

*(continues on page 918)*

## PROCEDURE 35-2 (continued)

| STEPS | PURPOSE |
|---|---|
| 14. **AFF** Explain how to respond to a patient who has dementia. | Solicit assistance from a caregiver or other staff member to help during the procedure. Give simple directions to the patient about what he or she should do. Speak clearly, not loudly. |
| 15. If a urine specimen was obtained, properly label the container and complete the laboratory requisition. Process the specimen according to the guidelines of the laboratory. | Specimens obtained to be sent to an outside laboratory should be labeled and accompanied by a completed request form. |
| 16. Remove your gloves and wash your hands. | Standard precautions must be followed throughout the procedure. |
| 17. Instruct the patient to dress and give any follow-up information regarding test results as necessary. | Telling the patient what to do and what to expect will reduce confusion and misunderstanding. |
| 18. **AFF** Log into the electronic medical record (EMR) using your username and secure password OR obtain the paper medical record from a secure location and assure it is kept away from public access. Document the procedure including the size of the catheter used and the amount and quality of the urine obtained. Your entry must include the date, time, and your name/credentials. | Procedures are considered not to have been done if they are not recorded. |
| 19. When finished, log out of the EMR and/or replace the paper medical record in an appropriate and secure location. | The integrity of the medical record must be protected at all times. |

Charting Example:

*6/17/20XX 3:00 PM Catheterization with 14-French straight cath, 600 mL light amber urine obtained, specimen to Acme lab for C & S* _____ *J. Jones, CMA.*

Note: *The medical assistant may sign his or her name in the patient record using only the "CMA" credential if the office has a signature log denoting the entire credential as "CMA(AAMA)."*

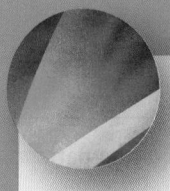

## PSY   PROCEDURE 35-3

# Instructing a Male Patient on the Testicular Self-Examination

**PSY** Instruct and prepare a patient for a procedure or treatment; coach patients regarding disease prevention and treatment plans; coach patients appropriately considering cultural diversity, developmental life stage, and communication barriers; and document patient care accurately in the medical record.

**Purpose:** Teach a male patient to perform the testicular self-examination

**Equipment:** A patient instruction sheet if available and testicular examination model or pictures

| STEPS | PURPOSE |
|---|---|
| **1.** Wash your hands. | Handwashing aids infection control. |
| **2.** Identify the patient and explain the procedure. | Identifying the patient prevents errors in the treatment. |
| **3.** Using the testicular model or pictures, explain the procedure, telling the patient to examine each testicle by gently rolling the testicle between the fingers and the thumb with both hands while checking for lumps or thickenings. | Both hands should be used to check each testicle to ensure complete palpation of all areas. Lumps and thickened areas are not normal and should be reported to the physician. |

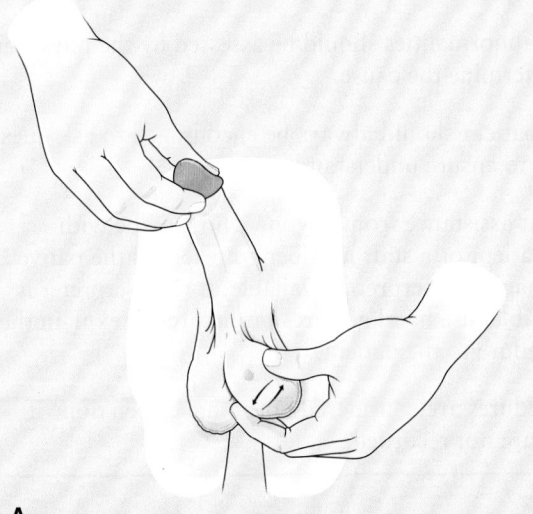
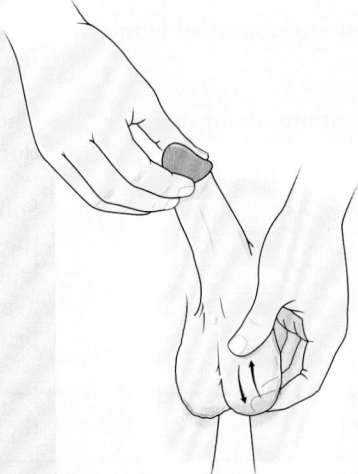

**A**    **B**

**Step 3. (A)** Gently roll the testes in a horizontal plane between the thumb and fingers.
        **(B)** Follow the same procedure and palpate upward along the testis.

*(continues on page 920)*

## PROCEDURE 35-3 (continued)

| STEPS | PURPOSE |
|---|---|
| 4. Explain that the epididymis is a structure on top of each testicle and should be palpated to avoid incorrectly identifying it as an abnormal growth or lump. | If the epididymis is not correctly identified, the patient may palpate it during the examination and erroneously believe it is an abnormal growth. |

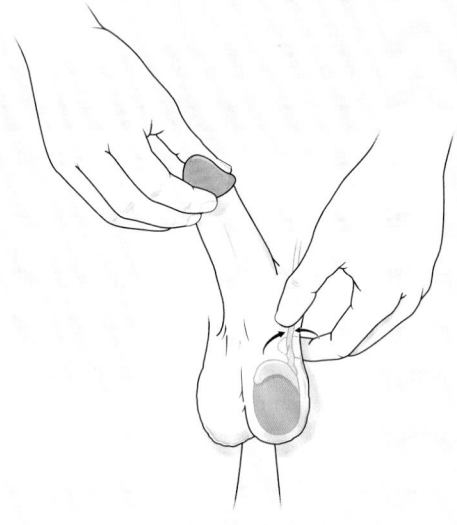

**Step 4.** Locate the epididymis, a cordlike structure on the top and back of the testicle that stores and transports sperm.

| STEPS | PURPOSE |
|---|---|
| 5. Instruct the patient to report any abnormal lumps or thickenings to the physician. | Any abnormalities should be assessed by the physician to determine the cause. |
| 6. Allow the patient to ask questions about the self-examination. | The patient should always be encouraged to ask questions to ensure understanding. |
| 7. **AFF** Explain how to respond to a patient who speaks limited English. | Solicit assistance from anyone who may be with the patient or a staff member who speaks the native language to interpret if available. If no interpreter is available, use hand gestures or pictures to explain the procedure to the patient. |
| 8. Document the procedure in the patient's medical record. | Procedures are considered not to have been done if they are not recorded. |

---

**Charting Example**

*12/13/2016 10:15 AM Pt. given verbal and written instructions on the testicular self-examination; verbalized understanding* _____ *C. Brook, CMA.*

---

**Note:** *The medical assistant may sign his or her name in the patient record using only the "CMA" credential if the office has a signature log denoting the entire credential as "CMA(AAMA)."*

# CHAPTER

# 36 Obstetrics and Gynecology

## Learning Outcomes

**COG Cognitive Domain***

1. Spell key terms
2. *Define medical terms and abbreviations related to all body systems*
3. *Describe structural organization of the human body*
4. *List major organs in each body system*
5. *Identify the anatomical location of major organs in each body system*
6. *Describe the normal function of each body system*
7. *Identify common pathology related to each body system including signs, symptoms, and etiology*
8. List and describe common gynecologic and obstetric disorders
9. Identify your role in the care of gynecologic and obstetric patients
10. Describe the components of prenatal and postpartum patient care
11. Explain the diagnostic and therapeutic procedures associated with the female reproductive system

12. Identify the various methods of contraception
13. Describe menopause

**PSY Psychomotor Domain***

1. Instruct the patient on the breast self-examination (Procedure 36-1)
   a. *Instruct and prepare a patient for a procedure or treatment*
   b. *Coach patients appropriately considering cultural diversity, developmental life stage, and communication barriers*
   c. *Coach patients regarding disease prevention and treatment plans*
   d. *Document patient care accurately in the medical record*
2. Assist with the pelvic examination and Pap smear (Procedure 36-2)
   a. *Instruct and prepare a patient for a procedure or treatment*
   b. *Coach patients appropriately considering cultural diversity, developmental life stage, and communication barriers*

*(continues on page 922)*

c. *Coach patients regarding disease prevention and treatment plans*

d. *Document patient care accurately in the medical record*

3. Assist with colposcopy and cervical biopsy (Procedure 36-3)

   a. *Instruct and prepare a patient for a procedure or treatment*

   b. *Coach patients appropriately considering cultural diversity, developmental life stage, and communication barriers*

   c. *Coach patients regarding disease prevention and treatment plans*

   d. *Document patient care accurately in the medical record*

### AFF Affective Domain*

1. *Incorporate critical thinking skills when performing patient assessment*

2. *Incorporate critical thinking skills when performing patient care*

3. *Show awareness of a patient's concerns related to the procedure being performed*

4. *Demonstrate empathy, active listening, and nonverbal communication*

5. *Demonstrate respect for individual diversity including gender, race, religion, age, economic status, and appearance*

6. *Explain to a patient the rationale for performance of a procedure*

7. *Demonstrate sensitivity to patient rights*

8. *Protect the integrity of the medical record*

***Note: AAMA/CAAHEP 2015 Standards are italicized.***

### ABHES Competencies

1. Assist the physician with the regimen of diagnostic and treatment modalities as they relate to each body system

2. Comply with federal, state, and local health laws and regulations

3. Communicate on the recipient's level of comprehension

4. Serve as a liaison between the physician and others

5. Show empathy and impartiality when dealing with patients

6. Document accurately

## Key Terms

| | | | |
|---|---|---|---|
| abortion | cystocele | laparoscopy | parity |
| amenorrhea | dysmenorrhea | lightening | pessary |
| amniocentesis | dyspareunia | lochia | polymenorrhea |
| Braxton Hicks contractions | Goodell sign | menarche | primigravida |
| Chadwick sign | gravid | menorrhagia | primipara |
| colpocleisis | gravida | menses | proteinuria |
| colporrhaphy | gravidity | metrorrhagia | puerperium |
| colposcopy | hirsutism | multipara | rectocele |
| culdocentesis | human chorionic gonadotropin (HCG) | nulligravida | salpingo-oophorectomy |
| curettage | hysterosalpingogram | nullipara | |
| | | oligomenorrhea | |

## Case Study

Great Falls Medical Center has a large specialty practice serving the needs of its female patients for obstetrics and gynecology. Christy Bolling, MD, is the OB/GYN specialist at GFMC, and she has given a standing order to Sarah Appleton, RMA, to obtain a urinalysis from all patients whose chief complaints include metrorrhagia, polymenorrhea, or amenorrhea. Why would it be necessary to get a urinalysis from these patients, and what diagnoses could be detected from an abnormal urinalysis result? What specific chemical would be present in a patient's urine that would indicate pregnancy? Other than pregnancy, what other female reproductive conditions might Dr. Bolling encounter when seeing patients in this specialty? This chapter answers these questions and covers the topic of pregnancy as well as other health-related issues involving the female reproductive organs.

The female reproductive system is responsible for the development and maintenance of primary and secondary sexual characteristics and for sexual reproduction. Gynecology and obstetrics are the two medical specialties concerned with female sexual and reproductive functions. Gynecology is a specialty of medicine that deals with development and disorders of the female reproductive system, including the internal and external organs. Obstetrics is the branch of medicine that cares for female patients through pregnancy, childbirth, and the postpartum period. The organs of the female internal reproductive system are shown in Figure 36-1.

Puberty is the onset of production of cyclical hormones that cause secondary sexual characteristics, including menses, or menstruation. The age at which a girl begins menses is **menarche**. The menstrual cycle, which is about 28 days, comprises a series of complex events in the internal organs controlled by hormones secreted by the anterior pituitary gland and the ovaries (Fig. 36-2). Always remind and encourage patients, especially adolescents, to record and track the menstrual cycle, since the regularity of the cycle is often critical to the physician's assessment of the patient's gynecologic health. In addition, the first day of the last menstrual period (LMP) is necessary for calculating an approximate due date in the pregnant patient. This chapter discusses some of the common disorders of the female reproductive system and caring for the obstetric patient in the medical office before and after delivery.

# GYNECOLOGIC DISORDERS

## Dysfunctional Uterine Bleeding

Dysfunctional uterine bleeding is abnormal or irregular uterine bleeding, including heavy, irregular, or light bleeding caused by an endocrine imbalance. Abnormal uterine bleeding includes the following:

- Menorrhagia: excessive bleeding during menses
- **Metrorrhagia**: irregular bleeding at times other than menses
- **Polymenorrhea**: abnormally frequent menses
- Postmenopausal bleeding: bleeding after menopause that is not associated with tumor, inflammation, or pregnancy

Diagnosis of dysfunctional uterine bleeding consists of ruling out other causes, such as hormonal imbalance,

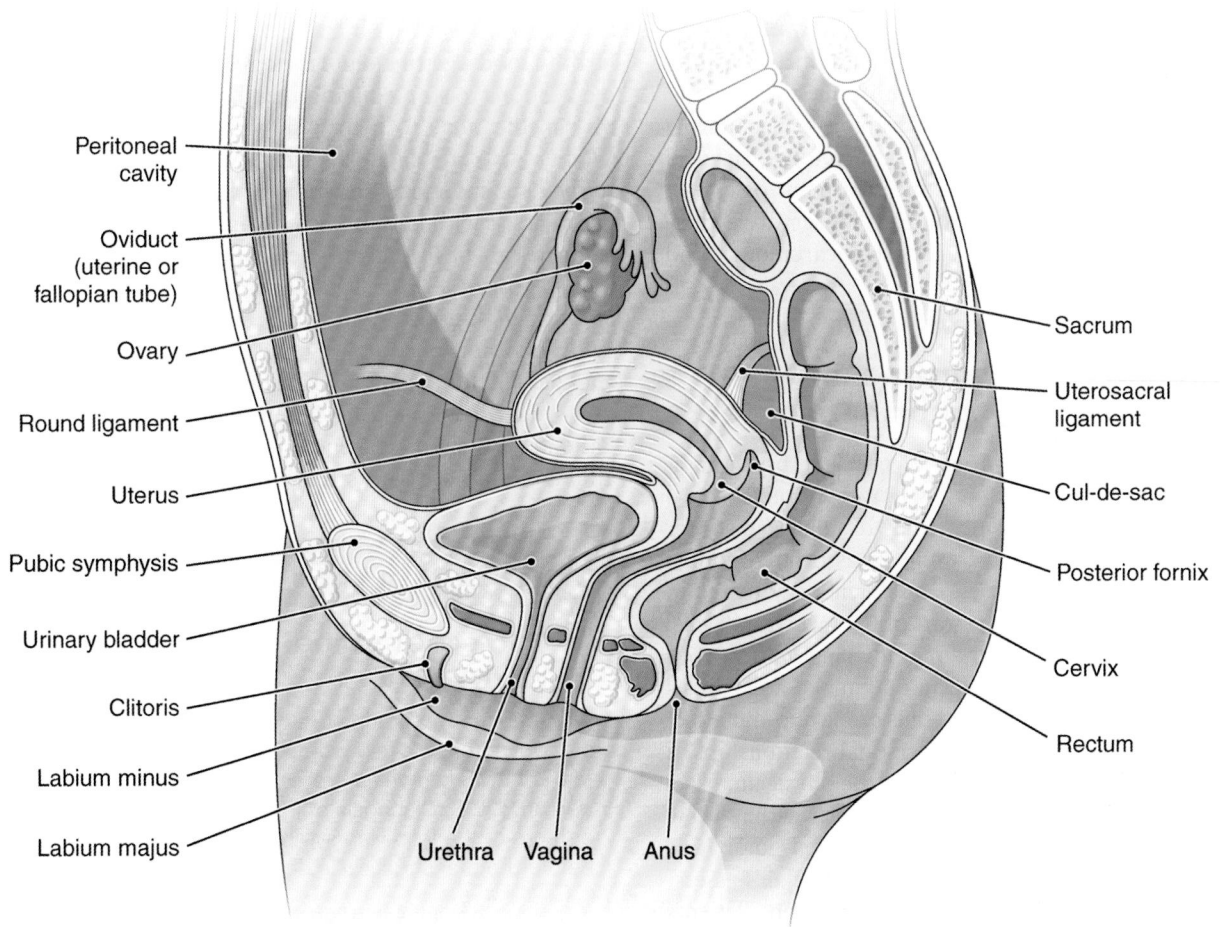

**Figure 36-1** • Female reproductive system. (Reprinted from Cohen BJ. *Memmler's The Human Body in Health and Disease*, 11th ed. Philadelphia, PA: Lippincott Williams & Wilkins, 2009, with permission.)

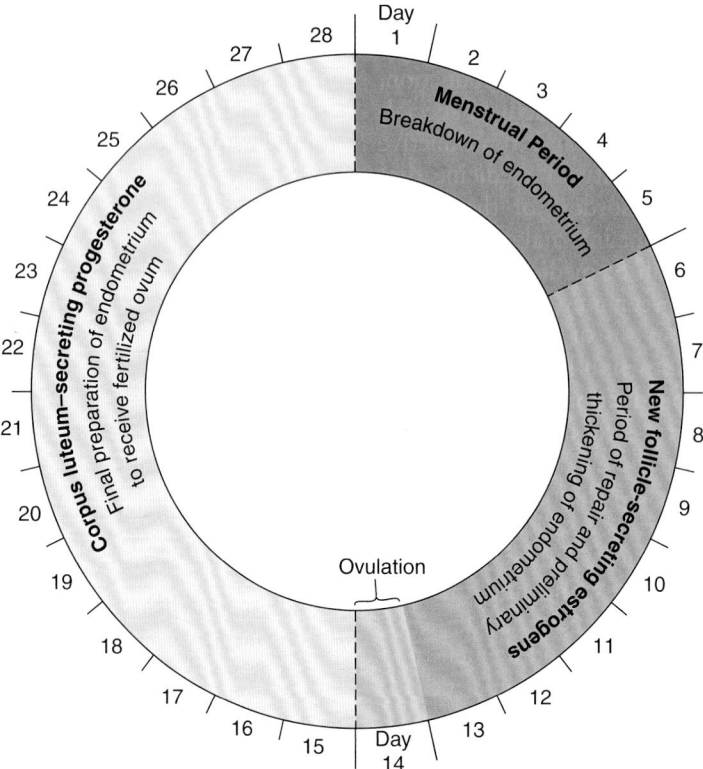

**Figure 36-2** • The menstrual cycle. (Reprinted from Cohen BJ, Wood DL. *Memmler's The Human Body in Health and Disease*, 11th ed. Philadelphia, PA: Lippincott Williams & Wilkins, 2009, with permission.)

tumor, or another condition of the endometrial lining of the uterus. Treatment includes hormone therapy and oral contraceptives or curettage (scraping) of the uterine cavity, depending on the cause. Hysterectomy, surgical removal of the uterus, may be the treatment of choice for patients who do not respond to conservative therapy, who are at increased risk for adenocarcinoma, and who do not desire pregnancy.

## Premenstrual Syndrome and Premenstrual Dysphoric Disorder

Characterized by a wide variety of physical, psychological, and behavioral signs and symptoms, premenstrual syndrome (PMS) and premenstrual dysphoric disorder (PMDD) occur on a regular, cyclic basis. Many women complain of breast tenderness and a tendency to retain fluids 7 to 10 days before the start of the menstrual cycle; however, when symptoms and mood changes affect routine daily activities, the physician may make a diagnosis of PMS (Box 36-1). When symptoms are severe and affect work, social activities, and interpersonal relationships, a diagnosis of PMDD may be made by the physician.

Both PMS and PMDD usually diminish within a few days after the onset of menses, and the cause is idiopathic (unknown). Diagnosis is based on the physician's assessment of the history and physical examination. Patients should chart their symptoms for several months on a calendar that includes the menstrual cycle. The treatment for both includes simple lifestyle changes, such as eating

healthy foods, getting regular exercise, using birth control medications to stop ovulation, and taking anti-inflammatory medications to help with any physical discomfort. Women who are diagnosed with PMDD may also be prescribed an antidepressant and may be referred to counseling to assist with developing coping strategies.

You can have a dramatic influence on the patient's ability to cope with PMS and PMDD by providing emotional support; educating the patient about the disorders; and encouraging the recommended lifestyle changes, including regular exercise and dietary restrictions, such as eliminating caffeine, salt, and animal fats. Patients also should be encouraged to get adequate rest and avoid unnecessary stress.

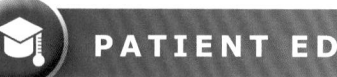

### PATIENT EDUCATION

#### Premenstrual Dysphoric Disorder

Although many women have symptoms of premenstrual syndrome, a few women have a more severe form of PMS known as *premenstrual dysphoric disorder*, or *PMDD*. Diagnosis of PMDD is made when five or more of the following symptoms are present a week before the menstrual cycle begins:

- Feelings of sadness or despair including possible suicidal thoughts
- Feelings of tension or anxiety

- Panic attacks
- Mood swings, crying
- Lasting irritability or anger that affects other people
- Disinterest in daily activities and relationships
- Trouble thinking or focusing
- Tiredness or low energy
- Food cravings or binge eating
- Difficulty sleeping
- Feeling out of control
- Physical symptoms such as bloating, breast tenderness, headaches, and joint or muscle pain

In addition to individual counseling and stress management, the physician may order antidepressants called *serotonin reuptake inhibitors*, which have been shown to help some women.

*Source: Office on Women's Health in the Department of Health and Human Services.*

 **CHECKPOINT QUESTION**

1. What is the difference between menorrhagia and metrorrhagia?

## Endometriosis

Endometriosis is a condition of unknown cause in which endometrial tissue grows outside the uterine cavity. Endometrial tissue may be found in the fallopian tubes, the ovaries, the uterosacral ligaments, and, in rare cases, in other parts of the abdominal cavity. The patient, who is often of reproductive age, complains of infertility, **dysmenorrhea**, pelvic pain, and **dyspareunia**. The patient's symptoms and physical findings may indicate endometriosis, but the diagnosis and the severity must be confirmed by direct visualization, usually by way of a **laparoscopy** (Fig. 36-3).

Treatment of endometriosis may relieve the pelvic pain, but some treatments reduce fertility. The type of therapy depends on the age of the patient, the severity of the symptoms, and the patient's desire for future pregnancy. Hormone and drug therapy to suppress the growth of the tissue and laparoscopic excision of the tissue using laser or cautery may be used to treat endometriosis. For patients with severe symptoms, the treatment of choice may be a hysterectomy with possible bilateral salpingo-oophorectomy, or surgical removal of the fallopian tubes and ovaries.

## Uterine Prolapse and Displacement

Prolapse of the uterus is an abnormal condition in which the uterus droops or protrudes down into the vagina. Often, the condition is accompanied by **cystocele**, **rectocele**, or both. Cystocele is herniation of the urinary bladder into the vagina, and rectocele is herniation of the rectum into the vagina. The degree of prolapse is usually described as mild, moderate, or severe, or grade I, II, or III. A commonly used method classifies the prolapse in degrees:

- First-degree prolapse occurs when the uterus has descended to the level of the vaginal orifice.

---

**BOX 36-1 Premenstrual Syndrome**

The hormonal flux associated with the menstrual cycle may affect body systems other than the reproductive system in some women. The cascade of events results in the following series of symptoms:

- Acne
- Breast swelling and tenderness
- Feeling tired
- Difficulty sleeping
- Upset stomach, bloating, constipation, or diarrhea
- Headache or backache
- Appetite changes or cravings
- Trouble concentrating or remembering
- Tension, irritability, mood swings, or crying spells
- Anxiety or depression

Although no treatment works the same on all women, the following are some common treatments for PMS that the physician may suggest:

- Take a multivitamin every day that includes 400 μg of folic acid.

- Include a calcium supplement with vitamin D to keep bones strong.
- Exercise regularly.
- Eat healthy foods, including fruits, vegetables, and whole grains.
- Avoid salt, sugary foods, caffeine, and alcohol.
- Get enough sleep.
- Find healthy ways to cope with stress.
- Don't smoke.

Over-the-counter medications such as ibuprofen, aspirin, or naproxen sodium may be ordered by the physician for the pain associated with PMS. Severe cases may require the physician to prescribe drugs to prevent ovulation such as birth control pills.

*From the Office on Women's Health in the Department of Health and Human Services, 2007, http://www.womenshealth.gov.*

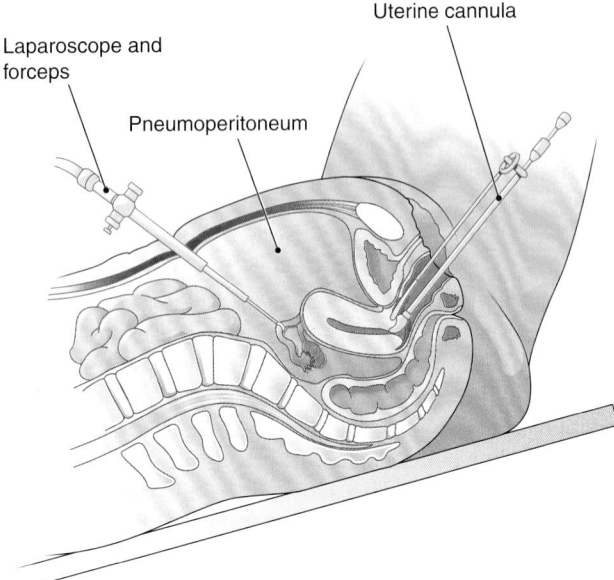

Laparoscope and forceps

Uterine cannula

Pneumoperitoneum

**Figure 36-3** • Laparoscopy. The laparoscope is inserted through a small incision in the abdomen. A pair of forceps is inserted through the scope to grasp the fallopian tube. To improve the view, a uterine cannula is inserted into the vagina to push the uterus upward. Insufflation of gas creates an air pocket, and the pelvis is raised, which forces the intestines higher into the abdomen. (Reprinted from Cohen BJ. *Medical Terminology: An Illustrated Guide.* Philadelphia, PA: Lippincott Williams & Wilkins, 2003, with permission.)

- Second-degree prolapse occurs when the uterine cervix protrudes through the vaginal orifice.
- Third-degree prolapse occurs when the entire cervix and uterus protrude beyond the vaginal orifice.

Diagnosis of uterine prolapse is made during a pelvic examination, at which time the degree of prolapse can be determined. While many women do not have symptoms, others complain of pelvic pressure, dyspareunia, urinary problems, or constipation. Surgical treatment may include vaginal hysterectomy, **colporrhaphy** (suture of the vagina), or **colpocleisis** (surgery to occlude the vagina). Medical management for patients who are elderly or a poor risk for surgery includes hormone therapy to strengthen the muscular floor of the pelvis and the use of a **pessary**. A pessary is a device that is inserted into the vagina and fits around the cervix to support the uterus. You should instruct the patient on the proper procedure for caring for the device by removing it according to the physician's orders and washing it with soap and warm water before reinserting it into the vagina.

The uterus is normally tilted slightly forward over the bladder with the cervix at a right angle to the direction of the vagina. The uterus is movable, and stress on the supporting ligaments occasionally tilts it from its natural position, known as **uterine displacement** (Fig. 36-4). The symptoms of uterine displacement may include pressure in the rectal area or against the bladder that is not usually severe, just troublesome to the patient. Treatment follows the same protocol as required for uterine prolapse. In some instances, the uterus may simply be stitched back into its original position in a hysteropexy.

## Leiomyomas

Leiomyomas are benign tumors of the uterus, including fibroid tumors, myomas, and fibromyomas. These tumors may be in any of the uterine tissue layers—endometrium, myometrium, or perimetrium—and they vary

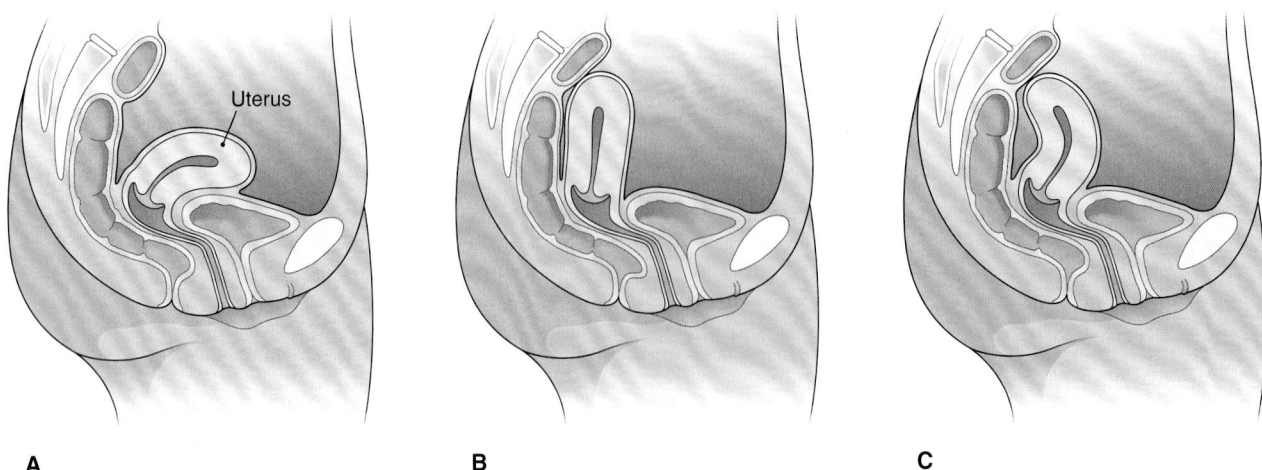

A    B    C

**Figure 36-4** • Retrodisplacements of the uterus. **(A)** The normal position of the uterus as detected on palpation. **(B)** In retroversion, the uterus turns posteriorly as a whole. **(C)** In retroflexion, the fundus bends posteriorly above the cervical end.

greatly in size. Most patients are asymptomatic, but large tumors tend to distort the uterus and are relatively likely to be symptomatic. Symptoms may include abnormal bleeding, pelvic pressure and discomfort, constipation, urinary frequency, and infertility.

A presumptive diagnosis is based on the patient's symptoms and physician's assessment, which initially includes bimanual examination and sounding of the uterus. Sounding of the uterus requires the physician to do a pelvic examination and possibly the insertion of a uterine sound (a long slender instrument; refer to Chapter 21) into the uterine cavity. Obstruction or resistance may be due to the tumor pressing into the uterine cavity. Most physicians request an ultrasound of the uterus to confirm the presence of these tumors.

Treatment of leiomyoma depends on the size of the tumor or tumors. Small asymptomatic tumors are monitored to detect excessive growth. Depending on the patient's age and desire for pregnancy, myomectomy or hysterectomy may be indicated.

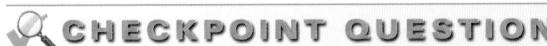

## CHECKPOINT QUESTION

2. What are some symptoms of endometriosis?

## Ovarian Cysts

Numerous types of ovarian cysts, including functional cysts and polycystic ovaries, are benign. Functional ovarian cysts, which are fairly common, include the follicular cyst. This is a fluid-filled sac that causes few if any problems. The patient is most often asymptomatic unless the cyst is large or ruptures. Functional cysts are usually detected during surgery, and treatment is simply puncture or excision.

In contrast, polycystic ovary syndrome (Stein-Leventhal syndrome) is a more troublesome and complex disorder. It affects both ovaries and is most often found in adolescent girls and young women, who have numerous symptoms of an endocrine imbalance. The signs include anovulation, irregular menses or **amenorrhea** (no menses), and **hirsutism**, an abnormal or excessive growth of hair. Diagnosis is based on pelvic examination, ultrasonography, laparoscopy, or exploratory laparotomy. Treatment is difficult and depends on the signs and symptoms and the patient's desire for future pregnancy. Management of this disorder includes hormone therapy or oral contraceptives.

## Gynecologic Cancers

The malignant tumors affecting the female reproductive system and their characteristics, diagnosis, and treatment are outlined in Table 36-1. For patient education, you should know the recommendations regarding the frequency of pelvic and breast examinations and Pap smears. You should obtain current brochures and literature on various types of cancers from either the American Cancer Society or the American College of Obstetrics and Gynecology and have them readily available to patients.

Cervical and breast cancers have an excellent prognosis when detected and treated early, but left untreated or diagnosed in later stages, these cancers are deadly. Instruct and encourage all female patients to perform a breast self-examination every month (Procedure 36-1). Patients should also be encouraged to have a complete physical that includes a breast examination by the physician and a pelvic examination and Papanicolaou (Pap) test, which is a screening test for early detection of cancer of the cervix. The American College of Obstetricians and Gynecologists (ACOG) recommends that the first Pap test and pelvic exam be performed about 3 years after the first sexual intercourse or by age 21 years, whichever comes first, and annually until age 30 years. Women over age 30 years who have had three negative Pap tests can be screened every 2 to 3 years or annually as recommended by the physician.

Initially, the abnormal growth of cancerous cells in the cervix is asymptomatic, which further necessitates early detection during the physical examination and Pap smear. The Pap test is a grading of any abnormal tissue scraped from the cervix using a classification system such as the one described in Table 36-2. Some laboratories use another classification, the Bethesda system, to provide a more descriptive narrative of the abnormal cells. Cervical cells in the Bethesda system are categorized as normal, atypical squamous cells (ASC), squamous intraepithelial lesions (SIL), atypical glandular cells, or cancer. In addition, the squamous intraepithelial lesions may be noted as high grade (HSIL) or low grade (LSIL) (Fig. 36-5). Regardless of the method used by the laboratory to classify the Pap test results, not all abnormal results indicate cancer. However, since this is a deadly disease, it must be ruled out using further diagnostic studies such as **colposcopy**, a magnified examination of the cervical tissue with a special instrument called a *colposcope*. Other reasons for an abnormal Pap result include inflammation of the cervix and some sexually transmitted diseases such as human papillomavirus (HPV) infection.

## Infertility

Female infertility is more difficult to diagnose than is male infertility. Most testing begins by eliminating the male as the infertile party and then focuses on the female partner. Testing is usually not started until after 1 year of unprotected intercourse without conception.

The causes of infertility may include uterine or cervical abnormalities, tubal occlusion or scarring, a hormonal imbalance, or psychological factors. Diagnosis

### TABLE 36-1   Cancers of the Female Reproductive System

| Cancer | Warning Signs | Risk Factors | Early Detection | Treatment |
|---|---|---|---|---|
| Breast | Breast changes: lumps, pain, thickening, swelling, retraction, dimpling | Over age 40, history of breast cancer, early menarche, nulliparity, first birth at late age | Monthly self-examination, mammogram by age 40 and yearly after age 40, yearly clinical breast exam, monthly self-breast exam | Lumpectomy, mastectomy, radiation, chemotherapy |
| Cervical | Often asymptomatic; irregular bleeding, abnormal vaginal discharge | Intercourse at early age, multiple sex partners, cigarette smoking, history of STDs such as HPV | Annual Pap smear | Cryotherapy, electrocoagulation, surgery, radiation, chemotherapy. New vaccine is available to prevent certain types of HPV that may cause cervical cancer. |
| Endometrial | Irregular bleeding outside menses, unusual vaginal discharge, excessive bleeding during menses, postmenopausal bleeding | Obesity, early menarche, multiple sex partners, late menopause, history of infertility, family history | Endometrial biopsy at menopause for high-risk women | Progesterone therapy, surgery, radiation, chemotherapy |
| Ovarian | Often asymptomatic; abdominal enlargement; vague digestive disorders, discomfort; gas, distention | Risk increases with age (esp. >60 years), nulliparity, history of breast cancer | Periodic complete pelvic examination | Surgery, radiation, chemotherapy |

requires a complete history and physical examination. An endometrial biopsy may diagnose anovulation; progesterone blood levels may indicate hormonal deficiencies; or hysterosalpingography may indicate tubal occlusion or uterine abnormalities. Treatment necessitates identifying and correcting the problem. Procedures such as in vitro fertilization may also be recommended, again, depending upon the nature of the problem.

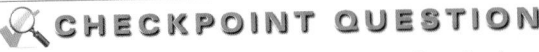

### CHECKPOINT QUESTION

3. Sarah Appleton was with Dr. Boling today when a patient was given the diagnosis of uterine cancer. What two factors greatly affect the prognosis of all cancers?

## Sexually Transmitted Diseases

Many of the diseases transmitted through sexual contact have serious consequences and may affect men or women. The most deadly of these is acquired immunodeficiency syndrome (AIDS), although other sexually transmitted diseases (STDs) also continue to be a problem.

Since STDs are easily transmitted, all STDs must be reported to the local health department by the medical office. This may be your responsibility, or the physician may be required to report the disease according to local policy or the policy of the medical office. In some areas, you may have to file a form or written report; others have a phone reporting system. You need to be familiar with your office policy and procedure manual regarding this requirement and the local

### TABLE 36-2   Classification of Papanicolaou Tests

| Class | Characteristics |
|---|---|
| I | Normal test, no atypical cells |
| II | Atypical cells but no evidence of malignancy |
| III | Atypical cells possible but not conclusive for malignancy |
| IV | Cells strongly suggest malignancy |
| V | Strong evidence of malignancy |

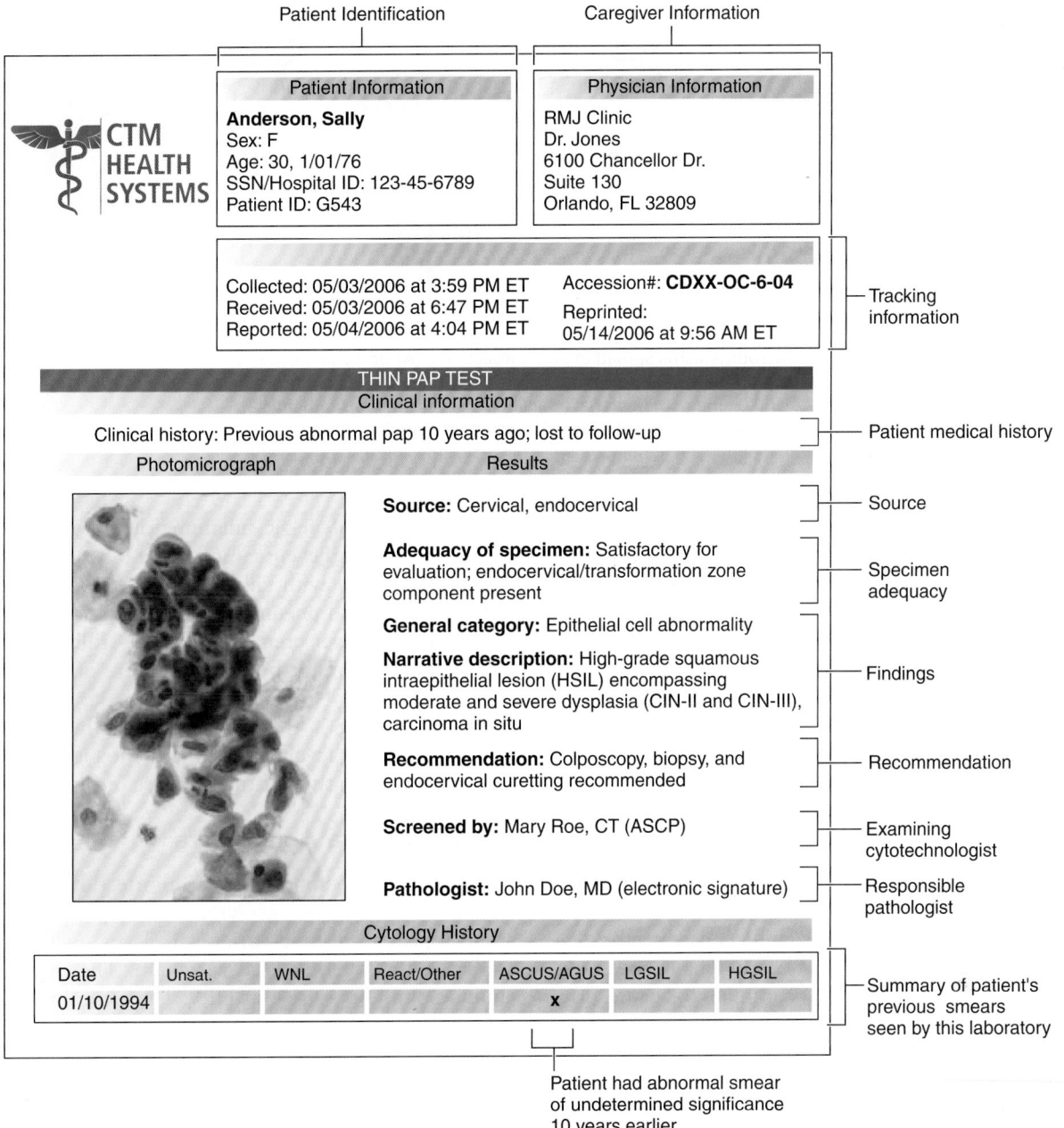

**Figure 36-5** • Typical Pap smear report. (From McConnell TH. *The Nature of Disease Pathology for the Health Professions*. Philadelphia, PA: Lippincott Williams & Wilkins, 2007.)

laws on reporting. The patient should be encouraged to notify sexual partners so that they may also receive treatment for the appropriate STD. Figure 36-6 outlines the pathway by which microorganisms spread in female pelvic infections regardless of the reason, but especially when sexually transmitted diseases are involved.

## AIDS

AIDS is an infectious disease that overwhelms the body's immune system. The pathogen that causes AIDS is the human immunodeficiency virus (HIV), which destroys T-helper cells, lowering the body's ability to

fight infection. Transmission of HIV most often occurs through an exchange of blood or body fluids, including a sexual act with an HIV-positive partner. A person who is HIV positive may go through the following stages as the infection progresses to AIDS:

1. Acute infectious state with generally mild flulike symptoms
2. Latent period without symptoms but still infectious
3. Weight loss, lymphadenopathy, fever, diarrhea, anorexia, fatigue, and skin rashes
4. Onset of immunodeficiency disorders, such as Kaposi sarcoma and *Pneumocystis carinii* pneumonia

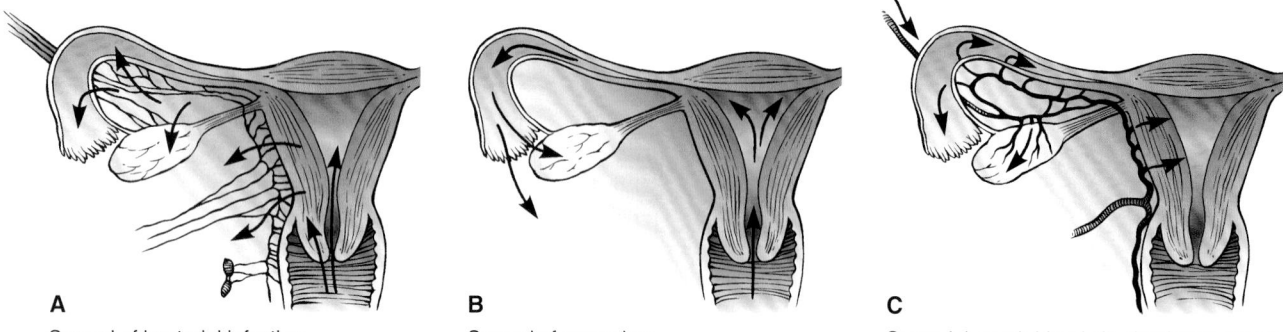

|   A   |   B   |   C   |
|-------|-------|-------|
| Spread of bacterial infection | Spread of gonorrhea | Spread through blood via circulatory system |

**Figure 36-6 •** Pathway by which microorganisms spread in pelvic infections. **(A)** Bacterial infection spreads up the vagina into the uterus and through the lymphatics. **(B)** Gonorrhea spreads up the vagina into the uterus and then to the tubes and ovaries. **(C)** Bacterial infection can reach the reproductive organs through the bloodstream (hematogenous spread). (From Smeltzer SC, Bare BG. *Textbook of Medical-Surgical Nursing*, 9th ed. Philadelphia, PA: Lippincott Williams & Wilkins, 2000.)

Although new treatments prolong the HIV-positive individual's life, there currently is no cure; however, research to find more effective treatments and a possible cure is ongoing.

### Syphilis

After AIDS, syphilis is the most serious STD. The cause of syphilis is a microorganism known as **Treponema pallidum,** a spirochete. The first sign is a chancre or ulcerated lesion at the primary site of infection on the genitalia. This chancre appears several days to several weeks after infection, heals very quickly, and may not be noticed. Although the chancre heals quickly, the spirochete spreads quickly through the bloodstream and becomes systemic, with far-reaching consequences. The second phase is identified by a rash that may appear anywhere on the body. The patient continues to be infectious at this stage, but treatment with penicillin will stop the progression of the disease to the next, or tertiary, phase. If left untreated, the rash will disappear, and the syphilis may lie dormant for years. At some point, however, the patient will experience cardiovascular damage, central nervous system involvement, and death (Fig. 36-7).

Infants born with syphilis caused by transplacental infection are commonly mentally retarded, deaf, blind, or deformed. Many babies spontaneously abort or are delivered stillborn.

### Chlamydia

Chlamydia infections cause urethritis in men, cervicitis in women, and lymphogranuloma venereum in both, all caused by the organism **Chlamydia trachomatis.** Chlamydia is the most common STD in the United States. Female patients may be asymptomatic or may have vague flulike symptoms that are difficult to diagnose without specific reason to suspect infection. In severe cases, there may be extensive lymph gland involvement known as *lymphogranuloma venereum.* Chlamydia is one of the leading causes of pelvic inflammatory disease, causing tubal scarring and eventual infertility in women. Infants born to mothers with chlamydial infections may have conjunctivitis and pneumonia. The fetus may spontaneously abort, deliver prematurely, or be stillborn.

Diagnosis is made by a swab culture of the site sent to the laboratory for identification of the microorganism. The disease is treated with an antibiotic such as doxycycline, tetracycline, or sulfamethoxazole until the patient tests negative for the presence of the pathogen.

### Condylomata Acuminata

Condylomata acuminata is a viral infection of the genital area causing the growth of soft, papillary warts that appear in a wide variety of places, including the vulva, vagina, cervix, and perineum. The cause is the human papillomavirus, or HPV. The genital warts usually appear about 3 months after exposure. Biopsy of the condyloma is appropriate to rule out the slight possibility of a malignancy. Although HPV is difficult

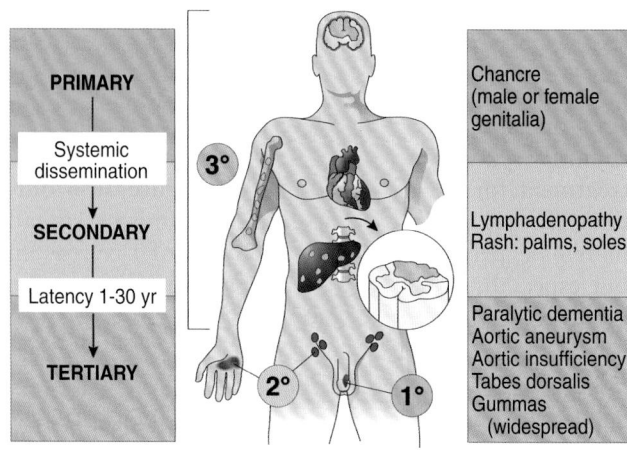

**Figure 36-7 •** Clinical characteristics of the various stages of syphilis. (Image from Rubin E, Farber JL. *Pathology*, 3rd ed. Philadelphia, PA: Lippincott Williams & Wilkins, 1999.)

to eradicate, cryotherapy (freezing the involved area) or laser ablation (burning with laser) has moderate success.

HPV has been implicated as a risk for cervical cancer in some women, but currently, there is a vaccine, Gardasil™, to protect against four types of HPV that are responsible for 70% of cervical cancers and 90% of genital warts (Centers for Disease Control and Prevention). The Advisory Committee on Immunization Practices (ACIP) recommends this vaccine for girls over the age of 9; however, there are no current federal laws requiring administration of this vaccine.

 **CHECKPOINT QUESTION**

4. Which sexually transmitted disease may cause conjunctivitis and pneumonia in newborns born to infected mothers?

## Gonorrhea

Gonorrhea is the second most common STD and is caused by a gram-negative diplococcus, **Neisseria gonorrhoeae.** The symptoms appear in the genitalia 2 to 8 days after exposure. In some female patients, the Bartholin and Skene glands fill with pus, and the infection may spread to the cervix. However, female patients may be asymptomatic and unaware of the disease. The disease may lead to salpingitis with scarring and adhesions or pelvic inflammatory disease. Infants born to mothers infected with gonorrhea may develop purulent conjunctivitis with corneal ulcerations that result in blindness. All infants are now treated prophylactically in the newborn nursery.

Diagnosis is based on the symptoms and through a culture of the drainage if present. Once diagnosed, gonorrhea may be treated with penicillin, although penicillin-resistant strains are now appearing.

## Herpes Genitalis

Herpes genitalis is caused by the herpes simplex virus 2 (HSV2) and is characterized by painful vesicular lesions in the vaginal, vulvar, or anorectal area. This genital infection usually appears within 3 to 7 days after exposure. The infected patient may present with painful vesicles in the genital region that rupture and leave equally painful ulcers that eventually heal in about 10 days. In addition, the patient may have swollen and tender lymph nodes and flulike symptoms. After the lesion heals, the patient may be in remission for years, or the symptoms may recur with each stressful situation. Patients with herpes genitalis should be advised to avoid sexual contact during episodes of vesiculation because the exudate is highly contagious. Although there is no cure, the condition is somewhat controlled with an antiviral agent such as acyclovir.

Infants born vaginally to mothers with active lesions may develop the disease within a few weeks of birth. The virus spreads rapidly to the organs of the infant and up to 90% of infected infants die.

## Vulvovaginitis, Salpingitis, and Pelvic Inflammatory Disease

Although vulvovaginitis, salpingitis, and pelvic inflammatory disease can be caused by any type of microorganism, these disorders are commonly caused by sexually transmitted infections (see Fig. 36-6). Vulvovaginitis is an inflammation of the vulva and vagina and is one of the common complaints of female patients. Symptoms often include pruritus, burning of the vulva or the vagina (or both), and increased vaginal discharge. On examination, the vulva and vagina are reddened. The type of discharge often indicates the cause of the disorder, and effective treatment depends on the cause. The causative agent is confirmed by a microscopic examination of a vaginal smear or by culture of the vaginal discharge and may include the following microorganisms:

- *Trichomonas vaginalis*: Known as *trich*, this protozoan causes an STD. The signs are a thin, frothy, greenish or gray vaginal discharge with an odor. Signs and symptoms include dysuria with urinary frequency and intense pruritus. Treatment is oral metronidazole for both partners.
- *Candida albicans*: Also known as *monilia*, this fungus grows best in the presence of glucose. The signs include a thick, curd-like discharge with white patches on the vaginal walls, usually with no odor. Intense itching is usual. The pathogen is found in the intestines and is most likely to affect the patient during the secretory phase of the menstrual cycle. It is very common during pregnancy and in patients receiving antibiotic therapy. Treatment requires nystatin vaginal suppositories, which may be purchased without a prescription.
- *Gardnerella vaginitis*: This gram-negative bacillus causes a gray discharge with a foul odor. It is treated with metronidazole.

Salpingitis is a bacterial infection of the fallopian tubes that is most often transmitted by sexual intercourse. Young sexually active women, women with multiple sexual partners, and women with intrauterine devices are at increased risk for salpingitis. Numerous microorganisms may cause salpingitis, but the most common microbes include N. gonorrhoeae, C. trachomatis, genital mycoplasma, and normal flora bacteria. Salpingitis is sometimes called *pelvic inflammatory disease* when the surrounding structures, including the pelvic peritoneum, uterus, ovaries, and surrounding tissues, are inflamed. Signs and symptoms include varying degrees of abdominal pain and tenderness with or without fever and leukocytosis, an abnormal increase in the white blood cell count.

Cultures for gonorrhea and tests for Chlamydia are essential for antibiotic therapy. **Culdocentesis** may be necessary to obtain purulent drainage and determine the exact cause of the infection. Laparoscopy may be performed to determine the extent of the infection. Treatment for mild infections includes antibiotic and analgesic therapy, bed rest, and removal of the source of infection. In patients with pyosalpinx (pus in the fallopian tubes), tubal obstruction, abscess, serious inflammation, and edema, treatment may be a hysterectomy with bilateral **salpingo-oophorectomy** or an incision and drainage.

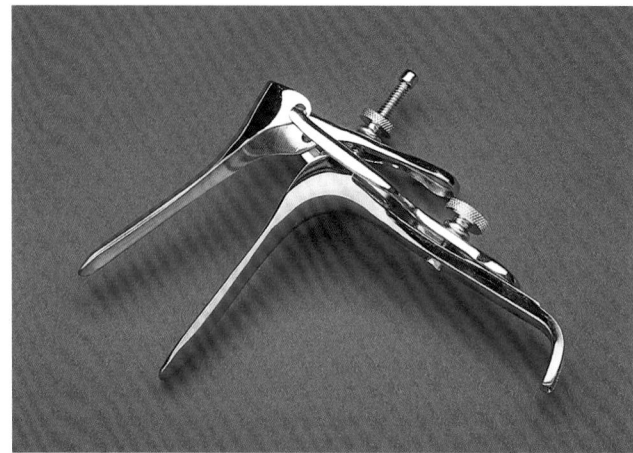

**Figure 36-8** • A stainless steel vaginal speculum. (LifeART image copyright © 2008 Lippincott Williams & Wilkins. All rights reserved.)

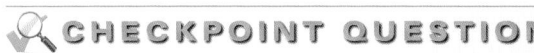

### CHECKPOINT QUESTION

5. Which sexually transmitted disease is associated with female reproductive cancer?

## COMMON DIAGNOSTIC AND THERAPEUTIC PROCEDURES

### The Gynecologic Examination

As part of the gynecologic examination, the physician examines the patient's breasts, performs a pelvic examination, and obtains a Pap smear. Because of the risk of contracting infection from body fluids, especially blood, you and the physician must observe standard precautions, wearing protective barriers such as gloves as appropriate during the examination. When scheduling the appointment, instruct the patient not to douche, use vaginal medication, or have sexual intercourse for 24 hours before the examination. If a Pap smear will be performed, the appointment should be scheduled about 1 week after the end of menses. When the patient arrives for the scheduled appointment, spend time with the patient to establish rapport, especially with new patients and patients with special needs, such as the young, elderly, and disabled. A procedure that is rushed or seems hurried to the patient may diminish the professional image of the office and the patient's attitude toward the physician and staff.

The physician usually begins the examination by examining the breast and surrounding tissue, including the axillae and chest tissue up to the clavicle. This tissue is inspected for dimpling or size disparity and palpated for lumps or thickenings. Next, the physician examines the external and internal female genitalia to identify or diagnose any abnormal conditions (Procedure 36-2). Although the dorsal lithotomy position provides the best visibility for the physician, this position may be difficult for elderly or some disabled persons. Elevating the head of the table to 30 degrees may be easier for the patient while allowing the physician to do a thorough examination.

The elevation of the table does not seem to have any disadvantages, and often, the patient finds this position more comfortable, but consult with the physician if the lithotomy position is not possible. If elevating the head of the examination table is not appropriate, an alternative position, such as the Sims position, may be necessary.

After visually inspecting the external genitalia, the physician examines the internal female structures. To begin, a vaginal speculum is inserted into the vagina. The vaginal speculum may come in a variety of sizes and is made of either stainless steel (Fig. 36-8) or plastic (Fig. 36-9). Selecting an appropriately sized vaginal speculum is important to maintain the patient's comfort and to facilitate the examination. Although the patient's age and size are the primary factors, the largest speculum that is comfortable for the patient provides the best visibility. Two sizes may be set out to give the physician a choice. Vaginal specula come in pediatric, small, medium, and large sizes, and a variety of sizes should be available in each examination room.

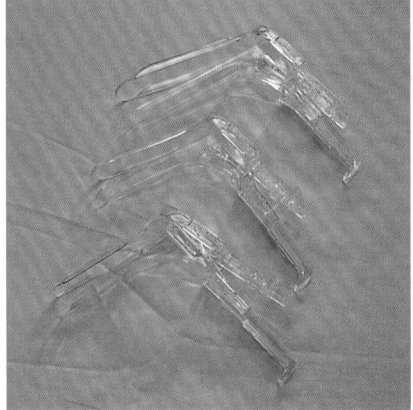

**Figure 36-9** • A variety of plastic, disposable vaginal specula. (From Weber J, Kelley J. *Health Assessment in Nursing*, 2nd ed. Philadelphia, PA: Lippincott Williams & Wilkins, 2003.)

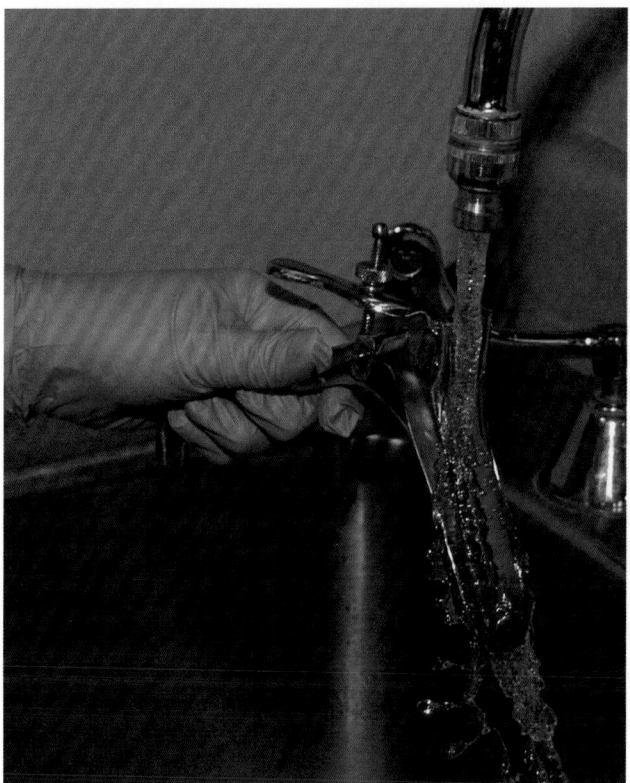

**Figure 36-10** • Warm the vaginal speculum with warm water.

In addition to having the correct size of vaginal speculum available for the physician, you should make sure the speculum is warmed for patient comfort. Warm the speculum by running it under warm water (Fig. 36-10) or by storing it on an electric heating pad set on a low setting. Some examination tables are equipped with a special warming drawer for the vaginal specula that heats them automatically as long as the examination table is plugged into an electrical outlet. Some physicians prefer that lubricant not be used on the speculum before insertion since it may interfere with obtaining the cells during the Pap smear. The water used to warm the speculum may serve as a lubricant for easier insertion. Always follow the instructions given by your physician to prepare the patient and the equipment and supplies for this examination.

Once the cervical cells are obtained, the physician will remove the vaginal speculum and perform a bimanual examination using gloved hands. During this part of the examination, the physician may want lubricant applied to gloved fingers for easier insertion into the vagina and rectum. Specifically, the physician will insert fingers into the vagina and the rectum to feel for the position and size of internal organs (Fig. 36-11). Your role during this part of the examination includes assisting the physician as necessary and supporting the patient. When this part of the examination is finished, you should assist the patient to a sitting position, prepare any specimens obtained for transport to the laboratory, and instruct the patient on the procedure for obtaining the results. You should also reinforce any instructions given by the physician before discharging the patient.

## WHAT IF?

**The first Pap smear or gynecologic examination for young women may cause great anxiety. What if an 18-year-old woman is to have her first Pap smear today? How should you handle the situation?**

Bring the patient into the room and encourage her to talk about her feelings. Do not have her change into an examining gown until she has had an opportunity to speak with the physician or practitioner about the procedure. The physician may require the presence of another health care worker, like the medical assistant, during the examination; however, some physicians feel comfortable performing the examination without assistance. If you remain in the room, you will have an opportunity to provide reassurance and information. Male physicians should have a female health care worker in the room during the examination as a legal precaution.

## Colposcopy

Colposcopy is visual examination of the vaginal and cervical surfaces using a stereoscopic microscope called a colposcope. It is often performed to evaluate patients with atypical Pap smear results to locate the origin of abnormal cells; to select areas for cervical, endocervical, or endometrial biopsy; to assess cervical lesions; or for follow-up in patients with a history of cervical dysplasia or cervical cancer.

If a biopsy is to be done, be sure that written consent has been obtained. When possible, label specimen containers and complete laboratory request forms before the procedure. Have the completed forms and labeled containers ready in the examination room for use after the specimen is obtained. Although there is usually very little or no bleeding from the biopsy, chemical cautery using silver nitrate or Monsel solution should be available to control bleeding as necessary. The patient preparation for colposcopy with cervical biopsy is similar to that required for the pelvic examination (Procedure 36-3).

## CHECKPOINT QUESTION

6. What procedures are normally included in the complete gynecologic examination?

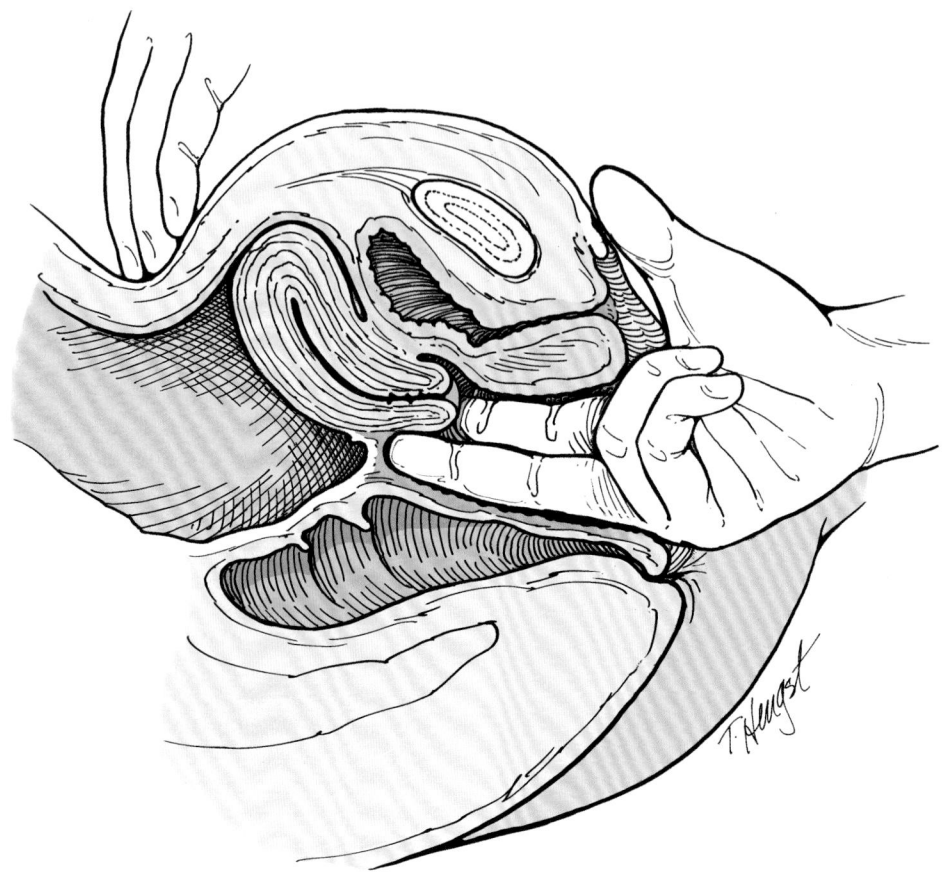

Figure 36-11 • The bimanual examination. (LifeART image copyright © 2008 Lippincott Williams & Wilkins. All rights reserved.)

## Hysterosalpingography

Hysterosalpingography is a diagnostic procedure in which the uterus and uterine tubes are radiographed after injection of a contrast medium. The radiograph is called a **hysterosalpingogram**. This test is often performed to determine the configuration of the uterus and the patency of the fallopian tubes for patients with infertility. Although this test is not usually performed in the physician's office, you may be responsible for scheduling the procedure and explaining to the patient any preparations including where to go and when the procedure will be performed.

## Dilation and Curettage

Dilation and **curettage** (D & C) may be performed to remove uterine tissue for diagnostic testing, to remove endometrial tissue, to prevent or treat **menorrhagia**, or to remove retained products of conception after a spontaneous **abortion** or miscarriage. During the procedure, the cervical canal is widened with a uterine sound, and the lining of the uterus is scraped with a curet (see Chapter 21 for a picture of a curet). This procedure usually requires anesthesia and may be performed as an inpatient or outpatient procedure. The patient must sign a preoperative consent form, and you may be asked to give any preoperative instructions as directed by the physician. Preoperative instructions may include advising

the patient of the need for a perineal pad, not a tampon, to be worn postoperatively and information regarding the signs of infection, hemorrhage, or other follow-up care according to the specifications of the physician.

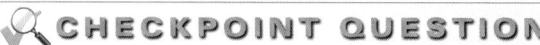

### CHECKPOINT QUESTION

7. Why would a hysterosalpingography be necessary?

## OBSTETRIC CARE

Unlike other physicians, obstetricians are frequently called to the hospital to deliver infants during regular office hours. In the absence of the physician, you must use good judgment when pregnant patients come into the office for a scheduled appointment or call with questions and concerns. For instance, you may have to determine whether a situation can wait for the physician's return, whether another physician should be consulted, whether the patient should go to the hospital, or whether, with the physician's permission, you should advise the patient how to manage the problem. Protocols listed in the policy and procedure manual for actions to be taken in specific situations help ensure that, in the physician's absence, safe procedures are followed for your patients and help protect you and your physician from errors in treatment.

## PATIENT EDUCATION

### Folic Acid Before and During Pregnancy

Women who are planning to get pregnant and those who are pregnant should take folic acid, a B vitamin to prevent neural tube defects. Although medical experts do not know how folic acid works, it is needed to make healthy new cells, like the ones that make up a baby's brain and spine. Taking folic acid every day, starting before and during pregnancy, can reduce the risk for these serious birth defects by 50% to 70%. Every woman who could possibly get pregnant should take 400 micrograms (400 mcg or 0.4 mg) of folic acid daily in a vitamin or in foods that have been enriched with folic acid. Many foods, including cereals, are enriched with folic acid. Encourage patients to check the label since some cereals provide 100% of the daily amount required.

## Diagnosis of Pregnancy

Many patients suspect that they are **gravid**, or pregnant, because they have signs; however, early signs of pregnancy may indicate other disorders and therefore are considered presumptive until a conclusive diagnostic procedure is done. Presumptive signs include amenorrhea, nausea, vomiting, breast enlargement and tenderness, fatigue, and urinary frequency. Probable signs include **human chorionic gonadotropin (HCG)** in the maternal urine or blood, changes in the uterus and cervix, **Braxton Hicks contractions**, and enlargement of the uterus (Table 36-3). Braxton Hicks contractions are irregular uterine contractions that occur fairly frequently but do not affect the cervix like the contractions of active labor. These contractions are normal, and although the patient may or may not be aware, the physician can feel the contractions during a bimanual examination or while palpating the abdomen. The diagnosis of pregnancy is confirmed by the physician or the image of a fetus on ultrasonography.

Cervical changes that occur during pregnancy include softening of the cervix, known as **Goodell sign**; increased vascularity of the cervix and vagina causing a bluish-violet color (**Chadwick sign**); and formation of a mucous plug. The mucous plug forms in the cervical os (opening) and protects the developing fetus and the amniotic sac from the external environment. With the onset of labor, the mucous plug is expelled with a small amount of blood and is often referred to as the bloody show.

## LEGAL TIP

### Fetal Protection

Many medications that might be considered beneficial to the pregnant female may be dangerous to the developing fetus. It is important, therefore, for the professional medical assistant to carefully question female patients who might be pregnant or who are known to be pregnant about any medications including drugs purchased over the counter. This information should be passed along to the physician. The U.S. Food and Drug Administration (FDA) has developed a method to classify drugs that are dangerous to the fetus. These categories are listed on package inserts that accompany prescription drugs and in various drug reference books such as the *Physician's Desk Reference*. The categories and a description of dangerous effects on the fetus are listed as follows:

- Category A: Research indicates that there is probably no risk at any point in the pregnancy.
- Category B: Animal research indicates no fetal risk, but human studies are not complete.
- Category C: Research on animals shows this drug to be a danger. Human studies are inconclusive, or no studies are available.
- Category D: There is clear precedence for risk, but the drug may be used if there is no substitution.
- Category X: There is clear evidence of risk, and the drug should not be used by pregnant women.

| TABLE 36-3 Signs and Symptoms of Pregnancy | | |
|---|---|---|
| **Presumptive Signs** | **Probable Signs** | **Conclusive Signs** |
| Cessation of menses | HCG in urine, blood | Fetal heart tone |
| Nausea and vomiting | Braxton Hicks contractions | Fetal movement detected by examiner |
| Breast tenderness | Enlargement of abdomen | Visualization of the fetus |
| Breast enlargement | Uterine changes | |
| Patient feels quickening or fetal movement | Goodell sign | |
| Fatigue | Chadwick sign | |
| Urinary frequency | | |

8. Why are presumptive signs and symptoms of pregnancy not considered to be conclusive?

## First Prenatal Visit

A pregnant patient's initial prenatal visit is extensive and critical to the ongoing assessment of the pregnancy. The first examination is done to establish a detailed baseline of the patient's physical condition and includes a confirmation of pregnancy, a complete history and physical, determination of the estimated date of delivery, assessment of gestational age, identification of risk factors, and patient education. To elicit complete and accurate information, the health history interview should be conducted in a private room where there will be no interruptions. This is a complete physical examination with a pelvic examination and screening for *N. gonorrhoeae*, chlamydial infection, cervical cancer, syphilis, and tuberculosis. The first prenatal visit also includes the following:

- Blood work: The Venereal Disease Research Laboratory, rapid plasma reagin, or other test for syphilis; complete blood count with hematocrit, hemoglobin, and white blood cell count with differential; and blood type with Rh factor. Blood for a rubella titer is also collected to determine maternal immunity to German measles, a disease that can result in serious birth defects if contracted during pregnancy.
- Tuberculosis screening: Tine test or purified protein derivative injection.
- Urinalysis: Glucose, albumin, and acetone testing.

The physical and pelvic examination will include laboratory tests such as the Pap smear, urine pregnancy test, clinical pelvimetry, and laboratory blood tests. Also, the estimated date of delivery will be calculated. This is a prediction of the due date, assuming the pregnancy progresses normally (Box 36-2). Normal gestation is 37 to 40 weeks. Infants born before the 37th week are considered to be premature. Those born after the 41st week are postmature.

Patients should be instructed to notify the physician if any of the following occurs:

- Vaginal bleeding or spotting
- Persistent vomiting
- Fever or chills
- Dysuria
- Abdominal or uterine cramping
- Leaking amniotic fluid
- Alteration in fetal movement
- Dizziness or blurred vision
- Other problems

In addition, advise the pregnant patient to avoid taking any medications or drugs, even over-the-counter preparations, without consulting the physician. Many factors, including medications, nicotine, and alcohol, can put the developing fetus at risk. Depending on maternal exposure to

---

**BOX 36-2    Determining the Estimated Date of Confinement or Expected Date of Delivery**

The estimated date of confinement (EDC) is also called the *expected date of delivery (EDD)*. Because of the negative connotations of the word "*confinement*" and because women are no longer confined during pregnancy or the postpartum period, terminology for the due date is changing to reflect current maternity trends. Many methods are used for determining this projected date. The Naegele rule requires an arithmetic calculation using the following formula:

The first day of the last menstrual period (LMP) −3 months + 7 days + 1 year

Example: LMP = May 3, 2007

| LMP = | 5 | 3 | 2007 |
|---|---|---|---|
| | −3 | +7 | +1 |
| Due date = | 2 | 10 | 2008 |

A simpler method is adding 9 months and 7 days to the first day of the LMP. Try that method with the example.

The third common method is to use a gestational wheel. Using the inner wheel, line up the first day of the LMP on the outer wheel with the appropriate arrow and read around the wheel to the indicated milestones in the pregnancy. Many wheels indicate the date of conception and times recommended for blood work and other testing, and all show the date that delivery is expected.

---

the substance and the stage of fetal development, development may be so altered as to cause deformities or damage to other internal organs and may threaten the life of the fetus.

### Parity versus Gravidity

You and the physician will obtain a thorough and detailed history of the patient, including information about previous pregnancies to help predict the outcome of this one. The term **parity** refers to the number of live births, and **gravidity** refers to any pregnancy, regardless of its length and outcome. The pregnant, or gravid, woman is a **gravida**, usually with an indicator of the number. A woman who has never been pregnant is a **nulligravida**, while the woman who is pregnant for the first time is a **primigravida**. The number of live births is also given a prefix indicator, such as **nullipara** (has never borne a living child), **primipara** (first living child), and **multipara** (many live births).

These numbers are listed for the physician's review as gr (or simply g), p, pret (preterm or premature), and ab (abortion, spontaneous or induced). For example, a woman who is pregnant for the third time, has lost no pregnancies, and carried her previous pregnancies to term is listed as gr iii, pret 0, ab 0, p ii. (Arabic numbers are also acceptable.) A woman who is pregnant for the fifth time and who has delivered one set of twins and two single infants, has had no premature infants, and has lost one pregnancy spontaneously would be listed as gr v, pret 0, ab i, p iv.

## Subsequent Prenatal Visits

If the pregnancy is progressing as expected and without complications (Fig. 36-12), then the patient is scheduled for office visits monthly at 4, 8, 12, 16, 20, 24, and

---

### FETAL DEVELOPMENT*

#### 1st Lunar Month (4 weeks)

The embryo is 4 to 5 mm in length.
Trophoblasts embed in decidua.
Chorionic villi form.
Foundations for nervous system, genitourinary system, skin, bones, and lungs are formed.
Buds of arms and legs begin to form.
Rudiments of eyes, ears, and nose appear.

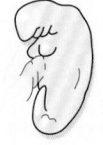

#### 2nd Lunar Month (8 weeks)

The fetus is 27 to 31 mm in length and weighs 2 to 4 g
Fetus is markedly bent.
Head is disproportionately large as a result of brain development.
Sex differentiation begins.
Centers of bone begin to ossify.

#### 3rd Lunar Month (3 months)

The fetus' average length is 6 to 9 cm, and weight is 45 g.
Fingers and toes are distinct.
Placenta is complete.
Fetal circulation is complete.

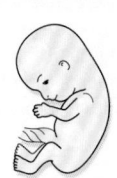

#### 4th Lunar Month (4 months)

The fetus is 12 cm in length and weighs 110 g.
Sex is differentiated.
Rudimentary kidneys secrete urine.
Heartbeat is present.
Nasal septum and palate close.

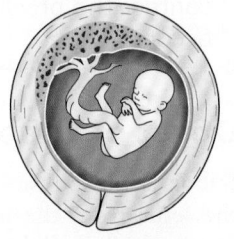

#### 5th Lunar Month (5 months)

The fetus is 19 cm in length and weighs approximately 300 g.
Lanugo covers entire body.
Fetal movements are felt by mother.
Heart sounds are perceptible by auscultation.

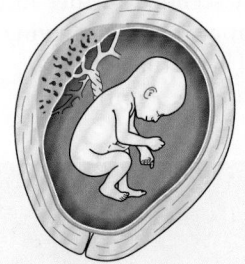

#### 6th Lunar Month (6 months)

The fetus is about 23 cm in length and weighs 630 g.
Skin appears wrinkled.
Vernix caseosa appears.
Eyebrows and fingernails develop.

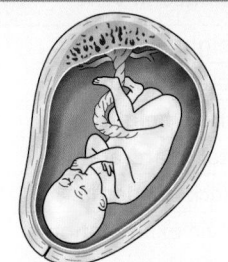

#### 7th Lunar Month (7 months)

The fetus is about 27 cm in length and weighs about 1100 g.
Skin is red.
Pupillary membrane disappears from eyes.
The fetus has an excellent chance of survival.

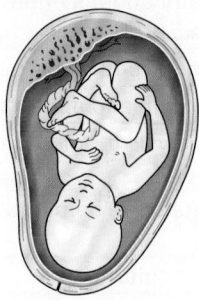

#### 8th Lunar Month (8 months)

The fetus is 28 to 30 cm in length and weighs 1.8 kg.
Fetus is viable.
Eyelids open.
Fingerprints are set.
Vigorous fetal movement occurs.

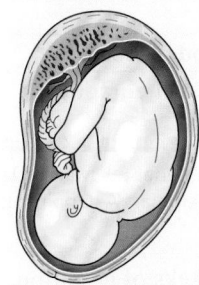

#### 9th Lunar Month (9 months)

The fetus' average length is 32 cm; weight is about 2500 g.
Face and body have a loose wrinkled appearance because of subcutaneous fat deposit.
Lanugo disappears.
Amniotic fluid decreases.

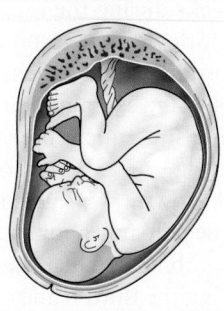

#### 10th Lunar Month

The average fetus is 36 cm in length and weighs 3000 to 3600 g.
Skin is smooth.
Eyes are uniformly slate colored.
Bones of skull are ossified and nearly together at sutures.

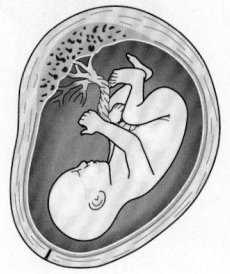

* All lengths given are crown to rump.

**Figure 36-12 •** Fetal development.

| TABLE 36-4 | Schedule of Prenatal Visits |
| --- | --- |
| **Month** | **Frequency** |
| 1–6 | Monthly |
| 7–8 | Every 2 weeks |
| 9 | Weekly |
| **Included in Visit** | **When Done** |
| Weight | Each visit |
| Blood pressure | Each visit |
| Fundal height | Each visit |
| Fetal heart rate | Each visit |
| Check of edema | Each visit |
| Pelvic examination | First visit, middle of ninth month, weekly as indicated |
| Inquiry about symptoms, signs, problems | Each visit |
| Prenatal education | Each visit |
| Nutrition and appetite | Each visit |
| Urinalysis for glucose, albumin | Each visit |
| Hematocrit, hemoglobin | First visit, at 32–34 weeks (more often for anemia) |
| Urine culture | Per signs, symptoms |
| Rh titer | First visit |
| AFP | 15–20 weeks |
| Blood glucose | First visit, 24–28 weeks |
| Ultrasonography | For fetal age, best 8–16 weeks |

From Reeder SJ, Martin LL, Koniak D. *Maternity Nursing*, 17th ed. Philadelphia, PA: Lippincott Williams & Wilkins, 1992:403.

28 weeks of gestation. The patient is usually seen every 2 weeks during the last 2 months and once a week after the 36th week of gestation. This schedule may be altered according to the patient's condition. Table 36-4 outlines the specific examination and procedures to be performed during subsequent prenatal visits. The height of the fundus (Fig. 36-13 ) is also palpated at each visit to assess fetal growth. Typically, the top of the uterus, the fundus, can be palpated at or slightly above the level of the maternal umbilicus when the fetus is at 5 months' gestation. During the third trimester, the abdomen will be palpated to determine fetal presentation and position, which are important details for a normal vaginal delivery.

The fetal heart tones (FHT) will also be recorded at the subsequent prenatal visits. Around the 10th week of gestation, the fetal heart rate can be heard with the aid of a Doppler device (Fig. 36-14 ), and after the 20th week, a fetoscope can be used. The fetoscope is a special nonelectronic stethoscope (Fig. 36-15 ). The fetal heart tones should fall within a range of 120 to 160 beats per minute.

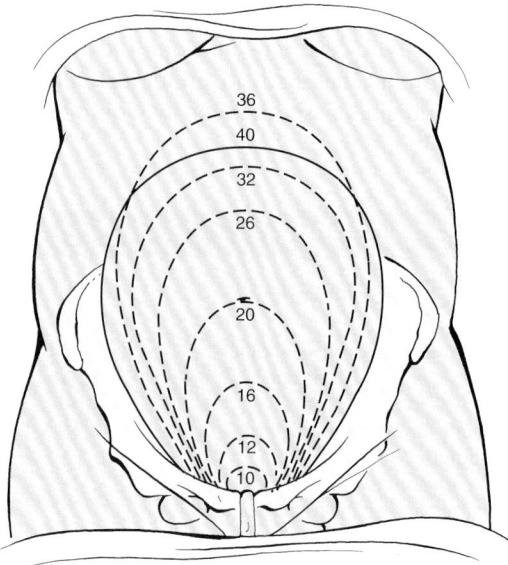

**Figure 36-13** • Height of the fundus at corresponding gestational dates varies greatly from patient to patient. Those shown are most common. A convenient rule of thumb is that at 5 months of gestation, the fundus is usually at or slightly above the umbilicus. (Reprinted from Weber J. *Health Assessment in Nursing*. Philadelphia, PA: Lippincott Williams & Wilkins, 2003, with permission.)

## CHECKPOINT QUESTION

9. The pregnant patient should be advised to contact the physician when what problems occur?

## Onset of Labor

Labor is the physiologic process leading to expelling the fetus from the uterus. About 4 weeks before the onset of labor, **lightening** indicates that the fetus has descended further into the pelvis, and the patient may appear to be carrying the baby lower in the abdomen. The actual onset of labor is characterized by regular uterine contractions that become more intense and

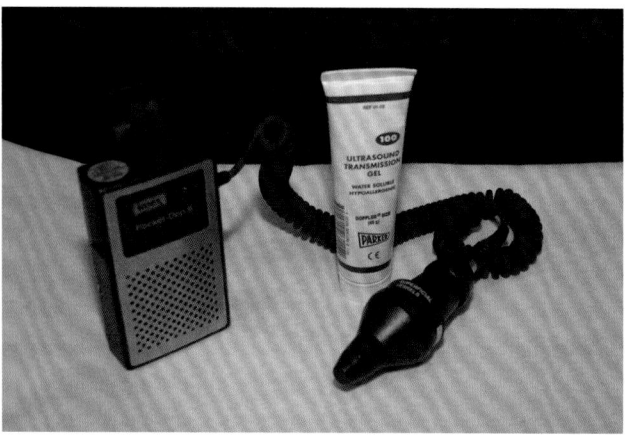

**Figure 36-14** • An electronic Doppler used to assess fetal heart tones before the 20th gestational week.

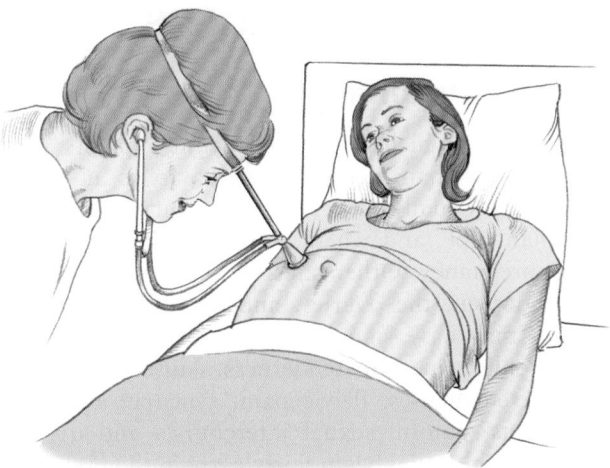

**Figure 36-15** • A fetoscope. (From *Nursing Procedures*, 4th ed. Ambler, PA: Lippincott Williams & Wilkins, 2004.)

more frequent with time. True labor is distinguished from false labor by its effect (dilation and effacement) on the cervix and the increased frequency and intensity of contractions. Another indication of true labor is bloody show, the expulsion of the mucous plug from the cervical os. The patient may call to say her water broke, which indicates rupture of the amniotic sac, another indication of impending labor and delivery.

Whatever signs or symptoms of labor occur, you should know how to advise the patient. The physician makes the decision to send the patient to the hospital, to come to the medical office, or to stay home and wait. You relay the information from the patient to the physician. The office's policy and procedure manual should include specific instructions regarding how the physician wants pregnant patients managed if the physician is not immediately available.

The onset of labor should be discussed with the patient so she knows what to expect and how to manage the situation. Always have the patient's medical record available when talking with the patient or the physician. It is critical to the decision-making process to know the patient's estimated date of delivery and physical condition. Many patients today are choosing options for delivery other than a standard hospital delivery with the physician present. Options include midwife assistance, a birthing center, water birth, and home delivery. The patient must be informed about the advantages and risks of all of these and, together with the physician, make a decision that takes into account the well-being of the mother and the newborn.

## Cesarean Section

Sometimes, a normal vaginal delivery is not possible or advisable, such as in the following situations:

- Cephalopelvic disproportion: the baby's head is too large for the birth canal.
- Placenta previa.

- Poor presentation other than an occipital presentation, such as transverse (the baby lying across the cervix) or breech (a buttocks first presentation).
- Failure to progress: inefficient labor or the cervix will not dilate.
- Infant or maternal distress

In these situations, the infant is delivered by cesarean section. An incision is made through the abdominal wall into the uterus, and the infant is removed. It was once believed that women who had delivered by cesarean section should not be allowed to deliver vaginally because it was feared that the uterine scar might rupture. Current surgical techniques have lessened that fear, and many women now deliver vaginally after a cesarean delivery.

## Postpartum Care

The postpartum period, the **puerperium**, runs from childbirth until involution, when the reproductive structures return to normal. It may take as long as 6 weeks. Once the patient is discharged from the hospital, her care will be managed at the medical office. Hospital reports received in the medical office for the patient's record usually contain certain acronyms and abbreviations related to labor and delivery and the postpartum period. Box 36-3 explains these special terms.

The time for the first postpartum visit depends on the type of delivery and the patient's condition when discharged from the hospital. The needs of postpartum

---

**BOX 36-3  Acronyms and Abbreviations Used in Labor and Delivery and the Postpartum Period**

Following is a brief list of terms frequently used in the medical record:

| | |
|---|---|
| AROM | Artificial rupture of membranes |
| AVD | Assisted vaginal delivery |
| CPD | Cephalopelvic disproportion |
| L & D | Labor and delivery |
| NSVD | Normal spontaneous vaginal delivery |
| PROM | Premature rupture of membranes |
| SROM | Spontaneous rupture of membranes |
| VBAC | Vaginal birth after cesarean |

*Terms for Presentations*

| | |
|---|---|
| LOA | Left occiput anterior |
| LOP | Left occiput posterior |
| ROA | Right occiput anterior |
| ROP | Right occiput posterior |

*Fetal Descriptors*

| | |
|---|---|
| AGA | Appropriate for gestational age |
| LBW | Low birth weight |
| LGA | Large for gestational age |
| SGA | Small for gestational age |

patients today may be greater than in the past because the length of stay in the hospital is typically shorter, with some patients discharged within 24 hours after delivery. Usually, the patient is scheduled for the postnatal visit within 4 to 6 weeks of delivery if there were no complications.

At the postpartum visit, the physician performs a complete gynecologic and breast examination. Allow plenty of time for counseling the patient regarding her new role as a parent. Many patients have questions and concerns regarding breastfeeding, birth control, menstruation, and parenting. Before the examination, obtain the patient's weight and vital signs and samples for urinalysis and possibly hematocrit and hemoglobin. During the examination, the physician assesses any uterine discharge. **Lochia**, a discharge from the uterus after delivery, progresses through the following stages:

- *Lochia rubra*: Blood-tinged discharge within 6 days of delivery
- *Lochia serosa*: Thin, brownish discharge lasting about 3 to 4 days after the lochia rubra
- *Lochia alba*: White postpartum discharge that has no evidence of blood and may last up to week 6

The amount of lochia should diminish considerably during the puerperium. The patient should be instructed to notify the physician if there is any abnormality of the lochial progression.

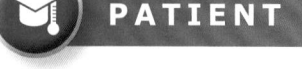 **CHECKPOINT QUESTION**

10. What is lochia? Name and describe the three types.

---

### PATIENT EDUCATION

#### Kegel Exercises

The patient's age, gravidity, and past childbearing take their toll on the muscles of the perineum. Kegel exercises can increase the tone of this area. Stronger perineal support helps eliminate stress incontinence and supports the vaginal walls to avoid uterine prolapse.

These exercises should be performed three times every day for 5 minutes each time. In addition, the exercises should be done in three positions: lying down, sitting, and standing. Explain to the patient that she can do Kegel exercises at any time, such as when standing in the grocery line, waiting at a stop light, or sitting in class. Essentially, the exercises involve tightening the pelvic muscles as if stopping the flow of urine. Advise the patient not to tighten the stomach, legs, or other muscles. Also, most patients do not feel bladder control results for 3 to 6 weeks.

## OBSTETRIC DISORDERS

### Ectopic Pregnancy

Gestation in which a fertilized ovum implants somewhere other than in the uterine cavity is an ectopic pregnancy. Usually, an ectopic pregnancy occurs in the fallopian tube, and when it does, it may be called a tubal pregnancy. Other sites of implantation include the abdomen, the ovaries, and the cervical os. The patient may have signs of early pregnancy, including breast enlargement or tenderness, nausea, and absent or delayed menses. Pelvic pain, syncope, abdominal symptoms, painful sexual intercourse, and irregular menstrual bleeding begin fairly early in the pregnancy. If an ectopic pregnancy is not diagnosed early, there is the potential for rupture of the fallopian tube, which causes hemorrhage into the abdominal cavity and the possibility of shock and death. Diagnostic procedures include urine or serum human chorionic gonadotropin pregnancy test, ultrasound to determine the location of the pregnancy, laparoscopy to visualize the enlarged tube, and perhaps culdocentesis to confirm abdominal bleeding. Treatment is surgical excision of the ectopic pregnancy through either a laparoscopy or laparotomy.

### Hyperemesis Gravidarum

Nausea and vomiting, commonly called morning sickness, are expected during early pregnancy and usually can be treated with small frequent meals, adequate hydration, and reassurance. However, if the vomiting becomes unrelenting and leads to dehydration, electrolyte imbalance, and weight loss, the diagnosis is hyperemesis gravidarum. Occasionally, the patient must be hospitalized. At early prenatal visits, you may have to discern between morning sickness and the more serious hyperemesis gravidarum by obtaining a complete description of the nausea and vomiting. Of course, the physician makes the diagnosis and orders appropriate treatment, including antiemetics or intravenous fluids if necessary.

### Abortion

One of the common disorders of pregnancy is first-trimester spontaneous abortion, also called an early pregnancy loss or miscarriage. With early diagnosis of pregnancy, it is now known whether the spontaneous abortion occurs more often than previously thought. An induced abortion is intentional, whereas a spontaneous abortion occurs because of fetal or maternal conditions without any outside interference in the pregnancy.

A spontaneous abortion is defined as the loss of pregnancy before the fetus is viable. You need to be familiar with the early signs and symptoms of an impending spontaneous abortion to advise a patient who calls until the physician can be contacted. The first symptom is usually vaginal bleeding, followed by uterine cramps and low back pain. Without telling the patient that she may be in danger of spontaneously aborting her pregnancy (this is diagnosing), you may instruct the patient to come to the medical office, go to the emergency room, or remain at home on bedrest until the physician returns the call, depending on the office policy and procedure.

## CHECKPOINT QUESTION

11. Where is the most common site of implantation for an ectopic pregnancy?

## Preeclampsia and Eclampsia

Hypertension that is directly related to the pregnancy is termed pregnancy-induced hypertension (PIH). The two types of PIH are preeclampsia and eclampsia. Preeclampsia is characterized by **proteinuria**, edema of the lower extremities, and hypertension after the 20th week of gestation. As the condition progresses, the patient may complain of blurred vision, headaches, edema, and vomiting. Medical management includes restricted activities, increased bedrest, sexual abstinence, antihypertensive therapy, and well-balanced meals with an increase in protein and a decrease in sodium. Close monitoring of the patient is important, and it requires scheduling the patient for more frequent office visits. The risk of developing eclampsia increases as the pregnancy advances.

Eclampsia is almost always preceded by preeclampsia but has a sudden onset. In eclampsia, the clinical signs of preeclampsia are still present but become more extreme. Eclampsia is always characterized by seizures that may be followed by coma, hypertensive crisis, and shock. The progression of preeclampsia to eclampsia constitutes a medical emergency. Management of eclampsia includes stabilizing the patient and may require induced delivery of the baby, regardless of gestational age.

## Placenta Previa and Abruptio Placentae

Placenta previa is a condition in which the placenta is implanted either partially or completely over the internal cervical os, making delivery of the fetus before the placenta difficult. During the second or third trimester of pregnancy, the patient may have painless vaginal bleeding, which may be minimal, such as spotting, or profuse. Placenta previa is easily diagnosed by prenatal ultrasound. Medical management includes bedrest and drug therapy if the patient is preterm. If the patient is near term and if the bleeding is severe and poses a danger to the mother or fetus, then delivery of the baby is essential, usually by cesarean.

The premature separation or detachment of the placenta from the uterus is abruptio placentae. Depending on the severity of the separation, symptoms include pain, uterine tenderness, bleeding, signs of impending shock, and fetal distress or death. If abruptio placentae is confirmed, the baby is usually delivered by cesarean section.

## CHECKPOINT QUESTION

12. What is placenta previa, and how is it managed in a preterm patient?

# COMMON OBSTETRIC TESTS AND PROCEDURES

## Pregnancy Tests

Many over-the-counter pregnancy tests check for HCG in the urine. Chapter 44 has more information about urine pregnancy tests.

## Alpha-Fetoprotein

Blood levels of alpha-fetoprotein (AFP) are obtained from maternal serum to screen the fetus for defects in the neural tube, a part of the fetus that develops into the brain and spinal cord. The test is performed at 16 to 18 weeks of gestation and is used for screening purposes. Elevated AFP levels may indicate nervous system deformities, including spina bifida, but falsely elevated tests can be caused by more than one fetus or incorrect gestational dates. AFP results that are below the normal range may indicate Down syndrome in the developing fetus. Abnormal results indicate the need for further studies, including **amniocentesis** and fetal ultrasound.

Amniocentesis is insertion of a needle through the abdomen and into the gravid uterus to remove fluid from the amniotic sac. This fluid is analyzed for a variety of nervous system disorders. It can also be used to diagnose genetic problems, estimate gestational age, or assess lung maturity of the fetus. It may be performed in the office, and if so, you are responsible for preparing the patient, assisting the physician, preparing the specimen for transportation to the laboratory, and giving the patient any postprocedural instructions from the physician.

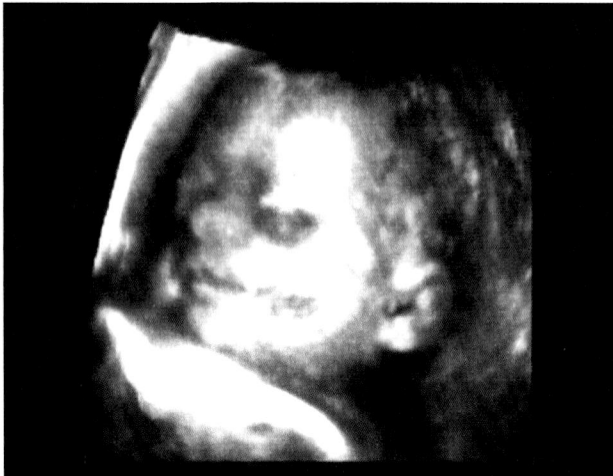

**Figure 36-16 •** A 3-D fetal ultrasound image showing clear details of facial and other physical features.

## Fetal Ultrasonography

An ultrasound of the fetus is performed using high-frequency sound waves to create an image of internal structures. Fetal ultrasound is performed to assess the size, gestational age, position, and number of fetuses as well as fetal structures and development (Fig. 36-16). Some abnormal maternal and fetal conditions, such as ectopic pregnancy, placenta previa, neural tube defects, and cardiac defects, may be diagnosed by ultrasound. The gender of the fetus may also be determined, although this is not typically a justification for performing an ultrasound. Although some obstetric offices have a sonographer on staff, fetal ultrasounds may have to be scheduled in an outpatient facility.

## Contraction Stress Test and Nonstress Test

A contraction stress test (CST) is performed in the third trimester to determine how the fetus will tolerate uterine contractions. Uterine contractions may be induced by the woman stimulating her nipples, known as the nipple-stimulating CST, or the contractions can be induced by the administration of oxytocin, called an oxytocin-stimulated CST. In both tests, the fetal heart tones and movement are monitored in relation to the uterine contractions. Although the contractions are meant to be temporary, the CST is usually performed in the hospital in case continued contractions and delivery occur.

The nonstress test (NST) is a noninvasive obstetric procedure used to evaluate the fetal heart tones and movement in relation to spontaneous uterine contractions. The NST may be safely performed in the medical office, whereas the CST is usually performed in the hospital setting.

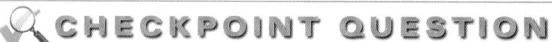

## CHECKPOINT QUESTION

13. In what instances might a fetal ultrasonography be ordered by the physician?

## CONTRACEPTION

Numerous methods of contraception (birth control) are available (Table 36-5). The decision to practice contraception and the selection of an appropriate method involves many factors, including the patient's religious, cultural, and personal beliefs. In addition, the health history, financial situation, and motivation of the patient may be important considerations for the patient, the spouse or partner, and the physician. To reinforce the physician's advice and instructions, you should understand the various methods, including the indications, risk factors, cost, and effectiveness. Both you and the physician should be prepared to educate and advise the patient regarding the choice of contraception.

## MENOPAUSE

Menopause, also called the climacteric period, is the stage of life during which ovulation ceases because of decreasing ovarian function. This period, characterized by the cessation of the menstrual cycle, usually occurs around 45 to 50 years of age. Changes in the menstrual cycle in early menopause include **oligomenorrhea**, amenorrhea, dysfunctional uterine bleeding, and hot flashes, flushing, or perspiration.

The use of supplemental estrogen, or hormonal replacement therapy (HRT), was prescribed a few years ago to relieve menopausal symptoms such as hot flashes and depression and was believed to also protect against cardiovascular and skeletal disorders. However, in 2002, a research study was published that revealed elevated health risks for women who took hormone replacement therapy. As a result, fewer women today are taking HRT, and most physicians only recommend these medications for women with severe symptoms of menopause. For women with only minor menopausal symptoms, weight-bearing exercises, a healthy diet, and vitamin and mineral supplements have eased the transition through the menopausal stage without the use of hormone replacement medications. In either case, women in this stage of life should continue to have regular pelvic examinations, Pap smears, breast examinations, and mammograms and should speak with the physician about any questions or concerns.

| TABLE 36-5 | Main Methods of Contraception | | |
|---|---|---|---|
| **Method** | **Description** | **Advantages** | **Disadvantages** |
| **Surgical** Vasectomy, tubal | Tubes carrying gametes cut | Nearly 100% effective; no chemical or mechanical devices | Not easily reversible; rare surgical complications |
| **Hormonal** Pill | Oral estrogen or progesterone to prevent ovulation | Highly effective; requires no last-minute preparation | Alters physiology; serious side effects possible |
| Injection | Inject synthetic progesterone every 3 months to prevent ovulation | Highly effective; lasts 3–4 months | Alters physiology; possible side effects are menstrual irregularity and amenorrhea. Expensive |
| Patch | Patch with progesterone and estrogen worn on skin 3 out of 4 weeks to prevent ovulation | Use is simple; does not require pill or injection | Should be replaced same day of week; pregnancy can occur if patch off for more than 24 hours or left on more than 1 week |
| Ring | Small, flexible ring in vagina releases synthetic progesterone and estrogen to prevent pregnancy for 1 month | Does not require pill or injection; does not interfere with sexual intercourse | Side effects may include bleeding between periods, breast tenderness, and other symptoms associated with hormone therapy |
| IUD | T-shaped plastic device with copper or progesterone | Spontaneous sexual intercourse | Heavy or long menstrual periods; cramping during and after insertion; periodic check for placement by feeling for string |
| **Barrier** Male condom | Sheath fits over erect penis, contains ejaculate | Easily available; does not affect physiology; protects from STDs | Must be applied before intercourse; may slip or tear |
| Female condom | Sheath that fits into vagina, held in place with rings | Easily available; protects from STDs | More expensive than male condom; must be inserted before intercourse |
| Diaphragm | Rubber cap fits over cervix; prevents entrance of sperm | Does not affect physiology; some protection from STDs | Must be inserted before intercourse; requires fitting by physician |
| **Other** Spermicide | Chemical to kill sperm; best used with a barrier method | Easily available; does not affect physiology; some protection from STDs | Local irritation; must be used just before intercourse |
| Fertility awareness | Abstinence while fertile per menstrual history, basal temperature, quality of cervical mucus | Does not affect physiology; accepted by certain religions | High failure rate; requires careful record keeping |
| Emergency contraception | Morning-after pill reduces risk of pregnancy up to 120 hours after unprotected sexual intercourse | May prevent pregnancy after unprotected sexual intercourse | Nausea, vomiting; no protection from STDs; may not prevent ectopic pregnancy; the closer to ovulation, the greater the chance of pregnancy |

Adapted from Cohen BJ. *Memmler's The Human Body in Health and Disease*, 11th ed. Baltimore, MD: Lippincott Williams & Wilkins, 2009.

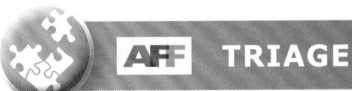

While you are working in a gynecology medical office, the following three situations arise:

A. Patient A calls wanting information about the vaginal ring contraception.
B. Patient B is pregnant, and this is the first prenatal visit.
C. Patient C has been seen by the physician and needs to have a hysterosalpingography scheduled at the outpatient ambulatory center.

**How do you sort these situations? What do you do first? Second? Third?**

First, have the receptionist take a message from patient A and call her back later. This is clearly not an emergency, and you can call her back at a more convenient time. Next, you should discharge patient C, letting her know that you will schedule the outpatient procedure later today and call her with the details tomorrow. Finally, call patient B to the examination room and take a thorough medical history and vital signs. Since patient B is new, she may require additional time and reassurance. She may also have questions and concerns about her pregnancy, and you do not want to be rushed during the patient education part of this initial visit.

## MEDICATION BOX

### Commonly Prescribed Female Reproductive System Medications

**Note:** *The generic name of the drug is listed first and is written in all lowercase letters. Brand names are in parentheses, and the first letter is capitalized.*

| | | |
|---|---|---|
| acyclovir (Zovirax) | Capsules: 200 mg<br>Suspension: 200 mg/5 mL<br>Tablets: 400 mg, 800 mg | Antiviral |
| citalopram hydrobromide (Celexa) | Tablets: 10 mg, 20 mg, 40 mg | Antidepressant |
| clomiphene citrate (Clomid, Milophene) | Tablets: 50 mg | Fertility |
| clindamycin phosphate (Cleocin, Clindesse) | Vaginal cream: 2%<br>Vaginal suppositories: 100 mg | Antibiotic |
| doxycycline hyclate (Atridox, Doryx, Vibramycin) | Capsules: 50 mg, 100 mg<br>Tablets: 20 mg, 100 mg | Antibiotic |
| drospirenone and ethinyl estradiol (YAZ) | Tablets (Yasmin): 3 mg drospirenone and 0.03 mg ethinyl estradiol as 21 yellow tablets and 7 white (inert) | Contraception |
| | Tablets (YAZ): 3 mg drospirenone and 0.02 mg ethinyl estradiol as 24 light pink tablets and 4 white (inert) | |
| escitalopram oxalate (Lexapro) | Tablets: 5 mg, 10 mg, 20 mg | Antidepressant |
| estradiol (Estrace, tablets) (Climara, patches) | Tablets: 0.5 mg, 1 mg, 1.5 mg, 2 mg<br>Transdermal: 0.014 mg/24 hours to 0.075 mg/24 hours | Hormone replacement |
| estrogen, conjugated (Premarin) | Injection: 25 mg/5 mL<br>Tablets: 0.3 mg, 0.45 mg, 0.625 mg | Hormone |
| etonogestrel and ethinyl estradiol (NuvaRing) | Vaginal ring: delivers 0.12 mg etonogestrel and 0.015 mg ethinyl estradiol daily | Contraception |
| fluoxetine hydrochloride (Prozac, Sarafem) | Capsules: 90 mg (delayed release)<br>Capsules: 10 mg, 20 mg, 40 mg<br>Tablets: 10 mg, 15 mg, 20 mg | Antidepressant |

## MEDICATION BOX (continued)

| | | |
|---|---|---|
| human papillomavirus recombinant vaccine (Gardasil) | Injection: 0.5 mL single-dose vial | Vaccine |
| imiquimod (Aldara) | Cream: 5% single-use packets, containing 12.5 mg | Immune response modifier |
| medroxyprogesterone acetate (Depo-Provera) | Injection: 104 mg/0.65 mL,150 mg/mL, 400 mg/mL | Contraceptive |
| paroxetine hydrochloride (Paxil) | Tablets: 10 mg, 20 mg, 30 mg, 40 mg | Antidepressant |
| valacyclovir hydrochloride (Valtrex) | Tablets: 500 mg, 1,000 mg | Antiviral |

## ROLE-PLAYING ACTIVITY

While working in the OB/GYN specialty office at Great Falls Medical Center, Sarah Appleton, RMA, assisted with a 16-year-old female patient who is approximately 7 weeks pregnant. The patient states that she is no longer "in a relationship" with the father and that her parents do not know about the pregnancy. She also indicates she attends high school full time and does not work. Role-play this activity as the medical assistant and think about the possible patient education that might be necessary for this patient to have a healthy pregnancy. What kinds of community resources might you be able to offer her, if needed? If you are playing the role of the patient, think about how you might feel and what assistance you might need if you were in this situation. Would you feel alone? Scared? Your instructor will give you additional information about this activity!

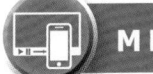

## MEDIA MENU

**Student Resources** on thePoint®
- **CMA/RMA Certification Exam Review**
- **English to Spanish Audio Glossary**

**Internet Resources**
**American College of Obstetricians and Gynecologists**
http://www.acog.org
**Center for Disease Control and Prevention, STDs**
http://www.cdc.gov/std/general
**American Social Health Association**
http://www.ashastd.org/sitemap.cfm
**American Fertility Association**
http://www.theafa.org
**American Cancer Society**
http://www.cancer.org
**National Women's Health Information Center**
http://www.womenshealth.gov

## español SPANISH TERMINOLOGY

**¿Cuál fue el primer día de su último periodo menstrual?**
When was the first day of your last menstrual period?

**¿Usa algún método anticonceptivo?**
Do you use a contraceptive device?

**¿Cuándo fue su última mamografía?**
When was your last mammogram?

**¿Ha alcanzado la menopausia?**
Have you gone through menopause?

**¿Cuando fué su último Papanicolau?**
When was your last Papanicolaou?

**¿Tiene vida sexual activa?**
Are you sexually active?

**¿Cuantas veces se ha embarazado?**
How many times you have been pregnant?

**DIU significa Dispositivo Intrauterino**
IUD means Intrauterine Device.

**¿Siente que se mueve su bebe?**
Do you feel the baby's movements?

**¿A qué edad tuvo su primera menstruación?**
How old were you when you had your first period?

# EMR Activity

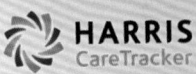

Harris CareTracker is a Web-based electronic medical record (EMR) application that you will use for the EMR activities included in this section at the end of each chapter. This application is actually used in physician offices but is provided to you through the publisher, Wolters Kluwer Health, to give you hands-on practice working with EMRs. Your instructor will have more information about accessing your username, log-in, and Quickstart guide.

Prerequisite Activities in Harris CareTracker

- *The Getting Started and Quickstart documents and EMR Activities Step-by-Step Instructions are available at* http://thePoint.lww.com/KronenbergerComp5e.

Activity Details

Patient Linda Bankston was seen by Dr. Dunn yesterday, for her annual checkup and birth control renewal. She phoned the office today and spoke to Sarah Appleton, RMA, stating that she forgot to get the prescription before she left yesterday. Using the *Rx Renewals* feature in the *Clinical Today* tab, document the LO Loestrin FE 1mg/10mcg as ordered by Dr. Dunn in the patient's EMR. Dr. Dunn authorized enough refills for 1 year

## Chapter Summary

- Assisting in obstetrics and gynecology is a challenging and fascinating area of medicine. This chapter:
- Describes the examination of the female reproductive system
- Explains your role in assisting the patient and the physician in the examination of the female reproductive system
- Describes a variety of disorders related to the female reproductive system
- Discusses normal physiologic functions such as menarche and menopause
- Addresses the care of the pregnant patient including disorders or conditions sometimes seen in pregnancy
- As a professional medical assistant, you will be responsible for:
- Providing reassurance and emotional support to the gynecologic patient
- Assisting the physician during the gynecologic exam if needed
- Processing any specimens for the laboratory using standard precautions
- Maintaining the examination room, equipment, and supplies

## Warm-Ups for Critical Thinking

1. A multiparous patient who is married and has a history of cigarette smoking desires a highly effective method of contraception. What are her best choices for contraception? Explain which choice is best and why.
2. Your patient has both genital herpes and condylomata acuminata. She wants to know whether these disorders are contagious and how they can be cured. How do you respond to these questions?
3. Research the effects of maternal exposure to alcohol, tobacco, and nicotine, and prepare a poster describing your findings that could be used to educate pregnant women and those considering pregnancy.
4. In addition to the contraceptives listed in this chapter, list the contraceptives available today, including the advantages and risks associated with each.
5. Using a drug reference book, research some of the newer drugs on the market to treat and/or prevent osteoporosis that may occur after menopause. What are the side effects of these medications?
6. Prepare a patient education poster for your medical office about breast cancer awareness.

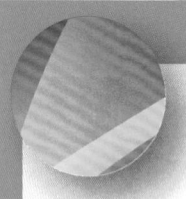

**PSY** PROCEDURE 36-1

## Instructing the Patient on the Breast Self-Examination

**AFF** Instruct and prepare a patient for a procedure or treatment; coach patients regarding disease prevention and treatment plans; coach patients appropriately considering cultural diversity, developmental life stage, and communication barriers; document patient care accurately in the medical record.

**Purpose:** Properly instruct the female patient on the procedure for performing a breast self-examination

**Equipment:** Patient education instruction sheet if available; breast examination model if available

| STEPS | PURPOSE |
|---|---|
| 1. Wash your hands. | Hand washing aids infection control. |
| 2. Explain the purpose and frequency of examining the breasts. | The purpose is to check for lumps, dimples, and thickened areas that can indicate malignancy and allow for early diagnosis and treatment. The patient should be encouraged to examine her breasts at the same time each month, about a week after the menstrual cycle. |
| 3. Describe the three positions necessary for the patient to examine the breasts: in front of a mirror, in the shower, and lying down. | Inspecting and palpating the breasts in a variety of positions allows for a thorough examination of all breast tissue. |
| 4. Explain that she should disrobe and inspect the breasts in front of a mirror with her hands on her hips and with her arms raised above her head. Advise the patient to look for any changes in contour, swelling, dimpling of the skin, or changes in the nipple. | Regular inspection shows what is normal and gives the patient confidence for the examination. |

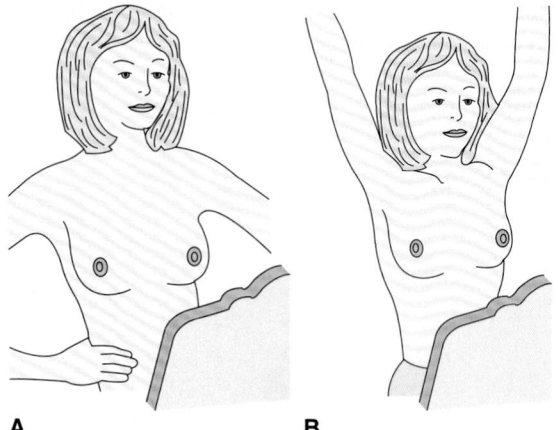

A    B

**Step 4** (**A**) Inspect both breasts in front of a mirror with the hands on the hips.
(**B**) Inspect both breasts with the arms raised over the head. (Reprinted from Pillitteri A. *Maternal and Child Health Nursing*. Philadelphia, PA: Lippincott Williams & Wilkins, 2007, with permission.)

| | |
|---|---|
| 5. In the shower, the patient should feel each breast with her hands over wet skin, using the flat part of the first three fingers. Instruct her to use her right hand to lightly press over all areas of her left breast and her left hand to examine her right breast, checking for any lumps, hard knots, or thickenings. | Palpating the breasts in the shower allows the hands to glide more easily over wet skin. |

## PROCEDURE 36-1 (continued)

| STEPS | PURPOSE |
|---|---|

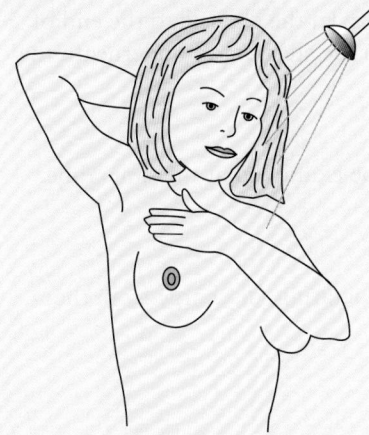

**Step 5.** Examine the breasts in the shower. (Reprinted from Pillitteri A. *Maternal and Child Health Nursing*. Philadelphia, PA: Lippincott Williams & Wilkins, 2007, with permission.)

6. After showering, the patient should lie down and examine her right breast after placing a pillow or folded towel under her right shoulder and placing her right hand behind her head. With her left hand, she should use the flat part of the fingers to palpate the breast tissue, using small circular motions beginning at the outermost top of her right breast and working clockwise around the breast.

Placing a pillow or folded towel under the right shoulder distributes the breast tissue more evenly on the chest.

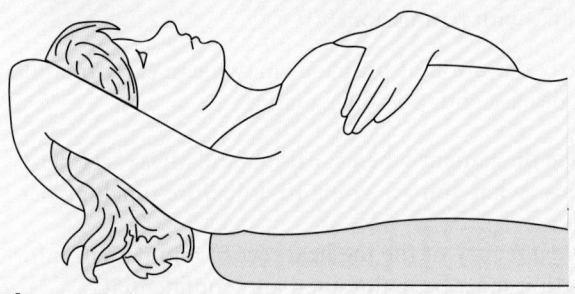

**A**

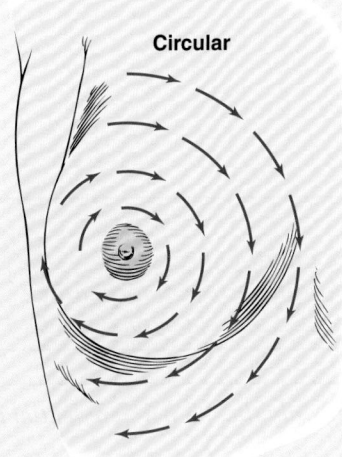

Circular

**B**

**Step 6.** (**A**) While lying down, palpate each breast carefully. (Reprinted from Pillitteri A. *Maternal and Child Health Nursing*. Philadelphia, PA: Lippincott Williams & Wilkins, 2007, with permission.) (**B**) Palpate the breast using the flat part of the fingers in a circular motion. (Reprinted from Weber J, Kelley J. *Health Assessment in Nursing*. Philadelphia, PA: Lippincott Williams & Wilkins, 2003, with permission.)

*(continues on page 950)*

## PROCEDURE 36-1 (continued)

| STEPS | PURPOSE |
|---|---|
| 7. Encourage the patient to palpate the breast carefully by moving her fingers in toward the nipple, while palpating every part of the breast, including the nipple. | Breast tissue extends from the clavicle to the end of the rib cage and from the sternum to underneath the axilla. |
| 8. Repeat the procedure for the left breast, placing a pillow or folded towel under the left shoulder and the left hand behind the head. | Both breasts should be examined at the same time. |
| 9. Gently squeeze each nipple between the thumb and index finger. Report any discharge to the physician. | Unless the patient is lactating, discharge from the nipple is not normal. |

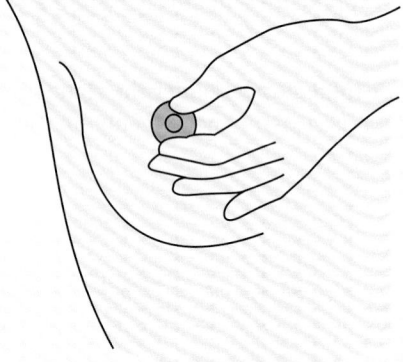

**Step 9**. Squeeze each nipple gently. (Reprinted from Pillitteri A. *Maternal and Child Health Nursing*. Philadelphia, PA: Lippincott Williams & Wilkins, 2007, with permission.)

| STEPS | PURPOSE |
|---|---|
| 10. Explain to the patient that she should promptly report any abnormalities to the physician. | Early detection of problems may mean early treatment of disease and, possibly, a cure. |
| 11. **AFF** Explain how to respond to a patient who is visually impaired. | Face the patient when speaking and always let her know what you are going to do before touching her. |
| 12. **AFF** Log into the electronic medical record (EMR) using your username and secure password OR obtain the paper medical record from a secure location and assure it is kept away from public access. Document the patient education including the date, time, and your name/credentials. | The integrity of the medical record and patient information must be maintained and confidential. Procedures are considered not to have been done if they are not recorded. |
| 13. When finished, log out of the EMR and/or replace the paper medical record in an appropriate and secure location. | |

Charting Example:
*4/12/2016 2:15 PM Pt. given written and verbal instructions on performing the monthly breast self-examination. Verbalized understanding. Advised to contact the office for any problems or abnormalities*
———————————————————————————————————— *S.Appleton, CMA*

Note: *The medical assistant may sign his or her name in the patient record using only the "CMA" credential if the office has a signature log denoting the entire credential as "CMA(AAMA)."*

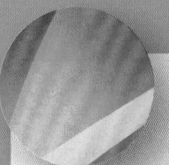

**PSY** Procedure 36-2

# Assisting with the Pelvic Examination and Pap Smear

**PSY** Instruct and prepare a patient for a procedure or treatment; coach patients regarding disease prevention and treatment plans; coach patients appropriately considering cultural diversity, developmental life stage, and communication barriers; document patient care accurately in the medical record.

**PSY** **Purpose:** Prepare the examination room and the female patient for a pelvic examination and Pap smear and assist the physician as needed

**Equipment:** Gown and drape; appropriate-size vaginal speculum; cotton-tipped applicators; water-soluble lubricant; examination gloves; examination light; tissues; materials for Pap smear: cervical brush, liquid-based preservative (SurePath®orThinPrep®), laboratory request form, identification labels, and other materials that may be required by laboratory; biohazard transport bag; and biohazard waste container

| STEPS | PURPOSE |
|---|---|
| **1.** Wash your hands. | Hand washing aids infection control. |
| **2.** Assemble the equipment and supplies. | The vaginal speculum can be warmed under warm running water (see Fig. 36-10 ), on a heating pad set on warm, or in a warming drawer found on some examination tables. Lubricant must not be used on the vaginal speculum before insertion because this will cause inaccurate Pap smear results. |
| **3.** Label the outside of the liquid-based preservative container. | |
| **4.** Greet and identify the patient. Explain the procedure. | Identifying the patient prevents errors. Explaining the procedure may reduce anxiety. |
| **5.** Ask the patient to empty her bladder and, if necessary, collect a urine specimen. | An empty bladder will make the examination more comfortable. |
| **6.** Provide the patient with a gown and drape and ask her to disrobe from the waist down. | If the patient is also having a breast examination, she should be instructed to disrobe completely and put the gown on with the opening in the front. This allows easier access for the breast examination. Allow the patient privacy for changing into the examination gown. |

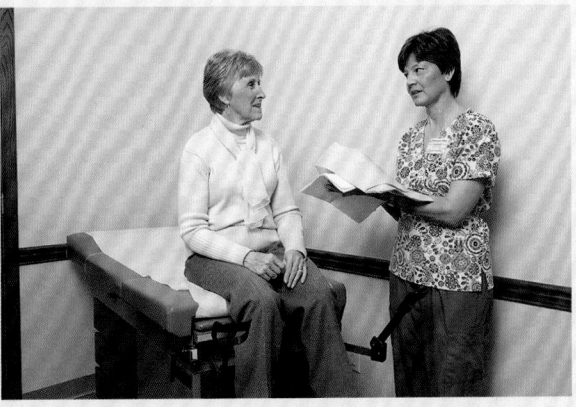

**Step 6.** Give the patient a gown and drape while explaining what to remove and how to put the gown on.

| | |
|---|---|
| **7.** Position the patient in the dorsal lithotomy position with her buttocks at the bottom edge of the table. | Because this position is embarrassing and may stress the legs and back, assist the patient into this position only when the physician is ready to do the examination. |

*(continues on page 952)*

## PROCEDURE 36-2 (continued)

| STEPS | PURPOSE |
|---|---|
| 8. Adjust the drape to cover the patient's abdomen and knees, exposing the genitalia, and adjust the light over the genitalia for maximum visibility. | Good visibility is essential for a thorough examination. |
| 9. Assist the physician with the examination by handing instruments and supplies as needed. | Anticipating the physician's needs during the procedure promotes a more thorough and efficient examination |
| 10. After applying examination gloves, hold the container of liquid medium while the physician obtains the specimen. | The physician may want you to assist once the specimen is obtained. |

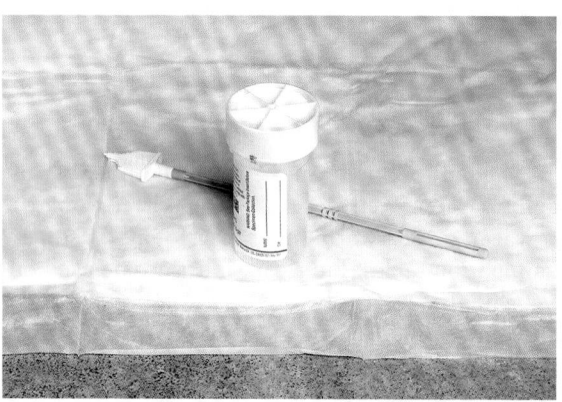

**Step 10.** Hold the container of liquid-based preservative while the physician swirls the brush with the cervical specimen in the solution 10 times. The physician may hand you the brush and have you swirl in the solution 10 times.

| STEPS | PURPOSE |
|---|---|
| 11. When the physician removes the vaginal speculum, have a basin or other container ready to receive it. | Disposable specula may be put into a biohazard trash container. Nondisposable specula need to be sanitized and sterilized between patients. |
| 12. Apply lubricant across the physician's two manual fingers without touching the end of the lubricant container to the physician's gloves. | Water-soluble lubricant helps make the examination more comfortable. |
| 13. Encourage the patient to relax during the bimanual examination as needed. | The patient may be more relaxed during the examination if you are supportive. |

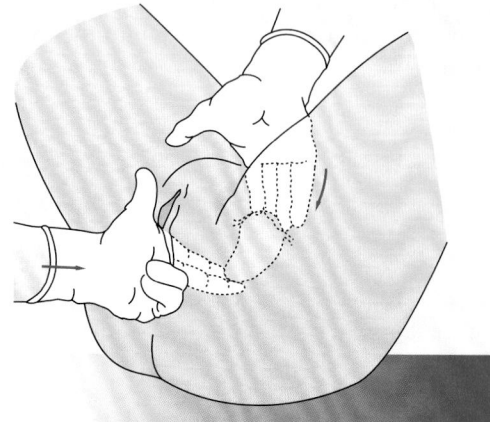

**Step 13.** Technique for bimanual examination of the pelvic organs in women. (Reprinted from Smeltzer SC, Bare BG. *Textbook of Medical-Surgical Nursing*. Philadelphia, PA: Lippincott Williams & Wilkins, 2008, with permission.)

## PROCEDURE 36-2 (continued)

| STEPS | PURPOSE |
|---|---|
| 14. After the examination, help the patient slide up to the top of the examination table and remove both feet at the same time from the stirrups. | Injury can be prevented if the patient moves up the table before removing feet from the stirrups. Removing both feet at the same time puts less strain on the patient. |
| 15. Offer the patient tissues to remove excess lubricant, and help her sit if necessary, watching for signs of vertigo. | Excess lubricant can be uncomfortable. Some patients, especially older adults, may be dizzy on sitting up. |
| 16. Ask the patient to get dressed and assist as needed. Provide for privacy as the patient dresses. | Telling the patient what to do will reduce confusion and misunderstanding. |
| 17. Reinforce any physician instructions regarding follow-up appointments and advise the patient on the procedure for obtaining the laboratory findings from the Pap smear. | For quality management, let the patient know when to schedule follow-up appointments and when and how laboratory findings will be obtained. |
| 18. **AFF** Explain how to respond to a patient who has dementia. | Solicit assistance from the caregiver or other staff member to help during the procedure. Give simple directions to the patient about what she should do. Speak clearly, not loudly. |
| 19. Properly care for or dispose of equipment and clean the examination room. Wash your hands. | Follow standard precautions when handling contaminated supplies and equipment. |
| 20. **AFF** Log into the electronic medical record (EMR) using your username and secure password OR obtain the paper medical record from a secure location and assure it is kept away from public access. Document your responsibilities during the procedures such as routing the specimen and patient education. You did not perform the Pap smear and pelvic exam so you do not document the procedure. Include the date, time, and your name/credentials for the information you document. | The integrity of the medical record and patient information must be maintained and confidential. Procedures are considered not to have been done if they are not recorded. |
| 21. When finished, log out of the EMR and/or replace the paper medical record in an appropriate and secure location. | |

---

**Charting Example:**

*2/27/2016 3:00 PM Pap and pelvic today per Dr. Todd. ThinPrep sent to Acme lab for cytology. Pt. given written and verbal instructions on obtaining results ———————————————————— S.Appleton, CMA*

---

Note: *The medical assistant may sign his or her name in the patient record using only the "CMA" credential if the office has a signature log denoting the entire credential as "CMA(AAMA)."*

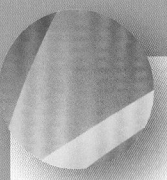

**PSY** PROCEDURE 36-3

## Assisting with the Colposcopy and Cervical Biopsy

**PSY** Instruct and prepare a patient for a procedure or treatment; coach patients regarding disease prevention and treatment plans; coach patients appropriately considering cultural diversity, developmental life stage, and communication barriers; document patient care accurately in the medical record.

**Purpose:** Prepare the examination room and the female patient for a colposcopy with cervical biopsy

**Equipment:** Gown and drape, vaginal speculum, colposcope, specimen container with preservative (10% formalin), sterile gloves in appropriate size, sterile cotton-tipped applicators, sterile normal saline solution, sterile 3% acetic acid, sterile povidone–iodine (Betadine), silver nitrate sticks or ferric subsulfate (Monsel solution), sterile biopsy forceps or punch biopsy instrument, sterile uterine curet, sterile uterine dressing forceps, sterile 4 × 4 gauze, sterile towel, sterile endocervical curet, sterile uterine tenaculum, sanitary napkin, examination gloves, examination light, tissues, biohazard container

| STEPS | PURPOSE |
|---|---|
| 1. Wash your hands. | Hand washing aids infection control. |
| 2. Verify that the patient has signed the consent form. | Colposcopy with biopsy is an invasive procedure that requires written consent. |
| 3. Assemble the equipment and supplies. | Anticipate and plan for necessary equipment and supplies before the procedure starts to avoid having delays during the procedure. |
| 4. Check the light on the colposcope. | Properly functioning equipment is crucial to the quality of the examination. |
| 5. Set up the sterile field without contaminating it. | A biopsy is an invasive procedure requiring surgical asepsis. |
| 6. Pour sterile normal saline and acetic acid into their sterile containers. Cover the field with a sterile drape. | Items that can be placed on the sterile field include the sterile cotton-tipped applicators and sterile containers for the solutions.<br>Covering the sterile field maintains sterility as you prepare the patient. |
| 7. Greet and identify the patient. Explain the procedure. | Identifying the patient prevents errors. Explaining the procedure may ease anxiety. |
| 8. When the physician is ready to proceed, assist the patient into the dorsal lithotomy position. If you are to assist the physician from the sterile field, put on sterile gloves after positioning the patient. | Correct positioning is essential for a clear view of the cervix. |

## PROCEDURE 36-3 (continued)

| STEPS | PURPOSE |
|---|---|

9. Hand the physician the applicator immersed in normal saline, followed by the applicator immersed in acetic acid.

Acetic acid swabbed on the area improves visualization and aids in identifying suspicious tissue.

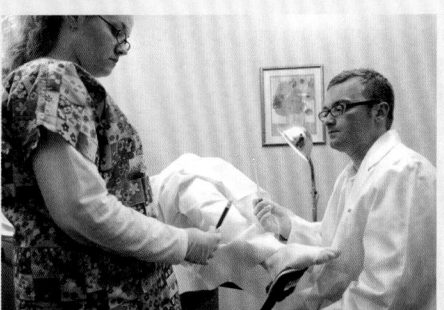

**Step 9.** Hand the physician an applicator that has been immersed in normal saline.

10. Hand the physician the applicator with the antiseptic solution.

The area to be sampled for biopsy must be swabbed with an antiseptic solution to reduce microorganisms and pathogens in the area.

11. If you did not apply sterile gloves to assist the physician, apply clean examination gloves and receive the biopsy specimen into the container of 10% formalin preservative.

Because the specimen may be hazardous, standard precautions must be observed.
The specimen container with preservative may be obtained from the laboratory.

12. Provide the physician with Monsel solution or silver nitrate sticks to stop any bleeding.

If bleeding occurs, a coagulant, such as Monsel solution or silver nitrate, may have to be applied if necessary.

13. When the physician is finished with the procedure, appropriately assist the patient from the stirrups and to a sitting position. Explain to the patient that a small amount of bleeding may occur. Have a sanitary napkin available.

Bleeding with a cervical biopsy is usually minimal, and a small sanitary pad should be sufficient.

14. Label the specimen container with the patient's name and date and prepare the laboratory request.

The specimen must be properly identified, and the laboratory request must be complete or the specimen may not be processed at the lab.

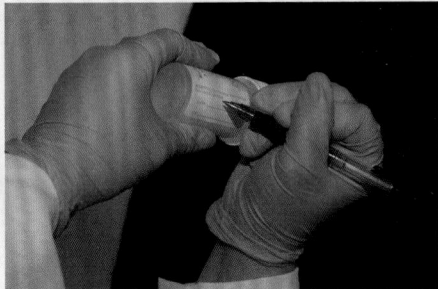

**Step 14.** Always label the specimen container before sending it to the lab.

15. Ask the patient to get dressed and assist as needed. Provide for privacy as the patient dresses.

Telling the patient what to do will reduce confusion and misunderstanding.

*(continues on page 956)*

## PROCEDURE 36-3 (continued)

| STEPS | PURPOSE |
|---|---|
| **16.** Reinforce any physician instructions regarding follow-up appointments and how to obtain the biopsy findings. | For quality management, let the patient know when to schedule follow-up appointments, and tell the patient when and how laboratory findings will be provided. |
| **17.** **AFF** Explain how to respond to a patient who does not speak English or is ESL. | Solicit assistance from anyone who may be with the patient or a staff member who speaks her native language to interpret if available. If no interpreter is available, use hand gestures or pictures to explain procedure to the patient. |
| **18.** Properly care for or dispose of equipment and clean the examination room. Wash your hands. | Standard precautions should be followed during and after this procedure. |
| **19.** **AFF** Log into the electronic medical record (EMR) using your username and secure password OR obtain the paper medical record from a secure location and assure it is kept away from public access. Document your responsibilities during the procedures such as routing the specimen and patient education. You did not perform the colposcopy and cervical biopsy so you do not document the procedure. Include the date, time, and your name/credentials for the information you document. | The integrity of the medical record and patient information must be maintained and confidential. Procedures are considered not to have been done if they are not recorded. |
| **20.** When finished, log out of the EMR and/or replace the paper medical record in an appropriate and secure location. | |

---

**Charting Example:**

*10/15/2016 10:45 AM Colposcopy performed per Dr. Lyttle; cervical biopsy obtained and sent to Acme lab for cytology. Minimal bleeding post procedure; pt. given sanitary pad, verbal and written instructions on postprocedure care _____ S.Appleton, CMA*

---

**Note:** *The medical assistant may sign his or her name in the patient record using only the "CMA" credential if the office has a signature log denoting the entire credential as "CMA(AAMA)."*

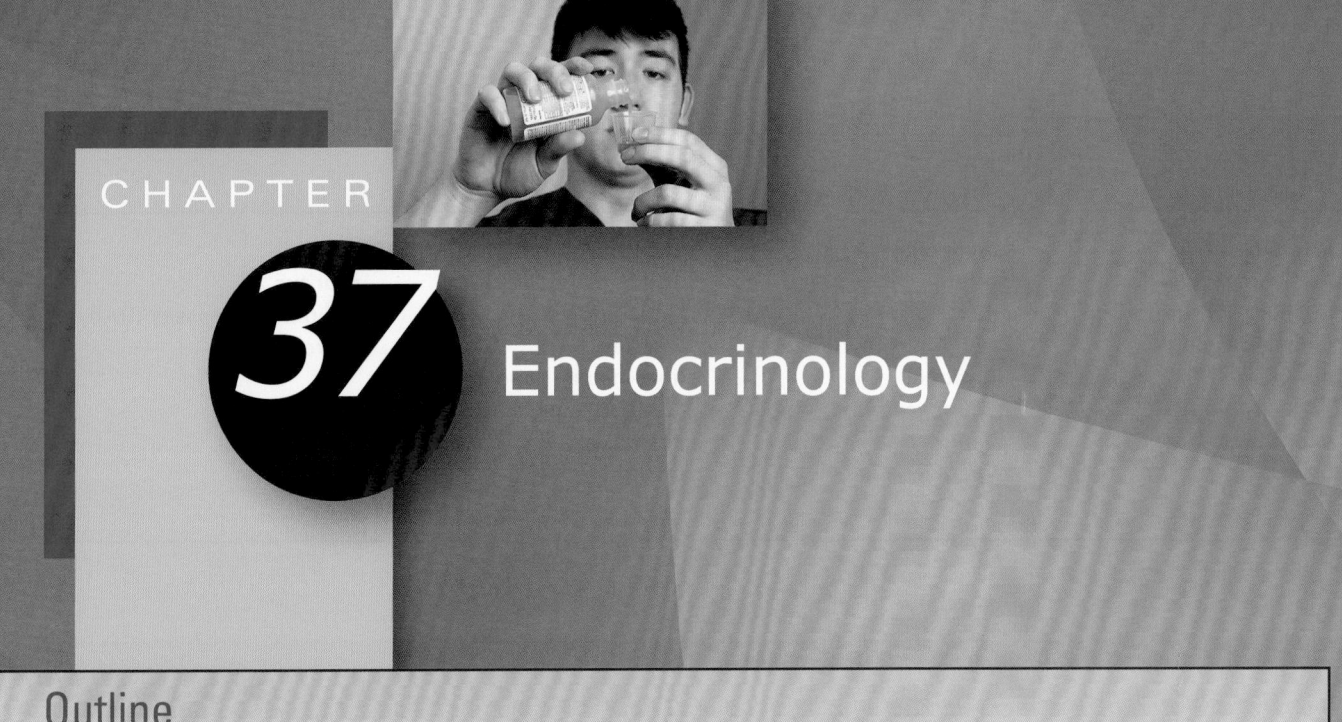

# CHAPTER 37 Endocrinology

## Outline

**Common Disorders of the Endocrine System**
  Disorders of the Thyroid

Disorders of the Pancreas
Disorders of the Adrenal Glands
Disorders of the Pituitary Gland

**Common Diagnostic and Therapeutic Procedures**

## Learning Outcomes

### COG Cognitive Domain*

1. Spell key terms
2. *Define medical terms and abbreviations related to all body systems*
3. *Describe structural organization of the human body*
4. *List major organs in each body system*
5. *Identify the anatomical location of major organs in each body system*
6. *Describe the normal function of each body system*
7. *Identify common pathology related to each body system including signs, symptoms, and etiology*
8. Identify abnormal conditions of the thyroid, pancreas, adrenal, and pituitary glands
9. Describe the tests commonly used to diagnose disorders of these endocrine system glands
10. Explain your role in working with patients with endocrine system disorders

### PSY Psychomotor Domain*

1. Manage a patient with a diabetic emergency (Procedure 37-1)
    a. *Instruct and prepare a patient for a procedure or treatment*
    b. *Coach patients appropriately considering cultural diversity, developmental life stage, and communication barriers*
    c. *Coach patients regarding disease prevention and treatment plans*
    d. *Document patient care accurately in the medical record*

### AFF Affective Domain*

1. *Incorporate critical thinking skills when performing patient assessment*
2. *Incorporate critical thinking skills when performing patient care*
3. *Show awareness of a patient's concerns related to the procedure being performed*
4. *Demonstrate empathy, active listening, and nonverbal communication*
5. *Demonstrate respect for individual diversity including gender, race, religion, age, economic status, and appearance*
6. *Explain to a patient the rationale for performance of a procedure*
7. *Demonstrate sensitivity to patient rights*
8. *Protect the integrity of the medical record*

*Note: AAMA/CAAHEP 2015 Standards are italicized.*

### ABHES Competencies

1. Assist the physician with the regimen of diagnostic and treatment modalities as they relate to each body system
2. Comply with federal, state, and local health laws and regulations
3. Communicate on the recipient's level of comprehension
4. Serve as a liaison between the physician and others
5. Show empathy and impartiality when dealing with patients
6. Document accurately

*(continues on page 958)*

# Key Terms

## Case Study

**D**r. Schroeder is the endocrinologist at Great Falls Medical Center who treats patients with problems pertaining to the endocrine glands. Patients seen in this specialty include those with metabolic disorders, thyroid diseases, diabetes, and other problems associated with hormone imbalances. The medical assistant, Laura Brewer, CMA (AAMA), is responsible for obtaining medical histories for new patients in this specialty office, and the first patient today was a 46-year-old female patient referred by her family physician for complaints of weight gain, fatigue, hair loss, and chronic constipation. The patient states that she suffers from bouts of memory loss and depression and that these problems have gotten progressively worse over the last four years. What tests will be used to determine the cause, if any, of this patient's symptoms, and what endocrine glands might be responsible? Are there any treatments available for diseases and disorders of the endocrine gland? What role can a medical assistant have in the management of patients with endocrine disorders? These and other questions about this specialty are addressed in this chapter.

Together with the nervous system, the endocrine system regulates most body functions. Although the control exerted by the nervous system is immediate and usually elicits a short-term response, the endocrine system regulates chemical metabolism for a longer acting, more widespread response. **Hormones** are the chemical regulators, or messengers, of the endocrine glands. Some hormones stimulate system-wide metabolic processes, whereas others target specific tissues or organs (Table 37-1).

The endocrine glands differ from the body's other glands, such as sweat glands, because they are ductless (Fig. 37-1). Endocrine glands secrete hormones directly into the bloodstream for transmission rather than having direct access to target tissues. The body regulates the release of hormones through negative feedback, which "tells" the appropriate gland how much hormone to release based on the need for increased or decreased secretion. Some endocrine glands release hormones to maintain a specific range in the blood (thyroid hormones), whereas others have cyclic or rhythmic fluctuations (estrogen or progesterone).

Although you may see patients with endocrine system disorders in any medical practice specialty, physicians who specialize in the treatment of these disorders specifically are known as **endocrinologists**. Many disorders of the endocrine system result from an oversecretion or undersecretion of hormones. This chapter will focus on some common disorders of the endocrine system and the role of the medical assistant in caring for these patients in the medical office.

## COMMON DISORDERS OF THE ENDOCRINE SYSTEM

### Disorders of the Thyroid

#### Hyperthyroidism

The most common form of hyperthyroidism, Graves disease, results from the hypersecretion of thyroid hormones. This condition, also known as **thyrotoxicosis** (Box 37-1), causes an increase in metabolism. In addition

## TABLE 37-1 The Major Endocrine Glands and Their Hormones

| Gland | Hormone | Principal Functions |
|-------|---------|---------------------|
| Anterior pituitary | HGH (human growth hormone) | Promotes growth of all body tissues |
| | TSH (thyroid-stimulating hormone) | Stimulates the thyroid gland to produce thyroid hormones |
| | ACTH (adrenocorticotropic hormone) | Stimulates adrenal cortex to produce cortical hormones |
| | FSH (follicle-stimulating hormone) | Stimulates growth and hormone activity of ovarian follicles; stimulates growth of testes |
| | LH (luteinizing hormone) | Causes development of corpus luteum in ruptured ovarian follicle in females; stimulates secretion of testosterone in males |
| Posterior pituitary kidney | ADH (antidiuretic hormone, vasopressin) | Promotes reabsorption of water in tubules |
| | Oxytocin | Causes contraction of uterus; causes ejection of milk from mammary glands |
| Thyroid | Thyroid hormone (thyroxine [$T_4$] and triiodothyronine [$T_3$]) | Increase metabolic rate; required for normal growth |
| | Calcitonin | Decreases calcium level in blood |
| Adrenal medulla | Epinephrine and norepinephrine | Increase blood pressure and heart rate |
| Adrenal cortex | Cortisol (95% of glucocorticoids) | Aids in metabolism of carbohydrates, proteins, fats; active during stress |
| | Aldosterone (95% of mineralocorticoids) | Aids in regulating electrolytes and water balance |
| Pancreatic islets | Insulin | Aids transport of glucose into cells; required for cellular metabolism of foods, especially glucose; decreases blood glucose levels |
| | Glucagon | Stimulates liver to release glucose, increasing blood glucose levels |
| Testes | Testosterone | Stimulates growth and development of male sexual organs |
| Ovaries | Estrogen | Stimulates growth of primary female sexual organs and development of secondary sexual characteristics |

to elevated blood levels of thyroid hormones (thyroxine [$T_4$] and triiodothyronine [$T_3$]), the patient may have an enlarged thyroid gland known as a **goiter** (Fig. 37-2) and unusual protrusion of the eyeballs known as **exophthalmia** (Fig. 37-3). Additional signs and symptoms of Graves disease include the following:

- Increased heart rate
- Increased body temperature
- Excessive sweating
- Inability to sleep
- Increased appetite
- Weight loss
- Excitability and nervousness

The treatment for hyperthyroidism includes destruction of part or all of the thyroid gland through the use of radioactive iodine or surgery. When seen in the medical office, these patients require frequent blood tests to check the thyroid hormone levels as ordered by the physician.

## Hypothyroidism

Hypothyroidism results from an undersecretion of thyroid hormones, which may be congenital or acquired. Infants with congenital hypothyroidism are usually diagnosed at birth and treated with appropriate thyroid hormones. However, if a diagnosis is not made in the infant, irreversible mental retardation will occur. In adults, hypothyroidism may occur because of surgical removal of thyroid tissue, radioactive destruction of the gland, the use of antithyroid medications, or a deficiency of iodine in the diet. One form of hypothyroidism, **Hashimoto thyroiditis**, is actually a disease of the immune system in which the tissue of the thyroid gland is replaced with fibrous tissue. Regardless of the cause, treatment of hypothyroidism is replacement of thyroid hormones, which must be taken by the patient for the remainder of his or her life.

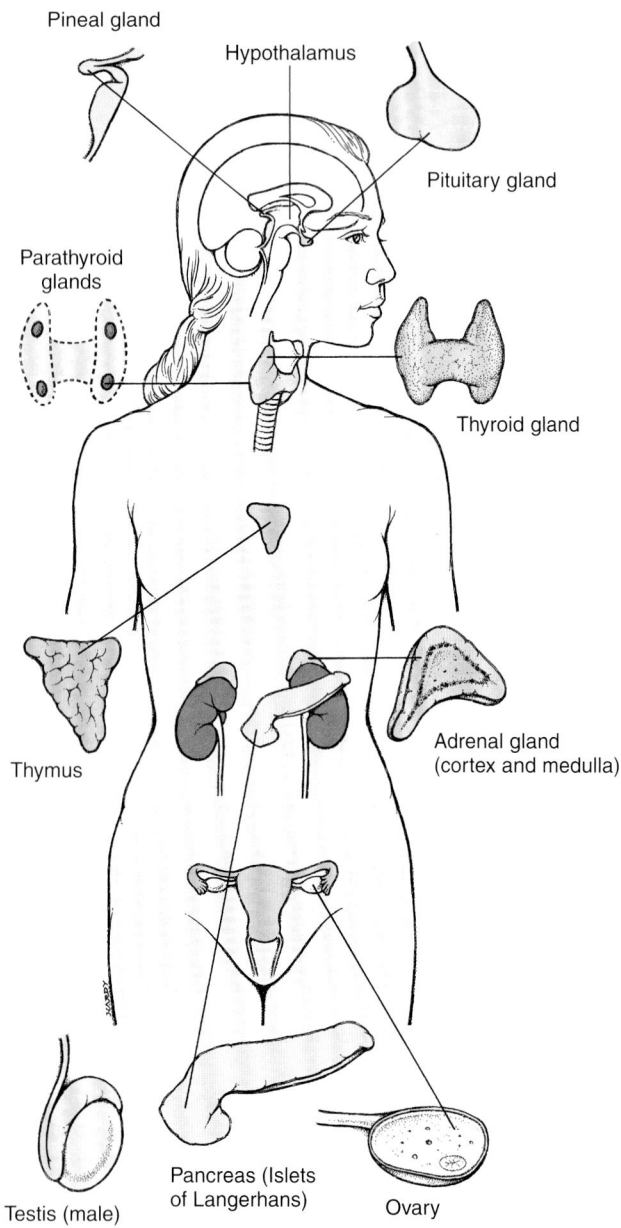

**Figure 37-1** • The main hormone-secreting glands of the endocrine system.

Pineal gland
Hypothalamus
Pituitary gland
Parathyroid glands
Thyroid gland
Thymus
Adrenal gland (cortex and medulla)
Testis (male)
Pancreas (Islets of Langerhans)
Ovary

Your role in the medical office includes assisting the physician with any tests or procedures to diagnose and treat thyroid disorders. These tasks may include performing venipuncture for blood specimens and sending these to the lab for testing, obtaining referrals as needed, and scheduling patients for thyroid surgery with a head or neck surgeon, educating patients about their disease, and encouraging compliance with any medications ordered by the physician.

### ✎ CHECKPOINT QUESTION

1. Why does the patient with hyperthyroidism have an increased appetite with weight loss?

---

### BOX 37-1   **Thyroid Storm**

A severe form of thyrotoxicosis is thyroid storm, or crisis, which may result in coma and death. Although very few patients suffer from thyroid storm today, symptoms include the following:

• Very high fever
• Dehydration
• Tachycardia
• Shortness of breath
• Productive cough
• Chest pain
• Agitation
• Mental confusion

Patients diagnosed with thyroid storm require immediate medical intervention to reduce the body temperature and replace fluids and electrolytes.

## Disorders of the Pancreas

### Diabetes Mellitus

Dysfunction of the islets of Langerhans cells within the pancreas results in diabetes mellitus, a disorder affecting carbohydrate metabolism. Although the exact cause of diabetes mellitus is not known, the result is a decrease in the production and secretion of insulin from the pancreas. Because insulin is necessary to carry glucose into the cells of the body, a decrease in insulin

Toxic goiter (Graves disease)

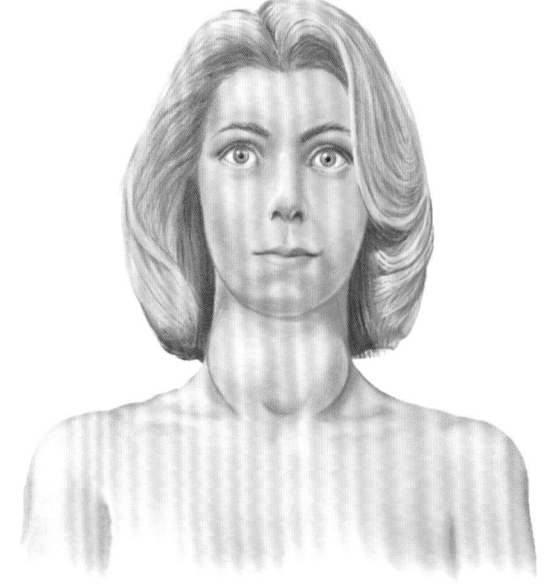

**Figure 37-2** • An enlarged thyroid gland or goiter. (Asset provided by Anatomical Chart Co.)

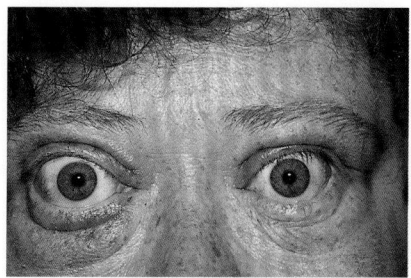

**Figure 37-3** • Exophthalmia. (From Goodheart HP. *Goodheart's Photoguide of Common Skin Disorders*, 2nd ed. Philadelphia, PA: Lippincott Williams & Wilkins, 2003).

results in **hyperglycemia** (an elevated blood glucose), which ultimately results in **glycosuria** (glucose in the urine).

### Type 1 Diabetes Mellitus

Type 1 diabetes mellitus is sometimes referred to as **insulin-dependent diabetes mellitus** and occurs most often in children and young adults. The signs and symptoms of hyperglycemia include the following:

- **Polydipsia** (increased thirst)
- **Polyuria** (excessive urination)
- **Polyphagia** (abnormal hunger)
- Weight loss

Usually, the young patient with type 1 diabetes develops symptoms abruptly without warning and may require hospitalization with intravenous insulin and frequent monitoring of blood glucose. Once diagnosed, these patients will require daily insulin and blood glucose monitoring for the remainder of their lives. Because these patients are often young, active, and still growing physically, managing blood glucose and diet may be challenging for both the patient and their caregivers. These patients should be encouraged to understand and manage their disease as independently as possible (Fig. 37-4).

### Type 2 Diabetes Mellitus

Type 2 diabetes mellitus may be referred to as **non–insulin-dependent diabetes mellitus**; however, many patients with this condition do require insulin to control elevated blood glucose levels. This type of diabetes mellitus occurs most often in adults over the age of 40 years and has a gradual onset. Although insulin is produced by the pancreas, it cannot exert its effect on cells because of a deficiency of insulin receptors on cell membranes. Risk factors for developing type 2 diabetes are obesity and a family history of diabetes mellitus.

The patient with type 2 diabetes will have symptoms of hyperglycemia similar to patients with type 1 diabetes including polydipsia and polyuria. However, patients with type 2 diabetes mellitus will also have **pruritus** (severe itching) and neuropathy (disorders of

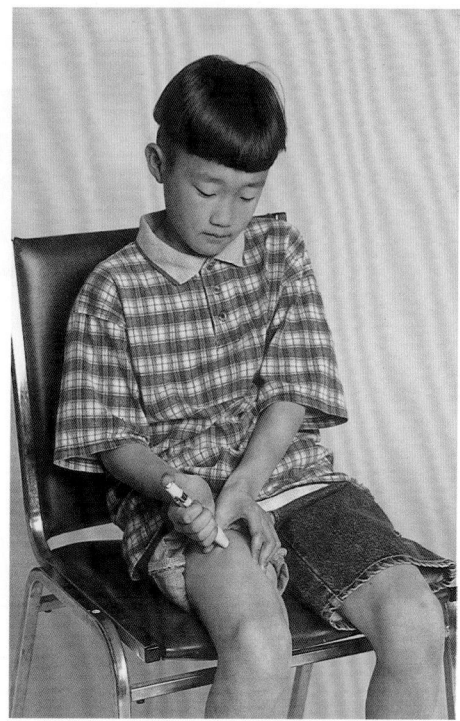

**Figure 37-4** • A young child with diabetes mellitus.

the nervous system). Usually, the physician will recommend that the patient lose weight and eat a well-balanced diet, which may help to control the elevated blood glucose levels and reduce the need for parenteral insulin. Oral medications that enable insulin to react with the remaining cell membrane receptors are used as necessary; however, elevated blood glucose that does not respond to diet control and oral medications must be treated with insulin, which is injected subcutaneously.

## Gestational Diabetes Mellitus

Another type of diabetes mellitus occurs only during pregnancy and is known as *gestational diabetes mellitus*. Although the pregnant patient may have all the signs and symptoms of type 1 or 2 diabetes mellitus, this condition disappears after the patient delivers the baby. It is important that the patient's urine be checked at every medical office visit for the presence of glucose; a blood specimen for glucose should be taken between 24 and 28 weeks of gestation. Early diagnosis of this condition is important to reduce complications, such as fetal abnormalities and death.

## Managing Diabetes Mellitus

Long-term complications from uncontrolled hyperglycemia include damage to the heart, kidneys, and eyes, usually resulting from vascular system (blood vessel) changes that affect many body systems (Fig. 37-5). Increased plaque buildup on the inside of arteries supplying blood to the heart and other organs causes a

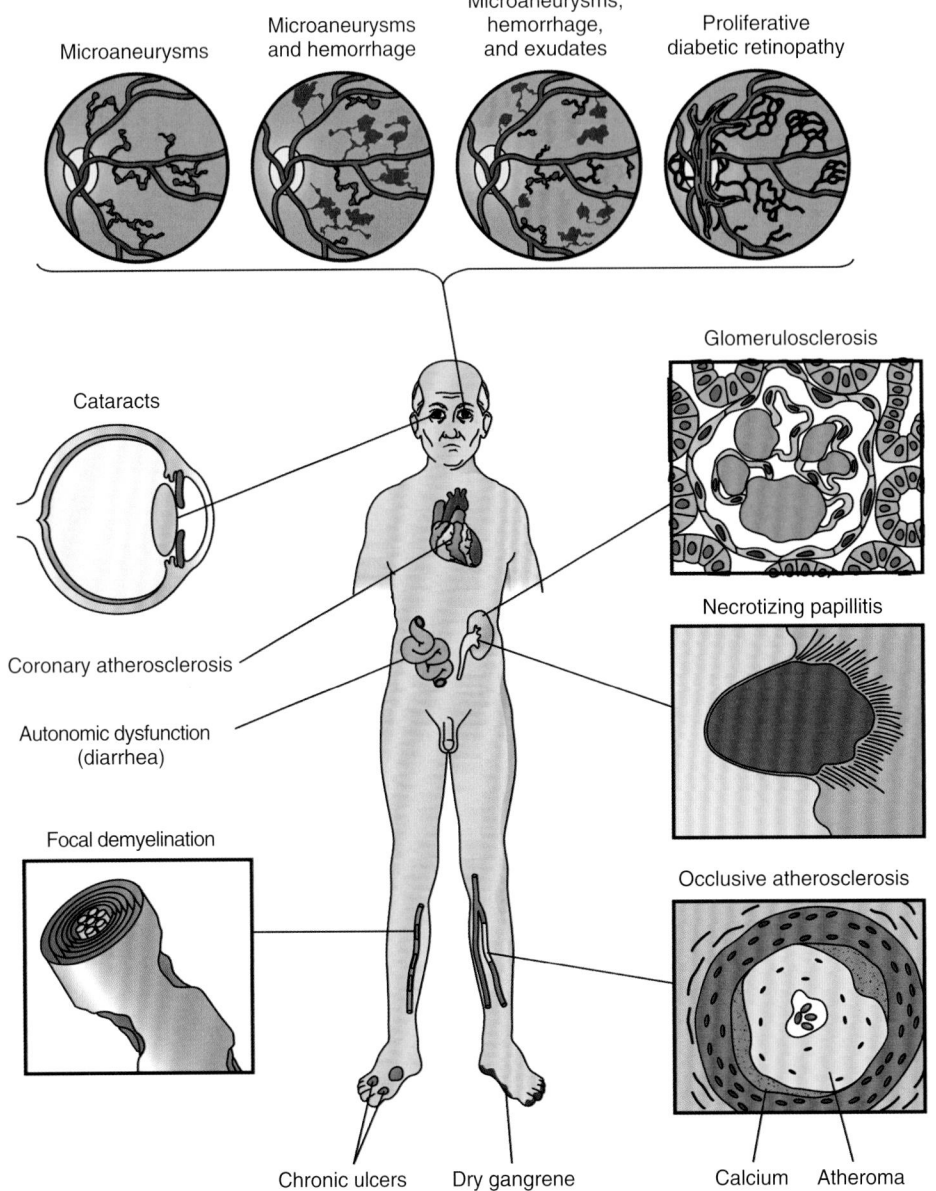

**Figure 37-5** • Secondary complications of diabetes. The effects of diabetes on a number of vital organs result in complications that may be incapacitating (cerebral and peripheral vascular disease), painful (neuropathy), or life threatening (coronary artery disease, pyelonephritis with necrotizing papillitis). (From Rubin R, Strayer DS. *Rubin's Pathology: Clinicopathologic Foundations of Medicine*, 5th ed. 2008.)

decreased blood supply to those organs and, over time, a loss of function. When this happens to the kidneys, the patient may develop kidney failure and require dialysis. Vascular changes to the eyes result in diabetic retinopathy (Box 37-2) with a decrease in visual acuity and blindness. Damage to the nervous system results in neuropathy and decreased sensation, particularly in the legs and feet. Combined with the decreased blood flow to the lower extremities, this neuropathy could result in ulcers on the feet and legs that do not heal, become infected, and require eventual limb amputation (Fig. 37-6). These complications are not only debilitating, but they can also be life threatening.

In addition to the dietary restrictions including carbohydrate intake, insulin injections are necessary for patients with type 1 diabetes and may be necessary for patients with type 2 diabetes. Insulin is measured in units and administered subcutaneously (refer to Chapter 24). An insulin syringe is identified by the calibration in units, not milliliters (mL), and the orange cap. When administering insulin, use only an insulin syringe and needle that are calibrated to the concentration of insulin ordered by the physician. Do not use an insulin syringe and needle for anything other than insulin (Fig. 37-7). Depending on the needs of the patient, the action of insulin may vary from rapid acting (onset 5 to 15 minutes), short

## BOX 37-2 Diabetic Retinopathy

Diabetic retinopathy is seen in patients with a history of diabetes mellitus and is caused by small hemorrhages from the capillaries supplying blood to the eye. After the capillaries rupture, scarring occurs that decreases the amount of oxygen to the eye. Over time, this scarring and decrease in oxygen result in permanent damage, causing a decrease in vision and eventual blindness. Controlling blood glucose levels can help control this devastating disease, which is currently the leading cause of blindness in the United States.

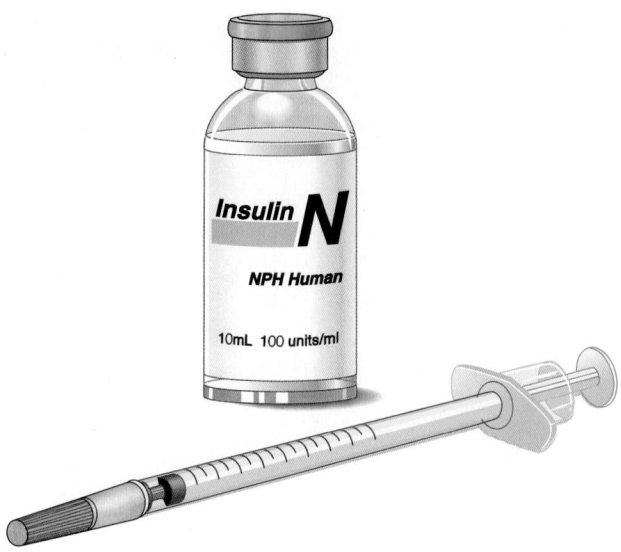

**Figure 37-7** • Only use an insulin syringe and needle to administer insulin. (LifeART image copyright © 2011. All rights reserved.)

acting (onset 30 minutes), intermediate acting (onset 2 hours), and long acting (onset 2 hours). Some diabetic patients may require more than one type of insulin to manage their blood glucose. Insulin can also be administered subcutaneously via an insulin pump (Fig. 37-8).

The role of the medical assistant includes working with the physician to diagnose and treat patients with diabetes mellitus while providing support and education to the patient and family members about this disease (Fig. 37-9). The lifestyle changes (e.g., dietary restrictions, weight management, exercise, frequent blood monitoring) that are necessary to control blood glucose levels are often new to the patient and difficult to manage alone. Once diagnosed, the medical record must clearly identify the diagnosed patient's diabetes because many other health care problems and treatments may exacerbate this disease. You should also be alert for patients who may be having a diabetic emergency and react according to physician orders and office policy and procedure with regard to these situations.

You may be asked by the physician to obtain frequent blood specimens, schedule patients to speak with a dietician as necessary, and educate patients about their oral hypoglycemic medications or insulin. Because of the decreased sensation and possibility of painless sores or ulcers on the feet that can lead to infection and amputation, it is important that diabetic patients remove their shoes and socks at each office visit so that a visual inspection may be made of the feet and lower legs. In some offices, the medical assistant may be asked to assist with evaluating sensation in the feet (Fig. 37-10A–C).

### WHAT IF?

**What if your older adult patient is having difficulty seeing the numbers on the insulin syringe?**

Although many elderly patients have visual difficulties that occur naturally with age, the patient with diabetes may have increased visual difficulties from the vascular changes in the eyes that result from the disease. Although you should always discuss these problems with the physician before advising the patient, there are visual aids that the patient can get from the pharmacist that fit onto the side of the syringe and magnify the image, making the numbers for "units of insulin" larger in appearance and easier to see. Perhaps a friend, neighbor, or other family member can assist the patient with filling the syringes. In some cases, the physician may want a visiting nurse to come to the patient's house during the week to prefill the syringes for the patient. Whatever the solution, always ask older adult patients about their medications and any difficulties they may be having with administering those medications, and work with the physician to come up with the best plan for the patient.

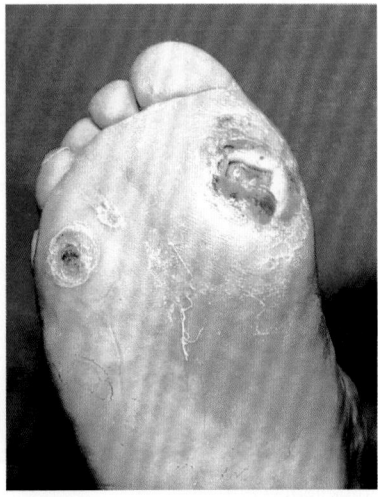

**Figure 37-6** • Neuropathic ulcers occur on pressure points in areas with diminished sensation in diabetic polyneuropathy. Because pain is absent, the ulcer may go unnoticed. (From Bates BB. *A Guide to Physical Examination and History Taking*, 6th ed. J.B. Lippincott, 1995.)

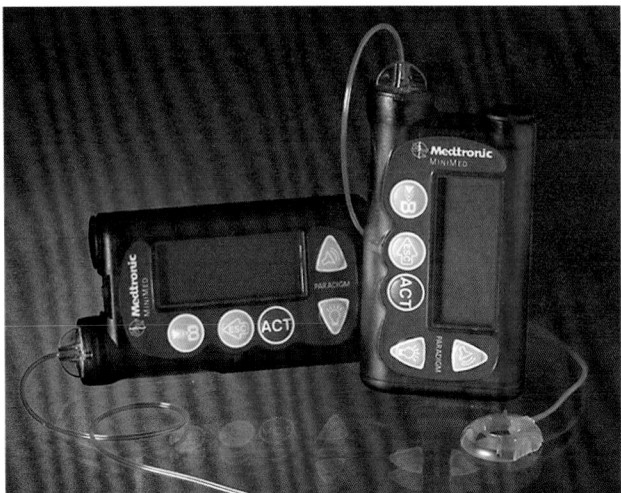

**Figure 37-8** • Medtronic (Northridge, CA) insulin pump system.

## Diabetic Emergencies

When glucose cannot be used for energy by the cells, the body turns to fats and proteins, which are converted to **ketones** by the liver. These ketones accumulate in the blood because the cells cannot use them rapidly. As these acids build up, they lower the pH of the blood, a condition known as **ketoacidosis.** Left untreated, ketoacidosis and hyperglycemia will progress to diabetic coma and death. The treatment is immediate intervention with parenterally administered fast-acting insulin. Symptoms of ketoacidosis and impending diabetic coma include the following:

• Flushed, dry skin
• A fruity (acetone) smell on the breath
• Thirst
• Deep respirations
• Rapid, weak pulse

| Foot Care Tips |
|---|
| 1. Check your bare feet every day. Look for cuts, sores, bumps, red spots. Use a mirror or ask a family member for help if you have trouble seeing the bottoms of you feet. |
| 2. Wash your feet in warm - not hot - water every day. Use a mild soap. Do not soak your feet. Dry your feet with a soft towel. Dry between your toes. |
| 3. Cover your feet with a lotion or petroleum jelly after washing them, before putting on your shoes and socks. Do not put the lotion or jelly between your toes. |
| 4. Cut your toenails straight across. Do not leave sharp edges that could cut the next toe. |
| 5. Use a dry towel to rub away dead skin. |
| 6. Do not try to cut calluses or corns yourself with a razor blade or knife. Do not use wart removers on your feet. If you have warts or painful corns or calluses, see a doctor who treats foot problems. This kind of doctor is called a podiatrist. |
| 7. Wear thick, soft socks. Do not wear mended socks or stockings with holes or seams that might rub into your feet. |
| 8. Check your shoes before you put them on to be sure they have no sharp edges or objects in them. |
| 9. Wear shoes that fit well and let your toes move. Break in new shoes slowly. Do not wear flip-flops, shoes with pointed toes or plastic shoes. Never go barefoot. |
| 10. Wear socks if your feet are cold at night. Do not use heating pads or hot water bottles on your feet. |
| 11. Have your doctor check your bare feet at least every visit. Take off your shoes and socks when you go in the exam room. This will remind the doctor to check your feet. |
| 12. See a podiatrist for help if you can't take care of your feet yourself. |

**Figure 37-9** • Foot care tips for people with diabetes.

• Abdominal pain
• Elevated blood glucose

Occasionally, a patient with diabetes mellitus has too much insulin in the blood, resulting in **hypoglycemia,** or

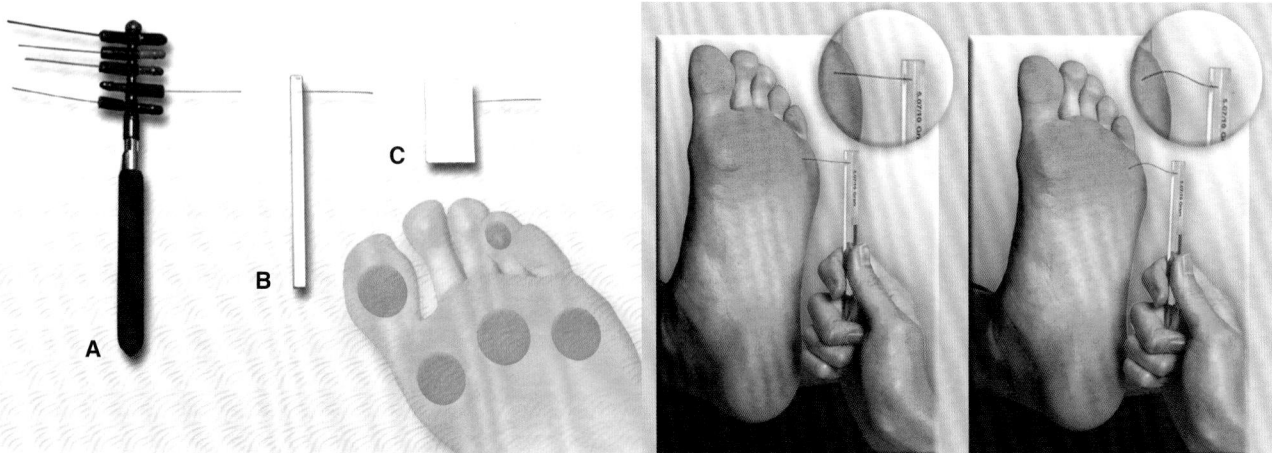

**Figure 37-10** • The monofilament test is used to assess the sensory threshold in patients with diabetes. The test instrument—a monofilament—is gently applied to about five pressure points on the foot (as shown in image on *left*). **(A)** Example of a monofilament used for advanced quantitative assessment. **(B)** Semmes-Weinstein monofilament used by clinicians. **(C)** Disposable monofilament used by patients. The examiner applies the monofilament to the test area to determine whether the patient feels the device. (Adapted from Cameron BL. Making diabetes management routine. *Am J Nurs* 2002;102(2):26–32, with permission.)

a decreased blood glucose level. This can result when the patient skips a meal or increases physical activity without making adjustments in insulin. The result can produce a condition known as *insulin shock* and includes the following symptoms:

• Pale, moist skin
• Shallow respirations
• Rapid, bounding pulse
• Subnormal blood glucose levels

Procedure 37-1 describes the management of a patient having a diabetic emergency, such as hyperglycemia and ketoacidosis or insulin shock.

 **CHECKPOINT QUESTION**

2. A patient in Laura Brewer's office asked her what is different between type 1 and type 2 diabetes. What is the difference between type 1 and type 2 diabetes mellitus?

 **PATIENT EDUCATION**

### Controlling Diabetes Mellitus

Use every opportunity to educate patients with diabetes about the importance of regulating blood glucose and eating sensibly. Also explain that, although these measures can control diabetes, the long-term effects of hyperglycemia can result in vascular changes that may cause blindness and kidney damage. Specifically, instruct patients how to:

• Maintain good personal hygiene to reduce secondary infections
• Manage their dietary intake of calories and carbohydrates
• Care for their feet properly because peripheral circulation may be poor
• Check blood glucose levels frequently and keep a log of the results
• Dispose of insulin syringes correctly
• Be aware of the signs and symptoms of diabetic ketoacidosis and insulin shock

## Disorders of the Adrenal Glands

### Addison disease

Hypoadrenocorticalism, or **Addison disease**, results from a deficiency of hormone secretion (mineralocorticoids and glucocorticoids) from the adrenal cortex. A decrease in these hormones causes an imbalance of electrolytes, specifically a loss of sodium and an increase in potassium. Other symptoms include weakness, lethargy,

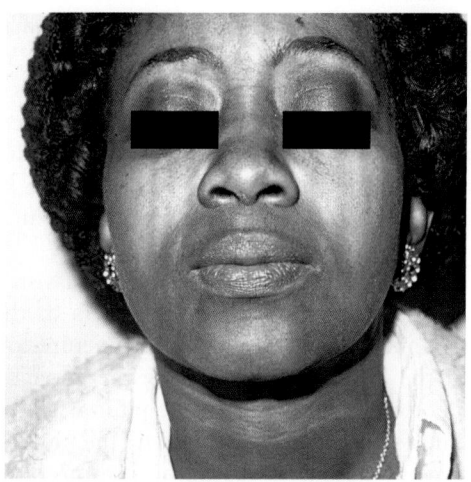
**Figure 37-11 •** Hyperpigmentation seen in Addison disease. (From Goodheart HP. *Goodheart's Photoguide of Common Skin Disorders*, 2nd ed. Philadelphia, PA: Lippincott Williams & Wilkins, 2003.)

weight loss, hypotension, anemia, and a poor tolerance to stress.

The adrenal insufficiency of this disease results in an increase in the release of adrenocorticotropic hormone (ACTH) from the anterior pituitary gland. As this hormone becomes elevated in the blood, the patient will have hyperpigmentation of the skin (Fig. 37-11). Treatment includes oral replacement of the deficient mineralocorticoid and glucocorticoid hormones.

### Cushing Syndrome

Hyperadrenocorticalism, also known as **Cushing syndrome**, may be caused by **hyperplasia** of the adrenal cortex or a tumor, resulting in an increased production of ACTH from the pituitary. Excessive cortisol promotes fat deposits in the trunk of the body, with the extremities remaining thin. Osteoporosis is accelerated, whereas the skin is fragile and heals slowly after injuries. The face is characteristically round (Fig. 37-12).

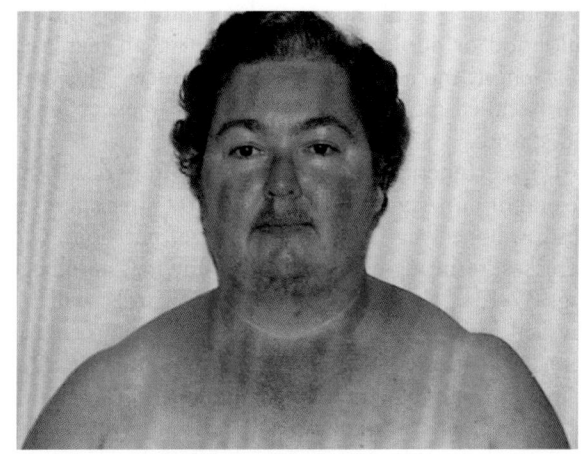
**Figure 37-12 •** The round face of Cushing syndrome. (From Weber J, Kelley J. *Health Assessment in Nursing*, 2nd ed. Philadelphia, PA: Lippincott Williams & Wilkins, 2003.)

Cushing syndrome may also be present in patients who are taking corticosteroids for medical reasons. Patients who may be prescribed corticosteroids include transplantation recipients and those with severe asthma or rheumatoid arthritis. Treatment for hyperadrenocorticalism requires removal of the cause of the hypersecretion, which could be either a pituitary or an adrenal tumor.

The role of the medical assistant in assisting with the diagnosis and treatment of disorders of the adrenal glands includes performing venipuncture for blood levels of the hormones secreted by the adrenal glands and supporting glands such as the pituitary. Diagnostic imaging tests may also be ordered by the physician and require you to obtain any preauthorizations or referrals if necessary and schedule the appropriate tests. Although the physician is responsible for advising patients on their diagnosis and treatment for adrenal gland disorders, your responsibilities may include supporting them through education and exhibiting a caring attitude to ensure compliance with any treatment prescribed by the physician.

 **CHECKPOINT QUESTION**

3. Which disorder of the adrenal gland results in elevated cortisol levels?

## Disorders of the Pituitary Gland

### Gigantism and Acromegaly

The pituitary gland, also known as the **hypophysis**, is the master gland responsible for controlling many aspects of the endocrine system. Hyperpituitarism is marked by an excess production of human growth hormone (HGH) secreted from the anterior lobe of the pituitary gland. Normally, HGH is secreted only up to the time of maturity when the epiphyseal lines on the long bones seal; however, hyperpituitarism during childhood or adolescence will result in an increase in bone length and a final height of 7 or 8 feet. This condition is called **gigantism** and is noted by excessive size and stature.

If hyperfunction of the anterior pituitary occurs near the end of puberty or during adulthood after epiphyseal closure, bone length does not change, but bone width increases, resulting in a condition known as **acromegaly** (Fig. 37-13). The patient with this disorder will have physical features such as a prominent jaw, an enlarged nose, and unusual thickening of the hands, feet, and skin. Unusual hyperactivity of the pituitary gland is associated with a tumor of the gland. Treatment of acromegaly requires surgical removal of the tumor or its destruction by radiation.

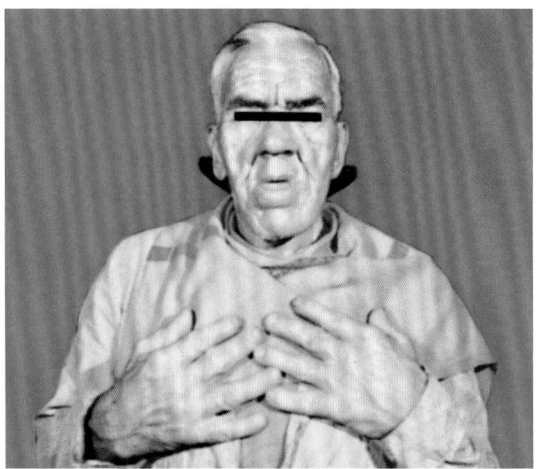

**Figure 37-13** • Acromegaly. (From Willis MC. *Medical Terminology: A Programmed Learning Approach to the Language of Health Care.* Baltimore, MD: Lippincott Williams & Wilkins, 2002.)

## Dwarfism

Hypopituitarism is a deficiency of the anterior pituitary hormones, which may be caused by injury, atrophy of the gland, or certain types of tumors. If this condition occurs early in life, growth will be retarded, and **dwarfism** will result. A person with dwarfism is extremely short but has normal body proportions. Children who are diagnosed with this disorder can be given human growth hormone (HGH) to stimulate growth.

Adult hypopituitarism may be classified according to whether the various anterior pituitary hormones are selectively or completely deficient. If all the hormones are deficient, the condition is called *panhypopituitarism*, and if only certain hormones are deficient, the condition is named for the specific deficiency.

 **CHECKPOINT QUESTION**

4. How are hypopituitarism and hyperpituitarism different?

## Diabetes Insipidus

**Diabetes insipidus** results from a deficiency of antidiuretic hormone (ADH) secreted by the posterior pituitary gland. A deficiency in this hormone causes the renal tubules in the kidneys to reabsorb water and salts, resulting in polyuria with an increased urine output between 5 and 10 L a day. Other clinical symptoms include polydipsia as the body tries to compensate for the dehydration caused by the increased urine production. Although the cause may be unknown, damage to the posterior pituitary gland from trauma or a pituitary tumor may result in this condition. Treatment involves correction of the causative factor if known and the administration of synthetic ADH by tablets, injection, or nasal spray.

As with other glandular disorders, your role in the medical office will be supportive, obtaining a thorough and complete history from the patient and performing any procedures or tests ordered by the physician to help with making an accurate diagnosis. Patients diagnosed with disorders of the pituitary gland will require patient education and emotional support to encourage compliance with any treatment prescribed by the physician.

## WHAT IF?

**What if your patient asks you if he or she should purchase and wear a medic alert bracelet?**

Many of the diseases of the endocrine system are chronic and require monitoring and appropriate administration of hormones for the remainder of the patient's life. Unfortunately, if these patients become unresponsive or unable to verbalize their condition in an emergency, the appropriate treatment may be overlooked and have serious consequences for the patient. Always encourage any patient with a chronic disease to wear a medic alert necklace or bracelet to avoid a delay in treatment should an emergency arise.

## COG COMMON DIAGNOSTIC AND THERAPEUTIC PROCEDURES

A variety of laboratory tests and diagnostic procedures may be ordered by the physician to assist in the correct identification of endocrine disorders. Your assistance with performing or scheduling these laboratory or other diagnostic procedures is important so that treatment may be initiated as quickly as possible. In most cases, testing of blood and urine can be used to measure the various hormone levels. Although the procedures for collecting these specimens are discussed in the clinical laboratory section of this text, you should be familiar with the procedures for collecting the specimen in addition to the procedure for processing the specimen appropriately. In some situations, you may have to schedule the patient for specimen collection at an outside laboratory facility.

Some examples of commonly performed tests for diabetes mellitus include the fasting glucose test and the glucose tolerance test (GTT), both using blood samples to check the levels of glucose. Although the urine glucose test is not used to diagnose or monitor diabetes

| TABLE 37-2 | Correlation of Hemoglobin A1C Values and Mean Blood Glucose Levels |
|---|---|
| **Hemoglobin A1C (%)** | **Mean Blood Glucose Levels (mg/dL)** |
| 6 | 135 |
| 7 | 170 |
| 8 | 205 |
| 9 | 240 |
| 10 | 275 |
| 11 | 310 |
| 12 | 345 |

mellitus, it is commonly part of the reagent strips used to check a variety of substances in the urine when performing a urinalysis (see Chapter 45). The glycohemoglobin, or hemoglobin A1C, blood test may be ordered by the physician to determine how well the blood glucose has been controlled in a patient with type 1 or type 2 diabetes mellitus during the previous 2 to 3 months. Ideally, a hemoglobin A1C level of 7% or lower is generally a good sign that the average blood glucose levels have been 170 mg/dL or less over the past 6 to 12 weeks. Table 37-2 describes the hemoglobin A1C levels and the corresponding mean glucose levels, and Table 37-3 describes other blood tests used to diagnose disorders of the endocrine system.

Thyroid functions tests measure the levels of T4, T3, and thyroid-stimulating hormone in the blood. In addition, the physician may order diagnostic imaging procedures to diagnose abnormalities with the thyroid gland. Specifically, a thyroid scan and the radioactive iodine uptake are ordered to diagnose thyroid disorders. During a thyroid scan, a radioactive compound

| TABLE 37-3 | Laboratory Tests for Endocrine System Disorders |
|---|---|
| **Endocrine Gland** | **Blood Test** |
| Thyroid | Thyroxine (T4) |
| | Triiodothyronine (T3) |
| Anterior pituitary | TSH (thyroid-stimulating hormone) |
| | GH (growth hormone) |
| | FSH (follicle-stimulating hormone) |
| | LH (luteinizing hormone) |
| Pancreas | Glucose |
| | Hemoglobin A1C |
| Adrenal cortex | Corticoids |

is administered and localizes in the thyroid gland. The gland is then visualized with a scanner device to detect tumors or nodules. The radioactive iodine uptake procedure determines the amount of thyroid function by having the patient take an oral dose of radioactive iodine and measuring the absorption of this iodine in the thyroid gland.

Another test for endocrine disorders is the **radioimmunoassay (RAI)**, which measures hormone levels in blood by introducing radioactive substances into the body. The test is based on the ability of antibodies to bind specifically to radioactively labeled hormone molecules and to nonradioactive molecules. Computed tomography (CT) scans, magnetic resonance imaging (MRI), and ultrasonography are also used in the diagnosis of pathologic conditions of the endocrine system. Although you will not be performing the imaging procedures used in diagnosing endocrine system disorders, your role will include scheduling the patient for these procedures as ordered by the physician.

 **CHECKPOINT QUESTION**

5. What is the purpose of the hemoglobin A1C blood test?

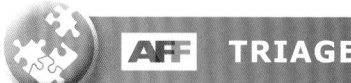 **TRIAGE**

While you are working in a medical office, the following three situations occur at the same time:

A. Patient A is a 62-year-old man who is waiting for you to obtain a blood specimen that the physician has ordered for $T_3$ and $T_4$.
B. Patient B is a new patient who has just been taken back to an examination room and needs to have vital signs taken.
C. Someone from the laboratory is on the phone with the results for a diabetic patient who had a hemoglobin A1C drawn yesterday.

**How do you sort these patients? What do you do first? Second? Third?**

First, have someone take the message from the laboratory personnel. Anyone from the clinical staff can take these results. Patient B should have his vital signs taken and recorded. After checking for completion of the necessary new patient paperwork, you should notify the physician that he is ready to be seen. While the physician is examining patient B, you should perform a venipuncture on patient A. Unless the physician has indicated a need to speak with patient A, he can be discharged after the blood specimen is taken.

 **MEDICATION BOX**

## Commonly Prescribed Endocrine System Medications

**Note:** *The generic name of the drug is listed first and is written in all lowercase letters. Brand names are in parentheses, and the first letter is capitalized.*

| | | |
|---|---|---|
| desmopressin acetate (DDAVP, Minirin) | Nasal solution: 0.1 mg/mL, 1.5 mg/mL<br>Tablets: 0.1 mg, 0.2 mg | Posterior pituitary hormone |
| glyburide (DiaBeta) | Tablets: 1.25 mg, 2.5 mg, 5 mg | Oral hypoglycemic |
| glimepiride (Amaryl) | Tablets: 1 mg, 2 mg, 4 mg | Oral hypoglycemic |
| glucagon (GlucaGen) | Powder for injection: 1 mg vial (mix with 1 mL of diluent) | Antihypoglycemic |
| hydrocortisone (Cortef) | Tablets: 5 mg, 10 mg, 20 mg | Glucocorticoid |
| insulin (Humulin R) | Injection: 100 units/mL | Antidiabetic/pancreatic hormone |
| insulin (Lispro, Humalog) | Injection: 100 units/mL | Antidiabetic/pancreatic hormone |
| insulin glargine (Lantus) | Injection: 100 units/mL | Antidiabetic/pancreatic hormone |
| levothyroxine sodium (Synthroid; Levoxyl) | Tablets: 25 mcg to 300 mcg | Thyroid hormone |
| metformin hydrochloride (Glucophage, Fortamet) | Tablets: 500 mg, 850 mg, 1,000 mg | Oral hypoglycemic |
| methylprednisolone (Medrol, Medrol Dosepak) | Tablets: 2 mg to 32 mg | Glucocorticoid |
| methylprednisolone acetate (Depo-Medrol) | Injection: 20 mg/mL; 40 mg/mL; 80 mg/mL | Glucocorticoid |
| somatropin (Accretropin, Genotropin, Humatrope) | Injection: 5 mg/mL (Accretropin)<br>Injection: 1.5 mg to 13.8 mg/vial<br>Injection: 5 mg to 24 mg/vial | Anterior pituitary hormone |
| triamcinolone acetonide (Kenalog-10, Kenalog-40) | Injection: 10 mg/mL, 40 mg/mL | Glucocorticoid |

## ROLE-PLAYING ACTIVITY

Laura Brewer, CMA (AAMA), enjoys her position working with the endocrinologist at Great Falls Medical Center and the opportunity to get to know many of the patients since they are seen on a regular basis. However, one patient in particular, Tammy Owens, has been a type 2 diabetic for nearly 15 years and takes oral medications as well as several insulin injections daily for her diabetes. Ms. Owens A1C is consistently in the 10 to 10.5 range, and she admits to not being compliant with diet restrictions and other healthy behaviors necessary to manage her diabetes effectively. What can Laura do to help this patient understand the seriousness of this disease and the consequences of unhealthy behaviors that contribute to her high blood glucose levels? Are there community resources Laura can use to help her work with this patient? If you are playing the role as the medical assistant, think about how you might feel in dealing with a patient with this chronic disease who is not doing what is necessary to control her blood glucose levels and putting her health at risk. Would you be frustrated? Angry? If you are playing the role of the patient, consider how you might feel with having a chronic disease that affects your lifestyle. Would you also be frustrated? Defeated? Your instructor will give you additional information about this activity!

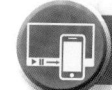
## MEDIA MENU

**Student Resources** on the**Point**®
- *Animation:* **Diabetes**
- **CMA/RMA Certification Exam Review**
- **English to Spanish Audio Glossary**

**Internet Resources**
**The Hormone Foundation**
http://www.hormone.org

**National Graves Disease Foundation**
http://www.ngdf.org

**American Diabetes Association**
http://www.diabetes.org

**American Dietetic Association**
http://www.eatright.org

**The Thyroid Foundation of America**
http://www.allthyroid.org

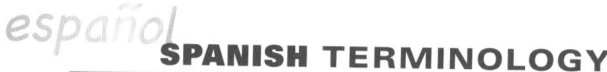
## español SPANISH TERMINOLOGY

**¿Le da mucha sed?**
Are you thirsty all the time?

**¿Le da mucha hambre?**
Are you hungry all the time?

**¿Cuantas veces orina al día?**
How many times do you urinate a day?

**Necesito una muestra de orina.**
I need a urine specimen.

**¿Cómo está su apetito?**
How is your appetite?

**Necesito tomarle una muestra de sangre.**
I need to take a blood sample.

**¿Siente palpitaciones?**
Do you feel your heart racing?

**Usted necesita un examen de sus pies.**
You need a foot exam.

**Le voy a enseñar como inyectarse.**
I will teach you how to inject yourself.

**Su glándula tiroides no produce suficientes hormonas.**
Your thyroid gland is not producing enough hormones.

**Usted necesita insulina de acción rápida.**
You need rapid-acting insulin.

## EMR Activity

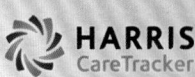
**HARRIS** CareTracker

Harris CareTracker is a Web-based electronic medical record (EMR) application that you will use for the EMR activities included in this section at the end of each chapter. This application is actually used in physician offices but is provided to you through the publisher, Wolters Kluwer Health, to give you hands-on practice working with EMRs. Your instructor will have more information about accessing your username, login, and Quickstart guide.

Prerequisite Activities in Harris CareTracker

• *The Getting Started and Quickstart documents and EMR Activities Step-by-Step Instructions are available at* http://thePoint.lww.com/KronenbergerComp5e.

Activity Details

Enter the following lab results in the EMR for patient Lonnie Taylor in the *Medical Record* module, in the *History* tab, *Preventative Care* section. Enter the results of this patient's lab work for A1C levels listed below:

| | |
|---|---|
| 06/05/2014 | 9.0 |
| 10/10/2014 | 8.0 |
| 2/03/2015 | 8.5 |
| 06/04/2015 | 7.5 |

## Chapter Summary

- The endocrine system controls many bodily processes indirectly through chemical messengers called *hormones*.
- Hormones are secreted directly into the blood stream.
- Disorders of the endocrine system include alterations in hormone secretion, and either too much hormone is secreted (hypersecretion or excess) or not enough hormone is secreted (hyposecretion or deficiency).
- Disorders of the thyroid gland include Graves disease and Hashimoto thyroiditis.
- Diabetes mellitus is a disorder of the pancreas involving the production of insulin and its ability to take glucose into the cells of the body.
- Depending on when the anterior pituitary gland secretes too much growth hormone, the patient may have gigantism or acromegaly.
- Your role in working with patients with endocrine system disorders includes emotional support to ensure compliance with treatments that are often required for the life of the patient.

## Warm-Ups for Critical Thinking

1. A 40-year-old female patient is seen in the office with a complaint of weight gain and hair loss. After the physical examination, she asks you why the physician felt the front of her neck. How would you respond? What gland is located there?
2. Your 56-year-old patient with diabetes cannot understand why his blood glucose levels are above 200 mg/dL, and he tells you that he "does not eat candy or sweets." Upon furthering questioning, you find out his diet consists of pasta and diet soda. What education does this patient need, if any? Create a brochure that would help this patient understand diabetes mellitus using language a patient would understand.
3. Research the transsphenoidal hypophysectomy surgical procedure used to remove pituitary gland tumors. How is this procedure performed? What hormone replacement medications will the patient have to take postoperatively?
4. Your patient is concerned about the thyroid function tests that the physician has ordered and asks you to explain what these tests involve. What could you say to this patient? Would you tell the patient that this test would determine the presence of a thyroid tumor? Why or why not?
5. Create a brochure for the newly diagnosed diabetic patient explaining the hemoglobin A1C test.

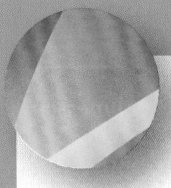

**PSY** PROCEDURE 37-1

## Manage a Patient with a Diabetic Emergency

**PSY** Instruct and prepare a patient for a procedure or treatment; coach patients regarding disease prevention and treatment plans; coach patients appropriately considering cultural diversity, developmental life stage, and communication barriers; document patient care accurately in the medical record.

**Purpose:** Respond to a patient who comes into the office with signs and symptoms consistent with a diabetic emergency, either hyperglycemia or hypoglycemia

**Equipment:** Gloves, blood glucose monitor and strips, fruit juice or oral glucose tablets

| STEPS | REASONS |
|---|---|
| 1. Wash your hands. | Hand washing aids infection control. |
| 2. Recognize the signs and symptoms of hyperglycemia and hypoglycemia.<br>*Hyperglycemia:*<br>• Flushed, dry skin<br>• A sweet, fruity smell on the breath<br>• Thirst<br>• Deep respirations<br>• Rapid, weak pulse<br>• Abdominal pain<br>*Hypoglycemia:*<br>• Pale, moist skin<br>• Shallow, fast respirations<br>• Rapid, bounding pulse<br>• Weakness<br>• Shakiness | |
| 3. Identify the patient and escort him or her into the examination room. | This prevents error in treatment, helps gain the patient's compliance, and eases anxiety. |
| 4. Determine whether the patient has been previously diagnosed with diabetes mellitus. | You may ask a patient if he or she is diabetic. However, if patients are confused, they may say "no" when they are, in fact, diabetic. You may also check the medical record or look for a medic alert bracelet or necklace, but the absence of a medic alert tag is not evidence that the patient is not diabetic. |
| 5. Ask the patient if he or she has eaten today and taken any medication. | The signs and symptoms of hyperglycemia or hypoglycemia may be difficult to distinguish. A patient who has eaten but has not taken insulin may be hyperglycemic. A patient who has not eaten but has taken insulin may be hypoglycemic. |

## PROCEDURE 37-1 (continued)

| STEPS | REASONS |
|---|---|
| **6.** Notify the physician about the patient and perform a stick for a blood glucose and measure as directed. | A patient experiencing hyperglycemia will have a capillary blood glucose between 250 and 800 mg/dL. A patient experiencing hypoglycemia will have a blood glucose of less than 70 mg/dL. |

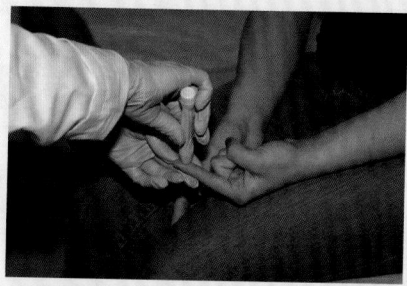

**Step 6.** Perform a fingerstick as directed by the physician or office policy and procedure.

**7.** Notify the physician of blood glucose results and treat the patient as ordered by the physician.
   **A.** Administer insulin subcutaneously to a patient with hyperglycemia.
   **B.** Administer a quick-acting sugar, such as an oral glucose tablet or fruit juice, for a patient with hypoglycemia.

It is important to act quickly while remaining calm when treating a patient having a diabetic emergency.

**8.** **AFF** Explain how to respond to a patient who is developmentally challenged.

Solicit information from anyone who may have accompanied the patient to the office. To avoid injury, assess for safety before completing a procedure when there is the possibility that the patient may not cooperate.

**9.** Be prepared to notify emergency medical services as directed by the physician if the symptoms do not improve or worsen.

In some situations, the patient requires insulin to be administered intravenously.

**10.** **AFF** Log into the electronic medical record (EMR) using your username and secure password OR obtain the paper medical record from a secure location and assure it is kept away from public access. Document all aspects of the emergency including the patient's signs, symptoms, and treatments or procedures ordered by the physician and performed by you. Do not diagnose the patient. Include the date, time, and your name/credentials in all entries.

The integrity of the medical record and patient information must be maintained and confidential. Procedures are considered not to have been done if they are not recorded.

*(continues on page 974)*

## PROCEDURE 37-1 (continued)

| STEPS | REASONS |
|---|---|

11. When finished, log out of the EMR and/or replace the paper medical record in an appropriate and secure location.

---

Charting Example:

10/14/2016 11:00 AM Pt. presented to office with complaint of weakness since last evening that has gotten worse this morning. Awake and answers questions appropriately, but seems lethargic. BP 110/62 (R) sitting, pulse 122. Skin pale, skin cool, moist. Denies being diabetic, but wearing a medic alert bracelet indicating that he is diabetic. Dr. Smith notified _____ L. Brewer, CMA

---

10/14/2016 11:05 AM Blood glucose 65 mg/dL. Pt. given 8 oz. orange juice orally and a glucose tablet as ordered _____ L. Brewer, CMA

---

10/14/2016 11:10 AM Pt. states he "feels better" but continues to look pale, pulse 110, BP 120/72. Given another 8 oz. orange juice as ordered. Repeat blood glucose 90 mg/dL _____ L. Brewer, CMA

---

Note: The medical assistant may sign his or her name in the patient record using only the "CMA" credential if the office has a signature log denoting the entire credential as "CMA(AAMA)."

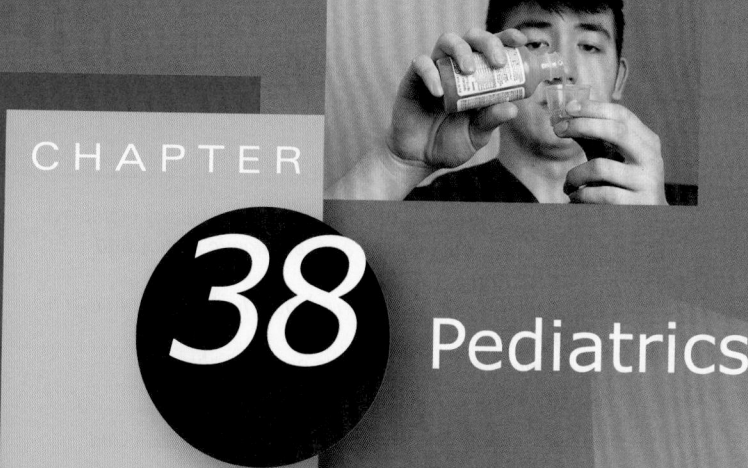

# CHAPTER

# 38 Pediatrics

## Learning Outcomes

### COG Cognitive Domain*

1. Spell key terms
2. Define medical terms and abbreviations related to all body systems
3. Compare structure and function of the human body across the life span
4. Analyze health care results as reported in graphs and tables
5. Identify common pathology related to each body system including signs, symptoms, and etiology
6. List safety precautions for the pediatric office
7. Explain the difference between a well-child and a sick-child visit
8. List types and schedule of immunizations
9. Describe the types of feelings a child might have during an office visit
10. List and explain how to record the anthropometric measurements obtained in a pediatric visit
11. Identify two injection sites to use on an infant and two used on a child
12. Describe the role of the parent during the office visit
13. List the names, symptoms, and treatments for common pediatric illnesses

### PSY Psychomotor Domain*

1. Obtain an infant's length and weight (Procedure 38-1)
   a. Instruct and prepare a patient for a procedure or treatment
   b. Coach patients appropriately considering cultural diversity, developmental life stage, and communication barriers
   c. Coach patients regarding disease prevention and treatment plans
   d. Document patient care accurately in the medical
   e. record
2. Obtain the head and chest circumference (Procedure 38-2)
   a. Instruct and prepare a patient for a procedure or treatment
   b. Coach patients appropriately considering cultural diversity, developmental life stage, and communication barriers
   c. Coach patients regarding disease prevention and treatment plans
   d. Document patient care accurately in the medical record

*(continues on page 976)*

**3.** Apply a urinary collection device (Procedure 38-3)
   **a.** *Instruct and prepare a patient for a procedure or treatment*
   **b.** *Coach patients appropriately considering cultural diversity, developmental life stage, and communication barriers*
   **c.** *Coach patients regarding disease prevention and treatment plans*
   **d.** *Document patient care accurately in the medical record*

**AFF Affective Domain\***

**1.** *Incorporate critical thinking skills when performing patient assessment*
**2.** *Incorporate critical thinking skills when performing patient care*
**3.** *Show awareness of a patient's concerns related to the procedure being performed*
**4.** *Demonstrate empathy, active listening, and nonverbal communication*

**5.** *Demonstrate respect for individual diversity including gender, race, religion, age, economic status, and appearance*
**6.** *Explain to a patient the rationale for performance of a procedure*
**7.** *Demonstrate sensitivity to patient rights*
**8.** *Protect the integrity of the medical record*

***Note: AAMA/CAAHEP 2015 Standards are italicized.***

**ABHES Competencies**

**1.** Assist the physician with the regimen of diagnostic and treatment modalities as they relate to each body system
**2.** Comply with federal, state, and local health laws and regulations
**3.** Communicate on the recipient's level of comprehension
**4.** Serve as a liaison between the physician and others
**5.** Show empathy and impartiality when dealing with patients
**6.** Document accurately

## Key Terms

| | | | |
|---|---|---|---|
| aspiration | immunization | pediatrics | sick-child visit |
| autonomous | neonatologist | psychosocial | well-child visit |
| congenital anomaly | pediatrician | restrain | |

## Case Study

*T*he pediatric specialty at Great Falls Medical Center focuses on taking care of children from birth through adolescence. They see children for all types of acute and chronic illnesses as well as visits for keeping children healthy and free from diseases when possible. Travis Haney, CMA (AAMA), enjoys working with the variety of ages of the pediatric patients. He especially enjoys working with families and caregivers in assisting the pediatrician to inform and educate them on helping their children deal with chronic illnesses. His knowledge and understanding of the stages of development for children is also greatly appreciated by the pediatrician, as Travis assists with well-child visits, taking medical histories, and getting accurate anthropometric measurements. What is a well visit, and how do you obtain anthropometric measurements? What are acute childhood illnesses, and what kinds of childhood illnesses are considered chronic? What treatments might chronic conditions require, and how can a medical assistant help? These and other questions will be covered in this chapter.

Medical assistants who work in an office where infants and children are seen must understand that the needs of children and adolescents are often different from those of adult patients. **Pediatrics** is the medical specialty devoted to the care of infants, children, and adolescents.

This care includes diagnosis and treatment of childhood diseases, prevention of accidents and trauma, and monitoring the physical and **psychosocial**, or mental and emotional, development of the child. These patients are not simply small adults; however, they may contract some of the illnesses that are seen in adult patients. Pediatric patients are also susceptible to a unique array of illnesses and problems not present in adults. Some young patients have **congenital anomalies** that are life threatening or debilitating. Because children have immature nervous systems, faster metabolism, and accelerated growth patterns, they are subject to complications that may not occur in adult patients.

A **pediatrician** is a physician who is specially trained to care for both the well child and diseases of infants, children, and adolescents. While most traditional pediatricians treat all children up through the teen years, pediatric specialists include **neonatologists**, physicians who treat only newborns, and physicians who specialize in the treatment of adolescents. In addition, the medical assistant working in the family practice office will see patients of all ages, including children.

## ⊙⊙G THE PEDIATRIC PRACTICE

### Safety

A pediatric office decorated and furnished in a manner appropriate to the physical and psychosocial needs of children creates an unthreatening and possibly even inviting environment (Fig. 38-1). Child-sized furniture helps these patients feel comfortable and welcome. Popular toys evoke happy associations. Safe toys allow for hands-on activity while the child is waiting to see the physician. Popular storybooks and magazines give parents an opportunity to read quietly to a child who may not feel well enough to play. Some offices provide waiting rooms that are designed to separate sick and well children to prevent the transmission of communicable diseases between patients.

Safety should be a prime concern for choosing toys and equipment for a pediatric office. Waiting room toys should be examined frequently and replaced when damaged or soiled. All toys should be washable and should be cleaned according to office policy to reduce the risk of disease transmission. Try to see the office from a child's

viewpoint. If necessary, get down to a child's level to discover dangers, such as sharp table corners and exposed electrical outlets, that an adult standing to observe and evaluate the environment might overlook.

The examination room should also be designed for children's safety. Keep all medical equipment out of a child's reach, and never leave a young child alone in the examining room. Follow these tips to ensure your patient's safety:

- Place infant scales on a sturdy table, and never leave an infant alone on a scale.
- Store any disinfectants away from patient care areas.
- Store and dispose of all sharps in proper containers.
- Practice stringent hand washing and standard precautions with every patient. Many childhood diseases are highly contagious and can be transmitted by poor medical asepsis.

### 🔍 CHECKPOINT QUESTION

1. What are the three safety precautions that should be used in a pediatric office?

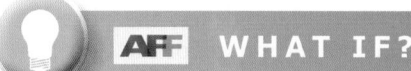

### WHAT IF?

**What if you have an uncooperative infant or child?**

During the examination and certain procedures, you may need to help restrain the child. Restraining is sometimes necessary to protect the child from injury and to help the physician complete the examination in a timely manner. Many children understandably resist the examination or procedure because they are frightened and do not want to be touched. Calm and gentle restraint is in the best interest of everyone involved.

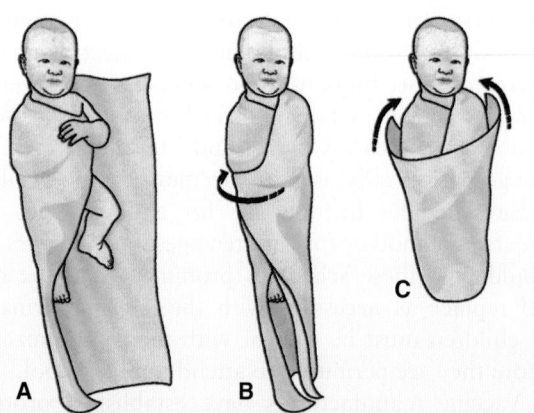

*Mummy restraint.* Place the child diagonally on a small receiving blanket. **(A)** Wrap the right corner across the torso, covering the right arm and shoulder. Pull it snugly under the child's left arm and tuck it under the child's body. **(B)** Pull the left corner across the child's left arm and shoulder, and tuck it snugly under the torso at the back so that the child's weight secures the end. **(C)** Wrap the end of the blanket up around the child.

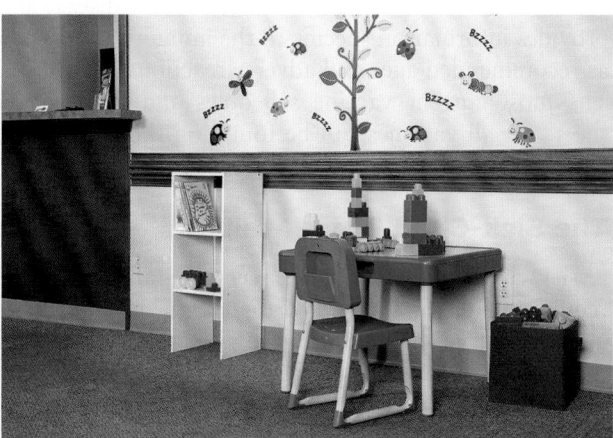

**Figure 38-1 •** The reception area for pediatric patients should be clean and safe.

# Types of Pediatric Office Visits

## The Well-Child Office Visit

Well-child visits are regularly scheduled office visits whose goal is to maintain the child's optimum health. Although these visits are typically scheduled to correspond with immunizations, the first newborn visit is often required within 1 week after birth. At this visit, you may be required to obtain a blood specimen from the newborn patient to check for the absence of the enzyme phenylalanine hydroxylase, also known as a *PKU test*. This test must be performed between 1 and 7 days after birth because an absence of this enzyme may result in mental retardation if not treated by 3 to 4 weeks of age. Treatment of the newborn with this deficiency includes a diet low in phenylalanine.

In addition to including a complete examination and an evaluation of the child's neurologic and psychosocial development, any other concerns on the part of the caregiver are also addressed at these visits (Fig. 38-2). The neurologic examination consists of the physician checking for the presence or absence of various reflexes. Table 38-1 describes various infant reflexes and the normal responses typically assessed at the well-child infant visit. In addition to the reflexes, the physician observes for development appropriate for the age of the infant or child. The child is observed or the caregiver is questioned about areas such as social development, fine motor development, gross motor development, language, and nutrition using a guide such as the Denver Developmental Screening Test II (DDST II).

The well-child visit also provides an opportunity to administer immunizations to protect children from diseases that in the past caused early death or long-term health problems. Immunizations produce immunity by slowly introducing an altered form of the disease-producing bacteria or virus into the body, which stimulates the body to produce antibodies to protect against the specific disease. Immunization schedules are developed by the American Academy of Pediatrics (AAP) and the Centers for Disease Control and Prevention, and they change periodically as new vaccines become available. These schedules include one for children ages 0 to 6 years and another for children ages 7 to 18 years. You should post these schedules prominently in the office and replace as necessary with the latest information. All children must be current with their immunizations before they are permitted to attend public school.

Vaccine manufacturers have established protocols that must be followed to ensure full immunity to the specific diseases. If you are responsible for administering vaccines, you must read all package inserts and become familiar with the correct administration and possible adverse effects before administering the medication. In addition, you must give the parent or caregiver of the child the written Vaccine Information Statement (VIS) about each vaccine you are administering (Fig. 38-3)

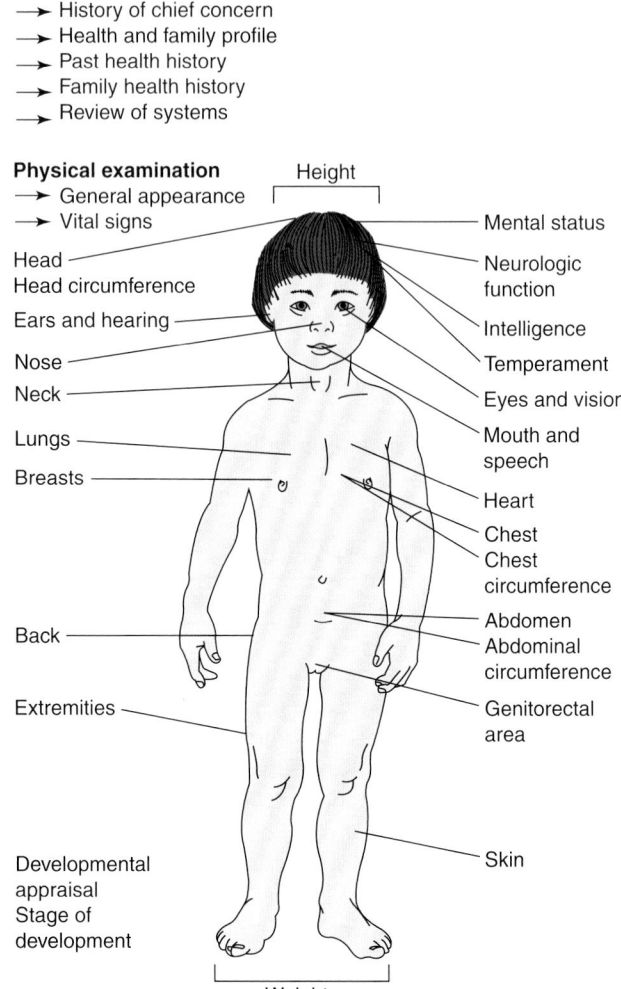

**History**
→ Demographic data
→ Chief concern
→ History of chief concern
→ Health and family profile
→ Past health history
→ Family health history
→ Review of systems

**Physical examination**
→ General appearance
→ Vital signs

Height

Mental status
Neurologic function
Intelligence
Temperament
Eyes and vision
Mouth and speech
Heart
Chest
Chest circumference
Abdomen
Abdominal circumference
Genitorectal area
Skin

Head
Head circumference
Ears and hearing
Nose
Neck
Lungs
Breasts
Back
Extremities
Developmental appraisal
Stage of development

Weight

**Figure 38-2** • Assessing the child overview: history and examination. (From Pillitteri A. *Maternal and Child Nursing*, 4th ed. Philadelphia, PA: Lippincott Williams & Wilkins, 2003.)

detailing the benefits and risks that may be associated with each vaccine. In some cases, it may be necessary to obtain written consent before administering the vaccine. The VIS for individual vaccines describes the disease and provides information specific to the immunization, such as recommended ages and adverse reactions (Fig. 38-4). The most current vaccine schedules and information sheets for all vaccines can be found on the Centers for Disease Control and Prevention Web site.

## The Sick-Child Office Visit

A **sick-child visit** occurs whenever an infant or child requires medical treatment for signs or symptoms of illness or injury. The goal of these visits is diagnosis and treatment of the child's immediate illness or injury. After examining the child, the physician may pursue diagnostic tests and treatments including radiography, laboratory tests, medication, or simply the reassurance that

| TABLE 38-1 | Infant Reflexes and Responses |
|---|---|
| **Reflex** | **Response** |
| Sucking or rooting | Stroking the cheek causes the infant to turn toward the stroke with its mouth open to suck. This reflex subsides by 3–6 months. |
| Moro or startle | A loud noise or sudden change in position causes the infant to look startled; the back arches, the arms and legs fly out and then quickly come back close to the body, and the infant cries. The Moro reflex results in the thumbs and forefingers forming a C while the other fingers spread open (in the startle reflex, the fingers remain clenched). Both reflexes disappear by 6 months. |
| Grasp | Stroking the infant's palm causes the fingers to grasp; stroking the plantar surface causes the toes to flex to grasp. The palmar grasp disappears by 3 months. The plantar grasp disappears by 9–12 months. |
| Tonic neck or fencing | With the infant supine, the physician turns the head to either side. The arm and leg on the side the infant is facing will flex, and the limbs on the opposite side will extend. This reflex disappears by 3–4 months. |
| Placing or stepping | The physician holds the infant upright at the edge of the examining table with the heel just below the edge. When the tops of the feet touch the table edge, the infant will place each foot up on the table and make walking movements. This reflex disappears by 6 weeks. |
| Babinski | When the plantar surface of the foot is stroked, the toes flare outward. This reflex disappears by 12 months. |

the illness will run a predictable and manageable course. Table 38-2 lists three common childhood illnesses and their causes, signs and symptoms, and treatments.

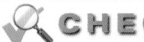 **CHECKPOINT QUESTION**

2. What is the difference between well-child and sick-child visits?

 **AFF  WHAT IF?**

**What if a child's mother complains that her baby vomits everything he eats?**

If the vomiting is projectile, the child may have pyloric stenosis, a disorder usually seen in infants several days to several months old. Diagnosis is usually made by parental history, physical examination, and radiography. The physician often can palpate an olive-shaped lump in the right upper quadrant of the abdomen while the child is supine. Surgery (pyloroplasty) is the treatment. Although pyloric stenosis is not an emergency, surgery is usually scheduled promptly to prevent dehydration. Inform the parents about the disorder and reassure them as needed.

Vomiting may also be caused by gastroenteritis, or an infection of the stomach and intestines caused by a bacterium or virus. These infants may also have diarrhea. Regardless of the cause, infants may dehydrate very quickly and should be seen by the physician without delay.

## **COG** CHILD DEVELOPMENT

### Psychological Aspects of Care

Understanding a child's psychological needs and development helps you provide safe and effective care. During an office visit, the patient may have the same feelings as adults: fear and powerlessness. However, depending on the child's age and ability to understand, the behaviors associated with these feelings are different from those of the adult patient. Specifically, children may have these feelings:

- Fear that something painful and frightening will be done
- Anxiety about repetition of a previous bad experience

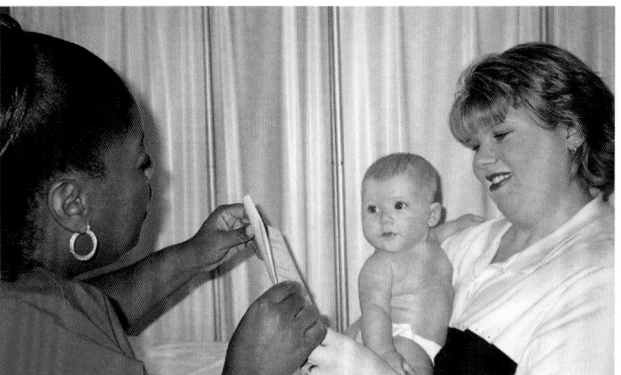

**Figure 38-3** • Provide VIS to the caregiver before administering any vaccines.

## VACCINE INFORMATION STATEMENT

# Td Vaccine

(Tetanus and Diphtheria)

## *What You Need to Know*

### 1 | Why get vaccinated?

**Tetanus** and **diphtheria** are very serious diseases. They are rare in the United States today, but people who do become infected often have severe complications. Td vaccine is used to protect adolescents and adults from both of these diseases.

Both tetanus and diphtheria are infections caused by bacteria. Diphtheria spreads from person to person through coughing or sneezing. Tetanus-causing bacteria enter the body through cuts, scratches, or wounds.

**TETANUS** (Lockjaw) causes painful muscle tightening and stiffness, usually all over the body.

- It can lead to tightening of muscles in the head and neck so you can't open your mouth, swallow, or sometimes even breathe. Tetanus kills about 1 out of every 5 people who are infected.

**DIPHTHERIA** can cause a thick coating to form in the back of the throat.

- It can lead to breathing problems, paralysis, heart failure, and death.

Before vaccines, the United States saw as many as 200,000 cases a year of diphtheria and hundreds of cases of tetanus. Since vaccination began, cases of both diseases have dropped by about 99%.

### 2 | Td vaccine

Td vaccine can protect adolescents and adults from tetanus and diphtheria. Td is usually given as a booster dose every 10 years but it can also be given earlier after a severe and dirty wound or burn.

Your doctor can give you more information.

Td may safely be given at the same time as other vaccines.

### 3 | Some people should not get this vaccine

- If you ever had a life-threatening allergic reaction after a dose of any tetanus or diphtheria containing vaccine, OR if you have a severe allergy to any part of this vaccine, you should not get Td. *Tell your doctor if you have any severe allergies.*

- Talk to your doctor if you:
  - have epilepsy or another nervous system problem,
  - had *severe* pain or swelling after any vaccine containing diphtheria or tetanus,
  - ever had Guillain Barré Syndrome (GBS),
  - aren't feeling well on the day the shot is scheduled.

### 4 | Risks of a vaccine reaction

With a vaccine, like any medicine, there is a chance of side effects. These are usually mild and go away on their own.

Serious side effects are also possible, but are very rare.

Most people who get Td vaccine do not have any problems with it.

**Mild Problems** following Td
*(Did not interfere with activities)*
- Pain where the shot was given (about 8 people in 10)
- Redness or swelling where the shot was given (about 1 person in 3)
- Mild fever (about 1 person in 15)
- Headache or Tiredness (uncommon)

**Moderate Problems** following Td
*(Interfered with activities, but did not require medical attention)*
- Fever over 102°F (rare)

**Severe Problems** following Td
*(Unable to perform usual activities; required medical attention)*
- Swelling, severe pain, bleeding and/or redness in the arm where the shot was given (rare).

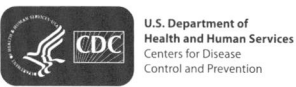

**U.S. Department of Health and Human Services**
Centers for Disease Control and Prevention

**Figure 38-4** • 2014 Td Vaccine Information Statement. (Accessed at http://www.cdc.gov/vaccines/hcp/vis/vis-statements/td.pdf)

**Problems that could happen after any vaccine:**

- Brief fainting spells can happen after any medical procedure, including vaccination. Sitting or lying down for about 15 minutes can help prevent fainting, and injuries caused by a fall. Tell your doctor if you feel dizzy, or have vision changes or ringing in the ears.

- Severe shoulder pain and reduced range of motion in the arm where a shot was given can happen, very rarely, after a vaccination.

- Severe allergic reactions from a vaccine are very rare, estimated at less than 1 in a million doses. If one were to occur, it would usually be within a few minutes to a few hours after the vaccination.

### 5 | What if there is a serious reaction?

**What should I look for?**

- Look for anything that concerns you, such as signs of a severe allergic reaction, very high fever, or behavior changes.

  Signs of a severe allergic reaction can include hives, swelling of the face and throat, difficulty breathing, a fast heartbeat, dizziness, and weakness. These would usually start a few minutes to a few hours after the vaccination.

**What should I do?**

- If you think it is a severe allergic reaction or other emergency that can't wait, call 9-1-1 or get the person to the nearest hospital. Otherwise, call your doctor.

- Afterward, the reaction should be reported to the Vaccine Adverse Event Reporting System (VAERS). Your doctor might file this report, or you can do it yourself through the VAERS web site at **www.vaers. hhs.gov**, or by calling **1-800-822-7967**.

*VAERS is only for reporting reactions. They do not give medical advice.*

### 6 | The National Vaccine Injury Compensation Program

The National Vaccine Injury Compensation Program (VICP) is a federal program that was created to compensate people who may have been injured by certain vaccines.

Persons who believe they may have been injured by a vaccine can learn about the program and about filing a claim by calling **1-800-338-2382** or visiting the VICP website at **www.hrsa.gov/vaccinecompensation**.

### 7 | How can I learn more?

- Ask your doctor.
- Call your local or state health department.
- Contact the Centers for Disease Control and Prevention (CDC):
  - Call **1-800-232-4636 (1-800-CDC-INFO)**
  - Visit CDC's website at **www.cdc.gov/vaccines**

Vaccine Information Statement (Interim)

## Td Vaccine

2/04/2014

42 U.S.C. § 300aa-26

Office Use Only

**Figure 38-4** • *(continued)*

| TABLE 38-2 | Common Childhood Illnesses | | |
|---|---|---|---|
| **Illness** | **Signs and Symptoms** | **Cause** | **Treatment** |
| Common cold | Congestion, cough, malaise, sore throat, fever | Virus | Increase oral fluids, rest, mist humidifier, cold medications if ordered by the physician |
| Gastroenteritis | Vomiting, diarrhea, fever | Virus *or* bacteria | Increase oral fluids, medications if ordered by the physician |
| Otitis media | Earache (may accompany or follow a cold), reduced the hearing, fever, tugging at the affected ear in infants | Virus *or* bacteria | Increased oral fluids, medications if ordered by physician |

- Guilt and feelings of being punished for being bad or misbehaving
- Powerlessness and loss of physical autonomy
- Curiosity about new surroundings and experiences

Some children verbalize these feelings, whereas others can express them only by crying and resisting the approach of the medical staff. As a professional medical assistant, you can reassure patients and family members by demonstrating your understanding of the child's feelings and displaying a kind and gentle manner. Include the child in the explanation of procedures on an age-appropriate level. Children who are encouraged to "help" during the examination or procedure (such as holding the adhesive bandage before receiving an injection) may also feel part of the examination and may be more cooperative.

## Physiologic Aspects of Care

To anticipate age-appropriate behavior and to provide proper psychological support and physical care, you must have a broad knowledge of child growth and development patterns. Never expect a child to react or respond beyond his or her developmental age. For example, a 2-year-old child is naturally reluctant to be examined and may resist your advances. Many 4- or 5-year-old children are curious and willing to cooperate if you turn the examination into a game. Children older than 4 years should understand the need to comply, but this age group may still have to be restrained during some procedures, such as injections. A normal child's growth and development of mind, body, and personality follow an orderly progression. Table 38-3 describes the stages of growth and development and lists special considerations for the medical assistant.

At birth, the nervous system is complete but immature. During regular visits to the pediatrician, the infant is tested for infantile automatisms—reflexes found in the newborn that disappear later in childhood (Fig. 38-5). Examples include the stepping reflex, the Moro (or startle) reflex, the Babinski reflex, and the rooting reflex. The absence of infantile automatisms after birth or the continuation of these reflexes beyond infancy suggests central nervous system dysfunction and requires further testing. A popular tool for evaluating specific gross and fine motor coordination in infants and children up to 6 years of age is the DDST II. This tool assists with

| TABLE 38-3 | Pediatric Growth and Developmental Stages | | | |
|---|---|---|---|---|
| **Age** | **Growth** | **Stage** | **Development** | **Medical Assistant Considerations** |
| Infancy (0–1 years) | Triples birth weight; increases physical control of body; may walk by first birthday | Trust | Newborn can see, hear, smell, feel pain, and communicate. Protective mechanisms include blink reflex, pulling in for warmth, and pulling away from pain or restraint. Development cephalic to caudal: head control; then full-body control (e.g., rolling over, crawling, walking); then motor (e.g., picking up small objects). Fastest period of growth and development, from total dependence to walking and talking | Involve parent; keep parent in child's view; approach child slowly; use soft, soothing voice; speak reassuringly. Advise parents to call for fever over 100.5°F, diarrhea, vomiting, failure to nurse or take a bottle. Encourage appropriate use of car seat as required by law in most states. |

**TABLE 38-3 Pediatric Growth and Developmental Stages (continued)**

| Age | Growth | Stage | Development | Medical Assistant Considerations |
|---|---|---|---|---|
| Toddler (1–3 years) | Growth rate slows; body proportions change; language skills begin | Autonomy | Growth levels off but exploration and social development continue. Negativism precedes autonomy. The child will begin to seek relationships and is acutely aware of strangers. | Use all skills above; explain procedures so child can understand; expect resistance; use firm, direct approach; ignore negative behavior; restrain to maintain child's safety; allow child to hold security object. Warn parents of increased potential for accidents. Continue to encourage use of car seat and proper restraint in motor vehicle. |
| Preschool (3–6 years) | Language and self-control develop; motor skills increase | Initiative | Socialization continues, with fairly clear-marked stages of social development in next 10 years. Many early-stage problems resolve. Except for usual communicable diseases, generally a time of good health. Diseases such as leukemia, Hodgkin disease, and various sarcomata may be present, but these are usually years spent establishing relationships with peers, exercising autonomy, and completing growth process. | Use all skills above. Encourage child to speak about feelings; explain why procedure is being done; have child help as much as possible (e.g., hold equipment). Advise parents to be alert for risks of accidents and trauma with riding toys such as tricycles and bicycles. Encourage the use of helmets. *Children over 40 pounds or 4 years can use booster seat until 8 years or 4 feet 9 inch tall. Check your state laws.* |
| School age (6–12 years) | Social skills develop; peer group becomes important; self-concept develops | Industry | | Involve child in decision making; involve child in care (e.g., collecting specimens, choosing which procedure is done first; encourage and support questions). Children may indicate what hurts and how they feel, so include child when asking questions. *Encourage use of booster seat to age 8 years and seat belt thereafter, according to state law.* |
| Adolescent (12–18 years) | Emotional changes; identity, place in world being defined | Identity | | Discuss procedures so adolescent can understand; adolescents may resist authority figures; be sure patient education includes smoking, alcohol, and perhaps birth control and sexually transmitted diseases. At physician's discretion, this information may be discussed without parent. As children in this age group begin to drive, encourage use of seat belts for self and passengers. |

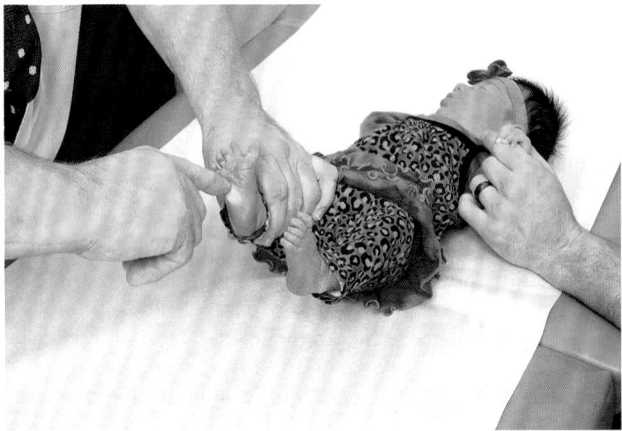

**Figure 38-5** • The presence or absence of reflexes such as the Babinski reflex in the newborn is determined during the pediatric examination.

evaluating children from the most basic reflexes to complex interpersonal reactions. If you perform the assessment, you should be trained in proper testing to evoke the most diagnostic response. Children should register within the normal range for their age. The DDST II does not measure intelligence levels.

## Role of the Parent

Parents are a source of support and comfort to a child. Their presence minimizes stress in unfamiliar surroundings. Encourage parents to remain with young children and to assist in care when appropriate. For instance, ask the parent to stand beside the child as you weigh him or her. Many children are more compliant if much of the preliminary workup is performed while the parent **restrains**, or holds, the child (Fig. 38-6).

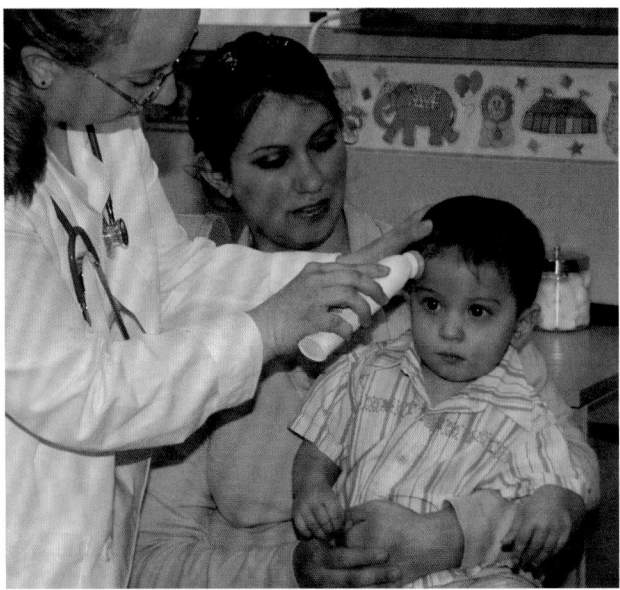

**Figure 38-6** • Much of the examination can be performed while the caregiver holds the infant or small child.

As a child develops and becomes more **autonomous**, or independent, a parent's immediate presence may be less meaningful as long as the child knows that the parent is close by. Many adolescent patients prefer to be alone with the physician to demonstrate their independence and to discuss matters that they may not be comfortable talking about with the parent present. Depending on the maturity of the adolescent, ask the patient, not the parent, if the parent should be present during the examination.

### CHECKPOINT QUESTION

3. What kinds of feelings might a pediatric patient experience during an office visit?

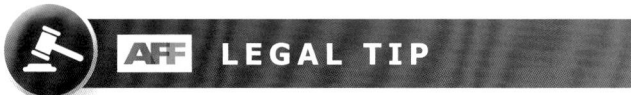

### LEGAL TIP

## Make Sure Your Interview Questions Are Appropriate

Some states require obtaining parental permission before treating a minor patient. The exceptions to this rule may include the following:

• Pregnancy or prenatal care
• Sexually transmitted disease
• Rape
• Life-threatening injury

Emancipated minors (children under age 18 years who support themselves financially), minors enlisted in the armed services, and married minors may obtain treatment without parental consent. You are responsible for knowing your state's laws regarding the treatment of minors. Refer to Chapter 2 for more information related to legal and ethical implications.

## COG THE PEDIATRIC PHYSICAL EXAMINATION

Typically, you prepare the pediatric patient for examination, and you may also assist with the examination by restraining the child. Often, you are responsible for documenting much of the history and the chief complaint and for collecting specimens for diagnostic testing. When approaching the patient, you should have a calm and cheerful manner and use a firm, but gentle, touch to increase the patient's feeling of security. Involve the parents as much as possible during the examination and keep them in the infant or child's view to reduce anxiety for both the patient and the parent.

During the examination, the physician will systematically review the body systems of the patient. The general appearance of the infant or child is assessed; the heart and lungs are auscultated; the eyes, ears, nose, and throat are inspected; and developmental issues appropriate for the age of the child are discussed with the parent or caregiver. The child who is preschool age or older will have vision and hearing tested. Your role includes obtaining relevant data from the parent, obtaining anthropometric measurements, and performing hearing and vision screening tests as appropriate. Of course, you will be responsible for recording this information in the patient's medical record.

## The Pediatric History

A child's medical history differs greatly from an adult patient's history. During the early years, it is important to know the prenatal history, including details of the mother's pregnancy, labor, and delivery. The length of the pregnancy, any maternal illnesses or complications, neonatal complications, and risk factors must be recorded as predictors of the infant's health and development. Most newborn charts contain a copy of the delivery record or birth summary outlining the delivery with the Apgar score and progress notes from the newborn nursery (Box 38-1). As the child grows, the history expands to include childhood illnesses, developmental milestones, immunizations, and nutritional status.

## Obtaining and Recording Measurements and Vital Signs

Before the physical examination is conducted, you should obtain some or all of the following measurements: height or length, head and chest circumference, weight, temperature, and the pulse and respiratory rate. The blood pressure may or may not be required, depending on the child's age and the preference of the examiner. The measurements and schedule for obtaining them should be detailed in the office policy and procedure manual.

For a well-child visit, you typically measure the child's height or length, head and chest circumference, and weight. These measurements show the child's growth and development patterns and are good indicators of health status. Weight is the most frequently obtained measurement in pediatrics; it is often needed by the physician to assess nutritional status and determine medication dosages. Head and chest measurements may alert the physician to cardiac or intracranial abnormalities. Procedures 38-1 and 38-2 describe the steps for obtaining the weight, length, and head and chest circumference.

After obtaining these measurements, you may be required to graph the weight, height or length, and head circumference on a separate growth chart that is placed into the patient's medical record (Fig. 38-7A, B). These charts are designed to show the child's growth patterns using data obtained at each well-child visit. Once the

---

**BOX 38-1    The Apgar Score**

Named for pediatrician Virginia Apgar, the Apgar score is a method for describing the general health of newborns at 1 minute and 5 minutes after delivery. Signs assessed include the following:

- Heart rate
- Respiratory effort
- Muscle tone
- Response to a suction catheter in the nostril
- Color

A perfect score for each sign is 2; a total absence of any sign is 0. A perfect score of 10 indicates the following:

- Heart rate is greater than 100 beats per minute.
- Respirations are eupneic, or the baby is crying.
- Muscle tone is good, and the baby is active.
- Baby coughs or sneezes in response to suction catheter.
- Skin is completely pink, with no acrocyanosis.

Most babies have 1-minute scores of 7 to 9 because many have a bit of acrocyanosis until respiration is fully established. Babies with 1-minute scores below 4 usually require medical assistance, particularly respiratory intervention with oxygen.

The Apgar score is not considered an indicator of future intelligence or health problems. Rather, it is used by the obstetrician, pediatrician, and delivery room personnel to assess newborns who may require closer observation or intervention.

---

measurements are plotted, the child's percentile can be determined. The percentile is used to compare the patient's growth with those of children of the same age. The head circumference is not included on growth charts for children older than 36 months, and chest circumference is usually not graphed.

### CHECKPOINT QUESTION

4. Why is it important to track a child's anthropometric measurements?

## Pediatric Vital Signs

### Temperature

A child's temperature may be measured by the axillary, oral, rectal, tympanic, or temporal artery method. If the child is compliant, the axillary route is satisfactory, but the tympanic and temporal artery methods have gained popularity because they are rapid, reliable, and most readily accepted at all ages (see Fig. 38-6). Oral measurement may be used with an older child but should not be used if

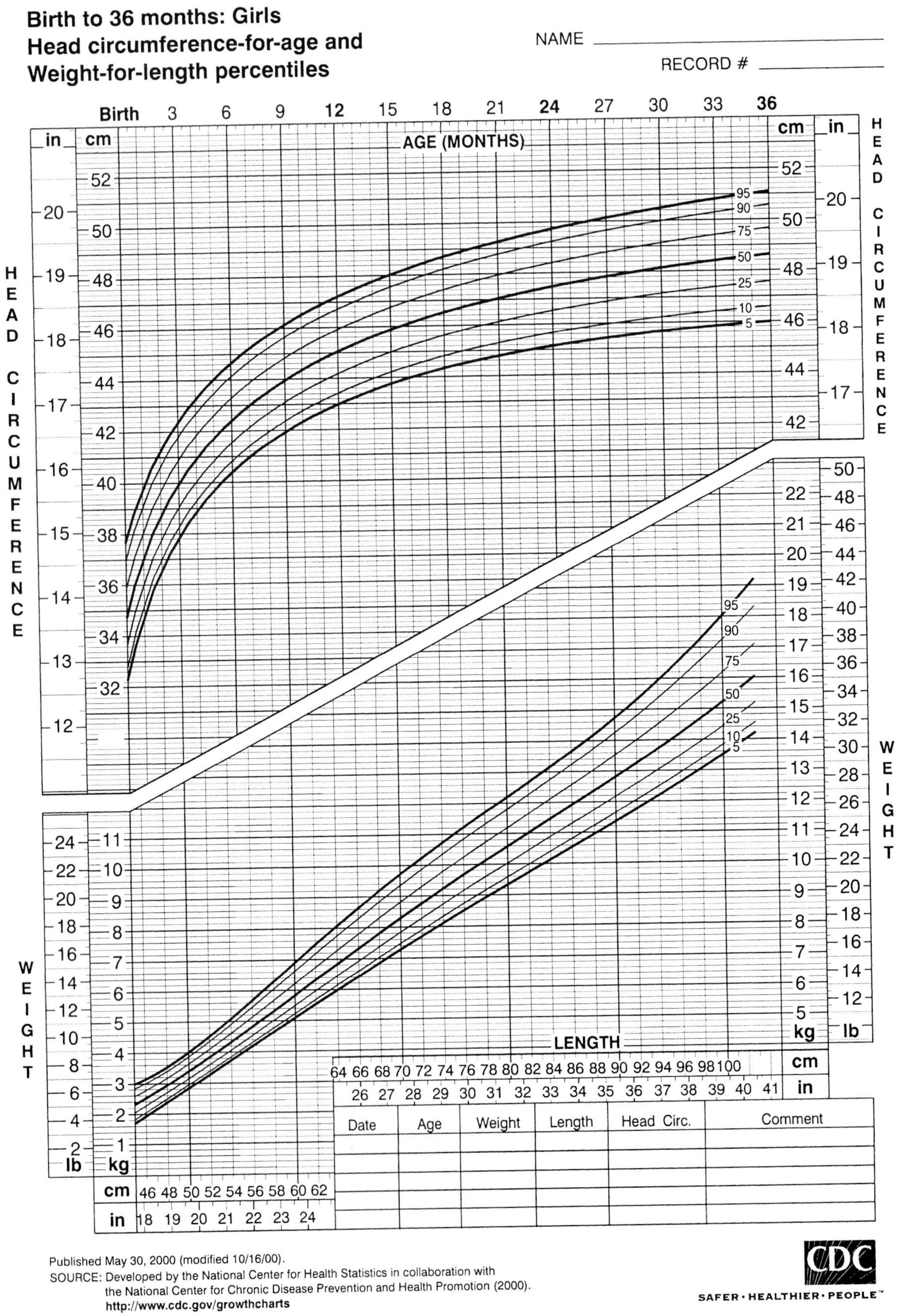

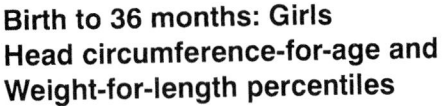

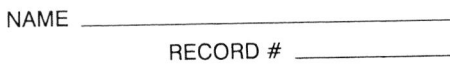

**Figure 38-7 •** Growth charts. **(A)** Birth to 36 months, girls. Growth charts.

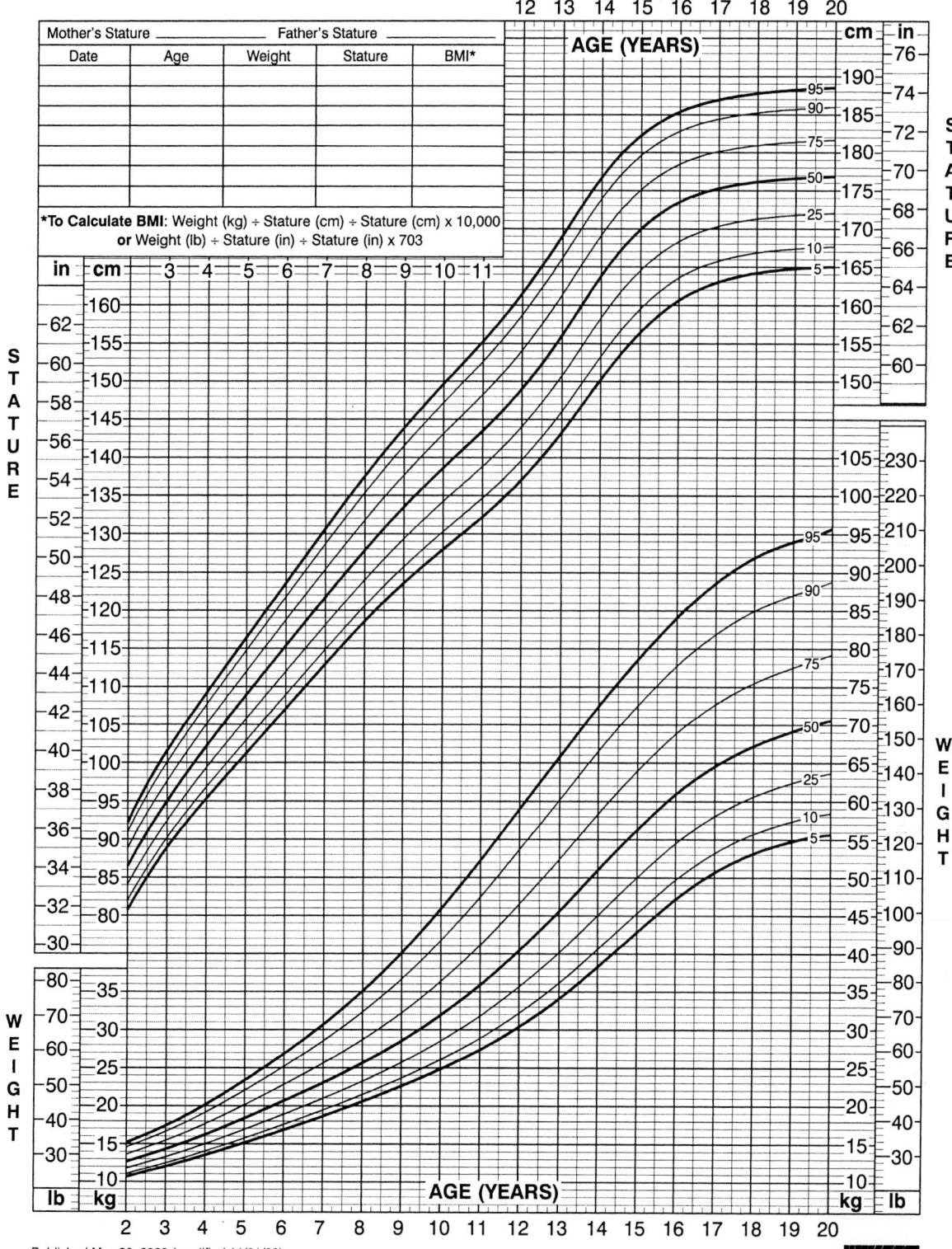

**2 to 20 years: Boys**
**Stature-for-age and Weight-for-age percentiles**

NAME _____

RECORD # _____

Published May 30, 2000 (modified 11/21/00).
SOURCE: Developed by the National Center for Health Statistics in collaboration with
the National Center for Chronic Disease Prevention and Health Promotion (2000).
http://www.cdc.gov/growthcharts

B

**Figure 38-7** • *(continued)* **(B)** Age 2 to 20 years, boys.

| TABLE 38-4 | Normal Pulse Rates for Children | |
|---|---|---|
| **Age** | **Rate/Minute** | |
| Newborn | 100–180 | |
| 3 months–2 years | 80–150 | |
| 2–10 years | 65–130 | |
| 10 years and older | 60–100 | |

| TABLE 38-6 | Normal Blood Pressure for Children | |
|---|---|---|
| **Age** | **Systolic** | **Diastolic** |
| Newborn | <90 | <70 |
| 1–5 years | <110 | <70 |
| 10 years and older | <120 | <84 |

Blood pressure measured in millimeters of mercury.

the child is congested, coughing, vomiting, or uncooperative. The rectal route should not be used for newborns and small infants or if the child has diarrhea.

### Pulse and Respirations

The pulse rate reflects the heart rate and usually is easily measured. Pulse rate can be affected by activity, body temperature, emotion, and illness. The pulse of children under 2 years of age should be assessed apically. To do this, place the stethoscope on the chest between the sternum and left nipple. Count the rate for 1 full minute. For children older than 2 years, take the radial pulse. Expect the child's heart rate to be considerably higher than an adult's rate. A newborn may have a pulse rate of 100 to 180 beats per minute, and with fever, a rate of 200 beats per minute or more is not unusual. As the child matures, the rate will slow. By age 2, a child's rate may range from 70 to 100 beats per minute. By puberty, the rate is comparable to that of an adult. Table 38-4 details normal pulse rates for children.

Measure respiratory rate by observing the rise and fall of the child's chest. It is not necessary to disguise the fact that you are counting respirations as with adults. Because infants breathe using the abdominal muscles more than the chest, observe abdominal movements and count for 1 full minute. For children over age 2 years, use the same method as adults: Count the respiratory rate for 30 seconds and multiply by two. Expect a newborn's respiratory rate to be as high as 35 per minute (Table 38-5). Like the pulse rate, the respiratory rate will slow as the child matures. At age 2 years, it will be about 25, and by puberty, it will be comparable to an adult's rate.

### Blood Pressure

Blood pressure measurements are not required for most pediatric patients but may be appropriate at times. Blood pressure is the most difficult measurement to obtain in an infant or child because it is so difficult to prevent movement. Infants and children have smaller extremities than adults and require a smaller cuff. Because of their soft, nonresistant vessels and smaller bodies, children have lower blood pressure than adults. You may have problems determining the diastolic pressure in some children using a standard sphygmomanometer. In children less than 1 year of age, expect a blood pressure of about 90/50. The blood pressure will gradually rise as the child matures. By age 10, a child's blood pressure will be in the low normal range of 110/60 (Table 38-6). Blood pressure checks become routine when children are about school age.

### CHECKPOINT QUESTION

5. How does a child's pulse and respiratory rate differ from an adult's?

## COG ADMINISTERING MEDICATIONS

Administering medications to children challenges you and the parents who are responsible for home administration. Medication dosages for children are calculated by weight or by body surface area. However, because children vary in weight, age, and fat-to-muscle ratio, they metabolize and absorb medication at varying rates. As a result, the physician prescribes medication according to how much the child weighs, and you must give only the amount prescribed. To prevent errors, always check drug dosage calculations for an infant or child with another staff member. The formulas for calculating pediatric dosages are described in Chapter 24. Before administering any medication, you should know the safe amount, correct administration procedure, intended actions, and side effects. In most pediatric practices, the physician uses only 50 or so medications that are suitable for children, making it relatively easy for you to learn all that is necessary about each medication. As for any medication, the seven "rights" of drug administration remain the same: the *right patient*, *right drug*, *right dose*, *right route*, *right time*, *right method*, and *right documentation*.

## Oral Medications

Use caution when administering oral medications to a child to prevent **aspiration**. Hold infants in a semireclining

| TABLE 38-5 | Normal Respiratory Rates for Children | |
|---|---|---|
| **Age** | **Rate/Minute** | |
| Newborn | 30–35 | |
| 1–2 years | 25–30 | |
| 4–6 years | 23–25 | |
| 8 years and older | 16–20 | |

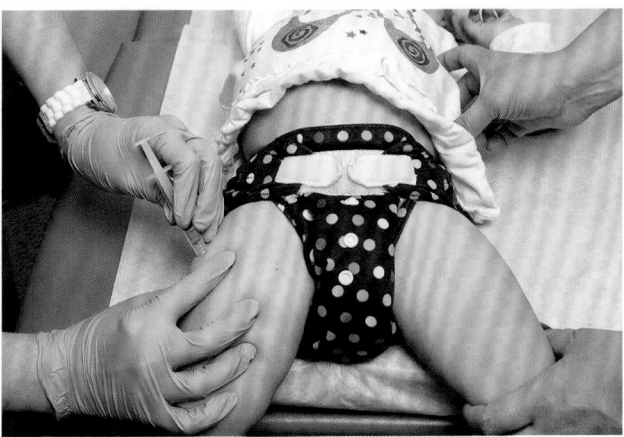

**Figure 38-8 •** The vastus lateralis is the site of choice for infant injections.

position, not lying down. Place the medication in the mouth beside the tongue. Depending on the child's age, use a medication spoon, syringe, dropper, or medicine cup. Many children will suck medication from a syringe easily and safely. Administer small amounts of medication, allowing the child time to swallow. Always explain to children who are old enough to understand why medications are important, and then proceed in a swift and safe manner to give the medication.

## Injections

Medications are given to infants and children by injection when there is no choice. Children commonly fear injections more than any other medical procedure. You should approach the child in a calm and firm manner, but never lie to the child or say that the injection will not hurt. Although it is important for the child to know that an injection is about to be given, you can prevent some anxiety by not letting the child see the syringe. Offer the child an age-appropriate explanation, and then quickly give the medication. After administering any medication, praise and comfort the child.

Most children's injections are given in the vastus lateralis, at least until age 2 years (Fig. 38-8). The dorsogluteal site is not used for children under age 2 years because the muscles have not developed well. Chapter 24 lists the steps in administering an intramuscular injection.

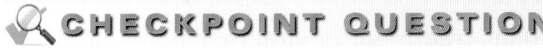

### CHECKPOINT QUESTION

6. How is medication dosage calculated for children?

## COLLECTING A URINE SPECIMEN

Because infants and small children cannot void into a specimen container on command, you must use a collection device if a urine specimen is needed. Procedure 38-3

describes the procedure for applying a urinary collection device. Once applied, the device should be left in place until the infant urinates. The infant may wear a diaper over the collection device until the specimen is obtained.

## UNDERSTANDING CHILD ABUSE

A child's social and physical well-being may be compromised by physical or emotional abuse or neglect or by sexual abuse. Abuse is thought to be the second most common cause of death in children under age 5 years. Although many children are permanently disabled or seriously injured as a result of physical abuse, many more carry emotional scars that will never heal. Medical assistants should be aware of the signs of abuse—either obvious indications or subtle warnings—that must be pursued for the child's safety.

These are the *obvious* indications of child abuse:

- Reports of physical or sexual abuse by the child
- Previous reports of abuse in the family with current indicators
- Conflicting stories about the "accident" or injury from the parents and the child
- Injuries inconsistent with the history
- Injuries blamed on siblings or someone other than the parent
- Repeated emergency room visits for injuries
- Fractures, burns, or skeletal injuries of a suspicious nature
- These indications of child abuse are *hidden* or not apparent:
- Dislocations
- Nervous system trauma, particularly shaken baby syndrome
- Internal injuries, particularly to the abdominal area
- These are *behavioral* indications of child abuse:
- Too-willing compliance, overeagerness to please
- Passive avoidance, such as refusing to make eye contact, shrinking from contact
- Extremely aggressive, demanding, rage-filled behavior
- Role reversal, parenting the parent
- Developmental delay (the child may be using energy needed for maturation to defend against abuse)

These are the *warning signs* of child abuse:

- Malnutrition
- Poor growth pattern
- Poor hygiene
- Gross dental disorders
- Unattended medical needs

If you suspect a child is being abused, approach the child and the parent in a calm and supportive manner. Discuss any suspicions about the cause of a child's injuries privately with the physician right away. State laws vary regarding the procedure for reporting abuse; local regulations should be outlined in the policies and procedures manual. As a medical assistant, you have an ethical and moral responsibility to report suspected cases of abuse or neglect.

## LEGAL TIP

### Reporting Suspected Child Abuse

The Federal Child Abuse Prevention and Treatment Act mandates that threats to a child's physical and mental welfare be reported by anyone having contact with children in a professional or employment setting (e.g., teachers, physicians, nurses, medical assistants, daycare workers). Health care workers, teachers, social workers, and others who work with children are protected against liability if they report their suspicions in good faith.

## COG PEDIATRIC ILLNESSES AND DISORDERS

Because children do not have a well-developed immune system, they are particularly susceptible to viral and bacterial infections. As a result, sick-child visits occur frequently during early childhood. Some infants and small children have febrile seizures during illness because of the child's immature nervous system. This does not mean that the child will be prone to seizures as he or she matures. Parents should be instructed how to obtain a child's temperature and be encouraged to call the office for any evidence of a fever. All parents should be advised never to give aspirin to young children with viral fever, since aspirin has been associated with Reye syndrome. This syndrome causes encephalopathy and fatty infiltration of the internal organs and may cause either mental retardation or death. Check with the physician about the type of medication to use before suggesting any medication or antipyretic, including over-the-counter medications.

### Impetigo

A common skin disorder in children is impetigo, a contagious bacterial infection that may be caused by either the *Staphylococcus* or *Streptococcus* bacteria. The lesions commonly occur on the face, neck, and other exposed areas of the body (Fig. 38-9). Patches of exudative vesicles produce honey-colored crusts. These vesicles leave red areas when the crusts are removed.

The treatment for impetigo is washing the area two to three times a day and applying a topical antibiotic. An oral antibiotic may be prescribed for severe cases. Discourage scratching and advise parents to keep separate and wash frequently any towels, washcloths, and bed linens to prevent the spread of the disease.

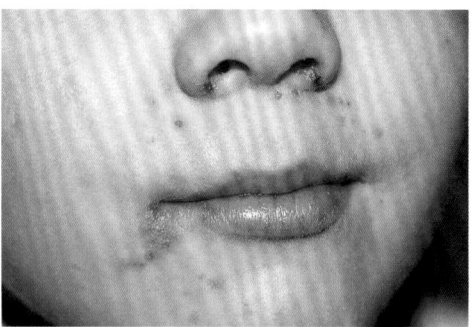

**Figure 38-9 •** Impetigo lesions are commonly found on the face and neck.

### Meningitis

Inflammation of the meninges covering the spinal cord and the brain, termed meningitis, can result from either a bacterial or a viral infection. Viral meningitis is usually not life threatening and is short-lived, but bacterial meningitis is often severe and may be fatal. The infectious process is usually precipitated by an upper respiratory, sinus, or ear infection, and since these infections commonly occur in children under age 5 years, they are the most likely age group to develop this disease. Meningitis can also result from head trauma in which an open area allows the microorganisms to enter the nervous system. Older adolescents living in college dormitories or residence halls are also at high risk for meningitis and should be immunized before leaving for college.

The signs and symptoms of meningitis include nausea, vomiting, fever, headaches, and a stiff neck. A rash with small, reddish-purple dots may appear on the body. As the patient becomes sicker, he or she may become comatose and develop seizures. To diagnose suspected meningitis, the patient is often sent to the emergency room where the physician orders a complete blood count. If the white blood cell count is elevated, a lumbar puncture is performed to withdraw cerebrospinal fluid for analysis. The treatment of meningitis is based on the microorganism. Bacterial and viral meningitis are treated with oral fluids and bed rest, and antibiotics are prescribed if the causative microorganism is bacterial. Although hospitalization is always required for bacterial meningitis, children with viral meningitis may also be admitted to the hospital for supportive care.

### CHECKPOINT QUESTION

7. How does treatment of viral meningitis differ from that of bacterial meningitis?

### Encephalitis

Encephalitis is inflammation of the brain that frequently results from a viral infection following chickenpox, measles, or mumps. A strain of the virus is transmitted by mosquitoes. This type is primarily seen on the East and Gulf coasts. Symptoms of all forms include drowsiness, headache, and fever in the early stages; however, seizures and coma may occur in the later stages. As with meningitis, patients suspected of having encephalitis are usually sent to the hospital emergency room for evaluation, including a lumbar puncture and analysis of the cerebrospinal fluid. A diagnosis of encephalitis requires hospitalization for intravenous therapy and supportive care, but the prognosis is usually good if the diagnosis is made early and treatment begins quickly.

## Tetanus

Tetanus, commonly called *lockjaw*, is an infection of nervous tissue caused by the tetanus bacillus, *Clostridium tetani*, which lives in the intestinal tract of animals and is excreted in their feces. The organisms are found in almost all soil. The bacilli enter the body through a puncture wound or open area in the skin. Wounds caused by farm equipment in which manure is present are especially susceptible to tetanus. All deep, dirty wounds should be treated as high risk for tetanus. You should make it a habit to always ask about previous tetanus immunization in patients with any type of accidental laceration or puncture wounds. The vaccine for tetanus is included in the schedule of pediatric immunizations as the diphtheria and tetanus toxoids and acellular pertussis vaccine (DTaP).

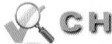 **CHECKPOINT QUESTION**

8. What is the best way to prevent tetanus?

## Cerebral Palsy

*Cerebral palsy* is a term for a group of neuromuscular disorders that result from central nervous system damage sustained during the prenatal, neonatal, or postnatal period of development. Although cerebral palsy is not progressive, the damage may become more obvious as developmental delays are discovered. Impairment may range from slight motor dysfunction to catastrophic physical and mental disabilities. Prognosis varies with the site of the damage and its severity, and, unfortunately, there is no cure. Treatment for patients with cerebral palsy is supportive and rehabilitative. Although the physical impairments may be obvious, you must determine the developmental level of each child individually and interact with the child accordingly. In addition, the physical challenges exhibited by the child with cerebral palsy may not reflect the cognitive abilities. These children may acquire the same pediatric illness and diseases of any child and require immunizations and follow-up expected for any patient. You may also be involved in obtaining preauthorizations and referrals for rehabilitative and supportive care as ordered by the physician.

## Croup

Laryngotracheobronchitis, also known as croup, is a disease primarily seen in children 3 months to 3 years of age.

This disease is caused by a viral infection of the larynx resulting in swelling and narrowing of the airway, which results in dyspnea (difficulty breathing). A child exhibiting signs of possible croup will often have stridor (high-pitched crowing wheeze) on inspiration and a sharp, barking cough. Although children diagnosed with croup may be seen in the office, some children may require hospitalization as determined by the physician. Whether treated at home or in the hospital, antibiotics are usually not ordered unless a secondary bacterial infection is suspected. A cool mist vaporizer and medication to decrease the swelling are often prescribed by the physician.

## Epiglottitis

Swelling of the epiglottis may resemble croup, but it is usually more serious and may be life threatening if it progresses to complete obstruction of the airway. It occurs most frequently in children aged 2 to 6 years, although it can be seen in all age groups. It is caused by a bacterial infection, usually *Haemophilus influenzae*. A child diagnosed with epiglottitis in the medical office must be transported immediately to the hospital, since the first priority is maintaining and possibly establishing an airway. As with any medical emergency in the office, you must be prepared to assist the physician as needed while contacting the emergency medical services for transport. In addition, the parents of the sick child will need support and guidance during this emotional time.

## Cystic Fibrosis

Cystic fibrosis is an inherited disease that affects the exocrine glands of the body, changing their secretions and making the mucus extremely thick and sticky. Although the disease affects several areas of the body, the most serious complications of cystic fibrosis are usually respiratory. Children with cystic fibrosis are prone to repeated respiratory infections because of the difficulty in clearing the mucus from their airways. Treatment of cystic fibrosis includes medication to reduce the thickness of secretions and frequent breathing treatments to maintain open airways. Many new treatments are being developed, and much exciting research into prevention and cure is underway.

 **CHECKPOINT QUESTION**

9. Why is epiglottitis considered a medical emergency?

## Asthma

As discussed in Chapter 31, asthma is a reversible inflammatory process of the bronchi and bronchioles. When a patient with asthma has dyspnea, it is due to bronchospasm and constriction of the smooth muscle lining the airways. Patients have an increase in mucus production with

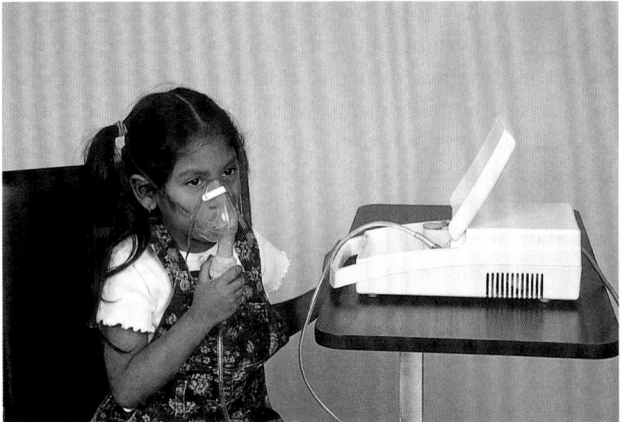

**Figure 38-10** • Breathing treatments may be administered through a mask.

a productive cough. It becomes difficult for the patient to move air into and out of the lungs. In children, asthma attacks may be triggered by exposure to an allergen in the environment such as mold or dust, an inhaled irritant such as cigarette smoke, or upper respiratory infection. Many children who develop asthma outgrow it by adulthood.

The treatment for asthma includes the administration of bronchodilators through an inhaler, which may not be appropriate for a small child or infant, or through a nebulizer machine (see Chapter 30 for more information about nebulized breathing treatments). An infant or small child will not be able to hold the mouthpiece tightly between the lips during the treatment; however, masks are available (Fig. 38-10). As with adult patients taking bronchodilators, the pulse rate should be monitored before, during, and after the treatment.

## Otitis Media

Otitis media, an inflammation or infection of the middle ear, is frequently caused by an upper respiratory infection (URI) in infants and children (Fig. 38-11). This

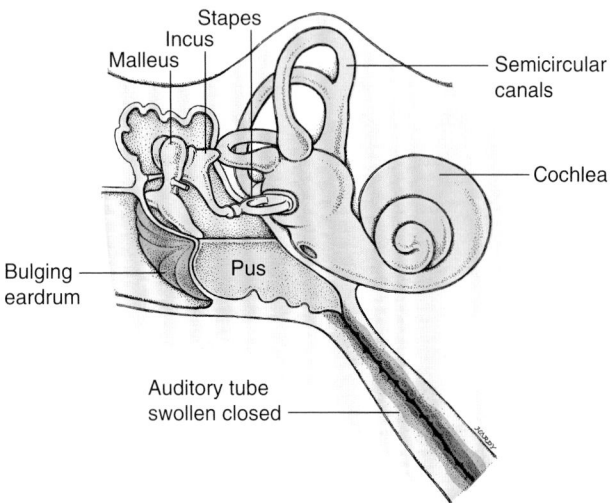

**Figure 38-11** • Internal structures of the ear with otitis media.

disorder is particularly common in infants and children because of the relatively horizontal position of the eustachian tube between the nasopharynx and middle ear (see Chapter 30). Symptoms include severe pain, fever of varying degrees, and mild to moderate hearing loss. Infants may be fussy and tug at their ears. Any elevation in a child's temperature should be a warning to check for otitis media.

Diagnosis is usually made by inspecting the tympanic membrane with an otoscope, which reveals a reddened, bulging tympanic membrane. If the suspected pathogen is bacterial, an antibiotic may be prescribed. With the exception of aspirin, analgesics are often recommended for the relief of the pain. If nasal congestion is present, a decongestant may reduce some of the swelling. In severe chronic cases, surgery may be performed to relieve pressure, and tubes may be inserted through the tympanic membrane to equalize the pressure.

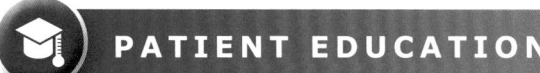

### PATIENT EDUCATION

## Middle Ear Infections

Explain to the child's parents that children have short, straight eustachian tubes. Upper respiratory infections, particularly with coughing, may force microorganisms into the middle ear spaces. As the infection grows, the eustachian tubes swell and eventually close. Exudate from the mucous membrane continues to be produced, causing fluid to build with resulting pressure and pain.

Although the infecting microorganism can be bacterial or viral, bacterial otitis media may be caused by putting the child to bed with a bottle of milk, juice, or formula. The drink and bacteria from the mouth set up a medium for growth within the eustachian tube. Provide patient education to caregivers whenever possible.

## Tonsillitis

Pharyngitis, or a sore throat, may be caused by inflammation of the tissues of the throat and/or the tonsils (see Chapter 30). Inspection of the throat may reveal the tissue to be red and swollen, possibly with pustules on the tonsils or in the throat. When a diagnosis of tonsillitis is made, you may be asked to take a sample for a throat culture to rule out *Streptococcus* bacteria as the causative pathogen. (Chapter 44 describes the steps for obtaining a throat culture.) If the throat culture is positive for *Streptococcus*, an antibiotic will be ordered. If the throat culture is negative but the infection appears bacterial, an antibiotic may still be prescribed. Chronic tonsillitis may be treated by surgical removal of the tonsils—a tonsillectomy—by a surgeon who specializes in disorders of the ears, nose, and throat. The medical assistant will often be responsible for obtaining a preauthorization and referral if needed and scheduling the consultation appointment with the referring ear, nose, and throat surgeon.

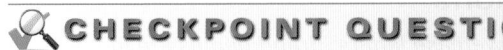

## CHECKPOINT QUESTION

10. Why is otitis media more common in children than adults?

## Obesity

According to the American Academy of Pediatrics (AAP), obesity in children has become an epidemic. The importance of assessing the weight and length of infants and children and plotting this information on the appropriate growth chart is essential in assisting the physician in early recognition; however, prevention of obesity is even more important in preventing long-term complications, such as heart disease and diabetes. You must ask parents or caregivers during each visit to the office about the eating patterns, nutritional status, and activity levels of the child and offer education and support when necessary or as indicated by the physician. Since children develop eating habits early in life and take these habits into adulthood, you should teach parents about eating in moderation and increasing physical activity as a means to reduce the weight of an overweight child or prevent abnormal gains in weight. If the physician prescribes a specific diet or reduces caloric intake, you should offer support and guidance to the caregiver as needed.

## Attention Deficit Hyperactivity Disorder

Attention deficit hyperactivity disorder (ADHD) is a condition of the brain affecting boys more frequently than girls and causing difficulty in controlling behavior. The problematic behavior in children with ADHD includes the following *signs of inattention* in the school-aged child:

- Daydreaming or difficulty paying attention
- Easy distraction
- Inability to complete tasks
- Forgetfulness
- Reluctance to perform tasks that require mental effort
- Low grades in school

The *signs of hyperactivity* are often seen in the following behaviors:

- Excessive talking
- Inability to sit quietly for any length of time
- Breaking rules regarding running or jumping

In addition to inattention and hyperactivity, children with ADHD are often impulsive and behave irrationally to others, even after being repeatedly warned about a specific behavior, dangerous or not. These children have difficulty taking turns and may be disruptive, shouting out answers before being called on in the classroom.

The diagnosis for a child with ADHD is often based on a thorough history of the child's behaviors, including reports from teachers or other professionals who work with the child. The AAP publishes guidelines for diagnosing ADHD in children ages 6 to 12 years. There is no one test for diagnosing this disorder; instead, the diagnosis is based on certain behaviors in several settings (i.e., school and home). Once the physician has made the diagnosis, an individual treatment plan is devised; it may include behavior therapy, psychological counseling for the child and the family, education about ADHD, coordination of the treatment plan with the family and involved teachers, and medications.

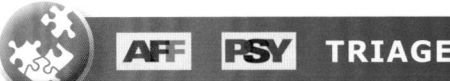

While working in a family practice office, you have to complete the following three tasks:

A. Patient A is a 2-month-old child who has just been placed in examination room 1. You are to take the vital signs and measurements, including length, weight, and head circumference.
B. Patient B is a 14-month-old child who was seen today and diagnosed with otitis media. The physician has asked you to give the parent a prescription for an antibiotic and schedule a referral with an ear, nose, and throat physician for possible myringectomy and tubes.
C. A mother is on the phone and is concerned because patient C, her newborn, is vomiting.

**How do you sort these tasks? What do you do first? Second? Third?**

First, speak to the mother of patient C. This infant will dehydrate very quickly, and the situation must be assessed promptly and efficiently. Give advice about increasing fluids or giving pediatric electrolyte solutions *only* after assessing the situation, consulting with the physician, and receiving instructions from the physician to pass along to the mother. Next, deal with patient B by giving the parent the prescription and clarifying any other orders from the physician. The information regarding the referral can be given to the parent to make the arrangements, or you may make the appointment later in the day, when time permits. Of course, the required paperwork for the referral must be faxed to the referral physician, and this may be delegated to an administrative assistant according to the office policy and procedure manual.

See patient A after patient B is discharged. When obtaining a history for a well-child checkup, you want to give the parent your undivided attention and take extra time to establish rapport with the parent and the infant.

## Medication Box

### Commonly Prescribed Pediatric Medications

**Note:** *The generic name of the drug is listed first and is written in all lowercase letters. Brand names are in parentheses, and the first letter is capitalized.*

| | | |
|---|---|---|
| Acetaminophen (Tylenol) | Oral syrup: 16 mg/mL<br>Oral solution: 48 mg/mL<br>Oral suspension: 80 mg/0.8 mL<br>Suppositories: 80 mg, 120 mg, 125 mg, 300 mg | Antipyretic<br>Analgesic |
| Acetylsalicylic acid (ASA, aspirin) (Bayer, St. Joseph's) | Tablets (chewable): 325 mg<br>Suppositories: 120 mg, 200 mg | Antipyretic<br>Analgesic (*do not give* to children with viral illness) |
| Amoxicillin trihydrate (Amoxil) | Oral suspension: 50 mg/mL, 125 mg/5 mL, 200 mg/5 mL<br>Tablets (chewable): 125 mg, 200 mg, 250 mg, 400 mg | Antibiotic |
| Atomoxetine (Strattera) | Capsules: 10 mg, 18 mg, 25 mg, 40 mg, 60 mg, 80 mg, 100 mg | Attention deficit hyperactivity disorder |
| Ceftriaxone sodium (Rocephin) | Injection: 250 mg, 500 mg, 1 g, 2 g | Antibiotic |
| Diphtheria and tetanus toxoids and acellular pertussis vaccine (DTaP) (Daptacel; Infanrix) | Injection: 0.5 mL | Vaccine (intramuscular [IM]) |
| *Haemophilus* b conjugate vaccine, meningococcal protein conjugate (PedvaxHIB) | Injection: 0.5 mL | Vaccine (IM) |
| *Haemophilus* b conjugate vaccine, meningococcal protein conjugate (PedvaxHIB) | Injection: 0.5 mL | Vaccine (IM) |
| Hepatitis B vaccine recombinant (Engerix-B; Recombivax HB) | Injection: 0.5 mL | Vaccine (IM) |
| Ibuprofen (Children's Motrin; Children's Advil; PediaCare Fever) | Oral drops: 40 mg/mL<br>Oral suspension: 100 mg/5 mL<br>Tablets (chewable): 50 mg, 100 mg | Antipyretic<br>Analgesic |
| Measles, mumps, and rubella virus, live (M-M-R II) | Injection: 0.5 mL | Vaccine (subcutaneous) |
| Methylphenidate (Concerta; Ritalin) | Tablets: 5 mg, 10 mg, 20 mg<br>Tablets: 18 mg, 27 mg, 36 mg, 54 mg | Attention deficit hyperactivity disorder |
| Pancreatin (Kutrase) | Capsules: 2,400 units lipase, 30,000 units protease, 30,000 units amylase | Pancreatic enzyme |
| Poliovirus vaccine, inactivated (IPV) rotavirus, live (Rotarix, RotaTeq) | Injection: 0.5 mL<br>Oral suspension: (Rotarix) 1 mL at age 6 weeks, 1 mL after 4 weeks (2 doses)<br>Oral suspension: (RotaTeq) 2 mL at age 6 weeks, 2 mL after 4 weeks, and 2 mL at 10 weeks (3 doses) | Vaccine (IM)<br>Vaccine |
| Simethicone (Mylicon) | Drops: 40 mg/0.6 mL | Antiflatulent |

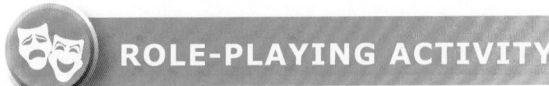

# ROLE-PLAYING ACTIVITY

The immunization policy at Great Falls Medical Center adheres strictly to the immunization guidelines of the American Academy of Pediatrics and the Centers for Disease Control and Prevention. GFMC believes that the risks of the diseases that the vaccines prevent are far greater than the unproven risks for their safety and that parents who delay or decline vaccines put their child and other susceptible children at risk. The immunization policy further states that although GFMC respects the rights of all parents/guardians to make decisions for their children, they are committed to the well-being of all patients and their families. The following policy will be followed regarding immunizations:

- All patients will be immunized according to the appropriate CDC immunization schedule.
- Immunizations will be started at the patient's first well visit.
- If parents/caregivers cannot comply with this policy, they must find another pediatrician immediately.

Naomi Turner brought her 2-year-old daughter for her first well visit and advised Travis Haney, CMA(AAMA), that she had never had the child immunized because she didn't feel they were safe. If you are playing the role as the medical assistant, consider how you might educate this patient on the necessity and safety of vaccines. What resources could you use to provide information about vaccines? Think about the GFMC immunization policy and how this might be brought up in your conversation with Ms. Turner. If you are playing the role as the mother of the child, consider how you might feel about having your child given injections for something you aren't comfortable with her receiving? Would you be nervous or afraid? Would you feel defensive? Consider her protective attitude with her child and only wanting what she thinks is best. Your instructor will give you additional information about this activity!

# *español* SPANISH TERMINOLOGY

**¿ El niño/la niña ha estado enfermo o se ha hecho algún daño?**
Has the child had any illnesses or injuries?

**Necesitamos una muestra de orina.**
We need a urine specimen.

**¿Qué vacunas ha recibido el niño/la niña?**
Which immunizations has the child received?

**¿Tose el niño por la noche?**
Does the child cough at night?

**¿Con qué frecuencia evacua el niño/la niña?**
How often does the child have a bowel movement?

**Vamos a medir la cabeza.**
We are going to measure the head.

**Su hijo/hija necesita un refuerzo de esta vacuna.**
Your child needs a booster of this vaccine.

**Es su hijo/hija alérgica al huevo?**
Is your child allergic to egg?

**Por favor lea la información referente a la vacuna (VIS).**
Please read the Vaccine Information Statement (VIS).

# MEDIA MENU

**Student Resources** on **thePoint®**
- **CMA/RMA Certification Exam Review**
- **English to Spanish Audio Glossary**

**Internet Resources**
**American Academy of Pediatrics**
http://www.aap.org

**About Pediatrics**
http://pediatrics.about.com

**Centers for Disease Control and Prevention, Vaccines and Immunizations**
http://www.cdc.gov/vaccines

**Denver Developmental Materials**
http://denverii.com/home.html

**United Cerebral Palsy**
http://www.ucp.org

**U.S. Department of Health and Human Services**
http://www.childwelfare.gov/can

**Mayo Clinic: Childhood Obesity**
http://www.mayoclinic.com/health/childhood-obesity/DS00698

# EMR Activity

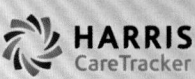

**HARRIS**
CareTracker

Harris CareTracker is a Web-based electronic medical record (EMR) application that you will use for the EMR activities included in this section at the end of each chapter. This application is actually used in physician offices, but is provided to you through the publisher, Wolters Kluwer Health, to give you hands-on practice working with EMRs. Your instructor will have more information about accessing your username, login, and Quickstart guide.

Prerequisite Activities in Harris CareTracker

- *The Getting Started and Quickstart documents and EMR Activities Step-by-Step Instructions are available at* http://thePoint.lww.com/KronenbergerComp5e
- *Note: You must first enter the patients into the EMR as new patients before completing the following EMR activity as given in the EMR Step-by-Step Instructions.*

Activity Details

Nancy Bolger left a copy of her daughter's immunization record from the local health department that must be entered into the EMR at Great Falls Medical Center. In the *Immunization* tool button in the *Clinical Toolbar*, enter Patty Bolger's immunizations as follows:

1. HepB given 7/16/2013
2. HepB, DTap, Hib, IPV, and RV given 9/20/2013
3. DTap, Hib, PCV, IPV, and RV given 11/21/2013
4. DTap, Hib, PCV, and RV given 1/25/2014

Also, indicate that this patient has an allergy to amoxicillin in the *Medical Record* module of the patient's EMR and click on *Allergy* under the *Chart Summary* module. The patient experienced an *anaphylaxis* reaction, so the *pop-up alert* should also be clicked.

# Chapter Summary

Working with children offers many rewards; however, the special developmental needs and unique physiology of children make these patients challenging and must always be taken into consideration. This chapter focuses on the following:

- The skills necessary to assist with a well-child visit including obtaining and recording normal growth information. It is important to record this information carefully to assist the physician in detecting problems as early as possible.
- Caring for the child who comes to the office for a sick-child visit. This includes maintaining the reception area by separating sick and well children if possible and disinfecting any toys to avoid cross-contamination in other children.
- Common diseases that may be seen in childhood including ear infections, upper respiratory infections, and gastrointestinal problems. Although these diseases are common, they are not pleasant for the child or the caregiver. You will have a role in reassuring anxious parents while caring for their sick children competently and professionally.
- Education of the pediatric patient caregiver including vaccine information. Parents should always be encouraged to ask questions and should expect to get honest and clear answers.
- Legal and ethical issues related to immunizations, child abuse, and neglect. You must always be alert for signs of neglect and/or abuse and be ready to report your suspicions to the physician.
- Your role in preventing disease in the pediatric patient and assisting with pediatric procedures. In addition to caring for children, you must also provide patient education to caregivers and older children to prevent the spread of disease. Also, your expertise in working with pediatric patients will be appreciated by the physician and the other staff who may find it necessary to have you assist with a variety of pediatric procedures.

# Warm-Ups for Critical Thinking

1. During years of practice, Dr. Hernandez has found that many new parents are unfamiliar with basic child care needs. He decides to publish a short booklet for his new parents describing various aspects of child care. The booklet should be informative and professional and show genuine concern for children. Using your creativity and your knowledge of child care, develop a sample booklet for Dr. Hernandez's patients after choosing two of the following topics:
   - General safety tips
   - Types of office visits
   - Immunizations (what they are, why they are important, at what ages they are given, side effects and adverse effects)
   - What a parent can expect during an office visit
   - Brief explanation of child development
   - Tips for administering oral medications to children
2. You obtained the weight on Lillian Parks, a 7-month-old girl. She weighs 16½ pounds according to your balanced pediatric scales. What percentile is this patient according to the growth chart? How would you explain a percentile to the mother of the infant?
3. The father of a toddler is insistent that you give the child an immunization in the arm rather than the thigh. How would you handle this situation?
4. Research one of the following conditions that may be found in pediatric patients and prepare a poster detailing the causes, signs and symptoms, and treatment. Include information for the caregivers or school personnel who may have questions about these conditions:
   - Strep throat
   - Pediculosis
   - Conjunctivitis
5. Compare the developmental skills of a 3-year-old and 5-year-old child. What are the similarities? What are the differences?

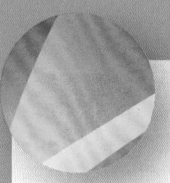

**PSY** PROCEDURE 38-1

# Obtaining an Infant's Length and Weight

**PSY** Instruct and prepare a patient for a procedure or treatment; coach patients appropriately considering cultural diversity, developmental life stage, and communication barriers; analyze health care results as reported in graphs; and document patient care accurately in the medical record.

**Purpose:** Accurately determine the length and weight of an infant

**Equipment:** Examination table with clean paper, tape measure, infant scale, protective paper for the scale, and appropriate growth chart

| STEPS | REASONS |
|---|---|
| 1. Wash your hands. | Hand washing aids infection control. |
| 2. Explain the procedure to the parent and ask him or her to remove the infant's clothing except for the diaper. | Explaining procedures encourages compliance. The diaper should be left on infants who involuntarily urinate. |
| 3. Place the child on a firm examination table covered with clean table paper. If using a measuring board, cover the board with clean paper. | Measurements may not be correct if the surface is not firm. Clean paper prevents cross infection. |
| 4. Fully extend the child's body by holding the head in the midline. Grasp the knees and press flat onto the table gently but firmly. Make a mark on the table paper with your pen at the top of the head and at the heel of the feet. | Most infants assume a flexed position, requiring you to extend the legs for accurate measurement. If you need assistance, ask the parent or a coworker to hold the child in position. A foot board against the soles will give the most accurate measurement. |

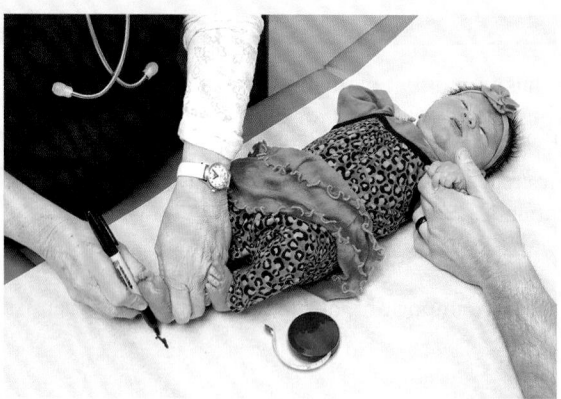

**Step 4.** Straighten the infant's leg.

| | |
|---|---|
| 5. Pick up the infant and give him or her to the caregiver, or ask the caregiver to pick the baby up. | Measurements cannot be taken with the baby lying on the paper. If a measuring board is used, it may not be necessary to move the baby. |
| 6. Measure between the marks in either inches or centimeters, according to the preference of the physician. | The length measured between the marks made at the infant's head and feet will determine the length. |
| 7. Record the child's length on the growth chart and in the patient's chart. | Procedures are considered not to have been done if they are not recorded. To plot the measurement on the growth chart, find the child's measurement in inches or centimeters and move in that line across to the age column. Make a mark where the two values intersect. |

# PROCEDURE 38-1 (continued)

| STEPS | REASONS |
|---|---|

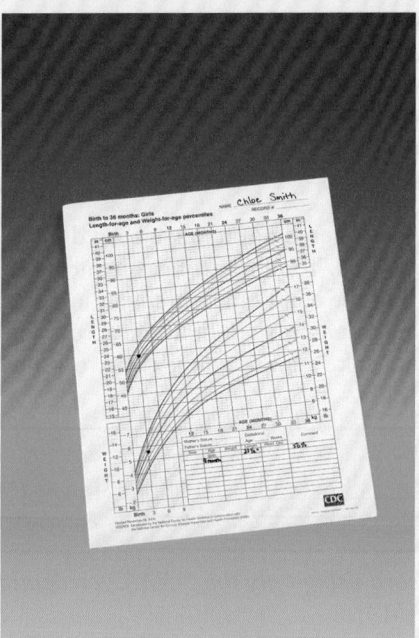

**Step 7.** Make a mark where the child's length and age intersect.

8. Either carry the infant or have the parent carry the infant to the scales.

The medical office may have only one infant scale located in a common area.

9. Place protective paper on the scale and microbalance the scale.

Protective paper prevents transmission of organisms. The balance beam must be centered before each use.

10. Remove the diaper just before laying the infant on the scale.

For the most accurate weight, infants should be weighed without any clothing. However, cool air against the infant's skin may cause the infant to void. Some offices permit the infant to be weighed in the diaper as long as it is dry and clean.

11. Place the child gently on the scale. Keep one of your hands over or near the child on the scale at all times.

Anticipate infant movement and prevent the infant from flipping off of the scale by having your hand ready to stop him or her. Avoid actually touching the infant as this will cause an inaccurate weight.

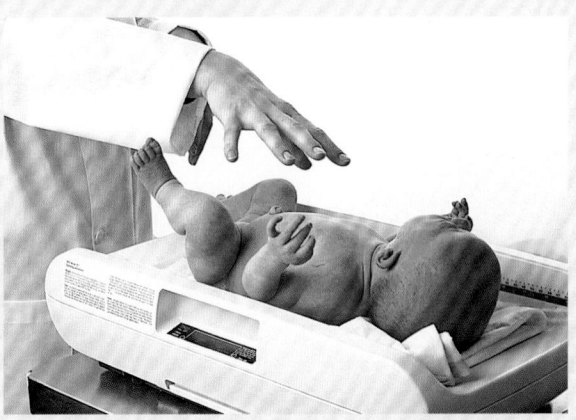

**Step 11.** Keep one hand close while weighing an infant.

(continues on page 1000)

## PROCEDURE 38-1 (continued)

| STEPS | REASONS |
|---|---|
| 12. Quickly but carefully move the counterweights to balance the apparatus exactly. | This will ensure accurate measurement. |
| 13. Pick up the infant and give to parent or have the parent pick up the child. Instruct the parent to replace the diaper if removed for the weight. | Parents should be encouraged to participate in the procedure whenever possible. |
| 14. Record the weight on the growth chart and in the patient's chart. | Procedures are considered not to have been done if they are not recorded. To plot the measurement on the growth chart, find the child's measurement in pounds or kilograms, and then move in that line across to the age column. Make a mark where the two values intersect. |

Charting Example:
*02/08/2016 10:00 AM 12-month-old, length 30 inches, wt. 22 lb. 6 oz. _____ T. Haney, CMA*

Note: *The medical assistant may sign his or her name in the patient record using only the "CMA" credential if the office has a signature log denoting the entire credential as "CMA(AAMA)."*

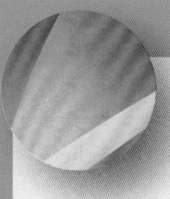

## PSY PROCEDURE 38-2

# Obtaining the Head and Chest Circumference

**PSY** Instruct and prepare a patient for a procedure or treatment; coach patients appropriately considering cultural diversity, developmental life stage, and communication barriers; analyze health care results as reported in graphs; and document patient care accurately in the medical record.

**Purpose:** Accurately determine the head and chest circumference of an infant

**Equipment:** Paper or cloth measuring tape and growth chart

| STEPS | REASONS |
|---|---|
| 1. Wash your hands. | Hand washing aids infection control. |
| 2. Place the infant supine on the examination table or ask the parent to hold the child. | This measurement does not require the infant to lie flat. |
| 3. Measure around the head above the eyebrow and posteriorly at the largest part of the occiput. For an accurate reading, measure the largest circumference. | Placing the tape measure low on the skull will result in an inaccurate head circumference. |

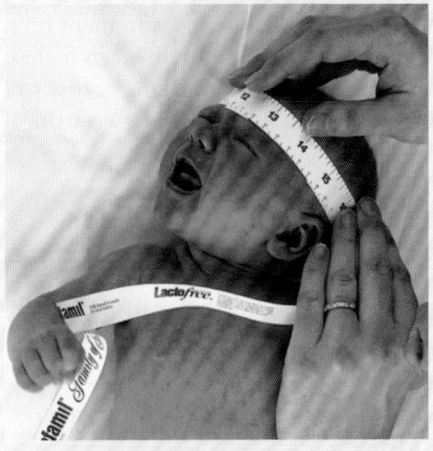

**Step 3.** Measure around the head above the eyebrow and posteriorly at the largest part of the occiput.

| STEPS | REASONS |
|---|---|
| 4. Record the child's head circumference on the growth chart and in the patient's chart. | Procedures are considered not to have been done if they are not recorded. To plot the measurement on the growth chart, find the child's measurement in inches or centimeters, and then move in that line across to the age column. Make a mark where the two values intersect. |

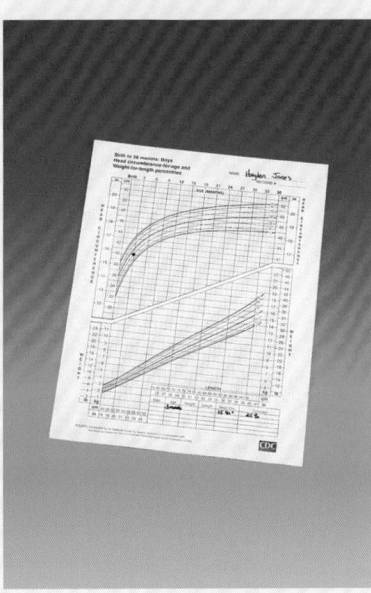

**Step 4.** Make a mark where the child's head circumference in inches or centimeters and age intersect.

*(continues on page 1002)*

## PROCEDURE 38-2 (continued)

| STEPS | REASONS |
|---|---|
| **5.** With the clothing removed from the chest, measure around the chest at the nipple line, keeping the measuring tape at the same level anteriorly and posteriorly. | The tape should be at the same level to ensure the most accurate reading. |

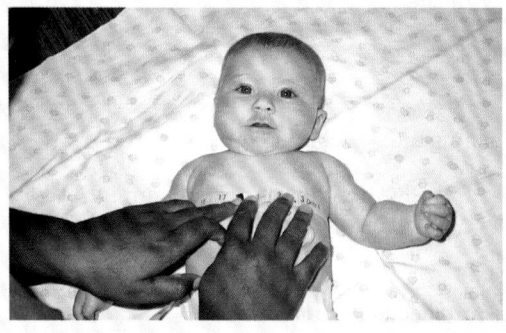

**Step 5.** Measure around the chest at the nipple line, keeping the measuring tape at the same level anteriorly and posteriorly.

| STEPS | REASONS |
|---|---|
| **6.** Record the child's chest circumference on the growth chart and in the patient chart. | Procedures are considered not to have been done if they are not recorded. To plot the measurement on the growth chart, find the child's measurement in inches or centimeters, and then move in that line across to the age column. Make a mark where the two values intersect. |

*Note:* If the head and chest growth are within normal limits, this measurement is not usually required after 12 months.

---

**Charting Example:**
*10/15/2016 9:45 AM Wt. 14 lb. Length 24 in., Head 15 in., Chest 17 in. _____ T. Haney, CMA*

---

Note: *The medical assistant may sign his or her name in the patient record using only the "CMA" credential if the office has a signature log denoting the entire credential as "CMA(AAMA)."*

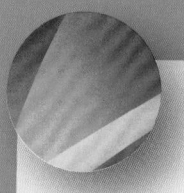

## PSY PROCEDURE 38-3

### Applying a Urinary Collection Device

**PSY** Instruct and prepare a patient for a procedure or treatment; coach patients appropriately considering cultural diversity, developmental life stage, and communication barriers; and document patient care accurately in the medical record.

**Purpose:** Correctly apply a urinary collection device to a child

**Equipment:** Gloves, personal antiseptic wipes, pediatric urine collection bag, completed laboratory request slip, and biohazard transport container

| STEPS | REASONS |
|---|---|
| 1. Wash your hands. | Hand washing aids infection control. |
| 2. Explain the procedure to the caregivers. | Informing caregivers of procedures aids in compliance and cooperation. |
| 3. Place the child supine. Ask for help from the parents as needed. | The child may be more cooperative if a parent helps. |
| 4. After putting on gloves, clean the genitalia with the antiseptic wipes:<br>A. For girls: Cleanse front to back with separate wipes for each downward stroke on the outer labia. The last clean wipe should be used between the inner labia.<br>B. For boys: Retract the foreskin if the baby has not been circumcised. Cleanse the meatus in an ever-widening circle. Discard the wipe and repeat the procedure. Return the foreskin to its proper position. | For girls, cleansing front to back will remove debris from the area and avoid introducing bacteria into the urethra. For boys, cleansing outward will avoid introducing bacteria into the urethra. Returning the foreskin to the correct position will prevent constriction of the penis. |
| 5. Holding the collection device, remove the upper portion of the paper backing and press it around the mons pubis. Remove the second section and press it against the perineum. Loosely attach the diaper. | The collection device must be securely attached to ensure collection of the next voiding. Reattaching the diaper will avoid soiling if the child has a stool. |

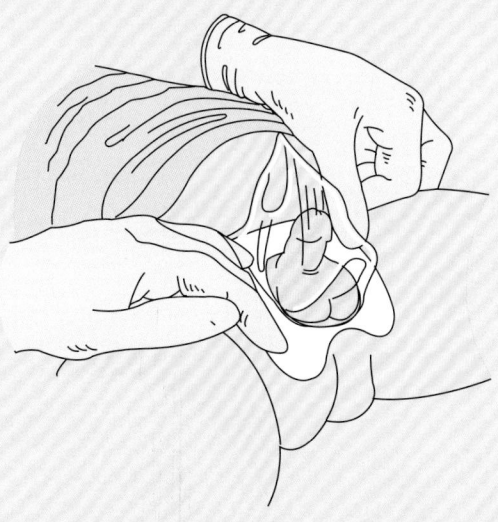

**Step 5.** The collection device fits over the genitalia.

| | |
|---|---|
| 6. Give the baby fluids unless contraindicated, and check the diaper frequently. | Giving the child fluids may stimulate voiding. |

## PROCEDURE 38-3 (continued)

| STEPS | REASONS |
|---|---|
| 7. When the child has voided, remove the device, clean the skin of residual adhesive, and diaper. | Adhesive left on the skin may be irritating. |
| 8. Prepare the specimen for transport to the laboratory or process it according to the office policy and procedure manual. | The specimen cannot be analyzed at the laboratory without proper processing. |
| 9. Remove your gloves and wash your hands. | Standard precautions must be followed when handling body fluids. |
| 10. Record the procedure. | Procedures are considered not to have been done if they are not recorded. |

Charting Example:
*08/16/2016 11:45 AM Urine collection device applied; approximately 50 mL clear amber urine obtained after 20 minutes. Specimen sent to GFMC lab for urinalysis* _____ *T. Haney, CMA*

Note: *The medical assistant may sign his or her name in the patient record using only the "CMA" credential if the office has a signature log denoting the entire credential as "CMA(AAMA)."*

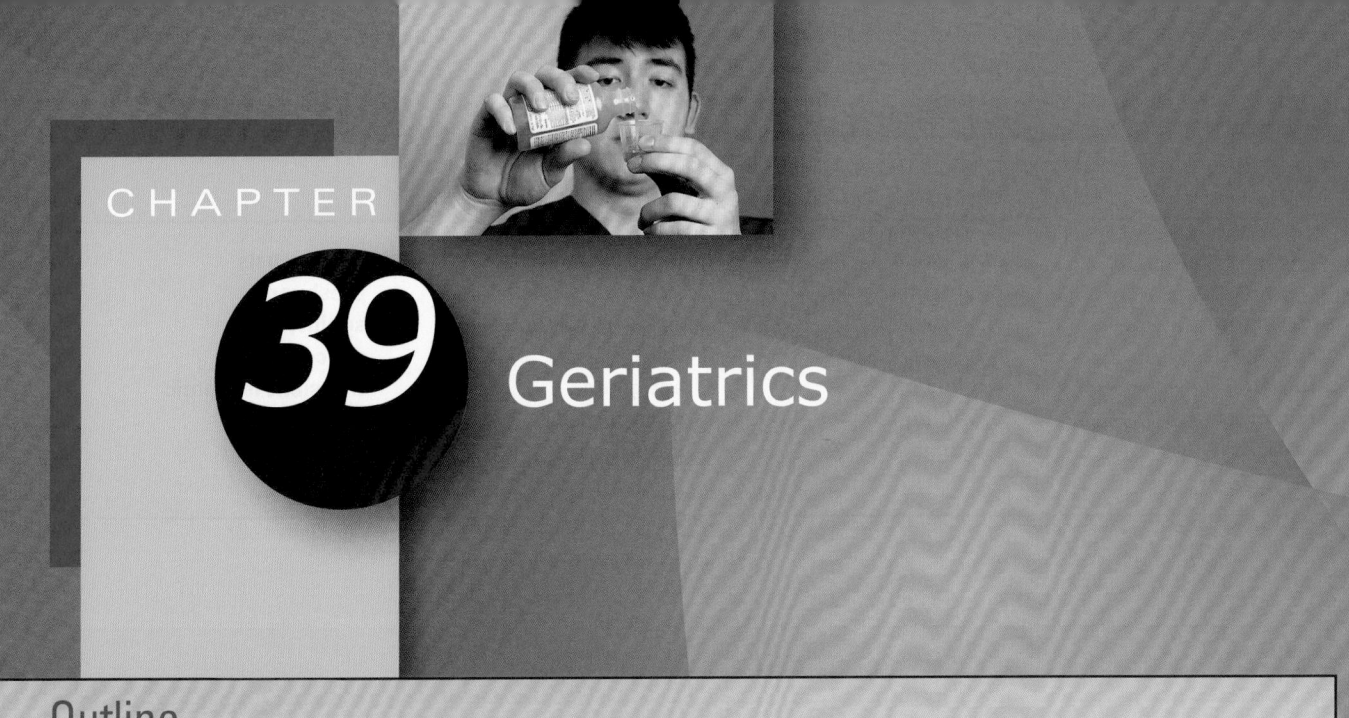

# 39 Geriatrics

## Outline

## Learning Outcomes

### COG Cognitive Domain*

1. Spell key terms
2. *Define medical terms and abbreviations related to all body systems*
3. *Compare structure and function of the human body across the life span*
4. *Identify common pathology related to each body system including signs, symptoms, and etiology*
5. Explain how aging affects thought processes
6. Describe methods to increase compliance with health maintenance programs among older adults
7. Discuss communication problems that may occur with the older adult and list steps to maintain open communication
8. Recognize and describe the coping mechanisms used by the older adult to deal with multiple losses
9. Name the risk factors and signs of elder abuse
10. Explain the types of long-term care facilities available
11. Describe the effects of aging on the way the body processes medication
12. Discuss the responsibility of medical assistants with regard to teaching older adult patients
13. List and describe physical changes and diseases common to the aging process

### AFF Affective Domain*

1. *Incorporate critical thinking skills when performing patient assessment*
2. *Incorporate critical thinking skills when performing patient care*
3. *Demonstrate empathy, active listening, and nonverbal communication*
4. *Demonstrate respect for individual diversity including gender, race, religion, age, economic status, and appearance*

***Note: AAMA/CAAHEP 2015 Standards are italicized.***

### ABHES Competencies

1. Assist the physician with the regimen of diagnostic and treatment modalities as they relate to each body system
2. Comply with federal, state, and local health laws and regulations
3. Communicate on the recipient's level of comprehension
4. Serve as a liaison between the physician and others
5. Show empathy and impartiality when dealing with patients
6. Document accurately

*(continues on page 1006)*

activities of daily
  living (ADL)
biotransform
bradykinesia
cataracts
cerebrovascular
  accident (CVA)

compliance
degenerative joint
  disease (DJD)
dementia
dysphagia
gerontologists
glaucoma

Kegel exercises
keratosis (senile)
kyphosis (dowager's
  hump)
lentigines
osteoporosis
potentiation

presbycusis
presbyopia
senility
syncope
transient ischemic
  attack (TIA)
vertigo

## Case Study

*T*he medical specialty of geriatrics focuses on the care of elderly patients. Geriatric patients include those who are very healthy and active to those who have several chronic conditions and on many medications. Ross Mason, CMA (AAMA), assists the physicians at Great Falls Medical Center with caring for geriatric patients and has gotten to know many of them and their families when they come into the office. Talking with and listening to the patients and their families helps him to determine if additional assistance or patient education might be necessary. When directed by the physician, Ross is able to offer community resources for patients who may need help, including assistance with activities of daily living. Why would geriatric patients need extra assistance, and what are the activities of daily living? Are there signs indicating an elderly patient is having difficulties? What kinds of resources would be available to an elderly patient? These and other questions are covered in this chapter.

As the older adult population has increased, established concepts about aging have also changed. The greeting card image of a cozy, gray-haired grandmother in her rocking chair is being replaced by a trim, active woman rushing out the door with a briefcase or tennis racket under her arm. **Gerontologists**, specialists in aging, describe many older adults today as healthy enough to maintain homes well into their 80s and 90s. The branch of medicine that deals with the older adult population is geriatrics, and while some physicians today are treating only geriatric patients, a family practice or internal medicine physician also treats older adult patients. Other specialties, such as ophthalmology, also see many geriatric patients daily. Box 39-1 outlines some myths and stereotypes about the older adult. How many are far from typical of this age group today?

Stereotyping the older adult is a subtle and usually unconscious way to disassociate ourselves from the prospect of growing old. Although other cultures respect their older adults for their wealth of wisdom and experience, the American media perpetuate myths and stereotypical reactions by implying that graying hair and wrinkles in the skin are repulsive and should

be avoided at all costs. Those costs include billions of dollars spent on delaying the physical signs of aging. Consider how the following situations take on new meaning when applied to different age groups.

- You are running late again. Dashing out of the door, you remember that you left the keys to the car on the kitchen table—again.
- You stride purposefully from the bedroom into the kitchen with a specific goal in mind, only to reach the kitchen without any idea why you were in such a hurry to get there.

We have all done these things and will no doubt do them again. However, if these things are done by an older adult person, they are considered to be a sign of approaching **senility** or **dementia**. While some memory loss and difficulty with thought processes are inevitable as a result of aging, memory loss in the older adult is often the result of various disease processes and medications. The next section describes some techniques that you can use to enhance **compliance** with patients who have difficulty with thought processes, whether the cause is natural aging or a specific disease or medication

## BOX 39-1   Myths and Stereotypes about the Older Adult

**Myths**

- Old people are weak and sick.
- Old people can no longer learn.
- Old people have no more contributions to make.
- Old people are boring.
- Old people are a drag on the economy.
- Old people are always lonely.
- Old people cannot live alone.
- Old people cannot be trusted to make rational decisions.
- Old people have lost all interest in life.

**Stereotypes**

- Old people have sensory losses.
- Old people have erratic sleep patterns and nap a lot.
- Old people do everything slower.
- Old people have lost stature and slump a lot.
- Old people cannot remember what happened this morning but can recall everything that happened 40 years ago.

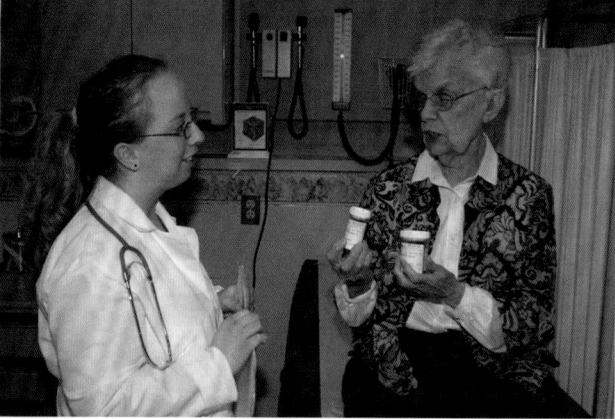

**Figure 39-1 •** Ask patients about medications at every visit.

regimen. You have a responsibility as a professional medical assistant to ensure that your interactions with older adults demonstrate dignity and respect, keeping in mind their individual abilities and uniqueness.

## REINFORCING MEDICAL COMPLIANCE IN THE OLDER ADULT

Working with older adult patients who may have problems with memory loss or thought processes is extremely important to ensure that they take their medications as prescribed and follow the physician's instructions precisely. A patient who has good rapport with the office staff is likely to be truthful about the need for memory aids, and compliance may be increased. A patient who has difficulties with memory may benefit from the following approaches:

- Write out instructions in easy-to-understand terms.
- Use large print.
- Have the patient repeat instructions to you for reinforcement.
- Ask the patient to show you how he or she will perform a procedure before leaving the office.
- Give the patient a copy of a large appointment calendar and list the times and days for treatments and medications, which should be crossed off as completed.

Many chronic illnesses that affect the older adult require medication or treatment for the remainder of the patient's life. In these situations, the patient may not notice much improvement, making compliance over a long period problematic. You should reinforce the fact that, although the patient may not return to his or her former health status, the prescribed treatment will maintain health at a manageable level. A patient's diabetes or heart disease will not be cured, but treatment will help the patient maintain a reasonable standard of health and independence.

It is important that, each time a patient visits the medical office, you ask for a complete account of all medications being taken, including prescribed and over-the-counter (OTC) medications, herbal supplements, and vitamins. To maintain a complete and accurate list of these medications, you may have patients bring all medications to the office at each visit and ask the patient to state how often each is taken (Fig. 39-1). If you ask, "Mrs. Jones, are you still taking your heart medicine?" she may answer yes whether or not she is actually taking the medication as prescribed. In addition to difficulty with thought processes and occasional forgetfulness, some patients simply grow tired of the constraints that illness and medications impose on their lives, and some must make the financial choice between medication and food on the table. Assisting the patient to find ways to fit health requirements into a fairly normal lifestyle or coordinating with community resources to relieve financial constraints will help to ensure that treatment plans are followed and that the patient achieves the best level of health possible.

### CHECKPOINT QUESTION

1. Ross Mason, the medical assistant in the case study, is having difficulty getting an elderly patient to follow the physician orders. What are some reasons a patient may not comply with a prescribed treatment plan?

## PATIENT EDUCATION

### Tips for Improving Memory in the Older Adult

Many research studies have been done regarding improving the forgetfulness that sometimes results from aging and that is not associated with an organic brain disorder such as Alzheimer disease or cerebrovascular disease. The factors that seem to play an important role in maintaining and improving memory include many of the same factors necessary for general good health:

• Regular physical exercise
• Maintaining a healthy body weight
• Eating a healthy diet that includes a variety of foods (grains, fruits, vegetables, etc.) and is low in fats

In addition, eating breakfast and regularly exercising the brain with puzzles, word searches, and other activities that require thinking skills may also affect cognitive function.

## REINFORCING MENTAL HEALTH IN THE OLDER ADULT

With the recognized correlation between physical and mental health, we must be acutely aware of the patient's mental status in patients who have acute or chronic physical problems. Some older adult patients are adapting to new roles of dependency after a lifetime of social interaction, career objectives, and family development. Some have been relieved of social responsibility whether they welcome it or not, and if they are ill, they must take on a dependent role. Adjusting to pain or disability is often easier than adjusting to loss of social interaction or dependency.

Paradoxically, if you open yourself to patients, including older adults, and you are accessible and caring, you are likely to be the object of anger simply because you are seen as a safe outlet for venting frustrations. A suffering patient is less likely to release pent-up anger at someone who may respond with hostility or corresponding anger; consequently, the patient may hold these feelings in, and the problem is compounded. Making yourself available to field these emotions can be as therapeutic as any treatment administered to this patient. To do this effectively:

1. Maintain open communication, freely discussing hopes and fears realistically, listening attentively, and offering advice without diagnosing or offering false hope.
2. By listening and being supportive to the patient and family members, help the patient to cope with and express feelings of guilt for being ill, anger at

self and others nearby, and the loss of health and independence.
3. Work toward maintaining the patient's positive self-image by reinforcing the positive qualities of the patient's physical health or personal situation as appropriate.
4. Assist family members to maintain a positive support system by listening to concerns and possibly serving as a liaison for outside social services or resources if available.
5. Without being discouraging or offering false hope, prepare the patient for the possibility that a return to the previous state of health may not be feasible.
6. Direct the patient and family to specific support groups, such as the American Heart Association, the American Cancer Society, or another group specific to the patient's problem, to assist them with acquiring information about the patient's condition.

 ## CHECKPOINT QUESTION

2. How can you help promote good mental health in your older adult patients?

## COPING WITH AGING

Although many older adult people are generally healthy and satisfied with their lives, those who live in long-term care facilities or whose health and economic situation are unstable have every right to feel overwhelming stress and grief. Stress will compromise the immune system, raise the blood pressure and blood sugar level, and strain the heart and lungs—all at a time when the patient needs all available resources to fight a debilitating disease process. You can help patients to cope with stress by listening to their fears and concerns, respecting their right to have these feelings, and helping them to reduce the stressors in their lives. Keep in mind that the coping mechanisms (e.g., denial, projection, repression) used to protect ourselves from stress may become more pronounced with age.

The ability of patients to cope with their losses is in direct relation to the importance of the losses and their own personal habits for coping with loss in the past. Be aware of a patient's loss of specific senses, abilities, or important things in life, such as sight, hearing, movement, perception, health, employment, home, and spouse. Also, be alert to the loss of nonspecific things, such as life purpose, goals, a sense of achievement, self-worth, recognition, and security. Some older adult patients react to these losses by disengaging emotionally and relinquishing all decision making to family members. This may compound their grieving and lead to a sense of hopelessness and resignation. To prevent this reaction, involve older adult patients, like all patients, as much as possible by allowing them to have a voice in decisions that will affect their care. The older adults who are encouraged to make decisions and take responsibility for themselves are happier, more sociable, and live longer than those who are not part of the decision-making process in issues that affect their lives.

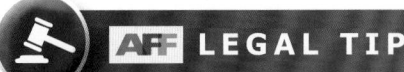

## LEGAL TIP

### Advance Directives

An advance directive is a legal document outlining the wishes of an adult should he/she become mentally incompetent or otherwise unable to communicate decisions about end-of-life care. Although physicians as medical professionals are dedicated to sustaining life, a patient's autonomy must be respected at all times, including decisions to avoid or terminate life-sustaining procedures or equipment. As unpleasant as the prospect of death may be, documenting and communicating the wishes of the patient to the physician will assist with avoiding any confusion about the wishes of the patient should a life-threatening situation arise. Also, if the patient has an advanced directive on file somewhere other than the medical office, this should be noted in the patient's medical record.

## Alcoholism

Some older adults, like individuals at any age, cope with loss and life changes by turning to alcohol. Because alcohol slows brain activity and impairs mental processes, coordination, and judgment, a patient who comes to the office under the influence of alcohol may be mistaken for having dementia (mental deterioration), a **transient ischemic attack (TIA)**, or central nervous system impairment. Also, many medications taken by the older adult affect the central nervous system and react badly with alcohol, compounding the problem. For example, alcohol increases the effect of opioids, barbiturates, and depressants of all types, and caretakers may not recognize this reason for the **potentiation**.

Identifying an older adult patient who is using or abusing alcohol may require the entire office to work as a team with the patient's family or caregiver to seek causes of various symptoms, such as impaired judgment or coordination. As often as necessary, you should reinforce with older adult patients and their caregivers the effects of alcohol on mental processes and undesirable interactions with medications. In addition, the patient and responsible caregivers may require a referral to a mental health professional or other community resource to deal effectively with alcohol abuse. You may be required to make this referral as ordered by the physician.

## Suicide

When ill health, multiple losses, and deep depression become too much for the patient to bear, suicide may seem preferable to life. Unlike suicide among younger people, suicide among the older adult is likely to be well planned and successful. Most older adult suicides are white men over age 65, especially those who have recently lost a spouse to death or divorce. These suicides are not usually a cry for help but a genuine effort to end life. Watch for these signs of intent:

- Deepening confusion and scattered attention
- Increasing anger, hostility, or isolation
- Increase in alcoholism or requests for opioids or sedatives
- Marked loss of interest in matters of health
- Secretive behavior
- Sharp mood swings from deep depression to euphoria
- Giving away favored objects

Always take seriously a patient who expresses an intent to commit suicide, and communicate this to the physician. You should work with the health care team to restore mental health as aggressively as to restore physical health.

### CHECKPOINT QUESTION

3. What are some signs of suicidal intent?

## LONG-TERM CARE

Although many older adults are able to live in their own homes, some enter long-term care facilities if they cannot return to health and independence or are simply tired of the tasks required to maintain a house. There are three main types of long-term care:

- *Group homes* or *assisted living facilities* are for the older adults who are able to tend to their own **activities of daily living (ADL)** (e.g., bathing, dressing, eating) but who may need companionship and light supervision for safety. Often, these facilities allow independent adults access to activities such as golf, swimming, and trips for those who are ready to enjoy life in the later years.
- *Long-term care facilities* are for those who need help with most areas of personal care and moderate medical supervision. Many of these patients are ambulatory but have a chronic disease that makes living at home difficult or impossible.

• *Skilled nursing facilities* are for those who are ill and need constant supervision or rehabilitation before returning home. If the illness is acute and short term, the patient may return to an intermediate stage of care after recovery and possibly to full independence. However, these facilities also provide support and resources to patients who may need end-of-life care.

Although fully independent adults moving to an assisted living facility may be relieved to leave behind the pressures of life and excited to remain active with fewer responsibilities, expect some older adult patients to react to a move to long-term care with sorrow and a deep sense of loss. The patient may show the signs and symptoms of grief: poor appetite, headaches, insomnia, deep depression, and vague aches and pains. Report all signs and symptoms to the physician. Many physicians continue to care for patients residing in long-term care facilities. You may be responsible for blocking time in the daily schedule for the physician to visit these patients, and you may receive phone calls at the medical office from facilities regarding changes in patient's care and physical condition.

---

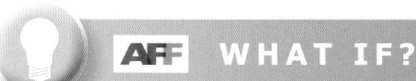

### CHECKPOINT QUESTION

4. How are long-term facilities and skilled nursing facilities different?

---

**AFF    WHAT IF?**

**What if a patient's relative asks you about options for home care for an older adult parent?**

Explain that many options allow patients to remain in their home. One option is the use of home health aides. Some insurance plans pay for this service. Home health aides do light housecleaning and cooking and promote patient safety. A second option is a community resource center. Some communities have senior citizen programs that provide transportation for shopping, doctor appointments, and entertainment. These programs get the older patient out of the house, preventing boredom and enhancing self-esteem. A third option is day care for the older adult. These programs keep the patient safe, entertained, and cared for during the day. The advantages of day care are that it relieves the caregiver of the need to place a parent in a long-term care facility, keeps the patient safe during the day, and allows the relative the freedom to continue employment or attend to personal needs. Community programs for senior citizens are good sources of information for caregivers or for relatives searching for respite or permanent care.

## OG   OLDER ADULT ABUSE

Although older adult abuse is not as widely publicized as child abuse, it is thought to be almost as prevalent. The following are common risk factors for older adult abuse:

• Multiple chronic illnesses that stress the family's physical, emotional, and financial resources
• Senile dementia that precludes reasoning or interaction
• Bladder or bowel incontinence
• Age-related sleep disturbances that interfere with the caretaker's rest
• Dependence on the caretaker for ADL

Older adult abuse and neglect may take several forms, but family members (adult children and spouses) are the typical perpetrators.

• Passive neglect may result from the caretaker's ignorance regarding the patient's physiologic and psychological needs.
• Active neglect may take many forms, including overmedicating to render the patient passive and easier to care for or depriving the victim of adequate nutrition to decrease physical resources.
• Psychological abuse may include threatening imprisonment in the home, perhaps locking in a room, or physical abuse, withholding food or medication, or physical isolation.
• Financial abuse may involve only small amounts of money or entire substantial estates. The patient's financial resources may be embezzled, squandered, or frankly stolen, leaving the victim destitute.
• Physical abuse may be as simple as pinches and slaps or may be life threatening, sexual, or so well concealed that even perceptive health care providers do not suspect it (Fig. 39-2).

Some older adult patients fear reprisal or abandonment by their caregivers, just as children do, and are reluctant to complain of any improprieties. Separate the caregiver from the patient for the examination if possible, and treat the patient with the utmost compassion and

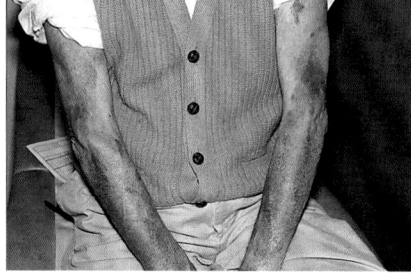

**Figure 39-2 •** You should always be alert to signs of older adult abuse. (From Weber J, Kelley J. *Health Assessment in Nursing*, 2nd ed. Philadelphia, PA: Lippincott Williams & Wilkins, 2003.)

care. Document all findings with full descriptions. It may be necessary to photograph the suspected injuries and report any suspicions to the local adult protective services. Always communicate your concerns with the physician, and, together, make decisions regarding how to proceed with any suspected abuse.

---

### CHECKPOINT QUESTION

5. What are the types of older adult abuse?

---

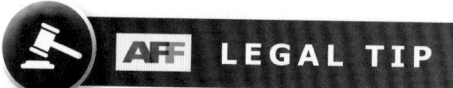 **LEGAL TIP**

### Older Adult Abuse

If you suspect abuse or neglect, you are responsible ethically and legally for bringing it to the attention of the physician, who should assess the situation and, if it is confirmed, notify the proper authorities. Most states require that health care professionals report all suspected cases of older adult abuse to the department of social services, just as is required for suspected child abuse. The entire medical staff may be held responsible if the abuse is not reported immediately. The following signs may indicate older adult abuse:

* Wound of suspicious origin in various stages of healing
* Signs of restraints having been used, such as wrist or ankle abrasions or bruising
* Neglected large, deep pressure ulcers
* Poor hygiene or poor nutrition with little or no effort at correction
* Dehydration not caused by a disease process
* Untreated injury or medical condition
* Excessive and unwarranted agitation or apathetic resignation

---

## MEDICATIONS AND THE OLDER ADULT

The need to teach some older adult patients about self-medication is a challenge that will become increasingly common as the general population ages. At the same time that older adult patients need more medications for various disorders, the body is coping with the stress of illness, disease, or injury along with slowing of many bodily functions. The gastrointestinal system is no longer moving medications along as efficiently because peristalsis has slowed. The circulatory system is not absorbing the dissolved medication from the intestines or the injection site and delivering it to the target tissue as quickly. The liver does not **biotransform** (convert) the medication as quickly, so that it remains in the body longer

than might be desirable and possibly adds to cumulative effect. Finally, the kidneys are receiving less blood, so that less medication is filtered and removed from the body. All of these decreases in body systems can result in possible toxic effects of medications in the older adult.

Your responsibility is to elicit information from the patient about all medications they are taking, including prescribed and OTC medications and herbal or vitamin supplements. Follow these guidelines to help ensure that your older adult patient adheres to the prescribed medication regimen:

1. Explain all side effects, precautions, interactions, and expected actions in a manner the patient can understand.
2. Explain the proper dosage and how to measure it. For patients with failing eyesight, mark plastic measuring cups with indelible ink at the correct level so they can easily see it.
3. Write out a schedule and suggest methods to help the patient remember. Suggestions may include a daily dose pack available at pharmacies, an egg carton with hours for taking the medications marked on the cups, and a calendar marked with the medications and hours, to be checked off after taking the medication.
4. Tell the patient to take the most important medication first and space out the other medications according to the physician's order. Medications that are ordered to be taken once a day may not have to be taken in the morning.
5. Encourage the patient not to rush when taking medications. The patient should be sitting or standing, not reclining. One pill should be taken at a time with lots of water. If the medication is difficult to swallow, have the patient try putting the pill on the back of the tongue and drinking water with a straw.
6. A patient who has difficulty reading or has failing eyesight can ask the pharmacist for large print on the label (Fig. 39-3). This makes medication errors less likely. Childproof containers are not necessary if there are no children in the home, and the patient may find them difficult to open.

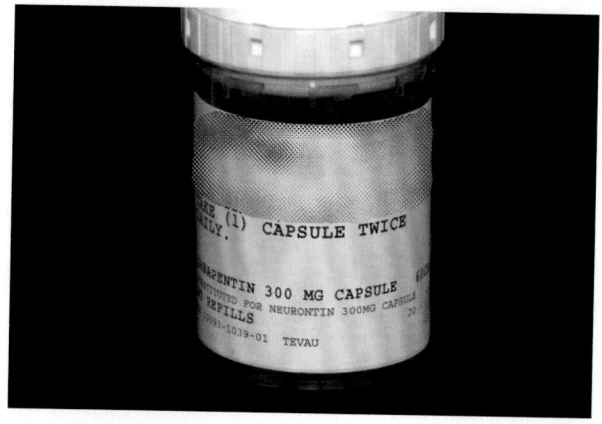

**Figure 39-3** • Large print on a medication label.

7. Explain that the medication must be taken until it is gone (if this is the case). No medication should be taken by other family members or saved for another illness.

8. Encourage patients to take an active role in therapy. Teach them to apply ointments or transdermal patches or to give themselves injections. A patient who feels in charge is more likely to complete a course of medication or to remain on the medication for the long term than one who feels passive.

## CHECKPOINT QUESTION

6. How can you help your older adult patients follow the medication regimen prescribed by the physician?

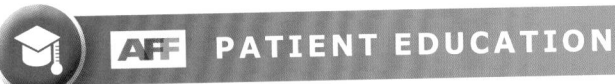

## PATIENT EDUCATION

### Herbal Supplements

The herb ginkgo, also known as *ginkgo biloba*, *maidenhair tree*, *kew tree*, *fossil tree*, *ginkyo*, and *yinhsing*, is advertised in the United States as a natural way to improve memory and concentration. It is for this reason that older adults have been targeted for the purchase of this product. After all, it can be purchased over the counter at many pharmacies and health food stores, and so many patients do not consider it a medication. However, it is extremely important that you obtain a thorough history from your patients each time they visit the office and specifically ask about any OTC medications, including herbs and vitamin supplements. This drug may improve memory in some patients, but it causes an increase in clotting time in anyone who takes it and should not be used by patients with bleeding or clotting disorders. Any patient being scheduled for a surgical procedure must also be asked about the use of herbs. Patients who are taking the following medications should avoid taking ginkgo:

- Warfarin (Coumadin)
- Aspirin
- Nonsteroidal anti-inflammatory drugs, such as ibuprofen, naproxen, and indomethacin

The physician should be informed of any patient taking this herbal supplement because reactions with other medications in addition to those listed could have serious consequences.

## SYSTEMIC CHANGES IN THE OLDER ADULT

Although longevity is considered largely hereditary, environmental factors play a significant part in how long and how well we will live. An obese, physically inactive smoker is much less likely to be in good health than a nonsmoker whose diet is well balanced and who exercises. In addition, certain occupational hazards, such as black lung disease from coal mining, may shorten a life that should have lasted for decades longer.

The aging changes are thought to be programmed into our cells along with our genetic material. Some experts suggest that when cells reach a specific reproduction level, they either do not replace themselves or replicate more slowly or ineffectively. These changes manifest themselves at varying rates for all persons but follow a recognized order as outlined in Table 39-1.

Some older adult patients develop disorders involving communication (Fig. 39-4); however, diseases affecting sight and hearing are common and may interfere with ADL for aging adults. Visually, conditions such as **presbyopia, cataracts,** and, possibly, **glaucoma** become evident with aging (refer to Chapter 30). All of these can affect sight, ranging from a decrease in visual acuity (presbyopia) to blindness if left untreated (cataracts and glaucoma). Having print materials available in large print, submitting preauthorizations and referrals to an ophthalmologist as ordered by the physician, and being alert for safety issues when assisting older adult patients are your responsibilities in the medical office.

Generalizing that all older adults cannot hear is not appropriate; however, as people age, conditions such as ceruminosis and presbycusis (see Chapter 30) are more common and cause hearing loss. Irrigating the ear and instilling otic solution to soften cerumen may be ordered by the physician to treat ceruminosis. Presbycusis is treated with a referral to an audiologist for evaluation and hearing aids (Fig. 39-5).

### WHAT IF?

**You are organizing your charts at the beginning of the day and you notice that one of your patients, an 88-year-old man, has HOH (hard of hearing) stamped inside his chart. How can you best communicate with him?**

When speaking to an older adult patient who is hearing impaired, it is important not to shout. Instead, get closer to the patient, face the patient directly, and speak slowly and distinctly. Try to give written instructions whenever possible, and encourage the patient to ask questions for clarification. Avoid speaking to the hard-of-hearing patient with your back to the light, since this may cast shadows and prevent the patient from being able to lip read.

## TABLE 39-1   Effects of Aging on Body Systems

| System | Physiologic Effects | Signs and Symptoms | Suggestions |
|---|---|---|---|
| Integumentary | Loss of subcutaneous fat<br>Loss of pigment<br>Loss of elasticity<br>Receding capillaries<br>Slower reproduction of hair, skin cells<br>Diminished oil, sweat production<br>Erratic pigment, cell production | Wrinkling, sagging, decreased ability to maintain hydration, reduced protection against temperature change<br>Less protection against sun damage, paler skin, graying hair<br>Increased skin dryness, risk of trauma<br>Sallow skin, thickened nails<br>Balding; thin, fine hair; slower healing<br>Dry, fragile skin; intolerance to heat<br>Senile lentigines, keratoses | Encourage drinking plenty of fluids, dressing appropriately for weather.<br>Encourage use of sunscreen with appropriate UV protection.<br>Suggest good lubricating lotion and bathing less often; caution to guard against injuries.<br>Suggest ways to avoid overheating.<br>Teach patient to conduct skin checks and to notify the physician of concerns. |
| Musculoskeletal | Loss of muscle strength, size<br>Loss of bone density, loss of height with osteoporosis<br>Degenerative joint cartilage | Loss of strength, flexibility, endurance<br>Vertebral compression with diminished height, kyphosis, osteoporosis with frequent fractures<br>Less clear margins with spurs of bone that restrict movement, degenerative joint disease (DJD), arthritis | Suggest frequent exercise appropriate to age and ability.<br>Explain weight-bearing exercises.<br>Encourage home safety check to avoid falls.<br>Physician may recommend calcium supplement, dietary consultation, estrogen replacement.<br>Physician may limit phosphorus intake. |

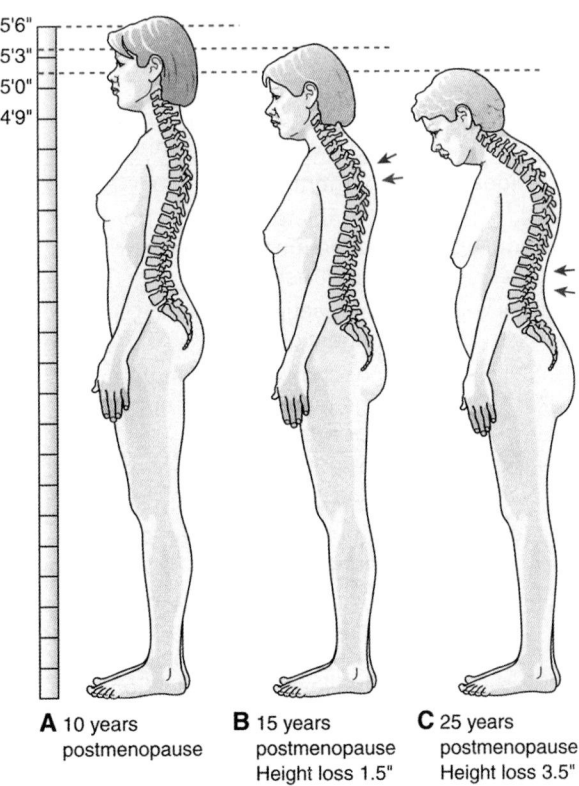

A  10 years postmenopause

B  15 years postmenopause Height loss 1.5"

C  25 years postmenopause Height loss 3.5"

Typical loss of height associated with osteoporosis and aging.

(continues on page 1014)

| TABLE 39-1 | Effects of Aging on Body Systems (continued) | | |
|---|---|---|---|
| System | Physiologic Effects | Signs and Symptoms | Suggestions |
| Nervous | Slow nerve conduction<br><br>Reduced cerebral reaction times<br><br>Referred circulatory problems | Slow reaction time, slow learning, slow perception of pain with resulting increase in injuries<br><br>Loss of balance, vertigo, frequent falls<br><br>Increase in cardiovascular diseases (atherosclerosis, arteriosclerosis) reflected as cerebrovascular accident (CVA), cerebral hypoxia, TIA | Allow extra time as needed and teach about hazards of delayed circulation. Aim at teaching to comprehension level. Encourage home safety checks.<br><br>Have patient install bath rails; remove throw rugs.<br><br>Encourage use of walking aid.<br><br>Teach patient and family about danger signs for CVA, TIA. |
| Cardiovascular | Atherosclerosis, arteriosclerosis, narrowing of blood vessels<br><br>Slow response to demands for increased output<br><br>Diminished function | Loss of peripheral circulation, fatty plaques with risk of MI, CVA, cold extremities, slow healing time, hypertension<br><br>Complaints of fatigue on exertion<br><br>Pulmonary involvement with edema, dyspnea | Encourage exercise; balanced low-fat, low-salt diet; dressing appropriately for weather; home safety check.<br><br>Help patient pace exercise and exertion.<br><br>Explain about low-salt diets and orthopneic positions.<br><br>Explain about smoking hazards, emphysema. Encourage moderate exercise. |
| Respiratory | Stiffening costal cartilage<br><br>Decreased gas exchange<br><br>General loss of muscle mass | Decreased expansion, contraction; barrel chest; decreased lung capacity<br><br>Fatigue, breathlessness on exertion; impaired healing due to insufficient oxygen, syncope<br><br>Difficulty coughing deeply, may lead to pneumonia | Encourage exercise as appropriate and use of walking aid. Caution about upper respiratory infection; encourage home safety check.<br><br>Encourage drinking adequate fluids to liquify respiratory secretions. |
| Gastrointestinal (GI) | Drying of secretions, including saliva<br><br>Decreased enzyme activity<br><br>Slower peristalsis<br><br>Loss of teeth | Dry mouth, dysphagia<br><br>Incomplete digestion, poor conversion of nutrients with malnourishment<br><br>Constipation, flatulence, indigestion<br><br>Poor chewing, choking on large pieces, loss of appetite, poor nutrition | Teach oral hygiene, adequate fluid intake.<br><br>Encourage small, frequent well-balanced meals.<br><br>Refer to a dentist.<br><br>Suggest dietary counseling. |
| Urinary | Decreased bladder capacity<br><br>Decreased bladder muscle tone<br><br>Fewer functioning nephrons | Urinary frequency<br><br>Urinary retention with urinary tract infection or incontinence<br><br>Less blood flowing through kidneys to be cleaned of wastes, creating possibly lethal levels of medications or normal body wastes | Encourage patient to respond to initial urge to void.<br><br>Suggest exercises for strengthening pelvic floor. Urge patient to empty bladder completely when voiding.<br><br>Suggest increase in fluid intake to maintain hydration. |

| TABLE 39-1 | Effects of Aging on Body Systems (continued) | | |
|---|---|---|---|
| **System** | **Physiologic Effects** | **Signs and Symptoms** | **Suggestions** |
| Endocrine | Decreased enzyme activity | Menopause, glucose intolerance with non-insulin–dependent diabetes mellitus, slower metabolism<br><br>Loss of resistance to illness | Physician will supplement as needed.<br><br>Encourage compliance with any prescribed medications. |
| Immune | Diminished production of T cells, B cells<br><br>Diminished ability of body to distinguish self from foreign substances<br><br>Diminished other defenses (e.g., GI enzymes) | Increase in autoimmune illnesses<br><br>Overload on compromised immune system | Encourage age-appropriate immunizations, guarding against communicable diseases.<br><br>Explain symptoms of autoimmunity. |
| Eyes | Less time spent in deep sleep<br><br>Diminished lens accommodation<br><br>Lens cloud<br><br>Loss of ciliary function | Less restful sleep, more frequent naps<br><br>Presbyopia<br><br>Cataracts (lens opacity) that dim vision as less light reaches the retina<br><br>Glaucoma (increased intraocular pressure), intolerance to light or glare, poor night vision | Encourage rest periods as needed.<br><br>Obtain referral to ophthalmologist.<br><br>Recommend adequate lighting, large print books, brochures, pamphlets.<br><br>Avoid night driving. |
| Ears | Loss of auditory hair cells (organ of Corti)<br><br>Ossicle becomes fixed. | Hearing loss in upper frequencies, problems distinguishing sounds Presbycusis | Obtain referral to otologist, audiologist.<br><br>Speak clearly, facing patient, in area with few distractions. |
| Other senses | Diminished sense of smell<br><br>Diminished sense of taste | Loss of appetite, poor nutrition<br><br>Increased use of salt, other seasonings | Suggest dietary consultation.<br><br>Encourage use of seasonings other than salt. |
| Reproductive (female) | Decreased egg production system<br><br>Decreased estrogen production<br><br>Poor perineal muscle tone<br><br>Rectocele, cystocele, stress incontinence | Menopause<br><br>Hot flashes; thinner, drier vaginal walls with itching<br><br>Painful intercourse; osteoporosis | Physician may prescribe supplemental estrogen.<br><br>Suggest **Kegel exercises** to strengthen pelvic floor. |
| Reproductive (male) | Smaller penis, testicles<br><br>Atherosclerosis, arteriosclerosis<br><br>Benign prostatic hypertrophy (BPH) | Loss of libido<br><br>Erectile dysfunction<br><br>Urgency, frequency, nocturia, retention | Physician may refer patient for counseling.<br><br>Explain good nutrition to avoid atherosclerosis.<br><br>Encourage patient to have yearly checks for BPH. |

SPEECH, LANGUAGE, AND HEARING DISORDERS

APHASIA: Aphasia is a complex problem which may result, in varying degrees, in a reduced ability to understand what others are saying, to express oneself, or to be understood. Some individuals with this disorder may have no speech, while others may have only mild difficulties recalling names or words. Others may have problems putting words in their proper order in a sentence. The ability to understand oral directions, to read, to write, and to deal with numbers may also be disturbed. Strokes are the major cause of aphasia in the older population. It has been estimated that there are over one million adults with aphasia in the United States today. Many can be helped to communicate more effectively.

DYSARTHRIA: Dysarthria interferes with normal control of the speech mechanism. Speech may be slurred or otherwise difficult to understand due to lack of ability to produce speech sounds correctly, maintain good breath control, and coordinate the movements of the lips, tongue, palate, and larynx. Diseases such as parkinsonism, multiple sclerosis, and bulbar palsy, as well as strokes and accidents, can cause dysarthria. Many individuals with dysarthria are over 65. Their communication skills often may be improved by appropriate treatment.

HEARING PROBLEMS: It is estimated that of the approximately 27 million Americans over the age of 65, as many as 50 percent may be affected by hearing impairment. The hearing loss observed as a part of the aging process is called "presbycusis." Many of those with presbycusis describe the problem as being able to "hear" what others are saying, but being unable to understand what is being said. This condition can lead to withdrawal from personal interactions of all types. Family or friends may confuse the disorder with "forgetfulness" or "senility." A hearing aid can often improve communication for older people with hearing loss.

VOICE PROBLEMS: Laryngectomy, the surgical removal of the larynx (voice box) due to cancer, affects approximately 9,000 individuals each year, most of whom are older. They can usually learn to speak again by learning esophageal speech, by using an electronic device or by surgical implant of voice prosthesis. Other forms of disease may result in complete or partial loss of the voice. Most of these problems can be treated.

OTHER COMMUNICATION PROBLEMS: Brain diseases that result in progressive loss of mental faculties may affect memory, orientation to time, place and people, and organization of thought processes, all of which may result in reduced ability to communicate.

**Figure 39-4 •** Focus on the older adult. What are the disorders of communication that most frequently affect older people? (From *Communication Disorders and Aging*. Rockville MD: American Speech-Language-Hearing Association. Reprinted with permission.)

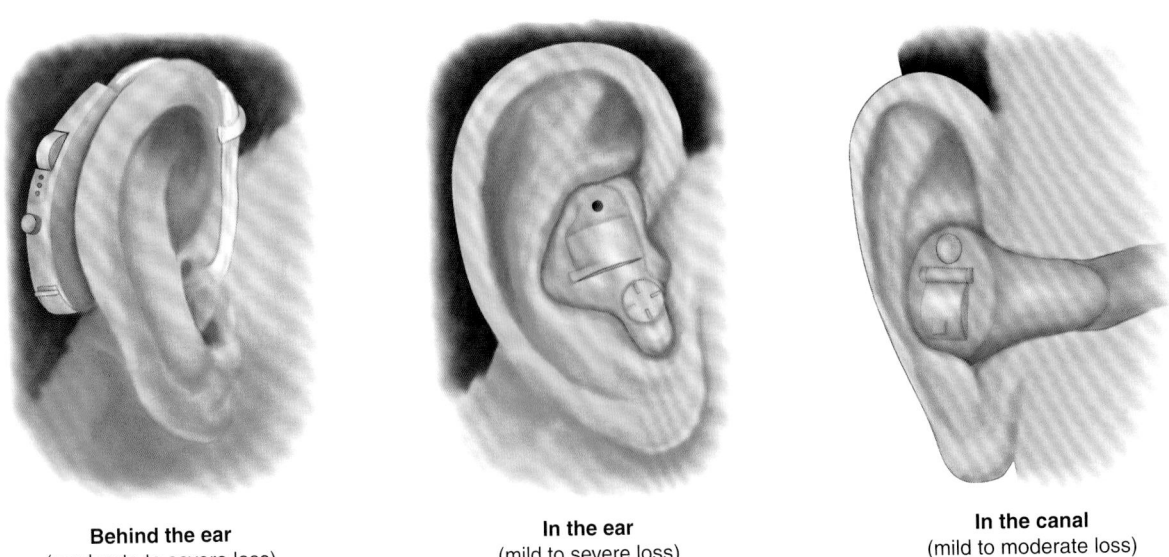

**Behind the ear**
(moderate to severe loss)

**In the ear**
(mild to severe loss)

**In the canal**
(mild to moderate loss)

**Figure 39-5 •** Several types of hearing aids. (From Carol R, Carol T, Lillis RN, et al. *Fundamentals of Nursing the Art and Science of Nursing Care*, 6th ed. Philadelphia, PA: Lippincott Williams & Wilkins, 2008.)

# DISEASES OF THE OLDER ADULT

The degenerative conditions noted in Table 39-1 are typically part of the aging process. Many of these changes cause problems that must be managed by the health care team; others are mere inconveniences for the patient. Diseases related to aging are described in the preceding chapters on specialties, and the disorders described previously also apply to older adults. However, there are some disorders that affect older patients more often than adults at younger ages. The following sections describe two conditions commonly associated with aging that may appear in the middle years as well.

## Parkinson Disease

Parkinson disease is a slow, progressive neurologic disorder affecting specific cells of the brain that produce the neurotransmitter dopamine. The initial symptoms frequently include muscle rigidity, involuntary tremors, and difficulty walking. Parkinson disease affects men more than women and is estimated to affect in some form approximately 1 in 100 persons over age 60 years. This disease may progress for 10 years or more before resulting in complete debilitation or death.

Normally, dopamine and acetylcholine, another neurotransmitter, are in balance and produce smooth, controlled muscle movement. With lower levels of dopamine, acetylcholine is not counterbalanced. This leads to involuntary movements of muscles and inability to control these movements. While the causes of Parkinson disease are unknown, researchers are working to determine whether there is a genetic component. Some evidence suggests that certain toxins may cause the disease. These toxins may be environmental or related to certain medications. The following are the signs and symptoms of Parkinson disease:

- Muscle rigidity
- **Bradykinesia** (abnormally slow voluntary movements)
- Difficulty walking, with a shuffling, mincing gait
- Forward-bending posture with no normal arm swing
- Laryngeal rigidity with a monotone voice
- Pharyngeal rigidity with dysphagia and drooling
- Facial muscle rigidity with a masklike, expressionless face and infrequent blinking reflex, causing frequent eye infections
- Small tremors in the fingers in a characteristic pill-rolling action. These start unilaterally and stop with purposeful action in the affected hand. Tremors are greatest during times of stress and anxiety and are diminished at sleep or rest. Muscles resist passive stretching and become rigid with passive manipulation (Fig. 39-6).

The diagnosis of Parkinson disease is usually made by excluding other causes; however, testing may show decreased levels of dopamine in the urine. A symptomatic history is the primary method of diagnosing after all other possibilities have been ruled out. Parkinson dis-

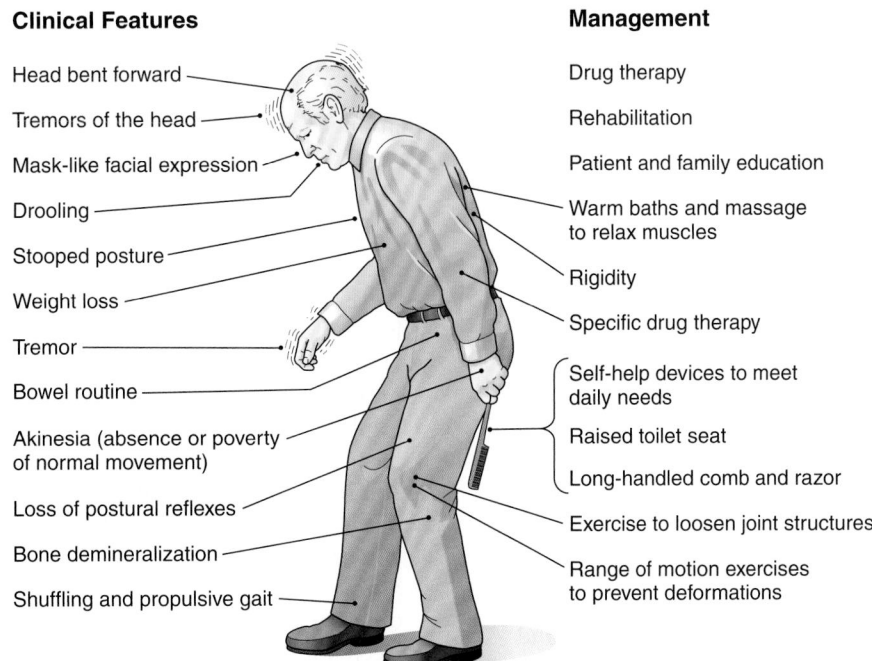

**Clinical Features**

- Head bent forward
- Tremors of the head
- Mask-like facial expression
- Drooling
- Stooped posture
- Weight loss
- Tremor
- Bowel routine
- Akinesia (absence or poverty of normal movement)
- Loss of postural reflexes
- Bone demineralization
- Shuffling and propulsive gait

**Management**

- Drug therapy
- Rehabilitation
- Patient and family education
- Warm baths and massage to relax muscles
- Rigidity
- Specific drug therapy
- Self-help devices to meet daily needs
- Raised toilet seat
- Long-handled comb and razor
- Exercise to loosen joint structures
- Range of motion exercises to prevent deformations

**Figure 39-6** • The Parkinson disease patient.

ease has no cure. Treatment is symptomatic, supportive, and palliative. Medications include the following:

- Levodopa (l-dopa). Dopamine replacement crosses the blood–brain barrier to restore balance with acetylcholine. Individualized doses are gradually increased as symptoms progress. Levodopa is fairly effective for a time but gradually loses its effectiveness. Unfortunately, levodopa has serious side effects, including nausea, vomiting, tachycardia, and arrhythmias. It has severe adverse reactions with alcohol.
- Anticholinergics. These drugs decrease the levels of acetylcholine so that depleted levels of dopamine are not so out of balance. This method works best in mild, early stages.
- Antihistamines with anticholinergic action. In the early, mild stages, this method of lowering acetylcholine levels to balance with low levels of dopamine alleviates symptoms.

A procedure known as *deep brain stimulation* is used to treat tremor and rigidity. In this procedure, electrodes are surgically placed in certain areas of the brain and are connected by wires to an impulse generator that is implanted under the skin of the chest. This transmitter sends electrical impulses to the electrodes in the brain, blocking the impulses that cause the tremors. Although this procedure is effective for controlling involuntary movements and tremors, it is generally not used if medication can control the patient's symptoms. Like all other methods, this treatment is palliative and not curative.

Parkinson patients retain their mental and cognitive functions unless an organic brain disturbance is also present. They are aware of the outward signs of the disease and may be embarrassed and emotionally depressed. They require great psychological support from the medical staff, family, and support groups. You can help in the following ways:

- Encourage the patient to participate in all ADL.
- Promote independence.
- Be aware that, because rigidity extends to the gastrointestinal tract, the patient may have dysphagia and constipation. Suggest that the patient increase fluid intake, eat a balanced diet, and increase fiber intake.
- Tell the patient that a decreased cough reflex can lead to choking. Suggest that the patient take small bites and chew each mouthful of food carefully before attempting to swallow.
- Encourage the patient to use eating aids such as a no-spill cup, plate with high sides, and special utensils. High toilet seats and handrails in the bath also help increase the patient's independence and safety.
- Listen to the patient. Intelligence is still intact and needs to be stimulated.
- Educate the patient about safety factors. The forward-bending posture and altered gait frequently lead to falls. Encourage these patients to hold on to handrails and pick up feet carefully to avoid falling. Also, the home should be free from rugs and loose cords that may cause accidental tripping.
- Enlist the help of support groups. Include the caregiver and urge respite care when exhaustion and stress become overwhelming.

---

### CHECKPOINT QUESTION

7. How can you assist a patient with Parkinson disease?

---

## Alzheimer Disease

Roughly half of the cases of dementia in the older adult are due to Alzheimer disease. The symptoms of Alzheimer disease may be similar to those caused by TIA, cerebral tumor, and dementia other than Alzheimer disease. Unfortunately, the cause of Alzheimer disease is not known.

The symptoms of Alzheimer disease may begin as early as age 40 years, with a gradual loss of memory and slight personality changes. The changes may occur over as long as 15 years and are frequently so gradual that diagnosis is difficult and may be made only by ruling out all other possibilities. Autopsy reveals organic brain changes, including a loss of neurons and neurotransmitters. Plaques or deposits may be present as a residue of the neural cell deterioration.

Alzheimer disease has seven recognized stages. The progression from one stage to the next may be gradual. Some stages may last for years, but a patient may pass through other stages so quickly that the progression goes unnoticed. Expect varying levels of response from patients in these different levels (Table 39-2). When caring for Alzheimer disease patients, you must remember that anger and hostility are often symptoms of the disease and should not to be taken personally. Be sure to do the following:

- Respond with the utmost patience and compassion.
- Speak calmly and without condescension.
- Never argue with the patient, even if the patient blames you unfairly for something the patient forgot.
- Do not expect the patient to remember you from previous visits. Reintroduce yourself.
- Explain even common procedures as if the patient has never had them explained.
- Approach the patient quietly and professionally in an unthreatening manner, and remind the patient who you are and what you must do.
- Speak in short, simple, direct sentences, and explain only one action at a time.
- Keep a list of support contacts for family members to call.

Home care agencies usually offer respite care, which can be vitally important for caregivers, who need to maintain

| TABLE 39-2 | Levels of Alzheimer Disease |
|---|---|
| **Level** | **Description** |
| I, II | Presenile dementia may end here, with no further progression. Brain changes insignificant; only remarkable symptom may be forgetfulness. ADL done with reasonable ease |
| III | Patient losing ability to remember facts, faces, and names but still aware enough to recognize problem and becomes increasingly frustrated and angry. Most ADL still performed reasonably well. |
| IV | Late confusional or mild Alzheimer disease. Patient beginning to misplace things, has increasing difficulty remembering, and neglects ADL. Most patients aware of a problem but deny any concern. |
| V | Early dementia or moderate Alzheimer disease. Patient must have custodial care, has severe memory lapses, disorientation, anger, and great frustration. |
| VI | Middle dementia or moderately severe Alzheimer disease with severe memory loss, no self-care at any level, disoriented most of the time with immense anger, hostility, and combativeness. Fear of water |
| VII | Late dementia. Patient requires full-time care and is rarely seen in the office. Unless home care is an option, physician will probably visit long-term care facility. Patient rarely speaks, almost never intelligibly; incontinent; may require tube feeding |

their own mental and physical health. An exhausted, distraught family member may not be thinking clearly. The most therapeutic action may be for you to assist the family with proper contacts to help make caring for a family member with this devastating disease less traumatic.

## MAINTAINING OPTIMUM HEALTH

No one realistically expects to have the same strength and agility at age 70 years as at age 20 years. With attention to exercise and good nutrition, however, it is possible to maintain a good level of fitness that adds to quality of life.

### Exercise

Exercise plays a vital role in maintaining overall physical and mental health (Table 39-3). Older patients should begin an exercise program only after a thorough physical examination and should follow the physician's recommendation. Provide the following guidelines for older adult patients who are starting an exercise program with the physician's approval:

1. Before exercise, always warm up cold muscles for at least 10 minutes. Slow and rhythmic movements, such as walking, raise the heart rate and increase metabolism. Then do slow, easy stretching to lengthen sluggish muscles.
2. Begin by exercising for brief periods. Exercise only 5 to 10 minutes a day the first week, then progress to 10 to 15 minutes a day the next week. Gradually work up to about 30 to 45 minutes of a pleasantly challenging strength and cardiovascular endurance activity after about a month. This routine reduces the chance of injury and is likely to be an attainable goal.

3. Stop if you feel pain, shortness of breath, or dizziness. Never try to work through pain.
4. Breathe deeply and evenly. If you cannot carry on a conversation, slow down. Never hold your breath while you exercise.
5. Rest when you get tired. Do not try to exercise to the point of exhaustion.
6. Keep a record of your progress. It is motivational to watch your performance improve.

| TABLE 39-3 | Benefits of Exercise | |
|---|---|
| **System** | **Benefits** |
| Cardiovascular | Increases endurance |
| | Lowers cholesterol to avoid atherosclerosis |
| | Maintains vascular elasticity to delay arteriosclerosis |
| Musculoskeletal | Increases bone mass to reduce osteoporosis |
| | Decreases fat-to-muscle ratio and increases metabolism |
| | Retains strength and flexibility to ensure mobility, improve posture |
| Nervous | Improves mental health by reducing stress, fatigue, tension, boredom |
| | Maintains or restores balance to reduce risk of falls |
| Endocrine | May decrease need for insulin or oral hypoglycemic medication in diabetes |

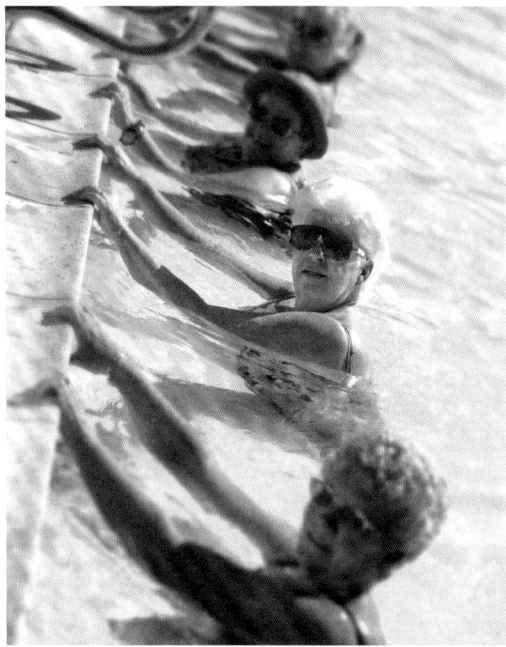

**Figure 39-7 •** Participating in group exercise helps to maintain overall physical and mental health.

7. Exercise with a friend, with a group, or to music that you enjoy (Fig. 39-7).
8. Make exercise a part of your daily routine, but do not make it a chore. Do something vigorous every day and take pride in it.

### CHECKPOINT QUESTION

8. What are the physical signs that indicate a patient should stop exercising?

## Diet

Many older adult patients have difficulty maintaining good nutrition. Reduced activity means a corresponding decrease in hunger. Decaying teeth or poorly fitting dentures cause pain, making it hard to chew. Saliva production decreases, making it harder to swallow. The senses of smell and taste diminish, interfering with the cephalic phase of digestion. Many older adult patients eat alone or are not able to enjoy the socializing that adds immeasurably to the pleasure of eating.

A balanced diet is vital to good health at any age. Although activity levels, and hence calorie requirements, are lower among older adults, vitamin and mineral requirements do not decrease with age. Efforts must be made to increase the nutritional level of older adults. Smaller, more frequent meals may be easier to digest than infrequent large meals. Water should be encouraged to maintain hydration and to aid digestion and elimination.

Talk to patients or their families about valuable social services that may deliver nutritious meals to the home daily or 5 days a week. These programs may ensure that at least one well-balanced meal a day is available. Most

services prepare meals to meet special dietary needs, such as low sodium or low fat. The program volunteer is alert to the needs of the patient and will report to a coordinator if the patient does not answer the door or seems ill or confused. These resources will help to reassure the family that the patient's nutritional and social needs are being met.

### PATIENT EDUCATION

#### Liquid Dietary Supplements

There are many liquid dietary supplements available on the market today, and some are specifically marketed for the older adult. When interviewing the older adult, always assess their nutritional status by asking about the frequency of meals and types of food eaten and obtaining a weight at each visit. Let the physician know if you notice a trend in weight loss or other signs of poor nutrition. With permission of the physician, encourage your patient with nutritional problems to get a liquid supplement in his or her favorite flavor; most come in vanilla, chocolate, and strawberry. Advise your patient that these supplements should not replace a meal, but rather provide extra nutrition between meals.

## Safety

Alert the patient and caregivers to hazards in the home of an older adult patient and offer the following suggestions:

• Remove any scatter rugs, especially on highly polished floors.
• Never allow electrical cords to cross passageways.
• Remove or reduce clutter as much as possible.
• Strengthen handrails on stairs and install them in tubs and near the commode.
• Install a telephone by the bedside and near a favorite chair.
• Install and carefully maintain smoke alarms and carbon monoxide detectors throughout the house.
• Establish a system in which someone calls and checks on the patient every day.

Many communities have programs in which volunteers call the sick or older adult daily to check on their needs and offer a few minutes of conversation. If the patient fails to answer, someone goes to the home to check on the patient. This service ensures that the patient is never without contact for long. Lifeline, an emergency service, is another option that increases the feeling of safety for patients who live alone.

### CHECKPOINT QUESTION

9. What are some reasons an older adult patient may have poor nutritional status?

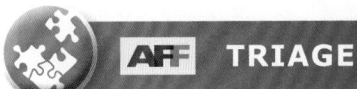 **TRIAGE**

While you are working in a medical office, the following three patients are waiting to be seen:

A. Patient A is a 76-year-old woman who is active but underweight, with a history of osteoporosis. She is here for a physical examination, and the doctor has just instructed you to obtain some blood work for laboratory analysis.

B. Patient B is an 87-year-old man brought in by his daughter, who takes care of him in her home since his stroke 3 years ago. His wife is deceased, and his daughter is concerned because his memory seems to be failing him.

C. Patient C is a 90-year-old man residing in an assisted living facility with his wife, who is 88. They were brought to the office today because the husband is due for a blood pressure check and possible medication adjustment. They are alert and sharp mentally, although both move more slowly than usual and the wife requires a walker.

**How would you sort these patients? Who do you see first? Second? Third?**

When working with older adult patients, it is important to remember not to rush them or appear inattentive. Since patient B is having new symptoms and may require a longer time with the physician, you should check him in first and get vital signs and any appropriate medical information from both the patient and his daughter. The husband and wife should be seen next, since all that is required is a brief chief complaint and obtaining vital signs. When both the husband and wife are comfortable and safely seated, you may leave them alone until the doctor is available to see them. Patient A should be seen last because obtaining blood from the older adult requires special attention to detail and patience. Once the blood sample is obtained, patient A may be discharged after checking the medical record to assure that no physician orders have been missed.

 **MEDICATION BOX**

## Commonly Prescribed Geriatric Medications

**Note:** *The generic name of the drug is listed first and is written in all lowercase letters. Brand names are in parentheses, and the first letter is capitalized.*

| | | |
|---|---|---|
| Adalimumab (Humira) | Injection: 40 mg/0.8 mL (subcutaneous [SC]) | Antirheumatic |
| Alendronate sodium (Fosamax) | Tablets: 5 mg, 10 mg, 35 mg, 40 mg, 70 mg<br>Oral solution: 70 mg/75 mL | Antiresorptive |
| Allopurinol (Zyloprim) | Tablets: 100 mg, 300 mg | Antigout |
| Alprazolam (Xanax) | Tablets: 0.25 mg, 0.5 mg, 1 mg, 2 mg<br>Oral solution: 1 mg/mL | Antianxiety |
| Benztropine mesylate (Cogentin) | Tablets: 0.5 mg, 1 mg, 2 mg<br>Injection: 1 mg/mL (intramuscular [IM]) | Antiparkinsonian |
| Celecoxib (Celebrex) | Capsules: 50 mg, 100 mg, 200 mg, 400 mg | Nonsteroidal anti-inflammatory |
| Diazepam (Valium) | Tablets: 2 mg, 5 mg, 10 mg<br>Oral solution: 5 mg/5 mL | Antianxiety |
| Donepezil hydrochloride (Aricept) | Tablets: 5 mg, 10 mg | Alzheimer disease |

*(continues on page 1022)*

## MEDICATION BOX (continued)

| | | |
|---|---|---|
| Enoxaparin (Lovenox) | Prefilled syringe: 60 mg/0.6 mL, (SC)<br>Injection: 80 mg/0.8 mL, 100 mg/mL<br>Injection: 120 mg/0.8 mL, 150 mg/mL<br>Vial: 300 mg/3 mL | Anticoagulant |
| Estrogen (Premarin, Cenestin) | Tablets: 0.3 mg, 0.45 mg, 0.625 mg<br>Vaginal cream: 0.625 mg/g | Hormone |
| Galantamine hydrobromide (Razadyne) | Capsules: 8 mg, 16 mg, 24 mg<br>Tablets: 4 mg, 8 mg, 12 mg<br>Oral solution: 4 mg/mL | Alzheimer disease |
| Gold sodium thiomalate (Aurolate; Myochrysine) | Injection: 50 mg/mL (IM) | Antirheumatic |
| Ibandronate sodium (Boniva) | Tablets: 2.5 mg, 150 mg<br>Injection: 3 mg/3 mL (intravenous) | Antiresorptive |
| Lorazepam (Ativan) | Tablets: 0.5 mg, 1 mg, 2 mg<br>Oral solution: 2 mg/mL | Antianxiety |
| Naproxen (Naprosyn) | Tablets: 200 mg, 250 mg, 375 mg, 500 mg<br>Oral suspension: 125 mg/5 mL | Nonsteroidal anti-inflammatory |
| Raloxifene hydrochloride (Evista) | Tablets: 60 mg | Antiresorptive |
| Sildenafil citrate (Viagra) | Tablets: 20 mg, 25 mg, 50 mg, 100 mg | Erectile dysfunction |
| Tadalafil (Cialis) | Tablets: 2.5 mg, 5 mg, 10 mg, 10 mg, 20 mg | Erectile dysfunction |
| Warfarin sodium (Coumadin) | Tablets: 1 mg, 2 mg, 2.5 mg, 3 mg, 4 mg, 5 mg, 6 mg, 7.5 mg, 10 mg | Anticoagulant |
| Zoster vaccine, live (Zostavax) | Injection: one vial (SC) | Vaccine |

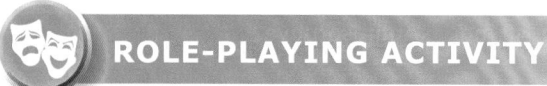

## ROLE-PLAYING ACTIVITY

When talking with an elderly patient this morning for a routine physical, Ross Mason CMA(AAMA), noticed that the patient seemed to be a little confused on several of occasions during the visit. Upon questioning the patient's unusual responses, the patient became aware that his answer was inappropriate and joked about his recent episodes of "forgetfulness." Although the patient's clothes seemed to be clean, they were not appropriate for today's weather and were very big for his stature. He was also wearing shoes that were dirty and appeared to be very large for him. The patient was unable to accurately identify several of his medications and was unable to describe his medication regimen to Ross. Role-play this scenario as the medical assistant attempting to gather information from an elderly patient who exhibits behaviors that might indicate additional help with ADLs may be warranted. What other indications might Ross note that this patient may have problems with living independently and taking his medications appropriately? How should Ross handle this patient, and what information should Ross document about this patient's behavior? What, if anything, should Ross communicate to the physician? If you are assuming the role of the patient, consider how you might feel as the elderly patient being questioned about these issues. Would you feel defensive or angry? Or would you feel a sense of loss with perhaps sadness? Your instructor will give you additional information about this activity!

## *español* SPANISH TERMINOLOGY

**Este medicamento se toma de esta manera.**
This is how you take this medication.

**Le duele donde esta rígido? Do you have pain and stiffness?**

**La/el asistente de salud a domicilio le ayudará con su cuidado personal.**
The home health aide will help with your personal care.

**¿Ha notado algún cambio en su habilidad para recordar las cosas?**
Have you noticed a change in your memory?

**El doctor recomienda buscar ayuda de un asistente personal para su familiar.**
The doctor recommends you look for home health aide services for your relative.

**El doctor recomienda preguntarle antes de comprar productos herbolarios o suplementos.**
The doctor recommends asking him first before you buy any herb product or supplements.

**Para evitar una ulcera, tienen que moverlo (a) frecuentemente.**
To avoid a bedsore, you have to change his/her position frequently.

**Ha firmado una Declaración de voluntad anticipada?**
Have you signed an advance directive form?

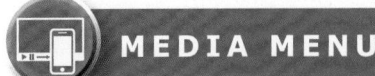

## MEDIA MENU

**Student Resources** on thePoint®
- **CMA/RMA Certification Exam Review**
- **English to Spanish Audio Glossary**

**Internet Resources**
**The Center for Social Gerontology**
http://www.tcsg.org

**American Association of Retired Persons**
http://www.aarp.org

**National Center on Elder Abuse**
http://www.ncea.aoa.gov/NCEAroot/Main_Site/Index.aspx

**National Institute on Aging**
http://www.nia.nih.gov

**Centers for Medicare and Medicaid Services**
http://www.cms.hhs.gov

## EMR Activity

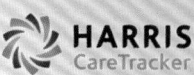

Prerequisite Activities in Harris CareTracker

- *The Getting Started and Quickstart documents and EMR Activities Step-by-Step Instructions are available at* http://thePoint.lww.com/KronenbergerComp5e

Activity Details

Create an outgoing referral from primary care physician Dr. Kyle Dunn in the EMR for patient Oscar Tinner to Alva Smith, psychiatrist. Mr. Tinner is suffering with depression as a result of the recent death of his wife of 52 years. Note that there is a transition of care where indicated in the EMR and that the patient's secondary insurance as authorized ten (10) visits under authorization number 87611PSY and the authorization starting today and for the next 3 months.

## Chapter Summary

Regardless of the type of specialty you work in, you will encounter the older adult patient. Some important things to remember about the older adult include the following:

- Avoid stereotyping the older adult into passive, dependent roles.
- Be alert to the normal physiologic changes of aging and adjust your communication techniques accordingly.
- Not all older adult patients are affected by diseases such as dementia, Alzheimer disease, or Parkinson disease.
- Having patients who are diagnosed with Parkinson or Alzheimer disease will require you to understand the disease process and develop excellent interpersonal skills.
- Use patient education opportunities to discuss issues of safety whenever possible.

## Warm-Ups for Critical Thinking

1. Mrs. Moss, age 78 years, lives with her son and daughter-in-law and their two school-aged children. She has dysphagia and a poor appetite. Identify ways in which Mrs. Moss can improve or maintain her nutritional status while participating in the family meals.
2. Mr. Brown is 90 years old, and his wife is 86 years old. They live alone, and Mrs. Brown is the primary caregiver. During the physical examination, Mr. Brown is found to have several large decubital ulcers. Summarize the various types of elder abuse or neglect. What is likely the problem in this case? Explain how you would handle this situation.
3. The pharmacist calls you at the office and says he has an older adult patient waiting to have a prescription for a high blood pressure medication filled. This prescription was filled just 2 weeks ago, but the patient says he is "all out of my medicine." What do you advise the pharmacist to do?
4. Your 68-year-old male patient tells you that he is thinking about joining the senior citizens exercise group at the local community college. He appears to be healthy and is not currently on any medications. How would you respond?
5. The daughter of an older adult woman comes to the office with her 76-year-old mother who lives alone. Would it be permissible to have the daughter present during the interview and physical exam? What about confidentiality?

PART

4

# The Clinical Laboratory

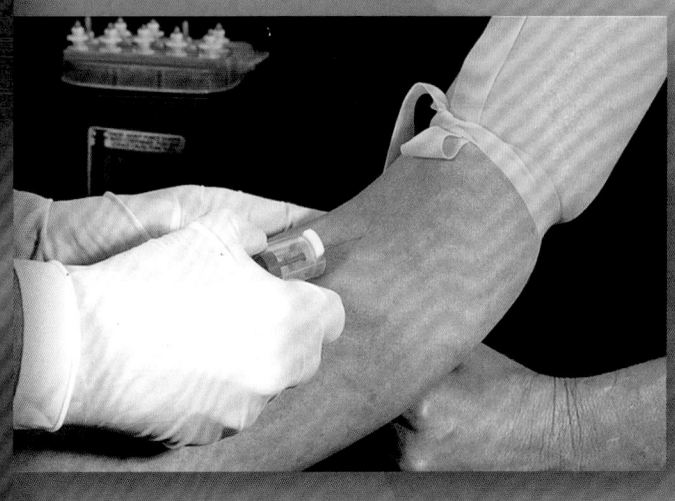

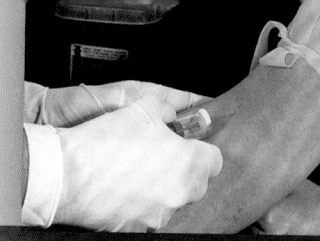

CHAPTER

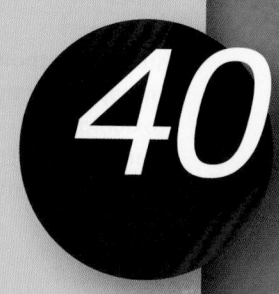

# *40* Introduction to the Physician Office Laboratory

## Outline

## Learning Outcomes

**COG Cognitive Domain***

1. Spell key terms
2. *Define medical terms and abbreviations related to all body systems*
3. List the various types of clinical laboratories including the physician office laboratory
4. Explain the types of departments found in most large laboratories
5. Describe common laboratory tests ordered to diagnose disease and illness
6. Explain the significance of CLIA and how to maintain compliance in the physician office laboratory
7. *Identify disease processes that are indications for CLIA-waived tests*
8. Identify equipment found in the physician office laboratory and routine maintenance
9. List and describe the parts of a microscope

10. Discuss the role of the medical assistant in clinical laboratory testing
11. Define critical values
12. *Analyze charts, graphs, and/or tables in the interpretation of health care results*

**PSY Psychomotor Domain***

1. Care of the microscope (Procedure 40-1)
2. Screen test results (Procedure 40-2)
3. *Maintain laboratory test results using flow sheets (Procedure 40-3)*

**AFF Affective Domain***

1. *Incorporate critical thinking skills when performing patient assessment*
2. *Distinguish between normal and abnormal test results*

**\*Note: AAMA/CAAHEP 2015 Standards are italicized.**

*(continues on page 1030)*

## Key Terms

aerosol
aliquots
analytes
antibody
anticoagulant
antigen
autoimmunity
calibration
centrifugation
chain of custody
Clinical and Laboratory
  Standards Institute
  (CLSI)
clinical chemistry
coagulation

Commission on Office
  Laboratory Accreditation
  (COLA)
confirmatory test
control
critical values
cytogenetics
cytology
external control
hematology
histology
immunodeficiency
immunohematology
immunology
internal control

microbiology
nonwaived testing
oncology
panels
physician office laboratory
  (POL)
plasma
product insert
provider-performed
  microscopy (PPM or
  PPMP)
qualitative test
quality assurance (QA)
quality control (QC)
quantitative test

reconstitution
reference intervals
referral laboratory
serum
shifts
specimen
surgical pathology
therapeutic range
toxicology
trends
unitized test device
urinalysis
whole blood

## Case Study

Melissa Miller, CMA (AAMA), works in a busy family practice office at Great Falls Medical Center. She was hired because of her ability to work in either the front office (scheduling appointments, answering the phone, collecting copayments and deductibles, etc.) or the back office, or clinical area. Today, she is assisting Dr. Singer in the clinical area and must obtain laboratory specimens to send to the hospital laboratory for testing or to be tested in the physician office laboratory. How does Melissa determine whether the laboratory tests ordered by Dr. Singer can be processed in the office or must be sent to the hospital laboratory? What is Melissa's role in obtaining test results and communicating those results to the physician and patient? These and other questions are addressed in this chapter.

## THE PURPOSE OF THE CLINICAL LABORATORY

When the physician orders laboratory tests in the medical office, the medical assistant must know how to obtain the **specimen** and process it for testing in the office or sending it to an outside laboratory for testing. Regardless of the type of specimen, the physician is requesting that a small sample taken from the patient be used to detect the presence, absence, or amount of a particular substance to make a diagnosis and provide appropriate treatment as necessary. While some tests can be performed in the physician office, others must be sent to an outside larger laboratory that employs professionals educated and trained to operate complex equipment and analyze a specimen or test result to report back to the physician.

Each professional position in a laboratory requires a particular level of education and training and has specific responsibilities (Box 40-1). The medical laboratory professionals analyze blood, urine, and other body samples to measure **analytes** (the substances a laboratory tests) that contribute to the diagnosis and treatment of disease. Results of laboratory testing are compared with normal or **reference intervals** (acceptable ranges for a healthy population) to determine the health of body systems or organs (refer to Appendix I for a list of commonly performed laboratory tests and their reference intervals). In some cases, patients take medications that must reach a certain blood level for effectiveness or the drug may become toxic if the level is excessive. In these situations, the physician will order blood levels of medications to adjust medication dosages. Some patients may have a

- Pathologist. A physician who studies disease processes. Commonly, a pathologist oversees the technical aspects of a laboratory.
- Chief technologist or laboratory manager. A supervisor who manages the day-to-day operations of a laboratory, including staffing, test menu and pricing, purchasing, and QC.
- Medical technologist or clinical laboratory scientist. A graduate of a bachelor's (4-year) degree program (or equivalent) in medical laboratory science, who has been certified by the American Society of Clinical Pathology. Laboratory technologists perform all levels of testing and supervise laboratory departments.
- Medical laboratory technician or clinical laboratory technician. A graduate of an associate (2-year) degree program (or equivalent) in medical laboratory science who is nationally certified.
- Laboratory assistant. A person with a high school diploma or equivalent who is a graduate of a vocational or on-the-job laboratory assistant training program. Laboratory assistants collect and process specimens and can perform some designated testing.
- Phlebotomist. A professional trained to draw blood and to process blood and other samples. A phlebotomist may be a laboratory assistant, medical assistant, or person trained specifically in phlebotomy. A nationally certified phlebotomist has a high school diploma or equivalent and either is a graduate of an approved training program or has a minimum of 1 year of full-time work in phlebotomy.
- Histologist. A technician trained to process and evaluate tissue samples, such as biopsy or surgical samples.
- Cytologist. A professional trained to examine cells under the microscope and to look for abnormal changes; Pap smears are generally examined by cytologists.
- Specimen processor or accessioner. A professional trained to accept shipments of specimens and to centrifuge, separate, or otherwise process the samples to prepare them for testing. In addition, this position usually includes numbering and labeling the specimens and entering specimen information into a computer.

Laboratory testing is most commonly used for the following:

- Diagnosing disease
- Monitoring a patient's medication and treatment
- Identifying the cause of an infection
- Preventing disease

# TYPES OF CLINICAL LABORATORIES

Laboratory testing is performed in three different kinds of laboratories including a **referral laboratory**, a hospital laboratory, and a **physician office laboratory** (POL).

A reference or referral laboratory is a large facility in which thousands of tests of various types are performed each day. Referral laboratories employ medical laboratory scientists and technicians who are educated and trained to perform testing that may be too expensive or complicated for other labs to perform. Because the referral lab performs such high volumes of each test, the cost is less than what might be charged to perform similar tests at a smaller laboratory. In addition to collecting the specimen in some cases, referral labs also receive specimens from smaller laboratories, physician offices, and clinics. Once the specimen is in the referral lab, specimen processors log patient data and specimen information into the laboratory information system. Processors also prepare **aliquots** (portions of specimens used for testing) if indicated and send them to the appropriate department for analysis. Specimens obtained off-site from the referral lab are often delivered by courier or, in some cases, sent via the mail. All specimens sent to referral laboratories must be packaged appropriately to withstand rough handling, pressure changes, or temperature extremes. Some specimens require refrigeration after obtaining, and these must be sent in a cooler. Packaging specimens also includes placement in a special leakproof secondary transport container approved for biohazardous materials and a completed laboratory request form (Fig. 40-1).

Some medical offices send laboratory specimens to a hospital lab for testing; however, the hospital lab may perform only the most commonly requested tests. Tests that are not commonly ordered by the physician may have to go to a referral lab. The professional medical assistant must be familiar with the type of specimen, test or tests ordered, and the appropriate lab to send the specimen to that will perform the requested tests. Whether the test is performed in a hospital lab or sent to a referral laboratory, results are generally available within 24 to 48 hours. Both hospital labs and referral labs require the medical lab professionals to adhere to **quality control** (QC) procedures or those procedures used to detect and correct errors that may occur. Quality

disease process caused by infection with microorganisms. Laboratory tests are done to identify bacteria, viruses, parasites, and other microorganisms to begin treatment. This chapter includes an introduction to the clinical laboratory including the physician office laboratory.

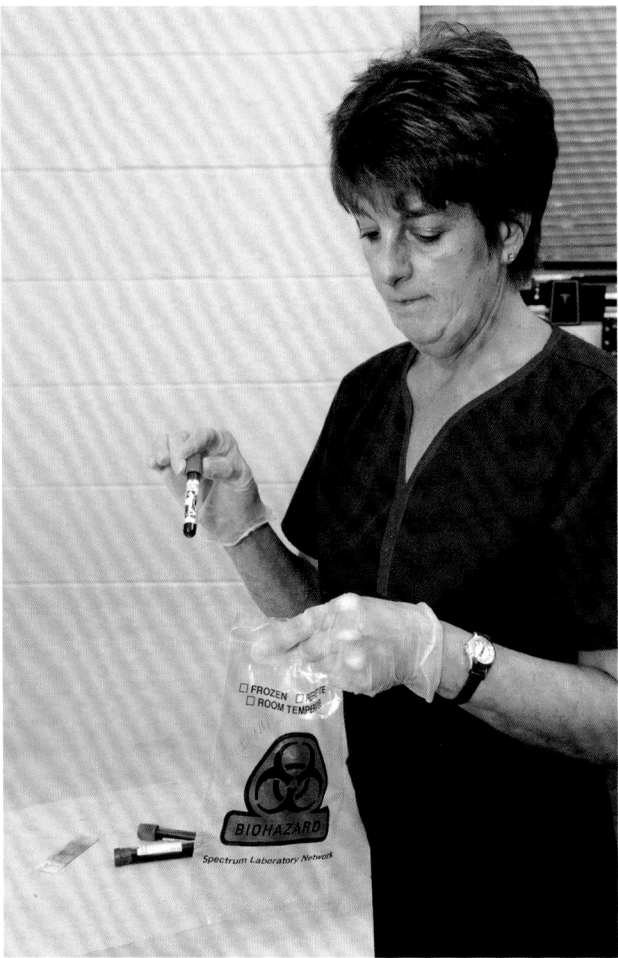

**Figure 40-1** • Transport containers are constructed to maintain the integrity of the specimen and to protect those who are responsible for the care and handling of possibly hazardous bodily fluids and substances.

control measures ensure the accuracy of the results, and acceptable quality control results must be achieved before laboratory test results can be reported.

## CHECKPOINT QUESTION

1. Melissa Miller must compare lab results with reference intervals each day as part of her medical assisting duties. What are reference intervals, and how are they significant to patient care?

## Laboratory Departments

Larger laboratory facilities typically include specialized departments that require special equipment and knowledge. Knowing the various departments in the larger laboratories is necessary when completing the laboratory request form as laboratory tests are often categorized by department on the form (Fig. 40-2). While

some larger laboratories may have many departments, the more common departments in a reference or hospital lab include those listed below.

## 1. Hematology

**Hematology** is the study of blood and blood-forming tissues and may include the specialty of **oncology**, the medical specialty that focuses on the diagnosis and treatment of cancer. Hematology tests are performed to evaluate diseases of the blood, including the evaluation of blood smears and bone marrow slides under the microscope. Hematology testing may be ordered to diagnose disease processes involving blood cells or blood-forming tissue such as bone marrow. Most hematology tests are performed on **whole blood** specimens or blood that contains all cellular components (Fig. 40-3). Common hematology tests include white blood cell count (WBC), red blood cell count (RBC), platelet count, hemoglobin, and hematocrit. These tests are discussed in more detail in Chapter 42, Hematology.

## 2. Coagulation

**Coagulation** testing includes evaluating how well the body's blood clotting process is performing. Tests that are considered coagulation studies include the measurement of prothrombin time (PT) or international normalized ratio (INR) and the activated partial thromboplastin time (APTT). Both tests may be ordered to monitor the effectiveness of **anticoagulant** drugs, such as heparin and Coumadin. **Plasma**, the liquid portion of a blood specimen that has not coagulated or clotted, is used for coagulation studies ordered by the physician (Fig. 40-3).

## 3. Clinical Chemistry

**Clinical chemistry** (also known as *chemical pathology*) is the area of the laboratory that analyzes body fluids. The tests are performed on any kind of body fluid but mostly on **serum** or plasma. Serum is the yellow liquid part of blood left after blood has been allowed to clot, and all blood cells have been removed. Separation of the serum from the cells is most easily done by **centrifugation**.

Chemistry tests can be further subcategorized into subspecialities of:

- General or routine chemistry
- Endocrinology—the study of hormones
- **Immunology**—the study of the immune system and antibodies
- Pharmacology—the study of drugs
- **Toxicology**—the study of drugs and poisons

Toxicology may be a separate department in the chemistry laboratory. In addition to detecting drugs of abuse, this lab is also used to detect poisoning. Drugs of abuse

**GREAT FALLS MEDICAL CENTER**
**LABORATORY SERVICES**

# LABORATORY OUTPATIENT FORM

**ORDERING PHYSICIAN:** _____

NPI: _____

OFFICE PHONE NUMBER: _____

PHONE: _____ FAX: _____

EMAIL: _____

**SPECIMEN COLLECTION DATE:** _____

**TIME:** _____

**COLLECTED BY:** _____

**PATIENT NAME:** _____

ADDRESS: _____

CITY/STATE/ZIP: _____

PHONE NUMBER: _____

PRIMARY INS: _____

MEMBER: _____ ID#: _____

RELATIONSHIP TO INSURED: _____

SECONDARY INS: _____

MEMBER: _____ ID# _____

RELATIONSHIP TO INSURED: _____

| √ | PANELS | TEST CODE | √ | URINES / SEROLOGY | TEST CODE | √ | SPECIAL CHEMISTRY | TEST CODE |
|---|---|---|---|---|---|---|---|---|
| | Basic Metabolic Panel | BMP | | Amino Acid - Urine | AAU | | **SPECIAL CHEMISTRY** | |
| | Comp Metabolic Panel | CPM | | Comprehensive Drug Screen | CDSU | | Amino Acid - Plasma | AAP |
| | Electrolyte Panel | LYT2 | | Drugs of Abuse Screen | BDSU | | Estradiol | ESTD |
| | Hepatitis Panel | ACHS | | Hepatitis B | HGAB | | Folate | FOLA |
| | Lipid Panel | FATS | | HIV Antibody | HIV | | FSH | FSH |
| | Liver Function Panel | LIVR | | IGE | IGE | | Hemoglobin Variants (HPLC) | HGBV |
| | Newborn Screen | SN | | Immunoglobulins | IMGL | | LH | LH |
| | Renal Function Panel | RNL | | Mono | IFM | | Organic Acid - Plasma | ORAP |
| | **ROUTINE CHEMISTRY** | | | Pregnancy, Qual. Serum | HCG | | Pregnancy, Quant HCG | HCGQ |
| | Albumin | ALB | | Pregnancy, Qual, Urine | UCG | | Prolactin | PROL |
| | Alk Phos | ALP | | Rubella Titer | RUBT | | Testosterone | TESC |
| | ALT / SGPT | GPT | | Stool Occult Blood | OCBL | | Free T4 | FT4 |
| | Ammonia | AMON | | Urinalysis (Dip Stick) | UAD | | T4 | T4 |
| | Amylase | AMY | | Urinalysis (Reflex Micro) | URA | | TSH | TSH |
| | AST / SGOT | GOT | | | | | Free T3 | T3FR |
| | BUN | BUN | | **MICROBIOLOGY** | | | T3 | T3T |
| | Bilirubin, Direct | DBIL | | Chlamydia | | | Vitamin B12 | VB12 |
| | Bilirubin, Total | TBIL | | Genital Culture (Routine) | GENC | | **TDM'S** | |
| | Calcium | CA | | Giardia –EIA | GIAR | | Cyclosporine | CYCB |
| | Calcium, Ionized | ICA | | Ova & Parasite (OP) | OP | | Digoxin | DIG |
| | Carbon Dioxide | CO2 | | Rapid Strep, Culture if negative | RSTR | | Dilantin (Phenytoin) | PTN |
| | Chloride | CL | | Rapid Strep, Screen Only | RSTRC | | Methotrexate | XATB |
| | Cholesterol | CHOL | | Strep Cultrue Only | THRC | | Phenobarbital | PHNO |
| | CPK / CK | CK | | Rotavirus EIA | ROTO | | Tegretol (Carbamazepine) | CRBA |
| | Creatinine | CREA | | RSV – EIA | RSVE | | Theophylline | THEO |
| | Glucose | GLU | | Stool Culture (Campylobacter) | STOC | | | |
| | Glucose, 2HR Post | GLUP | | Stool Culture (Routine) | STOR | | **HEMATOLOGY** | |
| | Hemoglobin A1c | HA1C | | Urine Culture | | | Hbg / Hct | HH |
| | Iron | IRN | | | | | Bloodcount, Hemogram + Plt | BCP |
| | IBC / TIBC | TIBC | | | | | Complete Bldct / Auto Diff | CBCP |
| | LDH / LD | LDH | | | | | Complete Bldct / Manual Diff | CBCM |
| | Magnesium | MG | | | | | Fibrinogen | FBG |
| | Phosphorus | PHOS | | | | | Protime / INR (PT) | PTX |
| | Potassium | K | | | | | PTT / APTT | PTTX |
| | Sodium | NA | | | | | Reticulocyte Count | RET |
| | Total Protein | TP | | | | | SedRate (Westergren) | SED |
| | Triglyceride | TRIG | | | | | | |
| | Uric Acid | URCA | | | | | **OTHER** | |

**PHYSICIAN'S SIGNATURE:** _____ **DATE:** _____

**Figure 40-2** • Sample laboratory request form.

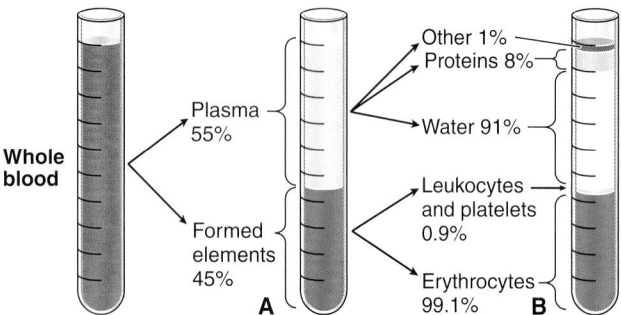

**Figure 40-3 •** Components of blood. **(A)** Whole blood is composed of formed elements and plasma, which can be separated by "spinning the blood" in a centrifuge. **(B)** Formed elements (platelets, leukocytes, and erythrocytes) as seen through a microscope (400×).

testing performed in the toxicology lab may be either for medical purposes or "for cause" scenarios such as requests from employers. Specimen testing requested by employers "for cause" and forensic specimens require a legal **chain of custody**, or procedures required for all aspects of specimen processing including the collection (See Chapter 45, Urinalysis, for more information about drug testing and chain of custody).

## 4. Urinalysis

The **urinalysis** department may stand alone or be a part of one of the other laboratory sections. Some laboratories include a microscopic examination of urinary sediment with all routine urinalysis tests. Urine pregnancy tests may also be performed in this department. Routine urine testing is performed for several reasons:

- To detect renal and metabolic diseases
- To diagnose diseases of the kidneys or urinary tract
- To monitor patients with diabetes

## 5. Immunology

Clinical immunology is the study of diseases caused by disorders of the immune system. Testing in the immunology department is based on the reactions of antibodies, or proteins formed in the body in response to foreign substances, such as bacteria or viruses. The foreign substances are proteins called **antigens**. Increased need for testing to evaluate the body's cellular immune response has resulted from treating autoimmune diseases and AIDS. The diseases caused by disorders of the immune system fall into two categories: **immunodeficiency** and **autoimmunity**. In immunodeficiency, parts of the immune system fail to respond normally, resulting in a patient who is susceptible to many communicable diseases as his or her body is unable to fight an invasion. In autoimmunity, the immune system of the patient recognizes "normal" tissues or structures as abnormal and attacks those tissues or structures. Examples of autoimmunity are systemic lupus erythematosus and rheumatoid arthritis.

Other immune system disorders include hypersensitivities—in which the immune system responds too much to harmless compounds in the environment. An example of hypersensitivity is asthma as a reaction to cat dander or dust.

## 6. Immunohematology

Commonly called the *blood bank*, some labs including hospitals and blood donor centers have an **immunohematology** department. The most common test performed in an immunohematology laboratory is cross-matching for compatibility of blood products for transfusion in patients. Blood products prepared, stored, and dispensed from the blood bank include whole blood, packed red cells, platelets, fresh-frozen plasma, and Rh immune globulin, such as RhoGAM. Other services may include autologous donation (donation of blood by prospective patients for their own use); however, the autologous service is not available in all blood banks.

## 7. Microbiology

The **microbiology** department identifies the microorganisms that cause disease. Once a microorganism causing disease or illness is identified, the physician may order a sensitivity test to determine the antibiotic that will successfully treat pathogens grown from a specimen. Microbiology may include one or more of the following:

- Bacteriology—the study of bacteria
- Virology—the study of viruses
- Mycology—the study of fungi and yeasts
- Parasitology—the study of parasites

## 8. Pathology

Anatomic pathology and surgical **pathology** are involved in the diagnosis of disease using the gross inspection and microscopic examination of tissues removed from the body during surgery. In surgical pathology, the pathologist, a physician, gives a diagnosis of the presence or absence of disease in tissue. **Histology**, the study of the microscopic structure of tissue, includes the preparation and staining of tissue by histotechnologists for the pathologist to review with a microscope. Types of histology specimens include tissue obtained through biopsy and surgical frozen sections that must be evaluated immediately to determine whether further surgery is needed.

## 9. Cytology

**Cytology** is the study of the microscopic structure of cells. Medical lab personnel working in cytology examine individual cells in body fluids and other specimens microscopically for the presence of disease such as cancer. The most common cytology test is the

Papanicolaou (Pap) test, in which vaginal cells scraped from the cervix are evaluated for the presence of cancerous cells. **Cytogenetics** is a type of cytology used to test the genetic structure of cells obtained from fluids such as amniotic fluid (Fig. 40-4). These cells are examined for chromosome deficiencies related to genetic disease. Cytotechnologists prepare the specimens for review and screen the slides for the test results. Pathologists confirm the accuracy of the cytologist reports.

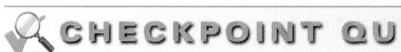 **CHECKPOINT QUESTION**

2. What is another name for the immunohematology department in a laboratory?

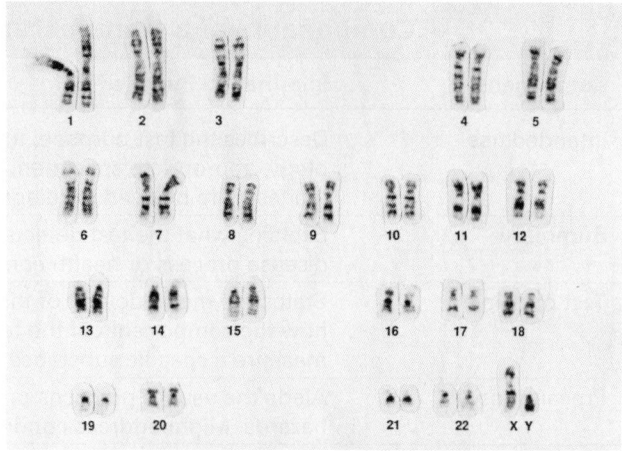

**Figure 40-4** • Human karyotype. The 46 chromosomes are in 23 pairs arranged according to size. The XY sex chromosomes, the 23rd pair at the lower right, indicate that the cell is from a male; a female cell has XX sex chromosomes.

 **PATIENT EDUCATION**

### Specimen Collection

Before collecting a specimen, instruct the patient on the proper preparation for testing. For instance, does the test require that the patient fast or follow a specific dietary regimen? Does the test require stopping any medications or modifying dose patterns? Is the timing of collection imperative, or will a random sample be sufficient? Failure to inform the patient properly before testing may result in erroneous (invalid) test results, which can cause a delay in treatment or incorrect diagnosis.

At the time of specimen collection, tell the patient:

• The name of the test (e.g., blood cell count)
• The type of specimen required (e.g., blood, stool, urine)

Be sure to tell the patient approximately how long it will take for the results to be available and how and by whom the patient will be contacted regarding the results.

Patient education requirements for drawing an HIV test vary from state to state, although most require pretest and posttest counseling. Most states do not allow HIV test results to be given over the telephone.

## The Physician Office Laboratory

The most common type of laboratory is the physician office laboratory, or the POL. The medical assistant working in the POL performs duties including collecting samples (blood, urine, etc.), performing tests, managing quality control, maintaining laboratory equipment, keeping accurate records, preparing specimens for transport to a hospital or reference lab, and reporting results. Tests performed at the point, or site, where patient care is given may be referred to as point-of-care tests (POC or POCT). In addition to the physician office, POC tests may be done by the patient in their home or other nonlaboratory locations. The duties of the medical assistant may also include educating patients on the use of these POC tests and machines including quality control procedures to assure accurate results. The most common tests performed by the medical assistant in the physician office lab are urinalysis, blood cell counts, hemoglobin, hematocrit, and blood glucose levels. Screening tests such as pregnancy tests and tests for diseases such as mononucleosis and strep throat are also available and performed regularly in the physician office.

Most tests performed in the POL fall into one of two general categories: tests performed on a semiautomated machine and tests conducted with a self-contained device known as a **unitized test device**, or a device that allows all steps of the testing process to occur in one container. The unitized test device is packaged as a test kit that includes all supplies and materials to perform a single test. Test kits vary among manufacturers and always include a **product insert**. This product insert is the best source of information for safe and accurate testing using that product or kit, and Table 40-1 describes the typical information found on this document. If necessary, the product insert can be used to write an office policy and procedure to place in the physician office policy and procedure manual.

Unitized test devices and test kits are single use only and must be discarded after each patient. These products also include an expiration date, and the medical assistant must not use any unitized test device or test kit that has expired as the results may not be accurate.

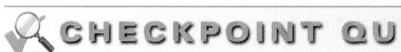 **CHECKPOINT QUESTION**

3. What POL laboratory duties may be performed by Melissa Miller in the family practice office?

| TABLE 40-1 | Components of a Manufacturer's Product Insert |
|---|---|
| **Component** | **Information Provided** |
| Intended use | Describes the test purpose, the substance being detected or measured, testing methodology, appropriate specimen, and the FDA-cleared conditions for use. It may address if the test is to be used for diagnosis or screening. |
| Summary | Explains what the test detects and a short history of the methodology, including the disease process or health condition being detected or monitored |
| Test principle | States the methodology of the test. Details the technical aspects of the test. Explains how the components of the test system interact with the patient's specimen to detect or measure a specific substance |
| Precautions | Alerts the user of practices or conditions that might affect the test and warns of potential hazards. Might address conditions for specimen acceptability |
| Storage/stability | Specifies conditions for storing reagents and test systems to protect their stability. It includes recommended temperature ranges and any physical requirements (e.g., protection from light or humidity.) Also addresses the stability of reagents and test systems when opened or after reconstitution. Describes indicators of reagent deterioration. |
| Reagents and materials supplied | Lists the reagents and materials provided in the test system kit and the concentration and major ingredients used to make the reagents |
| Materials required but not provided | Lists materials needed to perform the test, but not provided in the test system kit |
| Specimen collection and preparation | Details the procedures for specimen collection, handling, storage, and stability, including (as needed) the directions for performing a fingerstick, appropriate anticoagulant or swab type, and directions for specimen preparation. Might address conditions for specimen acceptability |
| Test procedure | Provides step-by-step instructions for performing the test, often with pictures or graphs. Includes critical information (e.g., the order of reagent addition, timing of test steps, mixing and temperature requirements, and reading of the test results) |
| Interpretation of results | Describes how to read and interpret the test results, often including visual aids. Alerts the user when results are invalid and gives instructions on what to do when the results cannot be interpreted. Might include precautions against reporting results unless supplementary and/or confirmatory testing is performed |
| Quality control | Explains what parts of the test system are monitored by QC procedures and provides instructions on how to perform QC. Includes recommendations on how frequently QC should be performed, acceptable QC results, and what to do when QC values are not acceptable. Might include information about external QC, and, if applicable, internal QC |
| Limitations | Describes conditions that might influence the test results or for which the test is not designed. Limitations should include:<br><br>• Possible interferences from medical conditions, drugs, or other substances<br>• Warning that the test is not approved with alternate specimen types or in alternate populations (e.g., pediatric)<br>• Indications of the need for additional testing that might be more specific or more sensitive. **Specificity** is the ability of a test to detect a particular substance or constituent without interference or false reactions by other substances. **Sensitivity** is the lowest concentration of an analyte that can reliably be detected or measured by a test system.<br>• Warning that the test does not differentiate between infection and the carrier state<br>• Statement that the test result should be considered in the context of clinical signs and symptoms, patient history, and other test results |
| Expected values | Describes the test result the user should expect. Explains how results might vary. Might contain study results conducted to derive the information |
| Performance characteristics | Details the results of studies conducted to evaluate test performance. Included are data used to determine accuracy, precision, sensitivity, specificity, and reproducibility of the test and results of studies of the impact of interfering substances |

From Good laboratory practices for waived testing sites. *Morbidity and Mortality Weekly Report*, Volume 54, November 11, 2005. (http://www.cdc.gov/mmwr/PDF/rr/rr5413.pdf)

# REQUESTING LABORATORY TESTS

Laboratory tests are ordered by the physician, physician assistant, or nurse practitioner to help identify the cause or screen for the presence of disease or illness. In some cases, a lab test reveals the specific cause, while in others, a test will only suggest the possibility of a specific cause or eliminate a suspected cause. Understanding the significance of laboratory test results as related to disease or body systems is the key to ordering the test or tests most significant for the patient's symptoms. Appendix J lists highlights of the body systems, associated diseases, and laboratory tests used in diagnosis.

Laboratories provide and utilize request forms appropriate to their individual operations (Fig. 40-2). All forms should be convenient to use, with clear instructions for complete patient and physician identification. Most request forms cover a variety of tests, so that a single form can be used for tests in hematology, chemistry, immunology, and so on. Some forms serve as both a request and report form and list expected values by test. Many requisitions now contain bar codes that allow fast, accurate processing and reduce specimen identification errors. Box 40-2 lists common information required on all laboratory request forms.

Common laboratory tests are organized into standard groups or **panels** to review the general health of an entire body system. In most cases, ordering a panel is more cost effective compared to ordering each test separately. The Centers for Medicare and Medicaid Services (CMS) require the use of panels defined by the American Medical Association (AMA). Table 40-2

---

**BOX 40-2  Laboratory Request Forms: Commonly Required Information**

- Patient's database. This includes name, address, and the medical office identification number to avoid errors with identical names. Other identifying information may be included.
- Patient's birth date and gender. Many test results vary with age and sex.
- Date and time of collection. Often test results are affected by the passage of time or the time of day the specimen was collected.
- Physician's name and address or identification number. Results may have to be reported immediately; this information also avoids errors in reporting.
- Checklist of the test or tests to be performed. These may be grouped under one heading as a panel, such as a renal panel or liver panel, which includes more than one test to determine the state of health of one organ, or a general health profile such as a complete blood count.
- Other required information may include the source of the specimen, such as culture swabs for microbiology tests; medications the patient is taking that may alter certain test results (e.g., anticoagulants affecting prothrombin time); directions for reporting (e.g., an immediate need should be marked "STAT"); and total volume of a 24-hour urine specimen.

---

**TABLE 40-2  Test Panels Defined by the AMA and Mandated by CMS**

| Comprehensive Metabolic | Basic Metabolic | Electrolyte | Hepatic Function | Lipid |
|---|---|---|---|---|
| Glucose | Glucose | Sodium | Albumin | Cholesterol |
| Calcium | Calcium | Potassium | Total protein | Triglycerides |
| Sodium | Sodium | Chloride | ALP | HDL |
| Potassium | Potassium | $CO_2$ | ALT | LDL |
| Chloride | Chloride | | AST | |
| $CO_2$ | $CO_2$ | | Total bilirubin | |
| BUN | BUN | | Direct bilirubin | |
| Creatinine | Creatinine | | | |
| Albumin | | | | |
| Total protein | | | | |
| ALP | | | | |
| ALT | | | | |
| AST | | | | |
| Total bilirubin | | | | |

$CO_2$, carbon dioxide; BUN, blood urea nitrogen; ALP, alkaline phosphatase; ALT, alanine aminotransferase; AST, aspartate aminotransferase; HDL, high-density lipoprotein; LDL, low-density lipoprotein.

lists tests included in various panels including the comprehensive metabolic panel, basic metabolic panel, electrolyte panel, hepatic function panel, and lipid panel.

 **CHECKPOINT QUESTION**

4. Who is authorized to order a laboratory test on patients in the physician office?

# LABORATORY QUALITY AND SAFETY

## Clinical Laboratory Improvement Amendments

In 1988, the federal government passed a law known as the **Clinical Laboratory Improvement Amendment, or CLIA,** established standards for the quality of laboratory testing for all facilities that perform lab procedures on human specimens. The Centers for Medicare and Medicaid Services (CMS) regulate all laboratory testing performed on humans through CLIA. All laboratories must have a CLIA certificate to meet federal requirements even if the lab only performs one test per year or performs tests at no cost to the patient. There are penalties for a laboratory that does not comply with CLIA regulations.

The goals of CLIA are to standardize laboratory testing and enforce quality protocols anywhere tests are performed on patients. Although CLIA is a federal law, there may be state regulations for laboratory testing also, and if state requirements are stricter than federal requirements, the state requirements must be followed. Specifically, CLIA established three levels of testing based on the complexity of the test referred to as waived tests, moderate-complexity tests, and high-complexity tests. Depending on the level of testing, health care professionals performing the tests are required to have specific education or training as regulated by CLIA. The levels of testing are monitored for compliance by agencies of the federal government including the **Commission on Office Laboratory Accreditation (COLA),** an organization that conducts laboratory inspections and also provides knowledge and resources for maintaining quality laboratory operations.

 **CHECKPOINT QUESTION**

5. What is the purpose of CLIA?

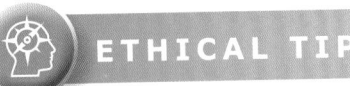 **ETHICAL TIP**

## Common Issues of Laboratory Noncompliance with CLIA Standards

Efforts to reduce medical errors, improve health care quality, and increase patient safety have been gaining national attention. It is the ethical responsibility of anyone performing laboratory tests to be informed of what testing he or she is allowed to perform and the performance requirements of each laboratory test.

The most common issues of noncompliance include the following:

- Performing nonwaived testing without using CLIA-required quality measures
- Performing nonwaived tests without proper credentials
- Not meeting CLIA requirements for personnel, quality control (QC), proficiency testing, or instrument maintenance; not having adequate records
- Not having the most recent instructions for the waived-test systems in use
- Not routinely checking the product insert for changes
- Not using correct terminology when reporting results
- Using expired reagents or control materials
- Not storing products as described in the product insert
- Not following up with **confirmatory tests** as specified in the test instructions (*Note*: A confirmatory test is an additional, more specific test performed to rule out or confirm a preliminary test result to provide a final result.)
- Not performing function checks or **calibration** checks to ensure the test system's operation (*Note*: Calibration is a method provided by the manufacturer to standardize a test or laboratory instrument.)

## Levels of Testing

### Moderate-Complexity and High-Complexity Levels

Moderate- and high-level complexity tests require the use of complex manual methods or instrumentation and are only approved for use by highly trained scientists inside the clinical laboratory. If the level of testing is in question, it must be considered high complexity. CMS publishes a list of all tests in all complexity categories. Most of the testing performed in large laboratories is considered moderate complexity and requires detailed **quality assurance** (QA) and quality control (QC) procedures. Some physician office laboratories may perform moderate-complexity level tests with moderate-complexity certification and medical laboratory scientists qualified to perform the tests. States may establish stricter rules than those set by the governing body, but they may not adopt less strict rules.

Examples of moderate-complexity level tests include the following:

- Urine and throat cultures
- Automated testing for cholesterol, high-density lipoproteins, and triglycerides
- Gram staining
- Microscopic urinalysis
- Automated hematology procedures
- Manual white blood cell count differentials
- Automated coagulation procedures
- Automated chemistry procedures
- Automated urinalyses

High-complexity tests, which are rarely performed in medical offices, include the following:

- Advanced cell studies (cytogenetics)
- Cytology (e.g., Pap tests)
- Histopathology
- Manual cell counts

### Waived Tests

Laboratory tests that are simple, one-step tests approved by CLIA for use in a physician office are called waived tests (Fig. 40-5). However, procedures for collecting specimens and processing waived tests must be followed precisely because performing them incorrectly can cause errors and endanger patient health.

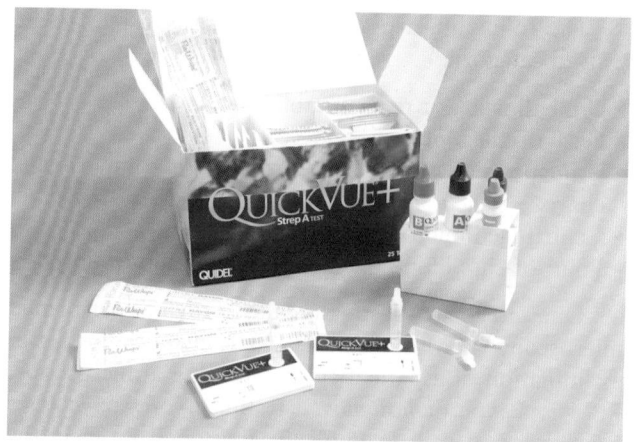

**Figure 40-5 •** A CLIA-waived strep A kit.

Consequently, the government requires a Certificate of Waiver (CW) to perform waived tests. Oversight of waived testing and Certificates of Waiver are controlled by the Department of Health and Human Services (HHS), an agency of the US government that regulates the protection of health of all Americans and provides essential human services.

Waived testing includes many tests simple enough for the patient to perform at home such as glucose monitoring. Even with the waiver, the physician office laboratory must follow all manufacturers' recommendations for each piece of equipment or product used for testing. These tests are often performed by the medical assistant in the POL. Disease processes that are indications for CLIA-waived tests are described in Table 40-3.

| **TABLE 40-3** | **Disease Processes That Indicate CLIA-Waived Tests** |
|---|---|
| **Waived Test** | **Some Related Disease Processes** |
| Urine dipstick or reagent tablets | Hematuria; metabolic disorders; kidney disorders; multiple myeloma; inflammation; diabetes mellitus; liver disease; urinary tract infection; hepatitis; hemolytic anemia |
| Fecal occult blood packets | Colon cancer |
| Urine pregnancy testing kits using color comparison charts | Pregnancy |
| Nonautomated erythrocyte sedimentation rate tests | Inflammation |
| Nonautomated copper sulfate testing for hemoglobin | Anemia; polycythemia; dehydration |
| Centrifuged microhematocrits | Anemia; polycythemia; dehydration |
| Low-complexity blood glucose determination testing | Hyperglycemia; hypoglycemia; diabetes; prediabetes |
| Hemoglobin by single analyte instruments with self-contained reagent and specimen interaction and direct measurement and readout | Anemia, polycythemia, dehydration |
| CLIA-waived strep test kits | Group A streptococcal infection |
| CLIA-waived mono test kits | Infectious mononucleosis |
| CLIA-waived influenza test kits | Influenza A or B |

The following are a few of the tests listed in the waived category:

- Urine dipstick or reagent tablets
- Fecal occult blood packets
- Urine pregnancy testing kits using color comparison charts
- Centrifuged microhematocrits
- Point-of-care blood glucose determination testing

One category of testing is called **provider-performed microscopy** (**PPM** or **PPMP**), which includes the direct examination of a patient specimen using a microscope. PPM is a type of **nonwaived testing**. Nonwaived tests are tests at a level of complexity that does not meet the CLIA criteria for waiver and are not within the scope of practice for the medical assistant in the POL. In the medical office laboratory, PPM can be performed only by a physician, dentist, nurse midwife, nurse practitioner, or physician assistant under the direct supervision of a physician. Provider-performed microscopy tests include the following:

- All direct wet-mount preparations
- All potassium hydroxide preparations
- Pinworm examinations
- Urine sediment examinations

Other tests, including those for rapid strep, have waived methodologies available, but the Food and Drug Administration (FDA) has not provided waived status for every lab test. Box 40-4 lists criteria to help understand waived testing.

 **CHECKPOINT QUESTION**

6. What are the three levels of laboratory testing defined by CLIA, and which level is approved for medical assistants working in the physician office lab?

## Laboratory Quality Assessment

All laboratories including the physician office lab are required by CLIA to have a quality assessment plan to ensure all areas of the laboratory's technical and support functions. This assessment plan should be written and communicated to everyone in the laboratory. The purpose of the QA policy is to prevent problems before they occur and to document procedures when an error or problem is detected. The plan must include corrective action that must be taken and how the information is documented. If the lab is inspected, the inspector will expect to see a well-written quality assessment plan and policy. The QA plan should monitor the following laboratory functions:

- Patient preparation procedures
- Specimen collection, processing, preservation, and transportation

- Test analysis, reporting, and interpretation
- Training and continuing education for lab personnel

## The Laboratory Procedure Manual

The laboratory procedure manual is the primary reference in operating the physician office laboratory. CLIA regulations require a procedure for every test performed in the laboratory, and procedures must follow the manufacturer's testing instructions. Many procedures require reagents and controls, and the requirements for using the controls are listed in the product insert. A **control** is a device or solution used to monitor the accurate performance of the test. A reagent is a substance that produces a reaction with a patient specimen so the analyte can be detected or measured.

## Quality Control Procedures

Quality control, or QC, testing is designed to detect problems that can happen because of operator error, reagent or test kit deterioration, instrument malfunction, or improper environmental conditions. The POL must have written policies and procedures for monitoring quality control including the accuracy, precision, and quality of each test in place. If a test has good precision, the medical assistant will get similar results if the test is repeated. If similar results are not obtained, the method is not in control and results are considered inaccurate and cannot be reported. When this happens, the medical assistant must investigate and resolve the problem with the test, also known as troubleshooting. When the problem is corrected, the patient specimen and controls can be tested again.

There are two types of controls in waived testing: the **internal control** and the **external control**. The internal control is built into the testing device and verifies that the device is in good working order. The internal control must measure acceptable results to get accurate test results on a patient specimen and must be recorded with each measurement.

An internal control does not prove that the results will be accurate when the specimen is added, whereas the external control acts just like a patient specimen. The external control monitors the test from applying the specimen to result interpretation. External controls are usually liquids similar to patient specimens. Documenting external control results is also a requirement of quality control.

The product insert or instrument manual describes the minimum requirement for internal and external control testing. The frequency for testing them cannot be less than what is specified by the manufacturer. At the very least, test external controls with each new shipment of reagents or kits, each new lot number, and each new operator. Companies that make the controls also make the sample specimens that will test like human specimens. These control samples come with known reference ranges. Quality control results that read within the known reference ranges indicate that the test system (reagents, instruments, or any components) performed as expected. Documenting and monitoring control testing results provides an indication that the test was properly performed by the medical assistant. Maintaining a record of each control sample result is a requirement of CLIA and may be referred to as the control log. The documentation on the control log must be consistent and the records should be retained for at least 2 years. The control log must show the following information:

- Date and time of the test
- Results expected
- Results obtained
- Action taken for correction, if any
- Initials of the person performing the test

Ideally, the control log should be reviewed monthly to detect shift and trend changes in performance over time. The Clinical and Laboratory Standards Institute (CLSI) establishes rules to ensure the safety, standards, and integrity of all testing performed on human specimens.

Figure 40-6 is an example of a quality control log form containing information recommended by CLSI on which control sample testing can be recorded. If the controls do not test as expected, then patient testing should not be performed or reported until the problem is identified and corrected.

If problems are detected when performing quality control, the product insert will provide information for troubleshooting. Start by checking the reagents and controls for expiration dates. Not all controls and test reagents come in liquid form and those that do not must have a liquid, usually water, added to the material. **Reconstitution** is the process of adding water to bring a material back to its liquid state. The water or other liquid added must be measured precisely and the date of reconstitution noted on the container. Troubleshooting errors when reconstituted controls and test reagents are used includes checking expiration dates once reconstituted. If there are no problems found after checking the expiration dates, the next step is checking the testing instrument to ensure it is clean and functioning properly. If all of this has been done, reconstitute or open a new control sample or reagent and begin the process again.

**QUALITATIVE QC LOG SHEET FOR** _____

RECORD LOT NUMBER IF DIFFERENT FROM LAST LOT NUMBER.

| TEST DATE | KIT LOT | POSITIVE CONTROL LOT # | NEGATIVE CONTROL LOT # | POSITIVE CONTROL RESULT | NEGATIVE CONTROL RESULT | OK TO USE? | IF NO, CORRECTIVE ACTION | INITIALS |
|-----------|---------|------------------------|------------------------|-------------------------|-------------------------|------------|--------------------------|----------|
|           |         |                        |                        |                         |                         |            |                          |          |
|           |         |                        |                        |                         |                         |            |                          |          |
|           |         |                        |                        |                         |                         |            |                          |          |
|           |         |                        |                        |                         |                         |            |                          |          |
|           |         |                        |                        |                         |                         |            |                          |          |
|           |         |                        |                        |                         |                         |            |                          |          |
|           |         |                        |                        |                         |                         |            |                          |          |
|           |         |                        |                        |                         |                         |            |                          |          |
|           |         |                        |                        |                         |                         |            |                          |          |
|           |         |                        |                        |                         |                         |            |                          |          |
|           |         |                        |                        |                         |                         |            |                          |          |
|           |         |                        |                        |                         |                         |            |                          |          |
|           |         |                        |                        |                         |                         |            |                          |          |
|           |         |                        |                        |                         |                         |            |                          |          |
|           |         |                        |                        |                         |                         |            |                          |          |
|           |         |                        |                        |                         |                         |            |                          |          |
|           |         |                        |                        |                         |                         |            |                          |          |
|           |         |                        |                        |                         |                         |            |                          |          |
|           |         |                        |                        |                         |                         |            |                          |          |
|           |         |                        |                        |                         |                         |            |                          |          |

**Figure 40-6 •** QC log sheet.

Use manufacturer contact information to get technical assistance if needed. If there is a delay in correcting the problems, specimens for this test can be sent to a referral laboratory for timely results.

### Qualitative and Quantitative Quality Control

Laboratory tests can be **qualitative**, while others are **quantitative**. A qualitative test has positive or negative results while the results of quantitative tests are measured and reported using a numeric value. A tool that may be used for manually recording quantitative quality control is the Levey-Jennings QC Chart. By completing this chart, a visual representation of **shifts** and **trends** will emerge that may give a warning that the test or instrument is not performing correctly (Fig. 40-7). A test is exhibiting a **shift** when quality control results make an obvious change in results, and a test is exhibiting a **trend** when results increase or decrease over time.

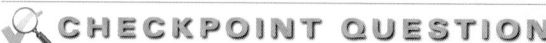

## CHECKPOINT QUESTION

7. How does a medical assistant such as Melissa Miller determine when to run quality controls on a test?

## Reagent Management

Reagents are chemicals used to perform a test, and all reagents have a manufacturer's lot number and expiration date. When the reagent reacts with the patient's specimen, it provides a test result. The lot number and expiration date must be recorded on the QC log sheet when quality control is tested. In addition, the date the package is opened and the initials of the person who opened the package should be documented on the outside of each package. Test kits may contain one reagent or several reagents. You must use only the reagents

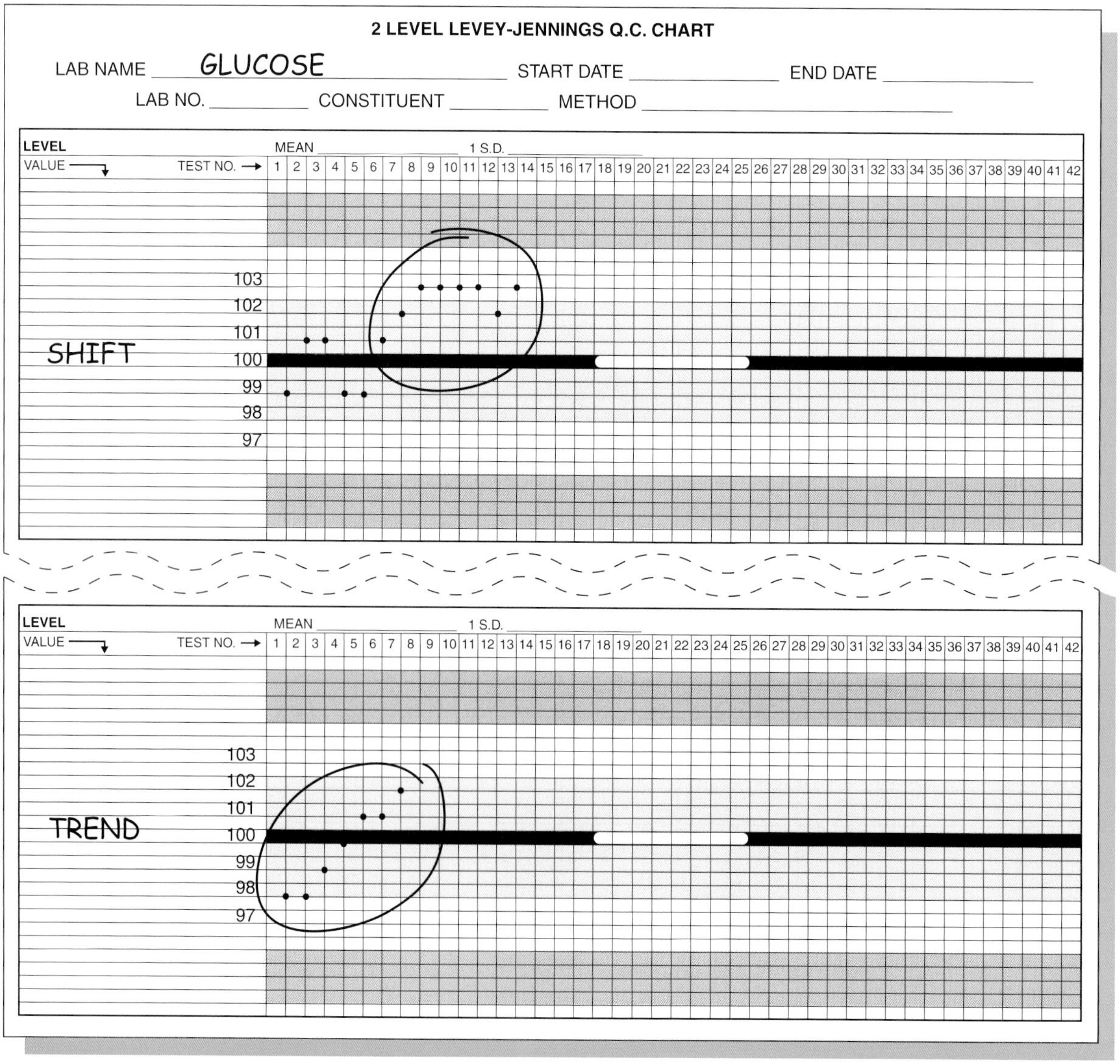

**Figure 40-7 •** QC charts representing a shift and a trend.

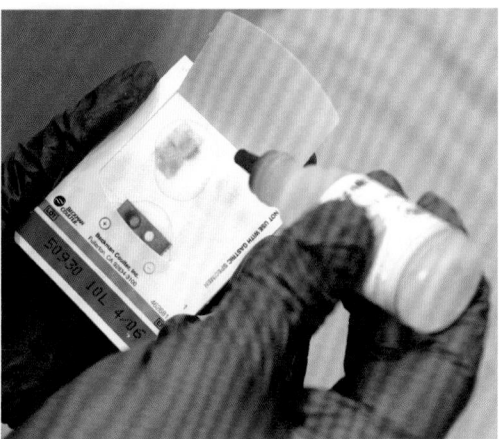

**Figure 40-8** • Fecal occult blood test card and reagent.

that come in the test kit—you should never mix or use reagents from one kit with another test kit, even when it is the same or a similar test. An example of this is fecal blood testing kit that contains cards for obtaining the stool specimen and a developer reagent for testing the stool sample on the card (Fig. 40-8). It is unacceptable to use fecal occult blood test cards from one kit and lot number and developer reagent solution from a different kit and lot number for testing.

## Laboratory Safety

All health care professionals including the medical assistant want to avoid exposure to health and safety risks in the medical office including the laboratory. Injuries affect morale and threaten the emotional and physical health of the injured person. Safe laboratory practice boils down to four skills:

• Common sense
• Safety-focused attitude
• Good personal behavior
• Good housekeeping

The Occupational Safety and Health Administration (OSHA) monitors and protects the health and safety of workers including health care professionals working in the physician office laboratory. Two OSHA standards of particular importance to medical laboratories are the Occupational Exposure to Bloodborne Pathogens Standard and the Hazardous Communication (HazCom) Standard, or the "right to know law." The OSHA Bloodborne Pathogens Standard requires all medical employers to provide training for their employees in techniques that will protect them from occupational exposure to infectious agents, including bloodborne pathogens. In addition, OSHA standards require that all workers who are at risk for exposure to potentially hazardous material wear personal protective equipment (PPE) supplied by the employer. A medical assistant performing phlebotomy or assisting with collection of most

samples is safe with glove protection; however, situations that may result in splashes, splatters, or spreading of an **aerosol** (particles suspended in gas or air) require full coverage, including a face shield and footwear.

Because of the increase in sensitivities and allergies to latex in employees and patients, most medical offices provide employees with latex-free gloves and tourniquets for phlebotomy procedures. Box 40-3 provides a review of the symptoms of latex allergies and evaluation criteria to determine their level of severity.

Another component of the Bloodborne Pathogens Standard is that all equipment and working surfaces be cleaned and decontaminated with disinfectant after contact with blood or other potentially infectious materials. The use of a hypochlorite, or bleach, solution (diluted 1:10 with water) is an acceptable disinfectant for cleaning surfaces that may be contaminated with bloodborne pathogens.

The OSHA HazCom Standard requires labeling by the manufacturer hazardous chemicals with warnings,

---

**BOX 40-3   Three Major Types of Latex Reactions**

1. *Irritant dermatitis*—skin irritation that is not an allergic response. Some causes include inadequate drying after hand washing, aggressive scrubbing technique or detergents, abrasive effect of glove powder, climatic irritation (cold climates can cause dry, chapped skin, and hot weather can cause excessive sweating), and emotional stress. Irritant hand dermatitis can cause breaks in the skin, which can allow easier entry of the sensitizing latex protein or glove chemicals, and, in turn, lead to latex allergy.

2. *Delayed cutaneous hypersensitivity (type IV allergy)*—contact (hand) dermatitis that is generally due to the chemicals used in latex glove production. It is mediated via T cells. The skin reaction is seen 6 to 48 hours after contact. The reaction is local and limited to the skin that has contacted the glove. Those with type IV allergy are at increased risk of developing type I allergy. One route of sensitization is that latex proteins more easily enter the body if the skin barrier is broken.

3. *Immediate reaction (type I allergy)*— systemic allergic reactions caused by circulating IgE antibodies to the proteins in natural latex. Symptoms include hives, rhinitis, conjunctivitis, asthma due to bronchoconstriction, and, in severe cases, anaphylaxis and hypotension. Symptoms occur within about 30 minutes of exposure to latex. Several routes of exposure that can lead to type I sensitivity are cutaneous, mucosal, parenteral, and aerosol (from inhaling latex glove powder).

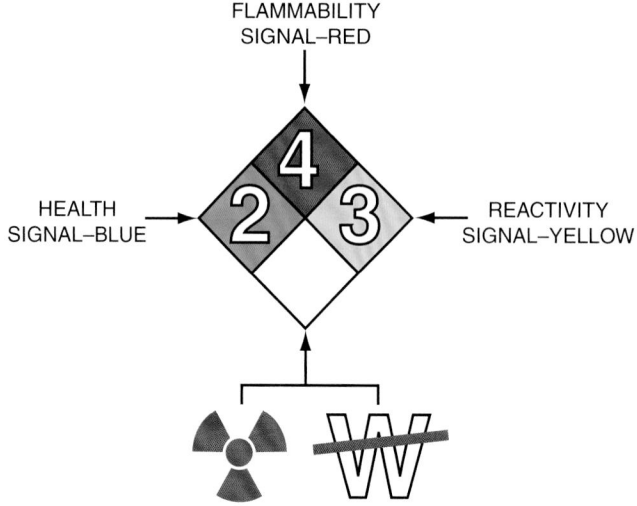

**Figure 40-9 •** Hazardous material rating system. (Reprinted from McCall R. *Phlebotomy Essentials.* Baltimore, MD: Lippincott Williams & Wilkins, 2007, with permission.)

| Identification of Health Hazard Color Code: **BLUE** | | Identification of Flammability Color Code: **RED** | | Identification of Reactivity (Stability) Color Code: **YELLOW** | |
|---|---|---|---|---|---|
| | Type of possible injury | | Susceptibility of materials to burning | | Susceptibility to release of energy |
| 4 | Materials that on very short exposure could cause death or major residual injury even though prompt medical treatment was given. | 4 | Materials that will rapidly or completely vaporize at atmospheric pressure and normal ambient temperature, or that are readily dispersed in air and that will burn readily. | 4 | Materials that in themselves are readily capable of detonation or of explosive decomposition or reaction at normal temperatures and pressures. |
| 3 | Materials that on short exposure could cause serious temporary or residual injury even though prompt medical treatment was given. | 3 | Liquids and solids that can be ignited under almost all ambient temperature conditions. | 3 | Materials that in themselves are capable of detonation or explosive reaction but require a strong initiating source or that must be heated under confinement before initiation or that react explosively with water. |
| 2 | Materials that on intense or continued exposure could cause temporary incapacitation or possible residual injury unless prompt medical treatment is given. | 2 | Materials that must be moderately heated or exposed to relatively high ambient temperatures before ignition can occur. | 2 | Materials that in themselves are normally unstable and readily undergo violent chemical change but do not detonate. Also materials that may react violently with water or that may form potentially explosive mixtures with water. |
| 1 | Materials that on exposure would cause irritation but only minor residual injury even if no treatment is given. | 1 | Materials that must be preheated before ignition can occur. | 1 | Materials that in themselves are normally stable, but that can become unstable at elevated temperatures and pressures or that may react with water with some release of energy, but not violently. |
| 0 | Materials that on exposure under fire conditions would offer no hazard beyond that of ordinary combustible material. | 0 | Materials that will not burn. | 0 | Materials that in themselves are normally stable, even under fire exposure conditions, and that are not reactive with water. |

precautions to avoid exposure, and first-aid measures for exposure (Fig. 40-9). In addition, manufacturers must supply a safety data sheet (SDS) for their products. These sheets should be maintained in a binder near the site of use and should be reviewed routinely by all office staff (refer to Chapter 17, Medical Asepsis and Infection Control).

### CHECKPOINT QUESTION

8. Which OSHA standard requires employers to provide gloves for the medical assistant working in the POL?

## General Safety Guidelines

The following guidelines are some important safety factors required in all laboratories. Follow them carefully to protect yourself, your coworkers, and your patients.

1. Never eat, drink, or smoke in the laboratory area.
2. Never touch your face, mouth, or eyes with your gloves or with items such as a pen or pencil used in the laboratory.
3. Do not apply makeup or lipstick or insert contact lenses in the laboratory.
4. Wear gloves and appropriate protective barriers whenever contact with blood, body fluids, secretions, excretions, broken skin, or mucous membranes is possible. If a splatter, splash, spill, or exposure to aerosols is possible, wear appropriate PPE.
5. Label all specimen containers with biohazard labels.
6. Store all chemicals according to the manufacturer's recommendations. Discard any container with an illegible label. Never store chemicals in unlabeled containers.
7. Wash hands frequently for infection control. Always wash hands before and after gloving and before leaving the work site.
8. Clean reusable glassware with recommended disinfectant or soap and dry thoroughly before reuse. Wear gloves to prevent cuts.
9. Avoid inhaling the fumes of any chemicals found in the laboratory or wearing contact lenses when working with these types of chemicals.
10. Know the location and operation of all safety equipment such as fire extinguishers.
11. Use safe practices when operating laboratory equipment. Read the manuals and know how to operate the equipment. Avoid contact with damaged electrical equipment.
12. Disinfect all laboratory surfaces after use and at the end of the day with a 10% bleach solution or appropriate disinfectant. Never allow clutter to accumulate.
13. Dispose of needles and broken glass in sharps containers. Use biohazard containers for any other contaminated articles.
14. Use mechanical pipetters, but never the mouth, to apply suction to a pipette.
15. Use the proper procedure for removing chemical or biological spills.
16. Avoid spills.
17. Use a splatter guard or splash shield whenever there is any risk of splatter or exposure to aerosols.
18. When removing a stopper, hold the opening away, use gauze around the cap, and twist gently. Avoid glove contact with the specimen.
19. Immediately report any work-related injury or biohazard exposure to your supervisor.
20. Follow all guidelines for standard precautions and the requirements of the various types of transmission-based precautions.
21. When opening a tube or container, hold the opening away from you to avoid aerosols, splashes, and spills.

A biologic spill is one that contains blood or body fluids that may be potentially infectious such as feces, nasal secretions, saliva, sputum, sweat, tears, urine, and vomitus. To clean a biohazardous spill, observe the following guidelines:

- Put on gloves and other PPE as indicated by the size of the spill.
- Cover the area with absorbent material, such as paper towels, to soak up the spill; discard in a biohazard container.
- Flood the area with disinfecting solution, such as a 10% bleach solution, and allow it to sit for 10 to 15 minutes.
- If a spill contains broken glass, use a mechanical means of picking up the glass. Do not use your hands.
- Wipe up the solution with disposable material.
- Dispose of all waste in a biohazard container.
- With gloves on, remove eyewear and discard or disinfect per office policy. Remove remaining PPE and place in a biohazard container or the biohazard laundry bag (for reusable linen).
- Remove and dispose of gloves. Wash your hands.

To prevent spilling nonbiohazardous chemicals, pour carefully while palming the label (refer to Chapter 24, Procedure 24-1), and pour the chemical or solution at eye level if possible or practical. Never pour close to your face and tighten all container lids or caps immediately after use.

# LABORATORY EQUIPMENT

Laboratory equipment and supplies for performing physician office tests come in a variety of types and sizes. It is not necessary to become familiar with every possible type of laboratory equipment; however, there are a few basic items that are common to most small laboratories including the following:

- Microscope
- Centrifuge
- Incubator
- Refrigerator or freezer

## Microscope

The microscope is used by the physician to identify and count cells and microorganisms in blood and other body specimens. The compound microscope is the type most commonly used in the medical office and is a two-lens system in which ocular and objective lenses together

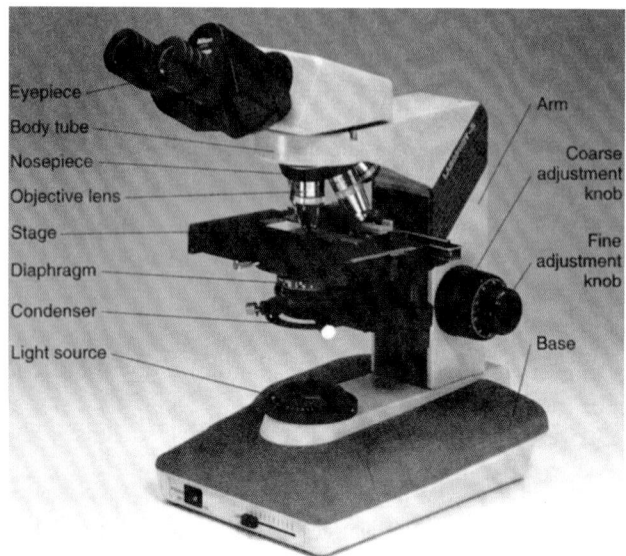

**Figure 40-10 •** Basic components of the standard light microscope. (Courtesy of Nikon, Melville, NY.)

provide the total magnification. A light source illuminates the objects as they are magnified. Figure 40-10 shows a microscope and its various parts.

The *frame*, which consists of the arm and base, is the basic structural component of the microscope. The *oculars* at the top of the instrument are for the user's eyes, and each is marked with its magnification, usually ×10. Binocular microscopes (two eyepieces) minimize eyestrain and have adjustments to allow for variations in spacing between the user's eyes.

To bring the object to be viewed into focus, the *coarse adjustment knob* is used with the lower-powered objective to focus on the object; the *fine adjustment knob* is used with the higher-powered objective or the oil immersion lens for the greatest definition. Always focus in two steps. First look at the slide and objective from the side (not through the ocular or oculars), bringing the slide very close to the lens using the coarse adjustment knob. Second, look through the ocular or oculars while moving the slide farther from the lens to bring it into focus using the fine adjustment knob. This procedure will prevent damage to the lens from contact with the slide.

The *nosepiece* houses three or four objective lenses and rotates to bring the objective into working position. Pressure to the objectives should never be used to rotate lenses. Only the grip should be used to make this adjustment. The magnification power is marked on each objective. The shorter, or low-power, objective magnifies ×10. The higher power magnifies ×40 for closer observation. With the use of oil, the third objective, called the *oil immersion lens*, magnifies ×100. Some microscopes have a fourth objective with a ×4 lens to scan larger specimens. To determine the total magnification of a specimen, multiply the magnification of the working objective by the magnification of the ocular lens (×10):

- Low power: $10 \times 10 = 100$
- High power: $40 \times 10 = 400$
- Oil immersion: $100 \times 10 = 1{,}000$

The *stage* is the flat surface that holds the slide for viewing. An opening in the solid surface allows illumination of the slide from below. Many stages have clips to hold the slide in place and to allow manual movement of the slide as needed. Some stages mechanically adjust the position vertically or horizontally by moving adjustment knobs, also called *x*- and *y-axis knobs*. The *condenser* concentrates the light rays to focus on the slide. The condenser is adjustable, and in the lower position, the light focus is reduced; in the higher position, it is increased. The *diaphragm*, in the condenser, consists of interlocking plates that adjust into a variable-sized opening, or iris, to regulate the amount of light from the source in conjunction with the condenser. The more highly magnified the slide, the greater the need for light. The *light source* is located in the base of the microscope.

Microscopes are delicate, expensive instruments. To ensure that the is kept in good working order, it must be handled properly (Box 40-4) and maintained according

---

**BOX 40-4    Proper Handling of a Microscope**

- Always lift your microscope with one hand holding the "arm" and the other hand under the base; avoid bumping or jarring the scope. This delicate instrument can easily go out of alignment if it is handled roughly. You will only be able to carry one microscope or lamp at a time if you are to avoid the possibility of damage.
- Use your microscope on a sturdy, solid surface and away from the edge. Vibrations can also cause the microscope to go out of alignment.
- Never touch the lenses of the eyepieces and objectives with your finger. Keep all glass and optical lenses clean. Use lens paper dipped in a lens cleaning solution to gently wipe dust and oils off the eyepieces, objectives, condenser, and illumination glass. (Never use a paper towel or tissue to wipe a lens—the fibers in them will scratch the lenses.)
- Keep the stage and the other metal parts free of excess oil. An alcohol wipe is best but is not recommended for use on the lenses.
- To keep your microscope in top condition for years, have the microscope professionally serviced once a year.
- When you are finished using your microscope, rotate the nosepiece so that it is on the low-power objective, roll the nosepiece so that it is all the way down to the stage, and then replace the dust cover.
- Always keep the dust cover on your scope when it is not in use.

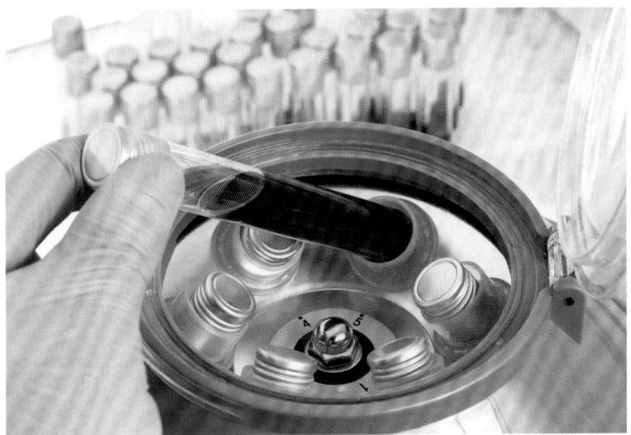

**Figure 40-11 •** StatSpin®CritSpin microhematocrit centrifuge. (Credit: IRIS International, Inc., Chatsworth, CA.)

**BOX 40-5   Quick Tips for Safe Centrifuge Operation**

1. Wear appropriate PPE including safety goggles.
2. Use the centrifuge on a level and firm work surface.
3. Balance the tubes in the rotor.
4. Do not open the lid while the rotor is moving.
5. If you see the centrifuge wobbling or shaking, pull the plug.
6. Do not bump, jar, or move the centrifuge while the rotor is spinning.

*Source*: United States Department of Agriculture, Centrifuge Safety, http://www.ars.usda.gov/Services/docs.htm?docid=14597&pf=1.

to the manufacturer's standards (Procedure 40-1). Be sure to place it in a low-traffic area and away from any source of vibration such as a centrifuge. It should always be covered when not in use.

## Centrifuge

A centrifuge rotates in a circular motion to swing its contents to separate liquids and solids into their component parts (Fig. 40-11). Centrifugation is the process of separating blood or other body fluid cells from liquid components using a centrifuge. For example, a specimen of **whole blood** (blood containing all its cellular components) is separated into a bottom layer of heavy RBCs, a thin middle layer of platelets and WBCs called the *buffy coat*, and a top liquid layer that is the lightest of the components when centrifuged (Fig. 40-12). The top layer is serum, if the specimen was allowed to clot before centrifuged or plasma if the specimen was anticoagulated and not allowed to clot.

When using a centrifuge, tubes must always be balanced (Box 40-5). If an uneven number of tubes is spun, a tube with water must balance the odd tube. Try to place tubes with approximately the same level of liquid in opposing spaces. All tubes must be securely capped. Never start centrifugation until the lid is locked and do not open the centrifuge until all motion has stopped. Do not stop the spinning centrifuge by hand. Follow the manufacturer's recommendations for cleaning, oiling, and maintaining the centrifuge. As with all equipment, read the instructions before operation.

## WHAT IF?

**What if a specimen tube breaks in the centrifuge?**

- If a specimen tube breaks in a centrifuge, do not open the lid. Avoid disturbing the centrifuge for 30 minutes so any aerosols can settle.
- Put on personal protective equipment (PPE), including face shield, impervious gown, and gloves.
- Remove rotors and buckets, seal in a plastic bag, and move aside to perform the cleaning procedure described below.
- Dispose of any sharp debris in a sharps container.
- Clean the inside of the centrifuge with paper towels and chemical disinfectant. (*Note*: Avoid bleach solution, which may be corrosive.)
- Soak removable parts in disinfectant for 30 minutes, rinse, dry, and replace them in the centrifuge.
- Discard liquid and other wastes using proper procedures.
- Clean the face shield and gown per lab protocol, and dispose of gloves appropriately.

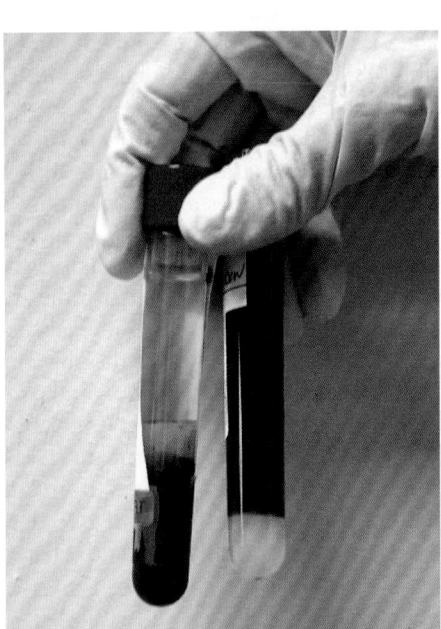

**Figure 40-12 •** Serum gel tubes before centrifuging (**right**) and after centrifuging (**left**).

## Incubator

Microbiology specimens require a suitable environment to thrive and reproduce. To grow one type of microorganism, bacteria, the specimen has to be placed in a special container that contains nutrients called **media** and then put into an incubator, an oven-like device, set at a temperature that reflects body temperature (99°F or 37°C) (Fig. 40-13). At this temperature, the bacteria will grow, allowing the microbes to reproduce to a large enough quantity for identification. The specimen must be allowed to grow in the incubator for approximately 24 hours and a daily log is maintained to record the incubator temperature. See Chapter 44, Microbiology and Immunology, for more information.

## Refrigerators and Freezers

Laboratory refrigerators and freezers are similar to those used in the home, but their uses are very different. In the clinical laboratory, the refrigerator and freezer should be used only to store reagents, kits, and specimens that require refrigeration or freezing. The temperature is critical and should be maintained at 4°C to 8°C to remain in service. The actual temperature in the refrigerator must be measured and recorded daily. Food should never be stored in these refrigerators because of the possibility of biohazard contamination. The refrigerator in the lab typically has a biohazard symbol on the front of the appliance and should clearly state that the refrigerator is not for storage of food and/or drinks for human consumption.

 **CHECKPOINT QUESTION**

9. How does the centrifuge work and what is the purpose of this machine in the POL?

# THE ROLE OF THE MEDICAL ASSISTANT AND THE POL

The medical assistant has an important role in the physician office laboratory. In addition to collecting samples for testing, the medical assistant is also responsible for the following:

- Informing patients of the proper procedure or preparation for obtaining laboratory specimens
- Obtaining a quality specimen
- Arranging for appropriate specimen transport to a hospital or reference lab if necessary
- Performing common CLIA-waived laboratory tests using standards to ensure the accuracy, reliability, and timeliness of patient results
- Documenting and maintaining a quality assurance (QA) program
- Maintaining laboratory instruments and equipment to manufacturers' standards
- Purchasing laboratory supplies and equipment
- Following OSHA and CDC guidelines with regard to handling biohazardous materials
- Working within the scope of practice for medical assistants in the clinical laboratory and following all state and federal guidelines and regulations

The medical assistant is also responsible for screening reported test results and performing follow-up actions. Screening a test result includes checking how it compares to the reference interval, which is usually listed on the report form from the hospital or reference lab or found in the package insert for CLIA-waived testing done in the POL. Reference intervals are the test results usually seen in a healthy population, and when screening a laboratory report, it is logical to start by noting test results that fall outside the listed normal values.

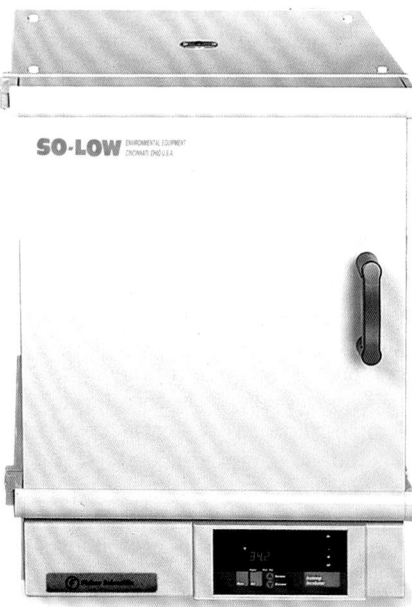

**Figure 40-13 •** Standard laboratory incubator. (Courtesy of So-Low Environmental Equipment, Cincinnati, OH.)

| TABLE 40-4 | Example Critical Values for Some Common Laboratory Tests | |
|---|---|---|
| | **Critical Values** | |
| **Analyte (Lab Test)** | **Low** | **High** |
| Serum glucose | <40 or 45 mg/dL | >500 mg/dL |
| Serum sodium | <120 mEq/L | >160 mEq/L |
| Serum potassium | <2.5 mEq/L | >6.0 mEq/L |
| Serum calcium (total) | <7.0 mg/dL | >13.0 mg/dL |
| White blood cell count | $<2 \times 10^{-9}$/L | $>50 \times 10^{-9}$/L |
| Platelet count | $<20 \times 10^{-9}$/L | $>1,000 \times 10^{-9}$/L |
| Prothrombin time | Not applicable | International normalized ratio (INR) >5 |
| Partial thromboplastin time | Not applicable | >100 seconds |

The follow-up actions on any report should be documented on the report and/or addressed with the physician. **Critical values**, also known as *alert values* or *critical limits*, are test results that are outside the reference intervals and are considered life-threatening test results. Table 40-4 lists results considered to be critical values for some common laboratory tests. Each medical office should establish a list of critical values agreed upon by the physician(s) in that office. The medical assistant must notify the physician of critical results measured in the POL or reported back from the referral laboratory. Documentation of the notification of critical test results is essential.

## LEGAL TIP

### Test Results

While working in a laboratory, you will have access to the results of many confidential blood tests, such as tests for HIV, drugs, pregnancy, and sexually transmitted diseases. You have an ethical responsibility not to communicate any results to unauthorized persons. Only patients and their physicians are entitled to the results. The only exception is the provision in state laws requiring the reporting of certain test results for public safety. Confidentiality is an HIPAA requirement in addition to an ethical responsibility.

## WHAT IF?

**What if the patient asks you why the physician is ordering a specific laboratory test?**

It is beyond any health care professional's scope of practice to answer a clinical question for a physician. The only exception is when the physician instructs the professional with a response for that particular patient. Some credible responses that may be shared with the patient include the following:

- "Your physician has ordered these tests to find out what is causing your symptoms."
- "These are the tests physicians order when you have a physical to be certain you are healthy."
- "This test is important to watch when you are taking this medication."

## Using Flow Sheets

A flow sheet may be used to collect important data regarding a patient's condition. Test results not recorded elsewhere in the patient medical record may be documented on this form, and it serves as a record to track results and follow-up actions. Using a flow sheet to document lab test results also assists the physician in providing quality care. Each time the patient makes an office visit, the flow sheet is reviewed, and additional testing or medication adjustments can be made based on recorded results. When a new test is performed, the medical assistant adds the newest results to the flow sheet. This allows the patient's progress to be monitored at a glance.

An example of a test often monitored by a flow sheet is the prothrombin time, or INR, test performed to monitor anticoagulant therapy (Fig. 40-14). The flow sheet

## ANTICOAGULATION FLOWSHEET

Patient's name: _____ Date of Birth: ___/___/_____

Target International Normalized Ratio (INR): ☐ 2.0-3.0 ☐ 2.5-3.5 ☐ Other:_____

| Date | Current Dose | INR | Complications | New Dose | Next INR | Initials |
|------|--------------|-----|---------------|----------|----------|----------|
|      |              |     |               |          |          |          |
|      |              |     |               |          |          |          |
|      |              |     |               |          |          |          |
|      |              |     |               |          |          |          |
|      |              |     |               |          |          |          |
|      |              |     |               |          |          |          |
|      |              |     |               |          |          |          |
|      |              |     |               |          |          |          |
|      |              |     |               |          |          |          |
|      |              |     |               |          |          |          |
|      |              |     |               |          |          |          |
|      |              |     |               |          |          |          |
|      |              |     |               |          |          |          |
|      |              |     |               |          |          |          |
|      |              |     |               |          |          |          |
|      |              |     |               |          |          |          |
|      |              |     |               |          |          |          |
|      |              |     |               |          |          |          |
|      |              |     |               |          |          |          |

**Figure 40-14 •** Anticoagulant flow sheet.

monitors the patient's results to maintain a certain **therapeutic range,** or the test result range of values the physician wants the patient to maintain. Using a flow sheet to record the results allows monitoring the stability of the result within the therapeutic range. Medication can be adjusted to an appropriate dose accordingly.

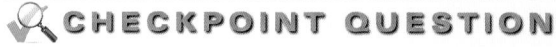

## CHECKPOINT QUESTION

10. Why would the physician want Melissa Miller to record lab test results on a flow sheet?

## ROLE-PLAYING ACTIVITY

Role-play these scenarios as if you are working with Melissa Miller in the family practice office (refer to the case study at the beginning of the chapter). You are preparing the office for the day, and while checking the small laboratory refrigerator and logging the daily temperature, you notice it is not the recommended temperature. In fact, it is 3 degrees lower than it was last week and has slowly been decreasing each day for the last month. Melissa comes into the room where you are reviewing the temperature log and proceeds to get a reagent for use in a test kit out of the refrigerator. What would you say to Melissa and why? How would you respond if she says you must tell the physician? What would you say to the physician about this situation? Your instructor will give you additional information about this activity!

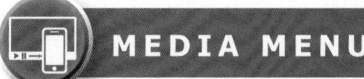

## MEDIA MENU

**Student Resources** on thePoint®
• **Video:** Caring for a Microscope
• **CMA/RMA Certification Exam Review**
• **English to Spanish Audio Glossary**

**Internet Resources**
**Commission on Office Laboratory Accreditation**
http://www.cola.org
**Centers for Medicare and Medicaid Services**
http://www.cms.hhs.gov
**Center for Disease Control and Prevention**
http://www.cdc.gov
**Clinical and Laboratory Standards Institute**
http://www.clsi.org
**Occupational Safety and Health Administration**
http://www.osha.gov
http://www.gpoaccess.gov/fr/index.html
**United States Department of Health and Human Services**
http://www.hhs.gov

## *español* SPANISH TERMINOLOGY

**Hola, mi nombre es Melissa Miller, le hablo de la oficina del doctor del Centro Médico Great Falls.**
Hello. This is Melissa Miller from Great Falls Medical Center physicians' office.

**¿Podría hablar con Carol acerca de sus más recientes resultados de laboratorio?**
May I speak with Carol about her recent laboratory tests?

**El doctor/la doctora me pidió que lo/la llamara con los resultados de su prueba.**
Dr. Singer asked me to call you about your test results.

**El médico quiere que usted siga estas instrucciones.**
The doctor wants you to follow these directions.

**El doctor quiere que haga una cita para discutir sobre sus resultados de laboratorio.**
The doctor wants you to come in for a follow-up appointment to discuss your lab results.

**¿Entiende usted lo que le pido que haga?**
Do you understand what I am asking you to do?

**Para estos examines usted necesita estar en ayuno por al menos 8 hours.**
For these exams, you need to be fasting for at least 8 hours.

## EMR Activity

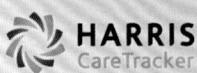

Harris CareTracker is a web-based electronic medical record (EMR) application that you will use for the EMR activities included in this section at the end of each chapter. This application is actually used in physician offices, but is provided to you through the publisher, Wolters Kluwer Health, to give you hands-on practice working with EMRs. Your instructor will have more information about accessing your username, login, and Quickstart guide.

Prerequisite Activities in Harris CareTracker

- *The Getting Started and Quickstart documents and EMR Activities Step-by-Step Instructions are available at* http://thePoint.lww.com/KronenbergerComp5e

Activity Details

Accurately document the following test results in the EMR for the following patients:

1. Patty Bolger: RBC 3.9 million/μL, WBC 10,500/μL, Platelets 350,000/μL
2. Tom Bankston: Hemoglobin 17 g/dL

# Chapter Summary

- Laboratory analysis of blood, urine, and other body samples provides the physician with powerful diagnostic tools to identify diseases and disorders.
- Hospital and referral laboratories are divided into departments named for the specialty testing done in that department. Knowledge of each of the specialty categories makes it easier to understand the nature of the tests and the diagnostic information they provide.** The product insert is the key tool for accurate testing and quality control. To obtain an accurate result from a test kit or reagent, the instructions in the product insert must be strictly followed.
- There are a few basic pieces of laboratory equipment that are standard in most laboratories including the physician office lab (POL). These include the microscope, the centrifuge, the incubator, and the refrigerator and freezer.
- The goals of CLIA are standardization of laboratory testing and enforcement of quality protocols.
- Only CLIA-waived tests are within the scope of practice for a medical assistant working in the POL. A comprehensive list of waived tests is available at http://www.cms.gov.
- Quality control testing is designed to detect problems that might arise because of operator error, reagent or test kit deterioration, instrument malfunction, or improper environmental conditions.
- Standard precautions are based on the principle that all blood, body fluids, secretions, excretions (except sweat), nonintact skin, and mucous membranes may contain transmissible infectious agents. Standard precautions include a group of infection prevention practices that apply to all patients.

# Warm-Ups for Critical Thinking

1. Ask your instructor for a copy of a package insert from a test kit you will be using in class. Locate each bulleted item listed in the box and find the corresponding information on your sample package insert.
2. Review the section of this chapter describing referral laboratories. The physician requests a laboratory test that is unfamiliar to you. You do not find the test listed in the referral laboratory's test catalogue. How would you get the appropriate patient preparation and specimen collection, processing, and transport instructions for the requested test?
3. Working with another student, develop a plan of action to use in case your controls do not come into range and how to go about correcting a problem.
4. Review the laboratory safety rules and create a poster summarizing these rules for display in the classroom.
5. Obtain a unitized test device for a test you will perform in your laboratory training. Demonstrate the internal control and the external control. Describe the purpose of each and why it is necessary to have both.

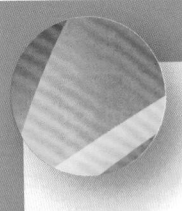

## PSY PROCEDURE 40-1

## Caring for a Microscope

**Purpose:** To protect the integrity and function of the microscope by performing routine care

**Equipment:** Lens paper, lens cleaner, gauze, mild soap solution, microscope, hand disinfectant, surface disinfectant

| STEPS | REASONS |
|---|---|
| 1. Wash your hands. | Hand washing aids infection control. |
| 2. Assemble the equipment and take the necessary items to the area where the microscope is located. | Equipment must be readily accessible and available before you start the procedure. |
| 3. If you need to move the microscope, carry it in both hands, one holding the base and the other holding the arm. | Jarring or dropping the microscope will damage the optics. |
| 4. Apply clean gloves and clean the optical areas following these steps:<br>**A.** Place a drop or two of lens cleaner on a piece of lens paper.<br>**B.** Wipe each eyepiece thoroughly with lens paper and lens cleaner. Do not touch the optical areas with your fingers | Do not use tissue or gauze because either may scratch the lenses. Direct contact will transfer oils from your skin to the optical surfaces. |

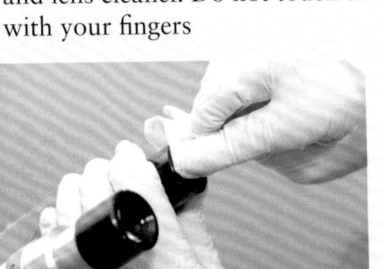

**Step 4B.** Wipe each eyepiece with lens paper and lens cleaner.

**C.** Wipe each objective lens starting with the lowest power and continuing to the highest power (usually an oil immersion lens). If the lens paper appears to have dirt or oil on it, use a clean section of the lens paper or a new piece of lens paper with cleaner.

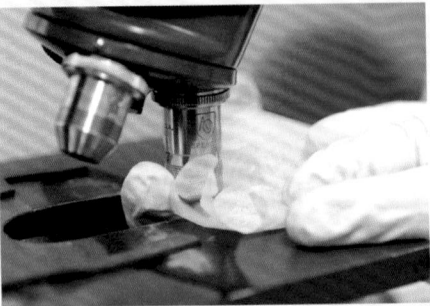

**Step 4C.** Wipe each objective lens with lens paper and lens cleaner. Clean the oil objective last so you won't carry its oil to the other objective lenses.

# PROCEDURE 40-1 (continued)

| STEPS | REASONS |
|---|---|

**STEPS**

D. Using a new piece of dry lens paper, wipe eyepiece and the objective lens so that no cleaner remains.

E. With a new piece of lens paper moistened with lens cleaner, clean the condenser and illuminator optics

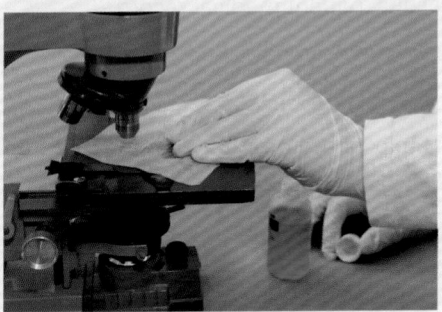

5. Clean areas other than the optics:
   A. Moisten gauze with mild soap solution or use an alcohol wipe and wipe all areas other than the optics including the stage, base, and adjustment knobs.
   B. Moisten another gauze with water and rinse the washed areas.

6. To store the cleaned microscope, ensure that the light source is turned off. Rotate the nosepiece so that the low-power objective is pointed down toward the stage. Cover the microscope with the plastic dust cover that came with it or a small trash bag.

7. Document microscope cleaning on the microscope maintenance log sheet.

| NAME OF LABORATORY: | | INSTRUMENT NAME AND ID: | | |
|---|---|---|---|---|
| Date of Maintenance | Action Performed | Comments | OK to Use? | Initials |
| | | | | |
| | | | | |
| | | | | |
| | | | | |
| | | | | |
| | | | | |
| | | | | |
| | | | | |
| | | | | |
| | | | | |
| | | | | |
| | | | | |
| | | | | |

**REASONS**

Removing the cleaner completely prevents distortion by residue.

**Step 4E.** Clean and dry the condenser and illuminator optics.

This removes oil and dirt from mechanical and structural surfaces.

This protects the mechanism and surfaces between uses.

Documentation of instrument service history is required for all laboratory equipment.

**Step 7.** Sample instrument log sheet.

*Note:* To maintain precision focusing, the microscope should be used in a low-traffic area and away from any source of vibration such as a centrifuge.

*Note:* Follow the manufacturer's recommendations for changing the light bulb and servicing the microscope.

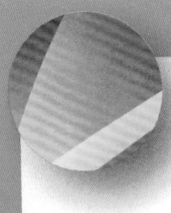

## PROCEDURE 40-2

# Screen and Follow Up Laboratory Test Results

**PSY** Perform patient screening using established protocols; differentiate between normal and abnormal test results; document patient care accurately in the medical record.

**Purpose:** To alert physician to a patient's critical lab results as soon as possible and document appropriately

**Equipment:** Laboratory report noting a patient's test results; patient medical record

| STEPS | REASONS |
|---|---|
| 1. Review laboratory reports received from reference laboratory. | Laboratory reports may contain results that require immediate intervention for patient safety. |
| 2. Note the results given, deciding which results are within normal limits and may be given to the physician for routine review and which results are critical and require immediate physician notification. | Critical results must be reported to the physician in a timely manner so that action can be taken to modify the patient's condition. |
| 3. After notifying the physician, follow any instructions given and take immediate action. | Lab results requiring immediate follow-up should be reported to the physician by the most direct method. |
| 4. Follow instructions and document notification and follow-up. | Relaying instructions to the physician is the first priority. Documenting physician notification and, if directed, the patient verifies that the process was completed. |
| 5. Document remaining reports appropriately. | All laboratory results should be routed according to office policy for timely follow-up with the patient. |

Charting Example:
*02/12/2016 10:00 AM Critical level glucose of 597 mg/dL reported to Dr. Singer. Pt. notified to come into office immediately as instructed by Dr. Singer. _____M. Miller, CMA*

Note: *The medical assistant may sign his or her name in the patient record using only the "CMA" credential if the office has a signature log denoting the entire credential as "CMA(AAMA)."*

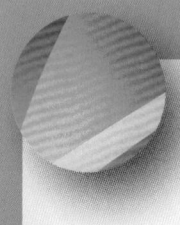

## PROCEDURE 40-3

## Use a Laboratory Flow Sheet

Maintain laboratory test results using flow sheet

**Purpose**: Document patient laboratory results using a flow sheet.

**Equipment**: Flow sheet for documenting a patient's anticoagulation therapy and test results.

| STEPS | REASONS |
|---|---|
| 1. Obtain flow sheet for specific laboratory test used by the physician office to document patient results and/or therapy. For this procedure, use the anticoagulant therapy flow sheet provided. | Flow sheets may vary depending on the laboratory test. Patient results should be recorded on the flow sheet immediately as reported by the laboratory or obtained in the physician office laboratory if a CLIA-waived test was performed. |
| 2. Record the patient's test results appropriately and accurately on the flow sheet. | The flow sheet must be completed accurately for a complete analysis of the results over time. |
| 3. Report any critical values immediately to the physician. | Lab results requiring immediate follow-up should be reported to the physician. |
| 4. Place the flow sheet in the patient medical record. | The flow sheet is part of the patient medical record whether using a paper record or an electronic medical record. |

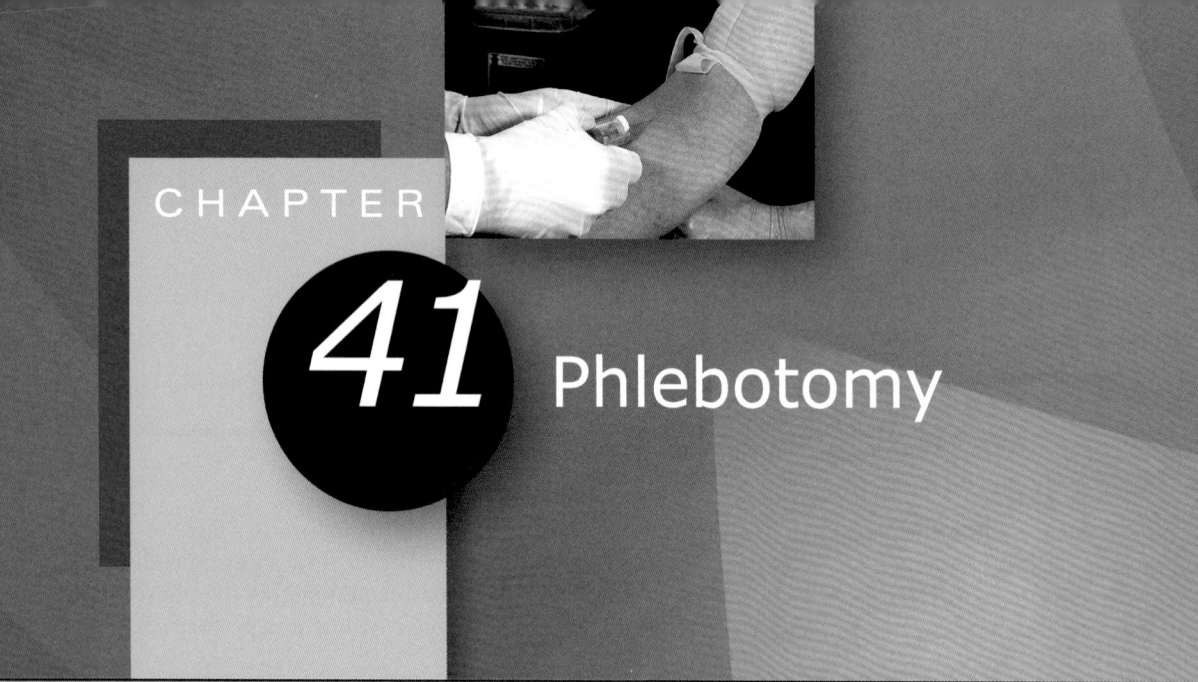

# CHAPTER 41 Phlebotomy

## Learning Outcomes

**COG Cognitive Domain***

1. Spell and define the key terms
2. *Define medical terms and abbreviations related to all body systems*
3. Identify equipment and supplies used to obtain a routine venous specimen and a routine capillary skin puncture
4. Describe proper use of specimen collection equipment
5. List the major anticoagulants, their color codes, and the suggested order in which they are filled during a venipuncture
6. Describe the location and selection of the blood collection sites using capillaries and veins
7. Differentiate between the feel of a vein, tendon, and artery
8. Describe care for a puncture site after blood has been drawn
9. Explain quality assessment issues in specimen collection procedures

**PSY Psychomotor Domain***

1. Obtain a blood specimen by evacuated tube or winged infusion set (Procedure 41-1)
   a. *Perform venipuncture*
   b. *Instruct and prepare a patient for a procedure or treatment*
   c. *Coach patients appropriately considering cultural diversity, developmental life stage, and communication barriers*
   d. *Document patient care accurately in the medical record*

2. Obtain a blood specimen by capillary puncture (Procedure 41-2)
   a. *Perform capillary puncture*
   b. *Instruct and prepare a patient for a procedure or treatment*
   c. *Coach patients appropriately considering cultural diversity, developmental life stage, and communication barriers*
   d. *Document patient care accurately in the medical record*

**AFF Affective Domain***

1. *Incorporate critical thinking skills when performing patient assessment*
2. *Incorporate critical thinking skills when performing patient care*
3. *Show awareness of a patient's concerns related to the procedure being performed*
4. *Demonstrate empathy, active listening, and nonverbal communication*
5. *Demonstrate respect for individual diversity including gender, race, religion, age, economic status, and appearance*
6. *Explain to a patient the rationale for performance of a procedure*
7. *Demonstrate sensitivity to patient rights*
8. *Protect the integrity of the medical record*

*Note: AAMA/CAAHEP 2015 Standards are italicized.*

### ABHES Competencies

1. Define and use entire basic structure of medical words and be able to accurately identify in the correct context, that is, root, prefix, suffix, combinations, spelling, and definitions
2. Build and dissect medical terms from roots/suffixes to understand the word element combinations that create medical terminology
3. Document accurately
4. Comply with federal, state, and local health laws and regulations

5. Identify and respond appropriately when working/caring for patients with special needs
6. Maintain inventory equipment and supplies
7. Communicate on the recipient's level of comprehension
8. Use pertinent medical terminology
9. Recognize and respond to verbal and nonverbal communication
10. Use standard precautions
11. Dispose of biohazardous materials
12. Collect, label, and process specimens
13. Perform venipuncture
14. Perform capillary puncture

## Key Terms

| | | | |
|---|---|---|---|
| antecubital space | gel separator | Luer adapter | thrombosed |
| anticoagulant | hematocrit | lymphedema | trough level |
| blood cultures | hematoma | multisample needle | venipuncture |
| butterfly | hemochromatosis | order of draw | |
| evacuated tube | hemoconcentration | peak level | |
| fasting | hemolysis | polycythemia vera | |

## Case Study

*T*om Carlisle, RMA, works in a large family practice office at Great Falls Medical Center. There are four physicians, two nurse practitioners, and two physician assistants in the office. On a typical day, Tom assists with many patient procedures, including collecting blood to either perform Clinical Laboratory Improvement Amendments (CLIA)–waived tests in the office or send to a reference laboratory for tests ordered that are not CLIA waived. Some tests require a venipuncture procedure, whereas others require a fingerstick or capillary puncture. If blood is collected during both of these procedures, what is the difference and why do some tests require one procedure and not the other? What should Tom do if he is collecting blood from a patient and during the procedure, the blood flow stops? Is it a problem to probe for a vein during a venipuncture to obtain a specimen? Why do the blood collection tubes have rubber tops that are different colors? These questions and others are addressed in this chapter.

Medical assistants are often responsible for collecting blood for testing in the office or sending to a larger laboratory or reference lab. In some patients, phlebotomy may also be a treatment for diseases such as **polycythemia vera** (an elevated red blood cell count) or **hemochromatosis** (too much iron in the blood). If used to treat these diseases, the procedure is referred to as **therapeutic phlebotomy**. However, most blood collection procedures performed in the physician office are done for diagnostic testing.

Although the successful **venipuncture** requires knowledge and skill, obtaining a blood specimen from a patient also requires empathy before, during, and after the procedure. The medical assistant who performs this procedure frequently will develop a comfortable routine that complies with office policy and procedure and conveys confidence to the patient. In addition, the blood specimen obtained by the skillful medical assistant will assure accurate results for the tests ordered by the physician or other qualified health care professional. The tests performed on the blood specimen you collect is only as good as the quality of the specimen collected. To ensure a high-quality specimen, you should give attention to several factors:

- Identifying the patient appropriately
- Verifying patient compliance with preparation requirements such as fasting or taking nothing by mouth before the test (NPO)
- Completing and checking the test requisition form for accuracy including the requested tests, patient information, and any special requirements if indicated
- Timing of collections is appropriate for the ordered test.
- Selecting a suitable site for the venipuncture or capillary puncture
- Preparing the equipment, the patient, and the puncture site
- Collecting the sample in the appropriate container
- Following all safety and quality control measures before, during, and after the procedure
- Recognizing complications from the phlebotomy
- Assessing the need for sample recollection and/or rejection
- Labeling the collection tubes at the drawing area
- Applying any special handling techniques as necessary

## PREPARING FOR BLOOD COLLECTION PROCEDURES

Before the blood collection procedure is performed, the location must be considered for appropriateness and safety. Some physician offices will have a specific location where patients needing blood drawn are taken while others require you to take the equipment and supplies to the patient in the exam room. If the office has a blood-drawing station, it should include a table close at hand for supplies and a phlebotomy chair with an adjustable armrest to allow proper positioning of either arms (Fig. 41-1). Patients who have a history of fainting or who appear unsteady or complaint of dizziness before the procedure should lie on an exam table. Phlebotomy chairs usually have a safety device on the armrest that locks it in place in front of the patient to prevent falling from the chair if fainting occurs.

Another important task that must be completed before collecting a blood specimen to send to a reference lab is the requisition form. This form accompanies the specimen to the laboratory and must be complete and accurate. It is the responsibility of the medical assistant to complete this

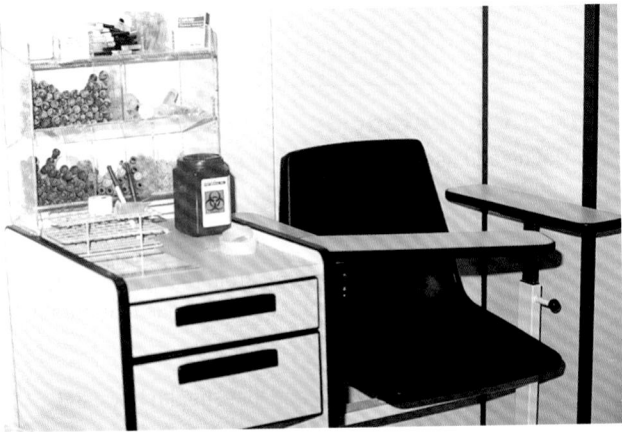

**Figure 41-1** • A well-stocked blood-drawing station in the physician office.

form using the physician order for the test or tests and the information required by the laboratory before the specimen is obtained. Many reference laboratories supply the laboratory requisition forms as hard copies, or the requisition completion and submission may be done electronically. It is also your responsibility to label the specimen container or blood tube by either writing the information with a permanent marker or pen on the tube or applying a label generated by the computer for offices that use an automated system. Relevant information required on the specimen container or blood tube includes the patient's first and last names, identification number if appropriate, date and time of collection, and the initials or name of the phlebotomist, which is the medical assistant in the physician office. The patient information must match the information supplied on the requisition form.

The equipment required for the phlebotomy procedure should be available and easily accessible before the procedure is started. You will need the following supplies to perform a venipuncture:

- **Evacuated tube**
- **Multisample needle** with a safety device
- A holder for the multisample needle
- Tourniquet
- 2- × 2-inch gauze pads and/or cotton balls
- Exam gloves
- Alcohol antiseptic pads or solution
- Adhesive bandage
- Sharps biohazard container
- Biohazard transport bag for sending specimens to a reference lab

### CHECKPOINT QUESTION

1. When preparing to do a venipuncture on a 22-year-old female patient, Tom notices her face looks pale and she complains of feeling "light-headed." How should Tom respond to this situation?

## Evacuated Collection Tubes

The evacuated tube system consists of a tube holder, also known as a **Luer adapter**, a multisample needle specifically for use with the evacuated tube, and the evacuated tube (Fig. 41-2). This system is a *closed system* allowing the patient's blood to flow from the vein through the needle and into the collection tube without exposure to the air and allows collecting multiple tubes with a one venipuncture.

Evacuated tubes are designed to fill with a predetermined volume of blood because of the vacuum inside the tube. The vacuum is premeasured by the manufacturer to draw the precise amount of blood into the tube, allowing blood to fill the tube until the vacuum is exhausted. A tube that has lost all or part of its vacuum will not fill completely, if at all. All blood tubes have an expiration date printed on the label, and tubes that expired should not be used to prevent using a tube that has lost all or part of its vacuum. *Troubleshooting tip*: If you are drawing a patient blood specimen and a tube does not fill, try another evacuated tube before withdrawing the needle from the vein.

Evacuated tubes are made of glass or plastic and range in size from 2 mL to 15 mL. The size is selected according to the patient's age, amount of blood required for the test ordered, and the size and condition of the patient's vein. The rubber stoppers on the evacuated tubes are self-sealing, meaning the needle puncture made when the tube is filling with blood seals afterwards to prevent blood from leaking out of the tube during processing or while being sent to the reference lab. The tubes are color coded according to the additive in the tube, and it is your responsibility to know the types of tests ordered and what type of additive is needed. Similar to an injection, the venipuncture procedure should be performed with medical and surgical asepsis in mind. Although you will practice medical asepsis when handling the outside of the tubes and other supplies, the multisample needle and area inside the evacuated tubes are considered sterile to prevent contamination of the specimen and the patient. Blood should *never* be poured from one tube to another because the tubes can have different additives or coatings.

### CHECKPOINT QUESTION

2. How does the evacuated tube fill with the correct measurement of blood?

### Tube Additives

Different laboratory tests require different types of blood specimens. For tests requiring serum samples, the blood is drawn into a tube that does not have coagulant added and allow the blood specimen to clot. After collecting the specimen in a tube that does not contain an additive, the tube is allowed to stand undisturbed while the specimen clots. The clotting process takes 30 to 60 minutes at 22°C to 25°C. When the specimen has clotted, it is placed into a centrifuge to separate the serum from the clot. The specimen should be allowed to complete the clotting process prior to being centrifuged for separation of the serum from the clot; this is required to attain the optimum specimen.

Other tests require whole blood or plasma, and these samples are drawn into a tube that contains an **anticoagulant** additive to prevent clotting. The following is a list of the most common additives found in evacuated tubes and their functions:

- Anticoagulants that prevent the blood from clotting.
- Clot activators that speed up coagulation.
- **Gel separators** that form a barrier between the cells and the serum or plasma portion after the specimen has been centrifuged. This protects the serum from interaction with the red blood cells (RBCs) that would alter test results.

The color-coded rubber stoppers on the evacuated tubes identify the additive contained in each type of tube (Table 41-1). It is necessary to use the tube with the correct anticoagulant to avoid altered or inaccurate test results. It is also necessary to fill the tube until the vacuum is exhausted because underfilled tubes will alter patient test results due to overdilution of the specimen by the tube additive.

### CHECKPOINT QUESTION

3. What type of blood specimen requires collecting in an evacuated tube that does not have an anticoagulant additive?

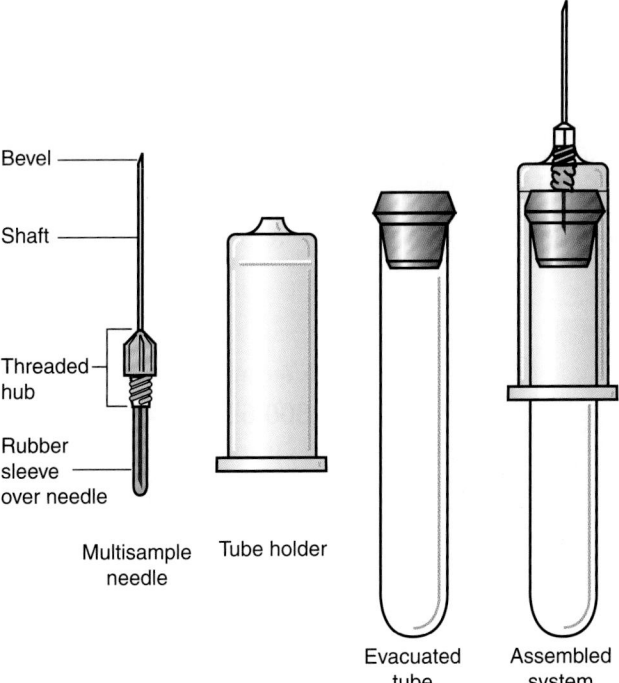

Bevel

Shaft

Threaded hub

Rubber sleeve over needle

Multisample needle

Tube holder

Evacuated tube

Assembled system

**Figure 41-2 •** Traditional components of the evacuated tube system. (Reprinted from McCall R. *Phlebotomy Essentials*. Baltimore, MD: Lippincott Williams & Wilkins, 2007, with permission.)

## TABLE 41-1    Evacuated Tube System: Color Coding

Helping all people
live healthy lives

# BD Vacutainer® Order of Draw for Multiple Tube Collections

*Designed for Your Safety*

Reflects change in CLSI recommended
Order of Draw (H3-A5, Vol 23, No 32, 8.10.2)

| Closure Color | Collection Tube | Mix by Inverting |
|---|---|---|
| **BD Vacutainer® Blood Collection Tubes** *(glass or plastic)* | | |
| | • Blood Cultures - SPS | 8 to 10 times |
| | • Citrate Tube* | 3 to 4 times |
| or | • BD Vacutainer® SST™ Gel Separator Tube | 5 times |
| | • Serum Tube *(glass or plastic)* | 5 times (plastic) none (glass) |
| | • BD Vacutainer® Rapid Serum Tube (RST) | 5 to 6 times |
| or | • BD Vacutainer® PST™ Gel Separator Tube With Heparin | 8 to 10 times |
| | • Heparin Tube | 8 to 10 times |
| or | • EDTA Tube | 8 to 10 times |
| | • BD Vacutainer® PPT™ Separator Tube K₂EDTA with Gel | 8 to 10 times |
| | • Fluoride (glucose) Tube | 8 to 10 times |

* When using a winged blood collection set for venipuncture and a coagulation (citrate) tube is the first specimen tube to be drawn, a discard tube should be drawn first. The discard tube must be used to fill the blood collection set tubing's "dead space" with blood but the discard tube does not need to be completely filled. This important step will ensure proper blood-to-additive ratio. The discard tube should be a nonadditive or coagulation tube.

## Note: Always follow your facility's protocol for order of draw

Handle all biologic samples and blood collection "sharps" (lancets, needles, luer adapters and blood collection sets) according to the policies and procedures of your facility. Obtain appropriate medical attention in the event of any exposure to biologic samples (for example, through a puncture injury) since they may transmit viral hepatitis, HIV (AIDS), or other infectious diseases. Utilize any built-in used needle protector if the blood collection device provides one. BD does not recommend reshielding used needles, but the policies and procedures of your facility may differ and must always be followed. Discard any blood collection "sharps" in biohazard containers approved for their disposal.

1 Becton Drive
Franklin Lakes, NJ 07417
www.bd.com/vacutainer

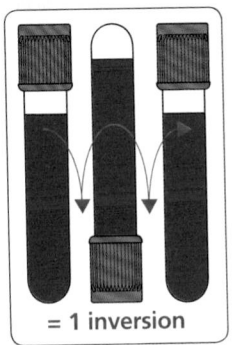

= 1 inversion

BD Technical Services
**1.800.631.0174**
BD Customer Service
**1.888.237.2762**
www.bd.com/vacutainer

BD, BD Logo and all other trademarks are property of Becton, Dickinson and Company. © 2010 BD
Franklin Lakes, NJ, 07417    1/10    VS5729-6

Courtesy Becton, Dickinson and Company.

## Order of Draw

In addition to patient safety during the phlebotomy procedure, there are additional concerns for the medical assistant collecting blood specimens including avoiding cross contamination between evacuated tubes that have a variety of additives or no additives. The chemicals added to evacuated blood tubes preserve the blood for various types of testing and have a possibility of carryover from one tube to the next if more than one tube of blood is collected during the venipuncture procedure. This possibility is low but must be considered because of the serious errors that may result in the test results if proper tube collection procedures are not followed. A specific **order of draw** during the procedure when obtaining multiple tubes from a single venipuncture avoids these concerns. The Clinical and Laboratory Standards Institute (CLSI) recommends an order of draw; however, each laboratory facility may slightly differ and you should follow protocol from the laboratory where the specimen is sent for testing. Table 41-2 lists the general order of draw for multiple tube collections

beginning with those that should be drawn first to those that should be drawn last and includes the rationale for collecting in this order:

- Culture (yellow)
- Light blue
- Red
- Red and gray; gold
- Green
- Lavender
- Gray

In addition to using the correct tube and following the order of draw, the additives should be thoroughly mixed with the blood in the tube. Mixing the additive and blood should be done gently by inverting the tube as noted in Table 41-1 depending on the additive.

**Blood culture** specimens are not a routine request in the physician office but may be ordered by the physician to check for the presence of microorganisms in the blood. As noted above, these specimens must be drawn first if multiple tubes of blood are also being drawn to

| TABLE 41-2 | CLSI Order of Draw and Rationale for Collection Order | |
|---|---|---|
| **Order of Draw** | **Tube Stopper Color** | **Rationale for Collection Order** |
| Blood cultures (sterile collections) | Yellow culture bottles (sterile media containers [SPS]) | Minimizes chance of microbial contamination |
| Coagulation tubes | Light blue | Second or third position in order of draw; prevents tissue thromboplastin contamination. Must be the first additive tube in the order because all other additive tubes affect coagulation tests |
| Plain (nonadditive) tubes | Red | Prevents contamination by additives in other tubes. Must be drawn prior to a light-blue top as a "throwaway tube" if not ordered |
| Serum separator gel tubes | Red and gray rubber; gold plastic | Prevents contamination by additives in other tubes. Comes after specimens drawn for coagulation tests because it contains silica particles to activate clotting in the tube. Carryover of the silica particles into the coagulation specimen would activate clotting and affect coagulation tests. Carryover of silica into subsequent tubes can override the anticoagulant in them. |
| Plasma tubes and plasma separator gel tubes | Green and light-green top | Contains heparin, which affects coagulation tests and interferes in collection of serum specimens. Causes the least interference in tests other than coagulation tests |
| Ethylenediaminetetraacetic acid (EDTA) tubes | Lavender; white | EDTA tubes have more carryover (EDTA) problems than any other additive. Elevates sodium and potassium levels. Chelates and decreases calcium and iron levels. Elevates prothrombin time and partial thromboplastin time results |
| Oxalate/fluoride tubes | Gray | Sodium fluoride and potassium oxalate elevate sodium and potassium levels, respectively. Comes after hematology tubes because oxalate damages cell membranes and causes abnormal red blood cell morphology |

avoid contamination of the specimen. In addition, the skin preparation before the venipuncture procedure requires additional steps including cleansing with an iodine solution to further reduce microorganisms normally found on the skin. If a mistake is made in the order of draw, record the actual order of draw on the request form or in the computer so that it is visible in the laboratory testing area. Findings are reviewed for evidence of contamination before they are reported. If interference is suspected, the laboratory can suggest recollection of the specimen to validate the original test results.

## CHECKPOINT QUESTION

4. What is the proper order of draw when using the evacuated tube system? Why is this important?

## Venipuncture Needles

The needles used during a venipuncture have similar features of needles used during injections including a shaft, hub, lumen, and bevel (refer to Chapter 24). These needles are also sterile, single use only, and silicon coated to penetrate the skin smoothly. However, venipuncture needles are used with a holder and have a needle at both ends, one to actually penetrate the vein during the procedure and the other end inserted in the rubber stopper on the evacuated tube. With beveled points on both ends, multisample needles are threaded in the middle to screw into the needle holder. One end of the needle is longer and is exposed for piercing the patient's skin and entering the vein. The shorter end penetrates the rubber stopper of the collection tube and, with its retractable rubber sleeve, prevents leakage of blood during tube changes. The sleeve is pushed back when it goes into the stopper, allowing blood to flow into the tube, and recovers the end of the needle when the tube is removed.

The open end of the holder is open so evacuation tubes can be inserted easily. The extensions, or flanges,

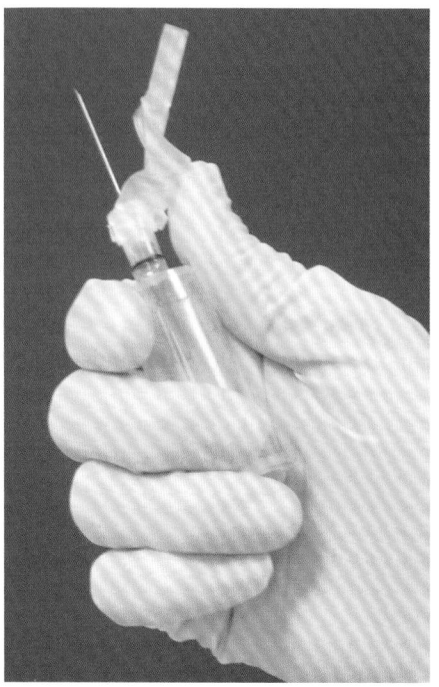

**Figure 41-3** • BD Eclipse multisample safety needle attached to traditional tube holder. (Courtesy of Becton-Dickinson, Franklin Lakes, NJ.)

on the side of the holder rim aid in tube placement and removal. A safety device is part of the holder and allows the immediate covering of the needle after it is withdrawn from the skin and vein to avoid accidental needlesticks to the phlebotomist (Fig. 41-3). The holder and the multisample needle are single use only and must be placed in a biohazard sharps container immediately after use. A safety needle-retracting device in the needle holder allows the safety to be provided as part of the needle holder rather than as part of the needle (Fig. 41-4).

When performing the venipuncture, the needle should be inserted into the skin with the bevel facing upward (Procedure 41-1). Selection of the needle

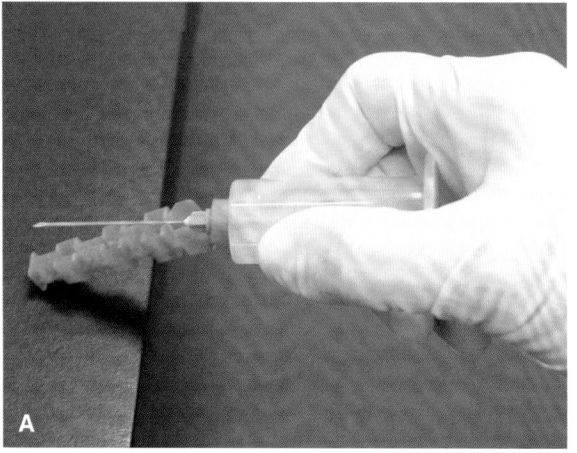
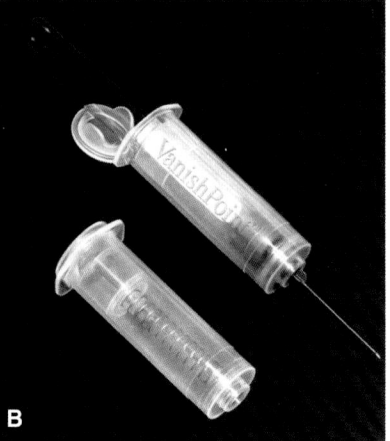

**Figure 41-4** • Safety tube holder. **(A)** Venipuncture Needle-Pro with needle-sheathing device. **(B)** VanishPoint tube syringe with needle-retracting device. (Retractable Technologies, Little Elm, TX.)

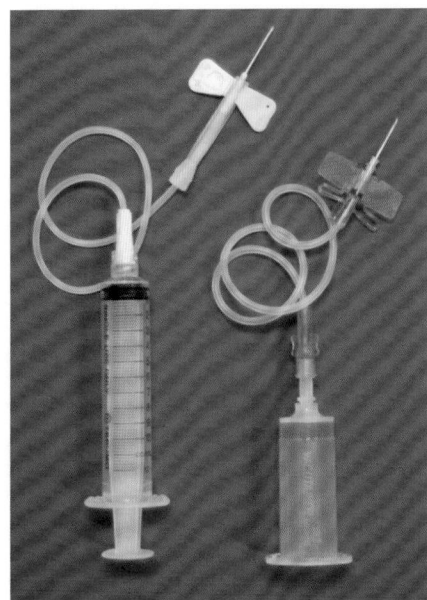

**Figure 41-5** • Winged infusion sets. **Left:** Attached to a syringe. **Right:** Attached to evacuated tube holder by means of a Luer adapter. (Reprinted from McCall R. *Phlebotomy Essentials.* Baltimore, MD: Lippincott Williams & Wilkins, 2003, with permission.)

size, or gauge, is based on the size and condition of the patient's vein; however, a needle size smaller than 23 gauge should never be used to collect blood because the lumen is too small and will rupture the erythrocytes, or red blood cells, causing **hemolysis** of the specimen and inaccurate test results.

In some situations, a winged infusion set, or **butterfly**, may be used to perform a venipuncture procedure. The winged infusion set may be attached to a syringe or an evacuated needle holder (Fig. 41-5). Winged sets should be used only for small, fragile, superficial veins such as those found in pediatric and geriatric patients or the posterior hand in other adults. The needle on a winged set is much shorter than a multisample needle and cannot reach deep veins. Figure 41-6 shows the procedure for using a winged infusion set during a venipuncture.

## CHECKPOINT QUESTION

5. When choosing a needle for venipuncture, why would Tom not choose a 23-gauge needle to draw a blood specimen for laboratory testing?

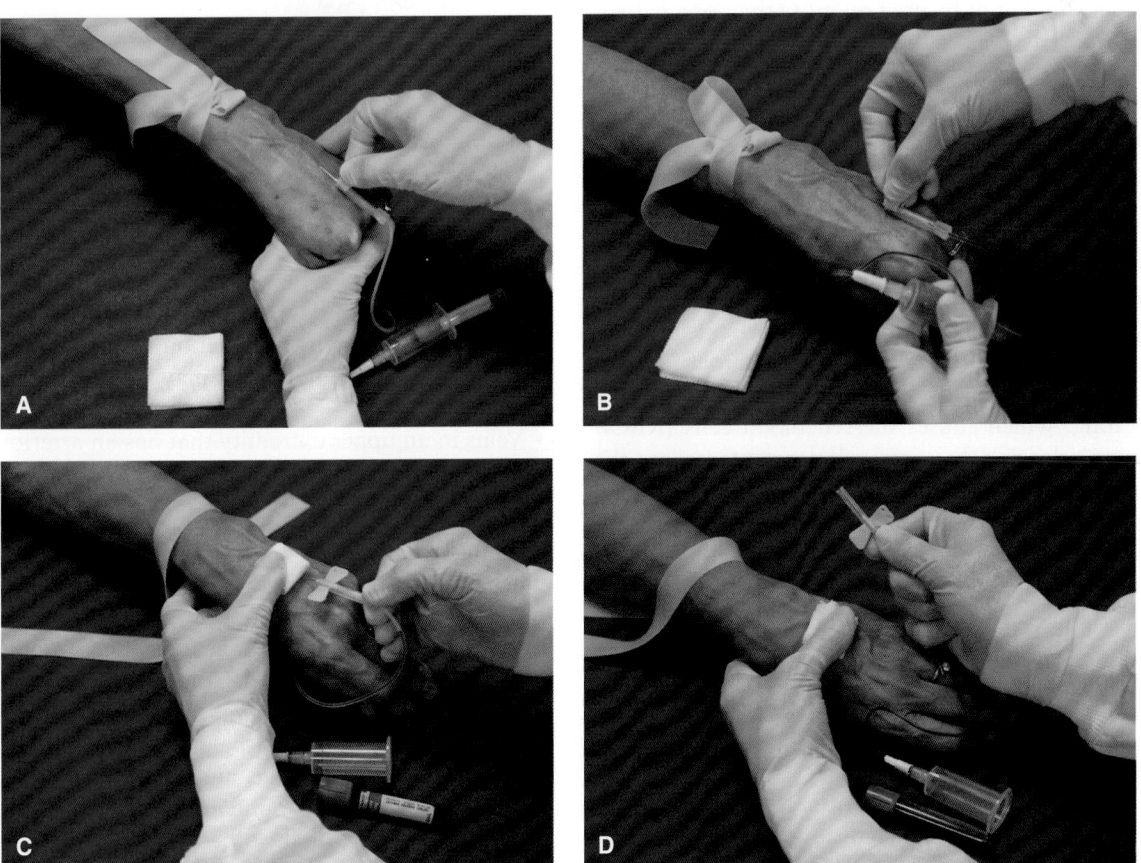

**Figure 41-6** • Procedure for using butterfly in a hand vein. **(A)** Hand with tourniquet in place reveals prominent vein. **(B)** With the skin pulled taut over the knuckles, the needle is inserted into the vein until there is a flash of blood in the tubing. **(C)** Using the nondominant hand, a wing of the butterfly is held against the patient's hand to steady the needle while the blood-collecting tube is pushed onto the blood-collecting needle. **(D)** Once the proper tubes have been drawn, gauze is placed over the vein, and the needle is removed. (Reprinted from McCall R. *Phlebotomy Essentials.* Baltimore, MD: Lippincott Williams & Wilkins, 2003, with permission.)

## ⦶OG **Venipuncture Site Selection**

The procedure should start with washing hands and putting on a new pair of exam gloves after selecting the equipment and supplies. Many patients know from experience where it is easiest to find an accessible vein and may tell you which arm is better for performing the venipuncture. Use the patient's experience and your own knowledge and skill to assist with choosing the best site for the procedure. Talk quietly with the patient and progress through the procedure including choosing an appropriate vein with confidence to minimize patient anxiety. To select a vein, a tourniquet is applied superior to the area of interest on the extremity, which constricts the flow of venous blood, making the veins more prominent so that they are easier to palpate and penetrate with a venipuncture needle.

Although the tourniquet is made of a pliable latex material that is typically 1 inch wide and 15 to 18 inches long, a nonlatex tourniquet should be used for patients who have known latex allergies. If tied correctly around the extremity, the tourniquet can be easily removed with one hand and should not cut into the patient's skin. The tourniquet should not be used on more than one patient and is disposed of after use according to office policy and procedure. After placing the tourniquet on the arm, do not leave it on for more than 1 minute. A tourniquet left on too long can result in **hemoconcentration** of the blood in the veins decreasing the fluid content of the blood and causing the blood to have more cells than usual for the amount of serum or plasma. This false elevation of cells results in inaccurate laboratory measurements of total protein, aspartate aminotransferase (AST), total lipids, cholesterol, iron, and calcium levels. Hemoconcentration also affects **hematocrit** levels. Hemolysis can also occur from leaving the tourniquet on too long, which causes the red blood cells (RBCs) to rupture, releasing their intracellular contents into the serum or plasma.

The anterior forearm veins in the **antecubital space**, or the inner aspect of the elbow, are commonly used for venipuncture. There are three veins in this area known as the cephalic, median cubital, and basilica (Fig. 41-7). Veins in the hand may also be used if a forearm vein is not easily palpable. The following areas should be avoided when choosing a site:

- Veins under a burn or scar.
- Veins under a hematoma or bruise. If that arm must be used, collect the specimen distal to the hematoma or bruise.
- Veins that are **thrombosed**, which will feel like rope or cord and roll easily.
- An area that is **edematous** that contains excess tissue fluid accumulation that may alter test results.
- Veins in an upper extremity on the side of a previous mastectomy may be affected by **lymphedema** due

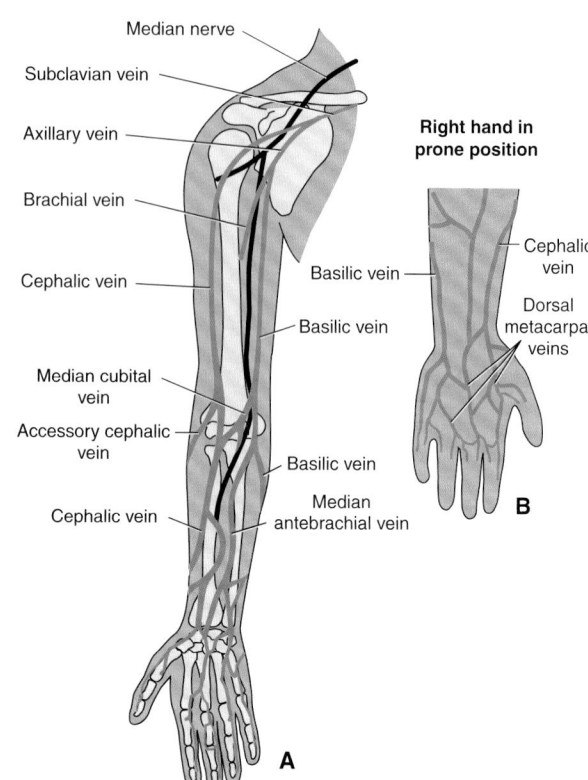

**Figure 41-7** • **(A)** Principal veins of the arm, including major antecubital veins subject to venipuncture. **(B)** Forearm, wrist, and hand veins subject to venipuncture. (Reprinted from McCall R. *Phlebotomy Essentials*. Baltimore, MD: Lippincott Williams & Wilkins, 2003, with permission.)

to the removal of lymph nodes during the mastectomy. The lymphatic obstruction that results from the removal of lymph nodes may affect test results.
- Veins in an upper extremity that has an arteriovenous shunt for renal dialysis.

Although some veins are visible, the best choice for venipuncture is found by touch. Do not slap the arm when trying to locate a vein because this can cause bruising in addition to altering test results from the specimen. Trace the path of veins with the index finger, noting their size, depth, and direction. Arteries are deeper than veins, pulsate, and have a thick wall. Veins are more superficial and may be seen and palpated. Thrombosed veins lack resilience, feel cordlike, and roll easily. If no suitable antecubital vein can be found in one extremity, repeat the selection procedure on the other arm. If suitable veins are not found in either antecubital space, force blood into the vein by massaging the arm from wrist to elbow; tap the site with the index and second fingers; apply a warm, damp washcloth to the site for 5 minutes; or lower the arm to allow the veins to fill. If necessary, veins in the posterior hand may be accessed using a winged infusion or butterfly set.

**CHECKPOINT QUESTIONS**

6. What areas are to be avoided when selecting the venipuncture site?

 **WHAT IF?**

**What if your patient feels faint while you are drawing blood?**

1. Remove the tourniquet and withdraw the needle as quickly as possible.
2. Talk to the patient to divert attention from the procedure and to help keep him or her alert.
3. Have the patient lower his or her head and breathe deeply while you physically support him or her to prevent injury in case of collapse.
4. Loosen a tight collar or tie if possible.
5. Apply a cold compress or washcloth to the forehead and back of the patient's neck.
6. Call for the physician if the patient does not respond.

Modified from McCall R. *Phlebotomy Essentials.* Baltimore, MD: Lippincott Williams & Wilkins, 2003, with permission.

## THE PHLEBOTOMY PROCEDURE

A medical assistant responsible for collecting blood via venipuncture needs to be thoroughly familiar with each step of the procedure. Procedure 41-1 details the procedure including the reasons or rationale for each step. Before performing the procedure, you must also verify patient compliance with any instructions necessary for accurate test results if applicable. For example, some tests require the patient fast or remain NPO for a specified time period before blood is collected while other test may have no special considerations. **Fasting** requires the patient to have no food or fluids except water for a specified amount of time before the specimen is collected. Patients who are fasting should be encouraged to drink plenty of water to stay hydrated, which will result in veins that are more easily palpated and accessible. A patient who is instructed to have nothing by mouth, or who is NPO, should not have anything including water. If the patient indicates that fasting or NPO instructions were not followed, notify the physician for a decision whether or not to proceed with the venipuncture. If you are instructed to proceed in obtaining the specimen, "nonfasting" should be written on both the test requisition and the specimen label to inform the laboratory personnel.

It is also appropriate to ask the patient about the use of medications such as "blood thinners" or anticoagulants including the use of aspirin that will cause additional bleeding after the procedure.

Verify that the necessary collection tubes are available and make sure you are aware of any special handling that may be required after the sample is obtained such as protect from light, place immediately on ice, etc. Always have extra supplies available because equipment such as the evacuation tubes can fail during the procedure and you will have to leave to obtain additional supplies before resticking the patient. Resticking the patient should be avoided if at all possible.

After cleansing the area with alcohol or another disinfectant, allow the cleansed site to air-dry. Do not blow on the site or wave the air with the hand above the site because this directs bacteria from the mouth back to the area that was just cleansed. Also, the cleansed venipuncture site should not be palpated again to avoid reintroducing microorganisms to the clean site. The vein should be anchored with the fingers of the opposite hand that holds the needle to prevent the vein from rolling or moving before being punctured with the needle. For personal protection, you should not use the forefinger to anchor the vein above the selected phlebotomy site because doing so increases the risk of a possible accidental needlestick.

After the procedure, apply adequate pressure to the site to avoid the formation of a hematoma. Rushing to complete the steps of the venipuncture can lead to a hematoma due to inadequate pressure at the site. Although asking the patient may be helpful in applying pressure after the venipuncture, this does not reduce the responsibility of the medical assistant for monitoring pressure on the site. A bandage should not be applied until the site has completely stopped bleeding. The patient who takes anticoagulants including aspirin regularly will have prolonged bleeding at the puncture site and pressure should be applied for a minimum of 5 minutes. The bandage should only be applied after the site has been monitored for adequate clotting.

 **CHECKPOINT QUESTION**

7. How do the patient instructions for fasting differ from having nothing by mouth?

### Troubleshooting Guidelines

#### No Blood Obtained during the Venipuncture Procedure

Probing, more commonly known as "fishing," is *not* the way to troubleshoot blood-drawing problems during the venipuncture procedure. If the needle is inserted and no blood is obtained, you should change the position of the needle including re-anchoring the needle and moving it forward as it may not have entered the vein as anticipated. In some cases, the vein rolls away from the point of the needle and re-anchoring before moving the needle forward allows the point of the needle to enter the vein. If you suspect you may have gone in too far, move the needle backward or out of the vein slightly. You may also slightly adjust the angle of the needle as the bevel could be against the vein wall. Figure 41-8 shows proper and improper needle positions.

If you are fairly certain you are in the vein but no blood enters the evacuation tube, try another tube in case the vacuum in the tube you originally chose is absent or minimal. In some cases, loosening the tourniquet may help as it may be obstructing blood flow. If none of these techniques work, you will have no choice but to restick the patient or have someone else attempt the venipuncture. Resticking the patient is not a sign of failure on the part of the medical assistant who is not successful but is often an indication that the veins have had multiple sticks and may be hardened from scarring or are thin and fragile. Even the most successful medical assistant who is competent in venipuncture has unsuccessful days or patients.

## Blood Flow Stops during the Venipuncture Procedure

If blood initially flows into the evacuation tube but then stops flowing, the vein may have collapsed. If possible, you should resecure the tourniquet to increase venous filling, but this will require assistance because you will not be able to let go of the needle holder inside the arm. If resecuring the tourniquet is not possible or successful, you should loosen the tourniquet, remove the needle, take care of the puncture site, and draw the specimen from another site. In some cases, the blood flow stops because the needle was pulled out of the vein when switching tubes during a multiple draw. Holding the needle holder firmly and placing fingers against patient's arm when removing and changing evacuation tubes will provide leverage and prevent movement of the needle within the vein.

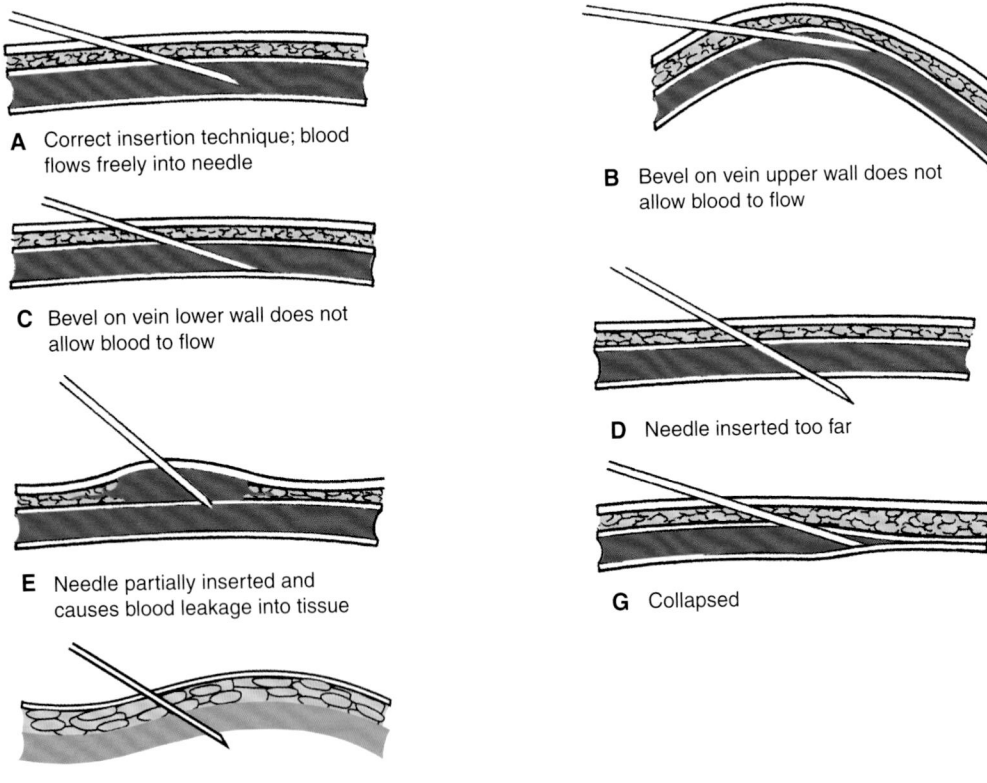

**A** Correct insertion technique; blood flows freely into needle

**C** Bevel on vein lower wall does not allow blood to flow

**E** Needle partially inserted and causes blood leakage into tissue

**F** When a vein rolls, the needle may slip to the side of the vein without penetrating it

**B** Bevel on vein upper wall does not allow blood to flow

**D** Needle inserted too far

**G** Collapsed

**Figure 41-8 •** Proper and improper needle positioning. **(A)** Needle correctly positioned in a vein; blood flows freely into the needle. **(B)** Bevel on the upper wall of the vein prevents blood flow. **(C)** Bevel on the lower wall of the vein prevents blood flow. **(D)** Needle inserted too deep runs through the vein. **(E)** Partially inserted needle causes blood to leak into tissue. **(F)** Needle slipped beside the vein, not into it; this occurs when a vein rolls to the side. **(G)** Collapsed vein prevents blood flow. (Reprinted from McCall R. *Phlebotomy Essentials*. Baltimore, MD: Lippincott Williams & Wilkins, 2007, with permission.)

## Problems Other Than an Incomplete Collection

The most common complication of venipuncture is **hematoma** formation caused by blood leaking into the tissues during or after venipuncture. Hematomas are painful, cause bruising, and can cause injuries to nerves. Box 41-1 describes situations that may trigger hematoma formation. If a hematoma begins to form during the venipuncture, release the tourniquet immediately, withdraw the needle, and hold pressure on the site for at least 2 minutes. Cold compresses reduce pain and swelling. Hematoma formation is especially a problem in older patients. To prevent a hematoma, make sure the needle fully penetrates the uppermost wall of the vein. Partial penetration may allow blood to leak into the soft tissue surrounding the vein by way of the needle bevel. Always remove the tourniquet before removing the needle to reduce the likelihood of a hematoma and use the major superficial veins when possible. Applying adequate pressure until bleeding has stopped also reduces hematoma formation.

If the needle is inserted too deeply, accidental puncture of an artery may occur. This is recognized by the blood's bright red color and the pulsing of the specimen into the tube. In this case, it is important to remove the tourniquet and needle and hold pressure over the site for a full 5 minutes after the needle is removed. The pressure of blood inside an artery is greater than the pressure inside a vein and therefore requires additional pressure to control or stop any bleeding.

Another consideration is permanent nerve damage from a venipuncture procedure. This may result from poor site selection, patient movement during needle insertion, inserting the needle too deeply or quickly, or excessive blind probing. Prolonged tourniquet application will not cause nerve damage but will result in hemoconcentration of the specimen.

To avoid hemolysis of the specimen, gently mix the evacuation tubes by inverting them to mix the blood and

---

**BOX 41-2** **Sources of Error in Venipuncture**

**Errors in Venipuncture Preparation**

- Improper patient identification
- Failure to check patient adherence to dietary restrictions
- Failure to calm patient prior to blood collection
- Use of improper equipment and supplies
- Inappropriate method of blood collection
- Failure to dry the site completely after cleansing with alcohol

**Errors in Venipuncture Procedure**

- Inserting needle bevel side down
- Use of needle that is too small, causing hemolysis of specimen
- Venipuncture in an unacceptable area
- Prolonged tourniquet application
- Wrong order of tube draw
- Failure to immediately mix blood collected in additive-containing tubes
- Pulling back on syringe plunger too forcefully
- Failure to release tourniquet prior to needle withdrawal

**Errors after Venipuncture Completion**

- Failure to apply pressure immediately to venipuncture site
- Vigorous shaking of anticoagulated blood specimens
- Forcing blood through a syringe needle into tube
- Mislabeling of tubes
- Failure to label appropriate specimens with infectious disease precaution
- Failure to put date, time, and initials on requisition
- Slow transport of specimens to laboratory

---

additives, avoid drawing blood from an area with a hematoma present, avoid forceful pulling back on the plunger if using a needle and syringe to obtain the specimen, and use a larger gauge needle. Box 41-2 lists some common errors to guard against in the venipuncture procedure.

## WHAT IF?

**What if, while drawing a blood specimen, the blood flow stops before collection of the required tubes is complete?**

While drawing a blood specimen, the blood flow may stop leaving a partially filled tube. The following steps may restart the blood flow. They should be

---

**BOX 41-1** **Situations That May Trigger Hematoma Formation**

1. The vein is fragile or too small for the needle.
2. The needle penetrates all the way through the vein.
3. The needle is only partly inserted into the vein.
4. Excessive or blind probing is used to find the vein.
5. The needle is removed while the tourniquet is still on.
6. Pressure is not adequately applied after venipuncture.

Reprinted from McCall R. *Phlebotomy Essentials.* Baltimore, MD: Lippincott Williams & Wilkins, 2003, with permission.

gently tried before discontinuing the collection and restricking the patient. Try each step, allowing a few seconds in between for the blood flow to respond. There should be no excessive or aggressive jabbing of the patient.

- Gently nudge the needle forward.
- Slightly pull the needle backward.
- Very slightly rotate the needle in the vein.
- Remove the vacuum tube and replace it with another tube.

If these attempts do not restart the blood flow, terminate the stick and follow up with postcare of the phlebotomy site. Another attempt should be made to complete the collection. Look for a site on the opposite arm. Do not tie the tourniquet around the same arm the second time. Perform the phlebotomy and complete the specimen collection.

Should the second attempt fail, *do not pour the specimen from tube to tube.* There is a reason why—it will critically ruin all test results.

Should a choice to pour off the specimen go unnoticed, there are several negative outcomes for the patient:

- If the tube collected contained no anticoagulant, the blood had begun to clot. What is poured off will be falsely diluted. The results of tests performed on that specimen will be abnormally low. The results of the tests performed on the original tube will be falsely elevated.
- If the tube collected contained no anticoagulant, again, the blood had begun to clot. Platelets are removed from the liquid part of the blood to make the clot. If the specimen is poured from a partially clotted tube into a lavender-top tube, it will be used to count blood cells. All of the cell counts will be abnormally low because some of the cells in the specimen have been tied up in the clot forming in the red-top tube. The platelet count will be critically low.
- The light-blue–top tube is used to test for blood-clotting factors. If the specimen just described is poured into a light-blue–top tube, the tests for clotting factors will be falsely abnormal because some of the clotting factors were left behind in the original tube with the forming clot.
- If the partially filled tube collected did contain an anticoagulant, the blood has been chemically altered. The poured-off blood will probably not clot and will require that the patient have another unnecessary stick. If the blood should clot and testing proceeds, the anticoagulant chemicals in the blood will ruin any chemistry tests that were ordered.

The patient is at risk from any testing performed on specimens poured off from the original tube.

## CHECKPOINT QUESTION

8. When performing a venipuncture procedure, what are some ways to avoid causing a hematoma?

## Patient Factors to Consider

In addition to the knowledge and skill necessary to perform a venipuncture procedure, you must also be aware of patient factors to consider including therapeutic drug monitoring, the effect of exercise and stress, **diurnal rhythms**, and postural changes. These factors are described below:

- *Therapeutic drug monitoring*: Drugs have different patterns of administration, body distribution, metabolism, and elimination that affect their concentration as measured in the blood. Some medications require monitoring blood levels to assure maximum effectiveness or monitor for toxicity. Many drugs will have a **peak** (the highest serum level of a drug based on the dosing schedule) and a **trough** (the lowest serum level of a drug drawn immediately before a dose is administered). If venipuncture is ordered by the physician for peak and/or trough levels of a medication, you should check with the patient to plan the time for drawing appropriate specimens.
- *Effects of exercise*: Muscular activity before a venipuncture may cause an increase in certain substances in the blood including creatine kinase (CK), AST, lactate dehydrogenase (LDH), and platelets.
- *Stress*: Stress may cause an elevation in white blood cells (WBCs). Anxiety that results in hyperventilation may cause acid–base imbalances.
- *Diurnal rhythms*: Many substances fluctuate in the blood throughout the day and evening hours. Serum iron levels tend to drop during the day. Check the timing of these variations for the desired collection point.
- *Posture*: Postural changes (supine to sitting, etc.) are known to vary the laboratory results of some analytes. The difference in these lab values has been attributed to shifts in body fluids. Fluids tend to stay in the bloodstream when the patient is recumbent or supine. There is a shift of fluids to the interstitial spaces upon standing or ambulation. The lab tests that are the most affected by this phenomenon are enzymes, albumin, triglycerides, cholesterol, calcium, and iron.

## CHECKPOINT QUESTION

9. What is the difference between a peak level and a trough level of a drug in the blood?

### Instructing Patients on Dietary Restrictions

Fasting and NPO are two common dietary restrictions. Because most patients will not understand the differences between these requirements, the medical assistant must provide clear explanations.

#### Fasting

Fasting, the most common dietary restriction, requires the patient to not eat for a certain period, usually from midnight until specimen collection the following morning. Fasting allows the patient to drink water; in fact, adequate hydration is necessary to ensure that veins are palpable and accessible for venipuncture. Dehydration by abstaining from all fluids can falsely elevate some test results, making them appear abnormal when they really are not.

#### NPO

NPO orders require that the patient have absolutely nothing by mouth for a certain period. This type of order is usually used if the patient is scheduled for surgery or for some radiology procedures. The purpose of an NPO order is to minimize secretions by reducing the body's fluid level.

## COG CAPILLARY PUNCTURE (MICROCOLLECTION)

The fingers in adults and children and heel in newborn infants are used to obtain smaller samples of blood from the capillaries. Adult capillary punctures are performed for several reasons including no veins are accessible, veins must be reserved for procedures such as intravenous therapy including chemotherapy, or POC (point of care) testing using technology that allows tests to be performed on small amounts of blood samples. The skin puncture is the preferred method to obtain blood from infants and children. Venipuncture on infants and children can damage veins and surrounding tissues.

Obtaining blood from a capillary puncture involves penetration of the capillary bed in the dermis of the skin with a puncture device instead of inserting a needle into a vein. The equipment used to collect the specimen depends on the patient's age and condition and on the test being performed including a puncture device, microhematocrit tubes or microcollection containers, and warming devices to increase blood flow to the heel or fingers before the procedure if necessary. The capillary puncture is done using the fingers on children and adults and the heel on infants.

## Microcollection Equipment

To perform a capillary puncture, you must use a sterile disposable puncture device to pierce the skin and obtain drops of blood for testing. These devices are designed to control depth of puncture and have a spring-loaded point or blade to reduce accidental sharps injuries. Manufacturers offer puncture devices in a range of lengths and depths to facilitate varying puncture situations and sample requirements. Figure 41-9A–C shows several types of puncture devices used for microcollection.

After the capillary puncture, the blood must be collected in a microhematocrit tube or container. Microhematocrit tubes are narrow glass or plastic disposable capillary tubes used for hematocrit determinations. The tubes may be plain or coated with the anticoagulant heparin and fill by capillary action, holding 50 to 75 mL of blood. Plain tubes have a blue band on one end of the capillary tube, and ammonium tubes have a red band. A plastic or clay sealant is used to close one end of the tube (Fig. 41-10).

Microcontainers are small plastic tubes with color-coded stoppers that indicate the additive. The color coding is the same as that for the tubes used in venipuncture, but the microcontainer contains no vacuum to remove the blood from the patient. Samples for light-sensitive

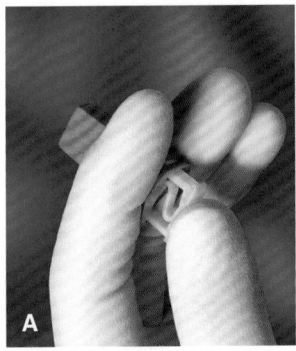
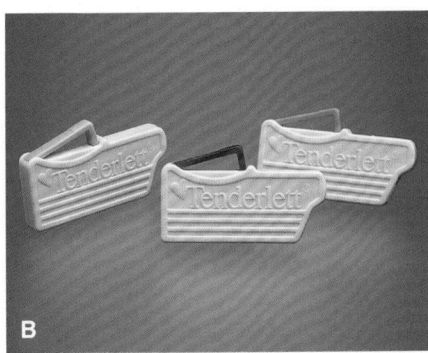
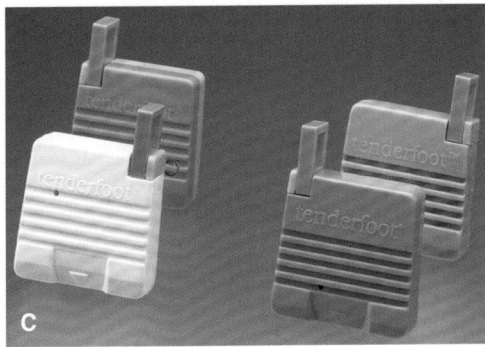

**Figure 41-9** • Several types of finger and heel puncture lancets. **(A)** Vacutainer Genie lancets. (Courtesy of Becton-Dickinson, Franklin Lakes, NJ.) **(B)** Tenderlett toddler, junior, and adult lancet devices. (Courtesy of ITC, Edison, NJ.) **(C)** Tenderfoot toddler, newborn, preemie, and micropreemie heel incision devices. (Courtesy of ITC, Edison, NJ.)

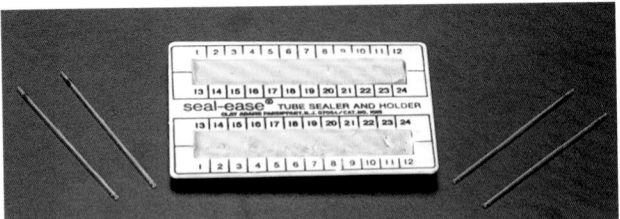

**Figure 41-10** • Microcollection tubes and clay sealant.

analytes, such as bilirubin, are collected in amber-colored plastic tubes that protect the blood from light exposure. Microcontainers are filled by blood droplets from a capillary puncture.

Microcollection may also be accomplished using filter paper attached to a test requisition. Filter paper is a special paper product made to be thick and absorbent. It is used to collect blood specimens to test newborns for genetic defects, such as hypothyroidism and phenylketonuria. The filter paper is printed with circles that must be filled with blood. Figure 41-11A, B shows an example of how the requisition and attached filter paper could look. The lateral surface of the newborn's heel is punctured and the blood droplet is absorbed into individual circles on a filter paper card. A large drop of blood must be applied from one side of the paper, and the blood must soak through to the other side. The specimen should air-dry in a horizontal position and not be stacked with other collection requisitions.

Applying heat to the fingers or heel in an infant before a capillary puncture increases blood flow to the area, allowing for an adequate blood sample. Warming devices such as a heel warmer (Fig. 41-12) may be used to increase blood flow before the skin is punctured. Heel-warming devices provide a temperature not exceeding 42°C and are used exclusively on newborns before a heel capillary puncture. Adults may wash their hands in warm water or rub the hands together vigorously, or you may apply a warm compress to the fingers if needed to obtain an adequate blood sample.

## CHECKPOINT QUESTION

10. Why are capillary punctures performed instead of venipuncture?

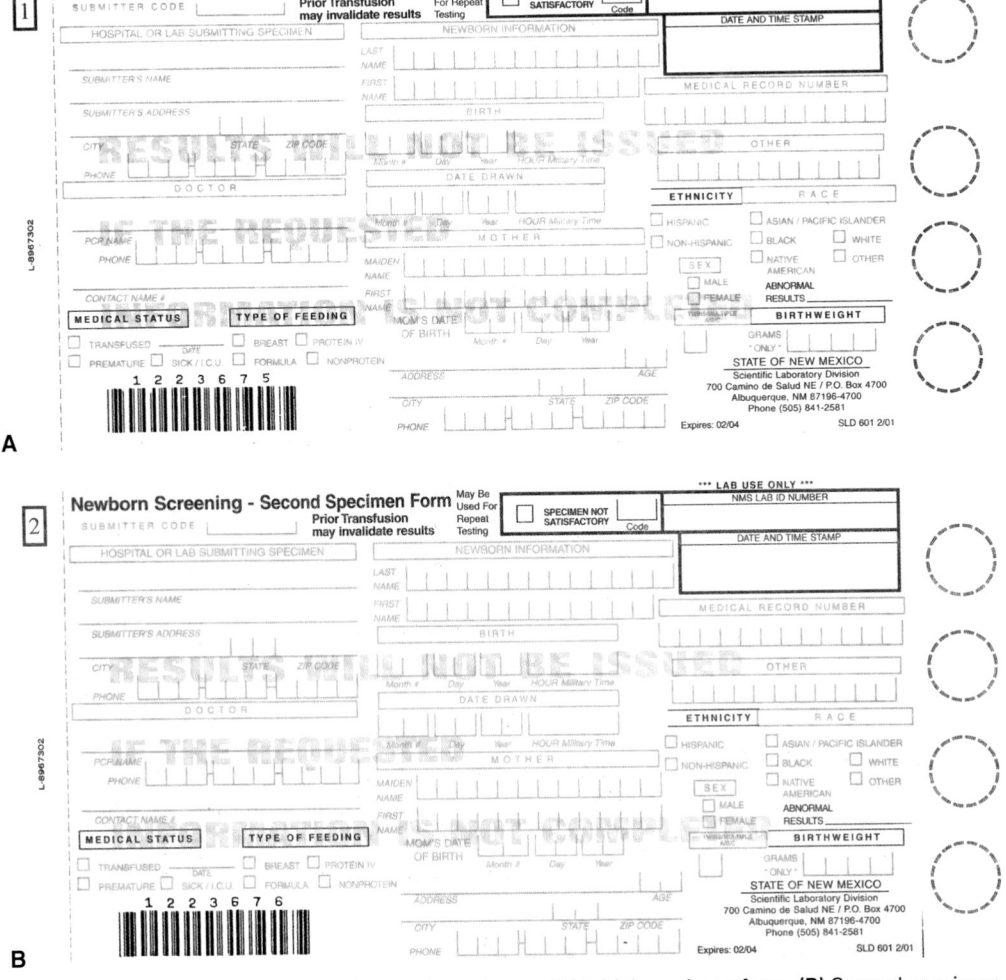

**Figure 41-11** • Newborn screening specimen forms. **(A)** Initial specimen form. **(B)** Second specimen form. (Courtesy of Daniel Gray, State of New Mexico Scientific Laboratory, Albuquerque, NM.)

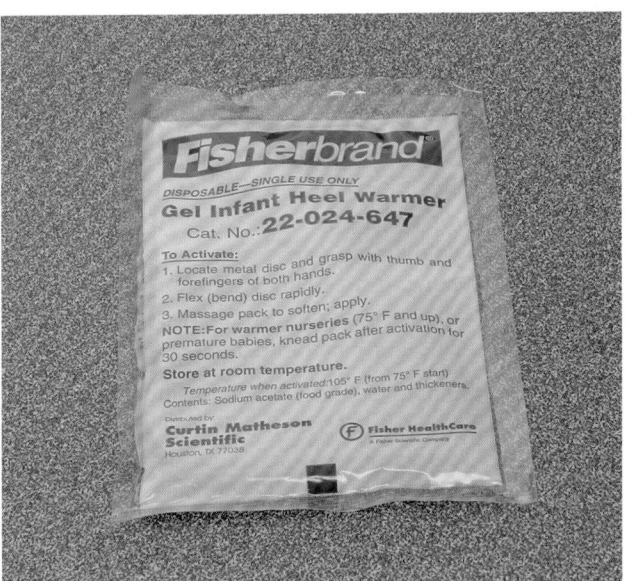

Figure 41-12 • Infant heel warmer. (Reprinted from McCall R. *Phlebotomy Essentials*. Baltimore, MD: Lippincott Williams & Wilkins, 2007, with permission.)

## Selection of the Capillary Puncture Site

The location of the capillary puncture must be carefully considered in addition to the patient's age, accessibility of acceptable sites, and the tests ordered. Skin puncture in adults and older children most often involves one of the fingers. Recommended sites are the fleshy pad of the third or fourth finger of the patient's nondominant hand only and it is best to have the hand below the heart during the puncture. Do not use the tip of the finger or the center of the finger. Avoid the side of the finger where there is less soft tissue, where vessels and nerves are located, and where the bone is closer to the surface.

For infant heel punctures in children under age 1 year, the CLSI set the standard of a maximum of 2.0 mm for heel punctures to avoid hitting bone. Because the thickness of the tissue on the side of an infant's heel can be as little as 2.0 mm and as little as 1.0 mm at the positive curvature of the heel, heel punctures on infants must never be performed on the back of the heel. If performed on the side of the heel, they must be no deeper than 2.0 mm. Prewarming the infant's heel (42°C for 3 to 5 minutes) increases the flow of blood for collection of heel punctures. Monitor the warming temperature to avoid burns to infants' thin skin.

Specific sites not recommended for capillary puncture include the following:

- Bruised, infected, swollen, or traumatized sites on fingers or heels
- The thumb because the skin is often too thick and difficult to puncture
- The second or index finger because it is much more sensitive than other fingers
- The fifth finger or pinky because the flesh may be so thin that the bone could be pierced

The complete procedure for performing a skin puncture is outlined in Procedure 41-2.

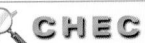

### CHECKPOINT QUESTION

11. Why must heel punctures on infants never be performed on the back of the heel?

## Performance of a Capillary Puncture

The introductory steps on the capillary collection process are the same as those for the venipuncture. Always start the procedure with clean hands, identify the patient, and verify the physician order. Use an antiseptic such as alcohol to cleanse the area in a circular motion, beginning at the site and working outward. Allow the cleansed site to air-dry; do not blow on the site or wave the air with the hand above the site. The puncture should be made perpendicular to the ridges of the fingerprint so that the drop of blood does not run down the ridges. Making the puncture perpendicular to the ridges of the fingerprint also prevents the pain of using that finger for touch. A puncture that is made horizontal with the ridges of the fingerprint causes that finger to feel like it has a paper cut when used later. Wipe away the first drop of blood, which tends to contain excess tissue fluid. Explaining this to the patient reduces surprise on seeing the first drop of blood "wasted." After obtaining the blood, apply pressure to the site with a sterile gauze as you would do for a venipuncture.

If microhematocrit tubes are used for the collection, put them inside a plain red-top tube and label the tube or process the blood as appropriate for a CLIA-waived microhematocrit test. If a microcontainer is used, write the information on a label and wrap it around the tube before processing to send to a reference laboratory for testing. Recheck the puncture site to verify that bleeding has stopped. Provide an adhesive bandage if necessary.

### Complications of Capillary Puncture

Obtaining a specimen before the blood begins clotting may be a challenge in performing a capillary puncture. The capillary puncture activates the body's clotting system to stop the bleeding as soon as the skin is punctured. If an anticoagulated specimen is required, it should be drawn first to get an adequate volume before the blood begins to clot. Any other additive specimens are collected next, and clotted specimens are collected last. If the blood has begun to produce microscopic clots while filling the last tube, this is not a problem because clotting is required in this tube.

Avoid excessive squeezing of the fingertip or heel because the RBCs will rupture and contaminate the specimen. If excessive squeezing is required because of inadequate blood flow, discontinue the puncture, choose another site, and warm the site prior to the puncture.

---

**BOX 41-3** **Sources of Error in Skin Puncture**

- Misidentification of patient
- Puncturing wrong area of infant heel
- Puncturing bone in infant heel
- Puncturing fingers of infants
- Puncturing wrong area of adult finger
- Contaminating specimen with alcohol or Betadine™
- Failure to discard first blood drop
- Excessive massaging of puncture site
- Collecting air bubbles in pH or blood gas specimen
- Hemolyzing specimen
- Failure to seal specimens adequately
- Failure to chill specimens requiring refrigeration
- Erroneous specimen labeling
- Failure to document skin puncture collection on the requisition or in the computer
- Failure to warm site
- Delaying specimen transport
- Bruising site as a result of excessive squeezing

---

Box 41-3 lists common sources of errors in microcollection that should be avoided.

### CHECKPOINT QUESTION

12. Why must anticoagulated specimens be drawn first when performing a capillary puncture?

 ## QUALITY CONTROL AND SAFETY IN BLOOD COLLECTION PROCEDURES

Many factors must be addressed to ensure specimen quality when performing venipuncture or capillary punctures. Quality control consists of methods practiced in every capillary puncture or venipuncture to optimize the quality of each specimen. Quality control begins with a thorough specimen collection manual that specifies the instructions for collecting every type of specimen. These methods include:

- Patient identification and preparation including noting the use of medications that increase bleeding times (i.e., anticoagulants and aspirin or products that contain aspirin)
- Selection of the venipuncture or capillary puncture site
- Type of collection and amount of specimen to be collected
- Need for special timing for collection
- Types and amounts of preservatives and anticoagulants
- Patient posture

- Duration of tourniquet use
- Actual time of specimen collection
- Choosing the correct equipment
- Order of draw
- Need for special handling between time of collection and time received by the laboratory (e.g., refrigeration, protection from light)
- Specimen labeling
- Accurate specimen processing, storage, and transport procedures when sending to a reference laboratory
- Needed clinical data when indicated

Because blood collection procedures involve working with potentially infectious body fluids, you should always follow OSHA standards to protect yourself, your patient, and others who could come into contact with the infectious substances. To protect yourself, you should practice standard precautions, use safety devices appropriately, dispose of needles immediately into a sharps biohazard container, disinfect work surfaces according to office policy and procedure, clean up any blood spills immediately with a commercial disinfectant or a 10% bleach solution, and take immediate action in case of an accidental needlestick with a contaminated needle. If stuck with a contaminated needle, most office policies include the following steps:

1. Remove gloves and allow the site to bleed for several minutes.
2. Wash the area well with soap and water.
3. Notify the office manager, clinical supervisor, or physician.
4. Follow the institution's guidelines regarding follow-up blood collection from the patient whose blood was involved in the accident, document the incident appropriately, and obtain treatment and follow-up care as directed.

Protect patients by placing blood collection equipment away from areas where patients will be left unattended, wear gloves during the procedure and dispose of them properly after each procedure, and wash your hands after removing gloves. For blood spills that may occur if an evacuation tube or microcollection container breaks, wear disposable gloves of sufficient sturdiness so they will not tear while cleaning. If the gloves develop holes, tears, or splits, remove them, wash your hands immediately, and put on fresh gloves. Disposable gloves must never be washed or reused. Although commercially prepared biohazard spill kits are available, the following items may be available in the office to clean up a blood spill:

- A copy of the biohazardous spill cleanup instructions, which may also be found in the office policy and procedure manual
- Nitrile disposable gloves
- Biohazard waste bags
- Absorbent material, such as absorbent paper towels or granular absorbent material
- All-purpose disinfectant such as normal household bleach (diluted 1:10)

## LEGAL TIP

### Assess the Risk of Phlebotomy Liability

To reduce a laboratory's exposure to phlebotomy liability, address the following issues in your policy manual, in your new employee training program, and in your employee competency assessments.

- Put the proper information on every tube of blood, including the time and date of collection and the phlebotomist's initials.
- Note that phlebotomy textbooks set a range between 15 degrees and 30 degrees for the angle of needle insertion.
- Require adherence to facility protocol regardless of an employee's experience.
- Perform regular competency evaluations on all phlebotomy staff members.
- In vein selection, the vein of choice is the medial vein, which typically lies in a depression in the center of the antecubital area. It is the vein of choice because it is usually larger, more stationary, closer to the surface of the skin, and more isolated from other underlying structures than the other veins.
- The error considered most critical for a medical office is misidentifying a patient. Avoiding this risk requires strict adherence to the facility's patient identification policy.

## ROLE-PLAYING ACTIVITY

Role-play these scenarios as if you are working with Tom Carlisle who works in the busy family practice at Great Falls Medical Center (refer to the case study at the beginning of the chapter). Today, Tom must obtain a blood specimen from a 19-year-old patient who has never had a venipuncture performed. The patient is very nervous and is criticizing all aspects of the procedure including the application of the tourniquet, complaining that it is "too tight." How would you respond to this patient? What if you are not successful on your first attempt to obtain a blood specimen? Your instructor will give you additional information about this activity!

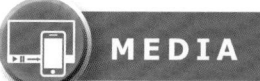

## *español* SPANISH TERMINOLOGY

**Le voy a tomar una muestra de sangre de su brazo.**
I will be drawing blood from your arm.

**¿Cuándo fue la última vez que se comió o tomó algo?**
When did you last eat or drink anything?

**Gracias**
Thank you

**Le voy a pinchar el dedo.**
I will be sticking your finger.

**¿Es alérgica (o) al latex?**
Are you allergic to latex?

**Puede poner hielo en una toalla sobre el sitio de la inyección.**
You can put some ice in a towel over the injection site.

**Si se siente mareado (a) por favor dígamelo.**
If you feel dizzy, please let me know.

## MEDIA MENU

**Student Resources** on thePoint®
- *Animation:* Intramuscular Injection
- *Animation:* Intravenous Injection
- *Video:* Obtaining a Blood Specimen by Evacuated Tube or Winged Infusion Set (Procedure 41-1)
- Video: Obtaining a Blood Specimen by Capillary Puncture (Procedure 41-2)
- CMA/RMA Certification Exam Review
- English to Spanish Audio Glossary

**Internet Resources**
**The University of Utah Eccles Health Sciences Library**
http://library.med.utah.edu/WebPath/TUTORIAL/PHLEB/PHLEB.html

**Centers for Disease Control and Prevention Health Care Associated Infections**
www.cdc.gov

**Occupational Safety and Health Administration— Disposal of Contaminated Needles and Blood Tube Holders Used for Phlebotomy**
https://www.osha.gov/dts/shib/shib101503.html

## EMR Activity

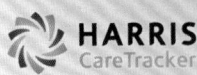

Harris CareTracker is a web-based electronic medical record (EMR) application that you will use for the EMR activities included in this section at the end of each chapter. This application is actually used in physician offices, but is provided to you through the publisher, Wolters Kluwer Health, to give you hands-on practice working with EMRs. Your instructor will have more information about accessing your username, login, and Quickstart guide.

Prerequisite Activities in Harris CareTracker

- *The Getting Started and Quickstart documents and EMR Activities Step-by-Step Instructions are available at* http://thePoint.lww.com/KronenbergerComp5e

Activity Details

Accurately document the following blood collection procedures in the EMR for the following patients:

1. Amanda Panci: Blood collected via venipuncture (right anterior forearm, antecubital space) and sent to Great Falls Medical Center laboratory for a complete blood count with differential.
2. Penelope Wringer: Capillary stick (left ring finger) and POC hemoglobin determined.

## Chapter Summary

Although blood collection procedures such as phlebotomy may be performed to treat diseases such as polycythemia vera or hemochromatosis, most blood collected in the physician office is used for testing or diagnostic purposes. This chapter included some of the following important points:

- The forearm veins (cephalic, median cubital, and basilica) in the antecubital space (the inside of the elbow) are commonly used for venipuncture.
- Avoid using areas for blood collection that have burns or scars, hematoma or bruising, thrombosed veins, edematous tissue, and the upper extremity on the side of a previous mastectomy or arteriovenous shunt used for renal dialysis.
- Skin puncture in adults and older children most often involves one of the fingers. Recommended sites are the fleshy pad of the third or fourth finger of the patient's nondominant hand only. Do not use the tip or the center of the finger. For infant heel punctures in children under age 1 year, the maximum of 2 mm for heel punctures is necessary to avoid hitting bone.
- Because the first step in quality of any laboratory test result is in the procurement of the specimen, quality assurance is critical in specimen collection procedures.
- Maintain a professional attitude and be sympathetic to the fears and anxieties of the patient in all areas of patient care. For many patients, venipuncture and capillary puncture are particularly frightening. Demonstrate compassion and understanding to allay their fears.

## Warm-Ups for Critical Thinking

1. What effects do hemoconcentration and hemolysis of the specimen have in test results?
2. Your patient complains of serious pain when you insert the needle into the vein. Explain the steps to improve the patient's comfort.
3. How can you help ease patient anxiety about venipuncture? List the steps to take.
4. Your patient asks you how long you have been drawing blood and whether you are "good." How do you respond? Justify your response.
5. Describe the steps you would take if you started a venipuncture and got no specimen in the tube. Explain how each step could result in a successful blood collection.
6. Your patient has come from the doctor with an order for you to draw and refer a specimen for HIV testing. The patient knows the doctor has specifically ordered a test for HIV. The patient wants to discuss with you all the questions she has about HIV testing. You are in a room with other medical assistants. What do you say to your patient?
7. Serious risk is created when specimens are poured from one collection tube to another. Describe these risks and how they are created.

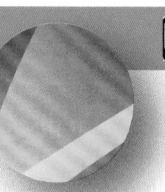  **PSY** PROCEDURE 41-1

## Obtaining a Blood Specimen by Evacuated Tube or Winged Infusion Set

**PSY** Perform venipuncture; instruct and prepare a patient for a procedure or treatment; coach patients appropriately considering cultural diversity, developmental life stage, and communication barriers; document patient care accurately in the medical record.

**Purpose:** To obtain blood for diagnostic purposes and/or monitoring of prescribed treatment.

**Equipment:** Multisample needle and adaptor or winged infusion set, evacuated tubes, tourniquet, sterile gauze pads, bandages, sharps container, 70% alcohol pad, permanent marker or pen, appropriate PPE (e.g., gloves, impervious gown, face shield)

| STEPS | REASONS |
|---|---|
| 1. Check the physician order and complete the requisition slip if appropriate. | This ensures proper specimen collection. |
| 2. Wash your hands and assemble the equipment. | Hand washing aids infection control. |
| 3. Check the expiration date on the tubes. Discard expired supplies according to office policy and procedure. | Assembling the equipment ensures that everything you need is available. Expired evacuation tubes may not have an adequate vacuum. |
| 4. **AFF** Greet and identify the patient and yourself including your title. Explain the procedure. | Identifying the patient maintains sample integrity. Explaining the procedure helps ease anxiety and ensure compliance. |
| 5. **AFF** Explain how you would respond to a patient who is visually impaired or blind. | A visually impaired patient cannot see actions taken to prepare for a phlebotomy procedure. Talking through each step builds the patient's confidence level by keeping him or her informed of what you are doing and why. |
| 6. Ask the patient about any dietary restrictions and the use of medications that increase bleeding time. If a fasting or NPO specimen is required, ask the patient for the last time he or she ate or drank anything. | For fasting specimens, the patient should not have eaten or consumed fluids other than water within at least the last 8 hours. Blood tests that require the patient to be NPO require the patient not to have consumed food or liquids for at least 8 hours or according to the test being performed. Medications such as anticoagulants and aspirin or aspirin-containing products will cause increased bleeding times and you can expect to apply pressure to the site for an extended amount of time. |
| 7. Apply nonsterile latex or vinyl gloves. | Standard precautions protect the phlebotomist and the patient. |

## PROCEDURE 41-1 (continued)

| STEPS | REASONS |
|---|---|
| 8. *For evacuated tube collection*: Break the seal of the needle cover and thread the sleeved needle into the adaptor, using the needle cover as a wrench. *For winged infusion set collection*: Extend the tubing. Thread the sleeved needle into the adaptor. *For both methods*: Tap the tubes that contain additives to ensure that the additive is dislodged from the stopper and wall of the tube. Insert the tube into the adaptor until the needle slightly enters the stopper. Do not push the top of the tube stopper beyond the indentation mark. If the tube retracts slightly, leave it in the retracted position. | This ensures proper needle placement and tube positioning and prevents loss of vacuum in the evacuated tubes. |
| 9. Instruct the patient to sit with the arms well supported. | Veins in the antecubital fossa are most easily located when the arm is straight and supported on a surface. |
| 10. After reviewing veins in both arms, choose one arm and apply the tourniquet 3 to 4 inches above the elbow. | The tourniquet makes the veins more prominent. |

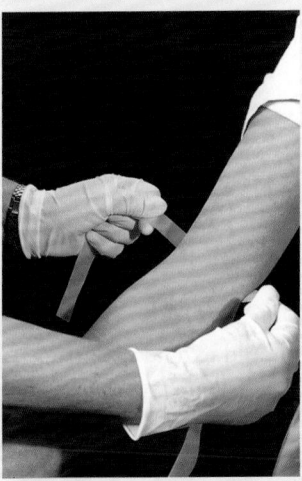

**A.** Apply the tourniquet snugly, but not too tightly.

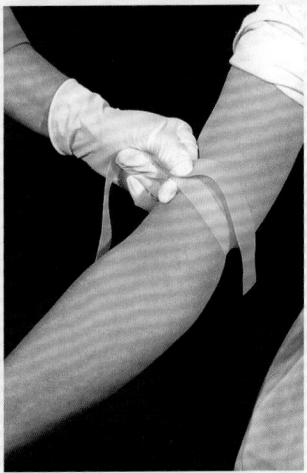

**Step 10.** Apply the tourniquet 3 to 4 inches above the elbow.

**Step 10A.** Apply the tourniquet snugly, but not tightly.

*(continues on page 1080)*

## PROCEDURE 41-1 (continued)

| STEPS | REASONS |
|---|---|

**B.** Secure the tourniquet by using the half-bow knot.

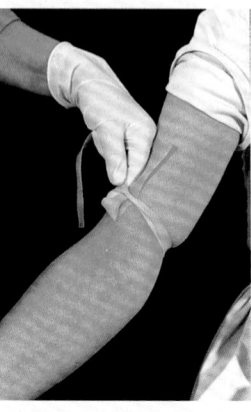

Step 10B. Secure the tourniquet by using a half-bow knot.

**C.** Make sure the tails of the tourniquet extend upward to avoid contaminating the puncture site.

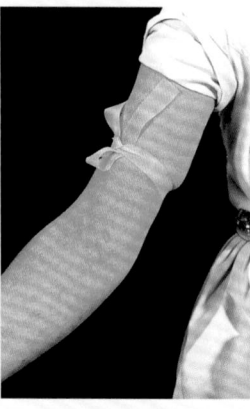

Step 10C. The tourniquet should extend upward.

**D.** Ask the patient to make a fist and hold it but not to pump the fist.

Making a fist raises the vessels out of the underlying tissues and muscles.

**11.** Select a vein by palpating the area with your gloved index finger to trace the path of the vein and judge its depth.

The index finger is the most sensitive for palpating.

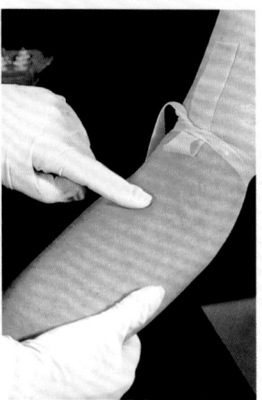

Step 11. Trace the path of the vein.

**12.** Release the tourniquet after palpating the vein if it has been left on for more than 1 minute. Have the patient release the fist.

The tourniquet should not be left on for more than 1 minute at a time during the procedure.

## PROCEDURE 41-1 (continued)

| STEPS | REASONS |
|---|---|
| **13.** Cleanse the venipuncture site with an alcohol pad, starting in the center of the puncture site working outward in a circular motion. Allow the site to dry, or dry the site with sterile gauze. Do not touch the area after cleansing. | The circular motion helps avoid recontamination of the area. Puncturing a wet area stings and can cause hemolysis of the sample. |
| **14.** If blood is being drawn for a blood culture, make sure the area is cleansed using a 2% iodine solution for 2 full minutes. | Ensuring sterility of the specimen will add in accurate identification of the pathogen, if present. |
| **15.** Reapply the tourniquet if it was removed after palpation. Ask the patient to make a fist. | Tourniquet time greater than 1 minute may alter test results. |
| **16.** Remove the needle cover. Hold the needle assembly in your dominant hand, with your thumb on top of the adaptor and your fingers under it. Grasp the patient's arm with the other hand, using your thumb to draw the skin taut over the site. This anchors the vein about 1 to 2 inches below the puncture site and helps keep it in place during needle insertion. | Anchoring the vein allows easier needle penetration and less pain. |
| **17.** With the bevel up, line up the needle with the vein approximately one quarter to half an inch below the site where the vein is to be entered. At a 15-degree to 30-degree angle, rapidly and smoothly insert the needle through the skin.<br><br>   Use a lesser angle for winged infusion set collections. Place two fingers on the flanges of the adapter, and with the thumb, push the tube onto the needle inside the adapter. Allow the tube to fill to capacity. | The sharpest point of the needle is inserted first. Proper tube filling ensures correct ratio of blood to additive. Removal of the tourniquet releases pressure on the vein and helps prevent blood from seeping into adjacent tissues and causing a hematoma. |
| **18.** Release the tourniquet and allow the patient to release the fist. When blood flow ceases, remove the tube from the adapter by gripping the tube with your nondominant hand and place your thumb against the flange during removal. Twist and gently pull out the tube. Steady the needle in the vein. Avoid pulling up or pressing down on the needle while it is in the vein. Insert any other necessary tubes into adapter and allow each to fill to capacity. | |

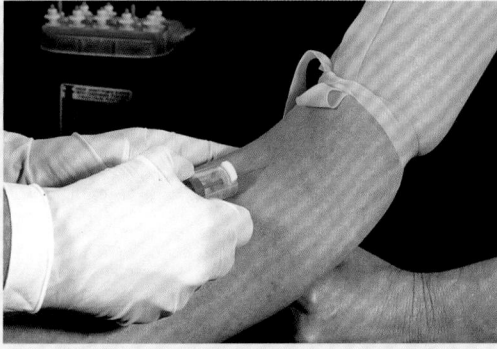

**Step 18.** Insert the needle at a 15-degree to 30-degree angle.

*(continues on page 1082)*

# PROCEDURE 41-1 (continued)

| STEPS | REASONS |
|---|---|
| 19. With the tourniquet released, remove the tube from the adapter before removing the needle from the arm. | Removing the last tube from the adapter before removing the needle from the vein prevents excess blood from dripping from the tip of the needle onto the patient. |
| 20. Place a sterile gauze pad over the puncture site. Do not apply any pressure to the site until the needle is completely removed. | Applying pressure before completely removing the needle will cause pain to the patient and most likely cause a hematoma. |

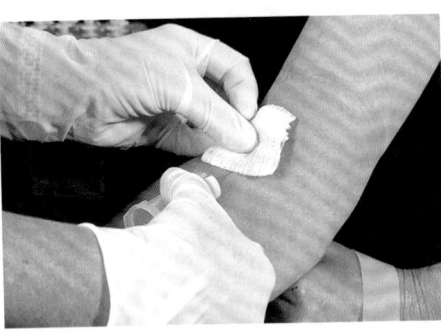

**Step 20.** Place a gauze pad over site.

21. After the needle is removed, immediately activate the safety device and apply pressure, or have the patient apply direct pressure for 3 to 5 minutes. Do not bend the arm at the elbow.

Pressure decreases the amount of blood escaping at the time of needle withdrawal. Bending the arm increases the chance of blood seeping into subcutaneous tissues. Unfolding the bent arm disturbs the clot forming at the puncture site and causes bleeding.

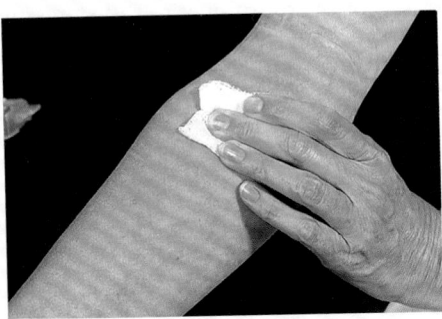

**Step 21.** Apply pressure for 3 to 5 minutes.

22. Activate needle safety device. Discard the used needle in a sharps container.

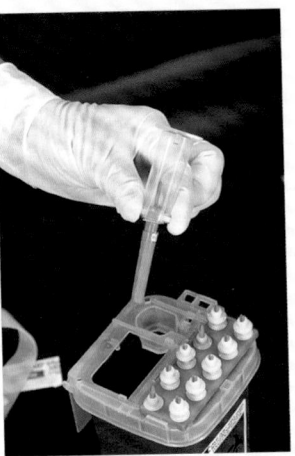

**Step 22.** Properly dispose of sharps.

PROCEDURE 41-1 (continued)

| STEPS | REASONS |
|---|---|
| 23. If the vacuum tubes contain an anticoagulant, they must be mixed immediately by gently inverting the tube 8 to 10 times. Do not shake the tube. | Mixing anticoagulated tubes prevents clotting of blood. |
| 24. Label the tubes with patient information as defined in facility protocol. | Proper labeling of blood specimens maintains accurate sample identification. |
| 25. Check the puncture site for bleeding. Apply a dressing, a clean 2 × 2 gauze pad folded in quarters, and hold in place using an adhesive bandage or 3-inch strip of tape. | |
| 26. **AFF** Thank the patient. Instruct the patient to leave the bandage in place for at least 15 minutes, not to carry a heavy object (such as a purse) or lift heavy objects with that arm for 1 hour. | Courtesy helps the patient have a positive attitude about the procedure and the physician office. |
| 27. Properly care for or dispose of all equipment and supplies. Clean the work area. Remove protective equipment and wash your hands. | Standard precautions must be followed throughout the procedure to prevent the spread of personal microorganisms. |
| 28. Test, transfer, or store the blood specimen according to the medical office policy. | |
| 29. **AFF** Log into the electronic medical record (EMR) using your username and secure password OR obtain the paper medical record from a secure location and assure it is kept away from public access. Record the procedure noting the date, time, site of the venipuncture, test results for CLIA-waived POC procedures or the name of the lab where the specimen was sent, and your name. | The integrity of the medical record must be maintained at all times to protect patient privacy. Procedures are considered not to have been performed if they are not recorded. |
| 30. When finished, log out of the EMR and/or replace the paper medical record in an appropriate and secure location. | |

Charting Example:

*05/31/2016 10:00 AM. venipuncture for platelet count per left anterior antecubital space. Specimen to Great Falls Laboratory _____ T. Carlisle, RMA*

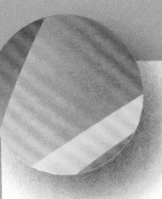 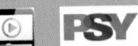 **PROCEDURE 41-2**

# Obtaining a Blood Specimen by Capillary Puncture

**PSY** Perform a capillary puncture; instruct and prepare a patient for a procedure or treatment; coach patients appropriately considering cultural diversity, developmental life stage, and communication barriers; document patient care accurately in the medical record.

**Purpose:** To obtain blood for diagnostic purposes and/or monitoring of prescribed treatment

**Equipment:** Skin puncture device, 70% alcohol pads, 2 × 2 gauze pads, microcollection tubes or containers, heel-warming device if needed, small bandages, pen or permanent marker, and PPE (e.g., gloves, impervious gown, face shield)

| STEPS | REASONS |
|---|---|
| 1. Check the physician order and complete the requisition slip if appropriate. | This ensures proper specimen collection. |
| 2. Wash your hands. | Hand washing aids infection control. |
| 3. Assemble the equipment. | Having the equipment ready will speed collection |
| 4. **AFF** Greet and identify the patient and yourself including your title. Explain the procedure. | Explaining the procedure helps ease anxiety and ensure compliance. |
| 5. **AFF** Explain how you would respond to an infant or small child. | Some children will respond well to distractions while most children become more upset the longer you drag out the procedure. Speak softly and move gently and with confidence. This will calm the child and the caregiver.<br><br>If the parent appears upset, suggest someone else such as another caregiver if present or another medical assistant hold the child while the blood is collected. The medical assistant will be more focused on positioning the child and maintaining that position than will an upset parent. |
| 6. Ask the caregiver about any dietary restrictions and the use of medications that increase bleeding time as appropriate. If a fasting or NPO specimen is required, ask the patient for the last time he or she ate or drank anything. | For fasting specimens, the patient should not have eaten or consumed fluids other than water within at least the last 8 hours. Blood tests that require the patient to be NPO require the patient not to have consumed food or liquids for at least 8 hours or according to the test being performed.<br><br>Medications such as anticoagulants and aspirin or aspirin-containing products will cause increased bleeding times and you can expect to apply pressure to the site for an extended amount of time. |
| 7. Apply nonsterile latex or vinyl gloves. | Standard precautions protect both the phlebotomist and the patient. |

**PROCEDURE 41-2** (continued)

| STEPS | REASONS |
|---|---|
| 8. Select the puncture site. The puncture should be made in the fleshy central portion of the second or third finger, slightly to the side of center and perpendicular to the grooves of the fingerprint. | The puncture should be made in the fleshy central portion of the second or third finger, slightly to the side of center and perpendicular to the grooves of the fingerprint. |

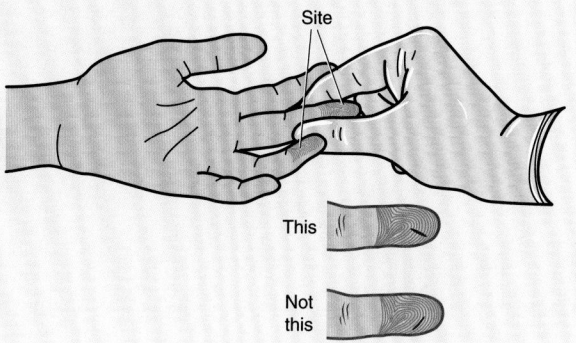

(continues on page 1086)

**Step 8A.** Recommended site and direction of finger puncture. (Reprinted from McCall R. *Phlebotomy Essentials*. Baltimore, MD: Lippincott Williams & Wilkins, 2003, with permission.)

Perform heel puncture only on the plantar surface of the heel, medial to an imaginary line extending from the middle of the great toe to the heel and lateral to an imaginary line drawn from between the fourth and fifth toes to the heel. Use the appropriate puncture device for the site selected.

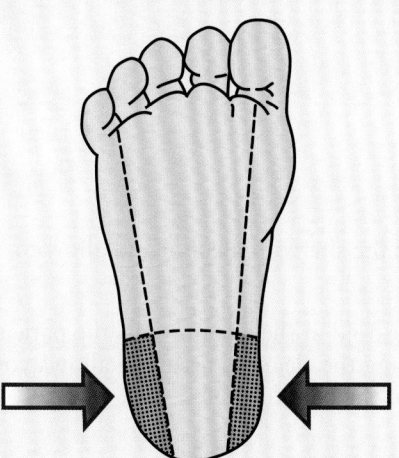

**Step 8B.** Acceptable areas for heel punctures on newborns. (Reprinted from McCall R. *Phlebotomy Essentials*. Baltimore, MD: Lippincott Williams & Wilkins, 2003, with permission.)

9. Make sure the site chosen is warm and not cyanotic or edematous. Gently massage the finger from the base to the tip, or massage the infant's heel.

Massaging the area increases the blood flow. Good circulation at the chosen site yields a better blood sample for analysis.

## PROCEDURE 41-2 (continued)

| STEPS | REASONS |
|---|---|
| 10. Grasp the finger firmly between your nondominant index finger and thumb, or grasp the infant's heel firmly with your index finger wrapped around the foot and your thumb wrapped around the ankle. | The area must be dry to eliminate alcohol residue, which can cause the patient discomfort and interfere with test results. |

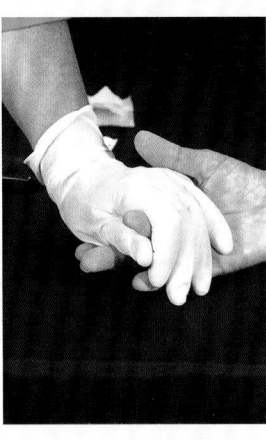 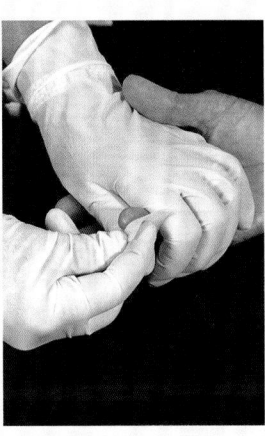

**Step 10A.** Grasp the finger firmly.

Cleanse the selected area with 70% isopropyl alcohol and allow to air-dry.

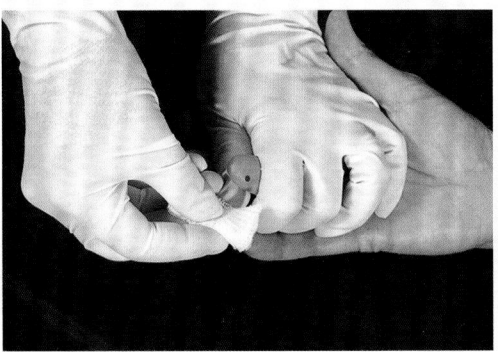

**Step 10B.** Cleanse the site with alcohol and allow to air-dry.

11. Hold the patient's finger or heel firmly and make a swift, firm puncture. Perform the puncture perpendicular to the whorls of the fingerprint or footprint. Dispose of the used puncture device in a sharps container.

Maintaining your hold at the site prevents the patient from contaminating the cleansed area and allows you to have control of the puncture site.

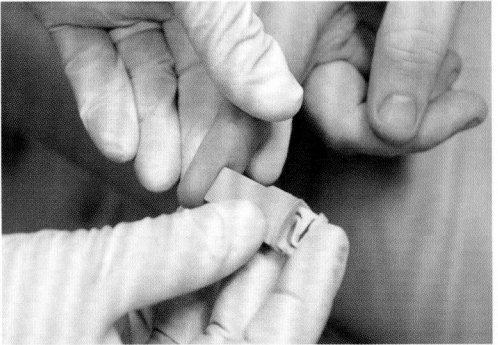

**Step 11.** Hold the patient's finger or heel firmly and make a swift, firm puncture.

# PROCEDURE 41-2 (continued)

| STEPS | REASONS |
|---|---|
| **12.** Obtain the first drop of blood and wipe it away with dry gauze. Apply pressure toward the site but do not milk the site. | The first discarded drop may be contaminated with tissue fluid or alcohol residue. Milking the site will dilute the specimen with tissue fluid. |

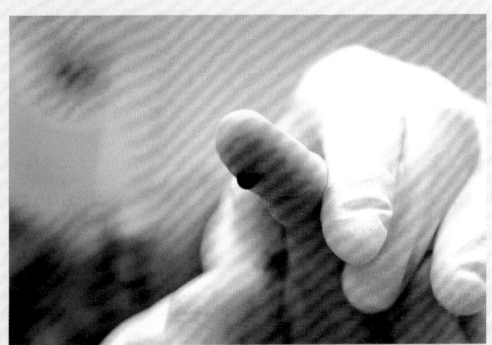

A

**Step 12A.** Obtain the first drop of blood.

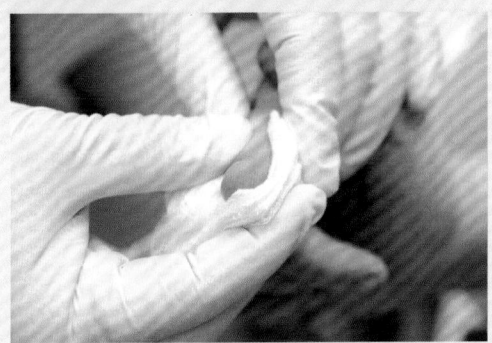

B

**Step 12B.** Wipe it away.

| STEPS | REASONS |
|---|---|
| **13.** Collect the specimen in the chosen container or on a slide. Touch only the tip of the collection device to the drop of blood. Blood flow is encouraged if the puncture site is held downward and gentle pressure is applied near the site. Cap microcollection tubes with the caps provided and mix the additives by gently tilting or inverting the tubes 8 to 10 times. | Scraping the collection device on the skin activates platelets and may cause hemolysis. Mixing the specimens prevents clotting. Touching the tube to the site may cause contamination. |
| **14.** When collection is complete, apply clean gauze to the site with pressure. Hold pressure or have the caregiver hold pressure until bleeding stops. Label the containers with the proper information. Do not apply a dressing to a skin puncture of an infant under age 2 years. Never release a patient until the bleeding has stopped. | Proper labeling of blood specimens maintains accurate sample identification. Younger children may develop a skin irritation from the adhesive bandage. Also, a young child may put the bandage in his or her mouth and choke. |
| **15.** Properly care for or dispose of equipment and supplies. Clean the work area. Remove gloves and wash your hands. | Standard precautions protect the phlebotomist and the patient. |
| **16.** Test, transfer, or store the specimen according to the medical office policy. | Specimens require immediate attention. |

*(continues on page 1088)*

## PROCEDURE 41-2 (continued)

| STEPS | REASONS |
|---|---|
| 17. **AFF** Log into the electronic medical record (EMR) using your username and secure password OR obtain the paper medical record from a secure location and assure it is kept away from public access. Record the procedure noting the date, time, site of the capillary puncture, test results for CLIA-waived POC procedures or the name of the lab where the specimen was sent, and your name. | The integrity of the medical record must be maintained at all times to protect patient privacy. |
| 18. When finished, log out of the EMR and/or replace the paper medical record in an appropriate and secure location. | Procedures are considered not to have been done if they are not recorded. |

Charting Example:

*07/12/2016 9:00 AM fingerstick for hemoglobin. Results in chart* _____ *T. Carlisle, RMA*

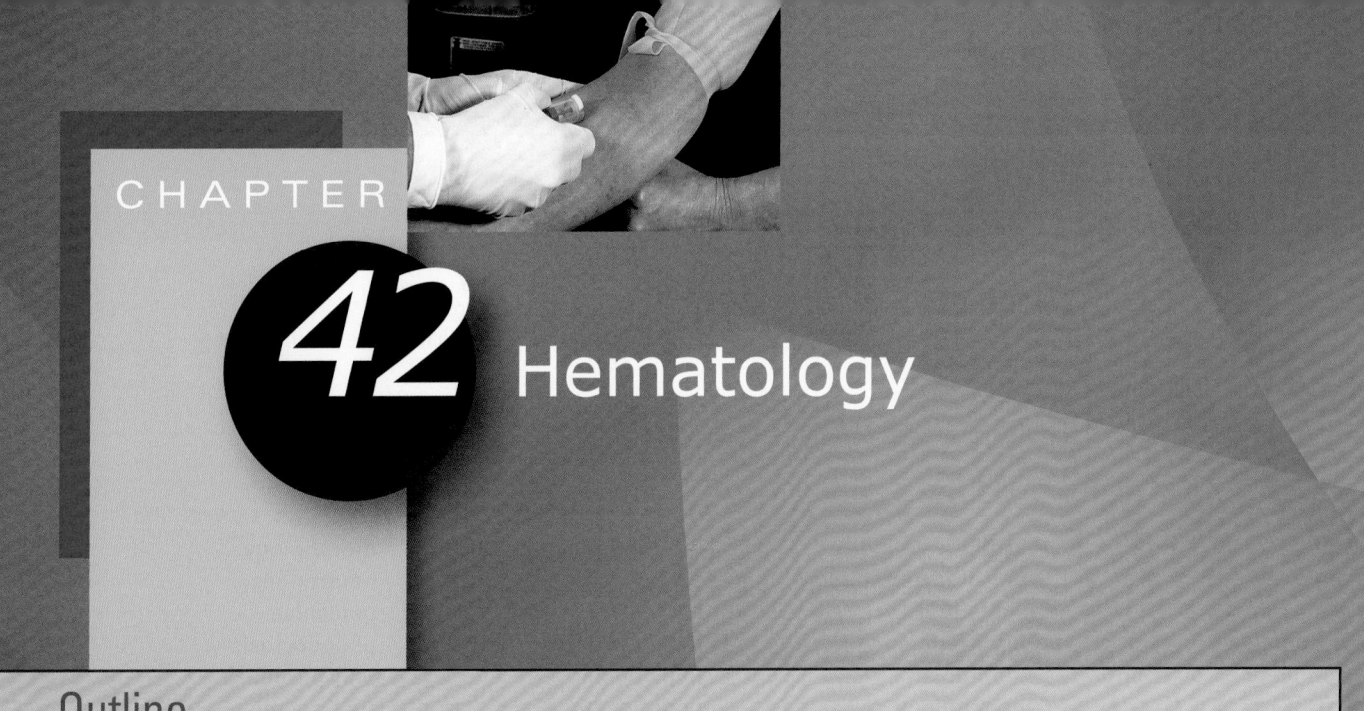

# CHAPTER

# 42 Hematology

## Learning Outcomes

### COG Cognitive Domain*

1. Spell key terms
2. *Define medical terms and abbreviations related to all body systems*
3. List the parameters measured in the complete blood count and their normal ranges
4. State the conditions associated with selected abnormal complete blood count findings
5. Explain the functions of the three types of blood cells
6. Discuss the purpose of testing for the erythrocyte sedimentation rate
7. List the leukocytes seen normally in the blood and the functions of each
8. *Analyze charts, graphs, and/or tables in the interpretation of health care results*

### PSY Psychomotor Domain*

1. Perform hemoglobin determination (Procedure 42-1)
   a. *Perform CLIA-waived hematology testing*
   b. *Instruct and prepare a patient for a procedure or treatment*
   c. *Coach patients appropriately considering cultural diversity, developmental life stage, and communication barriers*
   d. *Document patient care accurately in the medical record*
2. Perform microhematocrit determination (Procedure 42-2)
   a. *Perform CLIA-waived hematology testing*
   b. *Instruct and prepare a patient for a procedure or treatment*

   c. *Coach patients appropriately considering cultural diversity, developmental life stage, and communication barriers*
   d. *Document patient care accurately in the medical record*

### AFF Affective Domain*

1. *Incorporate critical thinking skills when performing patient assessment*
2. *Incorporate critical thinking skills when performing patient care*
3. *Show awareness of a patient's concerns related to the procedure being performed*
4. *Demonstrate empathy, active listening, and nonverbal communication*
5. *Demonstrate respect for individual diversity including gender, race, religion, age, economic status, and appearance*
6. *Explain to a patient the rationale for performance of a procedure*
7. *Demonstrate sensitivity to patient rights*
8. *Protect the integrity of the medical record*
9. *Distinguish between normal and abnormal test results*

**\*Note: AAMA/CAAHEP 2015 Standards are italicized.**

### ABHES Competencies

1. Apply principles of aseptic techniques and infection control
2. Collect, label, and process specimens

*(continues on page 1090)*

## Learning Outcomes (continued)

3. Perform selected CLIA-waived tests that assist with diagnosis and treatment
4. Dispose of biohazardous materials
5. Use standard precautions

6. Perform hematology testing
7. Document accurately
8. Practice quality control
9. Adhere to OSHA compliance rules and regulations

## Key Terms

| | | | |
|---|---|---|---|
| antibodies | erythrocyte indices | international normalized | morphology |
| antigens | erythrocyte sedimentation | ratio | neutrophils |
| band | rate (ESR) | leukocytes | petechiae |
| basophils | erythropoietin | leukocytosis | phagocytosis |
| complete blood count | hematocrit | leukopenia | polychromasia |
| (CBC) | hematology | lymphocytes | thalassemia |
| differential | hemoglobin | macrocytosis | thrombocytes |
| eosinophils | hyperchromia | microcytosis | thrombocytopenia |
| erythrocytes | hypochromia | monocytes | thrombocytosis |

## Case Study

Marilyn Mays, CMA (AAMA), works in an oncology office in Great Falls Medical Center. Although many of the patients seen in her office have various types of cancers, the physicians in this office also see patients with disorders of the blood. The chemotherapy agents used to treat various types of cancers also affect the blood, including blood cell counts. Today, one of the patients has been diagnosed with anemia and has an appointment to recheck her hemoglobin. Another patient was referred by his family physician for a review of abnormal white blood cells. In some situations, Marilyn must send blood specimens to the reference laboratory for testing, but in others, she may perform point-of-care testing. In addition to blood cell counts, what other laboratory tests are considered hematological testing? What are the criteria for donating blood or blood products if a transfusion is needed? These and other questions are answered in this chapter.

## HEMATOLOGY

**Hematology** is the study of blood cells including **erythrocytes** (RBCs), **leukocytes** (white blood cells [WBCs]), and **thrombocytes** (platelets) (Fig. 42-1). Most blood cells are erythrocytes, or red blood cells, that include a substance called **hemoglobin** to assist mature blood cells in carrying oxygen. Leukocytes, or white blood cells, assist in the ability of the body to fight inflammation and infection. Thrombocytes, also known as platelets, assist with the ability of the blood to clot. Although

some hematology tests must be performed on whole blood in a larger reference laboratory, others may be done using CLIA-waived point-of-care testing devices in the physician office. Hematology testing is done using whole blood specimens and is collected in an evacuation tube that contains an anticoagulant. Coagulation studies are done using plasma, the yellowish liquid part of an anticoagulated blood specimen.

Common hematology tests include the **complete blood count (CBC)**, **erythrocyte sedimentation rate (ESR)**, and coagulation tests with the CBC being the

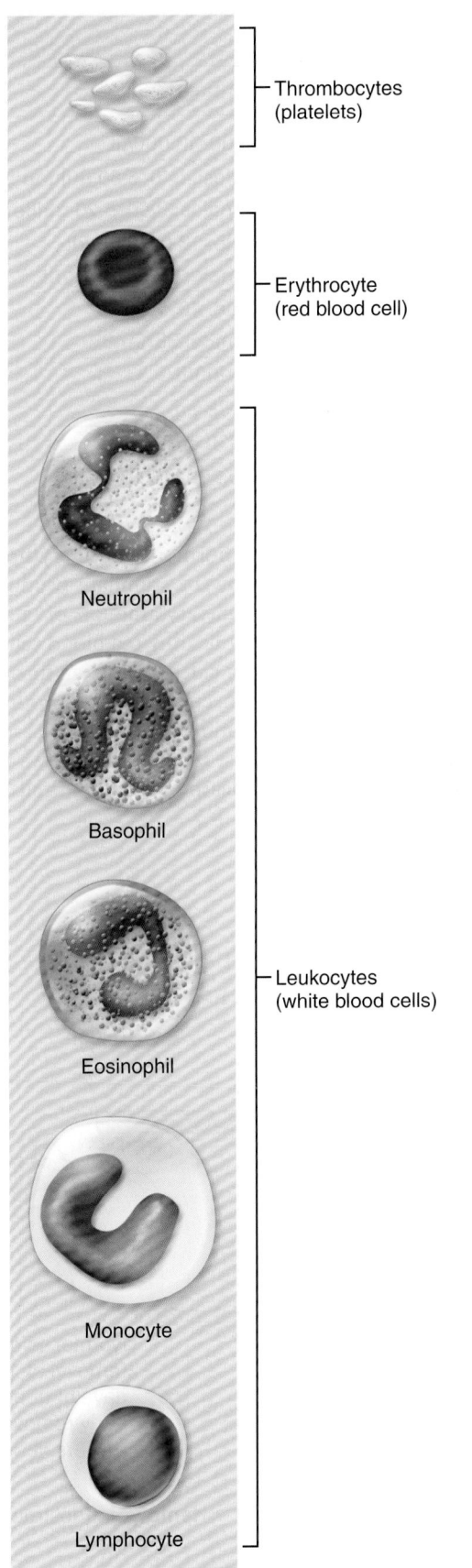

**Figure 42-1** • Formed elements of blood. Three types of cells make up the formed elements of blood: thrombocytes (platelets), erythrocytes (RBCs), and leukocytes (WBCs).

Thrombocytes (platelets)

Erythrocyte (red blood cell)

Neutrophil

Basophil

Eosinophil

Monocyte

Lymphocyte

Leukocytes (white blood cells)

---

**BOX 42-1 Automated Blood Cell Counters**

A number of biotechnology companies have instruments that can count and size blood cells. Although each has its own specific method, the main operating principles are similar.

A portion of whole blood (anticoagulated with EDTA) is taken in and diluted. These dilutions are moved into counting chambers, where they are drawn through tiny holes (apertures). As the cells pass through the holes, an electrical current, a light beam, or a laser beam is interrupted. The instrument registers the interruption as a cell. It can tell the size of the cell by the length of time the beam is interrupted or the amount of light scatter.

These instruments have become so sophisticated that a WBC differential now can be reported accurately. Hemoglobin is also measured, along with other parameters, such as mean corpuscular hemoglobin, adding to the diagnostic value of the complete blood count.

---

most frequently ordered laboratory test. The CBC consists of several parameters including

- White blood cell count
- Red blood cell count
- Hemoglobin
- Hematocrit
- Mean cell volume (MCV)
- Mean corpuscular hemoglobin (MCH)
- Mean corpuscular hemoglobin concentration (MCHC)
- Platelet count

Of course, these tests are also performed separately if the physician orders only a specific test. Box 42-1 describes automated blood cell counters found in larger reference labs and how these machines work to count blood cells. Table 42-1 is an example of a patient CBC report including patient results and the normal ranges for the various parameters included in a complete blood count. Results of laboratory tests are given in microliters (µL), deciliters (dL), or millimeters cubed (mm$^3$) depending on the test, laboratory, or equipment used to measure the test ordered. When documenting test results in the medical record, always indicate the results appropriately based on the CLIA-waived machine used or the laboratory report (Table 42-1).

### CHECKPOINT QUESTION

1. What is the function of thrombocytes?

**TABLE 42-1    Sample CBC Report**

| Analyte | Patient Result | Normal Range |
|---|---|---|
| White blood cells | 9,200/μL | 4,500–10,000/μL |
| Red blood cells | 3.9 million/mm³ | Males: 4.40–5.80 million/mm³<br>Females: 3.90–5.20 million/mm³ |
| Hemoglobin | 10.2 g/dL | Male: 13.0–18.0 g/dL<br>Female: 12.0–16.0 g/dL |
| Hematocrit | 35% | Male: 40%–50%<br>Female: 35%–46% |
| Mean cell volume (MCV) | 74/fL | 80–100/fL |
| Mean cell hemoglobin (MCH) | 23 pg | 27–32 pg |
| Mean cell hemoglobin concentration (MCHC) | 27 g/dL | 32–36 g/dL |
| Platelets | 279,000/μL | 150,000–400,000/μL |

## Erythrocytes

### The Function of Erythrocytes

Red blood cells, or RBCs, carry oxygen to tissues and organs in the body and pick up the waste product, carbon dioxide, to return to the heart and lungs. The hemoglobin in the RBCs actually carries the gases and is made up of protein. As blood filters through the kidneys, the amount of oxygen on the hemoglobin is detected, and if a low oxygen level is detected, a hormone called **erythropoietin** is sent to the bone marrow to stimulate production of red blood cells. Adequate dietary amounts of vitamin $B_{12}$ and folate are necessary for healthy red blood cells, which are curved inward on both sides to squeeze through tiny capillaries. Dietary iron is necessary for the production of hemoglobin, a protein found on RBCs that assists with carrying oxygen molecules. Figure 42-2 shows the production, circulation, and death of red blood cells.

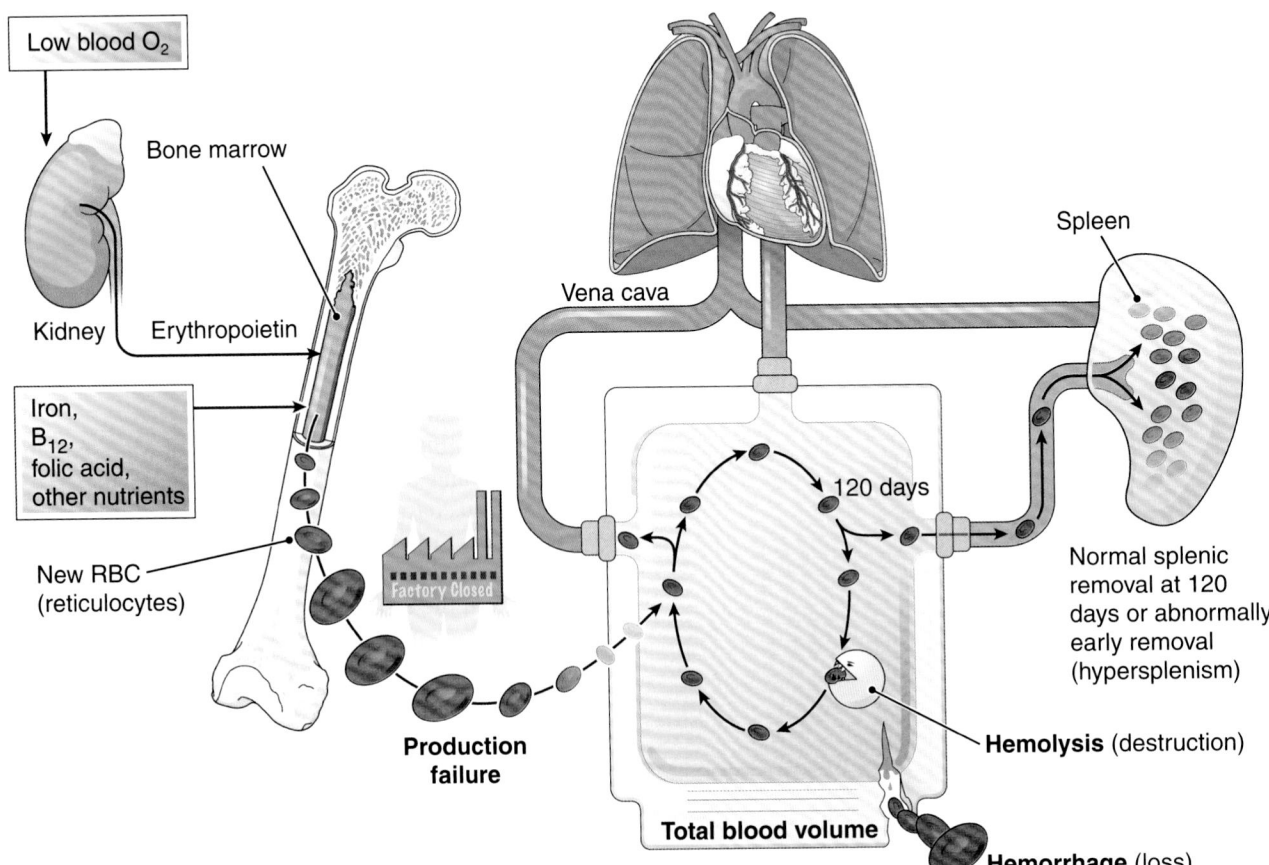

**Figure 42-2** • Production, circulation, and death of red blood cells. Every anemia is caused by at least one of three problems: (1) decreased red cell production, (2) loss of red cells by hemorrhage, or (3) early death (destruction) of red blood cells.

## Red Blood Cell Count

In the laboratory, red blood cells are counted using cell counter instruments such as those described in Box 42-1. Anemia, a condition in which there is an inadequate amount of oxygen-carrying RBCs in the blood, may have several causes including a low number of red blood cells due to blood loss from an accident or injury or destruction of RBCs due to illness or medications that affect the body's ability to produce red blood cells. The normal red blood cell count for adults differs based on gender and is generally a range, meaning a count within that range is "normal" for that gender. In males, the normal red blood cell count is 4.40 to 5.80 million per $mm^3$, and in females, it is 3.90 to 5.20 million per $mm^3$ (Table 42-1).

In some types of anemia, there are enough red blood cells but an inadequate amount of hemoglobin, preventing the red blood cells from the ability to carry oxygen. Other types of anemia may be caused by an abnormal **morphology**, or shape, of the red blood cells, also preventing them from carrying adequate amounts of oxygen. Sickle cell anemia is an example of anemia caused by an abnormally shaped red blood cell that is not able to carry oxygen because of its sickle shape. Figure 42-3 shows the appearance of a normal red blood cell and red blood cells in various forms of anemia. Table 42-2 describes some common erythrocyte abnormalities and their associated conditions. A red blood cell count that is higher than normal may also indicate disease such as polycythemia vera. This condition is treated by frequent phlebotomy or blood donations to remove the excess blood cells.

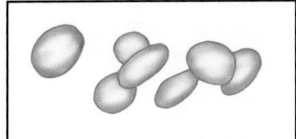
**A** Iron-deficiency anemia

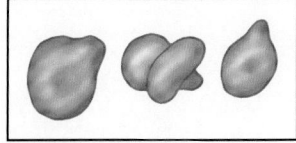
**B** Megaloblastic anemia

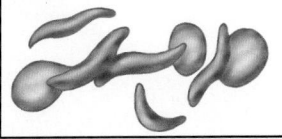
**C** Sickle cell disease

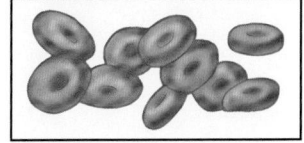
**D** Normal

**Figure 42-3** • Red cell characteristics seen in different types of anemia. **(A)** microcytic and hypochromic red cells, characteristic of iron deficiency anemia. **(B)** macrocytic and misshaped red blood cells, characteristic of megaloblastic anemia. **(C)** abnormally shaped red blood cells seen in sickle cell disease. **(D)** normocytic and normochromic red blood cells, as a comparison.

### Hemoglobin and Hematocrit

As already discussed, hemoglobin, also abbreviated Hgb, is made up of protein and includes iron consumed through the diet or by taking dietary supplements. The amount of hemoglobin found on red blood cells differs for men and women, including a normal range of 13.0 to 18.0 g/dL for men and 12.0 to 16.0 g/dL for women (Table 42-1). To measure the amount of hemoglobin in a blood specimen, you should collect the blood using an evacuated tube and send to the reference laboratory or

| TABLE 42-2 Erythrocyte Abnormalities | |
|---|---|
| **Abnormality** | **Associated Conditions** |
| **Hypochromia**—diminished hemoglobin in RBCs; appear paler with more area of central pallor | Anemias, especially iron deficiency anemia; thalassemia; hemolytic anemia |
| **Hyperchromia**—increased hemoglobin in RBCs; appear to have less or no area of central pallor | Megaloblastic anemia, characterized by large, dysfunctional RBCs, hereditary spherocytosis |
| **Polychromasia**—some RBCs have a blue color. | Hemolysis; acute blood loss |
| **Microcytosis**—RBCs are smaller than usual. | Iron deficiency anemia; thalassemia |
| **Macrocytosis**—RBCs are larger than usual. | Vitamin $B_{12}$ and folate deficiencies; megaloblastic anemias |
| **Elliptocytes/ovalocytes**—RBCs are distinctly oval in shape. | Hereditary elliptocytes, iron deficiency anemia, myelofibrosis (disorder in which bone marrow tissue develops in abnormal sites), sickle cell anemia |
| **Target cells**—RBCs resemble a target with light and dark rings. | Liver impairment, anemias, especially thalassemia and hemoglobin C disease (genetic blood disorder) |
| **Schistocytes**—RBCs are fragmented. | Hemolysis, burns, intravascular coagulation |
| **Spherocytes**—RBCs show no area of central pallor. | Hereditary spherocytosis; hemolytic anemias, burns |
| **Burr cells**—RBCs have small, regular spicules (sharp points). | Artifact as blood dries, hyperosmolarity (a condition of increased numbers of dissolved substances in the plasma) |

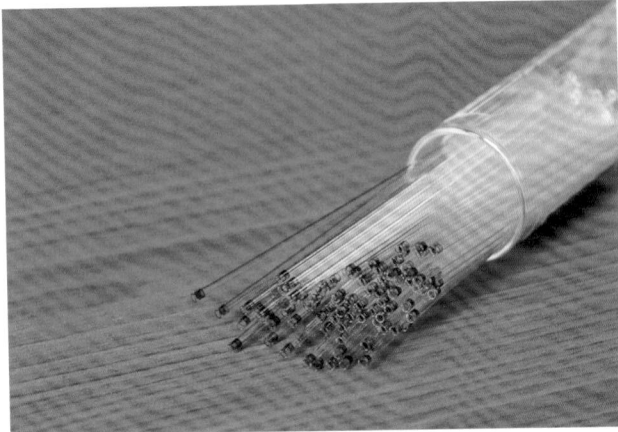

**Figure 42-4** • Microhematocrit capillary tubes.

use a CLIA-waived point-of-care machine such as the HemoCue Hb 201+ Analyzer or the Stat Site M Hgb Meter (Stanbio Laboratory).

Another test that is commonly performed along with the red blood cell count and hemoglobin to diagnose anemia is the **hematocrit**, also abbreviated Hct. This test is the *percentage* of RBCs in whole blood. This test is performed in a laboratory, or it may be done in the physician office using a microhematocrit capillary tube (Fig. 42-4) and a centrifuge such as the one shown in Figure 42-5. After collecting the specimen in the capillary tube and sealing one end of the tube with a sealant (refer to Procedure 42-2), the tube is put into the centrifuge and spun, causing the red blood cells to collect at one end of the tube and the plasma, or liquid portion, in the other end. The tube is held against the scale usually found on the centrifuge, and read according to the manufacturer's instructions. The results are always recorded as a percentage and differ for men and women, ranging from 40% to 50% for men and 35% to 46% for women.

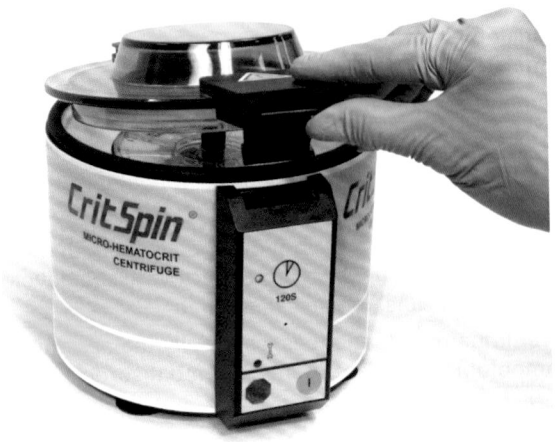

**Figure 42-5** • StatSpin® CritSpin microhematocrit centrifuge. (Photo used with permission from Beckman Coulter.)

**CHECKPOINT QUESTION**

2. Marilyn Mays, CMA(AAMA), is reviewing some laboratory results on a patient and notes that the hematocrit for a female patient is 20%. What conclusions should Marilyn have about this test result?

### Erythrocyte Indices

A complete blood count (CBC) also includes **erythrocyte indices**, calculations that measure the size of red blood cells and the amount of hemoglobin on the RBC. Because there are several types of anemia, the erythrocyte indices help with identifying the type of anemia so that the appropriate treatment can be prescribed.

There are three erythrocyte indices including the mean corpuscular volume (MCV), the mean corpuscular hemoglobin (MCH), and the mean corpuscular hemoglobin concentration (MCHC). The mean, or average, corpuscular volume (MCV) represents the average size of the red blood cells as either normal size (*normocytic*), smaller size (*microcytic*), or larger size (*macrocytic*). This test can indicate anemias caused by nutritional deficiencies with a normal result falling within the 80 to 100 fL (femtoliters) range. A femtoliter is a fraction of one-millionth of a liter. **Microcytosis**, a result below 80 fL, indicates an iron deficiency, while **macrocytosis**, a result above 100 fL, indicates a deficiency of folate or vitamin $B_{12}$.

The MCH calculation measures the average amount of hemoglobin on the average single red blood cell, while the MCHC calculation measures the concentration of hemoglobin in a given volume of red blood cells. The normal range for the mean corpuscular hemoglobin is 27 to 32 picograms (pg), and the normal range for mean corpuscular hemoglobin concentration is 32.0 to 36.0 g/dL (Table 42-1). Decreased values of MCH and MCHC, called **hypochromia**, may be due to:

- Iron deficiency anemia
- **Thalassemia**
- Blood loss
- Vitamin $B_6$ deficiency

There are disorders in which the erythrocyte indices differ such as pernicious anemia in which the body does not absorb enough vitamin $B_{12}$ to make red blood cells. In this type of anemia, the MCV is high, but the MCHC is normal. In iron deficiency anemia, the hemoglobin may be normal early in the disease but may decrease over time. The MCH and MCV values will be lower than normal. If iron deficiency anemia is suspected, the physician may order a blood test to determine the amount of ferritin in the blood. Ferritin is a protein that stores iron in the body and will be low in patients with anemia caused by a deficiency of iron.

## CHECKPOINT QUESTION

3. What is represented by the MCV value included in a complete blood count?

### The Erythrocyte Sedimentation Rate

The erythrocyte sedimentation rate (ESR) test measures how quickly red blood cells settle to the bottom of a tube, becoming sediment in the tube. It is sometimes referred to as a "sed rate" and is collected in a test tube specific to perform this test. Once the blood sample is obtained, the tube is placed in a holder and allowed to sit undisturbed for 1 hour, allowing the heavier red blood cells to fall in millimeters per hour to the bottom of the tube (Fig. 42-6). This test is not used to diagnose illness, but is used as a screening test for inflammation in the body or to monitor the effectiveness of treatment for inflammation.

The method used to perform the ESR in the physician office laboratory is called the Westergren method. To assure accurate results, the following conditions should be followed:

- Start the test within 2 hours of collecting the blood specimen.
- Conduct the test at room temperature.
- Make sure the column of blood in the tube does not contain bubbles.
- Keep the tube vertical during testing.
- Place the sedimentation rack on a counter with no vibrations. Do not place near a centrifuge.
- Keep the sedimentation rack away from all drafts and direct sunlight.
- Read the test results at exactly 60 minutes.

The normal range varies depending on gender and age. The normal sed rate for med under the age of 50 years is 0 to 15 mm/hour and less than 20 mm/hour for

men over the age of 50 years. Females under the age of 50 years have a normal ESR of 0 to 20 mm/hour and less than 30 mm/hour over the age of 50 years. The more rapidly the RBCs fall in the tube, the more inflammation is present in the body, but more tests are needed to determine the source of the inflammation. This test may be ordered to support a diagnosis or monitor inflammatory diseases such as rheumatoid arthritis or other autoimmune conditions. Conditions that may cause an elevated sed rate include infections, anemia, some cancers, pregnancy, and disorders of the thyroid. A low ESR rate may be found in conditions such as congestive heart failure, leukemia, and sickle cell anemia.

## PATIENT EDUCATION

### Iron Deficiency Anemia

Patients who have iron deficiency anemia may have all the symptoms of someone with anemia (fatigue, pallor, increased heart, and respiratory rates); however, the anemia may not be caused by a low red blood cell count. Instead, the patient with iron deficiency anemia has an inadequate amount of iron necessary for the body to make the protein hemoglobin. Depending on the patient's iron level, the physician may prescribe the patient to increase dietary iron including the consumption of the following foods, which are high in iron content such as:

- Liver
- Oysters
- Kidney beans
- Lean meats
- Turnips
- Egg yolks
- Whole-wheat bread
- Carrots
- Dark greens

Diagnosing iron deficiency anemia requires the measurement of serum iron in the blood, ferritin (a protein that stores iron in the body), transferrin (a protein that carries iron in the blood), and total iron-binding capacity (TIBC) or amount of transferrin available to bind to the iron. If the TIBC is low, the body could hold more iron if more were ingested or administered. A patient with iron deficiency anemia may have low levels of serum iron and ferritin but elevated levels of transferrin and TIBC.

The treatment for iron deficiency anemia includes increasing iron in the diet or supplements. In severe cases, the patient may be given iron supplements by injection, either intramuscular or intravenously. If the iron deficiency is due to blood loss, a blood transfusion may be ordered after the source of bleeding has been determined and treated appropriately. Patients who are prescribed oral iron supplements should be warned that iron may cause constipation and dark stools.

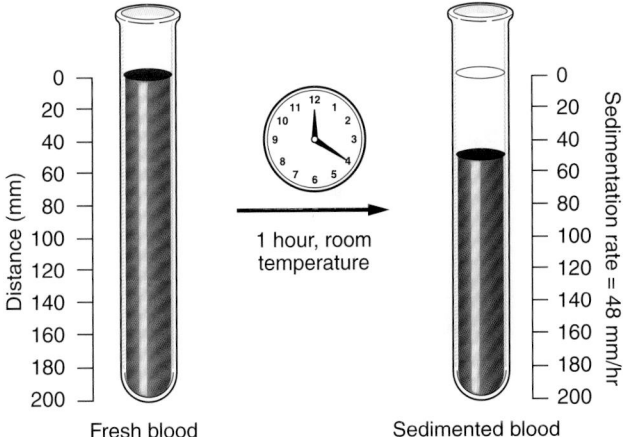

**Figure 42-6** • Determination of the erythrocyte sedimentation rate (ESR). Fresh, anticoagulated blood is allowed to settle at room temperature in a thin, graduated tube. After a fixed time interval (1 hour), the height (millimeters) that the erythrocytes sediment is measured.

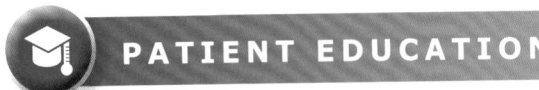

### Dietary Folate

The blood must contain enough folate to produce healthy RBCs. When there is not enough folate present, anemia develops. Folate in the blood comes from a person's diet. Some foods with folate are

- Leafy green vegetables
- Citrus fruits and juices
- Dried beans and peas

Folate may also be taken as a dietary supplement.

## Leukocytes

### The Function of Leukocytes

The primary function of leukocytes, or white blood cells, is defense against foreign substances that may cause illness or disease. There are two categories of leukocytes, agranular and granular, and five major types of leukocytes that make up white blood cells (Fig. 42-7). Agranular leukocytes include **lymphocytes** and **monocytes**. Lymphocytes are the smallest of the leukocytes and consist of T cells, B cells, and NK (natural killer) cells. Specifically, the B-cell lymphocytes respond to a bodily invasion of **antigens**, or cells considered foreign by releasing **antibodies**. These antibodies, or proteins

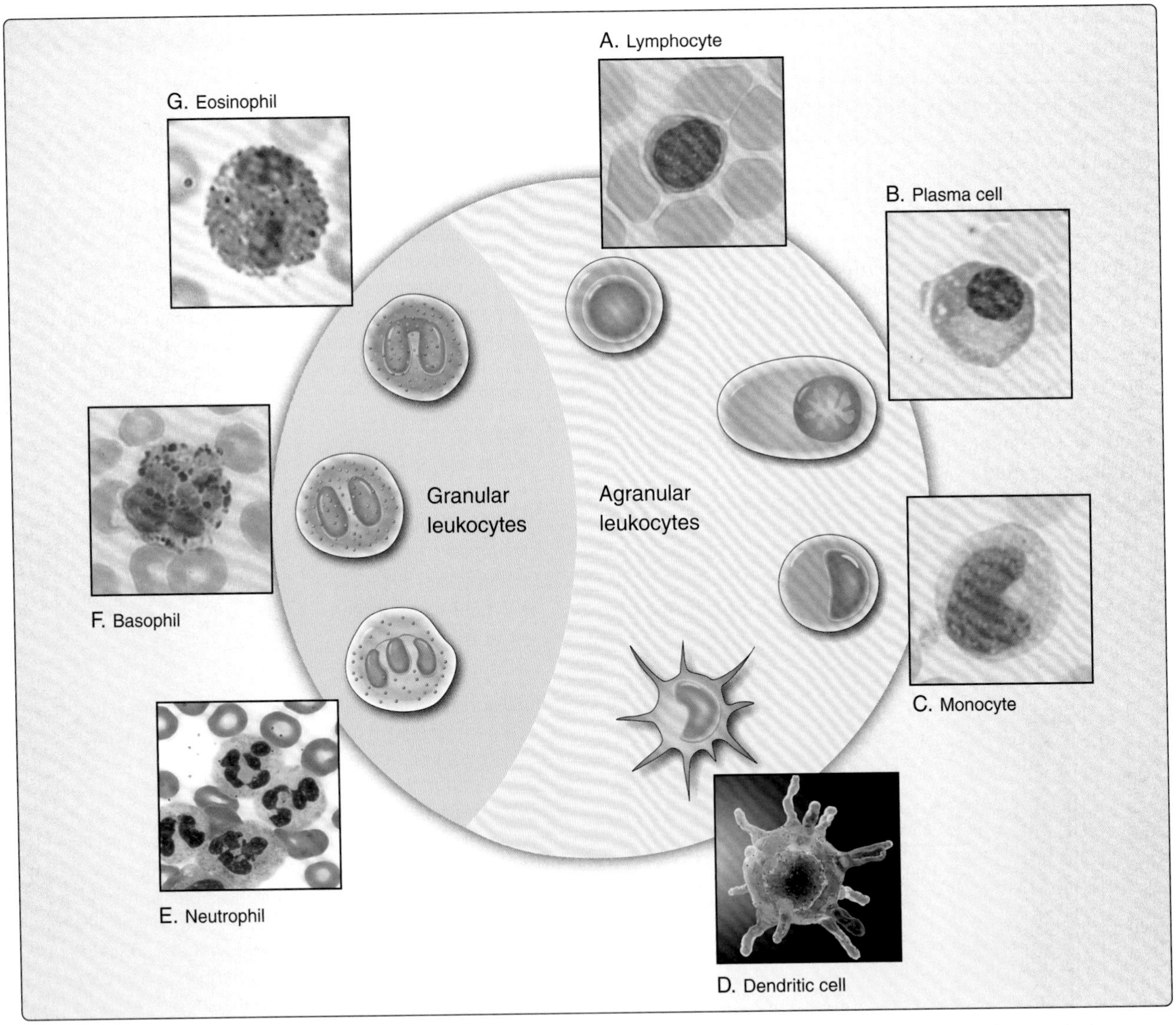

**Figure 42-7** • Types of leukocytes. White blood cells or leukocytes may be broadly classified by the absence (agranular) or presence (granular) of cytoplasmic inclusions or granules. **(A)** Lymphocytes include T, B, and natural killer (NK) cells. **(B)** B cells that enlarge and differentiate into immunoglobulin secretors are known as plasma cells. **(C)** Monocytes are phagocytic cells in the circulation and are called macrophages when they enter tissues. **(D)** Dendritic cells are phagocytic cells that bear treelike cytoplasmic processes. **(E)** Neutrophils have multilobed nuclei and cytoplasmic granules that stain with neutral (pH) dyes. **(F)** Basophils have bilobed nuclei and cytoplasmic granules that stain with basic (pH) dyes. **(G)** Eosinophils have bilobed nuclei and cytoplasmic granules that stain with acidic (pH) dyes.

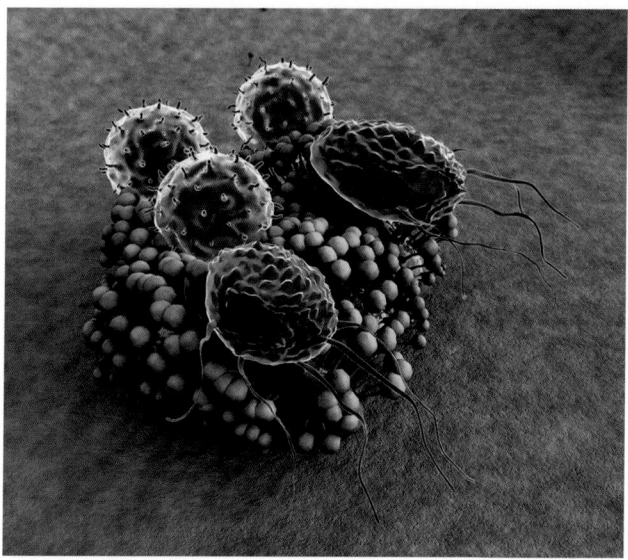

**Figure 42-8** • In this photograph, a white blood cell is killing a pathogen by eating it. This is a process called phagocytosis ("phago-" means "eat" and "cyt-" means "cell").

produced by the body in response to a specific antigen, coat the foreign cell and destroy it by puncturing holes in their membranes. Increased lymphocytes usually signal a viral infection. Monocytes also react to the antigens and react to the presence of foreign cells by engulfing and destroying the antigens through a process known as **phagocytosis** (Fig. 42-8).

Granular leukocytes include **neutrophils, basophils,** and **eosinophils.** At the first sign of an invasion by a foreign cell, lymphocytes respond as well as monocytes and neutrophils. Like monocytes, neutrophils also engulf and digest foreign substances; however, neutrophils release digestive enzymes that kill the foreign material and the neutrophil at the same time. A **band** is a young neutrophil, and increased amounts in the blood usually indicate an acute infection that needs immediate treatment.

The fourth type of white blood cells, basophils, have round, purple-black granules in their cytoplasm. These WBCs release a substance known as histamine as an immune response to antigens or substances recognized as foreign. The histamine causes inflammatory responses such as hives, asthma, and other allergy symptoms. Eosinophils, the fifth type of white blood cells, are also active in inflammatory responses such as allergies and may also be increased in parasite infections. These blood cells have red granules in their cytoplasm.

## CHECKPOINT QUESTION

4. What is the function of neutrophils in the immune system?

## White Blood Cell Counts

The normal range for a total WBC count is 4,500 to 10,000 cells per microliter of blood. A microliter is one one-thousandth of a milliliter and is represented by the symbol µ/L (see Table 42-2). **Leukopenia** is a white blood cell count below 4,500 µ/L and may be caused by a variety of conditions including bone marrow deficiencies, chemotherapy drugs, autoimmune disorders such as systemic lupus erythematosus (SLE), certain viral illnesses, and severe bacterial infections. In addition to chemotherapy agents, other drugs that decrease the white blood cell count include antibiotics, antithyroid medications, diuretics, and histamine-2 blockers such as those prescribed to decrease gastric secretions. **Leukocytosis** refers to an elevated white blood cell count, which may be caused by anemia, infections, cigarette smoking, and inflammatory diseases such as rheumatoid arthritis or allergies. Patients who have had a splenectomy may also have a slightly higher white blood cell count. Drugs that may increase the white blood cell count include corticosteroids, beta adrenergic agonists including albuterol, epinephrine, heparin, and lithium.

Because the white blood cell count is determined by using automated cell counters that are not CLIA waived, the hematology blood specimen to determine WBC count is drawn in the physician office and sent to the reference laboratory for testing. The laboratory request that accompanies the blood specimen must indicate a WBC count as ordered by the physician if a CBC is not ordered: a CBC will include a WBC count. In some situations, the physician will request total white blood cell count but will also want to know the amount of each of the five types of white blood cells. This test is known as a **differential** and may be ordered as a WBC and differential, CBC with differential. In addition, the word "differential" may be abbreviated as "diff." The normal range in percentages for each of the five types of WBCs includes the following:

- Lymphocytes = 20% to 30%
- Monocytes = 2% to 8%
- Neutrophils = 50% to 70%
- Basophils = 1%
- Eosinophils = 2% to 4%

## CHECKPOINT QUESTION

5. Marilyn Mays, CMA(AAMA), is reviewing the laboratory report for a patient that is scheduled to come into the office tomorrow for an appointment. The patient has a decreased WBC count. What is the medical term for a decreased WBC count and what are three possible causes?

## Thrombocytes

### The Function of Thrombocytes

The body uses thrombocytes, also known as platelets, to form clots and control bleeding. When there is an internal or external injury, platelets stick together on the injured vessel to form a plug and stop the bleeding. Compared to white blood cells and red blood cells, thrombocytes are smaller in size and are produced in the bone marrow. The physician may order a platelet count alone, or it will be part of the complete blood count or CBC.

### Platelet Count

A normal platelet count is 150,000 to 400,000 cells per microliter. Patients who have less than 150,000 have a condition called **thrombocytopenia**, which may be caused by an inadequate production by the bone marrow, destruction of platelets in the bloodstream, or destruction of the cells in an organ such as the spleen or liver. Some causes of thrombocytopenia include certain autoimmune disorders and drugs including chemotherapy agents, furosemide, nonsteroidal anti-inflammatory drugs (NSAIDs), and some antibiotics. Patients who do not have enough platelets may have abnormal bleeding with simple activities such as brushing the teeth. They may also bruise easily and have **petechiae**, bleeding under the skin that looks like small, pinpoint, red spots on the skin (Fig. 42-9).

An increased platelet count, **thrombocytosis**, is a platelet count above 400,000 microliters. Conditions that may cause an increased platelet count include anemia, cancer, certain medications, chronic myelogenous leukemia (CML), and polycythemia vera.

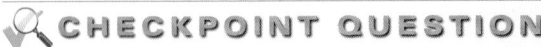

### CHECKPOINT QUESTION

6. What is the function of platelets?

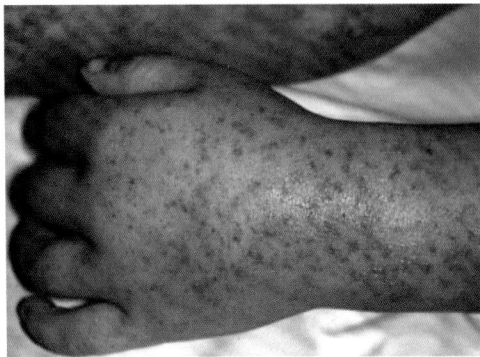

**Figure 42-9 •** Petechiae. These tiny skin hemorrhages occurred in a child with low platelet count (thrombocytopenia).

### WHAT IF?

**What if a patient asks you about the criteria for donating blood?**

The American Red Cross bases criteria for donating blood on recommendations from government agencies, the Centers for Disease Control and Prevention, and findings from research projects. In addition, each state has its own laws regulating the donation of blood or blood products. Generally, anyone donating blood or blood products must meet the following criteria:

- General good health and feeling well at the time of donation.
- Age 17 years or older. Donors who are 16 years may donate with parental consent.
- Weight of 110 lbs or more.
- Hemoglobin at least 12.5 g/dL.
- Pulse of 50 to 110 beats per minute.
- Blood pressure less than 180/100 mm Hg and higher than 80/50 mm Hg.
- Donors living in states that do not regulate tattoos must wait 12 months after getting a tattoo to donate.

The donor also must provide a brief history at the time of donation and may not qualify to donate based on criteria other than what is listed above. A donor should allow for approximately 1 hour for the entire process; however, the actual blood donation is about 10 minutes. Whole blood can be donated every 56 days but blood products such as platelets and plasma may be donated more frequently. All blood will be tested by the American Red Cross for HIV, hepatitis, and syphilis.

## COAGULATION STUDIES

Coagulation tests measure the ability of blood to clot. When the body receives an internal or external injury, coagulation proteins are activated in the body. The proteins initiate the formation of the clot, and as the clot gets bigger, it forms a plug that stops bleeding. The steps in the coagulation process include the following:

1. *Vasoconstriction.* The vein constricts to reduce blood loss.
2. *Platelet plug formation.* The platelets stick to each other and to the wound to form a plug.
3. *Fibrin clot formation.* The coagulation factors make the plug stable. (The two most common tests for testing clotting are prothrombin time and partial thromboplastin time.)

4. *Clot lysis and vascular repair.* The clot must lyse or it will cause other problems. The clot dissolving is called lysis. While the clot dissolves, the blood vessel heals.

About 20 seconds after an injury, platelets in the blood begin sticking together over the injury. While the platelets are sticking together, a protein produced by the liver called *fibrinogen* helps strengthen the plug. This clot assists with controlling bleeding from the injured site in the patient with normal coagulation processes. These normal processes are essential in preventing significant blood loss after an injury.

Unfortunately, some patients may produce clots within a blood vessel, and this results in increased risk for death of the tissue distal to blockage if blood flow in an artery is occluded. If the clot occurs in a vein, the condition is known as *venous thrombosis*, and if it occurs in an artery, it is known as an *arterial thrombosis*. If the arterial thrombosis affects an artery supplying blood to the heart, this is known as a *myocardial infarction* or heart attack (see Chapter 32, Cardiology). An arterial thrombosis affecting an artery supplying blood to the brain is a *cerebrovascular accident* or stroke (see Chapter 34, Neurology). Patients with a history of forming blood clots are often prescribed treatments such as a daily low dose aspirin or anticoagulant therapy such as warfarin or enoxaparin.

## Prothrombin Time, Partial Thromboplastin Time, and International Normalized Ratio (INR) Tests

If the physician suspects a coagulation problem or a patient is receiving anticoagulant therapy to prevent clot formation, a blood test for prothrombin time (PT), partial thromboplastin time (PTT), and/or **international normalized ratio** (INR) may be ordered. The two most common coagulation tests are the PT and the PTT, and in some offices, the blood must be collected and sent to a reference lab for testing. To perform the PT test in the lab, substances are added to the blood specimen and the clotting time is measured. The normal range for a PT is 10 to 14 seconds, but each laboratory establishes the range so the normal range may vary from laboratory to laboratory.

The partial thromboplastin time (PTT) uses a slightly different method to determine as compared to the PT. This test identifies some of the proteins, also known as factors, involved in the blood clotting process. The normal range for a PTT is 25 to 35 seconds, and like the PT, the laboratory establishes the range so it may vary. PT and PTT results that are higher than normal indicate the blood taking longer to clot. The higher the result, the

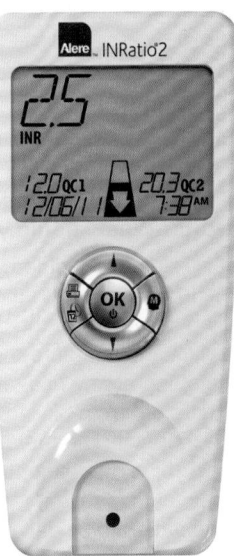

**Figure 42-10 •** The INRatio2 monitor for PT/INR testing from HemoSense provides PT and INR results in less than 1 minute using one drop of blood from a fingerstick.

longer it takes the blood to clot. A patient with hemophilia, a genetic disorder in which clotting factor VIII or IX are deficient, may have a normal PT but will have a higher PTT because of the low or missing coagulation factor.

For patients receiving anticoagulant therapy, the international normalized ratio, or INR, is the preferred test to monitor the effectiveness of the medications. This test is a standardized result calculated from the patient's PT and a reference standard and does not vary from laboratory to laboratory. Fortunately, CLIA-waived machines to accurately and easily measure the PT and INR in the physician office are available and typically use a small blood specimen from a capillary puncture (Fig. 42-10). Using CLIA-waived machines to monitor PT and INR results are an advantage to patients whose anticoagulant therapy must be adjusted according to the results. Otherwise, results must be obtained from a lab, and adjustments to medication may be delayed for a day or longer. A patient who is not taking anticoagulants should have an INR of 1.0. An INR of 2.0 means the blood is taking twice as long to clot as it normally would if the patient was not taking an anticoagulant. The higher the INR result, the "thinner" the patient's blood or the longer it will take for the patient to form a clot. A patient who is on anticoagulant therapy to prevent clot formation will typically maintain an INR between 2.0 and 3.0.

## CHECKPOINT QUESTION

7. Why is the INR a better result than the PT?

**Your patient requires anticoagulant therapy to treat a condition such as atrial fibrillation and does not keep follow-up appointments to check prothrombin time and INR results? What should you do?**

When the patient misses a scheduled appointment, you should always document this in the medical record and let the physician know. When the patient comes into the office, explain and reinforce the importance of monitoring blood clotting time while taking the medication including the dangers from having clotting times that are outside (low or high) the therapeutic range. If the PT or INR are too high, the patient may have uncontrolled bleeding that could result in death. If the PT or INR are too low, the patient may develop dangerous clots that result in a thrombosis in a major blood vessel such as those in the lungs (pulmonary embolism), the heart (myocardial infarction), or brain (cerebrovascular accident). While the goal is not to frighten the patient, the patient must be fully aware of the consequences of noncompliance. All patient education should be documented in the medical record.

## THE ROLE OF THE MEDICAL ASSISTANT IN HEMATOLOGY TESTING

Standard precautions are required in hematology as well as all other areas of the medical practice and physician office laboratory. In most cases, there are no pretesting requirements for basic hematology procedures, and most may be performed when ordered. When performing a phlebotomy procedure to obtain blood for hematology testing, you should remember to use a needle gauge that will not hemolyze or destroy the cells. Drawing blood specimens with a needle gauge that is too small will result in hemolysis and may result in inaccurate blood cell counts.

In addition to collecting blood for hematology testing and processing it to send to the laboratory if necessary, you may also be required to collect blood samples for hematology testing using CLIA-waived machines. Your responsibilities when using CLIA-waived machines includes being familiar with the machine including any calibration or quality control measures as determined by the manufacturer. Expired reagent strips or machines that are not working properly should not be used as these may give inaccurate results and lead to inappropriate treatment.

It is also your responsibility to be familiar with normal values for hematology tests. The physician should always be made aware of patient results according to office policies and procedures. Critical values, or those that are outside the normal range and may be life threatening, should always be reported to the physician immediately. You may also be responsible for reporting hematology results to patients, but only do so as directed by the physician. Patients on anticoagulant therapy are usually well aware of INR results and may have a physician order to adjust medication dosages according to the INR results without having to speak with the physician first. For other hematology tests, the physician may want to discuss the results directly with the patient.

## ROLE-PLAYING ACTIVITY

Role-play these scenarios as if you are working with Marilyn Mays, the CMA(AAMA) who works in the busy oncology practice at Great Falls Medical Center (refer to the case study at the beginning of the chapter). A 52-year-old female patient seen today has just been diagnosed with breast cancer and has been referred to the oncologist to begin chemotherapy. This is her first visit to the office, and the physician has ordered several blood tests including a CBC with differential. When you enter the exam room with the phlebotomy supplies, you notice she is crying quietly. How would you respond to this patient? She tells you she is "scared" of dying and is worried her blood results will be "abnormal." What would you say? Your instructor will give you additional information about this activity!

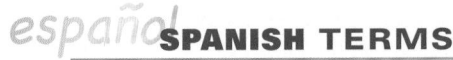 SPANISH TERMS

**El médico dice que usted está anémica (o) y que necesita aumentar el hierro en su dieta.**
The doctor says you have anemia and I need to talk to you about increasing iron in your diet.

**El médico quiere que le de sus resultados de su examen del conteo completo de células sanguíneas.**
The physician would like me to give you the results of your complete blood count.

**Su médico dice que su sangre está muy delgada y que necesita disminuir la cantidad de warfarina que esta tomando.**
Your INR is too high so the doctor wants you to decrease the amount of warfarin you are taking.

**¿Se siente cansado (a)?**
Are you tired?

**¿Cuando se dió cuenta de que aparecieron estas manchas en su piel?**
When did the bruising start?

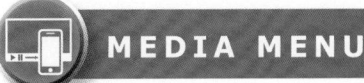 MEDIA MENU

**Student Resources** on thePoint®

- **Animation: Hemostasis**
- *Video:* **Performing a Microhematocrit Determination (Procedure 42-2)**
- **CMA/RMA Certification Exam Review**
- **English to Spanish Audio Glossary**

**Internet Resources**
**American Society of Hematology**
http://www.hematology.org
**Lab Tests Online**
http://www.labtestsonline.org/understanding/analytes/esr/test.html
**National Institutes of Health Hematology Test Guide**
http://cclnprod.cc.nih.gov/dlm/testguide.nsf/HematologyTests?OpenForm&Count=5000
**The Mayo Clinic**
http://www.mayoclinic.org/

# EMR Activity

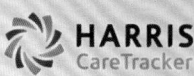

Harris CareTracker is a web-based electronic medical record (EMR) application that you will use for the EMR activities included in this section at the end of each chapter. This application is actually used in physician offices, but is provided to you through the publisher, Wolters Kluwer Health, to give you hands-on practice working with EMRs. Your instructor will have more information about accessing your username, login, and Quickstart guide.

Prerequisite Activities in Harris CareTracker

- *The Getting Started and Quickstart documents and EMR Activities Step-by-Step Instructions are available at* http://thePoint.lww.com/KronenbergerComp5e

Activity Details

Accurately document the following blood collection procedures and hematology results in each of the following patient's EMR:

1. Bobby Turner: Blood collected via venipuncture (left posterior hand using a winged infusion set) and sent to Great Falls Medical Center laboratory for a erythrocyte sedimentation rate.
2. Oscar Tinner: Capillary stick (right middle finger) for an INR (patient is on warfarin for atrial fibrillation). His results were 3.7.

# Chapter Summary

Hematology tests are ordered by the physician or other qualified health care provider to diagnose or monitor diseases of blood cells and the coagulation properties found within blood. This chapter focused on the following key points:

- Blood cells (erythrocytes, leukocytes, and thrombocytes) are produced in bone marrow. Red blood cells function to carry oxygen, white blood cells defend against infection and inflammation, and platelets are active in the blood clotting process.
- The physician may order a complete blood count (CBC), which includes the number of red blood cells, total white blood cells, and platelets in a given sample of blood. If the physician orders a CBC with differential blood count, the laboratory will count not only the total number of WBCs but also the number of each type of white blood cells.
- Dietary iron is essential in the formation of the protein hemoglobin, the substance on red blood cells responsible for carrying oxygen. Mature red blood cells are concave and do not have a nucleus, allowing the hemoglobin (Hgb) to carry as much oxygen as possible.
- A decreased red blood cell count is known as anemia, while a decreased white blood cell count is leukopenia. Decreased numbers of thrombocytes, or platelets, in the blood is called thrombocytopenia and will result in a decrease in the ability of the body to form a clot and stop internal or external bleeding.
- An erythrocyte sedimentation rate (ESR or sed rate) is the amount of time it takes red blood cells to settle to the bottom of a thin test tube. Patients with an infection or inflammatory process will have an elevated sed rate, meaning the cells settle to the bottom of the tube faster than expected.
- Patients with suspected bleeding disorders often have hematology coagulation studies including a prothrombin time (PT) and partial thromboplastin time (PTT) performed. Some disease conditions require anticoagulant therapy, and those patients require regular and frequent monitoring of bleeding times to adjust medication. The PT and international normalized ratio (INR) are the tests ordered to monitor anticoagulant therapy.
- Although some hematology tests must be performed in the reference laboratory, there are CLIA-waived machines available on the market to perform some hematology tests including the hematocrit, hemoglobin, ESR, and PT/INR. The medical assistant is responsible for collecting any blood specimens for hematology tests and preparing them for transport to the lab if necessary. If CLIA-waived testing is done in the office, it is the role of the medical assistant to be familiar with the machine and testing requirements according to the manufacturer. Calibration and quality control procedures must be followed to ensure accurate results.

# Warm-Ups for Critical Thinking

1. A patient was taking a medication that caused him to become neutropenic. To what might he be susceptible?
2. A patient lives at a very high elevation, where there is less oxygen than at sea level. Would you expect her hemoglobin to be greater than, less than, or the same as if she lived at sea level?
3. On microscopic review, a patient's RBCs are described as macrocytic. What impact would that characteristic have on the patient's MCV?
4. A patient with rheumatoid arthritis has an ESR of 77 mm/hour when she has her blood tested at the doctor's office; 2 weeks later, she returns, and now, the rate is 31 mm/hour. With her condition in mind, would you expect that she is improving or not?
5. A patient has a platelet count of 75,000/mm³. How would that impact the patient's coagulation studies?
6. Using the patient information in Box 42-1, use these steps to complete the exercise as a case study.

*(continues on page 1104)*

## Warm-Ups for Critical Thinking (continued)

To begin your evaluation:
*** *Research* the definitions of the morphology terms.
*Because of the initial test results, these tests were performed:*

Iron Studies

| | |
|---|---|
| Serum ferritin <10 ng/mL | (12–86) |
| Serum iron 24 mg/dL | (RI, 65–175) |
| TIBC 729 mg/dL | (RI, 250–410) |
| Saturation 3% | (RI, 20–55) |

**A.** Define the symptoms in the patient history and physical exam.
**B.** Use those definitions to develop areas of concern.
**C.** Why did the physician order a CBC with differential?
**D.** What are the RIs for the tests included in the CBC?
**E.** Define the terms used to describe the red cell morphology.
**F.** What are the possible causes of this morphology?
**G.** Why did the doctor choose the follow-up tests listed?
**H.** Predict the diagnosis for the patient.

*Let's take this to the next step:*

- The history and exam led to exploring a cause that would be the same for fatigue and for pallor. What causes can you list?
- Looking at the causes you listed, which ones would be evaluated using a CBC?
- Which tests on the CBC are abnormal? Are they elevated or decreased? Do these results eliminate any causes you listed?
- The patient's WBCs appear normal, so they are not involved in this disease process.
- After defining the terms used to describe the RBCs in the RBC morphology, the cells are determined to have very abnormal shapes with very little hemoglobin.
- Have you narrowed your list to iron deficiency anemia?
- For more information from this case study, evaluate the follow-up tests ordered by the physician. Do the results confirm the diagnosis of iron deficiency anemia?

## PSY   PROCEDURE 42-1

# Perform a Hemoglobin Determination

**PSY** Perform CLIA-waived hematology testing; instruct and prepare a patient for a procedure or treatment; coach patients appropriately considering cultural diversity, developmental life stage, and communication barriers; document patient care accurately in the medical record.

**Purpose:** To determine the oxygen-carrying capacity of the blood in a patient sample by performing a hemoglobin determination using CLIA-waived equipment

**Equipment:** Hemoglobinometer, applicator sticks, whole blood, hand disinfectant, surface disinfectant, gloves, biohazard container, medical record

| STEPS | PURPOSE |
|---|---|
| 1. Check the physician order and wash your hands. | The physician or other qualified health care professional must order a hemoglobin count. Hand washing aids infection control. |
| 2. Assemble the necessary equipment and supplies. Check the expiration dates on supplies that require this and ensure the equipment is in good working order. Perform any calibration or quality control procedures as required per the manufacturer and office policy and procedure. 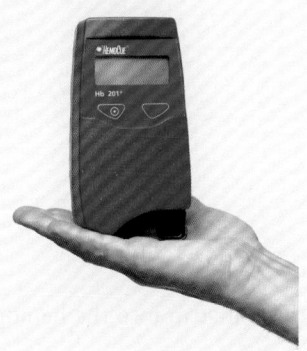 | Equipment must be readily accessible for the procedure to be done. The equipment and supplies must be checked and maintained to ensure accurate results. |
| | **Step 2:** A CLIA-waived machine for hemoglobin determination. (Photo used with permission from HemoCue America—A division of Radiometer America Inc., Brea, CA.) |
| 3. Take the equipment and supplies to the patient examination room or take the patient to the phlebotomy station if available. | PPE such as gloves prevents exposure to biohazardous materials. |
| 4. **AFF** Greet and identify the patient and yourself including your title. Explain the procedure. Explain the procedure and put on gloves. | Identifying the patient maintains sample integrity. Explaining the procedure helps ease anxiety and ensure compliance. |
| 5. **AFF** Explain how you would respond to an elderly patient. | An elderly patient should be treated with empathy, respect, and dignity as you would treat any other patient. Talking through each step builds the patient's confidence level by keeping him or her informed of what you are doing and why. |
| 6. Obtain a blood specimen from the patient by capillary puncture. | Hematology blood specimens obtained by venipuncture to send to an outside laboratory require evacuation tubes that contain EDTA. This is the anticoagulant additive required for hematology testing. |

*(continues on page 1106)*

## PROCEDURE 42-1 (continued)

**STEPS**                                                          **PURPOSE**

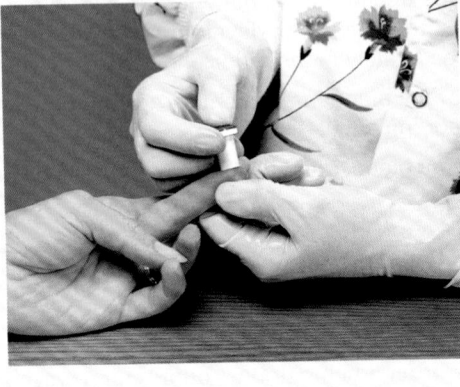

**Step 6:** Perform a capillary puncture.

7. Place well-mixed whole blood into the hemoglobinometer chamber or place the blood specimen on
   the reagent strip as described by the manufacturer.

This prepares the sample for the hemoglobin
determination.

8. Slide the chamber into the hemoglobinometer
   or process the specimen using the CLIA-waived
   machine as required by the manufacturer.

The chamber must be in the receiving slot for the reading. CLIA-waived hemoglobin devices should be operated according to the manufacturer's instructions.

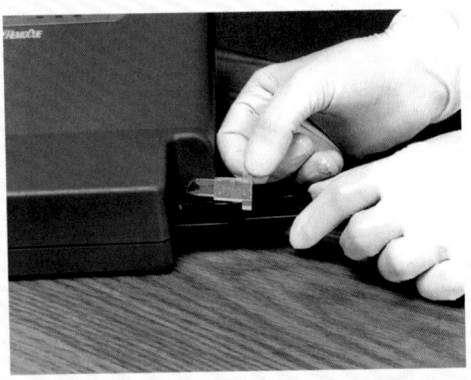

**Step 8:** Insert the test strip into the hemoglobin
machine.

9. Record the hemoglobin level from the digital
   readout.

The results should be read exactly as they appear on
the digital screen.

10. Dispose of the contaminated supplies into a bio-
    hazard waste receptacle according to office policy
    and procedure. Clean the work area with surface
    disinfectant. Dispose of equipment and supplies
    appropriately. Remove gloves and wash your
    hands.

Supplies that are contaminated with blood should be
disposed of properly. Maintaining a clean work space
limits exposure to biohazards.

11. **AFF** Log into the electronic medical record
    (EMR) using your username and secure password
    OR obtain the paper medical record from a secure
    location and assure it is kept away from public
    access. Record the procedure noting the date, time,
    site of the venipuncture, test results for CLIA-
    waived POC procedures or the name of the lab
    where the specimen was sent, and your name.

The integrity of the medical record must be maintained at all times to protect patient privacy.

Procedures are considered not to have been performed
if they are not recorded.

# PROCEDURE 42-1 (continued)

| STEPS | PURPOSE |
|---|---|
| 12. When finished, log out of the EMR and/or replace the paper medical record in an appropriate and secure location. | |

*Note:* This procedure may vary with the instrument. Some manufacturers offer a digital readout that is less subjective and is therefore considered more accurate and easier to use.

---

## Charting Example
*12/02/2016 10:30 AM Cap puncture L ring finger. Hgb 9.5. Dr. Royal notified of results*
_____*M. Mays, CMA*

---

**Note:** *The medical assistant may sign his or her name in the patient record using only the "CMA" credential if the office has a signature log denoting the entire credential as "CMA(AAMA)."*

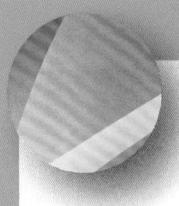

## PSY PROCEDURE 42-2

# Perform a Microhematocrit Determination

**PSY** Perform CLIA-waived hematology testing.

**Purpose:** To determine the percentage of erythrocytes in a centrifuged specimen of blood by performing a microhematocrit determination using CLIA-waived equipment

**Equipment:** Microcollection tubes, sealing clay, microhematocrit centrifuge, microhematocrit reading device, hand disinfectant, surface disinfectant, gloves, biohazard container, sharps container, and medical record

| STEPS | PURPOSE |
|---|---|
| 1. Check the physician order and wash your hands. | The physician or other qualified health care professional must order a microhematocrit. Hand washing aids infection control. |
| 2. Assemble the necessary equipment and supplies. Check the expiration dates on supplies that require this and ensure the equipment is in good working order. Perform any calibration or quality control procedures as required per the manufacturer and office policy and procedure. | Equipment must be readily accessible for the procedure to be done. <br><br> The equipment and supplies must be checked and maintained to ensure accurate results. |
| 3. Take the equipment and supplies to the patient examination room or take the patient to the phlebotomy station if available. | |
| 4. **AFF** Greet and identify the patient and yourself including your title. Explain the procedure. Explain the procedure and put on gloves. | Identifying the patient maintains sample integrity. Explaining the procedure helps ease anxiety and ensure compliance. PPE such as gloves prevents exposure to biohazardous materials. |
| 5. **AFF** Explain how you would respond to a patient who does not speak English as their first language. | A patient with limited English may be accompanied by a family member and, if so, speak to the patient but use the family member to interpret if necessary. Patients who request an interpreter and make this request before the date of the actual appointment must be provided one. If no interpreter or family member is present, speak slowly and use gestures or a picture chart if available. |
| 6. Obtain a blood specimen from the patient by capillary puncture. Draw blood into the capillary tube by holding the capillary microhematocrit tube horizontally and touching one end of the tube to the blood coming from the capillary puncture. Allow the tube to fill to ¾ or the indicated mark on the capillary tube. | Whole blood from a capillary puncture has not clotted and is acceptable. <br> Holding the microhematocrit tube in a horizontal position while filling will allow blood to fill the tube without spilling out the other end. |

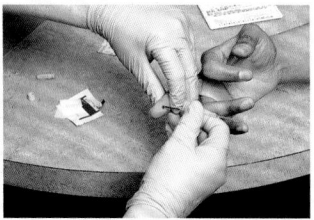

**Step 6:** Fill the microhematocrit tube to the indicated line on the tube.

# PROCEDURE 42-2 (continued)

| STEPS | PURPOSE |
|---|---|
| 7. With the microhematocrit tube in a horizontal position, place your forefinger over the opposite end of the tube, lift it up, and push the tube into the clay sealant with the blood side in the clay. | Holding the finger over the end of the tube while lifting it up and pushing into the clay sealant stops blood from dripping out the bottom. The clay seals one end of the tube to contain it during centrifugation. |

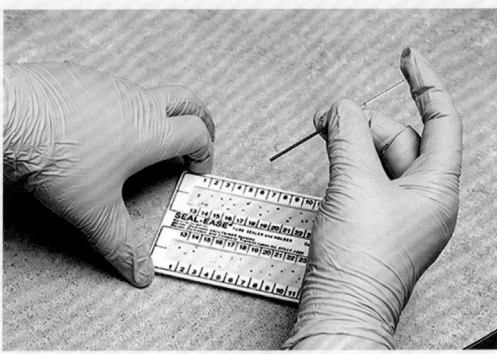

**Step 7:** Put your finger over the opposite end of the tube so the blood specimen does not spill out of the tube.

| STEPS | PURPOSE |
|---|---|
| 8. Draw a second specimen in the same manner using a second microhematocrit tube. | A second tube is necessary for duplicate testing as a quality control measure. |
| 9. Place the tubes, clay-sealed end out, in the radial grooves of the microhematocrit centrifuge opposite each other. Put the lid on the grooved area and tighten by turning the knob clockwise. Close the centrifuge lid. Spin for 5 minutes or as directed by the centrifuge manufacturer. | Specimens should always be placed opposite each other to balance the centrifuge. Read the manufacturer's directions for the specific centrifuge used in your facility; a 5-minute spin is normal. |

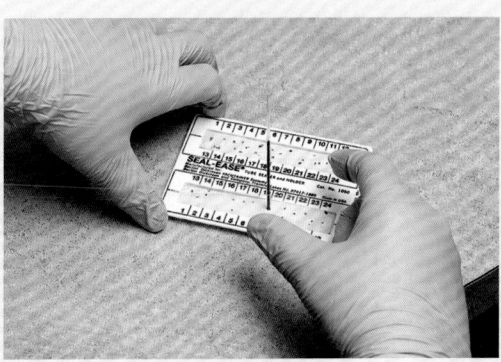

**Step 8:** Place the microhematocrit tubes in the centrifuge with the sealed clay end facing outward.

| STEPS | PURPOSE |
|---|---|
| 10. Remove the tubes from the centrifuge and read the results; instructions are printed on the device. Results should be within 5% of each other. Take the average and report as a percentage. | Results with greater than 5% variation have been found to offer unreliable results. |
| 11. Dispose of the contaminated supplies into a biohazard waste receptacle according to office policy and procedure. Clean the work area with surface disinfectant. Dispose of equipment and supplies appropriately. Remove gloves and wash your hands. | Supplies that are contaminated with blood should be disposed of properly. Maintaining a clean work space limits exposure to biohazards. |

*(continues on page 1110)*

# PROCEDURE 42-2 (continued)

| STEPS | PURPOSE |
|---|---|
| 12. **AFF** Log into the electronic medical record (EMR) using your username and secure password OR obtain the paper medical record from a secure location and assure it is kept away from public access. Record the procedure noting the date, time, site of the venipuncture, test results for CLIA-waived POC procedures or the name of the lab where the specimen was sent, and your name. | The integrity of the medical record must be maintained at all times to protect patient privacy. Procedures are considered not to have been performed if they are not recorded. |
| 13. When finished, log out of the EMR and/or replace the paper medical record in an appropriate and secure location. | |

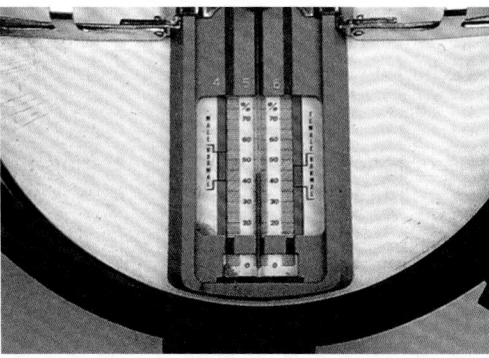

**Step 9:** Read results from the centrifuge reading device.

*Note:* Some microhematocrit centrifuges have the scale printed in the machine at the radial grooves.

---

**Charting Example**
*03/28/2016 4:20 PM Capillary puncture, left ring finger. Hct: 42%. Dr. notified of results*
_____ *M. Mays, CMA*

---

Note: *The medical assistant may sign his or her name in the patient record using only the "CMA" credential if the office has a signature log denoting the entire credential as "CMA(AAMA)."*

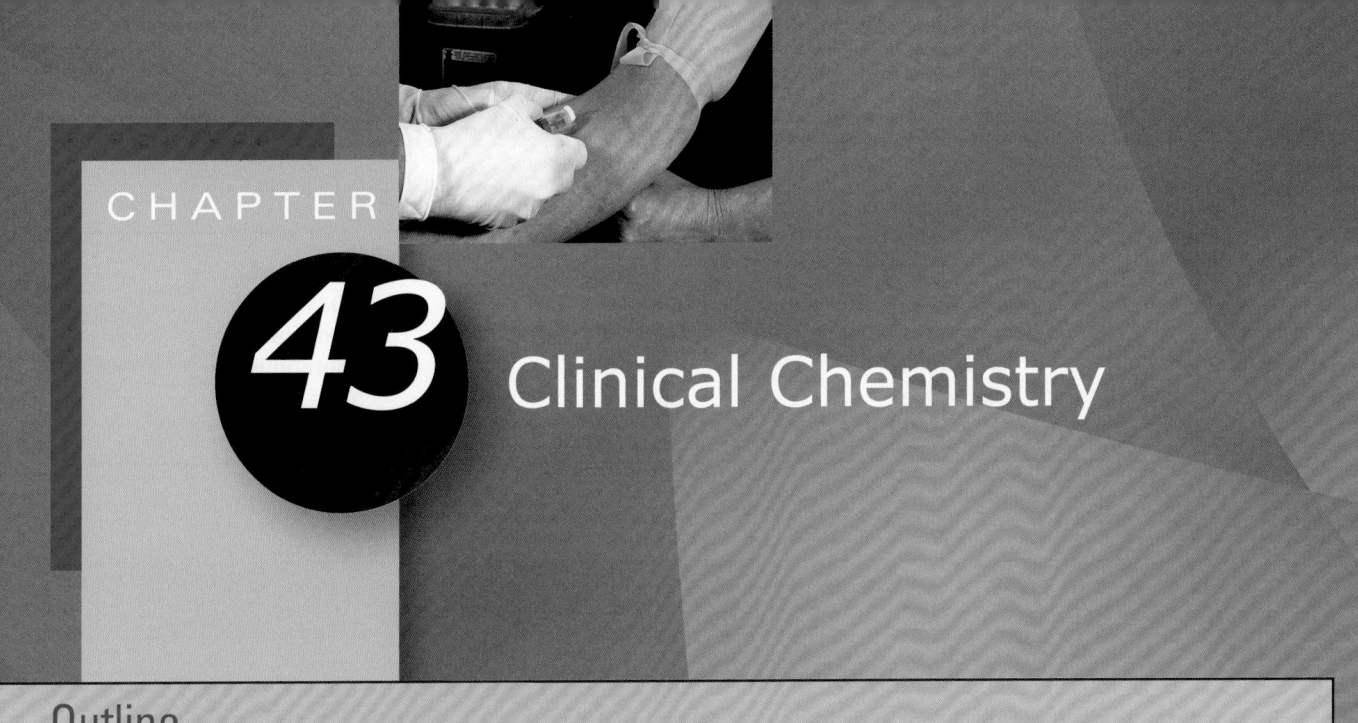

# CHAPTER 43

# Clinical Chemistry

## Outline

**Introduction to Clinical Chemistry**
Electrolytes
Nonprotein Nitrogenous Compounds

Acid–base Balance
Liver Function Tests
Thyroid Function

Cardiac Function
Pancreatic Function

## Learning Outcomes

### COG Cognitive Domain*

1. Spell key terms
2. *Define medical terms and abbreviations related to all body systems*
3. List the common electrolytes and explain the relationship of electrolytes to acid–base balance
4. Describe the nonprotein nitrogenous compounds and name conditions with abnormal values
5. *Identify CLIA-waived tests associated with common diseases*
6. *Analyze health care results as reported in graphs and tables*
7. List and describe the substances commonly tested in liver function assessment
8. Describe glucose use and regulation and the purpose of the various glucose tests
9. Describe the function of cholesterol and other lipids and their correlation to heart disease

### PSY Psychomotor Domain*

1. Perform blood glucose testing (Procedure 43-1)
   a. Obtain specimens and perform CLIA-waived chemistry testing
   b. Instruct and prepare a patient for a procedure or treatment
   c. Coach patients appropriately considering cultural diversity, developmental life stage, and communication barriers
   d. Document patient care accurately in the medical record

2. *Perform blood cholesterol testing (Procedure 43-2)*
   a. *Obtain specimens and perform CLIA-waived chemistry testing*
   b. *Instruct and prepare a patient for a procedure or treatment*
   c. *Coach patients appropriately considering cultural diversity, developmental life stage, and communication barriers*
   d. *Document patient care accurately in the medical record*

### AFF Affective Domain*

1. *Distinguish between normal and abnormal test results*

*\*Note: AAMA/CAAHEP 2015 Standards are italicized.*

### ABHES Competencies

1. *Incorporate critical thinking skills when performing patient assessment*
2. *Incorporate critical thinking skills when performing patient care*
3. *Show awareness of a patient's concerns related to the procedure being performed*
4. *Demonstrate empathy, active listening, and nonverbal communication*
5. *Demonstrate respect for individual diversity including gender, race, religion, age, economic status, and appearance*
6. *Explain to a patient the rationale for performance of a procedure*
7. *Demonstrate sensitivity to patient rights*
8. *Protect the integrity of the medical record*

## Key Terms

| | | | |
|---|---|---|---|
| acidosis | bicarbonate | electrolyte balance | jaundiced |
| alkalosis | bile | endocrine | lipase |
| amylase | buffer systems | enzyme | lipoproteins |
| atherosclerosis | creatinine | exocrine | metabolism |
| azotemia | electrolyte | ions | urea |

## Case Study

*T*he internal medicine office at Great Falls Medical Center has four physicians, one nurse practitioner, and a physician assistant. Amy Albers, CMA (AAMA), works for Dr. Schroeder, who has many elderly established patients who come to the office frequently for chronic health conditions such as diabetes. Today, the physician has ordered blood tests including uric acid for a middle-aged female patient who came in complaining of pain in her right big toe, which the doctor indicated could be gout. Another 77-year-old male patient with kidney disease takes a "water pill," or diuretic, daily and has come into the office today for a checkup. The physician has ordered electrolytes on this patient. How does uric acid affect joints like the one in the big toe, and is this substance made by the body? What are electrolytes and how are these affected by a diuretic? These and other questions will be addressed in this chapter.

## INTRODUCTION TO CLINICAL CHEMISTRY

While there are many chemicals found in the environment, body tissues and fluids also contain chemicals for normal functioning. Clinical chemistry is the science of using the chemical analysis of body fluids to obtain information about the clinical condition of the body. In addition to proteins, liver enzymes and lipids, or fats, other chemicals found in body fluids include electrically charged chemicals called **ions**, which include potassium ($K^+$), sodium ($Na^+$), and chlorine ($Cl^-$). As noted in Figure 43-1, chemicals are represented by an abbreviation that is the first 1 or 2 letters of the chemical name. The first letter is capitalized and ions have a superscript after the abbreviation, noting the type of electrical charge, positive or negative. Many of the chemicals have a Latin name, so the abbreviation may not be obvious to the name of the chemical in English. For example, natrium is the Latin word for sodium; hence, the abbreviation for sodium is Na and kalium is the Latin word for potassium that is abbreviated K. Not all chemicals on the periodic table of elements are found in the body; however, those that are important for good health can be measured in the blood or other body fluids and can assist the physician to assess organ function and understand the patient's health status.

In addition to chemicals, other substances that are measured or analyzed in the clinical chemistry lab include glucose, cholesterol, uric acid, creatinine, and ammonia. Only a few specific chemistry tests are CLIA-waived and may be performed in the physician's office laboratory (POL). However, specimen collection, processing specimens for transport to the laboratory, obtaining and reporting results, and follow-up of the patient as instructed by the physician are the responsibilities of the medical assistant. Because laboratories may use different analyzers and reagents, normal ranges for chemistry tests may vary from laboratory to laboratory. Chemistry tests may be ordered by the physician individually or grouped according to body system referred to as *panels* or *profiles*.

A summary of the common chemistry tests is presented in Table 43-1.

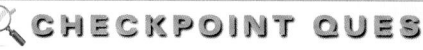 **CHECKPOINT QUESTION**

1. What is meant by clinical chemistry?

## Periodic Table

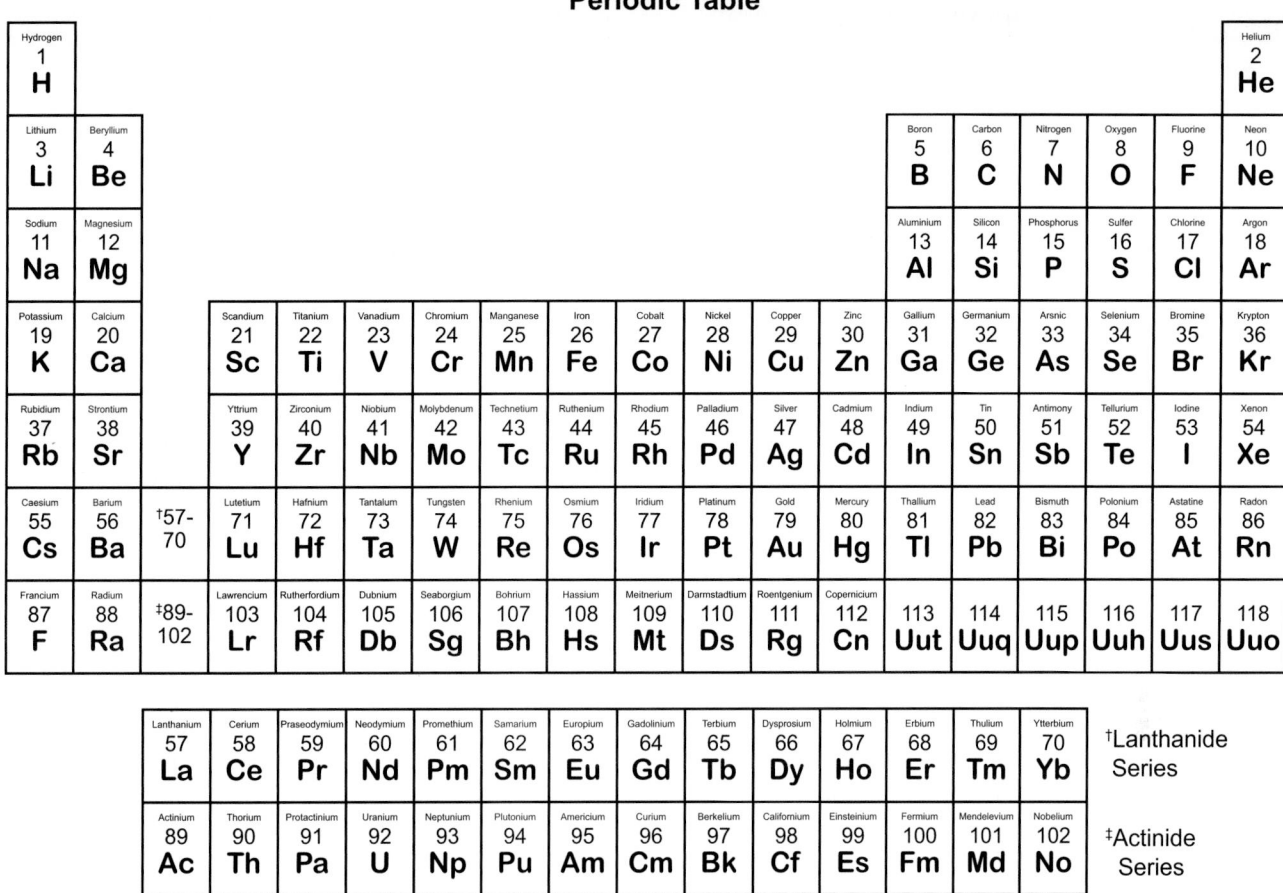

**Figure 43-1** • The periodic table of elements.

## Electrolytes

**Electrolytes** refer to any substance in the body containing ions, or chemicals that have an electrical charge. The body requires electricity to maintain many body functions including fluid balance, acid–base balance, and proper functioning of the cardiovascular and nervous systems. These substances are found in all body fluids, and if the levels are too low or too high, the patient may experience serious health issues including muscle weakness and death.

The kidneys play a major role in **electrolyte balance**, or keeping electrolytes at the right levels in the body. As the body moves electrolytes through the bloodstream, the blood flows through the kidneys, which remove waste products along with any excess electrolytes. When the kidneys cannot keep the electrolytes stable, disease develops. Conditions that can destabilize electrolytes include dehydration, certain medications, and the presence of heart, kidney, or liver disorders.

## Sodium

Water and various electrolytes are found both inside and outside all cells in the body. Sodium is the major electrolyte found in the water outside the cell in amounts that depend on how much water or fluids are consumed by the patient, how much water the kidneys allow into the urine, and the overall health status of the kidneys. Because sodium is the major electrolyte outside the cell, it causes the most problems when the level is not stable. *Hyponatremia* is the term when the sodium level is too low. Hyponatremia can result from vomiting, diarrhea, burns, and some medications such as diuretics. Symptoms of hyponatremia include headache, confusion, seizures, and muscle cramps. *Hypernatremia* is the term to describe a high sodium level in the blood. An elevated sodium level can result from factors such as too much sodium in the diet or not drinking an adequate amount of fluids, resulting in dehydration. Table salt, a source of dietary sodium, is made up of sodium and chloride (NaCl) and should be used sparingly, especially if the patient has an underlying heart condition such as congestive heart failure. When the body senses hypernatremia, healthy kidneys retain water to dilute the sodium in the body, which may result in edema of tissues and extra work for the heart.

The normal serum or blood levels of sodium are 135 to 145 milliequivalents per liter of blood (mEq/L). Some laboratories may indicate that the normal level is

| TABLE 43-1 | Common Chemistry Tests | | | |
|---|---|---|---|---|
| **Test** | **Body Function** | **Normal Values** | **Causes of Increase** | **Causes of Decrease** |
| BUN | Metabolic byproduct | 6–20 mg/dL | Kidney disease, kidney obstruction, dehydration | Liver failure, malnutrition |
| Calcium | Structural element for bones, teeth, muscles | 8.5–10.2 mg/dL | Hyperparathyroidism, hyperthyroidism, Addison disease, bone cancer, multiple myeloma, other malignancies | Hypoparathyroidism, renal failure |
| Chloride | Acid–base balance, component of stomach acid | 96–106 mEq/L | Dehydration, Cushing syndrome, hyperventilation | Severe vomiting, diarrhea, severe burns, pyloric obstruction, heat exhaustion |
| Cholesterol | Building block for cell membranes, steroid hormones, bile acids | <200 mg/dL | Atherosclerosis, heart disease, certain liver diseases with obstruction, hypothyroidism | Liver disease, hyperthyroidism, malabsorption syndrome |
| Creatinine | Metabolic byproduct | Men: 0.7–1.3 mg/dL Women: 0.6–1.1 mg/dL | Kidney disease, muscle disease | Muscular dystrophy |
| Glucose (fasting) | Energy source | FBS: 70–100 mg/dL Random: <125 mg/dL | Diabetes mellitus, Cushing syndrome, liver disease | Excessive insulin, Addison disease, bacterial sepsis, hypothyroidism |
| Phosphorus | Used in bone, endocrine processes | 2.4–4.1 mg/dL | Renal disease, hypoparathyroidism, hypocalcemia, Addison disease | Hyperparathyroidism, bone disease |
| Potassium | Acid–base balance | 3.5–5.2 mEq/L | Kidney disease, cell damage, Addison disease | Diarrhea, starvation, severe vomiting, severe burns, some liver diseases |
| Sodium | Fluid balance | 135–145 mEq/L | Dehydration, Cushing syndrome, diabetes insipidus | Severe burns, diarrhea, vomiting, Addison disease |
| Triglycerides | Energy source; lipid deposits for stored energy, organ support | <150 mg/dL | Atherosclerosis, liver disease, poorly controlled diabetes, pancreatitis | Malnutrition |
| Uric acid | Metabolic byproduct | 3.5–7.2 mg/dL | Renal failure, gout, leukemia, eclampsia | Drug therapy to lower uric acid levels |

135 to 145 millimoles per liter of blood (mmol/L), an international standard of measurement. Always report the results to the physician according to the measurement used by the laboratory. Table 43-2 lists the normal reference ranges for sodium in blood and urine.

| TABLE 43-2 | Reference Ranges for Sodium |
|---|---|
| **Measure** | **Range** |
| Serum, plasma | 135–145 mEq/L |
| 24-hour urine | 40–220 mEq/day , varies with diet |

## Potassium

Potassium is the major positive electrolyte *inside* the cell and supports the contraction of skeletal and cardiac muscles. This electrolyte is important in controlling the electrical activity of the heart muscle, building proteins, breaking down carbohydrates for energy, and maintaining acid–base balance. The normal range for a blood potassium is 3.5 mEq/L to 5.2 mEq/L. The condition to describe a potassium level that is too low in the blood is *hypokalemia*, which occurs in patients who take diuretics, overuse laxatives, or have severe or prolonged vomiting or diarrhea. The symptoms of hypokalemia include muscle weakness, fatigue, constipation, and abnormal heart rhythms.

*Hyperkalemia* is the term to describe a potassium level that is too high. The primary causes of hyperkalemia are high blood pressure and poor kidney function. Other factors that increase potassium levels in the blood are severe infections, some heart medications, and potassium-sparing diuretics. Increased blood levels of potassium are also seen in patients who have too much acid in their blood, which causes the potassium to leave the inside of the cells and into the blood. Symptoms of hyperkalemia include muscle weakness or numbness and abnormal and dangerous heart rhythms such as ventricular tachycardia (refer to Chapter 32, Cardiology).

One factor that will result in a false high potassium level is poor venipuncture techniques. Venipuncture techniques that cause red blood cells (RBCs) to lyse result in falsely elevated potassium levels. Those venipuncture techniques that cause lysis include a traumatic venipuncture (i.e., "fishing" for a vein after the needle is inserted into the skin) or inappropriate use of the tourniquet (i.e., it is left on the arm too long or applied too tightly). Symptoms of hyperkalemia are muscle weakness, numbness, mental confusion, and cardiac arrhythmias.

## Chloride

To produce and carry electricity in the body, electrolytes have either positive charges or negative charges. Chloride is the major electrolyte *outside* the cell that carries a negative charge. This electrolyte plays a major role in maintaining the acid–base, or alkaline, balance in the body. The normal range for chloride blood levels is 96 to 106 mEq/L. A chloride level that is lower than 96 mEq/L is known as *hypocholemia* and may occur in patients with severe burns, congestive heart failure, dehydration, or excessive vomiting. A patient in *metabolic alkalosis* will also have hypochloremia (refer to section on "Acid–base Balance").

*Hyperchloremia* is the term used to describe a chloride level that is higher than 106 mEq/L. Conditions that may cause an elevated blood chloride level include diarrhea, *metabolic acidosis*, renal disease, and some medications such as carbonic anhydrase inhibitors used to treat glaucoma. Although the body works very hard to maintain stability (also known as homeostasis), many factors affect the level of electrolytes such as chloride, which can also affect other body systems.

## Bicarbonate

Bicarbonate ($HCO_3^-$) is an electrolyte with a negative charge that is formed with carbon dioxide ($CO_2$) dissolved in the blood. This is the most important electrolyte used to maintain acid–base balance in the body including the pH (percentage of hydrogen) in the blood (Fig. 43-2). The amount of $CO_2$ in the blood is an indicator of the blood bicarbonate level and is the laboratory

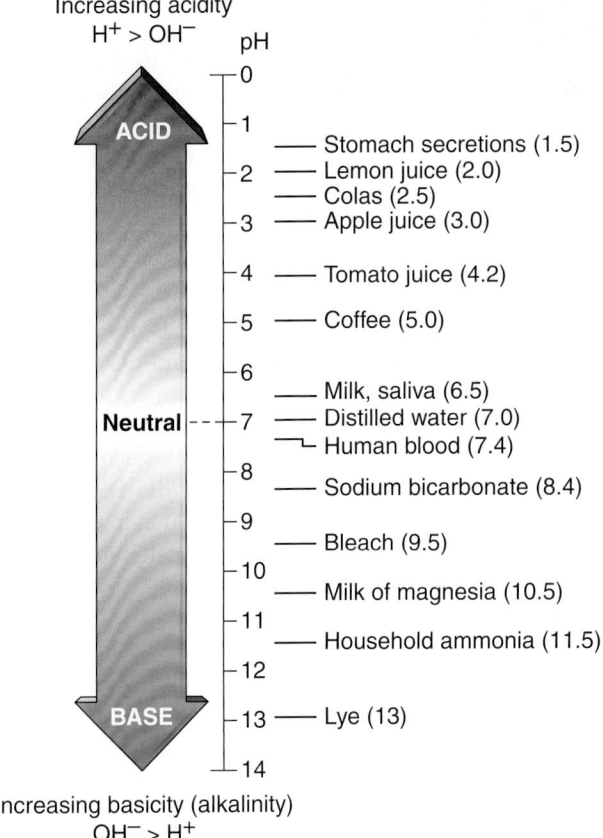

**Figure 43-2 •** The pH scale. Degree of acidity or alkalinity is shown in pH units. This scale also shows the pH of some common substances.

test used to measure this electrolyte. Normal blood carbon dioxide levels are 23 to 29 mEq/L, maintaining a blood pH range in the neutral range from 7.35 to 7.45. Refer to the section in this chapter "Acid–Base Balance" for more information on acid–base balance and pH levels of body fluids.

## Magnesium

Magnesium (Mg) is a mineral that is frequently found in the environment and the diet. Although magnesium dietary supplements are available over the counter, many foods including foods high in fiber contain magnesium. In the body, this electrolyte is found primarily *inside* the cell, and it carries a positive charge ($Mg^+$). Magnesium is necessary for bone development and strength, but is also necessary for proper functioning of nerves and muscles. Some laxatives and antacids contain magnesium because it is also used by the body naturally to neutralize stomach acids.

Serum magnesium levels range from 1.7 to 2.2 mg/dL. When the serum magnesium level is lower than normal, the condition is called *hypomagnesemia*. Decreased levels of magnesium may occur in patients with alcoholism, liver disease, pancreatitis, chronic diarrhea, ulcerative colitis, or toxemia in pregnancy (see Chapter 36, Obstetrics and Gynecology).

*Hypermagnesemia* is the term used to describe the condition when serum magnesium levels are higher than normal. The cause of hypermagnesemia is poor excretion due to kidney failure. Early symptoms of hypermagnesemia are low blood pressure, irregular heartbeat, nausea, vomiting, and fatigue.

## Calcium

Serum magnesium and calcium levels in the body are often related, carry positive charges, and play a part in teeth and bone health, nervous system function, and cardiac function. Most calcium in the body is stored in the bones, but blood levels, also known as serum calcium ($Ca^+$) levels, range from 8.5 to 10.2 mg/dL. Serum levels of calcium depend on the amount of calcium consumed in the diet, the intestinal absorption of calcium and vitamin D, and hormones such as calcitonin, a parathyroid hormone, and estrogen.

Again, *hypo* and *hyper* designate low and high calcium levels, respectively. Symptoms of a low serum calcium level, or *hypocalcemia*, include muscle cramps, twitching, tingling of the fingers or around the mouth, and cardiac arrhythmias. Causes of hypocalcemia include kidney failure, liver disease, low magnesium levels, vitamin D deficiencies, and pancreatitis. *Hypercalcemia*, an elevated calcium level, is primarily due to hyperparathyroidism or malignancies, but may also be caused by too much calcium or vitamin D in the diet, certain infections, and some medications such as lithium, tamoxifen, and thiazides. Symptoms of hypercalcemia include weakness, nausea and vomiting, constipation, and bone pain.

## Phosphorus

Phosphorus, or inorganic phosphate ($PO_4^-$), is the major negative electrolyte inside the cell. Like calcium, most of the phosphorus in the body is found in the bones, but some blood phosphorus is needed for nerve function and building genetic material. Normal serum phosphorus blood levels range from 2.4 to 4.1 mg/dL. Serum phosphorus and calcium levels are closely related, and when one is elevated, the other is decreased. A serum level that is lower than 4.1 is referred to as *hypophosphatemia* and may be caused by malnutrition, alcoholism, hypercalcemia, hyperparathyroidism, and a decreased intake of vitamin D in the diet.

*Hyperphosphatemia* may occur when the patient has hypocalcemia, hypoparathyroidism, kidney disease, too much vitamin D or phosphate in the diet, and overuse of some medications such as phosphate-containing laxatives. Although the symptoms of a low or high phosphorus level are associated with the abnormal calcium levels, an elevated phosphorus level may lead to cardiovascular disease and osteoporosis.

2. Which electrolyte has a positive charge and is important in controlling the electrical activity of the heart muscle, building proteins, breaking down carbohydrates for energy, and maintaining acid–base balance?

## **LOG** Nonprotein Nitrogenous Compounds

There are about 15 nonprotein nitrogenous (NPN) compounds in the body, but the blood levels of the three are commonly ordered by physicians to evaluate kidney function. The three nonprotein nitrogenous compounds include **urea**, **creatinine**, and **uric acid**. Each of these is described in more detail below.

### Urea

As protein is metabolized by the body, the waste products nitrogen and urea are produced and released into the blood. Although most of these waste products, known as blood urea nitrogen or BUN, are filtered by the kidneys and excreted in the urine, a certain amount remains in the blood. Measuring the blood urea nitrogen (BUN) is important to determine the filtering ability of the kidneys, and this blood test is often ordered by the physician to determine kidney function.

The normal range for blood urea nitrogen (BUN) is 6 to 20 mg/dL. Poor kidney function results in the body retaining urea nitrogen and an elevated BUN.

### Creatinine

The chemical creatinine is a waste product from the breakdown of creatine, a substance made by the body to supply energy to muscles. Like urea, creatinine is filtered out of the blood by the kidneys and increases in the blood if kidney function is decreased. Both the BUN and creatinine are used to assess kidney function; however, the creatinine level is more specific than a BUN for assessing kidney function and is ordered by the physician to determine the severity of kidney damage and to monitor the progression of kidney disease. Daily excretion of creatinine is fairly stable, and the normal range for creatinine in the blood is 0.6 to 1.3. The results may be lower in women because of the difference in muscle mass between women and men. **Azotemia** is the buildup of urea and creatinine in the blood, which may result in damage to kidneys and decrease in their inability to function normally.

When the kidneys are healthy, urinary excretion of creatinine is the same as the amount produced by the body. A healthy kidney filters creatinine to keep its secretion equal to its production. A test called *creatinine clearance* measures this filtering ability. To calculate the ability of the body to get rid of a substance requires measuring how much of the substance is removed in a given time frame. Measuring a creatinine clearance involves measuring the clearance of creatinine from urine in a 24-hour time period. To do this, urine must be collected over a 24-hour period, known as a 24-hour urine sample, because the excretion of creatinine varies throughout the day. A blood specimen for creatinine is also drawn during the 24-hour period that measures how much creatinine was cleared during the 24 hours. Arranging the collection of urine for 24 hours *and* collecting a blood specimen during the urine collection are critical to the completion of this test.

## CHECKPOINT QUESTION

3. Amy Albers, the CMA (AAMA) in the case study, is taking blood for a BUN and creatinine on an elderly woman who has diabetes. Why did the physician order these tests on this patient?

## Uric Acid

Uric acid is another nonprotein nitrogenous compound produced as a waste product from the breakdown of purine, a substance found in certain foods. Like urea and creatinine, uric acid is excreted in the urine. Although blood levels may be affected by kidney function, elevated levels of uric acid in the blood are more significant than low levels and usually result from a diet high in purine. Foods that contain purine include organ meats such as liver, dried beans and peas, gravies, and anchovies. Other causes for elevated uric acid levels include the use of certain drugs such as diuretics and immunosuppressant medications, obesity, renal disease, alcohol use, and genetics.

The normal blood uric acid ranges from 3.5 to 7.2 mg/dL, and elevated levels may cause uric acid crystals to form in certain body areas such as the kidneys and joints. If crystals form in the kidneys, the patient may suffer from kidney stones, and if the crystals form in the joints, the condition is called *gout* (Fig. 43-3).

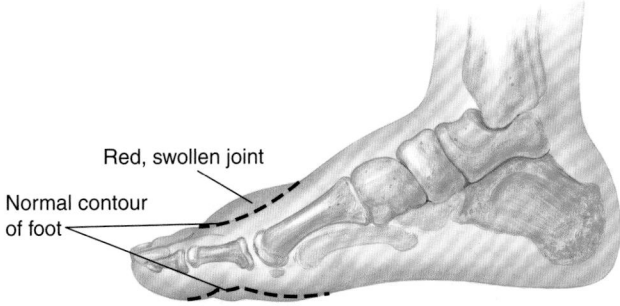

Red, swollen joint

Normal contour of foot

**Figure 43-3** • Gout of the foot.

Blood levels of uric acid are typically ordered by the physician to confirm a diagnosis and monitor treatment of gout, to assist in the diagnosis of kidney stones, and to detect kidney disease.

## Ammonia

As proteins are broken down in the intestines, ammonia ($NH_3$) is produced and is then converted to urea in the liver for excretion by the kidneys. Because the liver is essential in converting ammonia to urea, an ammonia blood level may be ordered by the physician to check liver function. However, ammonia is also part of the acid–base balance and may be ordered to diagnose metabolic alkalosis in which ammonia levels will be elevated. The normal range for blood ammonia is 15 to 45 mcg/dL, and if elevated, the condition is known as hyperammonemia. Causes of hyperammonemia include severe liver disease, Reye syndrome (see Chapter 38, Pediatrics), congestive heart failure, severe gastrointestinal bleeding, and metabolic alkalosis. High blood ammonia levels are neurotoxic and are often associated with encephalopathy, causing symptoms such as confusion and extreme lethargy.

Low blood ammonia levels are not as serious and may be seen in certain types of hypertension or some types of antibiotics.

## CHECKPOINT QUESTION

4. What are the three primary NPN compounds?

### WHAT IF?

**What if a patient is diagnosed with gout and asks you about dietary restrictions?**

Always speak to the physician to determine whether the patient has any other medical conditions that warrant a special diet. Most patients with gout are prescribed a diet low in foods containing purine. Foods that are high in purine include liver, kidneys, sardines, and anchovies. Diet and medications such as allopurinol and nonsteroidal anti-inflammatory medications (NSAIDs) can often keep gout under control.

## Acid–Base Balance

Body fluids including blood require stability of the acid and alkaline products produced by the body to promote adequate organ and body system function. The ability of the body to maintain this balance between acidity and alkalinity is referred to as acid–base balance. When the levels of the electrolytes carrying *positive* charges rise, so does the body's *alkalinity*. These ions can come from increased intake of acid foods and beverages or from decreased elimination in the urine. When the levels of the electrolytes carrying *negative* charges rise, so does the body's *acidity*. When acidity goes up, alkalinity comes down. When alkalinity goes up, acidity goes down. Because the acid levels and base levels are dependent on **metabolism**, imbalances show up when an organ or body system is not functioning well.

There are several mechanisms used by the body to control the acid–base balance. The first mechanism is the lungs and respiratory system. Blood picks up carbon dioxide waste, which is taken to the lungs to be exhaled. While in the blood, carbon dioxide is primarily bicarbonate, an alkaline product; however, part of the $CO_2$ gas is dissolved to become carbonic acid. As the carbonic acid increases in the blood, the pH of the blood lowers, causing the blood to become acidic. To control the $CO_2$ levels and decrease acidity of the blood, the brain increases the rate and depth of respirations, causing more $CO_2$ to be exhaled, resulting in the blood being less acidic. Likewise, the kidneys play a role in acid–base balance by filtering and excreting positive and negative ions (acids and bases) in the urine.

## Buffer Systems

While the lungs may change the pH of the blood rapidly, the kidneys change the pH slowly. The body manages the changes using a **buffer system**, which keeps the changes balanced. In addition to regular acids and bases that are produced by the body and are primary to acid–base balance, the body has other weak acids and weak bases that may be produced and used to maintain a neutral pH using carbon dioxide. The majority of carbon dioxide in the blood is made into bicarbonate, a weak base, but a small portion of the dissolved carbon dioxide gas becomes carbonic acid, a weak acid. Ideally, the body maintains a balance using bicarbonate and carbonic acid to keep the blood pH stable between 7.35 and 7.45. If everything is functioning normally, balance is maintained. But, when either the acid or the alkaline balance is out of balance, the pH of the blood is affected either becoming too acidic (**acidosis**) or too alkaline (**alkalosis**). In acidosis, the blood pH falls below 7.35 when there is either too much acid in the blood or too little alkaline products. Alkalosis results when the blood pH rises above 7.45 and is caused by too much alkaline products or too little acid in the blood.

Both acidosis and alkalosis indicate a serious problem and result in death if left untreated (Fig. 43-4). While the outcome may be the same, there are two types of acidosis and two types of alkalosis, *metabolic* or *respiratory* depending on the cause of the acidosis or alkalosis. The cause of metabolic acidosis may be caused by several factors including renal disease or failure when the kidneys are not able to filter wastes including acid from the urine effectively. In metabolic acidosis, the

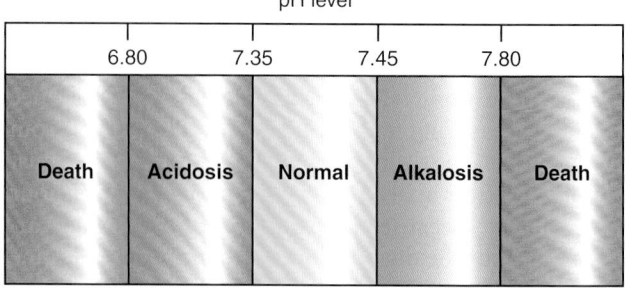

pH level

**Figure 43-4** • Acid–base balance. Note that acidosis is used to describe the condition when the pH falls below 7.35, and alkalosis describes a pH above 7.45. When the normal pH is exceeded in either direction, death can occur.

lungs cannot work quickly enough to produce bicarbonate to neutralize the acidosis coming from the kidneys. Other causes include poisoning from ethylene glycol, commonly found in antifreeze products, an overdose of medications that include salicylates such as aspirin, an increase in ketones in the blood from uncontrolled diabetes (also known as diabetic acidosis), and exercise (also known as lactic acidosis). Respiratory acidosis is a buildup of acid in the blood due to the inability of the body to remove $CO_2$ through adequate breathing. Causes of respiratory acidosis include chronic lung disease such as emphysema, chest injuries, and the overuse of sedative drugs that decrease respiratory effort.

Metabolic alkalosis is caused by too much bicarbonate in the blood that may be caused by the ingestion of sodium bicarbonate to relieve indigestion; an extreme loss of chloride due to vomiting, which removes hydrochloric acid; or a loss of potassium as seen in patients who may be taking diuretics. Respiratory alkalosis results from a decrease in $CO_2$ in the blood due to fever, lack of oxygen, and lung disease or conditions that increase the respiratory rate causing hyperventilation and excessive removal of $CO_2$ from the lungs.

## 🔍 CHECKPOINT QUESTION

5. What type of acid–base balance issue results from renal failure and what type is caused by vomiting?

The respiratory causes for acidosis and alkalosis are breathing disorders.

## Liver Function Tests

The liver is the largest organ in the body and has several important functions. First, the liver takes nutrients from the digestive system, processes them, stores the processed nutrients, and sends them to different parts of the body in the right form and quantity. It also regulates the level of sugars (glucose), protein, and fat entering

| TABLE 43-3 | Nonhepatic Sources of Abnormalities for Select Laboratory Tests |
|---|---|
| **Test** | **Nonhepatic Source** |
| Bilirubin | RBCs (e.g., hemolysis, intra-abdominal bleed, hematoma) |
| AST | Skeletal muscle, cardiac muscle |
| LDH | Heart, RBCs |
| ALP | Bone, first-trimester placenta, kidneys, intestines |

the blood. **Bile** and cholesterol are produced in the liver as well as substances to assist with blood clotting. Most importantly, the liver removes ammonia, bilirubin, and other toxins from the blood.

When the physician is interested in checking the overall function of the liver, a combination of tests may be ordered, sometimes referred to as liver function tests or LFTs. Liver function tests include the following:

- Bilirubin
- AST (aspartate aminotransferase)
- ALT (alanine aminotransferase)
- ALP (alkaline phosphatase)
- LD (lactate dehydrogenase)

One abnormal test result can cause a concern about the patient's liver function, but there are other causes besides the liver that can make these same test results abnormal. Some examples of causes for various liver function tests besides liver abnormalities are listed in Table 43-3. When several of the liver test results are out of the normal range, the source of the abnormal results becomes the liver.

An **enzyme** is a protein produced by living cells that speeds up chemical reactions. The liver has many enzymes including AST, ALT, ALP, and LD. ALT and AST are two of the most useful measures of liver function although elevated AST levels may also be seen in acute muscle injury. ALP is present in the bones, liver, intestines, kidneys, and placenta; however, blood levels of ALP come primarily from the liver and bone. Levels of ALP rise in bone and liver disorders such as bile duct obstruction and primary biliary cirrhosis.

Another enzyme, gamma glutamyl transpeptidase (GGT), is produced in the bile ducts and is usually elevated in bile duct illness. Certain drugs and alcohol use may also cause increased levels of GGT.

Because reference ranges for enzyme tests are the most sensitive to deviation among laboratories, always compare the results with the reference intervals (RIs) from the specific laboratory that performed the test. The reference intervals for the specific laboratory will be listed on the result report.

### CHECKPOINT QUESTION

6. What are the five primary liver function tests?

### Bilirubin

Bilirubin is produced by the normal breakdown of hemoglobin. As the liver and spleen remove old RBCs from the blood, these cells break down and hemoglobin is released. Bilirubin is formed as the hemoglobin breaks down and travels to the liver where the liver extracts the bilirubin and *conjugates* it, or combines it with specific types of sugars making it water soluble. The conjugated bilirubin is excreted into the bile where it moves to the intestines and is eliminated. This happens so quickly that the amount of conjugated bilirubin that stays in the blood is a small amount. Conjugated bilirubin may be referred to as a *direct bilirubin*, and if it is increased in the blood, it is due to liver disease. Conjugated bilirubin is the only form of bilirubin that can appear in urine, so finding a positive urine bilirubin result is also due to liver disease. Bilirubin is yellow–orange in color, and if an excess amount in the blood settles into the skin and sclera, it makes these tissues appear yellow, also known as **jaundiced**.

The laboratory can also measure *unconjugated bilirubin*, or bilirubin that has not been combined with certain sugars. This test may be referred to as an *indirect bilirubin* and is useful when all the liver test results are normal except the total bilirubin. When the total bilirubin level is elevated and more than 90% is unconjugated, liver disease is not indicated.

### CHECKPOINT QUESTION

7. What are the two types of bilirubin measured in the laboratory, and which one indicates liver disease?

### Cholesterol

Cholesterol is a substance produced in the liver and cells of all animals and is oil based with a waxy appearance. The function of cholesterol includes adding to the makeup of cell membranes and myelin sheath surrounding neurons, contributing to the digestive bile acids in the intestines, and assisting with the production of certain hormones such as estrogen, testosterone, cortisone, and aldosterone. Although the body produces an adequate amount of cholesterol necessary for good health, consumption of animal products increases the amount of cholesterol found in the body because cholesterol is produced by all animals and is found in their cells.

Because blood is water based, cholesterol must be carried in the blood by a special type of protein called a **lipoprotein**. These lipoproteins are further divided into 2 types: high-density lipoproteins (HDL) and low-density lipoproteins (LDL). The high-density lipoproteins carry cholesterol away from cells and back to the liver to be excreted in the bile. Therefore, HDLs are considered beneficial in reducing the amount of cholesterol in the blood. Low-density lipoproteins transport cholesterol from the liver to the arterial walls, increasing the risk of buildup on the inside of the blood vessels and causing narrowing and blockage. This condition is known as **atherosclerosis** and is a significant factor for heart disease. Although a total blood cholesterol test may be ordered as part of a routine physical examination or to monitor cholesterol-reducing medications, the physician may also want to know the blood levels of HDL and LDL cholesterol also. Triglycerides may also be ordered as these lipid molecules are stored in fat and are also a risk factor in heart disease.

Point-of-care testing instruments provide cholesterol levels on the spot (Figs. 45-7 and 45-8).

## Cholesterol and Lipid Testing

Lipid profiles include the measurement of total cholesterol, high-density lipoproteins, low-density lipoproteins, and triglycerides. The normal total blood cholesterol including HDL and LDL levels is less than 200 mg/dL. Table 43-4 shows the adult reference ranges for total cholesterol, high-density lipoproteins (HDL), low-density lipoproteins (LDL), and triglycerides. Although blood may be collected and sent to a lab for total cholesterol levels, there are point-of-care machines available to test cholesterol in the physician office (Fig. 43-5).

## PATIENT EDUCATION

### Good and *Bad Cholesterol*

There are two main types of cholesterol that affect health:

- **"Bad" cholesterol**: LDLs clog arteries and put patients at risk for heart disease.
- **"Good" cholesterol**: HDLs help remove bad cholesterol from the body.

Controlling diet and getting plenty of exercise are great ways to help get bad cholesterol down and get good cholesterol up. This well-known saying helps remember which is the "bad" or "good" cholesterol: Keep **L**DL **l**ow and keep **H**DL **h**igh.

How do you know if your bad cholesterol is high? Many people don't. *People with high LDL cholesterol usually do not have any symptoms.* That is why it is so important for adults to get a cholesterol screening at least every 5 years.

| TABLE 43-4 | Adult Reference Intervals for Lipids |
|---|---|
| Analyte | Reference Interval |
| Total cholesterol | <200 mg/dL |
| HDL cholesterol | >60 mg/dL |
| LDL cholesterol | <130 mg/dL |
| Triglyceride | <150 mg/dL |

Fasting for 9 to 12 hours before collecting blood and testing for cholesterol is required to obtain dependable results of lipid testing. Encourage the patient to drink water in the time leading up to the test but avoid any other food or beverages including coffee, chewing gum, and breath mints. The physician may have other requirements in addition to fasting including taking or not taking certain medications. Some medications such as birth control pills can increase cholesterol levels. Always check with the physician and the reference laboratory for additional patient instructions or collection procedures.

### CHECKPOINT QUESTION

8. What four tests are included in a lipid panel?

## Thyroid Function

The thyroid gland is a small gland, weighing less than 1 ounce that has two lobes that are joined together by a narrow band of thyroid tissue, known as the *isthmus*. Thyroid cells are the only cells in the body that can absorb iodine, which is necessary to make the hormones triiodothyronine ($T_3$) and thyroxine ($T_4$), or free thyroxine. These hormones regulate metabolism in all cells of the body.

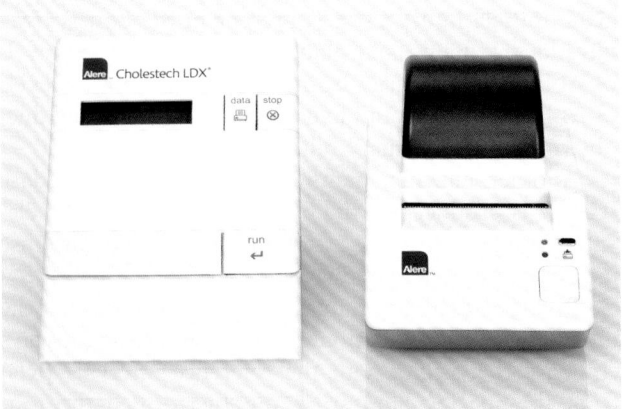

**Figure 43-5** • Alere Cholestech LDX. (Courtesy Alere Inc., Waltham, MA.)

| TABLE 43-5 | Thyroid Function Tests | |
|---|---|---|
| **Test** | **Common Name** | **RI** |
| Serum T$_4$ | T$_4$ | 4.5–11.2 mcg/dL |
| Serum T$_3$ | T$_3$ | 100–200 ng/dL |
| Thyroid-stimulating hormone | TSH | 0.4–4.0 mIU/L |

## Cardiac Function

### Cardiac Markers and Myocardial Infarction

No test is completely sensitive and specific for myocardial infarction (MI), but timing, patient symptoms, laboratory tests, and electrocardiogram results assist in the diagnosis and treatment of someone having an MI. Laboratory tests performed to assist with diagnosing an MI include measuring the blood levels of specific enzymes and proteins found in muscle tissue and released during muscle injury or death. One enzyme, creatine kinase (CK), is found in skeletal and cardiac muscle, and elevated levels do not always indicate myocardial damage. As a result, the physician may order more specific CK enzyme levels known as CKMM fraction, CKMB fraction, and CKBB fraction. The CKMM fraction is present in both cardiac and skeletal muscles, while the CKMB fraction is more specific to the cardiac muscle. The CKBB fraction enzyme is found in the brain, bowel, and bladder muscles and is not routinely measured for cardiac function. The CKMB fraction increases within 3 to 4 hours following an MI and indicates heart involvement when it is ≥6% of the total CK result.

Troponin I and T are proteins contained in cardiac muscle that are released into the bloodstream with myocardial injury. Troponins will begin to rise following MI within 3 to 12 hours. Troponin levels are the best indicator of MI. Myoglobin, a protein found in skeletal and cardiac muscle, is measured to determine the extent of the infarction or death of cardiac muscle. Another protein, C-reactive protein (CRP), is elevated in cases of inflammation, and because the cardiac muscle is inflamed during an MI, the blood levels of CRP may also be tested to diagnose an MI.

Patients with congestive heart failure have an enlarged heart and may have a blood test to determine the severity and prognosis of this condition. B-type natriuretic peptide (BNP) is released from the myocardium in response to excessive stretching of heart muscle cells and is a marker for heart failure. The level of BNP in the blood decreases when the heart failure condition is stable. BNP levels can be elevated even if the patient has no symptoms. BNP levels predict heart failure, atrial fibrillation, and stroke. Waived testing is available to make BNP levels easily available for patient treatment (Fig. 43-7).

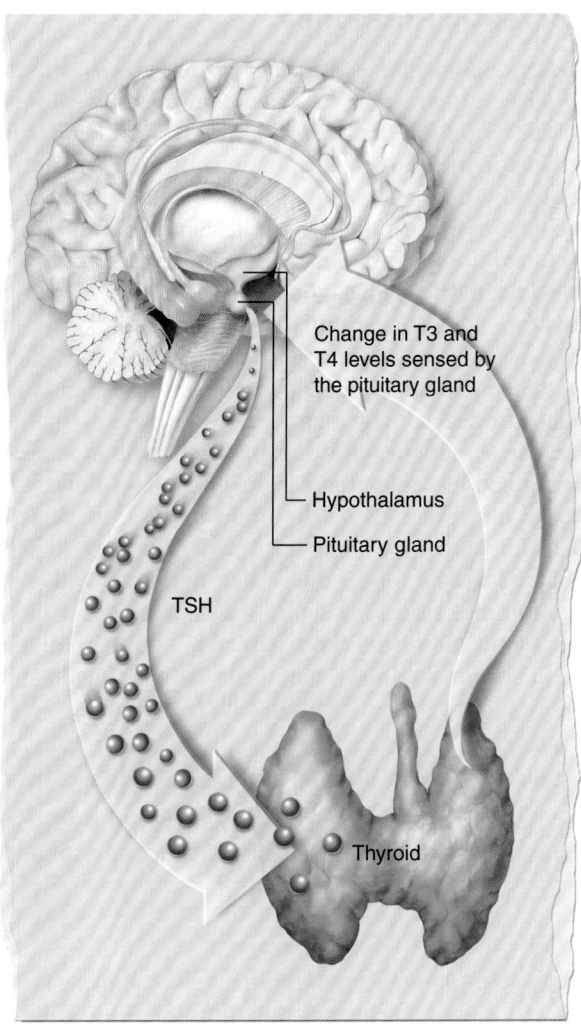

Change in T3 and T4 levels sensed by the pituitary gland

Hypothalamus

Pituitary gland

TSH

Thyroid

**Figure 43-6** • Thyroid-stimulating hormone production.

The thyroid gland is directed by the pituitary gland, a small gland the size of a peanut at the base of the brain. When the levels of T$_3$ and T$_4$ decrease, the pituitary gland is activated to produce and release TSH, or thyroid-stimulating hormone (Fig. 43-6; Fig. 45-2). TSH activates the thyroid gland to manufacture and secrete T$_3$ and T$_4$, which raises the T$_3$ and T$_4$ blood levels. When the pituitary senses that the T$_3$ and T$_4$ are increasing, it stops its TSH production. If the thyroid gland is malfunctioning, it cannot be activated regardless of the amount of TSH secreted. The normal TSH reference range is 0.4 to 4.0 mIU/L (milli-international units per liter). Table 43-5 lists various thyroid function tests and their associated reference intervals.

### CHECKPOINT QUESTION

9. What hormone levels are tested to determine thyroid functioning?

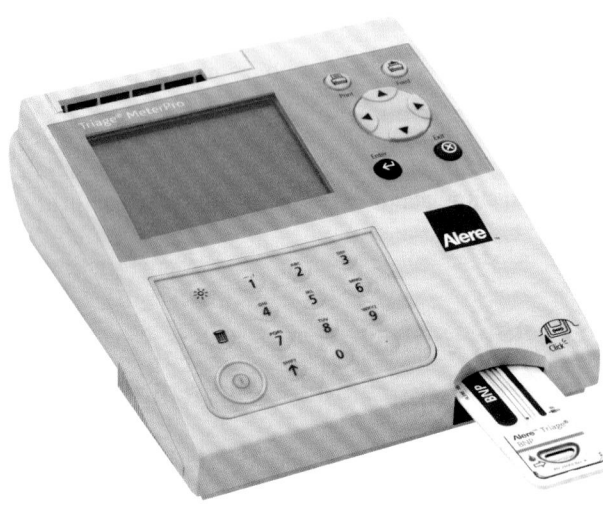

**Figure 43-7** • Alere Triage BNP. Waived testing instrument for measuring B-type natriuretic peptide. (Courtesy Alere Inc., Waltham, MA.)

### CHECKPOINT QUESTION

10. What is the most specific blood test to diagnose an MI?

## Pancreatic Function

### Pancreatic Enzymes

The pancreas is located behind the liver and mostly on the right side of the body. In addition to being an **endocrine** gland and secreting the hormone insulin, the pancreas is an **exocrine** gland. Exocrine glands release enzymes through ducts and include mammary glands, salivary glands, sweat glands, and glands that secrete digestive enzymes into the stomach and intestine such as the pancreas. This gland secretes two major digestive enzymes including **lipase**, which helps in the digestion of fats, and **amylase**, which breaks down starch into sugar.

Pancreatitis is an inflammation of the pancreas caused by an inflammation of the exocrine part of the pancreas. Although 25% of the cases of pancreatitis have no known cause, acute and chronic pancreatitis are often caused by alcohol abuse. Acute pancreatitis may also be caused by gallstones that block the pancreatic ducts, and this type of inflammation has a sudden onset and needs immediate medical intervention. In both types of pancreatitis, the enzymes secreted by the gland begin to digest the pancreas itself, and blood levels of amylase and lipase are elevated. Blood levels of amylase may also be increased in salivary gland diseases because this enzyme is also produced by salivary glands. Lipase levels stay elevated longer than amylase levels in patients with pancreatitis. Normal blood levels of amylase range from 23 to 85 U/L (units per liter), and normal lipase is 0 to 160 U/L.

## Pancreatic Hormones

As an endocrine gland, the *islets of Langerhans, specialized tissue in the pancreas*, make and release hormones into the blood that cause a response from other organs or tissues in the body. There are two hormones made and released by the pancreas that are important in metabolism. The first hormone is insulin, which is responsible for controlling the amount of glucose in the blood. The second hormone is glucagon, which works the opposite of insulin. Glucagon stimulates the liver, muscle, and fat to release stored glucose to make it available for energy.

Diabetes is a condition in which the amount of insulin produced by the pancreas is either low or does not exist. A patient with diabetes will have an elevated blood glucose because there is not enough insulin to take glucose into the cells of the body for use, leaving the glucose in the blood unable to provide energy to cells. Elevated levels of blood glucose left untreated will result in symptoms of thirst, weight loss, damage to the blood vessels, and death (refer to Chapter 37, Endocrinology). Patients control blood glucose levels with medication including hypoglycemic and insulin injections.

### CHECKPOINT QUESTION

11. What are the two hormones secreted by the pancreas that maintain blood glucose stability?

### Blood Glucose Testing

The glucose reflectance photometer (glucose meter) is an accurate, waived machine used to measure a blood glucose level. Glucose meters are sold under several names, including Accu-Chek™, Ascensia™, and OneTouch™, among others (Fig. 43-8). Testing includes application of whole blood from a capillary puncture to a reagent strip, which is read optically by the instrument after a designated time (Procedure 43-1). The amount of color change correlates with glucose concentration, and the value is measured and reported. Each type of blood glucose meter requires proper maintenance and storage. Always follow the manufacturer's

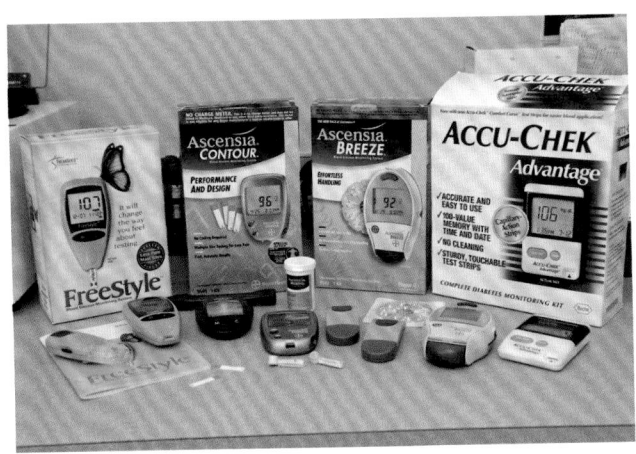

**Figure 43-8** • Various blood glucose monitoring systems.

instructions for using and maintaining the glucose meter. Blood may also be collected and sent to a reference laboratory for blood glucose testing. You should follow the physician order and office policy and procedure when obtaining a blood specimen for blood glucose testing. Although laboratory values may range, a normal blood glucose depends on when the patient last consumed carbohydrates.

The following lists various types of glucose testing that can be ordered by the physician including an explanation of each:

- *Fasting Glucose.* A fasting blood sugar (FBS) level requires the patient to fast 8 to 12 hours to detect either diabetes mellitus or hypoglycemia. The American Diabetes Association's (ADA) cutoff point for normal fasting blood glucose levels is 100 mg/dL. A value of 100 mg/dL or above indicates a diagnosis of prediabetes. Studies indicate that many people in the prediabetic range go on to develop diabetes within 10 years. Further testing by a 2-hour postprandial (PP) glucose test confirms a diagnosis of diabetes (see explanation below). An FBS level of 45 mg/dL confirms a diagnosis of hypoglycemia, or low blood glucose. The normal range for an FBS is 70 to 100 mg/dL. *Random Glucose.* The use of a random glucose level performed without fasting or any other special instructions is typically done for screening and does not result in a diagnosis. A random glucose is just that—done any time and not dependent on fasting or meals. Because the collection time is random, the reference interval varies but should be less than 125 mg/dL.

- *Two-Hour Postprandial Glucose.* A 2-hour postprandial glucose test, or PP glucose test, is diagnostic of diabetes. It is also the tool used to monitor insulin therapy and to screen for diabetes. Timing of the specimen collection is extremely important for this test result. "Good control" of diabetes has been defined as a 2-hour PP value of less than 140 mg/dL.

- *Oral Glucose Tolerance Test.* The ADA does not encourage the use of the glucose tolerance test (GTT) to diagnose diabetes. For those situations in which it is still used, the procedure should begin with effective patient preparation. For 3 days prior to the test, the patient should be mobile and eating a normal to high carbohydrate diet. The patient should fast for 10 to 16 hours prior to starting the test. The GTT should be performed in the morning because of diurnal variations in glucose levels. In preparation for the test and during the test, the patient should not exercise, smoke, or consume anything other than water.

  After an initial fasting blood specimen is collected for testing, the patient is given 100 grams of glucose in a flavored solution. Then, blood glucose levels are checked on a time schedule to determine how the body metabolizes the glucose. Blood is obtained 30 minutes, 1 hour, 2 hours, and 3 hours after the glucose has been consumed. Blood samples must be drawn on time. Urine specimens may also be

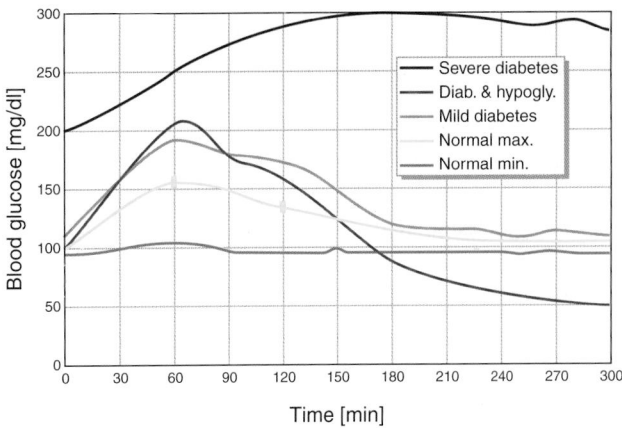

**Figure 43-9 •** GTT graphs by disease severity.

collected on the same timetable. Numerous methods are used to interpret the values obtained from a GTT. The criteria proposed by the National Diabetes Data Group and the World Health Organization and endorsed by the ADA recommend a diagnosis of diabetes if the fasting glucose level is greater than 110 mg/dL and the 2-hour measurement is equal to or above 155 mg/dL. See Figure 43-9 for a graph of various glucose tolerance responses.

- *Glucose Tolerance Testing in Obstetric Patients.* A lack of glucose tolerance has been frequently noted among pregnant patients in the second and third trimesters. This lack of glucose tolerance is called *gestational diabetes*, and because it endangers the life of the fetus and the mother, the pregnant patient's glucose level must be monitored. The screening method used for this type of diabetes is to have the patient consume a 50-g glucose liquid and draw blood 1 hour later. If the value exceeds 155 mg/dL, a GTT is indicated for a diagnosis of gestational diabetes. This screen is usually done during the second trimester.

- *Hemoglobin A1C.* The test for regulating glucose long term is hemoglobin A1C. The goal for a diabetic patient is to keep a steady glucose level below the cut off levels for diabetes. The physiology of glucose makes this type of measurement possible. Glucose molecules attach to the RBCs circulating in the blood. RBCs have a life span of about 120 days. The hemoglobin A1C is a test that measures just the glucose that is attached to hemoglobin molecules and gives information about how stable blood glucose levels have been over the past 3 months. A patient who is not diabetic has a hemoglobin A1C of less than 5.7%. A diabetic patient should have an A1C level of less than 7%, which is the goal desired by most physicians to show adequate control of blood glucose levels.

## CHECKPOINT QUESTION

12. What type of glucose measurement is used by the physician most often to confirm a diagnosis of diabetes?

## PATIENT EDUCATION

### Using a Glucose Meter

Many diabetic patients routinely monitor glucose levels at home. You can help reinforce the use of this procedure and help the patient get familiar with the machine. Instruct the patient to adhere to the manufacturer's instructions. Here are points to stress:

- Teach patients about the need to test and document glucose levels regularly.
- Instruct the patient in maintaining a quality control record for the instrument using control materials within the expiration date and as directed by the manufacturer.
- Offer instructions in the proper technique for obtaining a blood sample (e.g., cleanse the area well before beginning and do not milk the finger).
- Caution patients against self-regulating with insulin. Have patients call the physician if glucose levels are abnormal.
- Alert patients to the signs and symptoms of high and low glucose levels and the treatments for each.
- Most pharmacies and surgical supply stores that sell glucose meters will teach patients how to use them. The strips for glucose meters are expensive and may be covered by certain insurance companies if the physician clearly documents the need.

## ROLE-PLAYING ACTIVITY

Role-play these scenarios as if you are working with Amy Albers, CMA (AAMA), who works in the busy internal medicine practice at Great Falls Medical Center (refer to the case study at the beginning of the chapter). A 44-year-old male diabetic patient is seen today for follow-up and is ordered to have a hemoglobin A1C done today. The last one done 3 months ago was 8%, and when you ask the patient how he has been doing with following his low carbohydrate diet, he tells you he has done well and has not "eaten any candy bars" since his last visit. He is overweight and has actually gained 5 pounds since his last visit. How would you respond to this patient? Are there other questions you could ask about his diet and blood glucose levels? Give examples. Your instructor will give you additional information about this activity!

## SPANISH TERMINOLOGY

**Por favor, lávese las manos.**
Please wash your hands.

**¿Cuando fué la última vez que comió o bebió algo?**
When was the last time you had anything to eat or drink?

**Necesito una muestra de su sangre**
I need to get a blood sample.

**El doctor quiere revisar la función de su glándula tiroides.**
The doctor wants to check your thyroid function.

**Se siente mareado?**
Are you feeling light-headed?

**El doctor quiere estar seguro de que sus riñones están funcionando correctamente.**
The doctor wants to make sure your kidneys are working properly.

**El asistente médico le va a enseñar cómo usar el glucómetro.**
The medical assistant will teach you how to use the glucometer.

**Hay dos tipos de colesterol, uno malo que debe de evitar y otro bueno que debe consumir**
There are two types of cholesterol, one that is bad for your health and you have to avoid and one that is good that you are encouraged to consume.

**Las casas construidas antes de 1970 fueron hechas materiales que pueden tener plomo**
Houses built before 1970 were made with materials that could have contain lead.

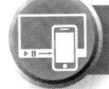

## MEDIA MENU

**Student Resources on** thePoint®
- *Video:* Performing a Glucose Test (Procedure 45-1)
- *Video:* Performing Routine Maintenance of a Glucose Meter (Procedure 45-3)
- CMA/RMA Certification Exam Review
- English to Spanish Audio Glossary

**Internet Resources**
**American Diabetes Association**
http://www.diabetes.org
**American Heart Association**
http://www.americanheart.org
**World Health Organization**
http://www.who.int/en
**National Diabetes Information Clearinghouse**
http://www.diabetes.niddk.nih.gov

## EMR Activity

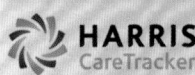

Harris CareTracker is a Web-based electronic medical record (EMR) application that you will use for the EMR activities included in this section at the end of each chapter. This application is actually used in physician offices, but is provided to you through the publisher, Wolters Kluwer Health, to give you hands-on practice working with EMRs. Your instructor will have more information about accessing your username, login, and Quickstart guide.

Prerequisite Activities in Harris CareTracker

• *The Getting Started and Quickstart documents and EMR Activities Step-by-Step Instructions are available at* http://thePoint.lww.com/KronenbergerComp5e

Activity Details

Accurately document the following blood collection procedures and chemistry results in each of the following patient's EMR:

1. Steve Sutter: Thyroid function panel ordered, venipuncture performed (left anterior forearm) and sent to Great Falls Medical Center laboratory.
2. Lawrence Black: Capillary stick (left ring finger) for a hemoglobin A1C. Results 7.4%.

## Chapter Summary

- Clinical chemistry is the science of using the chemical analysis of body fluids to obtain information regarding the clinical condition of the body.
- The kidneys rid the body of waste products and help maintain fluid balance and acid–base balance. When the kidneys begin to fail, waste products build up in the blood. The patient becomes edematous, and the acid–base balance is upset. Electrolytes are minerals in the body that have an electric charge. These minerals are ions (chemicals that carry an electrical charge) in the blood, urine, and body fluids.
- The acid–base system is extremely sensitive and cannot tolerate large pH fluctuations. The body's normal pH range is 7.35 to 7.45, very slightly basic (neutral = 7.0). The renal and respiratory systems work to regulate acid–base balance. Measurement of carbon dioxide is considered more useful for pH balance assessment than for measuring renal function, but it also aids in the overall assessment of renal function.
- The determination of nonprotein nitrogenous (NPN) compounds in the blood has traditionally been used to monitor renal function. Physicians most commonly request three NPN compounds for laboratory measurement: BUN, creatinine, and uric acid.
- Thyroid cells make $T_3$ and $T_4$. $T_3$ and $T_4$ are then released into the blood stream and are transported throughout the body where they control metabolism. Every cell in the body depends upon thyroid hormones for regulation of their metabolism.
- The pancreas as an endocrine gland makes two competing endocrine hormones that play an important role in diabetes: insulin and glucagon. As an exocrine gland, the pancreas secretes two enzymes: amylase and lipase.
- For diagnostic usefulness, the time a blood sample is taken for glucose testing must be related to the length of fasting or to the time of the previous meal.
- A cholesterol test can help determine the risk of atherosclerosis. Bile acids, partly formed by cholesterol, are produced in the liver, stored in the gallbladder, and released into the intestine as needed for the digestion of fats.

## Warm-Ups for Critical Thinking

1. A patient with edema is told by her physician to restrict her salt intake. Why may this help improve her condition?
2. A patient with diabetes gave herself too much insulin by mistake. Would you expect her glucose to be very high or very low? Why?
3. A patient's glucose level is repeatedly normal at routine office visits, but she continues to have worsening side effects of hyperglycemia. What test might the physician request that would reflect her glucose levels over a period of weeks?
4. A medical assistant draws a red top tube for a number of chemistry tests. Unfortunately, the tube is left on the counter for several hours before being centrifuged and refrigerated. Which chemistries may be affected by this? Why?
5. A physician needs to evaluate a patient's kidney function. Which chemistry measurements will the physician request? Which of these measurements is least impacted by the patient's diet?
6. Describe three ways cholesterol is beneficial to the body.

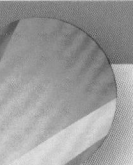

## PSY   PROCEDURE 43-1

# Perform Blood Glucose Testing

**PSY** Perform CLIA-waived chemistry testing; instruct and prepare a patient for a procedure or treatment; coach patients appropriately considering cultural diversity, developmental life stage, and communication barriers; and document patient care accurately in the medical record.

**Standard:** This task should take about 10 minutes.

**Purpose:** To determine a blood glucose as ordered by the physician

**Equipment:** Glucose meter, glucose reagent strips, control solutions, capillary puncture device, alcohol pad, gauze, paper towel, adhesive bandage, personal protective equipment (PPE), hand sanitizer, surface sanitizer, and contaminated waste container

| STEPS | PURPOSE |
|---|---|
| 1. Check the physician order and wash your hands. Wash your hands. | Hand washing aids in infection control. |
| 2. Assemble the equipment and supplies. | |
| 3. Review the instrument manual for your glucose meter. | Following the manufacturer's instructions ensures accurate testing. |
| 4. Turn on the instrument and verify that it is calibrated. | Calibration of the glucose meter is essential for accurate test results. |
| 5. Perform the test on the quality control (QC) material. Record results. Determine whether QC is within control limits. If yes, proceed with patient testing. If no, take corrective action and recheck controls. Document corrective action. Proceed with patient testing when acceptable QC results are obtained. | For waived testing, CLIA requires that quality control procedures be performed in compliance with the manufacturer's instructions. |
| 6. Remove one reagent strip, lay it on the paper towel, and recap the container. | The paper towel will serve as a disposable work surface and will absorb excess blood added to the strip. The strips are sensitive to humidity and will deteriorate if allowed to absorb moisture. |
| 7. **AFF** Greet and identify the patient. Identify yourself including your title. Explain the procedure. Ask for and answer any questions. | Help the patient feel at ease in an unfamiliar environment. |
| 8. Have the patient wash hands in warm water. Put on gloves. | Sugar residues on hands can falsely elevate glucose results if the strip is touched. Washing removes sugar residues from the skin, and the warm water stimulates blood flow. |
| 9. Cleanse the selected puncture site (finger) with alcohol. | Alcohol removes bacteria from the site. |

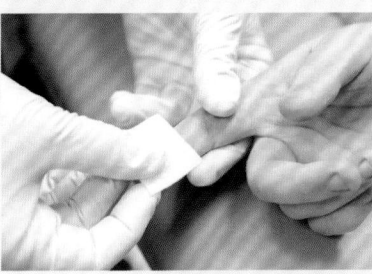

**Step 9.** Cleanse the selected puncture site with alcohol.

*(continues on page 1128)*

## PROCEDURE 43-1 (continued)

| STEPS | PURPOSE |
|---|---|

**STEPS**

10. Perform a capillary puncture and wipe away the first drop of blood.

11. Turn the patient's hand palm down and gently squeeze the finger to form a large drop of blood.

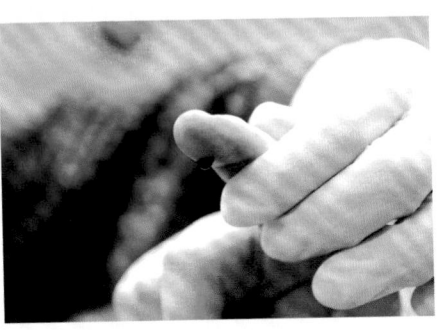

12. Bring the reagent strip up to the finger and touch the pad to the blood. Do not touch the finger. Completely cover the pad or fill the chamber with blood.

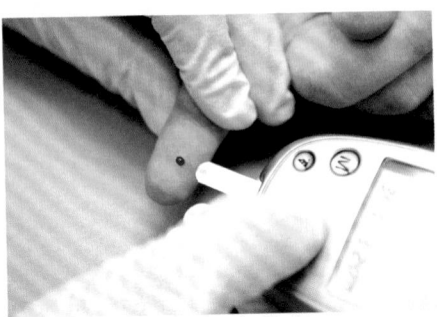

13. Insert reagent strip into analyzer, while applying pressure to the puncture wound with gauze. The meter will continue to incubate the strip and measure the reaction.

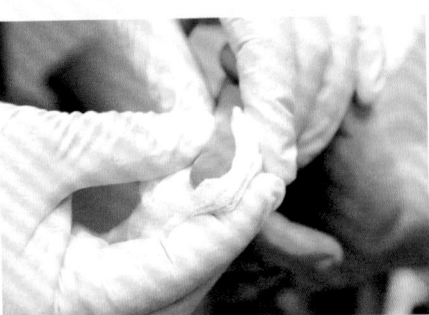

**PURPOSE**

The first drop of blood is contaminated with tissue fluid and will produce erroneous test first results.

Gentle squeezing obtains a blood specimen without diluting the sample with tissue fluid.

**Step 11.** Turn the patient's hand palm down and gently squeeze the finger to form a large drop of blood.

The entire pad must be covered or testing chamber filled for accurate reading. There is no chance of contamination by oils or other testing residue remaining on the finger if this surface is not touched.

**Step 12.** Touch the pad to the blood.

This allows time for the reaction.

**Step 13.** Apply pressure to puncture wound with gauze.

## PROCEDURE 43-1 (continued)

| STEPS | PURPOSE |
|---|---|
| **14.** The instrument reads the reaction strip and displays the result in milligrams per deciliter. | The reaction is now complete. The color change is photooptically measured and reported in milligrams per deciliter. |

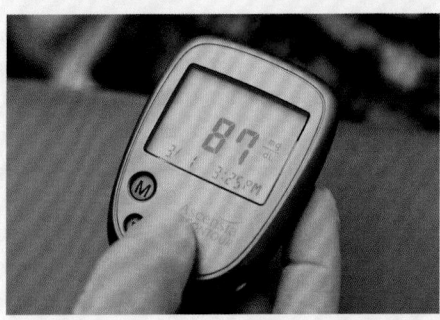

**Step 14.** Record the reading from the instrument display.

| STEPS | PURPOSE |
|---|---|
| **15.** Apply a small adhesive bandage to the patient's fingertip. | The bandage will protect the puncture site. |
| **16.** Properly care for or dispose of equipment and supplies. | Remove biohazards from the work space. |
| **17.** Clean the work area. Remove PPE and wash hands. | Washing hands is the key step in standard precautions. |
| **18.** **AFF** Log into the electronic medical record (EMR) using your username and secure password OR obtain the paper medical record from a secure location and assure it is kept away from public access. Record the procedure noting the date, time, test results for CLIA-waived POC procedure, and your name. | The integrity of the medical record must be maintained at all times to protect patient privacy. Procedures are considered not to have been performed if they are not recorded. |
| **19.** When finished, log out of the EMR and/or replace the paper medical record in an appropriate and secure location. | |

*Note:* These are generic instructions for using a glucose meter. Refer to the manufacturer's instructions for instructions specific to the particular instrument.

---

**Charting Example:**
*02/12/2016 10:00 AM. Capillary puncture left middle finger for glucose. Result 87 mg/dL _____
A. Albers, CMA*

---

Note: *The medical assistant may sign his or her name is the patient record using only the "CMA" credential if the office has a signature log denoting the entire credential as "CMA(AAMA)."*

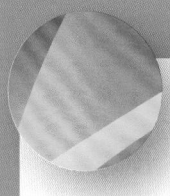

## PSY PROCEDURE 43-2

### Perform Blood Cholesterol Testing

**PSY** Perform CLIA-waived chemistry testing; instruct and prepare a patient for a procedure or treatment; coach patients appropriately considering cultural diversity, developmental life stage, and communication barriers; and document patient care accurately in the medical record.

**Standard:** This task should take about 10 minutes.

**Purpose:** To determine the blood cholesterol level

**Equipment:** Cholesterol meter and supplies or test kit, control solutions, capillary puncture equipment or blood specimen as indicated by manufacturer, PPE, hand sanitizer, surface sanitizer, and contaminated waste container

| STEPS | PURPOSE |
|---|---|
| 1. Check the physician order and wash your hands. Wash your hands. | Hand washing aids in infection control. |
| 2. Assemble the equipment and supplies. | |
| 3. Review the instrument manual for your cholesterol meter or kit. Put on gloves. | Following the manufacturer's instructions ensures accurate testing. |
| 4. Perform the test on the quality control material. Record results. Determine whether QC is within control limits. If yes, proceed with patient testing. If no, take corrective action and recheck controls. Document corrective action. Proceed with patient testing when acceptable QC results are obtained. | For waived testing, CLIA requires that quality control procedures be performed in compliance with the manufacturer's instructions. |
| 5. Follow manufacturer's instructions in using a patient specimen obtained by capillary puncture or from evacuation a tube. | CLIA requires that the manufacturer's instructions be followed on all procedures. |
| 6. Follow manufacturer's instructions for applying the sample to the testing device and inserting the device into the analyzer. Record results. | A written record is required for all laboratory test results. |
| 7. Properly care for or dispose of equipment and supplies. | Remove biohazards from the work space. |
| 8. Clean the work area. Remove PPE, and wash your hands. | Washing hands is the key factor of standard precautions. |
| 9. **AFF** Log into the electronic medical record (EMR) using your username and secure password OR obtain the paper medical record from a secure location and assure it is kept away from public access. Record the procedure noting the date, time, test results for CLIA-waived POC procedure, and your name. | The integrity of the medical record must be maintained at all times to protect patient privacy. Procedures are considered not to have been performed if they are not recorded. |

## PROCEDURE 43-2 (continued)

| STEPS | PURPOSE |
|---|---|
| 10. When finished, log out of the EMR and/or replace the paper medical record in an appropriate and secure location. | |

*Note:* These are generic instructions for performing cholesterol testing. Refer to the manufacturer's manual or package insert for instructions specific to the particular instrument or test kit.

Charting Example:
*02/12/2016 10:00 AM Cholesterol test performed. Results: 274 mg/dL. Dr. Peters notified* _____
*A. Albers, CMA*

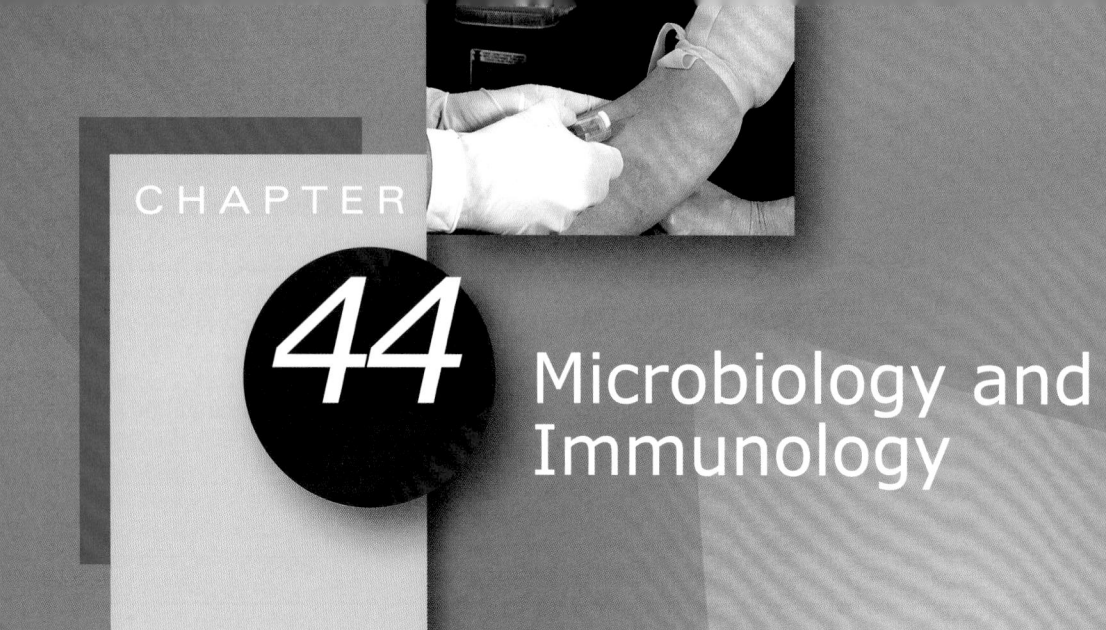

# 44 Microbiology and Immunology

## Outline

**Microbiology Specimen Collection**
 Quality Control in Microbiology
 Microbiology Cultures
**Types of Microorganisms**
 Bacteria

Viruses
Fungi
Protozoa and Helminthes

**The Immune System**
 Antigens and Antibodies
 Immunological Testing

## Learning Outcomes

**COG Cognitive Domain***

1. Spell the key terms
2. *Define medical terms and abbreviations related to all body systems*
3. *Identify CLIA-waived tests associated with common diseases*
4. *Analyze health care results as reported in graphs and tables*
5. List major types of infectious agents
6. Discuss quality control issues related to handling microbiological specimens

**PSY Psychomotor Domain***

1. Collect throat specimens (Procedure 44-1)
   a. *Obtain specimens and perform CLIA-waived microbiology testing*
   b. *Instruct and prepare a patient for a procedure or treatment*
   c. *Coach patients appropriately considering cultural diversity, developmental life stage, and communication barriers*
   d. *Document patient care accurately in the medical record*
2. Collect nasopharyngeal specimens (Procedure 44-2)
   a. *Obtain specimens and perform CLIA-waived microbiology testing*
   b. *Instruct and prepare a patient for a procedure or treatment*

   c. *Coach patients appropriately considering cultural diversity, developmental life stage, and communication barriers*
   d. *Document patient care accurately in the medical record*
3. Collect wound specimens (Procedure 44-3)
   a. *Obtain specimens and perform CLIA-waived microbiology testing*
   b. *Instruct and prepare a patient for a procedure or treatment*
   c. *Coach patients appropriately considering cultural diversity, developmental life stage, and communication barriers*
   d. *Document patient care accurately in the medical record*
4. Collect stool specimens for ova and parasites (Procedure 44-4)
   a. *Obtain specimens and perform CLIA-waived microbiology testing*
   b. *Instruct and prepare a patient for a procedure or treatment*
   c. *Coach patients appropriately considering cultural diversity, developmental life stage, and communication barriers*
   d. *Document patient care accurately in the medical record*
5. Inoculate a culture (Procedure 44-5)
   a. *Obtain specimens and perform CLIA-waived microbiology testing*
   b. *Instruct and prepare a patient for a procedure or treatment*

c. Coach patients appropriately considering cultural diversity, developmental life stage, and communication barriers

d. Document patient care accurately in the medical record

6. Perform mononucleosis testing (Procedure 44-6)

a. *Obtain specimens and perform CLIA-waived microbiology testing*

b. *Instruct and prepare a patient for a procedure or treatment*

c. Coach patients appropriately considering cultural diversity, developmental life stage, and communication barriers

d. *Document patient care accurately in the medical record*

7. Perform human chorionic gonadotropin pregnancy testing (Procedure 44-7)

a. *Obtain specimens and perform CLIA-waived immunology testing*

b. *Instruct and prepare a patient for a procedure or treatment*

c. Coach patients appropriately considering cultural diversity, developmental life stage, and communication barriers

d. *Document patient care accurately in the medical record*

8. Perform rapid group A strep testing (Procedure 44-8)

a. *Obtain specimens and perform CLIA-waived immunology testing*

b. *Instruct and prepare a patient for a procedure or treatment*

c. Coach patients appropriately considering cultural diversity, developmental life stage, and communication barriers

d. *Document patient care accurately in the medical record*

## AFF Affective Domain*

1. *Incorporate critical thinking skills when performing patient assessment*

2. *Incorporate critical thinking skills when performing patient care*

3. *Show awareness of a patient's concerns related to the procedure being performed*

4. *Demonstrate empathy, active listening, and nonverbal communication*

5. *Demonstrate respect for individual diversity including gender, race, religion, age, economic status, and appearance*

6. *Explain to a patient the rationale for performance of a procedure*

7. *Demonstrate sensitivity to patient rights*

8. *Protect the integrity of the medical record*

***Note: AAMA/CAAHEP 2015 Standards are italicized.***

### ABHES Competencies

1. Document patient care
2. Perform quality control measures
3. Screen test results
4. Perform immunology testing
5. Practice standard precautions
6. Perform handwashing
7. Obtain specimens for microbiology testing
8. Perform CLIA-waived microbiology testing
9. Perform pregnancy test
10. Perform strep A test
11. Instruct patients in the collection of fecal specimens

# Key Terms

| | | | |
|---|---|---|---|
| aerobes | diplococci | morphology | sensitivity testing |
| agar | Gram negative | mycology | smear |
| anaerobes | Gram positive | normal flora | specificity |
| antibodies | Gram stain | nosocomial infection | spirilla |
| antigens | helminthes | obligate intracellular | spirochetes |
| broth | immunity | parasite | virus |
| cocci | isolate | parasitology | virology |
| culture | media | resistant | |
| differential stain | mordant | sensitive | |

## Case Study

*R*amona Starr, RMA, works for Great Falls Medical Center Family physicians, where many patients of all ages are seen each day. This is flu season, and recently, the physician Ramona works for has seen at least four patients a day with flulike symptoms, including fever, cough, and lethargy. Today, a 3-year-old patient was brought in by his mother with sores around his mouth and nose that are crusty. The physician made a diagnosis of impetigo and ordered an oral antibiotic. Another patient came in with a complaint of a sore throat, and after performing a throat culture and testing the specimen for *Streptococcus*, the patient was diagnosed with a streptococcal throat infection and was also prescribed antibiotics. Six patients were seen for upper respiratory symptoms, and the physician did not prescribe antibiotics, but instead made a diagnosis of viral infection and gave instructions on treating the symptoms with rest, increased fluids, and an over-the-counter medication for nasal congestion. Why did the physician order antibiotics for some patients but not others? What are the different types of microorganisms that cause illness and disease that may be seen in the family practice office, and what is the role of the medical assistant in assisting the physician with diagnosis and treatment? These and other questions related to microbiology in the medical office are addressed in this chapter.

Microbiology is the study of organisms so small that they can only be seen with a microscope. These organisms are referred to as microorganisms or microbes and include some organisms that actually are visible without a microscope as they grow from microscopic eggs to adults. The goal of the microbiology department in a reference laboratory is to identify pathogens in the specimens submitted to the department so the physician can make a diagnosis and prescribe appropriate treatment. In some cases, specimens may contain **normal flora** or bacteria that normally live on the body and do not cause disease. Most specimens submitted to the laboratory for analysis contain the pathogen (if one is present) along with the normal flora growing at the site that was cultured. The role of the laboratory personnel who work in microbiology is to separate the pathogen and identify it from the midst of all the other microorganisms. The use of standard precautions in microbiology is to protect the medical assistant, the physician, patients, and all coworkers from **nosocomial infections**. Nosocomial infections are infections acquired in a medical setting.

Specimens submitted to the microbiology laboratory are collected from wounds, the throat, the vagina, the urethra, or the skin, using a swab. Specimens may be collected during surgery and also by venipuncture. Sputum, stool, and urine are other possible specimens. In all instances, aseptic technique must be practiced to ensure the integrity of the specimen (see Chapter 17).

## MICROBIOLOGY SPECIMEN COLLECTION

Microbiology reports give the physician a snapshot of the condition of the site used to obtain the specimen. For instance, a throat culture will identify pathogens present in the throat. For meaningful results, the specimen must be collected from the appropriate site using the proper method. The specimen must also be handled so that test results will be accurate (Box 44-1).

### BOX 44-1 Guidelines for Specimen Collection and Handling

- Follow standard precautions for specimen collection as outlined by the Centers for Disease Control and Prevention.
- Review the requirements for collecting and handling the specimen, including the equipment, the type of specimen to be collected (e.g., exudate, blood, mucus), the amount required for laboratory analysis, and the procedure to be followed for handling and storage.
- Assemble the equipment and supplies. Use only the appropriate specimen container as specified by the medical office or laboratory.
- Ensure that the specimen container is sterile to prevent contamination of the specimen by organisms not present at the collection site.
- Examine each container before use to make sure that it is not damaged, the medium is intact and moist, and it is well within the expiration date.
- Label each tube or specimen container with the patient's name and/or identification number, the date, the name or initials of the person collecting the specimen, the source or site of the specimen, and any other information required by the laboratory. Use an indelible pen or permanent marker. Make sure you print legibly, document accurately, and include all pertinent information.

Most microbiology specimens for culture in a physicians' office laboratory are referred to a reference laboratory although there are some CLIA-waived test kits available to perform some tests in the physician office. If the physician orders a specimen to be collected and it must be sent to a reference laboratory, refer to the laboratory specimen manual for information on the correct method for collecting and transporting these specimens. Table 44-1 is an example of various specimen collection guidelines that may be found in a laboratory specimen manual. The medical assistant must follow the guidelines listed in the charts to identify the correct methods for the specific specimen being referred.

## CHECKPOINT QUESTION

1. What is the appropriate transport media for drainage from a wound? Use Table 44-1 to help answer this question!

## Quality Control in Microbiology

The result of any laboratory test including microbiology tests is only as good as the specimen collected. Before collecting any specimen, you should positively identify the patient and prepare them for the collection procedure. Verify that you have the correct collection container and make sure you are collecting the specimen at the right time if appropriate. Once you have the correct collection container, you must label it according to the requirements of the reference laboratory, and most labs will generally want to see the name of the patient on the collection device, the date of the collection, and the time the specimen was collected. This information is also necessary to complete the laboratory request form that must be sent with the specimen in a biohazardous bag. If the specimen is not fully and correctly labeled, the laboratory may be required to dispose of the specimen and cancel the request.

**TABLE 44-1  Specimen Collection Guidelines by Specimen Type or Site**

| Specimen Type or Site | Volume or Method of Collection | Container or Transport |
|---|---|---|
| **Abscess** | | |
| Bacteria, fungal | 1–5 mL aspirate swab | Sterile no-additive tube, culturette, or transport medium |
| Acid-fast bacillus (AFB) (tuberculosis) | 1–5 mL aspirate | Sterile no-additive tube |
| **Blood** | | |
| Bacteria (1 culture = 1 set) | 10 mL | Aerobe (silver-top bottle) |
| Adult | 10 mL | Anaerobe (purple-top bottle) |
| Peds/short draw | 1–3 mL | Aerobe (blue-top bottle) |
| Fungal | 10 mL, adult | Isolator tube |
| | 1.5 mL, infant | |
| AFB | 10 mL | Isolator tube; can combine with fungal request |
| **Body fluids (sterile)** | | |
| Joint, pericardial, peritoneal, pleural, vitreous, etc. | 5 mL, optimal | Sterile no-additive tube |
| | 1 mL, minimum | |
| Bacteria, fungal, AFB | | |
| **Bronchial washing** | | |
| Bacteria, fungal, AFB | 1–5 mL | Sterile container |
| **Cervix** | | |
| Bacteria, fungal, AFB | Swab | Transport medium |
| **Cerebrospinal fluid** | | |
| Bacteria | 0.5 mL minimum | Sterile no-additive tube |
| Fungal (includes cryptococcal antigen) | 2 mL minimum | Sterile no-additive tube |
| AFB | 1 mL minimum | Sterile no-additive tube |
| **Cyst fluid** | | |
| Bacteria, fungal, AFB | 1–5 mL aspirate optimal, swab | Sterile tube; transport medium |

**TABLE 44-1   Specimen Collection Guidelines by Specimen Type or Site (continued)**

| Specimen Type or Site | Volume or Method of Collection | Container or Transport |
|---|---|---|
| **Dialysis fluid** | | |
| Bacteria | 1 mL minimum for Gram stain 10 mL per blood culture bottle | Sterile no-additive tube One aerobic (silver-top) tube and one anaerobic (purple-top) tube |
| **Ear** | | |
| Bacteria, fungal, AFB | Swab | Transport medium |
| **Exudate (pus)** | | |
| Bacteria, fungal, AFB | Aspirate optimal, swab | Sterile no-additive transport medium |
| Fungal, AFB | Aspirate, tissue, bone, pus, aspirated fluid | |
| **Eye** | | |
| Bacteria, fungal, AFB | Swab, ocular specimen | Transport medium |
| **Hair** | Hair shaft and base | Dry, sterile container |
| **Nail** | Nail shavings and debris | Dry, sterile container |
| **Skin scrapings** | Edge of lesion | Dry, sterile container |
| **Sinus** | | |
| Bacteria, fungal, AFB | Aspirate optimal, swab | Sterile tube; transport medium |
| Fungal, AFB | Aspirate, tissue, pus, bone | |
| **Sputum:** Three to five specimens, *collected on separate days,* will be accepted for culture (preferably first morning sputum). Additional specimens submitted after bronchoscopy or after therapy is initiated will be accepted. | 5 mL | Sterile screw-capped container |
| Bacteria, fungal AFB | 5 mL, minimum | Sterile screw-capped container |
| **Stool** | | |
| Bacteria (intestinal tract culture [ITC]) | 10-g minimum if delivery will be delayed | Container with sterile, leak-proof lid; deliver to lab within 1 hour via Cary Blair Transport (not suitable if looking for yeast). |
| Ova and parasite | 10-g minimum if delivery will be delayed | Container with sterile, leak-proof lid. Deliver to lab within 1 hour formalin/polyvinyl alcohol (PVA) vials. |
| *C. difficile* toxin | 10 g, minimum | Container with sterile, leak-proof lid; deliver to lab within 1 hour. |
| Fecal specimens for WBCs, occult, fecal fat | 10 g, minimum | Container with sterile, leak-proof lid; deliver to lab within 1 hour. |
| **Throat** | | |
| Bacteria, fungal | Swab | Transport medium |
| **Tracheal aspirate** Bacteria, fungal, AFB | 5 mL, minimum | Sterile screw-capped container |
| **Transtracheal** | As much as possible | Sterile tube or container; deliver to lab immediately. |
| **Ulcer** | | |
| Bacteria, fungal, AFB | Aspirate optimal, swab | Sterile tube; transport medium |
| Fungal, AFB | Aspirate, pus, tissue | |

| TABLE 44-1 | Specimen Collection Guidelines by Specimen Type or Site (continued) | |
|---|---|---|
| **Specimen Type or Site** | **Volume or Method of Collection** | **Container or Transport** |
| **Urethral cultures** | | |
| Bacteria, fungal, AFB | Exudate or drainage, swab | Sterile tube; transport medium |
| **Urine** | | |
| Bacteria, fungal | 10 mL, minimum | Urine-specific Vacutainer tube or a sterile screw-capped container |
| **Uterine cultures** | | |
| Bacteria, fungal | Exudate or drainage, swab | BD Vacutainer urine C&S Preservative Plus plastic tube |
| **Vaginal** | | |
| Bacteria | Swab | Transport medium |
| Fungal | Tissue, pus, aspirate | |
| **Wound** | | |
| Bacteria | Aspirate optimal, swab | Sterile tube; transport medium |
| Fungal, AFB | Aspirated fluid, pus, tissue, bone, ocular specimens | |

Always check the laboratory procedure manual for requirements to preserve the specimen and use the appropriate transport **media** as indicated. All specimens collected should be handled as if infectious, and standard precautions must be observed. Special handling instructions for the actual specimen may include refrigeration, freezing, and/or protection from light. The steps for handling a specimen for testing in microbiology are detailed and specific. It is detrimental to the patient if a specimen is mishandled or lost. Each step in the process is to keep the pathogen alive and the patient source correctly identified throughout the handling, transporting, testing, and reporting process. In addition to the patient medical record, your office may have additional documentation procedures for microbiological specimens collected to track the specimen from the time it is collected until it is picked up by a courier for transport to the laboratory for testing.

When performing CLIA-waived microbiology testing in the physician office, you will be responsible for being familiar with the testing kit and any quality control measures that must be taken to assure accurate results. Testing kits contain an expiration date, and you should make sure any testing performed is only done with nonexpired materials. After testing, follow office policy and procedures for disposing of the specimen collected and tested, keeping in mind the material is potentially infectious.

### Transporting Microbiological Specimens

Care must be taken to transport or process the specimen as soon as possible so the organisms do not die. For the most reliable results, laboratory tests should be performed in a fresh specimen within 1 hour after collection. When this is not possible, the specimen must be stored properly to preserve the physical and chemical properties

necessary for an accurate diagnosis. Specimens processed in outside or regional laboratories must be placed in a transport medium such as Culturette (Marion Scientific), which may also be used to collect the specimen (Fig. 44-1). Most transport systems are designed to be self-contained and include a plastic tube with a sterile swab and transport medium appropriate for the type of specimen and are stored at room temperature. Table 44-2 lists general guidelines for handling and storing specimens commonly collected in the medical office.

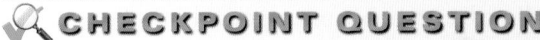

### CHECKPOINT QUESTION

2. List one reason that culture specimens must be processed as soon as possible after collection.

## Microbiology Cultures

### Culture Media

To identify a microorganism, the first requirement is to put it in a place it can grow. That supportive environment is created in a **culture**. To culture a specimen, a

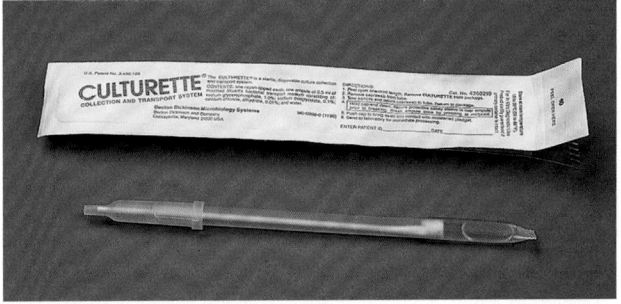

**Figure 44-1** • Transport media.

| TABLE 44-2 | Handling and Storing Commonly Collected Specimens | |
| --- | --- | --- |
| | **Handling** | **Storage** |
| Urine | Clean-catch midstream with care to avoid contaminating the inside of the container; must not stand more than 1 hour after collection. | Refrigerate if cannot be tested within 1 hour; add preservative at direction of laboratory; preservatives not usually used for urine culture. |
| Blood | Handle carefully, as hemolysis may destroy microorganisms; collect in anticoagulant tube at room temperature; specimen must remain free of contaminants; see laboratory manual for proper anticoagulant. | For most specimens, refrigerate at 4°C (39°F) to slow changes in physical and chemical composition. |
| Stool | Collect in clean container. To test for ova and parasites, keep warm. | Deliver to laboratory immediately. If delayed, mix with preservative provided or recommended by laboratory, or use transport medium. |
| Microbiology specimens | Do not contaminate swab or inside of specimen container by touching either to surface other than site of collection. Protect anaerobic specimens from exposure to air. | Transport specimen as soon as possible. If delayed, refrigerate at 4°C (39°F) to maintain integrity. |

Observe standard precautions while handling any of these specimens.

small sample is placed in or on the culture media, which are prepared with a mixture of substances that provide nourishment, water, and a neutral pH to support the growth of the microorganisms collected.

Liquid media are solutions that do not solidify at temperatures above freezing. The liquid media is most often poured into glass tubes or bottles and referred to as **broth**. A commonly used liquid media is nutrient broth, which contains beef extract and other nutrients.

Semisolid media have more **agar** or gelatin than the liquid media. Semisolid media provide information about the bacteria by observing its motility and growth pattern.

Solid media are most often poured into Petri dishes and offer a flat surface for growing bacteria or fungi (Fig. 44-2). The Petri dish is clear and allows visual examination of the culture as it grows, while the lid of the dish maintains the integrity of the specimen. Agar is the most widely used solid media, and the basic compo-

nent in agar comes from red algae. Various nutrients are added to agar to support the growth of different microorganisms. These agars are named in relation to their nutrients such as *nutrient agar* and *blood agar*. Observing the response of the organism to various agars offers information helpful in determining the organism's identity.

## Functional Types of Media

General purpose media are used to support the growth of a wide variety of microorganisms that do not have special growth requirements. The special media are called enriched, selective, and differential media and are described below.

• *Enriched media* contain added nutrients such as blood, serum, hemoglobin, or specific growth factors. Chocolate agar has heat-treated blood added that turns it a brown color, giving it the name chocolate agar.

• *Selective media* allow some organisms to grow by limiting the growth of other organisms. This is helpful in separating the pathogen from the normal flora. An example is mannitol salt agar. The salt additive inhibits most human pathogens other than *Staphylococcus*. So, if bacterial colonies grow on a mannitol salt agar plate when it is cultured from a specimen with mixed bacteria, those colonies are most likely one of the *Staphylococcus* species.

• *Differential media* grow several different organisms allowing them to show visible differences. Some of the differences make identification easier. Colonies of different bacteria grow a different color or cause the agar to change color. Some bacteria form gas bubbles in the agar. An example of a differential medium is MacConkey agar that contains neutral red, a dye that is yellow at a neutral pH and pink or red at an acidic pH. *Escherichia coli*, usually found in the intestinal

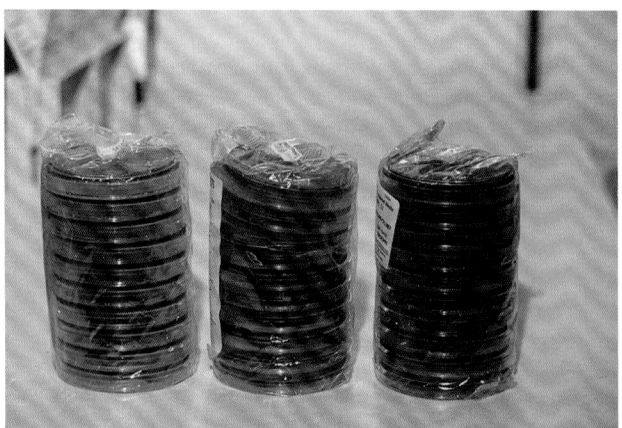

**Figure 44-2 •** Solid media are supplied on Petri plates wrapped in a plastic sleeve. Petri plates are always stored medium side up.

tract of animals, becomes acidic growing on this agar, so it appears pink or red. *Salmonella* remains a neutral pH growing on this agar, so it appears a natural off-white color.

### Caring for the Media

Culture media in disposable plastic Petri dishes can be purchased from medical supply companies and are supplied in a plastic sleeve that must be stored in the refrigerator with the side containing the medium on top. The plates should be stored in the plastic wrapper to keep the medium moist; however, they must be stored with the medium down to prevent condensation on the lids from dripping onto the media surface. If this happens, the surface of the media will be too moist for an accurate culture. Check the expiration date and the condition of the medium surface before using the plates. Discard any plates that are past the expiration date or any medium that has dried or cracked. When the shipment arrives, date each sleeve.

Transport media that is self-contained for collecting and transporting specimens to a laboratory also have an expiration date. Do not use a transport media that is compromised including expired, opened or torn package, or one in which the media appears dried.

### Incubation

Although agar must be refrigerated until needed, it must be warmed to room temperature before use. A cold plate or tube will kill many microorganisms. A warmer temperature for growth is provided by an incubator set at about 99°F (37°C), or just about body temperature (Fig. 44-3). If your office uses Petri dishes to grow collected specimens in the incubator, the temperature of the incubator must be recorded daily.

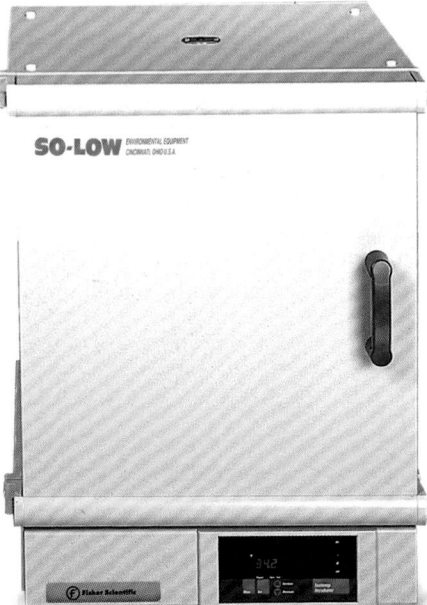

**Figure 44-3 •** Standard laboratory incubator. (Courtesy of So-Low Environmental Equipment, Cincinnati, OH.)

The incubator maintains optimal temperature, humidity, and other conditions, such as the carbon dioxide and oxygen content of the atmosphere inside.

### CHECKPOINT QUESTION

**3.** What is the purpose of a culture media?

## Microbiology Test Reports

The presence of pathogenic microorganisms is considered a positive culture. A culture that is reported as "no growth in 24 hours" usually indicates that there is no infection present, but the specimen is usually incubated another 24 hours to confirm there is no growth. Some pathogens require more than 24 hours to demonstrate growth on the culture medium. Box 44-2 describes the responsibilities of the medical assistant when reviewing microbiology results.

---

**BOX 44-2   Screening Laboratory Test Results**

When a laboratory test is reported, an expected range for the test is included on the report with the patient test result. The tests use a range because what is normal differs from person to person. Many factors affect test results. These include:

- Sex, age, and race
- Recent food and fluid intake
- Recent medications
- Compliance with any pretest instructions

The physician may also compare current test results to those from previous tests. Laboratory tests are often part of a routine checkup to look for changes in the patient's health status. They also help with the diagnosis of medical conditions, plan or the evaluation of treatments, and the monitoring of diseases.

The medical assistant will screen test results per the office policy manual. These duties may include:

- Comparing test results to those already in the patient's medical record and notifying the physician per his or her instructions
- Flagging abnormal test results for review by the physician. The physician may designate how abnormal the results must be to indict the need for follow-up.
- Screen for critical values. Each office must have a list of physician-approved critical levels that require immediate physician notification.
- Flagging new results posted in the medical record notifying the physician of the need to review and document
- Documentation of these functions must be noted on the report or in the medical record.
- Documentation must include the screener's initials and date.

Fecal Blood Testing

A screening test that is commonly performed in the microbiology laboratory is the fecal blood test. As discussed in Chapter 33 (Gastroenterology), the fecal test for blood is performed for several reasons. Blood in the stool is abnormal, but the cause may be simple or serious. Visible blood likely results from lesions in the lower colon or hemorrhoids. In some cases, the blood in stool is not visible and is referred to as *occult*. As a result, the test is often called "stool for occult blood." This test is CLIA waived, and after the patient collects the specimen, the medical assistant performs the testing (see Chapter 33). Positive results do not indicate a diagnosis, but usually require further testing such as a colonoscopy. Samples of abnormal tissue or lesions seen by the physician during a colonoscopy are sent to the laboratory for histology and pathology. The pathologist reports the final diagnosis of the biopsy specimen, and appropriate treatment is ordered by the physician.

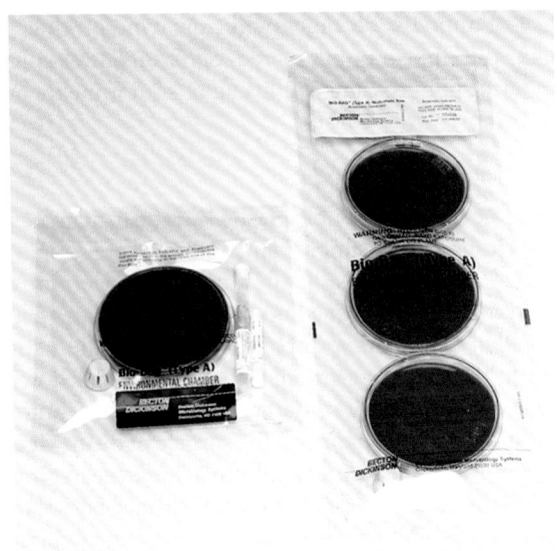

**Figure 44-4** • The BioBag anaerobic culture set. It includes a plate of CDC-anaerobic blood agar in an oxygen-impermeable bag. The system contains its own gas-generating kit and cold catalyst. (Courtesy of Becton Dickinson, Franklin Lakes, NJ.)

 **CHECKPOINT QUESTION**

4. What test result is indicated if a culture report reads "no growth in 24 to 48 hours?"

# TYPES OF MICROORGANISMS

## Bacteria

Bacteria are one type of microorganism that may cause disease and illness in humans. These microbes require nutrients, warmth, moisture, and darkness for survival and growth. Some bacteria require oxygen and are called **aerobes**, while some thrive in an environment without oxygen, known as **anaerobes**. The microbiology laboratory uses culture media, incubators, and techniques to control the specimen's exposure to oxygen to provide these conditions, causing the microorganism to grow and reproduce, allowing an accurate diagnosis.

Incubation containers designed for cultured specimens that may include anaerobic bacteria contain a tablet that generates carbon dioxide and eliminates oxygen in the closed environment of the medium container (Fig. 44-4).

### Bacterial Morphology

The size, shape, and arrangement of bacteria and other microbes is a defining characteristic called **morphology**. Bacteria come in a variety of sizes and shapes with the most common shapes including rod (**bacilli**), round (**cocci**), and spiral (**spirilla**) (Fig. 44-5). Within each of these groups are hundreds of variants. Bacteria may also exist as single cells or with other groupings such as chains, uneven clusters, pairs, tetrads, etc. Table 44-3 lists categories of bacteria by morphology.

Bacteria have two names including a genus and species name. The genus is the first name of a bacteria and is always spelled with a capital letter. The species name is the second name and begins with a lowercase letter (e.g., *Staphylococcus aureus*). In print, the entire name of the bacteria is noted in italics or underlined.

One species of cocci, a round bacteria, is the *Staphylococci* found on all surfaces of the skin and many mucous membranes. They are generally not pathogenic unless they reach an area that is usually sterile where they may cause some form of infection. Species of *Streptococci* may cause sore throat, scarlet fever, rheumatic fever, pneumonia, and various skin infections. **Diplococci**, spherical cocci in pairs, cause bacterial meningitis, gonorrhea, and some of the pneumonias.

Bacilli are rod shaped and are usually aerobic requiring oxygen to live. Most bacteria are bacilli and often found in soil. Diseases caused by bacilli include tetanus,

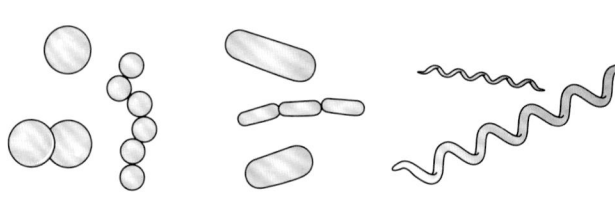

**A.** Cocci (spheres)    **B.** Bacilli (rods)    **C.** Spirilla (spirals)

**Figure 44-5** • Bacteria can be spherical **(A)**, rod shaped **(B)**, or spiral shaped **(C)**.

| TABLE 44-3 | Categorizing Bacteria |
|------------|----------------------|
| **Morphology** | **Types** |
| Round (spherical) | Cocci |
| Grapelike clusters | Staphylococci |
| Chain formations | Streptococci |
| Paired | Diplococci |
| Rod shaped | Bacilli |
| Somewhat oval | Coccobacilli |
| End-to-end chains | Streptobacilli |
| Spiral | Spirochetes |
| Flexible (usually with flagella, whiplike extremities that aid movement) | Spirilla |
| Rigid, curved rods (comma shaped) | Vibrios |

### BOX 44-3   Preparing a Wet Mount Slide

To prepare a wet mount, follow these steps:

1. Place a drop of the specimen on a glass slide with sterile saline or 10% potassium hydroxide (KOH).
2. Place a coverslip over the specimen to reduce evaporation.
3. To decrease evaporation, coat the rim of the coverslip with petrolatum.
4. Inspect the slide by microscope using the high-power objective lens with diminished light.

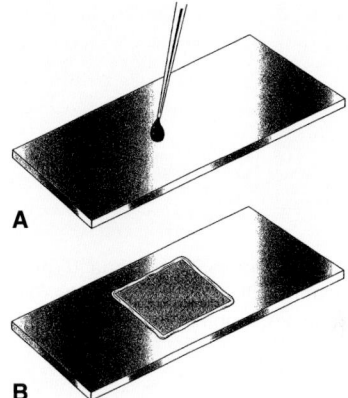

Wet mount slide preparation. **(A)** A drop of fluid containing the microorganism is placed on a glass slide. **(B)** The specimen is covered with a coverslip ringed with petroleum jelly.

botulism, gas gangrene, tuberculosis, pertussis, salmonellosis, certain pneumonias, and otitis media.

**Spirochetes** are long, spiral, flexible organisms. Spirochetes are responsible for syphilis and Lyme disease. *Vibrio* is a very motile comma-shaped bacteria. These bacteria cause the disease cholera.

### Slide Preparation and Staining

To observe microorganisms with a microscope, the specimen may require preparation on a slide as some pathogens are more easily identified if they are allowed to move freely in a solution. These types of microbes are best viewed immediately on a microscope slide, but at the latest, they should be viewed within 30 minutes of collection. When collected by the physician and put on a slide for observation and movement, the slide is referred to as a wet mount. Box 44-3 provides additional information about wet mount specimens.

Some bacterial specimens must be stained in order to be viewed under the microscope. First, the specimen must be dried on a glass slide, referred to as a **smear**. Once the specimen is put on the slide, it must be adhered to the slide, or fixed to the slide, by passing it quickly through a flame, causing a short exposure to heat. Once fixed to the slide, the smear must be stained to be visible under the microscope.

Most bacteria are hard to see or identify when viewed under a microscope without special treatment such as staining. The primary stain used in the microbiology lab is the **Gram stain**, which is considered a **differential stain** that allows differentiation between bacteria that take up the stain and those that do not absorb the stain. The Gram stain process is not typically performed in the physician office but may be ordered by the physician to be performed on a specimen in the laboratory. You would need to make sure the laboratory request that accompanies the specimen notes the Gram stain to be performed.

Each step of the staining procedure has a specific reason. The slide is first stained with crystal violet, a dye, followed by rinsing with water. At this point, Gram's iodine is applied, which is a **mordant** used to fix the dye on the smear to make it more intense. The iodine is removed from the slide with a water rinse. If viewed under the microscope at this point, all bacteria on the slide would appear purple. Next, 95% ethyl alcohol is applied to the slide to remove the color. **Gram-positive** bacteria will keep the purple color even when exposed to the ethyl alcohol. **Gram-negative** bacteria will lose the purple color when exposed to the ethyl alcohol. If viewed under the microscope now, the Gram-negative bacteria would be difficult to detect because they will be almost colorless. The slide is again rinsed with water and an intensely red stain, safranin, is applied. The slide is rinsed one last time with water to remove the excess safranin. Bacteria that retain the primary purple color of the crystal violet stain are called *Gram-positive bacteria*. The remaining bacteria appear red or pink due to the safranin stain. These are said to be **Gram negative** (Fig. 44-6).

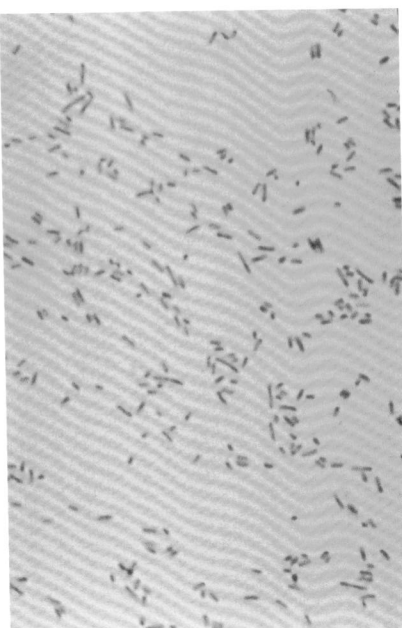

**Figure 44-6** • Gram-negative bacteria. (From Sweet RL, Gibbs RS. *Atlas of Infectious Diseases of the Female Genital Tract.* Philadelphia, PA: Lippincott Williams & Wilkins, 2005.)

## Sensitivity Testing

When microorganisms are unable to grow in the presence of one or more antimicrobial drugs, they are said to be *susceptible* to that drug. **Sensitivity testing** determines if an antibiotic will be effective in stopping the growth of a microorganism. It also identifies antibiotics that will *not* stop the growth of an organism. Organisms that are inhibited by an antimicrobial agent are called **sensitive**. Organisms that grow even in the presence of an antimicrobial agent are said to be **resistant** to that antimicrobial agent.

In sensitivity testing, the first step is to **isolate**, or separate, the microorganism from any other microorganisms present. Once it has been isolated and identified, the organism can be tested to determine its sensitivity to antibiotics that may be effective at killing the bacteria. The pathogen identified may respond to treatments that have already been established. If this is not the case, the physician will order the antibiotic that is effective.

To perform the sensitivity testing, the isolated pathogen is inoculated to a large agar plate. Paper disks impregnated with antibiotics are applied to the culture plate containing the organism and the prepared plate is incubated for 24 hours. When the plate is observed for growth, the antibiotic disks that exhibit a margin with no bacterial growth indicate that the pathogen is sensitive or susceptible to this medication. If there is no zone around the disk, the organism is said to be *resistant* to that antibiotic. If there is a small zone, it may be reported as *intermediate*. The antibiotic of choice will be the one with the largest zone of inhibition or no growth (Fig. 44-7). Automated instruments perform this testing in large laboratories.

Large area of growth inhibition – bacterium is <u>most sensitive</u> to antibiotic C

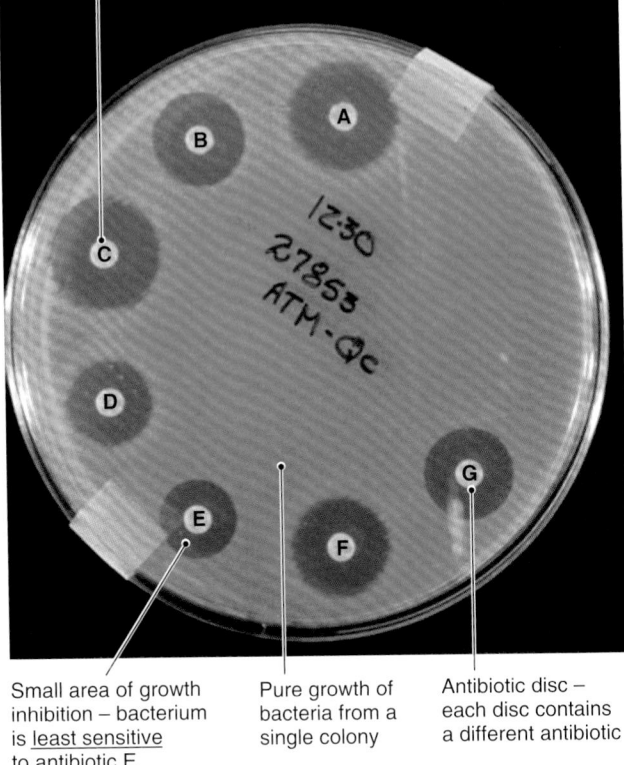

Small area of growth inhibition – bacterium is <u>least sensitive</u> to antibiotic E

Pure growth of bacteria from a single colony

Antibiotic disc – each disc contains a different antibiotic

**Figure 44-7** • Antibiotic sensitivity testing. The surface of the culture plate is overgrown by bacteria that were collected from a single colony and evenly spread across the surface. White paper disks soaked with different antibiotics are placed on the plate, and the plate is incubated 24 hours. Clear areas around disks are where bacterial growth has been inhibited. Bacterial sensitivity to a particular antibiotic is related to the size of the zone of inhibited: a large zone suggests the antibiotic may be effective in treating the patient's infection. (From McConnell TH. *The Nature of Disease Pathology for the Health Professions.* Philadelphia, PA: Lippincott Williams & Wilkins, 2007.)

## Rickettsias, Chlamydias, and Mycoplasma

Specialized forms of bacteria that fit in a category of their own are the rickettsias, chlamydiae, and mycoplasmas. They are smaller than bacteria but larger than viruses and stain negatively with the Gram stain. They cause disease in both animals and humans and require a living host for replication and survival, commonly referred to as **obligate intracellular parasites**. Due to the requirement for a living host, these microorganisms will not grow on laboratory culture media and must be collected using special procedures as indicated by the reference laboratory.

Organisms of the genus *Rickettsia* are carried on arthropods such as lice, fleas, and ticks and are transferred to humans by inhalation or direct contact. Diseases caused by *Rickettsia* species include Rocky Mountain spotted fever. *Chlamydia* species may cause blindness, pneumonia, and lymphogranuloma venereum, a prevalent sexually transmitted disease. Mycoplasmas cause diseases such as atypical pneumonia, a less severe form of pneumonia commonly referred to as "walking pneumonia," and genitourinary (GU) infections.

## CHECKPOINT QUESTION

5. The physician Ramona Starr works for ordered a culture and sensitivity on a patient with a wound that appears infected. What is a culture and sensitivity test?

## Viruses

One of the many diseases caused by a **virus** is chicken pox. **Virology** is the study of viruses, the smallest microorganisms that can only be seen with an electron microscope. Other diseases caused by viruses include influenza, infectious hepatitis, rabies, polio, and AIDS. These microbes require a living host for survival and replication and are referred to as *parasites*. Because viruses are not susceptible to antibiotics, most are extremely difficult to treat; however, antiviral medications are available to reduce the severity of symptoms and possibly prevent recurrent infections.

A virus is not a living cell, but is made up of a piece of genetic material, DNA or RNA. When a virus enters a cell, it takes over the cell and makes copies of itself until the cell bursts, releasing the replicated copies of the virus, which then take over other cells and the process continues. Viral diseases are detected by changes in how the host cells look and function. For a list of familiar diseases and the responsible common viral name, see Table 44-4.

## PATIENT EDUCATION

### What Do I Need To Know About The Flu Shot?

People get flu shots for protection from influenza, commonly referred to as the flu. Although the flu shot does not always provide total protection, many health care facilities now require all employees including medical assistants to get the vaccine each year as a condition of employment.

Influenza is an upper respiratory infection that can cause serious complications, particularly to young children and older adults. People including these high-risk groups die each year in the United States from influenza. Flu shots are the most effective way to prevent influenza and its complications. The Centers for Disease Control and Prevention (CDC) now recommends that everyone age 6 months or older be vaccinated annually against influenza. The nasal spray vaccine is recommended for healthy children 2 to 8 years of age.

Here are the answers to common questions about the flu vaccine:

*When should I get the flu vaccine?*
September through mid-November is when the vaccine is usually available and also when flu begins to be identified in the population. It takes up to 2 weeks to build immunity after the flu vaccine.

*Why do you get the flu vaccine every year?*
Influenza that is active one season can be different by the next season. Health officials use information about flu from all over the world to determine what the flu vaccine needs to during the next season. The vaccine usually lasts in the body about 6 months after receiving a flu shot.

*Should everyone get a flu vaccine?*
The CDC now recommends vaccinations for everyone age 6 months or older. Vaccination is important for people with conditions that could lead to complications from the flu, including:

- Pregnant women
- Older adults
- Young children

Chronic medical conditions can also increase your risk of influenza complications. Examples include:

- Asthma
- Cerebral palsy
- Chronic obstructive pulmonary disease
- Cystic fibrosis
- Epilepsy
- HIV/AIDS
- Kidney or liver disease
- Muscular dystrophy
- Obesity
- Sickle cell disease

*Who should not have the flu shot?*
Do not get a flu shot if you:

- Have had a bad reaction to the vaccine in the past
- Have a fever that day

## Fungi

**Mycology** is the study of fungi, small plantlike microorganisms with the potential to produce disease in susceptible hosts. Some fungi are microscopic, but some can be seen without the aid of a microscope. They usually become pathogenic when the host's normal flora cannot defend against them.

Diseases caused by fungal infections are referred to as **mycoses**, which are classified by the amount of tissue involved and the route of entry into the body. Mycoses that are superficial include fungal infections of the skin, hair, and nails. Subcutaneous fungal infections involve the dermis, subcutaneous issue, or adjacent structures. Fungal infections that affect internal organs are referred to as systemic, and those that occur due to immunosuppression are opportunistic. Human fungal infections are

| TABLE 44-4 | Familiar Medically Important Viruses |
|---|---|
| **Infection/Disease** | **Common or Typical Name** |
| Adult T-cell lymphoma, AIDS | Retroviridae HIV |
| Cervical cancer | Human papillomavirus Herpes simplex virus 2 (HSV2) |
| Common warts, plantar warts | Human papillomavirus |
| Oral herpes | Herpes simplex virus 1 |
| Chicken pox and shingles | Varicella zoster virus |
| Hepatitis B | Hepatitis B virus |
| Poliomyelitis | Poliovirus |
| Common cold | Human rhinovirus A |
| Gastroenteritis (one type) | Norovirus |
| Rubella | Rubella virus |
| Influenza | Influenza A and B |
| Measles | Rubeola virus |
| Respiratory trace infections (one type) | Respiratory syncytial virus |
| Rabies | Rabies virus |
| Smallpox | Smallpox (variola vera) |

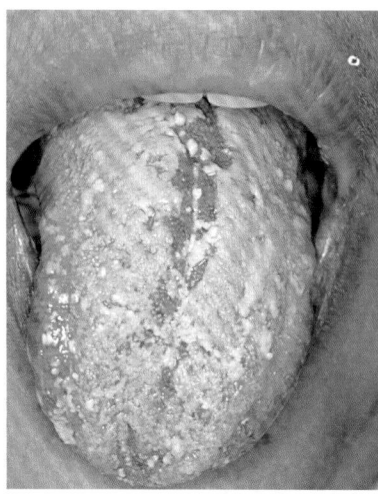

**Figure 44-8 •** Oral candidiasis. These curd-like lesions can easily be removed with gauze. (From Goodheart HP. *Goodheart's Photoguide of Common Skin Disorders*, 2nd ed. Philadelphia, PA: Lippincott Williams & Wilkins, 2003.)

usually limited to conditions such as candidiasis (thrush) and dermatophyte skin infections such as athlete's foot. Figure 44-8 is a photograph of the tongue of a patient with oral candidiasis, commonly referred to as thrush in infants who sometimes get this condition. If a patient does not have a strong immune system, nonpathogenic fungi can cause potentially fatal infections. Today's common travel in foreign countries transports unusual fungi into this country. Examples of fungal infections and the causative microorganism include:

- *Histoplasmosis.* This is caused by *Histoplasma capsulatum, or H. capsulatum, which is* common in many parts of the world including the United States. It spreads through contaminated soil and is usually asymptomatic. The lungs are the main site of infection, and the symptoms can resemble those of tuberculosis.
- *Opportunistic fungi.* These fungi grow where they have the opportunity, as in patients with weak immune systems. Because of the weak immune systems, other fungi that are normally not pathogenic cause infections. Examples of fungi that may cause opportunistic fungal infections include *Fusarium* (Fig. 44-9) or *Penicillium.*

- *Aspergillosis.* This is the name of several diseases caused by the mold *Aspergillus.* It occurs worldwide and often infects the lungs, inner ear, sinuses, and, rarely, the eye.
- *Candidiasis. C. albicans*, a part of the normal human flora, can grow and spread in patients having reduced immunity.
- *Cryptococcosis.* The yeast *Cryptococcus neoformans* can cause a systemic infection when inhaled. The microorganism may cause subacute meningitis or pulmonary infection. These diseases can affect a healthy person and is found globally. *C. neoformans* is commonly found in pigeon droppings.
- *Pneumocystis.* This is an infection of the lung caused by *Pneumocystis jiroveci.* The microorganism is a common cause of fatal pneumonia in AIDS patients.

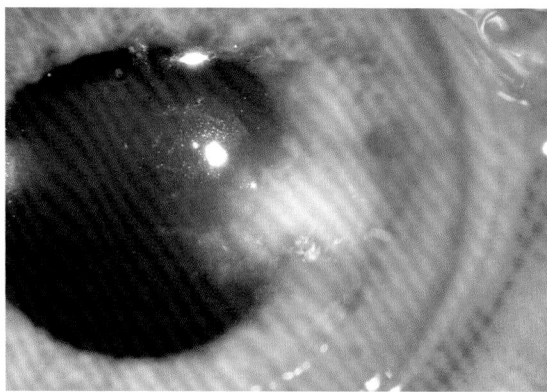

**Figure 44-9 •** This corneal ulcer in a patient using extended wear soft contact lenses was caused by a filamentous fungal organism, *Fusarium.* (From Tasman W, Jaeger E. *The Wills Eye Hospital Atlas of Clinical Ophthalmology*, 2nd ed. Lippincott Williams & Wilkins, 2001.)

**What if your patient asks you how to prevent a fungal infection such as athlete's foot?**

Explain to your patient that athlete's foot, also known as tinea pedis, is a common fungal infection that grows in a warm, dark, moist environment. Then offer the following suggestions, which can aid prevention:

- Practice good basic hygiene.
- Thoroughly dry between the toes.
- Do not share footwear.
- Use antifungal powder between the toes and in shoes.
- Wear foot protection when using public showers.

*Apply medication as ordered by the physician.

## Protozoa and Helminthes

**Parasitology** is the study of protozoa, one-celled animals, and **helminthes**, or worms. Parasites included in both of these categories can infect various body systems but primarily affect the gastrointestinal system. Although some parasites use a permanent host, others move through different animal or human hosts. Parasites must have a live host to live, grow, and reproduce and once the host organism is invaded, the parasite may disrupt the host's nutrient absorption, causing weakness and disease. Because parasites are often excreted in the feces of the infested human or animal, oral exposure to anything that has come into contact with the feces of the infected person or animal results in transmission of the parasite. These organisms may also be transmitted from host to host through contaminated food and water. Some common parasites and their related diseases include:

- *Entamoeba:* This parasite causes diarrhea, dysentery, and liver and lung disorders.
- *Giardia:* An infection with Giardia is often referred to as giardiasis. The symptoms of giardiasis include diarrhea and malabsorption of nutrients.
- *Trichomonas:* Trichomoniasis is the term to describe an infection with the parasite Trichomonas. This microorganism may cause vaginitis and urinary tract infections.
- *Plasmodium:* The disease malaria is caused by the parasite Plasmodium, which is transmitted by infected mosquitoes.
- *Toxoplasma:* The disease toxoplasmosis is caused by an infection with the parasite Toxoplasma, which may cause fetal abnormalities and lesions in the brain.

Helminths are parasitic worms that may infect animals including humans (Fig. 44-10). Although the worms can grow large enough to see without the aid of

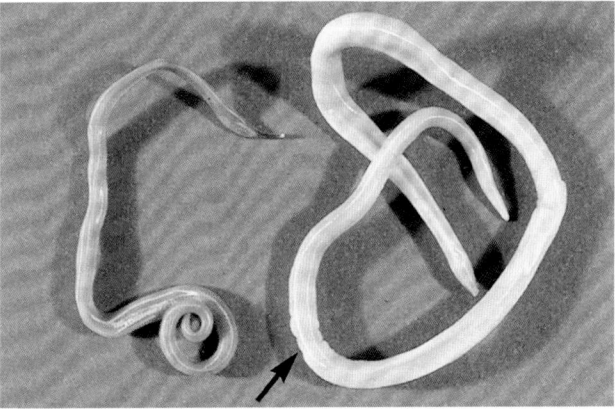

**Figure 44-10** • Female and male worms of *A. lumbricoides.*

a microscope, their eggs, or ova, are microscopic and are the source of transmission and infection. The ova of most helminthes are found in contaminated soil.

Examples of helminthes that cause disease in humans include:

- *Ascaris lumbricoides,* also referred to as roundworm
- *Ancylostoma duodenale* and *Necator americanus,* two types of hookworm
- *Trichuris trichiura,* commonly called whipworm
- *Enterobius vermicularis,* also known as pinworms (Fig. 44-11)

Another disease called Taeniasis is caused by a parasitic infection with one of several tapeworm species. The tapeworms that often infect humans include *Taenia saginata, Taenia solium, and Taenia asiatica.* Infections with these parasites are caused by eating undercooked beef (*T. saginata*) or pork (*T. solium*). *T. asiatica* infections are found in Asian countries.

Diagnosis of any infection with a helminth is done by identifying microscopic eggs in a stool specimen. Procedure 44-4 describes the steps involved in collecting a stool sample for ova and parasite testing. Box 44-4 outlines some tips for collecting a stool specimen for parasites.

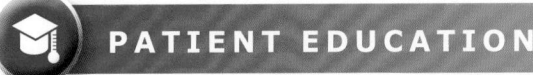

**CHECKPOINT QUESTION**

6. What parasite causes the disease malaria?

**PATIENT EDUCATION**

### Lyme Disease

The deer tick is an insect capable of transmitting *Borrelia burgdorferi*, the spirochete responsible for Lyme disease. When the infected deer tick bites a human, the organism enters the body and can produce mild to severe symptoms, including a rash, joint aches, fever, general body aches, and alterations in neurologic and cardiac function.

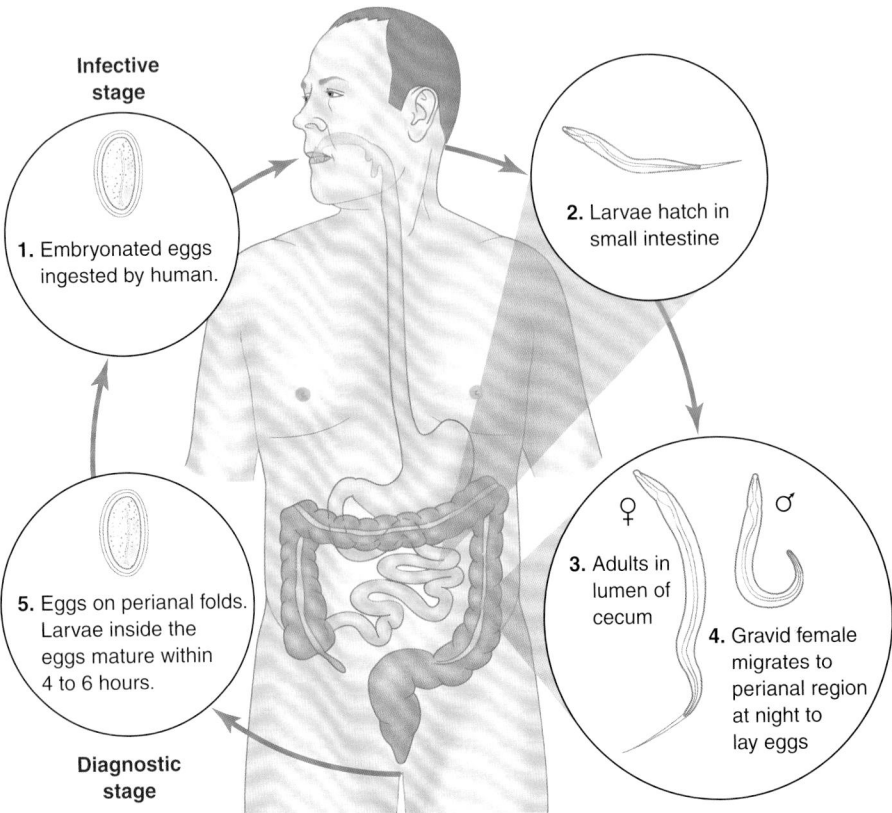

**Figure 44-11** • The life cycle of a pinworm infection begins (*1*) with hand-to-mouth transfer of pinworm eggs from a fecally contaminated environment; (*2*) once ingested, the eggs hatch in the small intestine of a human; (*3*) the eggs mature in the large intestine; (*4*) the mature female pinworms lay eggs in the perianal area and are shed by fecal elimination into the environment.

Lyme disease can be prevented. Instruct patients to avoid tick habitats, to apply insect repellent, and to wear shoes and light-colored clothing when working outside in wooded areas. Clothing should be checked for ticks and washed in hot water with strong soap. Stress the importance of looking for ticks and removing them properly when they are found.

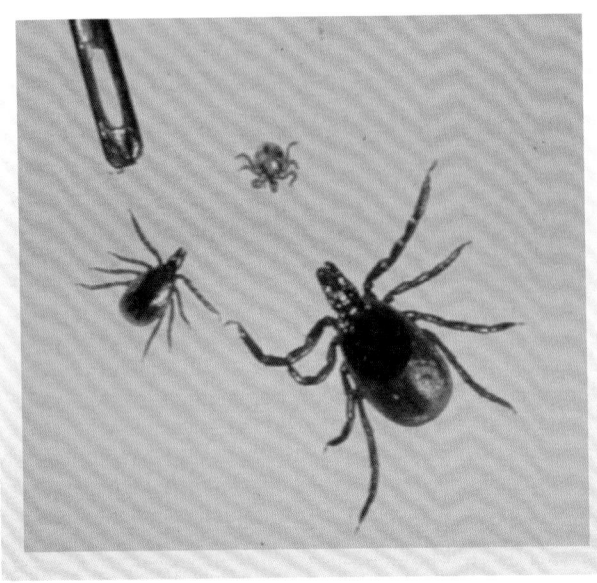

**BOX 44-4    Special Stool Specimens**

Follow these tips when collecting stool specimens to test for pinworms or parasites or to obtain a swab for culture. Remember to follow standard precautions.

- *Pinworms:* Schedule the appointment early in the morning, preferably before a bowel movement or bath. Pinworms tend to leave the rectum and lay eggs around the anus during the night. Press clear adhesive tape against the anal area. Remove it quickly and place it sticky side down on a glass slide for the physician to inspect.
- *Parasites:* Caution the patient not to use a laxative or enema before the test to avoid destroying the evidence of parasites. If the stool contains blood or mucus, include as much as possible in the specimen container because these substances are most likely to contain the suspected organism.
- *Stool culture:* A sterile cotton-tipped swab is passed into the rectal canal beyond the sphincter and rotated carefully. Place it in the appropriate culture container or process as directed for smear preparation.

## PATIENT EDUCATION

### Case Study Scenario

A 23-year-old white female came to the medical office at the end of summer (August) complaining of fatigue, tender joints, headache, stiff neck, and backache. Her temperature was 99.5°F. Upon examination, the physician noticed a circular "rash" on her right arm about 5 inches in diameter, with a bright-red leading edge and a dim center in the form of a "bull's eye."

The patient gave the following history: She is a graduate student in the wildlife program at the nearby university. She was in the field for 3 weeks in the Smoky Mountains during June. She tracks small mammals in the field and studies their behavior. She complained of a large number of biting flies, mosquitoes, and ticks in the area. She felt well until about 2 weeks after returning home.

- Although the physician is responsible for diagnosing the patient, what would you guess might be the problem with this patient given her symptoms and the physician observations?
- (Answer: Based on this patient's signs and symptoms, the physician may suspect Lyme disease.)
- What features are critical to a diagnosis of Lyme disease?

(Answer: The key symptom is the "bull's eye" rash and the possible exposure to ticks. The patient symptoms of a low-grade fever, joint pain, and aching are also indicative of a patient with Lyme disease.)

# THE IMMUNE SYSTEM

The immune system is the mechanism of the body to identify and destroy microorganisms that we encounter daily that have the potential to cause illness and disease. Immunology is the study of the actions of the immune system, while **immunity** is the response to foreign bodies or substances that the body recognizes as foreign.

## Antigens and Antibodies

**Antigens** are substances that are recognized as foreign by the body, which cause the body to begin the production of **antibodies**. Antibodies are proteins produced by the body in response to a specific antigen, and each antibody combines with only one antigen. The ability of the body to producer one antibody for each antigen is called **specificity**.

Because an antibody has a particularly strong attraction for its antigen, very little antigen need be present in

a sample for the antibody to find it; this is referred to as *sensitivity*. An antibody is named by using its specific antigen's name and adding the prefix *anti-*. In hepatitis, for instance, if the antigen is hepatitis A, then the antibody's name is antihepatitis A. If the antigen is hepatitis B, then the antibody is antihepatitis B. If the antigen is a bacteria, like *Streptococcus*, then the antibody's name is antistreptococcal antigen.

## Diseases Caused by the Immune System

Diseases caused by the immune system occur when there are problems with the immune reaction. The problem may be that the response is faulty, that it is too much, or that it is too little. The following list includes some common immune system diseases and a description of each:

- *Allergies and hypersensitivity reactions:* An allergen is a substance that is usually not harmful. This would be substances like pollen, mold, dust, cat dander, foods, insect stings, insect bites, certain foods, or medicines. When the immune system overacts and produces antibodies against these substances that are not normally harmful or pathogenic, symptoms occur and the resultant condition is known as allergy or hypersensitivity.
- *Autoimmune diseases:* These diseases occur when the body cannot distinguish between its own antigens and outside antigens. This causes the body to fight its own tissues. Examples of autoimmune diseases include systemic lupus erythematosus (SLE), rheumatoid arthritis, and polymyalgia rheumatica.
- *Myasthenia gravis* causes the patient to develop autoantibodies to attack neuromuscular function. The early stages involve the patient's eye and throat muscles. Later, there is complete loss of muscle function followed by death.
- *Multiple sclerosis (MS)* causes patient cells to attack the central nervous system. Triggers considered as causes of MS have been viral infection, environmental factors, or genetic predisposition.
- *Graves hyperthyroidism* is caused when autoantibodies bind to thyroid cells. This stimulates thyroid activity, which results in an enlarged thyroid gland, also known as a goiter.
- *Systemic lupus erythematosus (SLE)* is caused by autoantibodies damaging many body systems. The classic symptom of SLE is the characteristic "butterfly rash" across the cheeks and nose. SLE can destroy organs requiring organ transplants.
- Rheumatoid arthritis is an autoimmune disease that causes gradual debilitating damage to the joints. Treatment includes anti-inflammatory agents or immunosuppressive drugs.
- *Immune deficiency diseases:* Acquired immunodeficiency syndrome (AIDS) is caused by the human immunodeficiency virus. Once the disease progresses, symptoms vary because the infections that follow are by opportunistic organisms.

7. How do autoimmune diseases occur?

## Immunological Testing

Immunology testing uses the binding of a specific antibody to its specific antigen. The antigen is detected by use of a solution containing the antibody or the antibody is detected by using a solution containing the antigen. The way that an antigen–antibody reaction is identified is by detection of the complex reaction of the antigen and antibody.

Immunoassay test kits include reagents to extract the antigen from the specimen. The extraction is dripped onto the test strip or cartridge. The drops react with reagents in the test strip or cartridge. If the extracted specimen contains the antigen, a color change (usually blue or red) will indicate a positive result. Accuracy of testing is dependent upon following the specific manufacturer's instructions. These kits contain all of the reagents and most supplies, such as pipettes, tubes, and cups, needed to perform tests on a given number of samples. The kits must be stored at the temperature recommended on the kit box or package insert. Some kits are stored at room temperature, and some are stored in the refrigerator. It is important to follow the manufacturer's directions. If the kits are stored improperly, the reagents may deteriorate, and false results may be obtained.

Each kit package is marked with a lot number and expiration date. All reagents with the same lot number were made at the same time in the same manufacturing facility. The expiration date is the day past that the reagents are no longer guaranteed to perform correctly. Reagents from kits with different lot numbers should not be used together. The manufacturer will not guarantee that they will work correctly when components from different lots are mixed. Reagents should never be used past their expiration date.

Generally, the following guidelines should be followed when performing CLIA-waived immunoassay testing in the physician office:

- Follow any time limits precisely when performing the test.
- Add the proper reagents in the correct order.
- Use only the reagents that come from the kit and only use the exact amount as stated in the directions.
- Ensure the reagents and samples are at room temperature.
- Do not use reagents that have expired.

The three most common immunoassay tests include:

- *Infectious mononucleosis:* Infectious mononucleosis is caused by the Epstein–Barr virus. The symptoms are fever, sore throat, and swollen lymph glands. Because these symptoms are common to several

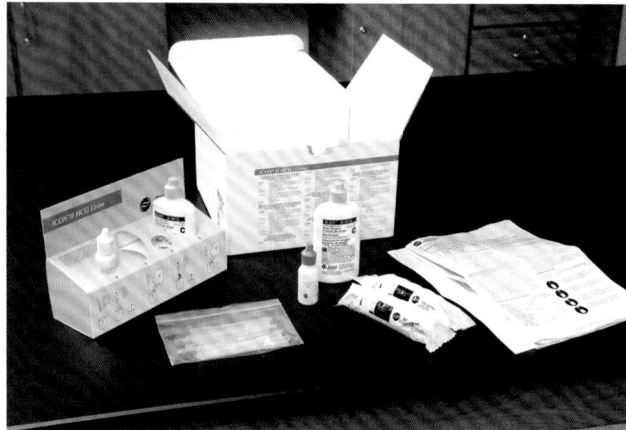

**Figure 44-12** • Pregnancy test kit.

illnesses, the immunoassay test is useful for a differential diagnosis (Procedure 44-6). False-negative results can occur early in the disease before antibodies are produced.

- *Pregnancy test:* The test for pregnancy (Procedure 44-7) is based on the detection of the hormone human chorionic gonadotropin (HCG). Today's tests are sensitive enough to determine pregnancy before the first missed menses (Fig. 44-12). A pregnancy test is frequently used to rule out pregnancy before a medical procedure that might harm the fetus. A urine specimen that is too dilute can give a false-negative reaction. The first morning urine specimen is the most likely to contain HCG if the patient is pregnant. Certain tumors (testicular and some fibroids) produce HCG and can cause a false-positive result.
- *Group A streptococcus:* Group A streptococcus (*Streptococcus pyogenes*) is one of the most common bacterial causes of sore throat and upper respiratory tract infections. Because of the need for rapid diagnosis to begin appropriate treatment, many immunoassay kits are available to test quickly for group A beta-hemolytic streptococcus or *S. pyogenes* (Fig. 44-13). If the test result is positive, treatment can begin at once.

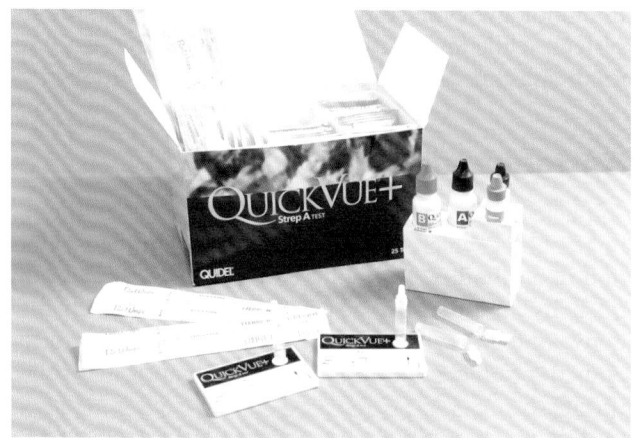

**Figure 44-13** • Rapid strep test kit.

## BOX 44-5 Waived Tests Based on Immunological Testing Principles

Streptococcus, group A (microbiology)
Helicobacter pylori (microbiology)
Urine HCG
Infectious mononucleosis
Influenza A/B (virology)
Respiratory syncytial virus (virology)
Adenovirus (virology)
HIV-1 and HIV-2 antibodies
Ovulation test (luteinizing hormone)
Follicle-stimulating hormone

Group A strep infection can be diagnosed by bacterial culture or immunoassay for the antigenic presence of the bacteria (Procedure 44-8). If improper technique is used in collecting the throat swab or an inadequate specimen is obtained, a false-negative result can occur. Culture testing is considered more sensitive and should be used to confirm negative immunoassay test results. Box 44-5 lists other waived tests that are based on testing principles, and Box 44-6 describes troubleshooting tips if an immunoassay control is not producing an acceptable result.

 **CHECKPOINT QUESTION**

8. What virus is the cause of infectious mononucleosis?

## BOX 44-6 Immunoassay Troubleshooting Tips

If an immunoassay control is not producing an acceptable result, try the following:

1. Reread the procedure to be sure a step was not omitted.
2. Check the labels of reagents to be sure the correct reagents were added in the correct order.
3. Visually check reagents for signs of contamination, such as cloudiness or color change.
4. Repeat the test with a new bottle of control.
5. Repeat the test with a new kit or reagent.
6. Call the manufacturer for assistance.

 **PATIENT EDUCATION**

### Case Study Scenario

A 5-year-old male was brought into the medical office with his mother who stated the child had a fever and had complained of a sore throat for about 24 hours. On physical examination, the patient had a fever of 102.3°F. The physician noted that he had considerable swelling and drainage of the pharynx, which was red in color, and that his tonsils were enlarged and coated with a white, patchy exudate.

- Although the physician is responsible for diagnosing the patient, what would you guess might be the problem with this patient given the symptoms and the physician observations?

  (Answer: A presumptive diagnosis for this child would be strep throat.)

- Why?

  (Answer: Signs of a streptococcal infection of the throat include a fever and enlarged tonsils with white patches.)

- What diagnostic testing might the physician order to make a diagnosis of strep throat?

  (Answer: The physician may want the medical assistant to obtain a throat culture and use a CLIA-waived immunoassay test to check for group A *Streptococcus*.)

- How would the test results be interpreted?

  (Answer: A positive test result indicates the presence of group A *Streptococcus*, whereas a negative test result indicates that group A strep is not present and is not the cause of the patient's sore throat.)

 **ROLE-PLAYING ACTIVITY**

Role-play these scenarios as if you are working with Ramona Starr, RMA, who works in the busy physician office that is part of the Great Falls Medical Center (refer to the case study at the beginning of the chapter). The mother of a 4-year-old boy comes into the office today complaining that her child was exposed to a neighbor boy who has had pinworms and has recently had a sleepover at her house. She is concerned that her child is now infected and is demanding medication for the entire family including her son. How would you respond to this patient? What questions would you ask to get more information about the potential infection? Your instructor will give you additional information about this activity!

*español* **SPANISH TERMINOLOGY**

**Voy a tomar una muestra en su garganta para enviarla a un cultivo.**
I am going to swab your throat to send for a culture.

**Por favor eche su cabeza hacia atrás.**
Please tilt your head back.

**Voy a tomar una muestra de mucosidad de su nariz.**
I am going to swab your nose to obtain a mucus sample.

**Usted tiene un virus. Los antibióticos no le sirven en este caso.**
You have a virus. Antibiotics will not help.

**Necesitamos que obtenga una muestra de su excremento.**
We will need you to collect a stool specimen.

**El doctor cree que usted puede tener faringitis bacteriana.**
The doctor believes you may have strep throat.

**Hay una epidemia de influenza en esta región del país, el doctor le recomienda vacunarse.**
There is an Influenza outbreak in this region of the country; the doctor recommends you get vaccinated.

**Voy a tomar una muestra de la secreción de su herida.**
I am going to swab the secretion of your wound.

**El pie de atleta es causado por un hongo que crece en áreas húmedas, sin luz pero es fácil de prevenir.**
Athlete's foot is caused by fungus that grows in moist and dark environments but is easy to prevent.

**Este procedimiento no le va a doler.**
This is a painless procedure.

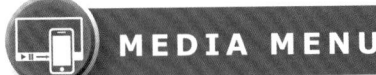

**MEDIA MENU**

**Student Resources** on thePoint®
- *Animation:* Immune Response
- *Video:* Collecting a Throat Specimen (Procedure 44-1)
- *Video:* Testing Stool Specimen for Occult Blood: Guaiac Method (Procedure 44-8)
- *Video:* Preparing a Smear for Microscopic Evaluation (Procedure 44-9)
- *Video:* HCG Pregnancy Test (Procedure 44-13)
- *Video:* Rapid Group A Strep Testing (Procedure 44-14)
- CMA/RMA Certification Exam Review
- English to Spanish Audio Glossary

**Internet Resources**
**MedlinePlus Health Information from the National Library of Medicine**
http://medlineplus.gov
**American College of Allergy, Asthma and Immunology (ACAAI)**
http://www.acaai.org
**Atlas of Microbiology**
www.medmaster.net/atlasofmicrobiol.html

# EMR Activity

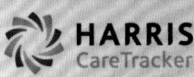

Harris CareTracker is a Web-based electronic medical record (EMR) application that you will use for the EMR activities included in this section at the end of each chapter. This application is actually used in physician offices but is provided to you through the publisher, Wolters Kluwer Health, to give you hands-on practice working with EMRs. Your instructor will have more information about accessing your username, log-in, and Quickstart guide.

Prerequisite Activities in Harris CareTracker

• *The Getting Started and Quickstart documents and EMR Activities Step-by-Step Instructions are available at* http://thePoint.lww.com/KronenbergerComp5e.

Activity Details

Accurately document the following microbiological procedures and results (if given) in each of the following patient's EMR:

1. Sarah Bankston: Throat specimen collected; group A strep test negative
2. Amanda Panci: Instructed on collecting stool sample for ova and parasites

## Chapter Summary

- Most microbiology specimens for culture in a physicians' office laboratory are referred to a reference laboratory. If a microbiology specimen collected is not fully and correctly labeled, the laboratory may be required to dispose of the specimen and cancel the request.
- Handle all specimens as if infectious. Care must be taken to transport or process the specimen as soon as possible so the organisms do not die. To observe microorganisms with a microscope, the specimen requires preparation on a slide and staining. The primary stain used in the microbiology lab is the Gram stain. The immune system is the biological mechanism for identifying and destroying pathogens within a larger organism. An antibody is named by using its specific antigen's name and adding the prefix *anti-*. An allergen is a substance that is usually not harmful. This would be substances like pollen or mold.
- In immunology, the substance to be tested is identified, or the amount present (quantity) is measured using the binding of a specific antibody to its specific antigen.

## Warm-Ups for Critical Thinking

1. You are asked to give a brief talk to a group of elementary school children on microbiological life forms. Develop an age-appropriate discussion of this topic. How would you make it possible for the children to correlate the presence of microbes with the need to wash their hands?
2. Write a policy that explains how to care for media and how to transport specimens.
3. Create a patient education brochure for streptococcal pharyngitis infections. Include information about what it is, how it is transmitted, signs and symptoms, and the testing procedure.
4. In performing an immunoassay, your controls do not give acceptable results. How would you resolve this problem and provide results for the patient?

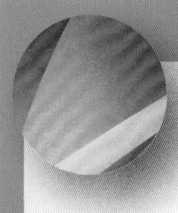

## PSY PROCEDURE 44-1

# Collect a Throat Specimen

**PSY** Obtain specimen and perform CLIA-waived microbiology tests; instruct and prepare a patient for a procedure or treatment; coach patients appropriately considering cultural diversity, developmental life stage, and communication barriers; and document patient care accurately in the medical record.

**Purpose:** This test is used to obtain a throat specimen for rapid strep testing or culture.

**Equipment:** Tongue blade, light source, sterile specimen container and swab, PPE, hand sanitizer, surface sanitizer, biohazard transport bag (if to be sent to the laboratory for analysis), gloves, and biohazard waste container

| STEPS | REASONS |
|---|---|
| 1. Check the physician order. Wash your hands. | Handwashing aids in infection control. |
| 2. Assemble the equipment and supplies. | Equipment must be readily accessible for the procedure to be done. |
| 3. Apply gloves. | Following standard precautions prevents the transmission of infectious microorganisms. |
| 4. **AFF** Greet and identify the patient. Identify yourself including your title. Explain the rationale of the performance of the collection to the patient | Identifying the patient prevents errors in treatment. |
| 5. **AFF** If the patient is hearing impaired, you need to speak clearly and distinctly in front of the patient's face. | Speaking clearly and distinctly to the patient's face will assist the patient in understanding spoken instructions. Have an easy-to-read instruction guide for the patient to follow and point out where there are questions. If the patient can sign and you cannot, have someone proficient in sign language assist you in instructing the patient. |
| 6. **AFF** Use active listening to observe patients' body language and detect a lack of understanding of instructions. Obtain assistance when you realize that you are not able to communicate with the patient. | Someone else in the office may have experience with sign language or may be more effective helping your patient understand. |
| 7. **AFF** Allow time for the adult or patient or caregiver if the patient is a child to ask questions. | Display sensitivity to patient feelings in collecting specimens. |
| 8. **AFF** Display empathy for the patient and family. | Offer this in a timely manner so as not to extend the discomfort of expectation of the procedure. |
| 9. Have the patient sit with a light source directed in the throat. | Enhancing visualization of specimen site improves accuracy of sampling. |
| 10. Carefully remove the sterile swab from the container. If performing both the rapid strep and culture or confirming negative results with a culture, swab with two swabs held together. | Swabbing with two swabs at once eliminates discomfort to the patient of having to perform the procedure twice. |

*(continues on page 1154)*

# PROCEDURE 44-1 (continued)

**STEPS**                                                          **REASONS**

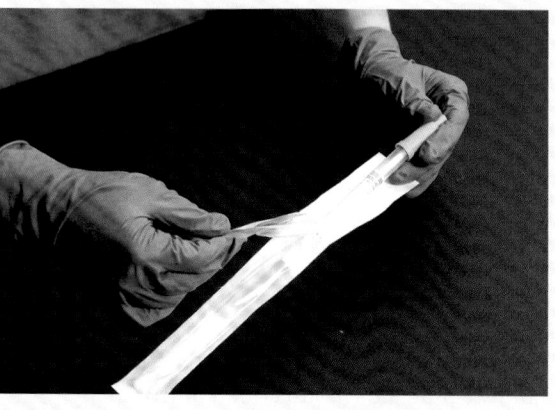

**Step 10.** Carefully remove the sterile swab from the container.

11. Have the patient say "Ah" as you press down on the midpoint of the tongue with the tongue depressor. If the tongue depressor is placed too far forward, it will not be effective; if it is placed too far back, the patient will gag unnecessarily.

Saying "Ah" raises the uvula to avoid contaminating the specimen and decreases the gag reflex.

12. Swab the mucous membranes, especially the tonsillar area, the crypts, and the posterior pharynx in a "figure 8" motion. Turn the swab to expose all of its surfaces to the membranes. Avoid touching the teeth, sides of the mouth, and the uvula.

Pathogens must be collected with a twisting motion for maximum collection. Touching the areas noted to avoid will contaminate the specimen with normal flora and inhibit testing accuracy.

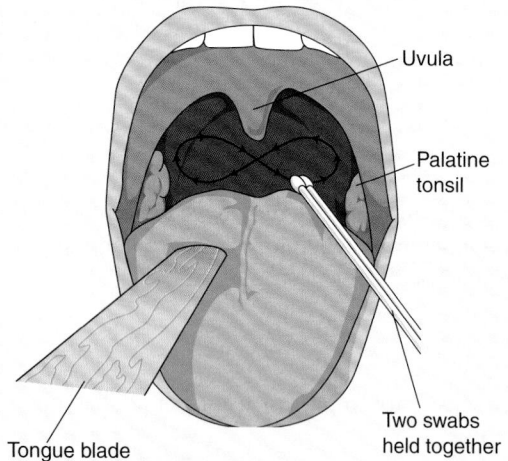

Uvula

Palatine tonsil

Tongue blade

Two swabs held together

**Step 12A.** Technique for obtaining a throat sample

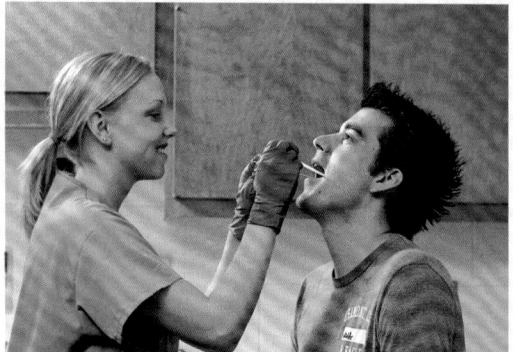

**Step 12B.** Avoid touching areas that will contaminate the specimen. Keeping the tongue down prevents contaminating the swab with normal flora.

## PROCEDURE 44-1 (continued)

| STEPS | REASONS |
|---|---|
| 13. Maintain the tongue depressor position while withdrawing the swab from the patient's mouth. | |
| 14. Follow the instructions on the specimen container for transferring the swab or processing the specimen in the office using a commercial kit. Label the specimen with the patient's name, the date and time of collection, and the origin of the material. | Improper handling of the specimen will compromise test results. Improper labeling will result in test delay and require the patient to have the procedure repeated. |
| 15. Properly dispose of the equipment and supplies in a biohazard waste container. Remove PPE and wash your hands. | This prevents the spread of microorganisms. |
| 16. Route the specimen or store it appropriately until routing can be completed. | Delay in transport to the testing site or improper storage will compromise test results. |
| 17. **AFF** Log into the electronic medical record (EMR) using your username and secure password OR obtain the paper medical record from a secure location and assure it is kept away from public access. Record the procedure noting the date, time, specimen collected, and specimen processing procedure (i.e., sent to lab, tested using CLIA-waived test, etc.). Include your name and title according to office policy and procedure. | The integrity of the medical record must be maintained at all times to protect patient privacy. Procedures that are not documented are considered to have not been performed. |

**Charting Example:**

*11/20/2016 10:30 AM Throat specimen obtained and sent to Great Falls Medical Center lab for C&S*

*———————————————————————————————— R. Starr, RMA*

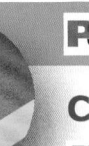

**PSY** P R O C E D U R E   4 4 - 2

## Collecting a Nasopharyngeal Specimen

**PSY** Obtain specimen and perform CLIA-waived microbiology tests; instruct and prepare a patient for a procedure or treatment; coach patients appropriately considering cultural diversity, developmental life stage, and communication barriers; and document patient care accurately in the medical record.

**Purpose:** This test is used to evaluate nasopharyngeal secretions for the presence of pathogenic organisms.

**Equipment:** Penlight, tongue blade, sterile flexible swab, transport media, PPE, hand sanitizer, surface sanitizer, biohazard transport bag (if to be sent to the laboratory for analysis), gloves, and biohazard waste container

| STEPS | REASONS |
|---|---|
| 1. Check the physician order. Wash your hands. | Handwashing aids in infection control. |
| 2. Assemble the equipment and supplies. | Equipment must be readily accessible for the procedure to be done. |
| 3. Put on gloves. | Following standard precautions prevents the transmission of infectious microorganisms. |
| 4. **AFF** Greet and identify the patient. Identify yourself including your title. Explain the rationale of the performance of the collection to the patient. | Identifying the patient prevents errors in treatment. |
| 5. **AFF** If your patient is developmentally challenged, have the individual who transported the patient to the office assist you with communicating with the patient. The developmentally challenged patient may struggle if you have to proceed with something he or she does not understand. Have another medical assistant available to help you should extra support be necessary to support the patient. | Two issues in working with a developmentally challenged patient are the patient's understanding and physically managing the patient's resistance. Securing help is safer for you and the patient. |
| 6. **AFF** Leave time for the adult patient or caregiver of a child to ask questions. | Display sensitivity to patient feelings in collecting specimens. Offer information in a timely manner so as not to extend the discomfort of the anticipated procedure. |
| 7. Position the patient with his head tilted back. | Tilting the head improves access to the interior of the nose. |
| 8. Using a penlight, inspect the nasopharyngeal area. | Enhancing visualization of specimen site improves accuracy of sampling. |

# PROCEDURE 44-2 (continued)

| STEPS | REASONS |
|---|---|
| 9. Gently pass the swab through the nostril and into the nasopharynx, keeping the swab near the septum and floor of the nose. Rotate the swab quickly, and then remove it and place it in the transport media. | Do not let the swab touch the sides of the patient's nostril or his or her tongue to prevent specimen contamination. |

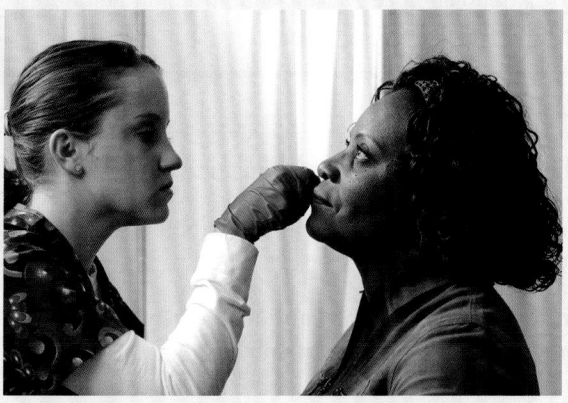

**Step 9.** Gently swab within the nostril.

| STEPS | REASONS |
|---|---|
| 10. Label the specimen with the patient's name, the date and time of collection, and the origin of the specimen. | Improper labeling will result in test delay and require the patient to have the procedure repeated. |
| 11. Properly dispose of the equipment and supplies in a biohazard waste container. Remove gloves and wash your hands. | This prevents the spread of microorganisms. |
| 12. Route the specimen or store it appropriately until routing can be completed. | Delay in transport to the testing site or improper storage will compromise test results. |
| 13. **AFF** Log into the electronic medical record (EMR) using your username and secure password OR obtain the paper medical record from a secure location and assure it is kept away from public access. Record the procedure noting the date, time, specimen collected, and specimen processing procedure (i.e., sent to lab, tested using CLIA-waived test, etc.). Include your name and title according to office policy and procedure. | The integrity of the medical record must be maintained at all times to protect patient privacy. Procedures not documented are considered not performed. |

**Charting Example:**
*11/20/2016 10:30 AM Nasopharyngeal specimen obtained and sent to Great Falls Medical Center laboratory for influenza testing _____ R. Starr, RMA*

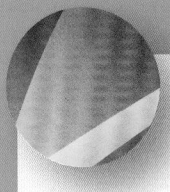

**PSY** PROCEDURE 44-3

## Collecting a Wound Specimen

**PSY** Obtain specimen and perform CLIA-waived microbiology tests; instruct and prepare a patient for a procedure or treatment; coach patients appropriately considering cultural diversity, developmental life stage, and communication barriers; and document patient care accurately in the medical record.

**Purpose:** This test is used to evaluate wound exudate for the presence of pathogenic organisms.

**Equipment:** Sterile swab, transport media, PPE, hand sanitizer, surface sanitizer, and biohazard transport bag (if to be sent to the laboratory for analysis)

| STEPS | REASONS |
|---|---|
| 1. Check the physician order. Wash your hands. | Handwashing aids in infection control. |
| 2. Assemble the equipment and supplies. | Equipment must be readily accessible for the procedure to be done. |
| 3. Put on gloves. | Following standard precautions prevents the transmission of infectious microorganisms. |
| 4. **AFF** Greet and identify the patient. Identify yourself including your title. Explain the procedure. | Identifying the patient prevents errors in treatment. |
| 5. **AFF** If your patient is struggling with dementia, be prepared to gently repeat yourself as necessary until you have collected your specimen. You may have to physically adjust your patient as necessary to collect the specimen. Be gentle but remember to speak to the patient as an adult. | The patient may forget what you just explained. He or she may have some trouble understanding immediately after you explained it. The patient may recognize when being spoken to rudely or as a child. |
| 6. If dressing is present, remove it and dispose of it in a biohazard container. Assess the wound by observing color, odor, and amount of exudate. Remove contaminated gloves and put on clean gloves. | Thorough visualization of specimen site improves accuracy of sampling. |
| 7. Use the sterile swab to sample the exudate. Saturate swab with exudate, avoiding the skin edge around the wound. | Skin around the wound will contain normal flora that may inhibit growth of the pathogen. |

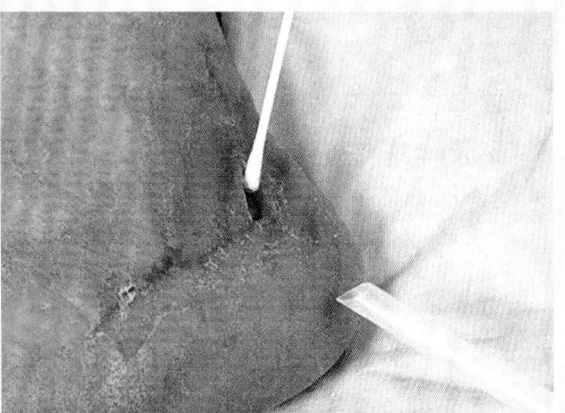

**Step 7.** Saturate swab with exudate.

## PROCEDURE 44-3 (continued)

| STEPS | REASONS |
|---|---|
| **8.** Place swab back into container and crush the ampule of transport medium. | Fastidious bacteria may require transport medium to maintain viability. |

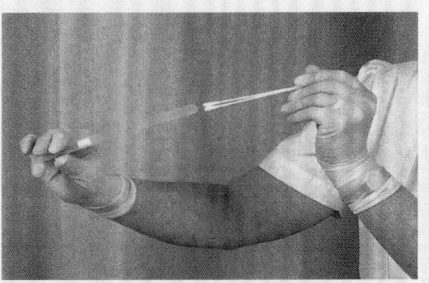

A

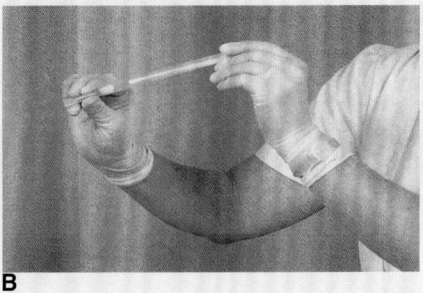

B

**Step 8.** (A) Place swab in culture tube. (B) Crush the ampule of media at the bottom of the tube.

| STEPS | REASONS |
|---|---|
| **9.** Label the specimen with the patient's name, the date and time of collection, and the origin of the specimen. | Improper labeling will result in test delay and require the patient to have the procedure repeated. |
| **10.** Route the specimen or store it appropriately until routing can be completed. | Delay in transport to the testing site or improper storage will compromise test results. |
| **11.** Clean the wound and apply a sterile dressing using sterile technique. | A sterile dressing protects the wound from infection. |
| **12.** Properly dispose of the equipment and supplies in a biohazard waste container. Remove gloves and wash your hands. | This prevents the spread of microorganisms. |
| **13.** **AFF** Log into the electronic medical record (EMR) using your username and secure password OR obtain the paper medical record from a secure location and assure it is kept away from public access. Record the procedure noting the date, time, specimen collected, and specimen processing procedure (i.e., sent to lab, tested using CLIA-waived test, etc.). Include your name and title according to office policy and procedure. | The integrity of the medical record must be maintained at all times to protect patient privacy. Procedures not documented are considered not performed. |

**Charting Example:**
*11/20/2016 10:30 AM Wound specimen obtained from right heel, sent to Great Falls Medical Center laboratory for C&S* _____ *R. Starr, RMA*

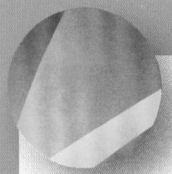

## PSY PROCEDURE 44-4

## Collecting a Stool Specimen

**PSY** Obtain specimen and perform CLIA-waived microbiology tests; instruct and prepare a patient for a procedure or treatment; coach patients appropriately considering cultural diversity, developmental life stage, and communication barriers; and document patient care accurately in the medical record.

**Purpose:** This test is used to evaluate stool for pathogens and/or blood.

**Equipment:** Specimen container dependent on test ordered (sterile container or Para-Pak collection system for C&S or ova and parasites), tongue blade or wooden spatula, gloves, hand sanitizer, surface sanitizer, biohazard transport bag, and biohazard waste container

| STEPS | REASONS |
|---|---|
| 1. Check the physician order. Wash your hands. | Handwashing aids in infection control. |
| 2. Assemble the equipment and supplies. | Equipment must be readily accessible for the procedure to be done. |
| 3. **AFF** Greet and identify the patient. Identify yourself including your title. Explain the procedure. Give the patient the proper specimen container and instruct them to defecate and return specimen to the office. | Identifying the patient prevents errors in treatment. Explanations will help gain compliance and ease anxiety. Noncompliance with preparation for specimen collection may cause unnecessary follow-up testing. |

**Step 3:** Para-Pak stool collection containers

| STEPS | REASONS |
|---|---|
| 4. **AFF** If you are in a significantly different generation than the patient, you will need to take extra precautions with communication. First, remember that collecting a stool specimen is embarrassing for most patients. Watch the patient's facial expressions to note if he or she is understanding your instructions. This is one of the times you may find that your patient does not understand professional terminology. | Patients prefer not to hear repeated instructions openly discussing body functions. Follow up with enough questions to validate the patient's understanding. |

## PROCEDURE 44-4 (continued)

| STEPS | REASONS |
|---|---|
| 5. When obtaining a stool specimen for C&S or ova and parasites, the patient should collect an amount of the first and last portion of the stool after the bowel movement with the wooden spatula or tongue blade and place it in the specimen container without contaminating the outside of the container. Fill Para-Pak until fluid reaches "fill" line, and recap the container. | Touching the inside of the container will contaminate the container and specimen. Stool on the outside of the container may be hazardous. The specimen is a biohazard, and capping the container immediately eliminates the danger of spreading microorganisms. |
| 6. Upon receipt of the specimen, you should put on gloves and place the specimen into the biohazard bag for transport to the reference laboratory. Fill out a laboratory requisition slip to accompany the specimen. | A laboratory requisition will tell the laboratory personnel the type of specimen and the specific tests ordered. |
| 7. Label the specimen with the patient's name, the date and time of collection, and the origin of the specimen. | Improper labeling will result in test delay and require the patient to have the procedure repeated. |
| 8. Transport the specimen to the laboratory or store the specimen as directed. Refer to the laboratory procedure manual since some samples require refrigeration; others are kept at room temperature, and some must be placed in an incubator at a laboratory as soon as possible after collecting. | Improper storage and/or delay in transport to the testing site will compromise test results. |
| 9. Properly dispose of the equipment and supplies in a biohazard waste container. Remove gloves and wash your hands. | This prevents the spread of microorganisms. |
| 10. **AFF** Log into the electronic medical record (EMR) using your username and secure password OR obtain the paper medical record from a secure location and assure it is kept away from public access. Record the procedure noting the date, time, specimen collected, and specimen processing procedure (i.e., sent to lab, tested using CLIA-waived test, etc.). Include your name and title according to office policy and procedure. | The integrity of the medical record must be maintained at all times to protect patient privacy. Procedures not documented are not considered to be performed. |

Charting Example:

*11/20/2016 10:30 AM Patient instructed on preparation for and collection of stool for occult blood. Patient demonstrated understanding and will return specimen to lab upon completion. _____ R. Starr, RMA*

*11/21/2016 8:00AM Stool specimen received from patient. Sent to Great Falls Medical Center lab for O&P testing _____ R. Starr, RMA*

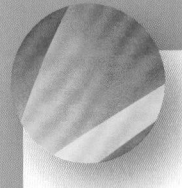

## PSY PROCEDURE 44-5

# Inoculating a Culture

**PSY** Obtain specimen and perform CLIA-waived microbiology tests; instruct and prepare a patient for a procedure or treatment; coach patients appropriately considering cultural diversity, developmental life stage, and communication barriers; and document patient care accurately in the medical record.

**Purpose:** This test is used to introduce a portion of a specimen into the culture medium for growth and replication of microorganisms and to produce isolated colonies.

**Equipment:** Specimen on a swab, permanent laboratory marker, Petri dish, gloves, hand sanitizer, surface sanitizer, and biohazard waste container

| STEPS | REASONS |
|---|---|
| 1. Check the physician order. Wash your hands. | Handwashing aids in infection control. |
| 2. Assemble the equipment. | Equipment must be readily accessible to perform the procedure. |
| 3. Put on gloves. | Following standard precautions prevents the transmission of infectious microorganisms. |
| 4. Label the medium side of the plate with the permanent marker. Include the patient's name, identification number, source of specimen, time collected, time inoculated, your initials, and date. | Because culture incubation may take 24–72 hours, dating ensures that the plate is read at the proper time. Labeling the medium side will prevent misplacing the culture. |

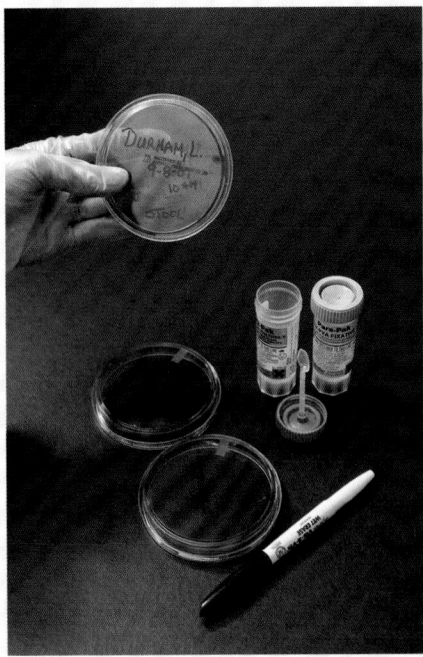

**Step 4.** Correctly labeled specimen plate

5. Remove the Petri plate from the cover (the Petri plate is always stored with the cover down), and place the cover on the work surface with the opening up. Do not open the cover unnecessarily.

Each time the cover is removed, there is a chance of contamination. Having the cover's opening upward avoids contamination from the work surface.

# PROCEDURE 44-5 (continued)

| STEPS | REASONS |
|---|---|

**STEPS**

6. Using a rolling and sliding motion, streak the specimen swab across one fourth of the plate, starting at the top and working to the center. Dispose of the swab in a biohazard container. The specimen will spread in gradually thinning colonies of bacteria.

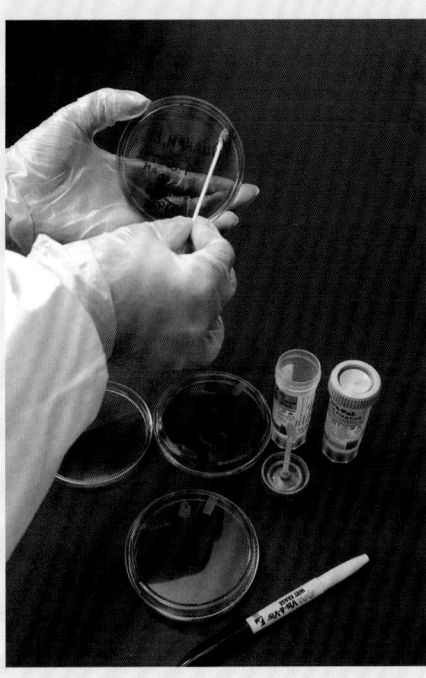

7. Use a disposable sterile loop and turn the plate a quarter turn from its previous position. Pass the loop a few times in the original inoculum and then across the medium approximately a quarter of the surface of the plate. Do not enter the originally streaked area after the first few sweeps.

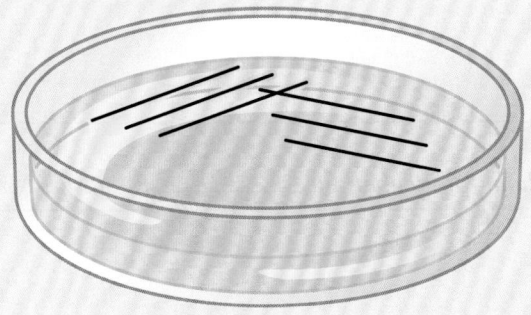

**REASONS**

**Step 6.** Use a rolling and sliding motion to apply specimen to plate.

The loop is the tool for spreading the specimen. The loop draws into the clean surface a bit of the specimen that was streaked in the first part of the procedure.

**Step 7.** Streak lightly from the original inoculum across the next quarter of the plate.

*(continues on page 1164)*

## PROCEDURE 44-5 (continued)

| STEPS | REASONS |
|---|---|
| 8. Turn the plate another quarter turn so that now it is 180° to the original smear. Working in the previous manner, draw the loop at right angles through the most recently streaked area. Again, do not enter the originally streaked area after the first few sweeps. | The loop pulls out gradually thinning bits of the specimen to isolate colonies. Large groups of colonies close together are more difficult to identify than isolated colonies. |

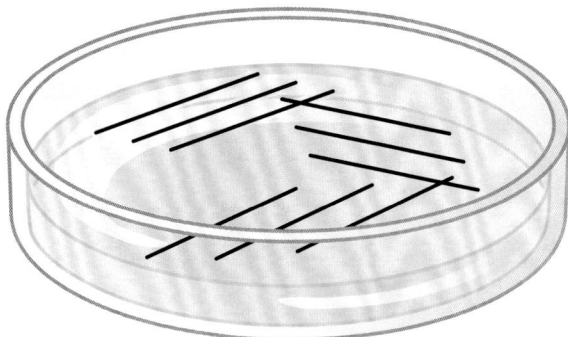

**Step 8.** Streak the third quadrant of the plate.

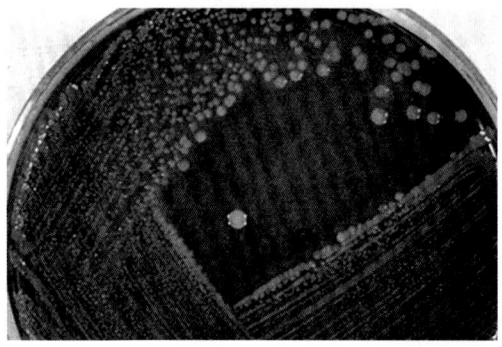

Pale yellow colonies of *Staphylococcus aureus.* Colonies demonstrate growth of the microbe on a properly streaked plate.

| STEPS | REASONS |
|---|---|
| 9. Place the prepared culture with the lid on in an incubator per office policy and procedure. Properly dispose of the contaminated supplies in a biohazard waste container. Remove gloves and wash your hands. | The inoculated Petri dish must be put into a warm environment to promote bacterial growth. Disposing of gloves properly and washing your hands prevents the spread of microorganisms. |
| 10. **AFF** Log into the electronic medical record (EMR) using your username and secure password OR obtain the paper medical record from a secure location and assure it is kept away from public access. Record the procedure noting the date, time, specimen collected, and specimen processing procedure (i.e., sent to lab, tested using CLIA-waived test, etc.). Include your name and title according to office policy and procedure. | The integrity of the medical record must be maintained at all times to protect patient privacy. Procedures not documented have not been performed. |

Charting Example:
*7/14/2016 9:15 AM Throat specimen transferred to culture medium for incubation. _____ R. Starr, RMA*

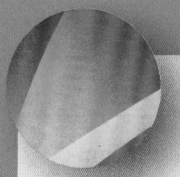

**PSY** PROCEDURE 44-6

# Mononucleosis Testing

**PSY** Obtain specimen and perform CLIA-waived immunology tests; instruct and prepare a patient for a procedure or treatment; coach patients appropriately considering cultural diversity, developmental life stage, and communication barriers; and document patient care accurately in the medical record.

**Purpose:** This test is used to determine the presence or absence of infectious mononucleosis using a CLIA-waived test kit.

**Equipment:** Patient's labeled specimen (whole blood, plasma, or serum, depending on the kit), CLIA-waived mononucleosis kit (slide or test strip) with instructions, stopwatch or timer, gloves, hand sanitizer, surface sanitizer, and biohazard waste container

| STEPS | REASONS |
|---|---|
| 1. Check the physician order. Wash your hands. | Handwashing aids in infection control. |
| 2. Assemble the equipment and ensure that the materials in the kit and the patient specimen are at room temperature. | Equipment must be easily accessible to perform the procedure. |
| 3. Label the test pack or test strip (depending on type of kit) with the patient's name, positive control, and negative control. Use one test pack or strip per patient and control. | This ensures accurate testing. |
| 4. Put on gloves. Collect the blood specimen according to the test kit instructions. | In most cases, a capillary stick is necessary to perform a CLIA-waived test for mononucleosis. If more blood is necessary, the instructions on the package insert for the test kit will explain the procedure. |
| 5. Perform the test as directed. Also, perform the controls according to the kit instructions. | Follow the instructions precisely for performing the procedure using the blood specimen obtained. Performing the control procedure satisfies quality assurance (QA) and QC standards. |
| 6. Set timer for the period indicated in package insert. | Timing is critical for an accurate test result. |
| 7. Read reaction results at the end of the time period. | Waiting the appropriate amount of time ensures that testing is complete. |
| 8. Verify the results of the controls before documenting the patient's results. Log the QC and patient information on any worksheet required per the office policy and procedure manual. | This satisfies documentation of QC and the patient's results. |
| 9. Properly dispose of the equipment and supplies in a biohazard waste container. | Using a biohazard container for disposal of biohazards prevents potential exposure. |
| 10. Remove your gloves and wash your hands. | This prevents the spread of microorganisms. |

*(continues on page 1166)*

## PROCEDURE 44-6 (continued)

| STEPS | REASONS |
|---|---|
| 11. **AFF** Log into the electronic medical record (EMR) using your username and secure password OR obtain the paper medical record from a secure location and assure it is kept away from public access. Record the procedure noting the date, time, specimen collected, and specimen processing procedure (i.e., sent to lab, tested using CLIA-waived test, etc.). Include your name and title according to office policy and procedure. | The integrity of the medical record must be maintained at all times to protect patient privacy. Procedures not documented have not been performed. |

*Note:* Kits vary with the manufacturer; read instructions carefully before beginning. Controls for test kits may be performed at different intervals depending on laboratory protocol. Follow procedures to ensure quality.

---

Charting Example:
*04/23/2016 10:00 AM Mono test performed, Results negative. Dr. Scott aware* _____ *R. Starr, RMA*

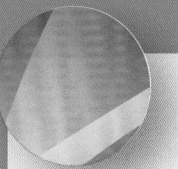

## PSY PROCEDURE 44-7

### HCG Pregnancy Test

**PSY** Obtain specimen and perform CLIA-waived immunology tests; instruct and prepare a patient for a procedure or treatment; coach patients appropriately considering cultural diversity, developmental life stage, and communication barriers; and document patient care accurately in the medical record.

**Purpose:** This test is used to detect the production of HCG to determine pregnancy using a CLIA-waived testing kit.

**Equipment:** Patient's labeled urine specimen, CLIA-waived HCG pregnancy kit, timer, gloves, hand sanitizer, surface sanitizer, and biohazard waste container

| STEPS | REASONS |
|---|---|
| **1.** Check the physician order. Wash your hands. | Handwashing aids in infection control. |
| **2.** Assemble the equipment. | Equipment must be readily accessible to perform the procedure. |

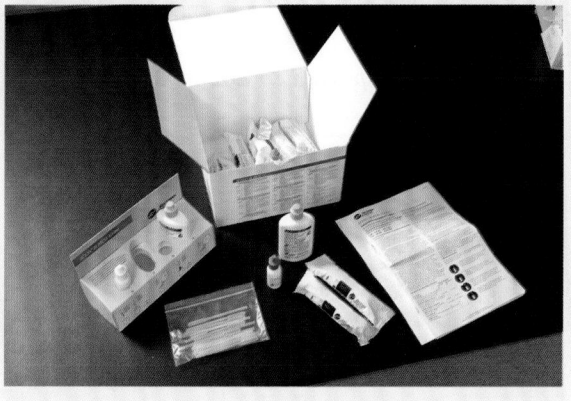

**Step 2.** Assembled equipment from an HCG pregnancy test kit

| STEPS | REASONS |
|---|---|
| **3.** Verify the urine specimen is for the correct patient. Verify the HCG test kit is not expired. | This validates the identity of the specimen and assures the results are for the correct patient. Do not use test kits or contents that are past the expired date noted on the containers. |
| **4.** Perform the test as indicated on the test kit package insert directions. | Follow the directions according to the test kit directions precisely. |
| **5.** Sample the positive and negative controls as directed for the test kit. | This satisfies QA and QC standards. |
| **6.** Set the timer for running the test as indicated in package insert. | CLIA requires performing the procedure as instructed by the manufacturer. |
| **7.** Read reaction results at the end of prescribed period of time. | Waiting the appropriate amount of time ensures that testing is complete. |
| **8.** Verify the results of the controls before documenting the patient's results. Log controls and patient information on the worksheet according to office policy and procedure. | This satisfies QA and QC standards. |
| **9.** Properly dispose of the equipment and supplies in a biohazard waste container. | Disposing biohazards appropriately reduces the risk of exposure. |

*(continues on page 1168)*

## PROCEDURE 44-7 (continued)

| STEPS | REASONS |
|---|---|
| 10. Remove gloves and wash your hands. | This prevents the spread of microorganisms. |
| 11. **AFF** Log into the electronic medical record (EMR) using your username and secure password OR obtain the paper medical record from a secure location and assure it is kept away from public access. Record the procedure noting the date, time, specimen collected, and specimen processing procedure (i.e., sent to lab, tested using CLIA-waived test, etc.). Include your name and title according to office policy and procedure. | The integrity of the medical record must be maintained at all times to protect patient privacy. Procedures not documented have not been performed. |

*Note:* Kits vary with the manufacturer; read instructions carefully before beginning. Controls for test kits may be performed at different intervals depending on laboratory protocol. Perform at least the minimum controls required in the product information to ensure quality. Your office protocol may require more frequent QC testing.

---

Charting Example:
*12/14/2016 9:30 AM Urine HCG test performed on urine, positive result reported to Dr. Schanzer*
*———————————————————————————— R. Starr, RMA*

**PSY** PROCEDURE 44-8

## Rapid Group A Strep Testing

**PSY** Obtain specimen and perform CLIA-waived immunology tests; instruct and prepare a patient for a procedure or treatment; coach patients appropriately considering cultural diversity, developmental life stage, and communication barriers; and document patient care accurately in the medical record.

**Purpose:** This test is used to determine the presence of *S. pyogenes* in a throat specimen using a CLIA-waived group A strep test kit.

**Equipment:** CLIA-waived group A strep kit (controls may be included, depending on the kit), timer, gloves, hand sanitizer, surface sanitizer, and biohazard waste container

| STEPS | REASONS |
|---|---|
| 1. Check the physician order. Wash your hands. | Handwashing aids in infection control. |
| 2. Assemble the equipment including the test kit. Familiarize yourself with the instructions before obtaining the specimen and performing the procedure. | |

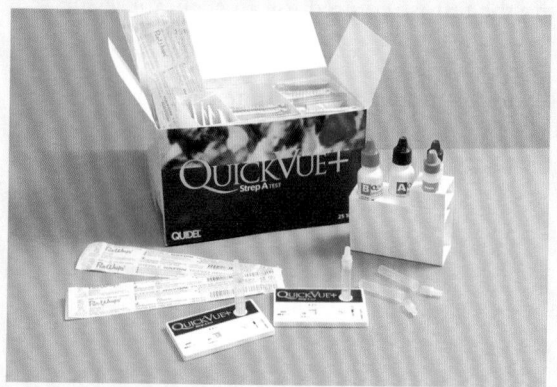

Step 2. Rapid strep kit

| | |
|---|---|
| 3. Apply gloves. Obtain the throat specimen from the patient after assuring you have the correct patient. Use the swabs that come with the testing kit. | |
| 4. Follow the directions for the kit. Add the appropriate reagents and drops to each of the extraction-appropriate test tubes. | Following the manufacturer's instructions exactly will ensure that you adhere to the guidelines. |
| 5. Insert the patient swab into the labeled extraction tube. | |

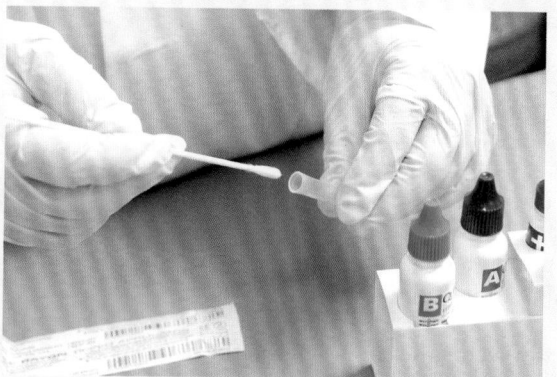

Step 5. Insert patient swab into extraction tube.

(continues on page 1170)

## PROCEDURE 44-8 (continued)

| STEPS | REASONS |
|---|---|
| 6. Add the appropriate controls to each of the labeled extraction tubes. | This begins the chemical reaction and provides the proper dilution factor for proper control results. |
| 7. Set the timer for the appropriate time to ensure accuracy. | Timing ensures accuracy. |
| 8. Add the appropriate reagent and drops to each of the extraction tubes. | |
| 9. Use the swab to mix the reagents. Then press out any excess fluid on the swab against the inside of the tube. | This maximizes the volume of the extraction solution for testing. |
| 10. Add the appropriate number of drops from the well-mixed extraction tube to the sample window of the strep A test unit. Do the same for each control. | |
| 11. Set the timer for the time indicated in the kit package insert. | Timing the test is required for an accurate result. |
| 12. Depending on the test kit used, a positive result may appear as a line in the result window within 5 minutes. The strep A test unit or strip has an internal control; if a line appears in the control window, the test is valid. | These are the instructions for interpreting the test results. |

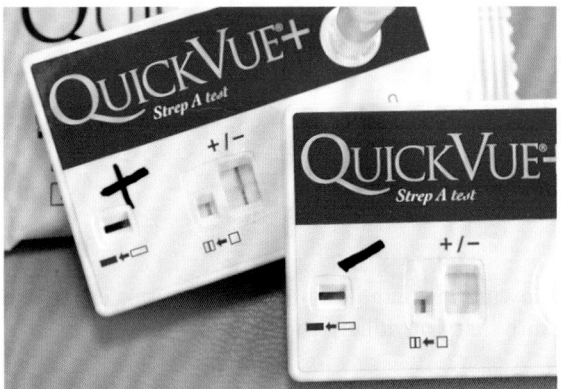

**Step 12.** Picture of positive- and negative-control packs

| STEPS | REASONS |
|---|---|
| 13. Read a negative result at exactly 5 minutes or as per the test kit instructions to avoid a false-negative result. | Waiting the correct amount of time will avoid false-negative results. |
| 14. Verify results of the controls before recording or reporting test results. Log the controls and the patient's information on the worksheet according to office policy and procedure. | This satisfies QA and QC standards. |
| 15. Properly dispose of the equipment and supplies in a biohazard waste container. | Disposing biohazards appropriately reduces the possibility of infection. |
| 16. Remove your gloves and wash your hands. | This prevents the spread of microorganisms. |

## PROCEDURE 44-8 (continued)

| STEPS | REASONS |
|---|---|
| 17. **AFF**  Log into the electronic medical record (EMR) using your username and secure password OR obtain the paper medical record from a secure location and assure it is kept away from public access. Record the procedure noting the date, time, specimen collected, and specimen processing procedure (i.e., sent to lab, tested using CLIA-waived test, etc.). Include your name and title according to office policy and procedure. | The integrity of the medical record must be maintained at all times to protect patient privacy. Procedures not documented have not been performed. |

*Note:* Kits vary with the manufacturer; read instructions carefully before beginning. Controls for test kits may be performed at different intervals depending on laboratory protocol. Follow procedures to ensure quality.

---

**Charting Example:**
*05/22/2016 11:15 AM Group A rapid strep test performed, positive results reported to Dr. Harrison.*
*—————————————————————————————————— B. White, CMA*

---

Note: *The medical assistant may sign his or her name in the patient record using only the "CMA" credential if the office has a signature log denoting the entire credential as "CMA(AAMA)."*

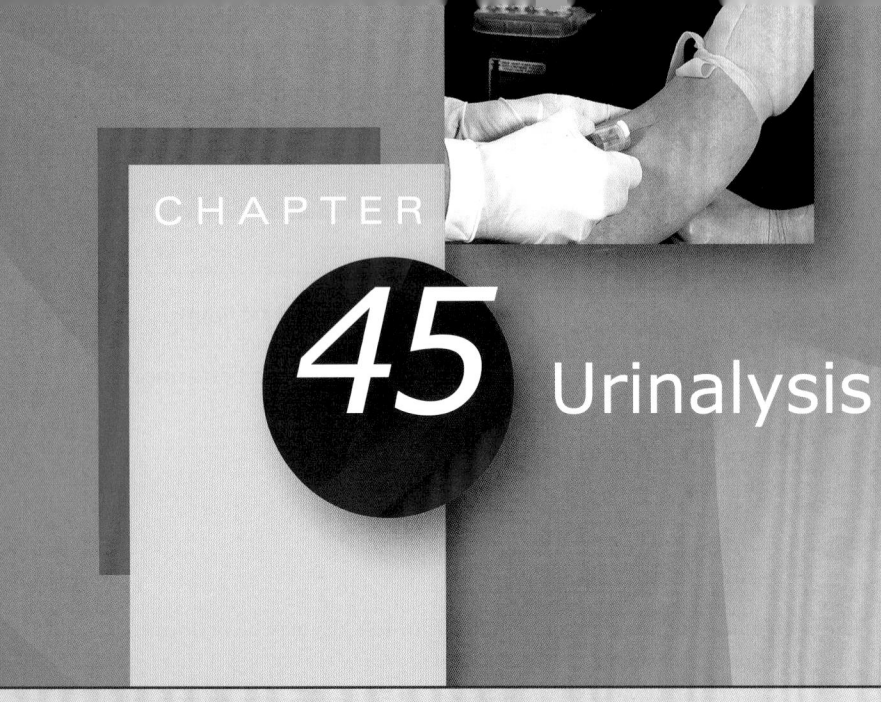

# 45 Urinalysis

## Outline

## Learning Outcomes

### COG Cognitive Domain*

1. Spell key terms
2. *Define medical terms and abbreviations related to all body systems*
3. *Identify CLIA-waived tests associated with common diseases*
4. *Analyze health care results as reported in graphs and tables*
5. Describe the methods of urine collection
6. List and explain the physical and chemical properties of urine
7. Describe the components that can be found in urine sediment and describe their relationships to chemical findings
8. Explain the procedures included in urine drug testing including chain of custody

### PSY Psychomotor Domain*

1. *Obtaining a clean-catch midstream urine specimen (Procedure 45-1)*
   a. *Obtain specimens and perform CLIA-waived urinalysis testing*
   b. *Instruct and prepare a patient for a procedure or treatment*
   c. *Coach patients appropriately considering cultural diversity, developmental life stage, and communication barriers*
   d. *Document patient care accurately in the medical record*
2. *Perform a physical and chemical urinalysis (Procedure 45-2)*
   a. *Obtain specimens and perform CLIA-waived urinalysis testing*
   b. *Instruct and prepare a patient for a procedure or treatment*

   c. *Coach patients appropriately considering cultural diversity, developmental life stage, and communication barriers*
   d. *Document patient care accurately in the medical record*

### AFF Affective Domain*

1. *Incorporate critical thinking skills when performing patient assessment*
2. *Incorporate critical thinking skills when performing patient care*
3. *Show awareness of a patient's concerns related to the procedure being performed*
4. *Demonstrate empathy, active listening, and nonverbal communication*
5. *Demonstrate respect for individual diversity including gender, race, religion, age, economic status, and appearance*
6. *Explain to a patient the rationale for performance of a procedure*
7. *Demonstrate sensitivity to patient rights*
8. *Protect the integrity of the medical record*

***Note: AAMA/CAAHEP 2015 Standards are italicized.***

### ABHES Competencies

1. Use standard precautions
2. Screen and follow up patient test results
3. Perform selected CLIA-waived urinalysis testing that assist with diagnosis and treatment
4. Instruct patients in the collection of a clean-catch midstream urine specimen

## Key Terms

| | | | |
|---|---|---|---|
| bacteriuria | glycosuria | lyse | proteinuria |
| bilirubin | hematuria | microalbumin | sediment |
| bilirubinuria | hematuria | microhematuria | specific gravity |
| chain-of-custody procedure | ketoacidosis | myoglobin | supernatant |
| | ketones | nitrite | turbidity |
| diurnal variation | leukocyte esterase | phagocytic | urobilinogen |

## Case Study

*H*eather Henderson, CMA (AAMA), works in a family practice office that is affiliated with Great Falls Medical Center. Each day, the physician orders urine samples for testing in the office for various reasons. Today, a patient has come into the office for a pre-employment physical examination including a urine drug test. What are the special procedures, if any, for collecting urine for drug testing? What drugs can be tested using a urine specimen? Why is the temperature of the urine recorded after collection? These and other questions are addressed in this chapter.

## THE URINALYSIS

A urinalysis is a physical and chemical examination of urine to assess renal function and other possible problems. Because the physical and chemical analysis of urine is a CLIA-waived test, the urinalysis is commonly performed in the physician office. Proficiency in collecting the urine specimen and performing the physical and chemical analysis is essential for the medical assistant. As indicated by clinical symptoms or physical and chemical findings in the urine, a microscopic examination may be ordered by the physician; however, this procedure is not CLIA-waived and may require a specimen to be sent to a reference laboratory.

The physician may order a urinalysis for several reasons:

- To assess overall health
- To diagnose a medical condition
- To monitor a medical condition

As with all body fluids, urine must be handled using Occupational Safety and Health Administration–mandated personal protective equipment and safety guidelines.

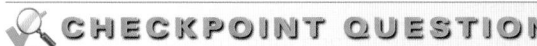

### CHECKPOINT QUESTION

1. What are the 2 reasons a physician might order a urinalysis?

## Physical Properties of Urine

The physical properties of the urine specimen include the urine's color, appearance, specific gravity, and odor. The first part of a urinalysis is direct visual observation. Color and clarity are assessed visually and are subjective, which means the individual performing the testing will determine whether these properties can be considered within the normal range (Table 45-1).

### Color

Urine color can be affected by many things including diet, drugs, diseases, and the concentration of the urine. Normal, fresh urine is pale to dark yellow or amber in color. The yellow color is due to the pigment urochrome. Pale urine is typically very dilute and is seen

| TABLE 45-1 | Expected Ranges for Urine Physical Properties |
|---|---|
| **Property** | **Expected Range** |
| Color | Pale yellow to amber |
| Clarity | Clear |
| Odor | Slightly aromatic but not fruity, no ammonia |
| Specific gravity | 1.001–1.035 |

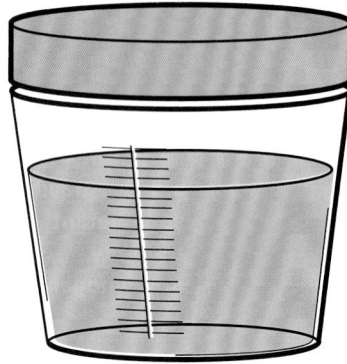

**Figure 45-1 •** Hematuria in a urine specimen.

after high fluid intake. Dark yellow color can signify highly concentrated urine such as when the patient is dehydrated. Red or red–brown color could be from a food dye, eating fresh beets, a drug, or the presence of either hemoglobin or **myoglobin** (a protein in the heart and skeletal muscle) (Fig. 45-1).

##  Clarity

Normal, freshly voided urine is usually clear. Haziness or **turbidity** (cloudiness) may be caused by cellular material or protein in the urine. It may also develop from precipitation of salts while standing. Red blood cells, WBCs, bacteria, or mucus can also cause turbidity. These are not considered normal. Laboratories vary in terminology used to express clarity or turbidity of urine. Common terminology dictates that when a small amount of turbidity is present so that black lines on white paper can be seen through the specimen, it is hazy. As turbidity increases and these black lines can no longer be seen, it is called *cloudy*. The three terms most

commonly used to describe clarity are *clear*, *hazy*, and *cloudy*. Table 45-2 summarizes the common causes of variations in the color and clarity of urine.

## Specific Gravity

The **specific gravity** reflects the ability of the kidney to concentrate or dilute the urine. Specific gravity is the weight of the urine compared to the weight of distilled water. Urine, which contains cells and elements such as sodium, potassium, and chloride, is heavier than water. Specific gravity for a normal urine specimen is 1.001 to 1.035.

Urine with low specific gravity is dilute, probably as the result of high fluid intake. Abnormal conditions that produce dilute urine are diabetes insipidus and kidney infection or inflammation. In end-stage renal disease, the kidney cannot concentrate urine above a specific gravity of 1.007 to 1.010.

Urine with high specific gravity is concentrated. A patient with a high specific gravity may be dehydrated. Sweating, vomiting, or diarrhea may produce a concentrated specimen because the body is trying to conserve water. A high specific gravity may also occur in diabetes mellitus. A urine specimen with a specific gravity of over 1.035 is contaminated, contains very high levels of glucose, or contains contrast media from radiographic studies.

Measuring a specific gravity can be determined by a variety of methods. The specific gravity pad on the reagent strip used for the chemical analysis takes a drop of urine, and the color change is compared to a chart to determine the value (Fig 45-2). This allows specific gravity to be determined in combination with the other chemical assays on the reagent strip and is the most common and efficient method of measurement. An older

| TABLE 45-2    Common Causes of Variations in the Color and Clarity of Urine | |
|---|---|
| **Color and Clarity** | **Possible Causes** |
| Yellow–brown or green–brown | Bile in urine (as in jaundice) |
| Dark yellow or orange | Concentrated urine, low fluid intake, dehydration, inability of kidney to dilute urine, fluorescein (intravenous dye), multivitamins, excessive carotene |
| Bright orange–red | Pyridium (urinary tract analgesic) |
| Red or reddish brown | Hemoglobin pigments, pyrvinium pamoate (Povan™) for intestinal worms, sulfonamides (sulfa-based antibiotics) |
| Green or blue | Artificial color in food or drugs |
| Blackish, grayish, smoky | Hemoglobin or remnants of old RBCs (indicating bleeding in upper urinary tract), chyle, prostatic fluid, yeasts |
| Cloudy | Phosphate precipitation (normal after sitting for a long time), urates (compound of uric acid), leukocytes, pus, blood, epithelial cells, fat droplets, strict vegetarian diet |

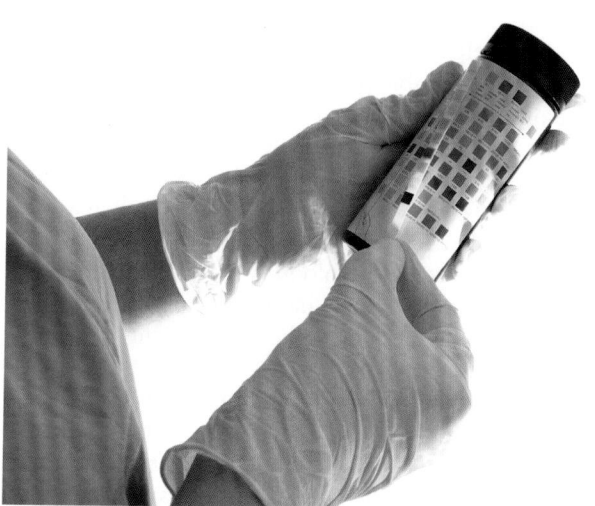

**Figure 45-2 •** Multistix reagent strip color pad.

tool for measuring specific gravity is the refractometer or total solids meter, which requires a drop of urine and is read using a scale that measures the amount of light bent by the particles in the urine (Fig. 45-3A, B). With the refractometer, the urine that contains more particles bends more light. That raises the specific gravity value registered by the refractometer.

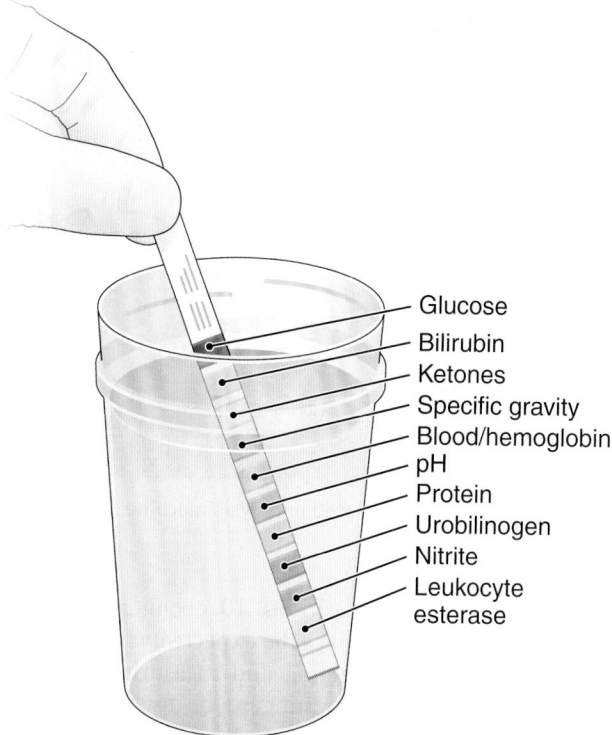

**Figure 45-4 •** Fresh or refrigerated urine tested by dipstick method. The intensity of color change is proportional to concentration.

The labels for Figure 45-4:
- Glucose
- Bilirubin
- Ketones
- Specific gravity
- Blood/hemoglobin
- pH
- Protein
- Urobilinogen
- Nitrite
- Leukocyte esterase

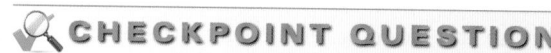

## CHECKPOINT QUESTION

2. Which physical properties of urine are assessed visually?

## Chemical Properties

Urine contains chemicals produced in the body and ingested from the environment. Reagent strips that can be dipped into urine have chemicals embedded in pads.

The chemicals in the pads react with the chemicals in the urine, and the reagent pad will change color as the chemical reaction takes place (Fig. 45-4). All reagent pad colors are compared with a color chart to interpret the reactions at the specific time indicated for each reaction. This color measurement may be performed visually or with a semiautomated strip-reading instrument (Fig. 45-5).

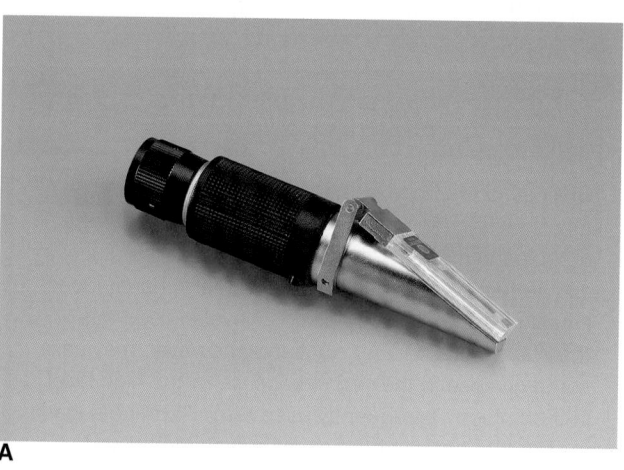

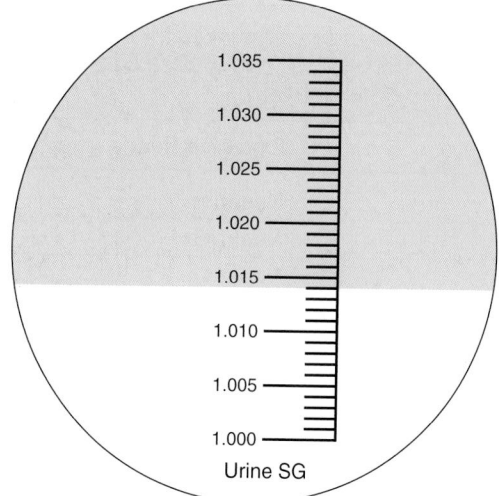

1.035
1.030
1.025
1.020
1.015
1.010
1.005
1.000

Urine SG

**A**  **B**

**Figure 45-3 • (A)** Clinical refractometer for measuring urine specific gravity. **(B)** This refractometer measurement represents a reading of 1.014.

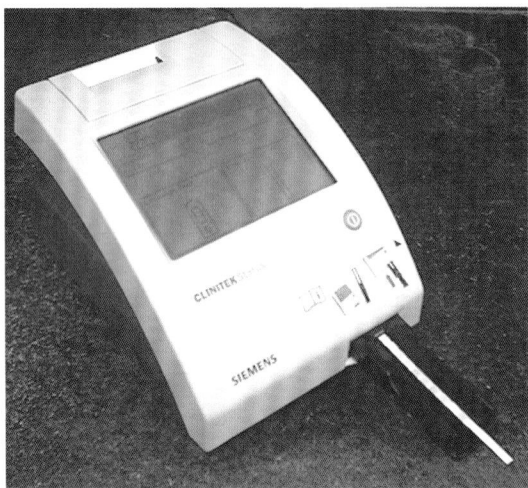

**Figure 45-5 •** An automated urinalysis machine.

The reagent strip performs 10 chemical measurements, and Table 45-3 gives the expected value for each chemical property. Detecting and measuring chemical properties allows urine testing to be used in diagnosis, and care must be taken to assure accurate results. Reagent strips should be tested with positive and negative controls on each day of use according to office policy and procedure. Each reagent pad on the strip must give a positive or negative test result as appropriate. Failure to observe color changes at the appropriate time intervals may cause inaccurate results. Reagents and reagent strips must be stored properly to retain reactivity. When using reagent strips, observe color changes and color charts under good lighting. Perform the chemical analysis on fresh urine specimens to ensure preservation of components, such as bilirubin and ketones, and do not allow the reagent pads of the strip to touch the fingers or other surfaces.

## pH

The kidney helps maintain the acid–base balance of the body. To keep a stable pH, the kidney must control the change of pH of the urine to balance the pH that results from diet and metabolism. If there is too much acid in the body (acidosis), then the kidney will excrete the acid. When the body does not contain enough acid, the kidney will not excrete as much acid so that more acid remains in the circulating blood.

A low pH, from 1 to 6, indicates more acid present in a solution. The less acid there is present in a solution, the higher the pH (8 to 14). A neutral pH is 7.0, making a solution neither an acid nor a base. Expected patient values for urine pH can range from 5.0 to 8.0 with the typical pH on a freshly voided urine specimen being 6.0. Slightly acidic urine is normal and may occur with a high-protein diet and uncontrolled diabetes. A pH above 7.0 can occur after meals and with a vegetarian diet, certain renal diseases, and a urinary tract infection (UTI).

## Glucose

Glucose is filtered and reabsorbed in the kidneys, with the renal threshold being 180 mg/dL. When the blood glucose goes over this threshold, the kidneys will not reabsorb all of it. The glucose that the kidney does not reabsorb into the blood is released into the urine (Box 45-1). This causes a positive result for the presence of glucose in the urine, or **glycosuria**. The threshold can vary and requires measuring the actual blood level in addition to the urine level for a diagnostic assessment. Normal urine does not contain glucose. When the glucose measured on the dipstick indicates that no glucose is present, the patient's blood level of glucose will be less than 180 mg/dL.

### CHECKPOINT QUESTION

3. In what disease process would monitoring glycosuria be useful?

| TABLE 45-3 | Expected Ranges of Chemical Properties |
|---|---|
| **Property** | **Expected Range** |
| Glucose | Negative |
| Bilirubin | Negative |
| Ketones | Negative |
| Blood | Negative |
| pH | 5.0–8.0 |
| Protein | Negative to trace |
| Urobilinogen | 0.1–1.0 mg/dL |
| Nitrite | Negative |
| Leukocyte esterase | Negative |
| Specific gravity | 1.001–1.035 |

**BOX 45-1    Renal Threshold and Glycosuria**

Glucose is resorbed in the proximal convoluted tubule. When blood glucose levels exceed 180 mg/dL, depending on the individual, not all of the glucose can be reabsorbed into the bloodstream. Rarely does a healthy person's blood glucose level exceed this threshold value. Diabetic patients, however, may pass some glucose in their urine because of the high level in their blood. A frequently used term, "spilling sugar," means that not all of the sugar is reabsorbed and some is excreted in the urine.

## Ketones

Energy is derived from carbohydrate metabolism, and without enough carbohydrates, fats are used by the body for energy. **Ketones** are chemicals produced during fat metabolism. Normally, ketones in urine are too low to measure, so a positive ketone test indicates the body is burning more fat than normal. This condition, **ketoacidosis**, may occur in patients with diabetes mellitus and is a sign that the disease is out of control.

## Proteins

It is not abnormal to have a small amount of protein in the urine, which may be recorded as a "trace" amount. However, an increased amount of protein in the urine, known as **proteinuria**, may be diagnostic of kidney disease. Other conditions that may cause protein in the urine include strenuous exercise, pregnancy, and a urinary tract infection, when there is blood or purulent material in the urine. The presence of vaginal discharge, semen, heavy mucus, pus, and blood in the urine can cause a false-positive urine protein results. To avoid a false-positive result, instruct the patient in the proper method for collecting a clean-catch specimen to avoid getting a contaminated urine sample.

## Erythrocytes

While small amounts of red blood cells are occasionally observed in urine, blood is not normally found in urine. There are two reasons why a urine specimen may contain RBCs with the first including blood getting into the specimen through contamination from menstrual bleeding, renal disorders, certain neoplasms, a urinary tract infection (UTI), or trauma to the urinary tract.

The second way blood appears in urine is as the contents of the RBCs rupture or **lyse**, resulting in hemoglobin being released into the urine and detected by the reagent strip that reacts to hemoglobin, the primary constituent of RBCs. Hemoglobinuria may occur with transfusion reactions, chemical toxicity, or severe burns. The strip also reacts to myoglobin, a protein found in muscles. Myoglobin may be released into the bloodstream from a crushing injury or other trauma and may then be excreted in the urine.

The color of urine that contains RBCs or hemoglobin may appear normal in samples that contain very small amounts, also known as **microhematuria**. Microhematuria can only be detected by testing the urine specimen with a reagent strip that detects blood. Gross **hematuria**, a large amount of urine in the blood, alters the color of the urine to a red or brownish red color. The presence of RBCs in the urine can result from multiple variations of kidney disorders, kidney stones, kidney trauma, and bleeding disorders.

## Bilirubin

**Bilirubin** is formed during breakdown of hemoglobin that occurs in the liver before being excreted into the intestines. With the exception of conjugated bilirubin, most bilirubin cannot dissolve, so urine contains very low levels of bilirubin. On the reagent test strip, bilirubin is either present (positive result) or not present (negative result) in the specimen. Although the reagent strip is designed to react to bilirubin, dark yellow urine can make it difficult to read the reaction because bilirubin is a yellow pigment.

**Bilirubinuria** (bilirubin in the urine) can occur with hepatitis, biliary tract obstruction, and hemolytic states such as transfusion reactions. Also, bilirubin is a highly unstable substance and will break down with exposure to light. The urine specimen must be shielded from light and processed as soon as possible to avoid deterioration of the specimen, which can alter the results of the bilirubin test.

## Urobilinogen

The bilirubin that goes to the intestines mixes with bacteria already in the intestinal tract. The enzymes in the bacteria break bilirubin into parts. One of the parts is called **urobilinogen**, which is primarily eliminated in the feces. About 15% of urobilinogen is reabsorbed into the blood, goes back to the liver, and is reexcreted into the intestines. A small amount is excreted by the kidneys usually 0.1 to 1.0 mg/dL. Like bilirubin, increased levels of urobilinogen can be found in patients who have conditions that cause a high rate of RBC destruction. Bowel obstructions cause the feces to remain in the intestines for longer periods, and during this retention, the intestines reabsorb urobilinogen, causing levels to rise in both urine and serum. Liver impairment can also lead to increased levels of urobilinogen.

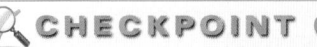 **CHECKPOINT QUESTION**

4. Heather Henderson, the CMA in the case study, performs a chemical urinalysis on a urine specimen, and the results show a positive result for protein. What factors may cause a false-positive test result?

## Nitrite

An enzyme produced by some types of bacteria reduces the chemical nitrate into **nitrite**, a substance that can be detected on the reagent strip. Because bacteria are not normally present in urine, the presence of nitrite indicates **bacteriuria**, or the presence of bacteria in the urine, which is diagnosed by the physician as a urinary tract infection, or UTI. Common bacteria that can cause UTIs and cause a positive nitrite test are *Escherichia coli, Enterobacter, Klebsiella,* and *Proteus* species. However, a negative nitrite test result does not indicate the absence of bacteriuria because not all types of bacteria that may cause a UTI reduce nitrate to nitrite, resulting in a test that is negative for nitrite when infection is present.

## Leukocyte Esterase

Leukocytes, or white blood cells, in the urine usually indicate an infection in the urinary tract. A positive **leukocyte esterase** test indicates that WBCs are present in the specimen. **Phagocytic** white blood cells including neutrophils are called to the kidney to fight an infection, and these leukocytes contain an enzyme called *esterase*. This enzyme is detected with the **leukocyte esterase** reaction on the reagent strip. Normal urine may contain a few WBCs but not in sufficient numbers to produce a positive leukocyte esterase test. A negative leukocyte esterase test means that an infection is not likely.

## Microalbumin

Commercially prepared reagent strips include the most commonly tested substances in the urine, but there may be variation depending on the manufacturer. Some urine reagent test strips contain a reagent pad for measuring specific type of protein known as **microalbumin,** or tiny bits of the protein albumin. When the kidneys are healthy, almost no proteins pass out of the kidneys and into the urine. However, if the kidneys become diseased or damaged, some proteins begin to filter through the kidneys and appear in the urine. In the very early stages of kidney disease, tiny bits of albumin, microalbumin, begin to appear in the urine. Once the microalbumin goes above 150 mg, the patient has reached early glomerular damage. Testing for microalbumin allows intervention to prevent additional damage to the kidneys. A patient with normal kidney function will have a urine protein range of 0 to 20 mg/dL and a urine albumin of 0 to 23 mg/dL. Higher values on protein and albumin indicate kidney disease.

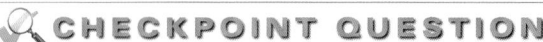

### CHECKPOINT QUESTION

5. A patient has a negative nitrite test on the urine reagent strip, but a positive leukocyte esterase test on the same specimen. How can this happen?

## Microscopic Properties

The microscopic examination of urine can corroborate the findings of the urinalysis and may produce additional data with diagnostic value. The solid material in the urine known as **sediment** is noted and counted during a microscopic examination. The microscopic examination of urine is not a CLIA-waived procedure, so examining and reporting results of the microscopic examination of urine is outside the scope of practice for a medical assistant. In most offices, a urine specimen for microscopic analysis will be collected and prepared for transport to a reference laboratory by the medical assistant. At the laboratory, the urine sample is put into a tube and centrifuged, causing a separation of the urine into solid material in the bottom of the tube and the **supernatant,** or liquid portion, above the sediment. The sediment is removed from the tube, placed on a microscope slide, and examined under a microscope by a physician or the medical laboratory technologist.

### Urine Sediment

Structures that may appear in the urine during the microscopic examination include red blood cells, white blood cells, bacteria, epithelial cells, crystals, and various types of casts (Fig. 45-6). Correlations with chemical properties of the urine are described as appropriate.

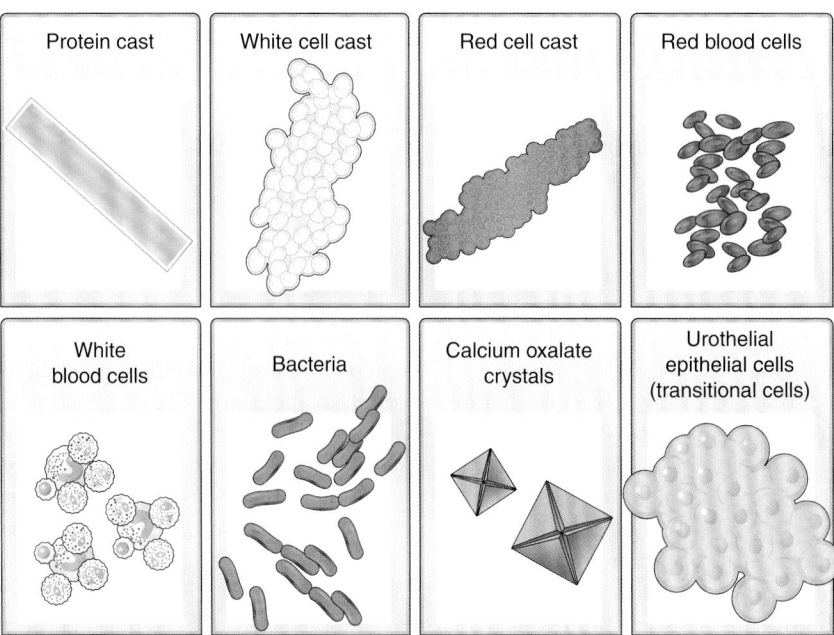

**Figure 45-6** • Microscopic examination of urinary sediment. Some of the more common formed elements found in urine are shown here.

## Red Blood Cells

Hematuria may indicate glomerular damage, tumors of the urinary tract, kidney trauma, urinary stones, renal infarcts, acute tubular necrosis, upper and lower UTIs, nephrotoxins, and physical distress. RBCs may also appear as a contaminant in urine from the vagina in menstruating women or from trauma from a bladder catheterization. When the urine sediment contains RBCs, the reagent strip should be positive for blood. A positive reagent strip test for blood with no RBCs seen microscopically may occur with various kinds of hemolysis. In hemolysis, the RBCs have ruptured and spilled their contents into the urine. The hemoglobin that remains turns the test blood positive, but there will not be visible red blood cells in the urine.

## White Blood Cells

As noted previously, leukocytes in urine sediment indicate an infection in the urinary tract, and the leukocyte esterase test on the reagent strip will be positive. These cells may also be seen microscopically if present (refer to Fig. 45-6).

## Bacteria

Bacteria are always present on the skin, but not usually in the urinary bladder if the urine specimen has been collected properly. The presence of significant amounts (more than a trace) of bacteria in a urine specimen is considered an indication of a UTI. A microscopic examination may reveal bacteria, and a culture may be indicated to further identify the type of bacteria causing the infection. Once a culture is done to identify the bacteria, a sensitivity may be indicated to determine the appropriate antibiotic to treat the infection. However, both the culture and the sensitivity must be ordered by the physician.

## Epithelial Cells

Epithelial cells cover the skin and organs and line the urinary tract. Their shapes vary according to their location of origin. Epithelial cells are normally found in the urine, but increased amounts can indicate an irritation such as inflammation somewhere in the urinary system. The three types of epithelial cells that are found in the urine are squamous, transitional, and renal. *Squamous epithelial cells* cover external skin surfaces and are considered a normal finding in urine, because urine comes in contact with skin during urination. *Transitional epithelial cells* line the bladder and are seen with infections of the lower urinary tract such as cystitis. *Renal epithelial cells* line the nephrons and are seen with infections and inflammations of the upper urinary tract. The presence of renal epithelial cells can also cause an increase of protein in the urine.

## CHECKPOINT QUESTION

6. A urinalysis report notes that renal epithelial cells were present when the specimen was examined microscopically. What reagent strip test may be positive?

## Crystals and Casts

Crystals are made up of a chemical substance in the urine in sufficient quantities to form a solid three-dimensional structure that can be seen microscopically. The three most common crystals found in urine sediment are calcium oxalate, uric acid, and triple phosphate. These are not independently pathologic; however, uric acid crystals in the urine may present in someone who has a fever, leukemia, or gout. Crystals can contribute to the formation of stones in the urinary tract.

Cast formation occurs in the distal convoluted tubule of the nephron or the collecting duct. When protein is present in sufficient quantities, it will cement together whatever solutes or cells are in the tubule as well, resulting in a *cast* (Fig. 45-7). Most casts eventually break free and flow into the urine, and identifying the type of cast can assist with diagnosing certain pathologies. For instance, WBC casts are present in pyelonephritis.

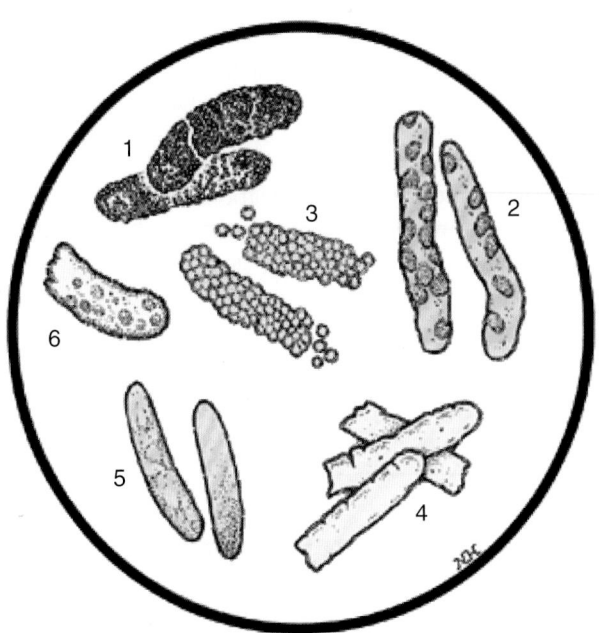

**Figure 45-7** • Urinary casts. (*1*) Coarse granular casts. (*2*) Epithelial casts. (*3*) RBC casts. (*4*) Waxy casts. (*5*) Hyaline casts. (*6*) Casts with pyocytes (pus corpuscles). (From Hardy NO, Wesport CT. *Stedman's Medical Dictionary*, 27th ed. Baltimore, MD: Lippincott Williams & Wilkins, 2000.)

### What Can I Do to Avoid a Kidney Stone?

Kidney stones may be hereditary or a function of the diet. To prevent dietary causes of renal calculi, the following guidelines may be helpful:

- *Drink more fluid.* Unless instructed by a physician not to do so, drink enough fluid to make your urine clear or pale yellow. In concentrated urine, crystals are more likely to grow and form a stone.
- *Eat less protein.* Americans eat much more protein than the body needs. The extra protein that the body does not need turns to fat, and an excess of fat in the diet makes kidney stones more likely to develop.
- *Cut the salt.* The average American consumes about twice the recommended amount of salt and five times more than the body needs. Sodium causes urine calcium levels to increase, making it more likely to have a kidney stone.
- *Take in more citrate.* Citrate is a chemical that inhibits the production of kidney stones. The more citrate in the urine, the less likely the formation of a stone. Citrate is found in citrus fruits such as lemons, oranges, and grapefruit.

### Other Types of Sediment

Other structures can be found in urine sediment including yeast, parasites, mucus, and spermatozoa. Yeast in the urine can result from vaginal contamination of the specimen or may be the causative agent of a urinary tract infection, especially in a diabetic patient. The parasite *Trichomonas vaginalis* is a contaminant from the genital tract of a person who is infected with this microorganism. Mucus may be present if there is an inflammation in the urinary tract and is seen as threads reported quantities such as few, moderate, or many. Spermatozoa may be found when there has been a recent emission or sexual activity in female patients.

 **CHECKPOINT QUESTION**

7. What is the difference between a crystal and a cast?

## SPECIMEN COLLECTION

A urine specimen may be tested for a variety of analytes. How the specimen is collected depends on the test that has been requested by the physician. To diagnose a urinary tract infection (UTI), the specimen is collected by either as a clean-catch midstream or by catheter and submitted to the laboratory in a sterile container with a

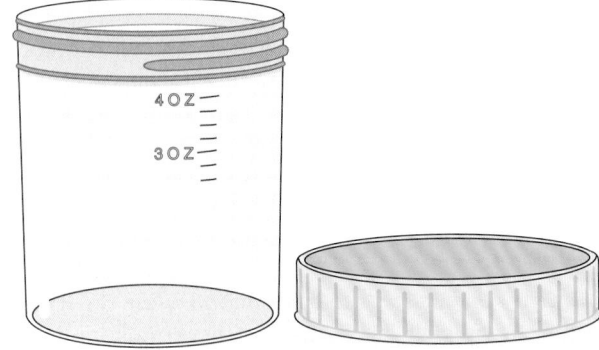

**Figure 45-8** • Sterile specimen cup with lid.

lid (Fig. 45-8). These methods are used to be sure any bacteria identified came from the urinary tract and not from a specimen that was contaminated during collection. If the physician needs to know the microorganism causing the disease, a culture must be performed to identify the causative bacteria. Some tests require urine collected over a period of time, often 24 hours. Patient instruction on each method of specimen collection is important to ensure compliance and reduce anxiety.

Once the urine is collected, many of its elements deteriorate within 1 hour. If testing cannot be performed within this time, the specimen must be refrigerated at 4°C to 8°C for up to 4 hours. Multiplication of microorganisms in an unrefrigerated specimen changes the pH from acidic to alkaline. Glucose in the urine may be used as a nutrient by the microorganisms, resulting in a false-negative or lowered glucose result. The timing of the collection is also an important consideration. During sleep, urine collects in the urinary bladder and is more concentrated, allowing for more accurate results for many tests that rely on a certain quantity of a substance for detection.

## Random Specimen

The most common type of urine specimen collected in the physician office is the *random specimen*. When a random specimen is indicated, the patient voids into a clean, dry container. No precautions are taken for any kind of contamination. The sample may contain white blood cells (WBCs), bacteria, and squamous epithelium cells as contaminants. Female patients may have urine contaminated with vaginal contaminants such as yeast. You should always ask female patient collecting urine if they are menstruating and note this on the laboratory requisition if the specimen is collected to send to a reference laboratory because the specimen may be contaminated with blood.

## First Morning and Postprandial Specimens

The timing of specimen collection may be important depending on the test ordered by the physician. A first morning voided specimen reflects the ability of the kidney to concentrate urine during dehydration, which occurs during sleep. Urine collected in the bladder over a 6- to 8-hour period provides the preferred concentration. It is easiest to identify urine abnormalities in a more concentrated urine specimen. This is called a *first morning specimen* or an *early morning void*. It may be necessary to clarify this term for the patient with alternative sleep patterns. A postprandial urine specimen is one that is collected exactly 2 hours after the patient eats a meal. The patient should be instructed to empty the bladder prior to eating the meal to ensure that the collected urine is entirely postprandial. Timing is essential including the exact time of the last meal consumed and the time of the collection. Instruct the patient not to urinate in the 2 hours between eating the meal and collecting the urine specimen.

## Clean-Catch Midstream Urine Specimen

A clean-catch midstream urine is useful when the physician suspects an infection and requires the patient to collect the specimen after cleansing the **urinary meatus** and surrounding tissue (Fig. 45-9). Once the meatus is cleansed properly, the patient begins urinating into the toilet then stops the flow to collect the specimen in a sterile container. The specimen is collected midstream, giving this method the title clean-catch midstream specimen. This specimen can be used for a culture if nothing has been allowed to contaminate the urine, such as a pipette or reagent strip. Procedure 45-1 outlines the patient instructions for obtaining a clean-catch midstream specimen for both male and female patients. Disabled or elderly patients may need assistance with this procedure as the container must not touch the genital area. The specimen must be labeled

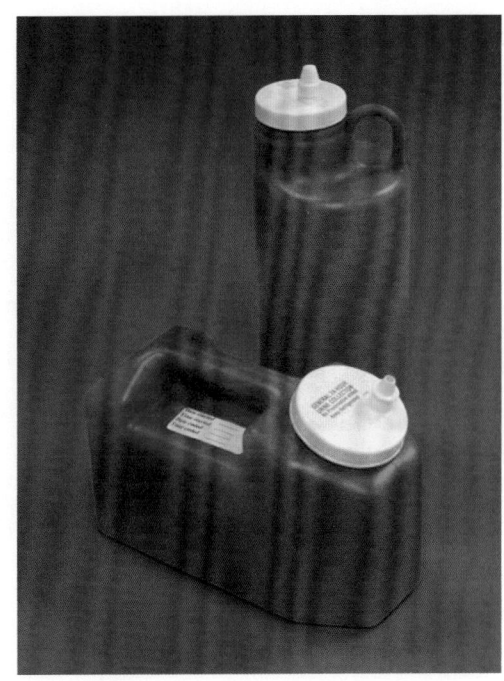

**Figure 45-10** • Two styles of 24-hour urine specimen collection containers

as established by office procedures and refrigerated immediately if it is not going to be tested right away.

## 24-Hour Collection

Because some substances including proteins are excreted with **diurnal variation** (variation during a 24-hour period), a 24-hour collection is a better indicator of values than a random specimen. To obtain this kind of specimen, the patient collects all voided urine within a 24-hour period in a special container provided by the office or laboratory (Fig. 45-10).

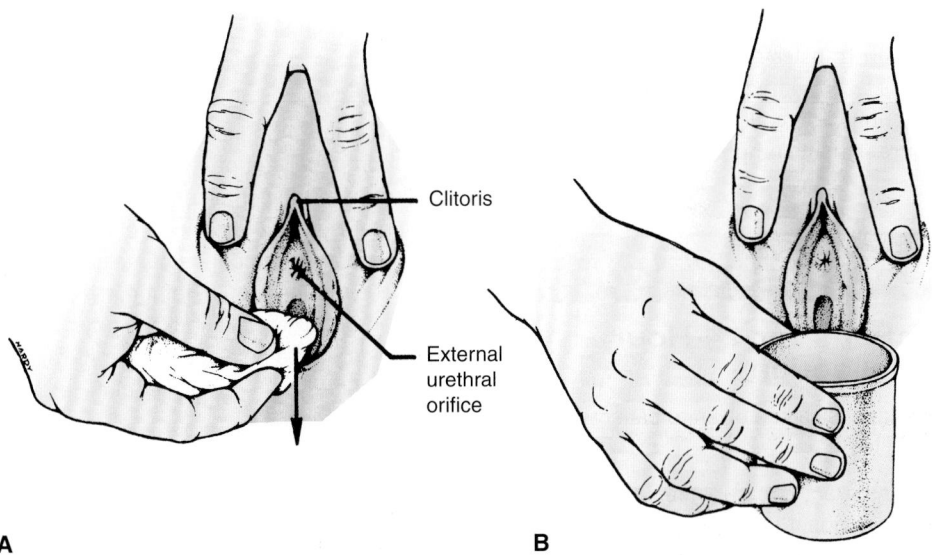

**A**  **B**

**Figure 45-9** • Obtaining a clean-catch midstream urine specimen in the female patient. Obtaining a clean-catch midstream urine specimen in the female patient. **(A)** Instruct the patient to hold the labia apart and wash from high up front toward the back with gauze soaked in soap. **(B)** The collection cup is held so that it does not touch the body, and the sample is obtained only while the patient is voiding with the labia held apart.

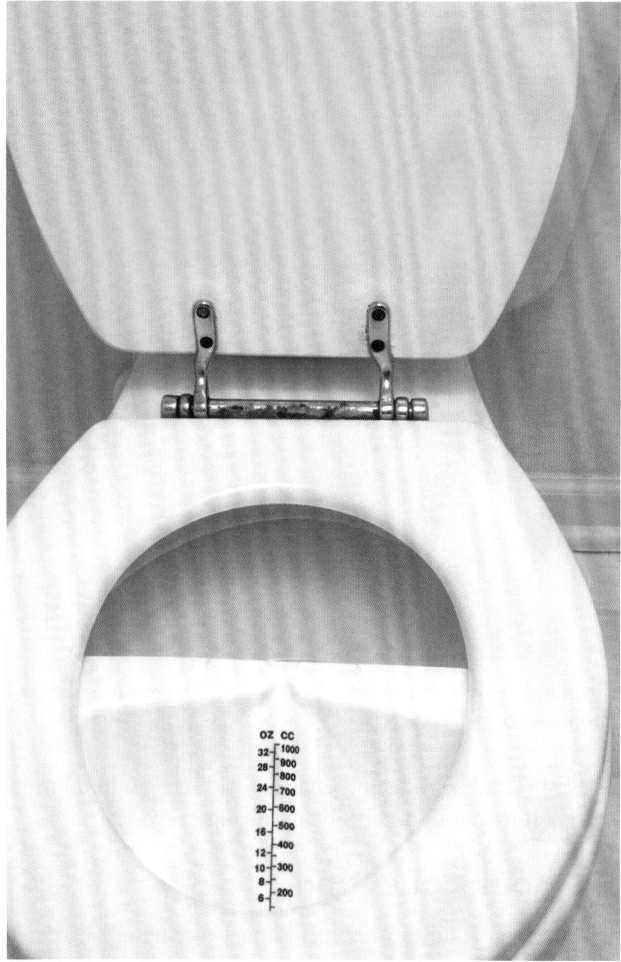

**Figure 45-11** • A collection device (sometimes called a "commode hat") is placed over the toilet seat before the person urinates, to contain and measure the amount of urine.

The patient must also be instructed not to urinate in the special container used to collect the urine over 24 hours, but they should urinate each time into a special device that is put on the toilet and transfer the urine into the special container (Fig. 45-11). Providing an information sheet with written instructions for collecting a 24-hour urine specimen helps ensure patient compliance.

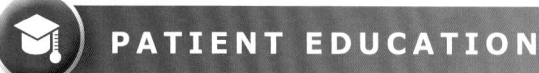

## PATIENT EDUCATION

### Instructions for 24-Hour Urine Collection

The following instructions can be given to patients to ensure proper collection:

- Follow instructions exactly. Your test results are based on the total amount of urine excreted by your body over a 24-hour period. Not following instructions will result in inaccurate results reported to your physician.

- The medical assistant will instruct you if the test requires any drug or dietary requirements.
- The medical assistant will give you a container to collect the urine. A preservative may be in the container. Do not throw away the preservative and avoid coming into contact with it as the preservative may be toxic.
- If you do spill the preservative, immediately wash the area with large amounts of water. You will have to get a new container from your physician or laboratory to collect the specimen.
- Do not void directly into the collection container. Be very careful not to spill the preservative. Refrigerate the container during collection or place the urine collection container in a larger device that holds crushed ice to keep the specimen cold. Refresh the ice as needed to ensure the specimen remains cold throughout the 24-hour period.

**Day 1**

- Empty your bladder into the toilet. Record the specific date and time on your 24-hour urine container. You will start your 24-hour collection after discarding this urine.
- Use the device given to you to place on the toilet. Transfer urine from this device to the collection container avoiding spilling any urine.
- Collect all urine voided during the day, evening, and night for the entire 24-hour period. Add all of the specimens to the container. Gently shake the container after each urine specimen is added to mix the urine with any preservatives in the collection container. Keep the urine container refrigerated or on ice during the collection period and until you take it to the physician or laboratory for testing.

**Day 2**

- Exactly 24 hours after you begin your collection, completely empty your bladder and add this specimen to the container. This last specimen completes your 24-hour collection. Record the ending date and time on the container. Replace the cap and tighten firmly. Refrigerate or ice the specimen until you can take it to the physician or laboratory.
- If you were on a special diet for this test, you may resume your normal diet after the specimen is collected.

## Urinary Catheterization

Another method for aseptic urine collection is urinary catheterization (refer to Chapter 35, Urology). A rubber or plastic catheter is inserted into the bladder

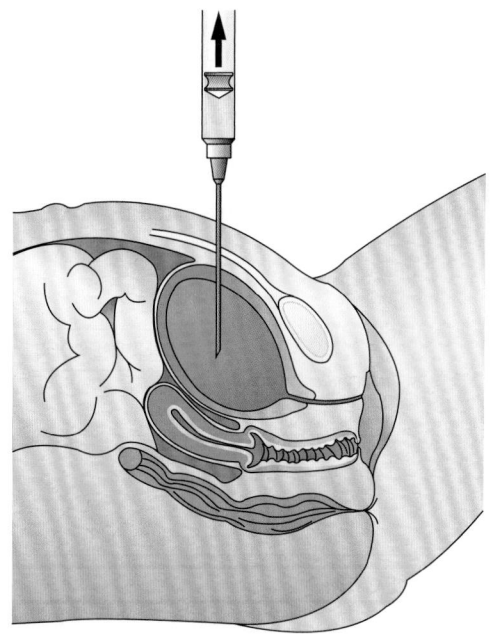

**Figure 45-12** • Suprapubic aspiration of urine. The full bladder is easily accessible by an abdominal puncture.

through the urethra using sterile technique. Although performing a urinary catheterization is not an entry-level skill for medical assistants, some medical assistants were trained to perform this procedure as part of their educational program. Urinary catheterization is recommended when the patient cannot give a urine specimen in an aseptic manner when using the clean-catch method or as ordered by the physician. If the patient has an indwelling catheter, the specimen must not be collected from a drainage bag that may be attached to the catheter to collect the urine continuously.

## Suprapubic Aspiration

Suprapubic aspiration is the least common method of urine collection and is only performed by a physician. In this procedure, a needle is inserted into the bladder through the skin of the abdominal wall above the symphysis pubis, and urine is withdrawn (aspirated) as shown in Figure 45-12. This method is not common and is performed by a physician. You may be asked to assist with the procedure.

### CHECKPOINT QUESTION

8. What is the time frame for testing urine that is not refrigerated, and why is this important?

## DRUG TESTING

Drug testing may be done for preemployment, to monitor pain medication use in pain management, when

there is an injury while on the job, or randomly on employees in occupations where personal or public safety is an issue. Although drug testing can be performed using blood or hair samples, many physician offices are involved in urine drug testing. Each urine specimen submitted for drug testing must be analyzed using an initial test approved for commercial use by the U.S. Food and Drug Administration, and while some of these are CLIA-waived, some are not waived (Fig. 45-13). It is your responsibility to be familiar with any CLIA-waived testing kits used in your office and the procedure for collecting the urine sample from the patient.

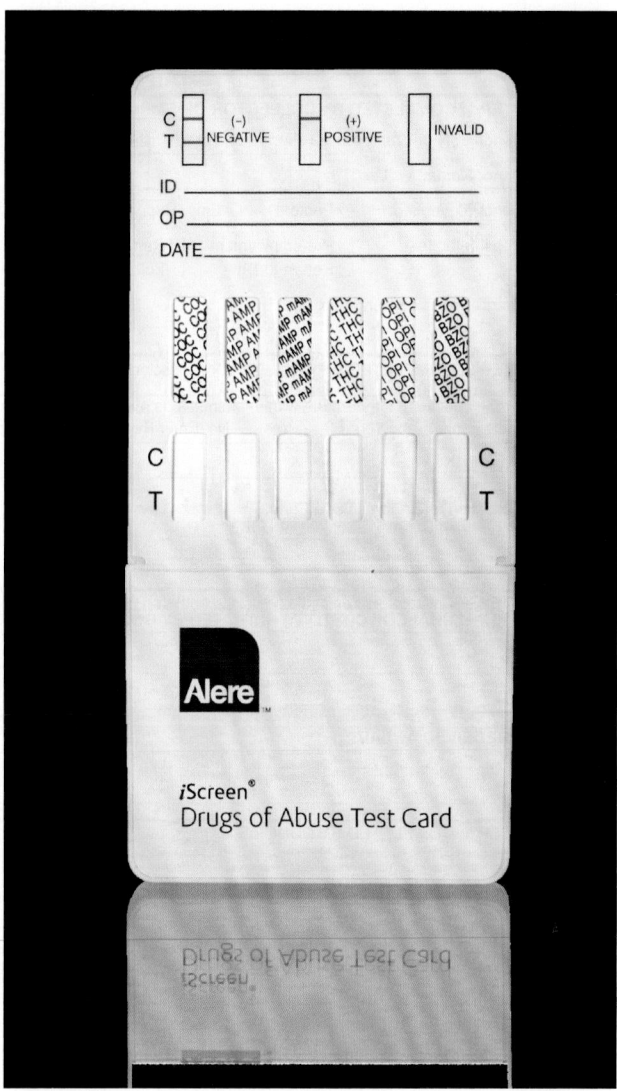

**Figure 45-13** • iScreen is a one-step urine drug detection card. The choice is from 15 commonly abused/used drugs. The program may choose 1 to 10 drugs to be placed on the test card. A simple dip in the urine sample and read provides results in minutes. The card also contains sample validity test zones for pH, specific gravity, oxidants, pyridinium chlorochromate, glutaraldehyde, and creatinine. (Permission granted courtesy of Alere Inc.)

## Chain-of-Custody Procedures

The **chain-of-custody** process is used to document that the sample has been in possession of, or secured by, a responsible person at all times. Legally, the laboratory results derived from the collection of specimens for drug or paternity testing must be defensible in court or to a government agency. Performed correctly, the chain-of-custody process eliminates doubt about sample identification or tampering. The chain-of-custody document should include the name or initials of the individual collecting the specimen, each person who subsequently had custody of it, and the date the specimen was received at the testing facility (Fig. 45-14). General guidelines of chain-of-custody procedures are listed in Box 45-2.

ORDERING PHYSICIAN/COMPANY OR FACILITY

SPECIMEN ID NO. 0000000

VARIABLE BARCODE

Sonora Quest Laboratories
A Subsidiary of Laboratory Sciences of Arizona
1255 West Washington Street
Tempe, Arizona 85281
602.685.5000 • 800.766.6721

LAB ACCESSION NO.

**CHAIN OF CUSTODY REQUISITION FORM**

**STEP 1: COMPLETED BY COLLECTOR OR EMPLOYER REPRESENTATIVE**

Donor SSN or Employee I.D. No.

Donor Name: Last: First:

Donor ID Verified: ☐ Photo ID ☐ Emp. Rep.

Reason for Test: ☐ Pre-employment ☐ Random ☐ Reasonable Suspicion/Cause ☐ Post-Accident ☐ Promotion ☐ Return to Duty ☐ Follow-up ☐ Other (specify)

Drug Tests to be Performed:

**STEP 2: COMPLETED BY COLLECTOR** (Collector Instructions)

Read specimen temperature within 4 minutes. Is temperature between 90° and 100° F? ☐ Yes ☐ No, Enter Remark

Specimen Collection: ☐ Split ☐ Single ☐ None Provided (Enter Remark) ☐ Observed (Enter Remark)

REMARKS

Collection Site Address/Site Code:

Collector Phone No.

Collector Fax No.

**STEP 3:** Collector affixes bottle seal(s) to bottle(s). Collector dates seal(s). Donor initials seal(s). Donor completes STEP 5

**STEP 4: CHAIN OF CUSTODY - INITIATED BY COLLECTOR AND COMPLETED BY LABORATORY**

*I certify that the specimen given to me by the donor identified in step 1 of this form was collected, labeled, sealed and released to the Delivery Service noted.*

X Signature of Collector — Time of Collection AM PM ▶ **SPECIMEN BOTTLE(S) RELEASED TO:**

(PRINT) Collector's Name (First, MI, Last) — Date (Mo./Day/Yr.) ▶ Name of Delivery Service Transferring Specimen to Lab

**RECEIVED AT LAB:**

X Signature of Accessioner ▶

(PRINT) Accessioner's Name (First, MI, Last) — Date (Mo./Day/Yr.) ▶

**Primary Specimen Bottle Seal Intact** ☐ Yes ☐ No, Enter Remark Below

**SPECIMEN BOTTLE(S) RELEASED TO:**

**STEP 5: COMPLETED BY DONOR**

*I certify that I provided my urine specimen to the collector; that I have not adulterated it in any manner; each specimen bottle used was sealed with a tamper-evident seal in my presence; and that the information numbers provided on this form and on the label affixed to each specimen bottle is correct.*

X Signature of Donor — (PRINT) Donor's Name (First, MI, Last) — Date (Mo./Day/Yr.)

Daytime Phone No. ( ) — Evening Phone No. ( ) — Date of Birth Mo. Day Yr.

Q7230 (Rev. 9/07) Sonora Quest Laboratories

COPY 1 - LABORATORY COPY 2 - COLLECTOR COPY COPY 3 - COMPANY/MRO COPY COPY 4 - LABORATORY-CONFIDENTIAL DONOR

**Figure 45-14** • Chain-of-custody requisition form.

## BOX 45-2 Chain-of-Custody Guidelines

1. Keep the number of people involved in collecting and handling samples to a minimum.
2. Always document the transfer of samples on a chain-of-custody form.
3. Always keep the chain-of-custody form together with the sample.
4. Identify samples legibly and written in permanent ink.

## Urine Collection and Chain of Custody

To perform a chain-of-custody specimen collection, the person collecting the specimen, also known as the collector, must escort the subject, or patient whose urine is being collected for testing, to the collection area. If you are the collector, you should be aware of body language and potential efforts to conceal a device to deliver clean urine. The only people permitted in the testing area are you and the patient during the collection process. Next, the collector should obtain the necessary supplies including the chain-of-custody form, specimen identification labels, tamper seals, and specimen bottle from a secured area or kit in view of the patient. You will fill out the appropriate parts of the chain-of-custody form. The subject is required to produce a form of photo identification (ID) issued by the subject's employer or the federal, state, or local government (e.g., a driver's license). Faxes or photocopies of ID are not acceptable. Positive ID by an employer representative (not a coworker or another employee being tested) is also acceptable. If the subject cannot produce positive ID, the specimen collection procedure cannot be performed. Once the appropriate chain-of-custody form is completed, you should instruct the patient to remove any outer clothing. Outer garments can conceal substances that could be used to tamper with a specimen. You, the collector, are responsible for examining all personal belongings brought by the patient including items that may be in pockets. Anything identified that could be used to contaminate the specimen must remain with the collector. The subject may return the items to his or her pockets once they are examined and approved by the medical assistant or placed in a locker according to office policy and procedure.

The following procedures must be followed to preserve the integrity of the specimen:

1. The patient, or subject, must witness the container being unwrapped and the seal broken. The subject signs a specimen ID label, places it on the specimen container, and places the matching ID label on the chain-of-custody form.

2. No water can be available to the subject in the restroom. The sink in the restroom may have the water disconnected, and blue dye is added to the toilet bowl to discourage specimen tampering. The subject is required to rinse and dry hands in front of the collector prior to specimen collection.

3. The patient can take nothing but the collection container into the bathroom used for urination, and you must escort the patient into the restroom. If the subject is wearing long sleeves, you should instruct the patient to roll up their sleeves. Instruct the patient to provide a specimen of at least 45 mL, do not flush the toilet, and bring the specimen to you as soon as he or she has completed the void. After collecting the urine sample, the patient should snap the cap tightly on the specimen container to prevent leakage. Do not accept an uncapped specimen container from the patient.

4. If the patient cannot provide a sample, all forms and containers must be destroyed. New supplies will be used if the subject returns to perform the collection again.

5. The patient places the tamper seal over the top of the specimen container. One end of the seal must attach to the ID label. Instruct the patient to write his or her initials on the seal after it is attached. The patient must read, sign, and date the chain-of-custody form. After the patient completes his or her part, you must record the temperature of the specimen, which is usually a strip found on the special container used to collect the specimen. Once the temperature of the specimen is recorded, you should review the form for completeness and sign/date the form as appropriate.

6. The patient must place the specimen into the specimen bag and the bag placed into the refrigerator until tested or picked up or shipped to the testing laboratory following specific procedures. If a courier picks up the specimen, the courier must sign the chain-of-custody form to document taking possession of the specimen. The form is placed in the bag with the specimen prior to leaving the office.

In addition to specific drugs, other substances may be included in the urine drug test to determine if methods were used to falsify the drug testing when the results might be detrimental. One substance tested is glutaraldehyde, a substance not normally found in urine, but present in synthetic urine. Creatinine, substance found normally in urine in constant levels, is tested, and if quantities are less than 20 mg/dL, the patient may have attempted to "flush" his or her system using diuretics. It is your responsibility to be familiar with drug testing procedures and the latest "fads" to falsify results. You are also responsible for maintaining chain-of-custody procedures and reporting accurate information on the chain-of-custody form.

## WHAT IF?

**A patient asks you what drugs can be detected in the urine. What do you say?**

Many employers are requiring routine urine drug testing for their employees. Urine tests are preferred to blood tests because they are less expensive and are noninvasive. The following drugs can be detected in the urine: amphetamines, barbiturates, benzodiazepines, cocaine, marijuana, opioids, phencyclidine (also known as *PCP*), methadone, methamphetamines, ecstasy, oxycodone, propoxyphene, and tricyclic antidepressants. Depending on the test kit used, one or more of these drugs can be tested using a urine specimen. You may tell or show the patient a list of these tests. If you must obtain urine specimens for drug testing, it is essential that you ensure security of the urine and confidentiality of the results.

## CHECKPOINT QUESTION

9. Why is the temperature of the urine specimen important to document when collecting urine for drug testing?

## ROLE-PLAYING ACTIVITY

Role-play these scenarios as if you are working with Heather Henderson, CMA (AAMA), who works in the busy physician office that is part of the Great Falls Medical Center (refer to the case study at the beginning of the chapter). A 28-year-old male patient comes into the office to have drug testing done for a preemployment physical examination. He tells you that he did "smoke pot" 2 days ago, and because he "really needs this job," he would like to go into the restroom by himself and refused to take off his jacket or empty his pockets. How would you respond to this patient? Is there a potential that this drug could show up in his urine test from 2 days ago? Your instructor will give you additional information about this activity!

## *español* SPANISH TERMINOLOGY

**Necesitamos que nos dé una prueba de orina.**
You will collect a urine specimen.

**Orine en el inhodoro por algunos segundos.**
Urinate in the toilet a few seconds.

**Pare, y orine en el envase para la muestra.**
Stop and urinate in the specimen cup.

**Necesita tomar una muestra de todo el orín que haga por 24 horas.**
You are going to save all of your urine for 24 hours.

**Devuelva la muestra de orina a la oficina tan pronto sea posible, luego de que haya terminado de tomar las muestras.**
Return the specimen to the office as soon as possible after collection is complete.

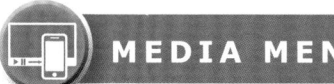

## MEDIA MENU

**Student Resources on** thePoint®

- *Video:* **Obtaining a Clean-Catch Midstream Urine Specimen (Procedure 45-1 )**
- *Video:* **Determining Color and Clarity of Urine (Procedure 45-2 )**
- *Video:* **Chemical Reagent Strip Analysis (Procedure 45-2 )**
- **CMA/RMA Certification Exam Review**
- **English to Spanish Audio Glossary**

**Internet Resources**
**National Institutes of Health—Urinalysis**
http://www.nlm.nih.gov/medlineplus/ency/article/003579.htm

**Lab Tests Online**
http://www.labtestsonline.org/understanding/analytes/urinalysis/test.html

**Medical Technology**
http://www.irvingcrowley.com/cls/urin.htm

## EMR Activity

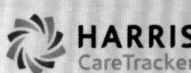

Harris CareTracker is a Web-based electronic medical record (EMR) application that you will use for the EMR activities included in this section at the end of each chapter. This application is actually used in physician offices, but is provided to you through the publisher, Wolters Kluwer Health, to give you hands-on practice working with EMRs. Your instructor will have more information about accessing your username, login, and Quickstart guide.

Prerequisite Activities in Harris CareTracker

- *The Getting Started and Quickstart documents and EMR Activities Step-by-Step Instructions are available at* http://thePoint.lww.com/KronenbergerComp5e

Activity Details

Accurately document the following urinalysis procedures in each of the following patient's EMR:

1. Sue Tamrick: UA, positive for leukocytes and blood
2. Kathy Newman: UA for C&S sent to Great Falls Medical Center Lab

## Chapter Summary

- Proper collection of a urine specimen varies with the test to be performed. Unless otherwise specified by the physician, a freshly voided specimen is all that is necessary. This is called a *random urine*. To diagnose a UTI, the specimen is collected either as a clean-catch midstream or by catheter and submitted to the laboratory in a sterile container with a lid. Once the urine is collected, many of its elements deteriorate within 1 hour. If testing cannot be performed within this time, the specimen is refrigerated at 4°C to 8°C for up to 4 hours.
- The physical properties of urine include color, appearance (such as clarity or turbidity), specific gravity, and odor.
- Urine contains chemicals produced in the body and ingested from the environment. The reagent strip produces 10 chemical measurements. Detecting and measuring chemical properties can facilitate the diagnosis of many conditions.
- The kidney helps maintain the acid–base balance of the body. To maintain a constant pH, the kidney must control the change of pH of the urine to balance the pH that results from diet and metabolism.
- Leukocytes in the urine indicate a UTI. A positive leukocyte esterase test indicates that WBCs are present in the specimen. Normal urine may contain a few WBCs but not in sufficient numbers to produce a positive leukocyte esterase test.
- The following structures may appear in the urine: RBCs, WBCs, bacteria, epithelial cells, crystals, casts, and others.
- Hematuria is the presence of RBCs in urine. This may indicate glomerular damage, tumors of the urinary tract, kidney trauma, urinary stones, renal infarcts, acute tubular necrosis, upper and lower UTIs, nephrotoxins, and physical distress.
- Bacteria are always present on the skin but not usually in the bladder. The presence of significant amounts (more than a trace) of bacteria in a urine specimen is considered an indication of a UTI.
- A urinalysis is a physical and chemical examination of urine to assess renal function and other possible problems. Because so many urinalyses are done in the office laboratory, proficiency in this skill is essential for the medical assistant.

## Warm-Ups for Critical Thinking

1. A patient was taking a medication that changed the color of his urine. How did this impact urine testing? What action should the medical assistant take?
2. What effects on test results are caused by leaving the urine specimen at room temperature for an extended length of time? How does this impact the usefulness of the test results?
3. Physicians frequently send orders back to the laboratory to have a culture and sensitivity done on a urine specimen that was collected earlier for urinalysis. What actions are necessary for the urine to still be acceptable for additional testing?
4. Create a patient education brochure for collecting a clean-catch midstream urine specimen. Remember that all patients may not understand clinical terms for laboratory specimens.
5. A urine specimen is left in the light for an extended period of time. What chemistry may be affected by this? Why?
6. A patient with kidney disease has a urinalysis. Which dipstick chemistry test will be elevated for this reason?

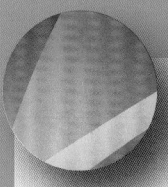

## PSY PROCEDURE 45-1

# Obtaining a Clean-Catch Midstream Urine Specimen

**PSY** Obtain specimen and perform CLIA-waived urinalysis tests; instruct and prepare a patient for a procedure or treatment; coach patients appropriately considering cultural diversity, developmental life stage, and communication barriers; and document patient care accurately in the medical record.

**Purpose:** To instruct a patient in collecting a clean-catch urine specimen and minimize contamination of a voided urine specimen

**Equipment:** Sterile urine container labeled with patient's name, cleansing towelettes (two for male patients, three for female patients), gloves if you are to assist patient, and hand sanitizer

| STEPS | REASONS |
|---|---|
| 1. Check the physician order. Wash your hands. If you are to assist the patient, put on gloves. | Hand washing aids infection control. |
| 2. Assemble the equipment. | Equipment must be readily accessible to perform the procedure. |
| 3. **AFF** Identify the patient and explain the procedure. Identify yourself including your title. Explain the rationale for performance of a procedure to the patient. | Show awareness of patients' concerns regarding their perceptions related to the procedure being performed. Ask for and answer any questions. |
| 4. **AFF** If the patient is hearing impaired, you may need to face the person and speak clearly, not loudly. You should have an easy-to-read instruction guide for the patient to follow and point out where there are questions. If the patient can sign and you cannot, have someone proficient in sign language assist you in instructing the patient. | Understanding the instructions is critical to obtaining a quality specimen. |
| 5. If the patient is to perform the procedure, provide the necessary supplies. | The patient will need the appropriate materials in order to do the collection properly. |
| 6. Have the patient perform the procedure properly with the following instructions:<br>A. Male patients:<br>  i. If uncircumcised, expose the glans penis by retracting the foreskin, and then clean the meatus with an antiseptic wipe. The glans should be cleaned in a circular motion away from the meatus. A new wipe should be used for each cleaning sweep.<br>  ii. Keeping the foreskin retracted, initially void a few seconds into the toilet or urinal.<br>  iii. Bring the sterile container into the urine stream and collect a sufficient amount (about 30–60 mL). Instruct the patient to avoid touching the inside of the container with the penis.<br>  iv. Finish voiding into the toilet or urinal. | The antiseptic solution removes bacteria from the urinary meatus and the surrounding skin. Wiping away from the meatus with an antiseptic wipe will remove bacteria from the area; wiping toward the meatus or returning to the area with a used wipe will reintroduce bacteria to the site<br>Organisms in the lower urethra and at the meatus will be washed away.<br>Collecting the middle of the stream ensures the least contamination with skin bacteria. Touching the inside with the penis may contaminate the specimen.<br><br>Prostatic fluid may be expressed at the end of the stream and may contaminate the specimen. |

*(continues on page 1190)*

| STEPS | REASONS |
|---|---|
| **B.** Female patients: | |
| i.  Kneel or squat over the toilet bowl. Spread the labia minora widely to expose the meatus. Using an antiseptic wipe, cleanse on either side of the meatus, and then cleanse the meatus itself. Use a wipe only once in a sweep from the anterior to the posterior surfaces, and then discard it. | The antiseptic solution removes bacteria from the urinary meatus. Bringing a wipe back to the surface already cleaned will recontaminate the area. The antiseptic solution is washed away before the specimen is collected at midstream. |
| ii.  Keeping the labia separated, initially void a few seconds into the toilet. | Organisms remaining in the meatus will be washed away. |
| iii.  Bring the sterile container into the urine stream and collect a sufficient amount (about 30–60 mL). | |
| iv.  Finish voiding into the toilet. | |
| **7.** Cap the filled container and place it in a designated area. | Cap the container to protect the specimen from contamination and to protect the handler from exposure. |
| **8.** Transport the specimen in a biohazard container for testing or test the urine specimen according to office policy and procedure. | Transporting in a biohazard container will protect those who handle it in transit. |
| **9.** Properly care for or dispose of equipment and supplies. Clean the work area. Remove gloves and wash your hands. | |
| **10.** **AFF** Log into the electronic medical record (EMR) using your username and secure password OR obtain the paper medical record from a secure location and assure it is kept away from public access. Record the procedure noting the date, time, specimen collected, and specimen processing procedure (i.e., sent to lab, tested using CLIA-waived test, etc.). Include your name and title according to office policy and procedure. | Caring for supplies and the work area provide a safe environment and a clean environment for future testing. Washing hands is the key step of standard precautions. <br><br> The integrity of the medical record must be maintained at all times to protect patient privacy. |

---

**Charting Example:**
*05/31/2016 1:30 PM Midstream clean-catch urine specimen obtain. . U/A: Color, straw; clarity, clear; specific gravity, 1.020; dipstick negative; pH 7.0. _____ S. Miller, CMA*

---

**Note:** *The medical assistant may sign his or her name in the patient record using only the "CMA" credential if the office has a signature log denoting the entire credential as "CMA (AAMA)."*

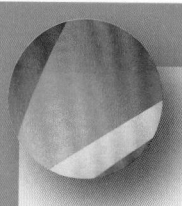

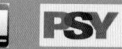 

# Perform a Physical and Chemical Urinalysis

**Purpose:** To determine the physical and chemical characteristics of a urine specimen

**Equipment:** Gloves, patient's labeled urine specimen, chemical reagent strips (such as Multistix™ or Chemstrip™) hand disinfectant, and biohazard waste container

| STEPS | REASONS |
|---|---|
| 1. Check the physician order. Wash your hands. | Hand washing aids infection control. |
| 2. Assemble the equipment. | Equipment must be readily accessible to perform the procedure. |
| 3. Put on gloves. | PPE is required for protection from biohazards. |
| 4. Verify the name on the specimen container and the physician order. | This prevents reporting errors. |
| 5. In bright light against a white background, examine the color of the specimen. The most common colors are straw (very pale yellow), yellow, dark yellow, and amber (brown–yellow). | The intensity of the yellow color, which is due to urochrome, depends on urine concentration. |
| 6. Determine clarity. Hold the specimen container in front of a surface with print such as blank print. If you see the image or print clearly (not obscured), record as clear. If you see the image or print but they are not well delineated, record as hazy. If you cannot see the image or print at all, record as cloudy. | The image or print helps discern clarity by providing contrast. |
| 7. Remove the reagent strip from its container and replace the lid to prevent deterioration of the strips by humidity. | Urine dipsticks are extremely sensitive to moisture. They will not provide accurate test results without protection from the moisture in the environment. |
| 8. Immerse the reagent strip in the urine completely, immediately remove it, sliding the edge of the strip along the lip of the container to remove excess urine. Pooling of excess urine on the dipstick causes cross-contamination among the reactions, possibly obscuring accurate color detection. | Immediate removal of the strip prevents colors from leaching during prolonged exposure to urine. |
| 9. Start your stopwatch or timer immediately. | |
| 10. Compare the reagent pads to the color chart, determining results at the intervals stated by the manufacturer. Example: Glucose is read at 30 seconds. To determine results, examine that pad 30 seconds after dipping and compare with color chart for glucose. | Reactions must be read at specific intervals as directed on the package insert and on the color comparison chart.<br><br>This adheres to strict time-sensitive protocol. |

*(continues on page 1192)*

## PROCEDURE 45.2 (continued)

| STEPS | REASONS |
|---|---|
| 11. Read all reactions at the times indicated and record the results. | |
| 12. Discard the reagent strips in the biohazard receptacle. Discard urine. | Test results are time specific. Failure to read with exact times will yield inaccurate test results. |
| 13. Remove your gloves and wash your hands. | |
| 14. **AFF** Log into the electronic medical record (EMR) using your username and secure password OR obtain the paper medical record from a secure location and assure it is kept away from public access. Record the procedure noting the date, time, specimen collected, and specimen processing procedure (i.e., sent to lab, tested using CLIA-waived test, etc.). Include your name and title according to office policy and procedure. | Discarding specimens maintains a biohazard-free environment. Washing hands is the key factor in standard precautions. The integrity of the medical record must be maintained at all times to protect patient. |

### Charting Example
*05/31/2016 2:45 PM Random urine collected. UA performed, pale yellow, clear, Multistix report in chart _____*
*_____ H. Henderson, CMA*

Note: *The medical assistant may sign his or her name in the patient record using only the "CMA" credential if the office has a signature log denoting the entire credential as "CMA (AAMA)."*

# PART

# 5

# Career
# Strategies

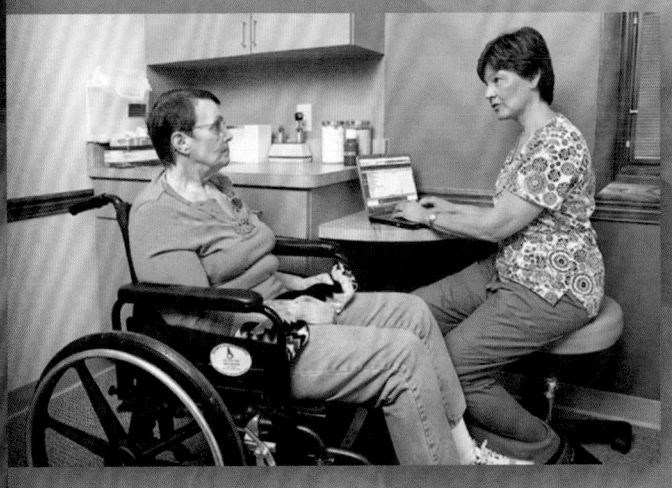

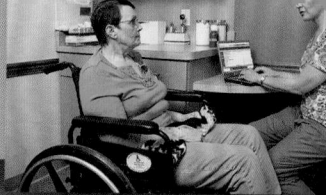

Congratulations! You have reached a pivotal point in your medical assisting career. This unit prepares you to make the transition from student to employee. The first chapter introduces you to the externship program. Your practicum is the springboard to starting your career. The remainder of Chapter 46 focuses on how to acquire the job that you have worked so hard to prepare for. The last chapter is a mock certification examination. You will now prepare for the next phase in your goal of becoming a medical assistant. You will be prepared to enter this fascinating and exciting career with confidence and professionalism while enjoying the rewards and accepting the challenges that face you. Good luck in your new adventure! Make it more than a job. Make it a profession and a career.

CHAPTER

# 46

# Making the Transition: Student to Employee

## Outline

## Learning Outcomes

**COG Cognitive Domain***

1. Spell and define the key terms
2. Explain the purpose of the practicum experience
3. Understand the importance of the evaluation process
4. List your professional responsibilities during your practicum
5. List personal and professional attributes necessary to ensure a successful practicum
6. Determine your best career direction based on your skills and strengths
7. Identify the steps necessary to apply for the right position and be able to accomplish those steps
8. Draft an appropriate cover letter
9. List the steps and guidelines in completing an employment application

10. List guidelines for an effective interview that will lead to employment
11. Identify the steps that you need to take to ensure proper career advancement
12. Explain the process for recertification of a medical assisting credential
13. Describe the importance of membership in a professional organization
14. *Recognize elements of fundamental writing skills*
15. *List and discuss legal and illegal applicant interview questions*
16. Discuss all levels of governmental legislation and regulation as they apply to medical assisting practice

*(continues on page 1196)*

**PSY** **Psychomotor Domain\***

**1.** Write a résumé to properly communicate skills and strengths (Procedure 46-1)
**2.** *Compose professional correspondence utilizing electronic technology (Procedure 46-1)*

**AFF** **Affective Domain\***

**1.** Apply local, state, and federal health care legislation
**2.** *Recognize the impacts of personal ethics and morals have on the delivery of health care*

*\*Note: AAMA/CAAHEP 2015 Standards are italicized.*

**ABHES Competencies**

1. Comply with federal, state, and local health laws and regulations.
2. Perform fundamental writing skills including correct grammar, spelling, and formatting techniques when writing prescriptions, documenting medical records, etc.

## Key Terms

| | | |
|---|---|---|
| **externship** | **portfolio** | **preceptor** |
| **networking** | **practicum** | **résumé** |

## Case Study

$C$arlos Zeller is a medical assistant student who just finished his practicum at Great Falls Medical Center. With guidance and supervision from his practicum supervisor, Carlos had many opportunities to practice the clinical and administrative skills he learned in school at his clinical site. This experience has made him confident in his knowledge as a professional medical assistant, and he is planning on taking his certification examination immediately upon graduation. Carlos is also gathering information to prepare his résumé and begin the search for a medical assistant position. What is a practicum and what are the responsibilities of the supervisor? What responsibilities does Carlos have at the practicum site? Who can Carlos contact for assistance in preparing his résumé? Are there any available resources for searching for a medical assistant position? How can Carlos prepare to answer questions that he will be asked at a job interview? This chapter answers these questions and others to help the medical assistant student enter this exciting career as an invaluable health care professional.

Graduation from a medical assisting program is an important milestone in your life. It is normal to have conflicting emotions ranging from excitement to anxiety. The purpose of this chapter is to help you make this transition from student to employee. The first part of the chapter discusses the practicum or **externship** experience. A practicum is your first opportunity to use your knowledge in a clinical setting. The chapter also discusses the benefits of practicum programs, how to get the most out of your practicum, and the documentation that accompanies the practicum. The later part of the chapter prepares you to begin searching for employment. Résumé preparation is discussed along with successful interviewing techniques. An introduction to key employment laws is also discussed.

## **COG** **PRACTICUM**

Accredited medical assisting programs are required to provide a **practicum** as part of the course requirement. A practicum is a training program that gives you the experience of working in a professional medical office

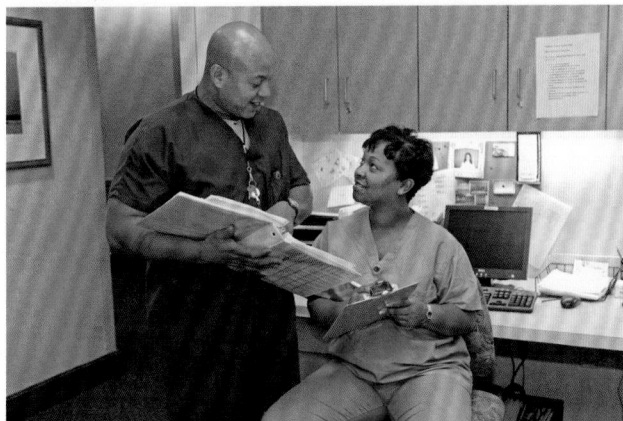

**FIGURE 46-1** • By working side by side with practicing allied health professionals, you will prepare for the real world in your extern site.

under the supervision of a supervisor who will help you to apply the theories and procedures you learned during classroom training. This is the opportunity for you to perform and perfect the skills that you have learned during the academic portion of your program.

In a practicum, you will discover areas of interest in certain types of practices or health care specialties (Fig. 46-1). Rotating through clinical sites will expose you to different offices you may pursue as possible opportunities for future employment. The length and schedule of your practicum will depend on your school's curriculum and the medical site where you will be working, but most practicums range from 160 to 240 hours in a semester. You are not paid for this experience, but you will receive curriculum credit based on the hours earned.

## Types of Facilities

The health care industry is diversified, with a wide variety of specialty offices and clinics. As a medical assisting student, you will experience an extensive scope of procedures during a practicum in a general or family practice clinic or office. Family practices are generally referred to as primary care providers. Patients range in age from newborns to the elderly and typically have a broad range of complaints and illnesses. General practice facilities provide the best exposure to all types of procedures performed by medical assistants.

Your practicum may be more limited in specialty practices. For example, staff members in obstetric offices usually do not perform electrocardiograms, and staff members in orthopedic offices wouldn't perform gynecologic examinations. Working in these types of practices, however, will give you experience in special examinations and procedures in areas that you might not observe in a general practice setting. Each specialty has advantages and disadvantages as a site, but all offer invaluable experience that cannot be adequately simulated in the classroom.

## Practicum Sites

Most schools have practicum sites they have used for years. Based on the experience of former students, personnel in these sites know what the student must do to complete the clinical experience. An ideal site should provide a variety of experiences, both in administrative (front office) and clinical (back office) procedures.

A **preceptor**, more commonly referred to as the practicum supervisor, works with students the same as the instructor in the classroom. Supervisors may be the practice manager or someone assigned by the practice manager to orient the student to the office procedures.

The school is careful to choose practicum sites who are willing to work with you and help you feel comfortable in the medical setting. They understand that all of your experience up to this point has been with fellow students in a protected classroom. They understand how nervous you are and will help you to ease the transition from classroom to the medical office. Your clinical sites are usually chosen within easy travel distance.

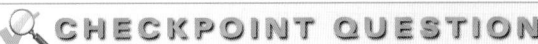

## CHECKPOINT QUESTION

1. What is the role of the supervisor?

## Practicum Benefits

### Benefits to the Student

The practicum is a vital part of medical assisting training. You will develop self-confidence and professionalism during this portion of your training. No amount of classroom training can compare with the experience of applying skills and knowledge in a medical facility. The practicum experience also allows you to broaden your knowledge base by learning new and different equipment and techniques. You will adapt your base of knowledge to your environment.

### Benefits to the Medical Assisting Program

As you gain experience from the practicum, the school also benefits from the affiliation, or connection, with the medical community. Many sites have a long history of training students. Schools rely on good training sites to enhance the medical assisting curriculum. Medical assisting programs also rely on the medical profession to aid in updating and revising the curriculum and course content to ensure that the methods and procedures presented to the students from year to year are current.

The school, the program director, and practicum supervisors review students' practicum experiences to change the program to reflect the needs of the community and the profession as health care constantly changes, such as with new technology. If students are routinely required to perform a procedure or examination that is not a part of the curriculum, for example, this will usually be considered for an addition to future lectures and laboratory sessions. If the accepted practice of a procedure has changed, changes will be made in the way it is taught to ensure that students are kept abreast of health care advances.

## Benefits to the Practicum Site

The student and the school are not the only ones to benefit from the practicum experience. The site also gains information about how well different areas of the facility are functioning. Site personnel may discover through the presence and questions of students that they should review certain policies or add others to help the office run more smoothly. Medical facilities must be updated on a continuing basis. Items may be deleted or added to policy, and procedure manuals or parts may have to be revised to provide clearer instructions.

As a student, you will be looking at the office as a newcomer, with a fresh perspective, and you may have many questions for the staff. As you become more familiar with the office routine, you will be more comfortable asking questions without the fear of appearing inexperienced. These questions may help point out to the office personnel things that should be changed or clarified.

## Practicum Responsibilities

### Responsibilities of the Student

You will develop many attributes, or characteristics, of a professional health care worker during the practicum. You should foster characteristics during this time to ensure that you continue to grow professionally and are an asset to the profession.

You must act in a professional manner. All concepts of professionalism include a positive, pleasant, confident attitude with a sincere desire to help the physician, the patient, and the staff. This image also includes being well groomed and following the dress code as required by your school policy (see Chapter 5). Professionalism also includes being dependable, which is a good sign of maturity. Students who are not at the site on time, who take excessive numbers of breaks, or who do not follow through on assignments cannot properly provide for the needs of the patients who rely on the medical staff of the facility.

Many programs require you to keep a journal listing the events of each day at the practicum site. Students will be expected to assist in the completion of the evaluation form and must therefore keep records of dates and procedures observed and performed. You will also keep a record of the time you spent at the site, which will be confirmed by your supervisor's signature on a daily time sheet.

## CHECKPOINT QUESTION

2. List three responsibilities that you have during your practicum.

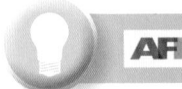 **WHAT IF?**

**You notice that on several occasions your site supervisor does not follow standard precautions. Why is this dangerous? Whom should you tell? Would you tell your instructor at school? Why or why not? How would you discuss this with your site supervisor?**

Not following standard precautions when handling body fluids may expose you to blood-borne pathogens like HIV and hepatitis. When you see dangerous practices, it is usually best to confront the employee first. As an extern, you may or may not feel comfortable doing that. You will have a faculty member who has been designated as the externship coordinator. This person needs to be notified. He or she will help you decide the best way to handle the situation. If necessary, the office manager or clinical supervisor might address the issue with everyone in an office meeting rather than singling out particular employees.

## Responsibilities of the Medical Assisting Program

The primary responsibility of the program is to arrange for the best possible clinical experience for students. The program usually has a coordinator who matches students to appropriate sites. Once a site has been chosen, you will meet with the practicum coordinator to discuss the particulars of the medical facility. An interview is sometimes held to acquaint you with your site practice manager or supervisor before the practicum begins.

After your site placement has begun, the program's practicum coordinator will visit or call frequently to follow your progress. If either you or the site has concerns, the coordinator will mediate to eliminate problems or concerns as they arise.

The practicum coordinator will make an evaluation, or appraisal, of your progress at the site. These evaluations, which are discussed later, will be used to determine whether you are prepared for the profession or your skills are deficient and need more reinforcement. The school is also responsible for maintaining liability insurance for students during clinical hours. You may pay a small premium when you pay your tuition. Students are required in most instances to provide proof of general immunizations and vaccination for hepatitis B. Some schools may provide the vaccine for students. Most programs require a current physical examination, a serology profile, and a tuberculin skin test before students are admitted to the program or before they make contact with patients.

## Responsibilities of the Practicum Site

The medical facility is, of course, responsible for providing opportunities for training. The staff will help orient you to the office and its policies. In some sites, students are allowed only to observe certain procedures but are given permission to perform some basic or routine procedures. Even if you are not allowed to perform specific procedures, the opportunity to observe and ask questions will be useful. In this way, you will become as familiar as possible with all clinical areas and functions. In many cases, the site supervisor will plan and oversee your practicum experience, verify time sheets and other documentation generated at the site, and report to the practicum coordinator from your school.

## Guidelines for a Successful Practicum

Success in your practicum is important for you to obtain employment and is evaluated according to certain standards, or criteria. The person or persons evaluating you during your practicum are professional medical personnel who know the standards for the health care field as they relate to medical assisting. These areas include the following:

- Procedural performance
- Preparedness
- Attendance
- Appearance
- Attitude

### Procedural Performance

You will be judged on your ability to measure up to the standard of care for an entry-level medical assistant. This means you are expected to perform at the level of a new employee in the field. Your supervisor is there to assist you, not to teach you the basics that you should have learned in the classroom. Come to your practicum site prepared, and ask questions, when in doubt, before starting any procedure.

### Preparedness

Preparation is the best insurance for success, regardless of the goal. Personal preparation for the practicum helps prevent losing time because of other extracurricular or personal obligations. Make sure in advance that you have prepared the following:

- Reliable transportation
- Reliable day care services
- Backup systems for a sick child, snow cancellations of school, or early dismissals from school
- Financial coverage and support for any hours that you are unable to work at your usual job because of your practicum site hours

## Attendance

If you have planned well for transportation, family considerations, and finances, you are more likely to attend all sessions at the clinical sites. You must also be healthy. A good diet, regular exercise, and proper rest help you maintain good health. Careful attention to hygiene and medical asepsis help ensure that you do not bring illnesses to home from the clinical sites.

If at any time you will be late or will not be able to attend the site for any reason, you must notify both the practicum coordinator and the site supervisor. Never be a no-call or no-show. Almost all sites have an answering service for leaving messages, as do most schools. There is no excuse for not notifying all parties involved if you will be unavoidably late or will not be able to attend the scheduled session.

Office hours vary from site to site; it is always a good practice, however, to arrive a few minutes before the scheduled opening. This allows time to check for telephone messages, arrange the day's appointments, turn on office equipment, and generally get into the routine of the office. Plan your transportation, leaving plenty of time for any problems that may occur. Arriving in a flurry, frustrated by traffic or home problems, with no time to ease into your day causes a high level of tension and anxiety. This makes it more difficult to have the caring and compassionate attitude necessary to deal with the complex problems in the medical office.

## Appearance

You have only one opportunity to make a first impression, which is usually based on appearance. Appearance is much more than looks. A beautiful face on a poorly groomed person is not seen as professional and does not inspire trust and confidence in patients or coworkers. The key to a professional appearance is careful preparation and planning.

You will, most likely, wear a uniform or scrubs mandated by your school for your practicum, and it must be freshly laundered and not wrinkled; clean but wrinkled is not acceptable. Plan your wardrobe for ease of care and a professional appearance. If you are not required to wear a uniform to your practicum site, keep in mind that fad or trendy clothing, suggestive clothing, and flashy clothing are not appropriate for clinical sites. All clothing should be in good repair, with no missing buttons, hanging hems, tears, rips, or stains. Shoes should be clean and kept in good condition. Laced shoes look better with fresh, clean shoelaces. You may wear laboratory coats in some programs; uniforms may be worn in others. The clinical supervisor preceptor or the practicum coordinator will inform you of the dress code in advance.

Professional appearance includes hair and makeup. Your hair should be conservatively styled, and long hair must be tied back and kept away from the face. Wash it frequently so that it is fresh and clean. Makeup should be minimal and tastefully applied. Never use perfume or cologne, which may be irritating to coworkers and patients. Keep fingernails short to avoid transferring pathogens or ripping gloves when you perform procedures.

Wear only minimal, tasteful jewelry. Rings can puncture gloves, possibly causing exposure to a pathogen. Therefore, it is a good idea to avoid wearing them in the clinical site. Small post earrings are usually acceptable, but dangling earrings pose a potential hazard and should not be worn in medical office. Most offices also have a policy that requires body piercings to be removed and visible tattoos covered with a bandage or long sleeves if necessary (see Chapter 5).

## CHECKPOINT QUESTION

3. Describe the proper attire for your practicum.

## ETHICAL TIP

### HIPAA and Students

The Health Insurance Portability and Accountability Act of 1996 (HIPAA) Privacy Rule does not prohibit students accessing patient medical information as part of their education. The wording of the privacy rules defines "health care operations" in a way that includes training of health care providers and professionals. Students are part of the covered entity's workforce for HIPAA compliance purposes. The rule does require that students receive training about the organization's policies and procedures related to protected health information. This training must be completed within a reasonable period of time after the student begins the practicum. Documentation of this training must be kept for 6 years.

## Attitude

Attitude is also part of appearance. Most patients and coworkers will see your emotions through facial expressions and body language. A person who looks eager is usually perceived as a good, diligent worker. Attitude is determined by how well you handle change and direction and how adaptable and flexible you are during difficult assignments.

The medical profession is constantly changing, making it imperative for all professionals to stay flexible. In the classroom, you learn generic methods for treatments and procedures. Because of the constantly changing technology, you may have to adjust to other methods in the field. If you learned a procedure one way in the classroom training but find that it is performed differently in the clinical site, the new method must be accepted and performed as well as possible. Frequently, there is more than career right way to do a procedure, and the classroom method you learned may be just one of

the accepted methods. The next physician or clinical site may use yet another equally correct procedural method.

## LEGAL TIP

### You're in the Real World Now!

In Chapter 2, you learned that a medical assistant practices under the license of a physician. As a student, you are not an employee of the physician; therefore, the legal doctrine of respondent superior does not apply. Since you are participating in a college activity, any liability issues are covered by the college's liability or malpractice insurance. Most colleges have a blanket policy to cover students who are taking courses conducted in a medical facility that has entered into a clinical affiliation with the college. Students pay a fee at the beginning of the semester of the clinical experience. Malpractice insurance covers any issues with patient care in the medical site. It is important that you identify yourself as a student. You must be wearing a name tag with your student status clearly visible. Patients have the right to know who is participating in their care. Most practicum sites will require criminal background and drug testing before allowing a student to begin an externship. In other words, students are put through the same hiring process as the permanent employees. Licensure and certification are discussed in Chapter 2.

Your attitude determines your altitude. Students who work with a positive attitude during their practicum are likely to reach higher levels of the profession than those who see the practicum as an imposition or a burden. Box 46-1 offers some additional suggestions.

### BOX 46-1    Strategies for a Successful Practicum

Your practicum will be successful if you:

- Show enthusiasm and interest in learning
- Are a team player
- Offer to assist with as many tasks as possible
- Ask questions or for clarification before doing any procedures or tasks about which you are unsure
- Immediately admit to any errors or mistakes that you make
- Accept corrections and suggestions by staff members
- Anticipate tasks that need to be done and do them before you are asked
- Do not make remarks such as: "I can't believe that you don't have that on the computer." "This office is outdated." "Don't you know about these new regulations?"

# Practicum Documentation

Most programs use a time sheet or record of some sort to document your hours in the practicum (Fig. 46-2). The beginning and ending hours of each day are recorded. How breaks are handled depends on the practicum coordinator, program requirements, and specific site. Some sites allow half an hour for lunch, and others allow an hour; some close for an hour or more midday, while others are open and staffed from morning until evening. Some programs make students responsible for time sheet signatures; others delegate the responsibility to the site preceptor. However the form is handled, it is used to validate your time in the practicum and is a requirement for completion of most programs.

Journals are required by many programs. These provide proof that tasks are performed and learning takes place. The student will list each day's activities, and this is reviewed by the practicum coordinator. Checklists serve as further documentation of tasks observed and performed. In many cases, the site supervisor actually assigns a grade to the student using criteria provided by the college. Site evaluations performed by the student are another form of practicum documentation and are discussed in the next section.

Every accredited school will use surveys to gather information from students. Sample evaluations are available through the American Association of Medical Assistants' (AAMA's) Web site. Evaluations are used to improve performance and services offered to students. Most medical assisting programs have advisory boards whose members use the results of such surveys to make necessary changes to existing programs. Your input is vital to this ongoing quest for excellence. Take these evaluations seriously and be honest. Do not take the opportunity to complain about individual problems that may have been encountered. It is more appropriate to

---

**CLINICAL EXPERIENCE
STUDENT'S TIME REPORT**

To obtain proper credit, an account of time and days in attendance must be recorded by each intern student. This report must be verified by the job supervisor and attached to the final 55-day roster. This information is kept strictly confidential.

Student's Name: _____   Course No.: _____

Program: _____   Course Title: _____

Minimum Contact Hrs. Required: _____   Quarter/Year: _____

| WEEK OF (DATES) | TIME OF DAY | | | | | | | TOTAL HOURS | SITE SUPERVISOR |
|---|---|---|---|---|---|---|---|---|---|
| | M | T | W | TH | F | S | | | |
| | | | | | | | | | |
| | | | | | | | | | |
| | | | | | | | | | |
| | | | | | | | | | |
| | | | | | | | | | |
| | | | | | | | | | |
| | | | | | | | | | |
| | | | | | | | | | |
| | | | | | | | | | |
| | | | | | | | | | |
| | | | | | | | | | |
| | | | | | | | | | |
| | | | | | | | | | |

**TOTAL HOURS FOR QUARTER:** _____

I certify that the above time report is a true statement of the hours worked.

I approve this statement of hours in attendance for the quarter covered.

_____   _____
Student's Signature          Date

_____   _____
Externship Coordinator's Signature          Date

**FIGURE 46-2** • Sample extern time sheet.

address these concerns under comments. For example, if a particular instructor's grading criteria are more strict than others' criteria, your evaluation of that instructor should not be based on the fact that you got a lower grade in his or her class. You should be fair and objective and evaluate the instructor on his or her actual performance in the classroom. Evaluations are not designed to prove popularity but to report strengths and deficiencies in areas that can be improved.

## Practicum Evaluations

The supervisor or office manager at your site will evaluate you on a completed form that contains detailed areas to be graded; these are equivalent to grades on a test or examination. The supervisor coordinator is responsible for compiling evaluations and keeping you abreast of your progress. Frequent conferences with your coordinator usually help accomplish this. After your practicum is completed, your input in the quality of your experience helps program administrators choose the best sites in the future.

Most schools use a site evaluation form to gather impressions of the program's practicum sites and the students' overall practicum experience (Fig. 46-3). This form helps determine the effectiveness of the site for training and whether any issues should be addressed before assigning other students. Be objective and honest

---

**Externship Site Evaluation**

**Pittsylvania Community College**
Medical Assisting Program

Name of externship site being evaluated: _____

> **INSTRUCTIONS:** Consider each item separately and rate each item independently of all others. Circle the rating that indicates the extent to which you agree with each statement. Please do not skip any rating.
> 5 = Strongly Agree   4 = Generally Agree   3 = Neutral (acceptable)   2 = Generally Disagree
> 1 = Strongly Disagree   N/A = This activity is Not Available at this site

At this externship site, I was:

| | | | | | | | |
|---|---|---|---|---|---|---|---|
| 1. | Provided orientation to the office/facility | 5 | 4 | 3 | 2 | 1 | N/A |
| 2. | Assigned to a supervisor/preceptor who actively participated in my learning experience | 5 | 4 | 3 | 2 | 1 | N/A |
| 3. | Allowed to perform the entry-level skills I had learned in school | 5 | 4 | 3 | 2 | 1 | N/A |
| 4. | Given the opportunity to perform administrative skills | 5 | 4 | 3 | 2 | 1 | N/A |
| 5. | Given the opportunity to perform clinical skills | 5 | 4 | 3 | 2 | 1 | N/A |
| 6. | Adequately supervised and knew who to ask for help if I needed it | 5 | 4 | 3 | 2 | 1 | N/A |
| 7. | Treated respectfully by healthcare providers and other staff | 5 | 4 | 3 | 2 | 1 | N/A |
| 8. | Provided with adequate personal protective equipment (e.g. gloves) to protect my health and safety | 5 | 4 | 3 | 2 | 1 | N/A |
| 9. | Able to communicate effectively with | | | | | | |
| | a.  supervisory personnel | 5 | 4 | 3 | 2 | 1 | N/A |
| | b.  staff and co-workers | 5 | 4 | 3 | 2 | 1 | N/A |
| | c.  physicians/health care professionals | 5 | 4 | 3 | 2 | 1 | N/A |
| | d.  patients/clients/family members | 5 | 4 | 3 | 2 | 1 | N/A |
| 10. | Not used to replace paid employees | 5 | 4 | 3 | 2 | 1 | N/A |
| 11. | Provided regular constructive verbal feedback from by supervisor | 5 | 4 | 3 | 2 | 1 | N/A |
| 12. | Provided a final written performance evaluation | 5 | 4 | 3 | 2 | 1 | N/A |

13. Were you asked to perform any skills for which you were not prepared by your medical assisting program?
   _____Yes   _____No

   If yes, please identify: _____

14. Would you recommend this site for future externship students?  ____Yes ____No   Why? _____
   _____

15. What part of the externship experience did you like best and/or least? _____
   _____

Student's name and signature _____ Date _____

**FIGURE 46-3 •** Sample site evaluation form.

in your evaluation of the site. When completing a site evaluation, consider these questions:

- Was the overall experience positive or negative?
- Were opportunities for learning abundant and freely offered or hard to obtain?
- Were staff personnel open and caring or unwelcoming?
- Was the site supervisor available and easily approachable or preoccupied and distant?

If the site is not providing a positive learning experience, the program should discontinue using it.

## Graduate Surveys

When you graduate, the college will want to know your opinion of its instruction and services. You will be asked to evaluate your experience at the college in general, your course work, and your practicum experience. Take the time to think back over your overall experience at the school. Information provided is tabulated and distributed to those evaluated. This is an integral part of the quality improvement and planning processes of educational institutions. Figure 46-4 illustrates a sample graduate survey.

## Employer Surveys

After you have been on a job for awhile, the college will survey your employer to assess his/her satisfaction with your performance, skills, and professionalism. Figure 46-5 is a sample of an employer evaluation. You must always do your best. Your performance is a reflection not only of you but also of your medical assisting program and the college you attended.

**CHECKPOINT QUESTION**

4. What is the purpose of having students evaluate their practicum experience?

## COG ESTABLISH THE JOB FOR YOU

Once your practicum is complete, you are one step closer to getting the job that you desire. Take an inventory of your qualifications, strengths, and weakness. Preparation will help you search for and find the perfect job.

**GRADUATE SURVEY**

**Pittsylvania Community College**
**MEDICAL ASSISTING PROGRAM**

**The primary goal of a Medical Assisting Education program is to prepare its graduates to function as competent Medical Assistants. This survey is designed to help your program faculty determine the strengths of your program as well as those areas that need improvement. All data will be kept confidential and will be used for program evaluation purposes only.**

**BACKGROUND INFORMATION:**

Job Title: ____________________ If not working, what are you doing? __________

Current Salary (optional): ____________________

Place of employment: ____________________

Length of employment at time of survey: ______ years and/or ______ months.

Name of graduate (Optional): ____________________

Certification/Registration Status (*check all that apply*): ☐ CMA __ RMA

**INSTRUCTIONS: Consider each item separately and rate each item independently of all others. Circle the rating that indicates the extent to which you agree with each statement. Please do not skip any rating.**
**5 = Strongly Agree 4 = Generally Agree 3 = Neutral (acceptable) 2 = Generally Disagree 1 = Strongly Disagree**

**I. KNOWLEDGE (Cognitive Learning Domain)**
**THE PROGRAM:**

| | | | | | |
|---|---|---|---|---|---|
| A. Helped me acquire the medical assisting knowledge appropriate to my level of training. | 5 | 4 | 3 | 2 | 1 |
| B. Helped me acquire the general medical knowledge base appropriate to my level of training | 5 | 4 | 3 | 2 | 1 |
| C. Prepared me to collect patient data effectively. | 5 | 4 | 3 | 2 | 1 |
| D. Prepared me to perform appropriate diagnostic and medical procedures. | 5 | 4 | 3 | 2 | 1 |
| E. Trained me to use sound judgment while functioning in the healthcare setting. | 5 | 4 | 3 | 2 | 1 |

Comments: ____________________

**II. SKILLS (Psychomotor Learning Domain)**
**THE PROGRAM:**

| | | | | | |
|---|---|---|---|---|---|
| A. Prepared me to perform all clinical skills appropriate to entry level medical assisting | 5 | 4 | 3 | 2 | 1 |
| B. Prepared me to perform all administrative skills appropriate to entry level medical assisting. | 5 | 4 | 3 | 2 | 1 |

Comments: ____________________

Februar y 2006, 2013 1

**III. BEHAVIORS (Affective Learning Domain)**
**THE PROGRAM:**

| | | | | | |
|---|---|---|---|---|---|
| A. Prepared me to communicate effectively in the healthcare setting. | 5 | 4 | 3 | 2 | 1 |
| B. Prepared me to conduct myself in an ethical and professional manner. | 5 | 4 | 3 | 2 | 1 |
| C. Taught me to manage my time efficiently while functioning in the healthcare setting. | 5 | 4 | 3 | 2 | 1 |
| D. Strongly encouraged me to apply for and pass my: | | | | | |
| CMA | 5 | 4 | 3 | 2 | 1 |
| RMA | 5 | 4 | 3 | 2 | 1 |

Comments: ____________________

**IV. GENERAL INFORMATION** ***(Check yes or no)***

| | | |
|---|---|---|
| A. I have attained CMA certification. | ☐ YES | ☐ NO |
| B. I have attained RMA registry. | ☐ YES | ☐ NO |
| C. I am a member of the American Association of Medical Assistants | ☐ YES | ☐ NO |
| D. I am a member of the American Medical Technology Association | ☐ YES | ☐ NO |
| E. I actively participate in continuing education activities. | ☐ YES | ☐ NO |

If you answered NO to any of the above questions, please explain why: ____________________

**V. ADDITIONAL COMMENTS**

**OVERALL RATING:**
Please rate and comment on the OVERALL quality of your preparation as a medical assistant:
5 = Excellent 4 = Very Good 3 = Good 2 = Fair 1 = Poor

Comments: ____________________

**Please identify two or three strengths of the program.**

**Please make two or three suggestions to further strengthen the program.**

**What qualities/skills were expected of you upon employment that were not included in the program?**

**Please provide comments and suggestions that would help to better prepare future graduates.**

**Thank You!** **Date:** __________

Februa ry 2006, 2013 2

**FIGURE 46-4** • Sample graduate survey.

**EMPLOYER SURVEY**

Pittsylvania Community College
**Medical Assisting Program**

**The primary goal of a Medical Assisting Education program is to prepare each graduate to function as a competent Medical Assistant. This survey is designed to help program faculty determine their program's strengths and those areas that need improvement. All data will be kept confidential and will be used for program evaluation purposes only. We request that this survey be completed by the graduate's immediate supervisor.**

**BACKGROUND INFORMATION:**

Name of Graduate (Optional): ____________________

Certification Status (*check all that apply*):

☐ CMA ☐ RMA

Length of employment at time of survey: __________ years and __________ months

Place of employment: ____________________

Name of evaluator completing this form: ____________________

**INSTRUCTIONS: Consider each item separately and rate each item independently of all others. Circle the rating that indicates the extent to which you agree with each statement. Please do not skip any rating.**
**5 = Strongly Agree 4 = Generally Agree 3 = Neutral (acceptable) 2 = Generally Disagree 1 = Strongly Disagree**

**I. KNOWLEDGE (Cognitive Learning Domain)**

**THE GRADUATE:**

| | | | | | | |
|---|---|---|---|---|---|---|
| A. | Has medical assisting knowledge appropriate to his/her level of training. | 5 | 4 | 3 | 2 | 1 |
| B. | Has general medical knowledge appropriate to his/her level of training. | 5 | 4 | 3 | 2 | 1 |
| C. | Is able to collect pertinent data accurately from charts and patients. | 5 | 4 | 3 | 2 | 1 |
| D. | Is able to perform appropriate diagnostic and medical procedures as directed. | 5 | 4 | 3 | 2 | 1 |
| E. | Uses good judgment while functioning in the ambulatory healthcare setting. | 5 | 4 | 3 | 2 | 1 |

Comments: ____________________

**II. SKILLS (Psychomotor Learning Domain)**

**THE PROGRAM:**

| | | | | | | |
|---|---|---|---|---|---|---|
| A. | Prepared the graduate to perform all clinical skills appropriate to entry level medical assisting | 5 | 4 | 3 | 2 | 1 |
| B. | Prepared the graduate to perform all administrative skills appropriate to entry level medical assisting. | 5 | 4 | 3 | 2 | 1 |

Comments: ____________________

February 2006, 2013

**III. BEHAVIORS (Affective Learning Domain)**

**THE GRADUATE:**

| | | | | | | |
|---|---|---|---|---|---|---|
| A. | Communicates effectively in the healthcare setting. | 5 | 4 | 3 | 2 | 1 |
| B. | Conducts himself/herself in an ethical and professional manner. | 5 | 4 | 3 | 2 | 1 |
| C. | Functions effectively as a member of the healthcare team. | 5 | 4 | 3 | 2 | 1 |
| D. | Accepts supervision and works effectively with supervisory personnel. | 5 | 4 | 3 | 2 | 1 |
| E. | Is self-directed and responsible for his/her actions. | 5 | 4 | 3 | 2 | 1 |
| F. | Arrives to work prepared and on time. | 5 | 4 | 3 | 2 | 1 |
| G. | Contributes to a positive environment in the department. | 5 | 4 | 3 | 2 | 1 |

Comments: ____________________

**IV. GENERAL INFORMATION** ***(Circle yes or no)***

| | | | |
|---|---|---|---|
| A. | Do you encourage/motivate employees to take and pass the CMA Certification exam? | Yes | No |
| B. | Do you encourage/motivate employees to take and pass the RMA Registry exams? | Yes | No |
| C. | If you answered NO to any of the above questions, please explain why: | | |

Comments: ____________________

**V. ADDITIONAL COMMENTS**

**OVERALL RATING:**

Please rate and comment on the OVERALL quality of this graduate:

5 = Excellent 4 = Very Good 3 = Good 2 = Fair 1 = Poor

Comments: ____________________

What qualities or skills did you expect of the graduate upon employment that he/she *did not* possess?

____________________

Please provide comments and suggestions that would help this program to better prepare future graduates.

____________________

What are strengths of the graduate(s) of this program?

____________________

Name and Title of Evaluator:

(Please Print) ____________________ Date: __________

Signature: ____________________

Thank you in advance

February 2006, 2013

**FIGURE 46-5** • Sample employer evaluation.

## Setting Employment Goals

Before beginning to search for a job, decide what you want and need from a job and make that your goal. People who do not set employment goals too often accept only what is presented to them. They often end up unhappy in their work because they did not choose their job in the first place. The average person approaches the job search with the attitude, "I wonder what is available," rather than, "Here is what I would like to do, and here is the facility where I would like to work." *That* is setting a goal. It is also a positive, proactive approach to the job market rather than a reactive position to what is available. In general, the medical field is looking for proactive people. You will work harder and more enthusiastically if you choose your workplace.

The best way to set a goal and eventually get what you want is to study your strengths and weaknesses and, from that self-knowledge, design the best job for you. Goal setting means describing the ideal job for you and deciding that this is the job that you will someday have.

On a sheet of paper, describe the best job for you if you had your choice. For example, you might describe these elements:

- Specialty area (e.g., obstetrics, pediatrics, surgery)
- Duties (clinical or administrative)
- Type of employer and supervisor
- Other employees and coworkers
- Type of facility
- Desired atmosphere (casual or formal)
- Ideal hours
- Availability of flextime (a system of scheduling that allows for a personal choice in hours or days worked)

Next, write down where you expect to be in 2 years and in 5 years, in terms of both position and income. Now you are more focused on where you want to work, what you want to do, and the direction you want to be going. The next question is how to get there.

To win the position you want, you have to learn to sell yourself. Generally, employers will not come looking for you; you will have to go to them. They will compare you with all of the other equally well-qualified candidates who are interested in the same position. If 25 people interview for a job, even if you are second best, you still lose. The one who is best suited for a job does not necessarily get it; instead, frequently the one who performs best in the interview does. Marketing yourself takes real effort.

## Self-Analysis

A good presentation of your qualifications begins with self-analysis. You must know what strengths you have to offer a potential employer as well as your weaknesses. Make an honest list of your strengths and weaknesses. Each of your strengths presents an opportunity to sell yourself and your value as an employee. When you are interviewing for a position, concentrate on projecting your strengths to the interviewer.

Just as your strengths give you a special advantage, each weakness is a reason someone may not want to offer you the position. Recognize and work to resolve your weaknesses. Recognizing your weaknesses as a threat to securing the position you want will help you develop strategies to eliminate these problems or turn them into strengths. As long as you are aware of your weaknesses, you are better prepared to handle them.

Once you know the type of job you want and have identified your positive and negative qualities, it is time to begin to look for the right job.

 **CHECKPOINT QUESTION**

5. What is the purpose of self-analysis?

##  FINDING THE RIGHT JOB

The Internet offers employment services that allow you to search for a certain type job in a specific geographic location. Even though searching the Internet is easier and less time consuming than the traditional ways of looking for a job, an Internet search may not be the best way to find a job. Keep in mind that many of the most desirable job openings are never advertised; they are posted internally and filled from within. Membership in your professional organization is an excellent way to network.

Many studies show that most positions are never advertised in the media. Open positions that are posted internally are often filled with current employees or by referrals from current employees. Any organization that looks within and obtains a recommendation from a current employee to fill an available position accomplishes two things: (1) it saves the cost of advertising, and (2) the recommendation itself is usually a good one because it comes from someone who presumably knows the demands and special needs of that particular organization.

It is important for someone seeking employment in the medical field to build as many contacts within the field as possible. These contacts help you with **networking**. Networking is using friends, family members, and professional colleagues to advance or obtain information in the workplace. It is impossible to have too many contacts. Everyone with whom you associate should know that you are looking for employment. Friends and acquaintances cannot tell you about a job or recommend you for a job if they do not know that you are searching.

Traditional sources of information for job openings:

- *Local, state, or federal government employment offices.* These agencies are designed to find work for the unemployed. They frequently have listings of

positions that are not found anywhere else. Rather than calling the office with inquiries, make an appointment to visit. Register with the service. Get to know the contact person with whom you will be contacting frequently.

- *School placement office.* If your school has a placement office, contact the coordinator or personnel officer and outline what you are looking for and where you want to work. Their job is to assist you in securing the position you want. If you establish a working relationship with a contact person, you will probably have better results.

- *Medical facilities.* Do not wait for an advertisement. Go to the office or facility where you would like to work and leave a résumé—a document summarizing your professional qualifications—and a cover letter explaining how much you want to work there. Find out the name of the office manager or personnel officer and call first for an appointment. This shows better planning and foresight and is more professional than dropping by unannounced.

- *Private agencies.* Many medical facilities solicit privately to avoid being swamped by applications from unqualified applicants. A fee is charged for the service but is usually paid by the employer. Call the agency to make an appointment with a representative who will interview you and tell you what steps to follow.

- *Temporary services.* These agencies fill short-term vacancies for medical offices. If you are new in an area, this is a good way to learn which facilities would be good choices for you. You may be assigned for several days or several weeks. If you work well as a temporary replacement and like the site, leave your résumé and let the appropriate individuals know that you would like to work in this place if an opening occurs. Check with the temporary agency regarding any fees that you may be charged or that the medical office may have to pay if it hires you, often called a finder's fee.

 **CHECKPOINT QUESTION**

6. List four resources that you may use to identify potential job opportunities.

##  APPLYING FOR THE JOB

### Answering Employment Advertisements

When responding to an employment advertisement, be sure to do exactly what the advertisement asks you to do; one of the qualities that many interviewers look for is the ability to follow directions. At the same time, try to make your response more distinctive (yet still professional) than others they may receive. The medical profession rarely responds well to those who do not fit its image and almost never accepts someone who does not conform at the entry level. Most employers will require you to submit a résumé. A well-prepared résumé and cover letter are essential to job hunting.

## Preparing Your Résumé

Many resources can help you write your **résumé**. Start with your school employment placement office for assistance. Your school library may also have books on how to create résumés. Numerous Web sites also offer this information. Caution: Many Web sites have free information, but some charge fees. Focus on free resources before paying for these services. Many word processing programs have templates for résumés. Save your résumé on a computer flash drive and be sure to personalize it for the position you are seeking. For example, if you give a career objective, try putting in the title a description of the particular job you are seeking. Keep changing this for every different position so that your résumé is personalized for each interview.

The résumé is a flash picture of yourself; if it is neat and professional, the reviewer will presume that it is a reflection of you. Procedure 46-1 outlines the steps in writing a résumé. Here are some guidelines that will help you create a résumé that will capture the reviewer's interest:

1. Evaluate your skills, goals, and what you have to offer. With this list in hand, you can better concentrate on highlighting your strengths.
2. Confine your résumé to one page, selecting carefully what you want to include. The résumé must state just what the reviewer needs to know and no more.
3. Include the following key information:
   • Name, address, and telephone number: Include these at the top of your résumé (usually centered). (Because you are including your telephone number, you should expect calls from prospective employers. Box 46-2 offers some tips for handling such calls.)

---

• Education: Start with the most recent and work backward.
• Affiliations or volunteer work (if appropriate): If this information shows that you have good organizational skills or have held an office for the group, you should include it.
• Experience: This may be listed in either of two standard forms: functional or chronological. A functional résumé focuses on skills and qualifications rather than employment and works well for those who recently graduated or who are reentering the job market after a period of years (Fig. 46-6). A chronological résumé is useful for those who have an employment history, particularly if the history is relevant to the position being sought. Start with the most recent employment and work backward. Include your title, position, and a few of your key responsibilities (Fig. 46-7). Explain any gaps such as pregnancy, schooling, relocations, and so on.
• References: You may or may not include your references on a separate sheet. When you have chosen the people you want to use as references, be sure to ask their permission. Start by asking your instructors if you can use them as references. Other medical professionals (physicians or nurses) will also make strong references. Previous employers also make very good references. You should have a minimum of three references. Do not bring a list of more than five people. Prospective employers are not interested in your neighbors, pastor, or relatives as references.
4. Do not include hobbies and personal interests unrelated to work. It is not relevant that you play the guitar, but it would be impressive to know that you volunteer at a free clinic.
5. Use action words (Box 46-3).
6. Center the résumé on white or off-white heavy bond or high rag content paper, 8.5 × 11 inches. (Colors are not acceptable, and cheap paper will not convey the professional impression you hope to make.) Keep a 1-inch margin around the text. Single space within the sections of information, but leave a blank line between the sections.
7. Use regular type. Avoid fonts that are cute or fancy. Use black ink. Do not print your résumé in color.
8. Have someone proofread your work. It is difficult to find your own errors or see areas that are not clearly worded.
9. Mail the résumé in an 8.5- × 11-inch manila envelope. This will present the interviewer with a résumé and cover letter that are smooth, with no fold lines. Many prefer to work with résumés that have not been folded for an envelope.

---

> **BOX 46-2    Handling Calls from Prospective Employers**
>
> Here are some tips for handling calls from prospective employers:
>
> • Tell family members or other household members that you are expecting important telephone calls.
> • Keep a pen and paper by the telephone.
> • Instruct people to take a complete message. Ask them to write down the person's name, phone number, message, and what time the call was received.
> • Leave a professional message on your answering machine. Avoid leaving cute or silly messages.

Tina Elmwood C.M.A.
22 Brandy Drive
Dayton, Ohio 00000
444-777-6666

**Employment Objective:** To use my medical assisting skills in a challenging position. My goal is to work with children. (*Change this sentence to reflect the type of office that you are applying to.*)

**Experience:**

Externship (160 hours) at Family Practice Associates, Bayview Drive, Dayton, Ohio (*If you have a positive evaluation from your preceptor, bring it with you to the interview. Do not attach it to the résumé.*)

**Education:**

Medical Assisting Program, Diploma. Graduated June 2008. West County Community College, Dayton Ohio (*Bring a copy of your diploma and transcripts to the interview. Do not attach them unless employer has specifically requested them.*)
Dayton High School, Diploma. Graduated June 2006. Dayton, Ohio

**Skills:**

Clinical and Laboratory skills listed on Role Delineation for Medical Assisting

Administrative skills listed on Role Delineation for Medical Assisting

Comfortable using all types of standard office equipment

Familiar with XYZ software programs (*List software programs that you are comfortable with. If you know what type of software the office uses, list that as well.*)

**Certifications:**

Certified Medical Assistant, American Association of Medical Assistants (*Bring copy to interview or attach to résumé.*)
Cardiopulmonary Resuscitation, American Heart Association (*Bring copy to interview or attach to résumé.*)

**FIGURE 46-6** • Sample functional résumé.

10. Many employers are now allowing applicants to send their résumés as an e-mail attachment. Use a well-known software to create your résumé, and keep it simple because some formatting may not transmit properly.
11. Be honest. Do not embellish your résumé or add fictional information. This could get you fired if discrepancies are discovered after you are employed.

### CHECKPOINT QUESTION

**7.** What is the difference between a functional résumé and a chronological résumé?

## Preparing Your Cover Letter

When contacting a prospective employer about a job, you need to send a résumé along with a cover letter. Keep your cover letter brief and meaningful. You want it to be read, and you want the reader to be impressed by what it says. Be sure that you mention the job itself in your letter. You may even consider a statement such as, "This is the type of position I would prefer." If you are applying to a pediatrician's office, you may write, "My goal is to work with children." If you know something favorable about the facility, include that in your letter. If you know anyone who works for the company, mention it. *Do not* mention the person by name unless you have secured his or her permission.

Make sure you address your letter to the right person. Call the personnel department or office manager and ask the name of the person handling the applications. Determine the correct spelling of the name and the preferred honorific, such as Mr., Ms., or Mrs.

The standard form for a cover letter has three brief paragraphs:

• First paragraph: State the position for which you are applying.

Beatrice Meza CMA
123 Main Street
West Harford, CT 00000
888-999-6666

**Employment Objective:** To use my medical assisting skills in a challenging position. My goal is to work in an obstetrical office. (*Change this sentence to reflect the type of office that you are applying to.*)

**Education:**

2013–2014 Medical Assisting Program; Mountain Laurel Community College, West Hartford, Connecticut (*Bring a copy of your diploma and transcripts to the interview. Do not attach them unless employer has specifically requested them.*)

**Externship:**

July 2014–(160 hours) Women's Health Care Center, Hartford, Connecticut (*If you have a positive evaluation from your preceptor, bring it with you to the interview. Do not attach it to the résumé.*)

**Work Experience:**

July 2013–present Receptionist, Dermatology Consultants, West Hartford, Connecticut. Worked part time while I was in school. Answered and triaged telephone calls. Assisted with various other medical administrative responsibilities. (*If you have a reference letter from this employer, bring it with you to the interview. Be prepared to answer questions about why you are leaving this position.*)
May 2010–July 2013 Cashier/Clerk for SuperMarket Grocers, West Hartford, Connecticut. Worked part time. Responsible for training new employees. Promoted to senior cashier.

**Skills:**

Clinical and Laboratory skills listed on the Role Delineation for Medical Assisting

Administrative skills listed on the Role Delineation for Medical Assisting

Comfortable using all types of standard office equipment

Familiar with XYZ software programs (*List software programs that you are comfortable with. If you know what type of software the office uses, list that as well.*)

**Activities/Honors**

Student Government representative

Most Improved Medical Assisting Student in 2013

**FIGURE 46-7** • Sample chronological résumé.

**BOX 46-3    Action Words**

| | | |
|---|---|---|
| Achieved | Established | Planned |
| Assisted | Filed | Prepared |
| Attained | Generated | Processed |
| Conducted | Handled | Scheduled |
| Completed | Implemented | Screened |
| Composed | Maintained | Selected |
| Created | Operated | Solved |
| Developed | Organized | Systemized |
| Directed | Participated | Wrote |
| Ensured | Performed | |

- Second paragraph: Stress your skills. Do not be redundant, since you will also send a résumé, but mention or highlight specifically the skills needed for this job.
- Third paragraph: Request an interview. Offer to call in a week to set up an interview (then do so). Keep a copy of your letter to refer to when calling.

Use the same good-quality paper for the cover letter that you use for your résumé. Include your name, address, and telephone number at the top of the page, centered or in block form. Single space the letter, and double space between paragraphs. Either block or modified block form is acceptable.

As mentioned earlier, many employers are now accepting résumés via e-mail. Although this may eliminate the need for a cover letter, the information included should still be communicated as an e-mail message. Accuracy is just as important in an electronic communication as in any other form. It is more professional to attach your résumé as a document instead of placing it in the body of an e-mail.

## Completing an Employment Application

Some sites will have you fill out an employment application while you wait for your interview; others may mail one to you to be filled out and taken to the interview. Although résumés have their place and are indispensable, many facilities rely more on an application form. Many organizations accept online applications. The guidelines for completing an online application are similar to those of manual completion of an application:

1. Read through completely before beginning.
2. Follow the instructions exactly. Prospective employers notice neatness, erasures, evasions, and indecision.
3. Answer every question. If the question does not apply to you, draw a line or write N/A so that the interviewer will know that you did not overlook the question.
4. In the line for wage or salary desired, write "negotiable" or find out before the interview what is usual for the area for this type of position.
5. In spaces requesting your reason for leaving a previous position, try to sound positive. Answers such as "to explore a new career direction" are general enough to fill many needs. If the reason for leaving was relocation, schooling, or pregnancy, say so.
6. Type, or print legibly, being as neat as possible.
7. Use a black or blue pen. Never use a pencil or colored pen (red, green, purple) to complete the application. It does not portray a professional image.
8. You may attach your résumé to the application if you did not mail one already.

## COG   THE INTERVIEW

Interviewing well is a skill that takes effort to develop. The résumé introduces you to potential employers, but the interview is how you "sell" yourself to them. As with any skill, if you want to stay proficient and keep your skills in good working order, you have to practice. Ask friends or family members to work with you to develop a relaxed approach to answering the questions most often asked during an interview. Have them try to trip you up or confuse you by throwing in tricky questions. Although the effect will not be the same with a friend or family member as with an interviewer, this practice can make a difference between getting the job and losing the chance. You can also rehearse in front of a mirror.

Usually, the person who interviews best is hired for the position. An excellent interview is absolutely crucial for obtaining any job. It is highly unlikely that you will get the job you want without doing well in the interview. Remember what the employer is looking for. Every employer is looking for something special from each employee. Medicine has special needs. The employer must believe that you possess a number of skills necessary to do the job:

- *Technical skills.* You must have the necessary proficiency to get the job done.
- *Confidentiality.* In medicine, you are exposed to sensitive information about patients. Is the interviewer convinced that you can be relied on to keep those confidences?
- *Human relations skills.* Will you get along with the others in the workplace?
- *Communication skills.* Do you have the verbal and writing skills that the job demands? Remember the importance of correct English. You will not be hired if your English and grammar are not exemplary.

If you fail to impress the interviewer with your grasp of these skills, you will never be considered for the position. The interviewer knows that whatever you display in the interview will also be displayed to the patients.

## Preparing for the Interview

Before the day of the interview, find out all you can about the facility. What is its reputation? Does it have a big turnover of employees? Review your textbooks that cover the specialty so that you can ask informed questions about procedures performed at the site. Think of questions to ask and write them down. Anticipate questions that might be asked of you. Find out the name of the interviewer; if it is a difficult name, practice saying it. Go to the site ahead of time to be sure of its location and time the trip so that you will not be late for your appointment. Do this ideally at the same time of day as your appointment to judge traffic delays, parking problems, and so on.

Dress appropriately for the interview. The general rule is to dress one step above what is required for the job. Do not overdress, as if for a party; make sure your outfit is professional. Your personal hygiene must be above reproach. Most medical practices prohibit smoking by their employees and test prospective employees for the presence of nicotine in their system. It is highly recommended that if you smoke, you quit as soon as possible for not only your health, but as a role model representing the health care industry. However, if you do smoke, avoid smoking before the interview. Those who do not smoke are acutely aware of the odor of smoke on one's clothes and breath. Avoid large, excessive jewelry and apply makeup carefully. Avoid perfumes; some people are very sensitive to scents.

Arrive on time or a few minutes early. Bring a few pens, a notepad, and your driver's license or official identification. Go alone; do not take a friend or family member for moral support. When you are introduced to the interviewer, offer your hand for a handshake and sit only when and where you are directed. Do not fidget, swing your foot, play with your hair, or tap your fingers on the chair arm. Make eye contact when the interviewer speaks with you and when you respond to the questions (Fig. 46-8). Sit up straight but relaxed, with your portfolio on your lap.

## Completing a Portfolio

A **portfolio** is a folder or binder containing documentation showing proof of your credentials, CPR certification, and other items that will verify the skills you have acquired. If you do not have a special folder or briefcase, a neat, new manila folder will be adequate. Procedure check-off sheets from your classes provide proof that you met the criteria needed to complete the tasks you will be expected to do on the job. Graded items known as "work products" or "competencies" in school are an excellent source as well. For example, a properly completed CMS-1500 from coding class will show an employer seeking a medical biller that you possess the knowledge to handle insurance claims.

Certificates of completion also make an impressive entry in a portfolio. They may be provided in your textbooks or from your instructors for specific training. For example, an instructor may give a certificate of completion for specific training for HIPAA, universal precautions, or blood-borne pathogens. Outside resources used in your medical assisting program may also provide certificates, like the use of a fire extinguisher from the fire department or aging sensitivity training from an agency on aging. Other documentation that will help you present yourself to a prospective employer includes

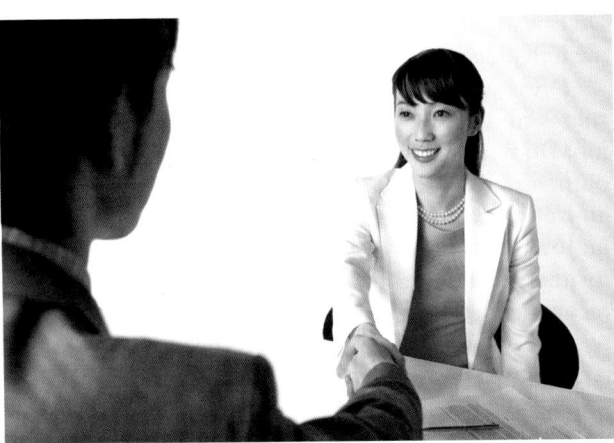

**FIGURE 46-8** • Dress and act professionally for the interview.

---

### BOX 46-4   Contents of a Portfolio

- Verification or at least the dates of immunizations (hepatitis B, TB test)
- Two copies of your résumé
- Two letters of reference
- Typed list of three references including names, phone numbers, and addresses
- Certificates of completion and awards received during the medical assisting program
- Graded "check offs," "work products," or "competencies"
- Proof of CPR certification

---

a copy of your current cardiopulmonary resuscitation certification and letters of recommendation. The items usually included in your portfolio are listed in Box 46-4.

## Crucial Interview Questions

Every interviewer must have the answers to three basic questions. When you respond to the interviewer's questions, keep these in mind:

1. Do you have the necessary skills to do the job? (Don't forget to include any foreign language skills; Box 46-5.)
2. Do you have the necessary drive, energy, and commitment to get the job done?
3. Will you work well with the rest of the team?

---

### BOX 46-5   Knowledge of a Foreign Language

If you are applying for a position that encourages bilingual applicants, be prepared for questions during the interview regarding your ability to speak another language. Know what languages are commonly spoken in your community. Whether it is Spanish, Polish, Italian, or any other language, take the time to become familiar with simple greetings: "Hello." "What is your name?" "Can I help you?" Tell the interviewer that you know a few words but are not fluent. It is not fair to the employer or to the patients to pretend otherwise if you are unable to communicate effectively. Most community colleges offer language courses. A local hospital may offer these courses with a focus on medical terms. Finally, the best way to learn a new language is to use it. If your classmates speak another language, ask them to tutor you. Being bilingual in the medical profession is always an asset.

A positive answer to all of these questions is not a guarantee that you will be offered the job, but a negative answer to any one of these will most assuredly mean that you will *not* get the job. Make sure that your comments make a positive impression regarding these three questions. In the medical field, the interviewer will need to establish your professionalism and ability to keep confidentiality. The interviewer will also want to know how interested you are in increasing and continuing your education and skills. Be sure that your answers will satisfy the interviewer.

Many interviewers use a prepared list of questions to direct the flow of the interview. Table 46-1 contains some commonly asked interview questions and guidance

| TABLE 46-1 Interview Questions and Responses | |
|---|---|
| **Common Interview Questions** | **Possible Responses and Points to Mention** |
| 1. Tell me about yourself. | "I enjoy working with other people." Stress the good points you wrote on your self-analysis. Keep the comments professional. Do not give long explanations about personal topics. ("I have three brothers." "I like basketball.") |
| 2. What are your strengths? | "My strengths are honesty and dependability." List any clinical or administrative skills in which you excel. |
| 3. What are your weaknesses? | Be honest; everyone has a weakness. "My weakness is phlebotomy skills," and add, "but I have improved my skills by reading magazine articles about blood drawing and by practicing in the school laboratory." Do not say, "I am perfect" or "I have no weaknesses." State one weakness and explain how you are trying to improve it. |
| 4. Why do you want this position? | "I like this office setting." "I always wanted to work for [as an example] a cardiologist." Mention that you are aware of the office's good reputation in the community, and if the location of the office is convenient, say so. |
| 5. What are your goals? | List two or three immediate goals: "My priority is to acquire a medical assisting position that will be challenging and rewarding." Have at least two goals in your mind for where you want to be in 5 years. |
| 6. Why did you leave your last position? | Always place a positive spin on why you left: "Looking for a new challenge." Never criticize past employers, their offices, or your coworkers. |
| 7. What salary rate are you looking for? | Know the average pay in your area. Check with your placement office if you are unsure of the typical salaries. Never demand a certain pay rate. |
| 8. How do you handle pressure? | Possible answers can include, "I set priorities" and "I remain calm and well organized." Avoid comments such as "I hate stress" or "I panic when I feel pressured." |
| 9. Do you work better alone or as also part of a team? | Stress that you can work as a team member but that you can function independently. |
| 10. Who was your best supervisor and why? | Possible remarks may include phrases such as "always fair," "supportive," and "encouraging." Avoid comments such as "She gave us long lunch breaks" or "She didn't make us work hard." |
| 11. How do you handle conflict? | Indicate that you begin trying to resolve any problems in a professional manner. Indicate that you are always open to constructive criticism. |
| 12. How would your classmates describe you? | Include remarks such as "good student," "team worker," and "helpful." |
| 13. I noticed your grades in computer class were poor. Why? | Be honest: "It was a tough course" or "Although my grade was poor, I have restudied the course material, and my computer skills have improved." If you have taken any additional studies or tutoring to help in this subject area, mention that. Never say the teacher was unfair, the class was boring, or you didn't care about the class. |
| 14. Describe the term "confidentiality" and how you would use it in our office. | Review the term. Stress to the interviewer that you know how important patient confidentiality is from a legal and ethical view point. |

for responses. Be prepared with answers that will reflect well on your professionalism and qualifications.

When the interviewer finishes asking questions, he or she will usually ask if you have any questions. Refer to your notepad, on which you have listed questions such as these:

- What are the responsibilities of the position offered?
- If it is not personal, why is the current employee leaving?
- What are the opportunities for future advancement?
- How long is the training or probation period?
- How does the facility feel about continuing education? Do they pay membership dues to your professional organization? Is time off offered to employees to upgrade their skills? Does the facility subsidize the expense?
- Is there a job performance or evaluation process?
- What is the benefit package? Is there access to a 401(k) plan or other retirement plan? Health insurance? Life insurance?

Make notes of the answers for future reference. Avoid asking about time off or vacations during the interview. These questions imply that you are more interested in being paid to avoid work than you are in contributing to the work at hand.

Make sure the interviewer knows how important continuing education is to you. Talk about the types of continuing education courses you would like to attend and the subjects you would like to study. Show that you realize that the only constant in medicine is change and that you expect to keep abreast of the information in your area. Thank the interviewer for the opportunity to apply for the position and ask the time frame for a decision. As you leave, offer your hand for a handshake and ask if you may call again before the decision date to clear up any questions that the interviewer may have during the decision-making process.

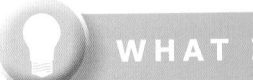

## WHAT IF?

**You become tongue-tied during an interview. What should you do?**

It's not unusual to feel nervous during the interview. To stay calm, take a deep breath and count to three before answering a question. Doing this also gives you time to think before you speak. Remember: Believe in yourself and your skills. Say to yourself, "I am going to get this job." Rehearse your answers to the common interview questions. Doing this exercise in front of a mirror is beneficial. Visit the Web sites listed in this chapter. Some of these sites offer virtual interviewing skills and have excellent tips for interviewing. Finally, arrive prepared and relaxed. Avoid excessive caffeine ingestion before the interview. Caffeine will increase your anxiety level.

---

September 15, 2014

Dear Dr. Whitten,

I would like to thank you for the opportunity to meet with you today to discuss employment. I enjoyed meeting everyone. Your employees made me feel welcome. After meeting with you and spending some time in your office, I feel that I would be a good addition to your team. Thank you for considering me in filling your CMA position. I look forward to hearing from you.

Sincerely,

Jan Joyce, CMA

**FIGURE 46-9 •** Sample thank-you letter.

## Follow-Up

The day of the interview or no later than the day after, write a short thank you note for the opportunity to be interviewed and restate how interested you are in the job (Fig. 46-9). Remind the interviewer that you are available for additional questions. Call several days after the interview. Reintroduce yourself politely and add any new information or ask any questions that might have occurred to you after the interview. Thank the interviewer again for this opportunity.

Think back to your performance in the interview. Determine what skills you still need to develop or enhance in order to improve your interview skills. Remember that experience is the best teacher and each interview helps you continue to improve.

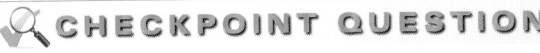

8. What are the three basic questions in every interviewer's mind?

## LEAVING A JOB

*Should you leave, or should you stay? Almost everyone comes to this question at some point in his or her career. Should I look for a new place to work and leave this place where I am safe and comfortable? Would another job be better or more satisfying? Would the benefits be better?*

An important factor in many relocations is salary. In addition to the financial aspects, however, employees today are looking for other elements that contribute to job satisfaction, such as:

- A sense of achievement
- Recognition
- Opportunity for growth and advancement
- Harmonious peer group relationships
- A good working relationship with supervisors
- Status
- Job security
- Comfortable working conditions
- Fair company policies

If you are no longer happy in your job, the reason probably lies in one or more of these elements. Before you make the decision to change jobs, do some internal soul searching to determine exactly what type of position would make you happy.

If you decide to leave your job, follow these steps:

- Always give adequate notice (minimum 2 weeks, optimal a month).
- Write a resignation letter. Keep the letter positive: "I am leaving this position to explore new opportunities." This is often the last item in your personnel file.
- Be positive during your exit interview. Do not criticize employees or the position.
- Clean and empty your locker, desk, and any other assigned space.
- Return your pager and any other equipment that has been assigned to you.
- Finish all duties and tie up any loose ends.
- Alert your supervisor to any unfinished business.
- Ask for a letter of reference.

## COG  BE A LIFELONG LEARNER

You are about to embark on the career you have spent time, money, and energy to prepare for. Even though your formal schooling is coming to an end, you must continue to learn. Be a lifelong learner. In the medical field, changes occur frequently. You must stay abreast of new technologies, procedures, and legal issues. In addition to facility training, inservices, and seminars, you will need to stay current with your CPR certification and recertify your credential.

### Recertification

You now face the process of acquiring certification in your field. As discussed in Chapter 1, whether you become a certified medical assistant or a registered medical assistant, you must keep your credential current. Both credentialing bodies require recertification. For AAMA, recertification is mandatory. A certified medical assistant (CMA) wishing to recertify must either retake the examination or complete 60 hours of continuing education units. A CMA who does not recertify by the end of the month of his or her birthday 5 years after the last date of certification loses the right to use the credential. Registered medical assistants (RMAs) are required to renew their certification each year by renewing their membership in the American Medical Technologists. If their membership lapses for more than 1 calendar year, the RMA must begin the process of becoming certified again. Both groups offer continuing education seminars and products. Information about the specific requirements and issues involving recertification is available on the organizations' Web sites.

To prepare for the process of recertifying, maintain a file with information about all educational sessions you attend. You should keep a brochure of the event with the following information: the topic, hours of session, learning objectives, and an outline of the program. You should also have proof of your attendance. When the time to apply for recertification comes, you will be prepared to complete the application.

## Professionalism

Experts say that professionalism is the one quality all employers seek. An allied health care career holds excitement, variety, and prestige. But with that comes a responsibility to the patients you serve. This requires professionalism and a commitment to excellence. As a member of the health care team, you are expected to conduct yourself professionally. One sign of professionalism and seriousness of purpose is membership in your professional organization. Whether you are a member of AAMA or American Medical Technologists, the benefits of membership will be invaluable to you and your future. Participation in a professional organization keeps you abreast of changes and issues facing your profession. If you are a student member, continue as an active member. If not, consider joining. Many employers will pay dues and other expenses for professional activities. Information about joining these organizations can be found at their Web sites.

### CHECKPOINT QUESTION

9. What is the policy of the AAMA regarding recertification of the CMA credential?

## ROLE-PLAYING ACTIVITY

Carlos Zeller, RMA, heard about a position in medical specialty office that has just been posted when he attended his local professional medical assistant meeting recently. This specialty is exactly what he has been looking for, so he got contact information from a medical assistant already working there who was at the meeting and updated his résumé accordingly. He also completed the online application process and is now awaiting an e-mail confirmation for an interview to be scheduled.

In the meantime, Carlos asked another medical assistant friend to help him prepare for the interview by role-playing the interview. If you are playing the role of the interviewer, think about the kinds of information that the employer may want from Carlos. Are there any questions that the employer may not ask him? If you are playing the role of the medical assistant seeking employment, think about your goals and how you might answer questions that may be asked by the interviewer. What are your strengths? Weaknesses? Are you a team player? How do you handle pressure? Your instructor will give you additional information about this activity!

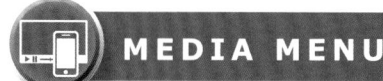

## MEDIA MENU

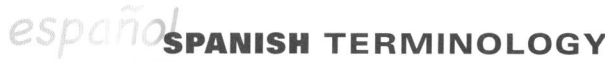

## español SPANISH TERMINOLOGY

**¿Que son los CEUs?**
What are the CEUs?

**¿Que tan frecuentemente me tengo que re-certificar?**
How often do I have to recertify?

**Usted necesita incluir en su curriculum vitae toda su experiencia laboral, incluyendo trabajo voluntario.**
You have to include in your résumé all your work experience, including volunteer work.

**¿Cuál es la diferencia entre el practicum y el internado?**
What is the difference between the practicum and the internship?

## Chapter Summary

- Your practicum is the transition from classroom to employment. A successful practicum helps lead to your ultimate goal—employment.
- During your practicum, you will perform in the workplace the skills that you have learned in the classroom and laboratory.
- There are many resources to help you locate job openings. A job should be fulfilling and rewarding in ways beyond just the income. Learn how to promote yourself and earn the position you want.
- A properly written cover letter, résumé, and thank you letter will enhance your chances of getting the job.
- Continuing education, recertification, and membership in a professional organization should be sought as you look to your future as a medical assistant.
- You will work hard, but there are many rewards. Welcome to the world of medical assisting!

## Warm-Ups for Critical Thinking

1. Search the Internet for local job openings for medical assistants. List any available positions and any other resources identified, and select a medical assisting position that interests you. Write a cover letter and résumé tailored to this position.
2. Assume you have been called for an interview for the position you selected in the above search. What questions do you ask the prospective employer? What questions do you expect to be asked? Explain your responses.
3. Obtain two employee application forms from a corporate physician office group. Complete one application form yourself and invite a fellow student to complete the other. Swap applications and evaluate each other's work. Determine which areas are appropriately addressed and which need further attention.
4. Visit the Equal Employment Opportunity Commission (EEOC) Web site. What is the purpose of the EEOC? Where is your nearest EEOC district office? Would you talk to your supervisor if you felt that you were discriminated against? Why or why not?
5. Suppose you were just hired into your dream position. On day 2, you overhear your supervisor telling another employee, "Don't report that billing error to Medicare. They won't catch us." What would you do? Whom would you tell, or would you pretend you didn't hear it? Would you report to Medicare? Why or why not?

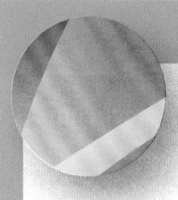

## PSY PROCEDURE 46-1

# Write a Résumé

**Purpose:** To summarize your skills and experience and to make yourself marketable in the medical assisting profession

**Equipment:** Word processor, paper, personal information

| STEPS | REASONS |
|---|---|
| 1. At the top of the page, center your name, address, and phone numbers. | The reader should be able to contact you easily. |
| 2. List your education, starting with the most current and working back. List graduation dates and areas of study. | Give the reader only the most vital information. |
| 3. For the chronological format, list your prior related work experience with dates, responsibilities, company, and supervisor's name. The most recent should be first. For the functional format, list skills and qualifications (refer to Figs. 46-6 and 46-7 for examples). | If you have a long work history, include only jobs that used skills needed for the job for which you are applying. Otherwise, your résumé will be too long. |
| 4. List any volunteer work with dates and places. | This will serve as proof of organizational and team-building skills. It will also show the reader that you are interested in helping others. |
| 5. List skills you possess including those acquired in your program and on your practicum. | This will show the prospective employer exactly what skills you possess. |
| 6. List any certifications or awards received. | This proves your competence. |
| 7. List any information relevant to a certain position. For example, list competence in spreadsheet applications for a job in a patient billing department. | Supplying information specific to a certain position shows your interest and attention to detail. |
| 8. After obtaining permission and/or notifying the people, prepare a list of references with addresses and phone contact information. | It is unprofessional to list someone for a reference without their knowledge and permission. |
| 9. Carefully proofread the résumé for accuracy and typographical errors. | Many employers will automatically reject a résumé with errors. |
| 10. Have someone else proofread the résumé for errors other than content. | Another set of eyes will ensure a perfect document. |
| 11. Print the résumé on high-quality paper. | The appearance and professionalism of your résumé is a direct reflection of you. |
| 12. **AFF** You have only had one job before finishing your medical assisting program. Should you try to "pad" your résumé by listing some anyway? Why or why not? | Honesty is one of the most important attributes sought by employers. |

*Note: This test is based on the information in this text-book only. Students should consult the content outline of the certification examination that they plan to take (Certified Medical Assistant or Registered Medical Assistant) to determine the possible content of the exam.*

1.  A medical assistant's training focuses on:

    A.  The hospital setting
    B.  Outpatient services
    C.  Nursing skills
    D.  Secretarial skills

2.  Maslow's hierarchy of human needs is based on the concept that:

    A.  Physiologic needs are the most basic and must be met first
    B.  Esteem must always come from people around us
    C.  A safe environment is placed above all other needs
    D.  People never really reach self-actualization

3.  A medical assistant's scope of practice is:

    A.  The same in every state
    B.  Determined by AAMA and/or AMT
    C.  Determined by their physician–employer
    D.  Not the concern of the CMA or RMA

4.  Which of the following medical specialists cares for people who are recovering from a stroke?

    A.  Endocrinologist
    B.  Internist
    C.  Neurologist
    D.  Emergency medicine

5.  Gathering information about a patient's present health care needs and abilities in preparation for teaching the patient a new diet is referred to as what?

    A.  Implementation
    B.  Planning
    C.  Assessment
    D.  Evaluation

6.  A system that selects the order of patients to receive urgent medical treatment is referred to as what?

    A.  Triage
    B.  Selection
    C.  Streamlining
    D.  Matrixing

7.  Which of the following is NOT required when taking a telephone message?

    A.  The caller's name and phone number
    B.  Time and date
    C.  The name of the person to whom the call is directed
    D.  The caller's account number

8.  The basic elements of communication include which of the following?

    A.  A message to be sent
    B.  A person to send the message
    C.  A person to receive the message
    D.  All of the above

9. Which of the following is NOT an example of nonverbal communication?

    A. Facial expression
    B. Touch
    C. Tone
    D. Posture

10. Patients should be given instructions in writing because:

    A. Most
       patients cannot read
    B. Most patients do not hear well
    C. Most patients do not really care to hear the details
    D. The human memory does not perform well in stressful situations

11. Why is understanding cultural differences important?

    A. Everyone is unique and their health care needs differ.
    B. One should never have predetermined notions.
    C. Perceptions may vary among nationalities.
    D. All of the above

12. A legally required disclosure is one that:

    A. Is given without the consent of the patient
    B. Is designed to protect the public
    C. Represents an exception to the rights of patients
    D. All of the above

13. A patient's medical record:

    A. Is considered a legal document
    B. Is only to be seen on a need-to-know basis
    C. Is the property of the physician
    D. All of the above

14. Medical ethics require physicians to:

    A. Be of good moral character
    B. Not accept money if they make a mistake
    C. Not charge a finance fee
    D. All of the above

15. A physician who treats a patient without his consent may be charged with:

    A. Assault
    B. Negligence
    C. Ethical behavior
    D. All of the above

16. Which of the following is considered an ethical issue?

    A. Long waits for patients in physician offices
    B. Certification of physicians
    C. Allocation of scarce resources such as donated organs
    D. Accepting a gift from a patient

17. A patient who is noncompliant is one who:

    A. Does not pay the bill in a timely fashion
    B. Has a difficult time understanding the physician's directions
    C. Should be given instructions in writing
    D. Does not follow the doctor's orders

18. When a hearing-impaired patient is communicating with the physician:

    A. Instructions should be given to a family member
    B. The office should require that they bring an interpreter
    C. The office is responsible for providing an interpreter
    D. The two of them can write back and forth to each other

19. A physician who dispenses narcotic drugs listed in the schedule of the Controlled Substances Act must keep the narcotic records:

    A. For 4 years
    B. For 6 years
    C. Forever
    D. For 2 years

20. An environmental safety plan should include all of the following EXCEPT:

    A. Procedures to notify families of staff and patients
    B. A plan to train employees on environmental safety guidelines
    C. Procedures to notify staff and patient in the event of an environmental emergency
    D. A plan for handling and disposing of hazardous waste

21. Among other things, HIPAA is concerned with:

    A. Protecting personal health information
    B. Patient safety
    C. Patient advocacy
    D. Patient compliance

22. Which of the following elements is NOT included in a memorandum?

    A. A heading
    B. A subject line
    C. To and from lines
    D. A complimentary close

23. A facsimile transmittal cover page:

    A. Is only necessary if you are sending the fax to someone you don't know
    B. Should include a confidentiality statement
    C. Should not be counted in the total number of pages being sent
    D. Requires postage

24. When sorting mail, you should:

    A. Place the physician's personal mail on top
    B. Dispose of any "junk mail"
    C. Place letters from other physicians in the appropriate chart
    D. Place all mail in the physician's mailbox

25. The minutes of a business meeting include all of the following, except:

    A. Motions passed
    B. Members present
    C. Members absent and the reasons for their absences
    D. A list of reports that were submitted

26. Missed appointments:

    A. Should be documented in two places
    B. Should be rescheduled by either the patient or the office
    C. Give the physician time to get caught up
    D. All of the above

27. In the following list of names, which one comes first in an alphabetical list?

    A. Stephen W. Long
    B. Jacqueline Stephens-Long
    C. Wilma Long-Adams
    D. Yolanda Long-Woodson

28. Your physician–employer is a participating provider with Mrs. Smith's insurance company. The difference in the fee for an office visit and the amount the insurance company "allows" for that service must be:

    A. Billed to the patient
    B. Adjusted off of the patient's account
    C. Collected at the patient's next visit
    D. Sent to a collection agency

29. A physician's fee schedule is determined by using UCRs, which means what?

    A. United compared resources
    B. Universal customary regulation
    C. Resource-based relative value scale
    D. Usual, customary, and reasonable

30. ICD-9-CM and ICD-10-CM are coding systems used to report what?

    A. Services provided by a nurse practitioner
    B. Services provided by a physician
    C. Medical necessity for services and procedures
    D. Procedures performed on the patient

31. CPT-4 codes include E&M codes, which are used to report what?

    A. Office procedures performed by a provider
    B. Anesthesia and surgeries
    C. Provider services and visits
    D. Medical necessity for services and procedures

32. In the ICD-9-CM and ICD-10-CM coding systems, a late effect is:

    A. A separately identifiable condition that is present during treatment of an acute illness or injury
    B. A symptom or condition arising from an acute illness that is still being treated after the acute illness has passed
    C. Always found by looking up "late effect" in the alphabetical index
    D. Left off of the CMS-1500 universal claim form after the acute illness is no longer being treated

33. The money owed to a physician for items such as rent, utilities, and payroll is referred to as what?

    A. Accounts receivable
    B. Business expenses
    C. Fixed accounts
    D. Accounts payable

34. What is the best way to ensure an accurate visual acuity exam?

    A. Provide adequate lighting
    B. Have the patient close one eye
    C. Ask the patient to speak up
    D. Allow the patient to sit down if necessary

35. At what age should children have their first MMR vaccination?

    A. Birth
    B. 12 to 15 months
    C. 2 to 3 months
    D. 12 months

36. At what age should children have their first hepatitis B vaccination?

    A. Birth
    B. 12 to 15 months
    C. 2 to 3 months
    D. 12 months

37. Which of the following is a normal rectal temperature?

    A. 99.6°F
    B. 98.6°F
    C. 97.6°F
    D. 95.6°F

38. Autoclaving is the only process that destroys all forms of living organisms, including:

    A. Spores
    B. Tuberculosis
    C. Viruses
    D. Bacteria

39. Following sterilization by autoclaving, the items remain sterile for how long?

    A. 21 days
    B. 2 weeks
    C. 30 days
    D. It depends on the item

40. In order to accomplish sterilization, the autoclave should reach what temperature?

    A. 250°F to 270°F
    B. 260°F to 270°F
    C. 35°C to 37°C
    D. 150°F

41. What is the most effective way to break the infection cycle?

    A. Wash your hands often
    B. Use only antibacterial soap
    C. Wash hands in Clorox
    D. Stay at home

42. Cross-contamination can be prevented by:

    A. Washing your hands between patients
    B. Washing the examination table with Clorox and water
    C. Sterilizing and/or disinfecting instruments
    D. All of the above

43. The most accurate way to measure the length of an infant is to:

    A. Use the measuring device on the back of the infant scale
    B. Make a mark on the exam table paper at the baby's head and bottom of the feet
    C. Use a yard stick
    D. Stand the infant up on the adult scale

44. Anaphylactic shock involves:

    A. Dysfunction of the nervous system following spinal injury
    B. General infection of the bloodstream
    C. Loss of blood and/or body fluids
    D. General allergic reaction to a foreign substance

45. In a physical examination, inspection refers to:

    A. Visual scanning of the patient
    B. Determining a patient's level of pain by his facial expression
    C. Feeling the patient's internal organs
    D. Looking over the patient's chart

46. Where is a Colles fracture located?

    A. Ankle
    B. Wrist
    C. Elbow
    D. Leg

47. Hepatitis B and rubella are examples of diseases caused by what?

    A. Yeasts
    B. Fungi
    C. Bacteria
    D. Viruses

48. Which of the following sutures does not usually require removal from the body?

    A. Catgut
    B. Silk
    C. Nylon
    D. Cotton

49. The first step performed to set up a sterile field is to do what?

    A. Open the sterile pack
    B. Wash your hands
    C. Prepare the local anesthetic in a syringe
    D. Put on gloves

50. In a standard EKG, lead V3 is located where?

    A. At the fourth intercostal space
    B. At the fifth intercostal space
    C. Midway between V2 and V4
    D. Anywhere on the right side of the chest

51. The EKG tracing is printed on graph paper at what standard speed?

    A. 10 cm/second
    B. 50 mm/second
    C. 35 cm/second
    D. 25 mm/second

52. A subcutaneous injection is given using which of the following techniques?

    A. A 45-degree angle with a 25-gauge needle
    B. A 15-degree angle with a 21-gauge needle
    C. A 90-degree angle with a 25-gauge needle
    D. A 10-degree angle with a 27-gauge needle

53. The reason you should aspirate before injecting a medication is to be sure:

    A. The patient receives all of the medication
    B. The needle is not in a blood vessel
    C. The injection is less painful
    D. The needle is in the muscle

54. An iron injection is administered by which of the following methods?

    A. Subcutaneous
    B. Z-track
    C. Intravenous
    D. Intradermal

55. The five phases of Korotkoff sounds may be heard when auscultating what?

    A. The pulse
    B. The carotid arteries
    C. The blood pressure
    D. The heart

56. Which classification of drugs prevents or decreases clotting?

    A. Anticoagulant
    B. Antiemetic
    C. Antineoplastic
    D. Antipyretic

57. The physician orders 500 mg of a medication tid for 10 days. The medication is available only in 250-mg capsules. How many capsules will the patient need to complete the course of medication?

    A. 60
    B. 45
    C. 30
    D. 20

58. Which organization developed guidelines to help people in making healthy diet decisions?

    A. FDA
    B. USDA
    C. CDC
    D. DEA

59. Which type of cholesterol is referred to as the "good cholesterol"?

    A. Unsaturated fats
    B. High-density lipoproteins
    C. Low-density lipoproteins
    D. Saturated fats

60. A clear liquid diet includes all of the following, except:

    A. Chicken broth
    B. Apple juice
    C. Tea
    D. Milk

61. Exercises performed with assistance are called what?

    A. Passive exercises
    B. Active exercises
    C. Range-of-motion exercises
    D. Aerobic exercises

62. Reasons a physician might order a 24-hour urine collection for a test include all of the following, except:

    A. Because of diurnal variation
    B. To compare the 24-hour value with the serum value
    C. For a culture and sensitivity
    D. To aid in the diagnosis of glomerular disease

63. Which of the following is the white blood cell count useful in determining?

    A. Anemia
    B. Coagulation factors
    C. Infection
    D. Platelet count

64. What information does a hemoglobin result provide about the patient?

    A. Helps to diagnose heart and liver diseases
    B. The amount of sugar in the blood
    C. The oxygen-carrying capacity of the blood
    D. The count of the number of cells that participate in blood clotting

65. A 9-year-old child falls off his skateboard going down a flight of concrete stairs. The child comes running home, where his mother notes some blood over the child's right knee and takes him to the emergency room. The ER doctor notes that the skin just below the knee has been scraped and irregularly broken to reveal underlying soft tissue over an area of 1 × 3 cm. This injury is best described as a/an:

    A. Abrasion
    B. Contusion
    C. Incision
    D. Laceration

66. A 54-year-old male has a long history of diabetes mellitus. Most of the time, his blood sugar was really high, causing damage to his kidneys. What laboratory result is most likely to be elevated?

    A. Creatinine
    B. Rheumatoid factor
    C. Calcium
    D. Prothrombin

67. The ability to repeatedly run a lab test and get the same result is called what?

    A. Accuracy
    B. Acceptability
    C. Calibration
    D. Precision

68. What action do you take if you have a critical value result on a patient?

    A. Get the information to the physician as soon as possible
    B. Record the information in the patient's chart
    C. Repeat the quality control before reporting the result
    D. Repeat the test

69. Two levels of quality control material must be analyzed:

   A. Annually
   B. By the policy you learned at school
   C. Following the manufacturer's instructions
   D. With each unknown specimen

70. The purpose of OSHA is:

   A. To protect all workers from occupational injury
   B. To identify epidemiology and track public health
   C. To establish policies on total quality management
   D. To provide tax relief for all laboratories

71. Anyone who has been thoroughly trained and demonstrates competency for the testing procedures regardless of educational background can perform which of the following?

   A. Complex tests
   B. Lab tests
   C. Waived tests
   D. Moderately complex tests

72. The first drop of a capillary puncture is removed with a clean gauze pad because it contains what?

   A. Bacteria
   B. Hemolysis
   C. Tissue thromboplastin
   D. Lipids

73. Blood-borne pathogens are:

   A. Human blood components and products made from human blood
   B. Disease-producing microorganisms transmitted by blood, body fluid, and tissue
   C. The presence of blood, body fluid, and tissue that can cause disease in humans
   D. Blood with potentially infectious materials that has soiled laundry

74. Why can latex gloves cause problems in providing patient care?

   A. They are easily perforated.
   B. They may cause allergic reactions.
   C. The powder frequently gets in workers' eyes.
   D. Most manufacturers cannot keep up with demand.

75. Which of the following vacuum tubes provides the least vacuum draw?

   A. 10 mL
   B. 7 mL
   C. 4.5 mL
   D. 2 mL

76. What is the reason why a 25-gauge needle is not recommended for blood collection?

   A. The red cells may be broken.
   B. The needle will be too painful for the patient.
   C. The bevel is too large.
   D. The needle is too short to reach deeper veins.

77. The fibrinogen-filled fluid that remains after centrifuging a tube of blood is:

   A. Plasma
   B. Anticoagulated blood
   C. Serum
   D. Whole blood

78. The primary veins located in the antecubital fossa are basilica, cephalic, and:

   A. Median cubital
   B. Brachial
   C. Median cephalic
   D. Median capital

79. All of the following are reasons for blood specimen rejection, except:

   A. Not enough blood collected
   B. Hemolysis
   C. Hematoma resulted
   D. Unlabeled tubes

80. What is the maximum time a tourniquet can be applied without jeopardizing the quality of the specimen?

   A. 2 minutes
   B. Two times
   C. 3 minutes with a difficult draw
   D. 1 minute

81. The process used to trace the direction of the vein is called what?

   A. Pumping
   B. Locating
   C. Anchoring
   D. Palpating

82. Which of the following is a glucose procedure that is collected 2 hours after consuming a carbohydrate meal?

   A. Stat glucose
   B. GTT
   C. 2-hour postprandial
   D. POCT glucose

83. The chemical examination of urine includes measurements of what?

   A. Color
   B. Bilirubin
   C. Clarity
   D. Odor

84. Some noncellular components of plasma are:

    A. Fats and hormones
    B. RBCs and WBCs
    C. Hormones and RBCs
    D. WBCs and serum

85. Oxygen is distributed in the cells of the body by which of the following?

    A. Platelets
    B. Leukocytes
    C. Erythrocytes
    D. Plasma

86. Where are erythrocytes formed?

    A. Liver
    B. Bone marrow
    C. Kidney
    D. Blood

87. Lipid tests include all of the following, except:

    A. HDL
    B. Bilirubin
    C. LDL
    D. Triglycerides

88. What hormone are you looking for in a pregnancy test?

    A. IgG
    B. hCG
    C. Estrogen
    D. Testosterone

89. What must laboratories provide for their employees?

    A. Safety and protection
    B. Education and training
    C. Health and welfare
    D. Retirement and health insurance

90. A patient's urine is yellow–orange. Which of the following substances would be found in the urine?

    A. Protein
    B. Glucose
    C. Nitrate
    D. Bilirubin

91. In the process of containing a blood sample by Vacutainer, a hematoma begins to form. Which is the most likely scenario?

    A. The bevel is inserted above the vein.
    B. The bevel is only partially inserted in the vein.
    C. The bevel is against the wall of the vein.
    D. The bevel is in the middle of the vein.

92. Which of the following tubes is used for RBC and WBC counts?

    A. Lavender
    B. Light blue
    C. Green
    D. Gray

93. What test is done by the Westergren method?

    A. CBC
    B. Sedimentation rate
    C. Coagulation test
    D. Hemoglobin

94. What is the best description of low-density lipoprotein?

    A. A complex molecule consisting of protein and a fat such as cholesterol
    B. The form in which carbohydrates are stored in the body
    C. A lipoprotein consisting of protein and cholesterol that removes excess cholesterol from blood vessel walls
    D. A lipoprotein consisting of protein and cholesterol that adheres to blood vessel walls, forming plaque

95. Which of the following is the causative agent of infectious mononucleosis?

    A. Variola major
    B. Epstein-Barr virus
    C. Cytomegalovirus
    D. Human immunodeficiency virus

96. The major purpose of an MSDS is:

    A. To provide information to clean up spills
    B. To provide information to protect employees and patients
    C. To complete all OSHA regulations
    D. To guide PPE use, identifying hazardous chemicals and procedures to follow for chemical exposure

97. Which laboratory department deals with disease-producing eggs present in specimens taken from the body?

    A. Parasitology
    B. Hematology
    C. Virology
    D. Chemistry

98. The presence of sugar in the urine is called what?

    A. Glycogen
    B. Hypoglycemia
    C. Glycosuria
    D. Hyperglycemia

99. What is the BEST way to avoid cross-contaminating patients who receive instillation of eye drops from the same bottle?

   A. Wash your hands after instillation.
   B. Wipe the tip of the dropper with a paper towel before and after each use.
   C. Avoid touching the tip of the dropper to the patient's eye.
   D. Have each patient bring their own bottle.

100. Which laboratory department deals with the identification of pathogens?

   A. Chemistry
   B. Hematology
   C. Microbiology
   D. Immunohematology

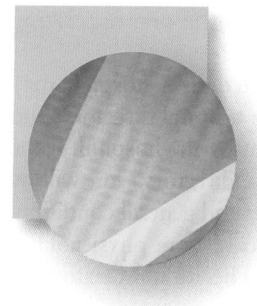

# Appendix A
# Health Insurance Portability and Accountability Act (HIPAA)

Throughout the text, the Health Insurance Portability and Accountability Act of 1996, known as HIPAA, is discussed. Chapters 2 and 8 discuss HIPAA's Privacy Ruling. The 104th US Congress had six goals in passing Public Law 104–191:

- To improve the portability of group and individual insurance companies by regulating such issues as refusal of coverage for preexisting conditions and continuing coverage when changing jobs
- To fight against fraud, abuse, and waste in the health care industry
- To promote the use of medical savings accounts
- To improve access to long-term care services and coverage
- To promote efficiency by simplifying the business of filing claims and processing of health insurance
- To provide funds for reforms and other related purposes

In keeping with the focus of this textbook, the discussion of HIPAA has been limited to issues related to the outpatient health care arena. Two areas directly influencing the medical office are found in Title II: Preventing Health Care Fraud and Abuse; Administrative Simplification; Medical Liability Reform. The Privacy Ruling from Title II addresses the issues of the rights of patients to protect their personally identifiable health information (PIHI). Information revealing physical and/or mental conditions and treatments that can be **directly linked** to a particular patient is considered personally identifiable health information (PIHI). Your goal is to protect the patient's privacy.

Following are some scenarios you might encounter in a typical day in a physician's office. An explanation follows:

1. A new patient refuses to sign the acknowledgment of receipt of a Notification of Privacy Practices (NOPP), the form requested by HIPAA's Privacy Ruling. Do you turn the patient away?

   No. You are only required to make a "good faith effort" to receive acknowledgment of an NOPP. Document the patient's refusal to sign.

2. One of your duties is to call patients to remind them of their appointments. Would leaving a message with the time and location of the appointment be a violation of the Privacy Ruling?

   No. "This is Terri at Dr. Smith's office calling to remind you of your appointment tomorrow at 10:00" does not disclose personal health information.

3. You have been asked to notify a patient with his test results. Can you leave a message?

   Maybe. Sensitive information should be treated as such. Patients should sign an authorization that gives you permission to leave any message on their voice mail. In the absence of that documentation, you would not leave test results on voice mail.

4. A hospital admissions representative calls and asks for a patient's insurance information. Is it okay to give her the patient's subscriber number, etc.?

   HIPAA was never meant to limit the sharing of information to the point that it interferes with the patient care or the financial issues involved. Only the minimum amount of information should be shared with only those who need to know. Giving the representative the information helps the patient in the long run.

5. A patient requests copies of her records. The chart contains letters and reports from other physicians and facilities. Should she be given these documents also, or would she need to request these from the physicians or facilities that generated them?

   Once the medical information becomes a part of a patient's chart in your office, it is okay to release it with proper authorization. Since all of the documents were used in the care and management of the patient in your office, all documents are now part of the record.

6. You need to request a radiology report on a patient coming in this afternoon. Is it okay to have it faxed over?

   Yes, it is okay as long as the fax machine is out of the view of patients and other visitors. The fax should have a cover sheet with the name of the person who should receive the fax. It should be delivered to that person by anyone who retrieves it.

7. You receive an operative report addressed to Dr. Richard Adams on your fax machine, but your physician is Dr. Robert Adams. As soon as you see the cover sheet, you realize you received it by mistake. What should you do?

Since you do not have a need to know, do not read the report. Call the number on the cover sheet, and tell them that you received the report in error. This alerts them to send another one to the correct Dr. Adams. Then, shred the copy you received by mistake.

8. What if the last scenario was reversed? You sent a fax to the wrong number. You realize it just as you push the "Send" button.

Call the party who received the information and ask them to shred it. Document the error in the patient's chart. If you do not know who received the misdirected fax, you should notify the patient of the possible breach.

9. Your boss asks you to check on the condition of his next door neighbor who is in the hospital. He tells you to let them know that he is the one requesting the information. Is this possible?

Yes. A patient being admitted to a hospital may choose to be excluded from the hospital directory, and no information can be given out by the hospital. If the neighbor did not opt out of the directory, you will be given the patient's room number and general condition. Unless involved in the patient's care, your physician has no special privileges to protected health information.

10. You work in a busy pediatric office. You are the PA as he examines a 2-year-old boy with a possible concussion. He tells you that he suspects abuse. Can you report this without authorization?

Not only can you report it, but you MUST report it. The Child Abuse Prevention and Treatment Act of 1974 (CAPTA) made reporting possible child abuse mandatory.

Adapted from Krager D, Krager C. *HIPAA for Medical Office Personnel*. New York: Thomson Delmar Learning, 2005.

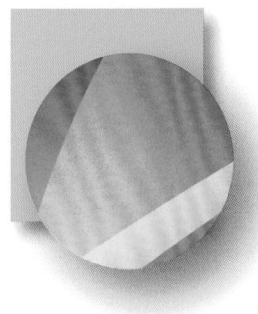

# Appendix B
# Key English-to-Spanish Health Care Phrases

Although English is the major language spoken in North America, a variety of languages are used in certain areas. Prominent among them is Spanish, representing Spain, the Caribbean Islands, Central and South America, and the Philippines. Rapport can be more easily established, and the patient and family will be at ease and feel more relaxed, if someone on the staff speaks their language. Some health care facilities, especially in areas with a large population of Spanish-speaking people, provide interpreters. In smaller hospitals or smaller communities, this may not be possible.

It is to your advantage to learn the second most prominent language in your community. For this reason, the following table of English-to-Spanish phrases has been prepared. Instructions for using it are simple. Look for the phrase in English in the first column of the table. The second column gives the phrase in Spanish. You can write this or point to it. The third column gives a phonetic pronunciation. The syllable in each word to be accented is printed in italic type. Even if you are not proficient in English-to-Spanish, your Spanish-speaking patients will appreciate your trying to converse in their language. Begin with "Buenos días. "¿Cómo se siente?" And remember "por favor."[a]

## Introductory Phrases

| please[a] | por favor | por fah-*vor* |
|---|---|---|
| thank you | gracias | *grah*-see-ahs |
| good morning | buenos días | *bway*-nos *dee*-ahs |
| good afternoon | buenas tárdes | *bway*-nas *tar*-days |
| good evening | buenas noches | *bway*-nas *noh*-chays |
| my name is | mi nombre es | me *nohm*-bray ays |
| yes/no | si/no | see/no |
| What is your name? | ¿Cómo se llama? | ¿Koh-moh say *jah*-mah? |
| How old are you? | ¿Cuántos años tienes? | ¿*Kwan*-tohs ahn-yos tee-*ayn*jays? |
| Do you understand me? | ¿Me entiende? | ¿Me ayn-tee-*ayn*-day? |
| Speak slower. | Habla más despacio. | Ah-blah mahs days-*pah*-see-oh |
| Say it once again. | Repítalo, por favor. | Ray-*pee*-tah-loh, por fah-*vor* |
| How do you feel? | ¿Cómo se siente? | ¿*Koh*-moh say see-*ayn*-tay? |
| good | bien | bee-ayn |
| bad | mal | *mah*l |
| physician | médico | *may*-dee-koh |
| hospital | hospital | *ooh*-spee-tall |
| midwife | comadre | koh-*mah*-dray |
| native healer | curandero | ku-ren-*day*-roh |

---

From Rosdahl CB. *Textbook of Basic Nursing*, 6th ed. Philadelphia, PA: J.B. Lippincott, 1995.
[a]You should begin or end any request with the word PLEASE (POR FAVOR).

# General

| zero | cero | *se*-roh |
| one | uno | *oo*-noh |
| two | dos | dohs |
| three | tres | trays |
| four | cuatro | *kwah*-troh |
| five | cinco | *sin*-koh |
| six | seis | says |
| seven | siete | see-*ay*-tay |
| eight | ocho | oh-choh |
| nine | nueve | new-*ay*-vay |
| ten | diez | *dee*-ays |
| hundred | ciento, cien | see-*en*-toh, see-*en* |
| hundred and one | ciento uno | see-*en*-toh *oo*-noh |
| Sunday | domingo | doh-*ming*-goh |
| Monday | lunes | *loo*-nays |
| Tuesday | martes | *mar*-tays |
| Wednesday | miércoles | mee-*er*-cohl-ays |
| Thursday | jueves | *hway*-vays |
| Friday | viernes | vee-*ayr*-nays |
| Saturday | sábado | *sah*-bah-doh |
| right | derecho | day-*ray*-choh |
| left | izqierdo | ees-kee-*ayr*-doh |
| early in the morning | temprano por la mañana | tehm-*prah*-noh por lah mah-*nyah*-na |
| in the daytime | en el dìa | ayn el *dee*-ah |
| at noon | a mediodía | ah meh-dee-oh-*dee*-ah |
| at bedtime | al acostarse | al ah-kos-*tar*-say |
| at night | por la noche | por la *noh*-chay |
| today | ñoy | oy |
| tomorrow | mañana | mah-*nyah*-nah |
| yesterday | ayer | ai-*yer* |
| week | semana | say-*may*-nah |
| month | mes | mace |

# Parts of the Body

| the head | la cabeza | la kah-*bay*-sah |
| the eye | el ojo | el *o*-hoh |
| the ears | los oídos | lohs o-*ee*-dohs |
| the nose | la nariz | la nah-*reez* |
| the mouth | la boca | lah *boh*-kah |
| the tongue | la lengua | la *len*-gwah |
| the neck | el cuello | el koo-*eh*-joh |
| the throat | la garganta | lah gar-*gan*-tah |
| the skin | la piel | la pee-el |
| the bones | los huesos | lohs hoo-*ay*-sos |
| the muscles | los músculos | lohs *moos*-koo-lohs |
| the nerves | los nervios | lohs *nayhr*-vee-ohs |
| the shoulder blades | las paletillas | lahs pah-lay-*tee*-jahs |
| the arm | el brazo | el *brah*-soh |
| the elbow | el codo | el *koh*-doh |
| the wrist | la muñeca | lah moon-*yeh*-kah |
| the hand | la mano | lah *mah*-noh |
| the chest | el pecho | el *pay*-choh |

| the lungs | los pulmones | lohs puhl-*moh*-nays |
| the heart | el corazón | el koh-rah-*son* |
| the ribs | las costillas | lahs kohs-*tee*-jahs |
| the side | el flanco | el *flahn*-koh |
| the back | la espalda | lay ays-*pahl*-dah |
| the abdomen | el abdomen | el ahb-*doh*-men |
| the stomach | el estómago | el ays-*toh*-mah-goh |
| the leg | la pierna | lah pee-ehr-nah |
| the thigh | el muslo | el *moos*-loh |
| the ankle | el tobillo | el toh-*bee*-joh |
| the foot | el pie | el *pee*-ay |
| urine | urino | u-*re*-noh |

## Diseases

| allergy | alergia | ah-*layr*-hee-ah |
| anemia | anemia | ah-*nay*-mee-ah |
| cancer | cancer | kahn-sayr |
| chickenpox | varicela | vah-ree-*say*-lah |
| diabetes | diabetes | dee-ah-bay-tees |
| diphtheria | difteria | deef-*tay*-ree-ah |
| German measles | rubéola | roo-*bay*-oh-lah |
| gonorrhea | gonorrea | gun-noh-*ree*-ah |
| heart disease | enfermedad del corazón | ayn-*fayr*-may-*dahd* dayl koh-rah-*sohn* |
| high blood pressure | presión alta | pray-see-*ohn* al-ta |
| influenza | gripe | *gree*-pay |
| lead poisoning | envenenamiento con plomo | ayn-vay-nay-nah-mee-*ayn*-toh kohn *ploh*-moh |
| liver disease | enfermedad del hígado | ayn-*fayr*-may-dahd del *ee*-gah-doh |
| measles | sarampión | sah-rahm-pee-*ohn* |
| mumps | paperas | pah-*pay*-rahs |
| nervous disease | enfermedades nerviosa | ayn-fayr-may-*dahd*-days nayr-vee-oh-sah |
| pleurisy | pleuresía | play-oo-ray-*see*-ah |
| pneumonia | pulmonía | pool-moh-*nee*-ah |
| rheumatic fever | reumatismo (fiebre reumatica) | ray-oo-mah-*tees*-moh (fee-*ay*-bray ray-oo-*mah*-tee-kah) |
| scarlet fever | escarlatina | ays-kahr-lah-*tee*-nah |
| syphilis | sífilis | *see*-fee-lees |
| tuberculosis | tuberculosis | too-*bayr*-koo-lohs-sees |

## Signs and Symptoms

| Do you have stomach cramps? | ¿Tiene calambres en el estómago? | ¿Tee-*ay*-nay kah-*lahm*-brays ayn el ays-*toh*-mah-goh? |
| chills? | escalofrios? | ays-kah-loh-*free*-ohs? |
| an attack of fever | un ataque de fiebre? | oon ah-*tah*-kay day fee-*ay*-bray? |
| hemorrhage? | hemoragia? | ay-moh-*rah*-hee-ah? |
| nosebleeds? | hemoragia por la nariz? | ay-moh-*rah*-hee-ah por-lah nah-*rees*? |
| unusual vaginal bleeding? | hemoragia vaginal fuera de los periodos? | ay-moh-*rah*-hee-ah *vah*-hee-nahl foo-*ay*-rah day lohs pay-ree-oh-*dohs*? |
| hoarseness? | ronquera? | rohn-*kay*-rah? |
| a sore throat? | le duele la garganta? | lay doo-*ay*-lay lah gahr-*gahn*-tah? |

| English | Spanish | Pronunciation |
|---|---|---|
| Does it hurt to swallow? | ¿Le duele al respirar? | ¿Lay doo-ay-lay ahl trah-gar? |
| Have you had any difficulty in breathing? | ¿Tiene difficultad al respirar? | ¿Tee-ay-nay dee-fee-kool-tahd ahl rays-pee-rahr? |
| Does it pain you to breathe? | ¿Le duele la cabeza? | ¿Lay doo-ay-lay ahl rays-pee-rahr? |
| How does your head feel? | ¿Cómo siente la cabeza? | ¿Koh-moh see-ayn-tay lah kah-bay-sah? |
| Is your memory good? | ¿Es buena su memoria? | ¿Ays bway-nah soo may-moh-ree-ah? |
| Have you had any pain in the head? | ¿Le duele al tragar? | ¿Lay doo-ay-lay lah Kah-bay-sah? |
| Do you feel dizzy? | ¿Tiene usted vértigo? | ¿Tee-ay-nay ood-stayd vehr-tee-goh? |
| Are you tired? | ¿Está usted cansado? | ¿Ay-stah ood-stayd kahn-sah-doh? |
| Can you eat? | ¿Puede comer? | ¿Pway-day koh-mer? |
| Have you had a good appetite? | ¿Tiene usted buen apetito? | ¿Tee-ay-nay ood-stayd bwayn ah-pay-tee-toh? |
| How are your stools? | ¿Cómo son sus heces fecales? | ¿Kog-moh sohn soos bay-says fay-kal-ays? |
| Are they regular? | ¿Son regulares? | ¿Sohn ray-goo-lah-rays? |
| Are you constipated? | ¿Está estreñido? | ¿Ay-stah ays-trayn-yee-do? |
| Do you have diarrhea? | ¿Tiene diarrea? | ¿Tee-ay-nay dee-ah-ray-ah? |
| Have you had any difficulty passing water? | ¿Tiene dificultad en orinar? | ¿Tee-ay-nay dee-fee-kool-tahd ayn oh-ree-nahr? |
| Do you pass water involuntarily? | ¿Orina sin querer? | ¿Oh-ree-nah seen kay-rayr? |
| How long have you felt this way? | ¿Desde cuándo se siente asi? | ¿Days-day Kwan-doh say see-ayn-tay ah-see? |
| What diseases have you had? | ¿Qué enfermedades ha tenido? | ¿Kay ayn-fer-may-dah-days hah tay-nee-doh? |
| Do you hear voices? | ¿Tiene los voces? | ¿Tee-ay-nay los vo-ses? |

## Examination

| English | Spanish | Pronunciation |
|---|---|---|
| Remove your clothing. | Quítese su ropa. | Key-tay-say soo roh-pah. |
| Put on this gown. | Pongáse la bata. | Phon-gah-say lah bah-tah. |
| We need a urine specimen. | Es necesário una muestra de su orina. | Ays nay-say-sar-ee-oh oo-nah moo-ay-strah day oh-ree-nah. |
| Be seated. | Siéntese. | See-ayn-tay-say. |
| Recline. | Acuestése. | Ah-cways-tay-say. |
| Sit up. | Siéntese. | See-ayn-tay-say. |
| Stand. | Parése. | Pah-ray-say. |
| Bend your knees. | Doble las rodíllas. | Doh-blay lahs roh-dee-yahs. |
| Relax your muscles. | Reláje los músculos. | Ray-lah-hay lohs moos-koo-lohs. |
| Try to … | Atente … | Ah-tayn-tay … |
| Try again. | Atente ótra vez. | Ah-tayn-tay oh-tra vays. |
| Do not move. | No se muéva. | Noh say moo-ay-vah. |
| Turn on (or to) your left side. | Voltese a su lado izquierdo. | Vohl-tay-say ah soo lah-doh is-key-ayr-doh. |
| Turn on (or to) your right side. | Voltése a su ládo derécho. | Vohl-tay-say ah soo lah-doh day-ray-choh. |
| Take a deep breath. | Respíra profúndo. | Ray-speer-rah pro-foon-doh. |
| Hold your breath. | Deténga su respiración. | Day-tayn-gah soo ray-speer-ah-see-ohn. |
| Don't hold your breath. | No deténga su respiración. | Noh day-tayn-gah soo ray-speer-ah-see-ohn. |
| Cough. | Tosa. | Toh-sah. |
| Open your mouth. | Abra la boca. | Ah-brah lah boh-kah. |

| Show me ... | Enséñeme ... | Ayn-*sayn*-yay-may ... |
| Here? | ¿Aqui? | ¿Ah-*kee*? |
| There? | ¿Allí? | ¿Ah-*jee*? |
| Which side? | ¿En qué lado? | ¿Ayn kay *lah*-doh? |
| Let me see your hand. | Enséñeme la mano. | Ayn-*sehn*-yay-may lah *mah*-noh. |
| Grasp my hand. | Apriete mi mano. | Ah-*pree*-it-tay mee *mah*-noh. |
| Raise your arm. | Levante el brazo. | Lay-*vahn*-tay el *brah*-soh. |
| Raise it more. | Más alto. | Mahs *ahl*-toh. |
| Now the other. | Ahora el otro. | Ah-*oh*-rah el *oh*-troh. |

## Treatment

| It is necessary. | Es necessario. | Ays neh-say-*sah*-ree-oh. |
| An operation is necessary. | Una operación es necesaria. | Oo-nah oh-peh-rah-see-*ohn* ays neh-say-*sah*-ree-ah. |
| a prescription | una receta | oo-na ray-say-tah |
| Use it regularly. | Tómelo con regularidad. | *Toh*-may-loh kohn ray-goo-*lah*-ree-dad. |
| Take one teaspoonful three times daily (in water). | Toma una cucharadita tres veces al dia, con agua. | *Toh*-may oo-na koo-chah-rah-*dee*-tah trays *vay*-says ahl *dee*-ah, kohn ah-gwah. |
| Gargle. | Haga gargaras. | *Ah*-gah gar-*gah*-rahs. |
| Use injection. | Use una inyección. | *Oo*-say oo-nah in-*yek*-see-ohn. |
| oral contraceptives | una pildora | oo-nah peel-*doh*-rah |
| a pill | una pastilla | oo-nah pahs-*tee*-yah |
| a powder | un polvo | oon *pohl*-voh |
| before meals | antes de las comidas | *ahn*-tays day lahs koh-*mee*-dahs |
| after meals | despues de las comidas | *days*-poo-ehs day lahs koh-mee-dahs |
| every day | todos los día | *toh*-dohs lohs *dee*-ah |
| every hour | cada hora | *kah*-dah *oh*-rah |
| Breathe slowly—like this (in this manner). | Respire despacio—asi. | Rays-*pee*-ray days-*pah*-see-oh—ah-*see*. |
| Remain on a diet. | Estar a dieta. | Ays-*tar* a dee-*ay*-tah. |

## General

| How do you feel? | ¿Cómo se siénte? | ¿*Koh*-moh say see-*ayn*-tay? |
| Do you have pain? | ¿Tiéne dolor? | ¿Tee-*ay*-nay doh-*lorh*? |
| Where is the pain? | ¿Adónde es el dolor? | ¿Ah-*dohn*-day ays ayl doh-*lorh*? |
| Do you want medication for your pain? | ¿Quiére medicación para su dolor? | ¿Kay-*ay*-ray may-dee-kah see-*ohn* *pak*-rah soo doh-*lorh*? |
| Are you comfortable? | ¿Está confortáble? | ¿Ay-*stah* kohn-for-*tah*-blay? |
| Are you thirsty? | ¿Tiéne sed? | ¿Tee-*ay*-nay sayd? |
| You may not eat/drink. | No cóma/béba. | Noh *koh*-mah/bay-*bah*. |
| You can only drink water. | Solo puede tomar agua. | Soh-loh *pway*-day toh-mar *ah*-gwah. |
| Apply bandage to ... | Ponga una vendaje a ... | *Pohn*-gah oo-nah vehn-*dah*-hay ah ... |
| Apply ointment. | Aplíquese unguento. | Ah-*plee*-kay-say oon-goo-*ayn*-toh. |
| Keep very quiet. | Estese muy quieto. | Ays-*tay*-say moo-ay key-*ay*-toh. |
| You must not speak. | No debe hablar. | Noh *day*-bay ha-*blahr* |
| It will be uncomfortable. | Séra incomódo. | *Say*-rah een-koh-*moh*-doh. |
| It will sting. | Va ardér. | Vah ahr-*dayr*. |
| You will feel pressure. | Vá a sentír presión. | Vah ah sayn-*teer* pray-see-*ohn*. |
| I am going to ... | Voy a ... | Voy ah ... |
| Count (take) your pulse. | Tomár su púlso. | Toh-*marh* soo *pool*-soh. |

Take your temperature.
Take your blood pressure.
Give you pain medicine.

You should (try to) …
Call for help/assistance.

Empty your bladder.
Do you still feel very weak?

It is important to …
Walk (ambulate).
Drink fluids.

Tomár su temperatúra.
Tomar su presión.
Dárle medicación para dolór.

Trate de …
Llamar para asisténcia.

Orinar.
¿Se siente muy débil todavía?

Es importánte que …
Caminar.
Beber líquidos.

Toh-*marh* soo taym-pay-rah-*too*-rah.
Toh-*mahr* soo pray-see-*ohn*.
*Dahr*-lay may dee-kah-see-*ohn* pah-
   rah doh-*lohr*.
*Tray*-tay day …
Yah-*marh* pah-rah
   ah-sees-*tayn*-see-ah.
Oh-ree-*narh*.
¿Say see-*ayn*-tay moo-ee *day*-beel
   toh-dah-*vee*-ah?
Ays eem-por-*tahn*-tay Kay …
Kah-mee-*narh*.
Bay-*bayr lee*-kay-dohs.

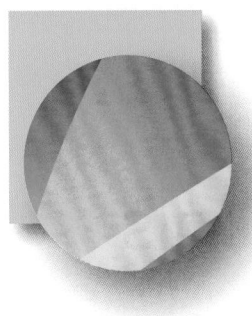

# Appendix C
# Two-Letter Postal ZIP Code Abbreviations

| | | | |
|---|---|---|---|
| Alabama | AL | Nebraska | NE |
| Alaska | AK | Nevada | NV |
| Arizona | AZ | New Hampshire | NH |
| Arkansas | AR | New Jersey | NJ |
| American Samoa | AS | New Mexico | NM |
| California | CA | New York | NY |
| Colorado | CO | North Carolina | NC |
| Connecticut | CT | North Dakota | ND |
| Delaware | DE | Northern Mariana Islands | MP |
| District of Columbia | DC | Ohio | OH |
| Federated States of Micronesia | FM | Oklahoma | OK |
| Florida | FL | Oregon | OR |
| Georgia | GA | Palau | PW |
| Guam | GU | Pennsylvania | PA |
| Hawaii | HI | Puerto Rico | PR |
| Idaho | ID | Rhode Island | RI |
| Illinois | IL | South Carolina | SC |
| Indiana | IN | South Dakota | SD |
| Iowa | IA | Tennessee | TN |
| Kansas | KS | Texas | TX |
| Kentucky | KY | Utah | UT |
| Louisiana | LA | Vermont | VT |
| Maine | ME | Virginia | VA |
| Marshall Islands | MH | Virgin Islands | VI |
| Maryland | MD | Washington | WA |
| Massachusetts | MA | West Virginia | WV |
| Michigan | MI | Wisconsin | WI |
| Minnesota | MN | Wyoming | WY |
| Mississippi | MS | Armed Forces of the Americas | AA |
| Missouri | MO | Armed Forces Europe | AE |
| Montana | MT | Armed Forces Pacific | AP |

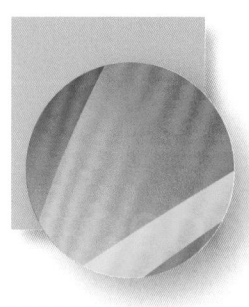

# Appendix D
# Abbreviations and Symbols

Abbreviations and symbols that appear in red font are considered "Dangerous Abbreviations" and should not be used.

| Abbreviation or Symbol | Meaning |
|---|---|
| ā | before |
| A | anterior; assessment |
| A&P | auscultation and percussion |
| A&W | alive and well |
| AB | abortion |
| ABG | arterial blood gas |
| a.c. | before meals |
| ACE | angiotensin-converting enzyme |
| ACS | acute coronary syndrome |
| ACTH | adrenocorticotropic hormone |
| AD | right ear |
| ad lib. | as desired |
| ADH | antidiuretic hormone |
| ADHD | attention deficit hyperactivity disorder |
| AIDS | acquired immunodeficiency syndrome |
| AKA | above-knee amputation |
| alb | albumin |
| ALS | amyotrophic lateral sclerosis |
| ALT | alanine aminotransferase (enzyme) |
| a.m. | morning |
| amt | amount |
| ANS | autonomic nervous system |
| AP | anterior-posterior |
| APKD | adult polycystic kidney disease |
| Aq | water |
| AS | left ear |
| ASD | atrial septal defect |
| AST | aspartate aminotransferase (enzyme) |
| AU | both ears |
| AV | atrioventricular |

| Abbreviation or Symbol | Meaning |
|---|---|
| Ⓑ | bilateral |
| B AEP | brainstem auditory evoked potential |
| BAER | brainstem auditory evoked response |
| BCC | basal cell carcinoma |
| BD | bipolar disorder |
| b.i.d. | twice a day |
| BKA | below-knee amputation |
| BM | bowel movement |
| BMP | basic metabolic panel |
| BP | blood pressure |
| BPH | benign prostatic hypertrophy; benign prostatic hyperplasia |
| BRP | bathroom privileges |
| BS | blood sugar |
| BUN | blood urea nitrogen |
| Bx | biopsy |
| c̄ | with |
| C | Celsius; centigrade |
| C&S | culture and sensitivity |
| CABG | coronary artery bypass graft |
| CAD | coronary artery disease |
| Cap | capsule |
| CAT | computed axial tomography |
| CBC | complete blood count |
| cc | cubic centimeter |
| CC | chief complaint |
| CCU | coronary (cardiac) care unit |
| CF | cystic fibrosis |
| CHF | congestive heart failure |
| CIN | cervical intraepithelial neoplasia |
| CIS | carcinoma in situ |
| cm | centimeter |

| Abbreviation or Symbol | Meaning |
|---|---|
| CMP | comprehensive metabolic panel |
| CNS | central nervous system |
| c/o | complains of |
| CO | cardiac output |
| $CO_2$ | carbon dioxide |
| COPD | chronic obstructive pulmonary disease |
| CP | cerebral palsy; chest pain |
| CPAP | continuous positive airway pressure |
| CPD | cephalopelvic disproportion |
| CPR | cardiopulmonary resuscitation |
| CSF | cerebrospinal fluid |
| CSII | continuous subcutaneous insulin infusion |
| CT | computed tomography |
| CTA | computed tomographic angiography |
| cu mm or $mm^3$ | cubic millimeter |
| CVA | cerebrovascular accident |
| CVS | chorionic villus sampling |
| CXR | chest x-ray |
| d | day |
| D&C | dilatation and curettage |
| D&E | dilation and evacuation |
| DC | discharge; discontinue; doctor of chiropractic |
| DDS | doctor of dental surgery |
| DJD | degenerative joint disease |
| DKA | diabetic ketoacidosis |
| DO | doctor of osteopathy |
| DPM | doctor of podiatric medicine |
| dr | dram |
| DRE | digital rectal exam |
| DTR | deep tendon reflex |
| DVT | deep vein thrombosis |
| Dx | diagnosis |
| ECG | electrocardiogram |
| echo | echocardiogram |
| ECT | electroconvulsive therapy |
| ECU | emergency care unit |
| ED | erectile dysfunction |
| EDC | estimated date of confinement |
| EDD | estimated date of delivery |
| EEG | electroencephalogram |
| EGD | esophagogastroduodenoscopy |
| EKG | electrocardiogram |

| Abbreviation or Symbol | Meaning |
|---|---|
| EMG | electromyogram |
| ENT | ear, nose, and throat |
| EPS | electrophysiologic study |
| ER | emergency room |
| ERCP | endoscopic retrograde cholangiopancreatography |
| ESR | erythrocyte sedimentation rate |
| ESWL | extracorporeal shockwave lithotripsy |
| ETOH | ethyl alcohol |
| EUS | endoscopic ultrasonography |
| F | Fahrenheit |
| FBS | fasting blood sugar |
| Fe | iron |
| FH | family history |
| fl oz | fluid ounce |
| FS | frozen section |
| FSH | follicle-stimulating hormone |
| Fx | fracture |
| g | gram |
| GAD | generalized anxiety disorder |
| GERD | gastroesophageal reflux disease |
| GH | growth hormone |
| GI | gastrointestinal |
| gm | gram |
| gr | grain |
| gt | drop |
| gtt | drops |
| GTT | glucose tolerance test |
| GYN | gynecology |
| h | hour |
| H&H | hemoglobin and hematocrit |
| H&P | history and physical |
| HAV | hepatitis A virus |
| HBV | hepatitis B virus |
| HCT or Hct | hematocrit |
| HCV | hepatitis C virus |
| HD | Huntington disease |
| HEENT | head, eyes, ears, nose, and throat |
| HGB or Hgb | hemoglobin |
| HIV | human immunodeficiency virus |
| hpf | high-power field |
| HPI | history of present illness |
| HPV | human papillomavirus |
| HRT | hormone replacement therapy |
| h.s. | hour of sleep |

| Abbreviation or Symbol | Meaning |
|---|---|
| HSV-1 | herpes simplex virus type 1 |
| HSV-2 | herpes simplex virus type 2 |
| Ht | height |
| HTN | hypertension |
| Hx | history |
| I&D | incision and drainage |
| ICD | implantable cardioverter–defibrillator |
| ICU | intensive care unit |
| ID | intradermal |
| IM | intramuscular |
| IMP | impression |
| IOL | intraocular lens |
| IP | inpatient |
| IUD | intrauterine device |
| I.V. | intravenous |
| IVP | intravenous pyelogram |
| IVU | intravenous urogram |
| JCAHO | Joint Commission on Accreditation of Healthcare Organizations |
| kg | kilogram |
| KUB | kidneys, ureters, bladder |
| L | liter |
| Ⓛ | left |
| L&W | living and well |
| LASIK | laser-assisted in situ keratomileusis |
| lb | pound |
| LEEP | loop electrosurgical excision procedure |
| LH | luteinizing hormone |
| LLETZ | large loop excision of transformation zone |
| LLQ | left lower quadrant |
| LP | lumbar puncture |
| lpf | low-power field |
| LTB | laryngotracheobronchitis |
| LUQ | left upper quadrant |
| m | meter |
| ⓜ | murmur |
| MCH | mean corpuscular (cell) hemoglobin |
| MCHC | mean corpuscular (cell) hemoglobin concentration |
| MCV | mean corpuscular (cell) volume |
| MD | medical doctor; muscular dystrophy |

| Abbreviation or Symbol | Meaning |
|---|---|
| mg | milligram |
| MI | myocardial infarction |
| ml or mL | milliliter |
| mm | millimeter |
| $mm^3$ or cu mm | cubic millimeter |
| MPI | myocardial perfusion image |
| MRA | magnetic resonance angiography |
| MRI | magnetic resonance imaging |
| MRSA | methicillin-resistant *Staphylococcus aureus* |
| MS | multiple sclerosis; musculoskeletal |
| MSH | melanocyte-stimulating hormone |
| MUGA | multiple-gated acquisition (scan) |
| MVP | mitral valve prolapse |
| NAD | no acute distress |
| NCV | nerve conduction velocity |
| NG | nasogastric |
| NK | natural killer (cell) |
| NKA | no known allergy |
| NKDA | no known drug allergy |
| noc. | night |
| NPO | nothing by mouth |
| NSAID | nonsteroidal anti-inflammatory drug |
| NSR | normal sinus rhythm |
| O | objective |
| $O_2$ | oxygen |
| OA | osteoarthritis |
| OB | obstetrics |
| OCD | obsessive–compulsive disorder |
| OCP | oral contraceptive pill |
| OD | right eye; doctor of optometry |
| OH | occupational history |
| OP | outpatient |
| OR | operating room |
| ORIF | open reduction, internal fixation |
| OS | left eye |
| OU | both eyes |
| oz | ounce |
| $\bar{p}$ | after |
| P | plan; posterior; pulse |
| PA | posterior-anterior |
| PACU | postanesthetic care unit |
| $PaCO_2$ | partial pressure of carbon dioxide |
| $PaO_2$ | partial pressure of oxygen |
| Pap | Papanicolaou (smear) |

| Abbreviation or Symbol | Meaning |
| --- | --- |
| PAR | postanesthetic recovery |
| p.c. | after meals |
| PCI | percutaneous coronary intervention |
| PD | panic disorder |
| PDA | patent ductus arteriosus |
| PE | physical examination; pulmonary embolism; polyethylene |
| PEFR | peak expiratory flow rate |
| per | by or through |
| PERRLA | pupils equal, round, reactive to light and accommodation |
| PET | positron emission tomography |
| PF | peak flow |
| PFT | pulmonary function testing |
| pH | potential of hydrogen |
| PH | past history |
| PI | present illness |
| PID | pelvic inflammatory disease |
| PIH | pregnancy-induced hypertension |
| p.m. | after noon |
| PLT | platelet |
| PMH | past medical history |
| PMN | polymorphonuclear (leukocyte) |
| PNS | peripheral nervous system |
| p.o. | by mouth |
| post-op or postop | postoperative |
| PPBS | postprandial blood sugar |
| PR | per rectum |
| pre-op or preop | preoperative |
| p.r.n. or prn | as needed |
| PSA | prostate-specific antigen |
| PSG | polysomnography |
| pt | patient |
| PT | physical therapy; prothrombin time |
| PTCA | percutaneous transluminal coronary angioplasty |
| PTH | parathyroid hormone |
| PTSD | posttraumatic stress disorder |
| PTT | partial thromboplastin time |
| PUD | peptic ulcer disease |
| PV | per vagina |
| PVC | premature ventricular contraction |
| Px | physical examination |
| q | every |
| q.d. | every day, daily |

| Abbreviation or Symbol | Meaning |
| --- | --- |
| qh | every hour |
| q2h | every 2 hours |
| q.i.d. | four times a day |
| q.o.d. | every other day |
| qt | quart |
| R | respiration |
| ® | right |
| RA | rheumatoid arthritis |
| RBC | red blood cell; red blood count |
| RLQ | right lower quadrant |
| R/O | rule out |
| ROM | range of motion |
| ROS | review of systems |
| RP | retrograde pyelogram |
| RRR | regular rate and rhythm |
| RTC | return to clinic |
| RTO | return to office |
| RUQ | right upper quadrant |
| Rx | recipe; prescription |
| $\bar{s}$ | without |
| S | subjective |
| SA | sinoatrial |
| SAB | spontaneous abortion |
| SAD | seasonal affective disorder |
| SC | subcutaneous |
| SCA | sudden cardiac arrest |
| SCC | squamous cell carcinoma |
| SH | social history |
| Sig: | instruction to patient |
| SLE | systemic lupus erythematosus |
| SOB | shortness of breath |
| SPECT | single-photon emission computed tomography |
| SpGr | specific gravity |
| SQ | subcutaneous |
| SR | systems review |
| $\overline{\overline{ss}}$ | one-half |
| STAT | immediately |
| STD | sexually transmitted disease |
| SUI | stress urinary incontinence |
| suppos | suppository |
| SV | stroke volume |
| Sx | symptom |
| T | temperature |
| $T_3$ | triiodothyronine |

| Abbreviation or Symbol | Meaning |
|---|---|
| T$_4$ | thyroxine |
| T&A | tonsillectomy and adenoidectomy |
| tab | tablet |
| TAB | therapeutic abortion |
| TB | tuberculosis |
| TEDS | thromboembolic disease stockings |
| TEE | transesophageal echocardiogram |
| TIA | transient ischemic attack |
| t.i.d. | three times a day |
| TM | tympanic membrane |
| TMR | transmyocardial revascularization |
| tPA or TPA | tissue plasminogen activator |
| Tr | treatment |
| TSH | thyroid-stimulating hormone |
| TURP | transurethral resection of the prostate |
| TV | tidal volume |
| Tx | treatment; traction |
| UA | urinalysis |
| UCHD | usual childhood diseases |
| URI | upper respiratory infection |
| US or U/S | ultrasound |
| UTI | urinary tract infection |
| VC | vital capacity |
| VCU or VCUG | voiding cystourethrogram |
| V/Q | ventilation/perfusion |
| VS | vital signs |
| VSD | ventricular septal defect |
| VT | tidal volume |
| w.a. | while awake |

| Abbreviation or Symbol | Meaning |
|---|---|
| WBC | white blood cell; white blood count |
| WDWN | well developed, well nourished |
| wk | week |
| WNL | within normal limits |
| Wt | weight |
| x | times; for |
| x-ray | radiography |
| y.o. or y/o | year old |
| yr | year |
| ♀ | female |
| ♂ | male |
| # | number; pound |
| ° | degree; hour |
| ↑ | increase; above |
| ↓ | decrease; below |
| ✓ | check |
| Ø | none; negative |
| ♀ | standing |
| ♀ | sitting |
| ⊶ | lying |
| x | times; for |
| > | greater than |
| < | less than |
| ı̇ | one |
| ı̇ı̇ | two |
| ı̇ı̇ı̇ | three |
| ı̇v | four |
| I, II, III, IV, V, VI, VII, VIII, IX, and X | uppercase Roman numerals 1–10 |

From Willis MC. *Medical Terminology: The Language of Health Care*, 2nd ed. Baltimore, MD: Lippincott Williams & Wilkins, 2006.

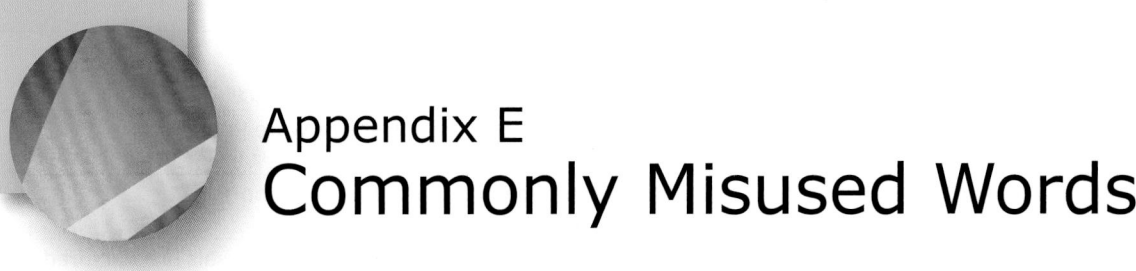

# Appendix E
# Commonly Misused Words

Because these words have similar spellings and pronunciation, they can easily be confused or misused. Watch your spelling carefully! Always proofread all business letters for accuracy and grammar.

| Word | Example of Correct Use |
|---|---|
| adverse (harmful)<br>averse (opposed to) | Some adverse reactions can be life threatening.<br>I am not averse to working on Mondays. |
| affect (verb, to influence, change)<br>effect (noun, result) | The protesters will not affect the outcome.<br>The effect of the antibiotics has been beneficial. |
| already (previously)<br>all ready (prepared, all set) | We already tried that approach.<br>Are we all ready to go? |
| anoxia (without oxygen)<br>anorexia (without appetite) | Anoxia will cause the brain cells to die quickly.<br>Anorexia is a serious illness that affects teenagers. |
| aphagia (without swallowing)<br>aphasia (without speech) | A feeding tube is needed because of her aphagia.<br>Her stroke caused aphasia. |
| appendices (end of book)<br>appendicitis (inflammation of appendix) | There are five appendices at the end of the book.<br>The patient was treated for appendicitis. |
| biannual (twice a year)<br>biennial (occurring every 2 years) | Productivity reports are printed on a biannual basis.<br>Staff contracts are renewed on a biennial basis. |
| bite (grip with teeth)<br>byte (character) | The patient's bite is poorly aligned.<br>Buy a computer with enough bytes for future growth. |
| bowl (container)<br>bowel (intestines, colon) | The jelly beans are in the bowl.<br>Instruct the patient to complete the bowel preparation. |
| emphysema (chronic lung disease)<br>empyema (accumulation of pus) | Smoking causes emphysema.<br>Empyema most commonly occurs in the pleural cavity. |
| ensure (be certain)<br>insure (protect against risk)<br>assure (provide confidence) | Call the patient to ensure that he comprehends the instructions.<br>Please insure this package for $200.<br>I assure you that he is getting the correct treatment. |
| everyday (adjective, routine, ordinary)<br>every day (adverbial phrase, each day) | Quality checks are an everyday procedure.<br>There can be legal ramifications if this is not done every day. |
| except (exclude)<br>expect (anticipate)<br>accept (agree) | All antibiotics except penicillin will work.<br>I expect this work to be completed by noon.<br>I accept this challenge. |
| farther (greater distance)<br>further (greater degree) | It is 1 mile farther down the road.<br>The process needs further refinement. |
| fundus (pertains to hollow organ)<br>fungus (organism that can lead to infection) | The fundus was firm after the baby's delivery.<br>A fungus was growing under her nails. |
| its (possessive pronoun)<br>it's (contraction of it and is) | The pharmacy must protect its supply of opioids.<br>It's time to take a break. |

*(Continues on page 1240)*

| Word | Example of Correct Use |
|---|---|
| lactose (type of sugar in milk)<br>lactase (enzyme) | I have a lactose allergy.<br>Lactase is responsible for dissolving lactose. |
| libel (written defamatory statement)<br>liable (legally responsible) | The statements about John Roberts were libel.<br>You are liable for your actions. |
| may be (compound verb)<br>maybe (adverb, perhaps) | Dr. Rogers may be in surgery this afternoon.<br>Maybe it will snow tomorrow. |
| metatarsals (bones in foot)<br>metacarpals (bones in palm) | Crutches are often needed when the metatarsals are fractured.<br>Typing is difficult for patients with a metacarpal fracture. |
| mucus (substance that is secreted)<br>mucous (membrane that secretes) | The patient had a mucus plug.<br>The mucous membrane secretes the mucus. |
| parental (pertaining to parent)<br>parenteral (not by mouth) | Follow parental guidelines for TV use.<br>Parenteral feedings will start on Monday. |
| postnatal (after birth)<br>postnasal (behind nose) | Complications can occur in the postnatal period.<br>Postnasal drainage can be uncomfortable. |
| principle (noun, law)<br>principal (noun, leader; adjective, most important) | A key principle of economics is understanding cash flow.<br>The principal's name is Tina Sefferin; her experience is the principal reason she was hired. |
| rubella (German measles)<br>rubeola (14-day measles) | You need a rubella vaccination.<br>There is an outbreak of rubeola at the middle school. |
| serum (liquid component of blood)<br>sebum (oily substance secreted by the sebaceous glands) | The patient's serum is used for various tests.<br>Sebum helps to lubricate the skin surface. |
| tact (behavior)<br>tack (different direction) | He handled his child with great tact.<br>A new tack may be needed for us to win that bid. |
| than (to show comparison)<br>then (next) | Salaries are higher now than they were a year ago.<br>Clean room 2; then go to lunch. |
| there (place, point)<br>their (possessive pronoun)<br>they're (pronoun plus verb) | You need to be there at 2:00 PM.<br>Leaving their bikes on the road caused the accident.<br>They're going to be late. |
| uvula (soft tissue at back of palate)<br>vulva (external female organ) | The patient's uvula was swollen.<br>A laceration of the vulva was noted during the gynecologic examination. |
| weather (climate)<br>whether (indicating a possibility) | The weather is unpredictable.<br>I wonder whether it will rain or snow. |

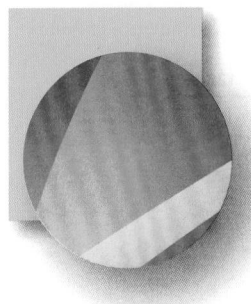

# Appendix F
# Sample Medical Reports

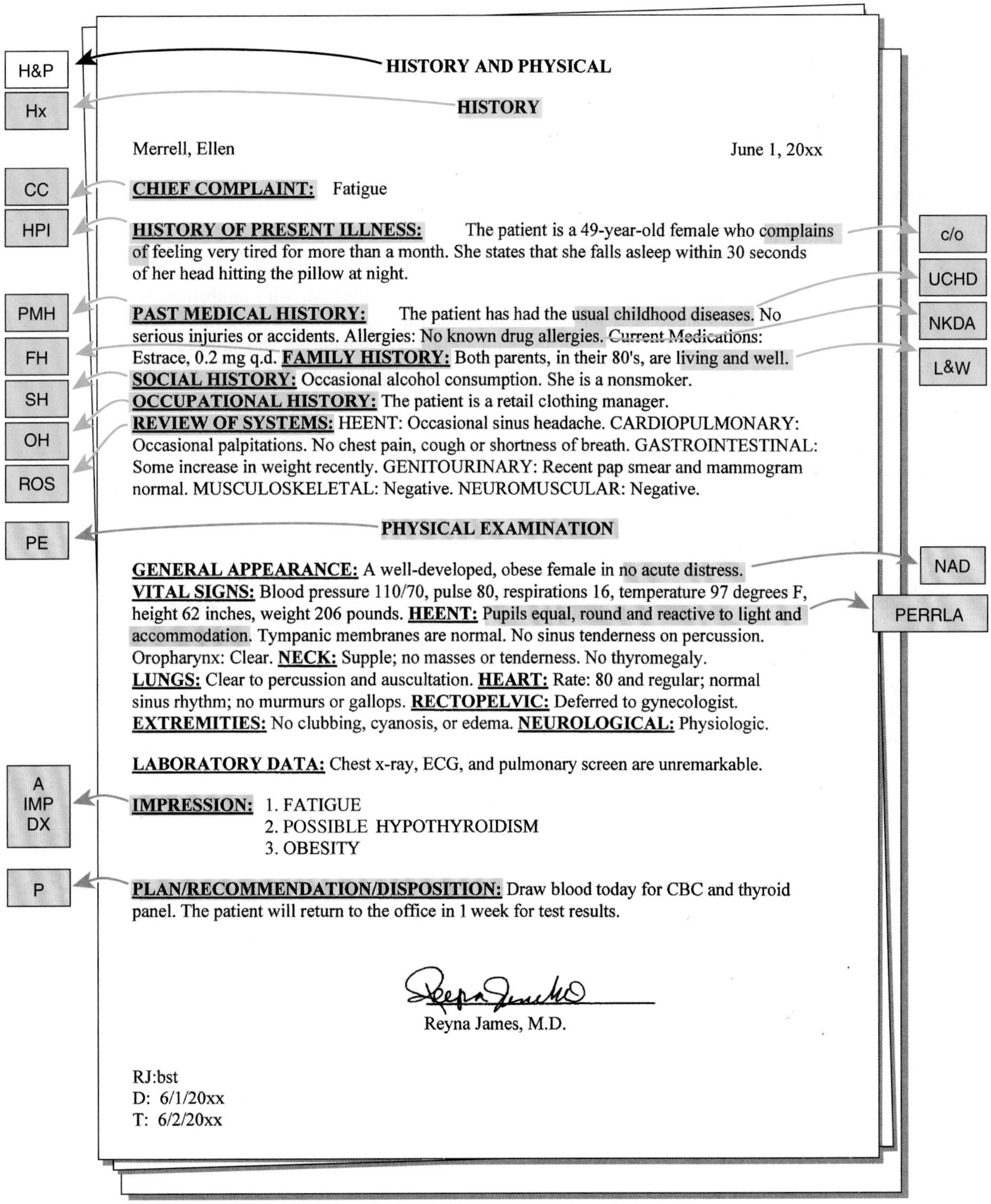

**HISTORY AND PHYSICAL**

**HISTORY**

Merrell, Ellen                                                    June 1, 20xx

**CHIEF COMPLAINT:**  Fatigue

**HISTORY OF PRESENT ILLNESS:**     The patient is a 49-year-old female who complains of feeling very tired for more than a month. She states that she falls asleep within 30 seconds of her head hitting the pillow at night.

**PAST MEDICAL HISTORY:**     The patient has had the usual childhood diseases. No serious injuries or accidents. Allergies: No known drug allergies. Current Medications: Estrace, 0.2 mg q.d. **FAMILY HISTORY:** Both parents, in their 80's, are living and well.

**SOCIAL HISTORY:** Occasional alcohol consumption. She is a nonsmoker.

**OCCUPATIONAL HISTORY:** The patient is a retail clothing manager.

**REVIEW OF SYSTEMS:** HEENT: Occasional sinus headache. CARDIOPULMONARY: Occasional palpitations. No chest pain, cough or shortness of breath. GASTROINTESTINAL: Some increase in weight recently. GENITOURINARY: Recent pap smear and mammogram normal. MUSCULOSKELETAL: Negative. NEUROMUSCULAR: Negative.

**PHYSICAL EXAMINATION**

**GENERAL APPEARANCE:** A well-developed, obese female in no acute distress.
**VITAL SIGNS:** Blood pressure 110/70, pulse 80, respirations 16, temperature 97 degrees F, height 62 inches, weight 206 pounds. **HEENT:** Pupils equal, round and reactive to light and accommodation. Tympanic membranes are normal. No sinus tenderness on percussion. Oropharynx: Clear. **NECK:** Supple; no masses or tenderness. No thyromegaly.
**LUNGS:** Clear to percussion and auscultation. **HEART:** Rate: 80 and regular; normal sinus rhythm; no murmurs or gallops. **RECTOPELVIC:** Deferred to gynecologist.
**EXTREMITIES:** No clubbing, cyanosis, or edema. **NEUROLOGICAL:** Physiologic.

**LABORATORY DATA:** Chest x-ray, ECG, and pulmonary screen are unremarkable.

**IMPRESSION:**   1. FATIGUE
                 2. POSSIBLE HYPOTHYROIDISM
                 3. OBESITY

**PLAN/RECOMMENDATION/DISPOSITION:** Draw blood today for CBC and thyroid panel. The patient will return to the office in 1 week for test results.

Reyna James, M.D.

RJ:bst
D: 6/1/20xx
T: 6/2/20xx

# CENTRAL MEDICAL CENTER

211 Medical Center Drive • Central City, US 90000-1234 • PHONE: (012) 125-6784 • FAX: (012) 125-9999

## OPERATIVE REPORT

**DATE OF OPERATION:** June 3, 20xx.

**PREOPERATIVE DIAGNOSIS:** Chronic tonsillitis.

**POSTOPERATIVE DIAGNOSIS:** Frequent, recurrent tonsillitis.

**SURGEON:** Patrick Rodden, M.D.

**ASSISTANT SURGEON:** None

**ANESTHESIOLOGIST:** Robert Jung, M.D.

**ANESTHESIA:** General.

**SURGERY PERFORMED:** Tonsillectomy.

**DESCRIPTION OF OPERATION:** After general anesthesia induction, with intubation, the McGivor mouth gag and tongue retractor were utilized for exposure of the oropharynx. Local anesthetic consisting of 6 mL of 0.5% Xylocaine with 1:100,000 epinephrine was utilized. Tonsillectomy was carried out using dissection and air technique. The right tonsillectomy electrocoagulation Bovie suction was utilized for hemostasis. Examination of the nasopharynx was normal.

The patient tolerated the procedure well and went to the recovery room in good condition.

*P. Rodden MD*

PATRICK RODDEN, M.D.

JR:as
D: 6/3/20xx
T: 6/4/20xx

| OPERATIVE REPORT | PT. NAME: | PERRON, CARLEEN |
|---|---|---|
| | ID NO: | 672894017 |
| | ROOM NO: | 312 |
| | ATT. PHYS: | PATRICK RODDEN, M.D. |

# CENTRAL MEDICAL CENTER

211 Medical Center Drive • Central City, US 90000-1234 • PHONE: (012) 125-6784 • FAX: (012) 125-9999

## PATHOLOGY REPORT

PATIENT:   PERRON, CARLEEN
                    28 Y (FEMALE)

DATE RECEIVED:  June 3, 20xx.                              DATE REPORTED:  June 4, 20xx

### GROSS:

Received are two tonsils each 2.5 cm in greatest diameter.

### MICROSCOPIC:

The sections show deep tonsilar crypts associated with follicular lymphoid hyperplasia.  No bacterial granules are seen.

### DIAGNOSIS:

CHRONIC LYMPHOID HYPERPLASIA OF RIGHT AND LEFT TONSILS.

_Mary Needham MD_
MARY NEEDHAM, M.D.

MN:gds


D:  6/4/20xx
T:  6/5/20xx

# CENTRAL MEDICAL CENTER

211 Medical Center Drive • Central City, US 90000-1234 • PHONE: (012) 125-6784 • FAX: (012) 125-9999

## DISCHARGE SUMMARY

DATE OF ADMISSION:      10/25/20xx      DATE OF DISCHARGE:      10/29/20xx

**ADMITTING DIAGNOSIS:**
Left ureteropelvic junction obstruction.

**DISCHARGE DIAGNOSIS:**
Left ureteropelvic junction obstruction.

**PROCEDURE PERFORMED:**
Left dismembered pyeloplasty and placement of stent.

**BRIEF SUMMARY:**
The patient is a 19-year-old male who was admitted to the hospital a month ago with left pyelonephritis. He was found to have a left ureteropelvic junction obstruction. The patient was brought to the hospital at this time for repair of the moderately to severely obstructed left kidney. A preoperative urine culture was sterile. The patient underwent the procedure without complication. A double-J stent was placed. The Jackson-Pratt drain was removed on the second postoperative day because of minimal drainage. The patient initially had urinary retention, but this resolved by the third postoperative day. He was doing fine at the time of discharge. His condition on discharge is good.

**INSTRUCTIONS TO THE PATIENT:**
1) Regular diet. 2) No heavy lifting, straining, or driving an automobile for six weeks from the day of surgery. He should also keep the incision relatively dry this week. 3) Follow up in my office in three weeks. 4) It is anticipated the stent will remain indwelling for six weeks and then will be removed cystoscopically at that time. 5) Discharge medication is Tylenol #3, 1-2 q 4 h p.r.n. pain.

L. Zlatkin, M.D.

LZ:mr

D:   10/29/20xx
T:   10/30/20xx

| DISCHARGE SUMMARY | PT. NAME:   MERCIER, CHARLES F. |
| | ID NO:      IP-392689 |
| | ROOM NO:    444 |
| | ATT. PHYS:  L.ZLATKIN, M.D. |

# CENTRAL MEDICAL CENTER

211 Medical Center Drive • Central City, US 90000-1234 • PHONE: (012) 125-6784 • FAX: (012) 125-9999

## OPERATIVE REPORT

DATE:  December 7, 20xx

**PREOPERATIVE DIAGNOSIS:**   Congenital left ureteropelvic junction obstruction status post pyeloplasty.  Indwelling left ureteral stent.

**POSTOPERATIVE DIAGNOSIS:**   Congenital left ureteropelvic junction obstruction status post pyeloplasty.  Indwelling left ureteral stent, removed

**OPERATION:**   Cystoscopy, removal of left ureteral stent, and left retrograde pyelogram.

**PROCEDURE:**   The patient was identified, was placed on the operating table, and was administered a general anesthetic.  He was placed in the lithotomy position, and a KUB was obtained.  The genitalia were prepped and draped in a sterile fashion.  After reviewing the KUB, it was noted at this time that the position of the stent was normal.  Cystoscopy was performed with a #22 French cystoscope.  The stent was identified coming from the left ureteral orifice, and the end was grasped with forceps and removed through the cystoscope.  A #8 French cone-tipped ureteral catheter was then placed in the left ureteral orifice and passed to 10 cm. Then, 20 cm$^3$ of contrast was injected into a left collecting system.  A film was exposed, and this showed patency without extravasation at the left ureteropelvic junction.  There was some filling of calyces and partial filling of the dilated renal pelvis.  A drainage film was subsequently obtained showing complete emptying of the pelvis and partial emptying of the mid and distal ureters.  Dilated calyces were noted in the kidney.  The patient was allowed to awaken and was returned to the recovery room in satisfactory condition.  There were no intraoperative complications.  He had no bleeding.  The patient did receive 1 gm Ancef one-half hour prior to the onset of the procedure.

L. Zlatkin, M.D.

LZ:mr
D:   12/07/20xx
T:   12/08/20xx

| OPERATIVE REPORT | PT. NAME:   MERCIER, CHARLES F. |
| --- | --- |
| | ID NO:   OP-912689 |
| | ROOM NO:   ASC |
| | ATT. PHYS:   L.ZLATKIN, M.D. |

# CENTRAL MEDICAL GROUP, INC.

*Department of Internal Medicine*

201 Medical Center Drive • Central City, US 90000-1234 • PHONE: (012) 125-8888 • FAX: (012) 125-3434

**PATIENT:  COHEN, SARA E.**                                              DATE:  April 8, 20xx

## HISTORY

**CHIEF COMPLAINT:**  Epigastric distress

**HISTORY OF PRESENT ILLNESS:**  This 33-year-old Caucasian female comes in because of excessive burping, epigastric distress and nausea for several weeks.  Coffee makes it worse.  She complains that it is worse at night when lying down.  She gets an acid-like taste in her mouth.  She has tried antacids, to no avail.

**PAST MEDICAL HISTORY:**  The patient states that she had the usual childhood diseases.  She has had no serious medical illnesses and has been involved in no accidents.  Family History:  There is some diabetes on her mother's side.  Her mother is 52 and has hypertension.  Her father, age 56, is living and well.  She has a sister who is anemic and a brother who has ulcers. Social History:  The patient discontinued smoking ten years ago.  Drinks alcohol socially.  Allergies:  NKDA. Current Medications:  Medications at this time consist of Entex, Guaifed, birth control pills, iron and vitamin supplements.

**REVIEW OF SYSTEMS:**  HEENT:  Chronic sinusitis.  She sees an ENT specialist and an allergist.  Respiratory:  Negative. Cardiac:  Occasional flutters.  Gastrointestinal:  As stated above.  Genitourinary:  Occasional infections.  Pap smear is up-to-date and negative.  She has had no mammogram at this point.  Neuromuscular:  Negative.

## PHYSICAL EXAMINATION

**GENERAL APPEARANCE:**  Reveals a well-developed, well-nourished female in no acute distress.

**VITAL SIGNS:**  Blood Pressure:  120/80.  Pulse:  76 and regular.

**HEENT**:  Head normocephalic.  Eyes:  Pupils are equal, round, and reactive to light and accommodation.  Fundi are benign.  Ears, nose and throat are negative.  NECK:  No thyromegaly.  No carotid bruits.

**CHEST**:  Clear to percussion and auscultation.  BREASTS:  Reveal no masses.  HEART:  Normal sinus rhythm.  No murmurs.

**ABDOMEN:**  Liver, spleen and kidneys could not be felt.  Femorals pulsate well, no bruits.

**EXTREMITIES:**  No edema.  Pulses are good and equal.

**PELVIC & RECTAL EXAMS:**  Deferred to gynecologist.

**NEUROLOGIC EXAM:**  Physiologic.

**IMPRESSION:**   1. PROBABLE PEPTIC ULCER DISEASE WITH GASTROESOPHAGEAL REFLUX.
                            2. POSSIBLE GALLBLADDER DISEASE.

**PLAN:**  Patient started on Pepcid 40 mg, 1 at night.  She is given Gaviscon tablets so she can carry them with her. Schedule routine lab work and upper GI series.  If negative, schedule ultrasound of the gallbladder.

D. Everley, M.D.

DE:mc
D:  4/8/20xx
T:  4/9/20xx

# CENTRAL MEDICAL GROUP, INC.
## Department of Otorhinolaryngology

201 Medical Center Drive • Central City, US 90000-1234 • PHONE: (012) 125-8888 • FAX: (012) 125-3434

**Patient: Perron, Carleen**                                          DATE: February 17, 20xx

Referring Physician: C. Camarillo, M.D.

## CONSULTATION

**REASON FOR CONSULTATION:** This 28-year-old white female presents with a one week history of upper respiratory infection (URI), sinusitis, and some periorbital headaches in recent weeks. She also has expectorated yellow-green mucus occasionally and has had a history of tonsillitis.

**MEDICATIONS:** None. **ALLERGIES:** No known allergies (NKA). **SURGERIES:** None. **HOSPITALIZATIONS:** None.

**PAST MEDICAL HISTORY/REVIEW OF SYSTEMS:** Cardiopulmonary: There is no history of angina, dyspnea, hemoptysis, emphysema, asthma, chronic obstructive pulmonary disease (COPD), hypertension, or heart murmurs. Cardiovascular: There is no history of high blood pressure. Renal: There is no history of dysuria, polyuria, nocturia, hematuria, or cystoliths. Gastrointestinal: There is no history of gallbladder disease, hepatitis, pancreatitis, or colitis. Musculoskeletal: There is no history of arthritis. Endocrine: There is no history of diabetes. Hematologic: There is no history of anemia, blood transfusion, or easy bruising. Gynecological: The patient states her menses are regular, and the start of her last menstrual cycle occurred 15 days ago.

**FAMILY HISTORY:** The patient states her maternal grandmother has diabetes.

**SOCIAL HISTORY:** The patient is single and has no children. She denies smoking tobacco. She denies drinking alcoholic beverages. She denies taking drugs.

**CHILDHOOD DISEASES:** The patient has had the usual childhood diseases.

**OTOLARYNGOLOGIC EXAMINATION:** Otoscopy: Tympanic membranes (TMs) are dull and slightly congested. Sinuses: There is maxillary fullness. Rhinoscopic examination reveals mild nasoseptal deviation (NSD). Pharynx: There is moderate inflammation; no exudates. Oropharynx: No masses. Nasopharynx: No masses. Larynx: Clear. Neck: Supple. Cervical Adenopathy: There is mild adenopathy.

**IMPRESSION:**
1. MAXILLARY SINUSITIS.
2. PHARYNGITIS.
3. CHRONIC TONSILLITIS.

**DISPOSITION:**
1. Warm salt water gargle (WSWG).
2. Ery-Tab 333, #24, 1 t.i.d. p.c.
3. Robitussin.
4. Return to office (RTO) in one week.

*P. Rodden MD*

PATRICK RODDEN, M.D.

JR:ti
D:  2/17/20xx
T:  2/18/20xx    9:50 a.m.

# CENTRAL MEDICAL GROUP, INC.
## Department of Otorhinolaryngology
201 Medical Center Drive • Central City, US 90000-1234 • PHONE: (012) 125-8888 • FAX: (012) 125-3434

### PROGRESS NOTES

Patient: PERRON, CARLEEN

03/30/20xx

**S:**     The patient presents with a sore throat × 2 weeks.

**O:**     Sinus exam: Maxillary and frontal congestion. Hypopharynx/adenoids: No inflammation.

**A:**     Recurrent pharyngitis/sinusitis × 2 weeks.

**P:**     1)   Ceftin 250 mg, #21, 1 t.i.d. p.o. p.c.

      2)   Entex LA, #30, 1 b.i.d. p.o.

      3)   Warm salt water gargle.

*P Rodden MD*
PATRICK RODDEN, M.D.

05/25/20xx

**S:**     Recurrent sore throat every month.

**O:**     Recurrent tonsillitis, cryptic tonsillitis. Sinus exam: Maxillary and frontal congestion. Neck: Supple; no masses. Hypopharynx/Adenoids: No inflammation. Paranasal Sinus X-ray: Bilateral frontal and maxillary sinusitis.

**A:**     Recurrent tonsillitis, 8-10 times per year. Chronic maxillary and frontal sinusitis.

**P:**     1)   Tonsillectomy discussed with the patient. The risks of general and local anesthesia, as well as the surgical procedure, were discussed with the patient. The consent form was signed.

      2)   An admitting order was given to the patient for CBC, UA, and basic metabolic panel to be done one day prior to being admitted.

      3)   Ceftin 250 mg, #21, 1 t.i.d. p.o. p.c.

      4)   Entex LA, #30, 1 b.i.d. p.o.

      5)   Flonase nasal inhaler, 2 sprays each nostril b.i.d.

      6)   Warm salt water gargle.

*P Rodden MD*
PATRICK RODDEN, M.D.

©2006, Lippincott Williams & Wilkins, Medical Terminology: The Language of Health Care, 2nd edition, by Marjorie Canfield Willis.

# CENTRAL MEDICAL CENTER

211 Medical Center Drive • Central City, US 90000-1234 • PHONE: (012) 125-6784 • FAX: (012) 125-9999

## X-RAY REPORT

**LUMBOSACRAL SPINE:**
Multiple views reveal no evidence of fracture.  There is slight lumbar spondylosis with slight lipping and minimal bridging.  The disc spaces appear maintained except for slight narrowing at L4-L5 and L5-S1.  There is also a Grade I spondylolisthesis of L5 on S1 and evidence of spondylolysis at L5 on the left.  There is also slight dextroscoliosis in the lumbar region and slight increased lordosis in the lumbosacral region.  The bony architecture is unremarkable except for eburnation between the articulating facets at L5-S1.  The SI joints appear unremarkable. Incidentally noted are slight osteoarthritic changes involving both hips.

**CONCLUSION:**

1. Slight lumbar spondylosis with hypertrophic lipping and slight narrowing of the L4-L5 and L5-S1 disc spaces, rule out discogenic disease.  If clinically indicated, CT of the lumbosacral spine may prove helpful in further evaluation.

2. Grade I spondylolisthesis of L5 on S1 with evidence of spondylolysis at L5 on the left.

3. Slight dextroscoliosis in the lumbar region and slight increased lordosis in the lumbosacral region.

*M. Volz MD*

M. Volz, M.D.

MV:ti

D:   10/19/20xx
T:   10/20/20xx

---

| X-RAY REPORT | PT. NAME: | DORN, JAY F. |
|---|---|---|
| | ID NO: | RL-483091 |
| | ATT. PHYS: | T. LIGHT, M.D. |

Medical reports courtesy of Willis M. *Medical Terminology: A Programmed Learning Approach to the Language of Health Care,* 2nd ed. Baltimore, MD: Lippincott Williams & Wilkins, 2007; and Willis MC. *Medical Terminology: The Language of Health Care,* 2nd ed. Baltimore, MD: Lippincott Williams & Wilkins, 2006.

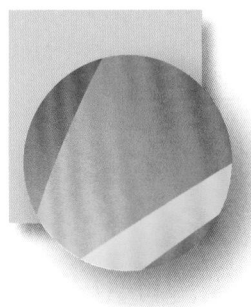

# Appendix G
# Metric Measurements

| Unit | Abbreviation | Metric Equivalent | US Equivalent |
| --- | --- | --- | --- |
| **Units of Length** | | | |
| kilometer | km | 1,000 meters | 0.62 miles; 1.6 km/mile |
| meter* | m | 100 cm; 1000 mm | 39.4 inches; 1.1 yards |
| centimeter | cm | 1/100 m; 0.01 m | 0.39 inches; 2.5 cm/inch |
| millimeter | mm | 1/1,000 m; 0.001 m | 0.039 inches; 2.5 mm/inch |
| micrometer | μm | 1/1,000 mm; 0.001 mm | |
| **Units of Weight** | | | |
| kilogram | kg | 1,000 g | 2.2 lb |
| gram* | g | 1,000 mg | 0.035 oz; 28.5 g/oz |
| milligram | mg | 1/1,000 g; 0.001 g | |
| microgram | μg, mcg | 1/1,000 mg; 0.001 mg | |
| **Units of Volume** | | | |
| liter* | L | 1,000 mL | 1.06 qt |
| deciliter | dL | 1/10 L; 0.1 L | |
| milliliter | mL | 1/1,000 L; 0.001 L | 0.034 oz; 29.4 mL/oz |
| microliter | μL | 1/1,000 mL; 0.001 mL | |

*Basic unit.

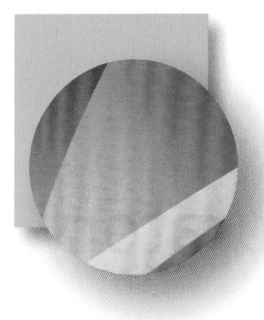

# Appendix H
# Celsius–Fahrenheit Temperature Conversion Scale

## Celsius to Fahrenheit

Use the following formula to convert Celsius readings to Fahrenheit readings:

$$°F = 9/5 × °C + 32$$

For example, if the Celsius reading is 37°:

$$°F = (9/5 × 37) + 32$$
$$= 66.6 + 32$$
$$= 98.6°F \text{ (normal body temperature)}$$

## Fahrenheit to Celsius

Use the following formula to convert Fahrenheit readings to Celsius readings:

$$°C = 5/9(°F − 32)$$

For example, if the Fahrenheit reading is 68°:

$$°C = 5/9(68 − 32)$$
$$= 5/9 × 36$$
$$= 20°C \text{ (a nice spring day)}$$

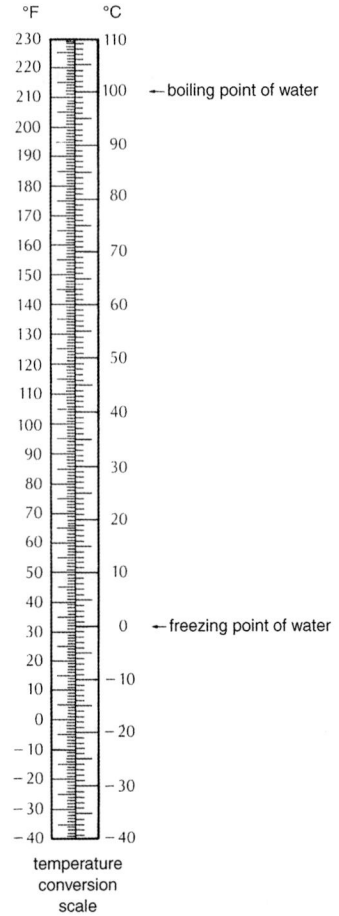

temperature
conversion
scale

From Memmler RL, Cohen BJ, Wood DL. *The Human Body in Health and Disease*, 10th ed. Baltimore, MD: Lippincott Williams & Wilkins, 2005.

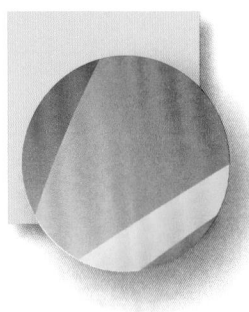

## Appendix I
# Body Systems and Laboratory Testing

| Body Systems and Laboratory Testing | | | |
|---|---|---|---|
| **System** | **Organs** | **Diseases** | **Laboratory Tests** |
| Cardiovascular | Heart<br>Blood vessels (i.e., arteries, capillaries, veins) | Coronary artery disease<br>Ischemic heart disease | Cholesterol<br>Triglycerides<br>LDL<br>HDL |
| | | Myocardial infarction | Sodium<br>Potassium<br>CKMB<br>Troponin<br>Myoglobin |
| | | Rheumatic fever<br>Rheumatic heart disease | WBC count<br>Hemoglobin<br>Hematocrit<br>Streptococcal antibody level |
| Circulatory | Heart, blood vessels | Arteriosclerosis | Cholesterol<br>Triglycerides<br>LDL<br>HDL |
| | | Anemias | RBC count<br>Hemoglobin<br>Hematocrit<br>MCV<br>MCHC<br>WBC count<br>Reticulocyte count<br>Platelet count<br>Bone marrow studies |
| | | Agranulocytosis | WBC count<br>Bone marrow studies<br>Blood cultures<br>Urine culture<br>Oral culture |
| | | Polycythemia | RBC count<br>Hemoglobin<br>Hematocrit<br>WBC count<br>Platelet count |

| Body Systems and Laboratory Testing (Continued) | | | |
|---|---|---|---|
| **System** | **Organs** | **Diseases** | **Laboratory Tests** |
| Digestive | Mouth | Oral tumor | Biopsy |
| | | Herpes simplex (cold sores) | Viral cultures |
| | | Thrush | Microscopic evaluation of lesion scrapings<br>RBC count<br>Hemoglobin<br>Hematocrit<br>Iron<br>TIBC<br>HIV |
| | | Necrotizing periodontal disease | Throat culture |
| | | Oral leukoplakia | Biopsy |
| | | Oral cancer | Biopsy |
| | Esophagus | Gastroesophageal reflux disease | Biopsy |
| | | Esophageal cancer | Biopsy |
| | Stomach | Peptic ulcer | *Helicobacter pylori* antibodies<br>Fecal occult blood<br>Hemoglobin<br>Hematocrit<br>Serum albumin<br>Transferrin |
| | | Gastritis | Biopsy<br>WBC count<br>Fecal occult blood |
| | | Gastric cancer | Biopsy |
| | Liver | Cirrhosis of the liver | AST<br>ALT<br>Total bilirubin |
| | | Hepatitis A | Hepatitis A antibody IgM<br>Hepatitis B core antibody IgM<br>Hepatitis B surface antigen<br>Hepatitis C virus antibody<br>Albumin<br>Total protein<br>ALP<br>ALT<br>AST<br>Total bilirubin<br>Direct bilirubin<br>Prothrombin time<br>Urinalysis |

*(Continued)*

## Body Systems and Laboratory Testing (Continued)

| System | Organs | Diseases | Laboratory Tests |
|---|---|---|---|
| | | Hepatitis B | Hepatitis A antibody IgM<br>Hepatitis B core antibody IgM<br>Hepatitis B surface antigen<br>Hepatitis C virus antibody<br>Albumin<br>Total protein<br>ALP<br>ALT<br>AST<br>Total bilirubin<br>Direct bilirubin<br>Prothrombin time<br>Urinalysis |
| | | Hepatitis C | Albumin<br>Total protein<br>ALP<br>ALT<br>AST<br>Total bilirubin<br>Direct bilirubin<br>Hepatitis C virus RNA test<br>Hepatitis C virus antibody |
| | | Cancer of the liver | Alpha-fetoprotein<br>Biopsy |
| | Gallbladder | Cholelithiasis<br>Cholecystitis | Total bilirubin<br>WBC count<br>Total bilirubin |
| | Pancreas | Pancreatitis | Serum amylase<br>Serum lipase<br>WBC count<br>Hematocrit<br>Glucose |
| | | Pancreatic cancer | CA 19-9<br>Biopsy |
| | Small intestine<br>Large intestine | Gastroenteritis | Stool culture<br>Fecal occult blood<br>Stool WBCs<br>Electrolytes |
| | | Acute appendicitis | CBC<br>Urinalysis |
| | | Crohn disease (any portion of the gastrointestinal tract from mouth to anus)<br>Ulcerative colitis | CBC<br>Serum albumin<br>Electrolytes<br>Fecal occult blood<br>Hemoglobin<br>WBC count<br>Stool culture<br>Biopsy |
| | | Intestinal obstruction | Electrolytes<br>WBC count |

## Body Systems and Laboratory Testing (Continued)

| System | Organs | Diseases | Laboratory Tests |
|---|---|---|---|
| Endocrine | Hypothalamus | Hypothalamic disease | TSH<br>Prolactin<br>Cortisol<br>ACTH<br>Testosterone<br>Growth hormone |
| | Pituitary | Gigantism | Growth hormone<br>Insulin-like growth factor |
| | | Acromegaly | Growth hormone |
| | | Hypopituitarism | Thyrotropin<br>Adrenocorticotropic hormone<br>Gonadotropin |
| | | Dwarfism | Growth hormone |
| | | Diabetes insipidus | Urinalysis<br>Osmolality<br>Antidiuretic hormone |
| | Thyroid | Goiter | Thyrotropin<br>$T_3$<br>$T_4$ |
| | | Hashimoto thyroiditis<br>Hyperthyroidism | TSH<br>$T_3$<br>$T_4$<br>TSH<br>Thyroid-stimulating hormone |
| | | Hypothyroidism | $T_3$<br>$T_4$<br>TSH |
| | | Cretinism | $T_4$<br>TSH |
| | | Myxedema | Total $T_4$<br>Total $T_3$<br>Free $T_4$<br>TSH |
| | | Thyroid cancer | Biopsy<br>Calcitonin<br>Carcinoembryonic antigen |
| | Parathyroids | Hyperparathyroidism | Serum-intact parathyroid hormone<br>Calcium<br>Phosphorus<br>ALP |
| | | Hypoparathyroidism | Calcium<br>Phosphorus<br>Parathyroid hormone |

*(Continued)*

## Body Systems and Laboratory Testing (Continued)

| System | Organs | Diseases | Laboratory Tests |
|---|---|---|---|
| | Adrenals | Cushing syndrome | Free cortisol |
| | | Addison disease | Blood cortisol<br>Urine cortisol<br>Sodium<br>Fasting glucose<br>CBC<br>Hematocrit |
| | Pancreas | Diabetes mellitus | Fasting glucose<br>Urinalysis<br>Insulin |
| | | Gestational diabetes | Urine glucose<br>Fasting glucose<br>Oral glucose tolerance tests<br>Two-hour postprandial glucose<br>Glycated hemoglobin |
| | | Hypoglycemia | Glucose |
| | Pineal body | Seasonal affective disorder | Serotonin<br>Melatonin |
| | Ovaries | Menopause | FSH<br>Estrogen |
| | | Polycystic ovary syndrome | Estrogen<br>FSH<br>Luteinizing hormone<br>Testosterone<br>17-Hydroxyketosteroids<br>Fasting glucose<br>Glucose tolerance<br>Insulin resistance<br>Cholesterol<br>Triglycerides<br>HDL<br>LDL<br>Serum HCG<br>Prolactin<br>$T_4$<br>TSH |
| | Testes | Epididymitis | Urinalysis<br>Urine culture<br>WBC count |
| Excretory | Small and large intestines | Diverticulitis | Fecal occult blood<br>CBC |
| | Rectum<br>Anus | Colorectal cancer | Fecal occult blood<br>Biopsy |

## Body Systems and Laboratory Testing (Continued)

| System | Organs | Diseases | Laboratory Tests |
|---|---|---|---|
| Immune | Bone marrow | Leukemia | Peripheral blood smear<br>Bone marrow aspiration |
| | | Anemia | CBC<br>Peripheral blood smear<br>Bone marrow aspiration |
| | | Lymphoma | Biopsy<br>CBC<br>ALP |
| | Thymus gland | Myasthenia gravis | Acetylcholine receptor antibodies |
| | | DiGeorge anomaly (thymic hypoplasia or aplasia) | T-cell count<br>Chromosome studies |
| | Spleen | Splenomegaly | Albumin<br>Total protein<br>ALP<br>ALT<br>AST<br>Total bilirubin<br>Direct bilirubin |
| | Lymph nodes | Lymphadenopathy | CBC |
| | | Lymphadenitis | WBC count<br>Throat culture<br>Sputum culture |
| | | Lymphoma | Lymph node biopsy<br>CBC<br>ESR<br>Bone marrow aspirate<br>Albumin<br>Total protein<br>ALP<br>ALT<br>AST<br>Total bilirubin<br>Direct bilirubin<br>BUN<br>Creatinine |
| Integumentary | Skin | Herpes zoster (shingles) | Vesicle scrapings culture<br>Varicella zoster antibodies |
| | | Impetigo | Gram stain |
| | | Cellulitis | Blood culture |
| | | Tinea cruris (jock itch) | Lesion culture |
| | | Decubitus ulcers | Culture and sensitivity |
| | Hair | Alopecia (baldness) | CBC<br>$T_4$<br>TSH |
| | | Folliculitis | Culture of purulent material |
| | Nails | Deformed or discolored nails | Comprehensive metabolic profile |
| | | Paronychia | Exudate culture |
| | Sweat glands | Sweat gland abscess | Culture |

*(Continued)*

## Body Systems and Laboratory Testing (Continued)

| System | Organs | Diseases | Laboratory Tests |
|---|---|---|---|
| Lymphatic | Ducts and lymph nodes | See "Lymph nodes" in the *Immune system* | |
| | Palatine tonsil | Tonsillitis | WBC count<br>Throat culture |
| | Thymus gland | See "Thymus gland" in the *Immune system* | |
| Muscular | Muscles (smooth, cardiac, and skeletal) | Muscle tumors | Core needle biopsy |
| | | Muscular dystrophy | Muscle biopsy<br>CK |
| | | Polymyositis | CK<br>Aldolase<br>AST<br>ALT<br>Lactate dehydrogenase<br>Muscle biopsy |
| Nervous | Brain | Epilepsy | Comprehensive metabolic panel |
| | Spinal cord | Meningitis | CSF levels of WBCs, protein, and glucose<br>CSF culture |
| | Nerves | Guillain–Barré syndrome | CSF protein |
| Reproductive | Male (penis and testes) | Klinefelter syndrome | Serum and urine gonadotropin<br>Semen analysis<br>Chromosome studies |
| | Female (vagina) | Vaginitis | Wet prep<br>KOH prep<br>Culture |
| | | Vaginal cancer | Pap smear<br>Biopsy |
| | | Trichomoniasis | Wet prep<br>Urinalysis |
| | Uterus | Endometrial cancer | Biopsy<br>CBC<br>Urinalysis<br>Creatinine<br>BUN<br>Albumin<br>Total protein<br>ALP<br>ALT<br>AST<br>Total bilirubin<br>Direct bilirubin |
| | Ovaries | Ovarian cancer | CA 125 |
| Respiratory | Nose | Leishmaniasis | Biopsy |
| | | Epistaxis | Platelet count |
| | Pharynx | Pharyngitis | CBC |
| | Larynx | Tumors of the larynx | Biopsy |
| | Trachea | Sarcoidosis | Biopsy<br>Serum angiotensin-converting enzyme |

## Body Systems and Laboratory Testing (Continued)

| System | Organs | Diseases | Laboratory Tests |
|---|---|---|---|
| | Bronchi | Hemoptysis | PT<br>PTT |
| | | Bronchiectasis | Sputum culture |
| | Alveoli | Fibrosing alveolitis | Biopsy |
| | Bronchioles | Cystic fibrosis | CF transmembrane conductance regulator<br>Sweat chloride |
| | Lungs | Pneumonia | Sputum culture<br>Blood culture |
| | | Pulmonary abscess | Sputum culture<br>Blood culture |
| | | Legionellosis | WBC count<br>ALP<br>ALT<br>AST<br>ESR<br>Sputum culture |
| | | Respiratory syncytial virus | Respiratory syncytial virus |
| | | Pneumonia<br>Pulmonary tuberculosis | Sputum culture |
| | | Lung cancer | Sputum cytology |
| Skeletal | Bone | Paget disease (osteitis deformans) | Bone marrow biopsy<br>ALP<br>Urine hydroxyproline |
| | | Bone tumors | ALP<br>Serum calcium<br>Bone marrow evaluation<br>Biopsy |
| | | Osteomalacia and rickets | Comprehensive metabolic panel<br>Vitamin D level<br>ESR |
| | Bone marrow | Leukemia | See *Immune system* |
| | | Anemia | See *Circulatory system* |
| | | Lymphoma | See *Immune system* |
| | Joints | Gout | Microscopy of synovial joint fluid<br>Serum uric acid |
| | Teeth | Dental diseases | Dental treatment |
| | Ligaments | Orthopedics | |
| | Cartilage | Costochondritis | WBC count |
| Urinary | Kidneys | Chronic glomerulonephritis | Urinalysis<br>Renal biopsy<br>BUN<br>Creatinine |
| | | Nephrotic syndrome (nephrosis) | Urinalysis with microscopic evaluation<br>Serum albumin<br>Cholesterol<br>Triglyceride<br>HDL<br>LDL<br>Renal biopsy |

*(Continued)*

## Body Systems and Laboratory Testing (Continued)

| System | Organs | Diseases | Laboratory Tests |
|---|---|---|---|
| | | Acute renal failure | Urinalysis<br>BUN<br>Creatinine<br>Potassium |
| | | Chronic renal failure | BUN<br>Creatinine<br>Potassium<br>Hematocrit<br>Urinalysis |
| | | Pyelonephritis | Clean-catch urinalysis<br>Blood culture<br>Urine culture |
| | Ureter | Ureteral obstruction (renal calculi) | Urinalysis<br>Renal calculi analysis |
| | Urethra | Urethritis | Clean-catch urinalysis with microscopic evaluation<br>Urine culture |
| Sensory | Sense of sight | Ophthalmology | |
| | Sense of hearing | Cancer of the ear | Biopsy |
| | Sense of feeling | Vitamin $B_{12}$ deficiency | Vitamin $B_{12}$<br>Serum folate<br>CBC |
| | Sense of smell | Anosmia | Neurology evaluation |
| | Sense of taste | Loss from gingivitis | Throat culture |
| | | Loss from strep throat | Rapid strep test<br>Throat culture |
| | | Sjögren syndrome | Antithyroglobulin antibody<br>Rheumatoid arthritis test<br>Antinuclear antibody test |
| | Sense of balance | Vitamin $B_{12}$ deficiency | See "Sense of feeling" |
| | | Hypoglycemia<br>Audiology evaluation | Glucose |

*Note*: Lists are representative, not comprehensive.

LDL, low-density lipoprotein; HDL, high-density lipoprotein; CKMB, creatine kinase-MB (muscle, brain); CK, creatine kinase; WBC, white blood cell; RBC, red blood cell; MCV, mean corpuscular volume; MCHC, mean corpuscular hemoglobin concentration; TIBC, total iron-binding capacity; HIV, human immunodeficiency virus; AST, aspartate aminotransferase; ALT, alanine aminotransferase; ALP, alkaline phosphatase; FSH, follicle-stimulating hormone; IgM, immunoglobulin M; CBC, complete blood count; $T_3$, tri-iodothyronine; $T_4$, thyroxine; TSH, thyroid-stimulating hormone; HCG, human chorionic gonadotropin; ESR, erythrocyte sedimentation rate; BUN, blood urea nitrogen; CSF, cerebrospinal fluid; KOH, potassium hydroxide; PT, prothrombin time; PTT, partial thromboplastin time; CF, cystic fibrosis.

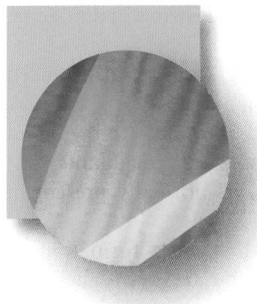

# Glossary

**A**

**abandonment** withdrawal by a physician from a contractual relationship with a patient without proper notification while the patient still needs treatment.

**abdominal regions** divisions of the abdomen into nine regions by two horizontal and two vertical lines; used to identify specific locations.

**ablation** removal or excision of a part; laser ablation is destruction/removal of tissue by use of laser.

**abortion** termination of pregnancy or products of conception prior to fetal viability and/or 20 weeks of gestation.

**Accountable Care Organizations (ACO)** groups of physicians, hospitals, and other providers who have joined together to provide coordinated care to their patients.

**accounting** the system of recording and summarizing business and financial transactions and analyzing, verifying, and reporting the results.

**accounting cycle** a consecutive 12-month period for financial record keeping following either a fiscal year (starting on a specified date) or the calendar year (January to December).

**accounts payable** a record of all monies owed.

**accounts receivable** a record of all monies due.

**accreditation** a nongovernmental professional peer review process that provides technical assistance and evaluates educational programs for quality based on pre-established academic and administrative standards.

**acidosis** condition in which there is too much acid in the body.

**acquired immunodeficiency syndrome (AIDS)** a cluster of disorders caused by HIV that specifically destroy cell-mediated immunity.

**acromegaly** a disorder marked by progressive enlargement of the head, face, hands, and feet, due to excessive secretion of growth hormone after puberty.

**acrosome** the superior surface of the head of the spermatozoon.

**activities of daily living (ADL)** activities usually performed in the course of the day, that is, bathing, dressing, and feeding oneself.

**acute** abrupt in onset.

**Addison disease** partial or complete failure of the adrenal cortex functions, causing general physical deterioration.

**adenosine triphosphate (ATP)** the energy currency used by the body; breaking down the phosphate bond of the compound releases high-energy potential.

**adipose** of or pertaining to fat.

**adjustment** a change in a posted account.

**administrative** pertaining to administration (e.g., office procedures and nonclinical tasks that a medical assistant will perform).

**adnexa** any part added to a main structure; an accessory part.

**advance beneficiary notice** document that informs covered patients that Medicare may not cover a certain service and the patient will be responsible for the bill.

**advance directive** a statement of a patient's wishes regarding health care prior to a critical medical event.

**aerobe** microorganism that requires oxygen to live and reproduce.

**aerosol** suspended particles in gas or air.

**afebrile** body temperature not elevated above normal.

**afferent** carrying impulses toward the center.

**affiliation** to connect or associate with, as a medical site would associate with a school to assist in completion of student training.

**Affordable Care Act (ACA)** the Patient Protection and Affordable Care Act was signed into law by President Barack Obama in March 2010 to reform health care through a series of regulations for coverage and benefits to Americans.

**agar** a gelatin-like substance made from red algae that is used in making solid culture media in a laboratory to grow bacteria and other microorganisms.

**agenda** a brief outline of the topics to be discussed at a meeting.

**agglutination** clumping of cells due to the presence of antibodies called *agglutinins*.

**aging schedule** a form used to track outstanding balances.

**albumin** because it is a small molecule, one of the first proteins able to pass through the kidneys into the urine when there are kidney problems.

**aliquots** portions of the original patient specimen that have been placed into a separate container to be routed to the appropriate laboratory work station for testing.

**alkalosis** condition in which the blood has too much base, resulting in an increase in blood pH.

**allergen** any substance that causes manifestations of an allergy, usually a protein to which the body has built antibodies.

**allergy** acquired abnormal response to a substance (allergen) that does not ordinarily cause a reaction.

**alopecia** baldness.

**alphabetic filing** arranging of names or titles according to the sequence of letters in the alphabet.

**alpha-fetoprotein** substance produced by the embryonic yolk sac.

**alternative** an option or substitute to the standard medical treatment plan, for example, herbal therapies, acupuncture, and hypnosis.

**alveolar–capillary membrane** the structure in the lung fields through which oxygen and carbon dioxide diffuse during the respiratory process.

**amenorrhea**    condition of not menstruating, without menses.

**American Association of Medical Assistants (AAMA)**    professional organization for medical assistants.

**Americans with Disabilities Act (ADA)**    a law designed to meet the needs of people with physical and mental challenges.

**American with Disabilities Act Amendments Act**    a law designed to meet the needs of people with physical and mental challenges that was updated to recognize and clarify other impairments not noted under the ADA.

**amino acids**    building blocks of protein.

**ammonia**    a common metabolic waste product.

**amniocentesis**    puncture of the amniotic sac in order to remove fluid for testing.

**amphiarthroses**    slightly movable joints.

**ampule**    small glass container that must be broken at the neck to aspirate the solution into the syringe.

**amylase**    an enzyme secreted by the pancreas into the intestines to aid in digestion; also secreted by the salivary glands.

**anabolism**    the constructive phase of metabolism, when smaller molecules are converted to large ones.

**anacusis**    complete hearing loss.

**anaerobe**    bacterium that requires the absence of oxygen for growth and reproduction.

**analyte**    substance or constituent for which a laboratory conducts testing.

**anaphylactic shock**    severe allergic reaction within minutes to hours after exposure to a foreign substance.

**anaphylaxis**    severe allergic reaction that may result in death.

**anatomic position**    a position used for reference in which the subject is standing erect, facing forward, feet are slightly apart and pointing forward, and the hands are down at the sides with palms forward and thumbs outward.

**anatomy**    the study of the structure of the body.

**anchor**    holding a vein in place so that it does not roll.

**anencephaly**    a neural tube defect in developing fetuses.

**aneroid**    sphygmomanometer that measures blood pressure without using mercury.

**aneurysm**    local dilation in a blood vessel wall.

**angina pectoris**    paroxysmal chest pain usually caused by a decrease in blood flow to the heart muscle due to coronary artery occlusion.

**angiotensin**    a substance occurring in the blood that works with renin to affect the blood pressure, usually increasing the pressure by vasoconstriction.

**anions**    chemicals that carry a negative charge.

**anisocytosis**    blood abnormality in which red blood cells are not equal in size (aniso = unequal).

**ankylosing spondylitis**    stiffening of the spine with inflammation.

**annotation**    the process of reading, highlighting, and summarizing a document for another person.

**anorexia**    loss of appetite.

**anovulation**    condition of not ovulating.

**antagonism**    mutual opposition or contrary action with something else; opposite of synergism.

**antagonist**    any muscle that opposes the action of the prime mover to balance movement (e.g., when the biceps contract and pull the forearm upward, the triceps oppose the motion and relax).

**antecubital space**    inner surface of the bend of the elbow where the major veins for venipuncture are located.

**antepartum**    period of time prior to labor.

**anthropometric**    pertaining to measurements of the human body.

**antibiotic**    a drug that inhibits or destroys pathogenic microorganisms.

**antibody/antibodies (pl)**    a complex glycoprotein produced by B lymphocytes in response to an antigen.

**anticoagulant**    a chemical compound introduced to the blood or blood sample to prevent clotting. Anticoagulants suppress the function of clotting factors normally present in the blood.

**antigen**    protein markers on cells that cause formation of antibodies and react specifically with those antibodies.

**antihistamine**    medication that opposes the action of a histamine.

**antiseptic**    any substance that inhibits the growth of bacteria; used on skin before any procedure that breaks the integumentary barrier.

**anuria**    failure of the kidneys to produce urine.

**apnea**    the absence of respirations.

**apothecary system of measurement**    old system that uses grains, minims, and drams.

**appeal**    process by which a higher court reviews the decision of a lower court.

**appendicular skeleton**    the parts of the skeleton added to the axial skeleton, including the shoulder and pelvic girdles and all of the bones of the upper and lower extremities.

**applicator**    device for applying local treatments and tests.

**approximate**    bring tissue surfaces as close as possible to their original positions.

**arachnoid**    weblike membrane covering the brain and spinal cord.

**arrector pili**    involuntary muscle attached to the hair follicle that, when contracted, causes "goose bumps."

**arteriole**    a small arterial branch that joins a capillary to an artery.

**arthrogram**    x-ray of a joint.

**arthroplasty**    surgical repair of a joint.

**arthroscopy**    examination of the inside of a joint through an arthroscope.

**artifact**    activity recorded in an electrocardiogram caused by extraneous activity such as patient movement, loose lead, or electrical interference.

**artifactual**    something added to a substance or structure, not belonging to it; in medicine, generally implies a negative connotation.

**ascites**    accumulation of serous fluid in the peritoneal cavity.

**asepsis**    a state of being sterile; a condition free from germs, infection, and any form of life, including spore forms.

**aspiration**    drawing in or out by suction; as in breathing objects into the respiratory tract or suctioning substances from a site.

**assault**    an attempt or threat to touch another person without his or her consent.

**assessment**    process of gathering information about the patient and the presenting condition.

**assignment of benefits**    transfer of the patient's legal right to collect third-party benefits for medical expenses to the provider of the services.

**astigmatism**    unfocused refraction of light rays on the retina.

**asymmetry**    lack or absence of symmetry; inequality of size or shape on opposite sides of the body.

**asymptomatic**    without any symptoms.

**atelectasis**    collapsed lung fields; incomplete expansion of the lungs, either partial or complete.

**atherosclerosis**    buildup of fatty plaque on the interior lining of arteries.

**atraumatic**  without injury; may pertain to treatments or instruments that are not likely to cause further damage.

**atria (plural)**  the upper chamber of each half of the heart; the atria receive blood from the great vessels (singular: atrium).

**atrioventricular (AV) node**  located on the floor of the right atrium on or close to the septum; receives the electrical impulse from the sinoatrial node after it is transmitted through the upper half of the heart; transmits the impulse to the bundle of His.

**attenuated**  diluted or weakened; pertaining to reduced virulence of a pathogenic microorganism.

**attitude**  a state of mind; how a person feels about a given subject or at a given time.

**attribute**  a characteristic or quality of a person; usually considered a positive feature.

**audit**  a review of an account; inspection of records to determine compliance and to detect fraud.

**aura**  a visual or other sensory warning experienced before an impending seizure.

**auscultation**  act of listening for sounds within the body, usually with a stethoscope, such as to evaluate the heart, lungs, intestines, or fetal heart tones.

**autoclave**  appliance used to sterilize medical instruments with steam under pressure.

**autoimmunity**  condition in which the immune system attacks its own host's body.

**autonomic**  self-controlling, spontaneous.

**autonomous**  existing or functioning independently.

**axial skeleton**  the bones forming the main skeleton around which the appendicular skeleton moves, including bones of the head, thorax, and trunk.

**axon**  part of the neuron that transmits impulses away from the cell body.

**azidothymidine (AZT)**  a drug used to treat AIDS by blocking the growth of the virus after it enters the T-cell lymphocyte.

**azotemia**  from the Latin *azote* meaning nitrogen, plus -emia, meaning blood; the condition of having excessive amounts of nitrogen in the blood.

## B

**Babinski reflex**  reflex (dorsiflexion of the great toe and extension and fanning of the other toes upon stroking the sole of the foot) exhibited normally by infants. This reflex is abnormal in children and adults.

**bacilli**  rod-shaped or cylindrical organisms.

**backup**  *noun*, a duplicate file made to a separate disk to protect information; *verb*, to make a duplicate file.

**bactericidal**  substance that kills or destroys bacteria.

**bacteriology**  the science and study of bacteria.

**bacteriuria**  the presence of bacteria in urine.

**balance**  equality between the debit and credit sides of an accounting equation; that which is left over after additions and subtractions have been made to an account; remainder; amount due.

**balance billing**  billing the patient for the balance or difference between the physician's charges and the Medicare-approved charges; prohibited by most managed care contracts.

**band**  younger, less mature neutrophil.

**bandage**  *noun*, a soft material applied to a body part to hold a dressing in place, immobilize a body part, or aid in controlling bleeding; *verb*, to apply a wrapping material for treatment.

**barrier precautions**  any device, including PPE, that provides an obstacle to minimize the risk of infection with blood-borne pathogens.

**Bartholin glands**  small mucous glands bilaterally in the vaginal vestibule.

**basal ganglia**  pertaining to the gray matter in the cerebral hemispheres.

**basal metabolic rate**  the amount of energy used in a unit of time to maintain vital functions by a fasting, resting subject.

**basic pH**  nonacidic pH 8 to 12.

**baseline**  original or initial measure with which other measurements will be compared.

**basophil**  a type of leukocyte.

**battery**  actual touching of a person without his or her consent.

**B cells**  lymphoid stem cells from the bone marrow that migrate to and become mature antigen-specific cells in the spleen and lymph nodes.

**beliefs**  ideas that are held to be true.

**bench trial**  trial in which the judge hears the case and renders a verdict; no jury is present.

**Benedict reaction**  the copper reduction test for measuring glucose.

**benign**  not cancerous or malignant.

**bevel**  the angled point of the needle cut on a slant to ease skin penetration.

**bias**  formation of an opinion without foundation or reason; prejudice.

**BiCaps**  words or phrases with unusual capitalization.

**bicarbonate**  the dissolved form of carbon dioxide; it combines with water to make carbonic acid, $H_2CO_3$. Carbonic acid loses one of its hydrogen (H) ions to then form bicarbonate, $HCO_3^-$.

**bile**  a bitter, yellow–green secretion of the liver stored by the gallbladder; derived from bilirubin, cholesterol, and other substances. Emulsifies fats in the small intestine so they can be further digested and absorbed.

**biliary obstruction**  blockage of one of the bile ducts (the tubes leading from liver and gallbladder into duodenum); common causes include cysts, tumors, and stones.

**bilirubin**  formed during the breakdown of hemoglobin.

**bilirubinuria**  bilirubin in the urine.

**bimanual**  pertaining to the use of both hands; an examination performed with both hands.

**bioethics**  moral issues and concerns that affect a person's life.

**biohazard**  biological agent that has the capacity to harm humans.

**biohazard symbol**  icon on the label for specimens containing potential biological agents.

**biohazardous**  describing a substance that is a risk to the health of living organisms.

**biohazardous waste**  infectious waste or biomedical waste; any waste containing infectious materials or potentially infectious substances such as blood.

**biological agent**  bacteria, viruses, fungi, other microorganisms, and their toxins.

**bioterrorism**  intentional release of a biologic agent with the intent to harm individuals.

**biotransform**  convert the molecules of a substance from one form to another, as in medications within the body.

**birthday rule**  determination of which policyholder's insurance is the first to pay when a patient is covered by two policies. The policyholder whose birth month and day comes first in the calendar is primary.

**blister**   a collection of fluid in or beneath the epidermis; a vesicle.

**block**   a type of letter format in which the date, subject line, closing, and signature are justified to the right margin; all other lines are justified left.

**blood cultures**   specimens drawn to culture the blood for pathogens.

**blood urea nitrogen (BUN)**   blood test to determine the amount of nitrogen in blood in the form of urea, a waste product normally excreted in urine.

**blood-borne pathogens**   viruses that can be spread through direct contact with blood or body fluids from an infected person.

**body fluids**   any of the fluids that accumulate in the compartments of the body, such as the blood plasma, and the intracellular and extracellular spaces.

**body mass index (BMI)**   a measurement of an individual's ratio of fat to lean body mass. It is calculated by using the following formula: [weight (pounds) ÷ height (inches)$^2$] × 703. A BMI over 30 is considered obese.

**body mechanics**   using the correct muscles and posture to complete a task safely and efficiently.

**boil**   an abscess of the subcutaneous tissues of the skin; a furuncle.

**bolus**   a mobile mass, for instance, a mass of food that passes into the upper gastrointestinal tract in one swallow, or a dose of medication injected intravenously.

**bookkeeping**   organized and accurate record keeping for financial transactions.

**boot**   to start up the computer.

**bore**   diameter of the interior of a needle.

**bradycardia**   heart rate of less than 60 beats per minute.

**bradykinesia**   abnormally slow voluntary movements.

**Braxton-Hicks contractions**   uterine contractions during pregnancy.

**breach**   an infraction, such as breach of contract, in which the agreed-on terms are violated.

**"breathing the syringe"**   pull back the plunger to about halfway up the barrel, then push it back; makes the plunger move more smoothly and reduces the tendency to jerk when it is first pulled after insertion into the vein.

**broth**   liquid media is most often poured into glass tubes or bottles.

**bruit**   abnormal sound or murmur in the blood vessels during auscultation.

**buccal**   describing medication administered between the cheek and gum of the mouth.

**budget**   financial planning tool that helps an organization estimate its anticipated expenditures and revenues.

**buffer**   extra time to accommodate emergencies, walk-ins, and other demands on the provider's daily time schedule that are not considered direct patient care.

**buffer system**   system that guards against sudden shifts in acidity and alkalinity depending on the body's own naturally occurring weak acids and weak bases.

**bulla**   large blister or vesicle.

**BUN**   *see* blood urea nitrogen.

**bundle of His**   a band of specialized cardiac muscle fibers that receives the electrical impulse from the atrioventricular node and transmits it through right and left branches to the Purkinje fibers.

**bursae**   small sacs filled with clear synovial fluid that surround some joints.

**butterfly**   winged infusion set.

**byte**   a unit of symbolic transfer; each character equals one byte.

## C

**caduceus**   a symbol using a wand or staff with two serpents coiled around it; sometimes used as the sign of the medical profession (the more appropriate symbol has only one snake).

**calibrated**   marked in units of measurement, as a thermometer calibrated in Celsius.

**calibration**   the standardization of any measuring instrument or testing procedure.

**callus**   in the musculoskeletal system, a deposit of new bone tissue that forms between the healing ends of broken bones; in the integumentary system, a thickened area of the epidermis caused by pressure or friction.

**calorie**   a unit of heat content or energy. The amount of heat necessary to raise 1 g of water from 14.5 to 15.5°C (small calorie).

**calyx (plural, calyces)**   a cuplike collecting structure of the kidney.

**cancellous**   porous, spongy bone inside the medulla of the bone, usually filled with marrow.

**capitation**   managed care plan that pays a certain amount to a provider over a specific time for caring for the patients in the plan regardless of what or how many services are performed.

**carbohydrates**   chemical elements in food that convert to sugar, providing energy.

**carbuncle**   infection of interconnected group of hair follicles or several furuncles forming a mass.

**cardiac cycle**   period from the beginning of one heartbeat to the beginning of the next; includes systole and diastole.

**cardiac output**   the amount of blood ejected from either ventricle per minute, either to the pulmonary or to the systemic circulation.

**cardinal signs**   usually, vital signs; signifies their importance in assessment.

**cardiogenic shock**   type of shock in which the left ventricle fails to pump enough blood for the body to function.

**cardiomegaly**   enlarged heart muscle.

**cardiomyopathy**   any disease affecting the myocardium.

**carina**   a ridgelike structure; that part of the trachea that projects from the lower end of the trachea.

**carrier**   person infected with a microorganism but without signs of disease; a company that assumes the risk of an insurance company.

**cassette**   lightproof holder in which x-ray film is exposed.

**catabolism**   the destructive phase of metabolism in which larger molecules are converted into smaller molecules.

**catabolize**   to break down fats.

**cataracts**   progressive loss of transparency of the lens of the eye, resulting in opacity and loss of sight.

**catheterization**   procedure for introducing a flexible tube into the body; urinary catheterization is for removal of urine from the bladder.

**cations**   chemicals that carry a positive charge.

**cautery**   means, device, or agent that destroys or coagulates tissue; may be electrical current, freezing or burning agent, or chemical solution (caustic).

**cell**   the most basic unit of all living organisms.

**cellulitis**   inflammation or infection of the skin and deeper tissues that may result in tissue destruction if not treated properly.

**Celsius, centigrade (C)**   a temperature scale on which 0 degrees is the freezing point of water and 100 degrees is the boiling point of water at sea level.

**Centers for Disease Control and Prevention (CDC)**   U.S. federal agency under the Department of Health and Human Services that works to protect public health and safety. CDC provides information to enhance health decisions.

**Centers for Medicare and Medicaid Services (CMS)**   government department that mandates the use of panels defined by the American Medical Association (AMA) for national standardization of nomenclature and testing.

**centesis**   surgical puncture made into a cavity.

**central processing unit (CPU)**   circuitry imprinted on a silicon chip that processes information; the "brain" of the computer.

**centrifugation**   process of separating blood or other body fluid cells from liquid components using a centrifuge.

**cephalalgia**   headache.

**cerebellum**   located in the posterior part of the brain, responsible for balance and muscle coordination.

**cerebrovascular accident (CVA)**   ischemia of the brain due to an occlusion of the blood vessels supplying the brain, resulting in varying degrees of debilitation.

**cerebrum**   largest part of the brain, divided into two hemispheres; responsible for thought processes, sensory and motor functions, speech, writing, memory, and emotions.

**Certificate of Waiver (CW)**   one of four types of certificates issued under CLIA; certifies the laboratory to perform waived testing.

**certification**   voluntary process that involves a testing procedure to prove an individual's baseline competency in a particular area.

**cerumen**   yellowish or brownish waxlike secretion in the external ear canal; earwax.

**cervix**   the part of the uterus that opens into the vagina.

**Chadwick sign**   sign of early pregnancy in which the vaginal, cervical, and vulvar tissues develop a bluish violet color.

**chain-of-custody procedure**   accurate written record to track the possession, handling, and location of chain-of-custody samples and data from collection through reporting.

**challenge**   a method of testing a patient's sensitivity or response to a substance by introducing it into the body and watching its effects.

**chancre**   a hard ulcer that appears 2 to 3 weeks after exposure to syphilis, near the site of infection.

**charge slip**   a preprinted three-part form that can be placed on a daysheet to record the patient's charges and payments along with other information in an encounter form.

**check register**   place to record checks that have been written.

**check stub**   indicates to whom a check was issued, in what amount, and on what date.

**Chemical Hygiene Plan (CHP)**   a part of the Occupational Safety and Health Administration's HazCom standard.

**chemical name**   exact chemical descriptor of a drug.

**chief complaint**   main reason for the visit to the medical office.

**chlamydia**   a parasitic microorganism with properties common to bacteria but unable to sustain life without a host, in the manner of a virus.

**chronic**   long-standing.

**chronic obstructive pulmonary disease (COPD)**   progressive, irreversible condition with diminished respiratory capacity.

**chronological order**   placing in the order of time; usually the most recent is placed foremost.

**chyle**   milky, fatty product of digestion absorbed through the small intestines and returned to circulation by the lymphatics.

**chyme**   the thick, semiliquid mass of ingested food mixed with gastric juices as it passes from the stomach.

**cilia**   hairlike projections on cells that propel either the cell or objects that come in contact with the cell.

**circumcision**   surgical removal of the prepuce.

**civil law**   a branch of law that focuses on issues between private citizens.

**claims**   requests to an insurance company for reimbursement of costs.

**claims administrator**   an individual who manages the third-party reimbursement policies for a medical practice.

**clarification**   explanation; removal of confusion or uncertainty.

**clearinghouse**   a company that receives, reviews, sends, and manages insurance claims for physicians.

**CLIA certification**   required by any group that performs even one test, including a waived test on materials derived from the human body for the purpose of providing information for the diagnosis, prevention, or treatment of any disease or impairment of, or the assessment of the health of, human beings to meet certain federal requirements. See *Clinical Laboratory Improvement Amendments*.

**climacteric period**   menopause; developmental phase in which a woman's reproductive ability ceases.

**clinical**   pertaining to direct patient care (e.g., nonadministrative tasks that a medical assistant will perform).

**clinical chemistry**   the study of the presence and measurement of substances in the blood.

**clinical diagnosis**   a diagnosis based only on the patient's clinical symptoms.

**Clinical Laboratory Improvement Amendments (CLIA)**   guidelines established by Congress in 1988 to standardize and improve laboratory testing.

**Clinical and Laboratory Standards Institute (CLSI)**   a committee appointed to establish rules to ensure the safety, standards, and integrity of all testing performed on human specimens.

**Clinitest™**   most common test for reducing sugars.

**cloning**   genetically identical replication of cells, an organ, or an organism in the laboratory.

**closed captioning**   printed words displayed on a television screen to help people with hearing disabilities or impairments.

**closing**   a one- to two-word phrase that precedes the sender's signature and indicates the end of the letter.

**cloud storage**   storing data on a third-party remote database through online capabilities.

**clustering**   grouping patients with similar problems or needs.

**coagulate**   change from a liquid to a solid or semisolid mass.

**coagulation**   the study of the blood's ability to clot.

**coagulopathies**   diseases associated with abnormal blood clotting functions.

**cocci**   spherical bacteria.

**coinsurance**   the agreed-upon amount paid to the provider by a policyholder. Also called *copayment*.

**collagen**   protein substance that gives structure to the connective tissue.

**collection** a process of acquiring funds that are due.

**colpocleisis** surgery to occlude the vagina.

**colporrhaphy** suturing of the vagina.

**colposcopy** visual examination of the vagina and cervix under magnification.

**Commission on Office Laboratory Accreditation (COLA)** works to support the health care industry by providing knowledge and resources for maintaining quality laboratory operations.

**common law** traditional laws that were established by the English legal system.

**comparative negligence** a percentage of damage awards based on the contribution of negligence between two parties.

**competency assessment** evaluation of a person's ability to perform a test and to use a testing device.

**complete blood count (CBC)** the CBC is a frequently ordered laboratory test consisting of white blood cell count and differential, red blood cell count, hemoglobin, hematocrit, erythrocyte indices, and platelet count.

**compliance** willingness of a patient to follow a prescribed course of treatment.

**compliance officer** person charged with ensuring that a facility follows laws, policies, and protocols.

**concierge medicine** is a new type of medicine in which a patient pays an annual fee or retainer in exchange for enhanced care by the primary care physician.

**computed tomography (CT)** a diagnostic procedure that uses x-rays to produce cross-sectional views of internal body structures.

**concussion** injury to the brain due to trauma.

**confidentiality** protection of patient data from unauthorized personnel.

**confirmatory test** an additional, more specific test performed to rule out or confirm a preliminary test result to provide a final result.

**congenital anomaly** abnormality, either structural or functional, present at birth.

**congestive heart failure** condition in which the heart cannot pump effectively.

**conjugated bilirubin** bilirubin that does dissolve into the bloodstream.

**consent** an agreement between a patient and physician to do a given medical procedure.

**constellation of symptoms** a group of clinical signs indicating a particular disease process.

**consultation** request for assistance from one physician to another.

**continuing education units (CEUs)** credits awarded for attendance at approved local and state AAMA meetings and seminars, completion of guided study courses, and journal articles designed to submit a posttest for CEU credit.

**contract** an agreement between two or more parties for a given act.

**contracture** abnormal shortening of muscles around a joint caused by atrophy of the muscles and resulting in flexion and fixation.

**contraindication** situation or condition that prohibits the prescribing or administering of a drug or medication.

**contrast medium** substance ingested or injected into the body to facilitate imaging of internal structures.

**contributory negligence** a defense strategy in which the defendant admits to negligence but claims that the plaintiff assisted in promoting the damages.

**control** a device or solution used to monitor the test to ensure correct test results.

**contusion** collection of blood in the tissues after an injury; a bruise.

**conventions** general notes, symbols, typeface, format, and punctuation that direct and guide the coder to the most complete and accurate ICD-9 code.

**convoluted tubules** the twisted portion of the nephron that connects the glomerulus to the collecting tubules; consists of a proximal and a distal portion connected by the loop of Henle.

**convulsion** sudden, involuntary muscle contraction of a voluntary muscle group.

**cookies** tiny files that are left on your computer's hard drive by a website without your permission.

**coordination of benefits** the method of designating the order in which multiple carriers pay benefits to avoid duplication of payment.

**copayments** that part of an insured service the patient must pay.

**coping mechanisms** unconscious methods of alleviating intense stressors.

**coronary artery bypass graft** surgical procedure that increases the blood flow to the heart by bypassing the occluded or blocked vessel with a graft.

**corpora cavernosa** the erectile bodies of the penis or clitoris.

**corpus spongiosum** erectile tissue around the male urethra.

**corticoid** any of the hormonal steroid substances obtained from the adrenal cortex.

**cortisol** a naturally occurring steroidal hormone that regulates metabolism and acts as an anti-inflammatory agent.

**coumarin** an anticoagulant prescribed for persons likely to form blood clots, such as valve replacement recipients; also called *Coumadin* (trade name) or *warfarin*.

**covered entity** anyone required to follow the Health Insurance Portability and Accountability Act's requirements. Health care providers, insurance companies, and insurance clearinghouses are covered entities.

**cranium** the portion of the skull that encloses the brain.

**creatinine** a breakdown product of creatine that aids in delivering energy to cells.

**credit** balance in one's favor on an account; promise to pay a bill at a later date; record of a payment received.

**cretinism** severe congenital hypothyroidism; signs include dwarfism, low intelligence, puffy features, dry skin, macroglossia, and poor muscle tone.

**criteria** the standard, rule, or test by which something or someone can be judged.

**critical values** considered to be life-threatening test results.

**crossover claim** a claim that crosses over automatically from one coverage to another for payment.

**cross-reference** notation in a file telling that a record is stored elsewhere and giving the reference; verification to another source; checking the tabular list against the alphabetic list in ICD-9 coding.

**cryosurgery** the surgical destruction of tissue using freezing temperature with liquid nitrogen or carbon dioxide.

**cryptorchidism** one or both testicles that have not moved into the scrotum before birth. Also known as *undescended testicles*.

**cul-de-sac** blind pouch or cavity, as in the cul-de-sac that lies between the rectum and the posterior uterus.

**culdocentesis**   surgical puncture and aspiration of fluid from the vaginal cul-de-sac for diagnosis or therapy.

**culture**   a laboratory process whereby microorganisms are grown in a special medium often for the purpose of identifying a causative agent in an infectious disease; also means the way of life, including commonly held beliefs, of a group of people.

**curettage**   scraping of a body cavity, such as the uterus.

**Current Procedural Terminology**   a comprehensive list of codes used by physicians to bill for procedures and services.

**cursor**   flashing line on the monitor indicating where data input will occur.

**Cushing syndrome**   a disorder resulting from increased adrenocortical secretion of cortisol.

**CW testing site**   location where CLIA-waived testing takes place. See *Clinical Laboratory Improvement Amendments* and *Certificate of Waiver*.

**cyanotic**   a bluish discoloration of the skin due to the lack of oxygen.

**cystocele**   herniation of the urinary bladder into the vagina.

**cystoscopy**   direct visualization of the urinary bladder through a cystoscope inserted through the urethra.

**cytogenetics**   a type of cytology in which the genetic structure of the cells obtained from tissue, blood, or body fluids, such as amniotic fluid, is examined or tested for chromosome deficiencies related to genetic disease.

**cytology**   study of the microscopic structure of cells.

## D

**DACUM**   a code of educational standards for medical assisting students developed by the American Association of Medical Assistants.

**damages**   the resulting injury or suffering that resulted from negligence.

**data**   information that are stored and processed by the computer.

**database**   accumulation of files on the computer.

**daysheet/daily journal**   a daily business record of charges and payments.

**debit**   a charge or money owed on an account.

**decibel (db)**   unit of intensity of sound.

**deciduous**   to fall or shed; deciduous teeth: the set of 20 teeth appearing during infancy and shedding during childhood.

**decongestant**   substance that reduces congestion or swelling.

**deductible**   a specified amount paid by the policyholder before the carrier begins paying.

**defamation of character**   making false or malicious statements about a person's character or reputation.

**defendant**   the party that is accused.

**degenerative joint disease (DJD)**   also known as *osteoarthritis*; arthritis characterized by degeneration of the bony structure of the joints, usually noninflammatory.

**deglutition**   the act of swallowing.

**dehiscence**   separation or opening of the edges of a wound.

**demeanor**   the way a person looks, behaves, and conducts himself or herself.

**dementia**   progressive organic mental deterioration with loss of intellectual function.

**demographic**   relating to the statistical characteristics of populations.

**dendrite**   part of the neuron that transmits impulses toward the cell body.

**denial**   saying that something is not true; refusing to acknowledge.

**dental cavities**   holes in the teeth.

**dentin**   the main component of the tooth structure, surrounds the inner pulp and lies just below the enamel.

**Department of Health and Human Services (HHS)**   U.S. government's agency for protecting the health of all Americans and providing essential human services.

**dependent**   spouse, children, and sometimes other individuals designated by the insured who are covered under a health care plan.

**depolarization**   progressive wave of stimulation causing contraction of the myocardium.

**deposition**   a process in which one party questions another party under oath.

**dermatophytosis**   fungal infection of the skin.

**dermis**   layer of the skin under the epidermis.

**descriptor**   description of a service listed with its code number.

**desiccation**   inhibits microbial growth by removing the water required for metabolism.

**detoxification**   clearing of drugs from the body and treating the withdrawal symptoms.

**dextrocardia**   the condition of having the heart in the right side of the thoracic cavity.

**diabetes insipidus**   a disorder of metabolism characterized by polyuria and polydipsia; caused by a deficiency in antidiuretic hormone (ADH) or an inability of the kidneys to respond to ADH.

**diagnosis**   identification of a disease or condition by evaluating physical signs and symptoms, health history, and laboratory tests; a disease or condition identified in a person.

**diagnostic test**   medical test performed to aid in the diagnosis or detection of disease.

**diagnostic-related group (DRG)**   categories used to determine hospital and physician reimbursement for Medicare patients' inpatient services.

**dialysis**   removal of waste in blood not filtered by kidneys by passing fluid through a semipermeable barrier that allows normal electrolytes to remain, either with a machine with circulatory access or by passing a balanced fluid through the peritoneal cavity.

**diaphoresis**   profuse sweating.

**diaphragmatic excursion**   the movement of the diaphragm during respiration.

**diarthroses**   freely movable joints; also called *synovial joints*.

**diastole**   relaxation phase of the cardiac cycle.

**diction**   the style of speaking and enunciating words.

**dideoxycytidine (ddC)**   a drug used to treat AIDS by blocking the growth of the virus after it enters the T-cell lymphocytes.

**dideoxyinosine (ddI)**   a drug used to treat AIDS by blocking the growth of the virus after it enters the T-cell lymphocytes.

**diencephalon**   part of the brain lying beneath the hemispheres, containing the thalamus and hypothalamus.

**differential**   a blood test in which total WBCs and the individual amounts of the five types of WBCs are measured and recorded for analysis; also see WBC with differential.

**differential diagnosis**   a diagnosis made by comparing the patient's symptoms to two or more diseases that have similar symptoms.

**differential stain**   staining process that uses more than one chemical stain to better differentiate between different microorganisms or structures/cellular components of a single organism.

**diluent**  specified liquid used to reconstitute powder medications for injection.

**diplococci**  spherical cocci in pairs.

**diplomacy**  the art of handling people with tact and genuine concern.

**direct microscopic examination**  examination of a patient specimen using a microscope; a type of nonwaived testing.

**directory**  a "table of contents" of a file system.

**disaster**  a sudden and unplanned event that has the potential to cause damage to property or life; may be caused by an accident or by nature including weather events such as a hurricane.

**discrimination**  making a difference in favor of or against someone.

**disease**  definite pathologic process having a distinctive set of symptoms and course of progression.

**disinfectant**  a chemical that can be applied to objects to destroy microorganisms; will not destroy bacterial spores.

**disinfection**  killing or rendering inert most but not all pathogenic microorganisms.

**disk drive**  a device that gets information on and off a floppy disk.

**dissemination**  the process of distributing information on community resources.

**distal**  away from the origin.

**diuretics**  substances that promote the formation and excretion of urine.

**diurnal variation**  variation over a 24-hour period.

**documentation**  the process of recording patient information.

**donor**  one who contributes something to another.

**double booking**  the practice of booking two patients for the same period with the same physician.

**dowager's hump**  exaggerated cervical curve with prominence of the top thoracic vertebrae found in some osteoporotic elderly women; a type of kyphosis.

**downcoding**  assigning a CPT code, usually an evaluation and management code, at a lower level by a provider or by an insurance company.

**downloading**  transferring information from an outside location to your computer.

**dressing**  a covering applied directly to a wound to apply pressure, give support, absorb secretions, protect from trauma or microorganisms, stop or slow bleeding, or hide disfigurement.

**drug**  any substance that may modify one or more of the functions of an organism.

**due process**  a formal proceeding in which the accused is considered not guilty until a verdict is reached.

**dura mater**  the outer covering of the brain.

**durable power of attorney**  a legal document giving another person the authority to act on one's behalf.

**duress**  the act of compelling or forcing someone to do something that they do not want to do.

**dwarfism (endocrine or pituitary)**  abnormal underdevelopment of the body with extreme shortness but normal proportions; achondroplastic dwarfism is an inherited growth disorder characterized by shortened limbs and a large head but almost normal trunk proportions.

**dysmenorrhea**  painful menstruation.

**dyspareunia**  painful coitus or sexual intercourse.

**dysphagia**  inability to swallow or difficulty in swallowing.

**dysphasia**  difficulty speaking.

**dysphonia**  impairment of voice; hoarseness.

**dyspnea**  difficulty breathing.

**dysuria**  painful or difficult urination.

## E

**E-codes**  codes indicating the external cause or reason for an injury or illness.

**ecchymosis**  characteristic black and blue mark that results from blood as it accumulates under the skin.

**eczema**  superficial dermatitis.

**edema**  an accumulation of fluid within the tissues.

**edematous**  describes a swollen area due to excess tissue fluid.

**efferent**  carrying impulses away from the center.

**elastin**  protein substance that gives elasticity and flexibility to the connective tissues.

**electrocardiography**  procedure that produces a record of the electrical activity of the heart.

**electrode**  medium for conducting or detecting electrical current.

**electroencephalogram (EEG)**  tracing of the electrical activity of the brain.

**electrolyte balance**  having electrolytes in the right concentrations in order to maintain fluid balance among the compartments.

**electrolytes**  certain chemical substances dissolved in the blood and having numerous basic functions such as conducting electrical currents; the principal electrolytes are sodium, potassium, chloride, and bicarbonate.

**electromyography**  recording of electrical nerve transmission in skeletal muscles.

**electronic health records**  information about patients that is recorded and stored on computer.

**element**  a substance that cannot be separated or broken down into substances with properties other than its own; a primary substance.

**eligibility**  the determination of an insured's right to receive benefits from a third-party payer based on such criteria as payment of premiums and date of start of coverage.

**emancipated minor**  a patient under the age of majority but who is legally considered to be an adult.

**embolus**  mass of matter (thrombus, air, fat globule) freely floating in the circulatory system.

**emergency medical services (EMS)**  a group of health care providers working as a team to care for sick or injured patients before they arrive at the hospital.

**empathy**  the ability to understand or to some extent share what someone else is feeling.

**employee**  a person hired to perform given duties in return for financial compensation.

**enclosure**  indication for the reader that an item is accompanying the letter.

**encounter form**  a preprinted statement that lists codes for basic office charges and has sections to record charges incurred in an office visit, the patient's current balance, and next appointment.

**encryption**  scrambling e-mail messages as they leave one site and unscrambling them when they arrive at the designated address.

**endemic**  a disease that occurs continuously in a particular population but has a low mortality; used in contrast to epidemic.

**endocarditis**  inflammation of the inner lining of the heart.

**endocardium**   the innermost part of the heart wall; it lines the heart chamber and covers the connective tissue skeleton of the heart valves.

**endocrine**   system of glands that secrete a type of hormone directly into the bloodstream to regulate the body.

**endocrinologist**   a physician who specializes in disorders of the endocrine system.

**endogenous**   having its origin within an organism.

**endometrium**   the inner layer of the uterine wall.

**endorphins**   chemicals that are often called the body's "natural painkillers" that tend to produce a euphoria, or "good feeling." Release of endorphins is often caused by physical movement or exercise.

**endotracheal tube**   a large instrument usually inserted through the mouth (may use the nose) and into the trachea to the point of the tracheal division to deliver oxygen under pressure.

**enumerated**   counted.

**enuresis**   bed wetting.

**enzyme**   a protein that begins (catalyzes) a chemical reaction.

**eosinophil**   a type of leukocyte increased in allergic reactions and parasitic infections.

**E-Prescribe**   a prescriber's ability to send prescriptions electronically to a pharmacy.

**epicardium**   the inner or visceral layer of the pericardium that forms the outermost layer of the heart wall.

**epidermis**   outer layer of the skin.

**epiglottis**   the leaflike flap that closes down over the glottis during swallowing.

**epiphyseal end plate**   a thin layer of cartilage at the end of long bones where new growth takes place.

**episiotomy**   incision of the perineum to accommodate vaginal delivery of fetus.

**eponym**   word derived from a personal name, for example, *Alzheimer* disease.

**erectile dysfunction**   the inability of a male to get and keep an erection. May also be referred to as *impotence* or *ED*.

**erector pili muscle**   muscle that causes the hair to stand up when it contracts.

**ergonomic**   describes a workstation designed to prevent work-related injuries and to promote work efficiency.

**ergonomics**   the study of human physical characteristics and their environment to minimize the risk for injury through the use of appropriate adaptive equipment.

**erythema**   redness of the skin.

**erythematous**   characterized by redness (erythema).

**erythrasma**   bacterial skin infection occurring where skin touches skin, like between toes, in armpits, or groin.

**erythrocyte**   a red blood cell.

**erythrocyte indices**   three measurements (mean cell volume, mean cell hemoglobin, and mean cell hemoglobin concentration) that indicate the size of the red blood cell and how much hemoglobin the red blood cell holds.

**erythrocyte sedimentation rate**   measures the rate in millimeters per hour at which red blood cells settle out in a tube.

**erythropoietin**   a hormone produced mainly by the kidney in response to lowered oxygen levels; stimulates the production of red blood cells to increase blood oxygen levels.

**essential amino acids**   amino acids nutritionally required by an organism and that must be supplied in its diet (i.e., cannot be synthesized by the organism).

**ethernet**   system that allows the computer to be connected to a cable or DSL system.

**ethics**   guidelines for moral behavior that are enforced by peer groups.

**ethylene oxide**   gas used to sterilize surgical instruments and other supplies.

**etiology**   cause of disease.

**eunuchoidism**   deficient production of male hormone by the testes, resulting in loss of the secondary male characteristics.

**euphoria**   a feeling of well-being.

**eustachian tubes**   a mucous membrane-lined tube between the nasopharynx and the middle ear bilaterally that equalizes the internal and external otic air pressure.

**euthanasia**   allowing a patient to die with minimal medical interventions.

**evacuated tube**   a type of blood collection tube that is sealed with a premeasured, partial vacuum. The tube receives the patient's blood during venipuncture.

**evaluation**   the process of indicating how well the patient or person is progressing toward a particular goal; to appraise; to determine the worth or quality of something or someone.

**exocrine**   glands that release enzymes through ducts, including mammary glands, salivary glands, sweat glands, and glands that secrete digestive enzymes into the stomach and intestine.

**exogenous**   having its origin outside of the organism; its opposite is endogenous.

**exophthalmia**   abnormal protrusion of the eyeballs.

**exophthalmic goiter**   abnormal protrusion of the eyeballs accompanied by goiter.

**expected threshold**   a numerical goal.

**expert witness**   a professional who testifies on the standard of care in a trial.

**explanation of benefits (EOB)**   a statement that accompanies a payment from an insurance carrier and outlines which dates and services are being paid.

**exposure control plan**   written plan required by the Occupational Safety and Health Administration that outlines an employer's system for preventing infection.

**exposure risk factors**   conditions that tend to put employees at risk for contact with biohazardous agents such as bloodborne pathogens.

**express consent**   a statement of approval from the patient for the physician to perform a given procedure after the patient has been educated about the risks and benefits of the particular procedure; also referred to as informed consent.

**express contracts**   formal agreements between two or more people.

**expulsion**   formal discharge from a professional organization.

**external control**   monitors the test from applying the specimen to result interpretation; controls the performance of the test.

**externship**   an educational course that allows the student to obtain hands-on experience. Also referred to as practicum.

**extracellular**   outside of the cell.

**extraocular**   outside the eye, as in extraocular eye movement.

**eyewashes**   used to irrigate and flush the eyes following a hazardous exposure.

**F**

**familial**   referring to a disorder that tends to occur more often in a family than would be anticipated solely by chance.

**Family and Medical Leave Act**   a law designed to allow an employee up to 12 weeks of unpaid leave from his or her job to meet family needs.

**fascia**  fibrous membrane tissue that covers and supports the muscles and joins the skin with underlying tissue.

**fast**  to abstain from eating or drinking anything but water; often done before a medical test or procedure.

**febrile**  having an above-normal body temperature.

**Federal Insurance Contributions Act (FICA)**  the law that established Social Security and that mandates Social Security tax payments and benefits.

*Federal Register*  official daily publication of the federal government; includes rules, proposed rules, notices of federal agencies and organizations, executive orders, and other presidential documents.

**federal unemployment tax**  tax used to finance all administrative expenses of the federal/state unemployment insurance system and the federal costs involved in extended benefits.

**fee-for-service**  an established set of fees charged for specific services and paid by the patient or insurance carrier.

**fee schedule**  a list of pre-established fee allowances set for specific services and procedures performed by a provider.

**fee splitting**  sharing of fees between physicians for patient referrals.

**feedback**  in communication, the response to input from another.

**fibrinolysis**  normal body process that keeps naturally occurring blood clots from growing and causing problems; the normal breakdown of clots.

**file**  grouping of data that is given a name for easy access.

**filing system**  a method for organizing records so that they can be found when needed.

**film**  raw material on which x-rays are projected through the body; prior to processing, it does not contain a visible image (similar to photographic film).

**fixative**  a chemical substance used to bind, fix, or stabilize specimens of tissue to slides for later examination.

**flagella**  hairlike extremity of a bacterium or protozoan; used to facilitate movement.

**flanges**  extensions on the sides of the rim of the needle holder to aid in tube placement and removal.

**floppy disk**  thin magnetic film on which to store data.

**flow sheet**  color-coded sheets that allow information to be recorded in graphic or tabular form for easy retrieval; form that gathers all the important data regarding a patient's condition and stays in the patient's chart as a reminder of care and a record of whether care expectations have been met.

**fluorescein angiography**  intravenous injection of fluorescent dye; photographing blood vessels of the eye as the dye moves through them.

**fluoroscopy**  special x-ray technique for examining a body part by immediate projection onto a fluorescent screen.

**folate**  a salt of folic acid; it acts to help enzymes that build structures such as blood cells.

**folliculitis**  inflammation of hair follicles.

**font**  a typeface; affects the way written messages look.

**Food and Drug Administration (FDA)**  responsible for protecting and promoting public health through the regulation and supervision of blood transfusions, medical devices, and other medically and nonmedically related products.

**for cause**  drug screening required by an employer following a questionable event.

**forced expiratory volume (FEV)**  volume of air forced out of the lungs.

**forceps**  surgical instrument used to grasp, handle, compress, pull, or join tissues, equipment, or supplies.

**fraud**  a deceitful act with the intention to conceal the truth.

**fulgurate**  destroy tissue by electrodessication.

**full block**  a type of letter format in which all letter components are justified left.

**full-thickness burn**  burn that has destroyed all skin layers.

**furuncle**  infection in a hair follicle or gland; characterized by pain, redness, and swelling with necrosis of tissue in the center.

## G

**gait**  manner or style of walking.

**galactosuria**  condition in newborns lacking an enzyme that metabolizes galactose; increased levels of galactose appear in the blood and urine (if proper therapy is not initiated, mental retardation and other difficulties will occur).

**gastroenteritis**  inflammation of the gastrointestinal tract caused by bacteria or viruses.

**gauge**  diameter of a needle lumen.

**gauze sponges**  pads that come in multiple sizes depending open their use in various clinical areas.

**gel separator**  a nonreacting substance located in an evacuated tube that forms a physical barrier between the cells and serum or plasma after the specimen has been centrifuged.

**generic name**  official name given to a drug whose patent has expired.

**Genetic Information Nondiscrimination Act**  a federal law to protect against discrimination based on a person or their family's genetic information.

**germicide**  chemical that kills most pathogenic microorganisms; disinfectant.

**gerontologist**  specialist who studies aging.

**gestation**  period of time from conception to birth; usually 37 to 41 weeks.

**gestational diabetes**  a disorder characterized by an impaired ability to metabolize carbohydrates, usually due to insulin deficiency, occurring in pregnancy and usually disappearing after delivery.

**gigantism**  excessive size and stature caused most frequently by hypersecretion of the human growth hormone (HGH).

**gingiva**  the gums; the mucous membrane–covered tissues that support the teeth.

**glaucoma**  abnormal increase in the fluid in the eye, usually as a result of obstructed outflow, resulting in degeneration of the intraocular components and blindness.

**glomerulus**  a small cluster of blood vessels within the Bowman capsule.

**glucose oxidase**  very specific testing method for measuring glucose.

**glycosuria**  the presence of glucose in the urine.

**goiter**  an enlargement of the thyroid gland.

**gonads**  a generic term referring to the sex glands of both sexes, either ovaries or testes.

**goniometer**  instrument used to measure the angle of joints for range of motion.

**Goodell sign**  softening of the cervix early in pregnancy.

**Gram negative**  describes bacteria that lose the purple color of the Gram stain when exposed to the ethyl alcohol and appear pink.

**Gram positive**  describes bacteria that keep the purple color of the Gram stain even when exposed to the ethyl alcohol.

**Gram stain**   primary stain used in the microbiology lab.

**granulocytes**   white blood cells that have visible granules when stained.

**Grave disease**   pronounced hyperthyroidism with signs of enlarged thyroid and exophthalmos.

**gravid**   pregnant.

**gravida**   pregnant woman.

**gravidity**   pregnancy.

**grief**   great sadness caused by loss.

**gross hematuria**   large amount of blood in the urine.

**gross income**   the amount of money earned by an employee before taxes are withheld.

**group member**   a policyholder who is a member of a group and covered by the group's insurance carrier.

**guaiac**   substance used in laboratory tests for occult blood in the stool.

**gyri**   the convolutions of the brain tissue.

## H

**hard drive**   a place where the computer stores programs and data files.

**hardship**   a circumstance or misfortune beyond the control of the patient or guarantor causing an unforeseen financial emergency resulting in suffering or deprivation.

**hardware**   equipment on the computer system, for example, keyboard, disk drive, monitor, and printer.

**Hashimoto thyroiditis**   diffuse infiltration of the thyroid gland with lymphocytes, resulting in diffuse goiter and hypothyroidism.

**HCFA**   *see* Health Care Financing Administration.

**HCPCS**   *see* Health Care Financing Administration Common Procedures Coding System.

**Healthcare Common Procedure Coding System**   American Medical Association's coding system based on CPT-4. Assigns alphabetic and numeric codes to items such as ambulance service, wheelchairs, and injections.

**Health Care Financing Administration (HCFA)**   a federal agency that regulates health care financing and the procedural classification (Volume 3 of the ICD-9-CM coding book).

**Health Care Financing Administration Common Procedures Coding System (HCPCS)**   a numerical system used by HCFA for services not covered by the CPT coding system.

**Health Information Technology for Economic and Clinical Health (HITECH) Act**   law enacted as part of the American Recovery and Reinvestment Act of 2009 to promote the adoption and meaningful use of health information technology.

**health care savings accounts (HSAs)**   a benefit offered by some employers that allows employees to save money through payroll deduction to accounts that can only be used for medical care.

**health insurance**   a policy that promises to pay some or all of a customer's medical bills.

**Health Insurance Portability and Accountability Act (HIPAA)**   federal law, originally passed as the Kassebaum–Kennedy Act, that requires all health care settings to ensure privacy and security of patient information. Also requires health insurance to be accessible for working Americans and available when changing employment.

**health maintenance organization (HMO)**   an organization that provides a wide range of services through a contract with a specified group at a predetermined payment.

**heat cramps**   type of hyperthermia that causes muscle cramping resulting from high-sodium heat exhaustion; hyperthermia resulting from physical exertion in heat without adequate fluid replacement.

**heat exhaustion**   a type of hyperthermia that causes an altered mental status due to inadequate fluid replacement.

**heat stroke**   most serious type of hyperthermia; body is no longer able to compensate for elevated temperature.

**helminthes**   a category of parasitic organisms whose eggs, or ova, are microscopic but the actual organism may be visible without the aid of a microscope; also referred to as worms.

**hemochromatosis**   disorder that increases the amount of iron in the patients' blood to dangerous levels.

**hematemesis**   vomiting blood or bloody vomitus.

**hematocrit**   the percentage of red blood cells in whole blood.

**hematology**   the study of blood and blood-forming tissues.

**hematoma**   blood clot that forms at an injury site.

**hematopoiesis**   blood cell production; also known as *hemopoiesis*.

**hematuria**   blood in the urine.

**hemoconcentration**   decrease in the volume of plasma in the blood causing an increase in blood components. Can be caused by excessive application of the tourniquet.

**hemoglobin**   the functioning unit of the red blood cell.

**hemoglobinuria**   presence of free hemoglobin in urine.

**hemolysis**   rupture of erythrocytes with the release of hemoglobin into the plasma or serum causing the specimen to appear pink or red in color.

**hemolytic anemia**   a disorder characterized by premature destruction of the red cells; this may be brought on by an infectious process, inherited red cell disorders, or as a response to certain drugs or toxins.

**hemoptysis**   coughing up blood from the respiratory tract.

**hemostasis**   process that results in control of bleeding after an injury.

**hemostat**   surgical instrument with slender jaws used for grasping blood vessels.

**heparin**   a naturally occurring anticoagulant given to prevent clot formation.

**hepatomegaly**   enlarged liver.

**hepatotoxin**   substance that can damage the liver.

**hereditary**   referring to traits or disorders that are transmitted from parent to offspring.

**hernia**   protrusion of an organ through the muscle wall of the cavity that normally surrounds it.

**herpes simplex**   infection caused by the herpes simplex virus.

**herpes zoster**   infection caused by reactivation of varicella zoster virus, which causes chickenpox.

**hiatus**   an opening or gap; hiatal hernia: a protrusion of part of the stomach upward through the diaphragm.

**HIPAA**   *see* Health Insurance Portability and Accountability Act.

**Hippocratic Oath**   a code of ethics written by Hippocrates.

**hirsutism**   abnormal or excessive growth of hair in women.

**histamine**   substance found normally in the body in response to injured cells, producing the inflammatory process: dilation of capillaries, increased gastric secretions, and contraction of smooth muscles.

**histology**   study of the microscopic structure of tissue.

**HITECH**   Health Information Technology for Economic and Clinical Health Act; law enacted as part of the American Recovery and Reinvestment Act of 2009 to promote the adoption and meaningful use of health information technology.

**homeopathic**   referring to an alternative type of medicine in which patients are treated with small doses of substances that produce similar symptoms and use the body's own healing abilities.

**homeostasis**   maintaining a constant internal environment by balancing positive and negative feedback.

**hordeolum**   an infection of any of the lacrimal glands of the eyelids, causing redness, swelling, and pain.

**hormone**   a substance that is produced by an endocrine gland and travels through the blood to a distant organ or gland where it acts to modify the structure or function of that gland or organ.

**human chorionic gonadotropin (hCG)**   hormone secreted by the placenta and found in the urine and blood of a pregnant female.

**human immunodeficiency virus (HIV)**   virus that causes acquired immunodeficiency syndrome (AIDS); the immune system begins to fail, leading to life-threatening opportunistic infections.

**humidifier**   appliance that increases the moisture content in the air.

**hydrocele**   a fluid-filled sac surrounding one or both testicles that results in swelling of the scrotum.

**hydrogen ion**   hydrogen that is missing an electron and therefore readily binds with substances having extra electrons; it is an important constituent of acids.

**hypercalcemia**   an excessive amount of calcium in the blood.

**hyperchromia**   increased hemoglobin in red blood cells.

**hyperextend**   extend beyond the normal range of motion.

**hyperglycemia**   an increase in blood sugar, as in diabetes mellitus.

**hyperopia**   farsightedness.

**hyperosmolarity**   a condition of having increased numbers of dissolved substances in the plasma.

**hyperplasia**   excessive proliferation of normal cells in the normal tissue arrangement of an organism.

**hyperpnea**   abnormally deep, gasping breaths.

**hyperpyrexia**   dangerously high temperature, 105° to 106°F.

**hypersensitivities**   the immune system responds inappropriately or too intensely to harmless compounds.

**hypertension**   morbidly high blood pressure.

**hyperthermia**   general condition of excessive body heat.

**hyperventilation**   a respiratory rate that greatly exceeds the body's oxygen demands.

**hypochromia**   red blood cells appearing paler with more area of central pallor.

**hypoglycemia**   deficiency of sugar (glucose) in the blood.

**hypopnea**   shallow respirations.

**hypothalamus**   part of the diencephalon; activates and controls the peripheral nervous system, endocrine system, and certain involuntary functions.

**hypothermia**   below-normal body temperature.

**hypovolemic shock**   shock caused by loss of blood or other body fluids.

**hysterosalpingogram**   radiograph of the uterus and fallopian tubes after injection with a contrast medium.

**hysteroscopy**   visual examination with magnification of the uterus.

**I**

**iatrogenic**   a condition caused by treatment or medical procedures.

**idiopathic**   unknown etiology.

**immune globulins**   proteins produced by plasma cells in response to foreign antigens; provide immediate antibody protection for a few weeks to a few months.

**immunity**   lack of susceptibility to a disease.

**immunization**   act or process of rendering an individual immune to specific disease.

**immunodeficiency**   parts of the immune system fail to provide an adequate response.

**immunohematology**   the study of blood typing and compatibility testing for transfusion.

**immunology**   the study of antigen–antibody reactions.

**impetigo**   highly infectious skin infection causing erythema and progressing to honey-colored crusts.

**implementation**   the process of initiating and carrying out an action such as a teaching plan or patient treatment.

**implied consent**   an informal agreement of approval from the patient to perform a given task.

**implied contracts**   contracts between physician and patient not written but assumed by the actions of the parties.

**impotence**   inability to achieve or maintain an erection.

**incident report**   a form used by an organization to document an unusual occurrence to a patient, visitor, or employee.

**incontinence**   inability to control elimination, either urine or feces or both.

**independent practice association (IPA)**   several independently practicing physicians contracted with a health maintenance organization to provide services to health maintenance organization members.

**indices (singular, index)**   numbers expressing a property or ratio.

**induration**   hardened area at the injection site after an intradermal screening test for tuberculosis.

**infarction**   death of tissues due to lack of oxygen.

**infection**   invasion by disease-producing microorganisms.

**infiltration**   leakage of intravenous fluids into surrounding tissues.

**informed consent**   a statement of approval from the patient for the physician to perform a given procedure after the patient has been educated about the risks and benefits of the procedure; also referred to as expressed consent.

**inguinal**   pertaining to the regions of the groin.

**inpatient**   a medical setting in which patients are admitted for diagnostic, radiographic, or treatment purposes.

**insertion**   a place of attachment, usually the freely movable portion of a muscle.

**inspection**   visual examination.

**installment**   partial payment of a bill.

**institutional review board**   internal committee that reviews ethical issues.

**insufflator**   device for blowing air, gas, or powder into a body cavity.

**insula**   fifth lobe of the cerebrum.

**insulin-dependent diabetes mellitus**   a deficiency in insulin production that leads to an inability to metabolize carbohydrates.

**insured**   an individual who owns a policy that promises to pay some or all of his or her medical bills.

**interaction**   effects, positive or negative, of two or more drugs taken by a patient.

**intercaps**   words or phrases with unusual capitalization.

**interferon**   group of proteins released by white blood cells and fibroblasts when the invading microorganism is a virus.

**intermittent**   occurring at intervals.

**internal control**   control built into the testing device.

**Internal Revenue Service (IRS)**   a federal agency that regulates and enforces various taxes.

**International Classification of Diseases, Ninth or Tenth Revision, Clinical Modification**   a system for transforming verbal descriptions of disease, injuries, and conditions to numeric (ICD-9) or alphanumeric (ICD-10) codes.

**international normalized ratio**   a standardized result calculated from the patient's prothrombin time (PT) and a reference standard used to measure blood clotting time; also known as an INR.

**Internet**   global system used to connect one computer to another.

**interosseous**   between bones.

**interstitial**   the spaces between the cells.

**intertrigo**   rash of the body folds.

**intracellular**   inside of the cell.

**intranet**   a private network system of computers.

**intraocular pressure**   pressure within the eyeball.

**intrauterine pregnancy (IUP)**   pregnancy located in the uterus.

**intravascular coagulation**   clot formation within the vessels; strands of fibrin may form from one wall of the vessel to the other and shear red cells as they pass by.

**intravenous pyelogram (IVP)**   radiography using contrast medium to evaluate kidney function.

**intrinsic**   found within a structure.

**introitus**   vaginal orifice.

**invoice**   a statement of debt owed; a bill.

**iodine**   an element that is an essential micronutrient used in the thyroid gland to manufacture its hormones; present in seafood, foods grown in iodized soil, iodized salt, and some dairy products.

**ion**   an atom or group of atoms that has become electrically charged by the loss or gain of one or more electrons.

**iontophoresis**   introduction of various chemical ions into the skin by means of electrical current.

**ischemia**   decrease in oxygen to tissues.

**isolate**   separate from any other microorganisms present.

## J

**jaundiced**   bilirubin settles into the skin and sclera, making the patient appear yellow.

**job description**   a statement that informs an employee about the duties and expectations for a given job.

**Joint Commission, The**   a voluntary organization that sets and evaluates the standards of care for health care institutions (formerly The Joint Commission on Accreditation of Healthcare Organizations); based on The Joint Commission evaluation, an accreditation title will be given to the organization.

## K

**Kaposi sarcoma**   cancer of the skin that is extremely rare except in AIDS patients.

**Kegel exercises**   isometric exercises in which the muscles of the pelvic floor are voluntarily contracted and relaxed while urinating.

**keratin**   a tough, insoluble protein substance of the stratum corneum, hair, and nails.

**keratoses (senile)**   premalignant overgrowth or thickening of the upper layer of epithelium or horny layer of the skin.

**keratosis**   skin condition characterized by overgrowth and thickening.

**ketoacidosis**   acidosis accompanied by an accumulation of ketones in the body.

**ketones**   the end products of fat and protein metabolism.

**key components**   the criteria or factors on which the selection of a CPT-4 evaluation and management is based.

**kinesics**   a form of nonverbal communication including gestures, body movements, and facial expressions.

**Kirby–Bauer method**   manual technique for sensitivity testing.

**kit**   a packaged set containing test devices, instructions, reagents, and supplies needed to perform a test and generate results.

**Krebs cycle**   a sequence of reactions within cells that metabolizes sugars and other energy sources, such as carbohydrates, proteins, and fats, into carbon dioxide, water, and adenosine triphosphate.

**kyphosis (dowager's hump)**   abnormally deep dorsal curvature of the thoracic spine; also known as *humpback* or *hunchback*.

## L

**laboratory**   a place where research, investigation, or scientific testing takes place.

**laboratory procedure manual**   Clinical Laboratory Improvement Amendments regulations require each laboratory to have its own procedure manual describing how to perform every test in the laboratory.

**laparoscopy**   process of viewing the internal abdominal cavity and its contents through a specialized endoscope.

**laparotomy**   incision of the abdominal cavity.

**laryngectomy**   surgical removal of the larynx.

**laser ablation**   destruction or removal of tissue by the use of laser.

**late effects**   conditions that result from another condition. For example, left-sided paralysis may be a *late effect* of a stroke.

**lead**   electrode or electrical connection attached to the body to record electrical impulses in the body, especially the heart or brain.

**learning objectives**   steps that need to be achieved to accomplish the learning goal.

**learning goal**   an agreed-upon outcome of the teaching process.

**ledger card**   a record of the patient's financial activities; a continuous record of business transactions with debits and credits.

**legally required disclosure**   reporting of certain events to governmental agencies without the patient's consent.

**lentigines**   brown skin macules occurring after exposure to the sun; freckles; tan or brown macules found on elderly skin after prolonged sun exposure; also known as *liver spots*.

**leukocyte**   a white blood cell.

**leukocyte esterase**   an enzyme present in the leukocytes; a reagent strip test that is positive for leukocyte esterase can identify a urinary tract infection.

**leukocytosis**   abnormal increase of leukocytes (white blood cells).

**leukopenia**   diminished numbers of leukocytes.

**leukoplakia**   white, thickened patches on the oral mucosa or tongue that are often precancerous.

**liabilities**   amounts the practice owes.

**libel**   written statements that defame a person's reputation or character.

**licensure**   granting of a license or legal permission to perform a certain profession.

**ligament**   a flexible band of tissue that holds joints together.

**lightening**   the descent of the fetus in the pelvis.

**limiting charge**   the total amount that can be charged for covered services by providers who do not participate with Medicare, which is 115% of the nonparticipating Medicare fee schedule.

**lipase**   any of several enzymes that begin the breakdown of fats in the digestive tract.

**lipids**   any of the free fatty acids (fats) in the body.

**lipoproteins**   a substance made up of a lipid and a protein.

**literary search**   finding professional journal articles on a given subject.

**lithotripsy**   crushing of a stone with sound waves.

**litigation**   process of filing or contesting a lawsuit.

**lochia**   uterine discharge following childbirth, composed of some blood, mucus, and tissue.

**locum tenens**   a substitute physician.

**log-in**   use of a password to gain access to the computer.

**loop of Henle**   a portion of the renal tubule that is shaped like a U and consisting of a thick ascending and thin descending vessels.

**lordosis**   abnormally deep ventral curve at the lumbar flexure of the spine; also known as *swayback.*

**lubricant**   agent that reduces friction.

**Luer adapter**   a device for connecting a syringe or evacuated holder to the needle to promote a secure fit.

**lumen**   bore; hollow interior of a needle.

**lymphedema**   obstruction of the lymphatic system.

**lymphocyte**   a type of leukocyte.

**lyse**   to cause disintegration; that is, destruction of adhesions or the breakdown of red blood cells.

## M

**macrocytosis**   abnormally large red blood cells with a mean corpuscular volume above 95 fL.

**macrophage**   a monocyte that has left the circulation and settled and matured in tissue; macrophages process antigens and present them to T cells, activating the immune-specific response.

**macule**   small, flat discoloration of the skin.

**magnetic resonance imaging**   imaging technique that uses a strong magnetic field.

**main terms**   words in a multiple-word diagnosis that a coder should locate in the alphabetic listing. They represent the condition (not the location) to be coded.

**mainframe**   central computer to which individual computers are connected; used in large institutions.

**malaise**   general feeling of illness without specific signs or symptoms.

**malignant**   cancerous.

**malocclusion**   abnormal contact between the teeth in the upper and lower jaw.

**malpractice**   a tort in which the patient is harmed by the actions of a health care worker.

**managed care**   the practice of third-party payers to control costs by requiring physicians to adhere to specific rules as a condition of payment.

**manipulation**   skillful use of the hands in diagnostic procedures.

**Mantoux**   intradermal injection screening test for tuberculosis.

**margin**   the blank space around the edges of a piece of paper, such as a letter or page of a book.

**masticate**   the act of chewing or grinding, as in chewing food.

**material safety Data sheet (MSDS)**   a detailed record of all characteristics and protection required from a hazardous substance.

**matrix**   a system for blocking off unavailable patient appointment times.

**media**   a liquid, semisolid, or solid nutrient used for growing bacteria from culture specimens.

**mediastinum**   the midportion of the thoracic cavity containing the heart, the great vessels, the upper esophagus, and the trachea.

**medical asepsis**   removal or destruction of microorganisms.

**medical assistant**   a multiskilled health professional who performs a variety of clinical and administrative tasks in a medical setting.

**medical history**   record containing information about a patient's past and present health status.

**medical necessity**   a determination made by a third party that a certain service or procedure was necessary based on sound medical practice.

**medical setting**   a place that is designed to meet the health care needs of patients; may be inpatient or outpatient.

**Medicare**   a federal health insurance coverage for individuals 65 years and older and disabled individuals.

**Medicare Administrative Contractors (MACs)**   companies contracted by CMS to process claims from providers for services rendered to Medicare beneficiaries.

**Medi–Medi Claim**   Medicare beneficiary with Medicaid as the secondary payer.

**medulla oblongata**   part of the brain that controls breathing, heart rate, and blood pressure.

**megabyte**   one million bytes; a way to measure the quantity of computer information that a particular device can hold.

**meiosis**   the cell division specific to sperm and ova that results in 23 chromosomes rather than 46 (23 pairs).

**melanin**   dark pigment that gives color to the skin, hair, and eyes.

**melanocyte**   cell that produces melanin.

**melena**   black, tarry stools caused by digested blood from the gastrointestinal tract.

**memorandum**   a type of written documentation used for interoffice communication.

**menarche**   onset of first menstruation.

**meninges**   membranes of the spinal cord and brain.

**meningocele**   meninges protruding though the spinal column.

**meniscus**   the curved upper surface of a liquid in a container.

**menorrhagia**   excessive bleeding during menstruation.

**menses**   menstruation; bloody discharge monthly or cyclically in the female when fertilization has not occurred.

**mensuration**   the act or process of measuring.

**message**   words sent from one person to another; information sent through spoken, written, or body language.

**metabolic acidosis**  an acidic condition of the body caused when excess acids are produced in the body's fluids (as in the metabolism of fats instead of glucose) or when the body's natural bicarbonates are lost or diminished.

**metabolism**  sum of chemical processes that result in growth, energy production, elimination of waste, and body functions performed as digested nutrients are distributed; conversion of oxygen and calories to energy.

**methicillin-resistant** *Staphylococcus aureus*  a strain of *Staphylococcus aureus* bacteria that is resistant to many antibiotics used to treat *Staphylococcus* skin infections. Commonly abbreviated MRSA.

**metric system**  system of measurement that uses grams, liters, and meters.

**metrorrhagia**  irregular uterine bleeding.

**microalbumin**  tiny bits of albumin that appear in the urine in early kidney disease.

**microbiology**  the study of pathogen identification and antibiotic susceptibility determination.

**microcytosis**  red blood cells are smaller than usual.

**microfiche**  sheets of microfilm.

**microfilm**  photographs of records in a reduced size.

**microhematuria**  the amount of blood in the urine is so small that the color of the specimen is not affected.

**microorganisms**  microscopic living organisms.

**microprocessor**  a chip that allows the computer to function.

**micturition**  also known as *voiding* or *urination*.

**midbrain**  part of the brainstem, responsible for relaying messages.

**migraine**  type of severe headache, usually unilateral; may appear in clusters.

**minerals**  inorganic substances (such as sodium, potassium, calcium, phosphorus, magnesium, iron, iodine, fluorine, zinc, copper, cobalt, and chromium) used in the formation of hard and soft body tissue; necessary for muscle contraction, nerve conduction, and blood clotting.

**mission statement**  a statement describing the goals of the medical office and those it serves.

**modem**  (modulator/demodulator) a communication device that connects a computer to the standard telephone system, allowing information exchange with other computers off-site.

**modifiers**  letters or numbers added to a code to clarify the service or procedure.

**monocyte**  a type of leukocyte.

**monosaccharide**  a simple sugar that cannot be broken down further.

**mordant**  a substance used to fix, or bind, dyes or stains.

**morphology**  description of the structural characteristics of blood cells.

**motherboard**  fiberglass board that contains the central processing unit (CPU), memory, and other pieces of circuitry.

**mourning**  to demonstrate signs of grief; grieving.

**multidisciplinary**  involving many disciplines; a group of health care professionals from various specialties brought together to meet the patient's needs.

**multimedia**  various forms of communication available on the computer, for example, stereophonic sound, animation, full motion video, and photographs.

**multipara**  woman who has given birth to more than one viable fetus.

**multisample needle**  used with the evacuated tube method of blood collection because multiple tubes of blood can be drawn during a multitube draw without removing the needle from the vein. The end of the needle that penetrates the stopper of the tube has a retractable rubber sleeve that covers it when the tube is removed and prevents leaks during tube changes.

**multiskilled health professional**  an individual with versatile training in the health care field.

**muscular dystrophies**  a group of genetically transmitted diseases characterized by progressive atrophy of skeletal muscles.

**mycology**  the science and study of fungi.

**mycoses**  diseases caused by fungi.

**myelofibrosis**  a disorder in which bone marrow tissue develops in abnormal sites such as the liver and spleen; signs include immature cells in the circulation, anemia, and splenomegaly.

**myelogram**  invasive radiologic test in which dye is injected into the spinal fluid.

**myelomeningocele**  protrusion of the spinal cord through the spinal defect; spina bifida.

**myocardial infarction (MI)**  death of cardiac muscle due to lack of blood flow to the muscle; also known as *heart attack*.

**myocarditis**  inflammation of the myocardial layer of the heart.

**myocardium**  the middle layer of the walls of the heart, composed of cardiac muscle.

**myofibrils**  a slender light/dark strand of muscle tissue in striated muscle.

**myoglobin**  protein found in skeletal and cardiac muscle; very sensitive indicator of muscle injury.

**myopia**  nearsightedness.

**myringotomy**  incision into the tympanic membrane to relieve pressure.

**myxedema**  the most severe form of hypothyroidism; signs include edema of the extremities and the face.

## N

**narrative**  a paragraph indicating the contact with the patient, what was done for the patient, and the outcome of any action.

**nasal septum**  wall or partition dividing the nostrils.

**National Provider Identifier (NPI)**  the 10-digit identification number assigned to all health care providers as part of the HIPAA Administration Simplification Standard.

**nebulizer**  device for administering respiratory medications as a fine inhaled spray.

**needle disposal unit**  container for the disposal of used needles, lancets, and other sharp objects in a puncture-resistant, leakproof disposable container.

**needle holder**  type of surgical forceps used to hold and pass suture through tissue.

**negative feedback**  a decrease in function in response to a stimulus.

**negative stress**  stress that does not allow for relaxation periods.

**negligence**  performance of an act that a reasonable health care worker would not have done or the omission of an act that a reasonable person would have done.

**neonatologist**  physician who specializes in the care and treatment of newborns.

**neoplasm**  abnormal growth of new tissue; tumor.

**nephron**   the portion of the kidney responsible for the production of urine.

**nephrostomy**   placement of a catheter in the kidney pelvis to drain urine from an obstructed kidney.

**net pay**   the amount of money an employee is paid after all taxes are withheld.

**networking**   a system of personal and professional relationships through which to share information.

**neurogenic shock**   shock that results from dysfunction of nervous system following spinal cord injury.

**neuron**   a nerve cell.

**neurotransmitter**   chemical needed to transmit a message between synapses.

**neutral pH**   pH = 7, neither an acid nor a base.

**neutrophil**   the most abundant leukocyte and the main granulocyte.

**nitrite**   a factor used to assess the presence of bacteria in urine.

**nitrogenous**   pertaining to or containing nitrogen, usually the end product of protein metabolism.

**nitroprusside**   a compound that reacts with ketones to produce a purple reaction.

**nocturia**   excessive urination at night.

**non compos mentis**   mental incompetence.

**noncompliance**   the patient's inability or refusal to follow prescribed orders.

**non–insulin-dependent diabetes mellitus (NIDDM)**   a type of diabetes in which patients do not require insulin to control the blood sugar.

**nonlanguage**   not expressed in spoken language, for example, laughing, sobbing, grunting, and sighing.

**nonwaived testing**   complex tests that do not meet the Clinical Laboratory Improvements Amendments' criteria for waiver and require training and specific quality measures to ensure the accuracy and reliability of test results.

**normal flora**   microorganisms normally found in the body; also known as *resident flora*.

**normal value**   acceptable range as established for an age, a population, or a sex; variations usually indicate a disorder.

**nosocomial infection**   infection acquired in a medical setting, generally presumed to be in a hospital setting but may also refer to the medical office.

**NPO**   patient must have nothing by mouth after midnight until the procedure is done; patient cannot have water.

**nuclear medicine**   branch of medicine that uses radioactive isotopes to diagnose and treat disease.

**nulligravida**   a woman who has never been pregnant.

**nullipara**   a woman who has never given birth to a viable fetus.

**numeric filing**   arranging files by a numbered order.

**nutrition**   the study of food and how it is used for growth, nourishment, and repair.

**O**

**obligate**   to require; a parasite that has no choice but to attach to a living organism.

**obligate intracellular parasite**   requires a living host for replication and survival.

**obstipation**   extreme constipation.

**obturator**   smooth, rounded, removable inner portion of a hollow tube, such as an anoscope, that allows for easier insertion.

**occult**   hidden or concealed from observation.

**Occupational Safety and Health Administration (OSHA)**   the federal agency that oversees working conditions, with the mission to protect employees from work-related hazards.

**olecranon fossa**   the depression in the posterior surface of the humerus that allows the arm to extend by receiving the olecranon process.

**olecranon process**   the proximal end of the ulna that becomes the point of the elbow that fits into the olecranon fossa.

**oligomenorrhea**   scanty menstruation.

**oliguria**   scanty urine production.

**oncology**   the medical treatment of cancer.

**online**   direct link to off-site computers.

**oophorectomy**   excision of an ovary.

**operating system**   the program that tells the computer how to interface with hardware and software.

**ophthalmia neonatorum**   eye infection acquired by infants passing through the birth canal of a mother infected with *Neisseria gonorrhoeae*.

**ophthalmic**   describing medication instilled into the eye.

**ophthalmologist**   physician who specializes in treatment of disorders of the eyes.

**ophthalmoscope**   lighted instrument used to examine the inner surfaces of the eye.

**opportunistic infection**   infection resulting from a defective immune system that cannot defend against pathogens normally found in the environment.

**optician**   specialist who grinds lenses to correct errors of refraction according to prescriptions written by optometrists or ophthalmologists.

**optometrist**   specialist who can measure for errors of refraction and prescribe lenses but who cannot treat diseases of the eye or perform surgery.

**order of draw**   guidelines for proper tube sequence to reduce cross-contamination from one tube to the next and to prevent tissue thromboplastin contamination on specimens for coagulation testing. Carryover of additives and/or tissue thromboplastin can cause erroneous test results.

**organ**   any part that is made up of cells and tissues that cause it to perform its specified function in conjunction with a body system.

**organizational chart**   a flow sheet depicting the members of a team in a structured or hierarchical manner.

**origin**   the source or starting point; (muscle) the more fixed end of a muscle, usually the proximal end.

**orthopnea**   inability to breathe lying down; the patient usually has to sit upright to breathe.

**OSHA**   *see* Occupational Safety and Health Administration.

**osteoporosis**   abnormal porosity of the bone, most often found in the elderly, predisposing the affected bony tissue to fracture.

**otic**   describing medication instilled into the ear.

**otolaryngologist**   physician who specializes in the treatment of diseases and disorders of the ears, nose, and throat.

**otoscope**   instrument used for visual examination of the ear canal and tympanic membrane.

**outlier**   a patient whose hospital stay is longer than allowed by the DRG.

**out-of-pocket**   payment for health care services that are the responsibility of the patient or guarantor.

**outpatient**   a medical setting in which patients receive care but are not admitted.

**overdraft protection**   protection against having insufficient funds to cover checks.

**over the counter (OTC)**   available without a prescription; includes herbal and vitamin supplements.

**ovulation**   the periodic rupture of the mature ovum from the ovary.

**ovum (plural, ova)**   the female reproductive cell; sex cell or egg.

## P

**packing slip**   a document that accompanies a supply order and lists the enclosed items.

**Paget disease**   degenerative bone disease usually in older persons with bone destruction and poor repair.

**palliative**   easing symptoms without curing.

**palmar**   the palm surface of the hand.

**palpate**   to examine by feeling or pressing, used in diagnostic procedures such as vein location for phlebotomy.

**palpation**   technique in which the examiner feels the texture, size, consistency, and location of parts of the body with the hands.

**palpitations**   feeling of an increased heart rate or pounding heart that may be felt during an emotional response or a cardiac disorder.

**panels**   laboratory tests organized into standard groups to effectively evaluate disease processes or organ systems.

**panic value**   critical limits defining the boundaries of the life-threatening values of laboratory test results.

**Papanicolaou (Pap) test or smear**   smear of tissue cells examined for abnormalities including cancer, especially of the cervix; named after George N. Papanicolaou, a physician, anatomist, and cytologist.

**papilla**   (plural, papillae) a small nipple-shaped projection.

**papillae lingua**   the taste buds.

**paralanguage**   factors connected with, but not essentially part of, language, for example, tone of voice, volume, and pitch.

**parameters**   values used to describe or measure a set of data representing a physiologic function or system.

**paraphrasing**   restating what you heard using your own words.

**parasite**   organism that derives nourishment and protection from other living organisms known as *hosts*.

**parasitology**   the science and study of parasites.

**parasympathetic**   the part of the autonomic nervous system involved in periods free from stress.

**parenteral**   describing medication administered by any method other than orally.

**parity**   pregnancy that resulted in a viable birth.

**partial-thickness burn**   burn that involves epidermis and varying levels of the dermis.

**participating providers**   those who agree to participate with managed care contracts and other third-party payers in exchange for building a solid patient base.

**passive range of motion**   assisted range-of-motion movements.

**pathogens**   disease-causing microorganisms.

**Patient-Centered Medical Home (PCMH)**   a model of health care delivery in which the primary health care provider coordinates the care for patients and refers patients to other providers for medical care as needed.

**patient copayment**   the part of an insured service that the patient must pay.

**patient education**   active participation of the patient in a process that will yield a change in behavior.

**patient navigator**   individuals trained to assist people in accessing the health care system.

**Patient Self-Determination Act**   a law requiring health care facilities to provide information to patients about their rights under state laws in the event they are unable to do so themselves.

**peak level**   the highest serum level of a free or unbound drug in a patient based on a dosing schedule that is usually measured about 60 minutes after the end of an infusion.

**pediatrician**   physician who specializes in the care of infants, children, and adolescents.

**pediatrics**   specialty of medicine that deals with the care of infants, children, and adolescents.

**pediculosis**   infestation with parasitic lice.

**peer review**   organization of a group of physicians and specialists that conducts a review of a disputed case and makes a final recommendation.

**percussion**   striking with the hands to evaluate the size, borders, consistency, and presence of fluid or air.

**percutaneous transluminal coronary angioplasty (PTCA)**   procedure that improves blood flow through a coronary artery by pressing the plaque against the wall of the artery with a balloon on a catheter, allowing for more blood flow.

**pericarditis**   inflammation of the sac that covers the heart.

**pericardium**   the double-layered serous, membranous sac that encloses the heart and the origins of the great vessels.

**peripheral**   pertaining to or situated away from the center.

**peristalsis**   contraction and relaxation of involuntary muscles of the alimentary canal producing wavelike movement of products through the digestive system.

**PERRLA**   abbreviation used in documentation to denote pupils equal, round, reactive to light, and accommodation if all findings are normal; refers to the size and shape of the pupils, their reaction to light, and their ability to adjust to distance.

**personal protective equipment (PPE)**   equipment used to protect a person from exposure to blood or other body fluids.

**pessary**   device that supports the uterus when inserted into the vagina.

**petechiae**   small, pinpoint broken blood vessels on the skin.

**Petri plate**   a shallow glass or plastic dish with a lid to hold solid media for cultures.

**pH**   abbreviation for potential hydrogen; pH is a scale representing the relative acidity or alkalinity of a substance in which 7.0 is neutral; numbers lower than 7.0 are acidic, and numbers above 7.0 are basic.

**phagocyte**   a cell that has the ability to ingest and destroy particular substances such as bacteria, protozoa, cells, and cell debris by ingesting them.

**phagocytosis**   the process by which certain cells engulf and dispose of microorganisms; to eat or ingest.

**pharmacodynamics**   study of how drugs act within the body.

**pharmacokinetics**   study of the action of drugs within the body from administration to excretion.

**pharmacology**   study of drugs and their origins, natures, properties, and effects upon living organisms.

**phimosis**   narrowing or tightening of the prepuce that prevents retraction over the glans penis.

**phonophoresis**   ultrasound treatment used to force medications into tissues.

**phosphates**   compounds containing phosphorus and oxygen; they are very important in living organisms, especially for the transfer of genetic information.

**physician hospital organization** a coalition of physicians and a hospital contracting with large employers, insurance carriers, and other benefit groups to provide discounted health services.

**physician's office laboratory (POL)** laboratory in a medical office.

**physiology** the study of the function of the body.

**pia mater** thin vascular covering that adheres to the surface of the brain.

**pilosebaceous unit** consists of the hair shaft, the hair follicle, the sebaceous gland, and the erector pili muscle, which causes the hair to stand up when it contracts.

**placebo** an inert substance given as a medicine for its suggestive effect; an inert compound identical in appearance to material being tested in experimental research, which may or may not be known to the physician and/or patient, administered to distinguish between drug action and suggestive effect of the material under study.

**plaintiff** the party who initiates a lawsuit.

**plan maximum** the highest amount paid by a third-party payer for any given service.

**planes** a point of reference made by a straight cut through the body at any given angle.

**planning** the process of using information gathered during the assessment phase to organize learning or patient care objectives in order to accomplish the specific learning or treatment goal.

**plasma** top liquid layer of a blood specimen if the specimen was anticoagulated and not allowed to clot.

**platelets** thrombocytes.

**pleura** the serous membrane enclosing the lungs (visceral pleura: the layer that covers the lungs most closely; parietal pleura: the layer that follows the contours and lines the chest wall, the diaphragm, and the mediastinum).

**poikilocytosis** abnormal variations in the shapes of red blood cells (*poikilo* = variation).

**point-of-care testing (POC or POCT)** testing at the point where patient care is given.

**policy** a statement that reflects the organization's rules on a given topic.

**polychromasia** some red blood cells (RBCs) have a blue color; bluish RBCs are more immature cells.

**polycythemia vera** a condition that causes an elevated hematocrit.

**polydipsia** excessive thirst.

**polymenorrhea** abnormally frequent menstrual periods.

**polyphagia** abnormal hunger.

**polyuria** excessive excretion and elimination of urine.

**pons** part of the brainstem, responsible for communication with the central nervous system.

**portfolio** a portable case containing documents.

**positive feedback** an increase in function in response to a stimulus.

**positive stress** stress that allows a person to perform at peak levels and then relax afterward.

**positron emission tomography (PET)** computerized radiography using radioactive substances to assess metabolic or physiologic functions within the body rather than anatomic structures.

**postexposure testing** laboratory tests that may be performed after a person comes into contact with a biohazard.

**posting** listing financial transactions in a ledger.

**postural hypotension** sudden drop in blood pressure upon standing.

**potentiation** describes the action of two drugs taken together in which the combined effects are greater than the sum of the independent effects.

**practicum** an educational course that allows the student to obtain hands-on experience; also referred to as externship.

**precedents** the use of previous court decisions as a legal foundation.

**preceptor** a teacher; one who gives direction, as in a technical matter.

**precertification** approved documentation prior to referrals to specialists and other facilities.

**precision** test results are similar when test is repeated.

**preexisting condition** medical problem treated by a physician before an insurance plan's effective date. A third-party payer may exclude coverage for pre-existing conditions.

**preferred provider organization (PPO)** an organization whose purpose is to contract with providers and then lease this network of contracted providers to health care plans.

**prepuce** a fold of skin that forms a cover.

**presbyacusis** (also: presbycusis) loss of hearing associated with aging.

**presbyopia** vision change (farsightedness) associated with aging.

**present illness** a specific account of the chief complaint, including time frames and characteristics.

**preservative** substance that delays decomposition.

**primary diagnosis** the condition or chief complaint that brings a person to a medical facility for treatment.

**primary survey** an initial assessment of an emergency patient for life-threatening problems.

**prime mover** the muscle most responsible for the desired muscle action or movement.

**primigravida** a woman who is pregnant for the first time.

**primipara** a woman who has given birth to one viable infant.

**probing** digging with the needle to locate a vein.

**problem-oriented medical record (POMR)** a common method of compiling information that lists each problem of the patient, usually at the beginning of the folder, and references each problem with a number throughout the folder.

**procedure** a series of steps required to perform a given task; a medical service or test that is coded for reimbursement.

**procedure manual** handbook that contains test methods and other information needed to perform testing, is suggested by the U.S. Department of Health and Human Services (HHS) and the Centers for Disease Control and Prevention (CDC) as a valuable resource for Certificate of Waiver sites.

**product insert** written product information usually supplied by the manufacturer with each test kit or test system containing instructions and critical details for performing the test; also referred to as the package insert.

**professional courtesy** a discount fee given to health care professionals.

**proficiency testing** program to assess tests and the testers' performance by providing challenge samples to test as if they were patient specimens.

**profit-and-loss statement** statement of income and expenditures; shows whether, in a given period, a business made or lost money and how much.

**proofreading** the part of editing a document in which the writer reads the draft for accuracy and clarity and corrects errors.

**prophylaxis** prevention of development of a disease or condition.

**proprietary** private school with preset curricula.

**prostate-specific antigen** normal protein produced by the prostate that usually elevates in the presence of prostate cancer.

**prosthesis** any artificial replacement for a missing body part, such as false teeth or an artificial limb.

**protected health information (PHI)** individually identifiable personal health information as defined by the Health Insurance Portability and Accountability Act. Information that can be linked to a particular individual by name, code, or number is PHI.

**proteinuria** the presence of large quantities of protein in the urine; usually a sign of renal dysfunction.

**prothrombin time (PT)** test that monitors a patient's blood clotting time.

**protocol** a code of proper conduct; a treatment plan.

**provider** a health care worker who delivers medical care.

**provider-performed microscopy (PPM)** direct examination of a patient specimen using a microscope; a type of non-waived testing.

**proxemic** having to do with the degree of physical closeness tolerated by humans.

**pruritus** itching.

**psoriasis** chronic skin disorder that appears as red patches covered by thick, dry, silvery scales.

**psychogenic** of psychological origin.

**psychomotor** describes a physical task.

**psychosocial** relating to mental and emotional aspects of social encounters.

**puerperium** period of time (about 6 weeks) from childbirth until reproductive structures return to normal.

**purchase order** a document that lists the required items to be purchased.

**Purkinje fibers** extensions of the bundle of His that branch through the myocardium to end the transmission of the electrical impulse and cause the ventricles to contract.

**purulent** describes drainage that is white, green, or yellow; characteristic of an infection.

**pyosalpinx** pus in the fallopian tube(s).

**pyrexia** body temperature of 102°F or higher rectally or 101°F or higher orally.

**pyuria** pus in the urine.

## Q

**quadrants** a division of the abdomen into four equal parts by one horizontal and one vertical line dissecting at the umbilicus.

**qualitative** has positive or negative results; not a specified amount.

**quality assessment** plan for ensuring the quality of all areas of the laboratory's technical and support functions.

**quality assurance (QA)** an evaluation of health care services as compared to accepted standards.

**quality control (QC)** method to evaluate the proper performance of testing procedures, supplies, or equipment in a laboratory.

**quality improvement** a plan that allows an organization to scientifically measure the quality of its product and service.

**quantification** the process of ascertaining the amount of something.

**quantitative** the measuring of an amount.

**quantitative test** quantity measured and reported in a number value.

**Queckenstedt test** test to determine presence of obstruction in the cerebrospinal fluid flow performed during a lumbar puncture.

## R

**radiograph** processed film that contains a visible image.

**radiographer** technical specialist who works to assist the radiologist in the performance of procedures and who is responsible for producing routine examination images for the radiologist to interpret.

**radiography** art and science of producing diagnostic images with x-rays.

**radiologist** physician who specializes in radiology; performs some procedures and interprets images to provide diagnostic information.

**radiology** branch of medicine including diagnostic and therapeutic applications of x-rays.

**radiolucent** permitting the passage of x-rays.

**radionuclide** radioactive material with a short life that is used in small amounts in nuclear medicine studies.

**radiopaque** not permeable to passage of x-rays.

**random access memory (RAM)** temporary memory; data are lost when the computer is turned off if it is not backed up on disk.

**range of motion (ROM)** range in degrees of angle through which a joint can be extended and flexed.

**ratchet** notched mechanism, usually at the handle end of an instrument, that clicks into position to maintain tension on the opposing blades or tips of the instrument.

**read-only memory (ROM)** permanent memory inside the computer.

**reagent** a substance used to react in a certain manner in the presence of specific chemicals to obtain a diagnosis.

**receptionist** a person who greets patients as they arrive at a medical office and performs various administrative tasks.

**recertification** certification renewed either by taking the examination again or by completing a specified number of continuing education units in a 5-year period.

**recommended dietary allowance (RDA)** the amount of a nutrient most people need each day to stay healthy.

**reconstitution** adding water to bring a material back to its liquid state.

**rectocele** herniation of the rectum into the vaginal area.

**rectovaginal** pertaining to the rectum and vagina.

**reducing sugars** sugars other than glucose.

**reduction** correcting a fracture by realigning the bones; may be closed (corrected by manipulation) or open (requires surgery).

**reference interval** a range established for test results assumed to be typical for a population asymptomatic for disease processes.

**referral** instruction to transfer a patient's care to a specialist.

**referral laboratory** a large facility in which thousands of tests of various types are performed each day.

**reflecting** repeat what one heard using open-ended questions.

**reflux** a return or backward flow of fluid.

**refraction** bending of light rays that enter the pupil to reflect exactly on the fovea centralis, the area of greatest visual acuity.

**registration**   enrollment in a particular professional entity that endorses one's skills and abilities.

**relapsing fever**   fever that returns after extended periods of being within normal limits.

**remittance advice**   a notice from the Medicare Administrative Contractor showing payments and adjustments made on Medicare claims with explanations for reimbursement decisions. RAs submitted electronically are known as ERAs.

**remittent**   fluctuating.

**renal cortex**   the portion of the kidney that contains the structures that form urine.

**renal medulla**   the inner portion of the kidney that contains the collecting structures.

**renal pelvis**   the funnel-shaped upper portion of the ureters that collects urine from the kidneys.

**renal pyramids**   situated in the renal medulla, part of the collecting structures.

**renin**   enzyme formed in the kidney that works with angiotensin to affect the blood pressure.

**repolarization**   the active process of restoring the cardiac fibers to the resting (polarized) state; re-establishment of the electrical polarized state in a muscle or nerve fiber following contraction or conduction of a nerve impulse.

**reportable range**   the very lowest and highest value the manufacturer has documented the test can determine.

**requisition**   an order form for laboratory tests; must accompany each sample submitted to the laboratory.

**res ipsa loquitur**   "the thing speaks for itself."

**res judicata**   "the thing has been decided."

**resident flora**   microorganisms normally found in the body; also known as *normal flora*.

**resistance**   body's immune response to prevent infections by invading pathogenic microorganisms.

**resistant**   describes organisms that grow even in the presence of an antimicrobial agent.

**resource-based relative value scale (RBRVS)**   a value scale designed to decrease Medicare Part B costs and establish national standards for coding and payment.

**respiration**   the exchange of oxygen and carbon dioxide (external respiration: the exchange between the alveoli and the bloodstream; internal respiration: the exchange between the cells and the bloodstream).

**respondeat superior**   "let the master answer."

**restrain**   control or confine movement.

**résumé**   document summarizing individual's work experience or professional qualifications.

**retinal degeneration**   pathologic changes in the cell structure of the retina that impair or destroy its function, resulting in blindness.

**retrograde pyelogram**   an x-ray of the urinary tract using contrast medium injected through the bladder and ureters; useful in diagnosing obstructions.

**retroperitoneal**   the space behind the peritoneal cavity that contains the kidneys.

**retrovirus**   virus containing reverse transcriptase, which allows the viral cell to replicate its DNA in the DNA of the host cell, thereby taking over the substance of the cell.

**returned check fee**   amount of money a bank or business charges for a check written with insufficient funds.

**reverse chronological order**   items placed with oldest first.

*Rickettsia*   organism that is smaller than bacteria, larger than viruses.

**ringworm**   lay term for tinea, a group of fungal diseases.

**risk factors**   any issue that possesses a safety or liability concern for an organization.

**role delineation chart**   a list of the areas of competence expected of the graduate.

**Romberg test**   test for inability to maintain body balance when eyes are closed and feet are together; indication of spinal cord disease.

**rugae**   ridges or folds in the skin or mucous membranes that allow for expansion of a part.

**rule of nines**   the most common method of determining the extent of burn injury; the body surface is divided into sections of 9% or multiples of 9%.

## S

**salpingectomy**   excision of the fallopian tube.

**salpingo-oophorectomy**   surgical excision of both the fallopian tube and the ovary.

**salutation**   an introductory phrase that greets the reader of a letter.

**sanitation**   maintenance of a healthful, disease-free environment.

**sanitization**   processes used to lower the number of microorganisms on a surface by cleansing with soap or detergent, water, and manual friction.

**sanitize**   reduce the number of microorganisms on a surface by the use of low-level disinfectant practices.

**scale**   a thin, dried flake of skin.

**scalpel**   small, pointed knife with a convex edge for surgical procedures.

**scanner**   a piece of office equipment that transfers a written document into a computer.

**scissors**   sharp instrument composed of two opposing cutting blades, held together by a central pin on which the blades pivot.

**sclera**   white fibrous tissue that covers the eye.

**sclerotherapy**   use of chemical agents to treat esophageal varices to produce fibrosis and hardening of the tissue.

**scoliosis**   lateral curve of the spine, usually in the thoracic area, with a corresponding curve in the lumbar region, causing uneven shoulders and hips.

**scope of practice**   the procedures, actions, and processes that are permitted for a particular health care profession.

**screening**   a preliminary procedure, such as a test or exam, to detect the more characteristic signs of a disorder.

**search engine**   program that allows you to find information on the Internet rapidly and effectively.

**sebaceous gland**   oil gland.

**seborrhea**   overproduction of sebum by the sebaceous glands.

**sebum**   fatty secretion of the sebaceous gland.

**secondary survey**   an assessment of an emergency victim for head to toe injuries.

**sediment**   the cells and other particulate matter that collect in the bottom of the tube when a urine sample is centrifuged.

**seizure**   abnormal discharge of electrical activity in the brain, resulting in involuntary contractions of voluntary muscles.

**self-boundaries**   the limits set on the relationships between health care professionals and their patients.

**semiblock**   a type of letter format that is styled the same as block, except the first sentence of each paragraph is indented five spaces.

**senility**   general mental deterioration associated with aging.

**sensitive**   describes organisms that are inhibited by an antimicrobial agent.

**sensitivity**   susceptibility to a certain substance.

**sensitivity testing**   testing to determine the antibiotic that will most effectively inhibit the pathogen.

**sentinel event**   an unexpected death or serious physical or psychological injury to a patient in a health care facility.

**septic shock**   shock that results from general infection in the bloodstream.

**septicemia**   presence of pathogenic bacteria in the blood.

**serration**   groove, either straight or crisscross, etched or cut into the blade or tip of an instrument to improve its bite or grasp.

**serum**   top liquid layer of a blood specimen if the specimen was allowed to clot.

**service**   medical interventions completed by a provider.

**service charge**   a charge by a bank for various services.

**sesamoid**   resembling the shape of a sesame seed.

**sharps container**   a rigid, leakproof, plastic container used to discard disposable sharp devices in a manner to reduce needlesticks.

**shift**   a situation in which quality control results make an obvious change in performance levels.

**shock**   lack of oxygen to individual cells of the body.

**sick-child visit**   a pediatric visit for the treatment of illness or injury.

**sickle cell anemia**   a condition in which the patient has both copies of the gene for hemoglobin S; the red cells become sickle shaped and nonflexible causing obstruction of small vessels and capillaries. Necrosis due to tissue hypoxia occurs beyond the obstruction. Most commonly seen in African Americans.

**signs**   objective indications of disease or bodily dysfunction as observed or measured by the health care professional.

**sinoatrial (SA) node**   considered the pacemaker of the heart, located in the upper portion of the right atrium; a specialized group of cells that initiate the electrical impulse of the heart.

**slander**   oral statements that defame a person's reputation or character.

**smear**   materials that have been dried on glass slides.

**smegma**   a cheesy secretion of the sebaceous glands in either the labia or the prepuce.

**SOAP**   a style of charting that includes subjective, objective, assessment, and planning notes.

**software**   application programs that direct the hardware to perform given tasks.

**sound**   long instrument for exploring or dilating body cavities or searching cavities for foreign bodies.

**specialty**   a subcategory of medicine, such as pediatrics, studied after completion of medical school.

**specific gravity**   density of a liquid, such as urine, compared with water.

**specificity**   relating to a definite result.

**specimen**   a small portion of anything used to evaluate the nature of the whole; samples, such as blood or urine, used to evaluate a patient's condition.

**speculum**   instrument that enlarges and separates the opening of a cavity to expose its interior for examination.

**spherocytosis**   red blood cells showing no area of central pallor.

**sphygmomanometer**   device used to measure blood pressure.

**spicules**   sharp points.

**spina bifida occulta, spina bifida**   congenital defect in the spinal column caused by lack of union of the vertebrae.

**spinal**   pertaining to the spine.

**spirilla**   a spiral-shaped bacteria.

**spirochete**   long, flexible, motile microorganisms.

**splint**   device used to immobilize a sprain, strain, fracture, or dislocated limb.

**spore**   bacterial life form that resists destruction by heat, drying, or chemicals. Spore-producing bacteria include botulism and tetanus.

**staff privileges**   hospital approval for a physician to admit patients for treatment.

**staghorn**   stone formation in the renal pelvis that fills the chamber and assumes the shape of the calyces.

**standard precautions**   usual steps to prevent injury or disease.

**staphylococci**   spherical microorganism found in grapelike clusters.

**stare decisis**   "the previous decision stands."

**STAT**   immediately.

**status asthmaticus**   asthma attack that is not responsive to treatment.

**statute of limitations**   a legal time limit; for example, the length of time in which a patient may file a lawsuit.

**statutes**   laws that are written by federal, state, or local legislators.

**stereotyping**   to place in a fixed mold, without consideration of differences.

**sterile field**   a specific area, such as within a tray or on a sterile towel, that is considered free of microorganisms.

**sterilization**   process, act, or technique for destroying microorganisms using heat, water, chemicals, or gases.

**stoma**   an opening to the surface; suggests that it is surgically created.

**stomatitis**   inflammation of the mucous membranes of the mouth.

**strabismus**   a misalignment of eye movements usually caused by muscle incoordination.

**stratum corneum**   outer layer of the epidermis.

**stratum germinativum**   innermost layer of the epidermis.

**streaming**   a method of allotting time for appointments based on the needs of the individual patient to minimize gaps in time and backups.

*Streptococcus*   genus of bacteria commonly implicated in infections of the skin.

**stress**   a factor that induces body tension; can be positive or negative.

**striated**   having a striped appearance with alternating light and dark bands.

**subcutaneous**   beneath the skin.

**subject filing**   arranging files according to their title, grouping similar subjects together.

**sublingual**   describing medication administered under the tongue.

**subpoena**   a court order requiring an individual to appear at court at a given date and time.

**subpoena duces tecum**   a court order requiring medical records to be submitted to the court at a given date and time.

**substrate**   an underlying layer; a substance acted upon, as by an enzyme or reagent.

**sudoriferous gland**   sweat gland.

**sulci**   a groove in the brain tissue.

**sulfosalicylic acid**    an acid used to test for protein.

**summarizing**    briefly reviewing the information discussed to determine the patient's comprehension.

**summation report**    any report that provides a summary of activities, such as a payroll report or a profit-and-loss statement.

**superbill**    preprinted patient bill that lists a variety of procedures.

**superficial**    describes fungal infections limited to skin, hair, and nails.

**superficial burn**    burn limited to the epidermis.

**supernatant**    the urine that rises above the sediment when the tube of urine is centrifuged.

**surfing**    navigating the Internet.

**surgical asepsis**    destruction of organisms before they enter the body.

**surgical pathology**    the primary subspecialty of anatomic pathology. Studies are performed on tissue and body fluid specimens from aspirations, autopsies, biopsies, organ removal, and other procedures to identify or evaluate the effects of cancer and other diseases.

**surrogate mother**    a woman who carries a baby to term for another female who is unable to carry a pregnancy to term.

**susceptibility testing**    determines the potential of an antimicrobial agent to be effective in inhibiting growth of an organism.

**suspension**    temporary removal of privileges.

**sustained fever**    fever that is constant or not fluctuating.

**swab**    *noun*, stick topped with cotton or other absorbent man-made fiber for cleaning areas, applying treatments, or obtaining specimens; *verb*, to wipe with a swab.

**swaged needle**    metal needle fused to suture material.

**symmetry**    equality in size or shape or position of parts on opposite sides of the body.

**sympathetic**    the part of the autonomic nervous system involved in stress reaction.

**sympathy**    feeling sorry for or pitying someone.

**symptoms**    subjective indications of disease or bodily dysfunction as sensed by the patient.

**synapse**    the junction of two neurons.

**synarthroses**    immovable joints.

**syncope**    sudden fall in blood pressure or cerebral hypoxia resulting in loss of consciousness.

**synergism**    harmonious action of two agents, such as drugs or organs, producing an effect that neither could produce alone nor that is greater than the total effects of each agent operating by itself.

**synergist**    muscles that work together for more efficient movement.

**syringe**    used for the phlebotomy of fragile veins because the vacuum can be applied slowly and gently, rather than all at once as with vacuum tubes.

**system**    a collection of organs that perform a certain function.

**systemic**    describes an infection of the internal organs.

**systole**    contraction phase of the cardiac cycle.

## T

**T cells**    lymphoid cells from bone marrow that migrate to the thymus gland where they mature into differentiated lymphocytes that circulate between blood and lymph.

**tachycardia**    heart rate of more than 100 beats per minute.

**tactile**    pertaining to the sense of touch.

**take back**    the process of withholding of reimbursement to a provider on a patient's account by an insurance company in order to apply it to a previous overpayment on another account.

**Tamm–Horsfall mucoprotein**    mucoprotein that cements urinary casts together.

**task force**    a group of employees that works together to solve a given problem.

**taut**    pull skin gently so that there is no give or slack.

**tax withholding**    the amount of tax that is withheld from a paycheck.

**telemedicine**    the use of electronic telecommunications technology for the delivery of health care

**teleradiology**    use of computed imaging and information systems to transmit diagnostic images to distant locations.

**teletypewriter (TTY)**    a special machine that allows communication on a telephone with a hearing-impaired person.

**template**    a skeleton of a letter or document with preset and prespaced elements.

**tendons**    tough, flexible fibers that bind muscle to bone.

**tetany**    severe cramping, convulsions, or muscle spasms due to an abnormality of calcium metabolism.

**texting**    the use of electronic telecommunications technology for the delivery of health care

**thalamus**    part of the diencephalon, responsible for sorting messages.

**thalassemia**    a hemolytic anemia caused by deficient hemoglobin synthesis; more commonly found in those of Mediterranean heritage.

**therapeutic**    having to do with treating or curing disease; curative.

**therapeutic phlebotomy**    phlebotomy done as part of the patient's treatment for certain blood disorders.

**therapeutic range**    test result range the physician wants for the patient.

**third-party administrator**    administrator who processes claims for the sponsor of self-funded benefit planning.

**thoracentesis**    surgical puncture into the pleural cavity for aspiration of serous fluid or for injection of medication.

**threshold**    the least amount of something that produces a response.

**thrombocytes**    platelets in the blood.

**thrombocytopenia**    decreased platelets.

**thrombocytosis**    increased platelets.

**thromboplastin**    a complex substance found in the blood and tissues that aids the clotting process.

**thrombosed**    veins that lack resilience, feel like rope or cord and roll easily.

**thrombosis**    blood clotting inside a blood vessel.

**thyrotoxicosis**    excess quantities of thyroid hormone in the tissues.

**tidal volume**    amount of air inhaled and exhaled during a normal respiration.

**tine test**    skin test for exposure to tuberculosis, involves pricking the skin with sharp tines coated with the tuberculin bacillus.

**tinnitus**    an extraneous noise heard in one or both ears, described as whirring, ringing, whistling, roaring, etc.; may be continuous or intermittent.

**titer**    measure of the amount of an antibody in serum.

**tomography**    procedure in which the x-ray tube and film move in relation to each other during exposure, blurring out all structures except those in the focal plane.

**tonometry**   measurement of intraocular pressure using a tonometer.

**tonsils**   a small mass of lymphoid tissue; includes the palatine, nasopharyngeal, and lingual tonsils.

**tonus**   the steady, partial contraction of skeletal muscles that allows the body to remain upright.

**topical**   describing medication applied directly to the skin or mucous membranes.

**tort**   the righting of wrongs or injuries suffered by someone because of another person's wrongdoing.

**total testing process**   multistep process that begins and ends with the needs of the patient.

**toxicology**   the study of the presence and measurement of drugs in the blood.

**toxoid**   toxin treated to destroy its toxicity but still capable of inducing formation of antibodies.

**trace minerals**   minerals needed by the body only in small amounts.

**tracheostomy**   permanent surgical stoma in the neck with an indwelling tube.

**tracheotomy**   incision into the trachea below the larynx to circumvent a blockage superior to this point; suggests an emergency situation and a reversible procedure.

**trade name**   name given to a medication by the company that owns the patent.

**transcription**   the process of typing a dictated message.

**transient flora**   microorganisms that do not normally reside in a given area; transient flora may or may not produce disease.

**transient ischemic attack (TIA)**   acute episode of cerebrovascular insufficiency, usually a result of narrowing of an artery by atherosclerotic plaques, emboli, or vasospasm; usually passes quickly but should be considered a warning for predisposition to cerebrovascular accidents.

**transillumination**   passage of light through body tissues for the purpose of examination.

**transition**   passing from one place or activity to another.

**traumatic**   causing or relating to tissue damage.

**trend**   when control results progressively increase or decrease over time.

**triage**   sorting of patients into categories based on their level of sickness or injury to ensure that life-threatening medical conditions are treated immediately.

**trigone**   the triangle formed in the base of the bladder by the entrance of the two ureters and the exit of the urethra.

**trough level**   the lowest serum level of a free or unbound drug remaining in the patient's circulation; drawn just prior to the next drug dose.

**truncated coding**   diagnosis coding that is not done at the highest level available for a particular diagnosis or problem.

**truss**   a device that presses against a hernia to keep it in place.

**turbid**   cloudy.

**turbidity**   cloudiness.

**turbinates**   mucous membrane–covered conchae, the three scroll-shaped bones that project into the nasal cavity bilaterally from the lateral walls; each covers a sinus meatus.

**turgor**   normal tension in a cell or the skin; normal skin turgor resists deformation and will resume its former position after being grasped or pulled.

**tympanic membrane**   thin, semitransparent membrane in the middle ear that transmits sound vibrations; the eardrum.

**tympanic thermometer**   device for measuring the temperature using the blood flow through the tympanic membrane, or eardrum.

## U

**ultrasound**   imaging technique that uses sound waves to diagnose or monitor various body structures.

**unbundling**   the practice of submitting a claim with several separate procedure codes rather than a single code that represents the services performed.

**unemployment tax**   federal tax paid by the employer based on each employee's gross income.

**unit**   each part of a name or title that is used in indexing; a quantity of a standard measurement.

**unitized test device**   a self-contained test device to which a specimen is added directly and in which all steps of the testing process occur. A unitized device is used for a single test and must be discarded after testing.

**universal precautions**   controlling infection by treating all human blood and certain human body fluids as if known to be infectious for HIV, hepatitis B virus, hepatitis C virus, and other blood-borne pathogens.

**upcoding**   billing more for a patient care service than it is worth by selecting a code that is higher on the coding scale; this is an illegal practice.

**upper respiratory infection (URI)**   infection of the nasopharynx, throat, and bronchi.

**urea**   the final product of protein metabolism in the body and the main nitrogenous component in the urine.

**uremic frost**   a frost-like deposit of uremic compounds on the skin of patients whose kidneys are no longer functional.

**ureterostomy**   surgical opening to the outside of the body from the ureter to facilitate drainage of urine from an obstructed kidney.

**ureters**   the pair of tubes designed to carry urine from the kidneys to the bladder.

**urethra**   the short tube that carries urine from the bladder to the outside of the body.

**urethral meatus**   the external opening of the urethra.

**uric acid**   a byproduct of protein metabolism present in the blood and excreted by the kidneys.

**urinalysis**   examination of the physical, chemical, and microscopic properties of urine.

**urinary frequency**   the urge to urinate occurring more often than is required for normal bladder elimination.

**urine dipstick**   urine reagent test strip.

**urobilinogen**   the chemical that results when bacterial action converts bilirubin when it is secreted in the bile.

**urticaria**   hives.

**usual, customary, and reasonable (UCR)**   the basis of a physician's fee schedule, the usual and customary cost of the same service or procedure in a similar geographic area and under the same or similar circumstances.

**utilization review**   an analysis of individual cases by a committee to make sure services and procedures being billed to a third-party payer are medically necessary and to ensure compliance with its rules and regulations regarding reimbursement.

## V

**V-codes**   codes assigned to patients who receive service but have no illness, injury, or disorder, for example, a vaccination or a screening mammogram.

**vaccine**   suspension of infectious agents or some part of them; given to establish resistance to an infectious disease.

**values**   established ideals of life, conduct, customs, etc., of an individual person or members of a society.

**varicella zoster**    viral infection manifested by characteristic rash of successive crops of vesicles that scab before resolution; also called *chicken pox*.

**vasopressin**    a hormone formed in the hypothalamus and transported to the posterior lobe of the pituitary through the hypothalamohypophyseal tract. It has an antidiuretic and a pressor effect that elevates the blood pressure.

**vector**    (biological) a living, nonhuman carrier of disease, usually an arthropod; (mechanical) a carrier of disease that does not support growth; examples include contaminated inanimate objects.

**ventricle**    either of the two lower chambers of the heart that, when filled with blood, contract to propel it into the arteries.

**venule**    the small vessel that joins a capillary to a vein.

**verruca**    wart.

**vertigo**    sensation of whirling of oneself or the environment; dizziness.

**vesicle**    skin lesion that appears as a small sac containing fluid; a blister.

**viable**    capable of growing and living.

**vial**    glass or plastic container sealed at the top by a rubber stopper.

**villus (plural, villi)**    tiny, almost microscopic projections in the mucous membrane of the small intestines.

**virology**    the science and study of viruses.

**virtual**    a paperless system or chart on your computer.

**virulent**    highly pathogenic and disease producing; describes a microorganism.

**virus**    a microorganism that is not affected by antibiotics and can only be seen with an electron microscope; a term that refers to a harmful attachment to electronics such as computers that can invade and damage your electronic device.

**visualization**    a relaxation technique that allows the mind to wander and the imagination to run free and focus on positive and relaxing situations.

**vitiligo**    depigmentation of patches of the skin.

**vulva**    external genitalia of females.

## W

**waived test**    determined by Clinical Laboratory Improvement Amendments to be so simple that there is little risk of error.

**WBC differential**    a blood test in which total WBCs and the individual amounts of the 5 types of WBCs are measured and recorded for analysis; also see "differential.".

**wave scheduling system**    a flexible scheduling method that allows time for procedures of varying lengths and the addition of unscheduled patients, as needed.

**well-child visit**    visit to the medical office for the administration of immunizations and evaluation of growth and development.

**Western blot**    specific confirmatory antibody test for presence of HIV in blood.

**whole blood**    blood containing all its cellular components.

**whorls**    a spiral arrangement, as in the ridges on the finger that make up a fingerprint.

**withdrawing**    the act of terminating a medical treatment that has already been initiated.

**withholding**    not initiating certain medical treatments.

**workers' compensation**    employer insurance for treatment of an employee's injury or illness related to the job.

**write-off**    cancelation of an unpaid debt.

## X

**x-rays**    invisible electromagnetic radiation waves used in diagnosis and treatment of various disorders.

## Y

**yolk sac**    a structure that develops in the inner zygotic cell mass and supplies nourishment for the embryo until the 7th week when the placenta takes over the function.

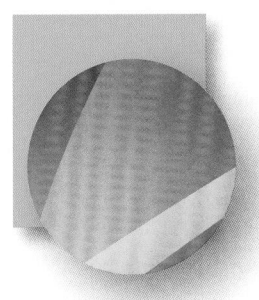

# Index

NOTE: Page numbers in *italics* denote figures; those followed by a t denote tables and b denote boxes.